CHICAGO PUBLIC LIBRARY

R00713 48918

Do Not Special Loan

D0212075

DISCARD

Anderson's
PATHOLOGY

VOLUME TWO

Anderson's
PATHOLOGY

Edited by

JOHN M. KISSANE, M.D.

Professor of Pathology and of Pathology in Pediatrics,
Washington University School of Medicine;
Pathologist, Barnes and Affiliated Hospitals,
St. Louis Children's Hospital, St. Louis, Missouri

NINTH EDITION

with **2269** *illustrations and* **8** *color plates*

The C. V. Mosby Company

ST. LOUIS • BALTIMORE • PHILADELPHIA • TORONTO   1990

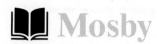

REF
RB
111
.P3
1989
v.2

Editor: George Stamathis
Developmental Editor: Elaine Steinborn
Assistant Editor: Jo Salway
Project Manager: Kathleen L. Teal
Production Editor: Carl Masthay
Book and Cover Design: Gail Morey Hudson
Production: Ginny Douglas, Teresa Breckwoldt

Two volumes

NINTH EDITION

Copyright © 1990 by The C.V. Mosby Company

All rights reserved. No part of this publication may be reproduced, stored in a retrieval system, or transmitted, in any form or by any means, electronic, mechanical, photocopying, recording, or otherwise, without prior written permission from the publisher.

Previous editions copyrighted 1948, 1953, 1957, 1961, 1966, 1971, 1977, 1985

Printed in the United States of America

The C.V. Mosby Company
11830 Westline Industrial Drive, St. Louis, Missouri 63146

Library of Congress Cataloging in Publication Data

Pathology (Saint Louis, Mo.)
  Anderson's pathology.—9th ed. / edited by John M. Kissane.
    p.   cm.
  Includes bibliographies and index.
  ISBN 0-8016-2772-9 (set)
    1. Pathology. I. Kissane, John M., 1928-   . II. Anderson,
W.A.D. (William Arnold Douglas), 1910-1986. III. Title. IV. Title:
Pathology.
    [DNLM: 1. Pathology. QZ 4 P2984]
RB111.P3 1990
616.07—dc19
DNLM/DLC   89-3072
for Library of Congress   CIP

C/VH/VH 9 8 7 6 5 4 3 2 1

Contributors

ARTHUR C. ALLEN, M.D.

Professor of Pathology, State University of New York,
Downstate Medical Center; Consultant Pathologist,
The Brooklyn Hospital–Caledonian Hospital,
Brooklyn, New York

ROBERT E. ANDERSON, M.D.

Frederick H. Harvey Professor and Chairman,
Department of Pathology, The University of New Mexico,
Albuquerque, New Mexico

FREDERIC B. ASKIN, M.D.

Professor of Pathology
University of North Carolina School of Medicine;
Director of Surgical Pathology,
North Carolina Memorial Hospital,
Chapel Hill, North Carolina

SAROJA BHARATI, MD.

Professor of Pathology, Department of Pathology,
Rush Medical School, Rush–Presbyterian–
St. Luke's Medical Center, Chicago;
Director, Congenital Heart and Conduction System Center,
Heart Institute for Children of Christ Hospital,
Palos Heights, Illinois

CHAPMAN H. BINFORD, M.D.

Formerly Chief, Special Mycobacterial Diseases Branch,
Geographic Pathology Division,
Armed Forces Institute of Pathology,
Washington, D.C.

FRANCIS W. CHANDLER, D.V.M., Ph.D.

Professor of Pathology, Department of Pathology,
Medical College of Georgia,
Augusta, Georgia

JOSÉ COSTA, M.D.

Professor of Pathology, Director, Institute of Pathology,
University of Lausanne,
Lausanne, Switzerland

JOHN REDFERND CRAIG, M.D., Ph.D.

Associate Clinical Professor, Department of Pathology,
University of Southern California School of Medicine,
Los Angeles;
Chief Pathologist, Department of Pathology,
St. Luke Medical Center, Pasadena;
St. Jude Hospital and Rehabilitation Center,
Fullerton, California

CHARLES J. DAVIS, Jr., M.D.

Associate Chairman, Department of Genitourinary
Pathology, Armed Forces Institute of Pathology,
Professor of Pathology,
Uniformed Services University of Health Sciences,
Washington, D.C.

KATHERINE De SCHRYVER-KECSKEMÉTI, M.D.

Professor of Pathology, Director, Anatomic and
Surgical Pathology, Case Western Reserve University,
Cleveland, Ohio

MICHAEL D. FALLON, M.D.

Associate Professor of Pathology and Cell Biology,
Department of Pathology,
Thomas Jefferson Medical College;
Attending Pathologist, Division of Surgical Pathology;
Director of the Division of Orthopaedic Pathology,
Department of Pathology,
Thomas Jefferson University Hospital,
Philadelphia, Pennsylvania

ROBERT E. FECHNER, M.D.

Royster Professor of Pathology and Director,
Division of Surgical Pathology,
University of Virginia Health Sciences Center,
Charlottesville, Virginia

GERALD FINE, M.D.

Formerly Chief, Division of Anatomic Pathology,
Henry Ford Hospital, Detroit;
Consulting Pathologist, Holy Cross Hospital, Detroit;
St. Joseph's Hospital,
Mt. Clemens, Michigan

KAARLE O. FRANSSILA, M.D. Ph.D.

Chief of Pathology Laboratory, Department of Radiotherapy and Oncology, Helsinki University Central Hospital, Helsinki, Finland

VICTOR E. GOULD, M.D.

Professor and Associate Chairman of Pathology, Rush Medical College, Chicago, Illinois

ROGERS C. GRIFFITH, M.D.

Assistant Professor of Pathology, Brown University, Providence, Rhode Island

JOHN G. GRUHN, M.D.

Associate Professor of Pathology, Rush Medical College, Chicago, Illinois

DONALD B. HACKEL, M.D.

Professor of Pathology, Department of Pathology, Duke University Medical Center, Durham, North Carolina

REID R. HEFFNER, Jr., M.D.

Professor of Pathology, Department of Pathology, State University of New York, Buffalo, New York

GORDON R. HENNIGAR, M.D.

Professor of Pathology, Department of Pathology and Laboratory Medicine, Medical University of South Carolina, Charleston, South Carolina

CHARLES S. HIRSCH, M.D.

Chief Medical Examiner, Suffolk County, New York; Professor of Forensic Pathology, SUNY Medical School at Stony Brook, Stony Brook, New York

PHILIP M. IANNACCONE, M.D., D.Phil. (Oxon)

Associate Professor of Pathology, Northwestern University, Chicago; Associate Staff Attending, Pathology, Northwestern Memorial Hospital, Chicago, Illinois

CHRISTINE G. JANNEY, M.D.

Assistant Professor of Pathology, St. Louis University School of Medicine, St. Louis, Missouri

HAN-SEOB KIM, M.D.

Associate Professor of Pathology, Baylor College of Medicine; Attending Pathologist, The Methodist Hospital, Harris County Hospital District, Houston, Texas

JOHN M. KISSANE, M.D.

Professor of Pathology and Pathology in Pediatrics, Washington University School of Medicine; Pathologist, Barnes and Affiliated Hospitals, St. Louis Children's Hospital at Washington University Medical Center, St. Louis, Missouri

FREDERICK T. KRAUS, M.D.

Professor of Pathology (Visiting Staff), Washington University School of Medicine; Director of Laboratory Medicine, St. John's Mercy Medical Center, St. Louis, Missouri

CHARLES KUHN III, M.D.

Professor of Pathology, Brown University, Providence, Rhode Island; Pathologist in Chief, Memorial Hospital of Rhode Island, Pawtucket, Rhode Island

MICHAEL KYRIAKOS, M.D.

Professor of Pathology, Washington University School of Medicine; Surgical Pathologist, Barnes Hospital; Consultant to St. Louis Children's Hospital at Washington University Medical Center and to Shriner's Hospital for Crippled Children, St. Louis, Missouri

PAUL E. LACY, M.D.

Mallinckrodt Professor and Chairman, Department of Pathology, Washington University School of Medicine, St. Louis, Missouri

RUSSELL M. LEBOVITZ, M.D., Ph.D.

Assistant Professor of Pathology, Baylor College of Medicine, Houston, Texas

MAURICE LEV, M.D.

Professor of Pathology, Department of Pathology, Rush Medical School, Rush–Presbyterian– St. Luke's Medical Center, Chicago; Associate Director, Congenital Heart and Conduction System Center, Heart Institute for Children of Christ Hospital, Palos Heights, Illinois

MICHAEL W. LIEBERMAN, M.D. Ph.D.

Professor and The W.L. Moody, Jr., Chairman, Department of Pathology, Baylor College of Medicine, Houston, Texas

CHAN K. MA, M.D.

Staff Pathologist, Department of Pathology, Henry Ford Hospital, Detroit, Michigan

JOSEPH A. MADRI, M.D., Ph.D.

Department of Pathology,
Yale University School of Medicine,
New Haven, Connecticut

MANUEL A. MARCIAL, M.D.

Associate Professor and Chairman,
Department of Pathology and Laboratory Medicine,
Universidad Central del Caribe, Escuela de Medicina,
Bayamón, Puerto Rico

RAÚL A. MARCIAL-ROJAS, M.D., J.D.

Professor and Dean, Universidad Central del Caribe,
Escuela de Medicina,
Bayamón, Puerto Rico

ROBERT W. McDIVITT, M.D.

Director, Division of Anatomic Pathology,
Department of Anatomic Pathology,
Washington University School of Medicine;
Chief of Anatomic Pathology,
Department of Anatomic Pathology, Barnes Hospital;
Consultant St. Louis Children's Hospital at Washington
University Medical Center, St. Louis, Missouri

WAYNE M. MEYERS, M.D., Ph.D.

Chief, Division of Microbiology,
Armed Forces Institute of Pathology,
Washington, D.C.

F. KASH MOSTOFI, M.D.

Chairman, Department of Genitourinary Pathology,
Armed Forces Institute of Pathology, Washington, D.C.;
Professor of Pathology,
Uniformed Services University of Health Sciences,
Bethesda, Maryland;
Associate Professor of Pathology,
Johns Hopkins University School of Medicine,
Clinical Professor of Pathology,
University of Maryland Medical School,
Baltimore, Maryland;
Clinical Professor of Pathology,
Georgetown University School of Medicine,
Washington, D.C.

JAMES S. NELSON, M.D.

Clinical Professor of Pathology, Department of Pathology,
University of Michigan, Ann Arbor, Michigan;
Division Head, Neuropathology, Department of Pathology,
Henry Ford Hospital, Detroit, Michigan

JAMES E. OERTEL, M.D.

Chairman, Department of Endocrine Pathology,
Armed Forces Institute of Pathology,
Washington, D.C.

JEFFREY M. OGORZALEK, M.D.

Major, US Air Force, Medical Corps;
Pathologist, Department of Endocrine Pathology,
Armed Forces Institute of Pathology,
Washington, D.C.

ALAN S. RABSON, M.D.

Director, Division of Cancer Biology and Diagnosis,
National Cancer Institute,
Bethesda, Maryland

KEITH A. REIMER, M.D., Ph.D.

Professor of Pathology, Department of Pathology,
Duke University Medical Center,
Durham, North Carolina

JUAN ROSAI, M.D.

Professor and Director of Anatomic Pathology,
Department of Pathology,
Yale University School of Medicine,
New Haven, Connecticut

DANTE G. SCARPELLI, M.D., Ph.D.

Ernest J. and Hattie H. Magerstadt Professor and Chairman,
Department of Pathology,
Northwestern University Medical School;
Chief of Service, Northwestern Memorial Hospital,
Chicago, Illinois

HARRY A. SCHWAMM, M.D.

Chairman, Department of Pathology,
The Graduate Hospital;
Clinical Professor of Orthopaedic Surgery (Pathology),
Department of Orthopaedic Surgery;
Clinical Professor of Pathology, Department of Pathology,
University of Pennsylvania School of Medicine,
Philadelphia, Pennsylvania

STEWART SELL, M.D.

Professor, Department of Pathology and Laboratory Medicine,
University of Texas Health Science Center at Houston,
Houston, Texas

GEORGE F. SCHREINER, M.D. Ph.D.

Assistant Professor of Medicine and Pathology,
Department of Medicine, Pathology,
Washington University School of Medicine;
Assistant Physician, Department of Medicine,
Barnes Hospital,
St. Louis, Missouri

HERSCHEL SIDRANSKY, M.D.

Professor and Chairman, Department of Pathology,
The George Washington University Medical Center,
Washington, D.C.

RUTH SILBERBERG, M.D.

Visiting Scientist,
Hadassah Hebrew University School of Medicine,
Jerusalem, Israel

MORTON E. SMITH, M.D.

Professor of Ophthalmology and Pathology,
Washington University School of Medicine,
St. Louis, Missouri

JACK L. TITUS, M.D., Ph.D.

Director, Jesse E. Edwards Registry of Cardiovascular
Disease, United Hospital;
Clinical Professor of Pathology, University of Minnesota,
St. Paul, Minnesota;
Formerly Professor and The W.L. Moody, Jr., Chairman,
Department of Pathology, Baylor College of Medicine;
Chief, Pathology Service, The Methodist Hospital;
Pathologist-in-Chief, Harris County Hospital District,
Houston, Texas

CHARLES A. WALDRON, D.D.S., M.S.D.

Professor Emeritus and Consultant, Oral Pathology,
Emory University School of Postgraduate Dentistry,
Atlanta, Georgia

DAVID H. WALKER, M.D.

Professor and Chairman, Department of Pathology,
The University of Texas Medical Branch at Galveston,
Galveston, Texas

NANCY E. WARNER, M.D.

Hastings Professor of Pathology,
University of Southern California School of Medicine,
Los Angeles, California

JOHN C. WATTS, M.D.

Attending Pathologist, Department of Anatomic Pathology,
William Beaumont Hospital, Royal Oak, Michigan;
Clinical Associate Professor of Pathology,
Wayne State University School of Medicine,
Detroit, Michigan

ROSS E. ZUMWALT, M.D.

Associate Professor, Department of Pathology,
University of New Mexico School of Medicine;
Assistant Chief Medical Investigator–State of New Mexico,
Office of the Medical Investigator,
Albuquerque, New Mexico

Preface to the Ninth Edition

My first responsibility, and it is a sad one, as editor of this ninth edition of *Anderson's Pathology*, is to mourn the loss of Dr. W.A.D. Anderson, creator and through nearly four decades guiding spirit of this book, which bears his name. He was an Emeritus Professor of Pathology and former Chairman of the Department of Pathology at the University of Miami School of Medicine in Miami, Florida. When he died on January 20, 1986, many of us lost a friend, and Pathology lost a scholarly spokesman. We will all miss him.

This edition continues the tradition of prior editions' concern. In the introductory chapters, mechanisms of human disease are addressed; these are followed by chapters that consider diseases of the several organ systems. Consideration of diseases of the various organ systems is deliberately made thorough so that the book can remain a useful and reliable source of information not only for medical students and trainees in pathology, but also for those training and practicing in other disciplines.

The eighth edition witnessed the emergence of acquired immunodeficiency syndrome (AIDS) as a major public health problem in industrialized societies as well as, by virtue of its protean clinical and morphologic manifestations, an important diagnostic consideration in specific patients. In preparing for this ninth edition, I considered allocating a separate chapter to AIDS. Eventually I decided to leave the consideration of AIDS within the several chapters addressing various organ systems, both for its basic aspects and for the descriptions of specific clinicopathologic features. Somewhat similar considerations related to the treatment of transplantation pathology, and the same decision was reached. These decisions remain very much open and may be amended in future revisions.

This edition of *Pathology* includes more than the usual number of chapters by new contributors. I welcome each of them and at the same time express my gratitude to their predecessors who have participated so importantly in the success this book has enjoyed throughout its long life.

John M. Kissane

Preface to First Edition

Pathology should form the basis of every physician's thinking about his patients. The study of the nature of disease, which constitutes pathology in the broad sense, has many facets. Any science or technique which contributes to our knowledge of the nature and constitution of disease belongs in the broad realm of pathology. Different aspects of a disease may be stressed by the geneticist, the cytologist, the biochemist, the clinical diagnostician, etc., and it is the difficult function of the pathologist to attempt to bring about a synthesis, and to present disease in as whole or as true an aspect as can be done with present knowledge. Pathologists often have been accused, and sometimes justly, of stressing the morphologic changes in disease to the neglect of functional effects. Nevertheless, pathologic anatomy and histology remain as an essential foundation of knowledge about disease, without which basis the concepts of many diseases are easily distorted.

In this volume is brought together the specialized knowledge of a number of pathologists in particular aspects or fields of pathology. A time-tested order of presentation is maintained, both because it has been found logical and effective in teaching medical students and because it facilitates study and reference by graduates. Although presented in an order and form to serve as a textbook, it is intended also to have sufficient comprehensiveness and completeness to be useful to the practicing or graduate physician. It is hoped that this book will be both a foundation and a useful tool for those who deal with the problems of disease.

For obvious reasons, the nature and effects of radiation have been given unusual relative prominence. The changing order of things, with increase of rapid, worldwide travel and communication, necessitates increased attention to certain viral, protozoal, parasitic, and other conditions often dismissed as "tropical," to bring them nearer their true relative importance. Also, given more than usual attention are diseases of the skin, of the organs of special senses, of the nervous system, and of the skeletal system. These are fields which often have not been given sufficient consideration in accordance with their true relative importance among diseases.

The Editor is highly appreciative of the spirit of the various contributors to this book. They are busy people, who, at the sacrifice of other duties and of leisure, freely cooperated in its production, uncomplainingly tolerated delays and difficulties, and were understanding in their willingness to work together for the good of the book as a whole. Particular thanks are due the directors of the Army Institute of Pathology and the American Registry of Pathology, for making available many illustrations. Dr. G.L. Duff, Strathcona Professor of Pathology, McGill University, Dr. H.A. Edmondson, Department of Pathology of the University of Southern California School of Medicine, Dr. J.S. Hirschboeck, Dean, and Dr. Harry Beckman, Professor of Pharmacology, Marquette University School of Medicine, all generously gave advice and assistance with certain parts.

To the members of the Department of Pathology and Bacteriology at Marquette University, the Editor wishes to express gratitude, both for tolerance and for assistance. Especially valuable has been the help of Dr. R.S. Haukohl, Dr. J.F. Kuzma, Dr. S.B. Pessin, and Dr. H. Everett. A large burden was assumed by the Editor's secretaries, Miss Charlotte Skacel and Miss Ann Cassady. Miss Patricia Blakeslee also assisted at various stages and with the index. To all of these the Editor's thanks, and also to the many others who at some time assisted by helpful and kindly acts, or by words of encouragement or interest.

W.A.D. Anderson

Contents

Color Plates

22 Upper Respiratory Tract and Ear

ROBERT E. FECHNER

The upper respiratory tract comprises the nose, paranasal sinuses, nasopharynx, larynx, and middle ear with its adjacent mastoid air cells. These structures encounter innumerable airborne agents that are potentially infectious, allergenic, or carcinogenic, Many of the reactive processes and neoplasms provoked by these agents are unique to the upper airway. In addition, diseases that involve multiple systems, such as Wegener's granulomatosis or malignant lymphoma, sometimes have their initial manifestation in the upper respiratory tract. The upper airway may also be secondarily affected by systemic diseases of diverse pathogeneses. Rheumatoid arthritis can damage the small joints in the larynx; tuberculosis or fungal infections can involve the upper airway by hematogenous spread from the lungs; hypothyroidism can produce laryngeal myxedema with resultant alterations in the voice.

This chapter is divided according to the anatomic areas of the upper respiratory tract just listed. A concluding section includes diseases that involve multiple parts of the upper airway.

NOSE
Malformations

Choanal atresia and choanal stenosis result from a membrane, which may contain bone or cartilage, that completely or partially occludes the nose at its junction with the nasopharynx. The defect is probably a persistence of the bucconasal membrane that ordinarily disappears at the seventh week of fetal development. Newborn infants with choanal malformations experience respiratory distress because they instinctively breathe through the nose, and they can be asphyxiated while nursing. The condition occurs in about 1 of 7000 births; there is a familial tendency.[14] About one half of infants with choanal atresia have other anomalies.[7]

Absence of the external nose can occur in association with choanal atresia.[8] Partial or complete duplication of the nose may be accompanied by duplications of foregut structures or may occur as an isolated malformation.[12]

Brain tissue can be located in the subcutaneous tissue of the glabella, with or without an intranasal component. In some patients the brain tissue connects with the cranial cavity through a defect in the skull—a meningoencephalocele. In others there is no communication, and the inaccurate term "nasal glioma" is applied to this heterotopic tissue. Nasal gliomas are not neoplasms, and any growth is commensurate with the growth of the child. Glial tissue dominates, and ganglion cells are rare.[9] Heterotopic brain tissue has also been found in the pharynx.[6]

Cysts of the nose are of two major types: dermoid and fissural. *Dermoid cysts* are developmental anomalies.[10] They are located beneath the skin at any point between the glabella and columella and are usually detected in childhood.[13] In addition to a cutaneous fistula, they can extend deep into the nasal septum or superiorly into the epidural space. The cysts are lined by squamous epithelium associated with hair follicles, sweat glands, and sebaceous glands in any combination.

Fissural cysts arise along the closure lines of the embryonic maxillary or globular processes and are often called nasolabial (nasoalveolar) or globulomaxillary, depending on the location. The cysts are lined mainly by squamous epithelium or columnar epithelium that may or may not be ciliated. Goblet cells are interspersed. Despite their presumed origin from entrapped embryonic epithelium, most do not appear until adulthood. Blacks have a predilection for these cysts.[11]

Skin

The skin of the nose is especially susceptible to solar damage and to inflammatory lesions that are centered in the sebaceous glands, for example, acne vulgaris. *Rhinophyma* is a term used for the hyperplastic glandular type of acne rosacea. Sebaceous glands are increased in number and size, the ducts are distended with keratinous debris, and dilated capillaries populate the dermis. This histologic complex is seen as an enlarged, lumpy, red nose. Although a variety of neoplasms have been reported in rhinophyma, there is no convincing evidence to indicate more than a chance association.[5]

NASAL CAVITY AND PARANASAL SINUSES
Infectious, allergic, and inflammatory processes

Acute rhinitis and sinusitis. The two most common causes of acute rhinitis are viral infections and allergic reactions. Mucosa reacting to an allergic insult is edematous and hyperemic with an inflammatory infiltrate rich in eosinophils.[67] In viral infections the virus replicates in the epithelial cells, and the degenerating epithelial cells are exfoliated.[22] The stroma becomes hyperemic, edematous, and infiltrated with neutrophils, lymphocytes, and plasma cells. Serous or mucinous fluid exudes through the epithelium. Clinically, these changes are manifest as nasal stuffiness and rhinorrhea. If a bacterial infection is superimposed, neutrophils dominate the inflammatory infiltrate and are evident clinically as a thick, purulent discharge.

Similar reactions to allergens or infectious agents occur in the mucosa of the paranasal sinuses and readily occlude the ostia. Retention of the exudate adds a sensation of facial fullness or pain to the nasal symptoms.

Bacterial infections of the sinuses can lead to serious complications. Infection of the ethmoid air cells may spread into the orbital soft tissues and the meninges. Sphenoiditis can lead to retrobulbar neuritis. Frontal sinusitis can be followed by meningitis or osteomyelitis of the frontal bone.

Nasal polyps. Nasal polyps are enlargements of the lamina propria mucosa caused by edema, inflammation, and the proliferation of fibroblasts (Fig. 22-1). Abnormal mucous glands form in about half of the polyps. The glands are often distended with mucus and form

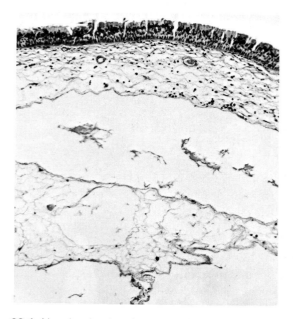

Fig. 22-1. Nasal polyp is edematous stroma with a few subepithelial inflammatory cells. It is covered with normal ciliated epithelium.

cysts, that contribute to the mass.[83] Polyps are covered with ciliated epithelium that sometimes undergoes squamous metaplasia. A thick, subepithelial basal lamina is often conspicuous. Ulceration of the surface or infarction can occur.

Nasal polyps are often called "allergic polyps" in patients with atopy. In the absence of atopy the polyps are usually attributed to infection. There are no constant histologic findings that permit this etiologic distinction. Eosinophils, traditionally viewed as a manifestation of allergic response, can be seen in polyps when no allergic basis can be identified clinically.

The pathogenesis of nasal polyps is not clearly understood. Polyps are uncommon before 20 years of age and are seen more frequently in asthmatics than in the general population.[76] It is likely that more than one mechanism exists, depending on different inciting factors and variables in the host's response. In some patients immunoglobulins have been found in polyps at a concentration higher than what can be explained by passive diffusion.[24] Eosinophils are especially prominent in these polyps.

A nasal polyp in a person younger than 20 years of age signals the likelihood of cystic fibrosis. Polyps from these patients differ from typical nasal polyps in lacking basement-membrane thickening and tissue eosinophilia. The mucus is also histochemically abnormal.[71]

Antrochoanal polyps arise from mucosa of the maxillary sinus and enter the nasal cavity through a large accessory ostium near the middle meatus. Approximately 10% of normal persons have an accessory ostium, which appears necessary for the development of the polyp. Once within the nasal cavity, the polyp protrudes posteriorly through the choana into the nasopharynx. In contrast to typical nasal polyps, approximately one third of the patients with antrochoanal polyps are younger than 20 years.[78] The lesions are almost always unilateral. Histologically antrochoanal polyps are similar to nasal polyps except that basement membrane thickening and eosinophilia are less pronounced. Stromal cells with pronounced nuclear abnormalities may be seen in antrochoanal polyps, as well as in typical nasal polyps.[27]

Mucocele and cholesterol granuloma. The epithelium of the paranasal sinuses secretes 1 to 2 liters of fluid daily as it humidifies the air. If the ostium of a sinus is blocked by inflamed mucosa, trauma, or an osteoma, the secretions accumulate. Two thirds of mucoceles are in the frontal sinus, and most of the remainder affect the anterior ethmoid sinus. The mucosal lining consists of normal or compressed ciliated epithelium that sometimes has squamous metaplasia. Mucus accumulates not only in the lumen but also in the lamina propria, where it can be phagocytosed by histiocytes (mucophages). The surrounding bone may be eroded.[69]

Hemorrhage into an obstructed sinus results in the accumulation of cholesterol from the breakdown of erythrocytes. The engulfment of cholesterol by histiocytes is termed "cholesterol granuloma."[45]

Rhinosporidiosis. Rhinosporidium seeberi is a fungus that has only recently been cultured.[61] Thick-walled sporangia contain several thousand spores that mature into trophocytes. The latter have clear cytoplasm and a distinct outer membrane and measure up to about 30 μm wide.[57] Rhinosporidiosis typically manifests as a friable, nasal polyp, but the nasopharynx, larynx, and conjunctiva are sometimes affected. The organisms elicit a nonspecific inflammatory response. The disease is most common in India and Sri Lanka, but rare cases have occurred in the United States.[54]

Rhinoscleroma. A gram-negative diplobacillus, *Klebsiella rhinoscleromatis*, induces chronic inflammation that includes plasma cells and foamy histiocytes. The histiocytes (Mikulicz cells) contain organisms and undigested mucopolysaccharides.[51] The inflammation produces nodular mucosal masses that obstruct the nose, nasopharynx, middle ear, larynx, or lower respiratory tract. Rhinoscleroma is endemic in well-demarcated areas of Africa, Central and South America, southern Asia, and eastern Europe. Sporadic cases occur elsewhere, including the United States.[17]

Mucormycosis (phycomycosis). Mucormycosis is an opportunistic infection by organisms of the order *Mucorales*. Nonseptate hyphae spread along nerves, across tissue planes, and into blood vessels.[81] There is thrombosis and infarction, and inflammation may be negligible. Complications include meningoencephalitis and cerebral infarction.[19]

Aspergillosis. Infections of the paranasal sinuses by *Aspergillus* can take several forms.[58] Septate hyphae can grow within the sinus and form a mass (aspergilloma) that elicits little reaction. At other times there is an indolent inflammatory reaction. In an immunosuppressed patient the clinical course can be fulminant with spread into the cranial fossa.[62]

Atrophic rhinitis. The nasal mucosa is dry, appears crusted, and emits a fetid odor. A loss of vascularity and seromucous glands contributes to the atrophy. Ciliated epithelium and mucous cells are replaced by squamous epithelium. Some patients give a history of repeated infections, but other patients yield no clues regarding the cause.[68]

Myospherulosis. Myspherulosis is an inflammatory and fibrous reaction that occurs after a surgical procedure on the nose or paranasal sinuses. If a hemostatic packing impregnated with antibiotic ointment is used postoperatively, the oil-based vehicle can produce a foreign-body reaction. This is accompanied by a peculiar encystment of degenerating erythrocytes. The recrudescence of symptoms that necessitates reoperation may be caused, at least in part, by the foreign body reaction.[86]

Destructive midline processes and Wegener's granulomatosis

The often-used rubric "lethal midline granuloma" is not an acceptable pathologic diagnosis. It is a clinical designation referring to a patient with a destructive lesion of unknown cause that involves the upper aerodigestive tract. Many entities cause midline destruction including infections, Wegener's granulomatosis, and neoplasms that are often difficult to diagnose such as lymphoma, lymphoepithelioma, or midline malignant reticulosis. To be sure, there is the rare patient with a destructive midline lesion that cannot be specifically diagnosed, even after exhaustive study. The term "idiopathic midline destructive disease" has been used for this clinicopathologic situation, and patients respond to radiation therapy.

Wegener's granulomatosis is characterized by vasculitis and, usually, granulomatous inflammation (Fig. 22-2). Although the changes may be an immune response, the inciting agent or agents are unknown. Patients have nonspecific symptoms interpreted as "chronic sinusitis" or "chronic otitis media." At its fullest expression, Wegener's granulomatosis can attack virtually every organ, but the upper respiratory tract, lung, and kidneys are usually the most severely affected. Localized forms occasionally occur in either the upper respiratory tract or the lung.[32]

Vasculitis is a prerequisite for the diagnosis, whereas granulomas are of secondary importance and may be absent. Vascular changes range from a transmural inflammation of an otherwise intact vessel to necrosis of

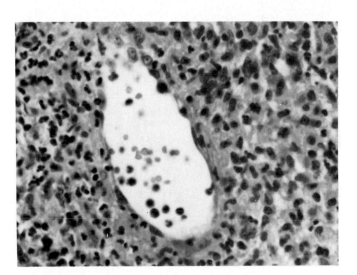

Fig. 22-2. Major alteration in Wegener's granulomatosis is acute inflammation and necrosis of vessel walls. Histiocytes are also seen *(right).*

either a sector or a segment of a vessel. Thrombosis and luminal fibrous obliteration also occur. The granulomas, when present, consist of mononuclear or multinucleated histiocytes. They may or may not be partly necrotic. Sometimes the only evidence of granuloma formation is small, poorly circumscribed collections of histiocytes.

Papillomas

Papillomas lined by normal or hyperkeratotic epidermis arise in the hair-bearing skin of the nasal vestibule. They are solitary and have no malignant potential.

Papillomas of the nasal cavity and paranasal sinuses have been given a bewildering number of names. The terms most widely employed are inverted papilloma, fungiform papilloma, and cylindrical cell papilloma. Sometimes they are collectively referred to as schneiderian papillomas. Although their cause is not known, they can be viewed as hyperplastic, reactive processes characterized by a proliferation of various epithelial types. Papillomas may erode bone but do not metastasize. They occur mainly in adults, especially middle-aged men. At least half recur locally unless major resections are performed to remove microscopic foci that extend beyond the grossly visible lesion.[23] Patients with fungiform papilloma are not at increased risk for malignancy, but about 5% of patients with inverted papilloma or cylindrical cell papillomas have synchronous or metachronous carcinoma, usually squamous. The carcinomas may be located in the papilloma itself or may arise at the site of a previous papilloma.[79]

The pattern seen with low-power microscopy distinguishes fungiform from inverted papillomas. Fungiform papilloma has an everted or exophytic configuration (Fig. 22-3); the inverted papilloma has invaginations or inversions of the epithelium into the underlying stroma (Fig. 22-4). Fungiform papillomas are nearly always located on the nasal septum. Inverted papillomas involve the lateral nasal wall, and often there is a paranasal sinus component. Both types of papillomas are lined with various combinations of normal ciliated epithelium, hyperplastic ciliated epithelium, mucous cells, squamous epithelium, or intermediate epithelium. The last derives its name because it is morphologically in-

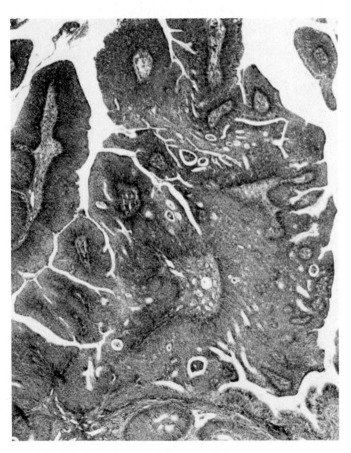

Fig. 22-3. Fungiform papilloma of nasal septum is lined predominantly by intermediate epithelium.

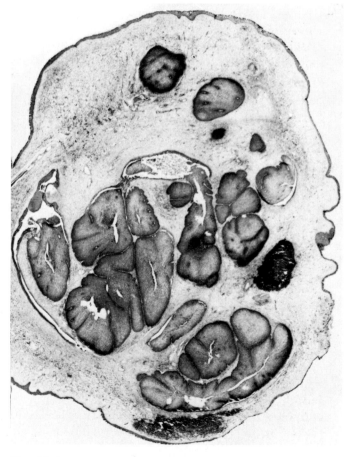

Fig. 22-4. Inverted papilloma has invaginations of intermediate epithelium into stroma. Lesion shown has normal ciliated epithelium on surface.

termediate between normal columnar and normal squamous epithelium. It has also been called "transitional epithelium," but this implies an unjustified relationship to transitional epithelium of the urinary bladder.[72]

Cylindrical cell papilloma has cells with eosinophilic granular cytoplasm attributable to mitochondrial hyperplasia.[15] Mucous cells are interspersed, and they may mimic fungal yeast forms when the mucus is inspissated (Fig. 22-5).

Benign lesions

Lobular capillary hemangioma (pyogenic granuloma). Lobular capillary hemangioma has a distinctive lobular arrangement of capillaries in an edematous, fibroblastic stroma (Fig. 22-6).[63] The surface may be ulcerated and have an inflammatory cell infiltrate as well as superimposed reactive granulation tissue. The term "pyogenic granuloma" is often used for the ulcerated lesions. This is a misnomer because they are neither pyogenic infections nor granulomas. Patients are 8 to 80 years of age. The lesions are rarely associated with trauma. Some occur in pregnant women ("pregnancy epulis," or "pregnancy tumor"). Other types of hemangiomas, hemangiopericytoma, and angiosarcoma are rare in the nose.[26,37]

Miscellaneous lesions. Necrotizing sialometaplasia occurs in the glands of the nose or paranasal sinuses after

surgery.[55] Other lesions include mixed tumors,[28] neural tumors,[73] fibromatosis,[70] and meningiomas without intracranial connections.[50] Osseous lesions that encroach on the airway include fibrous dysplasia, ossifying fibroma, osteoma, odontogenic tumors, giant cell granuloma, and myxoma.[38,42,33]

Malignant neoplasms

It is convenient to group some neoplasms of the nose and paranasal sinuses together because both areas are frequently involved when the patient is first seen, and

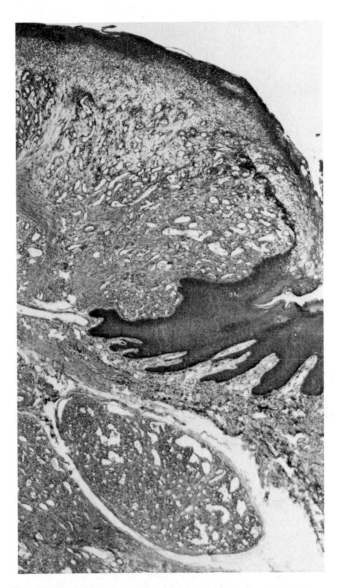

Fig. 22-6. Lobular capillary hemangioma (so-called pyogenic granuloma) has lobular pattern beneath epithelium. Lobular arrangement is lost in superficial, ulcerated portion. (From Fechner, R.E., Cooper, P.H., and Mills, S.E.: Arch. Otolaryngol. **107**:30, copyright 1981, American Medical Association.)

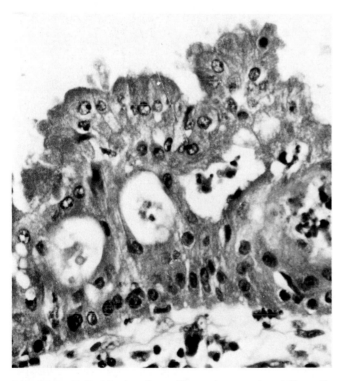

Fig. 22-5. Cylindrical cell papilloma has eosinophilic cells and spherical accumulations of mucus.

it is impossible to identify the precise site of origin. This is especially true for malignant lymphomas and undifferentiated carcinomas.

Malignant lymphoma. About 6% of sinonasal malignancies are lymphomas that are usually of the diffuse large-cell immunoblastic type. Most patients develop disseminated disease.[36]

Undifferentiated carcinoma. In recent years there have been several reports of carcinomas variously referred to as undifferentiated, anaplastic, small cell, or neuroendocrine. In one study, the patients had a histologically homogeneous undifferentiated carcinoma that followed a rapidly lethal course.[35] Other studies have discussed histologically more diverse tumors that also seem to be very aggressive.[49] The diagnosis of neuroendocrine carcinoma has been made on the ultrastructural finding of dense-core membrane-bound granules.[77] The tumors have well-demarcated groups of cells and may contain polypepetides.[56] Many of these patients have done well after therapy.[77] A few tumors have more closely resembled small-cell (oat cell) carcinoma of the lung.[85]

Nasal cavity carcinoma. Squamous carcinomas constitute the majority of cancers in the nasal cavity. Most patients are men beyond 50 years of age who are smokers; only about 25% survive.[20] Exposure to nickel fumes in refinery workers as well as other substances also are implicated.[16,74]

Adenocarcinoma is a rare tumor of the nasal mucosa but makes up a disproportionate number of carcinomas in woodworkers.[21,46] Specific carcinogens have not been identified. The tumors seldom metastasize but grow relentlessly and kill more than half of the patients. The microscopic pattern of the adenocarcinomas in woodworkers as well as patients with other occupations often resembles that of colonic carcinoma.[53,75] Extremely well-differentiated tumors may resemble normal intestinal mucosa.[64]

Paranasal sinus carcinoma. About 80% of cancers of the paranasal sinuses arise in the maxillary antrum, and most are squamous carcinoma. The patient often has had severe, chronic sinusitis. The diagnosis is rarely made before there is extension into surrounding structures. About 75% of patients die of their tumor, usually because of local extension, though 10% have widespread metastases.[25]

Adenocarcinomas comprise about 5% of sinus cancers. Adenoid cystic carcinoma, the most common, has a 90% 10-year mortality.[80] Adenocarcinoma similar to the colonic-like cancer of the nasal fossa occurs in any sinus,[44] but it is especially frequent in the ethmoid sinuses of woodworkers.[46] Mucoepidermoid carcinomas and small-cell ("oat cell") carcinomas also arise in the glands of the sinonasal region, as do low-grade adenocarcinomas.[47,60,85]

Olfactory neuroblastoma (esthesioneuroblastoma). The olfactory mucosa covers the superior one third of the nasal septum, the cribriform plate, and the superior turbinate. It has a mitotically active reserve cell layer from which olfactory neuroblastoma is probably derived. Clinically, there is a polypoid mass that may invade the paranasal sinuses and almost invariably destroys the cribriform plate. The tumors have variable amounts of intercellular neurofibrillary material interspersed between small cells. Rosettes are formed in about 10% to 30% of tumors. If the tumor lacks these features, a silver stain for neuronal processes may be helpful.[65] Ultrastructural examination shows neuritic

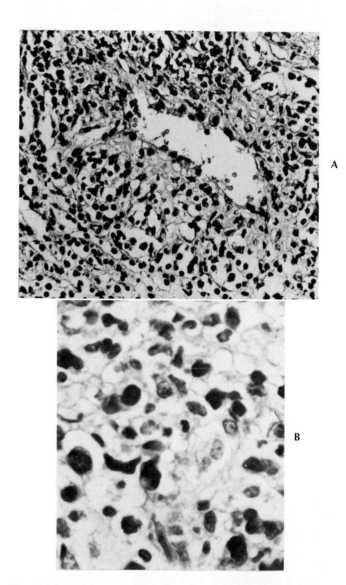

Fig. 22-7. Midline malignant reticulosis. **A,** Proliferating cells surround and invade vessel wall. **B,** Pleomorphic lymphocytes frequently have large quantity of clear cytoplasm. (**A** from Fechner, R.E., and Lamppin, D.W.: Arch. Otolaryngol. **95**:467, copyright 1972, American Medical Association.)

cell processes, neurofilaments, neurotubules, and dense core vesicles.[82]

Olfactory neuroblastoma occurs in all decades, with a peak incidence between 10 and 30 years of age. The disease is capricious. Some patients die quickly with widespread metastases, whereas others live for several years before metastases or local recurrence develop. A patient may live with symptomatic disease for many years.[52] Approximately 50% of patients survive, especially when the tumor can be completely excised.[65]

Midline malignant reticulosis (polymorphic reticulosis, lymphomatoid granulomatosis). Midline malignant reticulosis is a histologically distinctive lymphoproliferative disorder. The affected mucosa is thickened and ulcerated. Granulation tissue and inflammation may overlie the neoplastic component, and a deep biopsy is often necessary to reach the lesion. The lymphocytes are variable in size. Many cells have abundant clear cytoplasm and sharply defined cell membranes (Fig. 22-7). Some cells have features of immunoblasts. The tumor often is angiocentric with infiltration of vessel walls. This vascular invasion by abnormal cells must be differentiated from the inflammation of vessel walls seen in Wegener's granulomatosis.[34] The changes of midline malignant reticulosis are histologically similar, if not identical, to lymphomatoid granulomatosis. The two conditions probably represent the same process in different anatomic locations.[30,31]

Other malignant neoplasms. Malignant melanoma of the nasal cavity arises most often during the fourth to sixth decades of life.[18] Soft-tissue sarcomas are rare in the upper airway. Rhabdomyosarcoma is the most common (see discussion later in the chapter). A few cases of fibrosarcoma,[41] leiomyosarcoma,[40] malignant fibrous histiocytoma,[43] and synovial sarcoma[66] have been recorded. The most frequent malignant neoplasms of the facial bones are osteosarcoma and chondrosarcoma.[38,39] Teratocarcinoma, a histologically complex tumor, is a recently described neoplasm.[48]

NASOPHARYNX
Angiofibroma

Angiofibromas arise in the nasopharynx or extreme posterior portion of the nasal cavity. They can grow into paranasal sinuses, cheek, orbit, or base of the skull but do not metastasize.[93] With a few questionable exceptions, the lesion is confined to males. Nearly all occur between 10 and 20 years of age, suggestive of hormonal influences. In fact, the tumors contain testosterone-receptor proteins.[94]

The angiofibroma is a gray, rubbery mass that belies its vascularity and the risk of exsanguination. Microscopically, a fibrous stroma contains small vascular slits (Fig. 22-8). Ultrastructurally, the stromal cells are myofibroblasts, with distinctive electron-dense nuclear inclusions.[99]

Nasopharyngeal carcinoma

In ascending order of frequency, three histologic types of nasopharyngeal carcinoma can be recognized: nonkeratinizing squamous carcinoma, keratinizing squamous carcinoma, and undifferentiated carcinoma. Many tumors from the first and last groups are called "transitional cell carcinoma," but because of its inconsistent application, that term should be abandoned. Another time-hallowed term, "lymphoepithelioma," is useful as long as it is recognized as only a histologic variant of undifferentiated carcinoma with numerous lymphocytes that surround and intermix with the cancer. The lymphocytes are a nonneoplastic reaction to the carcinoma.

The keratinizing and nonkeratinizing carcinomas are microscopically similar to the commonplace squamous carcinomas that arise in other sites. On the other hand, undifferentiated carcinomas are characterized by cells with large vesicular nuclei, often arranged in a syncytium (Fig. 22-9). This carcinoma is frequently misdi-

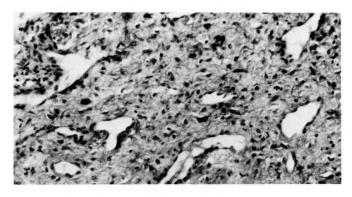

Fig. 22-8. Angiofibroma has capillaries scattered among myofibroblasts.

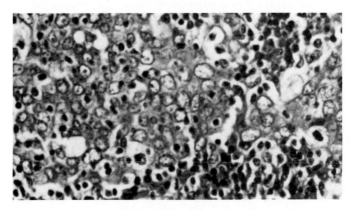

Fig. 22-9. Undifferentiated nasopharyngeal carcinoma is syncytium of cells with vesicular nuclei. This is lymphoepithelioma variant of undifferentiated carcinoma because of lymphocytic admixture.

agnosed as malignant lymphoma.[89] The keratinizing and nonkeratinizing carcinomas are almost invariably fatal; about 25% pf patients with undifferentiated carcinomas survive after radiation therapy.[87]

About one third of nasopharyngeal carcinomas, especially undifferentiated carcinomas, occur in teenagers and young adults. Many patients have no complaints referable to the nasopharynx. Cervical lymph node metastases are the first sign in half of the patients.

Genetic factors influence the risk of nasopharyngeal carcinoma. The Chinese are remarkably susceptible, especially before 45 years of age, and there is a significant association with the A2/sin HLA type.[98] Environmental factors are also important. Chinese immigrants to Hawaii and California have a decreased risk in succeeding generations that cannot be completely explained by genetic dilution.[91] In another study, all cases of nasopharyngeal carcinoma in American-blacks were undifferentiated cancers.[88] Most occurred before 45 years of age, but specific genetic or environmental factors have not been elucidated. The association with tobacco is less well established in patients with nasopharyngeal cancer than in other respiratory tract cancers. A history of recurrent otitis media, sinusitis, or tonsillitis is significantly more common in patients with nasopharyngeal carcinoma.[95] Long-standing inflammatory changes might alter nasal architecture and air currents, focally increasing concentrations of carcinogens.

The role of the Epstein-Barr virus in nasopharyngeal cancer is unclear. High titers of antibody to the viral capsid are found in most patients with nonkeratinizing carcinoma or lymphoepithelioma.[97] The titers often rise as the tumor burden increases.

Miscellaneous lesions

Other lesions in the nasopharynx include congenital teratomas, teratocarcinomas,[92] soft-tissue sarcomas,[41] and fibromatoses.[41] Chordomas, pituitary adenomas, and bone tumors arising in the base of the skull mimic carcinoma.[90,96]

LARYNX
Congenital malformations

The most common malformation is a fibrous tissue web between the true cords. The web usually leaves an adequate airway and may not be diagnosed until the child begins to talk, or even until middle age.[157]

Laryngeal atresia or stenosis occurs in the subglottic region, and both forms are usually incompatible with life. Laryngeal clefts represent a failure of the posterior larynx and trachea to become separated from the esophagus. The mortality is high because of aspiration. Moreover, infants with laryngeal clefts frequently have other major congenital defects.[150]

Victims of the sudden infant death syndrome have an excess of laryngeal mucous glands. Whether this is a congenital or an acquired condition is uncertain.[131]

Allergic and infectious processes

The larynx can be the site of an allergic response. The edematous component can lead to life-threatening airway obstruction.[180]

Acute laryngotracheobronchitis (croup) occurs almost exclusively during the first 3 years of life. Influenza A and B, parainfluenza, rhinovirus, and respiratory syncytical viruses are the most frequent causes. They damage the epithelium and excite an inflammatory infiltrate, edema, and congestion of the lamina propria. The stromal changes narrow or occlude the airway, especially in the subglottic area.[175] Viral infections can be localized to a portion of the larynx. Extensive ulceration and inflammatory exudate can mimic carcinoma.[161,167]

Infection confined to the epiglottis may be fatal. *Haemophilus influenzae* is the major cause. Acute epiglottis usually affects infants and children but occasionally strikes adults. Regardless of the patient's age, emergency treatment is required to prevent asphyxiation.

Corynebacterium diphtheriae multiplies in the pharyngeal mucus and elaborates a toxin that produces epithelial necrosis. A fibrinous exudate containing a few mononuclear cells, nuclear and epithelial fragments, and bacteria accumulates on the damaged mucosa. The membrane can extend to the larynx and obstruct it.

Tubercle bacilli or fungi involve the larynx as a part of disseminated disease and may be the initial manifestation. *Mycobacterium tuberculosis* usually but not always evokes a typical granulomatous inflammation.[177] By contrast, the granulomatous response to fungi is often absent, and the inflammation may consist of acute and chronic inflammatory cells with only a few mononuclear histiocytes intermixed. The organisms of *Histoplasma capsulatum* are likely to be imperceptible except on Gomori silver-methenamine stain.[110] One must think of fungal infection and perform the silver stain without the presence of granulomas to serve as a clue. Other fungi, such as *Cryptococcus*,[165] *Aspergillus*,[146] *Coccidioides*,[179] *Blastomyces*,[174] and *Candida*,[182] are usually visible on hematoxylin eosin−stained sections.

Laryngeal papillomatosis (juvenile papillomatosis)

Laryngeal papillomas are tiny proliferations of squamous epithelium supported by a delicate fibrovascular tree. The disease is a nonneoplastic reaction, presumably to a papillomavirus.[116] The offspring of mothers with genital condylomata acuminata seem to be at special risk.[164] A few papillomas cause hoarseness, but if hundreds are present, they compromise the airway. Sometimes there is progression down the trachea and bronchi. Papillomas of the larynx may deeply invade the mucosa but generally do not metastasize.[126] There are, however, a few examples of papillomatosis that have been followed by metastasizing carcinomas.[166]

Papillomatosis is usually first diagnosed in children between 1 and 6 years of age, but adult onset also occurs.[113,145] Careful removal is the most effective therapy, but there are nearly always one or more recurrences. About 25% of patients have no further episodes after 10 years of age, but approximately 20% have disease well into adulthood.[152]

Solitary squamous papilloma of the larynx is probably unrelated to papillomatosis. Solitary papillomas occur almost exclusively in adults and rarely recur. One must be certain that the squamous papilloma in an adult is not a papillary squamous carcinoma because invasive squamous carcinoma sometimes has a papillary surface. Many cases interpreted as papilloma evolving into invasive carcinoma were actually carcinomas from the start.[133]

Postintubation granulation tissue (intubation granuloma, pyogenic granuloma)

Endotracheal tubes invariably erode the epithelium.[123] Granulation tissue can form during the several days after the injury, resulting in a polypoid mass that is frequently referred to as "intubation granuloma" or "pyogenic granuloma." These are misnomers because there is no granuloma formation.[125] Long-standing intubation can lead to fibrous stenosis.[138]

Vocal nodule and polyp

Vocal nodules are 1 to 2 mm bulges of Reinke's space at the junction of the anterior and middle thirds of the true cord. The cause is believed to be trauma from vocal abuse. This is reflected in such terms as "screamer's node" and "preacher's node." Microscopically the nodules are extremely variable. Edema is usually prominent. Fibrous tissue may be sparse or dense. Newly formed, irregular, ectatic vascular channels are often numerous. There may be large deposits of fibrin that resemble amyloid (Fig. 22-10). A thickened subepithelial basement membrane contributes to the mimicry of amyloid. The epithelium can be hyperplastic, slightly keratotic, and disorganized slightly.[172] Atypical stromal cells may be found.[126]

Vocal polyps have the same microscopic spectrum as vocal nodules. However, they involve the entire cord. There is usually a history of heavy smoking and sometimes vocal abuse.[173]

Amyloid

Amyloid forms symptomatic, nonulcerated masses of the larynx in adults. The amyloid is deposited within vessel walls and mucous glands as well as amorphous masses. Plasma cells may be numerous or sparse. La-

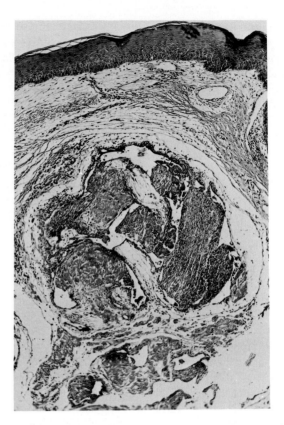

Fig. 22-10. Vocal nodule with edematous stroma, ectatic vessels, and fibrin deposits *(dark material).*

ryngeal amyloidosis usually occurs in the absence of systemic amyloidosis.[142]

Cysts

Laryngeal cysts form by retention of secretions in the occluded ducts of the mucous glands. Rarely they are multiple.[103] Hoarseness is the usual symptom, but there may be respiratory embarrassment by large cysts arising from the saccule of the ventricle.[121] The cysts are lined by squamous or ciliated columnar epithelium, the normal types of duct epithelium. Some cysts are lined by columnar cells with eosinophilic, granular cytoplasm (oncocytic cysts). The cytoplasmic appearance is caused by mitochondrial hyperplasia; hence the cells are true oncocytes.[158]

A laryngocele is an air-filled cyst that arises from the saccule of the ventricle. It can bulge into the supraglottic larynx or herniate beyond the larynx into the soft tissue of the neck. Laryngoceles may cause airway obstruction; they are also subject to infection (laryngopyocele).[111]

Keratosis and carcinoma in situ

Keratosis is found mainly in smokers and less often in those who abuse their voices. Microscopically a granular layer covered with keratin is present at the surface. The deeper epithelium may or may not have dysplastic nuclear changes. The patient who has keratosis without dysplasia is at a negligible risk of carcinoma though the keratosis may recur. On the other hand, patients with dysplastic cells have a small but increased risk of cancer. Cancer develops in about 3% of patients with keratosis, often several years later.[117] Moist keratin, whether covering a benign or a dysplastic lesion, causes a white patch called "leukoplakia." The term "leukoplakia" should never be used to describe the microscopic findings.

The diagnosis of carcinoma in situ (CIS) has been used for a wide variety of histologic lesions. The published images in the literature are so diverse that CIS is not a reproducible diagnosis.[124,139,140,141,163] It is extremely rare for the epithelium of the larynx to resemble the small-cell CIS of the uterine cervix. Because of the inconsistency with which CIS has been diagnosed, the diagnosis should be abandoned. The degree of aneuploidy rather than the severity of the histologic images is probably a more reliable guide to the risk for subsequent laryngeal malignancy.[108,118] The management of severely dysplastic lesions, including those designated as CIS, remains controversial.[144]

The meticulous autopsy studies by Auerbach suggest that dysplasia even in its severest form ("carcinoma in situ") is reversible in cigarette smokers who quit smoking.[104] Nearly 16% of smokers had "carcinoma in situ" and 99% had dysplasia. By contrast, none of the former cigarette smokers had "carcinoma in situ" and only 25% had mild dysplasia, a percentage similar to those who had never smoked.

Squamous carcinoma

About 99% of laryngeal malignancies are squamous carcinomas that arise almost exclusively in cigarette, cigar, or pipe smokers. Smokers who are ethanol abusers are at even greater risk, especially for cancer of the epiglottis and false cord.[181] The role of radiation, as of x rays used in dentistry, remains to be determined.[143]

The behavior of carcinomas of the larynx depends on the anatomic compartment of origin. Differences in access to lymphatics and routes of extension into the adjacent soft tissues influence the anatomic extent of tumor at the time of diagnosis. If the tumor is confined to the compartment of origin (and therefore is relatively small), the survival rate is around 90%. When there is extension into soft tissues, the rate is only 40%. If the invasion is sufficient to fix the larynx, that is, render it immobile on palpation, the survival rate is still lower. The presence of cervical lymph node metastases results in about a 40% survival rate. If the nodes are fixed, the rate is 20%.[168]

Two thirds of laryngeal cancers are in the glottis (true vocal cords and anterior commissure). The cord has minimal lymphatic drainage, and if the tumor is small and confined to the cord, more than 90% of patients are cured with radiation therapy or conservative laryngeal resection. Fixation of the cord, however, is evidence of extension into the vocal muscle where lymphatics are more numerous. Between 8% and 15% of the patients with glottic carcinoma have cervical node metastases.[168] One third of cancers are supraglottic tumors that involve the laryngeal surface of the epiglottis, the arytenoids, the false cords, or the ventricle. Between 30% and 40% have lymph node metastases when first seen.[148,168] The rare subglottic carcinoma arises inferior to the true cord. Lymph node metastases are found in about half of these patients, and the survival rate is correspondingly poor.[137] Transglottic carcinomas are either advanced glottic or supraglottic cancers that cross the ventricle and involve the other side. One third of these patients have lymph node involvement.[147] Carcinomas of the piriform sinus (properly a part of the hypopharynx rather than the larynx) have a poor prognosis, with fewer than one third of patients surviving. Most deaths occur within 2 years of the diagnosis.[154]

Death from laryngeal cancer is usually a result of uncontrolled local growth into vital structures such as the trachea or carotid artery. The patient's general status is also compromised by an inability to sustain adequate nutrition. Thirty percent to 60% of patients have distant metastases at the time of death, but most also have persistent growth of cancer in the neck.[101,159] Patients with carcinoma of the larynx are at high risk for primary carcinoma of the lung should they survive their laryngeal tumor.

Squamous carcinomas in the supraglottic and subglottic regions tend to be more poorly differentiated than glottic tumors. In addition to the conventional criteria of cellular maturity and keratin formation several other features can be assessed in determining the prognosis.[119]

Spindle cell carcinoma

Malignant tumors of the larynx can have a spindle cell component intermixed with conventional squamous carcinoma, or sometimes the tumors consist only of spindle cells. Immunocytochemical analysis of the spindle cells shows that they may have either epithelial or mesenchymal markers, and some cells contain filaments of both epithelial and mesenchymal cells. The term "spindle cell carcinoma" is still recommended for this histologically somewhat diverse group of tumors.[183] The tumor is often polypoid, and if there is a narrow base of attachment, the prognosis is favorable. Large infiltra-

60. Koss, L.G., Spiro, R.H., and Hajdu, S.: Small cell (oat cell) carcinoma of minor salivary gland origin, Cancer **30:**737, 1972.
61. Levy, M.G., Meuten, D.J., and Breitschwerdt, E.B.: Cultivation of *Rhinosporidium seeberi* in vitro: interaction with epithelial cells, Science **234:**474, 1986.
62. McGill, T.J., Simpson, G., and Healy, G.B.: Fulminant aspergillosis of the nose and paranasal sinuses: a new clinical entity, Laryngoscope **90:**748, 1980.
63. Mills, S.E., Cooper, P.H., and Fechner, R.E.: Lobular capillary hemangioma: underlying lesion of pyogenic granuloma; a study of 73 cases from the oral and nasal mucous membranes, Am. J. Surg. Pathol. **4:**471, 1980.
64. Mills, S.E., Fechner, R.E., and Cantrell, R.W.: Aggressive sinonasal lesion resembling normal intestinal mucosa, Am. J. Surg. Pathol. **6:**803, 1982.
65. Mills, S.E., and Frierson, H.F., Jr.: Olfactory neuroblastoma: a clinicopathologic study of 21 cases, Am. J. Surg. Pathol. **9:**317, 1985.
66. Moore, D.M., and Berke, G.S.: Synovial sarcoma of the head and neck, Arch. Otolaryngol. **113:**311, 1987.
67. Mygind, N.: Pathogenesis of allergic rhinitis, Acta Otolaryngol. **360**(suppl.):9, 1979.
68. Mygind, N., Thomsen, J., and Jorgensen, M.B.: Ultrastructure of the epithelium in atrophic rhinitis: transmission electron microscopic studies, Acta Otolaryngol. **78:**106, 1974.
69. Natvig, K., and Larsen, T.E.: Mucocele of paranasal sinuses: a retrospective clinical and histological study, J. Laryngol. Otol. **92:**1075, 1978.
70. Nieto, C.S., et al.: Aggressive fibromatosis of the sphenoid, Arch. Otolaryngol. **112:**326, 1986.
71. Oppenheimer, E.H., and Rosenstein, B.J.: Differential pathology of nasal polyps in cystic fibrosis and atopy, Lab. Invest. **40:**445, 1979.
72. Ridolfi, R.L., Lieberman, P.H., Erlandson, R.A., and Moore, O.S.: Schneiderian papillomas: a clinicopathologic study of 30 cases, Am. J. Surg. Pathol. **1:**43, 1977.
73. Robitaille, Y., Seemayer, T.A., and El Deiry, A.: Peripheral nerve tumors involving paranasal sinuses: a case report and review of the literature, Cancer **35:**1254, 1975.
74. Roush, G.C.: Epidemiology of cancer of the nose and paranasal sinuses: current concepts, Head Neck Surg. **2:**3, 1979.
75. Sanchez-Casis, G., Devine, K.D., and Weiland, L.H.: Nasal adenocarcinomas that closely stimulate colonic carcinomas, Cancer **28:**714, 1971.
76. Settipane, G.A., and Chafee, F.H.: Nasal polyps in asthma and rhinitis: a review of 6,037 patients, J. Allergy Clin. Immunol. **59:**17, 1977.
77. Silva, E.G., Butler, J.J., MacKay, B., and Goepfert, H.: Neuroblastomas and neuroendocrine carcinomas of the nasal cavity: a proposed new classification, Cancer **50:**2388, 1982.
78. Sirola, R.: Choanal polyps, Acta Otolaryngol. **61:**42, 1966.
79. Snyder, R.N., and Perzin, K.H.: Papillomatosis of nasal cavity and paranasal sinuses (inverted papilloma, squamous papilloma): a clinicopathologic study, Cancer **30:**668, 1972.
80. Spiro, R.H., Huvos, A.G., and Strong, E.W.: Adenoid cystic carcinoma of salivary origin: a clinicopathologic study of 242 cases, Am. J. Surg. **128:**512, 1974.
81. Straatsma, B.R., Zimmerman, L.E., and Gass, J.D.M.: Phycomycosis: a clinicopathologic study of fifty-one cases, Lab. Invest. **11:**963, 1962.
82. Taxy, J.B., Bharani, N.K., Mills, S.E., Frierson, H.F., Jr., and Gould, V.E.: The spectrum of olfactory neural tumors: a light-microscopic immunohistochemical and ultrastructural analysis, Am. J. Surg. Pathol. **10:**687, 1986.
83. Tos, M., and Mogensen, C.: Mucous glands in nasal polyps, Arch. Otolaryngol. **103:**407, 1977.
84. Tsokos, J., Fauci, A.S., and Costa, J.: Idiopathic midline destructive disease (IMDD): a subgroup of patients with the "midline granuloma" syndrome, Am. J. Clin. Pathol. **77:**162, 1982.
85. Weiss, M.D., de Fries, H.O., Taxy, J.B., and Braine, H.: Primary small cell carcinoma of the paranasal sinuses, Arch. Otolaryngol. **109:**341, 1983.
86. Wheeler, T.M., Sessions, R.B., and McGavran, M.H.: Myospherulosis: a preventable iatrogenic nasal and paranasal entity, Arch. Otolaryngol. **106:**272, 1980.

Nasopharynx

87. Baker, S.R.: Nasopharyngeal carcinoma: clinical course and results of therapy, Head Neck Surg. **3:**8, 1980.
88. Easton, J.M., Levine, P.H., and Hyams, V.J.: Nasopharyngeal carcinoma in the United States: a pathologic study of 177 U.S. and 30 foreign cases, Arch. Otolaryngol. **106:**88, 1980.
89. Giffler, R.F., et al.: Lymphoepithelioma in cervical lymph nodes of children and young adults, Am. J. Surg. Pathol. **1:**293, 1977.
90. Heffelfinger, M.J., Dahlin, D.C., MacCarty, C.S., et al.: Chordomas and cartilaginous tumors at the skull base, Cancer **32:**410, 1973.
91. Henderson, B.E., Louie, E., SooHoo Jing, J., et al.: Risk factors associated with nasopharyngeal carcinoma, N. Engl. J. Med. **295:**1101, 1976.
92. Hjertaas, R.J., Morrison, M.D., and Murray, R.B.: Teratomas of the nasopharynx, J. Otolaryngol. **8:**411, 1977.
93. Jones, G.C., DeSanto, L.W., Bremer, J.W., and Neel, H.B., III: Juvenile angiofibromas: behavior and treatment of extensive and residual tumors, Arch. Otolaryngol. **112:**1191, 1986.
94. Lee, D.A., Rao, B.R., Meyer, J.S., Prioleau, P.G., and Bauer, W.C.: Hormonal receptor determination in juvenile nasopharyngeal angiofibromas, Cancer **46:**547, 1980.
95. Lin, T.M., Yang, C.S., Tu, S.M., Chen, C.J., Kuo, K.C., and Harayama, T.: Interaction of factors associated with cancer of the nasopharynx, Cancer **44:**1419, 1979.
96. Lloyd, R.V., Chandler, W.F., Kovacs, K., and Ryan, N.: Ectopic pituitary adenomas with normal anterior pituitary glands, Am. J. Surg. Pathol. **10:**546, 1986.
97. Neel, H.B., III, Pearson, G.R., Weiland, L.H., Taylor, W.F., Goepfert, H.H., Pilch, B.Z., Lanier, A.P., Huang, A.T., Hyams, V.J., Levine, P.H., Henle, G., and Henle, W.: Anti-EBV serologic tests for nasopharyngeal carcinoma, Laryngoscope **90:**1981, 1980.
98. Shanmugaratnam, K., Chan, S.H., de-Thé, G., Goh, J.E., Khor, T.H., Simons, M.J., and Tye, C.Y.: Histopathology of nasopharyngeal carcinoma: correlations with epidemiology, survival rates and other biological characteristics, Cancer **44:**1029, 1979.
99. Taxy, J.B.: Juvenile nasopharyngeal angiofibroma: an ultrastructural study, Cancer **39:**1044, 1977.

Larynx

100. Abramson, A.L., Brandsma, J., Steinberg, B., and Winkler, B.: Verrucous carcinoma of the larynx: possible human papillomavirus etiology, Arch. Otolaryngol. **111:**709, 1985.
101. Abramson, A.L., Parisier, S.C., Zamansky, M.J., et al.: Distant metastases from carcinoma of the larynx, Laryngoscope **81:**1503, 1971.
102. Agarwal, R.K., Blitzer, A., and Perzin, K.H.: Granular cell tumors of the larynx, Otolaryngol. Head Neck Surg. **87:**807, 1979.
103. Altmeyer, V.L., and Fechner, R.E.: Multiple epiglottic cysts, Arch. Otolaryngol. **104:**673, 1978.
104. Auerbach, O., Hammond, E.C., and Garfinkel, L.: Histologic changes in the larynx in relation to smoking habits, Cancer **25:**92, 1970.
105. Babbitt, D.C., Yarington, C.T., Jr., and Yonders, A.J.: Malignant lymphoma of the larynx, J. Laryngol. Otol. **87:**807, 1973.
106. Bauer, W.C., and McGavran, M.H.: Carcinoma in situ and evaluation of epithelial changes in laryngopharyngeal biopsies, JAMA **221:**72, 1972.
107. Binder, W.J., Som, P., Kaneko, M., and Biller, H.F.: Mucoepidermoid carcinoma of the larynx: a case report and review of the literature, Ann. Otol. Rhinol. Laryngol. **89:**103, 1980.
108. Bjelkenkrantz, K., Lundgren, J., and Olofsson, J.: Single cell DNA measurements in hyperplastic, dysplastic and carcinomatous laryngeal epithelia, with special reference to the occurrence of hypertetraploid cell nuclei, Analyt. Quant. Cytol. **5:**184, 1983.

109. Bridges, G.P., Nassar, V.H., and Skinner, H.G.: Hemangioma in the adult larynx, Arch. Otolaryngol. **92**:493, 1970.

110. Calcaterra, T.C.: Orolaryngeal histoplasmosis, Laryngoscope **80**:111, 1970.

111. Canalis, R.F., Maxwell, D.S., and Hemenway, W.C.: Laryngocele: an updated review, J. Otolaryngol. **6**:191, 1977.

112. Cannon, C.R., Johns, M.E., and Fechner, R.E.: Immature teratoma of the larynx, Otolaryngol. Head Neck Surg. **96**:366, 1987.

113. Capper, J.W., Bailey, C.M., and Michaels, L.: Squamous papillomas of the larynx in adults: a review of 63 cases, Clin. Otolaryngol. **8**:109, 1983.

114. Chang-Lo, M.: Laryngeal involvement in von Recklinghausen's disease: a case report and review of the literature, Laryngoscope **87**:435, 1977.

115. Chung, C.K., Stryker, J.A., Abt, A.B., Cunningham, D.E., Strauss, M., and Connor, G.H.: Histologic grading in the clinical evaluation of laryngeal carcinoma, Arch. Otolaryngol. **106**:623, 1980.

116. Costa, J., Howley, P.M., Bowling, M.C., Howard, R., and Bauer, W.C.: Presence of human papilloma viral antigens in juvenile multiple laryngeal papilloma, Am. J. Clin. Pathol. **75**:194, 1981.

117. Crissman, J.D.: Laryngeal keratosis preceding laryngeal carcinoma: a report of four cases, Arch. Otolaryngol. **108**:445, 1982.

118. Crissman, J.D., and Fu, Y.-S.: Intraepithelial neoplasia of the larynx, Arch. Otolaryngol. **112**:522, 1986.

119. Crissman, J.D.: Squamous-cell carcinoma of the floor of the mouth, Head Neck Surg. **3**:2, 1980.

120. Crissman, J.D., Gnepp, D.R., Goodman, M.L., Hellquist, H., and Johns, M.E.: Preinvasive lesions of the upper aerodigestive tract: histologic definitions and clinical implications (a symposium), Pathol. Annu. **22**:311, 1987.

121. DeSanto, L.W., Devine, K.D., and Weiland, L.H.: Cysts of the larynx: classification, laryngoscope **80**:145, 1970.

122. Donaldson, K.: Fibrosarcoma in a previously irradiated larynx, J. Laryngol. Otol. **92**:425, 1978.

123. Dubick, M.N., and Wright, B.D.: Comparison of laryngeal pathology following long-term oral and nasal endotracheal intubations, Anesth. Analg. **57**:663, 1978.

124. Elman, A.J., Goodman, M., Wang, C.C., Pilch, B., and Busse, J.: In-situ carcinoma of the vocal cords, Cancer **43**:2422, 1979.

125. Fechner, R.E., Cooper, P.H., and Mills, S.E.: Pyogenic granuloma of the larynx and trachea: a causal and pathologic misnomer for granulation tissue, Arch. Otolaryngol. **107**:30, 1981.

126. Fechner, R.E., Goepfert, H., and Alford, B.R.: Invasive laryngeal papillomatosis, Arch. Otolaryngol. **99**:147, 1974.

127. Fechner, R.E., and Mills, S.E.: Verruca vulgaris of the larynx: a distinctive lesion of probable viral origin confused with verrucous carcinoma, Am. J. Surg. Pathol. **6**:357, 1982.

128. Fechner, R.E.: Pathologic quiz case 2: vocal nodule with atypical stromal cells, Arch. Otolaryngol. **110**:698, 1984.

129. Ferlito, A., and Recher, G.: Ackerman's tumor (verrucous carcinoma) of the larynx: a clinicopathologic study of 77 cases, Cancer **46**:1617, 1980.

130. Ferlito, A., Nicolai, P., Recher, G., and Narne, S.: Primary laryngeal malignant fibrous histiocytoma: review of the literature and report of seven cases, Laryngoscope **93**:1351, 1983.

131. Fink, B.R., and Beckwith, J.B.: Laryngeal mucous gland excess in victims of sudden infant death, Am. J. Dis. Child. **134**:144, 1980.

132. Freeland, A.P., Van Nostrand, A.W.P., and Jahn, F.F.: Metastases to the larynx, J. Otolaryngol. **8**:448, 1979.

133. Friedberg, S.A., Stagman, R., and Hass, G.M.: Papillary lesions of the larynx in adults: a pathologic study, Ann. Otol. Rhinol. Laryngol. **80**:683, 1971.

134. Gallivan, M.V.E., Chun, B., Rowden, G., and Lack, E.E.: Laryngeal paraganglioma: case report with ultrastructural analysis and literature review, Am. J. Surg. Pathol. **3**:85, 1979.

135. Gatti, W.M., Strom, C.G., and Orfei, E.L.: Synovial sarcoma of the laryngopharynx, Arch. Otolaryngol. **101**:633, 1975.

136. Gorenstein, A., Neel, H.B., Devine, K.D., et al.: Solitary extramedullary plasmacytoma of the larynx, Arch. Otolaryngol. **103**:159, 1977.

137. Harrison, D.F.N.: The pathology and management of subglottic cancer, Ann. Otol. Rhinol. Laryngol. **80**:6, 1971.

138. Hawkins, D.B., and Luxford, W.M.: Laryngeal stenosis from endotracheal intubation: a review of 58 cases, Ann. Otol. Rhinol. Laryngol. **89**:454, 1980.

139. Hellquist, H., Lundgren, J., and Olofsson, J.: Hyperplasia, keratosis, dysplasia and carcinoma in-situ of the vocal cords: a follow-up study, Clin. Otolaryngol. **7**:11, 1982.

140. Hellquist, H., Olofsson, J., and Gröntoft, O.: Carcinoma in-situ and severe dysplasia of the vocal cords: a clinicopathologic and photometric investigation, Acta Otolaryngol. **92**:543, 1981.

141. Hellquist, H., Olofsson, J., and Gröntoft, O.: Chondrosarcoma of the larynx, J. Laryngol. Otol. **93**:1037, 1979.

142. Hellquist, H., Olofsson, J., Sökjer, H., and Odkvist, L.M.: Amyloidosis of the larynx, Acta Otolaryngol. **88**:443, 1979.

143. Hinds, M.W., and Thomas, D.B.: Asbestos, dental x-rays, tobacco, and alcohol in the epidemiology of laryngeal cancer, Cancer **44**:1114, 1979.

144. Hintz, B.L., Kagan, A.R., Nussbaum, H., Rao, A.R., Chan, P.Y., and Miles, J.: A "watchful waiting" policy for in situ carcinoma of the vocal cords, Arch. Otolaryngol. **107**:746, 1981.

145. Johnson, J.T., Barnes, E.L., and Justice, W.: Adult onset laryngeal papillomatosis, Otolaryngol. Head Neck Surg. **89**:879, 1981.

146. Kheir, S.M., Flint, A., and Moss, J.A.: Primary aspergillosis of the larynx simulating carcinoma, Hum. Pathol. **14**:184, 1983.

147. Kirchner, J.A., Cornog, J.L., Jr., and Holmes, R.E.: Transglottic cancer: its growth and spread within the larynx, Arch. Otolaryngol. **99**:247, 1974.

148. Kirchner, J.A., and Som, M.L.: Clinical and histologic observations on supraglottic cancer, Ann. Otol. Rhinol. Laryngol. **80**:638, 1971.

149. Lambert, P.R., Ward, P.H., and Berci, G.: Pseudosarcoma of the larynx: a comprehensive analysis, Arch. Otolaryngol. **106**:700, 1980.

150. Lim, T.A., Spanier, S.S., and Kohut, R.I.: Laryngeal clefts: a histopathologic study and review, Ann. Otol. Rhinol. Laryngol. **88**:837, 1979.

151. MacMillan, R.J., and Fechner, R.E.: Pleomorphic adenoma of the larynx, Arch. Pathol. Lab. Med. **110**:254, 1986.

152. Majoros, M., Parkhill, E.M., and Devine, K.D.: Papilloma of the larynx in children: a clinicopathologic study, Am. J. Surg. **108**:470, 1964.

153. Markel, S.F., Magielski, J.E., and Beals, T.F.: Carcinoid tumor of the larynx, Arch. Otolaryngol. **106**:777, 1980.

154. Marks, J.E., Kurnik, B., Powers, W.E., and Ogura, J.H.: Carcinoma of the pyriform sinus: an analysis of treatment results and patterns of failure, Cancer **41**:1008, 1978.

155. Mills, S.E., Cooper, P.H., Garland, T.A., and Johns, M.E.: Small cell undifferentiated carcinoma of the larynx: report of two patients and review of 13 additional cases, Cancer **51**:116, 1983.

156. Mills, S.E., and Johns, M.E.: Atypical carcinoid tumor of the larynx: a light microscopic and ultrastructural study, Arch. Otolaryngol. **110**:58, 1984.

157. Montgomery, W.W., and Smith, S.A.: Congenital laryngeal defects in the adult, Ann. Otol. Rhinol. Laryngol. **85**:491, 1976.

158. Newman, B.H., Taxy, J.B., and Laker, H.K.: Laryngeal cysts in adults: a clinicopathologic study of 20 cases, Am. J. Clin. Pathol. **81**:715, 1984.

159. O'Brien, P.H., Carlson, R., Steubner, E.A., Jr., et al.: Distant metastases in epidermoid cell carcinoma of the head and neck, Cancer **27**:304, 1971.

160. Olafsson, J., and van Nostrand, A.W.P.: Adenoid cystic carcinoma of the larynx: a report of four cases and review of the literature, Cancer **40**:1307, 1977.

161. Pahor, A.L.: Herpes zoster of the larynx—how common? J. Laryngol. Otol. **93**:93, 1979.

162. Pellettiere, E.V., II, Holinger, L.D., and Schild, J.A.: Lymphoid hyperplasia of larynx simulating neoplasia, Ann. Otol. Rhinol. Laryngol. **89**:65, 1980.

163. Pene, F., and Fletcher, G.H.: Results of irradiation of the in-situ carcinomas of the vocal cords, Cancer 37:2586, 1976.

164. Quick, C.A., Watts, S.L., Krzyzek, R.A., and Faras, A.J.: Relationship between condylomata and laryngeal papilloma: clinical and molecular virological evidence, Ann. Otol. Rhinol. Laryngol. 89:467, 1980.

165. Reese, M.C., and Colclasure, J.B.: Cryptococcosis of the larynx, Arch. Otolaryngol. 101:698, 1975.

166. Schnadig, V.J., Clark, W.D., Clegg, T.J., and Yao, C.S.: Invasive papillomatosis and squamous carcinoma complicating juvenile laryngeal papillomatosis, Arch. Otolaryngol. 112:966, 1986.

167. Schwenzfeier, C.W., and Fechner, R.E.: Herpes simplex of the epiglottis, Arch. Otolaryngol. 102:374, 1976.

168. Smith, R.R., Caulk, R., Frazell, E., et al.: Revision of the clinical staging system for cancer of larynx, Cancer 31:72, 1973.

169. Snyderman, C., Johnson, J.T., and Barnes, L.: Carcinoid tumor of the larynx: case report and review of the world literature, Otolaryngol. Head Neck Surg. 95:158, 1986.

170. Spiro, R.H., Hajdu, S.I., Lewis, J.S., et al.: Mucus gland tumors of the larynx and laryngopharynx, Ann. Otol. Rhinol. Laryngol. 85:498, 1976.

171. Stanley, R.J., DeSanto, L.W., and Weiland, L.H.: Oncocytic and oncocytoid carcinoid tumors (well differentiated neuroendocrine carcinomas) of the larynx, Arch. Otolaryngol. 112:529, 1986.

172. Steinberg, B.M., Abramson, A.L., Kahn, L.B., and Hirschfield, L.: Vocal cord polyps: biochemical and histologic evaluation, Laryngoscope 95:1327, 1985.

173. Strong, M.S., and Vaughan, C.W.: Vocal cord nodules and polyps: the role of surgical treatment, Laryngoscope 81:911, 1971.

174. Suen, J.Y., Wetmore, S.J., Wetzel, W.J., and Craig, R.D.: Blastomycosis of the larynx, Ann. Otol. Rhinol. Laryngol. 89:563, 1980.

175. Szpunar, J., Glowacki, J., Laskowski, A., et al.: Fibrinous laryngotracheal bronchitis in children, Arch. Otolaryngol. 93:173, 1971.

176. Toker, C., and Peterson, D.W.: Lymphoepithelioma of the vocal cord, Arch. Otolaryngol. 104:161, 1978.

177. Travis, L.W., Hybels, R.L., and Newman, M.H.: Tuberculosis of the larynx, Laryngoscope 86:549, 1976.

178. Walker, G.K., Fechner, R.E., Johns, M.E., and Teja, K.: Necrotizing sialometaplasia of larynx secondary to atheromatous embolization, Am. J. Clin. Pathol. 77:221, 1982.

179. Ward, P.H., Berci, G., Morledge, D., and Schwartz, H.: Coccidioidomycosis in the larynx of infants and adults, Ann. Otol. Rhinol. Laryngol. 86:655, 1977.

180. Williams, R.I.: Allergic laryngitis, Ann. Otol. Rhinol. Laryngol. 81:558, 1972.

181. Wynder, E.L., Covey, L.S., Mabuchi, K., et al.: Environmental factors in cancer of the larynx: a second look, Cancer 38:1591, 1976.

182. Yonkers, A.J.: Candidiasis of the larynx, Ann. Otol. Rhinol. Laryngol. 82:812, 1973.

183. Zarbo, R.J., Crissman, J.A., Venkat, H., and Weiss, M.A.: Spindle-cell carcinoma of the upper aerodigestive tract mucosa: an immunohistologic and ultrastructural study of 18 biphasic tumors and comparison with seven monophasic spindle-cell tumors, Am. J. Surg. Pathol. 10:741, 1986.

Middle ear

184. Borley, J.E., and Kapur, Y.P.: Histopathologic changes in the temporal bone resulting from measles infection, Arch. Otolaryngol. 103:162, 1977.

185. Chevance, L.G., Bretlau, P., Jorgensen, M.B., et al.: Otosclerosis: an electron microscopic and cytochemical study, Acta Otolaryngol. 272(suppl.):1, 1970.

186. House, J.W., and Sheehy, J.L.: Cholesteatoma with intact tympanic membrane: a report of 41 cases, Laryngoscope 90:70, 1980.

187. Jahn, A.F., and Farkashidy, J.: New perspectives on the pathology of chronic otitis media, J. Otolaryngol. 9:131, 1980.

188. Juhn, S.K., et al.: Pathogenesis of otitis media, Ann. Otol. Rhinol. Laryngol. 86:481, 1977.

189. Mills, S.E., and Fechner, R.E.: Middle ear adenoma: a cytologically uniform neoplasm displaying a variety of architectural patterns, Am. J. Surg. Pathol. 8:677, 1984.

190. Rosenwasser, H.: Long-term results of therapy of glomus jugulare tumors, Arch. Otolaryngol. 97:49, 1973.

191. Saeed, Y.M., and Bassis, M.L.: Mixed tumor of the middle ear: a case report, Arch. Otolaryngol. 93:433, 1971.

192. Schiff, M., Poliquin, J.F., Catanzaro, A., and Ryan, A.F.: Tympanosclerosis: a theory of pathogenesis, Ann. Otol. Rhinol. Laryngol. 89(suppl.):70, 1980.

193. Shimada, T., and Lim, D.J.: Distribution of ciliated cells in the human middle ear: electron and light microscopic observations, Ann. Otol. Rhinol. Laryngol. 81:203, 1972.

194. Spector, G.J., Maisel, R.H., and Ogura, J.H.: Glomus jugulare tumors. II. A clinical pathologic analysis of the effects of radiotherapy, Ann. Otol. Rhinol. Laryngol. 83:26, 1974.

195. Stiller, D., Katenkamps, D., and Kuttner, K.: Jugular body tumors: hyperplasias or true neoplasms: light and electron microscopical investigations, Virchows Arch. [Pathol. Anat.] 365:163, 1975.

196. Tos, M.: Middle ear epithelia in chronic secretory otitis, Arch. Otolaryngol. 106:593, 1980.

197. Wine, C.J., and Metcalf, J.E.: Salivary gland choristoma of the middle ear and mastoid, Arch. Otolaryngol. 103:435, 1977.

External ear canal and auricle

198. Bailin, P.L., Levine, H.L., Wood, B.G., and Tucker, H.M.: Cutaneous carcinoma of the auricular and periauricular region, Arch. Otolaryngol. 106:692, 1980.

199. Chandler, J.R.: Malignant external otitis: further considerations, Ann. Otol. Rhinol. Laryngol. 86:417, 1977.

200. Dehner, L.P., and Chen, K.T.K.: Primary tumors of the external and middle ear: benign and malignant glandular neoplasms, Arch. Otolaryngol. 106:13, 1980.

201. Johns, M.E., and Headington, J.T.: Squamous cell carcinoma of the external auditory canal: a clinicopathologic study of 20 cases, Arch. Otolaryngol. 100:45, 1974.

202. Santos, V.V., Polisar, I.A., and Ruffy, M.L.: Bilateral pseudocysts of the auricle in a female, Ann. Otol. Rhinol. Laryngol. 83:9, 1974.

Temporal bone

203. Kobayashi, K., Igarashi, M., Ohashi, K., and McBride, R.A.: Metastatic seminoma of the temporal bone, Arch. Otolaryngol. 112:102, 1986.

204. Maniglia, A.J.: Intra and extracranial meningiomas involving the temporal bone, Laryngoscope 88:12, 1978.

205. Naufal, P.M.: Primary sarcomas of the temporal bone, Arch. Otolaryngol. 98:44, 1973.

206. Seftel, D.M.: Ear canal hyperostosis—surfer's ear, Arch. Otolaryngol 103:58, 1977.

207. Sweet, R.M., Kornblut, A.D., and Hyams, V.J.: Eosinophilic granuloma in the temporal bone, Laryngoscope 89:1545, 1979.

Diseases of diverse sites

208. Arkin, C.F., and Masi, A.T.: Relapsing polychondritis: review of current status and case report, Semin. Arthritis Rheum. 5:41, 1975.

209. Churg, A., and Ringus, J: Ultrastructural observations on the histogenesis of alveolar rhabdomyosarcoma, Cancer 41:1355, 1978.

210. Dehner, L.P., and Chen, K.T.K.: Primary tumors of the external and middle ear. III. A clinicopathologic study of embryonal rhabdomyosarcoma, Arch. Otolaryngol. 104:399, 1978.

211. Dehner, L.P., Enzinger, F.M., and Font, R.L.: Fetal rhabdomyoma: an analysis of nine cases, Cancer 30:160, 1972.

212. di Santi'Agnese, P.A. and Knowles, D.M., II: Extracardiac rhabdomyoma: a clinicopathologic study and review of the literature, Cancer 46:780, 1980.

213. Eusebi, V., Ceccarelli, C., Gorza, L., Schiaffino, S., and Bussolati, G.: Immunocytochemistry of rhabdomyosarcoma: the use of four different markers, Am. J. Surg. Pathol. **10:**293, 1986.

214. Fu, Y.-S., and Perzin, K.H.: Nonepithelial tumors of the nasal cavity, paranasal sinuses, and nasopharynx: a clinicopathologic study. V. Skeletal muscle tumors (rhabdomyoma and rhabdomyosarcoma), Cancer **37:**364, 1976.

215. Fu, Y.-S., and Perzin, K.H.: Nonepithelial tumors of the nasal cavity, paranasal sinuses, and nasopharynx: a clinicopathologic study. IX. Plasmacytomas, Cancer **42:**2399, 1978.

216. Kapadia, S.B., Desai, U., and Cheng, V.S.: Extramedullary plasmacytoma of the head and neck: a clinicopathologic study of 20 cases, Medicine **61:**317, 1982.

217. Kindblom, L.-G., Dalén, P., Edmar, G., and Kjelbo, H.: Relapsing polychondritis: a clinical, pathologic-anatomic and histochemical study of 2 cases, Acta Pathol. Microbiol. Scand. **85:**656, 1977.

218. Molenaar, W.M., Oosterhuis, J.W., Oosterhuis, A.M., and Ramaekers, F.C.: Mesenchymal and muscle-specific intermediate filaments (vimentin and desmin) in relation to differentiation in childhood rhabdomyosarcomas, Hum. Pathol. **16:**838, 1985.

219. Morales, A.R., Fine, G., and Horn, R.C., Jr.: Rhabdomyosarcoma: an ultrastructural appraisal, Pathol. Annu. **7:**81, 1972.

220. Noorani, M.A.: Plasmacytoma of middle ear and upper respiratory tract, J. Laryngol. Otol. **85:**125, 1975.

221. Wharam, M.D., Jr., Foulkes, M.A., Lawrence, W., Jr., Lindberg, R.D., Maurer, H.M., Newton, W.A., Jr., Ragab, A.H., Raney, R.B., Jr., and Tefft, M.: Soft tissue sarcoma of the head and neck in childhood: nonorbital and nonparameningeal sites: a report of the intergroup rhabdomyosarcoma study (IRS) — I, Cancer **53:**1016, 1984.

23 Face, Lips, Tongue, Teeth, Oral Soft Tissues, Jaws, Salivary Glands, and Neck

CHARLES A. WALDRON

FACE AND LIPS
Developmental anomalies including minor variations from normal

Facial clefts. Facial cleft, occurring in approximately 1 of every 800 births in whites, may exist as an isolated anomaly or in combination with other developmental disturbances (about 15% of clefts are so associated). Clefts have a racial predilection. They are most common in Native Americans (about 1 in 250) and least common in blacks (about 1 in 2500). Clefts in combination with other developmental disturbances may be so well known as to constitute a syndrome. Over 200 cleft syndromes are known; only a few are discussed here. Similarly, details of lateral and oblique facial clefts, cleft uvula, and microforms are left for comprehensive discussions elsewhere.[4]

Facial clefts arise from the failure of the ectomesenchyme to cross the junction of fusion of facial processes about the seventh week in utero. Thus cleft upper lip (harelip), the most common facial cleft, results from failure of fusion of the lower part of the median nasal (globular) process with the maxillary process. Unilateral cleft is about eight times more common than bilateral involvement. It is more common in males (about 60%) and on the left side (about 2:1). The degree of cleavage may vary from a slight notch at the lateral border of the philtrum to a complete separation extending into the nostril.

Commonly (in about 50% of cases), cleft lip is associated with cleft palate. When the cleft extends through the line of fusion between the primary and secondary palates, the area subsequently to be occupied by the developing lateral incisor frequently is disturbed. Supernumerary, impacted, or (most commonly) missing maxillary lateral incisors often are observed.

Cleft palate also may exist to varying degrees, ranging from bifid uvula to complete cleft. Not uncommonly, a submucous palatal cleft may remain undetected. Cleft palate unassociated with cleft lip (about 25%) is seen more commonly in females. Associated with abnormally small mandible (micrognathia) and tongue (microglossia) and posterior displacement of the tongue (glossoptosis), it is known as Pierre Robin syndrome. Cleft lip and cleft palate are commonly associated with chromosomal abnormalities; for example, cleft lip or cleft palate or both are seen in about 65% of infants with trisomy 13 and 4p-syndrome and in about 15% of the cases of trisomy 18.[3,4,16]

Congenital lip pits. Congenital paramedian pits of the lower lip vary in size from small bilateral dimples on the vermilion border to large snoutlike structures in the midline (Fig. 23-1). Resulting fistulas are lined by stratified squamous epithelium and are connected at the base with the mucous glands of the lip by means of communicating ducts. Mucus may exude from the openings.

The pits may occur alone or in combination with cleft palate or cleft lip and agenesis of second premolars as part of a syndrome. Inheritance is autosomal dominant with variable expressivity.[20] An unrelated condition, commissural lip pits, is observed on one or both sides in up to 15% of those examined.[13]

Fordyce's granules. Fordyce's granules are collections of sebaceous glands symmetrically located on the lateral vermilion part of the upper lip and on the buccal mucosa of approximately 65% of adults. They increase in number during mature adult life. The most common oral mucosal sites are lateral to the angle of the mouth about Stensen's papilla and lateral to the anterior pillar of the fauces.[19]

This chapter is a revision of the chapter authored by Dr. Robert J. Gorlin for the eighth edition of *Anderson's Pathology.* Some of the present material represents only a minor revision of Dr. Gorlin's text; other sections have been entirely rewritten by me. I thank Dr. Gorlin for his permission to use some of his original text here.

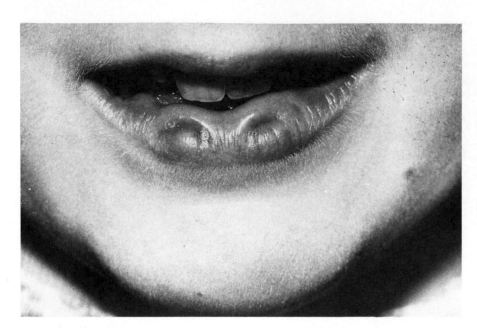

Fig. 23-1. Congenital lip pits (fistulas). Usually bilateral and symmetrically situated on vermilion border of lower lip, fistulas represent failure of closure of evanescent sulci that appear in 10 to 14 mm embryo. Congenital lip fistulas may occur alone or in association with facial clefts.

TONGUE
Developmental anomalies

Aglossia, microglossia, and macroglossia. Aglossia and its modification, microglossia, are rare congenital anomalies. Often, severe hypoglossia is associated with other defects, especially diminution of the extremities (hypoglossia-hypodactylia syndrome). The tongue, though apparently absent, is present as a small nubbin located posteriorly in the mouth and consisting essentially of that part normally developed from the copula. Cleft palate and bony fusion of the jaws have been associated with aglossia and microglossia.[4]

The term "macroglossia" is rather nonspecific, referring only to the presence of an enlarged tongue. In cases observed at birth or in the neonatal period, the usual cause is lymphangioma or hemangiolymphangioma, though rarely there may be true muscular hypertrophy or enlargement caused by congenital neurofibromatosis. Enlargement of half the tongue occurs in congenital hemifacial hypertrophy. The tongue may protrude from the mouth in trisomy 21 syndrome, congenital hypothyroidism, Hurler's syndrome, Beckwith-Wiedemann syndrome, glycogen storage disease type 2 (Pompe's disease), and many other conditions.[15]

Lingual thyroid gland. The presence of thyroid tissue within the tongue indicates arrested, partial, or incomplete embryologic descent of the gland. Approximately 10% of patients at autopsy have ectopic lingual thyroid tissue. Although the heterotopic tissue may occur anywhere along the normal path of the thyroglossal tract, the most frequent location is the base of the tongue at the foramen cecum. When superficial, the tissue is often raised, purplish, and crenulated and may be associated with hemorrhage. About 25% of patients are hy-

pothyroid. The incidence appears to be about 1 in 3000 patients with thyroid disease. Grossly, the heterotopic nodule measures about 2 to 3 cm and resembles the normal thyroid gland, though encapsulation is often less well defined.[18]

Median rhomboid "glossitis." This lesion is characterized by a roughly diamond-shaped reddish area devoid of papillae on the dorsum of the tongue, immediately anterior to the circumvallate papillae. Occurring in somewhat less than 1% of individuals, it has been traditionally considered to represent a developmental failure of coverage of the tuberculum impar by the lateral tubercles of the tongue. This concept, however, has been challenged by several investigators, and the term "central papillary atrophy" is probably more appropriate. *Candida albicans* infection has also been suggested as playing an etiologic role, but a direct cause-and-effect relationship has not been proved.[14,17,21]

Fissured tongue. Fissured tongue occurs in about 5% of the population, with the frequency increasing with age. It is noted more commonly in trisomy 21, being present in about 30% of affected individuals, and is also part of the Melkersson-Rosenthal syndrome (upper facial edema, facial palsy, cheilitis granulomatosa, buccal mucosal plication).[193]

TEETH
Developmental anomalies

Anomalies of number. Rarely is there complete absence of teeth (anodontia) or noticeable suppression in tooth formation (oligodontia). More commonly, a mild reduction in number (hypodontia) is observed.[10,26] The third molars and less commonly the maxillary lateral incisors and second premolars are the teeth most likely to be missing. Irradiation of the jaws may injure or inhibit developing tooth buds. Supernumerary teeth occasionally are observed—most commonly mesiodens in the midline of the maxilla and extra molars posterior to the third molars.

Anomalies of size. Rarely are all the teeth too large or too small. More frequently a single tooth is reduced in size (microdontia) or disproportionately enlarged (macrodontia).

Anomalies of shape. An anomaly called "dens invaginatus (dens in dente)" is manifest most commonly in the maxillary lateral permanent incisor.[10]

Anomalies of eruption. Rarely (1 in 2000 white infants) are teeth present at birth (natal teeth). This condition may occur idiopathically or occasionally in association with other anomalies (chondroectodermal dysplasia, pachyonychia congenita, oculomandibulodyscephaly) in the neonatal period. Delay in eruption may be related to physical obstruction (impaction), endocrine disturbances (cretinism), or a multitude of other causes (cleidocranial dysplasia, fibromatosis gingivae, and so on).[3,4]

Anomalies of dental pigmentation. The teeth may be discolored as a result of exogenous factors (usually chromogenic bacteria) or endogenous factors (usually altered blood pigments resulting from internal hemorrhage from trauma, congenital porphyria, erythroblastosis fetalis, and so on). Tetracyclines administered to the mother during the last trimester of pregnancy or to the infant are also incorporated in developing teeth, producing a yellow to gray color.[7,9] Their presence may be demonstrated by a noticeable yellow fluorescence under ultraviolet rays.[10]

Premature loss of teeth. Premature loss of a tooth or teeth may be attributable to trauma, histiocytosis X, or various genetic disorders such as hypophosphatasia, cyclic or chronic neutropenia, or premature periodontoclasia with hyperkeratosis of palms and soles (Papillon-Lefèvre syndrome).[4]

Hereditary enamel defects. Hereditary enamel defects occur in about 1 in 16,000 children, affecting both dentitions. According to Witkop and Rao,[31] there appear to be at least 10 distinct types.

In the hereditary enamel dysplasias, the teeth are frequently brown and the enamel has a tendency to flake off, but the enamel varies in hardness and thickness according to the specific type. The underlying dentin and the root formation are entirely normal, in contrast to dentinogenesis imperfecta and dentin dysplasia.

Hereditary dentin defects. Only two dentin defects are considered here: dentinogenesis imperfecta (hereditary opalescent dentin) and radicular dentin dysplasia. Both are transmitted as autosomal dominant traits.[27,32]

Dentinogenesis imperfecta usually occurs as an iso-

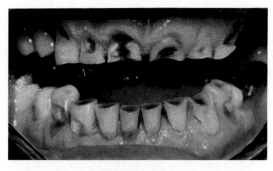

Fig. 23-2. Dental erosion characterized by smooth surface dissolution of enamel, especially at cervical position. Erosion may occur in persons who consume large quantities of highly acidic beverages, who habitually vomit, or who are exposed to vapors of inorganic acids. In many cases, however, the cause is unknown.

lated phenomenon (1 in 8000 individuals). A somewhat similar condition may occur as a component of osteogenesis imperfecta. Both deciduous and permanent teeth have an opalescent blue to brown color. Because of poor attachment at or near the dentinoenamel junction, the enamel fractures off. The roots are frequently thin and short and the canals obliterated. Microscopically, irregularly arranged dentinal tubules and defective matrix formation are noted.

Radicular dentin dysplasia is characterized by rootless teeth, generally exhibiting an absence of pulp chambers and canals but normal-appearing crowns.[11] Many teeth exhibit large periapical radiolucencies, and a pathognomonic half moon–shaped pulp chamber may be seen on radiographic examination.

Other enamel disturbances. Nonhereditary enamel disturbances may affect either dentition, and they may be widespread or involve only a single tooth. The disturbance may be severe, causing deep pitted grooves, or so mild as to be manifest by only a small chalky spot. Defective enamel may result from injury to the enamel organ at any time from the earliest period of matrix formation to the last stage when calcification is taking place or may result from acquired abnormalities as in dental erosion (Fig. 23-2).

Nutritional deficiencies (of calcium, phosphorus, vitamin D), endocrine and related disorders (hypoparathyroidism, pseudohypoparathyroidism, hypophosphatasia, rickets), congenital syphilis, infection of the deciduous precursor (Turner's tooth), ingestion of excessive fluoride (in excess of 1.5 ppm), and many miscellaneous conditions can injure the developing ameloblast, producing enamel hypoplasia.[10]

Other dentin disturbances. In rickets the developing dentin is hypocalcified, with a wide margin of predentin analogous to the wide osteoid seams in forming bone.

Vitamin D–resistant rickets, an X-linked dominant

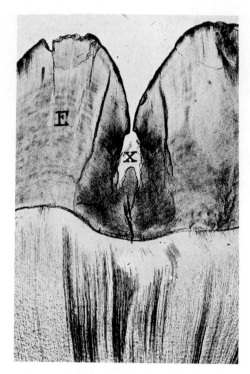

Fig. 23-3. Dental caries. Fissure lesion resulted in establishment of cavity, *X,* in enamel, *E.* Ground section of molar.

trait, is associated with defective dentin formation and resultant periapical abscess development. Similar changes have been reported in a variety of related metabolic disorders.[10]

Diseases of teeth

Dental caries. Dental caries is a disease of the enamel, dentin, and cementum that produces progressive demineralization of the calcified component and eventual destruction of the organic component, with the formation of a cavity in the tooth (Fig. 23-3). Microorganisms are present at all stages of the disease and, from the results of animal experiments, appear to be essential etiologic factors.[22-24] Specific strains of streptococci, especially *Streptococcus mutans* in its various serotypes, have been shown to induce dental caries in rats and hamsters. The etiologic process involves the metabolism of fermentable carbohydrates by these bacteria with the production of organic acids, which demineralize the tooth surface. Destruction of tooth structure by caries is easily differentiated from dental erosion and abrasion.

Tooth decay occurs or has occurred in the majority of individuals living in the United States, Canada, and Europe. Once a carious cavity has formed, the defect is permanent. The designation DMF (decayed, missing, filled) has proved useful in comparative studies of the frequency of dental caries, particularly in children and young adults.

Caries occurs in areas on tooth surfaces where saliva, food debris, and bacterial plaques accumulate. These areas are chiefly the pits and fissures, cervical part of the tooth, and interproximal surfaces. Surfaces that are cleansed by the excursion of food and the action of the tongue and cheeks are usually free of caries. If this process is disrupted (as by prosthetic appliances or lack of saliva), caries may develop rapidly.

The formation of bacterial plaques in areas of stagnation precedes cavity formation, especially in smooth dental surfaces. Acidogenic and aciduric bacteria, together with filamentous forms, are present in such plaques (Fig. 23-4).[23,24]

Studies throughout the world have given striking evidence of the efficiency of fluoridation of communal water supplies in reducing the rate of tooth decay in children.[10,25] After the introduction of fluoride to the drinking water (1 ppm) the DMF rate has generally decreased over a period of years by more than 50%.[25] Partial control of tooth decay by this method constitutes an important public health achievement. Topical applications of fluoride solutions to tooth surfaces and brushing the teeth with dentifrices containing fluoride appear to be effective in further reducing susceptibility to dental caries.

Excessive amounts of fluoride cause a condition called "mottled enamel." It occurs in children who have consumed drinking water containing 1.5 ppm fluoride or more during the time when tooth enamel is being formed in the developing, unerupted teeth.

Pulp and periapical periodontal disease. The tooth, projecting into the oral cavity through the mucous membrane and extending deep into the jawbone, affords a surprisingly direct pathway for infection after exposure and infection of the dental pulp and after ulceration or breakdown of the epithelial attachments.

Carious destruction of dental hard tissues frequently produces pulpitis or inflammation of dental soft tissues, including, by way of extension, those surrounding the apex of the tooth. An alternative, yet equally dentally threatening, pathway exists through the gingival attachment (see following discussion concerning periodontal disease).

Inflammation of the dental pulp may be noninfective. Trauma to the tooth from a blow, which may or may not fracture the tooth, from dental operations, or from excessive thermal changes may also induce inflammation. This may be minimal with recovery, particularly in teeth with incompletely formed roots, or it may be severe leading to necrosis.

Pulpitis, regardless of the etiologic agent, may be acute or chronic. In acute pulpitis, pain is usually severe and increased by heat or cold. Pulpitis, acute or chronic, may be asymptomatic or accompanied by a mild fever and leukocytosis. Periapical tissues become involved by extension.

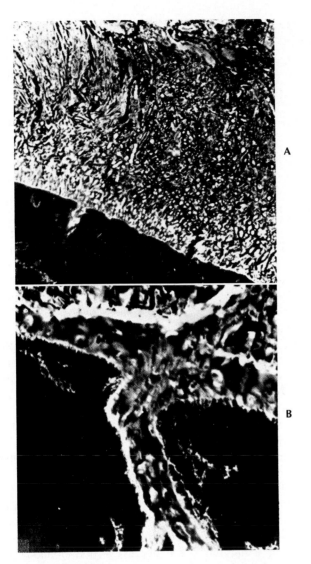

Fig. 23-4. A, Bacterial plaque isolated by acid flotation from clinically noncarious enamel. **B,** Mass of bacteria at enamel surface extending from plaque into lamella. (**A,** 2000×; **B,** 6000×; **A** and **B,** from Scott, D.B., and Albright, J.T.: Oral Surg. **7:**64, 1954.)

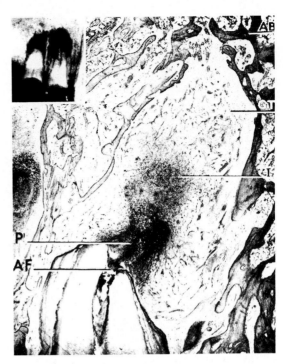

Fig. 23-5. Mesiodistal section through apex of maxillary first premolar with granuloma. *Inset,* Radiograph of specimen shows large areas of bone destruction around root ends of both maxillary premolars. *AB,* Alveolar bone; *AF,* apical foramen; *GT,* granulation tissue; *I,* dense cellular infiltration next to foramen; *P,* breaking down of tissue and formation of pus at foramen. (From Boyle, P.E., editor: Kronfeld's histopathology of the teeth and their surrounding structures, Philadelphia, 1955, Lea & Febiger.)

Acute alveolar or periapical abscess is usually the result of spread of suppurative infection from the tooth pulp through the root canals to the periodontal ligament about the tooth root apices. Drainage through the oral mucosa or to the adjacent skin of the face or neck may follow.

A more common sequela to dental pulp infection is the dental granuloma. Clinically, this may be completely symptomless. Radiographic examination frequently discloses an area of bone rarefaction about a tooth root apex, with a chronically infected or partially obliterated root canal. This area is usually spherical and well demarcated. Histologically, the tissue consists of fibrous connective tissue, often heavily infiltrated by lymphocytes and plasma cells, surrounding necrotic tissue at the apex of the root canal foramen or within the pulp canal. Peripherally, loose and dense connective tissue merges into the surrounding bone, which may develop a definite cortical layer (Fig. 23-5).

Remnants of epithelium (rests of Malassez) are found in the periodontal ligament, surrounding the teeth. In granulomas this epithelium may proliferate. The root end may become surrounded by fluid with epithelium lining the surface, thus forming a cyst. The cyst may enlarge to a considerable size. Although epithelium is present in practically all granulomas and often proliferates to line small cystic cavities, the development of large cysts is relatively uncommon (see also section on odontogenic cysts).

Periodontal disease. The inflammatory and degenerative processes that develop at the gingival margin and progress until the tooth-supporting structures are lost have much in common with periapical periodontal disease. In both instances, chronic asymptomatic infection by a variety of oral pathogens is usual, though episodes of acute suppuration may occur.

Anaerobic gram-negative bacteria are primary etiologic agents, but the destructive process is believed to be mediated in large part by immunologic reactions of

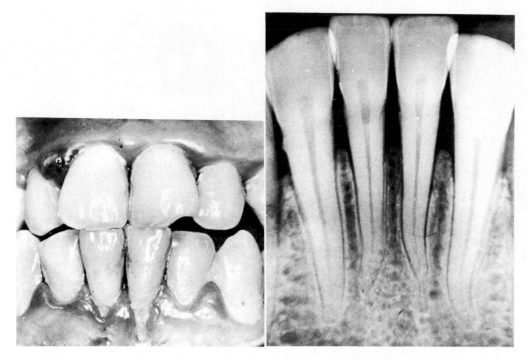

Fig. 23-6. Periodontitis. Edema, periodontal abscess, hemorrhage upon slight pressure, tissue recession with retraction of gingival margin, color change from light pink to deep red, loss of tissue in interdental area, horizontal bone loss, and widening of periodontal space. See Fig. 23-7.

the host.[28-30] The tissue response involves a walling-off process with a pronounced chronic inflammatory cell infiltration. The proliferation of epithelium is always present in the marginal form of periodontal disease. It represents an attempt to cover the surface of the chronic ulcer that develops about the involved tooth root area (Figs. 23-6 and 23-7).

The disease commonly begins as a gingivitis. Deposits of plaque and calculus on the tooth surfaces, impaction of food, decayed teeth, overhanging margins of dental restorations, and ill-fitting dental appliances are among the predisposing factors. With progression, a pocket is established below the gingival margin, thus prolonging and promoting the inflammatory process, with progressive resorption of tooth-supporting structures. Apical proliferation of epithelium to line the pocket occurs concomitantly with the loss of tissue. A purulent discharge from periodontal pockets can be elicited by digital pressure in many adult patients. Some individuals may show great resistance to the development of periodontal pockets despite adverse local factors, just as others have an extraordinary resistance to dental caries. Periodontal disease is more common in older individuals, and after middle age it becomes the chief cause of tooth loss.[10]

Juvenile forms of the disease can occur with a circumpubertal onset and a characteristic molar-incisor bone-loss pattern. Approximately 70% of patients with juvenile periodontitis have an associated neutrophil chemotactic defect.[30,33]

Pregnancy with its change in endocrine balance frequently is accompanied by gingivitis and hyperplastic inflammatory responses. Gingivitis may be somewhat more frequent during puberty.

Drug action may cause gingival response. The hyperplasia associated with the use of phenytoin (Dilantin) may be so extensive that the teeth are almost completely covered by gingival enlargement (Fig. 23-8).[37]

ORAL SOFT TISSUES
Mucocutaneous diseases

Although mucocutaneous disorders constitute a heterogeneous group, they are conveniently discussed together.

Lichen planus. Lichen planus usually appears as bilateral, irregular, lacelike whitening or keratosis of the buccal mucosa (Fig. 23-9), but other oral areas (gingiva, tongue, palate, and so on) also may be involved and the clinical appearance also may be bullous or erosive. Oral lesions are present in about 70% of patients with cutaneous lichen planus. Oral mucosal involvement in the absence of skin lesions may occur, but the reported incidence of lichen planus restricted to the oral cavity varies from 4% to 44% of patients seen in various clinics.[157] Mucosal surfaces of other body sites are much less frequently involved. The diagnosis may be sus-

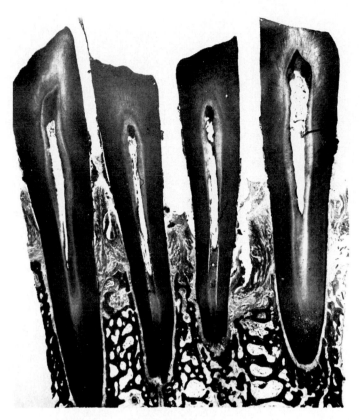

Fig. 23-7. Periodontitis (advanced). Mesiodistal section through mandibular incisors. Chronic inflammation of gingiva followed by proliferation of epithelium of gingival attachment along cementum, excessive osteoclastic resorption of interdental bone, and deep periodontal pocket formation between gingiva and surface of roots.

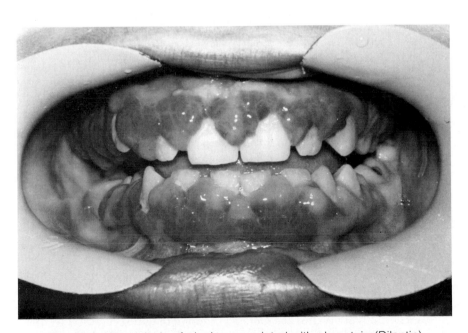

Fig. 23-8. Hyperplasia of gingiva associated with phenytoin (Dilantin).

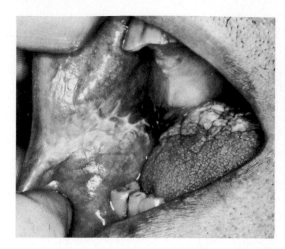

Fig. 23-9. Lichen planus of buccal mucosa. Dorsum of tongue is also involved. (Courtesy Jens O. Andreasen, Copenhagen.)

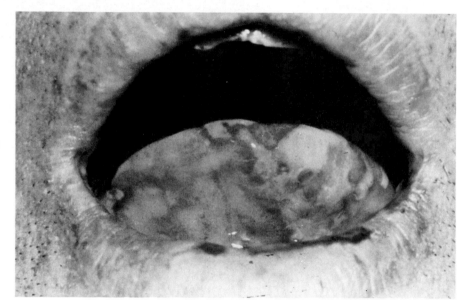

Fig. 23-10. Pemphigus involving lingual mucosa.

pected when the lacelike whitening of the surface of the buccal mucosa (Wickham striae) is seen. Lesions on the dorsum of the tongue are diffusely opaque. Biopsies and immunofluorescence of nonulcerated whitenings may be used in the diagnosis.[75,148,163,169]

The cause of lichen planus is not known. Patients are most frequently between 40 and 60 years of age. Oral lesions of the keratotic type of lichen planus are asymptomatic, but pain and discomfort have been observed with bullous or erosive types of the disease. There is considerable anecdotal evidence that lichen planus is "stress" related, but proof of this is difficult to establish.[35,99]

Pemphigus. Pemphigus, especially pemphigus vulgaris, characteristically involves the oral mucosa during its course and usually appears initially in this location. The oral tissues are very red, friable, and pebbly (Fig. 23-10). Vesicle and bulla formation is observed, but the blisters do not remain intact for long periods in the mouth. Smear preparations, biopsies of oral sites, and immunofluorescence (to detect intercellular IgG deposits)[116,117,197] are most useful in establishing the diagnosis (Fig. 23-11).

Benign mucous membrane pemphigoid. Benign mucous membrane pemphigoid is a vesicular or bullous disease involving the oral mucosa. It occurs most often in older women. Conjunctival tissues are frequently affected, and the associated inflammation and scarring of this site are the most serious sequelae.[142,164,170] Microscopically vesicle formation occurs immediately below the epithelium, and biopsy specimens of the short-lived vesicles are helpful in establishing the diagnosis, as are immunofluorescence studies that show complement and IgG deposits in the basement membrane zone.[117]

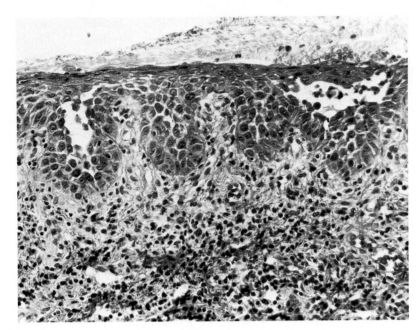

Fig. 23-11. Biopsy specimen of oral mucosa in pemphigus showing intraepithelial acantholysis.

Erythema multiforme. Erythema multiforme is characterized by large, vesiculobullous or erosive, frequently hemorrhagic lesions of the lips, buccal mucosa, and tongue. Oral and facial tissues are involved in approximately 25% of the patients.

Stevens-Johnson syndrome is a term applied to clinically severe examples of erythema multiforme, especially when the conjuctiva, genitalia, and, often, lungs are involved. The disorder appears to be a reaction to various medications (penicillin, sulfa drugs, phenobarbital) and the herpes simplex virus.[64,121,134]

Epidermolysis bullosa. Oral tissues are involved in several genetic types of epidermolysis bullosa. Microstomia, after the scarring of buccal mucosa, and dental abnormalities are complications of the dystrophic forms of this disease.[4,52]

Other mucocutaneous diseases. Keratosis follicularis (Darier's disease), lupus erythematosus, and herpes zoster are additional examples of so-called mucocutaneous conditions with oral manifestations.[133,138,189]

Hyalinosis cutis et mucosae (Urbach-Wiethe syndrome) causes induration of the oral mucosa, especially that of the lips and the tongue, which becomes atrophic and bound down to the oral floor.[89] In primary amyloidosis, infiltration of the tongue may be associated with macroglossia. Deposits of secondary amyloid in the gingiva are not clinically manifested. Scleroderma and acrosclerosis occasionally (about 7% of cases) are associated with a widening of the periodontal ligament of the teeth.

Hairy tongue is associated with proliferation of saprophytic organisms that cause extrinsic staining of elongated filiform papillae. Although the cause is unknown, hairy tongue may follow therapeutic use of antibiotics or radiation.[88] Benign migratory glossitis (geographic tongue), also of unknown cause is characterized by irregular superficial areas devoid of filiform papillae. It is more common in females and is seen in about 2% of the population.[45]

Oral and labial papillomatosis may be associated with the adult (malignant) form of acanthosis nigricans.[159] The oral lesions, in contrast to the cutaneous, are not pigmented.

Swelling of the lip and oral mucosa with facial palsy and plicated tongue is seen in the Melkersson-Rosenthal syndrome.[193]

Infections

Acute herpetic gingivostomatitis. Acute herpetic gingivostomatitis is the most common manifestation of primary infection with the herpes simplex virus, type 1. It is frequently misdiagnosed as necrotizing ulcerative gingivitis, or Vincent's stomatitis. Occurring clinically in less than 1% of the population, it is rarely if ever seen in a child under 1 year of age. It reaches its peak between the 1 and 3 years of age though it is also observed in older children and young adults. The incubation period is 4 to 8 days. The gingiva is red and swollen, is exquisitely tender, and bleeds easily. Numerous vesicles and bullae are present on the labial, lingual, and buccal mucosae.[65,96,173]

Microscopically the herpes simplex vesicle shows multinucleated giant cells having two to 15 nuclei per cell and eosinophilic inclusion bodies within the nuclei. Intraepithelial edema (ballooning degeneration) and intracellular edema are especially pronounced.

The incidence of oral infections related to type 2 herpes virus has increased in recent years and has been attributed to orogenital sex practices.[96]

Recurrent herpes (cold sore, fever blister). Recurrent herpes simplex infections occur most frequently about the face and lips and tend to recur at the same site in about 30% of the population. The condition is characterized by groups of small, clear vesicles on an erythematous base. The recurrent lesions seem to be induced by such agents as sunshine, fever, mechanical trauma, menses, and allergy. Intraoral involvement is rare but may involve the hard palate and fixed gingiva with pinhead-sized, grouped ulcers.[190]

Human immunodeficiency virus (HIV) infection–acquired immunodeficiency syndrome (AIDS). Oral lesions are prominent and important findings in patients with the acquired immunodeficiency syndrome (AIDS) and in the AIDS-related complex (ARC). Chronic candidiasis, often refractory to treatment and recurrent, is present in 70% to 90% of patients with AIDS and ARC. Herpes labialis and recurrent intraoral herpetic ulcerations are also seen with increased frequency.[38,143,166] Hairy leukoplakia is a common and apparently specific lesion representing an early clinical sign of exposure to HIV. This lesion occurs unilaterally or bilaterally on the lateral border of the tongue and occasionally on other oral mucosal surfaces. Most commonly hairy leukoplakia presents as a soft, white, corrugated, or "hairy"-appearing lesion. In about 20% of cases, however, the typical surface corrugations are not present. Microscopically the lesion shows hyperkeratosis, usually with keratinous hairlike projections on the surface, and acanthosis. Vacuolated epithelial cells with a clear cytoplasm and a pyknotic nucleus (koilocytes) are generally prominent in the superficial spinous layer. The underlying lamina propria is generally devoid of an inflammatory cell infiltrate. The presence of hairy leukoplakia appears to be a significant indicator of HIV infection, and the patients are almost invariably HIV-antibody positive. Current studies indicate that about 75% of patients with hairy leukoplakia will develop AIDS within 30 months.[97,152,155] Oral Kaposi's sarcoma is also not uncommon and is discussed on p. 1113.

Recurrent aphthae (canker sores). Although resembling the lesions of recurrent herpes, recurrent aphthae, which occur in about half of the population are not caused by the herpes simplex virus.[94,96,131] The lesions are larger than those of recurrent herpes and occur on freely movable mucosa. Circinate superficial lesions are seen on the oral mucosa in Reither's syndrome (arthritis, conjunctivitis, and urethritis).[4] The term *major aphthae* (Sutton's disease) refers to large chronic aphthae that scar. Similar lesions are seen in Behcet's syndrome (orogenital ulceration and iridocyclitis).[115]

Infectious mononucleosis. Infectious mononucleosis may present pronounced oral signs.[42] In addition to inflammation of the oral pharynx and lymphadenopathy, about one third of patients exhibit a grayish or grayish green membrane resembling that of diphtheria or Vincent's angina over the throat or posterior buccal mucosa. The gingiva bleeds easily and becomes enlarged. Petechiae are common on the soft palate.

Hand-foot-and-mouth disease. Generally unrecognized, hand-foot-and-mouth disease is a self-limited, febrile disease caused by group A coxsackieviruses, principally type 16 and less often types 5 and 10, and echovirus, type 6.[59] It is manifest by many small vesicles or punched-out ulcers of the lips and buccal mucosa. The gingiva characteristically is spared, in contrast to herpetic stomatitis. Those affected are principally under 10 years of age. Cutaneous involvement is usually limited to the palms, soles, and ventral surfaces and sides of fingers and toes.

Agranulocytosis. Agranulocytosis often is manifest by ragged necrotic ulcers of the gingiva, palate, tonsils, or oropharynx. Sialorrhea may be profuse. Drug sensitivity, especially to the barbiturates, chloramphenicol, antithyroid drugs, and the sulfonamides, is the best-known cause. Similar lesions are seen in cyclic neutropenia, an autosomal dominant disorder in which the neutrophils are decreased every 21 days.[10] Various autosomal recessive chronic neutropenias also result in oral ulceration and premature periodontal destruction. Cytotoxic agents employed in cancer chemotherapy produce severe oral ulceration.[46a]

Lethal granuloma (midline lethal granuloma). Probably a form of malignant reticulosis, lethal granuloma involves the palate, sinuses, and nasopharynx in a severe, progressive, ulcerative, destructive process.[135]

Wegener's granulomatosis. Considered to be a form of hypersensitivity, Wegener's granulomatosis, a possible variant of polyarteritis nodosa, may be heralded by multiple pyogenic granulomas of the interdental papillae of the gingiva.[79]

Crohn's disease. Oral lesions may occur in Crohn's disease. They are principally of three types. Most frequently involved is the buccal mucosa, which has a cobblestone appearance. In the mucobuccal fold are linear hyperplastic lesions and ulcers. Next most frequently involved are the lips, which may be diffusely swollen and indurated. Less frequently involved are the gingiva and alveolar mucosa. There the lesions are more granular and erythematous. The palate may be involved with multiple aphthous lesions. In contrast to intestinal lesions where there is no sexual predilection, oral lesions have at least a 4-to-1 male-to-female predilection.[47]

Eosinophilic ulcer of soft tissues. This lesion, albeit rare, is of sufficient interest for discussion. Most examples have involved the tongue of adults, though rarely other oral structures such as the gingiva or palate may be involved. It may be related to trauma of the tongue muscle. It is not related to either the cutaneous facial eosinophilic granuloma or the eosinophilic granuloma of bone (histiocytosis X). There is significant (7-to-1) male predilection. The cause is obscure and the lesion self-limiting.[84]

Acute necrotizing ulcerative gingivitis (Vincent's disease, fusospirochetosis). Acute necrotizing ulcerative gingivitis is far less common than supposed. Often the term "trench mouth" is used as a catchall to include primary herpetic gingivostomatitis, herpangina, infectious mononucleosis, and similar oral manifestations of disease. This is especially true in children, for fusospirochetosis is extremely uncommon in childhood (except in Africa), afflicting instead young and middle-aged adults. The disease is almost exclusively limited to the interdental papillae and the free gingival margin, rarely extending to the faucial area (Vincent's angina). Necrosis and ulceration of one or more interdental gingival papillae, mild fever, fetid breath, malaise, and local discomfort characterize the condition. Predisposing conditions seem to allow penetration of the oral tissues by several symbiotic organisms normally inhabiting the mouth, among these a fusiform bacillus and an oral spirochete, *Borrelia vincentii.*[10]

Noma (cancrum oris, gangrenous stomatitis). Noma may occur as a complication of acute necrotizing gingivitis in children or, rarely, in adults debilitated by infectious disease or possibly malnourishment. It is rare except in the Far East and Africa. The process usually begins in a gingival ulceration and rapidly spreads to involve the cheeks, lips, and jawbones. The tissues become blackened and necrotic. Pneumonia and toxemia are common sequelae.[172]

Syphilis. In both the prenatal and the acquired forms, syphilis may be manifest about the mouth.[129] In the acquired form, the primary lesion or chancre may appear on the lips or tongue, simulating a squamous cell carcinoma. The secondary stage is characterized by the mucous patch (a milky white, focal, superficial ulcer of the oral mucosa), sore throat, and occasionally a condyloma at the corner of the mouth (split papule). The hard palate may be perforated in the tertiary stage as a result of gumma formation. The tongue may be involved with a diffuse inflammatory process (syphilitic glossitis) that may predispose to the development of squamous cell carcinoma. Prenatal syphilis may be demonstrated by rhagades, or radiating scars about the mouth, and characteristic alteration in the form of the permanent teeth (Hutchinson's incisors and mulberry molars), in addition to the changes seen in the secondary and tertiary stages of acquired syphilis.[145]

Gonorrhea. The variable clinical conditions associated with oral, tonsillar, or pharyngeal infection by the gram-negative intracellular diplococcus *Neisseria gon-* *orrhoeae* are perhaps too poorly appreciated and diagnosed. Its identification, though rare, has been documented. Generally acute, erythematous, and ulcerative with associated systemic symptoms, it may also be pseudomembranous or even vesicular in its manifestations. Burning and itching have been early subjective symptoms.[109]

Granuloma inguinale. Oral lesions of granuloma inguinale are the most common extragenital (about 5% to 6%) manifestations of the disease.[146]

Actinomycosis. Actinomycosis of the cervicofacial type arises through invasion of oral mucous membranes or a tooth socket, spreading to involve the jawbones, musculature, and salivary glands. Multiple foci of suppuration lead into sinus tracts that drain to the cutaneous surface or oral mucosa, liberating pus containing the typical and diagnostic "sulfur granules" of *Actinomyces israelii.*[93]

Histoplasmosis. Oral lesions of histoplasmosis appear most frequently as nodular or ulcerated areas on the tongue or palate.[195]

Tuberculosis. Tuberculosis of the oral tissues is rare and usually is associated with advanced pulmonary disease. The typical lesion is an irregular, slowly enlarging, painful ulcer of the base of the tongue or palate.[91]

Other granulomatous infections

Many other fungal and tropical diseases have oral lesions, among them tropical sprue, leishmaniasis, scleroma, leprosy, and blastomycosis.[10,120,140,150]

Candidiasis (thrush). Candidiasis is a fungal disease occurring most often in debilitated persons, infants, or especially individuals who have been taking oral antibiotics. It also may be associated in the form of a syndrome with hypoparathyroidism, keratoconjunctivitis, and Addison's disease.[4] A chronic hyperplastic candidiasis is often present. It is characterized by a pseudo-epitheliomatous hyperplasia, with fungal invasion and a noticeable chronic inflammatory reaction. The fungus may invade the oral mucosa, skin, female genitalia, or urinary tract. Since the fungus *Candida albicans* is a normal oral inhabitant, the diagnosis cannot be based on smear alone. The presence of hyphae is more significant diagnostically. The clinical appearance is that of numerous milk-white plaques—that are easily stripped off, leaving a bleeding surface because of penetration of the mycelia.[70,105] Overclosure of the jaws in the edentulous patient or in the patient with poorly constructed dentures commonly results in low-grade chronic infection at the corners of the mouth, attributable at least in part to candidal organisms.[151] This is called perlèche, or angular cheilitis.[151] Cheilosis caused by deficiency of one or more of the B complex vitamins is rare.

Childhood exanthematous diseases. The childhood exanthematous disease frequently manifest oral lesions.

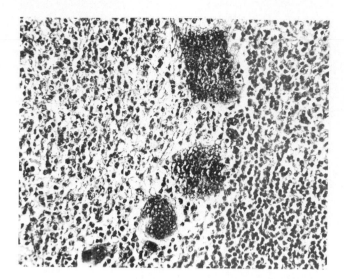

Fig. 23-12. Warthin-Finkeldey giant cells seen in lateral lingual tonsillar tissue during prodromal measles.

Koplik's spots, one of the prodromal signs of measles, are pinhead-sized, bluish white spots surrounded by erythematous halos. They appear in the buccal or labial mucosa about 18 hours before the skin rash. Warthin-Finkeldey giant cells may be histologically observed in the tonsils or other oral lymphatic lesions (Fig. 23-12).[119]

Disturbances of pigmentation

Melanotic pigmentation. Melanin may occur in the oral mucosa and about the lips under both normal and pathologic conditions.[78,104] Racial pigmentation, especially of the gingiva, is the most common type and appears to be directly related to skin color. It is present not only in nearly all blacks but also in Orientals and those of Mediterranean background. Even 10% of Scandinavians may have oral melanotic pigmentation. Little melanin is present at birth. It is deposited largely during the first decade.

Chronic adrenocortical insufficiency (Addison's disease), hemochromatosis, and Albright's syndrome (polyostotic fibrous dysplasia and precocious puberty)[4] may be associated with pigmentation of the oral mucosa and the skin. Pigmentation also is seen in chronic steatorrhea and in the Peutz-Jeghers syndrome. The latter is characterized by gastrointestinal polyposis, mucocutaneous pigmentation, and autosomal dominant inheritance.[3,4] Palatal melanotic pigmentation may be seen after extensive use of various antimalarial drugs, such as amodiaquin (Camoquin) or chloroquine. It also may be seen in patients with oral lichen planus ("melasmic" staining).

All types of melanotic nevi have been reported in oral tissues, as has malignant melanoma.[61,62]

Nonmelanotic pigmentation. Nonmelanotic pigmentation usually is caused by heavy metals. Amalgam tattoo results from implantation of particles of filling material under the mucosa at the time of dental procedures.[60] Lead, bismuth, arsenic, and mercury intoxications may be associated with a deposit of the metallic sulfide in the inflamed gingival margin.

Tumors and tumorlike lesions
Benign tumors and tumorlike lesions of the oral soft tissues

Generalized or localized enlargement of the gingiva should arouse clinical suspicion of neoplastic disease. Enlarged gingival papillae, with bleeding on slight pressure, are found in vitamin C deficiency (scorbutic gingivitis). Clinically similar appearances may indicate the local infiltration of the gingiva with immature leukocytes characteristic of one variety or another of leukemia.

Phenytoin (Dilantin) frequently causes a striking enlargement of the gingiva associated with a dense overgrowth of fibrous tissue (see Fig. 23-8).[37]

Fibromatosis gingivae. Fibromatosis gingivae represents a proliferation of the entire gingiva. Inflammation is characteristically absent, and the gingiva is of normal color and hard texture. The normal eruption of teeth is prevented. Fibromatosis gingivae may rarely be associated with hypertrichosis, seizures, and mental retardation. An autosomal dominant genetic pattern is common. There are several other varieties.[4,156]

Papilloma. Papilloma is an arborescent growth consisting of numerous squamous epithelial fingerlike projections, each of which contains a well-vascularized, fibrous, connective tissue core.[34] Although it may be seen throughout the mouth, the soft palate, tongue, and lips are common sites. There is no sex or age predilection.

Other oral papillary growths closely related to papillomas include condyloma acuminatum and verruca vulgaris. These may clinically be indistinguishable from papillomas and there are many histologic similarities.[95] Human papilloma virus (HPV) antigens have been detected in all these lesions, and it is possible that they represent variations of the same process.[158,178] Papillary hyperplasia (inflammatory papillary hyperplasia) is a relatively common and unique papillary lesion that is restricted to the oral cavity. It occurs almost exclusively on the hard palates of denture wearers. Clinically the lesion is characterized by numerous small (2 to 4 mm) papillary projections of hyperplastic squamous epithelium surrounding inflamed connective tissue. Although papillary hyperplasia is occasionally "overdiagnosed" by a pathologist who is unfamiliar with this lesion, it does not have a "premalignant" potential. Dramatic improvement is usually noted after various measures to correct denture irritation.[49]

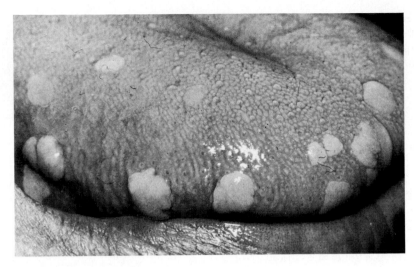

Fig. 23-13. Multiple lesions of focal epithelial hyperplasia on tongue. (From Praetorius-Clausen, F.: Pathol. Microbiol. **39**:204, 1973.)

Verruciform xanthoma. The verruciform xanthoma is often misdiagnosed as a papilloma. The most frequent site is the gingiva or alveolar ridge. About 75% of the patients are in the fifth to seventh decades of life. There may be a 3-to-2 female sex predilection. Microscopically the rough verrucous surface is covered by parakeratin, which forms invaginating crypts that extend deep into the epithelium. The latter exhibits acanthosis with uniform elongation of rete ridges. Numerous foamy xanthomatous cells fill the connective tissue papillae extending downward *only* to the tips of the rete ridges.[69,136]

Keratoacanthoma. Keratoacanthoma may involve the lower lip at the skin-mucosal junction. These appear as painless, exophytic crateriform lesions 1 to 2 cm in diameter. Clinical and microscopic differentiation from squamous cell carcinoma may be very difficult.[107] Most examples are seen in men over 50 years of age. Intraoral keratoacanthomas have also been rarely reported.[87] Most cases have been noted on the palate. Eruptive keratoacanthomas may rarely involve the oral mucosa as part of a generalized skin and mucosal dissemination. The lesions evolve over a period of 4 to 8 months and heal spontaneously with minimal scarring.[196]

Focal epithelial hyperplasia. This condition was first described by Heck as occurring on oral mucosal tissue of Navajo children and has since been observed in others, most prominently Greenlandic Eskimos. It is usually a soft, nonulcerated white or reddish papule approximately 0.5 cm in diameter (Fig. 23-13). The lesions are frequently multiple, are probably of viral cause, and have now been observed in the United States and other countries.[144,175,184]

Fibroma. The most common benign growth on the oral mucous membrane is fibroma that occurs as a dis-

crete, superficial, pedunculated or sessile mass. Such lesions appear to be nonneoplastic, arising as an exuberant response to physical trauma or other inflammatory agents. An example of this type of reaction is the so-called denture-injury tumor.[73] Some examples probably represent burnt-out pyogenic granulomas.[118] Microscopically these fibromas are composed of collagenic fibrous connective tissue covered by keratinized or parakeratinized stratified squamous epithelium.

Fibromas arising on the gingival mucosa are common lesions that often contain calcified elements. These are referred to as "peripheral ossifying fibromas." Histologically they are composed of a cellular fibroblastic tissue containing varying combinations of bone, cementum-like material, or dystrophic calcifications.[63,92]

Fibroproliferative lesions, generally classified as fibromatoses, also rarely involve the oral cavity or paraoral structures. These are characterized by fibroblasts and collagen fibers with varying degrees of cellularity. Included in this group as are nodular fasciitis, intravascular fasciitis, aggressive (juvenile) fibromatosis, and proliferative myositis. These lesion may be locally aggressive, invasive, and difficult to manage.[90,128,154]

Neuroma, neurilemoma, and neurofibroma. Neurilemoma and neurofibroma are also observed in oral environs, especially the tongue. Neurofibroma may occur as an isolated lesion or as part of neurofibromatosis.[4] The lesions of the latter condition may be of at least three types: discrete, diffuse, or plexiform.[194]

The traumatic neuroma occurs at the proximal end of crushed or severed peripheral nerves.[171] A history of extraction of teeth or prior soft tissue trauma is usually elicited. The lesion usually appears as a nodule having normal surface coloration. The most common sites are the mental foramen area, lower lip, and tongue, though any area of the oral mucosa may be involved. Microscopically the traumatic neuroma consists of a nonencapsulated tangled mass of axons, Schwann cells, and endoneural and perineural cells in a dense collagenous matrix. Similar lesions may be noted in the tongue and lips in multiple endocrine adenomatosis, type 3 (multiple mucosal neuroma syndrome).[67,110]

Rhabdomyoma and leiomyoma. Rhabdomyoma is a rare tumor and most oral cavity examples have been noted in the floor of the mouth, tongue, or soft palate. The tumor is found in males about twice as often as in females and most patients are over 50 years of age. Histologically the tumor is composed of large polyhedral cells with a granular cytoplasm. Occasional cross striations may be seen.[72] Leiomyoma is also an uncommon oral tumor. Most examples have been found in the tongue or lower lip. Both the solid and vascular form (angioleiomyoma) occur.[74] Epithelioid leiomyoma of the oral cavity has also been reported.[98] The phosphotungstic acid–hematoxylin stain is of value to demonstrate myofibrils to aid in differentiation of solid leiomyomas from other spindle cell tumors.

Granular cell tumor (granular cell "myoblastoma"). First described by Abrikossof in 1926 and assumed initially to be of striated muscle origin, granular cell tumor has in recent years been the subject of considerable controversy. Many investigators believe it to be of neural origin, whereas others suggest that it represents not a true noeplasm but a special type of muscle degeneration. Histochemical and electron microscopic investigations have added support to the neural (Schwann cell) theory of origin.[51,130,147,176]

Although having its origin in many tissues, especially the skin, about 30% arise in the tongue. There appears to be no age preference except for a possible variant that occurs at birth on the anterior alveolar ridges and has been called "congenital epulis of the newborn." It occurs predominantly (8:1) in female infants and twice as often in the upper jaw as in the lower jaw.[51]

Microscopically the tumor consists of large polyhedral cells with an acidophilic granular cytoplasm. Ultrastructural studies have demonstrated that the "granules" are lysosomal structures. The nucleus is small, somewhat pyknotic, and eccentrically placed. Pseudoepitheliomatous hyperplasia, characteristically absent in the congenital epulis, may be so pronounced in the tongue lesion that a diagnosis of squamous cell carcinoma is made (Fig. 23-14). Although the histologic features of this lesion are clear, its histogenesis is not.

Giant cell granuloma. The peripheral form of giant cell granuloma is similar to the central form discussed on p. 1115.

Hemangioma. Hemangioma of the oral mucous membranes is essentially similar to that of the skin and may occur in any area of the mouth with many appearances. Although it is most commonly of the capillary type, cav-

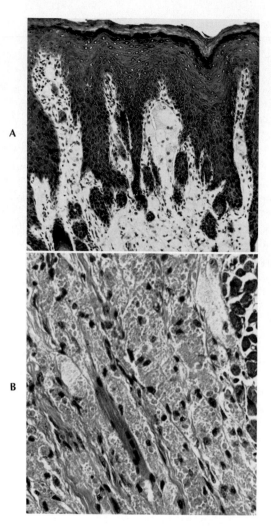

Fig. 23-14. Granular cell tumor (granular cell myoblastoma). Tongue and skin are two most frequent sites. **A,** Pseudoepitheliomatous proliferation may be pronounced, simulating squamous cell carcinoma. **B,** Tumor consists of sheet of large cells with granular eosinophilic cytoplasm and small hyperchromatic nuclei.

ernous and mixed types also are seen. These often congenital lesions should not be confused with the exuberant overgrowth of granulation tissue designated as pyogenic granuloma,[48,118] which apparently arises as the result of trauma and nonspecific infection. The pyogenic granuloma is indistinguishable microscopically from the so-called pregnancy tumor that arises on the gingiva during the secondary trimester of gestation in approximately 10% of gravid females. Consisting of new capillaries, fibroblasts, and polymorphonuclear neutrophils, these lesions frequently last long after termination of pregnancy, eventuating in a fibroma-like lesion.

Hemangiopericytoma,[111] glomangioma,[179] and epithelioid hemangioendothelioma[83] are uncommon vascular neoplasms that rarely may be encountered in the oral cavity. These show identical histologic features to their counterparts in other anatomic sites.

Hereditary hemorrhagic telangiectasia (Osler-Rendu-Weber disease). Hereditary hemorrhagic telangiectasia is manifest by numerous spiderlike angiomatoses of the lips and tongue. Nasal mucosal involvement results in frequent epistaxis. Usually noted at puberty, the condition has autosomal dominant inheritance. Microscopically the individual lesion is a superficial blood vessel surrounded by abnormal elastic fibers that permit dilatation.[4]

Encephalofacial angiomatosis (Sturge-Weber syndrome). Encephalofacial angiomatosis consists of superficial and deep-seated hemangiomas, usually of the upper two thirds or half of the face, associated with leptomeningeal angiomas, cerebral calcifications, seizures, glaucoma, and mental retardation. There are many clinical variations.[4]

Lymphangioma. The majority of lymphangiomas are found at birth in the head and neck region and may cause enlargement of the tongue (macroglossia) and the lip (macrocheilia). Cystic hygroma is a special type of lymphangioma occurring in the cervical region in the newborn.[125]

Lipoma. Although uncommon, lipoma occurs most frequently in the cheek, tongue, and oral floor. There is no sex or age predilection.[103,187]

Soft-tissue osteoma and chondroma (choristoma). Small circumscribed tumors composed of mature lamellated bone (osteoma) or mature cartilage (chondroma) may be rarely encountered in the oral cavity, mostly in the tongue. Chondromas are usually located on the lateral border and ventral surfaces of the tongue, whereas osteomas are mostly seen on the posterior dorsum in the region of the circumvallate papilla.[114]

Nevi. The intramucosal cellular nevus, pigmented or more often nonpigmented, is the most common nevus to occur on the oral mucosa. Next most frequent is the intraoral blue nevus. Over 65% of the nevi arise in the mucosa of the hard palate, and another 25% in the lips. There does not appear to be a sex predilection. The compound nevus and junctional nevus are both rare.[62]

White lesions of the oral mucosa

A change in color of the normally reddish or mucosa to white constitutes one of the most frequently encountered oral abnormalities. The term "leukoplakia" has been used for many years but has resulted in considerable confusion because of differing definitions of this term.

Leukoplakia. As currently defined by most oral pathologists, leukoplakia is a clinical term for a white patch or plaque on the oral mucosa that will not rub off and cannot be identified as any other disease process.[192]

It must be emphasized that this term does not carry any histologic connotation, and the lesion may microscopically show alterations ranging from simple hyperkeratosis to an early infiltrating carcinoma. Failure to identify the nature of a leukoplakic lesion may have serious consequences because the early stages of an oral squamous cell carcinoma may present as a rather innocuous-appearing area of leukoplakia.

Leukoplakia is a relatively common oral lesion. A recently reported epidemiologic study in Minnesota showed that it was the most commonly encountered mucosal lesion with an incidence rate of 28.9 cases per 1000 adults over 35 years of age.[54] Considerably higher incidence rates have been reported in other studies, particularly in India and Southeast Asia.[53,167] Leukoplakia is more common in males than in females, and most patients are between 40 and 60 years of age.[188] Any oral site may be involved, but lesions of the mandibular mucosa, mandibular sulcus, and buccal mucosa are the most common. The etiology appears to be multifactorial. Various tobacco habits, local irritation, and trauma appear to account for many examples, and dramatic resolution may be observed in some cases when tobacco is eliminated or other forms of local irritation are corrected.[46] However, in a significant number of cases no obvious etiologic factors are noted.

Microscopically leukoplakic lesions show varying combinations of hyperkeratosis and acanthosis. Morphologic alterations of a degree to warrant a designation of epithelial dysplasia are present in 16% to 24% of cases.[44,188] Lesions demonstrating the more severe degrees of epithelial dysplasia appear to have the greatest potential for progression to invasive carcinoma.[132] Leukoplakia is commonly regarded as a precancerous lesion, but estimates as to the frequency of malignant change vary. A number of prospective and retrospective studies have indicated a 2% to 6% rate of progression to carcinoma.[43,188] Leukoplakias of the floor of the mouth and ventral tongue are at greatest risk[58,112] (Fig. 23-15). A recent study by Silverman et al.[168] showed a 17% rate of malignant change in 257 patients followed for an average period of 7.2 years. Extensive lesions, particularly those described as proliferative verrucous leukoplakia are difficult to manage, are resistant to treatment, and show a frequent progression to invasive carcinoma.[101]

Erythroplakia. Although erythroplakia is not clinically a white lesion, it is conveniently discussed here. Erythroplakia is defined as a red, velvety plaque on the oral mucosa and cannot be characterized clinically or pathologically as any other condition. In this sense it is the red analog of leukoplakia.[192] In some cases the red lesion is interspersed with areas of leukoplakia, and these lesions are often designated as "speckled erythroplakia," or "speckled leukoplakia." There is little reli-

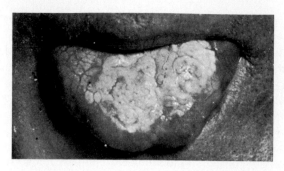

Fig. 23-15. Leathery and warty whitening (leukoplakia) of tongue associated with carcinoma of low-grade malignancy.

able epidemiologic data as to the incidence of erythroplakia, but it is far less common than leukoplakia.[161] Erythroplakia is somewhat more common in males than in females and most patients are in the sixth and seventh decades of life. Excessive use of tobacco and alcohol are suspected etiologic factors, but there are few detailed studies on etiologic factors. Erythroplakia is a significant oral lesion, and biopsy almost invariably shows severe degrees of epithelial dysplasia.[161] Erythroplakia is the most common clinical presentation for early, asymptomatic oral carcinoma.[123]

Nicotine stomatitis (leukokeratosis nicotina palati). Nicotine stomatitis is a specific keratotic lesion involving the hard and soft palates of tobacco users, particularly pipe and cigar smokers. There is a definite male predominance. In the early stages the mucosa shows a diffuse, grayish-white wrinkled appearance. In the later stages, white umbilicated nodules with depressed red centers develop. Microscopically the lesions show hyperkeratosis, acanthosis, and squamous metaplasia of the underlying ducts of the palatal mucous glands. Epithelial dysplasia is relatively uncommon in nicotine stomatitis, and carcinomatous change is quite uncommon.[192] Nicotine stomatitis is frequently a reversible lesion when tobacco use is discontinued.

Habitual cheek-biting (morsicatio buccarum). Chronic cheek-nibbling, which may be a conscious habit or performed unconsciously, results in rather characteristic white lesions of the buccal mucosa, most prominent opposite the occlusal plane of the teeth. The affected areas show a diffuse white thickening with an irregular frayed surface and alternating irregular areas of superficial erosion. Microscopic examination shows acanthosis with a rather characteristic irregular frayed hyperparakeratotic surface. Adherent colonies of microorganisms are often noted on the keratotic surface.[192]

Other white lesions. The white oral lesions of lichen planus were discussed previously (Fig. 23-9). Wickham's striae or lacelike patterns in this condition are characteristic. Several hereditary conditions feature whitening of the oral cavity. Hereditary benign intraepithelial dyskeratosis, white sponge nevus (leukokeratosis heredita), pachyonychia congenita, Darier's disease, and dyskeratosis congenita (Zinsser-Engman-Cole syndrome) are examples.[4]

Aspirin burns resulting from the unprescribed use of tablets as dental topical anesthetics or troches frequently are seen. Soft, focal, oral whitenings that peel away easily, leaving a raw, bleeding surface, occur in candidiasis.

Malignant tumors of oral cavity

Squamous cell carcinoma. Squamous cell carcinoma (epidermoid carcinoma) is the most common oral malignant neoplasm, accounting for over 90% of all oral malignancies.[113] It is responsible for about 5% of all cancer deaths in the United States.[36,53] Oral squamous cell carcinoma accounts for about 5% to 6% of all malignancies in the United States and most European countries. Significantly higher incidence of oral carcinomas have been reported in India and Southeast Asia.[141]

Squamous cell carcinomas of the lips and oral mucosa occur most often in males over 50 years of age. Although the incidence in males is generally stated to be three times greater than in females in the United States, several centers have noted a significant increase of oral carcinoma in females in the last several decades.[53,113] The clinical appearance of small, early oral squamous cell carcinomas may vary from a white, thickened, or verrucous lesion to a red velvety plaque or a chronic painless ulcer.

Leukoplakia is frequently observed in association with an oral carcinoma, and it is likely that many oral carcinomas evolve in this fashion.[55] Tobacco and alcohol have been etiologically implicated for many years. The role of oral sepsis, chronic irritation, sideropenic anemia, and so on are less certain.[50]

Histologically the majority of oral squamous cell carcinomas are well or moderately differentiated tumors. Metastasis generally occurs in a fairly predictable manner to the ipsilateral submandibular and cervical lymph nodes. The presence or absence of lymph node metastasis at the time of initial diagnosis and treatment is an important index of the clinical stage of disease and has a significant bearing on prognosis. Stage I tumors have an 83% 5-year survival that drops to 11% for stage IV tumors.[165,186] Patients with oral carcinoma have a significantly increased risk of developing a second or even third primary carcinoma of the upper aerodigestive tract.[162]

Carcinoma in situ. Carcinoma is situ of the oral mucosa is usually detected on histologic study of a biopsy specimen from a lesion clinically considered to be leukoplakia or erythroplakia. The frequency and rate of progression of oral carcinoma in situ to invasive carcinoma is not well established, but it is generally assumed that it is considerably more rapid than with carcinoma in situ of the uterine cervix. The floor of the mouth, ventral and lateral aras of the tongue, and lower lip vermilion are the principal sites of oral carcinoma in situ.[58,161]

Squamous cell carcinoma of lip. Squamous cell carcinoma of the lip is almost exclusively a male disease, with less than 3% of the cases occurring in women. It is rare in blacks. It originates most frequently in the sixth to eighth decades. The incidence of carcinoma of the vermilion of the lower lip in the United States has shown a remarkable decrease in recent years.[53] Approximately 90% arise on the vermilion border of the lower lip, usually on one side of the midline. It appears as a painless, characteristically indurated, ulcerated or exophytic lesion. Usually, lip carcinoma is well differentiated and slow to metastasize to the submental and submandibular nodes. Prognosis is good whether the lesion is treated by radiation or by surgery, with 5-year cure rates being about equal (90%). Carcinoma of the lip is more common in individuals of light complexion, especially those who, because of their occupation, receive an unusual amount of actinic radiation, such as farmers, sailors, and policemen. Some doubt has recently been expressed concerning the importance of the role of actinic radiation.[77]

Early or premalignant alterations of lip epithelium appear as localized keratotic plaques that may resolve, only to reappear. Alternatively, malignant degeneration is indicated by diffuse, thin whitening of superficial portions of the vermilion border of the lip.

Squamous cell carcinoma of the tongue. The tongue is the most common site for intraoral carcinoma, accounting for about 40% of all intraoral carcinomas.[113] Although it is predominantly a disease of males over 60 years of age, there is indication that the present male-to-female ratio is 2:1 instead of the former ratio of 4:1.[177] The positive correlation between carcinoma of the tongue and syphilitic glossitis appears to be less significant than formerly believed.[192] About two thirds of tongue carcinomas involve the oral (anterior two thirds) of the tongue, and one third are located in the base of the tongue. The lateral border and ventral surfaces are most commonly involved. About one third of patients with carcinoma of the oral tongue have regional node involvement at the time of hospital admission, and nodal involvement is present in over 70% of patients with carcinoma of the base of the tongue.[177]

Prognosis is greatly influenced by the stage of disease at the time of treatment. Five-year survival rates of 68% have been obtained in stage I (T1 N0) lesions, but curability drops greatly with more advanced disease. The presence or absence of regional node metastasis at the time of initial treatment is the most important factor

in prognosis.[174,191] Carcinoma of the tongue is occasionally seen in children and adults under 30 years of age. These patients usually have no history of tobacco or alcohol abuse, and the prognosis of these lesions is poor.[66,137]

Squamous cell carcinoma of the floor of the mouth. The floor of the mouth is the second most common site for oral carcinoma, accounting for about 30% of all intraoral carcinomas. The incidence appears to be increasing in relation to carcinoma of the tongue since 1970.[113] Although a definite male predominance was noted in most earlier reports, a four- to sixfold increase in females has been noted in recent decades.[102] Most patients are over age 60. The lesion is most often noted in the anterior floor of the mouth about the openings of the submandibular and sublingual gland ducts. Early lesions often present as an innocuous-appearing area of leukoplakia or erythroplakia, emphasizing the importance of investigation of such lesions.[123] More advanced lesions usually present as indurated ulcerations. Histologically most of these lesions are moderately differentiated tumors. Metastasis is common though as a rule this does not occur as early as noted with carcinoma of the tongue.

The tumor is often located in the midline area, and bilateral metastasis may occur. The incidence of cervical node metastasis varies from 20% to 60% in various reports. Carcinoma of the floor of the mouth has a slightly better prognosis than carcinoma of the tongue, with several rates of up to 70% being reported for stage I disease.[39]

Squamous cell carcinoma of gingiva. Squamous cell carcinoma of the gingiva constitutes about 10% of oral malignancy and is more common in men than in women (about 2:1). It occurs most commonly on the mandibular gingiva, and its early clinical resemblance to more common inflammatory conditions in this location may lead to delayed diagnosis. Early involvement of contiguous structures, such as bone and lymph nodes, characterizes the tumor.[139]

Squamous cell carcinoma of the buccal mucosa. The reported incidence of this tumor shows wide variation in various parts of the world. In India and Southeast Asia where betel-nut chewing is a common habit, the buccal mucosa is one of the most common sites for oral carcinoma. It is also relatively more common in the southeastern United States and has been related to use of smokeless tobacco.[126] There is a male predilection though some studies indicate that the carcinoma of the buccal mucosa is more common in females. Most patients are over 60 years of age. The tumors tend to be histologically well or moderately differentiated and often present a papillary configuration. The lesions are frequently associated with extensive leukoplakia of the buccal mucosa. Tumors arising in the retrocommissural region have a more favorable outlook than those arising in the posterior buccal mucosa. Cervical metastasis is present in about 25% of patients at the time of admission, and reported 5-year survivals range from 26% to 52%.[71,185]

Squamous cell carcinoma of the palate. Squamous cell carcinoma of the hard and soft palate comprises between 9% and 12% of intraoral carcinomas. The soft palate is more commonly involved, and these lesions may extend into the tonsillar area or nasopharynx. Carcinoma of the hard palate is relatively uncommon in the United States but is seen with greater frequency in parts of the world where reverse smoking is practiced. Most tumors are well to moderately differentiated. The prognosis is greatly influenced by the anatomic location. Stage I lesions of the hard palate demonstrate an excellent prognosis, whereas those arising on the soft palate often show metastasis at the time of initial diagnosis. Overall survival rates vary from 30% to 52%.[86,160]

Verrucous carcinoma. Verrucous carcinoma is a highly differentiated variety of squamous cell carcinoma that is seen chiefly in the oral cavity though identical tumors occur in the upper aerodigestive tract, genitalia, and other sites. In the mouth verrucous carcinoma most often occurs in the gingivobuccal sulcus, often at the site where a bolus of snuff or chewing tobacco is habitually held. The majority of patients are over 60 years of age. Most reports show a male predominance except in the southeastern United States where the disease is more common in females.[124,126] The typical presentation is a large, soft, papillary mass attached to the underlying mucosa by a broad base. Ulceration is uncommon. The tumors enlarge chiefly by lateral spread and slowly invade contiguous structures such as bone with a characteristic "pushing" border. Without an adequate, deep biopsy, microscopic diagnosis may be difficult because verrucous carcinoma presents a histologically well-differentiated pattern lacking the usual cytologic features of malignancy. Foci of conventional infiltrating squamous cell carcinoma may be present in large verrucous carcinomas emphasizing the need for careful sampling of the specimen.[127]

Lymph node metastasis of verrucous carcinoma is very rare. With adequate local excision, the disease can be controlled in up to 80% of cases, and survival rates of 90% have been reported. About one third of patients will subsequently develop a second primary carcinoma, often of conventional type, in the mouth or upper aerodigestive tract. Although there have been reports of anaplastic transformation of verrucous carcinoma after radiation therapy, the frequency and factors involved remain unsettled.[122]

Uncommon types of oral carcinoma

Adenoid squamous cell carcinoma. Adenoid squamous cell carcinoma is an unusual variant of squamous

cell carcinoma. Most examples have come from the head and neck. A few cases have involved the vermilion of the lower lip, rarely the upper lip. Most of the patients were middle-aged to old men. None developed regional lymph node spread, but almost 40% had local recurrence. Presumably the lesion is preceded by solar keratosis with acantholysis. Characteristic microscopic changes include downward proliferation, with the deeper islands of tumor cells exhibiting adenoid or tubular configuration. The ductlike structures are lined with cuboid cells, usually two layers thick. In the central portion the tumor masses exhibit acantholysis, shedding desquamated keratinized cells into the lumen. The adjacent stroma usually hosts a dense lymphocytic infiltrate.[108,182]

Spindle cell carcinoma. Spindle cell carcinoma (sarcomatoid carcinoma) is a rare tumor of the oral cavity and upper aerodigestive tract. These present as ulcerating polypoid or sessile masses with a bizarre sarcoma-like proliferation of neoplastic cells. Diligent search is often necessary to find convincing areas of recognizable areas of squamous cell carcinoma morphology, which are usually located at the base or stalk of the lesion. Males are most frequently affected, and the tumor may be seen in patients over a wide age range. The most common oral sites for this tumor are the lower lip, tongue, and alveolar ridge. Although the nature of this tumor has been controversial, current opinion indicates that this tumor is a squamous cell carcinoma with the unique ability to present as a largely anaplastic sarcomatoid histomorphology. This tumor has a serious prognosis with about a 30% survival rate.[82]

Nonkeratinizing and undifferentiated carcinomas. Nonkeratinizing and undifferentiated carcinomas (lymphoepithelial carcinomas) are occasionally located in the faucial area and base of the tongue. These lesions show the same histologic features as their counterparts in the nasopharynx. The primary tumor is often small and difficult to detect, and regional adenopathy is often the first indication of the disease.[1]

Malignant lymphoma. Non-Hodgkin's lymphoma (NHL) is the third most common form of oral cancer though it is very infrequent when compared to squamous cell carcinoma and carcinomas of salivary gland origin. Extranodal lymphomas of the oral soft tissues may present in any site, but the palate and vestibular mucosal and gingival areas are the most common sites. The majority of patients are over age 50. A painless submucosal mass, which may have a reddish or purplish coloration, is the most common clinical presentation. Although all histologic subtypes of NHL may be encountered, diffuse small cleaved cell and large cell types (international lymphoma formulation) are the most common.[80,81,100,106] There may be considerable difficulty in the differentiation of some oral NHL lesions from benign lymphoid hyperplasia, and large cell lymphomas may be difficult to differentiate from undifferentiated carcinomas. Hodgkin's lymphoma is very rare in the oral cavity but may involve the tonsils.[41]

Solitary plasmocytoma. About 80% of extramedullary plasmocytomas arise in the head and neck and are most common in the nasopharynx, nasal cavity, paranasal sinuses, and tonsillar area. Solitary plasmocytomas may also be located in the maxillar or mandible. Histologically these lesions show a monomorphic pattern indistinguishable from myeloma. These lesions are best considered as part of the spectrum of plasma cell dyscrasia, and prognosis is uncertain. Some patients will develop systemic myeloma after variable periods and others may respond to local treatment without dissemination. Plasmocytoma must be differentiated from plasma cell granulomas, which usually involve the alveolar mucosa.[68,76]

Soft-tissue sarcomas. About 15% of soft-tissue sarcomas involve the head and neck area with rhabdomyosarcoma accounting for about 45% of these lesions. Almost every type of soft-tissue sarcoma may occur in the oral soft tissues, but all are very uncommon.[56,153] Histologically these tumors are similar to their counterparts in other sites. Oral rhabdomyosarcomas are most commonly located on the soft palate or cheek. Most patients are under 10 years of age and the majority are of the embryonal histologic type.[57]

Oral Kaposi's sarcoma occurring in patients with the acquired immunodeficiency syndrome (AIDS) is being encountered with increasing frequency and is noted in about 15% of patients with AIDS. Kaposi's sarcoma is found in about 20% of all AIDS patients, and in approximately 50% of these cases the oral structures are involved.[166] Oral Kaposi's sarcoma, often clinically asymptomatic, may be the first clinical manifestation of AIDS. Microscopically the lesions are identical with Kaposi's sarcoma of the skin.

Malignant melanoma. Primary malignant melanoma of the oral mucosa comprises about 2% of all melanomas. Over 80% of these lesions arise on the palatal and maxillary alveolar mucosa. Both nodular and superficial spreading or lentiginous types occur. The latter are characterized by a prolonged intramucosal growth preceding the subsequent vertical growth and invasion. Contemporary concepts of surgical pathology of melanomas have not, however, been widely applied to oral melanomas. Most reports indicate a very poor prognosis for oral melanomas, with about 5% of patients surviving. However most tumors are advanced when first detected.[85,149,183]

JAWS
Developmental lesions

Exostoses (tori). Exostoses, or bony protuberances, are common about the mouth. The most frequent is to-rus palatinus, which occurs in the midline of the hard palate in about 25% of females and in 15% of males. Torus mandibularis is less frequent (about 7% of the population), generally bilateral (80%), and found on the lingual surface of the mandible, usually opposite the premolars.[260] Multiple exostoses are still less common and occur as small nodular outgrowths on the buccal surface of the maxilla and mandible, opposite the premolars and molars.[207]

Osteomatosis. Osteomatosis may be associated with polyposis and adenocarcinoma of the colon and multiple cutaneous and mesenteric fibromas and lipomas (Gardner's syndrome). Epidermoid inclusion cysts are scattered over the body. The syndrome is transmitted as an autosomal dominant trait.[248] Microscopically the bony growths consist of dense, irregular bone with well-marked haversian systems and fibrous medullary portions.

Inflammatory and metabolic lesions

Acute suppurative osteomyelitis. Acute suppurative osteomyelitis of the jaws has become a relatively rare disease with the advent of antibiotics.[268,284] Usually because of infection of the marrow cavity with *Staphylococcus aureus* subsequent to jaw fracture or severe periapical disease, the process spreads, especially in the lower jaw, causing severe pain and facial cellulitis. When the resistance of the host is high or the virulence of the organism low, a chronic focal sclerosing osteomyelitis or condensing osteitis is seen.

Osteomyelitis of jaw of newborn infants. A distinct clinical entity, osteomyelitis of the jaw of the newborn infant almost exclusively involves the upper jaw.[282]

Garré's chronic sclerosing osteomyelitis with proliferative periosteitis. Garré's chronic sclerosing osteomyelitis with proliferative periosteitis is a nonsuppurating type seen most often in the lower jaw in children and young adults. There may be a slight female predilection. The usual inciting factor is an abscessed mandibular first permanent molar. Histopathologic changes appear as supracortical but subperiosteal proliferation of reactive new bone with prominent osteoblastic rimming. Associated fibrous connective tissues are variably infiltrated with chronic inflammatory cells.[228,267]

Infantile cortical hyperostosis (Caffey's disease). Infantile cortical hyperostosis appears in infants, usually within the first 3 months of life, as a bilateral cortical thickening of the mandible.[208,233]

Osteoradionecrosis of the jaws. Osteoradionecrosis of the jaws, principally affecting the mandible, occurs after extensive therapeutic radiation in about 5% of patients. The severity seems to be proportional to the radiation dose, the presence of periodontal sepsis, the susceptibility of the host, and especially the presence of open mucosal wounds. When a patient is dentally

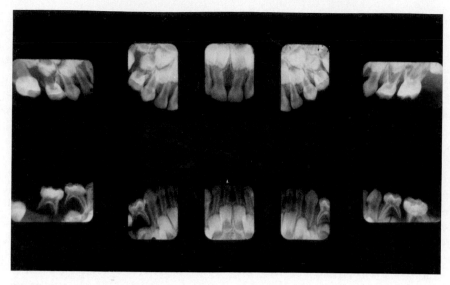

Fig. 23-16. Dental radiographs from patient with histiocytosis X. Molars appear to float in areas of bone loss.

healthy, there appears to be a low risk for osteoradione-crosis.[278]

Osteitis deformans (Paget's disease of bone). Osteitis deformans may involve the jaws, especially the maxilla, with progressive enlargement and displacement of teeth as part of the generalized disease.[277] This becomes especially apparent if the patient wears dentures. True giant cell tumors of the jaws or osteosarcoma may occasionally arise in Paget bone.[255,273]

Histiocytosis X. Histiocytosis X is a collective term for a spectrum of clinicopathologic disorders characterized by proliferation of distinctive histiocytes. These are generally considered to be Langerhans cells. The alveolar mucosa and jaws are involved in about 10% of cases, and oral lesions may be the first or only manifestation of the disease. Swollen, ulcerated gingiva, destruction of alveolar bone resulting in loosening or exfoliation of teeth, and intraosseous cystlike defects are the common findings[251,293] (Fig. 23-16).

Fibro-osseous lesions of the jaws. The term "benign fibro-osseous lesion" is widely applied to a group of lesions involving the craniofacial skeleton that are characterized by a fibrous stoma containing various combinations of bone and "cementum-like" material. A wide variety of lesions of developmental, dysplastic, or neoplastic origin with differing clinical and radiologic presentations and behavior have been included under this general designation. Proper diagnosis requires correlation of the history and clinical and radiologic findings. In the absence of this information, the pathologist can seldom be more specific than to report that the lesion in question represents a benign fibro-osseous lesion. The more important types of fibro-osseous lesions are discussed in this section.[304]

Fibrous dysplasia. The jaws may be involved in both monostotic and polyostotic forms of fibrous dysplasia. The monostotic form is more common and is most often seen in children and young adults. Maxillary lesions are the most common and may involve contiguous bones (that is, sphenoid, occiput, zygoma) and are not strictly monostotic. Clinically fibrous dysplasia is manifested by a painless swelling of the affected bone. Microscopically the jaw lesions of fibrous dysplasia tend to be more ossified than their counterparts in the extragnathic skeleton. Polyostotic fibrous dysplasia, in addition to manifestation in several or many bones, may be accompanied by melanotic pigmentation of the skin and various endocrine disturbances (McCune-Albright syndrome).[230,304]

Ossifying fibroma (cementifying fibroma, cemento-ossifying fibroma). Ossifying fibromas of the jaws and craniofacial skeleton are generally considered to be benign neoplasms. They occur most often in the mandible and present as circumscribed, expansile tumors that on occasion may grow to massive size. Grossly the tumor is well circumscribed and may be encapsulated. Microscopically the ossifying fibroma is composed of a cellular fibrous connective tissue containing varying combinations of trabecular woven or lamellar bone or relatively acellular calcifications that have been considered to represent cementum. Lesions of the latter type have been considered by the WHO[12] and others to be cementifying fibromas and classified as a type of odontogenic tumor. This appears to be an artibrary and unnecessary subdivision, and there is a growing tendency to include all these variations under the rubric of ossifying fibroma.[229,304] Most ossifying fibromas of the jaw respond well to simple enucleation with a low incidence of recurrence. Large lesions, however, may require resection and bone grafting. Ossifying fibromas also occur in the entragnathic craniofacial skeleton, particularly in the ethmoid and frontal bones. These tend to be larger, more radiographically diffuse, and often more histologically cellular than those in the mandible or maxilla.[236a] These lesions have been variously designated as aggressive, active, juvenile, or psammomatoid ossifying fibromas.[224,270] The relationship of craniofacial ossifying fibromas to ossifying fibroma of long bone, most often seen in the tibia, is uncertain.[286]

Other fibro-osseous lesions of the jaws. Periapical cemental dysplasia (periapical cementoma) is frequently encountered, particularly in middle-aged black women. This is a nonneoplastic, presumably dysplastic, condition. The anterior mandibular teeth are most often involved by asymptomatic periapical radiolucencies that in older lesions become increasingly calcified. In the early stages the lesion may be confused with periapical inflammatory disease. Treatment is not required.[312] Florid cemento-osseous dysplasia is less common and has been reported under various designations. This condition is usually seen in middle-aged or elderly black women and radiographically shows extensive, sclerotic areas often involving the posterior quadrants of the mandible and the maxilla symmetrically.[272]

Giant cell granuloma. The giant cell granuloma is generally considered to be a nonneoplastic lesion essentially limited to the jaws and oral mucosa. Although originally designated as "giant cell reparative granuloma," these lesions are clinically destructive and may be locally aggressive.[256] There has been an increasing tendency to drop the adjective "reparative." Giant cell granulomas may present as soft-tissue lesions of the alveolar mucosa (peripheral giant cell granuloma, giant cell epulis) or as an intraosseous lesion (central giant cell granuloma). Both types occur with about equal frequency.[202,242] Both the peripheral and central forms occur about twice as often in females, and the majority of patients are under age 30. The central type occurs about twice as often in the mandible as in the maxilla. The radiographic appearance is not diagnostic and shows a unilocular or multilocular, usually well-demarcated lucent lesion.

Microscopically the giant cell granuloma shows a well-vascularized stroma of spindle and ovoid mesenchymal cells containing variable numbers of multinucleated giant cells. Collagen formation is variable, and foci of osteoid may be present (Fig. 23-17). A considerable histologic variation may be noted. Some giant cell granulomas may be collagenized, with focal collections of giant cells often associated with areas of extravasated erythrocytes. Others may show an even distribution of large multinucleated giant cells in a cellular ovoid and spindle cell stroma without evidence of col-

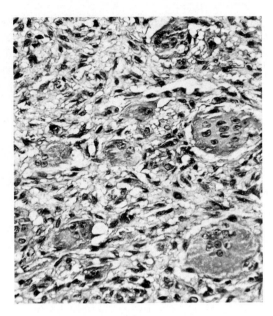

Fig. 23-17. Giant cell granuloma. Lesion is characterized by numerous multinucleated giant cells in fibrous cellular stroma. Collagen, osteoid, or bone is formed.

lagen formation or osteoid production. These are histologically indistinguishable from giant cell tumors of long bones.

The relationship between giant cell granuloma of the jaws and giant cell tumor of long bones has long been controversial. Many authorities in orthopedic pathology deny the existence of "true" giant cell tumors of the jaws or believe that they are exceedingly rare. Critical comparative study or series of giant cell granulomas of the jaws and giant cell tumors of long bones have been undertaken utilizing various types of quantitative analyses. These have shown that although the majority of giant cell granulomas of the jaws are histologically different from giant cell tumors of bone some jaw lesions clearly fall into the histologic characteristics of giant cell tumor. Most central giant cell granulomas of the jaws respond well to conservative surgical curettage with a low rate of recurrence. In a minority of cases, however, a central giant cell granuloma will show aggressive local behavior with rapid growth, resorption of tooth roots, perforation of the cortical plates, and frequent local recurrence. These lesions generally demonstrate histologic features similar to giant cell tumors of bone.[232]

Differential diagnosis includes cherubism, aneurysmal bone cyst, and brown tumor of hyperparathyroidism. The solid areas of an aneurysmal bone cyst are indistinguishable from giant cell granuloma, and distinction between the two may be arbitrary in some cases. Brown tumors of hyperparathyroidism occur in the jaws with some frequency and cannot be distinguised microscopically from a giant cell granuloma. It is wise to obtain blood calcium values in any case of central giant cell granuloma to rule out unsuspected hyperparathyroidism. These studies are mandatory in any case of recurrent giant cell granuloma. Loss of the lamina dura about the roots of teeth is also suggestive of hyperparathyroidism, but this is less common than generally believed.[258]

Cherubism. Cherubism is an autosomal dominant disease that is essentially limited to the jawbones. It has been imprecisely referred to as "familial fibrous dysplasia." The condition is characterized by bilateral enlargements of the jaws usually noted during the second or third years of life. The posterior body of the mandible and ascending ramus are the chief sites of involvement. Bony expansion increases for a few years and tends to stabilize or even regress in early adulthood. If the maxilla is extensively involved, a rim of sclera is exposed, giving rise to the cherubic facies. The microscopic findings are similar if not identical to those seen in the giant cell granuloma, and the two conditions often cannot be distinguished by microscopic study alone. In some cases the stroma in cherubism is more loose and fibrillar than usually present in giant cell granuloma with focal collections of giant cells surrounding capillaries that show a peculiar eosinophilic perivascular cuffing.[249,280]

Uncommon benign tumors of the jaws

Melanotic neuroectodermal tumor of infancy, a tumor of the jaws, is a rare benign lesion of neural crest origin, largely restricted to the maxilla of infants.[209] At the time of discovery of the tumor, the infant is nearly always under 6 months of age. There is no sex predilection. The local recurrence rate is about 15%. A few similar tumors have been reported in the shoulder, epididymis, mandible, calvaria, brain, and mediastinum. Borello and Gorlin[211] have demonstrated that a tumor elaborated vanillylmandelic acid, and neural crest origin appeared likely. Ultrastructural evidence supports this view.[252]

Grossly the tumor is often pigmented and well circumscribed, though no well-defined capsule is present. Microscopically the tumor consists of a fibrous connective tissue stroma in which tubules or spaces are present in large numbers (Fig. 23-18). The spaces are lined by a single layer of large cuboid cells with abundant cytoplasm in which are found numerous melanin granules. The spaces frequently are filled with many deeply staining neuroblast-like cells that are smaller than the duct cells and contain much less cytoplasm.

Osteoblastomas have been reported in the jaws, and the incidence is probably greater than indicated in the literature. The relationship between osteoblastoma of the jaws and some forms of ossifying fibroma and cementoblastoma are not well defined, and there are many overlapping histologic features.[275,292]

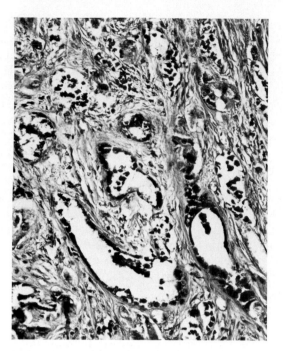

Fig. 23-18. Pigmented neuroectodermal tumor of infancy. This choristomatous lesion is composed of numerous tubules in fibrous connective tissue stroma. Tubules lined by large cuboid cells contain melanin. Within lumens are cells resembling neuroblasts.

Desmoplastic fibroma is an uncommon primary tumor of bone. A significant number of the reported cases have occurred in the mandible, most often in patients under 30 years of age. Histologically the lesion is identical to aggressive fibromatosis (extra-abdominal desmoid) of the soft tissues. Differentiation from low-grade fibrosarcoma may be difficult.[289] *Hemangiomas of bone* are particularly common in the craniofacial skeleton, and the jaws are involved in a significant number of cases. Severe and even fatal hemorrhage has been reported after biopsy or extraction of teeth involved in a hemangioma of the jaws.

Chondromyxoid fibromas,[269] *leiomyomas*,[245] and *neurilemomas*,[227] have rarely been noted as intraosseous jaw tumors. The histologic features are identical with their counterparts in other bones or in the soft tissues.

Malignant tumors of the jaws

Osteosarcoma (osteogenic sarcoma). About 7% of osteosarcomas are primary in the jawbones. The maxilla and mandible are involved with about equal frequency.[221] The average age for patients with osteosarcoma of the jaws is 10 to 15 years greater than that of patients with osteosarcoma of long bones.[253] Jaw osteosarcomas tend to be of a lower histologic grade of malignancy than those in long bones, and the lesion may be initially misdiagnosed as a benign process.[206] Local recurrence is a major problem, and distant metastasis is uncommon. Overall survival rates of 40% have been reported, but a survival rate of 80% has been reported in patients treated by initial radical surgery.[221] A few oral examples have been reported arising in Paget's disease or in benign fibro-osseous lesions that have been subjected to radiation treatment. Examples of juxtacortical[214] and periosteal osteosarcomas[311] have also been reported in the jaws.

Chondrosarcoma. Chondrosarcoma of the jaws is less common than osteosarcoma. It has been reported to occur in patients over a wide age range, and the average age of patients in the large series of cases at the Armed Forces Institute of Pathology is approximately the same as that for osteosarcoma.[253] In contrast to extragnathic chondrosarcoma, the jaw lesions appear to have no better prognosis than that seen in osteosarcoma.[241a] It has been suggested that failure to separate mesenchymal chondrosarcoma from the conventional forms of chondrosarcoma may account for differing reports concerning prognosis.[220] I also believe that some variations in reported incidence and prognosis of chondrosarcoma of the jaws may be attributable to differing criteria for separation of chondrogenic osteosarcoma from chondrosarcoma. A significant proportion of jaw osteosarcomas are of the chondrogenic type and may contain only small foci demonstrating osteoid production by the malignant cells. Rare reports of chondromas of the jaws may be found, but in my experience cartilage-producing tumors of the jaws invariably will prove to be malignant.[219,241a] Mesenchymal chondrosarcoma is an uncommon neoplasm, and in about one third of cases the lesion arises in soft tissues rather than in bone. In contrast to the usual type of chondrosarcoma, this lesion shows a striking predilection to involve patients between 10 and 30 years of age.[220] There is a relatively high incidence of facial bone involvement, particularly the maxilla. Microscopically the tumor is characterized by undifferentiated round or ovoid cells interspersed with islands of well-differentiated cartilage. It is generally agreed that mesenchymal chondrosarcoma has a poorer prognosis than conventional chondrosarcoma, but there is little reliable data on any large series of jaw lesions.

Fibrosarcoma. Fibrosarcomas of the jaws account for about 12% of all fibrosarcomas of bone. The posterior mandible is the most common site.[299] The tumor may arise endosteally or from the periosteum. Histopathologic interpretation and diagnosis are complicated by the numerous other fibrous and spindle cell neoplasms observed in the jaws.

Malignant lymphoma. About 35% to 45% of non-Hodgkin's lymphomas of the oral regions arise with the jawbones. The maxilla is more commonly involved than the mandible. Diffuse small cleaved cell and large cell types are the most common and occur with about equal frequency.[80,81] The African form of Burkitt's lymphoma involves the jaws in about 75% of cases and produces gross distortion of the mandible, maxilla, and orbital area. Jaw involvement in the American type of Burkitt's lymphoma is less frequent and the patients tend to be older.[40]

Multiple myeloma. Jaw involvement occurs in about 30% of cases, and occasionally jaw lesions are the first sign of the disease. About 10% of patients with multiple myeloma have amyloidosis, and macroglossia may occur.[68]

Rare primary malignant tumors of the jaws. Ewing's sarcoma uncommonly involves the jawbones, and less than 3% of cases are primary in the mandible or maxilla.[204,259] Malignant fibrous histiocytoma[295] and leiomyosarcoma[261] also have been reported as primary jaw tumors. It is of interest that 40% of reported instances of intraosseous leiomyosarcoma have occurred in the maxilla or mandible.

Malignant tumors metastatic to jaws. Malignant tumors metastatic to the jaws are uncommon. Spread probably takes place through the vertebral system of veins. In a survey of 150 cases, there was an indication of the following order of frequency: carcinoma of breast, lung, kidney, large intestine, thyroid gland, prostate, and stomach.[203]

The tooth-bearing area of the body and the molar regions of the mandible are the most frequent sites, possibly because of greater arterial blood supply in these regions. In about half the cases, the oral metastasis is the first sign of the generalized cancer. Swelling, pain, and anesthesia are the most common symptoms (Fig. 23-19).

Cysts

In contrast to their virtual nonexistence in other bones, epithelium-lined cysts of the jaws are common lesions and form an important aspect of oral pathology. Cysts of the jaws are classified into odontogenic and nonodontogenic types. The epithelial lining of odontogenic cysts is derived from odontogenic epithelium, whereas the lining of nonodontogenic cysts is presumably derived from remnants of the epithelium covering the primitive processes that participate in the embryonic development of the face and jaws. Odontogenic cysts are further subclassified as to whether they are of inflammatory or developmental origin.[12,288] The following is a classification of cysts of the jaws and oral soft tissues:

Odontogenic cysts
Inflammatory in origin
    Radicular cyst
    Residual cyst
    Paradental cyst

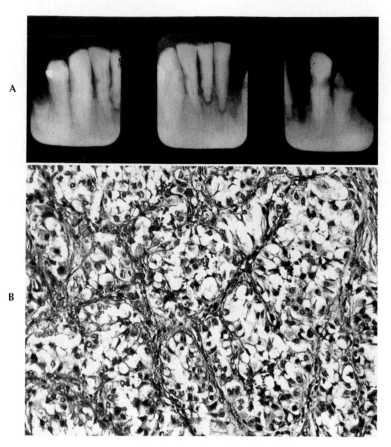

Fig. 23-19. Clinical radiographic, **A,** and histologic, **B,** appearance of metastatic adeno-carcinoma of kidney. Similarity to inflammatory conditions of dental tissue in radiograph may be striking.

Developmental cysts
  Odontogenic keratocyst
  Dentigerous cyst
  Eruption cyst
  Lateral periodontal cyst
  Gingival cyst of the adult
  Gingival cyst of infants
  Calcifying odontogenic cyst
Nonodontogenic cysts
  Nasopalatine duct cyst (incisive canal cyst)
  Median palatine, median alveolar, and median
    mandibular cysts
  Globulomaxillary cyst
  Nasolabial (nasoalveolar) cyst
Non–epithelium lined bone cysts
  Simple (traumatic, hemorrhagic) bone cyst
  Aneurysmal bone cyst
  Stafne cyst (latent, developmental cyst)
Cysts of the oral floor, neck, and salivary glands
  Lymphoepithelial cysts
  Dermoid and epidermoid cysts
  Thyroglossal duct cyst
  Branchiogenic cyst

  Oral cysts with gastric or intestinal epithelium
  Salivary gland cysts

Odontogenic cysts of inflammatory origin. The *radic-ular (apical periodontal) cyst* is the most common, ac-counting for over 60% of all jaw cysts.[287] The cyst is almost always located at the apex of a nonvital tooth though some examples are located laterally to the root at the site of an accessory pulp foramen. The cyst de-velops as a result of cystic degeneration of an epithe-lialized dental granuloma or chronic periapical abscess as a sequela to dental caries and pulpitis. The epithelial lining originates from the epithelial rests of Malassez, which are normally present in the periodontal ligament. The *residual cyst* is a radicular cyst that remains in the jaw after the responsible tooth has been lost. The *para-dental cyst* is a recently recognized type of inflamma-tory odontogenic cyst.[200] It is almost always located on the lateral root aspect of a partially erupted mandibular third molar. A history of repeated episodes of perico-ronal inflammation (pericoronitis) is usually noted. The epithelial lining is presumably derived from rests of Malassez or reduced enamel epithelium.

Developmental odontogenic cysts. The pathogenesis

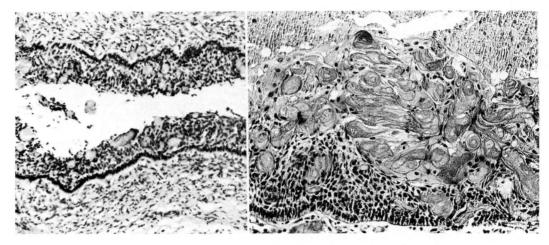

Fig. 23-20. Keratinizing and calcifying odontogenic cyst. Notice pronounced basal layer with palisaded cells and large masses of partially keratinized "ghost" cells.

of developmental odontogenic cysts is poorly understood but does not appear to be associated with inflammation or infection.

The *odontogenic keratocyst* shows specific histopathologic features and exhibits unique clinical behavior. Odontogenic keratocysts comprise between 3% and 12% of all jaw cysts.[201,212,213] These cysts arise from rests of the primitive dental lamina and possess greater growth potential and tendency to recur than is seen in other odontogenic cysts. About 80% are located in the mandible, particularly in the posterior body and ascending ramus. In about 25% of cases the cyst is associated with an unerupted tooth. Recurrence develops in about 30% of cases after enucleation. Multiple odontogenic keratocysts of the jaws are an important feature of the nevoid basal cell carcinoma syndrome, which has an autosomal dominant inheritance pattern. The jaw cysts in the syndrome are invariably keratocyts and tend to show more proliferative microscopic features than the isolated lesions not associated with the syndrome.[247,308]

The *dentigerous cyst* is the most common type of developmental odontogenic cyst. The cyst encloses the crown of an unerupted tooth and is attached to the tooth at the junction of the crown and root.[287] The epithelial lining is derived from the reduced enamel epithelium. Most cases are diagnosed before 30 years of age. Although any tooth may be involved, dentigerous cysts are most often seen associated with unerupted mandibular third molars and maxillary canines. Dentigerous cysts may occasionally grow to massive size before detection. Ameloblastomas may occasionally arise from neoplastic alteration of the epithelial lining, but the actual incidence of this has not been precisely determined.[301]

The *eruption cyst* is a special variant of the dentig-

erous cyst that occurs in the gingival mucosa over the crown of an erupting deciduous or permanent tooth.[287] The *lateral periodontal cyst* forms laterally to the root of an erupted vital tooth. Most examples are found in the mandibular premolar area. The etiology and pathogenesis are not completely clear, but proliferation of dental lamina rests or cystic degeneration of the enamel organ are the most likely possibilities.[310] The *gingival cyst of the adult* is considered to be the soft-tissue counterpart of the lateral periodontal cyst. Most examples are seen in the gingiva in the mandibular canine-premolar area.[216,310]

Gingival cysts of the newborn, which are usually multiple, occur on the alveolar process. They represent cystic degeneration of remnants of the dental lamina. These cysts rupture spontaneously and do not require treatment.[287] Similar cysts occur on the palates of newborns and are derived from epithelial remnants in the palatal mucosa. The *calcifying odontogenic cyst* (keratinizing and calcifying cyst, Gorlin cyst) is an uncommon lesion with unique histologic features. It is characterized by masses of "ghosts," or aberrantly keratinized epithelium lining the cyst cavity.[236] In about 35% of cases nontubular dentinoid substance has been noted in the connective tissue wall (Fig. 23-20). In about 20% of cases, the lesion occurs extraosseously in the gingival tissues. Some lesions are entirely solid with no gross cystic features. Some authorities consider the calcifying odontogenic cyst to be an odontogenic tumor rather than a cyst, and there is a wide spectrum of histologic features and clinical behavior.[281]

Nonodontogenic cysts. As the name implies, nonodontogenic cysts are not derived from the epithelium associated with tooth development. These cysts are believed to arise from epithelial rests entrapped along lines of fusion of embryonic processes. There is considerable question that some lesions formerly classified as nonodontogenic cysts actually represent specific entities. The *nasopalatine duct cyst* arises in the incisive canal from the remnants of the primitive nasopalatine duct. This cyst is located in the anterior maxilla between the roots of the maxillary central incisor teeth. It is the most common type of nonodontogenic cyst.[198] The *median palatine, median alveolar,* and *median mandibular cysts* are all very rare, and there is considerable doubt that any of these represent specific entities.[237] The *globulomaxillary cyst* has traditionally been considered to be an intraosseous cyst located between the maxillary lateral incisor and canine and arising from epithelial rests entrapped during development of the premaxilla. There is considerable doubt that this cyst exists as an entity, and most cysts in the location prove to be odontogenic keratocysts.[254,309]

The *nasolabial (nasoalveolar) cyst* develops at the junction of the median nasal, lateral nasal, and maxillary processes, being located at the ala of the nose and frequently extending into the nostril. It may resorb the alveolar bone but is not itself an intraosseous lesion. The pathogenesis is still unresolved, but origin from the lower part of the primitive nasolacrimal duct is favored.[241,287]

From a practical standpoint, few jaw cysts can be differentiated from one another on a microscopic basis alone. Specific diagnosis requires clinicoradiologic correlations as to the precise location of the cyst and its relationship to involved teeth. In the absence of this information the pathologist's diagnosis can seldom be more specific than benign epithelium-lined cyst. However, the following hints may be of help. Radicular, residual, paradental, and dentigerous cysts are usually lined by nonkeratinized stratified squamous epithelium overlying dense fibrous connective tissue containing a chronic inflammatory cell infiltrate. Dentigerous cysts may show islands of epithelial rests in the fibrous wall. Proliferation of these rests is responsible for an occasional misdiagnosis of ameloblastoma.

Lateral periodontal and gingival cysts of the adult are lined by a thin layer of stratified squamous or cuboid epithelium, and the fibrous wall tends to show little evidence of inflammation. The odontogenic keratocyst is lined by a uniform thin layer of stratified squamous epithelium showing a polarized hyperchromatic basal layer of columnar or cuboid cells. The luminal surface is composed of parakeratinized cells with a wavy or corrugated appearance. Satellite cysts, or islands of odontogenic epithelial rests resembling dental lamina, are found in the fibrous capsule in 7% to 25% of cases. The nasopalatine duct cyst is often lined by both stratified squamous and ciliated columnar epithelium. Mucous glands and congeries of blood vessels and nerves are frequently noted within the fibrous wall.

Malignant change in cysts. Squamous cell carcinoma arising in the lining of an odontogenic cyst is rare, but cases have been well documented. Most examples appear to be associated with residual or dentigerous cysts. The majority occur in the posterior mandibles of older males.[231,300]

Non–epithelium lined jaw cysts. The *simple (traumatic, hemorrhagic) bone cyst* of the jaws are probably the same lesion referred to as solitary or unicameral cyst in the long bones. Although commonly referred to as "traumatic cysts," there is little evidence that trauma is an etiologic factor, and the pathogenesis is obscure. Most examples are found in the mandibles of patients under 20 years of age. On surgical exploration the bone cavity is often empty or contains only a small amount of serosanguineous fluid. A thin layer of loose vascular connective tissue may be adjacent to the bony walls, but an epithelial lining is never present.[257]

Aneurysmal bone cysts rarely involve the jaws. These show identical histologic features with aneurysmal bone cysts of the extragnathic skeleton consisting of cavernous, blood-filled spaces surrounded by fibrous tissue containing giant cells and areas of new bone formation. Some aneurysmal bone cysts appear to arise anew, whereas others clearly represent some form of vascular accident in a preexisting intraosseous lesion.[294,296]

The *Stafne cyst* (lingual mandibular depression, static bone cavity) is not a cyst and represents a developmental defect of the lingual cortical plate of the mandible usually located near the angle. It occurs in 1 of 250 individuals. The condition is usually detected during a routine radiographic examination and may easily be confused with some type of bone cyst. Some of these cortical defects will contain a herniated lobule of submandibular gland tissue.[210]

Cysts of the oral floor, salivary glands, and neck. *Lymphoepithelial cysts* of the oral cavity appear as small, slightly elevated yellowish nodules in the floor of the mouth or ventral tongue. The lesion shows a central cystic cavity lined by squamous epithelium embedded in a circumscribed nodule of lymphoid tissue usually showing germinal centers. These cysts represent the intraoral counterpart of the lymphoepithelial (branchial cleft) cysts of the lateral area of the neck.[243] *Dermoid cysts* are relatively common in the head and neck area, with the floor of the mouth being the most common site. They probably arise from enclaves of epithelial debris in the midline during closure of the mandibular and other branchial arches.[279] *Gastric* or *intestinal epithelium-lined cysts* are rare and occur in the anterior floor of the mouth or tongue. This lesion corresponds to developmental anomalies (duplications) seen elsewhere in the gastrointestinal tract.[250] *Cysts of the salivary glands and neck* are discussed later in this chapter.

Odontogenic tumors

The odontogenic tumors, arising from tooth-forming tissues, form a complex group of lesions of diverse histologic patterns and clinical behavior. They are uncommon lesions, and even in the specialized oral pathology laboratory they comprise only about 1% or 2% of accessioned cases.[283] Odontogenesis is a complex process involving interaction of epithelium and mesenchyme with the eventual formation of mature calcified dental tissues. Neoplastic and hamartomatous aberrations can occur at any stage, resulting in lesions with varying proportions of proliferating odontogenic epithelium or odontogenic mesenchyme with or without calcified structures. A simplified classification of odontogenic tumors is presented here. This does not include some of the rare and transitional types, and more extensive works on the subject should be referred to for additional information.[12,246,303]

Benign odontogenic tumors
Epithelial origin
Ameloblastoma
Odontogenic adenomatoid tumor
Calcifying epithelial odontogenic tumor
Mesenchymal origin
Myxoma
Odontogenic fibroma
Cemental tumors
Mixed odontogenic tumors
Ameloblastic fibroma
Ameloblastic fibro-odontoma
Complex and compound odontomas
Malignant odontogenic tumors
Ameloblastic carcinoma
Ameloblastic fibrosarcoma

Benign odontogenic tumors
Epithelial origin

Ameloblastoma. The ameloblastoma is the most common of the significant odontogenic tumors. Its incidence is nearly equal to the combined incidence of all other odontogenic tumors, excluding odontomas. Although odontomas undoubtedly are more common in the general population, these generally small hamartomatous lesions are easily diagnosed and seldom are clinically significant. Ameloblastomas appear to originate from cell rests of enamel organ epithelium, from the epithelial lining of odontogenic cysts (chiefly dentigerous cysts), or occasionally from the basal layer of the oral mucosa.

Ameloblastoma appears most commonly in the third to fifth decades.[271,291,305] No sex or racial predilection is noted. Over 80% occur in the mandible, and 70% of these arise in the molar-ramus area. Rarely an extraosseous example is discovered.[217]

Traditionally ameloblastoma has been divided into solid and cystic types, but nearly all ameloblastomas demonstrate some cystic degeneration. Microscopically, many subtypes or patterns have been suggested: follicular, plexiform, acanthomatous, granular cell (Figs. 23-21 and 23-22), and basal cell varieties. However, two or more types may occur within the same tumor, and there is no evidence that any subtype is more aggressive than any other.

The majority of ameloblastomas demonstrate one of the two predominent patterns, follicular or plexiform, the former being the more common. In the follicular type there is an attempt to mimic the dental organ epithelium. The outermost cells resemble those of the inner dental epithelium of the developing tooth follicle, that is, the ameloblastic layer. The cells are tall columnar, with polarization of the nuclei away from the basement membrane.[301] These stringent criteria have recently been challenged.[239] The central portion of the epithelial island is composed of a loose network of cells resembling stellate reticulum. Squamous metaplasia within the stellate reticulum gives rise to the acanthomatous type. The epithelial islands demonstrate no inductive influence on the collagenized connective tissue stroma. Enamel and dentin are never formed by the ameloblastoma. The plexiform pattern demonstrates irregular masses and interdigitating cords of epithelial cells with a minimum of stroma.

Ameloblastomas tend to infiltrate the intertrabecular spaces of adjacent cancellous bone, and treatment by curettage is accompanied by a 55% to 90% incidence of recurrence.[276] Ameloblastomas may cause death by progressive infiltration into vital structures. Posterior maxillary tumors are particularly dangerous in this respect.[298]

Odontogenic adenomatoid tumor. A benign lesion, the odontogenic adenomatoid tumor probably arises from the preameloblast or from the inner enamel epithelium.[223,285] It appears to be more common in females, arises somewhat more often in the anterior region of the upper jaw, and occurs most frequently in the second decade of life. Frequently it is associated with an unerupted canine. Although the tumor expands, it is not invasive and does not recur even after extremely conservative surgical therapy.

Microscopically the lesion consists of congeries of ductlike structures, lined by medium to tall columnar epithelium, in an extremely scant fibrous connective tissue stroma (Fig. 23-23). Small calcified deposits are often seen scattered throughout the epithelial tissue.

Calcifying epithelial odontogenic tumor. The calcifying epithelial odontogenic tumor is a relatively rare lesion. The tumor may be invasive and locally recurrent, behaving like an ameloblastoma. It seems to occur most

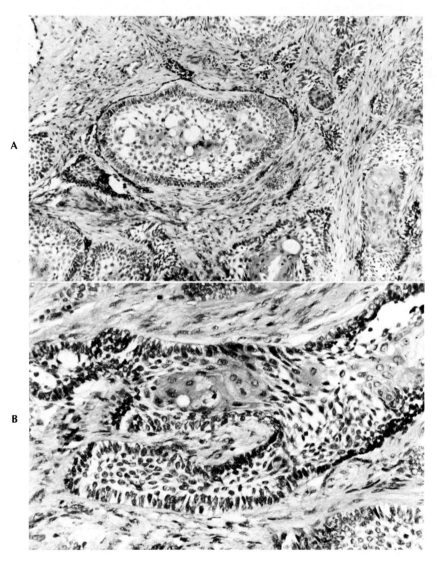

Fig. 23-21. Ameloblastoma. **A,** Numerous islands of odontogenic epithelium in mature fibrous connective tissue stroma. Notice resemblance to developing dental epithelial enamel organ. Within stellate reticular area are sites of squamous metaplasia. **B,** Higher-power view showing tendency of nuclei to polarize away from basement membrane. (Courtesy J. Sciubba, New Hyde Park, N.Y.)

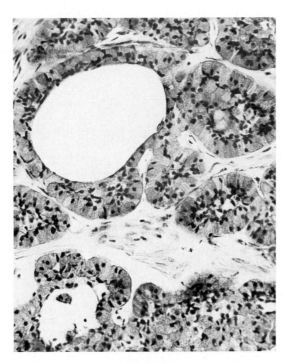

Fig. 23-22. Ameloblastoma exhibiting granular cell pattern. Occasionally, whole tumor may be composed of large granular cells with eosinophilic granular cytoplasm.

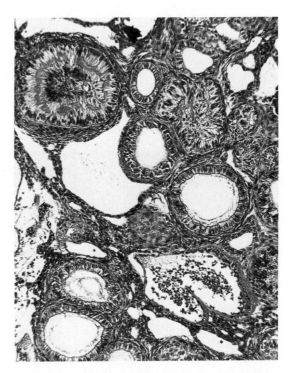

Fig. 23-23. Odontogenic adenomatoid tumor. Tumor consists of congeries of tubules and possibly arises from pre-ameloblast.

commonly in the fourth and fifth decades. There is no sex predilection. About 65% of reported cases have arisen in the mandibular premolar-molar area in association with an embedded tooth.[234,235,262] There is a 10% to 15% recurrence rate.

Microscopically, the tumor is composed of polyhedral epithelial cells with scanty stoma. The closely packed cells frequently demonstrate nuclear pleomorphism. Intracellular degeneration results in numerous spherical spaces filled with eosinophilic homogeneous material that in time becomes calcified. Although this substance stains like amyloid, ultrastructural studies have shown that it represents some fibrillar proserine secreted by the tumor epithelium (Fig. 23-24).

Mesenchymal odontogenic tumors

Myxoma. The myxoma is one of the more common odontogenic tumors. Since most investigators believe that myxomas do not occur in the extragnathic skeleton, all myxomas of the jaws represent odontogenic tumors. The myxoma presumably arises from primitive odontogenic mesenchyme and bears a close histologic resemblence to the mesodermal portion of a developing tooth (dental papilla). It is encountered most often in young adults and occurs in the mandible and maxilla with about equal frequency. In some instances tumor growth is fairly rapid and may result in noticeable bone

expansion. Microscopically the myxoma consists of loose stellate cells in an abundant mucoid stroma (Fig. 23-25). Some tumors contain small islands of odontogenic epithelial rests, but their presence is not required for the diagnosis. Myxomas may exhibit infiltrative growth, and recurrence rates of up to 25% have been reported after curettage. Some myxomas show a greater tendency to form collagen fibers, and these have been designated as myxofibromas.[205,245,307] On rare occasions a myxoma will be hypercellular and show atypical cytologic features and local aggressive behavior. These have been designated as myxosarcomas.[264] Since the myxoma is histologically identical to the dental papilla of a developing tooth, the latter may occasionally be "overdiagnosed" as a myxoma unless the clinical and radiologic situation is appreciated.

Odontogenic fibroma. The odontogenic fibroma is an uncommon, ill defined, and controversial lesion. Cases have been reported in patients over a wide age range, and the mandible is involved more often than the maxilla. The lesion designated in the World Health Organization (WHO) classification as odontogenic fibroma is composed of plump fibroblasts and collagen fibers arranged in an interlacing pattern. Stands of nests of odontogenic epithelium are scattered through the lesion and may be a prominent component. Calcified cementum-like structures, osteoid, or dysplastic dentin

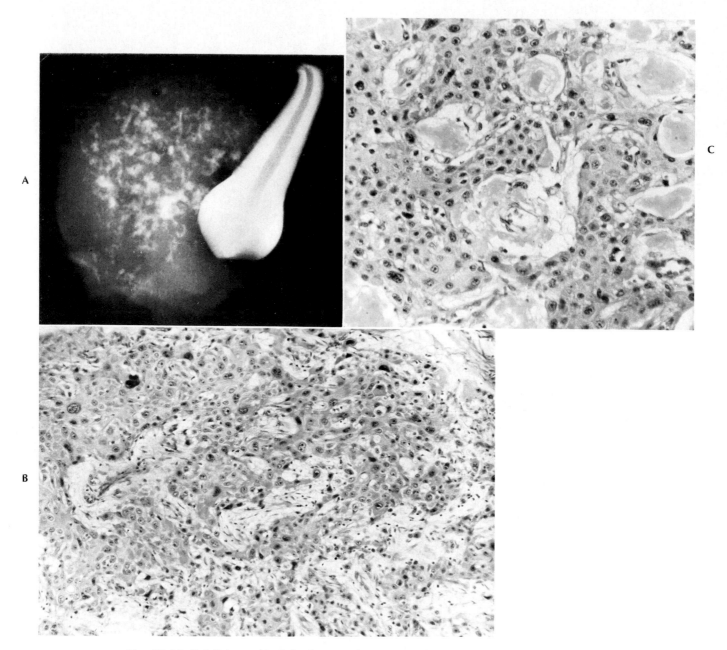

Fig. 23-24. Calcifying epithelial odontogenic tumor. **A,** Radiograph of upper canine tooth and tumor showing flecky calcification. **B,** Pleomorphic cells. **C,** Hyalinized amyloid-staining material. (Courtesy J. Sciubba, New Hyde Park, N.Y.)

Fig. 23-25. Odontogenic myxoma. Tumor consists of loose, embryonal connective tissue. Occasionally, strands of odontogenic epithelium are present.

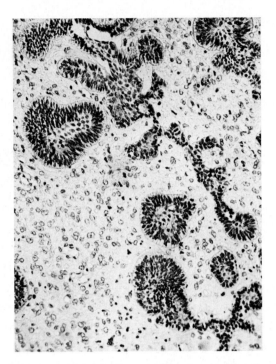

Fig. 23-26. Ameloblastic fibroma. Tumor consists of numerous islands of odontogenic epithelium in cellular mesenchymal matrix. This tumor is nonaggressive and must be differentiated from ameloblastomas, which lack the primitive mesenchymal matrix.

may be present.[225,238] An identical lesion occurs as an extraosseous lesion on the gingival mucosa and is designated as a "peripheral odontogenic fibroma."[215]

The other form of odontogenic fibroma is composed of plump stellate fibroblasts with fine collagen fibrils and considerable ground substance.[306] Occasional small islands of epithelial odontogenic rests may be observed. The relationship between these two lesions, both designated as "odontogenic fibroma," is as yet unresolved. Both types of odontogenic fibroma respond well to conservative enucleation.

Cemental tumors. Although four types of cemental tumors are recognized in the WHO classification of odontogenic tumors,[12] three of them (periapical cemental dysplasia, florid cemento-osseous dysplasia, and cementifying fibroma) are more logically considered with the fibro-osseous diseases of the jaws. These are discussed on p. 1114. The cementoblastoma is a rare benign neoplasm most often involving the roots of a mandibular first molar in young adult patients. It radiographically presents as a densely calcified mass intimately associated with and resorbing the roots of the involved tooth. Histologically the tumor is composed of sheets of mineralized material bordered by large blast-like cells. The histologic features are very similar to those of an osteoblastoma, and some investigators believe that cementoblastomas of the jaws are best classified as a form of osteoblastoma.[199,275]

Mixed odontogenic tumors

Ameloblastic fibroma. The ameloblastic fibroma is characterized by proliferation of both epithelial and mesenchymal elements in the absence of hard tooth structure (enamel or dentin). In contrast to ameloblastoma, the tumor for which it is most commonly mistaken, the ameloblastic fibroma usually occurs in a young age group, rarely being seen in persons over 21 years of age. Clinical behavior is entirely benign.[240,297]

Microscopically the ameloblastic fibroma is composed of strands and buds of epithelial cells in a very cellular connective tissue stroma (Fig. 23-26). The presence of this mesenchymal portion clearly differentiates this lesion from ameloblastoma. For the most part the cells composing the strands of epithelial cells are cuboid and are two cell layers thick. Occasionally a stellate reticulum is present. In contrast to ameloblastoma, simple curettage of the ameloblastic fibroma is usually adequate treatment though a comprehensive review showed an 18% incidence of local recurrence after curettage.[297]

Ameloblastic fibro-odontoma. This is a tumor showing the features of an ameloblastic fibroma but also containing a variably sized component of dentin and enamel. Undoubtedly some lesions diagnosed as ame-

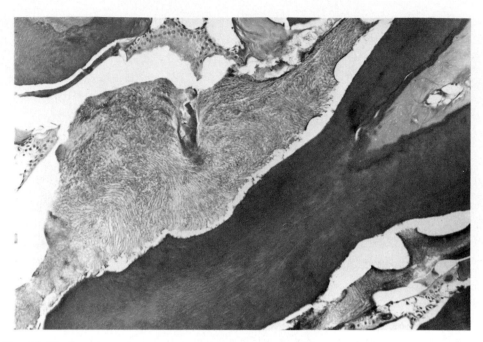

Fig. 23-27. Complex odontoma consists of unorganized mass of dentin, enamel, cementum, and pulpal tissue and occasional areas of enamel epithelium.

loblastic fibro-odontoma represent only a stage in the development of an odontoma. However others grow to considerable size, cause considerable bone destruction, and clearly represent benign neoplasms. The ameloblastic fibro-odontoma is a well-circumscribed lesion that responds readily to conservative enucleation.[240,274]

Odontoma. The odontomas are considered to be hamartomatous lesions that when fully developed consist of enamel and dentin. They are the most common odontogenic tumor. They are further subclassified into complex and compound types. *Complex odontomas* consist of a mass of irregularly arranged dentin enamel and cementum (Fig. 23-27). *Compound odontomas* are small, occasionally 100 or more, misshapen toothlike structures. Intermediate forms containing elements of both types are encountered and are referred to as *composite odontomas.*[218] Odontomas are somewhat more common in the maxilla than in the mandible and most patients are under 15 years of age. Compound odontomas are more commonly located in the anterior maxilla, whereas complex odontomas favor the posterior mandible. Most odontomas are small lesions that do not exceed the size of a tooth in the area in which they are located. Rarely, however, an odontoma may exceed 6 cm in diameter and cause expansion of the jaw. The majority of odontomas are detected during the course of a routine dental radiographic examination. They are completely benign lesions and cured by simple excision. A very rare lesion, the odontoameloblastoma

probably represents the simultaneous occurrence of an ameloblastoma and an odontoma.[263] These may be locally aggressive and behave in a manner similar to that of an ameloblastoma.

Malignant odontogenic tumors

Malignant behavior of odontogenic tumors is rare but has been well documented. These lesions are designated generically as "odontogenic carcinomas," or "odontogenic sarcomas."[12] The term "malignant ameloblastoma" is currently applied to the rare examples of a histologically typical ameloblastoma that metastasizes. Metastases have been demonstrated in regional lymph nodes, lungs, pleura, other bones, and occasionally other viscera. Both the primary tumor and metastatic deposits are histologically similar to most ameloblastomas that do not metastasize.

Ameloblastic carcinoma. The term "ameloblastic carcinoma" is applied to a tumor with the general features of ameloblastoma that shows cytologic evidence of malignancy in the primary tumor, in a recurrent tumor, or in a metastatic deposit. These lesions are characterized by aggressive local behavior, frequent recurrence, and occasional metastasis.[222,290]

Ameloblastic fibrosarcoma. The rare lesion ameloblastic fibrosarcoma appears to be the malignant counterpart of the ameloblastic fibroma. Some examples appear to arise anew, whereas others develop as a recurrence of a previously benign ameloblastic fibroma. The tumor demonstrates islands or strands of benign odontogenic epithelium similar to those seen in an ameloblastic fibroma together with a cell-rich mesenchymal component exhibiting the histologic features of fibrosarcoma. Pain, ulceration, and extensive bone destruction are usually present. The tumor is clinically aggressive with extension into adjacent tissue. Metastasis of ameloblastic fibrosarcoma, however, has not been convincingly documented.[266]

SALIVARY GLANDS
Development

Both the major and the minor salivary glands develop as buds of oral ectoderm, arising in much the same manner as teeth. The epithelial bud proliferates into the adjacent ectomesenchyme, enlarging at its most distal end to form alveoli, with the epithelial cords becoming hollow to form ducts. The parotid and submandibular gland anlagen first become apparent by the sixth fetal week (13 to 15 mm embryo), though acini are not developed until the fifth month in utero. During the eighth week (19 to 25 mm embryo) the buds of the sublingual gland become apparent. The minor salivary glands are initiated by the tenth week.

Labial glands arise as epithelial buds of the vestibular epithelial plate before the opening of the alveololabial sulcus. Buccal and molar glands arise at the same time, associated with the terminal portion of Stensen's duct. Retromolar glands develop in the fifth fetal month.

The major salivary glands are subject to many developmental anomalies. One or more lobes (rarely, whole glands) may be congenitally absent or aplastic. Total absence of all major glands also has been reported.[380] Accessory glands and glands ectopically placed within the mandible, tonsil, or neck have been noted.[374a,379] Major salivary ducts may be congenitally atretic or, rarely, imperforate or duplicated.[356,370]

Structure and types

The salivary glands, both major and minor, are tubuloalveolar structures. Both the parotid and submandibular glands are well encapsulated, though the sublingual is not. The adult parotid gland is serous in type, whereas the submandibular and sublingual glands are mixed, the former being predominantly serous and the latter mucous. Minor salivary glands are widespread, being scattered over the lips, buccal mucosa, palate, and tongue. Pure serous glands are seen about the circumvallate papillae (glands of von Ebner); pure mucous glands are located in the palate and base of the tongue (Weber's glands). All others are of the mixed type.

Disturbances of salivary flow

Increased salivary flow (sialorrhea, ptyalism) can result from many causes. It is most commonly associated with acute inflammation of the oral cavity, such as herpetic or aphthous stomatitis, and with "teething." It is often seen in mentally retarded individuals, in severe schizophrenics, and in patients with neurologic disturbances with lenticular involvement. Mercury poisoning, acrodynia, pemphigus, pregnancy, rabies, epilepsy, nausea, and ill-fitting dentures all may be accompanied by an increased degree of salivation. Also, increased gastric secretion is accompanied by increased salivary flow.

Xerostomia. Decreased salivary flow, xerostomia, is also associated with many conditions. Rarely there is congenital absence of one or more major glands or ducts. Epidemic parotitis (mumps) and sarcoidosis (uveoparotitis) are associated with reduced flow. Patients with Sjögren's syndrome exhibit xerostomia. Therapeutic radiation to the lateral cervical area commonly produces fibrotic changes after acinar destruction of the parotid glands. Megaloblastic anemias (pernicious anemia, anemia of pregnancy) are not uncommonly associated with decreased salivary output. The majority of cases of xerostomia appear to be medication related (tricyclic antidepressants, antihistamines, hypotensive drugs, and phenothiazines). Reduced salivary flow occurs with various disorders associated with fever or dehydration.

Enlargements

Enlargement of one or more salivary glands may be associated with sialorrhea, xerostomia, or normal salivary secretion. A single glandular enlargement may denote localized inflammation, cyst, or neoplasm. Bilateral enlargement may signify an inflammatory process, such as mumps or sarcoid, or a diffuse neoplastic infiltrate (leukemia or lymphoma), or it may be attributable to unknown factors related to malnutrition, alcoholic cirrhosis, or hormonal disturbance.

Cysts

Cysts of salivary gland origin fall into three categories: true cysts, ranulas, and mucoceles or mucus retention phenomena.

True cyst. The true cyst is usually small, 1 cm or less in diameter, and located within the body of the parotid or submandibular gland. It is lined by simple or stratified squamous epithelium.[357]

Ranula. Ranula is a term used rather loosely to indicate a thin-walled, cystic lesion located on the floor of the mouth.[323] It includes sublingual gland mucoceles and a deep burrowing lesion that frequently extends through the mylohyoid muscle. The so-called congenital ranula appears to represent the effect of atresia of the orifice of either the sublingual or submandibular ducts.[374]

Mucocele (mucus retention phenomenon). The extra-

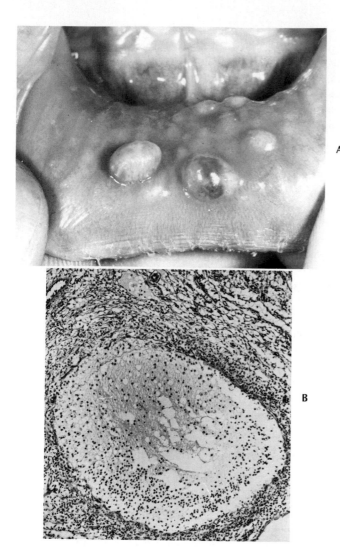

Fig. 23-28. Mucocele or minor salivary gland retention "cyst." **A,** Most commonly observed on lower lip, mucoceles are observed throughout oral cavity. They arise from spillage of mucus into surrounding connective tissue. The mucocele is usually a solitary lesion, and the multiple lesions in this patient are unusual. **B,** Low-power photomicrograph showing extraductal mucus surrounded by inflammation. Notice absence of epithelium.

vasation mucocele is a cavity lined by granulation tissue containing an eosinophilic hyaline material (mucus) composed of a variable number of mucus-laden macrophages (Fig. 23-28). Trauma, chiefly mechanical, appears to be responsible for damage to the ducts of minor salivary glands, resulting in the spillage of mucus into the lamina propria and submucous tissue.[354] The site is most commonly the lower lip and less often the buccal mucosa or oral floor. There is no sex predilection; most cases are seen in children or young adults, probably reflecting the role of trauma. This mucus pool may be localized and surrounded by a wall of granula-

tion tissue. The retention mucocele is lined by a single or double layer of oncocytic epithelium and probably represents cystic changes in an oncocyte-lined duct. It occurs most often in the oral floor and buccal mucosa of older patients.[381] It is much rarer than the extravasation type, constituting no more than 10% of all mucoceles. Mucocele of the glands near the ventral tip of the tongue is called cyst of Blandin-Nuhn. Mucocele of the maxillary sinus floor is not rare, being found in more than 1% of the population.[321,342]

Enlargements related to malnutrition, hormonal disturbances, and alcoholic cirrhosis (sialosis)

The relationship of parotid gland enlargement to malnutrition has been pointed out by many investigators.[332,389] Hypertrophy also has been noted in cases of alcoholism and cirrhosis. Enlargement of the submandibular glands also has been noted occasionally in these cases. It is well known that both alcohol consumption and restricted dietary intake contribute to hepatic cirrhosis. The enlargement may be associated with excessive salivation. Experimentally, parotid enlargement can be produced in rats on a protein-free diet or by feeding proteolytic enzymes.

Parotid enlargement has also been reported in mental patients and in patients with bulimia.[313,364]

Microscopic changes consist in enlarged acinar cells exhibiting a granular pattern, a numerical increase in secretory granules, or a vacuolar alteration of the cytoplasm (Fig. 23-29). No inflammatory changes are observed. The pathogenesis is unknown but is probably related to an alteration in the autonomic nervous system.

Inflammatory diseases

Acute parotitis (secondary suppurative type). Acute parotitis is caused by ascent of microorganisms, usually *Staphylococcus aureus*, up Stensen's duct when salivary flow is reduced by inadequate fluid balance as a result of fever, diuretics, starvation, and so on. It occurs most often in neonates,[363] the elderly, or postoperative patients.[392] It may become recurrent, leading to scarring and chronic parotitis.[359]

Microscopically there is widespread destruction of acini and replacement with fibrous connective tissue. Plasma cell and lymphocytic infiltration is usually considerable. Ducts and acini are frequently dilated.

Acute submandibular adenitis. This acute disorder nearly always follows acute obstruction from a salivary duct stone.

Chronic submandibular adenitis. Chronic submandibular adenitis is often attributable to blockage by stricture or calculi (sialoliths). This, in turn, renders the gland susceptible to retrograde bacterial invasion.

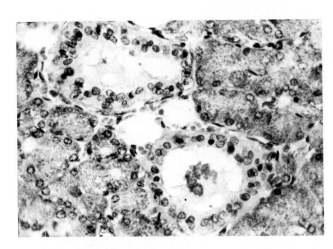

Fig. 23-29. Sialosis. Notice granular alterations in acinar cells of parotid glands. Patient had severe alcoholism. (Courtesy G. Seifert, Hamburg, Germany.)

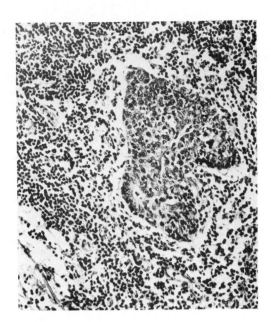

Fig. 23-30. Sjögren's syndrome (benign lymphoepithelial lesion). Acini are replaced by pronounced lymphocytic infiltrate. Differentiation from lymphosarcoma is made with difficulty.

Sjögren's syndrome. Sjögren, in 1933, first described a syndrome consisting of keratoconjunctivitis sicca, pharyngolaryngitis sicca, rhinitis sicca, rheumatoid arthritis with (about 35%) or without parotid (occasionally submanidublar) enlargement, and xerostomia. This syndrome subsequently was shown to accompany at times other disorders such as dermatomyositis, polyarteritis nodosa, systemic lupus erythematosus, chronic active hepatitis, primary biliary cirrhosis, purpura and hypergammaglobulinemia of Waldenström, scleroderma, Hashimoto's thyroiditis, Reiter's syndrome, and Behçet's syndrome.

The patient, usually a postmenopausal woman (about 90%), has red, burning eyes, photophobia, and lack of tears. The disorder has also been reported in children. The saliva is thick and ropy. Dysphagia and dysphonia may be pronounced, and the oral mucosa, especially that of the tongue, is atrophic and shiny. There is angular cheilitis and cracking of the lips. Dental caries, usually at the neck of the teeth, becomes widespread as the disease progresses.[331,369,375,377]

Sjögren's syndrome is believed to be a chronic inflammatory disease of autoimmune cause. It has been suggested that an antigen released from damaged acini coming into contact with lymphatic tissue (normally present with parotid gland) would result in the production of antibodies that in turn would damage more acinar epithelium, continuing the cycle. Arguing for the autoimmune nature of the disease are the following:

1. Associated rheumatoid arthritic changes in over 50%
2. Hypergammaglobulinemia
3. Rheumatoid factor in over 75%
4. Antithyroglobulin antibodies (about 35%) and antinuclear factors (about 65%)
5. Autoantibody reaction with salivary duct cytoplasm in over 50%
6. Association with other connective tissue disorders such as systemic lupus erythematosus, scleroderma, polymyositis, or polyarteritis

It has been suggested that there is impaired IgG autoantibody production.[368] Malignant lymphoma may develop late in the course of the disease. Microscopically there is initially a periductal mononuclear cell infiltrate consisting predominantly of small lymphocytes. Later, large lymphocytes and reticular cells appear. The acinar tissue is eventually totally replaced (Fig. 23-30). Epimyoepithelial islands arising from ductal proliferation are scattered throughout the tissue. Similar changes have been described in the lacrimal glands and the minor salivary glands of the lip and palate.[352]

Benign lymphoepithelial lesion. Benign lymphoepithelial lesion (sometimes referred to as Mikulicz's disease) is characterized by a lobular repalcement of salivary gland parenchyma by a lymphoid infiltrate containing epimyoepithelial islands. This lesion occurs independently of the other features of Sjögren's syndrome though the microscopic features are identical.[345,388] A rare malignant counterpart is characterized by islands of anaplastic carcinoma associated with a prominent benign lymphoid infiltrate. The parotid gland is the predominant site, and there is a noticeable prevalence of this lesion to occur in Arctic Eskimos or persons of Mongolian origin.[353]

Sialolithiasis. Sialolithiasis, the occurrence of salivary stones or calculus, is found most commonly in the submandibular gland or especially its duct. Involvement of the parotid gland is less common (estimated 4% to 21%). Calculus in the sublingual gland is relatively rare. For sialolithiasis of minor salivary glands, the two most common sites are the buccal mucosa and the upper lip. The disorder is not so rare as stated in most texts. For involvement of both major and minor glands there is a 2:1 male-to-female predilection. Most patients are middle aged.[358]

Although the cause is unknown, theories have been advanced that salivary retention, with resultant precipitation of calcium salts, is the significant factor. Whether the retention is preceded by inflammation of the duct because of a foreign body, bacteria, or other factor is debatable.

Because of the intermittent obstruction of the duct system, inflammation of the proximal portion of the gland occurs. Contrast media may be employed to demonstrate tortuous dilatation of the principal ducts and the presence of strictures. There is atrophy of the acinar cells, with replacement by scar tissue and fat cells if the obstruction process continues.

Cytomegalic inclusion disease. Cytomegalic inclusion disease is a widespread viral disease that becomes clinically manifest in only a small percentage of the population.[391] It appears to be largely harmless outside infancy but remains a risk to the fetus if first contracted by the mother during pregnancy.

Although initially believed to be limited to salivary and lacrimal glands, cytomegalic inclusion disease was subsequently shown to be generalized, producing a clinical picture resembling erythroblastosis or hepatitis in neonates and characterized by a train of events: mild jaundice, hepatosplenomegaly, bruising, and finally purpura. Interstitial pneumonitis, Addison's disease, or interstitial nephritis with hematuria also may occur. A high proportion of fatal cases have exhibited a peculiar laminar necrosis immediately beneath the ependyma of the brain. These areas become calcified and simulate congenital toxoplasmosis.

Microscopically the inclusions may be seen in the salivary glands, lacrimal glands, liver, kidney, lung, and so on. In the salivary gland the inclusions are round, highly refractile, homogeneous, eosinophilic bodies within the cytoplasm or nucleus of ductal cells (Fig. 23-31). These cells also may be seen with standard Wright's stain in gastric washings, subdural fluid, or sediment from freshly voided urine.

Epidemic parotitis (mumps). Epidemic parotitis is an acute, highly contagious viral disease. Despite the name, it is systemic, affecting many organs other than the parotid gland. It is probable that some degree of pancreatitis (and orchitis in men) occurs in nearly every case, but severe complication is rather uncommon. Oophoritis also may occur but is quite rare.

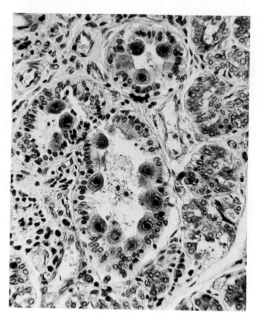

Fig. 23-31. Cytomegalic inclusion disease illustrating numerous, large, doubly contoured inclusion bodies within cytoplasm of duct cells of parotid gland. (Courtesy R. Marcial-Rojas, San Juan, Puerto Rico.)

There is diffuse tender enlargement of one or both parotid glands, accompanied by mild fever. Less commonly, the submandibular and sublingual glands are involved and, very rarely, the lacrimal glands. Examination of the buccal mucosa during the active state usually will reveal an erythematous halo about the opening of Stensen's duct.

In adolescent and adult males, clinical orchitis (usually unilateral) is present in about 25%. Only rarely is sterility produced, however. Pancreatitis, manifested by epigastric pain and nausea, though not very common as a severe complication, is probably a constant factor, causing elevated serum amylase and lipase levels.

Microscopically in the parotid glands there are degenerative changes of the ductal epithelium with infiltration of lymphocytes and macrophages about the ducts. The acini may undergo pressure atrophy.

Uveoparotid fever (Heerfordt's syndrome). Uveoparotid fever is a form of sarcoidosis originally described by Heerfordt in 1909. The syndrome consists in a triad of signs: parotid enlargement, uveitis, and facial paralysis. It usually is seen in the second and third decades and is decidedly more common in black women. It represents about 10% of the cases of sarcoidosis.

The parotid swelling, which is bilateral in over half of the cases, often is preceded by mild fever, lassitude, and anorexia. The swelling, in contrast to mumps, is not painful and is firm and nodular. Minor salivary glands may also be involved. The lacrimal glands occasionally are involved (Fig. 23-32). Ocular involvement, usually bilateral, may be severe and prolonged. Uveitis,

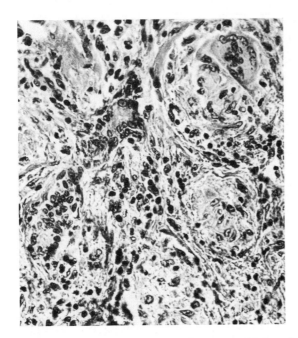

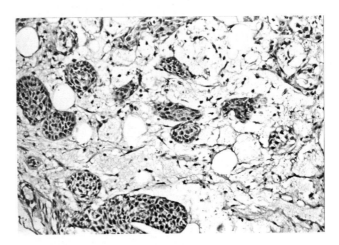

Fig. 23-33. Necrotizing sialometaplasia. Notice acinar necrosis with mucus pooling and squamous metaplasia with lack of cellular atypia. (From Lynch, D.P., et al.: Oral Surg. **47:**63, 1979.)

Fig. 23-32. Heerfordt's syndrome (uveoparotid fever) or sarcoidosis. Acini are replaced by multiple, usually discrete, sarcoidal granulomas. Lacrimal glands, as well as major salivary glands, are enlarged. This is associated with facial nerve paralysis.

iridocyclitis, and optic neuritis are not uncommon complications. Paralysis of the facial nerve occurs in about 25% of the patients with uveoparotid fever.[386]

Necrotizing sialometaplasia. This nonneoplastic self-healing inflammatory disorder of minor salivary glands may be confused clinically and microscopically with squamous cell carcinoma or mucoepidermoid carcinoma. The lesion is usually a single, rarely (15%) bilateral, elevated mass or crateriform ulcer, 1 to 2 cm in diameter, that most often involves the hard palate of adults. Rarely, lesions have been reported in the nasopharynx and parotid gland. There appears to be a 3:1 male sex predilection. The lesion heals spontaneously in 6 to 10 weeks. Characteristic microscopic features involve coagulative lobular necrosis of minor salivary glands, pronounced squamous metaplasia of mucous acini and ducts, pseudoepitheliomatous hyperplasia of the surrounding mucosa, maintenance of lobular morphology, and variable amounts of granulomatous tissue (Fig. 23-33). The squamous epithelium appears entirely benign. The basic lesion appears to be an infarct with subsequent ulceration and repair.[367]

Tumors
Epithelial tumors of salivary gland origin

Tumors of epithelial origin comprise most of the salivary gland neoplasms. These present a complex and diverse histomorphology. Most investigators believe that the basal cells of the excretory ducts and the inter-calated duct cells are the progenitor cells for most salivary gland tumors. Salivary gland tumors are most commonly located in the parotid gland (about 75% of all cases) followed by the minor oropharyngeal glands (about 14% of cases) and the submandibular gland (about 11%) of cases. The sublingual gland is a rare site, and less than 1% of salivary gland tumors occur in this site. Salivary gland tumors may occur in patients over a wide age range but are most commonly diagnosed in the sixth and seventh decades. The peak incidence for malignant salivary gland tumors is 5 to 10 years greater than that for patients with benign tumors. Most reports indicate a female preponderance varying from 1.2:1 to 1.8:1 for various histologic types.[336a,384]

The complex and diverse histologic features of salivary gland tumors presents problems in classification. Several classifications have been proposed, but none appears to be universally accepted. Most of these follow the general outlines of the classification present by Foote and Frazell.[340,388,389]

The classification of epithelial tumors of the salivary glands currently used at the Armed Forces Institute of Pathology (AFIP) is shown below. This classification includes several rare and as yet not widely recognized lesions.

Classification of epithelial salivary gland neoplasms*
  Benign
    Mixed tumor (pleomorphic adenoma)
    Papillary cystadenoma lymphomatosum (Warthin's tumor)
    Canalicular adenoma
    Basal cell adenoma

*From Ellis, G.L., and Gnepp, D.R.: In Gnepp, D.R., editor: Pathology of the head and neck, New York, 1988, Churchill Livingstone. By permission.

Oncocytoma

Myoepithelioma

Sebaceous adenoma

Sialadenoma papilliferum

Cystadenoma

Papilloma

Malignant

Carcinoma ex mixed tumors

Carcinosarcoma

Metastasizing mixed tumor

Adenoid cystic carcinoma

Mucoepidermoid carcinoma

Acinic cell adenocarcinoma

Epithelial-myoepithelial carcinoma

Clear cell carcinoma

Basal cell adenocarcinoma

Polymorphous low-grade adenocarcinoma

Malignant oncocytoma

Squamous cell carcinoma

Small-cell undifferentiated carcinoma

Malignant lymphoepithelial lesion

Sebaceous carcinoma

Sebaceous lymphadenocarcinoma

Adenosquamous carcinoma

Adenocarcinomas not otherwise specified

The ratio of benign to malignant histologic types of salivary gland tumors and the frequency with which various types are encountered vary in different anatomic sites. The majority of parotid tumors are benign, whereas in the submandibular and minor salivary glands a significantly higher percentage are malignant. Tumors of the sublingual gland are rare and almost always malignant (Table 23-1).

Pleomorphic adenoma (mixed tumor). Pleomorphic adenoma is the most common tumor of the parotid, submandibular, and minor salivary glands (Table 23-1). The palate is the most common site for pleomorphic adenomas arising from the minor salivary glands and occurring on the hard and soft palates with about equal frequency.[390] Grossly the tumor is rounded to bosselated and is surrounded by a fibrous capsule of varying thickness. Satellite nodules may be present outside the capsule, but these have been shown to represent extensions of the body of the tumor rather than true satellite spread. Even in the absence of a capsule, the tumor is clearly demarcated from the surrounding tissues.[335]

Histologic diversity is the hallmark of the pleomorphic adenoma with a variety of patterns showing varying combinations of epithelium and mesenchyme-like tissues. The epithelial component takes the form of ducts, sheets of myoepithelial cells, or squamous structures. The myoepithelial cells may form sheets of polygon-shaped cells or be present as eosinophilic spindle cells resembling smooth muscle (Fig. 23-34). Many pleomorphic adenomas show well-differentiated duct-

Table 23-1. Reported frequency of benign and malignant tumors and frequency of pleomorphic adenoma in different sites

	% benign	% malignant	% of all tumors that are pleomorphic adenoma
Parotid	80-85	15-20	60-76
Minor salivary glands	54-62	38-46	41-54
Submandibular	62-69	31-38	60-68
Sublingual	12-14	84-86	<1

Data compiled from various reports of large series of cases; reference numbers 336a, 340, 384, 388, and 390.

like structures consisting of an inner lining of single or double layers of cuboid or columnar cells surrounded by myoepithelial cells. The ductal lumens are clear or contain eosinophilic PAS-positive material. Hyaline, myxoid, or chondroid areas result from the accumulation of mucoid or hyaline material between myoepithelial cells, which alters their appearance. Accumulation of basophilic mucoid material separates the myoepithelial cells, and vacuolar degeneration of the myoepithelial cells results in an appearance very similar to cartilage. In other cases, accumulation of large amounts of mucoid material separates the epithelial cells into small groups or strands. In some instances careful search may be necessary to identify obvious epithelial structures.[388,389]

Although the majority of pleomorphic adenomas demonstrate the characteristic "mixed" appearance, some are highly cellular and the characteristic mesenchyme-like areas may be present in only limited fields. As a rule pleomorphic adenomas arising in the minor salivary glands tend to more cellular with less prominent mucoid, hyalin, and chondroid components than are seen in parotid tumors.[390] Some pleomorphic adenomas contain foci of epithelium in an adenoid arrangement simulating adenoid cystic carcinoma, but this does not influence prognosis. Variations in the microscopic patterns in pleomorphic adenomas do not appear to have any influence on behavior or prognosis. Bone, presumably arising by stromal metaplasia, is rarely noted in "old" pleomorphic adenomas. Islands of sebaceous glands and collections of tyrosine crystals are also rarely present.

Pleomorphic adenomas have an excellent prognosis after adequate surgical treatment and recurrence rates are essentially nil. In the parotid adequate treatment consists in partial parotidectomy with preservation of the facial nerve or total removal of the gland in the case of submandibular tumors. Minor salivary-gland pleomorphic adenomas also show a negligible incidence of recurrence after local excision including a margin of

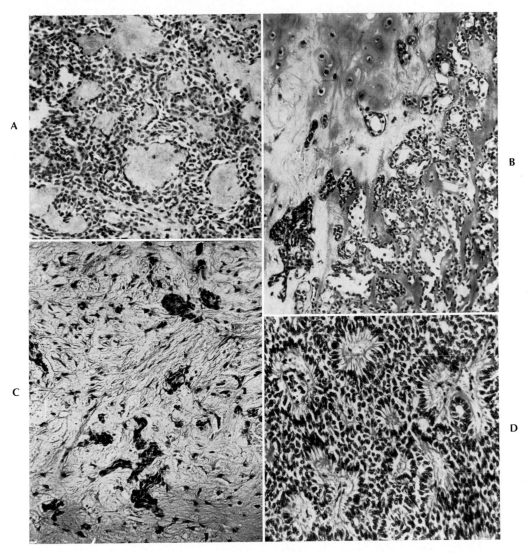

Fig. 23-34. Pleomorphic adenoma (mixed tumor). There is considerable variability of microscopic picture. **A,** Some tumors are exceedingly cellular, consisting of masses or sheets of small oval or rounded cells exhibiting little tendency to form ducts. **B,** Some tumors exhibit large masses of cartilage-like tissue. True cartilage is occasionally produced by metaplasia of fibrous connective tissue stroma. Numerous ductlike structures are manifest in this tumor. **C,** Certain tumors contain only few islands of epithelial cells in a sea of loose mucoid matrix. **D,** Unusual variant of pleomorphic adenoma, so-called adenomyoepithelioma.

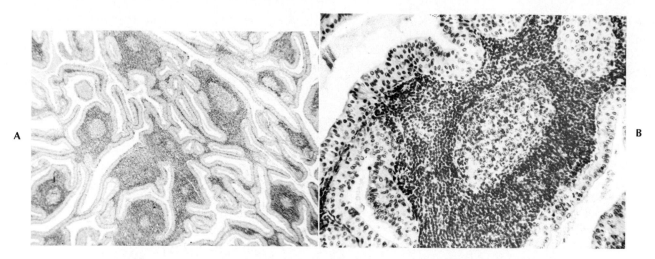

Fig. 23-35. Papillary cystadenoma lymphomatosum of parotid gland. **A,** Papillae extending into cavity contain lymphoid core covered by columnar epithelium. **B,** High magnification of area of **A** showing layer of columnar epithelium and lymphoid tissue.

surrounding tissue. The high incidence of recurrence of parotid tumors noted in the older literature was undoubtedly related to treatment by enucleation.[388]

Monomorphic adenoma. The term "monomorphic adenoma" has been widely used in recent years as a designation for a group of benign salivary gland tumors composed essentially of one type of epithelium and lacking the mesenchyme-like components of the pleomorphic adenoma. There is still disagreement as to further subclassification of monomorphic adenomas as evidenced by numerous proposed classifications. It is best to consider "monomorphic adenoma" as a generic term for benign adenomas of salivary gland origin that do not qualify as pleomorphic adenomas rather than as any specific diagnostic entity.[341a] The more important types of monomorphic adenomas are discussed here.

Papillary cystadenoma lymphomatosum (Warthin's tumor, adenolymphoma). Papillary cystadenoma lymphomatosum is a benign tumor arising in 99% of cases in the lower portion of the parotid gland over the angle of the mandible. Examples have rarely been reported in the submandibular and minor salivary glands. It comprises from 6% to 10% of all parotid neoplasms. It chiefly affects men (5:1) from 40 to 70 years of age. About 7% of the tumors occur bilaterally. The tumor may be superficial or deep to parotid fascia, or within the substance of the gland or occasionally posterior to it. Rarely, an extraparotid lesion is encountered.[337] The histogenesis of papillary cystadenoma lymphomatosum is controversial, but most evidence favors the concept that this tumor develops from heterotopic salivary gland ducts within preexisting intraparotid or paraparotid lymphoid tissue. Reactive changes, possibly in response to components of the neoplastic epithelium, causes an increase in the volume of the lymphoid tissue. Grossly

Warthin's tumors are well circumscribed and vary from partly to predominantly cystic.

Microscopically the essential components of the neoplasm are epithelial parenchyma and lymphoid stroma. The parenchymatous tissue is composed of tubules and dilated cystic spaces into whose lumens project slender, fingerlike, papillary processes, giving the neoplasm its characteristic appearance (Fig. 23-35). The lining epithelium is composed of two rows of cells, an inner row of tall nonciliated columnar cells with oxyphilic granular cytoplasm and an outer layer of cuboid, polygonal, or rounded cells. The cell nuclei of the inner layer tend to be deeply stained and are evenly arranged toward the luminal end. The nuclei of the basal layer are round or vesicular, with a distinct nuclear membrane and one or two nucleoli. Occasionally a mucous or goblet cell or sebaceous differentiation is observed. Within the tubular and cystic spaces, a pink, granular, or, more often, homogeneous substance is seen, probably a product of the lining epithelial cells. A thin basement membrane separates the epithelium from the lymphoid stroma. When present in abundant quantities, the lymphoid stroma contains numerous germinal centers.

Removal of the tumor with a margin of surrounding salivary tissue is curative. Small foci of "incipient" tumors are not rare in the surrounding salivary gland tissue, and continued growth of these may be responsible for the occasional reports of recurrence after enucleation. A primary Warthin's tumor developing in a cervical lymph node should not be mistaken for a metastatic deposit. The existence of a malignant papillary cystadenoma has been reported, but most investigators doubt that this lesion occurs.[365]

Cystadenoma. Cystadenoma of salivary gland origin is a poorly defined and controversial lesion that is not recognized in many classifications. Most reported examples have involved the minor salivary glands of the buccal mucosa, palate, and floor of the mouth. Histologically these lesions resemble papillary cystadenoma lymphomatosum but essentially lack the lymphoid component (Fig. 23-36). Whether this lesion actually represents an oncocytic salivary gland duct hyperplasia rather than a neoplasm is speculative.[361]

Oncocytoma (acidophilic adenoma, oxyphil adenoma). Oncocytoma is an uncommon benign lesion accounting for about 1% of parotid tumors. A few oncocytomas have been located in the submandibular gland, and rare examples have been noted in the minor salivary glands. Most oncocytomas are noted in older adults. Bilateral examples, either occurring synchronously or after an interval, have been reported. Microscopically the tumor is composed of uniform, plump polyhedral cells with a distinct eosinophilic cytoplasm and a centrally placed nucleus. The cells are arranged in broad parallel columns or a rounded grouping with a scant stroma (Fig. 23-37). Tubular formations are rare. The cells of an oncocytoma closely resemble oncocytes found in normal glands of older persons and the epithelial cells of the papillary cystadenoma lymphomatosum. Whether or not oncocytomas represent a hyperplasia of oncocytes rather than true neoplasms has been debated.[319,343] A clear-cell variant of the oncocytoma has been reported.[333] Most oncocytomas respond to simple local removal. Malignant oncocytoma is one of the rarest of all salivary gland tumors. These show cellular and nuclear pleomorphism, local and perineural infiltration, vascular invasion, and regional or distant metastasis.[344]

Basal cell and canalicular adenomas. These benign monomorphic adenomas share some common features though most authors consider them to be separate entities. Basal cell adenomas occur predominantly in the parotid gland (80%), with the remainder being located in the upper lip and submandibular gland. Grossly the basal cell adenoma is a well-circumscribed often encapsulated tumor. Microscopically it is composed of rela-

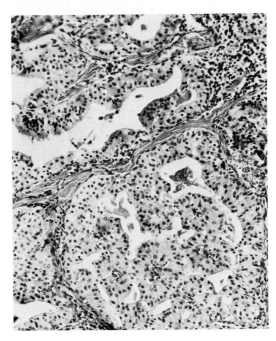

Fig. 23-36. Papillary cystadenoma. This tumor arises from neoplastic proliferation of ducts, being essentially a Warthin's tumor without lymphoid stroma.

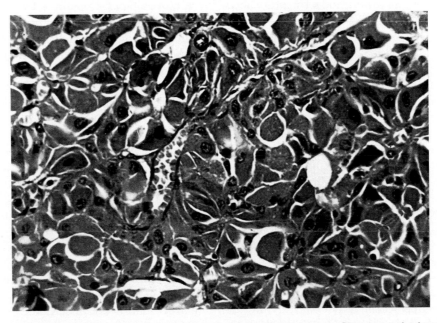

Fig. 23-37. Oxyphilic adenoma (oncocytoma) of parotid gland. Sheets and glandular formations of tall columnar cells with eosinophilic granular cytoplasm.

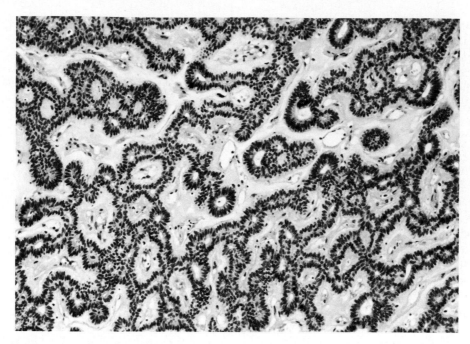

Fig. 23-38. Canalicular adenoma. Bilayered strands of columnar cells are present in a loose vascular stroma. (From Klein, H.Z.: Arch. Pathol. **95:**94, copyright 1973, American Medical Association.)

tively uniform basaloid cells. Ultrastructural and immunohistochemical studies, however, show that like many other salivary gland tumors, basal cell adenomas contain varying proportions of ductal and myoepithelial cells.[338,341a] Four histologic subtypes are recognized: (1) solid, (2) trabecular, (3) tubular, and (4) membranous. More than one pattern is commonly seen in an individual tumor. In the solid form, nests of basaloid cells, often showing palisading of the peripheral cells, are present in a fibrous stroma. The trabecular form shows anastomosing cords or islands of basaloid cells. The tubular form shows predominantly single-layered ductal structures. The membranous pattern shows solid nests of basaloid cells that are separated by a thick, eosinophilic PAS-positive hyaline lamina. Ultrastructurally this material appears to be replicated basil lamina. Some forms of membranous basal cell adenomas are histologically similar to dermal cylindromas and instances of synchronous salivary and dermal tumors have been reported. The salivary gland tumors have also been designated as dermal analog tumors of salivary gland.[317,354a] In contrast to other forms of basal cell adenoma, the membranous type is frequently multilobular and nonencapsulated. Tumor nodules separated by normal salivary tissue may be mistaken for invasion. Membranous basal cell adenomas may resemble and be mistaken for adenoid cystic carcinomas, particularly the solid variant.[333]

Canalicular adenomas occur predominantly in the upper lip (80%) with the remainder involving the buc-

cal mucosa and palate. The parotid is a rare location. Grossly canalicular adenomas are well circumscribed and frequently encapsulated. Microscopically the tumor is composed of bilayered strands or ribbons of columnar cells that contain focal nodular proliferations of basaloid cells. The stroma is vascular, is loosely arranged, and contains little collagen[330] (Fig. 23-38). The prognosis of both basal cell and canalicular adenomas is excellent after local excision, and few recurrences are encountered. A rare malignant analog of the basal cell adenoma, basal cell adenocarcinoma, has been reported. These lesions show an infiltrative growth pattern and a perineural and vascular invasion and may demonstrate nuclear and cellular pleomorphism.[326]

Myoepithelioma. Although myoepithelial cells are active participants in many salivary gland tumors, some salivary gland neoplasms are composed entirely or nearly entirely of myoepithelial cells. These rare lesions are classified separately as myoepitheliomas by some, whereas others consider them as only one end of the spectrum of pleomorphic adenoma.[376] Microscopically these tumors may show a spindle cell or plasmacytoid cell pattern or combinations of the two.

Sebaceous tumors. Although sebaceous differentiation is relatively common in parotid and submandibular glands, sebaceous neoplasms of the salivary glands are rare. The most common of these is the sebaceous lymphadenoma, which shows nests of sebaceous cells in a background of lymphoid follicles and lymphocytes (Fig. 23-39). It occurs most often in the parotid gland. Seba-

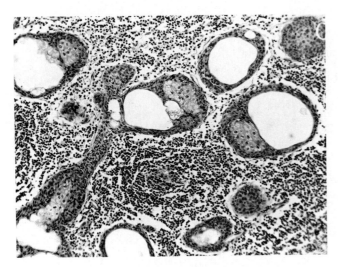

Fig. 23-39. Sebaceous lymphadenoma. Notice proliferated sebaceous glands in matrix of normal-appearing lymphoid tissue.

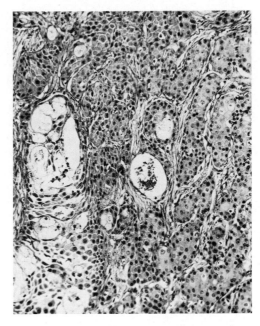

Fig. 23-40. Mucoepidermoid carcinoma of high-grade malignancy, strongly resembling squamous cell carcinoma. Careful search usually will reveal some cells that are producing mucus. Periodic acid–Schiff stain may aid in diagnosis.

ceous adenomas are composed of nests of sebaceous cells and are occasionally cystic. These have been reported in the parotid, the submandibular glands, and the buccal mucosa. Sebaceous carcinomas and sebaceous lymphadenocarcinomas are extremely rare.[347,348]

Sialadenoma papilliferum. Sialadenoma papilliferum is a rare salivary gland tumor that most often occurs on the palate. It presents as an exophytic, papillary growth usually clinically considered to be a papilloma. Histologically the tumor shows combinations of tortuous salivary ducts and papillary cystic structures composed of one or two layers of columnar epithelium. The tumor is surfaced by squamous epithelium that intermingles with the subjacent proliferating ductal epithelium. Local excision is curative.[339]

Malignant tumors

Mucoepidermoid carcinoma. Mucoepidermoid carcinoma is composed of epidermoid cells, mucus-secreting cells, and cells of intermediate type. Clear cells and columnar cells may also be present. The varied cell types show that the tumor may arise from ductal epithelium with great potential for varied differentiation and metaplasia.

Mucoepidermoid carcinomas comprise between 5% and 10% of tumors of the major salivary glands and between 10% and 30% of minor salivary gland tumors, representing the most common type of malignant minor salivary gland tumor.[390] In the major glands 90% of mucoepidermoid tumors occur in the parotid. Minor salivary gland mucoepidermoid tumors are most commonly located on the palate, but a significant number are found in the retromolar pad area, the floor of the mouth, and the buccal mucosa. These tumors also occur within the body of the mandible or in the maxilla.[320] The tumor is most common in the 40- to 60-year age group, but no age is exempt. Mucoepidermoid carcinomas usually present as a slowly growing, firm mass clinically indistinguishable from the more common pleomorphic adenoma. On gross examination the tumor may appear circumscribed but is seldom encapsulated. Cystic features are common and may be prominent.

Microscopically these tumors show great variability because of the varying proportions of mucus-producing, squamous, and intermediate cells present in an individual tumor. Mucoepidermoid tumors are often histologically classified into low-, intermediate,- and high-grade types. Low-grade tumors show a predominance of mucus-producing cells with formation of cystic spaces lined by mucous cells. Nuclear atypia and mitosis are not observed. Infiltrative growth is not a feature of low-grade tumors, and they tend to show a "pushing" margin. Intermediate-grade tumors show a greater tendency to form solid nests of squamous or intermediate cells with less prominent cystic spaces. Some degree of nuclear atypia and mitotic activity is present, and an infiltrative growth pattern is noted. High-grade tumors are predominantly solid and resemble squamous cell carcinomas of other anatomic sites (Fig. 23-40). Mucus-producing cells are relatively scarce and may require careful search and special stains for their identification. Keratin formation in mucoepidermoid carcinomas is relatively

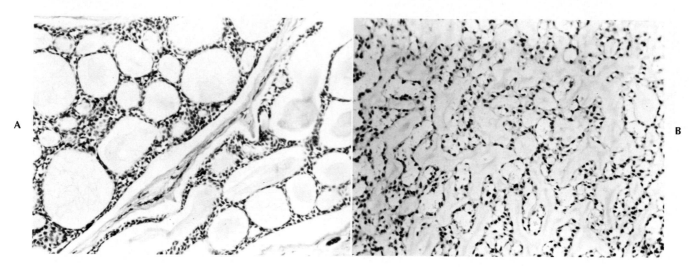

Fig. 23-41. Adenoid cystic carcinoma. **A,** Cribriform pattern. **B,** Hyaline or mucoid material with concomitant separation of tumor epithelium into strands.

uncommon. Clear cells are present in many mucoepidermoid tumors and in some cases are a prominent feature.[355,382] The histologic grading bears a relationship to prognosis and clinical staging. Low-grade tumors of the parotid and palate have a 90% to 100% survival rate after surgical excision including a margin of normal tissue. Although any mucoepidermoid carcinoma has the ability to metastasize, most examples of metastasis of low-grade tumors have been clinically associated with bulky recurrent tumors that have persisted after inadequate primary treatment. Intermediate- and high-grade tumors have a greater tendency to infiltrate, recur, and metastasize, and reported survival rates vary from 40% to 60%.

Adenoid cystic carcinoma. Adenoid cystic carcinoma accounts for about 4% of all salivary gland tumors. About 25% of these occur in the major glands, with the relative incidence being considerably higher in the submandibular and sublingual glands than in the parotid. About 75% of adenoid cystic carcinomas arise in the minor salivary glands, with the palate being the most common site. Histologically similar tumors occur in the nose, paranasal sinuses, lacrimal glands, ear canal, tracheobronchial tree, and other body sites.[324] There is considerable reported variation in the frequency of adenoid cystic carcinoma in relation to mucoepidermoid carcinoma. In the United States most reports indicate that mucoepidermoid carcinoma is more commonly encountered, whereas in England and Western Europe adenoid cystic carcinoma appears to be more common. Some have suggested that this may represent a true geographic variation in incidence.[336a]

Although adenoid cystic carcinomas may be noted over a wide age range, the peak incidence is in the sixth decade. The tumor is somewhat more common in fe-

males. It usually presents as a slowly growing mass that may have been present for some length of time. In contrast to most types of salivary gland neoplasms, pain is a fairly common symptom and is probably related to the propensity of the adenoid cystic carcinoma to infiltrate perineural spaces. Both myoepithelial and duct cells participate in the tumor.

Grossly the adenoid cystic carcinoma usually appears as a well-defined mass though careful inspection will often show infiltration of the surrounding tissues. Microscopically the tumor is composed of rather uniform basaloid cells. Three growth patterns—cribriform, solid, and tubular—are recognized and occur in varying proportions in many tumors. The cribriform pattern is the most characteristic.[322] The tumor cells are arranged in strands or clumps surrounding acellular spaces that contain a mucoid or hyaline material. The latter material is replicated basement membrane product. This arrangement imparts a "Swiss-cheese" appearance to the tumor (Fig. 23-41). Increasing amounts of formation of this material may result in the tumor cells being reduced to slender strands in an extensive hyaline background. The solid form of adenoid cystic carcinoma shows masses of fairly uniform basaloid cells containing a variable number of small ducts. The tubular pattern is characterized by tubular structures with a central lumen. There is some correlation between the predominant histologic pattern and prognosis.[373] Predominantly solid tumors have the poorest prognosis whereas the tubular pattern is associated with the most favorable outlook. Adenoid cystic carcinomas exhibit an infiltrative and invasive growth though in many cases growth is characteristically slow. Perineural invasion is a common and often conspicuous feature.

The adenoid cystic carcinoma has been aptly likened

to a "wolf in sheep's clothing." Despite slow and often deceptively benign clinical features and a "benign"-appearing histology, the long-term survival is poor. There is a strong tendency to develop late, distant metastasis. Although 5-year survival rates of up to 70% have been reported for parotid adenoid cystic carcinomas, this drops to 13% at 20 years. Tumors of the minor salivary glands, nose, and paranasal sinuses have a poorer outlook.[387] Lymph node involvement is relatively uncommon and when seen is usually attributable to direct invasion rather than embolic metastasis. Distant spread is usually by the hematogenous route with the lungs being the chief site for metastatic deposits.

Acinic cell carcinoma. The acinic cell carcinoma is relatively rare, accounting for only 2% to 3% of salivary gland tumors. Most examples are found in the parotid gland, but the tumor may occasionally be located in the submandibular or minor salivary glands. Acinic cell carcinomas have been recorded in patients from early childhood to old age. The highest incidence is in the fifth decade, and a female predilection is noted. Grossly acinic cell carcinomas usually appear circumscribed and may show a distinct capsule.

Histologically the tumor commonly consists of cells similar to the serous cells of the salivary gland and show a granular, basophilic cytoplasm. However, there is considerable microscopic variation, and vacuolated cells, nonspecific glandular cells, and clear cells may be conspicuous. About three fourths of all acinic cell carcinomas contain multiple cell types. Tumor growth demonstrates solid, microcystic, papillary cystic, and follicular patterns. The solid and microcystic are the most common, but about half of all tumors demonstrate multiple patterns. The solid pattern consists of sheets of tumor cells often showing an organoid arrangement (Fig. 23-42). The microcystic patterns shows numerous small cystic spaces, which presumably result from coalescence of intercellular vacuoles of ruptured cells. The uncommon papillary cystic and follicular patterns bear a resemblance to papillary and follicular thyroid carcinomas and may present problems in differential diagnosis. The use of special or histochemical stains is of little value in differentiating acinic cell carcinoma from other salivary gland neoplasms.[315]

The prognosis does not appear to be correlated with the histologic pattern. Infiltrative growth, multinodularity, and stromal hyalinization appear to indicate a more aggressive behavior. The reported prognosis of acinic cell adenocarcinoma varies widely and probably reflects the type of therapy employed. Local excision is accompanied by a high rate of recurrence. Follow-up data on 294 cases reviewed at the Armes Forces Institute of Pathology showed a 12% recurrence rate and an 8% metastatic rate. Six percent of the patients died of tumor over a mean follow-up period of 8.9 years. Acinic

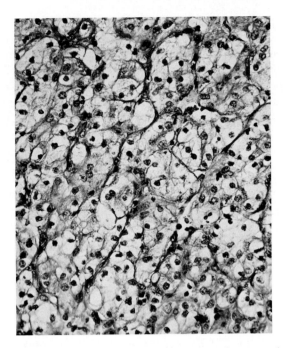

Fig. 23-42. Acinic cell carcinoma. Notice hypernephroid appearance.

cell carcinomas of minor salivary gland origin have a more favorable prognosis than those arising in the parotid.[334]

Malignant mixed tumor. The term "malignant mixed tumor" has been used for three distinct pathologic processes: carcinoma ex pleomorphic adenoma, carcinosarcoma, and metastasizing pleomorphic adenoma. *Carcinoma ex pleomorphic adenoma* is the most common of these. Incidence figures vary from 2% to 6% of all salivary gland tumors in various reports. The term implies a carcinoma that arises from or within a benign pleomorphic adenoma. The malignant epithelial element is most often a ductal or undifferentiated carcinoma. The diagnosis requires identification of areas of histologically benign pleomorphic adenoma within the tumor.[383] These areas may be small in relationship to the carcinomatous component, and sections from multiple tissue blocks may be necessary for identification of the pleomorphic adenoma component.[336a] In the majority of cases there is a long history (often 10 to 20 years) of a mass that then undergoes rapid increase in size. In a few instances the history of a mass that proves to be a carcinoma ex pleomorphic adenoma is relatively short. Carcinoma ex pleomorphic adenoma is most often encountered in the parotid but may involve the submandibular or minor salivary glands. The average age is about one decade greater than that for patients with pleomorphic adenoma. Patients with a short clinical history tend to be younger. Grossly the tumors may appear well circumscribed, but areas of disruption of the capsule and invasion of surrounding tissue may be present. Areas of necrosis or hemorrhage in a lesion considered to be a pleomorphic adenoma should arouse suspicion of carcinoma ex pleomorphic adenoma. These tumors demonstrate aggressive behavior, and the prognosis is serious. Regional and distant metastases occur in a high percentage of cases. Reported 5-year survival rates are 40% or less.

Carcinosarcoma (true malignant mixed tumor) is a rare and often lethal neoplasm. It exhibits epithelial malignancy, most often a ductal carcinoma and a sarcomatous component, most often a chondrosarcoma.[385] Fibrosarcomatous and malignant fibrous histiocytomatous elements may also be present. The putative origin of this tumor is from a preexisting pleomorphic adenoma, and a significant number of patients have evidence of a prior and often recurrent pleomorphic adenoma in the area. Most examples have occurred in the parotid. Carcinosarcomas are high-grade malignant neoplasms and the 5-year survival is about 50%. Metastatic deposits contain both the carcinomatous and sarcomatous elements. The third entity, *metastasizing pleomorphic adenoma*, is very rare. In these cases both the primary tumor, usually in the parotid, and metastatic deposits are cytologically benign pleomorphic adenoma.[325] There is usually a history of repeated recurrences of the primary tumor before eventual detection of metastasis. The lung is the chief site for metastasis. This tumor appears to run a slow, indolent course but is so rare that the long-term prognosis is not clear.

Adenocarcinoma. The term "adenocarcinoma" or "adenocarcinoma not otherwise specified" (NOS) is applied to a group of malignant epithelial tumors of salivary gland origin that cannot be histologically classified as one of the more specific forms of salivary gland carcinoma such as adenoid cystic, mucoepidermoid, and acinic cell. The incidence of adenocarcinoma of salivary glands is difficult to determine attributable in large measure to varying histologic classifications and criteria used for this diagnosis in reported series, and it ranges from less than 1% to over 10% of all salivary gland tumors. The relative frequency of minor salivary gland adenocarcinoma appears to be greater than that encountered in the major glands. Histologically these neoplasms show a wide range of features, some being similar to gastrointestinal adenocarcinomas whereas others resembling ductal carcinomas of the breast. Some of these lesions appear to be relatively low-grade neoplasms, whereas others are highly malignant. The polymorphous low-grade adenocarcinoma (lobular carcinoma) has recently been separated from the general group of salivary gland adenocarcinoma and deserves separate mention.[314,336,341]

This tumor appears to occur exclusively in the minor salivary glands, with the palate being the most common location. There is a female predilection with a peak incidence in the sixth decade. The tumor is characterized by a cytologically bland-appearing isomorphic cell population and an infiltrating growth. Several growth patterns exist, and multiple patterns may be seen in an individual lesion. These include solid tumor nests, tubular structures, interconnecting cords, streaming columns, cystic structures, and cribriform islands. An Indian-file pattern is often conspicuous about the periphery of the tumor. Perineural growth is a common feature. The tumor invariably shows infiltration into the surrounding tissue. In some instances differentiation from adenoid cystic carcinoma may be difficult. The prognosis appears better than that of most salivary gland carcinomas. There is less than a 20% incidence of recurrence, and only a few instances of regional lymph node metastasis have been reported. Although this lesion has been recognized only since 1983, retrospective studies up to now indicate a good prognosis with few tumor-related deaths.[314]

Squamous cell carcinoma. Primary squamous cell carcinoma of the salivary glands is uncommon, comprising 1% to 2% of salivary neoplasms. About 80% occur in the parotid, with the remainder involving the submandibular gland. Primary squamous cell carcinoma rarely if ever arises in minor salivary glands. It is predominantly found in males over 60 years of age. Most examples have been well to moderately differentiated tumors. Primary squamous cell carcinoma of salivary gland must be differentiated from a metastasis to the parotid or submandibular area and from mucoepidermoid carcinomas having only a minimal mucous component. The clinical course of primary squamous cell carcinoma is aggressive, and cervical node metastasis is seen in about 40% of cases. The 5-year survival rate is about 20% to 25%.[378]

Undifferentiated carcinoma. Undifferentiated carcinomas of the salivary glands are rare, and the true incidence is difficult to determine. These tumors are too poorly differentiated to be placed in any other category of salivary gland neoplasm. They have been subdivided into spheroid, spindle, and small-cell types. Small-cell carcinomas of salivary gland origin resemble small-cell carcinomas of the lung and appear to arise from ductal epithelium. Ultrastructural study has demonstrated neurosecretory granules in some tumors, and it has been suggested that two types of small-cell salivary carcinoma exist, a small-cell ductal carcinoma and a small-cell neuroendocrine carcinoma. The prognosis of small-cell salivary carcinoma is better than that of small-cell carcinoma of the lung or larynx. A 46% 5-year survival has been reported.[346,362]

Clear cell neoplasms. Clear cell neoplasms are uncommon and controversial lesions. Although mucoepidermoid carcinomas and acinic cell carcinomas may contain clear cells, which may uncommonly be a prominent component, some salivary neoplasms are essentially clear cell in nature. The clear cells have been identified in some instances as containing glycogen or mucin, and in other cases the clear cells probably result from fixation artifact. Although some salivary clear cell neoplasms have been designated as adenomas, accumulating evidence indicates that they should be considered as low-grade malignant tumors.[327,333] Primary clear cell tumors of the salivary glands may be confused with a metastasis of a renal cell carcinoma. The epithelial-myoepithelial carcinoma is a recently defined lesion that has a prominent clear cell component. This uncommon tumor has been most often located in the parotid gland, but examples have been reported in the submandibular and minor salivary glands. Most patients have been in the sixth and seventh decades of life, and women are affected twice as often as men. The most common microscopic pattern shows small ductal structures consisting of cells with a clear cytoplasm surrounding a layer of darkly staining ductal cells lining the lumen. Both electron microscopic and immunohistochemical studies have confirmed the epithelial and myoepithelial differentiation of the cells in this tumor. Some examples have shown large areas of clear cell differentiation without apparent ductal differentiation.[329] Epithelial-myoepithelial carcinomas show a 35% incidence of local recurrence, and a few patients have had regional and distant metastasis.[366]

Nonepithelial tumors. With the exception of hemangiomas, nonepithelial tumors of the salivary gland are very uncommon. The hemangioma is the most common tumor of the parotid gland during the first year of life, usually appearing within the first 3 months (Fig. 23-43). It is occasionally noted at birth. It may also arise in the submandibular gland. Skin hemangiomas overlie the salivary gland tumor in about 40% of patients. There is a 3:1 female predilection.[350,372]

Histologically the hemangioma is composed of capillary vessels lined by two or more layers of endothelial cells. The vessel lumens are often obscured as a result of the pronounced cellularity. The hemangioma is never encapsulated but infiltrates the gland, replaces the acini, and leaves only the ductal elements. Spontaneous regression is usual, and recurrence after surgical resection is very rare.

Lymphangiomas may also occur in the parotid gland but are considerably less common than hemangiomas.[371] Lipomas, neurofibromas, and neurilemomas rarely arise from the supporting connective tissue stroma of the major salivary glands, particularly the parotid.[388] Nonlymphoid soft tissue sarcomas of the major salivary glands are extremely rare.[316] Malignant schwannoma, undifferentiated sarcoma, malignant fibrous histiocytoma, and rhabdomyosarcoma have been

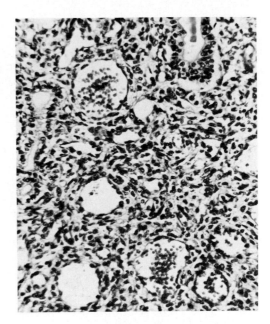

Fig. 23-43. Hemangioma of parotid gland, most common tumor of parotid gland in children under 1 year of age. Tumor is usually of capillary type, with few well-defined lumens.

reported. Malignant lymphoma also may arise in the major salivary glands, with the parotid being the predominant site.[328] Non-Hodgkin's lymphoma may arise in benign lymphoepithelial lesions and Sjögren's syndrome. Patients with Sjögren's syndrome have a greatly increase risk of developing malignant lymphoma.[360] Primary malignant melanoma of the parotid gland has been rarely reported.[351]

NECK
Tumors

Carotid body tumor. Carotid body tumor (chemodectoma) arises in the carotid bodies, small ovoid nodules situated on the medial aspect of the bifurcation of the common carotid arteries that mediate chemosensory reflexes sensing changes in pH and arterial oxygen tension. The carotid bodies are also involved in catecholamine storage. Histologically identical tumors are found in the aortic bodies, the glomus jugulare (paraganglion tympanicum), and the ganglion nodosum of the vagus nerve. All these structures are derived from neural crest cells and migrate to areas about the vessels of the embryonic branchial arches.[400,404]

The tumor may become manifest at any age but rarely before puberty.[408] There is a slight female predilection. About 5% are bilateral. In some cases there appears to be autosomal dominant inheritance.[410,417]

Microscopically the tumor is lobulated and thinly encapsulated or embedded in loose connective tissue. It consists of nests of rather large polyhedral cells grouped

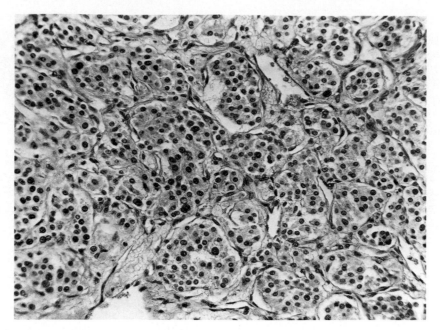

Fig. 23-44. Carotid body tumor. Notice classic "cell-ball" pattern. (From Abell, M.R., et al.: Hum. Pathol. **1**:503, 1970.)

together in an alveolar or organoid pattern (Fig. 23-44). The cell nests are separated by loose connective tissue and a richly vascular stroma. The individual cells are of two types: (1) large cell, with a rounded vesicular nucleus and a pronounced nucleolus, and (2) a smaller cell with a darker nucleus (less numerous). Its cytoplasm is pale, eosinophilic, and frequently vacuolated, with indistinct cell boundaries. Rarely, bizarre hyperchromatic cells, active mitoses, and capsular invasion may be observed. Spread to regional nodes or even distant dissemination has been noted in about 5% of the cases but rarely results in death of the patient.

Cervical thymus. There have been several case reports in which the thymus has failed to descend and appears as a cervical mass.[416]

Benign symmetric lipomatosis. Benign symmetric lipomatosis, also called "Madelung's disease," or "Launois-Bensaude syndrome," is characterized by slow, massive accumulation of fatty tissue in the cervical and supraclavicular regions, causing severe swelling about the neck and at times severe respiratory distress. There may be extensions of tonguelike projections of fatty tissue between the cervical and upper thoracic muscles, as well as a "buffalo hump" of fat over the cervical region. Involvement of the preauricular and postauricular regions may give the patient a chipmunk appearance. Similar masses may appear symmetrically in the axillae and groin.[403,414]

Benign symmetric lipomatosis appears in adult life, though onset in most patients is rather ill defined. Enlargement is intermittently progressive. In some pa-

tients, the size of the masses has remained relatively stationary for a long time and then increased rapidly within a few weeks. Not uncommonly the patient is an alcoholic. Microscopically the deposits appear to be normal, nonencapsulated, adipose tissue.

Fibromatosis colli. Fibromatosis colli (torticollis, wryneck) occurs both as a primary and as a secondary disease. Primary or congenital torticollis is manifest by a firm, fusiform swelling of the sternocleidomastoid muscle, especially in its lowest third, either at birth or within the first few weeks of life. The swelling usually increases for several weeks and then regresses, occasionally disappearing between the sixth and eighth months.[393,397]

Grossly the muscle is shortened, contracted, and fibrous. Clinically the chin becomes tilted upward and toward the unaffected side. If the disease is untreated, facial asymmetry results, with adaptive scoliosis of the lower cervical and upper thoracic spine, foreshortening of the skull, and flattening of the facial bones on the involved side. The cause is unknown, but theories have implicated uterine malposition. Often (35% to 50%) it is associated with breech delivery.

Microscopically the muscle fibers are widely separated by dense, scarlike fibrous connective tissue (Fig. 23-45). It should be differentiated from desmoid tumor. Secondary torticollis is usually caused by a myositis that is attributed to a "chill." Occasionally it occurs after a tumor of the cervical cord, or it may be a hysterical manifestation.

Congenital teratoma of neck. Congenital cervical ter-

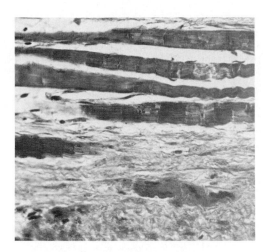

Fig. 23-45. Torticollis. Fibrous connective tissue replaces striated muscle fibers.

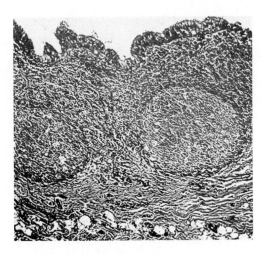

Fig. 23-46. Lymphoepithelial cyst lined by respiratory epithelium with lymphoid tissue in connective tissue wall.

atoma is relatively rare. There is argument for thyroid gland origin, but it is not entirely convincing. Some cervical teratomas assume massive dimensions. In over 40% of the patients the tumor is larger than 10 cm. A history of polyhydramnios is obtained in about half of this latter group. About 30% of the children are either stillborn or premature. Another third die of respiratory obstruction soon after birth. There is no sex predilection, but about half of the patients are black, suggestive of increased incidence in this racial group. Grossly the mass is usually semicystic but may be solid or multiloculated and is nearly always encapsulated. Microscopically all three embryonal layers are represented. Fetal brain tissue is especially common (about 70%). Nearly all congenital cervical teratomas as far reported have been benign. Teratoma of the neck in adults, which is extremely rare, is always malignant.[398,411,413]

Cysts

Thyroglossal tract cyst. The thyroid gland arises in the region of the foramen cecum of the tongue and begins descent into the anterior neck around the third intrauterine week. If it persists in its original embryonal position, it is spoken of as lingual thyroid. Rarely, a strand of epithelium persists and connects the base of the tongue with the normally positioned thyroid gland. The thyroglossal tract cyst results from cystic degeneration of this tract. It is in the midline of the neck usually at or below the level of the hyoid bone, through which the tract usually passes. The cyst is lined by respiratory or stratified squamous epithelium, or by both types. In about 35% of the cases the cyst may become infected and drain, becoming a thyroglossal tract fistula.[394,407]

Lymphoepithelial cyst. The lateral cervical cyst (branchial cyst) is located anterior to the sternocleidomastoid

muscle near the angle of the mandible. The alleged association of these cysts or sinuses with squamous carcinoma appears unwarranted. Microscopically the cyst is lined by either stratified squamous or pseudostratified ciliated columnar epithelium (Fig. 23-46). Beneath the epithelium is abundant lymphoid tissue with germinal centers. The cysts are believed to arise from cystic degeneration of epithelium enclaved in cervical lymph nodes. The cyst usually becomes apparent during the third decade. Similar lesions may occur in the parotid gland or in the oral floor beneath the tongue.[395,415]

Parathyroid cyst. Microscopic cysts of the parathyroid glands are seen in at least 50% of normal persons. At autopsy about 2% have true cysts. Nevertheless, cysts large enough to produce clinical symptoms are rare.

The parathyroid cyst is solitary and slow growing and if large may cause dysphagia and displacement of the trachea to the contralateral side, producing hoarseness by pressure on the recurrent laryngeal nerve. In several instances, this symptoms has led to a preoperative diagnosis of thyroid carcinoma. It is found anywhere in the lateral neck from the angle of the mandible deep to the sternocleidomastoid muscle to the mediastinum. Most of the patients are over 30 years of age, and a 3:1 female predilection is evident. About 60% of cysts occur on the left side.[396,406]

The cyst is usually very thin and filled with a clear, watery fluid. Microscopically it is lined by a somewhat flattened cuboid to low columnar epithelium. Within the collagenic connective tissue wall, one usually notes several types of parathyroid cells: water-clear cells, chief cells, and, occasionally, oxyphil cells. Not all three types are always present.

Cervical thymic cyst. Occasionally, remnants of thymus primordium are left in the neck, where they may remain undisturbed or, rarely, may undergo cystic alteration and subsequent enlargement. The cyst probably arises from degeneration of Hassall's corpuscles or from thyropharyngeal tubules. They occur clinically most often at about 7 years of age, and there appears to be a 2:1 male sex predilection. The cysts are usually elongated and may assume large proportions. They usually are located in the left (70%) lateral neck at the angle of the mandible just anterior to the sternocleidomastoid muscle.[401,405]

Microscopically the cysts are lined by stratified squamous epithelium and often contain a thick, reddish brown fluid. Rarely, cuboid epithelium is found. In the walls thymic structures (such as Hassall's corpuscles) may be identified. The cyst is well encapsulated and often exhibits cholesterol crystals among the connective tissue fibers.

Cystic hygroma. The cystic hygroma or diffuse lymphangioma is manifest as a rather poorly defined soft-tissue masses in the neck, usually behind the sternocleidomastoid muscle. It is either present at birth (50%) or manifested within the first 2 years of life. About 15% extend to involve the axilla, mediastinum, cheek, tongue, or oral floor, about 15% resolve spontaneously, and about 30% become infected. Microscopically the mass consists of numerous endothelium-lined lymphatic spaces of varied size in a loose connective tissue stroma.[399,409]

Inflammatory disease

Ludwig's angina. Ludwig's angina is a severe, board-like cellulitis of the neck involving all the submandibular spaces. Before the advent of antibiotics this was a rare complication of periapical infection of the mandibular molars or extension from an acute osteomyelitis occurring after compound fracture of the mandible. Drainage of pus through the lingual plate of the mandible into one or more spaces and subsequent extension with pronounced edema of the glottis commonly resulted in death from severe toxemia and asphyxiation.[402,412]

REFERENCES
General

1. Batsakis, J.G.: Tumors of the head and neck, ed. 2, Baltimore, 1979, The Williams & Wilkins Co.
2. Enzinger, F.M., and Weiss, S.: Soft tissue tumors, ed. 2, St. Louis, 1988, The C.V. Mosby Co.
3. Goodman, R.M., and Gorlin, R.J.: Atlas of the face in genetic disorders, ed. 2, St. Louis, 1977, The C.V. Mosby Co.
4. Gorlin, R.J., Pindborg, J.J., and Cohen, M.M.: Syndromes of the head and neck, ed. 2, New York, 1976, McGraw-Hill Book Co.
5. Ishikawa, G., and Waldron, C.A.: Color atlas of oral pathology, St. Louis, 1987, Ishiyaku EuroAmerica Inc.
6. Gnepp, D.R., editor: Pathology of the head and neck, New York, 1988, Churchill Livingstone.
7. Pindborg, J.J.: Pathology of the dental hard tissue, Philadelphia, 1970, W.B. Saunders Co.
8. Pindborg, J.J.: Atlas of diseases of the oral mucosa, ed. 3, Philadelphia, 1980, W.B. Saunders Co.
9. Pindborg, J.J., and Hjørting-Hansen, E.: Atlas of diseases of the jaws, Philadelphia, 1974, W.B. Saunders Co.
10. Shafer, W.G., Hine, M.K., and Levy, B.M.: A textbook of oral pathology, ed. 4, Philadelphia, 1983, W.B. Saunders Co.
11. Stewart, R.E., and Prescott, G.H., editors: Oral-facial genetics, St. Louis, 1976, The C.V. Mosby Co.
12. World Health Organization International Classification of Tumors No. 5, Histological typing of odontogenic tumors, jaw cysts and allied lesions, Geneva, 1971, World Health Organization.

Face, lips, and tongue

13. Baker, W.R.: Pits of the lip commissures in caucasoid males, Oral Surg. **21**:56, 1966.
14. Baughman, R.A.: Median rhomboid glossitis: a developmental anomaly? Oral Surg. **31**:56, 1971.
15. Cohen, M.M., Jr., Gorlin, R.J., Feingold, M., and tenBensel, R.W.: The Beckwith-Wiedermann syndrome: seven new cases, Am. J. Dis. Child. **122**:515, 1971.
16. Cohen, M.M., Jr.: Syndromes with cleft lip and cleft palate, Cleft Palate J. **15**:306, 1978.
17. Farman, A.G., van Wyk, C.W., Staz, J., Hugo, M., and Dreyer, W.P.: Central papillary atrophy of the tongue, Oral Surg. **43**:48, 1977.
18. Neinas, F.W.: Lingual thyroid: clinical characteristics in 15 cases, Ann. Intern. Med. **79**:205, 1973.
19. Sewerin, I.: The sebaceous glands in the vermilion border of the lip and in the oral mucosa, Acta Odontol. Scand. **33**(suppl. 68):1, 1975.
20. Shprintzen, R.J., Goldberg, R.B., and Sidoti, E.J.: The penetrance and variable expression of the Van der Woude syndrome: implications for genetic counseling, Cleft Palate J. **17**:52, 1980.
21. Wright, B.A.: Median rhomboid glossitis: not a misnomer, Oral Surg. **46**:806, 1978.

Teeth and periodontium

22. Gibbons, R.J., and van Houte, J.: Dental caries, Annu. Rev. Med. **26**:121, 1975.
23. Guggenheim, B.: Cariology Today: international congress in honour of Professor Hans Muhlemann, Basel, 1984, S. Karger AG.
24. Hamada, S., and Slade, H.D.: Biology, immunology and cariogenicity of *Streptococcus mutans*, Microbiol. Rev. **44**:331, 1980.
25. Horowitz, H.S.: A review of systemic and topical fluorides for the prevention of dental caries, Community Dent. Oral Epidemiol. **1**:104, 1973.
26. Schulze, C.: Developmental abnormalities of the teeth and jaws. In Gorlin, R.J., and Goldman, H.M., editors: Thoma's oral pathology, ed. 6, St. Louis, 1970, The C.V. Mosby Co.
27. Shields, E.D., Bixler, D., and El-Kafrawy, A.M.: A proposed classification for heritable human dentin defects with a description of a new entity, Arch. Oral Biol. **18**:543, 1973.
28. Socransky, S.S., Tanner, A.R.C., Haffajee, A.D., Hillman, J.D., and Goodson, J.M.: Present status of studies on the microbial etiology of periodontal disease. In Genco, R.J., and Mergenhagen, S.E., editors: Host-parasite interactions in periodontal disease, Washington, D.C., 1982, American Society for Microbiology.
29. Tanner, A.R.C., Haffer, C., Bratthall, G.T., Visconti, R.A., and Socransky, S.S.: A study of bacteria associated with advancing periodontitis in man, J. Clin. Periodontol. **6**:278, 1979.
30. Van Dyke, T.E., Levein, M.J., and Genco, R.J.: Periodontal diseases in neutrophil abnormalities. In Genco, R.J., and Mergenhagen, S.E., editors: Host-parasite interactions in periodontal disease, Washington, D.C., 1982, American Society for Microbiology.
31. Witkop, C.J., Jr., and Rao, S.: Inherited defects in tooth structures, Birth Defects **7**(7):153, 1971.
32. Wright, T., and Ganatt, D.G.: Dentinogenesis imperfecta, Arch. Oral Biol. **30**:201, 1985.
33. Zambon, J.J., Christersson, L.A., and Genco, R.J.: Diagnosis and treatment of localized juvenile periodontitis, J. Am. Dent. Assoc. **113**:295, 1986.

Oral soft tissues

34. Abbey, L.M., Page, D.G., and Sawyer, D.R.: The clinical and histopathologic features of a series of 426 oral squamous cell papillomas, Oral Surg. **49:**419, 1980.
35. Allen, C.M., Beck, F.M., Rossie, K.M., and Kaul, T.J.: Relation of stress and anxiety to oral lichen planus, Oral Surg. **61:**44, 1986.
36. American Cancer Society: Cancer statistics, 1988, CA **38:**5, 1988.
37. Angelopoulos, A.P., and Goaz, P.W.: Incidence of diphenylhydantoin gingival hyperplasia, Oral Surg. **34:**898, 1972.
38. Anneroth, G., Anneroth, I., and Lynch, D.P.: Acquired immune deficiency syndrome in the United States in 1986: etiology, epidemiology, clinical manifestations and dental implications, J. Oral Maxillofac. Surg. **44:**956, 1986.
39. Applebaum, E.L., Callins, W.P., and Bytell, D.E.: Carcinoma of the floor of the mouth, Arch. Otolaryngol. **106:**419, 1980.
40. Baden, E., and Carter, R.: Intraoral presentation of American Burkitt's lymphoma after extraction of a mandibular left third molar, J. Oral. Maxillofac. Surg. **45:**689, 1987.
41. Baden, E., Al Saati, T., Caverivière, P., Gorguet, B., and Delsol, G.: Hodgkin's lymphoma of the oropharyngeal region: report of four cases and diagnostic value of monoclonal antibodies in detecting antigens associated with Reed-Sternberg cells, Oral Surg. **64:**88, 1987.
42. Banks, P.: Infectious mononucleosis, Br. J. Oral Surg. **4:**227, 1967.
43. Bánóczy, J.: Follow-up studies in oral leukoplakia, J. Maxillofac. Surg. **5:**69, 1977.
44. Bánóczy, J., and Csiba, A.: Occurrence of epithelial dysplasia in oral leukoplakia: analysis and follow-up study of 120 cases, Oral Surg. **42:**766, 1976.
45. Bánóczy, J., Szabó, L., and Csiba, A.: Migratory glossitis: a clinical-histologic review of seventy cases, Oral Surg. **39:**113, 1975.
46. Bánóczy, J., and Sugár, L.: Progressive and regressive changes in Hungarian oral leukoplakias in the course of longitudinal studies, Community Dent. Oral Epidemiol. **3:**194, 1975.
46a. Barrett, A.P.: Clinical characteristics and mechanisms involved in chemotherapy-induced oral ulceration, Oral Surg. **63:**424, 1987.
47. Bernstein, M.L., and McDonald, J.S.: Oral lesions in Crohn's disease: report of two cases and update of the literature, Oral Surg. **46:**234, 1978.
48. Bhaskar, S.N., and Jacoway, J.R.: Pyogenic granuloma: clinical features, incidence, histology, and result of treatment, J. Oral Surg. **24:**391, 1966.
49. Bhaskar, S.N., Beasley, D., and Cutright, D.E.: Inflammatory papillary hyperplasia of the oral mucosa: report of 341 cases, J. Am. Dent. Assoc. **81:**949, 1970.
50. Binnie, W.H., Rankin, K.V., and Mackenzie, I.C.: Etiology of oral squamous cell carcinoma, J. Oral Pathol. **12:**11, 1983.
51. Blair, A.E., and Edwards, D.M.: Congenital epulis of the newborn, Oral Surg. **43:**687, 1977.
52. Block, M.S., and Gross, B.D.: Epidermolysis bullosa dystrophica recessive, J. Oral Maxillofac. Surg. **40:**753, 1982.
53. Bouquot, J.E.: Epidemiology. In Gnepp, D.G., editor: Pathology of the head and neck, New York, 1988, Churchill Livingstone.
54. Bouquot, J.E., and Gorlin, R.J.: Leukoplakia, lichen planus and other oral keratoses in 26,616 white Americans over the age of 35 years, Oral Surg. **61:**373, 1986.
55. Bouquot, J.E., Weiland, L.H., and Kurland, L.T.: Leukoplakia and carcinoma in situ synchronously associated with invasive oral/oropharyngeal carcinoma in Rochester, Minnesota, 1935-1984, Oral Surg. **65:**199, 1988.
56. Bras, J., Batsakis, J.G., and Luna, M.A.: Malignant fibrous histiocytoma of the oral soft tissues, Oral Surg. **64:**57, 1987.
57. Bras, J., Batsakis, J.G., and Luna, M.A.: Rhabdomyosarcoma of the oral soft tissues, Oral Surg. **64:**585, 1987.
58. Browne, R.M., and Potts, A.J.C.: Dysplasia in salivary gland ducts in sublingual leukoplakia and erythroplakia, Oral Surg. **62:**44, 1986.
59. Buchner, A.: Hand, foot and mouth disease, Oral Surg. **41:**333, 1976.
60. Buchner, A., and Hansen, L.S.: Amalgam pigmentation (amalgam tattoo) of the oral mucosa, Oral Surg. **49:**139, 1980.
61. Buchner, A., and Hansen, L.S.: Melanotic macule of the oral mucosa, Oral Surg. **48:**244, 1979.
62. Buchner, A., and Hansen, L.S.: Pigmented nevi of the oral mucosa: a clinicopathologic study of 36 new cases and a review of 155 cases from the literature. Part I. A clinicopathologic study of 36 new cases, Oral Surg. **63:**566, 1987; Part II. Analysis of 191 cases, Oral Surg. **63:**676, 1987.
63. Buchner, A., and Hansen, L.: The histomorphologic spectrum of peripheral ossifying fibroma, Oral Surg. **63:**452, 1987.
64. Buchner, A., Lozada, F., and Silverman, S., Jr.: Histopathologic aspects of oral erythema multiforme, Oral Surg. **49:**221, 1980.
65. Burns, J.C.: Diagnostic methods for herpes simplex infection: a review, Oral Surg. **50:**346, 1980.
66. Byers, R.M.: Squamous cell carcinoma of the oral tongue in patients less than thirty years of age, Am. J. Surg. **130:**475, 1975.
67. Carney, J.A., Sizemore, G.W., and Lovestadt, S.A.: Mucosal ganglioneuromatosis, medullary thyroid carcinoma and pheochromocytoma: multiple endocrine neoplasia type 2b, Oral Surg. **41:**739, 1976.
68. Cataldo, E., and Meyer, I.: Solitary and multiple plasma cell tumors of the jaws and oral cavity, Oral Surg. **22:**628, 1966.
69. Cobb, C.M., Holt, R., and Denys, F.R.: Ultrastructural features of the verruciform xanthoma, J. Oral Pathol. **5:**42, 1976.
70. Collins, J.R., and Van Sickles, J.E.: Chronic mucocutaneous candidiasis, J. Oral Maxillofac. Surg. **41:**814, 1983.
71. Conley, J., and Sadoyama, J.A.: Squamous cell carcinoma of the buccal mucosa, Arch. Otolaryngol. **97:**330, 1973.
72. Corio, R.L., and Lewis, D.M.: Intraoral rhabdomyoma, Oral Surg. **48:**525, 1979.
73. Cutright, D.E.: The histopathologic findings in 583 cases of epulis fissuratum, Oral Surg. **37:**401, 1974.
74. Damm, D.D., and Neville, B.W.: Oral leiomyomas, Oral Surg. **47:**343, 1979.
75. Daniels, T.E., and Quadra-White, C.: Direct immunofluorescence in oral mucosal disease: a diagnostic analysis of 130 cases, Oral Surg. **51:**38, 1981.
76. Dolin, S., and Dewar, J.P.: Extramedullary plasmocytoma, Am. J. Pathol. **51:**501, 1969.
77. Douglas, C.W., and Gammon, M.D.: Reassessing the epidemiology of lip cancer, Oral Surg. **57:**631, 1984.
78. Dummett, C.O., and Barens, G.: Pigmentation of the oral tissues: a review of the literature, J. Periodontol. **38:**369, 1967.
79. Edwards, M.., and Buckerfield, J.P.: Wegener's granulomatosis: a case with primary mucocutaneous lesions, Oral Surg. **46:**53, 1978.
80. Eisenbud, L., Sciubba, J., Mir, R., and Sachs, S.A.: Oral presentations in non-Hodgkin's lymphoma: a review of thirty-one cases. Part I. Data analysis, Oral Surg. **56:**151, 1983.
81. Eisenbud, L., Sciubba, J., Mir, R., and Sachs, S.A.: Oral presentations in non-Hodgkin's lymphoma: a review of thirty-one cases. Part II. Fourteen cases arising in bone, Oral Surg. **57:**272, 1984.
82. Ellis, G.L., and Corio, R.L.: Spindle cell carcinoma of the oral cavity, Oral Surg. **50:**523, 1980.
83. Ellis, G.L., and Kratochvil, F.J.: Epithelioid hemangioendothelioma of the head and neck: a clinicopathology report of twelve cases, Oral Surg. **61:**61, 1986.
84. Elzay, R.: Traumatic eosinophilic granuloma with stromal eosinophilia, Oral Surg. **55:**497, 1983.
85. Eneroth, C.M.: Malignant melanoma of the oral cavity, Int. J. Oral Surg. **4:**191, 1975.
86. Eneroth, C.M., Hjertman, L., and Moberger, G.: Squamous cell carcinoma of the palate, Acta Otolaryngol. **73:**418, 1972.
87. Eversole, L.R., Leider, A.S., and Alexander, G.: Intraoral and labial keratoacanthoma, Oral Surg. **54:**553, 1982.
88. Farman, A.G.: Hairy tongue (lingua villosa), J. Oral Med. **32:**85, 1977.
89. Finkelstein, M.W., Hammond, H.L., and Jones, R.B.: Hyalinosis cutis et mucosae, Oral Surg. **54:**49, 1982.

90. Freedman, P.D., and Lumerman, H.: Intravascular fasciitis: report of two cases and review of the literature, Oral Surg. **62**:549, 1986.

91. Fujibayashi, T., Takahashi, Y., Yoneda, T., Tagami, Y., and Kusama, M.: Tuberculosis of the tongue: a case report with immunological study, Oral Surg. **41**:427, 1979.

92. Gardner, D.G.: The peripheral odontogenic fibroma: an attempt at clarification, Oral Surg. **54**:40, 1982.

93. Goldstein, B.H., Sciubba, J.J., and Laskin, D.M.: Actinomycosis of the maxilla, J. Oral Surg. **30**:362, 1972.

94. Graykowski, E., and Hooks, J.: Summary of workshop on recurrent aphthous stomatitis and Behçet syndrome, J. Am. Dent. Assoc. **97**:599, 1978.

95. Green, T.L., Eversole, L.R., and Leider, A.S.: Oral and labial verruca vulgaris: clinical, histologic and immunohistochemical evaluation, Oral Surg. **62**:410, 1986.

96. Greenspan, J.S.: Infections and non-neoplastic diseases of the oral mucosa, J. Oral Pathol. **12**:139, 1983.

97. Greenspan, J.S., Greenspan, D., Conant, M., Petersen, V., Silverman, S., de Souzay, Y.: Oral "hairy" leukoplakia in male homosexuals: evidence of association with both papillomavirus and a herpes-group virus, Lancet **2**:831, 1984.

98. Hagy, D.M., Halperin, V., and Wood, C.: Leiomyoma of the oral cavity, Oral Surg. **17**:748, 1964.

99. Hampf, B.C.G, Malmström, M.J., Aalberg, V.A., Hannula, J.A., and Vikkula, J.: Psychiatric disturbances in patients with oral lichen planus, Oral Surg. **63**:429, 1987.

100. Handlers, J.P., Howell, R.E., Abrams, A.M., and Melrose, R.J.: Extranodal oral lymphoma. Part I. A morphologic and immunoperoxidase study of 34 cases, Oral Surg. **61**:362, 1986.

101. Hansen, L.S., Olson, J.A., and Silverman, S., Jr.: Proliferative verrucous leukoplakia, Oral Surg. **60**:285, 1985.

102. Hardingham, M.: Cancer of the floor of the mouth: clinical features and results of treatment, Clin. Oncol. **3**:227, 1977.

103. Hatziotis, J.C.: Lipoma of the oral cavity, Oral Surg. **31**:511, 1971.

104. Hedin, C.A., and Larsson, A.: Physiology and pathology of melanin pigmentation with special reference to the oral mucosa, Swed. Dent. J. **2**:113, 1978.

105. Holmstrup, P., and Bessermann, M.: Clinical, therapeutic and pathogenic features of chronic oral multifocal candidiasis, Oral Surg. **56**:388, 1983.

106. Howell, R.E., Handlers, J.P., Abrams, A.M., and Melrose, R.J.: Extranodal oral lymphoma. Part II. Relationships between clinical features and the Lukes-Collins classification of 34 cases, Oral Surg. **64**:597, 1987.

107. Iverson, R.E., Vistnes, L.M.: Keratoacanthoma is frequently a dangerous diagnosis, Am. J. Surg. **126**:359, 1973.

108. Jacoway, J.R., Nelson, J.F., and Boyers, R.C.: Adenoid squamous cell carcinoma (adenoacanthoma) of the oral labial mucosa, Oral Surg. **32**:444, 1971.

109. Jamsky, R.J., and Christen, A.G.: Oral gonococcal infections, Oral Surg. **53**:358, 1982.

110. Khari, M.R.A., Dexter, R.N., Burzynski, N.J., and Johnston, C.C.: Mucosal neuroma, pheochromocytoma and medullary thyroid carcinoma: multiple endocrine neoplasia, type 3, Medicine **54**:89, 1975.

111. Kwon, H.J., Browne, G.A., Posalaky, I.P., and Waite, D.E.: Hemangiopericytoma of the tongue: report of case, J. Am. Dent. Assoc. **109**:583, 1984.

112. Kramer, I.R.H., El-Labban, N., and Lee, K.W.: The clinical features and risk of malignant transformation in sublingual keratosis, Br. Dent. J. **144**:171, 1978.

113. Krolls, S.O., and Hoffman, S.: Squamous cell carcinoma of the oral soft tissues: a statistical analysis of 14,253, cases by age, sex and race of patients, J. Am. Dent. Assoc. **92**:571, 1976.

114. Krolls, S.O., Jacoway, J.R., and Alexander, W.N.: Osseous choristomas (osteomas) of intraoral soft tissues, Oral Surg. **32**:588, 1971.

115. Lakhanpal, S., Tani, K., Lie, J.T., Katoh, K., Ishigatsubo, Y., and Ohokubo, T.: Pathologic features of Behçet's syndrome: a review of Japanese autopsy data, Hum. Pathol. **16**:790, 1985.

116. Laskaris, G.: Oral pemphigus vulgaris: an immunofluorescence study of fifty-eight cases, Oral Surg. **51**:626, 1981.

117. Laskaris, G., Skavounou, A., and Stratigos, J.: Bullous pemphigoid, cicatricial pemphigoid and pemphigus vulgaris: a comparative study of 278 cases, Oral Surg. **54**:656, 1982.

118. Leyden, J.J., and Master, G.H.: Oral cavity pyogenic granuloma, Arch. Dermatol. **108**:226, 1973.

119. Lightwood, R., and Nolan, R.: Epithelial giant cells in measles as an aid in diagnosis, J. Pediatr. **77**:59, 1970.

120. Limongelli, W.A., Rothstein, S.S., Smith, L.G., and Clark, M.S.: Disseminated South American blastomycosis (paracoccidioidomycosis), J. Oral Surg. **36**:625, 1978.

121. Lozada, F., and Silverman, S., Jr.: Erythema multiforme, Oral Surg. **46**:628, 1978.

122. Luna, M.A., and Tortoledo, M.E.: Verrucous carcinoma. In Gnepp, D.R., editor: Pathology of the head and neck, New York, 1988, Churchill Livingstone.

123. Mashberg, A.: Erythroplasia: the earliest sign of asymptomatic oral cancer, J. Am. Dent. Assoc. **96**:615, 1978.

124. McCoy, J.M., and Waldron, C.A.: Verrucous carcinoma of the oral cavity, Oral Surg. **52**:613, 1981.

125. McDaniel, R.K., and Adcock, J.E.: Bilateral symmetrical lymphangiomas of the gingiva, Oral Surg. **63**:224, 1987.

126. McGuirt, W.F.: Snuff dipper's carcinoma, Arch. Otolaryngol. **190**:757, 1983.

127. Medina, J., Dichtel, W., and Luna, M.A.: Verrucous carcinoma of the oral cavity: a clinicopathologic study of 104 cases, Arch. Otolaryngol. **110**:437, 1984.

128. Melrose, R.J., and Abrams, A.M.: Juvenile fibromatosis affecting the jaws, Oral Surg. **49**:317, 1980.

129. Meyer, I., and Shklar, G.: The oral manifestations of acquired syphilis: the study of 81 cases, Oral Surg. **23**:45, 1967.

130. Miller, A.S., Leifer, C., Chen, S.Y., et al.: Oral granular-cell tumors: report of twenty-five cases with electron microscopy, Oral Surg. **44**:227, 1977.

131. Miller, M.F., Ship, I.I., and Ram, C.: A retrospective study of the prevalence and incidence of recurrent aphthous ulcerations in a professional population, 1958-1971, Oral Surg. **43**:532, 1977.

132. Mincer, H., Coleman, S.A., and Hopkins, K.P.: Observations on the clinical characteristics of oral lesions showing histologic epithelial dysplasia, Oral Surg. **33**:389, 1972.

133. Nally, F.F., and Ross, I.H.: Herpes zoster of the oral and facial structures, Oral Surg. **32**:221, 1971.

134. Nazif, M., and Randalli, D.N.: Stevens-Johnson syndrome, Oral Surg. **53**:263, 1982.

135. Nelson, J., Finkelstein, M.W., and Acevado, A., and Gonzáles, G.M.: Midline "non-healing" granuloma, Oral Surg. **58**:554, 1984.

136. Neville, B.W., and Weathers, D.R.: Verruciform xanthoma, Oral Surg. **49**:429, 1980.

137. Newman, A.N., Rice, D.H., Ossaff, R.H., and Sisson, G.A.: Carcinoma of the tongue in persons younger than 30 years of age, Arch. Otolaryngol. **109**:302, 1983.

138. Nisengard, R.J., Jablonska, S., Beutner, E.H., Shu, S., Chorzelski, T.P., Jarzabek, M., Blaszczyk, M., and Rzesa, G.: Diagnostic importance of immunofluorescence in oral bullous disease and lupus erythematosus, Oral Surg. **40**:365, 1975.

139. O'Brien, C.J., Carter, R.L., Soo, K.C., Barr, L.C., Hamlyn, P.J., and Shaw, H.J.: Invasion of the mandible by squamous carcinomas of the oral cavity and oropharynx, Head Neck Surg. **8**:247, 1986.

140. Page, L., Drummond, F., Daniels, H.T., Morrow, L.W., and Frazier, Q.Z.: Blastomycosis with oral lesions: report of two cases, Oral Surg. **47**:157, 1979.

141. Paymaster, J.S.: Some observations on oral and pharyngeal carcinomas in the state of Bombay, Cancer **15**:578, 1962.

142. Person, J.R., and Rogers, R.S.: Bullous cicatricial pemphigoid: clinical, histopathologic and immunopathologic correlations, Mayo Clin. Proc. **52**:54, 1977.

143. Phelan, J.A., Saltzman, B.R., Friedland, G.H., and Klein, R.S.: Oral findings in patients with acquired immune deficiency syndrome, Oral Surg. **64**:50, 1987.

144. Praetorius-Clausen, F.: Geographical aspects of oral focal epithelial hyperplasia, Pathol. Microbiol. **39**:204, 1973.

145. Putkonen, T.: Dental changes in congenital syphilis, Acta Derm. Venereol. **42**:44, 1962.

146. Rao, M.S., Kameswari, V.R., Ramula, C., and Reddy, C.R.R.M.: Oral lesions in granuloma inguinale, J. Oral Surg. **34**:1112, 1976.

147. Regezi, J.A., Batsakis, J.G., and Courtney, R.M.: Granular cell tumors of the head and neck, J. Oral Surg. **37**:402, 1979.

148. Regezi, J.A., Deegnan, M.J., and Hayward, J.R.: Lichen planus: immunologic and morphologic identification of the submucosal infiltrate, Oral Surg. **46**:44, 1978.

149. Regezi, J.A., Hayward, J.R., and Pickens, T.N.: Superficial melanomas of oral mucous membranes, Oral Surg. **45**:730, 1978.

150. Reichart, T.P.: Pathologic changes in the soft palate in lepromatous leprosy, Oral Surg. **38**:898, 1974.

151. Renner, R.P., Lee, M., Andors, L., and McNamara, T.F., and Brook, S.: The role of *C. albicans* in denture stomatitis, Oral Surg. **47**:323, 1979.

152. Rindum, J.L., Schiødt, M., and Scheibel, E.: Oral hairy leukoplakia in three hemophiliacs with human immunodeficiency virus infection, Oral Surg. **63**:437, 1987.

153. Russell, W.O., Cohen, J., Enzinger, F., Hajdu, S.I., Heise, H., Martin, R.G., Meissner, W., Miller, W.T., Schmitz, R.L., and Suit, H.D.: A clinical and pathologic staging system for soft tissue sarcomas, Cancer **40**:1562, 1977.

154. Sato, M., Yanagawa, T., Yoshida, H., Yura, Y., Shirasuna, K., and Miyozaki, T.: Submucosal nodular fasciitis arising within the buccal area, Int. J. Oral Surg. **10**:210, 1981.

155. Schiødt, M., Greenspan, D., Daniels, T., and Greenspan, J.S.: Clinical and histologic spectrum of oral hairy leukoplakia, Oral Surg. **64**:716, 1987.

156. Sciubba, J.J., and Niebloom, T.: Juvenile hyaline fibromatosis (Murray-Puretic-Diescher syndrome): oral and systemic findings in siblings, Oral Surg. **62**:397, 1986.

157. Scully, C., and El-Kom, M.: Lichen planus: review and update on pathogenesis, J. Oral Pathol. **14**:431, 1985.

158. Scully, C., Prime, S., and Maitland, N.: Papillomaviruses: their possible role in oral disease, Oral Surg. **60**:166, 1985.

159. Sedano, H., and Gorlin, R.J.: Acanthosis nigricans, Oral Surg. **63**:462, 1987.

160. Seydel, H.G., and School, H.: Carcinoma of the soft palate and uvula, Am. J. Roentgenol. **120**:603, 1974.

161. Shafer, W.G., and Waldron, C.A.: Erythroplakia of the oral cavity, Cancer **36**:1021, 1975.

162. Shikhani, A.H., Matanoski, G.M., Jones, M.M., Kashima, H.K., and Johns, M.E.: Multiple primary malignancies in head and neck cancer, Arch. Otolaryngol. Head Neck Surg. **112**:1172, 1986.

163. Shklar, G.: Lichen planus as an ulcerative disease, Oral Surg. **33**:376, 1972.

164. Shklar, G., and McCarthy, P.L.: Oral lesions of mucous membrane pemphigoid: a study of 85 cases, Arch. Otolaryngol. **93**:354, 1971.

165. Silver, C.E., Glackin, B.K., Brauer, R.J., and Lesser, M.L.: Surgical treatment of oral cavity carcinoma, Head Neck Surg. **9**:13, 1986.

166. Silverman, S., Jr.: AIDS update: oral findings, diagnosis and precautions, J. Am. Dent. Assoc. **115**:559, 1987.

167. Silverman, S., Jr., Bhargava, K., Smith, L.W., and Malaowalla, A.M.: Malignant transformation and natural history of oral leukoplakia in 57,518 industrial workers of Gujarat, India, Cancer **38**:1790, 1976.

168. Silverman, S., Jr., Gorsky, M., and Lozada, F.: Oral leukoplakia and malignant transformation: a follow-up study of 257 patients, Cancer **53**:563, 1984.

169. Silverman, S., Jr., Gorsky, M., and Lozada-Nur, F.: A prospective follow-up study on 570 patients with oral lichen planus: persistence, remission and malignant association, Oral Surg. **60**:30, 1985.

170. Silverman, S., Jr., Gorsky, M., Lozada-Nur, F., and Liu, A.: Oral mucous membrane pemphigoid, Oral Surg. **61**:233, 1986.

171. Sist, T.C., and Greene, G.W.: Traumatic neuromas of the oral cavity, Oral Surg. **51**:394, 1981.

172. Smith, I.: Cancrum oris, J. Maxillofac. Surg. **7**:293, 1979.

173. Southham, J.C., Colley, I.T., and Clarke, N.G.: Oral herpetic infection in adults: clinical, histologic and cytologic features, Br. J. Dermatol. **80**:248, 1968.

174. Spiro, A.H., Spiro, J.D., and Strong, E.W.: Surgical approach to squamous cell carcinoma confined to the tongue and floor of the mouth, Head Neck Surg. **9**:27, 1986.

175. Starink, T.M., and Woerdman, M.J.: Focal epithelial hyperplasia of the oral mucosa, Br. J. Dermatol. **95**:375, 1977.

176. Stewart, C.M., Watson, R.E., Eversole, L.R., Fischlschweiger, W., and Leider, A.S.: Oral granular cell tumors: a clinicopathologic and immunocytochemical study, Oral Surg. **65**:427, 1988.

177. Strong, E.W.: Carcinoma of the tongue, Otolaryngol. Clin. North Am. **12**:107, 1979.

178. Syrjänen, S.M., Syrjänen, K.I., and Lamberg, M.A.: Detection of human papillomavirus DNA in oral mucosal lesions using in situ DNA-hybridization applied on paraffin sections, Oral Surg. **62**:660, 1986.

179. Tajima, Y., Weathers, D.R., Neville, B.W., Benoit, P.W., and Pedley, D.M.: Glomus tumor (glomangioma) of the tongue, Oral Surg. **52**:288, 1981.

180. Teichgraber, J.F., and Clairmont, A.A.: The incidence of occult metastasis for cancer of the oral tongue and floor of the mouth: treatment rationale, Head Neck Surg. **7**:15, 1984.

181. Tohill, M.J., Green, J.G., and Cohen, D.M.: Intraoral osseous and cartilagenous choristomas: report of three cases and review of the literature, Oral Surg. **63**:506, 1987.

182. Tomich, C.E., and Hutton, C.E.: Adenoid squamous cell carcinoma of the lip, J. Oral Surg. **30**:592, 1972.

183. Trodahl, J.N., and Sprague, W.G.: Benign and malignant melanocytic lesions of the oral mucosa: an analysis of 135 cases, Cancer **25**:812, 1970.

184. Van Wyk, C.F., and Farman, A.G.: Focal epithelial hyperplasia in a group of South Africans: its clinical and microscopic features, J. Oral Pathol. **6**:1, 1977.

185. Vegers, J.W., Snow, G.B., and Van der Waal I.: Squamous cell carcinoma of the buccal mucosa: a review of 85 cases, Arch. Otolaryngol. **105**:192, 1979.

186. Vikram, B.: Changing patterns of failure in advanced head and neck cancer, Arch. Otolaryngol. **110**:564, 1984.

187. Vindenes, H.: Lipomas of the oral cavity, Int. J. Oral Surg. **7**:162, 1978.

188. Waldron, C.A., and Shafer, W.G.: Leukoplakia revisited: a clinico-pathologic study of 3256 oral leukoplakias, Cancer **36**:373, 1976.

189. Weathers, D.R., and Driscoll, R.M.: Darier's disease of the oral mucosa, Oral Surg. **37**:711, 1974.

190. Weathers, D.R., and Griffin, J.W.: Intraoral ulcerations of recurrent herps simplex and recurrent aphthae: two distinct clinical entities, J. Am. Dent. Assoc. **81**:81, 1970.

191. Whitehurst, J.O., and Droulias, C.A.: Surgical treatment of squamous cell carcinoma of the oral tongue: factors influencing survival, Arch. Otolaryngol. **103**:212, 1977.

192. WHO Collaborating Centre for Oral Precancerous Lesions: Definition of leukoplakia and related lesions: an aid to studies on oral precancer, Oral Surg. **46**:518, 1978.

193. Worsaae, N., Christensen, K.C., Schiødt, M., and Reibel, J.: Melkersson-Rosenthal syndrome and cheilitis granulomatosa: a clinicopathologic study of thirty-three patients with special reference to their oral lesions, Oral Surg. **54**:404, 1982.

194. Wright, B.A., and Jackson, D.: Neural tumors of the oral cavity, Oral Surg. **49**:509, 1980.

195. Young, L.L., Dolan, C.T., Sheridan, P.J., and Reeve, C.M.: Oral manifestations of histoplasmosis, Oral Surg. **33**:191, 1972.

196. Young, S.K., Larsen, P.E., and Markowitz, N.R.: Generalized eruptive keratoacanthoma, Oral Surg. **62**:422, 1986.

197. Zegarelli, D.J., and Zegarelli, E.V.: Intraoral pemphigus vulgaris, Oral Surg. **44**:384, 1977.

Jaws

198. Abrams, A.M., Howell, F.V., and Bullock, W.K.: Nasopalatine cysts, Oral Surg. **16**:306, 1963.

199. Abrams, A.M., Kirby, J.W., and Melrose, R.J.: Cementoblastoma: a clinical-pathologic study of seven new cases, Oral Surg. 38:394, 1974.
200. Ackerman, G., Cohen, M.A., and Altani, M.: The paradental cyst: a clinicopathologic study of 50 cases, Oral Surg. 64:308, 1987.
201. Alfors, E., Larson, A., and Sjögren, S.: The odontogenic keratocyst—a benign cystic tumor? J. Oral Maxillofac. Surg. 42:10, 1984.
202. Anderson, L., Fejerskov, O., and Philipsen, H.P.: Oral giant cell granulomas: a clinical and histologic study of 129 new cases, Acta Pathol. Microbiol. Scand. [A] 81:606, 1973.
203. Appenzeller, J., Weitzner, S., and Long, G.W.: Hepatocellular carcinoma metastatic to the mandible: report and review of the literature, J. Oral Surg. 29:668, 1971.
204. Arafat, A., Ellis, G.L., and Adrian, J.C.: Ewing's sarcoma of the jaws, Oral Surg. 55:589, 1983.
205. Barros, R.E., Domínguez, F.V., and Cabrini, R.L.: Myxomas of the jaws, Oral Surg. 27:225, 1969.
206. Bertoni, F., Unni, K.K., McLeod, R.A., and Dohlin, D.C.: Osteosarcoma resembling osteoblastoma, Cancer 55:416, 1985.
207. Blakemore, J.R., Eller, D.J., and Tomaro, A.J.: Maxillary exostoses, Oral Surg. 40:200, 1975.
208. Blank, E.: Recurrent Caffey's cortical hyperostosis and persistent deformity, Pediatrics 55:856, 1975.
209. Block, J.C., Waite, D.E., Dehner, L.P., Leonard, A.S., Ogle, R.G., and Gatto, D.J.: Pigmented neuroectodermal tumor of infancy: an example of rarely expressed malignant behavior, Oral Surg. 49:279, 1980.
210. Boerger, W.G.: Idiopathic bone cavities of the mandible, J. Oral Surg. 30:500, 1976.
211. Borello, E., and Gorlin, R.J.: Melanotic neuroectodermal tumor of infancy—a neoplasm of neural crest origin: report of case with high urinary excretion of vanilmandelic acid, Cancer 19:196, 1966.
212. Brannon, R.B.: The odontogenic keratocyst: a clinicopathologic study of 312 cases. Part I. Clinical features, Oral Surg. 42:54, 1976.
213. Brannon, R.B.: The odontogenic keratocyst: a clinicopathologic study of 312 cases. Part II. Histologic features, Oral Surg. 43:233, 1977.
214. Bras, J.M., Donner, R., van der Kwast, W.A.M., Snow, G.B., and van der Waal, I.: Juxtacortical osteogenic sarcoma, Oral Surg. 50:535, 1980.
215. Buchner, A., Ficarra, G., and Hansen, L.S.: Peripheral odontogenic fibroma, Oral Surg. 64:432, 1987.
216. Buchner, A., and Hansen, L.S.: The histomorphologic spectrum of the gingival cyst in the adult, Oral Surg. 48:532, 1979.
217. Buchner, A., and Sciubba, J.J.: Peripheral epithelial odontogenic tumors: a review, Oral Surg. 63:688, 1987.
218. Budnick, S.N.: Compound and complex odontomas, Oral Surg. 42:501, 1976.
219. Chaudhry, A.P., Rabinovich, M.R., Mitchell, D.F., and Vickers, R.A.: Chondrogenic tumors of the jaws, Am. J. Surg. 102:430, 1961.
220. Christensen, R.E.: Mesenchymal chondrosarcoma of the jaws, Oral Surg. 54:197, 1982.
221. Clark, J.L., Unni, K.K., Dahlin, D.C., and Devine, K.D.: Osteosarcoma of the jaws, Cancer 51:2311, 1983.
222. Corio, R.L., Goldblatt, L.I., Edwards, P.A., and Hartman, K.S.: Ameloblastic carcinoma: a clinicopathologic study and assessment of eight cases, Oral Surg. 64:570, 1987.
223. Courtney, R.M., and Kerr, D.A.: The odontogenic adenomatoid tumor: a comprehensive review of 21 cases, Oral Surg. 39:424, 1975.
224. Damjanov, I., Maenza, R.M., Snyder, G.G., Ruiz, J.W., and Toomey, J.M.: Juvenile ossifying fibroma, Cancer 42:2668, 1978.
225. Dunlap, C., and Barker, B.: Central odontogenic fibroma WHO type, Oral Surg. 57:390, 1984.
226. El-Lebban, N.G., Lee, K.W., Kramer, I.R.H., and Harris, M.: The nature of the amyloid-like material in a calcifying epithelial odontogenic tumor: an ultrastructural study, J. Oral Pathol. 12:366, 1983.

227. Ellis, G.L., Abrams, A.M., and Melrose, R.J.: Intraosseous benign nerve sheath tumors, Oral Surg. 44:731, 1977.
228. Eversole, L.R., Leider, A.S., Corwin, J.O., and Karian, B.K.: Proliferative periostitis of Garré: its differentiation from other neoperiostoses, J. Oral Surg. 37:725, 1979.
229. Eversole, L.R., Leider, A.S., and Nelson, K.: Ossifying fibroma: a clinicopathologic study of sixty-four cases, Oral Surg. 60:505, 1985.
230. Eversole, L.R., Sabes, W.R., and Rovin, S.: Fibrous dysplasia: a nosologic problem in the diagnosis of fibro-osseous lesions of the jaws, J. Oral Pathol. 1:189, 1972.
231. Eversole, L.R., Sabes, W.T.R., and Rovin, S.: Aggressive growth and neoplastic potential of odontogenic cysts, Cancer 35:270, 1975.
232. Ficarra, G., Kaban, L.B., and Hansen, L.S.: Central giant cell lesions of the maxilla and mandible: a clinicopathologic and cytometric study, Oral Surg. 64:44, 1987.
233. Finsterbush, A.A., and Rang, M.: Infantile cortical hyperostosis: follow-up of 29 cases, Acta Orthopaed. Scand. 46:727, 1975.
234. Franklin, C.D., Martin, M.V., Clark, A., Smith, C.J., and Hindle, M.O.: An investigation into the origin and nature of the "amyloid" in a calcifying epithelial odontogenic tumor, J. Oral Pathol. 10:417, 1981.
235. Franklin, C.D., and Pindborg, J.J.: The calcifying epithelial odontogenic tumor, Oral Surg. 42:753, 1976.
236. Freedman, P.D., Lumerman, H., and Gee, K.: Calcifying odontogenic cyst: a review and analysis of 70 cases, Oral Surg. 40:93, 1975.
236a. Fu, Y.S., and Perzin, K.H.: Non-epithelial tumors of the nasal cavity, paranasal sinuses, and nasopharynx: a clinicopathologic study. II. Osseous and fibro-osseous lesions, Cancer 33:1289, 1974.
237. Gardner, D.G.: An evaluation of reported cases of median mandibular cysts, Oral Surg. 65:208, 1988.
238. Gardner, D.G.: The central odontogenic fibroma: an attempt at clarification, Oral Surg. 50:425, 1980.
239. Gardner, D.G.: Plexiform unicystic ameloblastoma: a diagnostic problem in dentigerous cysts, Cancer 47:1358, 1981.
240. Gardner, D.G.: The mixed odontogenic tumors, Oral Surg. 58:166, 1984.
241. Gardner, D.G., Sapp, J.P., and Wysocki, G.P.: Odontogenic and fissural cysts of the jaws, Pathol. Annu. 13:177, 1978.
241a. Garrington, G.E., and Collett, W.D.: Chondrosarcoma II. Chondrosarcoma of the jaws: analysis of 37 cases, J. Oral Pathol. 17:12, 1988.
242. Giansanti, J.S., and Waldron, C.A.: Peripheral giant cell granuloma: review of 720 cases, J. Oral Surg. 27:787, 1969.
243. Giunta, J.: Lymphoepithelial cysts, Oral Surg. 16:306, 1963.
244. Goldblatt, L.I.: Ultrastructural study of an odontogenic myxoma, Oral Surg. 42:206, 1976.
245. Goldblatt, L.I., and Edesess, R.B.: Central leiomyoma of the mandible: report of a case with ultrastructural confirmation, Oral Surg. 43:591, 1977.
246. Gorlin, R.J., Chaudhry, A.P., and Pindborg, J.J.: Odontogenic tumors: classification, histopathology and clinical behavior in man and domesticated animals, Cancer 14:73, 1961.
247. Gorlin, R.J., Vickers, R.A., Kellen, E.: The multiple basal cell nevi syndrome: an analysis of a syndrome of multiple nevoid basal cell carcinomas, jaw cysts, skeletal anomalies, medulloblastoma and hyporesponsiveness to parathormone, Cancer 18:89, 1965.
248. Haggitt, R.C., and Reid, B.J.: Hereditary gastrointestinal polyposis syndromes, Am. J. Surg. Pathol. 10:871, 1986.
249. Hamner, J.E., and Ketcham, A.S.: Cherubism: an analysis of treatment, Cancer 23:1133, 1969.
250. Harris, C.M., and Courtmanche, A.D.: Gastric mucosal cyst of the tongue, Plast. Reconstr. Surg. 54:612, 1974.
251. Hartman, K.S.: Histiocytosis X: a review of 114 cases with oral involvement, Oral Surg. 49:38, 1980.
252. Hayward, A.F., Fickling, B.W., and Lucas, R.B.: An electron microscopic study of a pigmented tumour of the jaw of infants, Br. J. Cancer 23:702, 1969.

253. Hoffman, S., Jacoway, J.R., and Krolls, S.O.: Intraosseous and parosteal tumors of the jaws. In Atlas of tumor pathology, ser. 2, fascicle 24, Washington, D.C., 1985, Armed Forces Institute of Pathology.

254. Hollinshead, M.R., and Schneider, L.C.: A histologic and embryologic analysis of so-called globulomaxillary cysts, Int. J. Oral Surg. **9:**281, 1980.

255. Jacobs, T.P., Michelsen, J., Polay, J.S., D'Adamo, A.C., and Canfield, R.E.: Giant cell tumor in Paget's disease of bone: familial and geographic clustering, Cancer **44:**741, 1979.

256. Jaffe, H.L.: Giant-cell reparative granuloma, traumatic bone cyst and fibrous (fibro-osseous) dysplasia of the jawbones, Oral Surg. **6:**159, 1953.

257. Kaugars, G.E., and Cale, A.E.: Traumatic bone cyst, Oral Surg. **63:**318, 1987.

258. Kennett, S., and Pollack, H.: Jaw lesions in familial hyperparathyroidism, Oral Surg. **31:**502, 1971.

259. Kissane, J.M., Askin, F.B., Foulkes, M., Stratton, L.B., and Shirley, S.F.: Ewing's sarcoma of bone: clinicopathologic aspects of 303 cases from the intergroup Ewing's sarcoma study, Hum. Pathol. **14:**773, 1983.

260. Kolas, S., and Halperin, V.: The occurrence of torus palatinus and torus mandibularis in 2478 dental patterns, Oral Surg. **6:**1134, 1953.

261. Kratochvil, F.J., III, MacGregor, S.D., Budnick, S.D., Hewan-Lowe, K., and Allsup, H.W.: Leiomyosarcoma of the jaws, Oral Surg. **54:**647, 1982.

262. Krolls, S.O., and Pindborg, J.J.: Calcifying epithelial odontogenic tumor: a survey of 23 cases and discussion of histomorphologic variations, Arch. Pathol. **98:**206, 1974.

263. La Briola, J.D., Steiner, M., Bernstein, M., et al.: Odontoameloblastoma, J. Oral Surg. **38:**139, 1980.

264. Lamberg, M.A., Calonius, B., Makinen, J.E., Paavolainen, M.P., and Syrjänen, K.I.: A case of malignant myxoma (myxosarcoma) of the maxilla, Scand. J. Dent. Res. **92:**352, 1984.

265. Larson, A.K., Forsberg, O., and Sjögren, S.: Benign cementoblastoma—cementum analog of benign osteoblastoma? J. Oral Surg. **36:**299, 1978.

266. Leider, A.S., Nelson, J.P., and Trodahl, J.N.: Ameloblastic fibrosarcoma, Oral Surg. **33:**559, 1972.

267. Lichty, G., Langlis, R.P., and Aufdemorte, T.: Garré's osteomyelitis, Oral Surg. **50:**309, 1980.

268. Limongelli, W.A., Connaughton, B., and Williams, A.C.: Suppurative osteomyelitis of the mandible secondary to fracture, Oral Surg. **38:**850, 1974.

269. Lustman, J., Gazit, D., and Ulmansky, M.Y.: Chondromyxoid fibroma of jaws: a clinicopathologic study, J. Oral Pathol. **15:**343, 1986.

270. Makek, M.: Clinical pathology of fibro-osseous-cemental lesions in the cranio-facial and jaw bones, Basel, 1983, S. Karger AG.

271. Melisch, D.R., Dahlin, D.C., and Masson, J.K.: Ameloblastoma: a clinicopathologic report, J. Oral Surg. **30:**9, 1972.

272. Melrose, R.J., Abrams, A.M., and Mills, B.G.: Florid osseous dysplasia, Oral Surg. **41:**62, 1976.

273. Miller, A.S., Elzay, R.P., and Cuttino, C.L.: Giant cell tumor of the jaws associated with Paget disease of bone, Arch. Otolaryngol. **100:**233, 1974.

274. Miller, A.S., López, C.F., Pullon, P.A., and Elzay, R.P.: Ameloblastic fibro-odontoma, Oral Surg. **41:**354, 1976.

275. Monks, F.T., Bradley, J.C., and Turner, E.P.: Central osteoblastoma or cementoblastoma? a case report and 12 year review, Br. J. Oral Surg. **19:**29, 1981.

276. Müller, H., and Slootweg, P.J.: The ameloblastoma: the controversial approach to therapy, J. Maxillofac. Surg. **13:**79, 1984.

277. Murphy, J.B., Segelman, A., and Doku, C.: Osteitis deformans, Oral Surg. **46:**765, 1978.

278. Murray, G.C., Daly, T.E., and Zimmerman, S.O.: The relationship between dental disease and radiation necrosis of the mandible, Oral Surg. **49:**99, 1980.

279. Oatis, G.W., Hartman, G.L., Robertson, G.R., and Sugg, W.E.: Dermoid cyst of the floor of the mouth, Oral Surg. **39:**192, 1975.

280. Peters, W.J.N.: Cherubism: a study of 20 cases from one family, Oral Surg. **47:**307, 1979.

281. Praetorius, F., Hjørting-Hansen, E., Gorlin, R.J., and Vickers, R.A.: Calcifying odontogenic cyst: range, variations and neoplastic potential, Acta Odontol. Scand. **39:**227, 1981.

282. Ramon, Y., Oberman, M., Horovitz, I., and Freedman, A.: Osteomyelitis of the maxilla in the newborn, Int. J. Oral Surg. **6:**90, 1977.

283. Regezi, J.A., Kerr, D.A., and Courtney, R.M.: Odontogenic tumors: analysis of 706 cases, J. Oral Surg. **36:**771, 1978.

284. Royer, R.Q., and Neiblung, H.E.: Osteomyelitis of the jaws, Semin. Roentgenol. **6:**391, 1971.

285. Schlosnagle, D., and Someren, A.: The ultrastructure of the odontogenic adenomatoid tumor, Oral Surg. **52:**154, 1981.

286. Schoenecker, P.J., Swanson, K., and Sheridan, J.J.: Ossifying fibroma of the tibia, J. Bone Joint Surg. **63A:**483, 1981.

287. Shear, M.: Cysts of the jaws: recent advances, J. Oral Pathol. **14:**43, 1985.

288. Shear, M.: Cysts of the oral regions, ed. 2, Bristol, Eng., 1983, Wright PSG.

289. Slootweg, P.J., and Müller, H.: Central fibroma of the jaws, odontogenic or desmoplastic, Oral Surg. **56:**61, 1983.

290. Slootweg, P.J., and Müller, H.: Malignant ameloblastoma or ameloblastic carcinoma, Oral Surg. **57:**168, 1984.

291. Small, I.A., and Waldron, C.A.: Ameloblastomas of the jaws, Oral Surg. **8:**281, 1955.

292. Smith, R.A., Hansen, L.S., Resnick, D., and Chan, W.: Comparison of osteoblastoma of gnathic and extragnathic sites, Oral Surg. **54:**285, 1982.

293. Stewart, J.C., Regezi, J.A., Lloyd, R.V., and McClatchey, K.D.: Immunohistochemical study of idiopathic histiocytosis of the mandible and maxilla, Oral Surg. **61:**48, 1986.

294. Struthers, P.J., and Shear, M.: Aneurysmal bone cysts of the jaws, Int. J. Oral Surg. **13:**85, 1984.

295. Thompson, S.H., and Shear, M.: Fibrous histiocytoma of the oral and maxillofacial region, J. Oral Pathol. **13:**282, 1984.

296. Toljanic, J.A., Lechewski, E., Huvos, A.G., Strong, E.W., and Schweiger, J.W.: Aneurysmal bone cyst of the jaws: a case study and review of the literature, Oral Surg. **64:**72, 1987.

297. Trodahl, J.N.: Ameloblastic fibroma: a survey of cases from the Armed Forces Institute of Pathology, Oral Surg. **33:**547, 1972.

298. Tsaknis, P.J., and Nelson, J.F.: The maxillary ameloblastoma: an analysis of 24 cases, J. Oral Surg. **38:**336, 1980.

299. Van Blarcom, C.W., Masson, J.K., and Dahlin, D.C.: Fibrosarcoma of the mandible, Oral Surg. **32:**428, 1971.

300. Van der Waal, I., Rauhamaa, R., Van der Kwast, W.A.M., and Snow, G.B.: Squamous cell carcinoma arising in the lining of odontogenic cysts: report of 5 cases, Int. J. Oral Surg. **14:**140, 1985.

301. Vickers, R.A., and Gorlin, R.J.: Ameloblastoma: delineation of early histopathologic features of neoplasia, Cancer **26:**699, 1970.

302. Vincent, S.D., Hammond, H.L., Ellis, G.L., and Juhlin, J.P.: Central granular cell odontogenic fibroma, Oral Surg. **63:**715, 1987.

303. Waldron, C.A.: Odontogenic tumors and selected jaw cysts. In Gnepp, D.R., editor: Pathology of the head and neck, New York, 1988, Churchill Livingstone.

304. Waldron, C.A.: Fibro-osseous lesions of the jaws, J. Oral Maxillofac. Surg. **43:**249, 1985.

305. Waldron, C.A., and El-Mofty, S.: A histologic study of 116 ameloblastomas and special reference to the desmoplastic variant, Oral Surg. **63:**441, 1987.

306. Wesley, R.K., Wysocki, G.P., and Mintz, S.M.: The central odontogenic fibroma, Oral Surg. **40:**235, 1975.

307. White, D.K., Chen, S., Mohnac, A.M.: Odontogenic myxoma: a clinical and ultrastructural study, Oral Surg. **39:**901, 1975.

308. Woolgar, J.A., Rippin, J.W., and Browne, R.M.: The odontogenic keratocyst and its occurrence in the nevoid basal cell carcinoma syndrome, Oral Surg. **64:**727, 1987.

309. Wysocki, G.P.: The differential diagnosis of globulomaxillary radiolucencies, Oral Surg. **51:**281, 1981.

310. Wysocki, G.P., Brannon, R.B., Gardner, D.G., and Sapp, P.: Histogenesis of the lateral periodontal cyst and gingival cyst of the adult, Oral Surg. **50:**327, 1980.

311. Zarbo, R.J., Regezi, J.A., and Baker, S.R.: Periosteal osteogenic sarcoma of the mandible, Oral Surg. **57**:643, 1984.

312. Zegarelli, E.V., Kutscher, A.H., Napoli, N., Iurono, F., and Hoffman, P.: The cementoma: a study of 230 patients with cementomas, Oral Surg. **17**:219, 1967.

Salivary glands

313. Abelson, D.C., Mandel, I.D., and Karmoil, M.: Salivary studies in alcoholic cirrhosis, Oral Surg. **41**:186, 1976.

314. Aberle, A.M., Abrams, A.M., Bowe, R., Melrose, K.J., and Handlers, J.P.: Lobular (polymorphous low grade) carcinoma of minor salivary glands, Oral Surg. **60**:387, 1985.

315. Abrams, A.M., Cornyn, J., Schofield, H.H., and Hansen, L.S.: Acinic cell adenocarcinoma of the major salivary glands: a clinicopathologic study of 77 cases, Cancer **18**:1145, 1965.

316. Auclair, P.L., Langloss, J.M., Weiss, S.W., and Corio, R.L.: Sarcomas and sarcomatoid neoplasms of the major salivary glands: a clinico-pathologic study and immunocytochemical study of 67 cases and a review of the literature, Cancer **58**:1305, 1986.

317. Batsakis, J.G., and Brannon, R.B.: Dermal analogue tumors of major salivary glands, J. Laryngol. Otol. **95**:155, 1981.

318. Bernier, J.L., and Bhaskar, S.N.: Lymphoepithelial lesions of salivary glands: histogenesis and classification based on 186 cases, Cancer **11**:1156, 1958.

319. Blank, C., Eneroth, C.M., and Jakobsson, P.A.: Oncocytoma of the parotid gland: neoplasm or nodular hyperplasia? Cancer **26**:919, 1970.

320. Browand, B.C., and Waldron, C.A.: Central mucoepidermoid tumors of the jaws: report of 9 cases and review of the literature, Oral Surg. **40**:631, 1975.

321. Casamassimo, P.S., and Lilly, G.E.: Mucosal cysts of the maxillary sinus: a clinical and radiographic study, Oral Surg. **50**:282, 1980.

322. Caselitz, J., Schulze, J., and Seifert, G.: Adenoid cystic carcinoma of the salivary glands: an immunohistochemical study, J. Oral Pathol. **15**:308, 1986.

323. Catone, G.A., Merrill, R.G., and Henry, F.A.: Sublingual gland mucus-escape phenomenon: treatment by excision of the sublingual gland, J. Oral Surg. **27**:774, 1969.

324. Chen, J.C., Gnepp, D.R., and Bedrossian, C.W.M.: Adenoid cystic carcinoma of the salivary glands: an immunohistochemical analysis, Oral Surg. **65**:316, 1988.

325. Chen, K.T.K.: Metastasizing pleomorphic adenoma of the salivary gland, Cancer **42**:2407, 1978.

326. Chen, K.T.K.: Carcinoma arising in monomorphic adenoma of the salivary gland, Am. J. Otolaryngol. **6**:39, 1985.

327. Chen, K.T.K.: Clear cell carcinoma of the salivary gland, Hum. Pathol. **14**:91, 1983.

328. Colby, T.V., and Dorfman, R.F.: Malignant lymphomas involving the salivary glands, Pathol. Annu. **14**(part 2):307, 1979.

329. Corio, R.L., Sciubba, J.J., Brannon, R.B., and Batsakis, J.G.: Epithelial-myoepithelial carcinoma of intercalated duct origin: a clinicopathologic and ultrastructural assessment of sixteen cases, Oral Surg. **53**:280, 1982.

330. Daley, T.D., Gardner, D.G., and Smout, M.S.: Canalicular adenoma: not a basal cell adenoma, Oral Surg. **57**:181, 1984.

331. Daniels, T.E., Silverman, S., Jr., Michalski, J.P., Greenspan, J.S., Sylvester, R.A., and Talal, N.: The oral component of Sjögren's syndrome, Oral Surg. **39**:875, 1975.

332. Donath, K.: Wangenschwellung bei Sialadenose, HNO **27**:113, 1979.

333. Ellis, G.L., and Gnepp, D.R.: Unusual salivary gland tumors. In Gnepp, D.R., editor: Pathology of the head and neck, New York, 1988, Churchill Livingstone.

334. Ellis, G.L., and Corio, R.L.: Acinic cell adenocarcinoma: a clinicopathologic analysis of 294 cases, Cancer **52**:542, 1983.

335. Eneroth, C.M.: Mixed tumors of major salivary glands: prognostic role of capsular structure, Ann. Otol. Rhinol. Laryngol. **74**:944, 1965.

336. Evans, H.L., and Batsakis, J.G.: Polymorphous low-grade adenocarcinoma of the minor salivary glands: a study of 14 cases of a distinctive neoplasm, Cancer **53**:935, 1984.

336a. Eveson, J.W., and Cawson, R.A.: Salivary gland tumors: a review of 2410 cases with particular reference to histological types, site, age, and sex distribution, J. Pathol. **146**:51, 1985.

337. Eveson, J.W., and Cawson, R.A.: Warthin's tumor (cystadenolymphoma) of salivary glands: a clinicopathologic study of 278 cases, Oral Surg. **61**:256, 1986.

338. Fantasia, J.E., and Neville, B.W.: Basal cell adenomas of minor salivary glands, Oral Surg. **51**:433, 1980.

339. Fantasia, J.E., Nocco, C.F., and Lalley, E.T.: Ultrastructure of sialadenoma papilliferum, Arch. Pathol. Lab. Med. **110**:523, 1986.

340. Foote, F.W., and Frazell, E.L.: Tumors of the major salivary glands, Cancer **6**:1065, 1953.

341. Freedman, P.D., and Lumberman, H.: Lobular carcinoma of intraoral minor salivary glands, Oral Surg. **56**:157, 1983.

341a. Gardner, D.G., and Daley, T.D.: The use of the terms monomorphic adenoma, basal cell adenoma and canalicular adenoma as applied to salivary gland tumors, Oral Surg. **56**:608, 1983.

342. Gardner, D.G., and Gullane, P.J.: Mucoceles of the maxillary sinus, Oral Surg. **62**:538, 1986.

343. Ghandur-Mnaymneh, L.: Multinodular oncocytoma of the parotid gland: a benign lesion simulating malignancy, Hum. Pathol. **15**:485, 1984.

344. Goode, R.K., and Corio, R.L.: Oncocytic adenocarcinoma of salivary glands, Oral Surg. **65**:61, 1988.

345. Godwin, J.T.: Benign lymphoepithelial lesion of the parotid gland: report of eleven cases, Cancer **5**:1089, 1952.

346. Gnepp, D.R., Corio, R.L., and Brannon, R.B.: Small cell carcinoma of the major salivary glands, Cancer **58**:705, 1986.

347. Gnepp, D.R.: Sebaceous neoplasms of salivary gland origin: a review, Pathol. Annu. **18**:71, 1983.

348. Gnepp, D.R., and Brannon, R.B.: Sebaceous neoplasms of salivary gland origin: report of 21 cases, Cancer **53**:2155, 1984.

349. Gorman, J.M., and O'Brien, F.V.: Salivary inclusions on the mandible, Br. Dent. J. **133**:69, 1972.

350. Goldman, R.L., and Perzik, S.L.: Infantile hemangiomas of the parotid gland in children: a clinicopathologic study of 15 cases, Arch. Otolaryngol. **90**:605, 1969.

351. Greene, G.W., Jr., and Bernier, J.L.: Primary malignant melanomas of the parotid gland, Oral Surg. **14**:108, 1961.

352. Greenspan, J.S., Daniels, T.E., Talal, N., and Sylvester, R.A.: The histopathology of Sjögren's syndrome in labial salivary biopsies, Oral Surg. **37**:217, 1974.

353. Haji, D., and Gohao, L.: Malignant lymphoepithelial lesions of the salivary glands with anaplastic carcinomatous change: report of nine cases and review of the literature, Cancer **52**:2245, 1983.

354. Harrison, J.D.: Salivary mucoceles, Oral Surg. **39**:268, 1975.

354a. Headington, J.T., Batsakis, J.G., Beals, T.F., Campbell, T.E., Simmons, J.L., and Stone, W.D.: Membranous basal cell adenomas of parotid gland, dermal cylindroma and trichoepithelioma: comparative histochemistry and ultrastructure, Cancer **39**:2460, 1977.

355. Healey, W.V., Perzin, K.H., and Smith, L.: Mucoepidermoid carcinoma of salivary gland origin: classification, clinical-pathologic correlation and results of treatment, Cancer **26**:368, 1970.

356. Hoggins, G.S., and Hutton, J.B.: Congenital sublingual cystic swellings due to imperforate salivary ducts, Oral Surg. **37**:370, 1974.

357. Hooper, R., Saxon, R., and Troop, A.: Cysts of the parotid gland, J. Laryngol. Otol. **89**:427, 1975.

358. Jensen, J.L., Howell, F.V., Rick, G.M., and Correll, R.W.: Minor salivary gland calculi: a clinicopathologic study of 47 new cases, Oral Surg. **47**:44, 1979.

359. Kaban, L.B., Donoff, R.B., and Guralnick, W.C.: Acute parotitis, J. Oral Surg. **31**:377, 1973.

360. Kassan, S.S., Thomas, T.L., Moutsopoulos, H.M., Hoover, R., Kimberly, R.P., Budman, D.R., Costa, J., Decker, J.L., and Chused, T.M.: Increased risk of lymphoma in sicca syndrome, Ann Intern. Med. **89**:88, 1978.

361. Kerpel, S.M., Freedman, P.D., and Lumerman, H.: The papillary cystadenoma of minor salivary gland origin, Oral Surg. **46**:820, 1978.

362. Koss, L.C., Spiro, R.H., and Hajdu, S.: Small cell (oat cell) carcinoma of minor salivary gland origin, Cancer 30:737, 1972.
363. Leake, D., and Leake, R.: Neonatal suppurative parotitis, Pediatrics 46:203, 1970.
364. Levin, P.A., Falko, J.M., Dixon, K., Gallup, E.M., and Saunders, W.: Benign parotid enlargement in bulimia, Ann. Intern. Med. 93:827, 1980.
365. Little, J.W., and Rickles, N.H.: Malignant papillary cystadenoma lymphomatosum: report of a case with review of the literature, Cancer 18:851, 1965.
366. Luna, M.A., Ordóñez, N.G., Mackay, B., Batsakis, J.G., and Guillamondegui, O.: Salivary epithelial-myoepithelial carcinomas of intercalated ducts: a clinical, electron microscopic and immunohistochemical study, Oral Surg. 59:482, 1985.
367. Lynch, D.P., Crago, C.A., and Martínez, M.O.: Necrotizing sialometaplasia, Oral Surg. 47:63, 1979.
368. Martínez-Lavin, M., Vaughn, J.H., and Tan, E.M.: Autoantibodies and the spectrum of Sjögren's syndrome, Ann. Intern. Med. 91:185, 1979.
369. Moutsopoulos, H.M., moderator: Sjögren's syndrome (sicca syndrome): current issues, Ann. Intern. Med. 92:212, 1980.
370. Myerson, M., Crelin, E.S., and Smith, H.W.: Bilateral duplication of the submandibular ducts, Arch. Otolaryngol. 83:488, 1966.
371. Noone, R.B., and Brown, H.J.: Cystic hygroma of the parotid gland, Am. J. Surg. 120:404, 1970.
372. Nussbaum, M., Tan, S., and Som, M.L.: Hemangiomas of salivary glands, Laryngoscope 86:1015, 1976.
373. Perzin, K.H., Gullane, P., and Clairmont, A.C.: Adenoid cystic carcinomas arising in salivary glands: a correlation of histologic features and clinical course, Cancer 42:265, 1978.
374. Rees, R.T.: Congenital ranula, Br. Dent. J. 146:345, 1979.
374a. Samy, L.L., Girgis, I.H., and Wasef, S.A.: Ectopic salivary tissue in relation to the tonsil, Laryngoscope 82:247, 1968.
375. Sapiro, S.M., and Eisenberg, E.: Sjögren's syndrome (sicca complex), Oral Surg. 45:591, 1978.
376. Sciubba, J.J., and Brannon, R.B.: Myoepithelioma of salivary gland: report of 23 cases, Cancer 49:562, 1982.
377. Scully, C.: Sjögren's syndrome: clinical and laboratory features, immunopathogenesis and management, Oral Surg. 62:510, 1986.
378. Shemen, L.J., Huvos, A.G., and Spiro, R.H.: Squamous cell carcinoma of salivary gland origin, Head Neck Surg. 9:235, 1987.
379. Singer, M.I., Applebaum, E.L., and Loy, K.D.: Heterotopic salivary tissue in the neck, Laryngoscope 89:1772, 1979.
380. Smith, N.D.J., and Smith, P.B.: Congenital absence of major salivary glands, Br. Dent. J. 142:259, 1977.
381. Southam, J.C.: Retention mucoceles of the oral mucosa, J. Oral Pathol. 3:197, 1974.
382. Spiro, R.H., Huvos, A.G., Berk, R., and Strong, E.W.: Mucoepidermoid carcinoma of salivary gland origin, Am. J. Surg. 136:461, 1978.
383. Spiro, R.H., Huvos, A.G., and Strong, E.W.: Malignant mixed tumors of salivary origin: a clinicopathologic study of 146 cases, Cancer 39:388, 1977.
384. Spiro, R.H.: Salivary neoplasms: overview of 35-year experience with 2,807 patients, Head Neck Surg. 8:177, 1986.
385. Stephen, J., Batsakis, J.G., Luna, M.A., von der Hayden, U., and Byers, R.M.: True malignant mixed tumors (carcinosarcoma) of salivary glands, Oral Surg. 61:597, 1986.
386. Tarpley, T.M., Anderson, L., Lightbody, P., and Sheagren, J.N.: Minor salivary gland involvement in sarcoidosis, Oral Surg. 33:755, 1972.
387. Tarpley, T.M., Jr., and Giansanti, J.S.: Adenoid cystic carcinoma: analysis of fifty oral cases, Oral Surg. 41:484, 1976.
388. Thackray, A.C., and Lucas, R.B.: Tumors of the major salivary glands. In Atlas of tumor pathology, ser. 2, fascicle 10, Washington, D.C., 1974, Armed Forces Institute of Pathology.
389. Thackray, A.C., and Sobin, L.H.: Histologic typing of salivary gland tumors, Geneva, 1973, World Health Organization.
390. Waldron, C.A., El-Mofty, S., and Gnepp, D.R.: Tumors of the intra-oral minor salivary glands: a demographic and histologic study of 426 cases, Oral Surg. 66:323, 1988.
391. Wong, T., and Warner, N.E.: Cytomegalic inclusion disease in adults, Arch. Pathol. 74:403, 1962.
392. Yonkers, A.J., Krous, H.F., and Yarington, C.T.: Surgical parotitis, Laryngoscope 82:1239, 1972.

Neck

393. Armstrong, D., Pickrell, K., Fetter, B., and Pitts, W.: Torticollis: an analysis of 271 cases, Plast. Reconstr. Surg. 35:14, 1965.
394. Baughman, R.A.: Lingual thyroid and lingual thyroglossal duct remnants, Oral Surg. 34:781, 1972.
395. Buchner, A., and Hansen, L.S.: Lymphoepithelial cysts of the oral cavity, Oral Surg. 50:441, 1980.
396. Clark, O.H.: Parathyroid cysts, Am. J. Surg. 135:395, 1978.
397. Clark, R.N.: Diagnosis and management of torticollis, Pediatr. Ann. 5:43, 1976.
398. Devens, K., Holzmann, K., and Spier, J.: Teratomas in the cervical region, Z. Kinderchir. 30:119, 1980.
399. Farman, A.G., Katz, J., Eloff, J., and Cywes, S.: Mandibulofacial aspects of the cervical cystic lymphangioma (cystic hygroma), Br. J. Oral Surg. 16:125, 1978.
400. Glenner, G.G., and Grimley, P.M.: Tumors of the extra-adrenal paraganglion system (including chemoreceptors). In Atlas of tumor pathology, ser. 2, fascicle 9, Washington, D.C., 1973, Armed Forces Institute of Pathology.
401. Guba, A.M., Adam, A.E., Jacques, D.A., and Chambers, R.G.: Cervical presentation of thymic cysts, Am. J. Surg. 136:430, 1978.
402. Holland, C.S.: The management of Ludwig's angina, Br. J. Oral Surg. 13:153, 1975.
403. Hugo, N.E., and Conway, H.: Benign symmetrical lipomatosis, Plast. Reconstr. Surg. 37:69, 1966.
404. Irons, G.B., Weiland, L.H., and Brown, W.L.: Paragangliomas of the neck: clinical and pathologic analysis of 116 cases, Surg. Clin. North Am. 57:575, 1977.
405. Johnsen, N.J., and Bretlau, P.: Cervical thymic cysts, Acta Otolaryngol. 82:143, 1976.
406. Lack, E.E., Clark, M.A., Buck, D.R., and King, D.R.: Cysts of the parathyroid gland: report of two cases and review of the literature, Am. Surg. 44:376, 1978.
407. Macdonald, D.M.: Thyroglossal cysts and fistulae, Int. J. Oral Surg. 3:342, 1974.
408. McGuirt, W.F., and Harker, L.A.: Carotid body tumors, Arch. Otolaryngol. 101:58, 1975.
409. Ninh, T.N., and Ninh, T.X.: Cystic hygroma in children: a report of 126 cases, J. Pediatr. Surg. 9:191, 1974.
410. Pratt, L.W.: Familial carotid body tumors, Arch. Otolaryngol. 97:334, 1973.
411. Roediger, W.E., Spitz, L., and Schmaman, A.: Histogenesis of benign cervical teratomas, Teratology 10:111, 1974.
412. Rosen, E.A, Schulman, R.H., and Shaw, A.S.: Ludwig's angina: a complication of a mandibular fracture, J. Oral Surg. 30:1972.
413. Rundle, F.W.: Cervical teratoma, J. Otolaryngol. 5:513, 1976.
414. Schuler, F.A., Graham, J.K., and Horton, C.E.: Benign symmetrical lipomatosis (Madelung's disease), Plast. Reconstr. Surg. 57:662, 1976.
415. Toto, P.D., Wortel, J.P., and Joseph, G.: Lymphoepithelial cysts and associated immunoglobulins, Oral Surg. 54:59, 1982.
416. Tovi, R., and Mares, A.J.: The aberrant cervical thymus: embryology, pathology and clinical implications, Am. J. Surg. 136:631, 1978.
417. Wilson, H.: Carotid body tumors: familial and bilateral, Ann. Surg. 171:843, 1970.

24 Alimentary Tract

GERALD FINE
CHAN K. MA

CONGENITAL ANOMALIES
Atresia

Most malformations of the alimentary tract are congenital and are related to the formation of the bowel lumen or bowel rotation.[93,168] Interruption in the continuity of the bowel lumen, which may be partial (stenosis) or complete (atresia), manifests itself in early infancy and is incompatible with life without prompt surgical correction. The sites commonly involved are the esophagus, small intestine, and anus.[71] Esophageal atresia is frequently associated with tracheoesophageal fistulas and occasionally with one or more of a variety of other malformations—anal atresia, vertebral defect, and renal dysplasia or agenesis (Vater association).[18] Webs of vascularized fibrous tissue covered by mucosa may be the cause of narrowing of the upper or lower portion of the esophagus (Fig. 24-1).[278] Those in the former site are more often seen in women and frequently

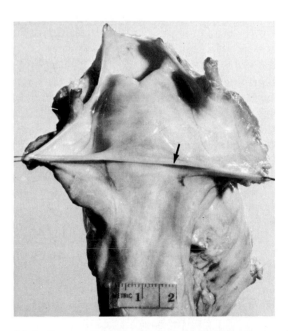

Fig. 24-1. Congenital esophageal web. Esophagus has been opened posteriorly.

are associated with atrophic glossitis, iron-deficiency anemia, and dysphagia (Plummer-Vinson syndrome). Intestinal atresia may be associated with meconium ileus (see discussion of cystic fibrosis, p. 1348), which some investigators have considered to be the cause of the atresia.[29] Faulty development of the hindgut, which is intimately related to the development of the cloacal septum, is frequently associated with fistulas between the rectum and urinary or genital tract or the perineum. Failure of the proctodeum to invaginate or of the anal plate to be absorbed results in imperforate rectum or anus.[165]

Heterotopia

Gastric mucous membrane may be found in the cervical esophagus[145,253] or associated with other malformations such as Meckel's diverticulum, duplications, or enteric cysts. Pancreatic tissue[308] in the form of discrete nodules of acinar and ductal tissue and occasionally islets of Langerhans, occurs most commonly in the stomach[196] and duodenum and less frequently in the jejunum, Meckel's diverticulum, and appendix. Pulmonary tissue has been found in the terminal ileum.[192] The adenomyoma, an admixture of ducts and smooth muscle, is encountered in the stomach and gallbladder.[180]

Duplications and enteric cysts

Duplications and enteric cysts are segments of gastrointestinal tube in apposition to any portion of the alimentary canal that may be completely independent of the adjacent normal intestine or share its lumen and mesentery and muscle coats. They develop in one of two ways—multicentric recanalization of the proliferated luminal gut epithelium or persistence, growth, and sequestration of diverticular buds of the developing intestine. The two are similar in makeup, but the cysts are more or less spherical and usually lack communication with the gut lumen. Duplications are most common in the region of the terminal ileum,[38] whereas cysts are most often intrathoracic and related to the esophagus. They may be lined by small intestinal, gastric, or even bronchial mucous membrane; if gastric, peptic ulceration with concomitant hemorrhage or perforation may occur.

Meckel's diverticulum

Meckel's diverticulum is a diverticulum on the antimesenteric aspect of the terminal ileum, 2.5 cm to 1.83 m proximal to the ileocecal valve, and possesses all the layers of small bowel (Fig. 24-2). It represents the most common of many possible residua of the omphalomesenteric duct; others are umbilical sinus, cyst between the ileum and umbilicus, and ileoumbilical fistula. Its mucosa is usually that of the small intestine, but in 25% of the cases gastric mucosa with or without pancreatic tissue may be present. It may be manifested clinically by peptic ulceration and hemorrhage, obstruction of its lumen, intussusception, or diverticulitis.[150,277,327]

Aganglionic megacolon (Hirschsprung's disease)[204]

Aganglionic megacolon is characterized by symptoms of partial or complete intestinal obstruction, usually from birth or very early in life, with great dilatation and hypertrophy of the colon. The underlying anatomic defect is a lack of ganglion cells in Auerbach's (myenteric) plexus and Meissner's (submucous) plexus in a narrowed, nonhypertrophied segment of intestine distal to the extremely dilated and hypertrophied colon, which is innervated normally (Plate 2, A). The aganglionic area usually does not extend higher than the sigmoid colon, but instances of involvement of the entire colon and even the small intestine occur. The diagnosis can be based on the failure to find ganglion cells in adequate rectal biopsy specimens. Surgical resection of the aganglionic segment relieves the condition. Adynamic bowel syndrome may simulate Hirschsprung's disease clinically and roentgenographically, but there are no morphologic changes in the bowel ganglia.[156]

Pyloric stenosis

Congenital pyloric stenosis is gross narrowing of the pylorus as a result of an unexplained hypertrophy of the pyloric muscle, usually in male infants. It is manifested by vomiting with attendant dehydration and malnutrition.[25] Surgical relief is obtained by incision of the hypertrophied muscle. A similar condition is occasionally seen in adults and is usually associated with a gastric or duodenal ulcer.

Achalasia of esophagus

Loss of normal esophageal peristalsis and impaired relaxation of the lower esophageal sphincter result in progressive dysphagia and dilatation of the esophagus. Loss of ganglion cells in Auerbach's plexus is a consistent finding in the body of the esophagus; in the sphincter such cells have been reported to be normal in number, reduced, or absent. Alterations in the vagus nerves and their motor nuclei have also been implicated in the esophageal dysfunction, but some authors have considered these changes to be the result of the esophageal ganglion cell changes.[48,85]

Miscellaneous anomalies

A variety of anomalies of position may involve the gastrointestinal tract: the presence of portions of the tract in internal or external or diaphragmatic hernial sacs, malrotation or failure of descent of the intestine, transposition associated with transposition of other viscera, and variations in development or attachment of the mesentery. Any or all of these anomalies may be responsible for volvulus and intestinal obstruction.

Abnormal peritoneal bands also may produce obstruction. A congenitally short esophagus may be associated with herniation of a portion of gastric cardia into the thoracic cavity, so-called hiatus hernia (p. 1156).

Multilocular rectal cysts with variable epithelial lining—squamous, columnar with mucin, or transitional—presumably having their origin from the neurenteric

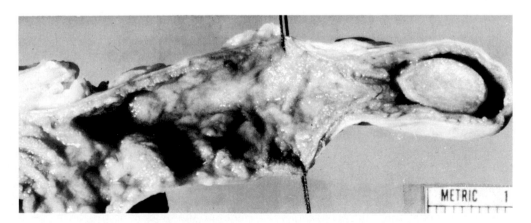

Fig. 24-2. Meckel's diverticulum. Notice fruit pit in tip of diverticulum.

canal or postanal gut, may be responsible for intestinal obstruction, abscesses, or fistulas.[90] Association of the cysts with a dimple of the anal mucous membrane in its posterior midline has been reported.

ACQUIRED MALFORMATIONS
Diverticula

Acquired diverticula of the gastrointestinal tract are for the most part "false" (pulsion diverticula), representing herniations of the mucous membrane and muscularis mucosae through weakened areas or defects in the muscularis propria. Their walls do not have all the layers of the segment of alimentary tract from which they arise but are composed of mucous membrane, muscularis mucosae, and areolar tissue (Fig. 24-3). They occur at the junction of the esophagus and hypopharynx (Zenker's diverticulum),[166,173] in the second portion of the duodenum, in the small intestine,[36,89] and in the appendix, but they are most common and clinically significant in the colon.[6,238] In the last site, they are frequently multiple and most prevalent in the descending and sigmoid colon. They occur on the convexity of the intestine opposite the mesenteric attachment and between the long muscle bands (taenias). Although numerous, they may be difficult to discern, being hidden externally by epiploic appendages and in-

ternally by muscle contraction, which diminishes their luminal orifice. Clinical manifestations may be acute or chronic and related to one or a combination of conditions, such as bowel spasms, diverticulitis, hemorrhage, fistulas, perforation, and intestinal obstruction.[307]

The less commonly acquired diverticula, "true" (traction) diverticula, occur in the esophagus and first portion of the duodenum just distal to the pylorus. In both sites they are the result of inflammation and scarring; those in the esophagus are related to hilar and mediastinal lymph node disease, whereas those in the pylorus result from duodenal or pyloric ulcers.

Pneumatosis cystoides intestinalis[87]

In pneumatosis intestinalis, gas-filled cysts are found in the submucosa or wall of the small intestine, less frequently in the colon, and rarely in the stomach[174] and esophagus at necropsy (Fig. 24-4). The process is associated with gastric or duodenal ulcers, enterocolitis, or respiratory disease, notably asthma. It now appears that the condition can be explained on a mechanical basis in association with (1) obstruction with ulceration, (2) trauma from biopsy, sigmoidoscopic examination, and so on, or (3) respiratory disease with severe cough. In the last case it is postulated that pneumomediastinum occurs after pulmonary alveolar rupture, since the air

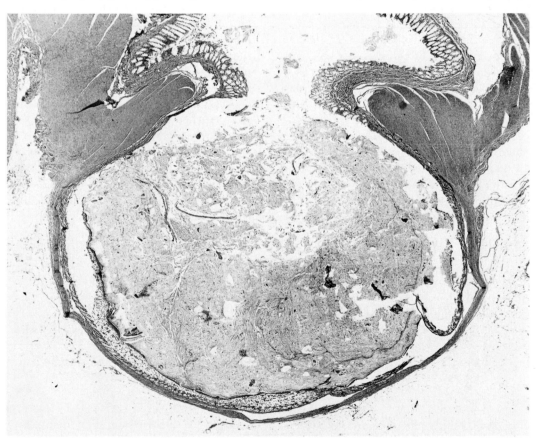

Fig. 24-3. Diverticulum of sigmoid colon, demonstrating hernia-like nature. Notice fecal content. (17×.)

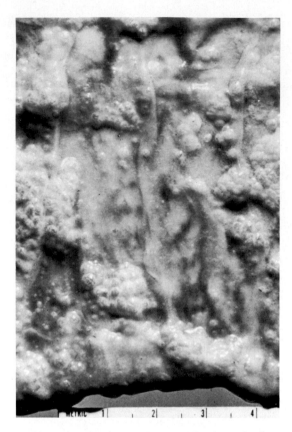

Fig. 24-4. Pneumatosis cystoides intestinalis.

then dissects retroperitoneally and reaches the intestine along the path of the mesenteric blood vessels.[164] A bacterial cause has also been proposed.[24,337] The gas cysts range in diameter from a few millimeters to a centimeter or more and may be lined by flattened endothelium-like cells resembling lymphatic spaces or multinucleated giant cells, or they may have no visible lining.[285] The cysts do not communicate with the intestinal lumen or with each other. The symptoms of pneumatosis are generally nonspecific. Spontaneous resolution with roentgenographic clearing can and does occur.

Melanosis of colon

The mucous membrane of the colon and appendix may acquire a brown color because of the accumulation of brown granular pigment in phagocytes in the lamina propria. Although the pigment is referred to as melanin, its exact nature is unknown. The condition is not of clinical significance. One suggestion is that it is related to colonic stasis and the habitual use of anthracene laxatives.[86]

Endometriosis

Foci of endometrial glands and endometrial stroma may involve the colon,[297] usually the sigmoid or rectum, appendix, or small bowel. It may be responsible

for obstructive symptoms, colic, and diarrhea, or even rectal bleeding. Obstruction is the result of fibrosis or muscle spasm, and cancer can be simulated both roentgenographically and at operation. Less commonly a decidual reaction associated with pregnancy may be found involving the serosa of the bowel.

MECHANICAL DISTURBANCES
Obstruction

The relative incidence of the various causes of intestinal obstruction varies, but hernias, adhesions, and neoplasms are the common causes. Other causes are volvulus, foreign objects, inflammatory disease, stricture, and external compression by tumors, cysts, enlarged viscera, and so on, as well as such congenital lesions as annular pancreas, meconium ileus, and the atresias, bands, and the like previously noted.

Hernia

Hernia is the protrusion of tissue, organ, or part of an organ through an abnormal opening in the wall of the body cavity in which it is normally confined. The majority of hernias are abdominal, resulting from herniation of abdominal contents through the internal or external inguinal rings, femoral ring, or defects in the abdominal wall resulting from trauma or improper healing after a surgical procedure.[199] Less common are internal hernias, wherein loops of intestine penetrate normally small peritoneal recesses, such as the fossa at the junction of the duodenum and jejunum. Diaphragmatic hernias are not a significant cause of intestinal obstruction. Herniation of abdominal viscera through congenital defects in the diaphragm is infrequent compared to hiatus hernia, which is the protrusion, often intermittent ("sliding" hernia), of a portion of the stomach and abdominal esophagus through the esophageal hiatus of the diaphragm into the thoracic cavity.[17,126,190] Symptoms in the latter—a disease of obese, middle-aged individuals—are related to the reflux of gastric secretions into the esophagus, with resultant so-called peptic esophagitis, ulceration, and hemorrhage. Herniation of the gastric cardia through the esophageal hiatus also may occur alongside the esophagus; this is called paraesophageal hernia.

Adhesions

In addition to congenital bands, peritoneal adhesions resulting from inflammation and after laparotomy may be responsible for intestinal obstruction, usually in the small intestine.

Neoplasms

Intestinal obstruction may result from primary or secondary bowel involvement by neoplasm. The most common obstructing primary tumors are the encircling

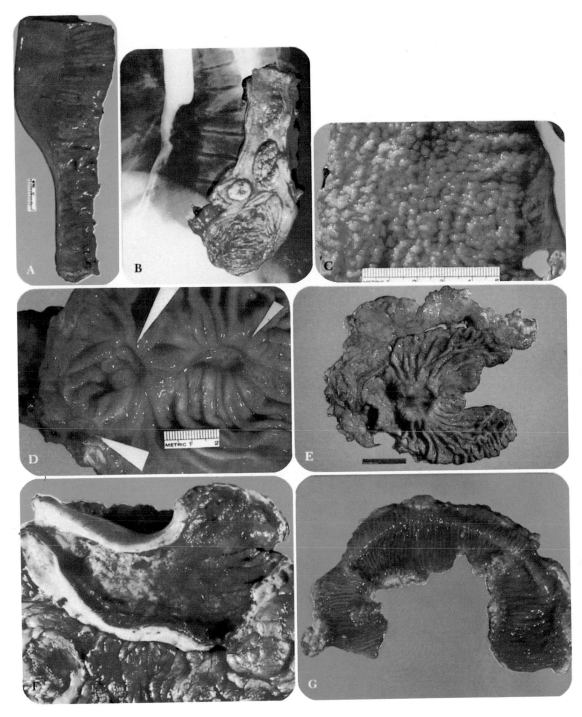

Plate 2

A, Congenital aganglionic megacolon (Hirschsprung's disease).

B, Multifocal epidermoid carcinoma of esophagus. Photograph of gross specimen superimposed on roentgenogram demonstrating lesion with aid of contrast medium.

C, Familial polyposis coli. Entire colon is carpeted by similar-appearing polyps.

D, Multiple gastric ulcers. Notice mucosal folds converging on ulcer edge without interruption.

E, Malignant gastric ulcer. Mucosal folds are interrupted toward crater.

F, Carcinoma of stomach, linitis plastica type. Surgically resected specimen.

G, Multiple carcinoid tumors of ileum. Patient had lymph node and liver metastases and demonstrated carcinoid syndrome.

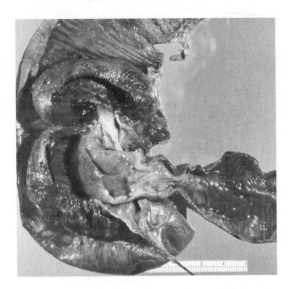

Fig. 24-5. Ileocecal intussusception with infarction.

carcinomas that occur in the left half of the colon where the intestinal is semisolid.

Intussusception

Intussusception is the invagination of a segment of intestinal tract (the intussusceptum) into the immediately adjacent (almost always distal) intestine (the intussuscipiens). It is primarily a disease of infants and young children,[26] but it does occur in adults, in whom it may be initiated by a pedunculated benign or malignant primary tumor or a metastatic growth. In children it is more common in the ileocecal region, with the ileum telescoping into the colon and the ileocecal valve retaining its normal position (Fig. 24-5). Less common are ileoileal and colocolonic intussusception. Masses of lymphoid tissue, polyps, or the ileocecal valve itself may form the advancing head of the intussusception, or the lesion may be the result of uncoordinated muscle contractions of the bowel. Bowel obstruction or compromise of blood supply to the involved intestine requires surgical intervention if spontaneous correction does not occur. Multiple foci of intussusception, unassociated with any reaction, are seen occasionally at necropsy and are believed to be agonal.

Volvulus

Volvulus is the twisting of a loop (or loops) of intestine upon itself through 180 degrees or more, producing obstruction of both the intestine and the blood supply of the affected loop. Causative factors are usually long mesenteric attachment, redundant intestine, abnormal bands (congenital or acquired), or abdominal attachments of the intestine. The lesion is most common in the sigmoid colon and has a preponderance in men. Because strangulation occurs almost simultaneously with obstruction, operative treatment must be prompt to avoid death of the patient.

Obturation obstruction

A foreign body, exogenous or endogenous, large or small, may obstruct the intestinal lumen by inducing bowel spasm or becoming entrapped in areas of anatomic or pathologic narrowing of the intestinal lumen. Gallstone obstruction of the small intestine complicating cholecystogastric or cholecystoduodenal fistula, large-bowel obstruction by enteroliths, and appendiceal obstruction by fecaliths are examples of common endogenous obstruction. Almost any conceivable ingested foreign body may produce bowel obstruction.[233] Fruit pits and bezoars—masses of ingested hair (trichobezoars) or vegetable residues (phytobezoars), most notably persimmons—are worthy of mention. Parasites, particularly *Ascaris lumbricoides*, are also causes of intestinal obstruction.

Stricture

Intrinsic narrowing of the intestinal lumen may be the result of scarring in one or more of its layers as a result of chemical injury (for example, lye in the esophagus), peptic ulceration of the esophagus or duodenum, x-ray irradiation,[244] scarring at the sites of surgical anastomosis or intestinal resection, or scleroderma.

Adynamic (paralytic) ileus

The clinical picture of acute intestinal obstruction may occur in the absence of mechanical or organic obstruction as a result of paralysis of the musculature of a portion or all of the intestinal tract. Abdominal distension and accumulation of gas and fluid in the intestine may be extreme, producing the same effects as mechanical obstruction. It frequently occurs after laparotomy, usually in a mild form. It may be associated with intra-abdominal infection, trauma, or other disease (such as ureteral stone) or systemic infection (such as pneumonia in children).[235] Peritonitis resulting from acute appendicitis with perforation, perforated peptic ulcer, and so on is probably the most important single underlying cause. A related condition is acute dilatation of the stomach, which occasionally complicates surgery, usually abdominal.

Effects of intestinal obstruction

The systemic effects of bowel obstruction are variable in their severity, being dependent on the site involved and the degree of obstruction. They are related to fluid and electrolyte loss, distension with fluid and gas, and damage to the bowel wall and resulting permeability to bacteria and, potentially, peritonitis.[313] One or more of the following may be associated with the obstruction: dehydration, acidosis, alkalosis, hemoconcentration, decrease in intracellular fluid, and finally renal suppression. The bowel proximal to the obstruction shows varying degrees of dilatation and hypertrophy depending on the location and the completeness of the obstruction, as well as the duration.

Mallory-Weiss syndrome[63]

Any action that increases intra-abdominal pressure, but particularly bouts of repeated and forceful vomiting, may produce longitudinally oriented lacerations in the gastric cardia, distal esophagus, or esophagogastric junction, which may be the source of gastrointestinal hemorrhage. Alcoholism, aspirin ingestion, gastritis, and hiatus hernia have been commonly associated with the syndrome.[172]

VASCULAR DISTURBANCES
Esophageal varices

Elevated pressure in the portal venous system, most often the result of cirrhosis of the liver but at times caused by other lesions such as portal vein thrombosis, commonly results in esophageal varices.[14] The esophageal venous plexus receives blood from the gastric and coronary veins of the stomach, forming part of one of the routes by which portal venous blood may bypass the liver to reach the right atrium. As a result, the submucosal veins of the lower part of the esophagus, and sometimes of the upper part of the stomach as well, become greatly dilated, tortuous, and engorged. They are covered by a thin mucous membrane. The increased venous pressure, with or without inflammation or ulceration, often results in massive and frequently fatal hemorrhage.[183]

Ischemic bowel disease[234]

Compromise of the blood supply to the gastrointestinal tract may occur in a variety of ways and be responsible for a variety of bowel changes. The complex control of the mesenteric circulation[193] (cardiac, autonomic nervous system, peripheral collateral circulation, and peripheral autoregulation), coupled with the degree of local vascular disease, makes the bowel vulnerable to ischemia in a variety of ways. Abundant collateral blood supply to the stomach, duodenum, and rectum from extracoelomic vessels makes these sites less vulnerable than others to ischemia. Excluding strangulation, as discussed previously, the causes of bowel ischemia in order of decreasing frequency are sclerosis of the mesenteric arteries with or without associated thrombosis[305]; embolism (thrombotic, atherosclerotic plaques, or tumor); venous thrombosis, sometimes associated with contraceptive drugs[52,125]; hypotension generally associated with nonocclusive atheromatous

disease,[255] which by itself has compromised the blood supply short of producing necrosis; and vascular diseases such as thromboangiitis obliterans and vasculitis of various types. The superior mesenteric vessels and consequently the jejunum and proximal part of the ileum are involved most frequently though any part of the gastrointestinal tract may be affected.

Complete arterial occlusion results in full-thickness infarction of the bowel, which is usually anemic initially but with time becomes hemorrhagic. Venous occlusion preceding arterial blockage causes infarction that is hemorrhagic from its inception. The bowel becomes dusky and purple-red because of hemorrhage into the bowel wall and lumen and subsequent necrosis and inflammatory cell infiltration. The resulting paralysis of the bowel muscle produces an intestinal obstruction with its attendant physiologic alterations.

Reduction in blood flow to the intestine insufficient to produce a full-thickness infarct may result in a variety of nonspecific lesions (ischemic enteritis and colitis): ulceration, inflammation, cicatrization with stricture formation,[331] and "intestinal angina." The distinction between such lesions and those believed to be related to potassium ingestion is not always clear.[335]

Hemorrhoids

Hemorrhoids are varicosities of the hemorrhoidal vein—"internal" and covered by mucous membrane if of the superior hemorrhoidal plexus and "external" and covered by skin if of the inferior hemorrhoidal plexus. The former are the more important and the more troublesome. They result from increased venous pressure related to such causes as portal hypertension, cardiac failure, carcinoma of the rectum, or myomatous or pregnant uterus, but chronic constipation appears to be far more important in their pathogenesis.

The coincidence of hemorrhoids and rectal carcinoma is sufficiently great to make search for the latter mandatory in every patient with hemorrhoids.

Complications of hemorrhoids are thrombosis with associated inflammation, scarring, pain, and hemorrhage in the form of bright red blood passed by rectum. Organization of a thrombus may produce a histologic picture that may mimic the malignant hemangioendothelioma.

Gastrointestinal hemorrhage

Bleeding into the gastrointestinal tract may be the result of a wide variety of lesions and may be minimal, producing anemia, or massive and life threatening.[41] If the blood is eliminated orally or rectally soon after escaping from the vascular system, it is bright red, but if it is confined to the alimentary tract for a period of time before being eliminated, it is brown or black (coffee-ground vomitus and tarry stools—melena). The most important sources of massive hematemesis (vomiting of blood) are esophageal varices,[101] gastric or duodenal (peptic) ulcers, and leiomyoma. Other tumors (benign or malignant), hiatus hernia, gastritis, and so on usually produce bleeding of lesser degree. Massive bleeding from the rectum or anus is less common than massive hematemesis. Hemorrhoids, diverticular disease,[209] or the polyps of the Peutz-Jeghers syndrome may cause it. However, these lesions also may be associated with bleeding of small amount, as is commonly found in carcinoma of the large intestine and, less often, with other tumors, regional enteritis, ulcerative colitis, and anal fissure.[306] The lesions causing hematemesis are also associated with blood in the stool, which may be occult.

The site and cause of gastrointestinal bleeding is often not discerned in a high percentage of cases. However, with the advent of fiberoptic endoscopy and angiography, a variety of vascular anomalies are being increasingly recognized as important causes of idiopathic gastrointestinal hemorrhage.[220] "Vascular ectasia" (angiodysplasia), usually occurring in the cecum and ascending colon of elderly women, is an important cause of lower intestinal hemorrhage.[35] Other vascular anomalies include gastric antral vascular extasia (watermelon stomach),[144] Dieulafoy's aneurysm (arterial caliber persistence),[218,317] and hereditary hemorrhagic telangiectasia (Rendu-Osler-Weber disease).[88,286]

INFLAMMATIONS
Esophagitis

Esophageal inflammation most commonly results from secretion—reflux or peptic esophagitis—associated with hiatus hernia, achalasia, or scleroderma. Less common causes are corrosive substances (lye) and infectious agents—viral (herpes simplex and varicella) and fungous (*Candida*).[197,226] Scarring and stricture generally result from lye ingestion, prolonged gastric juice reflux, or neoplasms. Initially gastric juice produces basal cell hyperplasia of the esophageal epithelium, with elongation of the connective tissue papillae with or without neutrophilic infiltrates.[143] Persistent reflux leads to one or more complications—ulceration, stricture, or columnar epithelial metaplasia of the squamous mucosa (Barrett's esophagus),[96,237] in which there has been a 10% incidence of adenocarcinoma.[45,229]

Esophageal pseudodiverticulosis is a condition that roentgenographically mimics diverticula but that pathologically is dissimilar.[49] The x-ray changes are attributable to dilatation and tortuosity of the esophageal glands and their ducts, but there is no abnormal extension of mucosa beyond the confines of the esophageal submucosa.[186] The process appears to be the result of inflammation and obstruction of the increased number of esophageal glands and ducts, with dilatation and squamous metaplasia of their lining epithelium (Fig. 24-6).

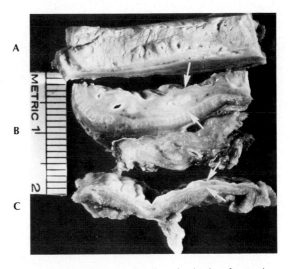

Fig. 24-6. A and **B,** Pseudodiverticulosis of esophagus. **C,** Normal esophagus. Ducts of esophageal glands are prominent in thickened submucosa *(arrows)* in pseudodiverticulosis, and their openings on mucosal surface are accentuated, **A.** (Courtesy Dr. Aaron Lupovitch, Detroit, Mich.)

Gastritis and gastroenteritis

The gastritis and gastroenteritis that are such common clinical complaints rarely come to the attention of the pathologist. They are the result of exogenous agents, such as ethanol, therapeutic drugs (salicylates and so on), irradiation, and corrosive agents, or endogenous agents, such as bacterial and viral agents involving the bowel or other organs and allergy. Phlegmonous gastritis,[120] usually of streptococcal origin, results from inflammation elsewhere in the body, such as osteomyelitis.

Inflammatory fibroid polyp and eosinophilic gastroenteritis

Inflammatory fibroid polyp and eosinophilic gastroenteritis manifest themselves as either a localized, fibrotic, polypoid, tumorlike mass (inflammatory fibroid polyp[153]; Fig. 24-7), or a diffuse infiltration throughout all coats of the gut wall.[152] Eosinophils are a prominent part of the histopathologic picture in both lesions, but blood eosinophilia and a history of allergy are associated only with the diffuse lesion. Sites of involvement in order of frequency include the stomach, jejunum, ileum, and cecum. The colon and rectum are rarely involved. No relationship between these conditions and histiocytosis X has been found.[31]

Ulcers of stomach and duodenum

Ulcers, usually small and multiple and not penetrating the muscularis mucosae (erosions), are frequently encountered in the stomach as a terminal event in a

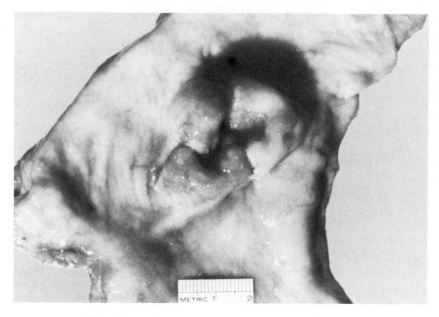

Fig. 24-7. Inflammatory fibroid polyp of stomach.

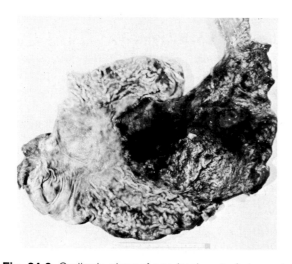

Fig. 24-8. Curling's ulcer of proximal part of stomach.

variety of conditions.[116] Acute ulcers of the stomach or duodenum may be associated with extensive burns (Curling's ulcers, Fig. 24-8),[62,247] Cushing's disease, hypothalamic lesions, stress, or trauma; they may also be iatrogenic (resulting from corticosteroid therapy or gastric tubes). They may be fatal as a result of uncontrolled hemorrhage or spontaneous perforation and peritonitis.

Nonspecific ulcers in the small intestine have been encountered with increasing frequency. They may be complicated by scarring and partial intestinal obstruction. Vascular changes and potassium, a known tissue irritant therapeutically employed in enteric-coated tablets, have been implicated in their pathogenesis.[325]

Peptic ulcer

Incidence and pathogenesis. Chronic ulcers having certain similarities and distinct differences occur in the stomach and duodenum, with a frequency of 2.5% and 1.4%, respectively, among men and women.[206] Duodenal ulcers are more common and more often found in young and middle-aged men of blood group O, particularly in nonsecretors. Gastric ulcers are more frequent at an older age, with a preponderance among blood group A. Duodenal ulcer has been associated with tension, stress, and anxiety, but this is by no means always the case and there is no agreement on the importance of stress in its pathogenesis.[97] Peptic ulcers occur only in the environment of acid gastric secretions: the stomach, duodenum, lower esophagus, jejunum just distal to the site of surgical gastroenteric anastomosis, and malformations containing gastric mucosa. The mucous membrane not accustomed to the acid-pepsin environment is the site involved. Thus gastric ulcers occur in the antrum and infrequently in the cardia, whereas the acid secretion is usually limited to the fundus.

Hypersecretion of gastric juice and emotional factors have been considered to be important in the pathogenesis of peptic ulcers. The gastroduodenal mucous membrane is protected against digestion of normal gastric secretions not only by its mucus coating but also by dilution and neutralization with swallowed food, saliva, and regurgitated duodenal fluids. Hypersecretion of hydrochloric acid into the fasting stomach at night is regarded by Dragstedt[80] as the cause of duodenal ulcer. This is considered to be the result of vagal stimulation and can be abolished by section of the vagus nerve. He regards the gastric ulcer also to be the result of increased hydrochloric acid secretion attributable to a humoral (gastrin) stimulation brought about by stasis of ingested food in an atonic stomach.[81]

Although hyperacidity is common among patients with peptic ulcers, hypoacidity is not uncommon with gastric ulcers, particularly those on the lesser curvature unassociated with ulcers in the duodenum or pylorus.[151,207] To explain the latter, it has been postulated that several factors singly or in combination—bile reflux, gastritis, and reduced mucus production by the gastric mucosa—may alter local tissue resistance to hydrochloric acid.[107,130,257] The spiral bacterium *Campylobacter pylori* has been frequently isolated from patients with gastritis or peptic ulcer disease, but its pathogenetic role remains to be determined.[121] Prostaglandin deficiency has also been implicated as a possible cause of peptic ulcer disease.[64]

Emotional factors responsible for vagal stimulation through the hypothalamus–anterior pituitary–adrenal cortex stress mechanism have been shown by Wolf[336] to affect gastric function. Cortisone, which may be the cause of ulcers, usually gastric, may also activate a preexisting ulcer and be responsible for perforation or hemorrhage.

Morbid anatomy and histology. Gastric ulcers most commonly occur on or near the lesser curvature of the stomach, usually within about 5 cm of the pylorus. They are more numerous on the posterior than the anterior wall. A few occur in the cardia, and a few seemingly straddle the pylorus, making it difficult to assign them definitely to either stomach or duodenum. Duodenal ulcers usually occur in the first centimeter or two distal to the pylorus on the anterior or posterior wall rather than laterally.

Although some gastric ulcers are large and irregular, the typical peptic ulcer is small (about 1 cm in the duodenum; 1 to 2.5 cm in the stomach). It is characteristically "punched out," with sharply defined margins, and has overhanging mucosa producing a flashlike appearance. Its edges are not raised, and the mucosal folds converging on the ulcer are distinct to its edge (Plate 2, *D*). Malignant gastric ulcers are generally bowl shaped, with margins that are usually sloped and generally without overhanging mucosa. The edges are raised and indurated, and the mucosal folds toward the crater are interrupted by nodular mucosal or submucosal thickenings (Plate 2, *E*).

Microscopically the bed of the ulcer is seen to be covered by fibrinous exudate containing fragmented leukocytes. Separating this from the scar tissue base is fibrotic granulation tissue with a plasma cell and lymphocytic infiltrate. Occasionally, eosinophils are prominent. The scar tissue is dense and avascular and occupies a full-thickness defect in the muscularis.

Hypertrophic nerve bundles may be conspicuous, and in some cases a large artery, often thrombosed or sclerotic, may be seen. In some bleeding ulcers, such a vessel may be recognized on gross examination.

Many ulcers heal, and epithelium grows over the defect in a single layer. In time, glandlike structures may develop, but a completely normal mucous membrane is not regenerated. Because of the dense scar, the muscle does not regenerate, and evidence of the ulcer remains indefinitely.

Complications. The principal complications of peptic ulcer are hemorrhage, perforation, and obstruction. Which, if any, occurs is dependent in part on the location of the ulcer. Both gastric and duodenal ulcers are subject to massive hemorrhage. Duodenal ulcers are especially prone to perforation. Any ulcer, but especially those located posteriorly, may bleed in smaller amounts, producing melena or evidence of occult blood in the stool.

Anterior duodenal ulcers may perforate into the free peritoneal cavity, with resultant generalized peritonitis. Perforating posterior ulcers more often penetrate the pancreas, producing intractable pain. Posterior perforation also may occur into the lesser peritoneal sac, leading to localized peritonitis. The omentum or adhesions to adjacent organs also may serve to localize peritoneal inflammation. The peritonitis from perforated peptic ulcer is initially a chemical inflammation, but bacterial contamination soon follows.

Pyloric obstruction may be a complication of an ulcer, gastric or duodenal, situated near the pylorus. It usually results from a combination of cicatricial narrowing and spasm. The stomach becomes greatly dilated and hypertrophied.

The development of carcinoma has been referred to as one of the complications of peptic ulcer. It seems probable that carcinoma can develop in a preexisting ulcer, but it is equally probable that it is a rare event. It is extremely difficult to establish the occurrence of such a sequence of events in any particular case.

A complication of surgical treatment of ulcer is the development of a marginal (stomal) ulcer—peptic ulceration of the jejunum just distal to the site of anastomosis with the stomach after gastroenterostomy or gastric resection with gastrojejunostomy. Such ulcers may perforate. If perforation into the transverse colon takes place, gastrojejunocolic fistula is the result.

Inflammatory bowel disease

The term *inflammatory bowel disease* (IBD) includes regional enteritis (Crohn's disease, CD) and ulcerative colitis (UC). Although they have many common features, most cases can be classified as either CD or UC on the basis of clinical, roentgenographic, and pathologic findings. The incidence of IBD is obscured because of inaccuracies in diagnosis. There is a preponderance in whites, especially Jews. Men and women are about equally affected, with a slightly greater incidence of UC in women. Both diseases can occur at any age but are more common in young adults, with a peak incidence at 20 to 30 years of age.

Etiology. Although much has been written regarding the cause of IBD, it remains unknown.[265] Search for infectious agents has not been fruitful, but injecting homogenates of UC or CD tissue into animals has produced pathologic changes in their bowel.[50,213] A genetic role has been considered important in view of a familial incidence and an association with ankylosing spondylitis, which is known to have genetic transmission. Psychogenic factors have been considered important in UC. More recently an immune-mediated mechanism for both diseases has been given much attention.[78,147,187,188]

Clinical features. The onset of both diseases may be acute or insidious; their course is protracted. UC is characterized by exacerbation and remission, whereas CD is chronic and progressive. Diarrhea and rectal bleeding occur in both diseases but are less frequent and less severe in CD. Perirectal abscesses, fistulas, and bowel strictures are common in CD.

Ulcerative colitis

It is frequently stated that UC begins in the rectum or sigmoid and progresses to involve part or all of the colon. This is not universally accepted, and it is possible that the theory is based on the relative ease of establishing the diagnosis by proctoscopic examination.

When the whole colon is examined, almost all of it is affected in the majority of cases. When a limited segment is involved, it is usually in the left half. It is probable that some of the instances of segmental distribution really represent regional enteritis or enterocolitis. The terminal ileum is involved in approximately one fourth of cases, almost always in direct continuity with colonic disease. The appearance of the colon varies greatly in different stages of the disease. Invariably there is hyperemia, and the mucosa is dark red or purplish red and velvety (Fig. 24-9). At first tiny erosions

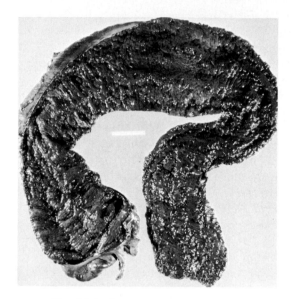

Fig. 24-9. Chronic ulcerative colitis.

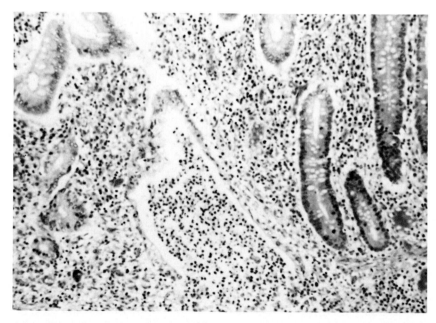

Fig. 24-10. Acute ulcerative colitis showing crypt abscess *(center)* and depletion of mucin production by epithelial cells. (63×.)

appear, later becoming deeper and coalescing to form linear ulcers, which have the appearance of longitudinal furrows distributed in the long axis of the colon. The ulcers are often undermining, partially freeing ragged remnants of mucous membrane. In occasional acutely progressing cases, the entire colon is extremely friable and bleeds freely. The muscle is thickened, apparently by contraction, and rigid, having lost all or part of its distensibility. This produces shortening as well as narrowing, and as the disease progresses, the colon increasingly resembles a garden hose. Inasmuch as chronic UC is a disease of remissions and exacerbations, periods of relative quiescence and healing alternate with periods of activity.

The earliest histologic lesion in most cases is a crypt abscess, the accumulation of neutrophils in the crypts of Lieberkühn (Fig. 24-10). The abscesses tend to coalesce to form enlarging, shallow ulcers. Other usual changes of inflammation, that is, hyperemia, edema, hemorrhage, and, more deeply, accumulation of lymphocytes and plasma cells, are present. Frequently, eosinophils and basophils are present in impressive numbers. Some authors have emphasized vasculitis as an early feature, but this is striking only in occasional cases. UC is primarily a mucosal disease, with infrequent and usually limited involvement of the other layers, whereas regional enteritis is a disease of the submucosa and deeper tissues. Also, the inflammation of UC is not characteristically productive of abundant fibrous scar tissue. Granulomas with giant cells, so frequently found in regional enteritis, are only an occasional finding in UC. When the ulcers heal, they are covered by a single layer of epithelium. Although there is an attempt to re-form crypts, regeneration is not complete, and structural abnormalities persist. In the quiescent chronic stage, the mucosa remains red and granular. As noted in the discussion of regional enteritis, chronic UC is to be distinguished from granulomatous colitis.

Pseudopolyps are a frequent and striking finding in UC. They consist of polypoid masses of granulation tissue that include distorted, inflamed crypts, often with hyperplastic epithelium. In contrast to adenomatous polyps, they vary greatly in size and shape, may be long and pendulous, and show no clear distinction between stalk and main body of the polyp. True adenomatous polyps do occur, however, in association with these inflammatory pseudopolyps.

Crohn's disease

Unlike UC, Crohn's disease may involve any portion of the gastrointestinal tract, though it is most commonly found in the terminal ileum, often with extension into the cecum and sometimes into the ascending colon as well. In more than half of the cases, multiple areas of both small and large intestine are involved in segmental fashion; that is, lengths of normal intestine separate areas of disease (so-called skip areas). Changes may be limited to the colon segmentally or may involve the whole organ. Crohn's disease of the colon (granulomatous colitis) is being recognized with greater frequency (Fig. 24-11). Anal lesions are often associated with lesions of the small and large bowel and may be the first manifestation of the disease. The inflammatory changes

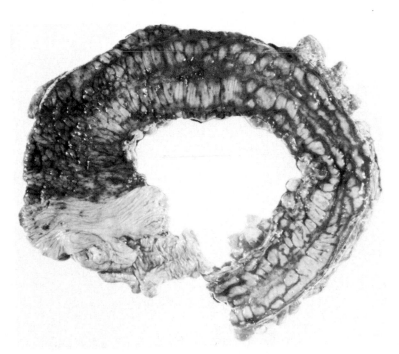

Fig. 24-11. Granulomatous colitis (Crohn's disease of colon) involving almost entire large bowel.

are nonspecific and more or less granulomatous. The mucosal surface has a red, nodular, cobblestone-like appearance, with multiple linear and serpiginous ulcerations often extending varying distances into the bowel wall. All coats of the diseased intestine are thickened— the mucosa by inflammatory infiltration, chiefly lymphocytes and plasma cells, the submucosa and subserosa by fibrosis, and the muscularis by hypertrophy (Fig. 24-12).

Histologically, irregular ulceration with a neutrophilic reaction is seen. Crypt abscesses are not so conspicuous as in UC. In the preserved mucous membrane, the glands are dilated, goblet cells are absent or

decreased in number, and Paneth cells are more prominent than usual. Glands resembling Brunner's glands of the duodenum or pyloric glands are frequently seen. The muscularis mucosae is hypertrophied, and nerves in the involved segment are increased in number, size, and prominence. Lymphoid nodules are conspicuous in the submucosa and often in the subserosa as well (Fig. 24-13). Noncaseating tubercles composed of epithelioid cells, with occasional multinucleated giant cells, are conspicuous in some areas. They gave rise to speculation of an etiologic identity with Boeck's sarcoid, an idea that has since been abandoned. It has been suggested that the recurrence rate is less in cases with granulomas.[112] Deep ulcers may give rise to sinus tracts and perforations, which usually are walled off by omentum or adhesions. Fistulas may complicate long-standing cases. They may be internal, involving other organs or other segments of intestine, or external, opening on the skin of the abdomen after surgical procedures. The lymph nodes are enlarged and usually show nonspecific inflammatory changes but may contain granulomas like those in the intestine.

Complications

Intestinal and extraintestinal complications occur frequently with CD and UC, some being common to both but with greater frequency in one. Bowel obstruction from stricture or adhesions, fistulas, or perforation is more frequent in CD. Acute toxic megacolon resulting in bowel perforation occurs in a small percentage of cases of IBD and is more common in UC. Carcinoma is a well-known complication of UC, the incidence being 3% to 5% of patients with long-standing disease.[221] Un-

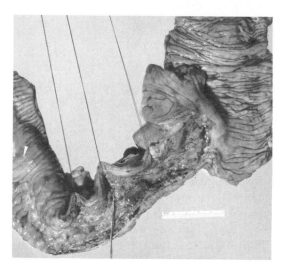

Fig. 24-12. Regional enteritis of terminal ileum. Notice abrupt cessation of pathologic change at ileocecal valve.

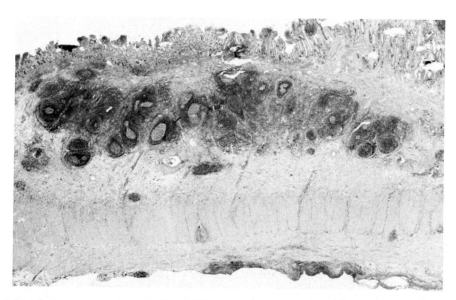

Fig. 24-13. Crohn's disease. Wall is thickened with conspicuous lymphoid nodules in the submucosa and subserosa. (75×.)

like bowel carcinoma unassociated with UC, the tumors are often multiple and uniformly distributed throughout the colon, tend to be flat and infiltrative, and histologically are of a higher-grade malignancy. The frequency of carcinoma in these patients has prompted repeated examinations for its early detection and treatment.[258,338] Carcinoma associated with CD occurs, but its frequency is not so great as with UC.[55,132,326]

Extraintestinal complications develop in a significant proportion of patients with IBD during the course of their disease.[5] Among these are hepatobiliary tract abnormalities, that is, fatty metamorphosis, pericholangitis, primary sclerosing cholangitis, chronic active hepatitis, cirrhosis, and bile duct carcinoma[72,163]; arthritis; ankylosing spondylitis; erythema nodosum; pyoderma gangrenosum; and iritis.

Appendicitis

Acute appendicitis is uncommon at the extremes of age and is most frequently seen in older children and young adults.[56] The most important factor in its pathogenesis is obstruction of the lumen,[322] with the most frequent cause being a fecalith, a molded mass of inspissated fecal material that may develop rock-hard consistency. Fecaliths are found in at least three fourths of acutely inflamed appendices and in virtually all that are gangrenous. In youth the lymphoid tissue of the mucous membrane may become sufficiently hyperplastic, at times in association with systemic infection, to produce obstruction leading to appendicitis or to cause symptoms and signs indistinguishable from those of mild acute appendiceal inflammation. Other causes of obstruction are scars representing a residuum of previous attacks of appendicitis, tumors, external bands, adhesions, rarely masses of parasites[273] (especially pinworms), foreign bodies, and possibly spasm of the muscle at the base of the appendix. The immediate cause of acute appendicitis is bacterial infection from the intestinal lumen, though bacterial invasion from the bloodstream in systemic disease is possible. All species of bacteria common to the intestinal tract can be identified, and usually multiple organisms can be isolated from an individual case.[7]

Inflammation of limited extent may manifest itself grossly only by mild hyperemia. Microscopic examination[302] may show only small amounts of purulent exudate in the lumen, though careful study may reveal one or more foci of inflammation with ulceration of the mucosa. Many examples of focal appendicitis are not merely an early phase of diffuse inflammation but also a milder form of the disease, perhaps dependent on temporary or incomplete obstruction by such mechanisms as lymphoid hyperplasia or muscle spasm. The inflammation may appear to be limited to the muscle coat or subserosa, or both, but careful search usually shows mucosal involvement.

Hyperemia and margination of leukocytes in the peripheral blood vessels of the appendix or even infiltration of polymorphonuclear leukocytes into the subserosal tissues may occur as a result of trauma during a surgical procedure, particularly if appendectomy is performed incidentally after a complex operation. Inflammatory change in the serosa and subserosa (periappendicitis) may be associated with disease primarily outside the appendix (such as salpingitis). At times a few neutrophilic leukocytes may be found in the lumen of an incidentally removed appendix without any evidence of inflammation of the appendiceal wall.

Diffuse acute appendicitis almost always occurs in an obstructed appendix. Increased intraluminal pressure compromises the blood supply, and thus the effects of ischemia and bacterial infection contribute to an anatomic picture that is dependent on the time when the appendix is removed. Degrees of ulceration of the mucous membrane, infiltration of leukocytes, and hemorrhagic necrosis result in a distended appendix whose vessels are engorged and whose surface is dulled by a fibrinopurulent exudate. Perforation[100] or sloughing of part or all of the appendix may result in peritonitis, which may be generalized, or walled off to form an appendiceal abscess. Infrequently encountered complications are pylephlebitis and liver abscess.

Not every instance of appendicitis follows this course. If tissue destruction is minimal, resolution or cicatrization occurs. Occasionally, true chronic inflammation of the appendix occurs, usually associated with fistula formation or a foreign body (intestinal content) after acute appendicitis with perforation. Otherwise true chronic appendicitis as a distinct entity does not exist.

Obliteration of part or all of the appendiceal lumen by a mixture of fibrous tissue, lymphocytes, lymphoid follicles, and nerve bundles is common. Although frequently referred to as obliterative appendicitis, there is no evidence that it is the result of inflammatory disease.

The appendix may be involved in diseases primarily affecting other portions of the gastrointestinal tract, such as Crohn's disease, typhoid fever, and amebiasis and in certain systemic diseases (such as measles). In the prodromal stage of measles, characteristic Warthin-Finkeldey giant cells may be seen in the lymphoid tissue of the appendix, as well as in the lymphoid tissues of the rest of the body.[66]

Many parasites may be found in the appendix. *Enterobius vermicularis* is the parasite most often encountered and may be noted on gross and histologic examination.[273] Ordinarily they merely inhabit the appendix and have no relationship to appendiceal disease. On oc-

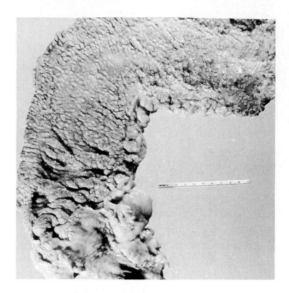

Fig. 24-14. Pseudomembranous enterocolitis.

casion, however, they may penetrate the wall and become the center of granulomatous inflammatory reaction.

Pseudomembranous enterocolitis

Pseudomembranous enterocolitis is a term used to describe an often lethal gastrointestinal lesion characterized by discrete, raised, yellow-green, adherent, sometime coalescing plaques separated by normal or edematous congested mucosa (Fig. 24-14). Any part of the intestinal tract may be involved, but the ileum and colon are more common. The pseudomembrane is composed of mucin, fibrin, nuclear debris, and neutrophils. The mucosa underlying the pseudomembrane may be partially or completely necrotic.[246]

Its occurrence in a variety of situations indicates that more than one cause may be involved. There has been an association with major surgical procedures (usually of the intestinal tract); ischemic cardiovascular disease; hypotension; staphylococcal infection; heavy metal poisoning; septicemia; uremia; colonic neoplasm with obstruction[123]; and a variety of antibiotics.[19] Studies indicate the toxin of *Clostridium difficile* to be the cause among the antibiotic group.[20,21,179]

Tuberculosis

Primary intestinal tuberculosis, ordinarily the result of ingestion of foods (especially dairy products) infected with the bovine tubercle bacillus, has become rare in the United States. Tuberculosis of the gastrointestinal tract is almost invariably associated with advanced open pulmonary disease with discharge from the lung lesions, and subsequent swallowing, of large numbers of bacilli. In fatal pulmonary tuberculosis, gastrointestinal involvement is quite common, and in disseminated disease, gastrointestinal lesions may be widespread.[2]

The usual isolated gastrointestinal lesion involves the ileocecal or anal region.[61] Rarely the esophagus, stomach, or intestine may be involved. Differentiation must be made from other granulomatous conditions—Crohn's disease,[300] sarcoidosis, syphilis, fungal and parasitic infestations, and talc and barium granuloma.

Necrotizing enterocolitis

Necrotizing enterocolitis is an inflammatory process that involves primarily the mucosa and submucosa or the entire wall of the terminal ileum and varying lengths of the colon, principally of premature infants within the first few days of life and less commonly full-term infants or children in the first 2 months of life. Air, either superficial in the bowel wall or in the peritoneum, is sometimes an accompaniment and in the latter site may be an aid in recognizing the condition by x-ray examination.[309] Factors considered important in the etiology of the condition are ischemia resulting from a Shwartzman-like reaction, shunting of blood from the involved areas as might occur with hypoxia and anoxia that is commonly seen in these infants, bacterial infections, and endotoxins. The disease is rapidly progressive and requires aggressive supportive therapy and surgical intervention in some instances if a cure is to be effected.

Fungal infections

Involvement of the gastrointestinal tract, in particular the esophagus and stomach, by fungi of the genus *Candida* is not an uncommon finding at necropsy in patients who had chronic debilitating diseases or received prolonged intensive antibiotic therapy. Other fungi, for example, *Mucor* and *Cryptococcus*, are rarely seen.

Intestinal histoplasmosis[263] may mimic tuberculosis in histopathologic detail, and its differentiation is made by demonstration of the causative organism either in microscopic sections or in cultures. It is most common in the ileocecal region, but widespread gastrointestinal lesions may be present as part of a generalized histoplasmosis.

When actinomycosis involves the gastrointestinal tract, it too shows predilection for the ileocecal region or appendix.[248]

Parasitic infestations

Amebiasis. Entamoeba histolytica most frequently involves the cecal or rectal region and less commonly extensive segments of the large intestine.[159] In the earliest lesions there is a minimal mononuclear and eosinophilic leukocytic infiltration associated with the

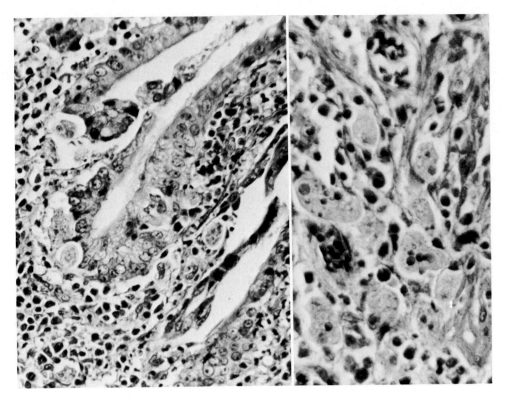

Fig. 24-15. Amebic colitis. Higher magnification demonstrates erythrocyte ingestion by trophozoites.

trophozoites penetrating the colonic epithelium.[240] This produces tiny, yellow, nodular elevations that eventuate in flask-shaped ulcerations. Organisms may be variable in number and difficult to identify without special staining procedures (Fig. 24-15). In advanced cases the mucosa may have a shaggy appearance with shreds of fibrin and tags of underlying mucous membrane attached to the margins of the ulcers. The colon may be greatly thickened, and there may be many adhesions to adjacent loops of intestine or to the mesentery. Amebic granulomas may develop.

Schistosomiasis. Ova of the parasite *Schistosoma mansoni* or *S. japonicum* in the mucosa and submocosa may excite a tubercle-like reaction and a polypoid adenomatoid hyperplasia of the mucous membrane of the colon or rectum.[74] Less often, adult worms may be found in the submucosal veins. Various other parasites that inhabit the intestinal tract are considered in Chapter 11.

Malakoplakia

A disease of unknown cause[1] generally affecting the urinary tract has been reported in the appendix and colon.[270] The histopathologic condition is identical to that seen in the urinary tract—macrophages harboring calcium-containing Michaelis-Gutmann bodies and periodic acid–Schiff–positive granules.

Acquired immunodeficiency syndrome (AIDS)

The manifestations of AIDS in the gastrointestinal tract are Kaposi's sarcoma and opportunistic infections. "Kaposi's sarcoma" involves the gastrointestinal tract in about 50% of the AIDS patients who have documented Kaposi's sarcoma of the skin.[105] The lesions, red-purple macules, plaques, or nodules, are found throughout the gastrointestinal tract and are often multiple.[320] Opportunistic infections by cytomegaloviruses,[110,205] *Cryptosporidium*,[232] *Isospora belli*,[333] *Mycobacterium avium-intracellulare* complex,[124] *Candida*,[170] and herpes simplex[279] frequently occur in the gastrointestinal tract either as primary or part of a more systemic infection. In *Mycobacterium avium-intracellulare* infection, the mucosa is filled with organisms containing foamy histiocytes with little or no inflammation. The histopathology is very similar to that of Whipple's disease and must be distinguished from it.[261,296] Homosexual men also have a high incidence of amebiasis,[274] anorectal lymphogranuloma venereum,[251] and anal condyloma and carcinoma.[60]

Other causes of gastrointestinal inflammation

Radiation. Ionizing radiation given for treatment of cancer, usually of the female generative organs, may be responsible for inflammation in one or more focal areas of the small intestine or colon. Telangiectasia, edema and inflammatory cell infiltration of the submucosa, and necrosis of mucous membrane are early changes.[108] Chronic or delayed radiation injury may not manifest itself until many years after irradiation.[30] Radiation fibrosis, endarteritis, and vascular fibrosis may lead to bowel stricture or mucosal ulceration.

Poisons. Mercury and arsenic may be responsible for nonspecific inflammation or necrosis in the colon, with the changes being less apparent and less extensive with arsenic. In addition, consumption of inorganic arsenical compounds such as Paris green may produce similar changes in the stomach and small intestine[119]

Metabolites. Accumulation of metabolic products as occurs in patients dying of uremia may be responsible for changes ranging from minimal nonspecific inflammation to extensive necrotizing colitis. Some of the lesions may represent pseudomembranous enterocolitis or other specific infection.

Collagenous colitis. Collagenous colitis, a disease of unknown cause and pathogenesis, is characterized clinically by intermittent or persistent chronic water diarrhea and histologically by a thick eosinophilic collagenous band in the subepithelial region (Fig. 24-16) throughout the colon and rectum.[103] Endoscopically the mucosa is normal. The collagenous nature of the eosinophilic collagenous band has been confirmed by ultrastructural study and immunotyping.[102] Effective therapy is not available.[321]

ANORECTAL LESIONS

Stercoraceous (stercoral) ulcers[128] are irregular and involve the mucous membrane of the rectum and less often of the colon. They result from trauma caused by impacted, inspissated fecal masses. They may be associated with perforation and peritonitis or with hemorrhage.

Colitis cystica profunda may be diffuse and involve extensive areas of the large intestine, but it usually is confined to the rectum.[324] It is characterized by mucous cysts and glands lined by goblet cells in the submucosa. It is often associated with chronic inflammatory change and extraglandular accumulation of mucin. The condition may result from extension of surface epithelium along granulation tissue tracts after deep ulceration. Colitis cystica profunda localized to the rectum is considered by some authors to be identical to "solitary rectal ulcer syndrome."[181] Lesions with a similar appearance are infrequently encountered in the stomach.

The crypts of Morgagni have traditionally been implicated in the causation of most anorectal inflammatory disease, specifically perirectal abscesses and anorectal fistulas.[241] Corresponding to the columns in the sinuses of Morgagni is a circular band, 0.3 to 1.1 cm wide of "transitional" or "cloacogenic" epithelium interposed between rectal and anal mucus membrane. This transitional epithelium, often including mucus-secreting cells, lines the sinuses of Morgagni and the anal ducts or glands that communicate with them. The distribution of the ducts and glands varies greatly. They may extend caudally penetrating the internal anal sphincter or cephalad beneath the rectal mucosa and may branch in complex fashion (Fig. 24-17). It is infection in the crypts of Morgagni and of these anal ducts that is re-

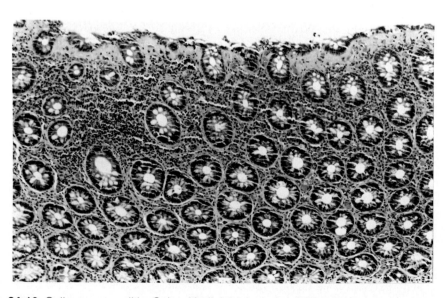

Fig. 24-16. Collagenous colitis. Subepithelial thick eosinophilic collagenous band. (87×.)

sponsible for the troublesome perianal and ischiorectal abscesses, which in turn are responsible for anal fistulas that may open internally in the region of the anorectal junction or externally on the perianal skin. Histologically, inflammation in this area is nonspecific, often with a foreign-body reaction, no doubt because of contamination with fecal matter.

Anal fissures are acute or chronic ulcers situated posteriorly in the anal canal just distal to the anorectal junction. These various anal, perianal, and anorectal lesions are insignificant in themselves, but they may be the source of great discomfort and disability.

FUNCTIONAL STATES
Gastric atrophy (atrophic gastritis)

So-called atrophic gastritis is not properly classified as an inflammatory condition. The term is used by some as a synonym for gastric atrophy. Others consider the two to be different stages of the same pathologic process.

In atrophic gastritis the mucous membrane is greatly thinned, and the gastric glands are correspondingly shortened and also widely separated.[332] On inspection

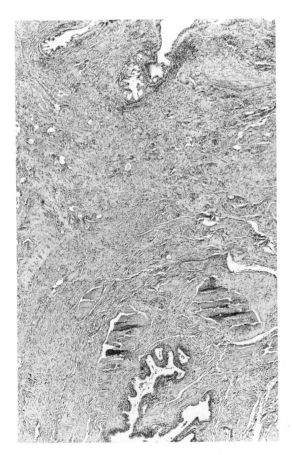

Fig. 24-17. Anal ducts. Small portion of epithelial lining of anal canal is visible above, and anal ducts occur both superficially and deep within muscle. (55×.)

with the unassisted eye, the mucosa in advanced atrophy is smooth, is patently thinned, and has a waxy cast. The striking cellular changes in the gastric glands are two: (1) a decrease in number or, in the fully developed case, complete absence of parietal cells and (2) the occurrence, usually in the deeper part of the mucosa of glands identical to those of the small intestine (Fig. 24-18, *C*). All cell types normally found in the glands of the small intestine may be represented. This change has been regarded as intestinal metaplasia by some and as heterotopia by others. The decrease or absence of parietal cells, which has been demonstrated to be associated with autoantibody in a high precentage of patients with atrophic gastritis, accounts for deficient hydrochloric acid secretion or complete achlorhydria. Large numbers of lymphocytes and plasma cells are present in the lamina propria, but the increase may be more apparent than real. The changes described occur focally in many stomachs without overt disease. They are seen more often and in more widespread and advanced degree with increased age.

Atrophic gastritis commonly is associated with gastric carcinoma,[92] but a postulated predisposing role has not been demonstrated. Advanced atrophy regularly accompanies polypoid carcinoma and adenomatous polyp. Indeed, the appearance of many of the latter and of some polypoid carcinomas strongly indicates origin from glands typical of the small intestine. Gastric atrophy, increased serum gastrin levels, and G-cell hyperplasia in the gastric antrum are frequently encountered in pernicious anemia,[182] a disease associated with achlorhydria and a high incidence of gastric carcinoma. Antibodies to parietal cells and intrinsic factor have been demonstrated in a proportion of patients with atrophic gastritis. These patients are predisposed to pernicious anemia, in contrast to those in whom the antibody cannot be demonstrated.[295] However, in general, it has been difficult to correlate the pathologic findings of atrophic gastritis with clinical disease or with roentgenographic or gastroscopic findings.

Hypertrophic gastropathy

Gastric rugal hypertrophy, called hypertrophic gastritis by some, is characterized by enlargement of the gastric mucosal folds in both length and breadth, producing thickening and convolution of the mucous membrane reminiscent of the appearance of the cerebral convolutions (Fig. 24-19). In some instances this appearance is not caused by mucosal thickening but by an increase in the submucosal connective tissue. The changes may be diffuse and pronounced or localized and of limited degree, sparing the antrum. Histologic and clinical differences have been observed in gastric rugal hypertrophy, permitting recognition of entities based on clinical and pathologic findings. Hyperchlorhydria (in some instances with extreme gastric hypersecretion), hypoproteinemia, hypochlorhydria and achlorhydria, and tumors or hyperplasias of multiple endocrine glands have been associated with gastric rugal hypertrophy. It is postulated that it is one manifestation of a syndrome consisting also in islet cell tumor, primary chief cell hyperplasia of parathyroid glands, and at times abnormalities of other endocrine glands, especially the adrenal cortex and pituitary, and having different modes of clinical expression.[217,223,227] The principal one is the Zollinger-Ellison syndrome, with

intractable peptic ulcer often in an unusual location and islet cell tumor of the pancreas or duodenum.

Mucosal alterations in hypertrophic gastropathy may be of two types, both lacking in significant inflammatory cell infiltration, thus supporting the use of the term *gastropathy* rather than gastritis: (1) Glandular hyperplasia with increased parietal and chief cells and normal or reduced surface and foveolar mucous epithelium (see Fig. 24-18, *D*) has been observed in the Zollinger-Ellison syndrome but may occur without clinical manifestations.[292] (2) In hyperplasia of the surface and foveolar

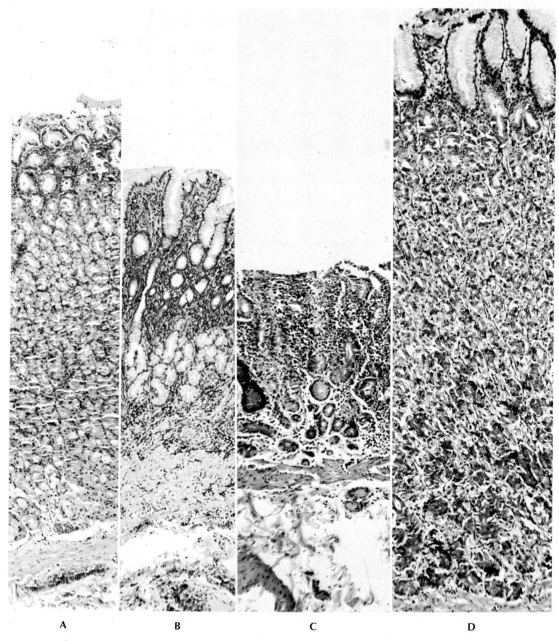

A   B   C   D

Fig. 24-18. A and **B,** Normal stomach. **A,** Fundus. **B,** Antrum. **C,** Atrophic gastritis. **D,** Gastric rugal hypertrophy. (**A** to **D,** 90×.)

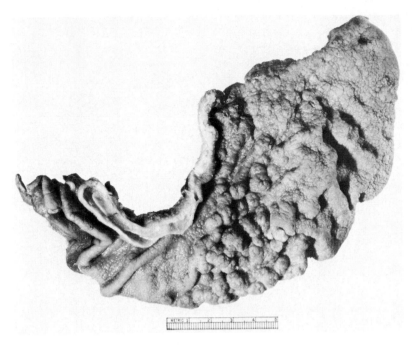

Fig. 24-19. Gastric rugal hypertrophy.

mucous cells with increased depth of the foveolas, parietal and chief cells may be normal, atrophic, or hyperplastic. This change has been observed in Ménétrier's disease, characterized by hypochlorhydria or achlorhydria and hypoproteinemia caused by albumin loss into the gastric juice.[69]

Malabsorption syndrome

The malabsorption syndrome is characterized by impaired intestinal absorption, especially of fats, and is manifested by diarrhea with bulky, foul stools, abdominal distension, and malnutrition with attendant vitamin deficiencies, all in varying degree. The clinical picture may be associated with a wide variety of underlying diseases, and the cases may be conveniently subdivided into primary and secondary groups. Among the numerous causes of secondary malabsorption are cystic fibrosis of the pancreas, chronic incomplete intestinal obstruction, surgical resection of significant segments of the gastrointestinal tract, infections (especially enteric), antibiotics, biliary tract disease, scleroderma, Whipple's disease parasitic infestations, regional enteritis, diabetes, neoplasms (notably lymphoma), and possible allergy.

Celiac sprue (nontropical sprue)

The names given to primary malabsorption or steatorrhea are celiac disease in infants and children, nontropical sprue in adults, and tropical sprue. In the first two conditions there seems to be an identical, genetically controlled abnormality resulting in sensitivity to gluten (gluten-sensitive enteropathy, GSE).[94] Elimination of gluten from the diet usually relieves the symptoms, though it does not cure the underlying defect. Refractoriness to gluten withdrawal occurs in a small percentage of cases, some of which may be associated with collagen deposition in the subepithelial portion of the lamina propria.[328] The small intestine mucosa, of the upper jejunum in particular and to a lesser extent of the duodenum and ileum, has a flat surface partially or completely lacking in villi. The mucosal crypts appear elongated, dilated, and more widely spaced than normal. The surface epithelial cells are cuboid or low columnar with irregular nuclei (Fig. 24-20, B). Numerous plasma cells and lymphocytes and fewer eosinophils and neutrophils are present in the lamina propria. Two theories of pathogenesis for the mucosal changes have been suggested: (1) toxic effect on the mucosa by increased gluten resulting from an enzyme deficiency in intestinal mucosal cells and (2) damage to mucosal cells by gluten-stimulated antibodies and lymphokines produced in the intestinal lymphoid tissue.[311] Clinical remissions and reversal of the bowel changes, though usually not complete, can be induced by a gluten-free diet. The pathologic changes are not specific for celiac disease or nontropical sprue and may be seen in tropical sprue, infectious gastroenteritis, giardiasis, and allergy to cow's milk and soybean protein.[243] A very small percentage of patients with GSE have IgA deficiency, with absence of plasma cells in the lamina propria.[8] An

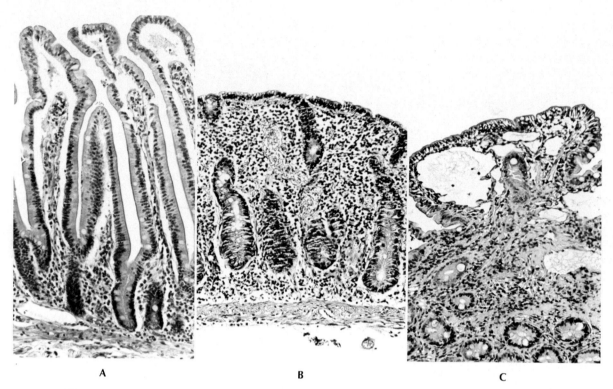

A   B   C

Fig. 24-20. A, Normal jejunum. **B,** Jejunum in nontropical sprue. **C,** Lymphangiectases of jejunum in protein-losing enteropathy. (**A** to **C,** 150×.)

association between celiac sprue of long duration and intestinal lymphoma, esophageal and small bowel carcinoma, and dermatitis herpetiformis has been noted.[42]

Tropical sprue, endemic in the topics and probably infectious in nature, is similar to celiac sprue in its clinical and morphologic expressions. The pathologic changes are usually not so noticeable and are reversible with broad-spectrum antibiotic and folic acid therapy, but they are unaffected by elimination of gluten from the diet. Macrocytic anemia is usually a feature of the disease.

Protein-losing enteropathy (exudative enteropathy)

In protein-losing enteropathy, which also may be associated with steatorrhea, large amounts of serum protein are lost in the intestine, and serum levels of both globulin and albumin are abnormally low. Like the malabsorption state, it may result from some specific gastroenteric disease state or congestive heart failure, or it may be idiopathic.[67,319]

Some of the gastrointestinal diseases that may be associated with considerable protein loss are gastric rugal hypertrophy, sprue, regional enteritis, and ulcerative colitis. Constrictive pericarditis is the most important underlying cardiac lesion. In some patients with "idiopathic" protein-losing enteropathy, dilatation of lym-

phatic channels (lymphangiectasia) in the intestinal mucosa and mesentery has been demonstrated (Fig. 24-20, C). Some of these latter patients have had systemic lymphatic abnormalities,[245] but in others no cause of lymphatic obstruction is found.

GASTROINTESTINAL MANIFESTATIONS OF SYSTEMIC DISEASE

The gastrointestinal tract may be the site of involvement in some diseases involving multiple organs. Such involvement may produce symptoms, which are the first manifestations of the disease, or it may be occult. In both situations biopsy of the intestinal tract may be helpful and an easily accessible means of establishing the diagnosis. Symptoms that may be present—diarrhea, steatorrhea, and those of malabsorption—may be unassociated with histologic changes in the gut or there may be degrees of villous mucosal atrophy. Gastrointestinal manifestations may be seen in a variety of endocrine diseases (diabetes,[10] thyrotoxicosis, hyperparathyroidism, and hypoparathyroidism), skin diseases[191] (dermatitis herpetiformis), pseudoxanthoma elasticum, Ehlers-Danlos syndrome, and mastocytosis.

Cystic fibrosis

The most important gastrointestinal manifestation is malabsorption with steatorrhea and azotorrhea, resulting from pancreatic achylia, and deficient secretion of the intestinal glands. Approximately 10% of patients have intestinal obstruction in the newborn period as the result of meconium ileus.[73] The abnormal accumulations of meconium distend the loops of intestine, which in one third of the cases rotate upon themselves producing a volvulus. Another complication is intestinal perforation in utero with the development of sterile peritonitis, so-called meconium peritonitis.[77] The escape of epithelial cells, mucus, and cellular debris usually stimulates a foreign body reaction, and calcification, visible roentgenographically, frequently takes place (see also p. 1348).

Progressive systemic sclerosis (scleroderma)

Although any portion of the intestinal tract may be involved, the esophagus is the most frequent site.[115] There is hyaline sclerosis of the submucosa with lymphocytic infiltration, as well as atrophy and fibrosis of the muscularis. The overlying mucous membrane may be thin and become ulcerated.[140] In the esophagus the rigidity of the wall may predispose the patient to regurgitation of acidic gastric juice from which there may be further complications.

Other collagen diseases, dermatomyositis and lupus erythematosus,[329] may also involve the gastrointestinal tract, affecting the musculature in the former condition and blood vessels in both instances.

Whipple's disease (intestinal lipodystrophy)

Originally considered to be a disorder of intestinal function involving lipid metabolism, Whipple's disease is now recognized as a systemic disease.[23,280] Aggregates of large macrophages bearing intracytoplasmic sickle-shaped inclusions in the intestinal mucous membrane (Fig. 24-21, A). and mesenteric lymph nodes that react strongly with the periodic acid–Schiff stain dominate the microscopic picture, but similar deposits have also been described in virtually every organ of the body. Lipid deposits in virtually every organ of the body. Lipid deposits are striking in lymph nodes, especially those of the mesentery, but not in the other organs. Whipple's disease is generally a condition of adult white men and may be familial. The manifestations are diarrhea, gradual wasting, and migratory polyarthritis.[189] An infectious cause has replaced the concept of a disorder of lipid metabolism. This is based on data generated from electron microscopic studies,[222,310] indicating that the "inclusions" are in fact bacilliform microorganisms (Fig. 24-21, B and C); bacterial cultures and production of the disease in rabbits[53]; and favorable response of the disease to antibiotic therapy. Many types of bacteria have been isolated from the lesions of Whipple's disease. However, when immunohistochem-

ical techniques are used, the microorganism that causes Whipple's disease contains antigens found mainly on streptococci and *Shigella* group B.[162] Host factors have also been suggested to be important in the pathogenesis of this disease, and immunologic defects have been described.[76,129,195]

Storage disease

Deposits of one of a number of substances seen in a variety of diseases—Tay-Sachs, Niemann-Pick, Fabry's, Hurler's, Gaucher's glycogen storage, and metachromatic leukoencephalopathy—may be found in ganglion cells, histiocytes, or nerve fibers in the gut.

Tangier disease is an autosomal recessive inherited disease in which there is deposition of cholesterol esters in the reticuloendothelial system as well as in histiocytes of the mucous membrane of the pharynx and intestine.[15] The disorder is benign except for a possible predisposition to atherosclerosis.

Wolman's disease[185] is also inherited as an autosomal recessive disease in which cholesterol esters may be found deposited in histiocytes in the lamina propria of the intestine as well as in the reticuloendothelial system of the liver, spleen, lymph nodes, and bone marrow. Calcification of the adrenal glands is a common accompaniment. The central nervous system appears not to be involved. The patients reported have died before attaining 6 months of age.

Congenital beta-lipoprotein deficiency, an autosomal recessive disease, manifests itself in the intestinal tract by deposition of lipid droplets in the mucosal epithelial cells with practically no fat droplets in the lamina propria and submucosa.[75] It usually manifests itself within the first 2 years of life as a mild steatorrhea and neurologic symptoms resembling Friedreich's ataxia.

The frequent involvement of the intestinal tract in these storage diseases has made biopsy of the gut an easy approach to diagnosis.[39]

Rectal biopsy has also proved useful for obtaining diagnostic information in a large number of other disease entities—schistosomiasis, amyloidosis, amebiasis, Crohn's disease, Hirschsprung's disease, melanosis coli, ulcerative colitis, pneumatosis, hemochromatosis, and the changes produced by chemotherapeutic agents and antibiotics. The finding of colonic macrophages (muciphages),[11] however, must be carefully evaluated. The variation in interpretation given to them by different authors—early phase of Whipple's disease, ceroid-containing phages, and so on—appears to be in part the result of nonuniformity in the histochemical methods employed in their study. Recent investigations carried out on surgical and necropsy specimens indicate their frequent occurrence and lack of clinical significance.[184] It appears that they are unrelated to the many storage diseases cited previously and that they are the result of

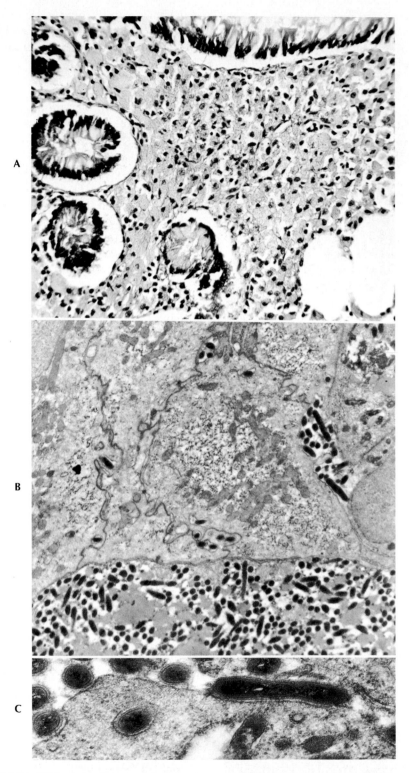

Fig. 24-21. Whipple's disease involving mucous membrane of small intestine. **A,** Pale macrophages in mucosa. **B,** Bacilliform bodies are extracellular. **C,** Encapsulated bodies are seen both intracellularly and extracellularly. (**A,** 300×; **B,** 8100×; **C,** 45,000×.)

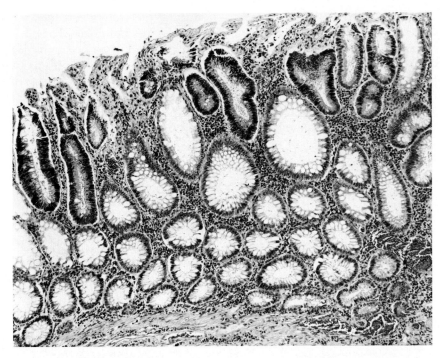

Fig. 24-22. Adenomatous (neoplastic) change in gland of colon *(upper part of field)* in contrast to normal glands. (115×.)

phagocytosis of mucin released from the goblet cells of the colonic mucous membrane.

NEOPLASMS
Adenomatous polyps, papillary adenomas, and miscellaneous polyps

Luminal projections of the gastrointestinal mucosa may result from a variety of neoplastic and nonneoplastic changes ultimately detected only by microscopic examination. Most commonly they are epithelial alterations, but they may result from submucosal mesenchymal lesions. The polypoid glandular neoplasms, adenomatous (tubular), papillary (villous), or mixed tubulopapillary, occur throughout the gastrointestinal tract from the stomach to the rectum but are most frequent in the colon and rectum.[160] Their incidence increases after 30 years of age; estimates of incidence range as high as 25% to 50% in an autopsy population of the older age groups (60 to 80 years). In one fourth or more of cases the polyps are multiple, frequently but not always limited to one part of the intestine. Approximately 75% of adenomatous polyps occur in the rectum and sigmoid colon, though their exact incidence in various segments of the large intestine varies from one reported series to another.

The earliest adenomatous change that can be recognized is the replacement of lining cells of the crypts, beginning at the base, by cells that are generally taller, more slender, and more deeply staining than the nor-

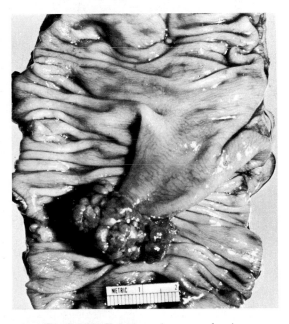

Fig. 24-23. Tubular adenoma of colon.

mal. They have hyperchromatic nuclei and lack vacuoles, indicative of mucin secretion (Fig. 24-22). Mitotic figures may be numerous. Proliferation progresses to the formation of epithelial tubular aggregates, grossly manifested as a lobulated, berrylike, tubular adenoma that is usually less than 2 cm in diameter and attached to the intestinal wall by a pedicle of varying length, composed of normal mucous membrane (Fig. 24-23). Villous adenomas are usually larger and sessile and have a papillary configuration (Fig. 24-24, *B*). The papillae consist of fingerlike projections with a core of lamina propria covered by epithelial cells (Fig. 24-24, *A*). Large villous adenomas have been recognized as the occasional cause of severe fluid and electrolyte loss pro-

ducing electrolyte imbalance, which may threaten life.[330] The glandular changes are usually confined to the mucosa but on occasion may be seen in fibrovascular stalk, sometimes associated with recent or old hemorrhage (Fig. 24-25). This has been regarded as pseudoinvasion, possibly resulting from twisting of the polyp's stalk.[228,249] These foci are not to be confused with invasive carcinoma, from which they differ in hav-

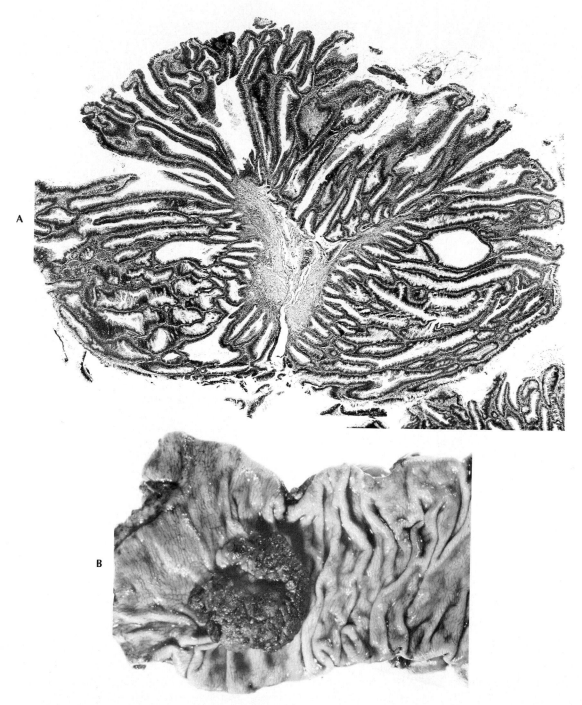

Fig. 24-24. A, Papillary (villous) adenoma of rectum. Papillary configuration readily apparent. **B,** Papillary adenoma of colon. (**A,** 25×.)

ing benign cytologic characteristics. Some polypoid epithelial lesions of the colon bear a resemblance to the adenomatous polyp and are commonly confused with it. Abnormal folds or minute elevations of the mucous membrane are sometimes mistaken for adenomas on proctoscopic or sigmoidoscopic examination. Rather frequently occurring polyps, best termed hyperplastic or metaplastic, are small, flat lesions composed of en-

larged, regular glands with scalloped luminal borders showing excessive mucin secretion but lacking the neoplastic change and malignant potential of the adenomatous polyp described previously (Fig. 24-26). Another lesion that must be distinguished from the adenomatous polyp and does not have any relationship to cancer is the juvenile polyp. Also referred to as a retention polyp, it is usually a single, smooth, rounded nodule, 1

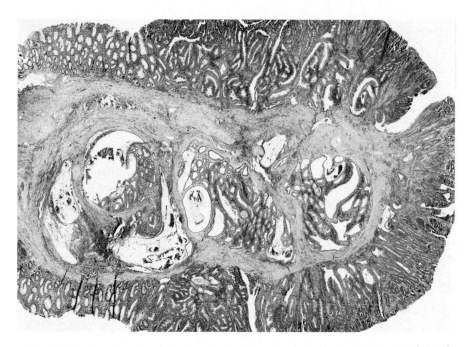

Fig. 24-25. Misplaced epithelium (pseudoinvasion) in tubular adenoma. (15×.)

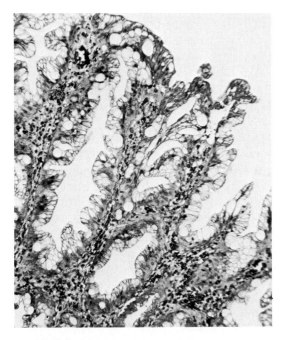

Fig. 24-26. Hyperplastic polyp of colon. (175×.)

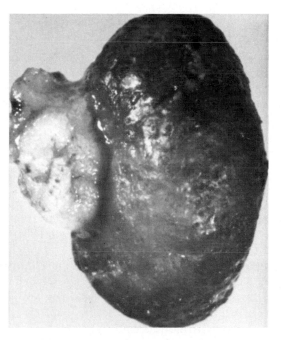

Fig. 24-27. Juvenile polyp of rectum.

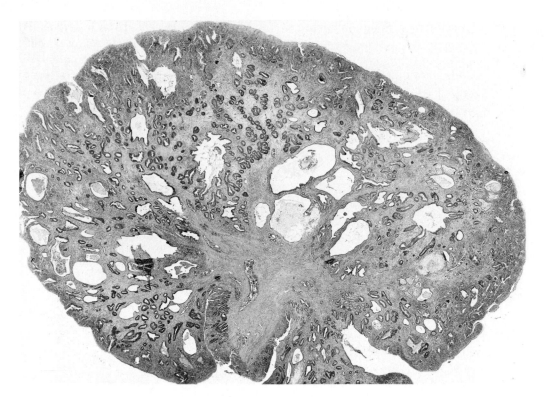

Fig. 24-28. Juvenile polyp of rectum. Cystic dilatation of glands and abundant stroma. (13×.)

to 3 cm in diameter (Fig. 24-27), composed of large, hyperplastic or cystic glands with an abundant, well-vascularized fibrous stroma infiltrated by inflammatory cells (Fig. 24-28). Multiple lesions in the gastrointestinal tract or colon alone, sometimes familial, have been reported.[44,266] The nodules are supported on a stalk of normal mucous manifestation. Bleeding is the most frequent clinical manifestation. Juvenile polyp is a lesion of children, though similar polyps occasionally occur in adults.[200] They have been regarded as hamartomas or the result of inflammation.[262] Polypoid inflammatory or nonspecific granuloma-like nodules, inflammatory polyps, are occasionally seen as solitary lesions, but the inflammatory polyp or pseudopolyp is generally seen in chronic ulcerative colitis.

Polyps may be associated with other abnormalities. In Gardner's syndrome polyposis of the colon is associated with neoplasms of both bone and soft tissues elsewhere in the body—epidermoid cyst, fibroma, and osteomas (in the mandible and maxilla)—and sometimes with polyps in other portions in the gastrointestinal tract.

In the Cronkhite-Canada syndrome one finds multiple polyposis of the colon associated with ectodermal changes—alopecia, nail atrophy, and hyperpigmentation—as well as polyps in the stomach and small intestine. The polyps morphologically have the features of

juvenile (retention) polyps. In Turcot's syndrome polyps of the colon are present with brain tumors.[314]

In the Peutz-Jeghers syndrome, melanin spots on the buccal mucosa, lips, and digits are associated with polyps occurring almost anywhere in the gastrointestinal tract but most commonly in the upper small intestine. The disease is transmitted as a simple mendelian dominant trait, but cases without familial history have been recorded. The polyps differ from those generally found in the intestinal tract in that they are hamartomatous (that is, composed of normal-looking but irregularly arranged glands of any of the types normally occurring in the mucous membrane of origin) and may include bands of smooth muscle (Fig. 24-29). Thus parietal cells may be present in gastric polyps, Brunner's glands in duodenal lesions, and so on. The polyps of the large intestine are not always readily distinguishable from adenomatous polyps. The principal clinical manifestations of the Peutz-Jeghers syndrome are hemorrhage and intussusception. Instances of development of gastrointestinal carcinoma in patients with this syndrome have been documented, but progression of the Peutz-Jeghers polyps to cancer must be rare, as is the association of sex cord ovarian tumors with this syndrome.[231,276] Cytologic atypia is frequent but is apparently not significant.

In familial polyposis (Plate 2, C), the entire colon is studded with polyps, usually tiny and sessile. The disease is transmitted as an autosomal dominant trait and usually is manifested in childhood or adolescence. The incidence of carcinoma in this disease is so high and the cancers occur so often in young adults (or even adolescents) that total colectomy is geneally regarded as the treatment of choice once the diagnosis has been established.

Relationship of tubular and papillary adenomas to carcinoma of colon

Epidemiologic, histologic, and experimental studies support the concept of the precancerous nature of both tubular and villous adenomas, with the incidence of malignant transformation being greater among the latter tumors.[178] The malignant potential of the colonic adenomas has been found to be related to size, histologic type (tubular or villous), and degree of epithelial dysplasia.[131,224]

GASTRIC POLYPS

Benign epithelial proliferations in the stomach are of three varieties: hyperplastic, adenomatous, and hamartomatous, in that order of frequency.[211] The hyperplastic polyp, which is small and pedunculated or sessile and smooth surfaced, is often multiple, occurs anywhere in the stomach, and represents approximately 75% to 95% of the polyps. Polyps are composed of the foveolar portion of the gland, dilated with mucin and lined by a mucin-producing epithelium with fewer parietal and chief cells or pyloric glands, depending on their location in the stomach (Fig. 24-30). They merge imperceptibly with the surrounding mucosa and are considered to be regenerative rather than neoplastic. They have no significant malignant potential, but carcinoma in other portions of the stomach is frequently associated with them. Adenomatous polyps, on the other hand, are not only commonly associated with carcinoma elsewhere in the stomach but are often the site of malignant transformation. They may be tubular or villous and are formed of poorly differentiated epithelium, resembling the colonic adenoma and differing from the adjacent gastric mucosa, which may be atrophic with intestinal metaplasia. Despite the fact that some gastric cancers may arise in adenomatous polyps, not all polyps become invasive cancers, and relatively few cancers can be traced to polyps as precursors. Hamartomatous polyps, composed of differentiated glandular or stromal cells normally present in the area of origin, are least frequently encountered. They and the adenomatous polyps may be associated with polyps in other portions of the gastrointestinal tract: hereditary Peutz-Jeghers syndrome, familial or juvenile polyposis, Gardner's syndrome, and nonhereditary Cronkhite-Canada syndrome.

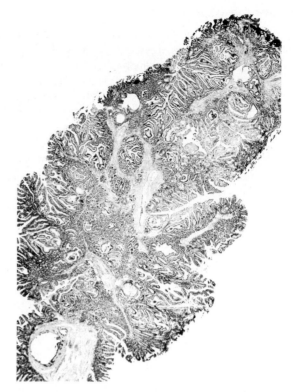

Fig. 24-29. Polyp of ileum from patient with Peutz-Jeghers syndrome. Notice irregularities and variegated appearance. (16×; from Horn, R.C., Jr., Payne, W.A., and Fine, G.: Arch. Pathol. **76:**29, 1963.)

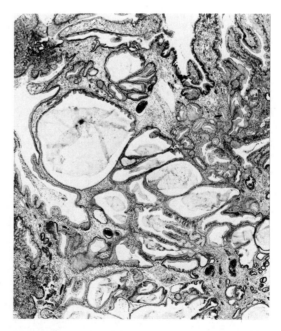

Fig. 24-30. Hyperplastic polyp of stomach. (15×.)

Carcinoma of the colon and rectum

Incidence. The incidence of cancer is higher in the colon and rectum than in any part of the body except the skin. Roughly three fourths of carcinomas of the large intestine occur in the rectum and sigmoid colon. Of the remainder, a majority arise in the cecum and ascending and descending colon, with the flexures and transverse colon being least often affected.

Histology and morbid anatomy. Generally they are well-differentiated tumors that reproduce the appearance of normal colonic glands more or less faithfully (Fig. 24-31). The usual cellular aberrations of neoplasia are generally obvious. Mucin production by tumors is variable, but tumors are sometimes capable of secreting very large amounts of mucin. Signet-ring cells (cells in which a large vacuole of mucin pushes the nucleus off to one side) may be conspicuous in some of these tumors (Fig. 24-32). In others, signet-ring cells may grow within the colonic wall without any readily apparent mucosal lesions, thus producing a linitis plastica type of growth.[283]

Distinct differences between the growth patterns of carcinoma of the right and left half of the colon can be observed. Those in the right colon are usually bulky and may show extensive necrosis because they outgrow their blood supply (Fig. 24-33, *A*). Occult bleeding is common, and the initial symptoms may be generalized weakness and anemia. In the more distal portions of the colon, the tumor frequently has a napkin-ring configuration (Fig. 24-33, *B*). Considerable fibrous tissue stroma accompanies the tumor and accounts for contraction and narrowing of the bowel lumen and thus a higher incidence of obstruction than carcinoma in the right side of the colon. Carcinomas of the rectum do not have a characteristic gross anatomic pattern. Bleeding is a common symptom. Many are discovered on routine proctoscopic or digital examination. Not uncommon in the rectum is the bulky "colloid" carcinoma, a varicolored mass with extensive ulceration. The smaller, more or less flat carcinomas that occur in the rectum and sigmoid colon commonly undermine the peripheral normal mucous membrane as they grow centrifugally. It is thus possible to obtain only overlying normal mucosa by a proctoscopic or a sigmoidoscopic biopsy, if the forceps bite is not deep enough.

Spread.[127] By the time the lesion is first observed, penetration of the muscular wall with involvement of the serosa and subserosa has usually occurred. Of greatest significance to the patient's longevity is spread via the lymphatics.[111] Extension is generally to anatomically predictable lymph nodes proximal to the growth. Knowledge of the anatomy of the lymphatic circulation and associated lymph nodes is the basis for properly planned surgical treatment of carcinoma in general, as well as specifically of carcinoma of the colon and rectum. Metastatic spread bypasses uninvolved nodes infrequently. In the laboratory the isolation of lymph nodes and demonstration of lymph node metastases are facilitated by clearing techniques.

Blood-vascular spread of colonic cancer is also highly significant.[219] Cancer cells have been found circulating in the bloodstream, but their significance remains incompletely understood. The finding of cancer cells in the circulating blood and the establishment of metastatic foci are not synonymous. In general, when venous invasion and blood-borne metastases are present, local growth and lymphatic spread are also extensive. However, striking examples are encountered of extensive venous dissemination of otherwise localized carcinomas and of locally far-advanced highly invasive tumors without significant lymphatic or venous spread.

The bulky tumors producing large amounts of mucin are prone to spread widely over the peritoneal surface and are in contrast to the usual carcinomas of the large intestine. This type of spread may result in the formation of a metastatic tumor mass palpable on rectal examination in the rectovesical or rectouterine space, the so-called rectal shelf. Implantation of cancer cells at the suture line of intestinal anastomosis or in the peritoneum is another mode of tumor spread.[288]

Several classifications of colonic and rectal carcinoma, the most important of which are based on degree of differentiation and on the extent of spread both directly through the intestinal wall and via the lymphatics, as proposed by Dukes,[82,83] correlate reasonably well with the results of surgical treatment. The 5-year survival rates after intestinal resection vary from 15% to 20% to better than 60% depending on the parts of the intestine involved and the extent of the disease at the time of diagnosis and treatment. The foregoing figures take into account only tumors not so far advanced as to be considered inoperable.

Carcinoma of the stomach

Incidence. The incidence of carcinoma of the stomach varies greatly in various parts of the world and among various peoples. It is known to be particularly frequent in Japan and is very rare among the Malay population of Java but not rare among the Chinese inhabitants of Java. In Iceland it accounts for 35% to 45% of all fatal cancers in males. This high incidence has been attributed to the consumption of considerable amounts of smoked fish and meat, particularly the former.[84] It thus appears that the geographic variation in the incidence of gastric carcinoma may depend, at least in part, on the dietary customs and resultant exposure to carcinogens. The incidence in women is about half that in men.

Classification. Most carcinomas of the stomach arise from the mucus-secreting cells. Differentiation is vari-

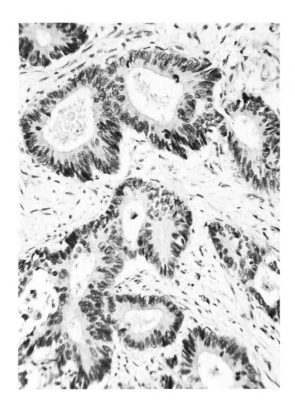

Fig. 24-31. Typical well-differentiated adenocarcinoma of colon. (300×.)

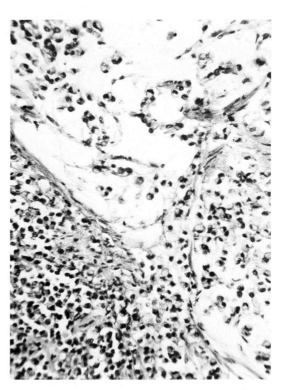

Fig. 24-32. Colloid (mucinous) carcinoma of cecum. Both patterns of pools of mucin and of sheets of individual signet-ring cells are seen. (300×.)

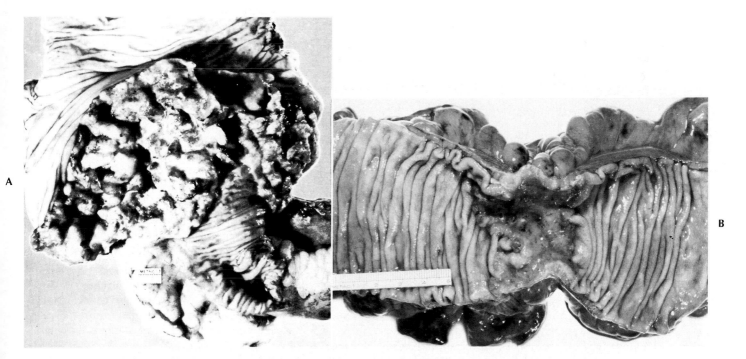

Fig. 24-33. A, Characteristic bulky, ulcerated carcinoma of right side of colon. Lesion in cecum. **B,** Characteristic constricting, "napkin-ring" carcinoma of left side of colon.

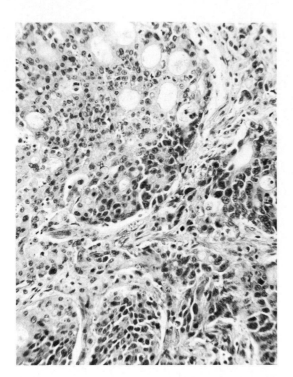

Fig. 24-34. Carcinoma of stomach showing limited degree of glandular differentiation. (300×.)

able as to the extent and regularity of gland formation, mucus secretion, cytologic features, and so on, but in general they tend to be less well differentiated and less characteristic than the carcinomas of the colon and rectum (Fig. 24-34). The most common site of involvement is the antrum on or near the greater curvature. Ulcerative cancers in particular have a predilection for location in proximity to the greater curvature or to the pylorus.

Their association with several mucosal changes—atrophic gastritis, intestinal epithelial metaplasia, mucosal hypertrophy, peptic ulcer, and polyps—has been noted, but, except for the adenomatous polyp, a causal relationship is controversial.

Of the many classifications of gastric carcinoma, a large proportion lack the merit of clinical significance. An exception is that of Borrman. It is based upon the extensiveness of the lesion as judged by gross examination, showing a gradual gradation between the less malignant tumors that grow mainly within the lumen of the stomach and those prognostically less favorable, which are deeply invasive and penetratee the gastric wall. Stout's classification[294] is somewhat similar, being basd upon direction of growth and the resultant gross configuration of the tumor. He recognized (1) a fungating or polypoid type, (2) an ulcerating type (ulcer cancer), (3) a superficial spreading type, and (4) a diffusely spreading type (linitis plastica).

Polypoid or fungating gastric carcinomas have a particularly favorable prognosis. An exception is the fungating carcinoma of the cardioesophageal junction, which is prone to become very extensive, both locally and in terms of lymph node spread, before giving rise to symptoms. Superficial spreading is also a relatively favorable type. Unfortunately these two forms of gastric carcinoma are relatively infrequent varieities. Linitis plastica type, equally or more rare, is hopeless in its outlook.

The various classifications and their clinical correlations support the concept that tumor growth by frank infiltration offers a greater and more immediate threat to the life of the host than does the gastric cancer that grows expansively, essentially pushing aside the host tissue.[212] Defects in the classification of gastric carcinomas arise in the fact that they often cannot be assigned to any of the categories, either because they are too far advanced to yield a clue to their initial gross configuration or because they show features of tumors of two or more growth types.

Morbid anatomy. Polypoid gastric carcinomas resemble adenomatous polyps except that they are usually larger and have a less delicate and often less distinct pedicle because of carcinomatous invasion. Hyperplastic polyps are commonly seen, and atrophic gastritis is always present in stomachs that are the site of polypoid carcinomas. Pernicious anemia may be associated. Polypoid carcinomas usually show good glandular differentiation, and the neoplasic glands very often resemble those of the small intestine.

The macroscopic differences between ulcer cancers and peptic ulcers have been described in the discussion of peptic ulcer (Plate 2, *D* and *E*). The old controversy over how many gastric cancers have their origin in peptic ulcers seems to have been largely resolved. Current opinion is that a small number of gastric carcinomas may arise in preexisting ulcers. Confirmation of such an occurrence must rest on demonstration of a characteristic peptic ulcer with cancer limited to one portion of its base or margin. Caution must be exercised not to misinterpret cytologically atypical, proliferative epithelial changes in the mucous membrane at the edge of an ulcer as malignant. A majority of ulcer cancers are malignant lesions from their inception, either because of primarily deeply penetrating growth or because of early peptic ulcerations of a small cancer. Ulcerative cancer has no specific histologic features.

The superficial spreading type is a distinctive variety of gastric carcinoma that spreads superficially in the mucosa or submucosa of the stomach forming a serpiginous lesion that may cover a large portion of the mucosal surface. Even without deeper penetration, lymph node metastases may take place. This type of tumor may be multicentric.[106,114]

In the linitis plastica or diffusely spreading type of carcinoma, the wall of the entire stomach is thickened, more or less uniformly, by neoplastic infiltration and new fibrous tissue production. The shrunken stomach with its relatively rigid wall has earned the descriptive term "leather-bottle stomach" (Plate 2, *F*). Characteristically the mucosa displays no focal lesion, though it may show thickening and irregularities, with flattening and distortion of its folds. Tumor infiltration involves all layers, but the submucosa and subserosa are chiefly affected. Lymphatic permeation is usual within the gastric wall proper, as well as into the adjacent omentum. Extension into the duodenum is generally sharply limited, though the subserosa may be involved to some extent.

Histologically carcinomas of the linitis plastica type tend to be undifferentiated, and at times distinction from malignant lymphoma is difficult or impossible. If a tumor secretes mucin, this may be a helpful diagnostic feature. At times, mucin secretion may be abundant, and signet-ring cells may be the predominant cells. Desmoplasia often is pronounced and dominates the histologic picture, making recognition of cancer cells difficult. The prognosis is essentially hopeless in this variety of gastric cancer because of the extent of the disease by the time it is clinically recognized.[271] Occasionally, focal fibrotic thickening of the antrum, apparently of inflammatory nature, may simulate cancer clinically and on unassisted-eye inspection of the specimen.

The majority of gastric carcinomas, which do not meet the criteria of any one of these groups, are extremely variable in gross appearance and histologic pattern. Again, because they are usually far advanced before an opportunity for treatment is offered, the outlook is poor.

Spread. Direct spread and spread by way of the lymphatics are of foremost importance in dictating principles of surgical treatment and in assessing the individual patient's prognosis. Metastasis to lymph nodes along the greater and lesser curvatures of the stomach is frequent. Extension to the para-aortic and celiac lymph nodes is also often seen. Metastasis to the left supraclavicular lymph nodes by way of the thoracic duct may be an initial sign of gastric carcinoma, so-called Virchow's (Ewald's) node. Spread into the esophagus, especially submucosal, and to the mediastinal lymph nodes may be a feature. In occasional cases there may be permeation of pulmonary lymphatics and the bone marrow (with clinically unexplained anemia) as early manifestations of the disease.

Liver metastasis, common even in cases believed to be "early," results from invasion of the tributaries of the portal venous system.[139] Peritoneal spread and carcinomatosis occur, and gastric cancer is an important di-

agnostic consideration when a rectal shelf is demonstrated clinically. Carcinoma of the stomach, as well as other parts of the gastrointestinal tract, may metastasize early to the ovaries so that the ovarian tumor dominates the clinical picture, the so-called Krükenberg tumors. The typical Krükenberg tumor is characterized by signet-ring cancer cells with abundant fibrous tissue stroma.

Carcinoma of the esophagus

Among gastrointestinal cancer, epidermoid carcinoma of the esophagus ranks behind only carcinoma of the colon and rectum and carcinoma of the stomach in frequency. It is a disease of older age groups, affecting men more often than women.[43] Half of the cancers arise in the middle third of the esophagus, the remainder being approximately equally distributed between the upper and lower thirds. It is generally an ovoid growth with its long axis parallel to the long axis of the esophagus (Plate 2, *B*). Central ulceration of the elevated plaquelike growth undermines the peripheral mucous membrane. It may extend to involve the full circumference of the esophagus and commonly infiltrates the full thickness of the esophageal wall. Lymphatic spread and mediastinal invasion are frequent. As a result, carcinoma of the esophagus is generally well established when recognized, and the results of treatment, as measured in terms of 5-year survivals, are quite poor.[157]

Although epidermoid carcinomas are by far the most common in the esophagus, glandular carcinomas and small-cell carcinomas indistinguishable from those of the lung and having the propensity for squamous and glandular differentiation are occasionally seen.[137] Although most of the adenocarcinomas are primary tumors of the gastric cardia with extension into the esophagus,[32] occasionally they originate in esophageal glands and may grow in an adenoid cystic pattern.

Carcinoma of the small intestine

Carcinoma of the small intestine is an infrequent primary malignant tumor,[65] and when it occurs in the duodenum, one may have difficulty in distinguishing it from pancreatic carcinoma or carcinoma of the common bile duct secondarily infiltrating the duodenum.[289] Except for some of the periampullary carcinomas, many of which resemble the biliary duct system tumors morphologically, carcinomas of the small intestine are similar in appearance and behavior to those of the large intestine, though their clinical diagnosis may be more difficult and their evolutionary stage more advanced when they are diagnosed. An occasional carcinoma of the small intestine may originate in a papillary adenoma.[40]

Carcinoma of the anal region

Several different epithelial tumors originate in the vicinity of the anus and anorectal junction. The epidermoid carcinoma arising from the squamous epithelium of the anal mucous membrane appears and behaves similarly to epidermoid carcinomas of other squamous epithelial mucous membranes. They spread freely by way of the rich perianal lymphatic plexuses to the lymph nodes of the groin.

The so-called basaloid tumors, which histologically resemble the basal cell epitheliomas of the skin and presumably arise from the mucosa of the transitional or cloacogenic zone separating the rectal and anal mucous membranes, spread similarly to the epidermoid carcinoma. A more favorable prognosis of the basaloid tumors has been reported but has not been observed in all studies.[79,171]

Occasional epidermoid tumors in this area include some glandular elements or individual cells with mucin secretions—mucoepidermoid carcinomas.[225]

Anal duct carcinoma is an infrequent tumor, usually glandular and mucin secreting, that occurs in the anorectal area without apparent involvement of the anal skin or anal or rectal mucous membrane. It arises from anal glands or ducts and usually is not recognized as being malignant until some time has elapsed, often while treatment has been directed toward such conditions as fistula in ano.

Rarely, epidermoid carcinomas arise in the rectum without anatomic continiuty with the anus.[318] They also occur, but even more rarely, in the stomach as do mixed glandular and epidermoid tumors—adenoacanthomas.[37]

Malignant melanoma

Malignant melanomas have been encountered in many parts of the gastrointestinal tract, and except for those primary in the anus and esophagus, they are considered to be metastatic. Unlike the metastases from carcinoma, they are infrequently accompanied by peritoneal spread. The appearance and behavior of the primary tumors do not differ from those of the corresponding skin lesions. Anal malignant melanomas may occur primarily as rectal lesions because anal sphincteric action may cause them to grow cephalad initially.

Establishment of the primary nature of gastrointestinal malignant melanomas rests on demonstration of junctional change, with the recognition of neoplastic proliferation in the area of the junction of epithelium and subepithelial stroma.[250]

Carcinoid tumor

Carcinoid (argentaffin) tumors are relatively uncommon neoplasms whose endocrine secretion may produce systemic effects. They are found throughout the gastrointestinal tract, from the stomach to the rectum, as well as in the gallbladder and in teratoid ovarian tumors. Morphologically and functionally identical tumors arise in the bronchial and tracheal mucous membranes. The cell of origin is believed to be the Kulchitsky cell, one of the cell types occurring in the crypts of Lieberkühn, characterized morphologially by the presence of cytoplasmic granules capable of reducing ammoniacal silver nitrate (argentaffin granules).

The origin of Kulchitsky cells—endodermal or neuroectodermal—is in dispute, but current data support the latter. It has been suggested that more than one cell type may be involved, since argentaffin granules are found frequently in the midgut carcinoids and rarely, if at all, in tumors of the bronchi, stomach, and hindgut.[194] Argyrophil granules, which stain with metallic silver after the addition of exogenous reducing agent, have a distribution pattern similar to that of argentaffin granules but are seen with greater frequency in tumors of the bronchi, stomach, and hindgut than the argentaffin granules are. The argentaffin cells secrete serotonin (5-hydroxytryptamine), a hormone also found in blood platelets and concerned with blood coagulation, probably through a vasoconstrictive action. Serotonin has also been shown to have a normal central nervous system function, and these facts, together with its pathologic role in the development of cardiovascular lesions and the "carcinoid syndrome," account for the widespread interest it has generated.

A variety of clinically evident endocrine dysfunctions have also been manifested by tumors with argyrophil cells from other sites (such as bronchus), lending support for the proposed name *neuroendocrine tumor* for these neoplasms.[122] Some carcinoids are grossly indistinguishable from carcinomas, but generally the lesions are small submucosal nodules or merely focal areas of submucosal thickening. Their yellow color has been emphasized, but many are actually gray or gray-white. Muscle hypertrophy is often considerable in the involved area, and this, together with the characteristic fibrosis and perhaps peritoneal adhesions, may produce kinking and partial obstruction (Plate 2, *G*).

Two histologic types of carcinoid tumors ar recognized. The "classic" variety, composed of solid nests of uniform small cells with round or oval nuclei that are usually regular, is more commonly encountered. The less common histologic pattern is trabeculas of interanastomosing bands or ribbons of tumor cells. Rosettelike formation may occur with either type of tumor, and both patterns may be seen in some tumors (Fig. 24-35). Mucus-secreting cells may be found in either variety of tumor,[138] and in some instances when they are in great numbers, the diagnosis of mucus-producing carcinoma may be suggested.[134,135] The argentaffin granules when present appear to be concentrated at the periphery of

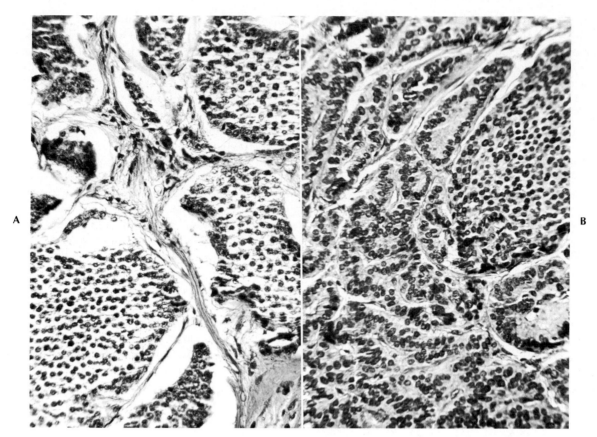

Fig. 24-35. Carcinoid (argentaffin) tumor. **A,** "Classic" pattern, **B,** Trabecular pattern. (**A** and **B,** 300 ×.)

the cell about one pole of the nucleus. The tumors tend to grow invasively and have the potential for metastasizing by way of lymphatics and bloodstream. However, even when metastases occur, it is not uncommon for a patient to live with essentially asymptomatic tumors for many years. Carcinoid tumor combined with adenocarcinoma has occurred rarely in several gastrointestinal sites.[169]

Carcinoid tumors occur more frequently in the appendix and rectum than elsewhere and are usually asymptomatic, being found during the course of proctoscopic examination or in the appendix removed surgically for acute inflammation or other reasons.[113] However, roughly 10% to 15% of rectal carcinoid tumors, usually those more than 2 cm in diameter, invade the lamina muscularis propria and behave like rectal carcinomas, though perhaps progressing more slowly.[216] Occasionally, very small tumors may be associated with distant, even widespread, metastases. Carcinoid tumors that metastasize and prove fatal, as well as those associated with the "carcinoid syndrome," most often are encountered in the ileum and commonly are multiple. The carcinoid syndrome consists in diarrhea, a peculiar cyanotic flushing of the skin, and right-sided heart fail-

ure, the last being based on organic disease of the tricuspid or pulmonic valve. Almost invariably, extensive liver metastases are present in patients with the syndrome. In the usual functioning carcinoid tumor, 5-hydroxyindoleacetic acid (5-HIAA), a degradation product of 5-hydroxytryptamine (5-HT), can be demonstrated in the urine. The cardiac lesion consists of dense, fibrous endocardial thickening, the fibrous tissue apparently being deposited on the surface of the endocardium of the pulmonic valve, tricuspid valve, or endocardium of the auricle. Less commonly other chambers of the heart, the great vessels, and coronary sinus may be involved. As the result of these changes, functional pulmonary stenosis and tricuspid insufficiency may occur. Normally, serotonin is destroyed in the lungs by monoamine oxidase, accounting for the preponderance of right-sided cardiac disease.

The fibrosis seen in the heart and in the vicinity of the primary carcinoid tumor has been considered to be the result of histamine and mucopolysaccharides from mast cells, which in turn produce local edema, and fibrin deposition with organization of the latter resulting in fibrosis.[22]

Williams and Sandler[334] have subdivided carcinoid

tumors into three groups: (1) those of the bronchus and stomach, arising from the foregut; (2) those of the jejunum, ileum, and cecum, arising from the midgut; and (3) those of the rectum, developing from the hindgut. They point out that those from the foregut are often of trabecular pattern and sometimes secrete 5-hydroxytryptophan, a precursor of serotonin, and store the latter poorly; those of midgut origin are the classic lesions morphologically, tinctorially (positive argentaffin reaction), and in the ability to store large amounts of serotonin; those of the hindgut are usually of trabecular pattern and lack secretory function. The syndrome, as well as 5-HIAA excretion, is more frequent with midgut tumors than those from the foregut and hindgut.

Neoplasms of smooth muscle

Except for the uterus, the muscle of gastrointestinal tract gives rise to more tumors of smooth muscle than any other organ or organ system of the body. As is true of the uterus, leiomyomas far outnumber leiomyosarcomas. They arise in any portion of the alimentary tract from the esophagus[34,46] to the rectum but are most common in the stomach.[28,284] The small intestine is next most frequently involved.[290] They may grow primarily into the gut lumen (Fig. 24-36), and in that part of the intestine supported on a mesentery, they may become pedunculated and form the head of an intussusception. They also may project primarily from the serosa and grow to a large size without producing gastrointestinal symptoms. Some tumors are dumbbell-shaped lesions projecting in both directions. It is common for gastrointestinal muscle tumors to ulcerate and undergo extensive central necrosis, accounting for the frequency of hematemesis (or melena). A small leiomyoma of the intestine may be the cryptic source of massive, even exsanguinating, hemorrhage.

These neoplasms are most frequently composed of interlacing bundles of fusiform cells with long processes

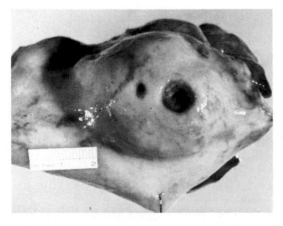

Fig. 24-36. Leiomyoma of stomach. Growth essentially endogastric.

and nuclei with blunted ends, often bearing a striking resemblance to normal smooth muscle. Less commonly they feature round or polygonal cells that are frequently vacuolated and sometimes associated with spindle cells more characteristic of smooth muscle. This pattern is now generally considered to represent an atypical growth pattern of smooth muscle tumors and is referred to as bizarre leiomyoma, leiomyoblastoma, and epithelioid leiomyoma.[9,299] Although they appear well delineated grossly, under the microscope no capsule is seen, and tumor muscle fibers usually can be seen to interdigitate with those of the lamina muscularis propria or, occasionally, the lamina muscularis mucosae. The histologic distinction between leiomyoma and leiomyosarcoma may be difficult regardless of the tumor's microscopic pattern; the atypical appearance of the leiomyoblastoma by itself is not indicative of malignancy. Occasional sarcomas appear very orderly and well differentiated, giving no hint of malignancy until metastasis occurs. More often, however, completely benign tumors show great cellularity and nuclear pleomorphism, even to the presence of bizarre giant cells. The presence of mitotic figures in appreciable numbers is generally a reliable indication of malignancy.[252]

Distant metastases of leiomyosarcomas are usually blood borne, but some display a tendency to spread over the peritoneal surface and some are only locally invasive.[4] Local invasion, particularly of those arising in the retroperitoneum, makes complete removal and thus cure less likely.

Lymphoma

A benign lesion, often referred to as lymphoma of the rectum but also known as lymphoid polyp or rectal tonsil, is occasionally encountered on proctoscopic examination and removed as a "polyp." It is usually only a few millimeters in diameter but may reach a dimension as great as 1.5 cm. It can be recognized microscopically as benign by its excellent organization with "germinal centers" and its usual limitation to the mucosa and submucosa without invasion of the muscle coat. It is of significance only in differential diagnosis.[58] With this exception, the lymphomas of the gastrointestinal tract are malignant. Such malignant lymphomas may arise as primary, or apparently primary, gastrointestinal tumors or may be but one manifestation of generalized disease. The latter situation is more common, and all varieties of malignant lymphoma encountered in the lymphoid tissue of the body generally may involve the alimentary tract. The same varieties also occur as "primary" lesions, but Hodgkin's disease and plasmacytoma are very rare.[70] Gastrointestinal lesions in generalized malignant lymphoma (including the leukemias) are of importance in themselves, and they may demand treatment when they are responsible for problems relative to gastrointestinal hemorrahge or obstruction. Malignant lymphomas readily perforate, occasionally at multiple sites, especially after radiotherapy.

"Primary" malignant lymphoma of the gastrointestinal tract is most often seen in the stomach, less commonly in the rectum, cecum, and ascending colon, and infrequently elsewhere.[12] Gastric malignant lymphomas usually simulate carcinoma in their clinical manifestations and sometimes their gross pathologic appearance

as well. However, many characteristically appear as flat, disclike or plateaulike elevations with rather sharply defined borders (Fig. 24-37, *A*). They are raised a few millimeters or a centimeter or so above the surrounding mucous membrane, and if they involve the antrum, their pyloric margin is abrupt. Frequently involvement is multifocal, and ulceration is usual, producing shallow, saucerlike lesions. In the intestine, involvement of submucosa rather than mucosa is a

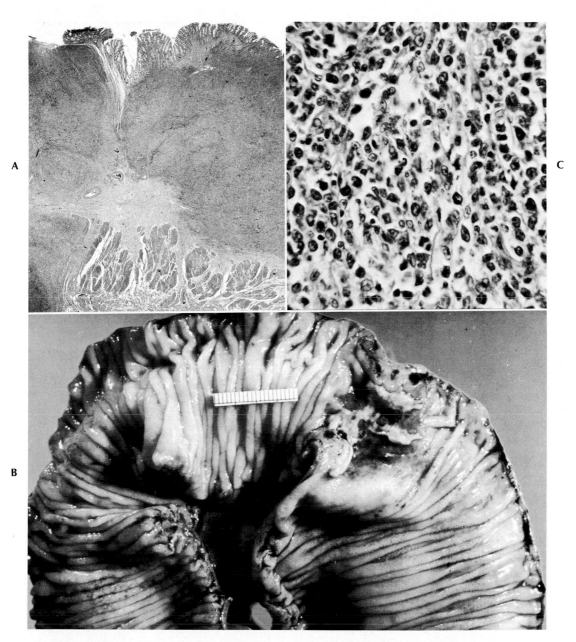

Fig. 24-37. A, Malignant lymphoma of stomach. Characteristic plateaulike elevation of mucosa and pronounced thickening of submucosa are well demonstrated. At left, muscle has been freely invaded. **B,** Malignant lymphoma of small intestine, with multiple sites of involvement. Notice similarity to gross appearance of carcinoid tumor illustrated in Plate 2, *G.* **C,** Malignant lymphoma of stomach showing considerable pleomorphism. **(A,** 13×; **C,** 625×.)

prominent feature, and again multicentric origin is frequent. As with carcinoid tumors, kinking and incomplete obstruction may bring the disease to the patient's attention (Fig. 24-37, B).

Lymphomas may be difficult to distinguish histologically from carcinoma (Fig. 24-37, C) and benign lymphoid lesions of the gastrointestinal tract (so-called pseudolymphomas).[57,146] Immunocytochemistry has aided in these distinctions.[142]

Although malignant lymphomas of the gastrointestinal tract have their greatest incidence in the same age range as carcinoma, they have a greater incidence during early ages, including childhood. Primary malignant lymphoma of the stomach, the most common malignant gastric tumor next to carcinoma, has a distinctly better prognosis than carcinoma does in terms of 5-year survival after surgical treatment.[154] On the other hand, so-called primary malignant lymphomas of the colon and rectum in the majority of instances prove to be manifestations of systemic disease, though the extraintestinal involvement may not be apparent at the time of recognition of the colonic or rectal lesion.

Local excision of lymphoma may be curative but extraabdominal recurrences are not infrequent. Histologic typing and clinicopathological staging have been found to be useful in the identification of those cases with high risk of systemic recurrence, which probably are best treated with chemotherapy in addition to surgery and radiotherapy.[98]

Miscellaneous rare tumors

Mucocele of the appendix is a cystic distension of the organ with thick, glairy mucus. Although there may be a cicatricial structure proximal to the dilated portion, often there is not. The normal mucous membrane is replaced by focal or diffuse hyperplasia of the glands resembling those of the hyperplastic colonic polyp, a mucinous cystadenoma with epithelial atypia, or a mucinous cystadenocarcinoma.[136] In some cases there are associated mucinous ovarian tumors or carcinoma of the large bowel.

Lipomas occasionally are encountered in various parts of the gastrointestinal tract, most often in the colon and rectum and particularly in the vicinity of the ileocecal valve, where appreciable submucosal adipose tissue is usually present.[268] They are submucosal, often superficially ulcerated, and may lead to an intussusception (Fig. 24-38). In instances of incipient intussusception, there may be puckering of the overlying serosa, and this, coupled with induration as the result of inflammation, accounts for their occasionally being mistaken for carcinoma at operation.

Vascular tumors, especially cavernous hemangiomas, have been reported as occurring in various parts of the gastrointestinal tract. Multiple hemangiomas may be seen as part of Osler-Weber-Rendu disease.[141] Lym-

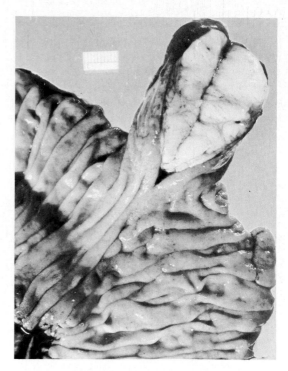

Fig. 24-38. Lipoma of jejunum.

phangiomas occur less frequently. Characteristic glomus tumors may form polypoid, sometimes painful, gastric tumors.[158] Rarely gastrointestinal lesions occur in Kaposi's sarcoma.

Tumors of nerve origin—neurofibroma, ganglioneuroma and paraganglioma, teratoma, and choriocarcinoma—are rare in the gastrointestinal tract.[161,242,254] Stromal tumors have been reported in von Recklinghausen's disease and resemble leiomyoma by light microscopy but not completely by electron microscopy.[272] Adenomas, or papillary cystadenomas, arise from the apocrine sweat glands in the region of the anus and may give rise to Paget's disease. Granular cell myoblastomas have been encountered in the stomach, rectum, and esophagus.[54]

Carcinosarcoma is a rare but spectacular tumor of the esophagus incorporating both epithelial growth (usually epidermoid) and a sarcomatous or sarcoma-like stroma, which may dominate the picture.[177] Many such tumors are polypoid. There is no agreement as to the nature of the stromal change—whether it is genuinely malignant or pseudosarcomatous.[198] The carcinosarcomas are distinctly less malignant than the much more common epidermoid carcinomas. Although they may be grossly simulated by the polypoid fibrovascular tumors occurring most commonly in the upper one third of the esophagus,[148] their malignant histologic features should serve adequately to distinguish the two growths. Metastases, which are relatively infrequent, may be carcinomatous, sarcomatous, or mixed.

DISEASES OF THE PERITONEUM, RETROPERITONEUM, MESENTERY, AND OMENTUM
Peritoneum
Peritonitis

Inflammation of the peritoneum is an acute or chronic response, diffuse or localized, to a variety of agents—bacterial, viral, chemical, parasites and their ova, fungi, or foreign material.[16,51,68,303] The acute variety is most frequent and is usually associated with inflammation of abdominal organs with or without perforation, such as appendicitis, cholecystitis, intestinal infarction, diverticulitis, perforated peptic ulcer, and hemorrhage attributed to ruptured ectopic pregnancy. Less common is the "primary" form caused by a pneumococcus or hemolytic streptococcus. The organisms causing acute peritonitis are numerous and most commonly include one or more of the normal flora of the gastrointestinal tract, usually *Escherichia coli*, *Proteus*, and *Enterococcus*, though *Bacteroides* and *Clostridium* are also important. Initially there is hyperemia, edema, and extravasation of red blood cells followed by exudation of leukocytes and fibrin. The plastic exudate may cause adhesions between loops of intestine, omentum, and abdominal parietes, forming abscesses in localized areas rather than permitting general spread of the process. Such abscesses, most likely to develop in the lumbar gutters, right subdiaphragmatic or subhepatic area, and the pelvic cul-de-sac, may persist and require surgical drainage.

Tuberculous peritonitis may occur as a manifestation of disseminated tuberculosis, miliary or otherwise, or in association with involvement of intestinal or female generative organs.[118] The disease process is the same as in other parts of the body. It may produce widespread, dense adhesions.

A variety of irritants may be responsible for peritonitis—bile, hydrochloric acid, and other intestinal contents that gain access to the peritoneum as a result of rupture of a viscus (gallbladder, bile duct, duodenum, and so on), hemorrhage from an ectopic pregnancy or corpus luteum, and other foreign materials such as *Lycopodium* spores and talc.

Bile may produce a profound initial systemic reaction in the host, but the nature of the resulting pathologic process is dependent on the source of the contaminating bile and the type and number of associated bacteria.[203] Foreign-body granulomas may result from *Lycopodium* spores and talc crystals—material used as dusting powders for surgical rubber gloves in the past.[91] The use of absorbable starch has eliminated such granulomas, but the starch does not appear to be completely innocuous. Instances of peritonitis and foreign-body granuloma have been reported, presumably developing as the result of hypersensitivity to the starch.[287]

Infrequently, oily materials used in salpingography, parasites or their ova, barium sulfate administered for diagnostic roentgenographic study and escaping into the peritoneum as a result of perforation, and sclerosing agents used in the treatment of hernia may incite a foreign-body reaction.

Adhesions

Intraperitoneal adhesions result from abdominal operations and the inflammatory processes described. The former are related to drying of the serosal surfaces, blood in the peritoneal cavity, and a local depression of plasminogen activator.[33,264] Less frequently, an extensive peritoneal fibrosis (sclerosing peritonitis), which has been attributed to asbestos, carcinoid tumor, and beta-adrenergic receptor blocking drugs may be observed.[13]

Periodic disease (familial Mediterranean fever, familial recurring polyserositis)

Periodic bouts of pain occur particularly in the abdomen, but they may also be noted in the chest and joints. During intervals between attacks, the patients are in excellent health. The disease is a genetic disorder of unknown cause and pathogenesis affecting persons of Armenian, Arab, or Jewish ethnic origin, the last being predominantly the non-Ashkenazi Jews—the Sephardi and Iraqi ethnic groups.[208] Sterile exudates in the involved serous surfaces are minimal, consisting of focal collections of neutrophils, fibrin strands, and ecchymoses, and only rarely are fibrinous adhesions and scars produced despite the many attacks. Amyloid of the perireticular type, described in the kidneys, spleen, adrenals, pulmonary alveolar capillaries, and hepatic sinusoids but not in other organs, may result in the patient's death. Otherwise the course is a protracted one.

Ascites

Ascites is the condition of transudation of clear, low-specific-gravity fluid into the peritoneal cavity. The protein content is less than 3%. Ascites is most commonly seen with cirrhosis of the liver but may result from other causes of hypertension in the portal venous system, such as thrombosis or cardiac decompensation, or from hypoalbuminemia. Chylous ascites, in which the fluid appears milky and has a high fat content, is related to obstruction of the thoracic duct, usually neoplastic.

Splenosis

Asymptomatic nodules of spleen may be implanted in the peritoneum after laceration of the spleen and in women may grossly be interpreted as endometriosis because of their red color. They are correctly identified by microscopic examination.[323]

Hyperplasia

Proliferation of the peritoneal lining cells or underlying stroma, or both, in response to irritants may produce solid or cystic growths that grossly and microscopically mimic primary or secondary neoplasm. The former are more commonly seen in hernia sacs of men and boys, whereas the latter are frequently associated with and attached to inflamed pelvic organs in women; rarely, they are free in the abdominal cavity.[202,259]

Metaplasia

A transformation of the mesothelial cells or stromal cells, or both, of the peritoneum in women, attributable to their sensitivity to sex hormones, results in a variety of benign and malignant growths not observed in men. Cystic, glandular, or papillary nodules of müllerian type of epithelium—tubal, cervical, or endometrial not associated with endometrial stroma thus distinguishing it from endometriosis—may be found on any peritoneal surface and in pelvic lymph nodes, but there is a predilection for the pelvic peritoneum, omentum, and surfaces of the ovaries, uterus, and fallopian tubes. The term *endosalpingiosis*, originally employed for those lesions with tubal epithelium, has been expanded by some authors to include all varieties of müllerian epithelium.[95,339] Unlike endometriosis, endosalpingiosis is asymptomatic and generally is discovered during the course of surgery for other abdominal conditions. Their banal behavior with occasional spontaneous regression is common, and rarely a malignant tumor has arisen in glandular lymph node inclusions. Distinction from malignant tumor, principally metastatic carcinoma from the ovary, is based on their banal epithelium, often tubal and partly ciliated, which lacks destructive stromal invasion. Although metaplasia can be demonstrated to be a mode for their formation, pathogenetic factors considered causative in endometriosis also appear to contribute to their formation.

Walthard cell rests in the serosa of the fallopian tube represent another benign form of mesothelial cell metaplasia found frequently as incidental microscopic and rarely as gross findings. Their microscopic and ultrastructural features are those of transitional-urothelial cells.[260]

Mutation of the peritoneal stroma cells, generally associated with pregnancy or consumption of contraceptive steroids, results in the formation of extrauterine foci of *decidual cells*, or *leiomyomatosis peritonealis disseminata*, consisting of multiple nodules of fibrous tissue and smooth muscle sometimes with decidual cells or endometrial glands that grossly may mimic metastatic tumor and microscopically may be misdeemed as leiomyosarcoma.[175,301,316] Its course has been benign with instances of spontaneous regression and recurrence after respectively the cessation and recurrence of pregnancy, suggestive of a pathogenetic role for the hormonal imbalance associated with pregnancy.

Endometriosis may result from a combined stromal and epithelial peritoneal mutation consisting of glands and stroma identical to uterine endometrium. More frequently it affects the pelvic peritoneum, but the ovaries, fallopian tubes, bowel, or urinary tract may also be involved. The pathogenesis of endometriosis is by no means settled by the metaplastic theory. Implantation of endometrium from the uterus and lymphatic or hematogenous dissemination must be considered along with other factors—hormonal, heredity, and immunologic.[117] The response of endometriosis to hormones is similar to that of the endometrium. Symptoms are variable: some cases are asymptomatic, but others cause pain connected with the menstrual cycle or compression of involved organs. Although they are not life threatening as such, malignant transformation, most commonly carcinoma and exceptionally sarcoma or carcinosarcoma, may occur infrequently and result in the patient's death.

Retroperitoneum and mesentery

The retroperitoneum is an ill-defined area that may share in the complications of diseases of the many organs that lie within it or impinge on it. Hemorrhage, infections, and extensions of neoplasms are the important complications and may be related to the urinary tract, retroperitoneal lymph nodes, and blood vessels, including the aorta and vena cava.

Several possibly related conditions involve the mesenteric and retroperitoneal adipose tissue. At one end of the spectrum is a self-limited, chronic, productive inflammation of the mesentery, usually of the small intestine. This has been variously termed mesenteric panniculitis, lipogranuloma, and isolated lipodystrophy and likened to Weber-Christian disease.[167] It may produce a significant mass and may or may not be symptomatic. Retractile mesenteritis is a similar condition, distinguished by fibrosis and hyalin scarring and retraction of the mesentery, with distortion of intestinal loops producing episodes of pain, constipation, and obstruction.[304]

Idiopathic retroperitoneal fibrosis is a lesion characterized by dense fibrosis and a limited, nonspecific inflammatory reaction that frequently is manifested by ureteral obstruction.[214] An association with fibrotic processes in other areas lends credence for its being part of a systemic disease.[293] Drugs, methysergide,[275] beta blockers, alpha-1-antitrypsin deficiency, and autoallergy to ceroid have been considered etiologic factors.[149,215,239]

Cysts

Cysts are encountered in the mesentery, omentum, and retroperitoneum in order of decreasing frequency and occur in children and adults as acute problems or incidental operative findings.[176] Most are lymphatic, arising principally in the mesentery of the small bowel. Enteric cysts, frequently intra-abdominal, may also be retroperitoneal.[27] Urogenital cysts of mesonephric or paramesonephric origin are less common than others cysts and are retroperitoneal.[291] Parasitic cysts of Echinococcus have been rarely encountered in the retroperitoneum.[282]

Omentum
Torsion

Omental torsion, resulting from adhesions, tumors, and so on or at times of unknown cause, may result in infarction and give rise to signs and symptoms simulating those of acute appendicitis but usually without vomiting.[47] Similarly, epiploic appendages may become infarcted. Fat necrosis of an appendage, presumably a late result, is not uncommon. Rarely the omentum may be involved by parasitic or fungal disease and endometriosis.[230,256]

PRIMARY NEOPLASMS OF THE PERITONEUM, RETROPERITONEUM, MESENTERY, AND OMENTUM
Peritoneum

Primary peritoneal tumors differ in type and frequency in men and women because of the capability of the female peritoneum to undergo müllerian metaplasia. *Mesotheliomas* arise from the serosal lining cells as benign and malignant tumors. Benign tumors occur as papillary, cystic, and adenomatoid variants more frequently in women than in men and rarely in children.[59,104,210,281] The solitary benign fibrous mesothelioma, common in the pleura, is rarely seen in the peritoneum. Malignant mesotheliomas, much more frequent in men than in women and rare in children, have been associated with asbestos exposure.[104,155,201,298] Papillary and tubulopapillary diffuse tumors predominate over the mixed epithelial-fibrous variety, and both are generally associated with recurrent ascites and rarely witth hypoglycemia.[267]

Papillary tumors arising from a simultaneous or sequential process of peritoneal metaplasia and neoplasia of the mesothelium in women may have any of the histologic patterns of ovarian epithelial tumors, but most are serous type, solitary or multifocal.[104,109,201] Rarely, mixed müllerian tumors or endometrial stroma tumors, identical to those of uterine origin, are encountered.[133,315]

Histologic distinction between mesothelioma, mesothelial cell hyperplasia, metastatic adenocarcinoma, and primary peritoneal carcinoma may be difficult and requires knowledge of the distribution of the peritoneal tumor and the histopathology of the extraperitoneal tumor being considered as a primary site.

Retroperitoneum, mesentery, and omentum

Primary benign and malignant tumors, exclusive of those arising in contiguous organs and lymph nodes, involve the retroperitoneum, mesentery, and omentum in order of decreasing frequency.[99] They are more commonly malignant in the retroperitoneum, benign in the mesentery, and essentially equally distributed between benign and malignant in the omentum. Mesenchymal tumors are most frequently arising from adipose, muscle, fibrous, and vascular tissue in order of decreasing frequency. Retroperitoneal teratomas, most frequent in the sacrococcygeal region of children, and tumors arising from nerve tissue in that order constitute most of the remaining tumors in these areas.

METASTATIC TUMORS OF THE PERITONEUM, RETROPERITONEUM, MESENTERY, AND OMENTUM

Secondary tumors in the gastrointestinal tract are rare in the absence of peritoneal, mesenteric, or omental involvement. Rarely, isolated melanoma, lung, or female breast carcinoma may be observed in the gastrointestinal tract. Metastases, common in the peritoneum, mesentery, and omentum, are more frequently from tumors in the abdominal organs than in distant sites. Two rare forms of secondary peritoneal involvement by tumor are *pseudomyxoma peritonei* and *gliomatosis peritonei*. The former represents a spread of mucus-secreting cells over the peritoneal surfaces with accumulation of mucoid material in the peritoneal cavity.[269] Most commonly it follows rupture of an appendiceal or ovarian mucinous cystadenocarcinoma, but it may result from malignant mucinous tumors of other abdominal organs; in some instances the source cannot be determined. The behavior of pseudomyxoma peritonei is one of a locally infiltrating surface growth that generally cannot be eradicated.

Gliomatosis peritonei represents benign glial implants on peritoneal surfaces in association with immature ovarian teratoma.[312] The implants may remain without change, undergo malignant change, or regress.

Secondary tumor in the retroperitoneum can occur from extension of primary bone neoplasms, notably sacrococcygeal chordoma, and pancreatic carcinoma, but generally it is secondary to retroperitoneal lymph node metastases, principally from the testis, prostate, pancreas, kidney, urinary bladder, uterine cervix, and endometrium.

REFERENCES

1. Abdou, N.I., NaPombejara, C., Sagawa, A., et al: Malakoplakia: evidence for monocytic lysosomal abnormality correctable for cholinergic agonist in vitro and in vivo, N. Engl. J. Med. **297**:1413, 1977.
2. Abrams, J.S., and Holden, W.D.: Tuberculosis of the gastrointestinal tract, Arch. Surg. (Chicago) **89**:282, 1964.
3. Akwari, O.E., Van Heerden, J.A., Foulk, W.T., et al.: Cancer of the bile ducts associated with ulcerative colitis, Ann. Surg. **181**:303, 1975.
4. Akwari, O.E., Dozois, R.R., Weiland, L.H., and Beahrs, O.H.: Leiomyosarcoma of the small and large bowel, Cancer **42**:1375, 1978.
5. Allan, R.N.; Extra-intestinal manifestations of inflammatory bowel disease, Clin. Gastroenterol. **12**:617, 1983.
6. Almy, T.P., and Howell, D.A.: Diverticular disease of the colon, N. Engl. J. Med. **302**:324, 1980.
7. Altemeier, W.A: Bacterial flora of acute perforated appendicitis with peritonitis: bacteriologic study based upon 100 cases, Ann. Surg. **107**:517, 1938.
8. Anderson, K.E., Finlayson, N.D.C., and Deschner, E.E.: Intractable malabsorption with a flat jejunal mucosa and selective IgA deficiency, Gastroenterology **67**:709, 1974.
9. Appelman, H.D., and Helwig, E.B.: Gastric epithelioid leiomyoma and leiomyosarcoma (leiomyoblastoma), Cancer **38**:708, 1976.
10. Atkinson, M., and Hosking, D.J.: Gastrointestinal complication of diabetes mellitus, Clin. Gastroenterol. **12**:633, 1983.
11. Azzopardi, J.G., and Evans, D.J.: Mucoprotein-containing histiocytes (muciphages) in the rectum, J. Clin. Pathol. **19**:368, 1966.
12. Azzopardi, J.G., and Menzies, T.: Primary malignant lymphoma of the alimentary tract, Br. J. Surg. **47**:358, 1960.
13. Baddeley, H., Lee, R.E.J., Marshall, A.J., et al.: Sclerosing peritonitis due to practolol, Br. Med. J. **2**:192, 1977.
14. Baker, L.A., Smith, C., and Lieberman, G.: The natural history of esophageal varices: a study of 115 cirrhotic patients in whom varices were diagnosed prior to bleeding, Am. J. Med. **26**:228, 1959.
15. Bale, P.M., Clifton-Bright, P., Benjamin, B.N.P., et al.: Pathology of Tangier disease, J. Clin. Pathol. **24**:609, 1971.
16. Barnett, L.: Hydatid cysts: their location in various organs and tissues of body, Aust. NZ J. Surg. **12**:240, 1943.
17. Baret, N.R.: Hiatus hernia: a review of some controversial points, J. Surg. **42**:231, 1954.
18. Barry, J.E., and Auldist, A.W.: The Vater Association: one end of a spectrum of anomalies, Am. J. Dis. Child. **128**:769, 1974.
19. Bartlett, J.G.: Antibiotic-associated colitis, Clin. Gastroenterol. **8**:783, 1979.
20. Bartlett, J.G., Chang, T.W., Gurwith, M., et al.: Antibiotic-associated pseudomembranous colitis due to toxin-producing clostridia, N. Engl. J. Med. **298**:531, 1978.
21. Bartlett, J.G., Taylor, N.S., Chang, T., and Dzink, J.: Clinical and laboratory observations in *Clostridium difficile* colitis, Am. J. Clin. Nutr. **33**:2521, 1980.
22. Bates, H.R., Jr., and Clark, R.F.: Observations on the pathogenesis of carcinoid heart disease and the tanning of fluorescent fibrin by 5-hydroxytryptamine and ceruloplasmin, Am. J. Clin. Pathol. **39**:46, 1963.
23. Bayless, T.M., and Knox, D.L.: Whipple's disease: a multisystem infection, N. Engl. J. Med. **300**:920, 1979.
24. Beart, R.W.: Pneumatosis cystoides intestinalis: a review of the literature, Dis. Colon Rectum **29**:358, 1986.
25. Benson, C.D., and Lloyd, J.R.: Infantile pyloric stenosis: a review of 1,120 cases, Am. J. Surg. **107**:429, 1964.
26. Benson, C.D., Lloyd, J.R., and Fischer, H.: Intussusception in infants and children: an analysis of 300 cases, Arch. Surg. (Chicago) **86**:745, 1963.
27. Bentley, J.F.R., and Smith, J.R.: Developmental posterior enteric remnants and spinal malformations: the split notochord syndrome, Arch. Dis. Child. **35**:76, 1960.
28. Berg, J., and McNeer, G.: Leiomyosarcoma of the stomach, Cancer **13**:25, 1960.
29. Bernstein, J., Vawter, G., Harris, G.B., Young, V., and Hillman, L.S.: The occurrence of intestinal atresia in newborns with meconium ileus: the pathogenesis of an acquired anomaly, AMA J. Dis. Child. **99**:804, 1960.
30. Berthrong, M., and Fajardo, L.F.: Radiation injury in surgical pathology. Part II. Alimentary tract, Am. J. Surg. Pathol. **5**:153, 1981.
31. Blackshaw, A.J., and Levison, D.A.: Eosinophilic infiltrates of the gastrointestinal tract, J. Clin. Pathol. **39**:1, 1986.
32. Block, G.E., and Lancaster, J.R.: Adenocarcinoma of the cardioesophageal junction, Arch. Surg. (Chicago) **88**:852, 1964.
33. Bockman, R.F., Woods, M., Sargent, L., et al.: A unifying pathogenetic mechanism in the etiology of intraperitoneal adhesions, J. Surg. Res. **20**:1, 1976.
34. Bogedain, W., Carpathios, J., and Najib, A.: Leiomyoma of the esophagus, Dis. Chest **44**:391, 1963.
35. Boley, S.J., Sammartano, R., Adams, A., et al: On the nature and etiology of vascular ectasias of the colon: degenerative lesions of aging, Gastroenterology **72**:650, 1977.
36. Borow, M., Smith, M., Jr., and Soto, D., Jr.: Diverticular disease of the duodenum, Am. Surg. **33**:373, 1967.
37. Boswell, J.T., and Helwig, E.B.: Squamous cell carcinoma and adenoacanthoma of the stomach: a clinicopathologic study, Cancer **18**:181, 1965.
38. Bremer, J.L.: Diverticulas and duplications of the intestinal tract, Arch. Pathol. (Chicago) **38**:132, 1944.
39. Brett, E.M., and Berry, C.L.: Value of rectal biopsy in pediatric neurology: report of 165 biopsies, Br. Med. J. **2**:400, 1967.
40. Bridge, M.F., and Perzin, K.H.: Primary adenocarcinoma of the jejunum and ileum: a clinicopathologic study, Cancer **36**:1876, 1975.
41. Brief, D.K., and Botsford, T.W.: Primary bleeding from the small intestine in adult: the surgical management, JAMA **184**:18, 1963.
42. Brow, J.R., Parker, F., Weinstein, W.M., et al.: The small intestinal mucosa in dermatitis herpetiformis. I. Severity and distribution of the small intestinal lesion and associated malabsorption, Gastroenterology **60**:355, 1971.
43. Burgess, H.M., Baggenstoss, A.H., Moersch, H.J., and Clagett, O.T.: Cancer of the esophagus: a clinicopathological study, Surg. Clin. North Am. **31**:965, 1951.
44. Bussey, H.J.R.: Gastrointestinal polyposis, Gut **11**:970, 1970.
45. Camerson, A.J., Ott, B.J., and Payne, W.S.: The incidence of adenocarcinoma in columnar-lined (Barrett's) esophagus, N. Engl. J. Med. **313**:857, 1985.
46. Camishion, R.C., Gibbon, J.H., Jr., and Templeton, J.Y., III: Leiomyosarcoma of the esophagus: review of the literature and report of 2 cases, Ann. Surg. **153**:951, 1961.
47. Carmichael, D.H., and Organ, C.H.: Epiploic disorders, Arch. Surg. **120**:1167, 1985.
48. Cassella, R.R., Brown, A.L., Jr., Sayre, G.P., et al.: Achalasia of esophagus: pathologic and etiology consideration, Ann. Surg. **160**:474, 1964.
49. Castillo, S., Aburashed, A., Kimmelman, J., et al.: Diffuse intramural esophageal pseudodiverticulosis: new cases and review, Gastroenterology **72**:541, 1977.
50. Cave, D.R., Mitchell, D.N., and Brooke, B.N.: Evidence of an agent transmissible from ulcerative colitis tissue, Lancet **1**:1311, 1976.
51. Chandrasoma, P.T., and Mendis, K.N.: *Enterobius vermicularis* in ectopic sites, Am. J. Trop. Med. Hyg. **26**:644, 1977.
52. Civetta, J.M., and Kolodny, M.: Mesenteric venous thrombosis associated with oral contraceptives, Gastroenterology **58**:713, 1970.
53. Clancy, R.L., Tomkins, W.A., Muckle, T.J., et al.: Isolation and characterization of an aetiological agent in Whipple's disease, Br. Med. J. **3**:568, 1975.
54. Cohen, R.S., and Cramm, R.E.: Granular cell myoblastoma—an unusual rectal neoplasm: report of a case, Dis. Colon Rectum **12**:120, 1969.
55. Collier, P.E., Turowski, P., and Diamond, D.L.: Small intestinal adenocarcinoma complicating regional enteritis, Cancer **55**:516, 1985.

56. Collins, D.C.: A study of 50,000 specimens of human vermiform appendix, Surg. Gynecol. Obstet. **101**:437, 1955.

57. Cornes, J.S.: Multiple lymphomatous polyposis of the gastrointestinal tract, Cancer **14**:249, 1961.

58. Cornes, J.S., Wallace, M.H., and Morson, B.C.: Benign lymphoma of the rectum and anal canal: a study of 100 cases, J. Pathol. Bacteriol. **82**:371, 1961.

59. Craig, J.R., and Hart, W.R.: Extragenital adenomatoid tumor: evidence for the mesothelial theory of origin, Cancer **43**:1678, 1978.

60. Croxson, T., Chabon, A.B., Rorat, E., and Barash, I.M.: Intraepithelial carcinoma of the anus in homosexual men, Dis. Colon Rectum **27**:325, 1984.

61. Cullen, J.H.: Intestinal tuberculosis: a clinical pathological study, Q. Bull. Sea View Hosp. **5**:143, 1940.

62. Czaja, A.J., McAlhany, J.C., and Pruitt, B.A., Jr.: Acute duodenitis and duodenal ulceration after burns: clinical and pathological characteristics, JAMA **232**:621, 1975.

63. Dagradi, A.E., Broderick, J.T., Juler, G., et al.: The Mallory-Weiss syndrome and lesion: a study of 30 cases, Am. J. Dig. Dis. **11**:710, 1966.

64. Dajani, E.Z.: Is peptic ulcer a prostaglandin deficiency disease? Hum. Pathol. **17**:106, 1986.

65. Darling, R.C., and Welch, C.E.: Tumors of the small intestine, N. Engl. J. Med. **260**:397, 1959.

66. Davidsohn, I., and Mora, J.M.: Appendicitis in measles, Arch. Pathol. (Chicago) **14**:757, 1932.

67. Davidson, J.D., Waldmann, T.A., Goodman, D.S., and Gordon, R.S., Jr.: Protein-losing gastroenteropathy in congestive heart failure, Lancet **1**:899, 1961.

68. Davis, J.H.: Current concepts of peritonitis, Am. Surg. **33**:673, 1967.

69. Davis, J.M., Gray, G.F., and Thorbjarnarson, B.: Ménétrier's disease: a clinicopathologic study of 6 cases, Am. Surg. **185**:456, 1977.

70. Dawson, I.M.P., Cornes, J.S., and Morson, B.C.: Primary malignant lymphoid tumors of the intestinal tract: report of 37 cases with a study of factors influencing prognosis, Br. J. Surg. **49**:80, 1961.

71. DeLorimer, A.A., Fonkalsrud, E.W., and Hays, D.M.: Congenital atresia and stenosis of the jejunum and ileum, Surgery **65**:819, 1969.

72. Dew, M.J., Thompson, H., and Allan, R.N.: The spectrum of hepatic dysfunction in inflammatory bowel disease, Q. J. Med. **48**:113, 1979.

73. di Sant'Agnese, P.A., and Lepore, M.J.: Involvement of abdominal organs in cystic fibrosis of the pancreas, Gastroenterology **40**:64, 1961.

74. Dimmette, R.M., Elwi, A.M., and Sproat, H.F.: Relationship of schistosomiasis to polyposis and adenocarcinoma of large intestine, Am. J. Clin. Pathol. **26**:266, 1956.

75. Dobbins, W.O., III: An ultrastructural study of the intestinal mucosa in congenital beta-lipoprotein deficiency with particular emphasis upon the intestinal absorptive cell, Gastroenterology **50**:195, 1966.

76. Dobbins, W.O., III: Is there an immune deficit in Whipple's disease? Dig. Dis. Sci. **26**:247, 1981.

77. Donnison, A.B., Schwachman, H., and Gross, R.E.: A review of 164 children with meconium ileus seen at the Children's Hospital Medical Center, Boston, Pediatrics **37**:833, 1966.

78. Dopp, A.C., Mutchnik, M.G., and Goldstein, A.L.: Thymosin-dependent T-lymphocyte response in inflammatory bowel disease, Gastroenterology **79**:276, 1980.

79. Dougherty, B.G., and Evans, H.L.: Carcinoma of the anal canal: a study of 79 cases, Am. J. Clin. Pathol. **83**:159, 1985.

80. Dragstedt, L.R.: Cause of peptic ulcer, JAMA **169**:203, 1959.

81. Dragstedt, L.R., and Woodward, E.R.: Gastric stasis: a cause of gastric ulcer, Scand. J. Gastroenterol. **5**(suppl. 6):243, 1970.

82. Dukes, C.E.: The classification of cancer of the rectum, J. Pathol. Bacteriol. **35**:323, 1932.

83. Dukes, C.E.: Cancer of the rectum: an analysis of 1,000 cases, J. Pathol. Bacteriol. **50**:527, 1940.

84. Dungal, N., and Sigurjonsson, J.: Gastric cancer and diet: a pilot study of dietary habits in two districts differing markedly in respect of mortality from gastric cancer, Br. J. Cancer **21**:270, 1967.

85. Earlam, R.; Pathophysiology and clinical presentation of achalasia, Clin. Gastroenterol. **5**:73, 1976.

86. Ecker, J.A., and Dickson, D.R.: Melanosis proctocoli—the so-called "brown-bowel," etiology and significance, Am. J. Gastroenterol. **39**:362, 1963.

87. Ecker, J.A., Williams, R.G., and Clay, K.L.: Pneumatosis cystoides intestinalis—bullous emphysema of the intestine: a review of the literature, Am. J. Gastroenterol. **56**:125, 1971.

88. Ecker, J.A., Doane, W.A., Dickson, D.R., Gebhardt, W.F., and Hardham, J.: Gastrointestinal bleeding in hereditary hemorrhagic telangiectasia: review of the literature and report of a case with massive recurrent hemorrhage necessitating right colectomy, Am. J. Gastroenterol. **33**:411, 1960.

89. Edwards, H.C.: Diverticulosis of small intestine, Ann. Surg. **103**:230, 1936.

90. Edwards, M.: Multilocular retrorectal cystic disease—cysthamartoma: report of 12 cases, Dis. Colon Rectum **4**:103, 1961.

91. Eisman, B., Seelig, M.G., and Womack, N.A.: Talcum powder granuloma: frequent and serious postoperative complication, Ann. Surg. **126**:820, 1947.

92. Elsborg, L., and Mosbech, J.: Pernicious anemia as a risk factor in gastric cancer, Acta Med. Scand. **206**:315, 1979.

93. Estrada, R.L.: Anomalies of intestinal rotation and fixation, Springfield, Ill., 1958, Charles C Thomas, Publisher.

94. Falchuk, Z.M.: Gluten-sensitive enteropathy, Clin. Gastroenterol. **12**:475, 1983.

95. Farhi, D.C., and Silverberg, S.G.: Pseudometastases in female genital cancer, Pathol. Annu. **17**(1):47, 1982.

96. Feczko, P.J., Ma, C.K., Halpert, R.D., and Batra, S.K.: Barrett's metaplasia and dysplasia in postmyotomy achalasia patients, Am. J. Gastroenterol. **78**:265, 1983.

97. Feldman, E.J., and Sabovich, K.A.: Stress and peptic ulcer disease, Gastroenterology **78**:1087, 1980.

98. Fillippa, D.A., Lieberman, P.H., Weingard, D.N., et al.: Primary lymphomas of the gastrointestinal tract: analysis of prognostic factors with emphasis on histologic type, Am. J. Surg. Pathol. **7**:363, 1983.

99. Fine, G., and Raju, U.B.: Retroperitoneum, mesentery, omentum, and peritoneum: principles and practice of surgical pathology, ed. 2, New York, 1989, Churchill Livingstone.

100. Fitz, R.H.: Perforating inflammation of the vermiform appendix with special reference to its early diagnosis and treatment, Am. J. Med. Sci. **92**:321, 1886.

101. Fleischer, D.: Etiology and prevalence of severe persistent upper gastrointestinal bleeding, Gastroenterology **84**:538, 1983.

102. Flejou, J.F., Grimaud, J.A., Molas, G., Baviera, E., and Potet, F.: Collagenous colitis: ultrastructural study and collagen immunotyping of four cases, Arch. Pathol. Lab. Med. **108**:977, 1984.

103. Foerster, O.F., and Hovig, T.: Collagenous colitis: a clinical, histological, and ultrastructural study, Scand. J. Gastroenterol. **20**:8, 1985.

104. Foyle, A., Al-Jobi, M., and McCaughey, W.T.E.: Papillary peritoneal tumors in women, Am. J. Surg. Pathol. **5**:241, 1981.

105. Friedman, S.L., Wright, T.L., and Altman, D.F.: Gastrointestinal Kaposi's sarcoma in patients with acquired immunodeficiency syndrome: endoscopic and autopsy findings, Gastroenterology **89**:102, 1985.

106. Friesen, G., Dockerty, M.B., and ReMine, W.H.: Superficial carcinoma of the stomach, Surgery **51**:300, 1962.

107. Gear, M.W.L., Truelove, S.C., and Whitehead, R.: Gastric ulcer and gastritis. Gut **12**:639, 1971.

108. Gelfand, M.D., Tepper, M., Katz, L.A., et al.: Acute radiation proctitis in man: development of eosinophilic crypt abscesses, Gastroenterology **54**:401, 1968.

109. Genadry, R., Poliakoff, S., Rotmensch, J., et al.: Primary papillary peritoneal neoplasia, Obstet. Gynecol. **58**:730, 1981.

110. Gertler, S.L., Pressman, J., Price, P., Brozinsky, S., and Miyai, K.: Gastrointestinal cytomegalovirus infection in a homosexual man with severe acquired immunodeficiency syndrome, Gastroenterology **85**:1403, 1983.

111. Gilchrist, R.K.: Lymphatic spread of carcinoma of the colon, Dis. Colon Rectum **2**:69, 1959.

112. Glass, R.E., and Baker, W.N.W.: Role of the granuloma in recurrent Crohn's disease, Gut **17**:75, 1976.

113. Godwin, J.D., II: Carcinoid tumors: an analysis of 2,837 cases, Cancer **36**:560, 1975.

114. Golden, R., and Stout, A.P.: Superficial spreading carcinoma of the stomach, Am. J. Roentgenol. **59**:157, 1948.

115. Goldgraber, M.B., and Kirsner, J.B.: Scleroderma of the gastrointestinal tract: a review, Arch. Pathol. (Chicago) **64**:255, 1957.

116. Goldman, H., and Rosoff, C.B.: Pathogenesis of acute gastric stress ulcers, Am. J. Pathol. **52**:227, 1968.

117. Gompel, C., and Silverberg, S.G.: Pathology in gynecology and obstetrics, Philadelphia, 1985, J.B. Lippincott Co.

118. Gonnella, J.S., and Hudson, E.K.: Clinical pattern of tuberculous peritonitis, Arch. Intern. Med. **117**:164, 1966.

119. Gonzales, T.A., Vance, M., and Helpern, M.: Legal medicine, pathology and toxicology, ed. 2, New York, 1954, Appleton-Century-Crofts.

120. González-Crussi, F., and Hackett, R.L.: Phlegmonous gastritis, Arch. Surg. **93**:990, 1966.

121. Goodwin, C.S., Armstrong, J.A., and Marshall, B.J.: *Campylobacter pyloridis*, gastritis and peptic ulceration, J. Clin. Pathol. **39**:353, 1986.

122. Gould, V.E.: Neuroendocrinomas and neuroendocrine carcinomas: APUD cell system neoplasms and their aberrant secretory activities, Pathol. Annu. **12**(Pt. 2):33, 1977.

123. Goulston, S.J.M., and McGovern, V.J.: Pseudo-membranous colitis, Gut **6**:207, 1965.

124. Greene, J.B., Sidhu, G.S., Lewin, S., et al.: *Mycobacterium avium-intracellulare*: a cause of disseminated life-threatening infection in homosexuals and drug abusers, Ann. Intern. Med. **97**:539, 1982.

125. Grendell, J.H., and Ockner, R.K.: Mesenteric venous thrombosis, Gastroenterology **82**:358, 1982.

126. Grimes, O.F., and Stephens, B.H.: Surgical management of acquired short esophagus, Ann. Surg. **152**:743, 1960.

127. Grinnell, R.S.: The spread of carcinoma of the colon and the rectum, Cancer **3**:641, 1950.

128. Grinvalsky, H.T., and Bowerman, C.I.: Stercoraceous ulcers of the colon: relatively neglected medical and surgical problems, JAMA **171**:1941, 1959.

129. Groll, A., Valberg, L.S., Simon, J.B., et al.: Immunologic defect in Whipple's disease, Gastroenterology **63**:943, 1972.

130. Grossman, M.I., Guth, P.H., Isenberg, J.I., et al.: A new look at peptic ulcer, Ann. Intern. Med. **84**:57, 1976.

131. Haggitt, R.C., Glotzbach, R.E., Soffer, E.E., et al.: Prognostic factors in colorectal carcinomas arising in adenomas: implications for lesions removed by endoscopic polypectomy, Gastroenterology **89**:328, 1985.

132. Hamilton, S.R.: Colorectal carcinoma in patients with Crohn's disease, Gastroenterology **89**:398, 1985.

133. Hasiuk, A.S., Peterson, R.O., Hanjani, P.H., et al.: Extragenital malignant mixed müllerian tumor: case report and review of the literature, Am. J. Clin. Pathol. **78**:726, 1984.

134. Hernández, F.J., and Fernández, B.B.: Mucus-secreting colonic carcinoid tumors: light and electron microscopic study of 3 cases, Dis. Colon Rectum **17**:387, 1974.

135. Hernández, F.J., and Reid, J.D.: Mixed carcinoid and mucus-secreting intestinal tumor, Arch. Pathol. (Chicago) **88**:489, 1969.

136. Higa, E., Rosai, J., Pizzimbono, C.A., et al.: Mucosal hyperplasia, mucinous cystadenoma, and mucinous cystadenocarcinoma of the appendix: a re-evaluation of appendiceal "mucocele," Cancer **32**:1525, 1973.

137. Ho, K.J., Herrera, G.A., Jones, J.M., et al.: Small cell carcinoma of the esophagus: evidence for a unified histogenesis, Hum. Pathol. **15**:460, 1984.

138. Horn, R.C., Jr.: Carcinoid tumors of the colon and rectum, Cancer **2**:819, 1949.

139. Horn, R.C., Jr.: Carcinoma of stomach: autopsy findings in untreated cases, Gastroenterology **29**:515, 1955.

140. Hoskins, L.C., Norris, H.T., Gottlieb, L.S., and Zamcheck, N.: Functional and morphologic alterations of the gastrointestinal tract in progressive systemic sclerosis (scleroderma), Am. J. Med. **33**:459, 1962.

141. Hyun, B.H., Palumbo, V.N., and Null, R.H.: Hemangioma of the small intestine with gastrointestinal bleeding, JAMA **208**:1903, 1969.

142. Isaacson, P.G., Spencer, J.O., and Finn, T.: Primary B-cell lymphoma, Hum. Pathol. **17**:72, 1986.

143. Ismail-Beigi, F., Horton, P.F., and Pope, C.E., II: Histological consequences of gastroesophageal reflux in man, Gastroenterology **58**:163, 1970.

144. Jabbari, M., Cherry, R., Lough, J.O., et al.: Gastric antral vascular ectasia: the watermelon stomach, Gastroenterology **87**:1165, 1984.

145. Jabbari, M., Goresky, C.A., Lough, J., et al.: The inlet patch: heterotopic gastric mucosa in the upper esophagus, Gastroenterology **89**:352, 1985.

146. Jacobs, D.S.: Primary gastric malignant lymphoma and pseudolymphoma, Am. J. Clin. Pathol. **40**:379, 1963.

147. James, S.P., Fiocchi, C., Graeff, A.S., and Strober, W.: Immunoregulatory function of lamina propria T cells in Crohn's disease, Gastroenterology **88**:1143, 1985.

148. Jang, G.C., Clouse, M.E., and Fleischner, F.G.: Fibrovascular polyp: a benign intraluminal tumor of the esophagus, Radiology **92**:1196, 1969.

149. Jeffries, J.J., Lyall, W.A., Bezchlibnyk, K., et al.: Retroperitoneal fibrosis and haloperidol, Am. J. Psychiatry **139**:1524, 1984.

150. Johns, T.N.P., Wheeler, J.R., and Johns, F.S.: Meckel's diverticulum and Meckel's disease: a study of 154 cases, Ann. Surg. **150**:241, 1959.

151. Johnson, H.D.: Gastric ulcer: classification, blood group characteristics, secretion patterns and pathogenesis, Ann. Surg. **162**:996, 1965.

152. Johnstone, J.M., and Morson, B.C.: Eosinophilic gastroenteritis, Histopathology **2**:335, 1978.

153. Johnstone, J.M., and Morson, B.C.: Inflammatory fibroid polyp of the gastrointestinal tract, Histopathology **2**:349, 1978.

154. Joseph, J.I., and Lattes, R.: Gastrolymphosarcoma: clinicopathologic analysis of 71 cases and its relation to disseminated lymphosarcoma, Am. J. Clin. Pathol. **45**:653, 1966.

155. Kannerstein, M., Churg, J., McCaughey, W.T.E.: et al.: Papillary tumors of the peritoneum in women: mesothelioma or papillary carcinoma, Am. J. Obstet. Gynecol. **127**:306, 1977.

156. Kapila, L., Haberkorn, S., and Nixon, H.H.: Chronic adynamic bowel simulating Hirschsprung's disease, J. Pediatr. Surg. **10**:885, 1975.

157. Kay, S.: A 10-year appraisal of the treatment of squamous cell carcinoma of the esophagus, Surg. Gynecol. Obstet. **117**:167, 1963.

158. Kay, S., et al.: Glomus tumors of stomach, Cancer **4**:726, 1951.

159. Kean, B.H., Gilmore, H.R., Jr., and Van Stone, W.W.: Fatal amebiasis: report of 148 fatal cases from the Armed Forces Institute of Pathology, Ann. Intern. Med. **44**:831, 1956.

160. Keeley, A.F., and Gottlieb, L.S.: Villous adenoma of the small bowel: an unusual lesion, Gastroenterology **57**:185, 1969.

161. Kepes, J.J., and Zacharias, D.L.: Gangliocytic paragangliomas of the duodenum: a report of two cases with light and electron microscopic examination, Cancer **27**:61, 1971.

162. Keren, D.F.: Whipple's disease: a review emphasizing immunology and microbiology, Crit. Rev. Clin. Lab. Sci. **14**:75, 1981.

163. Kern, F., Jr.: Hepatobiliary disorders in inflammatory bowel disease, Prog. Liver Dis. **5**:575, 1976.

164. Keyting, W.S., McCarver, R.R., Kovarik, J.L., and Daywitt, A.L.: Pneumatosis intestinalis: a new concept, Radiology **76**:733, 1961.

165. Kiesewetter, W.B., Turner, C.R., and Sieber, W.K.: Imperforate anus: review of a 16 year experience with 146 patients, Am. J. Surg. **107**:412, 1964.

166. King, B.T.: New concepts of etiology and treatment of diverticula of esophagus, Surg. Gynecol. Obstet. **85**:93, 1947.

167. Kipfer, R.E., Moertel, C.G., and Dahlin, D.C.: Mesenteric lipodystrophy, Ann. Intern. Med. **80**:582, 1974.

168. Kissane, J.M.: Pathology of infancy and childhood, ed. 2, St. Louis, 1975, The C.V. Mosby Co.

169. Klappenbach, R.S., Kurman, R.J., Sinclair, C.F., et al.: Composite carcinoma-carcinoid tumors of the gastrointestinal tract: a morphologic, histochemical, and immunocytochemical study, Am. J. Clin. Pathol. **84**:137, 1985.

170. Klein, R.S., Harris, C.A., Small, C.B., Moll, B., Lesser, M., and Friedland, G.M.: Oral candidiasis in high-risk patients as the initial manifestation of the acquired immunodeficiency syndrome, N. Engl. J. Med. **311**:354, 1984.

171. Klotz, R.G., Jr., Pamukcoglu, T., and Souilliard, D.H.: Transitional cloacogenic carcinoma of the anal canal: clinicopathologic study of 373 cases, Cancer **20**:1727, 1967.

172. Knauer, C.M.: Mallory-Weiss syndrome: characterization of 75 Mallory-Weiss lacerations in 528 patients with upper gastrointestinal hemorrhage, Gastroenterology **71**:5, 1976.

173. Knuff, T.E., Benjamin, S.B., and Castell, D.O.: Pharyngoesophageal (Zenker's) diverticulum: a reappraisal, Gastroenterology **82**:734, 1982.

174. Kussin, S.Z., Henry, C., Navarro, C., Stenson, W., and Clain, D.J.: Gas within the wall of the stomach: report of a case and review of the literature, Dig. Dis. Sci. **27**:949, 1982.

175. Kwan, D., and Pang, L.S.: Deciduosis peritonei, J. Obstet. Gynaecol. Br. Cmwlth. **71**:804, 1964.

176. Kyrtz, R.J., Heimann, T.M., Holt, J., et al.: Mesenteric and retroperitoneal cysts, Ann. Surg. **203**:109, 1986.

177. Lane, N.: Pseudosarcoma (polypoid sarcoma–like masses) associated with squamous cell carcinoma of the mouth, fauces, and larynx, Cancer **10**:19, 1957.

178. Lane, N.: The precursor tissue of ordinary large bowel cancer, Cancer Res. **36**:2669, 1976.

179. Larson, H.E., Price, A.B., and Honour, P.: *Clostridium difficile* and the etiology of pseudomembranous colitis, Lancet **1**:1063, 1978.

180. Lasser, A., and Koufman, W.B.: Adenomyoma of the stoamch, Am. J. Dig. Dis. **22**:965, 1977.

181. Levine, D.S.: "Solitary" rectal ulcer syndrome: Are "solitary rectal ulcer syndrome and "localized" colitis cystica profunda analogous syndromes caused by rectal prolapse? Gastroenterology **92**:243, 1987.

182. Lewin, K.J., Dowling, F., Wright, J.P., et al.: Gastric morphology and serum gastrin levels in pernicious anemia, Gut **17**:551, 1976.

183. Liebowitz, H.R.: Pathogenesis of esophageal varix rupture, JAMA **175**:874, 1961.

184. Lou, T.Y., Teplitz, C., and Thayer, W.R.: Ultrastructural morphogenesis of colonic PAS-positive macrophages ("colonic histiocytosis"), Hum. Pathol. **2**:421, 1971.

185. Lough, J., Fawcett, J., and Wiegensberg, B.: Wolman's disease: an electron microscopic, histochemical, and biochemical study, Arch. Pathol. **89**:103, 1970.

186. Lupovitch, A., and Tippins, R.: Esophageal intramural pseudodiverticulosis: a disease of adnexal gland, Radiology **113**:271, 1974.

187. MacDermott, R.P.: Cell-mediated immunity in gastrointestinal disease, Hum. Pathol. **17**:219, 1986.

188. MacDermott, R.P., Bragdon, M.J., Kodner, I.J., and Bertovich, M.J.: Deficient cell-mediated cytotoxicity and hyporesponsiveness to interferon and mitogenic lectin activation by inflammatory bowel disease, peripheral blood and intestinal mononuclear cells, Gastroenterology **90**:6, 1986.

189. Maizel, H., Ruffin, J.M., and Dobbins, W.O., III: Whipple's disease: a review of 19 patients from one hospital and a review of the literature since 1950, Medicine (Balt.) **49**:175, 1970.

190. Marchand, P.: The anatomy of esophageal hiatus of the diaphragm and the pathogenesis of hiatus herniation, J. Thorac. Surg. **37**:81, 1959.

191. Marks, J.: The relationship of gastrointestinal disease and the skin, Clin. Gastroenterol. **12**:693, 1983.

192. Marsden, H.B., and Gilchrist, W.: Pulmonary heterotopia in the terminal ileum, J. Pathol. Bacteriol. **86**:532, 1963.

193. Marston, A.: Basic structure and function of the intestinal circulation, Clin. Gastroenterol. **1**:539, 1972.

194. Martin, E.D., and Potet, F.: Pathology of endocrine tumors of the GI tract, Clin. Gastroenterol. **3**:511, 1974.

195. Martin, F.F., Vilseck, J., Dobbins, W.O., III, et al.: Immunological alterations in patients with treated Whipple's disease, Gastroenterology **63**:6, 1972.

196. Martínez, N.S., Morlock, C.G., Dockerty, M.B., Waugh, J.M., and Weber, H.M.: Heterotopic pancreatic tissue involving the stomach, Ann. Surg. **147**:1, 1958.

197. Mathieson, R., and Dutta, S.K.: *Candida* esophagitis, Dig. Dis. Sci. **28**:365, 1983.

198. Matsusaka, T., Watanabe, H., and Enjoji, M.: Pseudosarcoma and carcinosarcoma of the esophagus, Cancer **37**:1546, 1976.

199. Mayo, C.W., Stalker, L.K., and Miller, J.M.: Intra-abdominal hernia: review of 39 cases in which treatment was surgical, Ann. Surg. **114**:875, 1941.

200. Mazier, W.P., Bowman, H.E., Sun, K.M., et al.: Juvenile polyps of the colon and rectum, Dis. Colon Rectum **17**:523, 1974.

201. McCaughey, W.T.E.: Papillary peritoneal neoplasms in females, Pathol. Annu. **20**(2):387, 1985.

202. McFadden, D.E., and Clement, P.B.: Peritoneal inclusion cysts with mural mesothelial proliferation, Am. J. Surg. Pathol. **10**:844, 1986.

203. Means, R.L.: Bile peritonitis, Am. Surg. **30**:583, 1964.

204. Meier-Ruge, W.: Hirschsprung's disease: its aetiology, pathogenesis and differential diagnosis, Curr. Top. Pathol. **59**:131, 1974.

205. Meiselman, M.C., Cello, J.P., and Margaretten, W.: Cytomegalovirus colitis: report of the clinical, endoscopic, and pathologic findings in two patients with the acquired immune deficiency syndrome, Gastroenterology **88**:171, 1985.

206. Mendeloff, A.I., and Dunn, J.P.: Digestive disease, vital and health statistics monographs, Cambridge, 1971, American Public Health Association, Harvard Univeristy Press.

207. Menguy, R.: Pathophysiology of peptic ulcer, Am. J. Surg. **120**:282, 1970.

208. Meyerhoff, J.: Familial Mediterranean fever: report of a large family, review of the literature, and discussion of the frequency of amyloidosis, Medicine **59**:66, 1980.

209. Meyers, M.A., Alonso, D.R., Gray, G.F., and Baer, J.W.: Pathogenesis of bleeding colonic diverticulosis, Gastroenterology **71**:577, 1976.

210. Miles, J.M., Hart, W.R., and McMahon, J.T.: Cystic mesothelioma of the peritoneum: report of a case with multiple recurrences and review of the literature, Cleveland Clin. Q. **53**:109, 1986.

211. Ming, S.C.: The classification and significance of gastric polyps, International Academy of Pathology monograph, The gastrointestinal tract, Baltimore, 1977, The Williams & Wilkins Co.

212. Ming, S.C.: Gastric carcinoma: a pathological classification, Cancer **39**:2475, 1977.

213. Mitchell, D.N., Rees, R.J.W., and Goswami, K.K.A.: Transmissible agents from human sarcoid and Crohn's disease tissue, Lancet **11**:761, 1976.

214. Mitchinson, M.J.: The pathology of idiopathic retroperitoneal fibrosis, J. Clin. Pathol. **23**:681, 1970.

215. Mitchinson, M.J.: Retroperitoneal fibrosis revisited, Arch. Pathol. Lab. Med. **110**:784, 1986.

216. Moertel, C.G., Sauer, W.G., Dockerty, M.B., and Baggenstoss, A.H.: Life history of the carcinoid tumor of the small intestine, Cancer **14**:901, 1961.

217. Moldawer, M.: Multiple endocrine tumors and Zollinger-Ellison syndrome in families: one or two syndromes? A report of two families, Metabolism **11**:153, 1962.

218. Molnar, P., and Miko, T.: Multiple arterial caliber persistence resulting in hematomas and fatal rupture of the gastric wall, Am. J. Surg. Pathol. **6**:83, 1982.

219. Moore, G.E., and Sako, K.: The spread of carcinoma of the colon and rectum: a study of invasion of blood vessels, lymph nodes and the peritoneum by tumor cells, Dis. Colon Rectum **2**:92, 1959.

220. Moore, J.D., Thompson, N.W., Appelman, H.D., and Foley, D.: Arteriovenous malformations of the gastrointestinal tract, Arch. Surg. **111**:381, 1976.

221. Morgan, C.N.: Malignancy in inflammatory disease of the large intestine, Cancer **28**:41, 1971.

222. Morningstar, W.A.: Whipple's disease: an example of the value of the electron microscope in diagnosis, follow-up, and correlation of a pathologic process, Hum. Pathol. **6**:443, 1975.

223. Morrison, A.B., Rawson, A.J., and Fitts, W.T., Jr.: The syndrome of refractory watery diarrhea and hypokalemia in patients with a non-insulin-secreting islet cell tumor: a further case study and review of the literature, Am. J. Med. **32**:119, 1962.

224. Morson, B.C.: Polyps and cancer of the large bowel, International Academy of Pathology monograph, The gastrointestinal tract, Baltimore, 1977, The Williams & Wilkins Co.

225. Morson, B.C., and Volkstadt, H.: Mucoepidermoid tumors of the anal canal, J. Clin. Pathol. **16**:200, 1963.

226. Moses, H.L., and Cheatham, W.J.: The frequency and significance of human herpetic esophagitis: an autopsy study, Lab. Invest. **12**:663, 1963.

227. Murphy, R.T., Goodsitt, E., Morales, H., and Biltons, J.L.: Peptic ulceration with associated endocrine tumors: collective review and report of a case, Am. J. Surg. **100**:764, 1960.

228. Muto, T., Bussey, H.J.R., and Morson, B.C.: Pseudocarcinomatous invasion in adenomatous polyps of the colon and rectum, J. Clin. Pathol. **26**:25, 1973.

229. Naef, A.P., Savary, M., and Ozzelo, L.: Columnar-lined lower esophagus: an acquired lesion with malignant predisposition: report on 140 cases of Barrett's esophagus with 12 adenocarcinomas, J. Thorac. Cardiovasc. Surg. **70**:826, 1975.

230. Naraynsingh, V., Raju, G.C., Ratan, P., and Wong, J.: Massive ascites due to omental endometriosis, Postgrad. Med. J. **61**:539, 1985.

231. Narita, T., Eto, T., and Ito, T.: Peutz-Jeghers syndrome with adenomas and adenocarcinomas in colonic polyps, Am. J. Surg. Pathol. **11**(1):76, 1987.

232. Navin, T.R., and Juranek, D.D.: Cryptosporidiosis: clinical, epidemiologic, and parasitologic review, Rev. Infect. Dis. **6**:313, 1984.

233. Norberg, P.B.: Food as a cause of intestinal obstruction, Am. J. Surg. **104**:444, 1962.

234. Norris, H.T.: Ischemic bowel disease: its spectrum, International Academy of Pathology monograph, The gastrointestinal tract, Baltimore, 1977, The Williams & Wilkins Co.

235. Ochsner, A., and Gage, I.M.: Adynamic ileus, Am. J. Surg. **20**:378, 1933.

236. Ogden. W.W., Bradburn, D.M., and Rines, J.D.: Mesenteric panniculitis: review of 27 cases, Ann. Surg. **161**:864, 1965.

237. Ozzello, L., Savary, M., and Roethlisberger, B.: Columnar mucosa of the distal esophagus in patients with gastroesophageal reflux, Pathol. Ann. **12**:41, 1977.

238. Painter, N.S., and Burkitt, D.P.: Diverticular disease of the colon: a 20th century problem, Clin. Gastroenterol. **4**:3, 1975.

239. Palmer, P.E., Wolfe, H.J., and Kostas, C.I.: Multisystem fibrosis in alpha-1-antitrypsin deficiency, Lancet **1**:221, 1978.

240. Parathap, K., and Gilman, R.: The histopathology of acute intestinal amebiasis: a rectal biopsy study, Am. J. Pathol. **60**:229, 1970.

241. Parks, A.G.: Pathogenesis and treatment of fistula-in-ano, Br. Med. J. **1**:463, 1961.

242. Perea, V.D., and Gregory, L.J., Jr.: Neurofibromatosis of the stomach: report of a case associated with von Recklinghausen's disease and review of the literature, JAMA **182**:259, 1962.

243. Perera, D.R., Weinstein, W.M., and Rubin, C.E.: Small intestinal biopsy, Hum. Pathol. **6**:157, 1975.

244. Perkins, D.E., and Spjut, H.J.: Intestinal stenosis following radiation therapy, Am. J. Roentgenol. **88**:953, 1962.

245. Pomerantz, M., and Waldmann, T.A.: Systemic lymphatic abnormalities associated with gastrointestinal protein loss secondary to intestinal lymphangiectasia, Gastroenterology **45**:703, 1963.

246. Price, A.B., and Davies, D.R.: Pseudomembranous colitis, J. Clin. Pathol. **30**:1, 1977.

247. Pruitt, B.A., Jr., Foley, F.D., and Moncrief, J.A.: Curling's ulcer: a clinical pathological study of 323 cases, Ann. Surg. **172**:523, 1970.

248. Putman, H.C., Jr., Dockerty, M.B., and Waugh, J.M.: Abdominal actinomycosis: analysis of 122 cases, Surgery **28**:781, 1950.

249. Qizilbash, A.H., Meghji, M., and Castelli, M.: Pseudocarcinomatous invasion in adenomas of the colon and rectum, Dis. Colon Rectum **23**:529, 1980.

250. Quan, S.H.Q., White, J.E., and Deddish, M.R.: Malignant melanoma of the anorectum, Dis. Colon Rectum **2**:275, 1959.

251. Quinn, T.C., Goodell, S.E., Mkrtichian, E., et al.: *Chlamydia trachomatis* proctitis, N. Engl. J. Med. **305**:195, 1981.

252. Ranchod, M., and Kempson, L.: Smooth muscle tumors of the gastrointestinal tract and retroperitoneum: a pathologic analysis of 100 cases, Cancer **39**:255, 1977.

253. Rector, L.E., and Connerley, M.L.: Aberrant mucosa in esophagus in infants and in children, Arch. Pathol. (Chicago) **31**:285, 1941.

254. Regan, J.F., and Cremin, J.H.: Chorionepithelioma of the stomach, Am. J. Surg. **100**:224, 1960.

255. Renton, C.J.C.: Non-occlusive intestinal infarction, Clin. Gastroenterol. **1**:655, 1972.

256. Reyes, C.V., Foy, B.K., Aranha, G.V., et al.: Omental oxyuriasis: case report, Milit. Med. **149**:682, 1984.

257. Rhodes, J., and Calcraft, B.: Aetiology of gastric ulcer with special reference to the roles of reflux and mucosal damage, Clin. Gastroenterol. **2**:227, 1973.

258. Riddell, R.H., Goldman, H., Ransohoff, D.F., et al.: Dysplasia in inflammatory bowel disease: standardized classification with provisional clinical applications, Hum. Pathol. **14**:931, 1983.

259. Rosai, J., and Dehner, L.P.: Nodular mesothelial hyperplasia in hernial sacs: a benign reactive condition simulating a neoplastic process, Cancer **35**:165, 1975.

260. Roth, L.M.: The Brenner tumor and the Walthard cell nest: an electron-microscopic study, Lab. Invest. **31**:15, 1974.

261. Roth, R.I., Owen, R.L., Keren, D.F., and Volberding, P.A.: Intestinal infection with *Mycobacterium avium* in acquired immune deficiency syndrome (AIDS): histological and clinical comparison with Whipple's disease, Dig. Dis. Sci. **30**:497, 1985.

262. Roth, S.I., and Helwig, E.B.: Juvenile polyps of the colon and rectum, Cancer **16**:468, 1963.

263. Rubin, H., Furcolow, M.L., Yates, J.L., and Brasher, C.A.: The course and prognosis of histoplasmosis, Am. J. Med. **27**:278, 1959.

264. Ryan, G.B., Grobety, J., and Majno, G.: Postoperative peritoneal adhesions: a study of the mechanisms, Am. J. Pathol. **65**:117, 1971.

265. Sachar, D.B., Auslander, M.O., and Walfish, J.S.: Aetiological theories of inflammatory bowel disease, Clin. Gastroenterol. **9**:231, 1980.

266. Sachatello, C.R., Pickren, J.W., and Grace, J.T., Jr.: Generalized juvenile gastrointestinal polyposis: a hereditary syndrome, Gastroenterology **58**:699, 1970.

267. Saeed, S.M., Fine, G., and Horn, R.C., Jr.: Hypoglycemia associated with extrapancreatic tumors: an immunofluorescent study, Cancer **24**:158, 1969.

268. Sahai, D.B., Palmer, J.D., and Hampson, L.G.: Submucosal lipomas of the large bowel, Can. J. Surg. **11**:23, 1968.

269. Sandenberg, H.A., and Woodruff, J.D.: Histogenesis of pseudomyxoma peritonei: review of 9 cases, Obstet. Gynecol. **49**:339, 1977.

270. Sanusi, I.D., and Tio, F.O.: Gastrointestinal malakoplakia: report of a case and a review of the literature, Am. J. Gastroenterol. **62**:356, 1974.

271. Saphir, O., and Parker, M.L.: Linitis plastica type of carcinoma, Surg. Gynecol. Obstet. **76**:206, 1943.

272. Schaldenbrand, J.D., and Appelman, H.D.: Solitary solid stroma gastrointestinal tumors in von Recklinghausen's disease with minimal smooth muscle differentiation, Hum. Pathol. **15**:229, 1984.

273. Schenken, J.R., and Moss, E.S.: *Enterobius vermicularis* in appendix: report of study on 1,000 surgically removed appendices, Am. J. Clin. Pathol. **12**:509, 1942.

274. Schmerin, M.J., Gelston, A., and Jones, T.C.: Amebiasis: an increasing problem among homosexuals in New York City, JAMA **238**:1386, 1977.

275. Schwartz, F.D., Dunea, G., and Kark, R.M.: Methysergide and retroperitoneal fibrosis, Am. Heart J. **72**:843, 1966.

276. Scully, R.E.: Sex cord tumor with annular tubules: a distinctive ovarian tumor of the Peutz-Jeghers syndrome, Cancer **25**:1107, 1970.

277. Seagram, C.G.F., Louch, R.E., Stephens, C.A., et al.: Meckel's diverticulum: a 10-year review of 218 cases, Can. J. Surg. **11**:369, 1968.

278. Shamma'a, M.H., and Benedict, E.B.: Esophageal webs, N. Engl. J. Med. **259**:378, 1958.

279. Siegal, F.P., Lopez, C., Hammer, G.S., Brown, A.E., Kornfeld, S.J., et al.: Severe acquired immunodeficiency in male homosexuals, manifested by chronic perianal ulcerative herpes simplex lesions, N. Engl. J. Med. **305**:1439, 1981.

280. Sieracki, J.C., and Fine, G.: Whipple's disease: observations on systemic involvement. II. Gross and histologic observations, Arch. Pathol. (Chicago) **67**:81, 1959.

281. Silberstein, M.J., Lewis, J.E., Blair, J.D., et al.: Congenital peritoneal mesothelioma, J. Pediatr. Surg. **18**:243, 1983.

282. Singh, R.S., and Sahay, S.: Retroperitoneal primary hydatid cyst of pelvis, J. Indian Med. Assoc. **83**:64, 1985.

283. Sizer, J.S., Frederick, P.L., and Osborne, M.P.: Primary linitis plastica of the colon: report of a case and review of the literature, Dis. Colon Rectum **10**:339, 1967.

284. Skandalakis, J.E., Gray, S.W., and Shepard, D.: Smooth muscle tumor of the stomach, Int. Abst. Surg. **110**:209, 1960.

285. Smith, B.H., and Welter, E.H.: Pneumatosis intestinalis, Am. J. Clin. Pathol. **48**:455, 1967.

286. Smith, C.R., Jr., Bartholomew, L.G., and Cain, J.C.: Hereditary hemorrhagic telangiectasia and gastrointestinal hemorrhage, Gastroenterology **44**:1, 1963.

287. Sobel, H.J., Schiffman, R.J., and Schwartz, R., et al.: Granulomas and peritonitis due to starch glove powder, Arch. Pathol. (Chicago) **91**:559, 1971.

288. Southwick, H.W., Harridge, W.H., and Cole, W.H.: Recurrence at the suture line following resection for carcinoma of the colon: incidence following preventive measure, Am. J. Surg. **103**:86, 1962.

289. Spira, I.A., Ghazi, A., and Wolff, W.I.: Primary adenocarcinoma of the duodenum, Cancer **39**:1721, 1977.

290. Starr, G.F., and Dockerty, M.B.: Leiomyomas and leiomyosarcoma of the small intestine, Cancer **8**:101, 1955.

291. Steinberg, L., Rothman, D., and Drey, N.W.: Müllerian cyst of the retroperitoneum, Am. J. Obstet. Gynecol. **107**:963, 1970.

292. Stempien, S.J., Dagradi, A.E., Reingold, I.M., et al.: Hypertrophic hypersecretory gastropathy: analysis of 15 cases and a review of the pertinent literature, Am. J. Dig. Dis. **9**:471, 1964.

293. Stewart, T.W., Jr., and Finberg, T.R.: Idiopathic retroperitoneal fibrosis with diffuse involvement: further evidence of systemic idiopathic fibrosis, South. Med. J. **77**:1185, 1985.

294. Stout, A.P.: Pathology of carcinoma of the stomach, Arch. Surg. (Chicago) **46**:807, 1943.

295. Strickland, R.J., and Mackay, I.R.: A reappraisal of the nature and significance of chronic atrophic gastritis, Am. J. Dig. Dis. **18**:426, 1973.

296. Strom, R.L., and Gruninger, R.P.: AIDS with *Mycobacterium avium-intracellulare* lesions resembling those of Whipple's disease, N. Engl. J. Med. **309**:1323, 1983.

297. Tagart, R.E.B.: Endometriosis of the large intestine, Br. J. Surg. **47**:27, 1959.

298. Talerman, A., Montero, J.R., Chilcote, R.R., et al.: Diffuse malignant peritoneal mesothelioma in a 13 year old girl: report of a case and review of the literature, Am. J. Surg. Pathol. **9**:73, 1985.

299. Tallqvist, A., Salmela, H., and Lindström, B.L.: Leiomyoblastoma of the stomach, Acta Pathol. Microbiol. Scand. **71**:194, 1967.

300. Tandon, H.D., and Prakash, A.: Pathology of intestinal tuberculosis and its distinction from Crohn's disease, Gut **13**:260, 1972.

301. Tavassoli, F.A., and Norris, H.G.: Peritoneal leiomyomatosis (leiomyomatosis peritonealis disseminata): a clinicopathologic study of 20 cases with ultrastructural observations, Int. J. Gynecol. Pathol. **1**:59, 1982.

302. Therkelsen, F.: On histological diagnosis of appendicitis, Acta Chir. Scand. **94**(suppl. 108):1, 1946.

303. Thieme, G.A., Bundy, A.L., Fleischer, A.C., et al.: Blastomycosis presenting as a peritoneal inflammatory cyst, J. Clin. Ultrasound **13**:205, 1985.

304. Thompson, G.T., Fitzgerald, E.F., and Somers, S.S.: Retractile mesenteric of the sigmoid colon, Br. J. Radiol. **58**:266, 1985.

305. Thompson, H.: Vascular pathology of the splanchnic circulation, Clin. Gastroenterol. **1**:597, 1972.

306. Thompson, H.L., and McGuffin, D.W.: Melena: study of underlying causes, JAMA **141**:1208, 1949.

307. Thompson, W.G., and Patel, D.G.: Clinical picture of diverticular disease of the colon, Clin. Gastroenterol. **15**:903, 1986.

308. Tonkin, R.D., Field, T.E., and Wykes, P.R.: Pancreatic heterotopia as a cause of dyspepsia, Gut **3**:135, 1962.

309. Torma, M.J., DeLemos, R.A., Rogers, J.R., Jr., et al.: Necrotizing enterocolitis in infants: analysis of forty-five consecutive cases, Am. J. Surg. **126**:758, 1973.

310. Trier, J.S., Phelps, P.C., Eidelman, S., et al.: Whipple's disease: light and electron microscope correlation of jejunal mucosal histology with antibiotic treatment and clinical status, Gastroenterology **48**:684, 1965.

311. Trier, J.S., Falchuk, Z.M., Carey, M.C., and Schreiber, D.S.: Celiac sprue and refractory sprue, Gastroenterology **75**:307, 1978.

312. Truong, L.D., Jurco, S., and McGavran, M.H.: Gliomatosis peritonei, Am. J. Surg. Pathol. **6**:443, 1982.

313. Tumen, H.J.: In Bockus, H.L.: Gastroenterology, vol. 2, Intestinal obstruction, ed. 2, Philadelphia, 1964, W.B. Saunders Co.

314. Turcot, J., Despres, M.P., and St. Pierre, F.: Malignant tumors of the central nervous system associated with familial polyposis of the colon, Dis. Colon Rectum **2**:465, 1959.

315. Ulbright, T.M., and Kraus, F.T.: Endometrial stromal tumors of extrauterine tissue, Am. J. Clin. Pathol. **76**:371, 1981.

316. Valente, P.T.: Leiomyomatosis peritonealis disseminata: a report of two cases and review of the literature, Arch. Pathol. Lab. Med. **108**:669, 1984.

317. Veldhuyzen van Zanten, S.J.O., Bartelsman, J.F.W.M., Schipper, M.E.I., and Tytgat, G.N.J.: Recurrent massive hematemesis from Dieulafoy vascular malformation: a review of 101 cases, Gut **27**:213, 1986.

318. Vezeridis, M.P., Herrera, L.O., López, G.E., et al.: Squamous cell carcinoma of the colon and rectum, Dis. Colon Rectum **26**:188, 1983.

319. Waldmann, T.A., Steinfeld, J.L., Dutcher, T.F., Davidson, J.D., and Gordon, R.S., Jr.: The role of the gastrointestinal system in "idiopathic hypoproteinemia," Gastroenterology **41**:197, 1961.

320. Wall, S.D., Friedman, S.L., and Margulis, A.R.: Gastrointestinal Kaposi's sarcoma in AIDS: radiographic manifestations, J. Clin. Gastroenterol. **6**:165, 1984.

321. Wang, K.K., Perrault, J., Carpenter, H.A., Schroeder, K.W., and Tremaine, W.J.: Collagenous colitis: a clinicopathologic correlation, Mayo Clin. Proc. **62**:665, 1987.

322. Wangensteen, O.H., and Dennis, C.: Experimental proof of the obstructive origin of appendicitis in man, Ann. Surg. **110**:629, 1939.

323. Watson, W.J., Sundwall, D.A., and Bensen, W.L.: Splenosis mimicking endometriosis, Obstet. Gynecol. **59**(suppl.):518, 1982.

324. Wayte, D.M., and Helwig, E.B.: Colitis cystica profunda, Am. J. Clin. Pathol. **48**:159, 1967.

325. Wayte, D.M., and Helwig, E.B.: Small bowel ulceration—iatrogenic or multifactorial origin? Am. J. Clin. Pathol. **49**:26, 1968.

326. Weedon, D.D., Shorter, R.G., Ilstrup, D.M., et al.: Crohn's disease and cancer, N. Engl. J. Med. **289**:1099, 1973.

327. Weinstein, E.C., Cain, J.C., and ReMine, W.H.: Meckel's diverticulum, 55 years of clinical and surgical experience, JAMA **182**:251, 1962.

328. Weinstein, W.M., Saunders, D.R., Tytgat, G.N., et al.: Collagenous sprue: an unrecognized type of malabsorption, N. Engl. J. Med. **283**:1297, 1970.

329. Weiser, M.M., Andres, G.A., Brentjens, J.R., Evans, J.T., and Reichlin, M.: Systemic lupus erythematosus and intestinal venulitis, Gastroenterology **81**:570, 1981.

330. Wells, C.L., Moran, T.J., and Cooper, W.M.: Villous tumors of the rectosigmoid colon, with severe electrolyte imbalance: a cause of unexplained morbidity and sudden mortality, Am. J. Clin. Pathol. **37**:507, 1962.

331. Whitehead, R.: The pathology of ischemia of the intestines, Pathol. Annu. **11**:1, 1976.

332. Whitehead, R., Truelove, S.C., and Gear, W.L.: The histological diagnosis of chronic gastritis in fibreoptic gastroscope biopsy specimens, J. Clin. Pathol. **25**:1, 1972.

333. Whiteside, M.E., Barkin, J.S., May, R.G., Weiss, S.D., Fischl, M.A., and Macleod, C.L.: Enteric coccidiosis among patients with the acquired immunodeficiency syndrome, Am. J. Trop. Med. Hyg. **33**:1065, 1984.

334. Williams, E.D., and Sandler, M.: The classification of carcinoid tumors, Lancet **1**:238, 1963.

335. Windsor, C.W.O.: Ischemic strictures of the small bowel, Clin. Gastroenterol. **1**:707, 1972.

336. Wolf, S.: Summary of evidence relating life situation and emotional response to peptic ulcer, Ann. Intern. Med. **31**:637, 1949.

337. Yale, C.E., Balish, E., and Wu, J.P.: The bacterial etiology of pneumatosis cystoides intestinalis, Arch. Surg. **109**:89, 1974.

338. Yardley, J.H., Bayless, T.M., and Diamond, M.P.: Cancer in ulcerative colitis, Gastroenterology **76**:221, 1979.

339. Zinsser, K.R., and Wheeler, J.E.: Endosalpingiosis in the omentum: a study of autopsy and surgical material, Am. J. Surg. Pathol. **6**:109, 1982.

25 Liver

JOHN REDFERND CRAIG

GENERAL CONSIDERATIONS: EMBRYOLOGY AND STRUCTURE

The liver arises from the hepatic diverticulum in the 20- to 25-somite embryo. The primitive hepatic cells grow into the septum transversum, where the endodermal cells proliferate rapidly. At the same time, rapid growth of the mesoderm produces angioblasts and sinusoids.[57] The formation of hepatocytes is determined by an interaction between the endodermal cells and the precardiac mesoderm.[39] Glycogen granules are noted at 8 weeks. The development of intrahepatic bile ducts is complete at 3 months,[37] at which time bile secretion is said to begin. In the third month the liver begins to store iron and concurrently becomes the chief blood-forming organ of the embryo. The site of hematopoiesis is in the extravascular component of the lobule.[28] This hematopoietic function is gradually transferred to the bone marrow as it develops so that by birth only an occasional focus of hematopoiesis remains in the liver. In premature infants, areas of hematopoiesis are abundant. Sinusoids appear at 5 weeks' gestation as do Kupffer cells apparently derived from extrahepatic sources.[13] Circulating macrophages settle in the sinusoids and become Kupffer cells before marrow hematopoiesis is established. Ito cells probably develop from the septum transversum and are established in the sinusoids also.[13] In the full-term baby the liver weight is 135 g and the range is 75 to 180 g. The liver projects well below the costal margin. The left lobe is relatively large in the neonate and during fetal life. This lobe receives well-oxygenated blood from the umbilical vein. This vein atrophies after parturition and becomes the round ligament. The omphalomesenteric veins drain predominantly into the large right lobe of the liver, and from these veins evolves the portal vein.

The vascular and biliary supply of the liver has many anatomic variations, which require special study prior to major hepatic surgery. Traditionally, the liver may be divided anatomically into a right and left lobe with the division 1 to 1.5 cm to the right of the falciform ligament, approximately the gall bladder/vena cava line. However, further study reveals that there are eight segments of the two lobes and a caudate segment (lobe), each segment with a separate blood supply and biliary drainage. Whereas the portal vein, hepatic artery, and bile ducts form a unified vascular mesenchymal stalk in the liver structure, the hepatic venous drainage follows a slightly different course and has its own variations.[47]

The liver grows at a relatively slower rate than the rest of the body and reaches approximately 1350 g in the adult. At maturity the liver is located most commonly at or above the right costal margin, and the right lobe is larger than the left. The organ is held in place by the falciform and triangular ligaments. A thin, firm, and smooth fibrous capsule (Glisson's capsule) covers the liver and is continuous with the porta hepatis, which is the combined portal vein, hepatic artery, and common bile duct as they enter the liver at the hilum. A connective tissue sheath surrounds the subdivisions of the portal veins, biliary ducts, and hepatic arteries as they divide and supply the segments.

The microscopic anatomy of the liver reveals a lobular structure that in the classic terminology was composed of a portal triad and central vein. However, in vivo microcirculatory studies have demonstrated that the functioning liver unit is the acinus. Blood flow is a rhythmic pattern of varying flow to different portal areas and into the lobules and thus variable flow into the associated central vein. Furthermore, the most oxygenated blood is in the portal areas and periportal areas, and the least oxygenated blood is centrilobular. Therefore Rappaport has advocated that the portal area is central; the central vein is peripheral (in reference to oxygenation) and better called the terminal hepatic venule.[53] An acinus is composed of hepatocytes arranged in plates of two cells with bile canaliculi between them along with a sinusoid at the vascular side.

There are four types of hepatic sinusoid lining cells: (1) Kupffer cells (a major function is phagocytosis), (2) endothelial cells (a major function is pinocytosis), (3) Ito cells (vitamin A storage), and (4) the pit cells (unknown function[14,32]). Although the Kupffer cells may appear similar throughout the lobule, there is also functional heterogeneity, with the periportal Kupffer cells possessing greater endocytotic activity than the perivenular

Kupffer cells. Other functions of the lining cells are pinocytosis, phagocytosis, erythrophagocytosis and iron metabolism, clearance of immune complexes and antigens, and secretion of endogenous pyrogen, collagenase, lysosomal hydrolases, and erythropoietin.[32] The arrangement of these sinusoid lining cells has been clarified by scanning electron microscopy and rapid-freeze fixation. The endothelial cells form a lining with many small fenestrae (average diameter of 100 nm[26]) in clusters called a sieve plate, and thus a sieve for plasma is present. Microvilli of the hepatocyte protrude into the sinusoid through the fenestrae especially during transit of blood cells through the sinusoid. As a relatively large blood cell passes through the small sinusoid, the blood cells push the endothelium aside and next to the hepatocyte (a "massage"), thus promoting the circulation of blood plasma along the space of Disse. The space of Disse resides behind the endothelial lining cells and is next to the hepatocyte. These endothelial fenestrae change in response to hormones, anoxia, drugs, and location, with a higher density at zone 3 (perivenular) than zone 1 (periportal[26]). The sinusoid cells perform many functions integrated with the hepatocytes. The integrated relationship is also demonstrated by the longer survival of cultured hepatocytes if grown with the sinusoid lining cells compared to their absence. Pathologic fenestrae diminish in number and increase in size with alcohol injury. Disruption and injury of the sinusoid endothelium, caused by carbon tetrachloride, paracetamol, anoxia, virus, and so forth, precede injury and death of hepatocytes.[14] Whereas the endothelial lining cells form a barrier to the blood (so-called blood-hepatocytic barrier), the Kupffer cell resides within the sinusoid, and the Ito cell (the original Kupffer cell as first described) resides within the perisinusoidal space (that is, between the endothelial cell and the hepatocyte and called the space of Disse). The reticulin stain reveals by light microscopy the thin fibers that form the framework for the sinusoid cells to be supported. These thin fibers are relatively inapparent by routine light microscopy.[27] By scanning electron microscopy, microfilaments and granular material are noted encircling the sinusoids.[27] The role of Ito cells in the normal liver appears to be storage of vitamin A, and they are likely the major site of collagen production.[35] Pit cells, a fourth type of nonhepatocytic lobular component, appear to be lymphocytes and have been identified in human liver.[34]

Biliary drainage begins by secretion of fluid into the small biliary canaliculi formed by adjacent hepatocytes. These small biliary canaliculi form a channel continuous with the short duct of Hering, which joins the cholangiole at the limiting plate of the portal area. These cholangioles merge into large bile ducts (which are recognized by the adjacent hepatic arteriole) and then the channel progresses to large sublobular bile ducts and to large major bile ducts. Biliary casts of human liver indicate a biliary plexus is formed around large (1 to 1.5 mm diameter) bile ducts and that this pattern differs from the biliary channels in rabbit and dog.[64] Aberration in development of this plexus may account for "limiting plate anomalies."

Each portal tract has a branch of the hepatic artery with a high pressure, and the sphincter activity allows a reduction in pressure as the arterial blood is passed onto the sinusoid. Microvascular casts of the hepatic artery in human liver has revealed that small arterioles terminate in sinusoids adjacent to the portal tracts and that no arterioportal anastomoses exist in the normal state.[65] Lymph flow extends from the space of Disse to portal lymphatic vessels to the hilum of the liver.

Each portal tract contains connective tissue and inflammatory cells as well as the branches of hepatic artery, portal vein, and bile duct. The connective tissue is mainly collagen type I, which is thick blue fiber by trichrome stain. Thin blue fibers are collagen type III. Subcapsular portal tracts often contain considerable fibrous branches from the adjacent Glisson's capsule, which may simulate significant fibrosis even though deeper sections reveal no true functional portal fibrosis. The number of portal lymphocytes changes with systemic inflammatory activity and appears to increase with age.[18]

The hepatocyte, which is 60% of the liver cell population and is 80% of the cell volume, has been extensively studied by electron microscopy in healthy human volunteers as well as a variety of disease states.[40,50,54] The hepatocellular sinusoid border, 40% of the total surface, is specialized microvilli, and the bile canaliculi are 15% of the plasma membrane (Fig. 25-1). The content of organelles within the hepatocytes varies with location within the acinar zone. Hepatocytes with greater oxygen exposure in the periportal area (zone 1 of Rappaport) have more mitochondria, and they are oval and oblong, whereas the perivenular hepatocytes have fewer mitochondria and they are round.[50] The nuclear envelope, with its 3000- to 4000-pore complexes demonstrated by freeze fracture, is bilayered, with the outer bilayer continuous with the rough endoplasmic reticulum. Nuclear glycogen, densely packed, clumped granules, are common in diabetes, glycogen storage disease, and Wilson's disease. A cytoplasmic invagination into the nucleus, recognized by its nuclear membrane surrounding a small collection of cytoplasmic organelles, may be noted by light microscopy as well. The nucleus is 7% of the hepatocyte volume, and the endoplasmic reticulum (both rough and smooth types) constitutes 19% of the total volume. The endoplasmic reticulum is 60% ribosome-coated membrane, and it has been estimated that the hepatocyte has more than

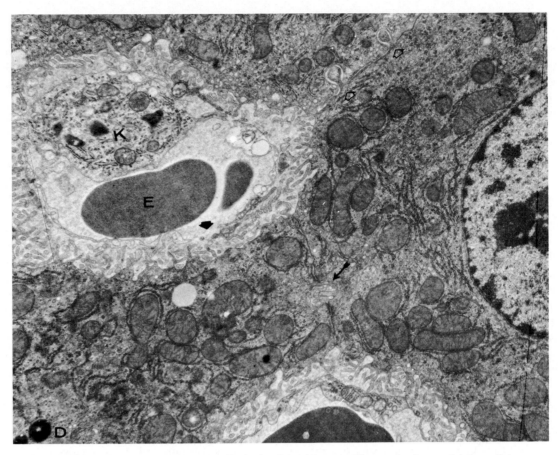

Fig. 25-1. Interlocking of liver cells is furnished by studlike projections of intercellular membrane *(open arrowheads)*. *E,* Erythrocyte in sinusoid; *K,* Kupffer cell; *D,* dense body; *arrow,* bile canaliculus; *black arrowhead,* pore in endothelium lining.

10 million ribosomes. Mitochondria account for 17% of the volume and are the most numerous of the organelles with about 2200 per hepatocyte. They are highly mobile and change shape rapidly. Peroxisomes are 1% to 2% of the hepatocyte volume and are named to reflect their role in hydrogen peroxide metabolism. They are more numerous in the perivenular zones and are important in oxidation of fatty acids and detoxification. Secretion of macromolecules is accomplished by the Golgi apparatus, which is a small part of the total volume. Ground substance is 51% of the hepatocellular volume and includes microfilaments (actin filaments), intermediate filaments, and microtubules. Visualization of intermediate filaments required development of special techniques including perfusion with detergent solution. This allowed recognition of the physical connection the intermediate filaments made with the various subcellular organelles, including the nuclei, centrioles, microtubules, vesicles, and rough endoplasmic reticulum.[16] Lysosomes are membrane-bound bodies containing many hydrolases as well as degradative products including ferritin (then called siderosomes), coarse

electron-dense granules (lipofuchsin granules), and many other vacuolated vesicles. Glycogen particles are diffusely distributed, clumped granules that vary in number according to the metabolic state of the entire organ. Small lipid droplets are common and in abnormal metabolic conditions become very numerous and even coalesce into large droplets.

CONGENITAL AND ACQUIRED ABNORMALITIES OF FORM

Developmental anomalies may produce atypical clinical findings including hepatomegaly. Noticeable enlargement and downward growth of the right lobe is called Reidel's lobe and may be attributable to adhesion to the mesocolon during development. An accessory lobe may protrude through a defect in the abdominal wall and be visible externally.[30] Abnormal development of primordial liver rests may result in ectopic hepatic tissue located in the gallbladder, spleen, pancreas, umbilicus, adrenal, mesentery, and lung.[42] However, ectopic tissue "trapped" within the liver includes pancreas, adrenal cortex, and presumable germ cell tissue from which teratoma arise.[20] Fusion of the right adrenal gland and liver is recognized by the lack of a fibrous capsule between the two structures in contrast to adhesion of the two organs.[11] Functioning adrenal tumors apparently derived from aberrant adrenocortical tissue have been reported.[7] Inflammatory conditions within the abdomen may promote adhesion of an epiploic appendage from the colon and thus forms a pseudolipoma of liver and is recognized by the separation of the fat by a fibrous capsule (Glisson's capsule). Other acquired anomalies may be attributable to infection, infarction, or tumor. Hepar lobatum is a coarsely lobulated liver caused by broad fibrous scars that have contracted around large macroregenerative nodules and in recent years has been associated with chemotherapy though traditionally it occurred with hepatic syphilis.[52] Deep transverse, oblique, or sagittal grooves on the anterior liver surface have been attributed to pressure from ribs perhaps aggravated by repeated coughing, or hypertrophied diaphramatic muscles from lung disease. Glisson's capsule is thickened in the grooves, and no functional significance is known. Atrophy of a liver segment or lobe occurs in inflammatory conditions such as alcoholic liver disease, which often has a dense fibrous scar near the hilum usually in the midline on the anterior region and seems to promote left lobe atrophy. Severe atrophy of one lobe may occur with vascular or bile duct occlusion of a major vessel or bile duct feeding or draining the lobe.[23,46] Cirrhosis (either alcoholic or cryptogenic), cholangiocarcinoma of a major bile duct, and severe repeated attacks of cholangiohepatitis with abscess formation and secondary pyelophlebitis are common causes of left-lobe atrophy.

BASIC HEPATIC HISTOPATHOLOGY

Microscopic assessment of the liver requires systematic review of the hepatic components and a knowledge of the cellular changes. I describe below an approach to histologic analysis of the liver in simple terms and more precise details follow in the sections of specific diseases. Although each reader may utilize a specific method of review, a systematic and thorough review of the hepatic microscopic structure is essential for complete evaluation and correlation with the clinical state. Final conclusion regarding the type and activity of hepatic disease requires correlation with clinical information, special tests (often immunologic and serologic), and often special stains for specific agents or markers. I prefer to describe the hepatic architecture in sequence from a low-power to a high-power view through the microscope and then also to follow the blood flow.[49a] Thus my descriptive approach is to observe the low-power overall lobular architecture including the relationship of the portal areas to terminal hepatic veins, the presence of apparently normal liver, in contrast to large areas of tumor (either hepatocellular or other cellular origin), and the number of major vessels and ducts. Then I proceed into the lobule and describe the hepatic cords and terminal hepatic venule as well as search for pertinent structures such as granuloma or tumor as suggested by clinical or other information.

The "normal" portal area has approximately one portal vein and one cholangiole and one hepatic arteriole though, frequency attributable to branching, two channels of any of the structures are common. In some diseases numerous bile ducts or vessels occur, and in other diseases their absence is a helpful clue. The components of the portal area also include lymphocytes, macrophages (sometimes filled with pigment such as iron), and abnormal portal areas may include neoplastic cells or granuloma formation. The limiting plate that separates the portal area from the adjacent hepatic cords of hepatocytes is sharp in contrast to some chronic liver disease with prominent lymphocytic hyperplasia and extension of these lymphocytes and also of macrophages into the adjacent cords. This extension of inflammatory cells and associated hepatocellular necrosis is called "piecemeal necrosis." Such change is noted in a wide variety of acute and chronic inflammatory conditions and is not diagnostic of previous or current viral hepatitis but is commonly noted in viral hepatitis. Because the portal areas include a significant lymphocyte population, a systemic inflammatory response includes portal lymphoid hyperplasia (not infiltration). Such hyperplasia should not be considered a hepatic disease. Conditions predisposing to portal lymphoid hyperplasia include rheumatoid arthritis, systemic lupus erythematosus, intravenous drug use, sepsis, and inflammatory bowel disease. This portal hyperplasia includes lymphocytes, macrophages, immunoblasts, and plasma cells.

The density of the collagen (whether portal or lobular) is very hard in the chronic alcoholic, whereas in the normal portal area the density and closeness of the collagen bundles appears less hard. The number of portal vessels increases in most chronic liver diseases and is a reflection of the abnormal blood flow (portal hypertension). Bile duct proliferation is common in biliary tract obstruction in the early stages but is reduced in the late stages.

Hepatocellular changes

Hydropic change is a descriptive term applied to the hepatocyte with pale, watery cytoplasm and a normal nucleus. A wide variety of conditions produce this relative lack of cytoplasmic staining. Mitochondria and ribosomes of the rough endoplasmic reticulum are the principal eosinophilic components of hepatocytes, and increased eosinophilia may occur with drug-related hyperplasia of the smooth endoplasmic reticulum. Physiologic causes for reduction in cytoplasmic eosinophilia include an increased glycogen storage, which may be prominent after high levels of carbohydrate feeding. Such a diet also stimulates proliferation of smooth endoplasmic reticulum, but the usual light-microscopic expression of the abundant glycogen is pale cytoplasmic staining. Active regeneration of hepatocytes after necrosis as in severe viral hepatitis, or recovery phase of fatty liver, produces a widespread hepatocellular hydropic change as well as a *cobblestone pattern* of the liver cords, in which the sinusoids are obliterated by the hepatocellular swelling and the cells are "packed" together and appear as stones of a cobblestone street. Hydropic change is also an indicator of hepatocellular damage and is noted in acute viral hepatitis (which also has inflammatory reaction), and drug-induced hepatic injury including alcohol injury, in which case interference with microfilament function is postulated.[91]

Atrophy of hepatocytes characterized by smaller cells and slightly more eosinophilic cytoplasm is common in cachectic states and old age and by circulatory impairment such as may occur with a large tumor-producing pressure on the adjacent hepatic vessels. The sinusoids are usually expanded, and careful fixation is necessary to avoid mistaking poor fixation for true atrophy.

Hepatocellular fat accumulation may be either large cytoplasmic bodies *(macrovesicular fatty change)* or foamy fat *(macrovesicular fatty change)* composed of minute fine foamy vesicles of fat within a hepatocyte. Normal liver contains 5% fat (by weight) and with pronounced fatty liver nearly 50% of the weight is triglyceride. Lipid droplets form in the endoplasmic reticulum and coalesce into larger masses. Fatty liver occurs because of (1) sudden increase in mobilization of fat from the periphery to the liver, (2) relative lack of protein necessary for hepatocellular fat release, (3) increased hepatocellular fat formation by metabolic changes, and (4) decrease hepatocellular fat degradation. Fatty liver is common in alcohol ingestion, parenteral nutrition, tuberculosis, starvation, certain drugs (tetracycline, steroids), diabetes mellitus, and obesity. *Kwashiorkor,* caused by protein-calorie malnutrition, produces a noticeable fatty change in hepatocytes, first in the periportal areas and later in the perivenular region.[117] Electron microscopy shows that the cytoplasmic fat is not membrane bound[158] and lysosomes are greatly increased.

Alcoholic hyaline body (or Mallory body, MB) is a distinctive, irregularly clumped cytoplasmic mass that stains deeply with eosin, red with Masson's trichrome, and blue with aniline blue and does not stain with acid-fast or PAS.[133] MBs have been isolated from human liver and are composed of at least five polypeptide bands. By electron microscopy, large mitochondria were believed responsible for the MB structure. With more careful study, MB have been classified into three morphologic types and are clumps of thin filaments.[163] MBs are derived from intermediate filaments (IF), which are so named because they are intermediate in size compared to the thinner actin filaments and the thicker microtubules.[91] IF function is apparently to mechanically organize the cytoplasmic space, and major classes of IF include prekeratin, vimentin, desmin, neurofilaments, and glial IF. MBs were recognized as prekeratin type by immunofluorescence.[83] The origin of MB remains unknown, and three major theories have been proposed. "Microtubular failure," "preneoplasia marker," and "vitamin A deficiency" have been studied, and currently the last hypothesis is most convincing.[131] MBs occur primarily in hydropic hepatocytes of the alcoholic and were named Mallory body in honor of F.B. Mallory, who first described them in the liver of patients with alcoholic cirrhosis.[111] However, MBs are recognized in many primary hepatic conditions (of which alcoholic liver disease is the most common), in the liver secondary to nonhepatic disease, and also in organs outside the liver such as renal cell carcinoma (Table 25-1). The location of the MBs may be helpful in the determination of the likely cause as is presented in the subsequent sections on alcoholic liver disease and primary biliary cirrhosis.

Table 25-1. Clinical conditions associated with alcoholic hyalin (Mallory bodies)

Liver diseases	Alcoholic liver disease
	Chronic active hepatitis
	Primary biliary cirrhosis
	Chronic biliary obstruction
	Wilson's disease
	Indian childhood cirrhosis
	Hepatocellular carcinoma
	Steatohepatitis of unknown cause
	Focal nodular hyperplasia
	Hepatocellular adenoma
Secondary to other diseases	Weber-Christian disease
	Diabetes mellitus
	Obesity
	Jejunoileal bypass
	Small intestinal resection
	Gastroplasty for morbid obesity
Organs other than liver	Asbestosis in lung
	Chronic interstitial pneumonitis
	Radiation pneumonitis
	Renal cell carcinoma
	Scar adenocarcinoma of lung
Hepatic: secondary to drugs	Amiodarone
	Glucocorticoids
	Perhexiline maleate

Enlarged *(giant) mitochondria* (GM) are relatively common in alcoholic liver disease,[79,156] and three classes have been described. Giant mitochondria are defined as eosinophilic (by routine hematoxylin and eosin stain) spheroid cytoplasmic bodies more than one third the hepatocyte nuclear diameter and red stained with Masson's trichrome, blue stained with toluidine blue, and no stain with digested periodic acid–Schiff (PAS), the last distinguishes them from lysosomes and alpha$_1$-antitrypsin globules. The three morphologic types are large round GM, spindle GM, and irregular GM with several surveys of liver disease indicating the increased prevalence of GM in alcoholic liver disease, especially in acute foamy degeneration, and likely have a milder clinical course.[79,156] Another type of distinctive eosinophilic cytoplasmic globule is attributable to *alpha$_1$-antitrypsin deficiency* with a Z allele. In such patients, periportal small to large globules (single or multiple) that are PAS positive can be found in numerous lobules. These globules have a slight halo around them in contrast to megamitochondria (GM).

Hepatocellular lysosomes are not prominent in normal conditions, but increased iron storage involves increased numbers of siderosomes (iron-containing lysosomes), which are visible by light microscopy. Furthermore, other hepatocellular pigments are stored in lysosomes, including Dubin-Johnson pigment, lipofuchsin, and bilirubin in obstructive biliary tract disease.[87] However, prominent lysosomes are recognized by the residual staining after digestion by periodic acid–Schiff stain, and they are very numerous after hepatocellular necrosis, in which case the numerous PAS-positive bodies are from lysosomes in the macrophages having engulfed dead hepatocytes. *Thorotrast* pigment is dark brown granules (of thorium dioxide) noted within portal macrophages and are a radioactive compound injected to assist in radiographic imaging of the liver but long since discarded because of the health risk of long-term exposure to the radioactive compound.

Common hepatocellular pigments include iron (glistening hard particles that stain with iron stain such as Prussian blue), lipofuchsin (light brown usually more prominent in the perivenular cells of older patients), bile (often light green if the sections are thick and more prominent in severe biliary tract obstruction), and Dubin-Johnson pigment. The cellular distribution of iron pigment is helpful in elucidating the mechanism of storage. The iron storage of hemochromatosis is within the hepatocytes, whereas Kupffer cell iron is a feature of hemolytic anemia.

Cholestasis has many morphologic features and refers to the retention of bile pigments. The earliest manifestation of cholestasis is canalicular plugs of bile, "pure" cholestasis, which occur in a variety of clinical settings, including sepsis, total parenteral nutrition, drugs (such as estrogen, testosterone) hypoxia, postoperative conditions, and a rare condition called benign jaundice of pregnancy. In contrast to pure cholestasis, "mixed" cholestasis occurs with a portal reaction and is discussed in the biliary disease section. The mechanism for perivenular cholestasis is not well explained, but the zonal predilection is possibly related to oxygen tension or drug-metabolizing activity of hepatocytes in the zone 1 versus zone 3 hepatocytes.

Hepatocytes with a finely granular cytoplasm are called *ground-glass cell* of Hadziyannis, which is attributable to the proliferation of hepatitis B surface antigen and smooth endoplasmic reticulum.[98] This distinctive cytoplasmic change is scattered throughout the lobule and usually is only a few cells but seems to increase in number with the duration of chronic hepatitis B. If such a finely granular cytoplasmic change is noted in a patient with no evidence of hepatitis B (that is, lacks serologic evidence or the cells are not stainable by orcein) and the cells stain with phosphotungstic acid–hematoxylin, the hepatocytes are oncocytes and the cytoplasmic change is attributable to abundant mitochondria.[95] Occasionally, nodules of oncocytes occur though usually the cells are scattered in the lobule or concentrated at the periphery of nodules. No specific significance of hepatic oncocytes is recognized. A similar uniform globular staining may be noted in *globular amyloid*,[105] and the eosinophilic mass is extracellular within the sinusoid rather than in a hepatocyte. Furthermore, the Shikata, or orcein, stain identifes the ground glass cell but not the amyloid. Similar cytoplasmic staining changes are noted in LaFora bodies and after some drugs such as cynamide which are PAS positive and orcein negative.[76]

Pale nuclei caused by glycogen deposition *(glycogen nuclei)* are common in diabetes, congestion, and nonspecific reaction. A similar pale intranuclear appearance occurs with cytoplasmic invagination in which with thin sections, a membrane may be noted around the vacuole.

Hepatocellular necrosis

Necrosis may be classified in many ways, including location (zonal, periportal, perivenular, and so on), mechanism (lytic, coagulative), amount (submassive versus focal), cellular type (lymphocytotoxic versus hyaline necrosis) and various patterns are associated with different etiologic factors.[136] *Zonal necrosis* is a common pattern of injury after an acute hepatic injury. Sharply demarcated perivenular (zone 3) coagulative necrosis is typical of severe anoxic injury or acetaminophen injury and may be explained by differences in oxygenation and activity of drug-metabolizing enzymes. Periportal necrosis (zone 1) is not common and is noted in eclampsia. Midzonal injury is reported for yellow fever.

Hepatocellular necrosis *(hepatocytolysis)* of the lytic

type, with the associated macrophage activity that is so complete and rapid that dead hepatocytes are rarely noted, is recognized by only the clumping of mononuclear cells in a cord, indicating that a hepatocyte formerly existed at the site. Such necrosis is common in viral hepatitis, alcoholic liver disease, and many hepatotoxic reactions, and the type of inflammatory reactions varies in these conditions. Coagulative necrosis in the liver is characterized by dying hepatocytes that retain some staining of the cytoplasm, and the nuclei lose basophilia and gradually disappear. The cells become shrunken and slowly disappear because of the action of inflammatory cells. Coagulative necrosis occurs commonly in anoxic damage because of poor hepatic circulatory states, acetaminophen injury, and the early phase of halothane injury. The lack of an inflammatory response is striking in contrast to lytic necrosis. *Acidophilic necrosis* usually occurs in an isolated hepatocyte and is similar to coagulative necrosis except that the cytoplasm becomes more eosinophilic and waxy, and the nucleus may be retained and be a dark basophilic mass. Acidophilic bodies are common in acute viral hepatitis of various causes (hepatitis A, B, and non-A, non-B), as well as unusual viral hepatitis (such as Bolivian hemorrhagic fever[80], chronic active hepatitis, severe burns, and occasionally many other liver diseases (Fig. 25-2). *Confluent necrosis* is attributable to fusion of focal or zonal necrosis and may result from intensive necrosis that "bridges" between different zones (such as zone 1 to zone 3, that is, periportal to perivenular; or zone 3 on one acinus to zone 3 of an adjacent acinus). "Bridging hepatic necrosis" has been ascribed to have prognostic significance, but numerous studies have not agreed on the significance. Bridging hepatic necrosis is extensive necrosis and does indicate severe liver disease, but the prognosis is related to the overall setting of the liver condition. *Submassive hepatic necrosis* is recognized by confluent necrosis that usually involves many perivenular areas and occurs most commonly in severe acute viral hepatitis, autoimmune chronic active hepatitis, drug injury (halothane, acetaminophen), and those of unknown cause. *Massive hepatic necrosis* is distinguished from submassive hepatic necrosis by the presence of a thin rim of viable-appearing hepatocytes around each portal tract. However, exact classification is difficult as multiple areas of the liver have different degrees of necrosis and the most altered area is recommended for classification.

Postmortem autolysis develops rapidly, and if the patient was febrile at death, the softening of the parenchyma proceeds more rapidly. If submassive hepatic necrosis is present ante mortem, then postmortem autolysis is even more advanced. Bacteria may grow in the liver after sepsis and death. The ground-glass cell change of the hepatocyte cytoplasm is gradually "lost" by autolysis during the first 8 hours and then immunoperoxidase stains are needed to identify the presence of HBsAg.

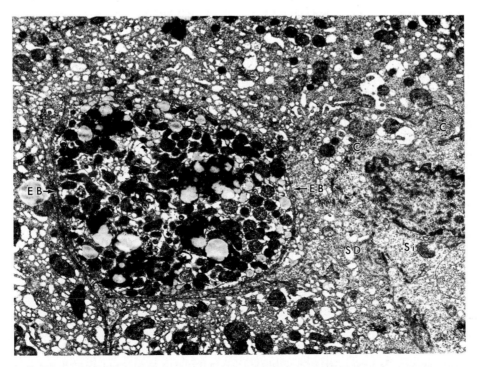

Fig. 25-2. Electron photomicrograph of acidophilic body just before extrusion into sinusoid. Notice collagen in Disse's space, which is not generally detectable on light microscopy. *C,* Collagen; *EB,* eosinophilic (acidophilic) body; *SD,* Disse's space; *Si,* sinusoid. (Courtesy Dr. Hisando Kobayashi, Nagoya, Japan.)

Inflammation: portal and lobular

Inflammatory reaction in the liver has many appearances, including differences in the type of cell involved, location, and extent of change. Portal tracts normally contain T-lymphocytes during development (12- to 17-week embryo) and in adult life also include some lymphocytes in the normal condition (B- and T-lymphocytes). Some sinusoid cells are also lymphocytes (such as pit cells), and the Kupffer cells are derived from the monocyte-macrophage system and are stationary in the liver in adult life. Portal lymphoid hyperplasia is a common hepatic reaction to system illnesses, including rheumatoid arthritis, pneumonia, viral infections elsewhere, infectious mononucleosis (EB virus, cytomegalovirus), sepsis, and repeated challenge with foreign materials as with intravenous drug use. Such portal lymphoid hyperplasia is not sufficient evidence for chronic hepatitis, but lobular changes are essential as well. Follicular lymphoid hyperplasia is unusual but may occur. Repeated portal inflammatory reactions (as with recurrent biliary tract obstruction as in common bile duct calculi) may produce a portal fibrous reaction, and the collagen fibers appear condensed and acellular and lack bile-duct proliferation as well as lack lymphocytes. Another common inflammatory reaction besides portal lymphoid hyperplasia is Kupffer cell hyperplasia in the lobule, and this occurs in response to sepsis and circulating toxins and is common in acute viral hepatitis as well. Distinction of primary hepatic disease especially in an early phase from nonspecific reactive hyperplasia can be challenging. The periodic acid–Schiff stain will assist in recognizing the lysosomes of macrophages and Kupffer cells that increase in case of focal hepatocellular necrosis, which if abundant indicates a primary hepatic disease.

Circulatory changes in the liver can be dramatic, and with severe congestive heart failure or hepatic vein obstruction, the perivenular areas have widened sinusoids stuffed with red blood cells. Dilated sinusoids are noted in a variety of states including hepatic tissue adjacent to a mass lesion such as metastatic cancer, after exposure to oral contraceptives or anabolic steroids, in renal transplantation, and in pregnancy. In addition, small cytoplasmic blebs emerge from the hepatocytes into the sinusoids in hypoxic states.

Regeneration

The liver has a remarkable capacity for regeneration, as occurs after surgical resection (which may be up to 70% of the human liver) and during recovery from submassive hepatic necrosis. In the normal adult rat liver, the hepatocytes have an annual turnover of one mitosis per year, and after partial hepatectomy there is a burst of mitotic activity so that the liver weight doubles at 48 hours and has returned to normal weight at 3 to 6 days.

The DNA synthesis can be measured at 15 to 18 hours and reaches a peak at 24 hours. The periportal hepatocytes have the maximal labeling for DNA synthesis in the initial period, but at 34 hours the zone of maximal proliferation has shifted to the perivenular area. In human liver, regeneration also occurs rapidly and also even in cirrhotic liver.[123] After major hepatic resection for tumor, regeneration of normal hepatic volume occurs by 3 to 6 months, and liver function appears normal at 2 to 3 weeks after surgery. Diminution of the regenerative capacity with advancing age correlates with the increased mortality by submassive hepatic necrosis in older patients. The mechanism for such a burst of hepatocellular regeneration is a subject of great interest because the molecular understanding of the process has promise in stimulating recovery from severe hepatic necrosis from a variety of situations. Although earlier concepts of regeneration reflected the "dedifferentiation" of the young regenerating hepatocytes, recent evidence indicates that very few new proteins or messenger-RNA species are detected during regeneration, and thus the regenerating hepatocytes have the same proteins as mature hepatocytes.[89]

The search for humoral factors that initiate, potentiate, and finally inhibit hepatocyte proliferation after complete regeneration has led to numerous substances. It has long been known that nonhepatic portal blood from the splanchnic area supplies important humoral factors, called "portal hepatotrophic factors," of which the best known is insulin. Glucagon and epidermal growth factor (urogastrone–eosinophil chemotactic factor) from the gut are also considered essential.[110] Nonportal hepatotrophic factors include parathyroid hormone, calcitonin, and insulin-like substances produced by the liver somatomedin c. Purification of hepatic stimulator substance from the cytosol of regenerating rat liver indicates that it is a highly charged protein that is stable and is organ specific but not species specific.[109]

After regeneration to the normal mass of liver, some factors inhibit continued growth. The regenerative response does not produce new lobes but is a hyperplasia of existing lobes. There is concomitant lengthening of blood vessels and bile ducts.

Morphologic features of regeneration indicate that mitosis are common in the early phases and the growth of hepatocellular components is fairly rapid. However, the normal sinusoidal-hepatocyte pattern is not as readily established. The liver plate is ballooned, and the hepatocytes form nodules in which the sinusoids are inapparent in the fixed state. The liver lobular architecture after regeneration in humans after submassive hepatic necrosis or after regeneration of hepatocellular cytoplasm as in recovery from severe fatty liver is devoid of apparent sinusoid spaces and has a cobblestone appearance, thus mimicking a street of cobblestone that fit together in a jagged irregular pattern. This cobble-stone pattern persists for many months in the human liver and, before 1 year, has readjusted to the normal cell-plate architecture of one to two hepatocytes per cell plate. Atypical regenerative changes also occur in several human diseases, and the hepatocellular meta-plasia to ductlike epithelium is a common observation in submassive hepatic necrosis as well as severe chronic alcoholic liver disease. The presence of alcoholic hya-line within the cytoplasm of some of these small duc-tules as well as the histochemical demonstration of gly-cogen and glucose-6-phosphatase indicate that the ductules are transformed hepatocytes.[155] The ductules have a small or absent lumen, are called "atypical bile ductules," "pseudocholangioles," or "neocholangioles," and are also noted within focal nodular hyperplasia.

Fibrosis

Hepatic fibrosis is the most important feature of chronic liver disease and leads to cirrhosis and irrevers-ible physiologic changes in the liver that account for many clinical manifestations of fatal liver disease. Fi-brosis of the liver is a common response to chronic in-flammatory conditions as well as a variety of tumors (primary and metastatic), and such fibrosis has many patterns of growth, which may aid in recognition of the cause.

Normally 4% of the liver protein is collagen, and in cirrhosis there is a four- to sevenfold increase.[143] Hu-mans have a far more exuberant response by collagen formation than other animals do, and an equivalent col-lagenosis in the liver of humans is not duplicated even in other primates. Experimental cirrhosis in the carbon tetrachloride–treated rat and mouse have served as models, but the adequacy of the morphologic and bio-chemical lesion has been doubted compared to human cirrhosis.[152] Collagen is a family of similar compounds that may be classified into several types of chemical and immunologic differences of which type III is the new collagen formed in response to injury and type I colla-gen is the major structural protein in normal organs in-cluding the liver. Type I and type III collagen is pres-ent in the portal tracts, within the reticulin fibrils of the sinusoids, and around the terminal hepatic venules. Collagen types IV and V is normally present in the basement membranes surrounding the portal vessels, bile ducts, and nerves but not in the interstitium of the portal tracts.

Patterns of fibrosis. Simple hepatocellular necrosis does not result in collagen formation, but in severe he-patic necrosis a collapsed stroma may form a framework for collagen retention. Repeated or continuous necrosis is associated with fibrosis, and the most striking fibrosis within the lobule is noted in chronic alcoholic liver dis-ease. The collagen is deposited within the perivenular

area, space of Disse, and sinusoids and may obliterate the terminal hepatic vein. This fibrosis may occur even with a very mild inflammatory response. As this fibrosis continues, one may apply the term *"progressive peri-venular alcoholic fibrosis"* to it. In the early phases, pericellular fibrosis occurs, and this fibrous tissue con-denses in time to form larger aggregates.

Another common pattern of fibrosis occurs in the portal areas in chronic active hepatitis, which tends to be more confined to the portal tracts and does not ex-tend into the lobule as much as portal fibrosis does in the alcoholic. Periductular fibrosis is common in re-peated chronic biliary tract obstruction. Portal tract fi-brosis of a distinctive nature is noted in congenital he-patic fibrosis in which numerous dilated bile ducts are noted and contain bile concretions. These various pat-terns of fibrosis can be distinctive, and the diseases are discussed elsewhere in the specific-disease category.

Neoplastic disease is associated with a variety of fi-brous reactions; some metastatic tumors promote fibro-sis, and some benign hepatic tumors occur with prom-inent fibrosis such as focal nodular hyperplasia and bile duct adenoma. Curiously, bile duct carcinoma is strik-ingly fibrogenic, and yet hepatocellular carcinoma is not. In fibrolamellar carcinoma a distinctive pattern of fibrosis is noted even in the metastatic lesions, an in-dication that the hepatocyte may be the collagen-pro-ducing cell.

The cell of origin of collagen and its precursors has been the subject of much debate. Whereas collagen production by fibroblasts has long been recognized, the source of sinusoid collagen has been difficult to eluci-date. The fat-storing cells (Ito cells) have been the sub-ject of continued research and are the likely candidates for collagen production in the space of Disse.[35,119] How-ever, additional recent evidence using monoclonal an-tibodies to type II collage and procollagen indicates that the hepatocyte may produce collagen.[145] Molecular hy-bridization technology is available to measure procolla-gen mRNA content in human liver, and thus the mech-anism of collagen production may be more readily explained.[160] Increased transcription rates may be a likely mechanism for the increased production com-pared to increased translation. The detection of human hepatic fibrosis by serologic tests has also been a sub-ject of great interest, with numerous serum assays being tested. Serum procollagen III measurement by radioimmunoassay has been applied to patients with al-coholic fatty liver and alcoholic fibrosis.[93] Differences in techniques may account for some disagreement in reli-ability, but the Fab radioimmunoassay of procollagen III did correlate with the degree of fibrosis but in an individual patient did not reflect the exact degree of hepatic fibrosis noted in a liver biopsy speciman.[147] Fifty-five percent of patients with perivenular fibrosis had elevated levels of procollagen III, 62% of patients with septal (portal) fibrosis had elevated levels, and the highest levels were noted in cirrhosis (95%). However, there was considerable overlap of values in the difference groups, and a single test was not a reliable indicator of hepatic histology. Experimental studies in carbon tetrachloride hepatic fibrosis indicate that serum procollagen III assays may reflect collagen degradation as well as secretion and thus not be useful in allowing prediction of hepatic fibrosis.[85]

Non–collagen matrix components have been investigated for a possible role in fibrosis. Fibronectin both is a plasma protein and may produce a cellular form in injury.[116] Immunochemical staining reveals a continuous layer of fibronectin in the space of Disse in human liver.[82] During the development of cirrhosis, collagen production increases as does acidic glycosaminoglycans (AGAGs), which also are important intercellular components.[122] These high-molecular-weight components increase as fibrosis and cirrhosis advance, and during this process higher-molecular-weight fractions are synthesized. AGAGs promote cell adhesion to collagen and regulate collagen fibril formation. Current concepts of fibrosis indicate that the production of collagen and associated matrical components is proceeding at a higher rate than the normally present degradation steps for these components.

Cirrhosis

The currently accepted definition of cirrhosis requires the term be applied to a liver with a *diffuse fibrosis* (that is, the entire liver and not focal) and contain *regenerative nodules*, which are masses of hepatocytes lacking the normal blood flow because of the lack of terminal hepatic venules.[70] One form of diffuse fibrosis and nodularity is congenital hepatic fibrosis, but it is not considered cirrhosis because true regenerative nodules are not formed. The nodularity is attributable to the retraction of portal areas by fibrosis, and the remaining hepatic parenchyma has normal lobular growth pattern with terminal hepatic veins. Regenerative or hyperplastic nodules are required for the definition of cirrhosis because altered blood flow and portal hypertension correlates with their presence. In contrast, hepatic fibrosis, which is usually a precursor to cirrhosis, is not associated as frequently with portal hypertension as diffuse fibrosis is. In addition, the development of hepatocellular carcinoma is relatively common in cirrhosis with the required regenerative nodules and is not as frequent as it is in fibrosis. Thus the two major reasons to require the definition of cirrhosis to have regenerative nodules reflect the common clinical and pathologic complications of portal hypertension and hepatocellular carcinoma. In recent decades, many pathologists applied the term "cirrhosis" to a condition that most would refer to as "fibrosis." Major terms of various cirrhosis are listed in Table 25-2.

Classification of cirrhosis has been confusing and unproved over the years, and numerous terms that cannot be proved with more modern technology are applied. The classification terms have reflected pathogenesis, etiology, morphology, and eponyms. Pathogenesis is often difficult to determine in the advance quiescent state often noted at autopsy, and yet morphologic appearance has been used to relate the autopsy appearance to a specific pathogenesis. Clearly a variety of agents can produce a similar morphologic pattern, and furthermore the morphologic pattern changes in a patient as the disease progresses. Nonetheless, it is still conventional to classify cirrhosis on the basis of nodule size and also etiology if well proved (such as hepatitis B viral cirrhosis). *Micronodular cirrhosis* applies to the liver in which nearly all the nodules are less than 3 mm in diameter[70] though some have used 1.5 mm as the maximum diameter because that is the diameter of a normal lobule.[88] However, "hyperplastic nodule" has also been used for the micronodular cirrhosis with nodules greater than 1.5 mm diameter.[96] Examples of common micronodular cirrhosis include alcoholic cirrhosis, biliary tract obstruction, and hepatic venous obstruction. *Macronodular cirrhosis* applies if most of the nodules are greater than 3 mm in diameter, and it occurs in two forms. The more common form of macronodular cirrhosis has nodules divided by thin septa that are often incomplete and have linking portal tracts. This pattern is common in so-called posthepatitic cirrhosis even though the evidence for hepatitis is not usually proved. Another form of macronodular cirrhosis has some large nodules that include smaller regenerative nodules as well as large areas of collapse, and this is often called "postnecrotic cirrhosis," or "postcollapse cirrhosis." This may occur in the setting of established cirrhosis with continued necrosis of other nodules and growth of remaining nodules. It is commonly believed that macronodular cirrhosis evolves from micronodular cirrhosis especially in the alcoholic with abstinence, but conversion occurs with alcohol consumption as well.[88] The median time interval for conversion of micronodular cirrhosis to macronodular type is 2.25 years, and the majority of patients have such progression.[88]

Liver weight is commonly measured, and guidelines for normal weight are based on age, sex, and body length.[112] As a rough guideline, a normal adult liver is 1400 to 1600 g; one with a greater weight is hypertrophy, and a small liver is hypotrophy or atrophy. As the fibrous tissue is increased in cirrhosis, the parenchyma (that is, lobular portions and not the portal areas) may be decreased or even increased by weight. Alcoholic cirrhosis often contains fat within the hepatocytes, and the parenchyma is increased in weight. However, in cirrhosis with little fat, as after chronic active hepatitis, the liver parenchyma may be reduced.

Classification of cirrhosis by cause is preferred, but the pathogenesis may not be understood. Etiologic factors related to cirrhosis include alcoholism, hepatitis B virus, various metabolic disease such as hemochromatosis, Wilson's disease, alpha$_1$-antitrypsin deficiency, galactosemia and glycogen storage disease (type IV), long-standing biliary tract obstruction, and specific toxins and drugs (very rare and difficult to demonstrate). Suggested etiologic factors that are not well proved but have been suggested include autoimmunity, mycotoxins, schistosomiasis, and malnutrition. Cirrhosis without recognizable cause is called "cryptogenic cirrhosis" and, with additional study including immunoperoxidase stains, "HBV in situ hybridization," and with additional techniques some cirrhosis may be classified by etiology. With the development of HBV and delta-hepatitis staining we have reclassified a large number of previously "cryptogenic" cirrhoses, and it is likely that additional etiologic factors will be identified in the future. The morphologic patterns of cirrhosis are discussed in the disease category in later sections.

The *microcirculatory effects* of cirrhosis are dramatic because the acinar blood flow is redirected.[141] Serial sections of cirrhotic nodule show many interconnections of the smaller micronodules so that some larger macronodules have many extensions. In serial section, the fibrous bands at the margins contain complex vascular tracts that are the altered collateral circulation. Although the histologic appearance of these "portal" areas in cirrhosis contains small vessels that may appear to be portal venous tracts, it is possible that such vessels are hepatic veins that are "misplaced," and thus so-called portal cirrhosis may not be portal at all but the result of hepatic venous occlusion and the development of additional collateral circulation. The location of the vascular resistance that produces portal hypertension is a subject of great interest. In the experimental animal (carbon tetrachloride cirrhosis), micropuncture studies reveal that the major vascular resistance occurs near the portal vein branches and not within the hepatic vein branches.[148] Thus a major degree of vascular resistance may occur within the sinusoid, and such resistance may correlate with the fibrosis noted within the sinusoid and space of Disse. Correlation between the amount of collagen in the space of Disse, and the intrahepatic pressure has been correlated.[74]

The *irreversibility* of cirrhosis has been emphasized in several experimental and clinical studies.[128] Although there are a few scattered reports of human liver biopsies that showed possible irreversibility after some treatment, many reports are suspect for inadequate sampling of the liver by a small-needle biopsy. If cirrhosis is reversible, it must be very rare, though the most convincing patients have biliary obstruction that has been corrected surgically.[159] However, hepatic fibrosis is reversible and collagen resorption is well recognized as a dynamic process during the development of cirrhosis. Thus the passage of hepatic fibrosis to the irreversible stage of cirrhosis is not easily defined or recognized.

The *incidence* of cirrhosis appears to be increasing in the Western countries and in large part attributable to an increase in female acquisition of the disease.[114] A large autopsy series of 520 patients recorded in a 70-year review from Scotland reflects the etiologic distribution noted in many Western countries (Table 25-2). New techniques for immunostaining and in situ hybridization were not applied, and thus the cryptogenic category is larger than is likely to be determined in an ideal study with current methodology. It may be difficult to recognize a cirrhotic liver as alcoholic in type when the alcoholic cirrhotic person has stopped drinking for 3 or 4 years. Alternatively the patient whose drinking pattern is steady and substantial, day by day, throughout many years but who maintains a good diet may never show signs of acute alcoholic liver disease, but cirrhosis may develop insidiously. Such a patient may seldom or never have been intoxicated.

Cirrhosis after chronic active hepatitis has a pathogenesis different from that of alcoholic cirrhosis. Although initially characterized grossly by a uniform finely granular pattern that represents the widened portal areas, chronic active hepatitis becomes quiescent, with respect to continuing necrosis, several years before clinical signs of cirrhosis appear. Because the collagen deposition within nodules in the liver is far less in chronic active hepatitis than in alcoholism, hepatic nodules in the former grow to a much larger size by the time of death. Thus nodular size and discreteness are the result of both density of collagen and freedom of continued regeneration, without disrupting necrotizing activity. Functionally more important than nodular size in cirrhosis is the size of the entire hepatic mass, which can be estimated with radioisotope scans. The more common types of cirrhosis are listed in Table 25-2. Their causes and key tests are listed in Table 25-3.

Table 25-2. Etiology of cirrhosis: large autopsy review

Alcoholic	96	18.5%
Posticteric	54	10.4%
Hemochromatosis	42	7.9%
Familial	3	0.6%
Primary biliary cirrhosis	4	0.8%
Cryptogenic	322	61.9%
TOTAL SERIES	520	100%

Adapted from MacSween, R.N.M., and Scott, A.R.: J. Clin. Pathol. **26**:936, 1973, which covers the period 1900 to 1969. Notice that HBV test results are absent and posticteric cirrhosis includes hepatitis B viral cirrhosis, but most B viral cirrhosis are within the cryptogenic group because the majority evolve without icteric experience.

Table 25-3. Major causes of cirrhosis and their tests

Alcoholic cirrhosis	Clinical information, biopsy with alcoholic hepatitis
B viral cirrhosis	Hepatitis B surface antigen (HbsAg), hepatitis B virus integration
Non-A, non-B viral cirrhosis	History, lab, and negative hepatitis B virus tests
Autoimmune cirrhosis	Antinuclear antibody, smooth muscle antibody
Primary biliary cirrhosis	Mitochondrial antibody, serum alkaline phosphatase
Secondary biliary cirrhosis	History, cholangiogram
Hemochromatosis	Iron (serum, liver), iron-binding capacity, ferritin
Wilson's disease cirrhosis	Ceruloplasmin, liver copper
Alpha₁-antitrypsin (AAT) deficiency cirrhosis	Serum alpha₁-antitrypsin phenotype

INFECTIOUS DISORDERS
Viral hepatitis

Viral hepatitis is a necrotizing inflammatory lesion of the liver produced by multiple viral agents of which three have been isolated and their nucleic acid sequence has been determined and much information about the serologic response and viral replication is known. In common usage, the term "viral hepatitis" refers to a clinical pathosis with common features of a prodrome phase, often icteric phase, and a recovery phase, which may also lead to associated chronic disease in the non–hepatitis A virus types or to complete recovery. Acute viral hepatitis A (AVH-A) is the most common acute liver disease in children and adolescents and may occur in epidemics from poor hygenic conditions. Furthermore, hepatitis B virus is a very common infection on a worldwide basis, with an estimated 200 million persons infected and annually more than 250,000 to 500,000 persons succumbing to hepatocellular carcinoma associated with the chronic hepatitis B virus (HBV) infection. Because hepatocellular carcinoma is the commonest fatal human cancer in the world, and the majority of patients are chronically infected with HBV, the virus is the most common cause of cancer in the world.

The viruses that produce classical acute viral hepatitis are hepatitis A virus (HAV), hepatitis B virus (HBV), delta-hepatitis virus (DHV), and two or more varieties of non-A, non-B viral hepatitis viruses (NAB). The clinical features of the viral infections are so typical and similar that few clinical signs allow accurate distinction, and serologic testing is required for accurate classification. With the widespread use of a serologic test, the Centers for Disease Control records indicate the distribution of the viral agents in the 57,557 reported United States cases of acute viral hepatitis as follows for 1984: HAV 38%, HBV 45%, NAB 7%, hepatitis not specified 10%, and testing for DHV not performed reliably but likely representing less than 1%.

Other viruses infect the liver and produce hepatic symptoms but are not included in the clinical and pathologic discussions of classical viral hepatitis. These other hepatic viral illnesses are called by the virus name and include yellow fever, Lassa fever, Marburg virus infection, Ebola virus, and many other viruses that produce systemic illness such as herpes simplex, variola, varicella-zoster, measles, cytomegalovirus, and Epstein-Barr virus (infectious mononucleosis).

Hepatitis A

Etiologic agent. Viral hepatitis A (also known as VH-A, epidemic hepatitis, infectious hepatitis, infective hepatitis, Botkin's disease, and, in older usage, catarrhal jaundice) is caused by an orally acquired, fecally excreted RNA virus that is 27 nm in diameter[180] (Fig. 25-3) and has been demonstrated in cytoplasm of hepatocytes of infected humans, marmosets, and chimpanzees.[241,242,258,276] No other organ has been shown to be a source of HAV proliferation. The agent can be inoculated and passed into tissue culture of green-monkey kidney cells,[184] in which it produces no cytopathic effect.

HAV infectivity is totally destroyed by heating to 100° C for 5 minutes, reduced in infectivity by heating to 60° C for 1 hour, almost completely inactivated by ultraviolet irradiation, and destroyed after 3 days of incubation at 37° C in 1:4000 formalin.[258] Infectivity is neutralized by addition of convalescent serum. HAV infection in the subhuman primate produces mild histologic hepatic changes, but rarely significantly illness.[198,202]

Hepatitis A particles have been demonstrated in sera of infected persons, but their brief presence in serum is inferred because, experimentally, serum taken from a patient in the prodrome of VH-A is infective for a second susceptible human. Although HAV theoretically can be transmitted by percutaneous routes, it is not, for practical purposes, an agent that produces posttransfusion hepatitis (PTH).[257,286] Hepatitis A particles are demonstrable for a brief period in the stool of infected patients[199]; the viral particles in ultracentrifugal fractions of the stool are agglutinated by convalescent sera, allowing the electron microscopic visualization of not only the clusters of the 27 nm round structures but also the halo of antibodies attached to the viral bodies. The particles appear in the stool about 2 weeks before symptoms and 5 days before development of abnormal transaminase levels and remain until nearly peak serum transaminase levels are reached.[198,233]

Clinical and immunologic aspects. HAV is highly in-

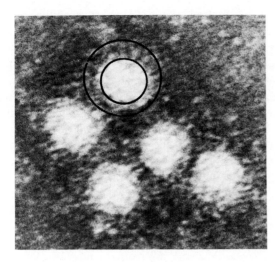

Fig. 25-3. Hepatitis A particles from stool of infected patient, agglutinated by anti-HA. Notice fuzzy halo around particles representing antibodies. (One particle and halo are encircled.) (Courtesy Dr. Jorge Rakela, Rochester, Minn.)

fective, and infection confers lifetime immunity with no chronic carrier or chronic disease state. Thus it occurs in epidemics, in densely populated areas, and predominantly in children. The disease is usually overlooked because it may be symptomless or appear as a mild influenza-like illness. When a clinical illness does develop after a 15- to 45-day incubation period, it is ushered in with fatigue, nausea, vomiting, and anorexia. A distaste for cigarettes often develops. Patients with symptomatic acute viral hepatitis type A (AcVH-A) also usually have fever, lymphadenopathy, and tender hepatomegaly. Biliuria is followed by icterus; the highest serum bilirubin level is usually reached 1 to 2 weeks after onset of jaundice, at which time the patient usually becomes subjectively improved. All the signs and symptoms usually disappear by 6 weeks after onset of jaundice. Fatalities are uncommon; between 1% and 13% of deaths from viral hepatitis can be attributed to HAV.[243,259] Chronic liver disease caused by HAV has not been demonstrated.

Patients with AcVH-A rapidly produce a specific IgM type of antibody that appears about 2 weeks after infection and usually persists for 2 months but may last for several months.[226] Its presence is considered diagnostic of acute or recent VH-A. A specific IgG type of antibody is produced about 5 weeks after infection, rising in titer as the titer of IgM falls. The IgG antibody persists throughout the patient's life, conferring immunity.[179,270]

Passive transfer of small amounts of convalescent serum to a patient at risk protects the patient from clinically evident infection for about 6 months. Commercially available "hyperimmune" gamma globulin contains antibody to HAV of titers between 1:2000 and 1:8000.

Epidemiology. VH-A has a worldwide distribution and apparently is primarily a disease of humans; other primates are only occasional secondary hosts, deriving the disease from humans.[202] In 1960 it was found that certain mollusks harvested from polluted seawater concentrated the virus, and ingestion of raw or partially cooked mollusks was associated with an occasional epidemic. Because of its high infectivity, its mode of transmission, the apparent rarity of either animal vectors or a chronic carrier state, and the immunity conferred by HAV infection, VH-A tends to occur in epidemics only as a susceptible population reaches an age at which there is intimate contact with older children. The continual entry of new susceptible persons is necessary for the maintenance of the virus. For unknown reasons, incidence figures for VH-A also show seasonal variation. In most countries of the world the incidence of AcVH-A is decreasing, but in certain countries, including Yugoslavia, Taiwan, and Israel, nearly 100% infection rate has been acquired by midadult life.[287] In New York City, 72% to 80% of adults in lower socioeconomic groups have acquired an immune status, compared with 18% to 30% of persons in upper-middle socioeconomic groups.[285] The disease is common in homosexual men, particularly those participating in oral-anal sexual activities.[199]

Hepatitis B

Structure. Hepatitis B virus produces acute viral hepatitis as recognized in the classical clinical tradition and accounts for serum jaundice as demonstrated in the remarkable yellow fever vaccine experience of World War II.[273] The virus is spread by parenteral means in the majority of patients but also by sexual and mother-to-fetus modes as well. The virus is a small complex double-stranded DNA virus with unusual properties that with other related viruses have been classified as *hepadnaviruses* (Fig. 25-4). These viruses include woodchuck hepatitis virus (WHV), Beechey ground squirrel virus (GSHV), and Peking duck hepatitis virus (DHBV). All infect the liver of the appropriate species and have considerable nucleic acid homology.[269] These four viruses share similar structure and patterns of infection and disease. The woodchuck hepatitis virus is naturally occurring and has been found in 45% of wild animals in Pennsylvania.[281] Experimental production of WHV infection results in similar antigenic changes as noted in human HBV acute infection, and 50% of animals develop chronic disease and hepatocellular carcinoma.

The HBV genome nucleotide base sequence is known to be approximately 3200 bases, and various subtypes have different lengths. The complete long minus strand is the primer for viral DNA synthesis, and the complete virus particle is circular.[208] Four genes are known for HBV DNA and they code for a surface protein (S gene, HBsAG), a nucleocapsid coat protein

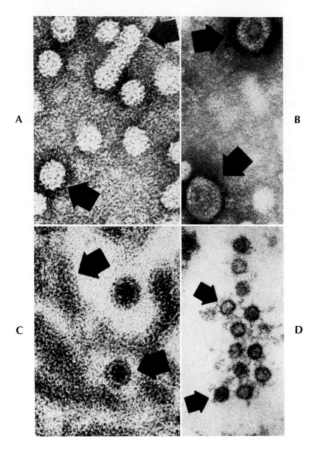

Fig. 25-4. Electron microscopic appearance of components of hepatitis B virus. HBsAg is found in serum, **A**, as 20 nm spheres *(left arrow)* or tubular structures *(right arrow)* but is also found sparsely in serum, **B**, as the Dane particle *(arrow)*, apparently the complete virion. In hepatocyte cytoplasm, **C**, HBsAg is form of long filamentous structures; rarely a spherical shell surrounds a hexagonal core, apparently the complete virus *(arrow)*. Liver cell nuclei contain core, which is inner part of Dane particle without HBsAg envelope, **D**. (Courtesy Alfred E.G. Dunn, Los Angeles.)

(C gene, HBcAg), a DNA polymerase (probably P gene, DNA P), and a protein of unknown function (gene X). These genes are arranged with an overlap so that the minus strand is read 1½ times, which allows HBV, the smallest known mammalian DNA virus, to increase its coding capacity.[245] The complete virus particle is a 40 nm particle called a "Dane particle," and the replication cycle has not been entirely proved. The virus seems to require a specific HBV attachment site to the hepatocyte plasma membrane, possible related to serum albumin, and then replication of HBV DNA occurs by means of a proviral DNA, messenger RNA, followed by assembly by the virion possible by budding from the endoplasmic reticulum. Cell culture of HBV has recently been accomplished with introduction of a cloned HBV DNA into a human hepatocellular carcinoma (HepG2) culture, and HBV proteins were synthesized and released into the culture medium.[283]

Integration of the HBV into the host DNA has been proved in numerous laboratories since the initial report by Brechot. The Southern blot technique with cloned HBV DNA probe allows recognition of HBV integration into human host DNA. The pattern of integration is specific for each person, and unique patterns exist for each carcinoma, implying a monoclonal origin of hepatocellular carcinoma.[204] Integration of HBV DNA does not include necessarily the entire HBV genome sequence but seems to be random and involve incomplete sequences. Retroviruses readily integrate into DNA and do so at random sites.[269] Integration of other hepadnaviruses into the appropriate host has been demonstrated. Patients with HBV integration may not express all HBV genomic material yet have progressive HBV-related chronic liver disease. Earlier immunohistochemical HBV studies indicated that some patients with advanced cirrhosis (so-called cryptogenic cirrhosis) and lacking serologic markers of HBV may have HBV as the cause of their chronic liver diease.[252] It has not been shown that some HBsAg-negative patients have their chronic liver disease and hepatocellular carcinoma associated with HBV integration.[222] HBV in situ hybridization has confirmed that the integration occurs within hepatocytes and not other cells of the liver parenchyma.[266] HBV may occur as free DNA or integrated viral DNA or both in patients with chronic liver disease, and HBcAg was highly correlated with the presence of free viral DNA rather than integrated forms.[252] The amount of stainable HBcAg correlated with the amount of free HBV DNA whereas HBsAg was well expressed with either free or integrated HBV DNA.

Clinical and immunologic aspects. HBV infection involves adults more frequently than VH-A does and is more often associated with serious liver disease. Whether the diseases differ in severity in age-matched individuals is unclear, but many clinicians believe that even in age-matched patients, VH-B is still a more severe illness than VH-A.

Prodromal influenza-like symptoms, joint swelling, and effusion, all apparently manifestations of acute immune-complex disease, are more common in the prodrome of AcVH-B than in VH-A or viral hepatitis non-A, non-B (VH-NAB).[246] Prodromal skin rashes and pruritus occur in about equal frequency in AcVH-B and in acute viral hepatitis non-A, non-B (AcVH-NAB). Some patients develop no prodrome with AcVH-B. Patients with VH-B may have fewer gastrointestinal symptoms than patients with VH-A do, but nausea, vomiting, and fatigue are the principal symptoms of VH-B.

The laboratory and serologic changes in acute viral

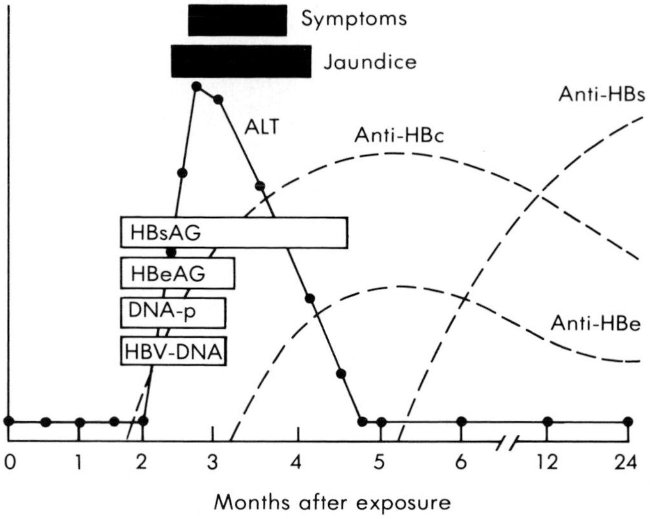

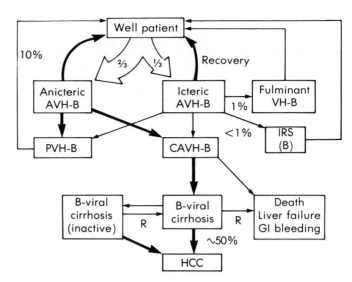

Fig. 25-5. The clinical, serologic, and biochemical course of typical acute type B hepatitis. *ALT,* Alanine aminotransferase; *Anti-HBc,* antibody to hepatitis B core antigen; *Anti-HBe,* antibody to HBeAG; *Anti-HBs,* antibody to HBsAg; *DNA-p,* serum hepatitis B virus DNA polymerase activity; *HBeAg,* hepatitis B e antigen; *HBsAg,* hepatitis B surface antigen; *HBV-DNA,* serum hepatitis B virus DNA. (From Hoofnagle, J.: Viral hepatitis, North Chicago, Abbott Laboratories Monograph.)

Fig. 25-6. Typical course of group of healthy adults with acute viral hepatitis B. Infection in immune impaired, in chronically ill, or in infants has different course. Notice that the arrow size reflects generally the number of patients in a given pathway. Thus a major number of patients with B viral cirrhosis evolve by anicteric acute disease and chronic active hepatitis. *AVH,* Acute viral hepatitis; *CAVH,* chronic active viral hepatitis; *HCC,* hepatocellular carcinoma; *IRS,* impaired regeneration syndrome; *PVH,* persistent viral hepatitis; *R,* reactivation.

hepatitis B are shown in Fig. 25-5. The HBsAg is the surface-coat antigen and is present at the time of jaundice but may be detected 1 to 2 months before jaundice. This protein is the stimulus for protective antibody and is useful in conferring immunity by vaccination. The HBc antigen is derived from the C gene and is a major polypeptide that binds to the HBV DNA, and antibody to this protein appears early in the course of AVH. Numerous tests of anti-HBc IgM have been devised to distinguish acute viral hepatitis from chronic hepatitis by serologic means. Usually serum HBcIgM identifies acute viral hepatitis, but in severe reactivation of chronic active hepatitis the test is positive also. A few patients may be tested in the early phase of AVH with serum positive for HBs and yet not have developed anti-HBc IgM.[238] Furthermore, after recovery of AVH, the anti-HBc IgM may remain detectable for a long time, the range in one study being 2 to 134 weeks and 14% having levels measured after 1 year.[238] The anti-HBc IgM declines and is replaced by IgG-class antibody during the recovery phase. Another protein of clinical importance is HBe (hepatitis B e) antigen because of the close correlation with infectivity and complete virions. The availability of serum HBV DNA is a better marker of infectivity, and serum HBV does not always correlate with HBe antigen. Serum HBV DNA was not detected in 11 of 25 serum HBeAg–

positive patients. However, HBeAg appears related to HBcAg because proteolytic digestion converts purified HBcAg to HBeAg.[268] The lack of serum HBV DNA in fulminant hepatitis reflects lower infectivity of such patients.[197] The rise of serum bilirubin lags behind the elevation of serum transaminases and often remains elevated longer.

The course of acute viral hepatitis B in otherwise healthy United States persons is diagrammed in Fig. 25-6. Previously published diagrams indicated up to a range of 10% to 12% of patients with acute viral hepatitis who developed chronic hepatitis from acute infection, but more recent follow-up studies from the 1942 United States Army yellow fever vaccine experience[273] and from Greece[290] indicate that less than 1% of patients with AVH develop chronic hepatitis.[273,290] This lower chronicity rate (1% not 10%) depends on a healthy patient with AVH. Newborns of HBV-carrier mothers have very high chronic disease rates (90+%) as do immunocompromised patients (such as patients having renal dialysis, 50% to 70%). Furthermore it is clear that the majority of patients with chronic hepatitis B evolve from anicteric silent acute infection.

After active HBV infection, anti-HBc in particular remains in the serum, probably indefinitely. One study has shown that 98% of drug addicts in the United States have serologic evidence of previous HBV infection; of those with evidence of prior infection, 11% have chronic HBs antigenemia, 67% have both anti-HBs and anti-HBc, 20% have anti-HBc alone, and only 2% have anti-HBs alone.[250] However, in a population survey a relatively larger number of persons who have never had clinically evident HBV infection may be shown to have anti-HBs without anti-HBc. It is possible that subclinical infection with HBV may result in a serologic pattern that differs from that found in patients who have had clinically evident disease. Since successful vaccination against HBV results in the appearance of anti-HBs only,[244,289] the question has been raised that perhaps persons with anti-HBs but without anti-HBc may have been naturally immunized but not actually infected by the HBV agent.

Epidemiology. VH-B has a worldwide distribution but, in contrast to VH-A, a large reservoir of asymptomatic carriers exists. Although transmission of HBV in the United States is often by inoculation of human blood products, HBV is not dependent on such artificial techniques for its propagation. Since HBsAg has been encountered in saliva,[272,296] tears, ascitic fluid, sneeze droplets,[296] blood-sucking insects,[254,256] menstrual fluid,[187] semen,[272] gingival and anorectal mucosa,[264] and, rarely, urine,[291] many mechanisms of person-to-person transmission have been suggested. These have included kissing,[294] biting,[237] sharing of razors and toothbrushes,[246] homosexual and heterosexual activities,[215] and transmission transplacentally or perinatally.[270]

The incidence of VH-B increased in large cities at alarming rates until 1970, mostly because of the practice of needle sharing by parenteral drug users. It is uncertain whether a recent decrease has resulted from diminished percutaneous drug abuse or the creation of immunity among drug users.

In the late 1970s the number of patients with VH-B related to illicit drug use declined (Fig. 25-7), and the high incidence of VH-B in male homosexuals became apparent. The high transmission rate of HBV among homosexuals led to the use of the homosexual community in controlled vaccine studies.[289] Approximately 8.2% of homosexuals in the Los Angeles area are chronic carriers of HBV, between 20- and 40-fold more than the remaining population. Transmission of the infection among homosexual men is correlated with punctate anal and gingival mucosal lesions.[264]

An important discovery of worldwide significance was the demonstration that HBV could be transmitted in the perinatal period and, occasionally, transplacentally from infected mother to offspring. The transmissibility in the perinatal period is strongly associated with the positive HBeAg status. Infants who acquire HBV in this fashion seldom develop a clinical illness; only 17% become icteric; 25% develop aminotransferase levels rising above 500 units, without icterus; whereas 58% develop a low-level persistent elevation of aminotransferase activities. Most infants infected in the first month of extrauterine life who develop icteric disease lose the virus on recovery from the acute illness. In contrast,

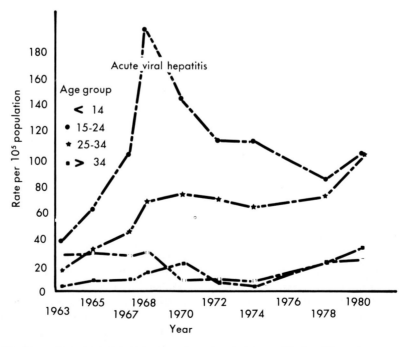

Fig. 25-7. Changing annual incidence of acute viral hepatitis in different age groups in California, 1963-1980. Despite increased incidence in 15- to 24-year-olds, age group with hepatitis most often related to transfusion has no change of incidence over 10-year period.

those whose hepatitis is asymptomatic retain the virus and often the HBeAg into adult life; consequently, the women transmit HBV to their subsequent offspring. Thus perinatal infection is the leading cause for a high incidence of chronic HBV infections, including cirrhosis and resulting hepatocellular carcinoma in the Orient and, probably, in Africa.

Offspring of women with AcVH-A do not develop an infection during the neonatal period. It is unclear whether they would do so if born while the mother was in the prodrome of hepatitis A, that is, when fecal viral content is high and before transplacentally acquired or breast-secreted HAV antibody is available.

Screening candidate blood donors for HBsAg reduced the total incidence of posttransfusion hepatitis by about 25%. Despite sensitive screening of donor blood, a few cases of posttransfusion hepatitis are still type B. Pooling of blood products may increase the risk of transmitting the agent; however, pooling also adds anti-HBs, which is protective. Were it not for the addition of anti-HBs, every large pool of human blood products used in the past would have been infective. Blood fibrinogen carries a particularly high risk of transmitting HBV,[175] a risk reduced but not eliminated by HBsAg screening of donors. However, heat-treated serum albumin and Cohn-fractionated gamma globulin are free of infectivity.[249] Passive protection against HBV has been achieved by inoculation of high-titer anti-HBs.[234,284] Inoculation of heated HBsAg, as in some lots of human albumin, confers active immunization against HBV.[218,232,289] Protection is conferred apparently because of the immune response that develops to HBsAg, even though HBsAg itself is not infective.

A vaccine made from plasma-derived HBsAg was produced and tested, and such production indicated that effective antibody was stimulated in immune-competent persons.[288] The duration of the antibody remains to be determined, and some patients may require booster doses to stimulate the antibody. Recombinant-made HBV vaccine has been tested as well and released for use in the United States.[271] Despite considerable concern about possible contamination of the plasma-derived HBV vaccine, the manufacturing steps have proved to be effective in eliminating HIV viability in the final product. Prime candidates for HBV vaccination include high-risk health care workers (physicians with blood exposure, laboratory technologists, nursing personnel, dialysis staff, dental workers, and so on), sexual partners of chronic HBV carriers and homosexual males with active sexual practice, institutionalized mentally retarded persons, travelers to endemic areas, and newborn infants of mothers with infection.

Delta hepatitis virus

Structure. Delta hepatitis virus (DHV) is a highly infectious small single-stranded circular RNA virus that requires concurrent hepatitis B virus infection to assist its own replication. Immunofluorescence of liver tissue led Rizzetto to the discovery of another antigen-antibody system in a patient with chronic hepatitis B.[267] Isolation of the virus and sequence analysis of the 1678 nucleotides has been completed, and there is no homology with HBV.[298] The virion is a spherical 36 nm particle with chimeric structure having a coat of HBsAg and the inner core of DHV RNA. The hepatitis delta antigen is composed of two major proteins with a molecular weight of 27 and 29 kilodaltons. Immunoelectron microscopy has revealed the viral antigen staining within the nucleus and in scattered hepatocellular cytoplasm, but not complete viral particles were identified.[231] It is suggested that the lack of finding intracellular DHV particles may be attributable to their formation by budding from the HBsAg-positive surface membrane and thus not be formed until extrusion into the extracellular area. By routine light microscopy, scattered hepatocellular nuclei stain for the antigen.

Clinical features and immunologic aspects. The serum ALT (alanine aminotransferase) and immunologic events in AVH-DHV are shown in Fig. 25-8, *B*, and indicate that in the prodrome phase the DHV antigen (virus) is circulating. At the time of icterus and clinical recognition the DHV antigen is below detectable limits in most patients, and anti-HDV is present. The first antibody is IgM followed by IgG, but in some patients the IgM antibody is not detectable. Serum HDV RNA is present in patients with IgM HDV.[176] As recovery occurs, the HDV antibody falls to low and undetectable levels, which unfortunately makes serologic surveys of populations reflect a falsely low experience with the virus. A radioimmunoassay for antibody to HDV is available commercially, and the test identifies total antibody levels, but separation into IgM and IgG levels is helpful in the classification of the infection as acute or chronic. The serologic changes in chronic HDV are persistence of IgG antibody with change in level of antibody and at times increased levels of IgM antibody.

The clinical course of AVH DHV, if it occurs with acute hepatitis B, is healing of the acute illness with loss of antibody to DHV (Fig. 25-9). Antibody to HBs occurs with the recovery of AVH HBV, and that antibody protects against future contact with DHV because its coat is HBsAg. The relapse of AVH seen as biphasic illness also usually leads to recovery.[215]

Fulminant DHV occurs after AVH with both viruses or after acquisition of DHV in the chronic carrier of HBV (either with persistent HBV or chronic active HBV). In a survey of 126 patients in the Los Angeles area (1967-1982), two thirds of the DHV infections occurred in patients with chronic hepatitis B infection, and one third were dual acute infections.[195] Fulminant hepatitis DHV accounted for 17 of 29 fatal cases.

Epidemiology. HDV infection is worldwide but has

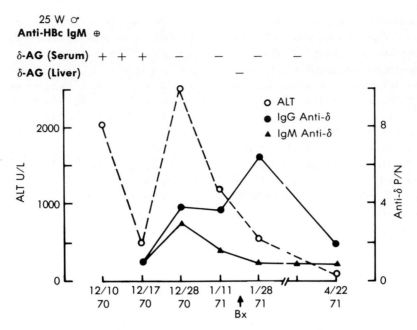

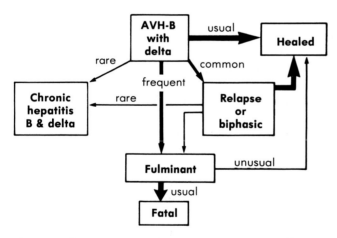

Fig. 25-8. Serologic and serum alanine aminotransferase (ALT) values in intravenous drug addict with acute viral hepatitis attributable to both hepatitis B virus and hepatitis D virus with biphasic icterus and ultimate healing of both viral infections. *AG,* Antigen; *Bx,* biopsy; *P/N,* ratio of counts per minute of control positive sample to counts per minute of control negative sample; *U/L,* units per liter; *25 W ♂,* 25-year-old white male.

Fig. 25-9. Typical course of acute delta hepatitis with acute viral hepatitis B in adult patient. (From Craig, J.R., Govindarajan, A.S., and DeCode, K.M.: Pathol. Annu. **2:**1-21, 1986.)

very irregular prevalence. Epidemiologic surveys indicate that the virus is endemic in southern Europe, Africa, and the Middle East especially around Turkey and Saudi Arabia, and it occurs in epidemic proportions in South America.[278] In the tropics, Lábrea hepatitis in the Amazon basin is principally caused by the DHV.[171] In Italy, up to 50% of chronic B carriers have antibody

to HDV, whereas in China and Taiwan there is a low prevalence of HDV despite the abundance of HBV.[187] HDV occurs in the United States primarily in intravenous drug users but is also noted in the male homosexual community. In the University of Southern California Liver Unit series of 126 patients with DHV, male homosexual DHV was a risk factor in 21.4% of 126 patients recorded in the period 1967 to 1982.[195]

The DHV is spread primarily through parenteral means and thus is common in intravenous drug addicts. The virus is also spread in close contacts and sexual transmission in countries with intermediate and high HBV experience. Maternal-infant spread occurs in HBeAg-positive HDV-infected mothers and is not common presumably because many HBV-infected patients have low levels of HBV replication.[176] Because blood products are screened for HBsAg, much HDV-contaminated material is also removed from the recipient pool.

Hepatitis non-A, non-B

Hepatitis non-A, non-B (NAB) is clinically identical to AVH attributable to HAV and HBV but lacks the serologic markers of either virus. There is ample clinical, epidemiologic, and experimental evidence that at least two viral agents are responsible.[200] In 1982, 24% of our patients with AVH were NAB, and yet only 7% of AVH reported to the Centers for Disease Control in

1984 was so classified and thus may reflect the well-known underreporting of AVH. Spread of NAB is both parenteral and nonparental with sporadic cases as well as a major number identified after blood transfusion. The mean incubation period in posttransfusion cases is 7.8 weeks and is less than the 11.6-week mean time for hepatitis B.[200] In the posttransfusion group of NAB compared to posttransfusion HBV, the NAB illness is milder with lower peak serum enzyme and bilirubin values, and more patients are asymptomatic. One form of epidemic waterborne NAB is unusually virulent, with mortality of up to 10% and even higher in pregnant women. Epidemics have been reported from Kashmir Valley in India. Of our fatal AVH at the University of Southern California Liver Unit, 42% is recognized as NAB. Two outbreaks of enterically transmitted NAB viral hepatitis were recognized in Mexico in the summer and fall of 1986.[290a] Epidemic NAB hepatitis has been noted in Pakistani travelers to the United States.[194a] Development of an accurate serologic test is anxiously awaited so that better epidemiologic data and accurate clinical diagnosis may be developed. Chronicity develops at a higher rate in the posttransfusion group than in NAB from other sources (that is, sporadic cases, intravenous drug users, and so on) and estimates of chronic hepatitis (carriers) in the United States are 20 to 100 higher than the carrier rate for HBV.

Pathology of viral hepatitis

AcVH is associated with histologic changes that vary considerably, depending on the temporal stage of the disease, severity of the process, and individual cellular and reparative response. Any differences in morphology produced by the various hepatitis agents are less than the variation in severity, response, or regeneration seen with any one of the virus infections. Comparison of hepatic histopathologic characteristics of patients with HAV, HBV, and NAB acute viral hepatitis have produced mixed results, and the features are so overlapping that specific etiology cannot be reliably determined by light microscopy.[235] Some features may indicate one cause, but other studies fail to corroborate such findings. See Plate 3, A.

In a liver biopsy specimen taken before the onset of symptoms and before there is biochemical evidence of cell necrosis, there is only nonspecific change. The hepatic cords are straight and regular; the hepatocytes have slightly enlarged nuclei and sharp nuclear membranes. The size and number of Kupffer cells, as well as the number of lymphocytes in the sinusoids, are increased, but portal lymphoid hyperplasia is lacking. Sparse foci of cell dropout of hepatocytolysis may be seen, but generalized liver cell hydropic swelling develops just before the onset of symptoms and simultaneously with serum biochemical abnormalities.

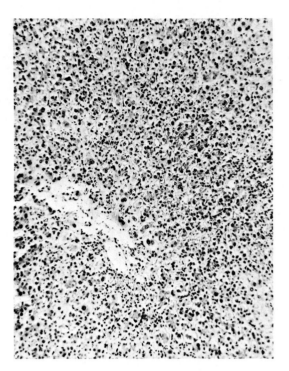

Fig. 25-10. Acute viral hepatitis. Appearance is that generally seen on needle biopsy. Notice swollen liver cells, lack of cord pattern, and focal necrosis.

Three nearly concurrent, independently variable, morphologic changes characterize viral hepatitis at the height of clinical disease: (1) hepatocyte damage, (2) lymphoid and reticuloendothelial reaction, and (3) hepatocyte regeneration.

The hepatocyte damage is generalized. All the cells become swollen with a watery-appearing cytoplasm; this change is most severe in the perivenular regions, where the hydropic change at the sinusoidal margin of the hepatocyte contrasts sharply with the perinuclear and pericanalicular condensation of cytoplasm. In the early stage the hepatocyte cord arrangement becomes disrupted because of the cytoplasmic swelling and onset of hepatocyte regeneration (Fig. 25-10). The nuclei are slightly, but uniformly, enlarged with finely divided, granular nuclear chromatin, a prominent nucleolus, and a sharp nuclear membrane. Hepatocytolysis is not randomly distributed throughout but is most prominent in the perivenular regions, where the intercellular membranes often become indistinct and structures that resemble syncytial giant cells are often seen. Rarely, severe confluent cell destruction may leave only a spongy stromal network in the perivenular areas. The lysis of dying cells is rapid, and dead liver cells are not identifiable on biopsy. An exception is the type of cell death that results in the acidophilic body, examples of which are often scattered throughout the lobule.

The hepatic lymphoid and reticuloendothelial response usually produces the most prominent histologic change in acute viral hepatitis. Kupffer cell activity is greatly increased, and unicellular foci of hepatocytolysis usually are identified by the histiocytes, which along with Kupffer cells phagocytose cell debris. The histocytes usually are filled with glycoprotein, apparently representing activated lysosomes, and also contain lipochrome pigment. The foci of hepatocytolysis are further marked by numerous lymphocytes and a few plasma cells, which also are in sinusoids and spaces of Disse, often forming a cuff around hepatocytes. In the portal areas proliferative cholangiolar epithelium and poorly formed duct structures are found; lymphocytes, plasma cells, and mononuclear cells often transverse the limiting plates of portal zones, producing a sawtoothed effect, often referred to as piecemeal necrosis. Although piecemeal necrosis has often been described as a feature of chronic liver disease, it is usually present in acute viral hepatitis.

Concurrently with acute damage and necrosis, regeneration without nodularity occurs. Regeneration is manifest by zones of clustered hepatocytes without the regular contiguous relationship of hepatocytes to sinusoids. The periportal cells, particularly, have a solid pavement appearance early in the disease and form closely packed clusters of pale, swollen cells. Histochemical studies indicate the mitochondrial and endoplasmic reticulum–associated enzyme activity in periportal hepatocytes is reduced, which reduction correlates with the ultrastructural appearance by diminished endoplasmic reticulum.[293]

Perivenular canalicular cholestasis is variable, but even when extensive, there is poor correlation with clinical features that usually characterize cholestatic disease. In contrast, patients who have unusually high elevations of alkaline phosphatase activity in association with acute viral hepatitis do not have unusual cholestasis on biopsy. If jaundice is prolonged, the Kupffer cells also contain bile pigment, but there is usually little bile staining of the cytoplasm of the swollen hepatocytes.

Late histologic changes. After a patient's clinical recovery, though the serum transaminase levels approach normalcy, histologic changes persist. Pigment-laden and glycoprotein-rich histocytes remain in scattered foci of previous cell necrosis, and hepatic parenchymal cells develop a cobblestone configuration, whereas the perivenular accentuation of cell damage disappears. A slow establishment of the sinusoidal and cord pattern often requires a year, and the portal lymphoid hyperplasia often remains prominent for months.

Electron microscopic studies. HAV, which is associated with cytoplasmic antigenic material in the liver even after the virus becomes undetectable in stool,[241] has been associated with cytoplasmic, viruslike, round bodies packaged in a saclike structure.[276] Although HAV antigenic material is found in Kupffer cells by immunofluorescent microscopy, there are no reports that these cells contain hepatitis A viral particles when studied under the electron microscope.

Electron microscopic studies disclose that viral particles are extremely sparse during AcVH-B, but the opposite is true of the liver of the patient who is a chronic carrier or who has HBsAg-positive chronic liver disease.

At least two electron microscopically different viruslike structures have been described in AcVH-NAB. Except for one report, however, these particles have been described only in studies of VH-NAB in chimpanzees. One type of particle has a tubular ultrastructure with double-membrane walls enclosing electron-dense material found in hepatocyte cytoplasm during acute viral hepatitis[212,235,277,303] and is said to have an incubation period of 2 to 4 weeks in chimpanzees. An agent with an incubation time of 5 weeks in a chimpanzee produces a disease without cytoplasmic tubular structures but with poorly defined spherical structures that apparently develop in hepatocyte nuclei. Equivocal cytoplasmic tubules and nuclear particles have been described in humans, occurring simultaneously in both acute and chronic VH-NA, but the development of well-formed cytoplasmic and nuclear forms in humans has not been demonstrated. One study in chimpanzees showed that the same inoculum produced nuclear particles in one chimpanzee and cytoplasmic particles in another. Thus the electron microscopic features of viruses responsible for VH-NAB remain controversial and unsettled.

Other ultrastructural changes observed in liver cells and Kupffer cells are nonspecific[291] and are apparently similar for hepatitis A, B, and NAB. Early in the disease the endoplasmic reticulum becomes irregularly dilated and vesicular and often is separated or destroyed by ballooning of the cytosol. The nuclei enlarge, and nucleoli are prominent. Free ribosomes increase in the cytoplasm, and glycogen deposition is irregular. The intercellular membranes, instead of disappearing as one would anticipate from light microscopy, actually develop microvilli. The space between adjacent cells is widened. Fine stands of collagen are occasionally found in Disse's space and in the intercellular space (Fig. 25-2).

The acidophilic, or Councilman-like, body is observed often in viral hepatitis though it may be seen in many other diseases in humans and animals. Councilman described the bodies in yellow fever.[282] Although some doubt has been expressed as to whether the bodies are the same as those seen in viral hepatitis, most hepatopathologists use the terms *acidophilic body* and *Councilman's body* interchangeably. The acidophilic body is composed of condensed cytoplasm from which ribosomes have largely disappeared but in which the shadowy, electron-dense remains of many cell organelles are still visible.[174,183]

Pathogenesis of acute viral hepatitis

The pathogenesis of acute viral hepatitis is likely different for the different viral agents and is not easily understood even though the morphologic appearances are similar. T-lymphocytes of the OKT8 type (cytotoxic-suppressor type) are reported to be the predominant lymphocyte in AVH of all three major viral agents.[211] Others have evidence that HBV is not directly cytopathic but requires a relatively intact immune system.[208] Fulminant viral hepatitis B is associated in a few patients with recent removal of immune suppression. Also, HBV carriers have little cytotoxic activity despite high levels of HBV replication. Furthermore, there is little correlation between circulating HBV-related antigens and severity of liver damage. Surprisingly, in fulminant hepatitis there is little or no HBV viral components identified at the time of necrosis. The lack of any serum HBV DNA in patients with fulminant fatal hepatitis B in contrast with the presence of the HBV DNA in serum of nonfulminant AVH-B indicates that viral replication itself is not cytopathic.[197] Because AVH occurs after some weeks of incubation and viral replication, it seems likely that the host immune response as well as viral replication are essential for cytopathic effect. Recent studies have also indicated that HBV is in nonhepatocytes including pancreas, skin, and kidney.[191]

Viral hepatitis in homosexuals

A leading reservoir for HAV and HBV in large American cities is the male homosexual. Of the hepatitis agents, HBV has been studied most thoroughly. In Los Angeles 8.2% of homosexual men have a chronic HBV infection, whereas many more have serologic evidence of previous HBV infection. In Boston 70% of acute hepatitis infections in homosexuals in 1981 were type A. Of the remainder of homosexual men tested, 70% had serologic evidence of previous HAV infection.[206]

In New York over a 2-year period, 34.5% of the homosexual men studied developed serologic evidence of new HBV infection.[288] The high rate of infectivity is apparently related in part to promiscuity. Heterosexual contact between an acutely infected and a susceptible person results in as high as a 40% transmission rate[262]; heterosexual transmission rarely becomes epidemic, however. Experimental transmission studies have shown semen of HBV-infected persons to transmit HBV and have demonstrated that HBV can be acquired transvaginally. When there are breaks in oral mucosa, as can occur after brushing of teeth, HBV may be transmitted orally. There is evidence that the infection can be transmitted rectally, apparently through asymptomatic rectal mucosal abrasions[264]; whether the agent traverses intact mucosa is unclear.

Viral hepatitis in intravenous drug users

Although it appears that AcVH-B is on the decrease, as perhaps is the illicit use of intravenous drugs, an increased frequency of viral hepatitis among drug addicts has been recognized for many years, reaching a peak during the late 1960s.[236] In one study in 1981, 97% of the intravenous drug users had serologic evidence of chronic or healed VH-B.[250]

In some studies, up to 82% of intravenous drug users have heavy alcoholic consumption; thus assessment of the liver disease in this group is often difficult. Chronic HBs antigenemia has been reported to occur in over 10% of chronic intravenous drug users.[250]

Some intravenous drug users develop icteric hepatitis on more than one occasion; some have had four or five episodes; many have had three. The multiple attacks led to the recognition that there were indeed several types of virus involved, even before discovery of the B virus or demonstration of HAV. Occurrence of multiple bouts of icteric viral hepatitis is rare in non–drug users, including individuals who receive hundreds of units of blood or blood products. Immunoglobulin levels in addicts who have multiple attacks of hepatitis are not depressed.

On biopsy the liver of the percutaneous drug user with hepatitis often has more lymphoid proliferation in the portal areas than that seen in typical AcVH; occasionally, formation of lymph follicles occurs. The lymphoid hyperplasia may be related to the repeated inoculations of foreign material. After the patient has had multiple bouts of hepatitis, the portal areas may become widened, but nodular regeneration does not develop. At one time in many cities, heroin and other opiates were often adulterated, or "cut," with substances that included talclike particles; the repeated intravenous injection of these drugs resulted in accumulation of polarizable crystals in the portal areas and in Kupffer cells. The crystals rarely cause true granulomas but are often associated with mild nonprogressive increase of connective tissue. In addition, the high incidence of alcoholism in drug users is reflected by the large proportion of liver biopsy specimens that show increased collagen, which confuses the diagnosis.

Fatal viral hepatitis

Fulminant viral hepatitis. Fulminant hepatic failure is the clinical designation for the abrupt onset of liver failure with coma that always results from acute massive hepatic necrosis and usually occurs after severe submassive hepatic necrosis. The most common cause of severe, coma-producing hepatic necrosis in the United

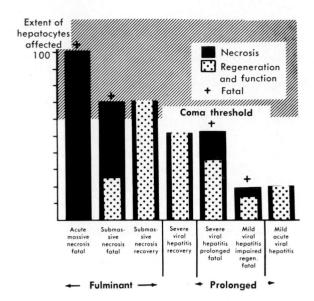

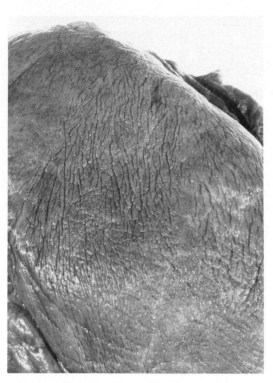

Fig. 25-11. Schematic relationship between extent of necrosis, regeneration and function, and survival. First three bars reflect extensive necrosis to extent that coma develops (fulminant). First bar depicts total destruction (thus no regeneration or function). Second bar has regeneration and function inadequate to regain original mass. Third bar reflects recovery because of greater regeneration, despite amount of necrosis similar to that of second bar. Remaining bars indicate that, with less necrosis, death may still occur if regeneration and function are impaired.

Fig. 25-12. Fulminant viral hepatitis occurring after blood transfusions given 140 days before onset of jaundice. Notice typical wrinkling of capsule of liver when flexed.

States is viral hepatitis. About 1% of patients hospitalized with viral hepatitis during the 1960s and 1970s developed abrupt and severe liver cell necrosis, producing hepatic insufficiency. During the early 1980s the percentage of patients with overt hepatitis who developed fulminant disease was about 3%, with about 66% mortality (Fig. 25-11, *bars 1-3*). In patients designated as having fulminant viral hepatitis, coma usually develops after less than 4 weeks of symptoms. Death usually follows coma within 24 hours to a few days. The liver morphology is determined by the extent of necrosis, amount of regeneration, and duration of survival of the patient after onset of fulminant disease.

Recovery of patients with AcVH is based on a balance of four semi-independent factors: (1) extent of hepatocellular loss, (2) extent and rapidity of regeneration of residual hepatocytes, (3) adequacy of functional activity of residual hepatocytes, and (4) adequacy of mechanisms of defense against continued viral replication and activity.

Patients with fatal fulminant hepatitis are divided into two major groups based on morphology: those who have less than a single layer of hepatocytes around the portal areas and no islands if viable parenchyma are classified as having acute massive necrosis; those with larger numbers of hepatocytes, either as islands of regenerating tissue or as evenly distributed periportal cells, are classified as having acute submassive necrosis.

In acute massive necrosis the liver weighs about 1 to 1.2 kg, only slightly less than normal. The liver capsule is smooth, but the liver is limp. When the liver is sectioned, the portal connective is accentuated; the remaining tissue is deep red and retracted. The liver in acute massive necrosis simulates the appearance of spleen, a pattern once referred to as acute red atrophy (Fig. 25-12). With complete necrosis there has usually not been sufficient time for bile pigment to accumulate, and there are no hepatocytes to extract it from blood; thus neither the patient nor the liver is deeply icteric.

Microscopic study reveals the destruction of hepatocytes. The Kupffer cells are large and numerous, and there is a minimum amount of lymphocytic infiltrate and hyperplasia. The liver stroma is intact, and little collapse is noted. The bile ducts show little hyperplasia unless the fulminant episode occurred late in the course of ordinary hepatitis. Since all hepatocytes are destroyed, the factors of regeneration, function, and continued viral activity are not a consideration (Fig. 25-11, *bar 1*).

A patient with submassive necrosis (Fig. 25-11, *bars*

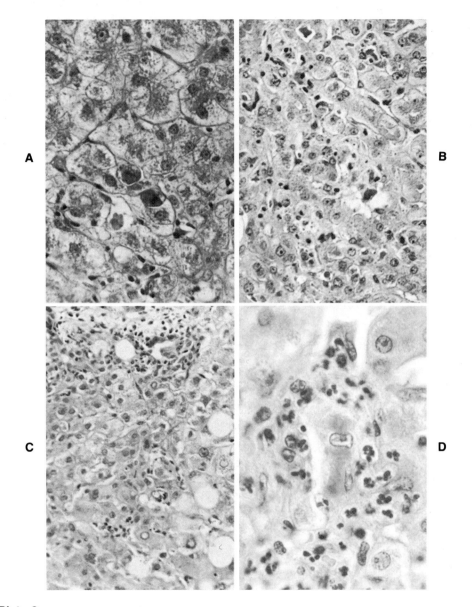

Plate 3
A, Needle biopsy in acute hepatitis A. Two acidophilic bodies are present near bottom. Cytoplasm is swollen and granular and cell membranes are indistinct.
B, Perivenular bile stasis in patient taking oral contraceptive.
C, Acute pericholangitis and cholestasis in needle biopsy. Large at surgery, stone was removed from common bile duct.
D, Hyaline necrosis in alcoholic patient. Many neutrophils are in sinusoids.

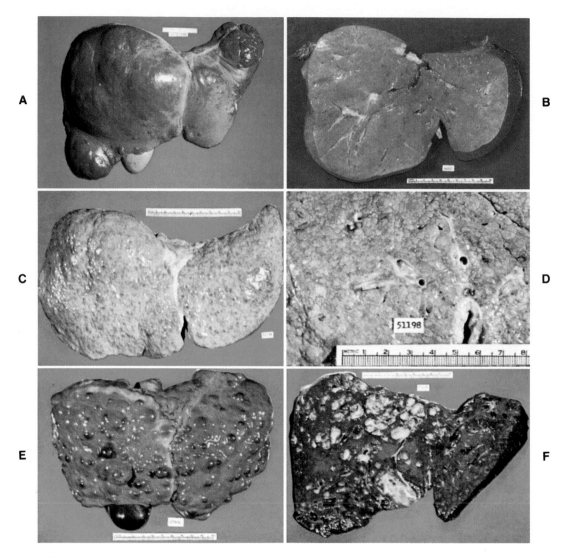

Plate 4

A, Submassive hepatic necrosis from viral hepatitis, with bulging areas of residual liver and much shrinkage and collapse of left lobe. Patient lived 24 days after onset of clinical symptoms.

B, Hypertrophic, firm, smooth alcoholic fatty liver.

C, Eutrophic, hard, finely pseudolobular alcoholic cirrhosis in 65-year-old man.

D, Cut surface of alcoholic cirrhosis showing pseudolobular pattern.

E, Atrophic, firm, megalonodular lupoid cirrhosis, quiescent in 20-year-old woman.

F, Suppurative cholangitis with multiple abscesses resulting from carcinomatous obstruction of common duct.

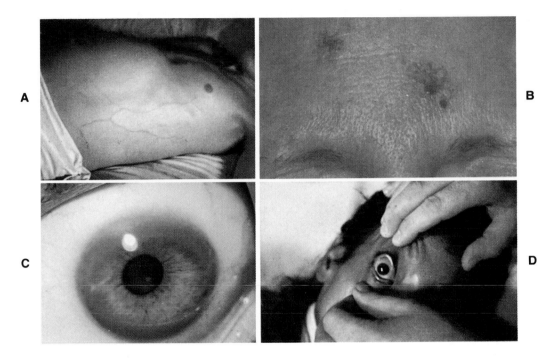

Plate 5

A, Hepatic cirrhosis. Ascites, congested veins, pigmented male nipple, axillary alopecia, and absence of striae.

B, Arteriovenous fistulas (vascular spiders) in diabetic cirrhosis. Arterial blood supply in center of lesion.

C, Kayser-Fleischer ring in Wilson's disease.

D, Jaundice and biliary cirrhosis after ligation of common bile duct.

(**A** and **D,** From Wiener, K.: Skin manifestations of internal disorders, St. Louis, 1947, The C.V. Mosby Co.)

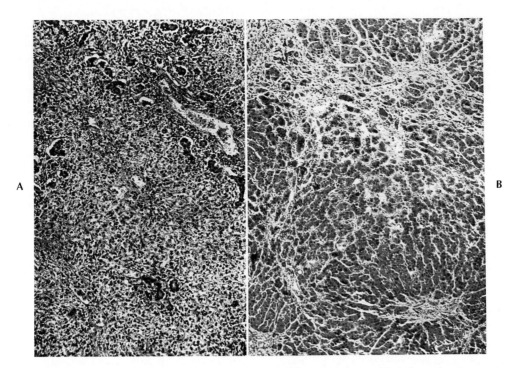

Fig. 25-13. Fatal viral hepatitis. **A,** Appearance of liver on ninety-third day, showing collapsed areas. **B,** Residual liver. (From Lucké, B.: Am. J. Pathol. **20:**595, 1944.)

2 and 3) of the liver may die in less than 1 week but may live for 2 or 3 weeks when there is enough surviving liver parenchyma or greater regenerative and functional capacity.

The livers of patients who survive less than a week (stage I) are slightly shrunken, limp, and finely mottled. The deeply icteric swollen parenchymal cells remaining in periportal areas impart a golden yellow color that caused Rokitansky in 1842 to use the term "acute yellow atrophy" to describe such a liver. If the patient survives more than a week after developing hepatic coma from submassive necrosis, all the parenchymal cells may disappear in some large zones, whereas the other areas yellow periportal parenchymal remains and replicates (Fig. 25-13).

The pattern of collapse and regeneration may become irregular. There may be some areas of considerable residual periportal liver parenchyma fading into zones of sharply defined perivenular collapse. These areas gradually merge into those where the periportal rims of residual hepatocytes are narrower or nonexistent and the corresponding stromal collapse of the remaining lobules more extensive (stage II). The liver is shrunken to a weight of about 800 to 900 g. It is wrinkled and deeply icteric (Fig. 25-12), particularly in the areas of less collapse. See Plate 4, *A*.

In patients who survive 3 weeks or more (stage III), the liver is characterized grossly by islands of yellow liver parenchyma bulging above the surrounding back collapsed stroma. In the past, this stage was called subacute yellow atrophy. However, the necrosis is acute, even though the patient may have survived longer because there was enough functionally active residual liver. If the patient lives for several weeks after the episode of submassive hepatic necrosis, the blood channels in the collapsed stroma of the liver may sclerose, and areas of collapse may become pale and lose the congested "splenic" appearance. The residual and regenerating liver is nearly devoid of inflammatory exudate (Fig. 25-13, *B*).

These patterns, often misinterpreted as cirrhosis or precursors to cirrhosis, are called early (I), middle (II), and late (III) stages of submassive necrosis. Microscopically in late submassive necrosis there are striking numbers of bile plugs and microconcretions of bile in periportal canaliculi.

In both massive and submassive necrosis, changes such as minimal ascites, pleural effusion, and peripheral edema are often present. The regional lymph nodes and spleen are generally enlarged at autopsy. Hemorrhagic areas often are found in various tissues because of deficiency of coagulation factors normally produced by the liver. Hemorrhages are often present in the intestine, lungs, and mesentery, and gastrointestinal bleeding occasionally contributes to death.

Mortality. The survival rate in patients with fulminant viral hepatitis has varied in different studies. One important factor in outcome has been the age of the patient. Chance of survival is greater in younger individuals; of 81 patients with fulminant hepatitis admitted to our liver unit from 1965 to 1972, there was a 47.3% survival of the 11- to 20-year age group, 25% survival in the 21- to 40-year age group, and none in those over 40 years.[263] Since 1965, all but one of 22 survivors of fulminant hepatitis at our liver unit have been under 30 years of age. None of 22 survivors of the 81 cases of clinically fulminant hepatitis has developed cirrhosis or any other hepatic sequela.[225]

However, a report from the National Acute Hepatic Failure Study Group indicated a difference in prognosis for patients with fulminant hepatitis B, in contrast to those with fulminant hepatitis non-A, non-B (NAB). Patients with fulminant hepatitis NAB had only a 13% overall survival, in contrast to a 33% survival in the patients with fulminant hepatitis B. In addition, patients under 24 years of age with fulminant hepatitis NAB had a 21% survival; those 25 to 44 years, a 5% survival; those over 45 years, a 16% survival.[257] Since 60% of the patiens with fulminant hepatitis at the USC Liver Unit had type B hepatitis, compared with 31% in the national study group,[172] survival expectations might be expected to differ not only with respect to patient age but also with respect to the infective agent. All these studies were completed before DHV testing was available and need reevaluation with more detailed testing.

Infectivity. Patients with fulminant hepatitis B are HBeAg positive, but, of the fatal cases, none (of 14) had HBV DNA in the serum at autopsy an indication of lower infectivity at death than nonfatal cases.[197] Thus they have much lower infectivity than patients with ordinary AcVH or, for that matter, many patients with chronic active hepatitis or B viral cirrhosis. There is neither documentation of needle-stick transmission of hepatitis B from a patient with fulminant hepatitis nor evidence of an autopsy prosector contracting hepatitis B after being cut during the course of autopsy of such a patient. Although data are less complete regarding infectivity of fulminant hepatitis NAB, there is no evidence of greater risk to medical personnel by patients with more serious illness. Since HAV is demonstrable in the liver of patients dying of fulminant hepatitis A, one might suspect a greater hazard at autopsy from fulminant hepatitis A than B, but there are no data to clarify that point, and only about 1% or less of fulminant hepatitis in the United States is caused by HAV.

Viral hepatitis with impaired regeneration syndrome (VH-IRS), protracted viral hepatitis, and subacute hepatic necrosis. A small but significant segment of the patients who die after AcVH undergo a protracted nonfulminant form of the disease. Twenty-two percent of

the patients who have died of viral hepatitis at the USC Liver Unit have had such a protracted, rather than fulminant, pattern. Because the basic difficulty appears to be related more to the failure to regenerate than to the amount of necrosis, we have called this pattern the "impaired regeneration syndrome" (VH-IRS).[253] Patients who fit into the category average 60 years of age, in contrast to the 20- to 30-year-old patients dying of fulminant disease; the average duration of illness of patients with VH-IRS is 75 days rather than 14 and 20 days for acute massive and submassive necrosis, respectively. The percentage of patients who survive after developing the IRS is unclear because there is a degree of impaired regeneration in the clinical pattern of most elderly patients with viral hepatitis; viral hepatitis in older patients is regularly protracted and the cholestasis more prominent even after transaminase activities have dropped to nearly normal range.

Liver biopsy specimens from patients with IRS who ultimately recover show regular, straight liver cords that are frequently somewhat shrunken, apparently a reflection of the failure of those cells to proliferate at an accelerated rate. Otherwise, in initial aspects of the disease the histologic appearance is similar to AcVH. However, when the necrosis is more severe, areas of confluent hepatocellular destruction are not replaced by rapidly regenerating hepatocytes, as they are in younger persons with hepatitis, but are characterized by collapsed stroma. When this stroma produces "bridging" bands that connect adjacent portal areas or perivenular regions throughout the biopsy specimen, the pattern has been referred to as subacute hepatic necrosis (SHN).[178] Bridging, however, can be seen as a result of severe acute necrosis if biopsies are performed as early as it is safe to do so; it also may be seen in chronic active hepatitis and after there has been only an ordinary degree of necrosis with impaired regeneration. Thus the prognosis of patients with the bridging lesion depends on the underlying hepatic disorder in which the bridging is recognized.[299]

The liver of the patient who dies with the bridging lesion of VH-IRS is shrunken and slightly toughened but limp. Its surface is bumpy or irregular with few regenerative areas. Microscopic examination shows shrunken hepatocytes and little exudate in the parenchyma; hyperplasia of the lymphoid and reticuloendothelial system within widened portal areas is somewhat less than in ordinary viral hepatitis. There is also considerable collapse within each lobule. Thin fingers of collapsed stroma and collagen extend from both the portal and the perivenular areas. Regeneration is minimal; thus the hepatic cords are straight and obvious. Cholestasis is striking in the liver of many patients with VH-IRS, producing periportal biliary concretions that may result in acute cholangitis around the plugged interlobular duct radicals. Of survivors in an older group of patients with late-onset hepatic failure, several patients had chronic active hepatitis.[209] Liver transplantation has been successfully complete in one patient with late-onset hepatic failure.

Relapse of viral hepatitis

DHV may occur as a dual infection with two viruses (such as DHV and HBV) producing a single icteric illness recognized clinically as acute viral hepatitis or as a biphasic illness (Fig. 25-8). Approximately one half of the biphasic AVH type B in our series were attributable to HBV and DHV, and so possibly the other half were attributable to another agent or agents. In the past this event was considered a relapse of acute viral hepatitis, but now it can be diagnosed as acute viral hepatitis caused by both agents with the first icteric peak caused by HBV and the second peak caused by DHV.[215]

Role of DHV in fulminant hepatitis

Delta-hepatitis virus is common in our patients with fulminant viral hepatitis B because many are intravenous drug users or male homosexual patients. The prevalence of the DHV markers was 33.8% in a review of 71 patients with fulminant hepatitis, and the majority had acute viral hepatitis with dual infection of HBV and DHV though 5 of 24 had chronic hepatitis B infection and a clinical illness recognized as fulminant acute viral hepatitis-DHV.[212] Before the serologic testing for DHV, these patients were all classified as fulminant hepatitis type B, and thus without testing one third were misidentified. Morphologic features were compared in fulminant data and fulminant HBV infection and no specific features were noted by routine light microscopy.[213] However, in contrast to the lack of identifying features of fatal DHV in the United States, the Santa Marta hepatitis (also called Lábrea hepatitis) in South America has microsteatosis and pronounced eosinophilic degeneration as distinctive typified morphologic features.[184]

Chronic hepatitis

Chronic hepatitis is defined as continuing and prolonged hepatitis with either active liver destruction (so called *chronic active hepatitis*) or with very mild inflammatory change and a benign course called *chronic persistent hepatitis* (which our group calls "persistent viral hepatitis" to avoid the redundancy of chronic and persistent). It is customary to classify chronic hepatitis by cause if known or suspected based on epidemiologic grounds. *Chronic carrier* of hepatitis B virus is a term that applies to the patient with 6 or more months of known HBV infection who fails to be classified into another category (that is, chronic active hepatitis, B viral cirrhosis, or persistent viral hepatitis) because of lack of

biopsy evidence or clinical evidence for progressive liver disease. Carriers of HBV have silent infection and by definition are asymptomatic.[221] However, because many patients with chronic active viral hepatitis B have indolent silent infection and progressive destruction of the liver, they may appear to be carriers also (that is, lack signs of serious liver disease) until liver tissue is available for microscopic analysis or until more detailed hepatic examination is concluded. Not only is clinical classification of chronic hepatitis difficult because of the lack of symptoms and signs of progressive liver disease, but also there are considerable differences in the course of chronic hepatitis because of the various viral agents. However, most of our information about course and pathogenesis comes from following chronic hepatitis B or delta viral hepatitis, and these principles may not apply to the several NAB viral agents that also appear to cause chronic hepatitis. Clearly the lack of accurate serologic tests for NAB agents interferes with defining the course and effect of treatment of chronic NAB hepatitis. Chronic active (type B or NAB), autoimmune or lupoid chronic active hepatitis, drug-induced chronic active hepatitis, and cryptogenic chronic active hepatitis for the patient with no known cause but with clinical features of chronic destructive progressive liver disease resembling chronic active viral hepatitis. The term "chronic active hepatitis" was originally applied to the patient with recurrent bouts of inflammatory activity and jaundice appearing to be recurrent hepatitis, with the result usually being cirrhosis and liver failure. With better screening tests and HBV markers available, it has become clear that the majority of patients with chronic hepatitis have clinically silent initial infection and clinically silent progression to advanced liver disease (that is, cirrhosis) with a jaundice or bleeding episode appearing late in the disease course. Conversion of silent chronic active hepatitis to active inflammatory disease is called *reactivation* and occurs intermittently in the lifetime and bouts may last for a few weeks to many months.[193] Progression of liver disease is believed to occur during these episodes though some patients will succumb to hepatic failure during reactivation. Acquisition of DHV infection (so-called *superinfection*) in a patient with persistent viral hepatitis B usually results in conversion to chronic activie hepatitis B and chronic delta, and fairly progressive liver disease ensues.

In a large population, between 0.1% (United States) and 15% (Taiwan) of the population asymptomatically have HBsAg in their sera. Most have had no signs or symptoms of AcVH. The initial infection was therefore subclinical by definition. A small percentage of these "asymptomatic" carriers have AVH-B, but most have the clinical and histologic features of PVH-B. Persistent viral hepatitis type B, as I define it, rarely progresses to the more serious chronic active hepatitis unless superimposed delta viral hepatitis occurs. Many investigators believe that patients vacillate between the benign and the progressive forms of chronic hepatitis B, which is not our group's experience. Many investigators have demonstrated HBsAg in hepatocyte cytoplasm and HBcAg in hepatocytic nuclei of such carriers. The worldwide incidence of chronic hepatitis B is estimated at 200 million persons and in the United States at 1.5 million persons.[220] This large reservoir of chronically infected persons is the source of virus for the susceptible population.

Most patients chronically infected with HBV are HBeAg positive early in the course but, over the years, lost HBeAg and acquire anti-HBe.[219] From a practical standpoint, HBeAg-positive persons represent the important transmitters of HBV, doing so by sexual contact, perhaps by kissing, by percutaneous inoculation of various sorts, or during the birth process. Chronically HBV-infected persons who are HBeAg negative have distinctly lower infectivity, requiring a substantial percutaneous inoculation of blood or fluid into a susceptible person to bring about infection. In the Orient and probably in Africa and the Pacific Islands, the major source of chronic hepatitis B is perinatal infection. Individuals who have acquired their hepatitis at birth apparently retain not only their infection but also their infectivity (HBeAg) longer, even into the childbearing age. In the United States most of the 0.1% to 0.4% of chronically HBsAg-positive women have acquired the virus in adolescence or young adulthood, and many more become HBeAg negative at an earlier age. Thus a low incidence of HBeAg positivity in the women of childbearing age is critical in a population, since the HBsAg-positive childbearers who are also HBeAg positive are responsible for perpetuating the infection from generation to generation. The advent of immunoglobulin and vaccine and the apparent effectiveness in aborting the perinatal transmission may bring about resolution of this worldwide problem though the economic barriers are formidable.

Persistent viral hepatitis type B

PVH-B is the most common form of chronic disease caused by VH-B. In our special hepatitis clinic patient population (with many intravenous drug users and male homosexual patients), up to 10% of clinically evident AVH patients developed "asymptomatic" chronic hepatitis B, which for the majority is a benign "carrier" state. However, several recent reviews of large HBV-infected populations (United States Army 1942 yellow fever vaccine experience[273] and 821 Greek patients[290]) indicate that otherwise healthy adults have a much lower chronic infection rate that approaches 1% or less. Patients with persistent viral hepatitis B are asympto-

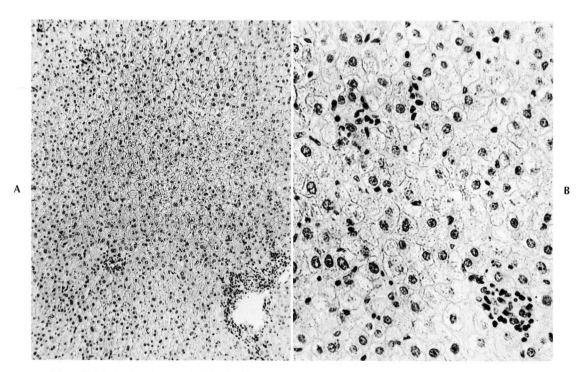

Fig. 25-14. A, Persistent viral hepatitis. Notice cobblestone pattern of liver cells and scattered areas of focal necrosis. **B,** Higher magnification, emphasizing focal necrosis.

matic, have serum HBsAg, and have intermittently elevated serum transaminases in the low range of 50 to 300 IU/liter primarily during the first 5 years after the acute episode (if the episode is identified, which is not usually the case). Recurrence of jaundice or progression of the condition does not occur. Ultimately, transaminase activities return to normal, and about 10% of the patients lose HBsAg and acquire anti-HBs over the years.[237] While HBsAg is present, however, the titer is always high.

The morphologic pattern of the liver in PVH-B changes somewhat with time. The changes are minimal, initially resembling healed hepatitis. Uniformity is maintained within the lobule and from one lobule to another. For the first few years the hydropic appearance of hepatocytes and lack of distinct cord pattern is present throughout the lobule. There are usually unicellular foci of hepatocytolysis, only one to four per lobule, replaced by accumulation of lymphocytes and macrophages condensed into the site of a lysed hepatocyte (Fig. 25-14). About one third of the patients with PVH-B have portal lymphoid hyperplasia, one third have patchy lymphoid hyperplasia in portal areas, and one third have normal portal areas. Clearly the reticuloendothelial component of the liver is not reacting similarly in all patients. In time, usually years, the hydropic change diminishes, and a regular cord pattern may be

recognized. The HBsAg accumulates in some hepatocytes and produces a characteristic body that occupies part or nearly all of the cytoplasm of scattered hepatocytes. These faintly granular cells are called ground-glass (GG) cells or Hadziyannis cells, after the person who described them and recognized their relationship to VH-B (Fig. 25-15).[216] GG cells are found in any type of chronic hepatitis B and never in AcVH-B. In PVH-B, GG cells, when present, are regularly distributed throughout the liver, unlike the distribution in AVH-B, in which they are frequently in clusters and quite irregular in distribution. The GG cells actually consist of closely packed smooth endoplasmic reticulum with tubular structures composed of HBsAg. Specific immunoperoxidase stains[166] or orcein stains for disulfide bonds[275] establish the presence of large amounts of HBsAg (Fig. 25-16).

Acquisition of HDV by a patient with PVH-B has resulted in dramatic change in course. At the time of acquisition, AVH is apparent, with high levels of serum bilirubin and transaminases. The liver biopsy specimen will reflect acute viral hepatitis, and no sign of persistent viral hepatitis B is usually present, though ground-glass cells may be present if the necroinflammatory activity is mild. The course of acquired DHV superinfection is shown in Fig. 25-21 and indicates that a significant number of patients develop fulminant and fatal hepatitis.

Chronic active hepatitis B and B viral cirrhosis

Chronic active viral hepatitis type B (CAVH-B) evolves in most people by a recurrent slow necroinflammatory reaction in the liver that over a few years time, progresses to cirrhosis, and remains clinically si-

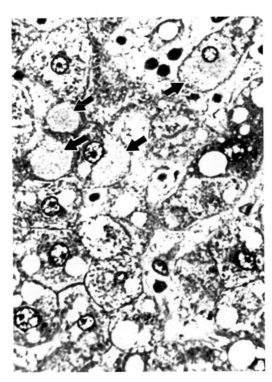

Fig. 25-15. "Ground-glass" hepatocytes of Hadziyannis *(arrows)* may be found either in persistent viral hepatitis B or in chronic active viral hepatitis B.

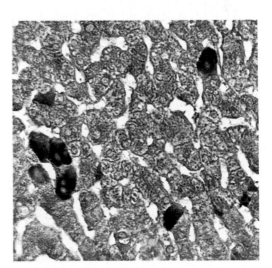

Fig. 25-16. Immunoperoxidase stains reveal HBsAg in "ground-glass" cells of Hadziyannis. (Courtesy Dr. Angelos Afroudakis, Athens, Greece.)

lent from initial infection until advanced cirrhosis has been established. Integration of HBV occurs early in the course, and as time passes, the serologic markers of HBV infection may be below detectable levels and thus the patient may be classified as cryptogenic CAH.[252]

Routine screening tests such as serum transaminases or HBsAg testing in blood donors or high-risk personnel may lead to a liver biopsy of an asymptomatic person who has histologic evidence of B viral cirrhosis, or CAVH-B. Elevated serum transaminases correlate with histologic disease activity though CAVH may progress to cirrhosis with no obvious elevation in serum transaminases. The active phases of CAVH are characterized by variation in necroinflammatory activity in different lobules with ballooned hepatocytes and lymphoid hyperplasia within the portal areas. In the quiescent phase, lobular necroinflammatory activity is minimal, and portal lymphoid cells may be minimal, but the presence of portal fibrosis is helpful. Piecemeal necrosis, which is destruction of the limiting plate by portal lymphoid hyperplasia, and periportal hepatocellular necrosis are common in active phases of CAVH but are also seen in acute viral hepatitis. Acute viral hepatitis may appear similar in a patient with portal widening caused by recurrent infection (as in intravenous drug users). In AVH the ballooned heptocytes are uniformly involved in all lobules, whereas in CAVH the involve-

ment is irregular (Fig. 25-17). Regeneration of hepatocytes may involve only parts of lobules and be irregularly distributed in different lobules. Regenerative nodule with the absence of a terminal hepatic venule and a fibrous capsule are the hallmark of cirrhosis and, if ground-glass (GG) cells are present, indicates B viral cirrhosis (Fig. 25-18). Piecemeal necrosis has been emphasized by many as essential for CAVH; however, it is common in numerous other hepatic conditions, including acute viral hepatitis. The overall lobular necroinflammatory activity and the regenerative features are also important in recognition of chronic active hepatitis. To classify the hepatitis reaction on the portal reaction alone will often lead to overdiagnosis of chronic active hepatitis, which is relatively easy to do because of the abundance of portal fibrosis and suggestion of true regenerative nodules as well as widespread lobular inflammation. However, the desire to identify the earliest stage of chronic active hepatitis and to institute treatment has pressed the histopathologist to elucidate criteria to make the distinction of chronic active hepatitis from active viral hepatitis.[190]

The *pathogenesis* of chronic active viral hepatitis B is poorly understood. Hepatitis B virus alone is not sufficient because the virus proliferates in patients with persistent viral hepatitis and no significant cytopathic or fibrosing reaction is noted. The hallmark of chronic active viral hepatitis in the necroinflammatory reaction, but how the virus induces such necrosis is puzzling. The major hypothesis involves the lymphocytotoxicity

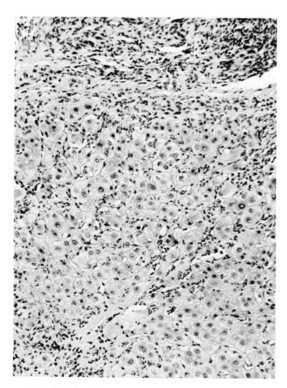

Fig. 25-17. Diffuse inflammation and liver cell necrosis in regenerative nodule from liver in chronic active hepatitis.

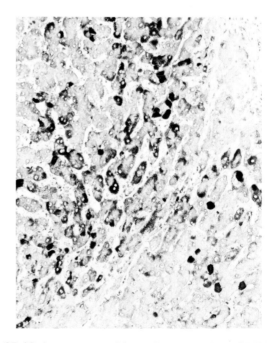

Fig. 25-18. Immunoperoxidase demonstration of HBsAg in chronic active viral hepatitis B. (Courtesy Dr. Angelos Afroudakis, Athens, Greece.)

of replicating virus and proposes that host immune differences account for the variation in individual response to the agent.[208,295] Withdrawal of chemotherapy in HBV carriers has resulted in massive hepatic necrosis, an indication that removal of immune suppression may have stimulated the necrosis.[292] Furthermore, cessation of prednisone (which produces mild immune suppression) in patients with chronic active hepatitis B usually results in rebound elevation in serum transaminases, a marker of hepatocellular necrosis. The lymphocyte target for the immune reaction may be cytoplasmic membrane expression of HBc.[189]

During the quiescent phases of CAVH-B, when the patient is asymptomatic and the serum aminotransferase levels are normal or nearly so, necrosis and exudate are reduced or absent. Morphologic abnormalities may be restricted to irregularly distributed, poorly defined zones of regenerating hepatocytes that subtly compress adjacent hepatocytes. Some areas have hepatocytes with dysplastic or polyploid nuclei, and others are interspersed with increased Kupffer cells. Portal areas are usually larger than normal with increased amounts of collagen or lymphoid tissue. HBsAg-containing heptocytes or ground-glass (GG) cells are irregularly distributed, usually sparing zones of the more actively regenerating hepatocytes. GG cells may be extremely abundant or nonexistent. The hepatic morphologic changes during the early, inactive phase of CAVH-B are so vague and nonspecific that the diagnosis often cannot be made during quiescent phases on morphologic changes alone unless the HBsAg-containing GG cells are recognized, allowing identification of the disease as a form of CAVH-B. The distinction from PVH-B is based on the uniformity of cell arrangement of the latter. Changes similar to those of the quiescent phase of an early CAVH-B may, except for the GG cells, be seen in nonprogressive hepatic disorders.

Despite the paucity of necrosis and inflammation that may be a feature of CAVH-B, progression to cirrhosis proceeds relentlessly in both the subclinical (quiescent) and the clinically apparent (active) forms of the disease, with cirrhosis developing between 1 and 3 years after acquisition of the infection. Serologic studies of chronic active hepatitis B indicate that most patients convert from HBe antigen to anti-HBe, which coincides with quiescence (that is, low or normal serum transaminases and lack of symptoms). *Spontaneous reactivation* occurs in many patients with chronic active hepatitis B (more than one third) manifested by appearance of serum HBV DNA, HBe antigen, and symptoms including ascites, jaundice, and gastrointestinal bleeding.[193] Spontaneous reactivation may be fatal and may appear as fulminant acute hepatitis with serum reappearance of anti-HBc IGM. Previous experience with the patient allows recognition of spontaneous reactivation in chronic active hepatitis B, whereas if the patient appears with icterus for the first time the clinical impression may be acute disease rather than reactivation of a chronic destructive lesion.[196]

After the development of frank cirrhosis, even the disease of those patients with earlier episodes of jaundice and elevated aminotransferase activities tends to become quiescent, and a latent period of 5 to as much as 50 years may elapse before either hepatocellular carcinoma or the consequences of portal hypertension supervene. From 40% to 45% of patients dying of B viral cirrhosis have hepatocellular carcinoma; in the United States, where B viral cirrhosis is relatively uncommon, this results in relatively low incidence of hepatocellular carcinoma. However, in the Orient and in Africa, where B viral cirrhosis is the leading form of cirrhosis, the resultant neoplastic development makes hepatocellular carcinoma one of the most common neoplasms in the world.

The cirrhosis that develops from CAVH-B is called B viral cirrhosis. Although the nodules in B viral cirrhosis have their origin in small, poorly defined areas of regeneration, the nodules are usually large by the time symptoms of portal hypertension or hepatic failure develop (Fig. 25-19). However, hepatocellular carcinoma may develop while the nodules are still small or poorly defined. The average weight of the liver involved at the end stage of B viral cirrhosis at autopsy is 860 g, ranging from 400 to 1600 g. Nodules are from 0.3 to 1 cm in diameter, septa are usually thin, and the collagen is loose (Fig. 25-20) rather than hard and leathery as it is in the alcoholic person. On cut surface the nodules bulge, reflecting the paucity of collagen within them.

The 5-year survival for chronic persistent hepatitis was reported as 97% and was 86% for chronic active hepatitis B but only 55% for B viral cirrhosis.[300] High-

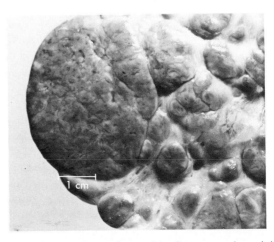

Fig. 25-19. Cut surface of atrophic, firm, megalonodular B-viral cirrhosis.

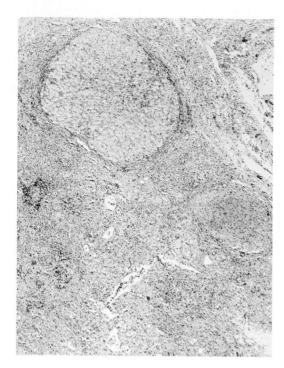

Fig. 25-20. Well-defined regenerative nodule amid collapsed inflamed stroma in coarsely nodular cryptogenic cirrhosis.

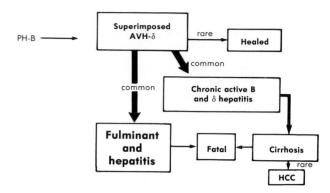

Fig. 25-21. Course of acute delta hepatitis in patients with superinfection occurring in setting of persistent viral hepatitis B. The most common pathways are to chronic active hepatitis and fulminant delta hepatitis.

risk factors included age over 40 years, total serum bilirubin over 1.5 mg/dl, ascites, and spider nevi. Antiviral treatment of chronic hepatitis B is under investigation, but if integration of the HBV occurs early, elimination of the virus will likely not be possible.[274]

Interferon treatment after prednisone withdrawal in chronic B hepatitis has produced sustained loss at HBV-DNA and thus is a promising treatment to eradicate the chronic viral infection.[252a]

Chronic active hepatitis and delta hepatitis

Of my selected patients with delta hepatitis (that is, abundant intravenous drug users and male homosexual patients), two thirds had chronic hepatitis B, and one half of that group had chronic delta and the other half had acute delta hepatitis.[195] Fig. 25-21 shows several pathways for the AVH DHV type occurring in chronic B hepatitis (usually PVH-B). This dual infection is called "superinfection." Although fulminant acute DHV may occur in a fourth of patients with chronic hepatitis B, most of the survivors end up with chronic BHV also. Futhermore, acquisition of DHV with chronic B usually produces progressive chronic active hepatitis and cirrhosis because the chronic DHV infection is active and has abundant necroinflammatory activity.[214] With immune staining, chronic delta hepatitis usually shows prominent nuclear staining, which does not correlate in intensity with inflammatory activity. However, without

immune staining for HDV, the presence of the agent may be suspected by unusually active forms of chronic active hepatitis B.[225] The development of hepatocellular carcinoma in this setting is uncommon possibly because of the occurrence of liver failure before oncogenesis. The typical course of serology and serum ALT in acute delta hepatitis in patients with persistent hepatitis B are shown in Fig. 25-22. A liver biopsy specimen at the time of acute viral hepatitis will show only the changes of acute viral hepatitis, and the chronic B viral infection cannot be detected by routine light microscopy. Serologic tests such as anti-HBc IgG indicate the chronicity of the hepatitis B infection.

Lobular hepatitis

"Lobular hepatitis" was a term introduced by Popper and Schaffner[255] for the unusual patient with histologic features of acute viral hepatitis more than 6 months after the onset of disease. The histologic hallmarks of AVH are lobular changes rather than portal and reflect a hepatocellular necrotizing reaction. The course of patients with chronic lobular hepatitis is not well described, but it appears that some have progression of disease and others a complete healing. This condition is rare enough in my experience to make prognostication of its course difficult.

Chronic forms of hepatitis non-A, non-B

Although by 1988 there were not reliable serologic or tissue markers to identify chronic forms of VH-NAB, there is substantial evidence that chronicity exists.[200,260] Since the number of H-NAB-V agents that may be responsible for chronicity is unknown and the differing characteristics (if they do differ) of the chronic disorders associated with each H-NAB-V agent are similarly unclear, prediction of events in individual instances is not based on well-defined criteria. Follow-up serum trans-

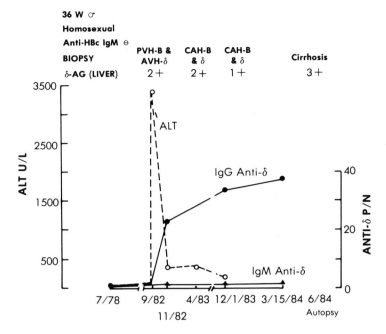

Fig. 25-22. Serologic, liver biopsy, and serum ALT changes in acute delta hepatitis occurring in persistent hepatitis B. *AVH,* Acute viral hepatitis; *CAH,* chronic active hepatitis; *PVH,* persistent viral hepatitis; *P/N,* ratio of counts per minute of control positive sample to counts per minute of control negative sample; *U/L,* units per liter; *36 W ♂,* 36-year-old white male.

aminase values on patients with posttransfusion hepatitis indicates an astounding frequency of persistent elevated values.[169] The NIH study showed that 68% of 75 patients with posttransfusion hepatitis had persistent and fluctuating ALT (transaminase) values for more than 1 year and most for more than 3 years. Furthermore, when liver biopsy is available, there is considerable difficulty by experienced hepatopathologists to be consistent and classify the chronic hepatitis lesions into mild, early chronic active hepatitis (that will progress), persistent viral hepatitis (nonprogressive), and severe chronic active hepatitis.[168]

Persistent viral hepatitis non-A, non-B (PVH-NAB)

The persistent form of non-A, non-B hepatitis is more common but more elusive than PVH-B. More than 50% of the patients who develop AcVH-NAB related to percutaneous injections of illicit drugs continue to have elevated serum levels of aminotransferases for longer than 6 months. Very few, less than 1%, develop progressive liver disease. A similar percentage of patients who develop VH-NAB after transfusion have protracted elevation of aminotransferase activities, but about 40% of the patients who develop chronically elevated serum aminotransferase levels after transfusion-transmitted VH-NAB progress to cirrhosis. Of patients who have no obvious source for the acquisition of hepatitis, only 20%

have continued elevation of serum aminotransferase levels, and few (less than 1%) of these patients develop progressive hepatic lesions.[260] It is unclear whether the differences in course are a result of different viral infection or infections or are related to the means of acquisition. As with PVH-B, patients with PVH-NAB have a slow diminution of serum aminotransferase levels and of histologic alterations. There is no way, at present, to know whether PVH-NAB has healed.

The pathologic changes of PVH-NAB are difficult to separate from the changes associated with continued intravenous drug use, which in itself results in reactive inflammatory hyperplasia. However, the changes in PVH-NAB include portal lymphoid hyperplasia and Kupffer cell hyperplasia, with scattered focal hepatocytolysis. The cobblestone pattern often associated with PVH-B may be lacking. There is no regenerative activity or nodularity, but the portal areas are often somewhat widened. This histologic appearance is not so bland as it is with PVH-B. Because of the lack of a serologic marker for PVH-NAB, we cannot tell if the lesion heals, if it progresses to cirrhosis, or, as with PVH-B, if the patient has no progressive disease but is part of an infective pool. It has been suggested that transmission of the H-NAB-V agents from mother to newborn occurs, but conclusive evidence of continued H-NAB-V infection of the children is lacking.

Chronic active hepatitis, non-A, non-B, and NAB viral cirrhosis

Chronic active hepatitis non-A, non-B (CAVH-NAB) is a lesion whose cause is difficult to establish. The lack of serologic or tissue markers restricts the use of the term *chronic active viral hepatitis non-A, non-B* to patients whose chronic disease follows an episode of acute hepatitis. If, as with hepatitis B, most chronic illness is derived from initially mild or subclinical acute disease, a substantial number of cases would be anticipated. Instead, HBsAg-negative chronic active hepatitis is uncommon in both drug users and male homosexuals, though both groups of individuals have a high incidence of acute viral hepatitis A, B, and NAB. But CAVH-NAB is common as a sequela to posttransfusion hepatitis NAB. In brief, it seems that either a large inoculum is necessary for the induction of CAVH-NAB or a different agent is inoculated in blood transfusion than is transmitted by illicit drug use.

Pathology. Although livers of many patients with CAVH-NAB have changes indistinguishable from those of CAVH-B, often the converse is true. CAVH-NAB often features less regenerative activity, a tendency toward more intrasinusoid and pericellular fibrosis, and scattered fat droplets. Other features of CAVH-B such as randomly distributed focal hepatocytolysis, irregular distribution of regeneration, and portal widening are present. The rate of progression of CAVH-NAB is unclear. In at least some instances the progression is more rapid than in CAVH-B and results in a cirrhotic liver that, at time of death from hepatic failure, has small, poorly defined nodules. The nodules are invaded by fine collagen fibers, but the connective tissue is loose, thus differing from the dense, hard liver in cirrhosis of the alcoholic person. However, since there are no markers to identify H-NAB-V agents, it is uncertain whether progression of CAVH-NAB is, at times, self-limiting; it is possible that the H-NAB-V agent or agents may not persist as tenaciously as the HBV agent does in CAVH-B. On the contrary, it is not clear how many of the patients with cryptogenic cirrhosis or with cryptogenic chronic active hepatitis derive their diseases from the H-NAB-V agent or agents.

The prognosis of CAVH-NAB is suggested in several reports of liver biopsy in posttransfusion hepatitis in which cirrhosis evolved in 11% of the patients with chronic elevation in serum transaminase and in 20% of those biopsied.[169] The cirrhosis appeared to be indolent, but of the 6 patients in the NIH study, two died of liver failure and a third was ill. Therefore cirrhosis seems to evolve and progress to liver failure in a surprisingly high number of posttransfusion patients.

Chronic active autoimmune (lupoid) hepatitis (CALH)

Autoimmune (lupoid) hepatitis is a variety of chronic active hepatitis in which the patient has one or more immunologic abnormalities. Although the disease has no known viral relationship, the possibility of a viral-host interaction to produce a "foreign" antigen has been proposed by some investigators.

Some 85% to 90% of patients with autoimmune hepatitis are women, principally those of childbearing age. Early symptoms include the development of amenorrhea or systemic complaints long before liver disease is manifest. The name "lupoid" was based on the finding of positive lupus erythematosus preparations (LE "preps") in peripheral blood. In addition to positive LE preps, biologic false-positive tests for syphilis occur in 25% of patients with lupoid hepatitis.[238,265] 50% have positive latex-fixation reaction for rheumatoid arthritis, 75% have antinuclear antibodies,[240] and 90% or more have a positive reaction for IgG type of smooth muscle antibodies.[301]

Autoimmune hepatitis responds to immunosuppressant therapy in a fashion not paralleled by other forms of CAH. Without such therapy, fatal submassive hepatic necrosis often develops, a complication rarely found in other forms of CAH. At the USC Liver Unit, 50% of patients with autoimmune hepatitis died in fulminant failure after submassive necrosis, whereas only one of 63 patients dying of CAVH-B had a terminal fulminant course. Although immunosuppressants are effective in aborting such episodes in autoimmune hepatitis, the effect on the ultimate course is unclear, and the oncogenic potential of protracted immunosuppression is still an unsettled question. Recently, two patients with autoimmune hepatitis who had taken steroids for years developed hepatocellular carcinoma. The infrequency of hepatocellular carcinoma in patients with CALH may be related to the preponderance of females with autoimmune hepatitis, whereas hepatocellular carcinoma is far more common in men. See Plate 4, *E*.

Chronic active hepatitis may result from certain idiosyncratic drug reactions and must be considered in the differential diagnosis. Some patients develop abnormal serologic findings, usually associated with chronic active autoimmune hepatitis, when administered certain drugs to which they are sensitive. Very few drugs truly initiate chronic active hepatitis, though many cases of submassive necrosis have been considered incorrectly to be chronic active hepatitis (see discussion of drug necrosis).

Cryptogenic chronic active hepatitis (CCAH)

The cryptogenic form of CAH includes those cases of CAH and even cirrhosis in which all other causes have been excluded. As this group is reviewed and new causes are elucidated, the category designated *cryptogenic* should shrink. In some livers previously classified as showing CCAH, HBV infection may be present in hepatocytes without HBsAg in serum.[167,228,230,251] In my series of previously diagnosed cryptogenic cirrhosis patients, one third had demonstrable HBcAg in hepatocyte nuclei. In addition, some persons with CCAH undoubtedly have CAVH-NAB infection. Certain other diseases of specific causes must also be excluded, such as Wilson's disease (p. 1269) and alpha$_1$-antitrypsin aberrant types (p. 1264). The gross and microscopic changes of CCAH and cirrhosis are similar to those of B viral cirrhosis.

Other acute infections

There are other acute infectious diseases of the liver that occur much less frequently than viral hepatitis. In this group are certain viral, bacterial, rickettsial, and other diseases that involve the liver primarily or in some secondary fashion.

Other viral infections may involve the liver, some producing extensive hepatic necrosis with high incidence of fatality.[305] Most of these diseases are uncommon (Lassa fever,[199,245,300] yellow fever, Ebola virus,[177,229,286] and Marburg viral hepatitis).[168,277] Other viral infections may involve the liver of patients who have systemic infection, but rarely do such viruses produce hepatic symptoms.[297] An exception is herpes simplex, which in the immunosuppressed patient may produce extensive fatal hepatic necrosis. Varicella, rubeola, and hemorrhagic fevers[203,297] may produce incidental hepatic lesions that are usually asymptomatic.

The involvement of the liver by Epstein-Barr virus (EBV) in patients with the clinical features of infectious mononucleosis has long been recognized. The hepatic involvement is usually clinically mild but may be associated with hyperbilirubinemia. The liver has noticeably atypical mononuclear cell hyperplasia in the portal areas, with striking atypical lymphocytosis and Kupffer cell hyperplasia in the lobules. The hepatocytes are not ordinarily swollen or in disarray, as they are in viral hepatitis, but there may be punched-out foci of non-epithelioid granulomatous necrosis. Patients with symptomatic infectious mononucleosis almost always have histologic hepatic involvement whether hepatic symptoms are found. Abnormal findings in hepatic tests are usually present in such patients. The liver does not progress to cirrhosis; fatal fulminant disease, though reported, is a rarity.[181]

Cytomegalovirus (CMV) infections in the liver have grown in incidence with increased blood usage, homosexuality,[223] and treatment modalities that reduce immune response but may be contracted by normal persons who have no obvious source and no apparent immune defect. CMV disease may be associated with fatigue or only with chronic fever; rarely are aminotransferase activities above 300 units, and jaundice is not a feature. Microscopically there may be only Kupffer cell hyperplasia or a pattern indistinguishable from infectious mononucleosis. CMV nuclear inclusions and CMV antigen are rarely found, and immunoperoxidase technique is of little value.[280] There is no evidence of progression of CMV liver disease to cirrhosis.

Herpes simplex viruses, both type 1 and type 2, have become important etiologic agents of severe hepatic necrosis. Hepatic herpes simplex infection is usually restricted to neonates, malnourished infants, pregnant women, and patients undergoing immunosuppressive therapy or with diseases associated with depressed immune response[173] but also occurs in apparently immunocompetent adults.[210] Systemic symptoms are nonspecific, but the disease is generalized, with death occurring in 90% of patients 1 to 2 weeks after onset. The involved liver is enlarged and mottled with sharply defined yellow areas or multiple 0.1 to 0.2 cm yellowish foci. Microscopically the yellow areas represent coagulative necrosis of hepatocytes. The margins of the areas of necrosis are made up of deeply eosinophilic degenerated hepatocytes. Many viable hepatocytes at the margins of the areas of necrosis have nuclei with large eosinophilic inclusion bodies. The inclusions can be identified as herpes simplex type 1 or 2 by immunoperoxidase or immunofluorescence techniques.

Bacterial infections arising in nonhepatic locations may cause jaundice, the exact mechanism of which is unknown. Infections caused by gram-negative organisms may affect both the neonate (see p. 1265) and the adult.[304] In both age groups cholestasis is the chief microscopic finding, usually with some degree of Kupffer cell hyperplasia. There is little or no necrosis. Experimental evidence indicates that the effect of endotoxin on cell membranes may be the causative factor.[304] Typhoid fever is accompanied by hyperbilirubinemia in a sizable percentage of cases. Focal necrosis (typhoid nodules) of the liver is common in typhoid fever, but microscopically the diffuse cholestasis bears no relationship to the foci of necrosis. The cause of jaundice is unclear.[189] In adults, septicemia caused by both gram-negative and gram-positive organisms may cause jaundice within a few days after onset of sepsis. A large number of organisms and sources of infections have been reported.[305] It has been suggested that jaundice accompanying severe bacterial infection is caused by a selective defect in the excretion of conjugated bilirubin because there is a disproportionate increase in serum bilirubin as compared to serum alkaline phosphatase and AST. Jaundice is also known to occur in patients with lobar pneumonia, probably caused by hepatocellular injury. This type of jaundice is more common in

Africa and the southwestern Pacific area.[304]

The principal rickettsial disease that may cause hepatic symptoms is Q fever, discussed on p. 1284. Although rare, Weil's disease (p. 328), caused by a spirochete,[269a] should be suspected when there is jaundice, high fever, and sore muscles.

Treponema pallidum as a liver pathogen is not well documented because many older reports may be related to chronic liver disease secondary to viral hepatitis agents not well characterized at the time of reporting.[294]

CHEMICAL AND DRUG INJURY

Hundreds of compounds, both inorganic and organic, are capable of causing liver injury when they gain access to the body. This may be by inhalation, by injection, or, most commonly, through the intestinal tract. Among the inorganic compounds are arsenic, phosphorus, copper, and iron salts. The organic agents include certain naturally occurring plant toxins, such as the pyrrolizidine alkaloids; mycotoxins, of which aflatoxin is an example; and bacterial toxins. The synthetic group of organic compounds is by far the most important, especially the medicinal agents used for the diagnosis and treatment of disease. In addition, exposure to hepatotoxic compounds[368] may be occupational, environmental, or domestic, including accidental, homicidal, or suicidal ingestion.

The incidence of heptotoxic injury is low compared with other forms of acute liver disease, being far less than viral hepatitis or alcoholic liver disease. However, among patients with fatal hepatocellular disease, the percentage who have drug-related injury is much higher. All patients with acute liver disease should be questioned regarding drug usage and exposure to known hepatotoxins. Furthermore, in patients receiving the drugs that are most commonly hepatotoxic, it is worthwhile to check liver enzyme and serum bilirubin levels routinely for the first few months. This is especially true of drugs, such as isoniazid, that are capable of causing fatal liver cell necrosis.

The role of the liver in drug metabolism and the mechanism of drug-related injury have been the subject of intensive research. Most synthetic drugs are lipid soluble and easily absorbed from the intestines, but their elimination from the body requires the addition of polar groups to make them water soluble. This conjugation occurs in the liver. The enzyme systems responsible for the metabolism of the lipid-soluble drugs are located in the smooth endoplasmic reticulum (SER). These enzymes, present in the SER fragments (microsomal fraction), may be isolated by centrifugation at high speeds and are known as microsomal enzymes. Because of the diversity of the reactions attributed to microsomal enzymes, the term *mixed-function oxidase*

system (MFO system) has been used to describe them. The MFO system includes cytochrome P-450, NADPH-cytochrome c reductase, and phosphatidylcholine, a lipid. Apparently the key component is cytochrome P-450, and there is strong evidence of its important role in the metabolism of drugs in humans.[317] Two reactions are necessary for the biotransformation of the lipid-soluble drugs. In phase 1, a polar group, either oxygen or a hydroxyl, is added. This is known as a nonsynthetic reaction. In phase 2 conjugation with a glucuronide, a sulfate group, or other anions makes the compound soluble in water and thus excretable in the urine or the bile. The metabolite formed by the addition of a polar group may make the activity of the metabolite less than, the same as, or greater than that of the parent compound.

Some drugs, such as barbiturates and phenytoin, when taken over a long period are enzyme inducers, increasing the amount of SER and of cytochrome P-450. The metabolic pathway is nonspecific, however, and any one of many drugs or chemicals can be detoxified at an increased rate. These increase the rate of drug oxidation and may result in toxic metabolites. The sharp increase in SER is prominent on electron microscopic examination. A biopsy discloses enlarged hepatocytes with abundant, finely reticular cytoplasm and a thickened cell membrane. These changes are most noticeable in the perivenular (zone 3) areas.[361] The lobules and even the liver may become enlarged.

Many classifications of hepatotoxic injury have been proposed.[368] One of the more recent and all inclusive has first a group of intrinsic agents that act directly on the liver cells, such as carbon tetrachloride, or indirectly, such as acetaminophen. In the second group are the idiosyncratic reactions, either by hypersensitivity or through a secondary metabolite. The greatest advances have been made in the study of the latter group.

A condensed clinicopathologic approach is used in this chapter, with emphasis on the pathologic changes (Table 25-4). Occasionally some overlap from one group to another occurs. The changes produced by hepatotoxins vary from mild disease that is diagnosed only by a rise in serum enzymes to instances of massive necrosis and death. Some reactions are relatively innocuous, even though the patient is jaundiced. Two clinical groups are recognized: drugs that are administered for diagnosis or therapy and those that are not. In the latter the injurious agent may be taken accidentally or for suicidal or homicidal purposes. Also in the latter group are compounds that have a direct toxic reaction on the liver of humans and experimental animals that is dose related and fairly prompt. The morphologic expression commonly known as toxic hepatitis is usually uniform and predictable. Among these organic and inorganic hepatotoxins are carbon tetrachloride, chloroform,[361] chlorinated naphthalenes, phosphorus, and the toxins of mushrooms, all of which usually produce a zonal type of hepatic necrosis accompanied by fatty change. Other body organs may also be affected. If death from the acute exposure does not occur, hepatic recovery is complete. The best-known hepatotoxin in this group, often used in experimental pathology, is carbon tetrachloride. It is postulated that this compound is split by microsomal enzymes into the free radicals —CCl$_3$ and —Cl. These attack methylene bonds of the unsaturated fatty acids of microsome membranes, producing lipoperoxidases, which cause severe membrane alterations.[49,350] The free radicals also damage microsomal proteins and cytochrome P-450. Cysteine protects the liver cell from necrosis, possibly by reducing the binding of the free radical to the microsomal proteins.[324] The ultrastructural changes in carbon tetrachloride injury include the dislocation of ribosomes and dilatation of cisternae.[310] An early morphologic change in the plasma membrane of isolated rat hepatocytes has also been demonstrated.[343]

Amanita phalloides mushrooms produce several cyclopeptides, or amanitins, that are among the most lethal poisons known.[335] The structural formula and mode of action of these toxins have been extensively studied.[367] The cyclopeptides act by inhibiting nuclear RNA polymerase B, and thus they interfere with RNA and DNA transcription. This results in necrosis of liver cells. Damage occurs to both nuclei and cytoplasm at the ultrastructural level, particularly in the periportal zone.[341] Fatty change has been observed in fatal cases.[341] Nonfatal cases are characterized by perivenular (zone 3) necrosis and collapse.[366] Many cases of nonlethal mushroom poisoning have been reported.[333]

Poisoning by inorganic compounds is rare, but the accidental ingestion of a large quantity of ferrous sulfate by children is a cause of periportal necrosis and jaundice[354] and may be fatal. Many hepatic features of copper poisoning are similar to results of iron toxicity, except that the perivenular zone (zone 3) is damaged.[318]

The largest and most important group of toxic reactions are those that occasionally follow the use of pharmaceutical compounds usually given for treatment but that may also be ingested in large quantities accidentally or for suicidal purposes. Some drugs taken in excessive amounts are intrinsic hepatotoxins; others act in an idiosyncratic fashion. The deleterious action of this group of compounds has been termed "drug-induced jaundice," or "drug-induced liver disease." An important advance in knowledge occurred when it was shown that with many drugs the mechanism of injury was indirect and caused by the metabolites that, after oxidation, form covalent linkages to macromolecules that are vital to cell function. It was first shown in experimental animals that the drug metabolites would often bind to glutathione rather than structural macromolecules as long as glutathione was available, thus preventing hepatocellular necrosis. Cysteamine and other agents have been used successfully in therapy for patients with overdose of acetaminophen. The mode of action results either from the binding capacity of cysteamine[338,342,347,348] or because the toxic metabolite is reconverted to acetaminophen. Pretreatment of experimental animals with enzyme inducers causes an increased severity of the hepatic necrosis, presumably because of the increased production of toxic metabolite along the proliferated smooth endoplasmic reticulum.[319] Experimental studies have shown that various drugs form covalent linkage to macromolecules.[336]

Liver disease resulting from hypersensitivity is usually assumed when a drug causes injury in only a small percentage of patients, is not dose related, and is accompanied by allergic manifestations such as skin rash, fever, and eosinophilia.[336] The microscopic findings often include eosinophilic infiltrate or a granulomatous reaction.[367]

Genetic factors may also influence drug hepatotoxicity. For example, some patients are rapid acetylators, and others are slow acetylators. Acetylation rate has a genetic basis, and since many drugs are acetylated, genetic factors may play a part in toxic reactions noted when patients who are rapid acetylators are given isoniazid for the treatment of tuberculosis.

The pathologic changes include two large categories. In one there is acute liver disease characterized by one or more of the following: cholestasis, hepatocellular necrosis with or without inflammatory reaction, fatty change, and granulomatous formation. In the second category there is a chronic reaction with variable degrees of fibrosis and, rarely, cirrhosis or neoplasia.

Acute liver disease

The first group (Table 25-4) is usually characterized by simple cholestasis without cell necrosis or inflammation. It is likely that in simple cholestasis more than one defect exists in the normal steps of the physiologic flow of bile. Normally, the flow of bile depends on (1) transport of the basic constituents from sinusoid blood into the hepatocytes, (2) the metabolic alteration of some of these constituents by the hepatocytes, (3) transport into the canaliculi, (4) passage along the bile ductules and ducts during which a varying degree of modification occurs, and (5) exit from the liver.[369] Cholestasis results from physiologic defects distal to the conjugation within the hepatocyte. The formation of canalicular bile follows its active transport across the cell membrane. First, a bile salt–dependent flow results from the osmotic pull of the bile salts after active transport into the canaliculi. Second, a bile salt–independent flow results from the osmotic pull of Na$^+$ (so-

Table 25-4. Drug hepatotoxicity

Common examples of drug action	Incidence	Pathologic condition	Symptoms	Bilirubin	Transaminases	Alkaline phosphatase	Prothrombin activity
CHOLESTATIC ACTION							
Anabolic steroids with a 17-alkyl group, methyltestosterone	High	Perivenular cholestasis	Uncomplicated jaundice	Elevated, usually 15 mg	Normal	Elevated often above 20 BL units	Normal
Oral contraceptives	1:10,000	Perivenular cholestasis	Itching and jaundice	Mild elevation	Mild increase	Elevation mild to moderate	Normal
CHOLESTASIS WITH NECROSIS							
Phenothiazine drugs Sulfonamides Thiouracil Mercaptopurine Sulfonylureas	1% 0.6% Rare 5% <1%	Perivenular bile stasis and focal necrosis; lymphoid hyperplasia of portal areas in many instances	In addition to jaundice, may be fever, rash, and eosinophilia	Elevated, usually 15 mg	Mild rise, 500 units; occasionally 1000 units or more	Elevated	Normal
NECROSIS							
Isoniazid	Very rare	Necrosis, inflammation	Jaundice	Increased	Increased	Variable	Decreased
Acetaminophen	Suicide, variable	Coagulative necrosis	Jaundice	Moderate elevation	Rise, 1000 to 2000	Normal	Often decreased
Phenytoin	Rare	Varies—necrosis to granulomas	Jaundice usually	Usually high	High		
Alpha-methyldopa	F:M = 9:1	Necrosis, inflammation	Jaundice	Increased	High	Usually increased	Decreased
Halothane	1:10,000	Liver cell injury—massive necrosis or zonal necrosis	Severe usually; may proceed to hepatic coma and death	Moderate to high	Rise, 500 to 2000	Normal to mild elevation	Decreased
Phenylbutazone	Rare	Necrosis or mild reaction with granulomas	Jaundice	Increased	High	Slight to moderate increase	Decreased

CHRONIC ACTIVE HEPATITIS

Drug						
Alpha-methyldopa	Rare	Usually submassive necrosis at autopsy, cirrhosis rare	Jaundice	High	High	Variable	Decreased
Isoniazid	Rare	Same as above	Insidious, weakness	Normal or high	High	Variable	Decreased
Nitrofurantoin	Rare	Fibrosis and chronic inflammation	None	Normal	Increased	Normal	Decreased
OTHER						
Tetracycline, especially in pregnancy	Unknown	Fine, foamy fatty change	Jaundice, coma	Elevated	Rise, 500	Elevated	Moderate decrease
Novobiocin	Unknown	Cholestasis	Newborn infants more susceptible	Elevated unconjugated bilirubin	Normal	Normal	Normal
Methotrexate	Uncommon	Fibrosis, inflammation	Insidious	Normally not elevated	Often a mild increase	Variable	Decreased late

dium pump). This occurs after the active transport of sodium into the canaliculus under the influence of canalicular Na^+, K^+-adenosine triphosphatase (ATPase).[323]

As a group, the cholestatic drugs produce reversible injury to the secretory mechanism that prevents bilirubin glucuronide from normally entering the canaliculi. The bilirubin that does enter the canaliculi tends to accumulate and form bile plugs, which are obvious on microscopic examination, especially in the perivenular zones (Plate 3, *B*). Mild swelling or hydropic change of the hepatocytes is a usual finding. An occasional focus of liver cell necrosis may occur, and on rare occasions severe necrosis has been reported. The electron microscope discloses a distortion and disappearance of the canalicular microvilli and widening of the canalicular ectoplasm. Damage to the pericanalicular microfilaments has been shown in experimental cholestasis. This may be important in the etiology of simple cholestasis.[345]

Women who have had a condition known as benign jaundice of pregnancy, presumably because of excess production of sex hormones, often have a recurrence of jaundice when they take one of the oral contraceptives.[320] The estrogens appear to be responsible for the rare instances of jaundice that follow the use of oral contraceptives.[357] The 17α-alkyl-19-norsteroids cause the most difficulty with bile secretion.[334]

In the second and largest group of acute drug-related reactions (Table 25-4), there is liver cell injury as well as cholestasis, and so the laboratory findings often include a rise in the serum transaminase levels. This type of injury has been referred to as hepatocanalicular injury.[367] Among the drugs that cause it are the phenothiazines, sulfonamides, mercaptopurines, and organic arsenical drugs. On microscopic examination the findings are variable, but cell ballooning, focal necrosis of hepatocytes, cholestasis, and inflammation along the portal tracts are usually present. The reaction in the portal areas varies greatly. In some biopsy specimens there is an increase in connective tissue and inflammatory exudate in which round cells, neutrophils, or eosinophils may predominate. Ductular proliferation may also be seen. Granulomas with eosinophilic infiltrate may result from sensitivity to one of the sulfonamide drugs. Most patients in the second group recover when the offending drug is discontinued.

In the third pattern of acute drug reaction (Table 25-4) liver cell necrosis occurs with a minimal to moderate inflammatory response accompanied by hyperbilirubinemia and high serum transaminase activity. Many commonly used drugs are included in this group. One of these is isoniazid, the most widely used drug in the treatment of tuberculosis. Mild subclinical liver injury, characterized by mild elevations of serum transferase activities, may occur within the first 3 months of treatment in 12% to 20% of patients, but the damage never progresses in most of the patients throughout the period of treatment. Most patients spontaneously improve, even while treatment continues. However, in about 0.5% of patients treated, a more serious reaction occurs in which there is hepatocellular necrosis. The occurrence of necrosis is distinctly age related; it is extremely rare in those under 20 years of age and occurs in about 0.3% of patients 30 to 40 years of age, 1.2% of patients 35 to 45 years of age, and 2.3% of patients over 50 years.[337] The extent of necrosis varies from a moderately severe disease that resembles viral hepatitis, both clinically and pathologically, to submassive or massive hepatocellular necrosis, also resembling hepatitis. In patients with the latter the mortality is high. Isoniazid-related hepatic necrosis, when it occurs, almost always develops within the first year of therapy; half of the time it is within the first 8 weeks of therapy.[337] It has been suggested that isoniazid liver injury is related to the rapid acetylation of the drug. Patients who are of the rapid acetylator phenotype hydrolyze a larger percentage of isoniazid to isonicotinic acid and the free hydrazine compound.[337] However, this theory has been questioned.[332]

Quinidine produces a common and reversible hypersensitivity reaction that occurs in 2% to 3% of patients. Increased serum enzymes occur within 2 weeks of beginning the drug and resolve rapidly with cessation.[330]

Acetaminophen is another widely used drug that is assumed to be safe when used in recommended doses. When used to excess, as for suicidal purposes, there is a dose-related type of perivenular liver cell necrosis. Prognosis has been linked to the total quantity taken, rate of disposition, activity of the MFO system, and glutathione stores.[331,353,368] Moderately severe injury may occur with therapeutic doses when the MFO system has been stimulated by other drugs or alcohol.[355] Unlike isoniazid-indirect hepatic necrosis, acetaminophen toxicity is associated with little inflammatory reaction and is characterized by coagulative necrosis of perivenular hepatocytes. Dead hepatocytes are slowly removed by histiocytes over approximately a 1-week period.[346] Toxic hepatitis has also been claimed to result from long-term, moderate to excessive self-therapeutic use of acetaminophen.[309,314] Treatment with alternative binding agents, such as N-acetylcysteine, is very effective if these agents are administered within 12 hours after ingestion, before hepatic necrosis develops.[338,348]

Although phenytoin is widely used in the treatment of seizure disorders, hepatotoxic reactions are rare. Adverse reactions usually occur within 1 to 6 weeks after the beginning of therapy. The microscopic findings vary widely and include hepatocellular necrosis, granulomatous reaction, bile duct injury,[358] and ground-glass

transformation of the hepatocytes.[339] The reaction appears to be caused by hepatic hypersensitivity, since most of the patients have fever, skin rash, chills, pruritus, and hepatomegaly associated with jaundice. Most hepatic reactions resemble hepatic involvement in infectious mononucleosis.

Alpha-methyldopa, an antihypertensive drugs, occasionally causes acute necrosis of the liver as a short-term effect, especially in women. The clinical features are similar to those of acute viral hepatitis. In about 10% of the patients the disease is fatal, submassive necrosis being noted at autopsy. Long-term effects have also been reported.[307,308] These include fatty change and fibrous septa formation.

One drug, allopurinol, is unique in that the toxic reactions are of the hypersensitivity type, but the microscopic change varies greatly from patient to patient. Most patients have perivenular necrosis, whereas others may have a granulomatous change along the portal tracts.[306] Halothane and similar compounds, such as methoxyflurane (Penthrane), occasionally are associated with liver necrosis.[329,344,356] It has been reporteed that the serum of patients with fulminant hepatic failure after halothane-induced anesthesia contains a circulating antibody that reacts specifically with the cell membrane of hepatocytes isolated from halothane-anesthetized rabbits.[363] The nature of the antigenic substance on the membrane of the hepatocytes is yet to be determined. The biotransformation of halothane has been extensively studied in rats, and it seems possible that liver cell necrosis may result from some reactive intermediary, particularly by means of a reductive or oxygen-deficient pathway.[316] A possible genetic factor in halothane-producing injury has also been proposed.[325] In most instances halothane-associated liver damage occurs after more than one exposure, usually in a patient who has had an unexplained fever after the first halothane-induced anesthesia.

In fatal massive necrosis after halothane anesthesia, three stages can be recognized: necrotic, absorptive, and regenerative. In the necrotic stage, dead liver cells are still recognizable and occur in the first 5 days after onset of jaundice (Fig. 25-23). In the absorptive stage the liver cells have disappeared, leaving areas of collapse. This is the period in which most of the patients die, usually 1 to 2 weeks after the onset of jaundice. In the regenerative stage submassive necrosis has occurred, and the patients live from 2 weeks to a month. These patients are older and have insufficient regenerative capacity to restore the liver parenchyma. Patients under 30 years of age who survive 3 weeks after the onset of jaundice may be expected to recover. Nonfatal, mild hepatic injury has also been noted with halothane.[312]

Phenylbutazone may cause a severe reaction with hepatocellular necrosis or a milder illness characterized by granulomas.[313] The toxic manifestations usually occur within 6 weeks after drug use begins. Clinical evidence indicates that drug sensitivity is a major factor.

A mild nonfatal hepatotoxic injury may follow the use of aspirin, sometimes with a pronounced hypertransaminasemia.[368] Hepatic injury is most likely to follow when the blood levels of salicylate are higher than 25 mg/dl.[370]

Effect of chronic drug use

After the chronic use of certain drugs, the histologic, clinical, and laboratory findings may closely resemble those of chronic active hepatitis of the immune or lupoid type (fourth group in Table 25-4). Relatively few drugs produce chronic active hepatitis, since most agents that produce hepatocellular necrosis will bring about massive necrosis and death if not discontinued when signs of liver disease develop. Production of drug-induced chronic active hepatitis requires either that the drug cause only a low level of necrosis with continued use, so that much of the disease is subclinical, or that repeated small doses of the hepatotoxin are administered with sufficient time between exposures to allow partial recovery. An example of the latter may occur in sensitive anesthesiologists who sniff halothane to assure themselves of adequate flow of the agent when administering anesthesia.[327] Chronic active hepatitis after self-medication with minimal toxic doses of acetamin-

ophen[314] has been reported in a few patients.

The histologic findings of drug-related chronic active hepatitis may be essentially the same as those described on p. 1225. The drug oxyphenisatin, not now in use in the United States but still available in some countries, was a frequent cause of this disorder. Alpha-methyldopa,[332,351] sulfonamides,[362] and isoniazid[313] have also been implicated, but the reported cases actually seem to represent examples of submassive necrosis. Nitrofurantoin, a drug used to treat urinary tract infections, may cause an acute cholestatic reaction with fever, skin rash, an eosinophilia in some patients and a more subtle chronic active hepatitis in others.[328] On withdrawal of the offending drug, patients with chronic active hepatitis–like disease almost invariably recover.

In addition to the chronic changes mentioned, a primary biliary cirrhosis–like disease may rarely occur in patients taking chlorpromazine, tolbutamide, or organic arsenical drugs. This disorder slowly resolved after cessation of drug therapy in nearly every case.[362]

In a small miscellaneous group (fifth group in Table 25-4), the abnormalities produced are distinctive for each drug.[321] There are no common findings in the liver. A charactristic foamy type of fatty change occurs in the liver after intravenous administration of large amounts of tetracycline (Fig. 25-24).[315] In this disorder the nucleus is not displaced as it is in the macrovesicular type of fatty change. The tetracycline interferes with the production of protein by RNA. Thus formation

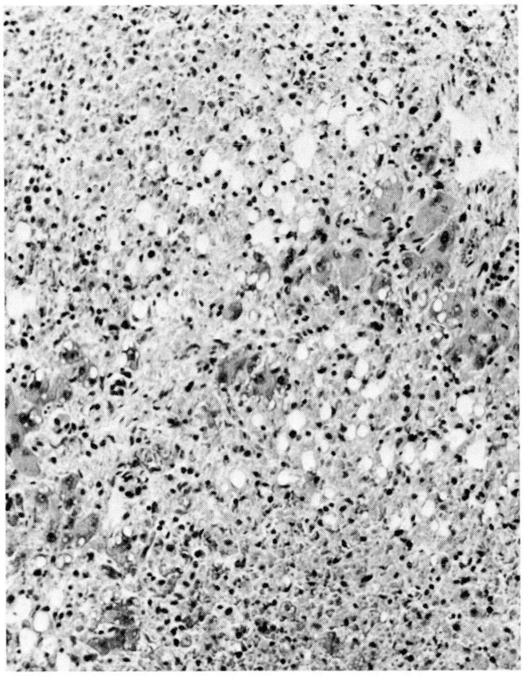

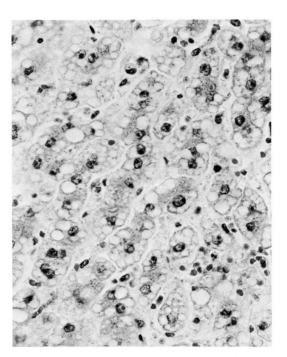

Fig. 25-23. Massive hepatocellular necrosis after halothane anesthesia. (From Peters, R.L., et al.: Am. J. Med. **47:**748, 1969.)

Fig. 25-24. Fine foamy vacuolization of liver after large amounts of intravenously administered tetracycline. (From Peters, R.L., et al.: Am. J. Surg. **113:**622, 1967.)

of lipoprotein, necessary for the transfer of fat from the liver, is blocked. Amiodarone hepatoxicity often has no symptoms but produces a laboratory and biopsy change suggestive of alcoholic liver disease because of mild fatty change, hepatocellular necrosis, and occasionally alcoholic hyaline.[352] Novobiocin inhibits the action of glucuronyl transferase, producing an unconjugated hyperbilirubinemia.

A true toxic cirrhosis caused by drugs has rarely been reported except in patients taking methotrexate.[326,340,365] A difference of opinion exists as to whether methotrexate is soley responsible for cirrhosis that may be seen in psoriatic persons taking the drug. In my patients I have observed diffuse fibrosis along the sinusoid walls, and the presence of megalohepatocytes is a characteristic change in patients taking methotrexate for a protracted period. Total parenteral nutrition has been associated with pronounced cholestasis, with mild fatty change, and with portal fibrosis in patients with long-term use often associated with massive loss of intestine.[359]

Several other adverse reactions to drugs and chemicals are more appropriately discussed elsewhere in this chapter. Among these are peliosis hepatis, thrombosis of the hepatic veins or Budd-Chiari syndrome, neoplasms, and granulomas.

ALCOHOLIC LIVER DISEASE

Since prehistoric times, alcohol has been the most widely used euphoriant. Probably the first alcoholic drink was mead made from fermented honey.[384] The long history of alcohol use and alcoholism has recently been reviewed.[391] The rise in the use of distilled liquor began in the eighteenth century and led to the early recognition of chronic liver disease, first by Matthew Baillie[371] in 1793 and by René Laënnec[395] in 1819. Since Laënnec introduced the term *cirrhosis* (from Gr. *kirrhos,* 'tawny'), a multitude of diagnostic terms have been used for this most common type of cirrhosis. They include Laënnec's cirrhosis, alcoholic cirrhosis, portal cirrhosis, septal cirrhosis, diffuse cirrhosis, and hobnail cirrhosis.

Of the approximately 100 million of the U.S. population who use alcoholic beverages, about 10% become alcoholics. The definition of alcoholism is still controversial, but certain major and minor criteria have been established for its diagnosis by the National Council on Alcoholism.[377]

The frequency of cirrhosis at autopsy from all causes is alleged to vary between 1% to 10% throughout the world. In various centers in the United States the range is from 1.6% to 11%. Although alcoholic liver disease (ALD) may occur anytime from the third decade to senility, the peak incidence is in middle life (50 to 55 years), with most patients between 40 and 65 years of age. Men are affected more frequently than women; in the latter the peak age incidence is about a decade earlier than in men. In the Los Angeles County–University of Southern California Medical Center in 1970, at a time when 25% of deaths were caused by alcohol-associated diseases, the frequency of cirrhosis at autopsy was 11%, principally of the alcoholic type. Furthermore, ALD was the leading cause of death in those under 50 years of age.

Alcoholic cirrhosis follows the long-continued consumption of alcohol. The epidemiologic evidence indicates that the mortality for cirrhosis is directly related to the per capita consumption of alcohol from wine and spirits.[411] In India, Africa, and certain other parts of the world in which B viral cirrhosis is common, alcoholism is not etiologically important. However, in some countries an increase in alcoholic consumption has been followed by an increase in alcoholic cirrhosis,[389] though there are differences in male-to-female ratio and the frequency of acute alcoholic hepatitis as compared with the United States. A relationship between alcoholism and cirrhosis is unquestionable, but the exact mechanism of the injurious effect of alcohol is unknown. Among patients with cirrhosis, a history of excessive use of alcohol has been found in 30% to 92% in various series in the United States. About 90% of patients have a history of 5 to 15 years of heavy consumption of alcohol. Many consume as much as a quart of whiskey or a gallon of wine per day. In addition to steady drinking, most patients periodically drink excessively for 1 to 2 weeks, during which time they eat little or no food. These bouts often terminate in an attack of jaundice, pneumonia, pancreatitis, or delirium tremens. The drinking patterns of alcoholics differ from one country to another and even within one country.

Ethanol metabolism

After ingestion and absorption from the stomach and small bowel, ethanol is distributed in the water space of the body. As ethanol circulates through the liver, it is removed by the hepatocytes where, by a two-step enzymatic process, some 90% of it is oxidized to acetate. Studies in humans indicate that 50% to 100% of ethanol entering the liver appears in the hepatic venous outflow as acetate.[400] Only a small percentage is oxidized elsewhere so that within 24 hours 90% of the ingested ethanol is oxidized finally to carbon dioxide and water and a small amount (2% to 10%) is excreted unchanged by the lungs and kidneys.

The major pathway for hepatic ethanol oxidation is shown in Fig. 25-25. The enzyme alcohol dehydrogenase (ADH) present in the cytosol is sufficient to account for the maximal rate of ethanol metabolism. Because ADH has a wide range of substances, the physiologic role of the enzyme has been debated. The

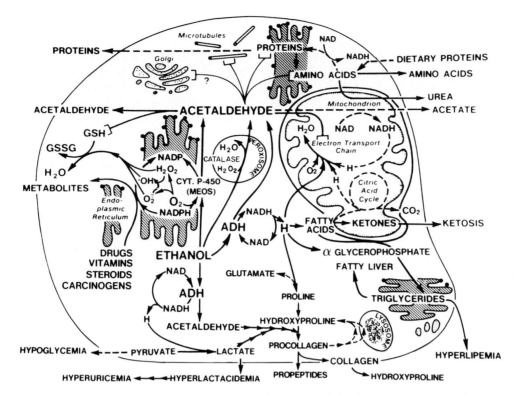

Fig. 25-25. Oxidation of ethanol in the hepatocyte and link of the two products (acetaldehyde and H) to disturbances in intermediary metabolism. *MEOS,* Microsomal ethanol-oxidizing system; *NAD,* nicotinamide adenine dinucleotide; *NADH,* reduced NAD; *NADP,* nicotinamide adenine dinucleotide phosphate; *NADPH,* reduced NADP; *GSH,* reduced glutathione; *GSSG,* oxidized GSH. *Broken lines,* Pathways that are depressed by ethanol. Symbol –[denotes interference or binding; →→→, stimulation or activation. (From Lieber, C.A.: Hepatology **4**(6):1243, 1984.)

finding of measurable levels of ethanol in the portal blood of nondrinking rats supports the concept that the primary function of ADH is ethanol oxidation.[393] As ethanol is oxidized to acetaldehyde by ADH, the cofactor nicotinamide-adenine dinucleotide (NAD) is reduced to NADH. The second enzymatic step occurs in the mitochondria where acetaldehyde is oxidized to acetate by acetaldehyde dehydrogenase (AcDH) and the same cofactor NAD is reduced to NADH. The acetate leaves the liver to be oxidized further to carbon dioxide and water in other tissues. Reduction in the NAD/NADH redox ratio is the fundamental biochemical alteration that occurs during ethanol metabolism. The free NAD/NADH ratio cannot be measured because of the binding of the pyridine nucleotides; therefore the ratio of oxidized and reduced metabolites is measured by showing that the lactate/pyruvate ratio and the beta-hydroxybutyrate/acetoacetate ratios are both increased, the former in the cytoplasm and the latter in mitochondria. In persons who drink excessively, the amount of NADH that is reoxidized becomes the rate-limiting fac-

tor for the oxidation of ethanol. Because the mitochondrial membranes are impenetrable to NADH, the reoxidation of this substance is accomplished by a shuttle system, whereby reducing equivalents enter the mitochondria. These shuttles are (1) the alpha-glycerophosphate shuttle, (2) the malate-asparate shuttle, and (3) the fatty acid elongation shuttle.[375] The mitochondrial respiratory chain is therefore ultimately responsible for the oxidation of NADH. As long as ethanol is available to the hepatocytes, it may replace up to 90% of all the substrates that are normally used by the liver, taking over almost the entire intermediary metabolism. Many of these substrates therefore cannot be metabolized by the liver. Furthermore, the continuous presence of alcohol causes a strong depression in the Krebs cycle. This particularly affects the metabolism of fat and leads to fatty liver, the most common microscopic observation in alcoholism. The disturbed lactate/pyruvate ratio probably decreases gluconeogenesis and could be partially responsible for the hypoglycemia that is sometimes seen in persons with alcoholism.

The total activity of ADH varies considerably in normal humans because of the presence of isoenzymes and enzyme polymorphisms.[397,412,421] A genetic model has been proposed that includes three autosomal gene loci that code for three subunits: alpha, beta, and gamma. Atypical subunits give rise to isoenzymes that show a higher specific activity. Among whites, only 5% to 20% are atypical phenotypes, whereas Orientals are predominantly atypical. Thus Orientals may oxidize alcohol at a faster rate on ingestion, leading to higher blood aldehyde levels; this may in turn be responsible for the well-known flushing syndrome that is so frequently recognized in some Orientals when they consume alcoholic beverages.

The oxidation of acetaldehyde to acetate occurs for the most part in the mitochondria. In the chronic alcoholic this second step in the metabolism of alcohol may be overburdened by the production of NADH. Under these circumstances it is believed that aldehyde may enter the bloodstream. The quantity, however, is unclear, primarily because of difficulty in its chemical determination. Furthermore, the pathologic significance of acetaldehyde that is not immediately oxidized to acetate but remains in the liver is unknown.

In chronic alcoholism there is an increase in SER, and alcohol is metabolized at an increased rate. This has led to the study of other pathways for the oxidation of alcohol. One of these is the microsomal ethanol-oxidizing system (MEOS), which is associated with the degradation of ethanol by microsomes.[375,399] Another alternative pathway is by means of catalase present in the peroxisomes.[399] The MEOS system may be of considerable importance in the chronic alcoholic. An additional metabolic pathway has been recently described in which acetaldehyde is converted to acetoin by the brain.[420] This substance undergoes reduction to 2,3-butanediol by the liver.

In advanced cirrhosis, poor nutrition and poor blood supply to the hepatocytes may alter the rate of oxidation of alcohol.[419]

Pathology

The chronic use of ethanol may produce one or more morphologic changes in the liver that are characteristic and allow a presumptive diagnosis of ALD to be made on these grounds alone. The spectrum of alterations includes hydropic change, fatty change, necrosis, regeneration, inflammation, and fibrosis. Some of these may occur singly, but often more than one microscopic change is seen. A major advance in the study of ethanol hepatoxicity was the production of the morphologic lesion of acute and chronic ALD in baboons given an alcoholic diet supplemented with adequate nutritional factors.[407] Therefore ethanol and its metabolites may produce both acute and chronic damage, but deficient diet is not required for liver injury in the person with chronic alcoholism. Among the millions of persons with chronic alcoholism, it has been estimated that only 5% to 15% will develop cirrhosis.[392] The exact percentage who develop some form of symptomatic or asymptomatic disease is unknown. Other factors that have been given consideration include genetic and constitutional status of the patient. It has been shown that children born of a biologic alcoholic parent have a significant increase in alcoholic-related problems.[378] Furthermore, it has been reported that patients with alcoholic cirrhosis have a higher frequency of HLA-B40 than (1) those patients with ALD but without cirrhosis, (2) those with miscellaneous liver disease, or (3) alcoholic persons without liver disease.[372] It is possible that severe dietary deficiency has an additive effect in ALD.[401] The observation that severe liver disease, indistinguishable from ALD, often occurs after a jejunoileal bypass for morbid obesity is an example of the role that other factors, possibly nutrition, play in another indistinguishable form of liver disease.[394]

The term *alcoholic liver disease* may be used for all lesions of the liver associated with excessive use of ethanol that cannot be ascribed to any other etiologic factor. Persons with chronic alcoholism may have liver disease, sometimes severe, that has a nonalcoholic cause, or even a combination of alcoholic and nonalcoholic disease.[396] A clinicopathologic classification of ALD that I have found useful includes the following:

A. Asymptomatic alcoholic disease
B. Acute alcoholic liver disease
  1. Fatty liver
  2. Fatty liver with lytic necrosis
  3. Acute foamy degeneration
  4. Sclerosing hyaline necrosis
  5. Acute portal fibrosis
C. Chronic alcoholic liver disease
  1. Alcoholic fibrosis: portal perivenular (chronic sclerosing hyaline necrosis)
  2. Cirrhosis

Alcoholic fibrosis is difficult to classify because overlapping patterns are present in a single biopsy. Fig. 25-26 illustrates the relationship of the various predominant patterns, and the result is usually cirrhosis unless death occurs from hepatic failure or complications of portal hypertension.

Classification of alcoholic liver disease does not fit easily into distinct categories of clinical or pathologic entities. Broad overlap and mixtures of symptoms, laboratories findings, and pathologic features are common, and predominant features are utilized for classification. Acceptance and recognition of some features as changes have brought new categories to focus in hopes of sim-

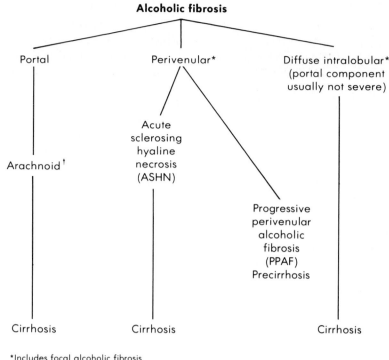

Fig. 25-26. Pattern and course of alcoholic fibrosis. (From Edmondson, H.A.: In Peters, R.L., and Craig, J.R., editors: Liver pathology, New York, 1986, Churchill Livingstone.)

plifying the system to allow better scientific study of alcoholic liver disease. A simplified classification of alcoholic liver disease was presented by an international group, and it included four broad categories of fatty liver, alcoholic hepatitis (an ill-defined syndrome), cirrhosis, and hepatocellular carcinoma.[388] Multiple biopsy specimens do indicate that some patients progress from fatty liver to alcoholic hepatitis to cirrhosis over several years, but it is also apparent that many patients are relatively asymptomatic and present for medical care, with advanced cirrhosis as the first clinical problem.

Early asymptomatic alcoholic liver disease

Before clinical disease is manifest, usually after a few years of heavy drinking, hepatomegaly may occur. This is caused by fatty or hydropic change. Although usually considered a benign disorder, a fatty liver may be associated with sudden death, the exact cause of which is uncertain. Hypoglycemia, hypomagnesemia, and the withdrawal syndrome have been considered.[394] Many patients with fatty liver are seen by the physician or hospitalized for any one of several nonhepatic complications of alcoholism. These include delirium tremens, nausea and vomiting, trauma, acute infection, and al-

coholic pancreatitis. More severe changes, including alcoholic hepatitis and cirrhosis, have been noted in a small percentage of persons with asymptomatic alcoholism.[373] Hepatomegaly in asymptomatic alcoholism has been ascribed to hydropic change and excess protein in the hepatocytes.[398]

The time between the onset of heavy drinking and microscopic abnormalities in the liver is unknown. Alcohol given to young nonalcoholic volunteers produced fatty vacuolation in 2 days.[410] However, the fat was uniformly distributed throughout the lobule, and droplets were relatively small (usually from 5 to 15 μm) and different from the fat deposition of sympatomatic stages of alcoholic liver disease.

A biopsy performed in the asymptomatic stage usually reveals fatty change or hydropic vacuolization or both. Sometimes the hydropic change noted in the perivenular hepatocytes may be extreme. The nucleus is still apparent, but the cytoplasm is so watery that it is difficult to find any granular material (Fig. 25-27).

Another helpful finding in some biopsies performed in the early stages of ALD is the presence of giant mitochondria. These are easily seen with a light microscope because they are in the cytoplasm and are often approximately the size of an erythrocyte (Fig. 25-28).[376]

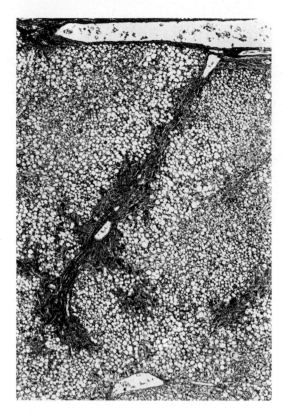

Fig. 25-27. Early stage of cirrhosis in fatty liver of alcoholic patient. Fibrosis and bile duct proliferation can be seen along small branch of portal tree. Irregular manner in which connective tissue invades periphery of lobules is clearly shown. There is little change around sublobular and terminal hepatic vein at bottom.

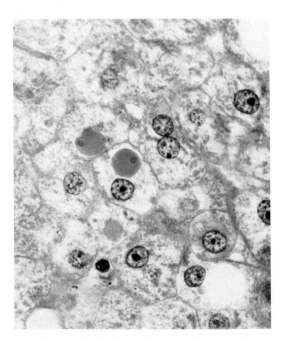

Fig. 25-28. Megamitochondria in hepatocytes of chronically alcoholic patient.

Acute liver disease

The onset of acute liver disease in alcoholism is difficult to predict but is usually associated with an increased intake of ethanol and poor eating habits. The symptoms differ somewhat, depending on the morphologic abnormalities in the liver, but most commonly the patient has a more or less sudden onset of jaundice that often is accompanied by fever. In the literature these patients have been described as having alcoholic hepatitis. A liver biopsy specimen usually discloses one of four structural changes, each of which has certain identifiable features: (1) fatty liver with cholestasis; (2) fatty liver with foamy change, which in more severe cases undergoes a lytic type of necrosis; (3) sclerosing hyaline necrosis; and (4) acute portal sclerosis. There may be some overlap between the first of these and the other three.

The simplest microscopic change is a fatty liver with cholestasis. A mild thickening of sinusoid and central vein walls is common, but little or no increase of portal connective tissue is seen. On hospitalization, the patients usually recover in a period of a few weeks. It is remarkable how rapidly a large fatty liver shrinks when the patient partakes of an adequate diet and abstains from alcohol. In addition to hyperbilirubinemia, the hepatic tests usually show a moderate rise in alkaline phosphatase levels. Rarely a patient with severe fatty change and cholestasis may die of liver failure.[402] The cause or causes of fatty liver in the person with alcoholism are still under discussion.[413] It seems likely that the major factor is concerned with beta oxidation of fatty acids.[420]

A second acute clinicopathologic syndrome in the precirrhotic alcoholic patient is alcoholic foamy degeneration (AFD). Patients with AFD may have very transient elevations of both the ALT and AST activities to over 300 units; the elevated ALT level is often missed because it may be an elevated range for only 24 hours. The perivenular hepatocytes are bloated with fine, fatty vacuoles, separated by a delicate cytoplasmic interface (Fig. 25-29). The hepatocytes are deficient in mitochondrial enzyme activity and by electron microscopic study are virtually lacking in mitochondria.[416] The nuclei of these foamy cells are often pyknotic. The foamy cell change may be the early change, still reversible, that when severe leads to lytic necrosis.

On rare occasions, a fatty liver may undergo a lytic type of necrosis.[379] Most patients who die in hepatic failure with only fatty livers or fatty livers with fibrosis have severe perivenular lytic necrosis of the hepatocytes. The lytic foci are devoid of inflammatory exudate. Cholestasis, bile staining of cytoplasm, and bile in Kupffer cells are uniformly present. Some of the patients become critically ill and die in hepatic coma. At autopsy the liver is hypertrophic, weighing as much as 5000 g; the capsule is smooth and usually tautly stretched around bulging, fatty icteric parenchyma. However, if lytic necrosis is sufficiently severe and the patient has survived for more than a week or so in coma, the parenchyma is limp and soft. In such instances of severe necrosis there is perivenular depression and deep bile staining. Microscopically the bloated, hydropic perivenular hepatocytes appear foamy and partially autolyzed; the periportal cells usually contain a large single fat globule. The laboratory findings are similar to those in patients with fatty liver and cholestasis alone, except that the AST level may reach 300 units, and the ALT remains normal. The prothrombin activity may be decreased to the range of 20%. Since prothrombin activity precludes early biopsy, it has not been proved that lytic necrosis is a more severe stage of acute foamy degeneration, but clinically it would appear to be so.

A third type of microscopic change is now known as alcoholic hepatitis, though I continue to use the term *sclerosing hyaline necrosis*.[380] In this disorder the perivenular hepatocytes undergo hydropic and hyaline change that precedes necrosis. This change is most striking in a liver with few fat vacuoles, though fatty livers are not spared. The hyalin first appears as clumps in the cytoplasm and then as large masses that often have an eccentric location in the cell (Plate 3, *D*). Usually there are many neutrophils in the sinusoids around the necrotic cells that may even penetrate the cytoplasm of the cell and possibly assist in its death or liquefaction.[417] The latter appears to be a slow process. Various stages in the progression of hyaline necrosis are seen in the liver at any one time. A remarkable increase in collagen occurs in the perivenular areas (Fig. 25-30). The cell of origin of the collagen has been debated, and the Ito cell is a likely candidate as is the hepatocyte. The conversion of the Ito cell into a myofibroblast has been suggested.[398] However, scanning electron microscopy has revealed that in alcoholic liver disease, the normal number of endothelial fenestrae are greatly reduced (so-called defenestration), and this reduction in "porosity" may reduce the exchange between hepatocyte and blood within the sinusoid.[26,27] A highly significant correlation has been noted between the amount of collagen and the intrahepatic portal venous pressure.[403] The increased connective tissue leads to obliteration of many of the perivenular sinusoids and terminal hepatic veins. The changes in sclerosing hyaline necrosis may be so severe that death ensues, but many patients recover. The necrotic cells finally disappear; the connective tissue condenses, and although the regenerative response is poor, the remaining cells in the altered lobules resume their functions. In the acute phase the patients often have jaundice, ascites, abdominal pain, and an exceptional neutrophilic leukocy-

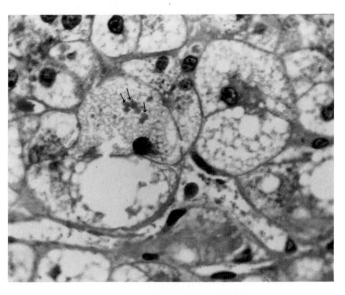

Fig. 25-29. Acute foamy degeneration in alcoholic patient. Notice foamy vesicles and pale cytoplasm. This pattern may be found in liver of patient with acute alcoholism. Notice megamitochondria *(arrows)*, somewhat smaller than those in Fig. 25-28.

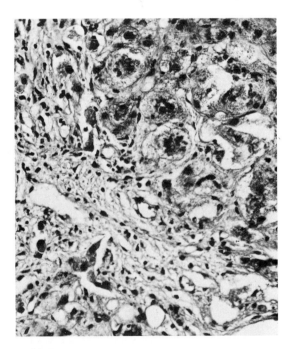

Fig. 25-30. Cytoplasm of hepatic cells contains eosinophilic granular material, so-called alcoholic hyalin. Cells appear swollen, and cell borders are indistinguishable. Sclerosis of vascular walls has begun. Needle biopsy of liver of 42-year-old Native American chronic alcoholic who had been on long drinking spree before entering hospital.

tosis.[380] Ultrastructural studies have shown that hyaline bodies are composed of light and dark conglomerate filaments. These are surrounded by proliferated rough endoplasmic reticulum (RER) from which ribosomes have been shed, hypertrophied Golgi complex, and enlarged mitochondria that often contain matrical granules.[406] Almost always there is a cuff of the detached ribosomes around the hyaline bodies. Similar changes may be seen in hepatocytes without alcoholic hyalin but which probably represent an early stage in the development of the disease. Branching and tubular microfilaments have been recognized. Electrophoretic and immunologic studies of the isolated and homogenized hyaline bodies show several bands identical to protein bands in normal liver. Mallory bodies are antigenic and contain similar antigenic determinants in common with the axial filaments of the hepatocyte.[381] The exact role of any antigen-antibody reaction in the pathogenesis of acute alcoholic hepatitis remains to be proved. Deposition of IgA in a continuous pattern was considered specific for ALD,[390] and subsequent studies noted that this finding correlated with progression of disease and may be an effect of alcohol on IgA metabolism.[415,418]

It has been shown that when Mallory bodies are present, T-lymphocytes in the liver are increased as compared with their numbers in the peripheral blood, an indication that a cell-mediated immune response has occurred.[382]

Acute portal fibrosis is a rare complication of alcoholism we have recognized in recent years. The portal tracts are moderately enlarged by a profuse increase of connective tissue that obliterates many of the portal vein and hepatic artery branches. Fatty change is usually present. The patients are jaundiced and have an elevated alkaline phosphatase.

The prognosis of acute alcoholic hepatitis varies considerably, and some follow-up studies indicate cirrhosis may develop even with no obvious alcohol consumption, and alcoholic hepatitis may occur superimposed on cirrhosis, which as a poorer prognosis than without cirrhosis.[404,405]

Fatty liver

Fatty liver is a common finding with mild chronic alcohol use, and the routine screening of donated blood for elevated transaminase levels to remove potential non-A, non-B viral hepatitis–contaminated blood has lead to study of large populations of blood donors with mild elevation of serum transaminase.[383] Whereas such blood donors are asymptomatic for liver disease, mild alcohol use may account for 45% of the elevated transaminases. Also, elevated serum transaminases are identified in routine screening of outpatients, and fatty liver is the most common histologic diagnosis identified by liver biopsy.[387] In a large review of such asymptomatic adults in Sweden, other causes associated with mild transaminase elevation were diabetes mellitus and obesity. Cirrhosis accounted for only 6% of the 149 patients.[387] The mechanism of the transaminase elevation with fatty liver is obscure. See Plate 4, B.

Chronic alcoholic liver disease

As the early changes of alcoholic liver disease revolve toward cirrhosis, several patterns of fibrosis can be recognized even though overlap of features are present in the same patient. For example, multiple sections of an autopsied liver will reveal different degrees of fibrosis whereby one area will be cirrhotic with true regenerative nodules and another area will have predominantly perivenular fibrosis (so-called progressive perivenular alcoholic fibrosis). Acute sclerosing hyaline necrosis may be a precursor to advanced fibrosis, but more often alcoholic fibrosis seems to evolve in a subclinical fashion with patients experiencing ascites and portal hypertension as first manifestations of alcoholic liver disease. Fig. 25-26 shows the three major patterns of alcoholic fibrosis.

Progressive perivenular alcoholic fibrosis (PPAF), previously called "chronic sclerosing hyaline disease," is intense sclerosis that ultimately obliterates the venous outflow tract at the level of the terminal hepatic venules and sublobular veins (Fig. 25-31). In the advanced and purest form of PPAF, veno-occlusive disease is noted. Milder forms are common in alcoholic hepatitis and play a role in progressive alcoholic injury.[374,385] A higher incidence of hepatic veno-occlusive lesions in alcoholic cirrhosis than alcoholic hepatitis indicates that the venous lesion is likely a progressive lesion.[385] Patients with PPAF have an indolent clinical course characterized by muscle wasting, resistant ascites, and, frequently, functional renal failure. Jaundice is not usually present. Wedged hepatic vein pressure is nearly always elevated.[409] At autopsy the liver may be eutrophic or atrophic but has a smooth or fine sandstone-like thickened capsule that encloses a tough hard parenchyma (Fig. 25-31, B). The presence of dense perivenular fibrosis at biopsy in patients with acute alcoholic hepatitis may be the forerunner of progressive perivenular alcoholic fibrosis.

Precirrhosis and cirrhosis

In some patients precirrhotic changes occur in a fatty liver in which the portal tracts have an increase in amount and density of connective tissue, along with bile duct proliferation. There is little or no perivenular change. The widened portal area assumes an arachnoid configuration as the limiting plate disappears. Irregular prolongation of the portal connective tissue encroaches on the periphery of the lobules and may extend directly along the sinusoids (Fig. 25-22). In this type of portal

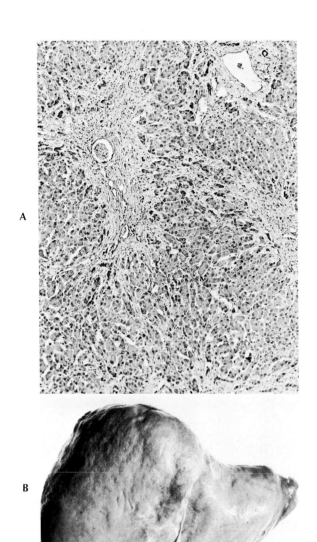

Fig. 25-31. Progressive perivenular alcoholic fibrosis (PPAF) with eutrophic, hard, granular, precirrhotic pattern. **A,** Fibrous destruction of centrilobular areas and slight widening of portal areas. **B,** Surface has sandstone appearance.

fibrosis there is little or no necrosis and not necessarily any regenerative nodules. The liver is always hypertrophic, sometimes weighing as much as 2000 to 5000 g. The capsule has finely granular regular areas of retraction and is unthickened but taut. The liver is yellow with fat or is yellow-green with bile and fat. There is slight to moderate increased resistance on cutting, to a degree that would be characterized as firm. The bulging parenchyma is greasy, and thin sections of the liver may float in water. The lobules are enlarged, and the terminal hepatic venules may be indistinct.

In the most common precirrhotic pattern there is both a perivenular and a portal component, and both fatty change and perivenular sclerosis are observed. The lobular pattern is altered, small regenerative nodules are seen, and communicating septa often connect perivenular and portal areas. This stage is called "alcoholic fatty liver with perivenular and portal fibrosis." Should the patient discontinue alcohol consumption, the fat will disappear in about 3 months; however, the fibrosis will remain, displaced somewhat by the concomitant hepatocellular regeneration that begins about a week after alcohol consumption is discontinued.

Although there are all degrees of severity in the cirrhotic process, the next step in progression may be called "cirrhosis." The morphologic pattern that develops in the alcoholic patient is a result of the continual encroachment of collagen fibers into regenerating nodules that proliferate most exuberantly during periods of improved nutrition and cessation of alcoholic intake. The outcome is a cirrhotic liver, usually made up of poorly defined, irregularly sized nodules with thin collagen fibers insinuated between the hepatocytes. In this early stage the liver is hypertrophic, weighs 2000 to 4000 g, and has a firm rubbery quality. It is more resistant to cutting, and the fibrous septa delineate fairly uniform-sized nodules 1 to 2 mm in diameter. As the cirrhosis progresses to the moderate stage, one or more areas of dense scarring may develop. The scars are irregular in configuration and are up to about 1.5 cm in greatest dimension. At the margin of the scars the pseudolobules are smaller than those in liver remote from the scar. Near the center of the scar the pseudolobules are absent. The pathogenesis of these scars is unknown; the area most frequently involved is in a line between the gallbladder bed and the hepatic vein orifices, a less vascular area, in that the line drawn between these structures represents the boundary separating the true median portion of left lobe from the true right lobe. Often the scarring results in a U-shaped area of retraction of the capsule over the dome of the liver. In alcoholic cirrhosis, severe obliterative change along the hepatic venous outflow tract is noted in nearly all cases. The terminal hepatic veins disappear or are in the process of obliteration (Fig. 25-32). The small hepatic veins (sublobular veins) are severely damaged, and even larger veins are sclerosed in some areas, particularly where there is gross scarring. The vascular sclerosis probably occurs after earlier subclinical attacks of sclerosing hyaline necrosis, though a milder degree of connective tissue proliferation about hepatic venous tributaries does occur in fatty livers in which there has been no demonstrable sclerosing hyaline necrosis. There are no lobules with a normal pattern. Instead, arachnoid connective tissue septa surround and invade pseudolobules of various sizes. Regeneration occurs in some portions of the liver, and this further distorts the normal architecture so that the hepatic and portal veins

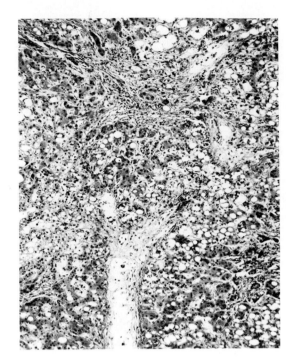

Fig. 25-32. Moderate cirrhosis. There is fatty change and early obliteration of central and subhepatic veins. This is granular fatty liver of 25-year-old Mexican man with history of chronic alcoholism.

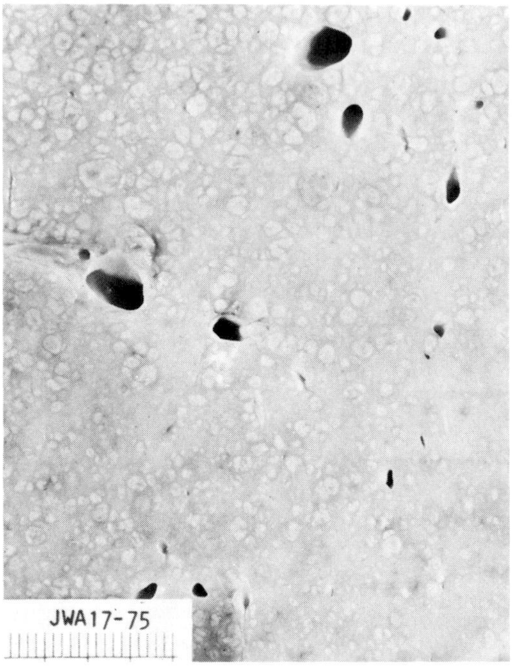

Fig. 25-33. Cut surface of liver of alcoholic cirrhotic patient with atrophic, sclerotic, finely insular alcoholic cirrhosis. Notice denser scarring on right of photograph.

may come to occupy positions near one another in the fibrous septa. Infiltration with round cells and occasionally neutrophils may occur in the septa. Fatty change is usually found in the early stages of alcoholic cirrhosis; however, if alcoholism is discontinued at any stage, the fat is diminished and parenchymal regeneration becomes prominent, resulting in the formation of larger, more discrete regenerative nodules.

In the histogenesis of moderately advanced stages of cirrhosis, there is both portal and perivenular sclerosis. Attacks of necrosis may result in subdivision of preexisting nodules. The necrosis in turn acts as a stimulus to further regeneration, and larger nodules form, particularly if there is cessation of alcoholic intake for a while. The patients who die in this stage of cirrhosis are most often in hepatic coma but may also die of bleeding or intercurrent infection, especially pneumonia.

In the advanced stage of alcoholic cirrhosis the liver is atrophic, weighing between 800 and 1200 g. The nodules are usually well defined and are described as nodular if they bulge hemispherically and as insular if the cut surface is flat (Fig. 25-33). Nodules are usually between 1 and 4 mm in diameter (referred to as finely nodular or insular), but occasionally individual nodules may be as large as 1 cm (referred to as coarsely nodular between 0.3 and 1 cm). The capsular surface is deformed by the projecting nodules. The liver is resistant

to cutting, and after sectioning, the characteristic yellow–mahogany brown nodules are sharply outlined and appear to have been embedded in the pale gray bands of connective tissue. In some irregular areas parenchymal tissue may be completely absent. On microscopic examination the liver is composed entirely of pseudolobules and wide bands of connective tissue (Fig. 25-34). Much of the outflow tract is obliterated, especially its smaller radicles. The larger and thick-walled hepatic veins that remain may be near some of the larger portal triads, the two being separated only by the connective tissue bands. See Plate 4, *C* and *D*.

There is usually diminution or absence of fat in the atrophic stage. The collagenous connective tissue is dense, but there may be small foci of hyaline necrosis, usually without inflammatory exudate or sclerosis of sinusoids. Focal areas of cholestasis resulting from loss of communication between the regenerative nodules and functioning bile ducts may be observed. Often the liver cells in the hyperplastic nodules have abnormally large hyperchromic nuclei or even two nuclei. The cells in areas of recent regeneration lack any lipochromic pigment. In the atrophic stage the cord pattern usually becomes reestablished and regular within the nodules; apparently the stimulus for or the response to regeneration was abated. Adenomatous hyperplasia occasionally occurs in quiescent alcoholic cirrhosis, and the scat-

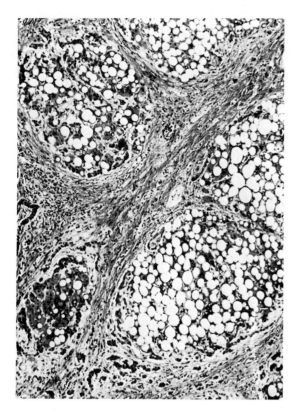

Fig. 25-34. Advanced stage of cirrhosis in 49-year-old white woman, known alcoholic for many years. Increase of connective tissue forms septa that subdivide liver into many small pseudolobules. Patient died in hepatic coma. Portacaval shunt was done 1 year before death, but patient continued to drink excessively.

tered nodules are two or three times larger than their neighbors and are dark brown. Since such nodules are more common in patients who have a hepatocellular carcinoma elsewhere, it is possible that the adenomatous nodules are preneoplastic.

Some cirrhotic patients after portacaval anastomosis will abstain from further use of alcohol, and the biopsy specimens taken at surgery may be compared with autopsy material many years later. There is usually considerable improvement or at least an increase in regenerated liver parenchyma at the expense of the connective tissue septa, which after revascularization have become thinner and less cellular. The portal lymphatics are less prominent, the liver cells in the pseudolobules often are normal in appearance, and the liver cord pattern is reestablished. The person with alcoholism with early or moderate cirrhosis who discontinues alcohol consumption will demonstrate similar improvement. The degree of reversibility after cessation of drinking is of clinical importance. The lack of further episodes of necrosis and jaundice as a result of excessive alcohol use plus the disappearance of fat and any acute

change provides maximal opportunity for limited recovery. These patients, with or without portacaval shunt, may enter the phase of compensated cirrhosis. Even those who continue to drink much less may survive many years with few or no symptoms of cirrhosis.

In some patients with alcoholism the first symptoms of hepatic disease may not develop until the advanced stage of atrophic cirrhosis. There may be nothing in the history to indicate that a patient with an attack of jaundice ever had a large fatty liver that would cause necrosis of liver cells. It would seem that in some of these individuals the cirrhotic process may progress through various stages of severity to the atrophic and coarsely nodular liver with little or no fat demonstrable on biopsy. The quantitative aspects of alcohol consumption and malnutrition may well determine whether fibrosis and pseudolobules occur with or without fatty changes. Certainly in the presence of severe fatty change, the sequence of necrosis of hepatic cells, jaundice, and coma is more likely to develop. Also, alcoholic patients who develop fatal infections, pancreatitis, and delirium tremens seem to have such occurrences at the fatty liver stage more often than not.

It has been shown by injection-corrosion casts of normal and cirrhotic livers that in cirrhosis the hepatic arteries and arterial bed are enlarged, with an increased number of communications between the hepatic arteries and portal veins.[386] The portal and hepatic venous systems are reduced in size, the change being much more severe on the hepatic vein side. The reduction of venous systems often is associated with fibrosis. Anastomotic channels are occasionally seen between portal and hepatic veins, but no significant differences were observed in the vascular pattern of alcoholic liver disease when compared with that of coarsely nodular cryptogenic cirrhosis.

In the advanced stages of alcohol cirrhosis, portal hypertension with variceal bleeding, hepatic failure with encephalopathy, and functional renal failure are the most common causes of death. An increased frequency of peptic ulcer also occurs in these patients, and bleeding from this source must always be considered. In some patients, ascites may become chronic and resistant to treatment, whereas in others the ascites is easily controlled or spontaneously disappears. Hepatic encephalopathy is easily precipitated by hemorrhage, infection, or further insults to the liver.

PATHOPHYSIOLOGY OF CHRONIC LIVER DISEASE

Many pathophysiologic phenomena are associated with chronic liver disease. Although some of these are the direct results of hepatic disease, others are unexplained. The concept that hepatic failure or insufficiency may occur to a variable degree is important. The most severe form of hepatic failure is coma. Only occasionally does the cirrhotic patient die in deep coma without some complication. The patient may from time to time have episodes of encephalopathy that are reversible. Some of these mild forms of encephalopathy are indicated by an inability to perform simple mental tests. More severe forms include flapping tremor, agitation, and disorientation.

In addition to encephalopathy, the more common complications of chronic liver disease in its progression to cirrhosis are portal hypertension, esophageal varices, and ascites.

Encephalopathy

The chief manifestation of hepatic failure is encephalopathy. This occurs in both acute and chronic liver disease. In fulminant hepatitis the onset is sudden and the mortality high.[426] In chronic liver disease the symptoms are more likely to be mild and the onset gradual. The manifestations are of a neuropsychiatric nature, varying from minor disturbances of consciousness and behavior to drowsiness, confusion, and coma. Often a flapping tremor of the extremities is evident. Despite the severe neurologic features that may develop, histopathologic changes at autopsy are minimal, apparently limited to enlargement and increased numbers of protoplasmic astrocytes.[429] One of the surprising aspects of hepatic coma is the rapid and complete recovery that may occur if hepatic failure is ameliorated.

The cause of hepatic encephalopathy is unknown, but four major hypotheses have been developed, each of which has devoted adherents.[465]

The first and foremost hypothesis is concerned with certain toxic metabolites formed in the gut or in the process of intestinal absorption that are usually removed by a normal liver but accumulate when there is hepatic malfunction. These substances interact, synergistically producing alteration of neural transmission and ultimately coma. The foremost of the toxic metabolites is ammonia, produced excessively in the breakdown of animal proteins and also by urea-splitting organisms in the gut. Reduction of meat in diet and sterilization of the gut have been the principal effective methods of reducing the development of encephalopathy.

Although ammonia is considered the most important toxic metabolite, methylmercaptan and short- and medium-chain fatty acids are believed to be contributory, and hypoxia, hypoglycemia, and electrolyte imbalances also offer synergistic effects. Methylmercaptan with its metabolites is believed to be the source of hepatic fetor, the peculiar breath odor of patients in hepatic coma or impending coma. Patients who have had surgical anastomoses of the portal vein to the vena cava to reduce the pressure in the splanchnic bed (portacaval

shunt), particularly those patients who are over 60 years of age, are at high risk of encephalopathy. The encephalopathy develops because the blood is deviated from the gut into the systemic circulation without passing through the liver.

A second hypothesis is that efflux of aliphatic amino acids and glutamine from brain tissue is associated with an influx of aromatic amino acids, resulting in increased production of inhibitory transmitter (serotinin) and decreased synthesis of excitatory neurotransmitters such as dopamine and norepinephrine. However, efflux of glutamine may be the result of increased levels of blood ammonia that will increase brain glutamine severalfold.

A third hypothesis holds that gamma-aminobutyric acid (GABA), synthesized by gut bacteria, also becomes increased in serum when an intact liver is not available for adequate removal. At the same time, the permeability of the blood-brain barrier is increased, and larger numbers of central nervous system–binding sites for GABA form. GABA is a major component of the inhibitory neurotransmitter system of the mammalian brain. In excessive amounts it is alleged to induce coma.[457]

The fourth hypothesis proposes that encephalopathy is a result of impaired energy metabolism by the brain, based on the observation that oxygen consumption and glucose use by the brain are greatly reduced. However, the impaired metabolism is only measurably diminished after 24 hours or more of encephalopathy or coma.[465]

Meager but demonstrable morphologic changes occur in the brains of patients with encephalopathy. Alzheimer II astrocytes form in brains of these patients (Chapter 42).[429] Changes in astrocytes, indistinguishable from those found in the brain of a patient in hepatic coma, can be induced by ammonia,[465] by portacaval shunts in normal chimpanzees,[460] or by inducing ischemic hepatic necrosis in animals.[447]

Portal hypertension

Resistance to the flow of blood within the liver in chronic liver disease is the most common cause of portal hypertension. Such portal hypertension is intrahepatic, in contrast to the posthepatic type caused by lesions of the hepatic veins or the prehepatic type in which the obstruction is caused by disease of the portal vein or its radicles.

Intrahepatic portal hypertension. Any form of cirrhosis may be associated with intrahepatic portal hypertension. The mechanism of obstruction was once attributed to compression by regenerative nodules.[434] However, at least in the alcoholic patient, a significant portal hypertension develops in response to perivenular intrasinusoidal collagen deposition before the development of regenerative nodules.[454] Whether or not small arterioportal shunts contribute to portal hypertension in cirrhotic livers is not established, but in the patient with hepatocellular carcinoma (HCC), arterial supply to the tumor associated with egress of blood from the tumor into the portal venous system is apparently the usual flow pattern.[446] How much the arterial portal shunt contributes to portal hypertension in the patient with HCC is unclear. The normal pressure in the portal vein is 6 to 10 mm Hg.[453] In cirrhosis it may rise to 20 to 30 mm Hg. The rise in pressure is directly related to the resistance to blood flow within the liver.

In about 15% of patients in whom portacaval shunt has been performed, the pressure on the hepatic side of a clamp placed on the vein is higher than it is on the splanchnic side, indicating that there is a reversal of portal vein blood flow in these patients. The pressure within the portal system may be measured indirectly with a fair degree of accuracy by introduction of a catheter through the inferior vena cava into a small branch of the hepatic venous system. The catheter, when wedged into the vein, gives a pressure reading similar to the pressure within the portal vein system.[455] The so-called wedged hepatic vein pressure is helpful in determining whether the point of obstruction is within the liver or is extrahepatic. In the latter, normal wedged pressures are observed.

The portal pressure can also be measured directly, either by threading a firm catheter through the loose connective tissue of the closed umbilical vein into the left portal vein branch or by thin-needle insertion into the liver percutaneously, directly into one of the major portal vein branches. The latter has become the more popular method of measurement of portal pressure.

The portal vein averages 7 cm in length and is formed by the confluence of the superior mesenteric and splenic veins. The inferior mesenteric vein joins the latter about 3 cm from its junction point. Thus the portal blood is received from the gastrointestinal tract, mesentery, spleen, gallbladder, and pancreas. Obstruction to the flow of blood through the portal trunk results in hypertension throughout the system. In cirrhosis this develops slowly but finally results in chronic passive hyperemia of the tissues drained by the portal vein. The intestines and peritoneum appear congested and edematous. The spleen is usually enlarged in portal hypertension, though how much of the cause is fibrocongestive, as once stated, is not clear. In the alcoholic cirrhotic patients who regularly have splenic lymphoid atrophy, only 23% have spleens weighing more than 400 g. Patients with cirrhosis of other types, however, may have spleens that weigh as much as 1000 g, and occasionally even more. There is poor correlation between spleen size and the severity of portal hypertension.

Posthepatic portal hypertension. Posthepatic portal hypertension is rare. It results from impeded egress of blood from the hepatic vein into the vena cava. Neoplastic obstruction, thrombosis of the hepatic veins or of the inferior vena cava, and prolonged congestive heart failure may transmit elevated pressure through the hepatic vascular bed to the portal vein.

Prehepatic portal hypertension. Prehepatic portal hypertension is an uncommon condition in which a block is hypothesized to occur before the portal blood reaches the sinusoidal bed. The liver is presumed not to be involved. Idiopathic portal hypertension is the principal example (see p. 1281). Classically, extrahepatic portal vein thrombosis has been considered a cause of prehepatic portal hypertension. However, neoplastic occlusion of the extrahepatic portal vein produces neither portal hypertension nor splenomegaly. When thrombosis of the portal vein associated with splanchnic portal hypertension occurs, quite possibly sludged blood already under increased pressure allowed the thrombus to form.[444] Congenital absence of the portal vein has been reported.[448]

Myelofibrosis rarely produces portal hypertension, probably because of the fibrous involvement of all the intrahepatic portal structures rather than increased blood flow through the enlarged spleen.

A condition known as nodular regenerative hyperplasia is often associated with portal hypertension believed to be prehepatic. Patients with Felty's syndrome (arthritis, leukopenia, and splenomegaly) often have nodular regenerative hyperplasia.

Esophageal varices. As a result of the increase in pressure within the portal system, the blood tends to bypass the liver and return to the heart by various collaterals (Fig. 25-35). These develop more prominently cephalad than caudad. Although hemorrhoids are common, they do not cause serious complications. More important are the large varices, susceptible to erosion and fatal bleeding, that arise in the mucosa at the lower end of the eosphagus (Fig. 25-36). The blood entering these veins is short-circuited from the portal system through the coronary veins of the stomach and also the left gastroepiploic vein and vasa brevia. In the lower third of the esophagus the submucosal veins are poorly supported and are subjected to trauma by the passage of food. They may also be eroded by regurgitation of gastric juice. However, microscopic analyses of varices that have ruptured do not show overlying esophagitis or ulceration. It is unknown why the precipitating event that causes repeated variceal bleeding in some patients may seldom cause it in other patients who have even higher portal pressures. In patients with cirrhosis both esophagoscopy and roentgenograms are used to demonstrate the presence of varices. The exsanguination that follows rupture of the esophageal varices is a precipitating cause of death in 15% of cirrhotic patients. An additional 35% die of liver failure after esophageal hemorrhage.

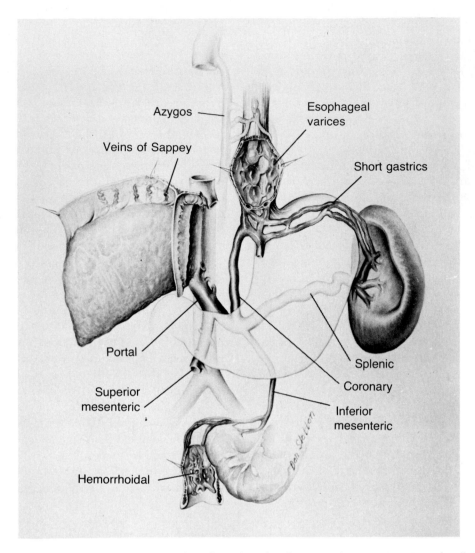

Fig. 25-35. Portal vein and its major tributaries showing most important routes of collateral circulation between portal and caval systems.

Other anastomoses between the portal circulation and systemic veins may develop between the hilum of the liver and the umbilicus along the paraumbilical plexus of veins. These may cause enlargement of the umbilicus (caput medusae). When paraumbilical veins are greatly enlarged, the term *Cruveilhier-Baumgarten syndrome* sometimes is applied, especially when a murmur is heard. The cutaneous vessels over the upper abdomen may be enlarged. Other communications may be established through the veins of Retzius in the posterior mesentery and directly through the diaphragm via the veins of Sappey. It has been demonstrated that blood may even find its way through the periesophageal veins directly to the pulmonary veins and left atrium.[428] See Plate 5, *A* and *B*.

In patients who have esophageal varices demonstrable by esophagoscopy or by roentgenograms and who may or may not have had an episode of hemorrhage,

the construction of a portal-systemic shunt[442] is often performed to decompress the portal system. This is usually of the portacaval type. If an end-to-side anatomosis is used, it prevents any possible retrograde flow in the portal vein through anastomoses with branches of the hepatic artery within the liver. Patients with thrombosed hepatic veins profit by side-by-side anastomosis, which helps the nutrition of the liver by allowing more hepatic artery blood to circulate through the parenchyma and then out through the portal vein (reversed flow). In the past several years a selective portacaval shunt, reducing pressure in the esophagus and stomach without forcing blood from the small and large intestines by bypass the liver, has been popular. This procedure, a distal splenorenal shunt, achieves selective amelioration by dividing the splenic vein and swinging its splenic end to an end-to-side anastomosis into the renal vein. The hepatic side of the divided

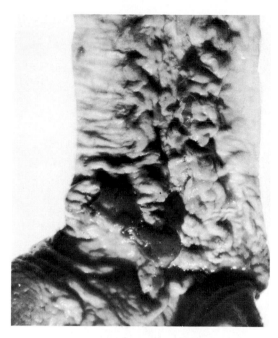

Fig. 25-36. Large esophageal varices on mucosal surface of opened esophagus.

splenic vein is ligated, as is the coronary vein. After the shunting procedure, the varices tend to decrease in size, as the spleen does in about one half the patients. Further variceal hemorrhage is rare. The status of the fibrotic process in the liver is unaffected by surgery. Proper diet and abstinence from ethanol are of most value in slowing the progress of the disease. In extra-hepatic portal vein thrombosis a portcaval shunt is usually impossible, and a splenorenal shunt may be done. In recent years injection of sclerosing agents into varices through the esophagoscope has had a resurgence of popularity. Repeated injections, as needed, are an effective therapeutical and more cost effective means than shunting. Whether further patient survival is actually increased by portal system shunt procedures remains undetermined. Clearly, however, such procedures greatly reduce the demands for scarce blood for transfusions.

Ascites. Ascites often accompanies portal hypertension, especially in the advanced stages of cirrhosis. The ascitic fluid, by definition, is a transudate, having a specific gravity of around 1.01. The mechanism of formation is complex, and many factors are involved: (1) portal hypertension and increased capillary filtration pressure, (2) postsinusoidal block, (3) hypoalbuminemia, (4) impaired renal function, (5) inferior vena cava hypertension, and (6) hyperaldosteronism.

The simple elevation of portal pressure and increased capillary filtration pressure may produce a soft-tissue transudate from the entire splanchnic bed and liver sur-face. Postsinusoidal block is believed to be the fundamental mechanism of ascites formation. Not only does increased lymph form, but also the liver surface tends to weep considerable amounts of fluid. Hypoalbuminemia may contribute to ascites by reduction of osmotic pressure in plasma, and its importance is believed to be significant.

Impaired renal function. Impaired renal function in cirrhosis may be caused by pooling of splanchnic blood, which results in a diminution of effective blood volume, reduced glomerular filtration rate, and sodium retention. There is also evidence that renal dysfunction is related to hepatic disease by changes other than blood flow. It has been suggested that in some unexplained fashion the liver may have a direct effect on the ability of the kidney to excrete sodium. The failure to excrete sodium would be responsible for increased blood volume and partially responsible for ascites.[436]

Other changes

Inferior vena cava hypertension. Inferior vena cava hypertension has been proposed as a contributing feature in the formation of ascites.[445] Frequently in cirrhosis an enlarged caudate lobe compresses the inferior vena cava into an elliptical shape, which may lead to a pressure differential between the abdominal and the thoracic inferior vena cava. It has been suggested that such narrowing may impair both the hepatic venous and the renal venous returns, thus accentuating hepatic postsinusoidal portal hypertension and renal sodium clearance.

Aldosterone has strong sodium-retaining properties and is frequently increased in the plasma and urine of the cirrhotic patients, particularly those with ascites.[439,449] Whether the elevated levels are a primary or secondary feature in relation to ascites is unknown. Certainly hyperaldosteronism is not a prerequisite for ascites.

On occasion ascites may be associated with right-sided hydrothorax as a result of small defects that develop in the diaphragm.[437,438]

Arteriovenous fistulas of skin. Arteriovenous fistulas of skin, also called vascular spiders, are often observed in chronic liver disease. Similar lesions in the lung have been described and recognized as a possible cause of finger clubbing and cyanosis, which are common in patients with alcoholic cirrhosis.[427] Other findings in the cirrhotic patient may include palmar erythema,[423] pallor of the fingernails, enlargement of the salivary glands, and Dupuytren's contractures of the palmar fascia. In women with alcoholic cirrhosis a decrease in menstruation or amenorrhea is frequent.

Testicular atrophy. Testicular atrophy almost invariably accompanies cirrhosis in the patient with alcoholism but not most other types of cirrhosis.[424] This is often accompanied by signs of feminization in those with alcoholic liver disease.[461] These include a decrease in beard, development of gynecomastia, and impotence. The plasma levels of testosterone are decreased, and those of estradiol are normal or slightly increased. Plasma gonadotropin levels are elevated. It appears that the testicular dysfunction and anatomic changes are the product of alcoholism, not of cirrhosis.[462]

Renal failure. Renal failure is a common cause of death in cirrhotic patients or patients with fulminant hepatic necrosis; 80% of patients with terminal cirrhosis or fulminant necrosis have elevated levels of blood urea.[424] Elevated creatinine levels, followed by a less striking rise of serum urea, often develop in patients with ascites. Although it is well established that functional renal failure occurs after reduced renal plasma flow and an even more pronounced decrease in glomerular filtration rate, the pathogenesis is unknown. The total plasma volume actually is increased, though it is possible that splanchnic pooling of blood, resulting from portal hypertension, may reduce effective plasma volume.[430,451] The liver disease is linked somehow with the impaired renal capacity to excrete sodium and with consequent fluid retention.

It is believed that there are two varieties of renal failure in patients with advanced liver disease. In the first type urinary sodium levels are low because of accentuated renal tubular absorption that results from reduced glomerular infiltration rate. This is called functional renal failure. A second type of renal failure is hypothesized to represent acute tubular necrosis because of the failure to conserve sodium.[440,456] The kidneys at autopsy in either type of renal failure have unusually well-preserved but slightly dilated tubules.

Proximal convoluted tubular epithelial proliferation. Proximal convoluted tubular epithelial proliferation occurs in patients who die of hepatic failure. The parietal layer of Bowman's capsule may be involved by a peculiar proliferation of the proximal convoluted tubules. Only scattered glomeruli may be involved. The cause of hepatic failure seems unimportant.

Spur cell hemolytic anemia and cirrhosis. Spur cell hemolytic anemia occurs in patients with either cirrhosis or other liver diseases. These patients may develop a hemolytic process with large numbers of circulating erythrocytes that have spurlike projections from their surface, producing distortion. The spurlike formation is accentuated by absence of the spleen. The syndrome is associated with anemia and hyperbilirubinemia, predominantly in the indirect fraction. Conflicting experimental results have been reported regarding whether the defect is in the erythrocytic cell membrane[458] or in a plasma fraction.[431] The prognosis is poor. Occasionally, hypersplenism is associated with portal hypertension.

Folate deficiency. Folate deficiency is relatively common in alcoholic liver disease, producing anemia but only rarely significant megaloblastosis. Usually folate deficiency is blamed on inadequate dietary intake,[433] but possibly the damaged liver may be incapable of adequate storage.

Hemorrhagic phenomena. Hemorrhagic phenomena are common in patients with hepatic disease. Several defects in the clotting mechanism have been studied.[452] Fibrinogen, prothombin, and factors VII, IX, X, and V are all produced by the liver parenchymal cell, and the platelet count may be reduced by hypersplenism. In addition, an abnormal fibrinogen molecule may be produced,[459] and defects of fibrin polymerization have been reported.[432]

Immunologic defects. Immunologic defects are widely known in patients with cirrhosis, particularly those with the alcoholic type who often die of severe bacterial infection. A severe leukotactic defect attributable to the presence of abnormally high levels of chemotactic factor activator has been reported.[441] An increase in the number of T-cells and a failure to develop delayed hypersensitivity have been noted.[425] Hyperglobulinemia is commonly observed. It has been suggested that this may be caused by the failure of the liver to sequester antigens absorbed from the intestine, since these circulate through the rest of the body because of the collateral circulation in cirrhosis.

CHOLESTATIC DISORDERS
Biliary tract disease and liver abscess

Many important diseases involve the intrahepatic biliary tract in adults: they may be primary or secondary. The latter are much more common, occurring when the extrahepatic flow of bile is obstructed, usually by stone, cancer, or stricture. Primary disease of the intrahepatic ducts, principally primary biliary cirrhosis (PBC), is now being diagnosed more frequently because of the use of laboratory screening that on occasion shows a high alkaline phosphatase activity or mitochondrial antibodies in an asymptomatic patient.

Biliary tract disease, either primary or secondary, is usually manifested by jaundice sometime in the course of the disease. The use of ultrasonography and cholangiograms, either transhepatic cholangiography or endoscopic retrograde cholangiopancreatography (ERCP), has resulted in a high degree of accuracy in the diagnosis of biliary tract disease in its various stages. Both PBC and secondary biliary tract disease may lead to cirrhosis.

Biliary obstruction

The extrahepatic biliary tract may be obstructed at any point from the hilus of the liver to the papilla of Vater by stone, carcinoma, or stricture. Taken as a group, these obstructive diseases produce many common features, though individual differences in clinical course, laboratory findings, and cholangiograms exist. Since jaundice is the outstanding symptom, mechanical obstruction of the biliary tree is also referred to as surgical jaundice. See Plate 5, D.

Carcinoma of the bile ducts or the head of the pancreas usually produces complete obstruction with pronounced dilatation of the biliary tree, easily seen on cholangiograms (Fig. 25-37). There is jaundice accompanied by little or no pain. In obstruction caused by choledocholithiasis there is often a history of gallbladder disease, and jaundice is usually accompanied by pain. Although a calculus impacted in the papilla of Vater may produce complete obstruction, stones in the common duct are usually mobile and jaundice tends to fluctuate or even disappear for varying periods of time. Cholangiograms are often diagnostic. Benign stricture of the extrahepatic bile ducts may follow surgical mishaps during cholecystectomy[521] or arise in the intrapancreatic portion of the common bile duct as a result of chronic alcoholic pancreatitis.[528] In the former the common hepatic duct is clamped or injured during surgery. Such surgical damage is followed by excessive drainage and usually jaundice within 1 week. Repair of the stricture is often difficult, and many of the patients have chronic jaundice and ultimately other complications, such as cholangitis and biliary cirrhosis. Obstruction of

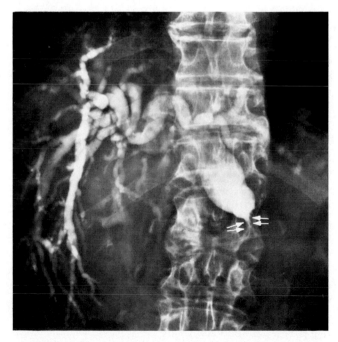

Fig. 25-37. Transhepatic cholangiogram showing extreme dilatation of extrahepatic and intrahepatic bile ducts caused by carcinoma of head of pancreas, narrowing intrapancreatic portion *(arrows)*.

the common duct attributable to carcinoma causes a prompt rise in the serum alkaline phosphatase, which precedes the rise in serum bilirubin, which with complete obstruction, can reach levels of 20 to 25 mg/dl and even higher if there is renal failure. The blood prothrombin activity decreases, the preprothrombin activity rises after parenteral administration of vitamin K. Bile appears in the urine, and there is an absence of stercobilin in the stool. In choledocholithiasis the serum bilirubin level often fluctuates and usually does not go as high as it does when the duct is obstructed by carcinoma. Serum bilirubin levels are stable at a high level with neoplastic obstruction. The alkaline phosphatase level likewise does not show the constant elevated level in choledocholithiasis that is usually seen in cancerous obstruction. Since patients with postoperative strictures are usually subjected to multiple attempts at surgical repair, from time to time the laboratory and physical findings vary considerably. Chronic alcoholic pancreatitis may cause stricture of the common duct with jaundice and a bilirubin level that is usually less than 10 mg/dl.[524,528] Calcific alcoholic pancreatitis may produce partial obstruction only, characterized by a very high alkaline phosphatase and little if any elevation of serum bilirubin.

The bile acids in the serum have been studied extensively in patients with biliary obstruction and other forms of chronic liver disease. An increased level of serum bile acids is held responsible for the pruritus that is common in patients with chronic biliary obstruction.[505]

The sequence of events that follows obstruction of the bile duct depends to some extent on the severity of obstruction and infection that so often occurs in the stagnant column of bile in the dilated ducts behind the obstructing lesion. The early microscopic changes seen soon after obstruction include dilatation of the small ducts and, particularly, prominence of the ductules where they penetrate the limiting plate to join the canaliculi. The dilated ductules are usually outlined by neutrophils just beneath their basement membranes. Bile accumulates in the perivenular canaliculi, forming green-yellow to brown plugs (Plate 3, C). Later in unrelieved obstruction the ducts enlarge further and may proliferate. The bile canaliculi become more distended with bile plugs. In this state clinical symptoms of acute cholangitis may supervene, characterized by chills and fever in addition to the jaundice. The periductal neutrophils become more numerous and penetrate the lumen of the ducts. The cholangitis is of bacterial origin. Organisms often are found in stagnant bile when obstruction is attributable to stone or stricture, but only rarely are they present in surgical specimens when the obstruction is caused by tumor. The same morphologic features of acute cholangitis occur without biliary obstruction in sepsis and the toxic shock syndrome.[489] Electron microscopic studies of the livers of patients with duct obstruction show flattening of the canalicular microvilli and condensation of the pericanalicular ectoplasm.[470]

Studies of the intercellular junctions by the freeze-fracture method in biopsy material from patients with extrahepatic obstruction have shown discontinuities that might well allow the leakage of the bile directly from the canaliculi into the sinusoidal system.[513] The liver cells often contain intracytoplasmic bile, and Kupffer cells are enlarged by easily discernible masses of bile pigment. Foci of necrosis may appear within the lobules, with transformation to bile lakes and a rise in the serum transaminase levels. Often a feathery type of degeneration of liver cells is noted.[485] Increased connective tissue around the bile ducts may assume a lamellar arrangement, and small prolongations enter the periphery of the lobules. The patient with calculous obstruction, in particular, may have repeated attacks of chills, fever, and jaundice that last only a few days, a triad known as Charcot's intermittent hepatic fever.[476] In some patients with obstruction a more severe and life-threatening situation arises, characterized by fever, chills, a serum bilirubin level above 4 mg/dl, systemic sepsis, and a fall in blood pressure. These are caused by suppurative cholangitis, which is treated as a surgical emergency. Suppurative cholangitis is most often a complication of cancerous obstruction.[473] It is less often seen in calculous obstruction and is rarely seen in patients with a benign stricture. The actual presence of pus in the obstructed ducts is not always noted at surgery. See Plate 4, F.

The borderline between suppurative cholangitis and multiple liver abscesses, particularly microabscesses, is indistinct because both may be present. In addition to surgical intervention and drainage of the common duct, percutaneous transhepatic cholangiography and drainage have been used successfully in diagnosis and treatment at this stage of the disease.[525] Thus the spectrum of changes that follow obstruction begins with a mild pericholangitis and includes the various stages of infectious cholangitis, multiple liver abscesses, and even biliary cirrhosis. The severity of infection and abscess formation may vary considerably from one part of the liver to another. A clinicopathologic syndrome, *recurrent pyogenic cholangiohepatitis*, common in Oriental populations, illustrates the advanced features of severe acute and chronic cholangitis. These patients have multiple attacks of biliary tract obstruction beginning early in life (age 10 to 20 years) and involving initially the left lobe. Complications include hepatic abscesses, intrahepatic calculi, and cholangiocarcinoma.[479]

The prognosis in obstructive disease varies with the cause: cancerous obstruction has a poor prognosis, with the patients dying of their disease or of cholangitis. Choledocholithiasis is usually relieved by surgery though occasionally death is caused by cholangitis or, rarely, biliary cirrhosis. Postoperative benign strictures are difficult to treat with bypass surgery and often lead to biliary fibrosis or cirrhosis. Bypass procedures for strictures caused by calcific pancreatitis may be successful.

Among the unusual types of cholangitis is massive hepatobiliary ascariasis in childhood. This disease is characterized by severe right upper quadrant pain accompanied by vomiting, fever, and often findings indicative of right upper quadrant (local) peritonitis. A diagnosis of massive intrahepatic involvement of the bile duct by the worms can be made by ultrasonography. In some cases conservative management fails and surgical drainage of the liver lesion is necessary. Cholangitis and multiple small abscesses are usually present.[496]

Because fatal cholangitis may occur quickly after obstruction by a stone in the duct of the diabetic patient, the screening of all diabetics past 40 years of age for cholelithiasis by ultrasonography should be a clinical consideration. In a small percentage of patients with choledocholithiasis, clinical features of acute cholangitis occur in the absence of jaundice.

Biliary cirrhosis

Obstruction of the biliary tract (either extrahepatic or intrahepatic) may, if prolonged, lead to cirrhosis of the liver. The causes of biliary obstruction have already been discussed (p. 1252). The appearance of the liver in extrahepatic obstruction depends on the degree of blockage and the time factor. Neoplastic obstruction is usually complete, and the patient dies before a true cirrhosis develops. The biliary tree proximal to the neoplasm is greatly dilated. The liver is green to greenish brown and finely granular. An increase of connective tissue along the large bile ducts near the hilus of the liver usually is noted. The organ is often increased in size and palpable before death though there is little increase in weight. Occasionally a carcinoma obstructing the ducts grows very slowly; the increase in connective tissue is such that the diagnosis of early biliary cirrhosis is justified. Obstruction of the common duct caused by a calculus or a benign stricture is usually incomplete. Therefore the distension of the ducts and bile stasis in the liver are not as extreme as with cancerous obstruction. On occasion a stone or a stricture may obstruct the common duct for years and leads to true biliary cirrhosis. I have observed several such cases caused by inapparent choledocholithiasis.

The liver in biliary cirrhosis has a granular appearance or may even be nodular. Fibrosis is as pronounced as it is in alcoholic cirrhosis. Biliary cirrhosis of this type may on rare occsions cause portal hypertension, splenomegaly, and hemorrhage from esophageal varices. A portacaval shunt may become necessary.[467]

In the early stage of extrahepatic obstruction, microscopic examination reveals that dilatation of the large ducts near the hilus is constant, whereas the size of the smaller ducts is variable. Some increase of fibroblastic activity with the formation of spurs is seen within 30 to 50 days. Bile stasis is predominantly perivenular. In the intermediate stage, between 60 and 100 days, connective tissue is more abundant and often has a concentric configuration around the bile ducts. Both at this stage and in the later cirrhotic phase, the arrangement of the connective tissue may give a "pipestem" effect (Fig. 25-38). Bile duct proliferation is present in only a small percentage of the total. The mononuclear type of exudate may be increased. Focal necrosis of hepatic cells of either the lytic or the eosinophilic type is frequent. As the result of necrosis, particularly of cells in the peripheries of the lobules, bile lakes may form. The terminal hepatic veins are present, and a normal lobular architecture can be seen throughout most of the liver. A few abnormal hyperplastic nodules may make their appearance at this stage. Later, especially in patients with calculous obstruction or stricture, a well-developed cirrhosis is noted, with connective tissue septa outlining pseudolobules. Intralobular bile stasis is irregular but is now both perivenular and peripheral. There is usually no bile stasis within the interlobular ducts, probably because bile is absorbed within the lobule. Occasionally a liver may exhibit wide connective tissue septa with abundant bile duct proliferation. Fatty changes, extensive necrosis of parenchyma, and even abscesses may complicate the disease.

Primary biliary tract disease

There are three slowly progressive primary diseases of the intrahepatic biliary tract: primary biliary cirrhosis (PBC), primary sclerosing cholangitis (PSC), and Caroli's disease. The first two are of unknown cause and are often associated with diseases of other organ systems, whereas Caroli's disease is a congenital disorder.

Primary biliary cirrhosis

Primary biliary cirrhosis (PBC), or chronic nonsuppurative destructive cholangitis, is a complex autoimmune disorder that is characterized by destruction of the interlobular bile ducts. The name "PBC" is somewhat misleading because the end stage of cirrhosis may not be reached until 5 to 10 years or more after diagnosis. Hanot first recognized the disorder in 1876, using the term *hypertropic cirrhosis with jaundice*.[515] PBC accounts for 0.6% to 2% of deaths from cirrhosis worldwide.[492]

Little attention has been given to the geographic aspects of PBC, since most studies of the disease have been in the United States and Europe. In the United States about 94% of the PBC patients are women with a mean age of 52, 95% between 32 and 72 years of age.[510] PBC in patients under 30 years of age is rare. The frequency in the general population is unknown; however, the routine use of biochemical screening that includes determination of serum alkaline phosphatase levels has resulted in an increased number of cases being diagnosed in the asymptomatic stage. In about 20% of all patients with PBC the disease is diagnosed at this stage. Liver biopsy in this subclinical stage have shown that any one of the various pathologic stages of PBC may be present, even cirrhosis.

The onset is generally insidious, beginning with pruritus that may be present for several months to years before the onset of dark urine or icterus.[478] A few pa-

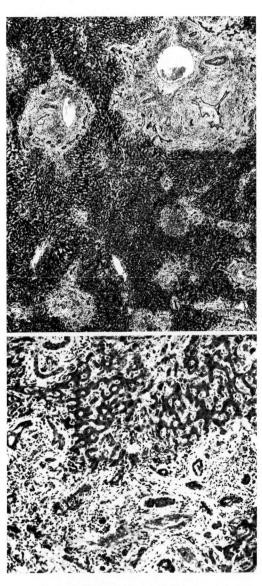

Fig. 25-38. Biliary cirrhosis.

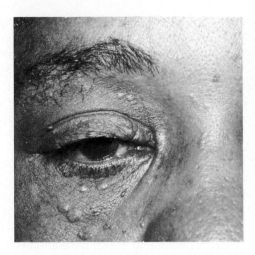

Fig. 25-39. Xanthomas of eyelid in primary biliary cirrhosis.

tients have darkening of the skin well before the onset of pruritus and jaundice. After jaundice has been present for months, the patient may notice foul fatty stools, and slowly over the years the skin manifestations of hyperlipemia may become noticeable as xanthomas or fine yellowish deposits in the creases of the palms of the hands, anticubital spaces, and elsewhere (Fig. 25-39).

From the outset there is hepatomegaly, and about one half of the patients have splenomegaly. The impaired flow of bile into the intestine causes a deficiency of the absorption of vitamin D and calcium, which results in osteomalacia, often with bone pain and even compression fractures of the vertebrae. Weight loss is noted as greater amounts of ingested fat are excreted in the stool, and a defect in glucose absorption occurs. The course is one of slow deterioration, with a duration of life from 5 to 15 years after the diagnosis is established. In the end stage of cirrhosis, ascites, hepatic coma, and bleeding from esophageal varices are common features.

The laboratory findings consist in positive results of a properly performed mitochondrial antibody test, an increase in IgM, and an elevated alkaline phosphatase. A variety of mitochondrial antibody tests are available, and prognostic value of the various subtypes is in review.[523] Multiple mitochondrial antibodies can be detected in PBC, and these are directed to different components of the inner and outer mitochondrial membrane. The most common mitochondrial antibody is anti-M2, which reacts with several antigens on the inner mitochondrial membrane.[492] Other mitochondrial antibodies are found in syphilis (anti-M1), drug-induced disorders (anti-M3 and anti-M6), and collagen vascular diseases (anti-M5). In PBC there is often a familial type of hypergammaglobulinemia.[490] The serum copper level is moderately elevated in symptomatic PBC. Abnormalities of serum complement levels have been noted.

Immune complexes are common in PBC but appear to be of secondary importance.[492] The withered biliary tree seen on cholangiograms is characteristic of the disease.

More than any other liver disease, PBC is associated with several immune type of disorders. Among these are Sjögren's syndrome, scleroderma, arthritis, lupus erythematosus, interstitial pneumonitis, and thyroiditis.[480] Sjögren's syndrome (dry eyes and mouth) is the most common autoimmune type of disorder noted. Rheumatoid arthritis occurs in a relatively small percentage of patients.[472] An additional asymptomatic erosive type of arthritis involving the distal small joints of the hands has been described.[501] The arthritis is usually symptomless and is accompanied by osteopenia in a majority of patients. Association with thyroiditis has been noted in about one third of patients with PBC.[521] Scleroderma may occur alone or with Raynaud's phenomenon, calcinosis cutis, sclerodactyly, and telangiectasia; the latter four are known as the CRST syndrome.[512]

Four pathologic stages, from the earliest changes seen on biopsy to the end stages of cirrhosis, have been described[497] in my patients, now consisting of over 140 cases in the last 5 years, and there is considerable overlap of staging features within the same biopsy specimen. Thus in the biopsy diagnosis I use only rough approximations and find staging, as described, inexact with respect to the clinical course of disease.

In the early stages of the disease there is destruction of interlobular bile ducts as well as obliteration of the limiting plate (Fig. 25-40). The ducts show various stages of damage and are surrounded by a dense infiltrate of lymphocytes, plasma, cells, and a few eosinophils. The lymphocytes often form follicles that impinge on or surround the affected ducts. In the destructive process the ductal epithelium shows cytoplasmic vacuolization, nuclear pyknosis, and karyorrhexis, along with some degree of atypical epithelial proliferation. The limiting plate is infiltrated with mononuclear cells and is difficult to define. The periportal hepatocytes may show degenerative hydropic change, and about 10% of the patients have scanty alcoholic hyalin in the hydropic periportal hepatocytes. Histiocytes may form granulomatous collections, more often in the portal areas than within the lobules. True epithelioid granulomas with giant cells are rare, occurring in about 10% to 20% of cases. With progression the portal areas become wider and fibrotic. The inflammtory reaction tends to regress, and the interlobular bile ducts disappear. More than 60% of the portal tracts ultimately become devoid of interlobular bile ducts, whereas the liver in other hepatic diseases shows less than 15% destruction.[468] Along with the reduction of the interlobular bile ducts, the proliferation of atypical "pseudoductules" is prominent. These little ducts have flat

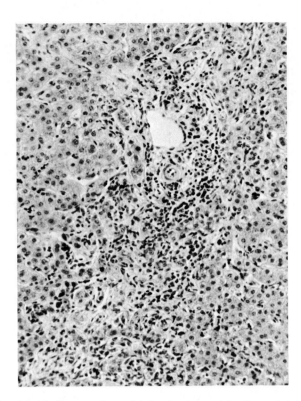

Fig. 25-40. Destruction of bile ducts and limiting plate in primary biliary cirrhosis.

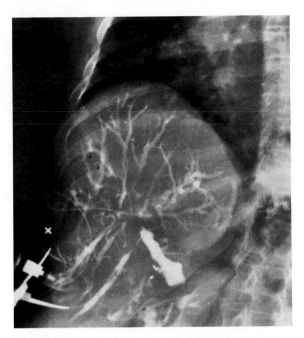

Fig. 25-41. Cholangiogram of patient with intrahepatic sclerosing cholangitis. Notice irregular diameter of intrahepatic duct radicals, some of which appear amputated.

irregular epithelium and a tiny or absent lumen, are located at the peripheral zone of the portal tract, and probably represent transformed hepatic cords. The hepatic cords show little damage except for those in the periportal areas, where necrosis, fibrosis (stage 3 or 4), and periportal cholestasis are often apparent. In the later stages of PBC, fibrous septa connect adjacent portal areas and also split the lobules. Finally, encircled nodules join to form biliary cirrhosis. In the final stages of the disease, perivenular cholestasis may occur. Considerable copper accumulation may occur in livers of patients with chronic jaundice. Appropriate stains on either biopsy or autopsy material disclose large quantities of copper, fairly uniformly distributed in the periportal hepatocytes.

Primary sclerosing cholangitis

Primary sclerosing cholangitis (PSC) is predominantly a disease of men (80%) with an average age range of 25 to 45 years. It is characterized by jaundice, pruritus, and hepatomegaly.[494,527] In about one half to three fourths of the patients the disease coexists with chronic ulcerative colitis but not or only rarely with Crohn's disease[475,527] It has occurred with an immunodeficiency syndrome[470] and AIDS. PSC has a moderately progressive course, and many patients die of biliary cirrhosis within 5 years. Grossly the extrahepatic bile ducts are usually sclerosed and hard; the intrahepatic ducts are likewise affected, but increased numbers of patients with only intrahepatic PSC and "normal" extrahepatic ducts are now being recognized.[471] In the liver there is bile duct proliferation, fibrosis, and cholestasis that progresses to biliary fibrosis, often to cirrhosis. The ductal involvement has a very irregular distribution; thus the biopsy pattern is highly variable from one area to another. Some areas resemble the changes from mechanical obstruction; others simulate the changes of primary biliary cirrhosis. The regions of intrahepatic sclerosis have prominent thickening of ducts with intramural inflammation, and some areas have practically no changes. As with other types of biliary cirrhosis, a large amount of copper is present in hepatocytes of protracted cases but less than that found in patients with PBC. Cholangiograms in PSC are diagnostic (Fig. 25-41). Cholangiograms in PSC are diagnostic because of the "beading" of bile ducts. Only a third of the liver biopsy specimens reflect features suggestive of the disease,[487] and in advanced cases not only are obliterated ducts noted (which correspond to the "beading"), but ectatic ducts are also common.[498] Improved survival of PSC has been recognized.[487]

Caroli's disease

Congenital cystic dilatation of the intrahepatic bile duct (choledochal cyst, or Caroli's disease) is a rare familial disorder. The cystic dilatations are easily seen on cholangiograms and may involve many intrahepatic bile ducts. The dilatations are filled with bile and have a characteristic gross and microscopic appearance.[526] Calculi may form within the cystic areas. Cholangitis and liver abscesses may be fatal. The disease may consist only of an isolated choledochal cyst or may be associated with renal tubular ectasia and other forms of cystic diseases of the kidneys. Carcinoma of the intrahepatic bile ducts has also been noted.[486] A form of the disease may be associated with congenital hepatic fibrosis.[484]

Other diseases

Other diseases of the intrahepatic bile ducts include hemobilia and pneumobilia. The clinical entity of hemobilia or hemorrhage into the biliary tract is characterized by biliary colic, gastrointestinal hemorrhage, and often bilirubinuria and clinical jaundice. Both melena and hematemesis may be present. Unrecognized hemobilia has a high mortality. Among the causes of hemobilia are trauma (p. 1275), needle biopsy of the liver,[469] transhepatic cholangiography,[482] neoplasms of the intrahepatic bile ducts or of the hepatic parenchyma, and aneurysms (hemocholecyst)[518] of the hepatic artery. Diseases of the gallbladder and extrahepatic ducts may also give rise to hemobilia. Superior mesenteric angiography is considered the best diagnostic procedure for the diagnosis of hemobilia. Air in the intrahepatic biliary tract, or pneumobilia, in the patient who has not had surgery may be associated with emphysematous cholecystitis, incompetence of the sphincter of Oddi, or biliary enteric fistula or may result from blunt abdominal trauma. Pneumobilia is a common finding in patients who have undergone biliary bypass surgery. In addition to ultrasonography, radionuclide scans, and plain abdominal roentgenograms, computerized tomography is an excellent means of diagnosing air in the intrahepatic biliary tract. Acquired bile duct cysts that result from liver infarcts caused by polyarteritis nodosa have been reported.[482a]

Abscesses

Since the study by Ochsner, DeBakey, and Murray[504] on liver abscesses in 1938, there has been a considerable change in the etiologic background, diagnosis, and treatment of liver abscesses. Most abscesses are of bacterial pyogenic origin, a lesser number by *Entamoeba histolytica*, and rarely by actinomycosis. They can be diagnosed by liver scans, computerized tomography, and angiography. The occurrence of liver abscesses may constitute a severe clinical disorder, often with a delay in diagnosis and treatment and a high mortality. However, the symptoms may be rather subtle and systemic manifestations mild.[466,507]

Pyogenic abscesses

Liver abscesses of pyogenic origin are far more common than those caused by amebas, though cases of the latter do occur in the southern United States and also in travelers to parts of the world where amebic dysentery is endemic. Pyogenic liver abscesses have been classified on the basis of the mode of entry, that is, (1) through ascension of the biliary tract (acute cholangitis), (2) by means of the hepatic artery (septicemia), (3) through the portal vein (pylephlebitis), (4) by direct extension (subphrenic abscess), (5) after trauma, and (6) from unknown sources. The pathologic changes vary from multiple microscopic lesions to single or multiple macroscopic abscesses.[516] The gross pattern of pyogenic abscess depends primarily on the source of infection and the accompanying pathologic changes in the liver and elsewhere.

Acute cholangitis. Multiple abscesses most often occur after acute cholangitis as the result of obstruction of the common duct. These abscesses are intimately associated with the biliary tree, often causing destruction of the walls of the dilated bile ducts.

Septicemias. Septicemias may produce multiple liver abscesses of variable size and abscesses of other organs in adults, infants, and children. In children they usually occur before 5 years of age, particularly in patients with acute blastic leukemia.[481] In the neonate, liver abscesses may complicate umbilical infections or sepsis.[503] Chronic granulomatous disease (CGD) caused by an inherited defect in the bactericidal capacity of polymorphonuclear neutrophils may occur in both children and adults.[506] and may result in hepatic abscesses.

Pylephlebitis. Pylephlebitis in the early part of the century was a well-known complication of acute appendicitis. This source of infection is now almost nonexistent in the United States but still occurs in some parts of the world. Pylephlebitis may complicate other types of intra-abdominal suppuration, such as diverticulitis. However, in recent decades suppurative pylephlebitis that extends from the source of the infection to involve the major portion of the extrahepatic portal system is rare indeed. In autopsy material, pylephlebitis that involves the hilar areas of the liver or portions of the intrahepatic portal branches still occurs, especially after attacks of acute cholangitis caused by obstructive biliary tract disease. Extensive involvement of the intrahepatic portal venous system is a common complication of recurrent pyogenic cholangitis, seen primarily in Asians.[529] Intrahepatic phylephlebitis may be present without liver abscesses; often, however suppuration follows and microscopic or gross abscesses develop. Pylephlebitis with or without abscesses may occur in one lobe only. Thrombosis of intrahepatic branches of the portal vein may accompany carcinomas of the biliary tract or the head of the pancreas and produce multiple infarcts. If obstructive cholangitis is present, some infarcts may suppurate.

Suppurative abdominal disease. Suppurative abdominal disease with or without pylephlebitis may result in emboli or bacteria being carried to the liver by the portal vein, giving rise to liver abscesses. These most often occur in the right lobe when the suppurative disorder is drained by the superior mesenteric vein, whereas disease on the left side of the abdomen may cause suppuration in one or both lobes.[495]

Solitary abscesses. Solitary abscesses may complicate both penetrating and nonpenetrating injuries to the liver or arise from contiguous infections.[516] These abscesses are often anticipated and clinical diagnosis is easily made. A much more difficult problem is the patient with a solitary abscess or multiple large abscesses, in which case there is no recognizable source of infection. In the distant past, fever, chills, septicemia, and a large tender liver pointed the way toward the diagnosis of liver abscess. However, in recent years there appears to be milder reaction to pyogenic liver abscess.[505,522] Most abscesses are now seen in the elderly, are of bacterial origin, and can be diagnosed with liver scans.[516] The symptoms may be rather subtle and the systemic manifestations mild.[505] In many patients with solitary hepatic abscesses, no recognizable source can be found. Such abscesses have been reported in diabetic patients.[488]

Laboratory examination reveals a leukocytosis, elevated alkaline phosphatase level, hypoalbuminemia, and often a positive blood culture.[477] Chest roentgenograms may disclose basilar atelectasis or pneumonitis, an elevated right diaphragm, and a pleural effusion. A high degree of accuracy in diagnosis is achieved by the use of sonograms and scintiscans. Ultrasonography discloses a round to ovoid lesion with discrete, irregular, echo-poor margins. The walls are rather ragged. Liver scans are also used; however, lesions less than 2 cm in diameter are difficult to demonstrate.[493] In nonicteric patients with a solitary hepatic abscess, a filling defect is demonstrable on scintiscan far more often than in patients with multiple small hepatic abscesses. Some abscesses are characterized by gas formation, which is easily recognized on a plain film of the abdomen.[491]

A wide variety of organisms have been cultured both from pyogenic abscesses and from the blood. Although *Escherichia coli* seems to be the most common, many other organisms have been noted. Among these are streptococci, staphylococci, and *Klebsiella pneumoniae.*[517] Septicemia caused by melioidosis is another cause of liver abscesses.[509] Anaerobic cultures should always be performed on any aspirate. Although surgery is the generally accepted treatment for large abscesses, medical treatment has also proved successful.[499]

Amebic abscesses

Amebic abscesses of the liver are much less common than pyogenic abscesses but have many similar features. They are caused by the spread of *Entamoeba histolytica* from intestinal lesions by way of the portal vein. It is predominantly a disease of men, about 4:1, occurs before the age of 50 years, and is one of the serious diseases noted among travelers exposed to the organism. It is rare in persons who have not been outside the United States but does occur in some areas. Children are also susceptible to abscess formation.[507] A history of diarrhea weeks or months before onset of symptoms is obtained from approximately 50% of patients with hepatic amebic abscess. However, trophozoites are usually not demonstrable in the stools. Fever, leukocytosis, pain in the upper right quadrant, and a tender enlarged liver are common findings. In the diagnosis of amebic liver abscess the indirect hemagglutination test is highly sensitive, with a positive titer of at least 1:128 in 90% of patients. Effective demonstration of the organism in aspirated abscess contents is difficult but should be attempted on the last few drops of the aspirate.[507] Ultrasonography can also determine the size and number of the abscesses and is of great value in early diagnosis. Antiamebic therapy usually leads to rapid recovery. Scintiscans show that healing takes 2 to 4 months in most patients.[520]

The amebic abscesses recognized clinically may vary greatly in size but are usually solitary and often located in the superoposterior portion of the right lobe (Fig. 25-42). However, in autopsy series as many as 57% of the cases are reported to be multiple, attesting in part to a higher mortality in patients with multiple abscesses.[471] Left lobe abscesses have the highest incidence of rupture, especially into the pericardial and pleural cavities. The contents of an abscess vary in appearance, probably depending on age and degree of parenchymal necrosis. Some observers have noted the contents to be more liquid early but becoming thick with age. This is not entirely in accord with my experience in autopsy material. The aspirate may vary in appearance from light tan to chocolate or "anchovy sauce." The lining of the abscess is usually gray-white and round, and small ne-

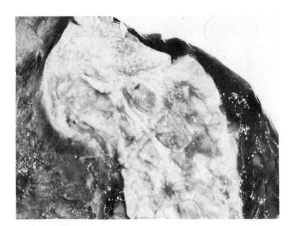

Fig. 25-42. Amebic liver abscess with rough, irregular lining of necrotic tissue.

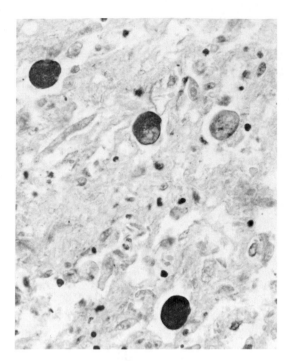

Fig. 25-43. Amebas in necrotic wall of liver abscess. (Periodic acid–Schiff stain.)

crotic penetrations into the surrounding liver are seen. A striking "foam rubber" lining has been noted in much of our material. The abscess wall has an irregular lining composed of exudate and necrotic liver tissue. The contents usually stain deeply with hematoxylin, in contrast to pyogenic abscess. Amebas are most easily found in the marginal liver tissue, often in colonies with a clear zone about each ameba. A periodic acid–Schiff stain accentuates the contrast between ameba and body cells (Fig. 25-43). The amebic infection may involve the branches of the portal and hepatic veins, producing an amebic phlebitis and thrombosis, thus accentuating the necrotic process.

Actinomycotic abscesses of the liver usually have a pathogenesis similar to that of pyogenic pylephlebitic abscesses. Spread to the liver from intestinal lesions is by the portal venous channels. Multiple, small ragged abscess cavities are produced in which the actinomycotic colonies can be found.[502] A honeycomb type of calcification is sometimes seen on roentgenograms.

LIVER DISEASES IN INFANTS AND CHILDREN

The differential diagnosis of liver disease in a neonate, infant, or child includes a multitude of disorders. When age, symptoms, and etiology are considered, most of the disease entities may be discussed in a few broad categories, though there is a considerable overlap. One group is made up of neonates and those up to 3 months of age with jaundice. A second group includes older infants and children with acute or chronic liver disease. Finally, there is a small group of infants and children in whom the chief finding is hepatomegaly. In general the etiologic factors include infections, genetic or familial diseases, and congenital anatomic disorders, and there is a sizable group in which the cause is unknown. The relative incidence and frequency of the various clinical forms of neonatal cholestasis is shown in Table 25-5.

Neonatal jaundice

Neonatal jaundice may arise from any one of many disturbances of bilirubin metabolism, varying from physiologic jaundice to fatal disease of the liver.[534] The various diseases are now included in one of two groups that consist of the indirect-acting (approximately unconjugated) and the direct-acting (approximately conjugated) hyperbilirubinemias. However, this separation does not become too evident until the fifth to seventh days of life when the liver has enough glucuronyl transferase to conjugate bilirubin.

Physiologic neonatal hyperbilirubinemia

Normally an acholuric indirect-acting type of hyperbilirubinemia is noted in most full-term infants on the second to fourth days of life and in premature infants on the fifth or sixth days of life. A maximum level of approximately 6 mg/dl is present in the full-term neonate and 10 to 12 mg/dl in the premature neonate. Levels exceeding 12 mg/dl in the full-term neonate and 15 mg/dl in the premature neonate require further studies as to the cause of jaundice.[532] In the full-term baby the hyperbilirubinemia usually disappears by the seventh day and in the premature baby by the ninth or tenth day. Many factors may contribute to physiologic jaundice. One of these is an increased bilirubin load caused by the erythrocyte volume in the neonate and a shorter life span of the erythrocytes. Second is the decreased amount of glucuronyl transferase necessary for bilirubin conjugation. This is most noticeable in premature babies. A third factor is the lack of ligandins, the intracellular acceptors of bilirubin.[581] These proteins, also termed Y and Z, are the organic anion-binding proteins that facilitate the transfer of both bilirubin and sulfobromophthalein. A change in hepatic blood supply during transit from fetal to newborn life may also transiently impair hepatic function. It has been suggested that there is a correlation between elevated levels of alpha-fetoprotein and physiologic jaundice.[561]

In indirect-acting hyperbilirubinemia less than 15% of the total bilirubin is of the direct-reacting type. When the serum bilirubin rises above 20 mg/dl, irreversible damage to the central nervous system, called kernicterus, may be caused by unconjugated bilirubin

Table 25-5. Neonatal and childhood cholestasis

Disease	Features	Diagnostic tests
Biliary atresia	25% to 30% of neonatal jaundice; surgically treated (Kasai procedure)	Technetium-dye, biopsy of the liver
Neonatal "hepatitis"	Most familial cases progress; most nonfamilial heal; 35% to 40% of jaundice	Biopsy of the liver
Choledochal cyst	2% of neonatal jaundice; surgically treated	Mass on ultrasound testing
Alpha$_1$-antitrypsin deficiency	7% to 10% of neonatal jaundice; Only in Pi ZZ (0.07% of population)	Alpha$_1$-antitrypsin level
intrahepatic familial cholestatic syndromes	5% to 6% of jaundice	Liver biopsy and family history
infections		
Sepsis	*Escherichia coli;* beta-hemolytic streptococci groups A and B 2%	Blood cultures
Syphilis	Rash, anemia	Cord blood/infant VDRL test
Viral hepatitis A and B	Birth to 8 to 12 weeks; mother HBsAg positive	HBsAg, HAV-Ab
Toxoplasmosis	Progressive liver dysfunction	Sabin-Feldman dye test positive
Rubella	Congenital heart disease, hepatomegaly, occasionally jaundice (15%)	Fluorescent antibody test
Cytomegalovirus (CMV)	Jaundice, hepatosplenomegaly, hemolytic anemia	Fetal viruria by culture, fluorescent antibody test for CMV-specific IgM antibody
Herpes simplex	Usually jaundice and hypoprothrombinemia; liver may not be palpable; skin vesicles	Viral culture
Metabolic diseases		
Galactosemia	Cataracts, ascites, cirrhosis	Clinistix/Galactostix
Endocrine (hypothyroidism, panhypopituitarism)	1% of neonatal jaundice	Thyroid-stimulating hormone, etc.
Fructosemia	Hypoglycemia, seizures	Enzyme assay, liver biopsy, serum and urine levels
Tyrosinemia type 1	Aminoaciduria, aminoacidemia; autosomal recessive; liver cell carcinoma	Serum level of tyrosine
Parenteral nutrition	Cholestasis, fibrosis	Biopsy

From Balistreri, W.F.: Prenatal cholestasis lessons from the past, issues for the future, Semin. Liver Dis. **7**(2):Foreword, 1987.

entering nerve cells, particularly those in the basal ganglia. Despite extensive research, the exact mechanism of brain damage in kernicterus is still unknown.[575] Inasmuch as unconjugated bilirubin circulates bound to albumin, a low level of serum albumin or drug therapy that replaces the bilirubin bound to albumin will allow central nervous system damage at levels lower than 20 mg/dl. This is especially true in premature infants[582]; the presence of pulmonary hyaline membrane disease accentuates the risk. Ethnic differences in the frequency of neonatal jaundice have been observed.[569]

Because of the danger of kernicterus, severe hyperbilirubinemia often is treated by exchange transfusions with good results. The indications for exchange transfusions include (1) bilirubin level approaching 20 mg/dl at any time during the first few days of life in a full-term infant without evidence of acidosis or respiratory distress; (2) bilirubin level of 10 to 15 mg/dl at any time in a premature infant with evidence of hypoxia, acidosis, or respiratory distress; (3) severe erythroblastosis fetalis and severe anemia (hemoglobin value of less than 10 g/dl), with or without evidence of fetal hydrops at birth; (4) clinical signs suggestive of kernicterus at any time or at any bilirubin level; and (5) low unsaturated albumin binding level as determined by a reliable method, irrespective of serum bilirubin level at any age.[532] Phototherapy of the infant and phenobarbital treatment before delivery have also proved useful.[532,544]

Many disorders must be considered in the etiology of indirect-acting hyperbilirubinemia. At one time the most important was hemolytic anemia of the newborn caused by an isoimmunization syndrome that occurred when Rh-positive infants produced anti-Rh factors in

Rh-negative mothers. The disease condition occurs only after an earlier sensitization, either an earlier pregnancy or a transfusion of Rh-positive blood. In the past, this disease was known as erythroblastosis fetalis or icterus gravis neonatorum; it has been largely prevented by administration of anti-Rh serum (anti-D) to Rh-negative mothers after they delivered their first Rh-positive infant and after the delivery of each subsequent Rh-positive infant.[625] Usually in erythroblastosis the liver is unable to secrete the large amount of unconjugated bilirubin that results from the hemolysis of erythrocytes, and jaundice appears in the first 24 hours. In fatal instances there is an even distribution of bile in canaliculi and also in the hepatic cells. Liver cell necrosis of variable degree may occur and could account for the increase in conjugated bilirubin that is sometimes seen in hemolytic disease of the newborn. However, additional factors may be involved.[563] Extramedullary erythropoiesis is common and may be extensive, not only in the liver but also in other organs. When hemolytic disease is caused by ABO incompatibility, the jaundice is usually mild though kernicterus can occur if the serum bilirubin level rises excessively. ABO hemolytic disease is now the most common cause of neonatal jaundice, occurring almost exclusively in infants of group A or B having mothers of group O. The highest percentage of jaundiced babies are those who have a positive direct antiglobulin test. These infants also have the most severe jaundice.[550]

Maternal diabetes mellitus, newborn infection, glucose-6-phosphate dehydrogenase defect,[559] polycythemia, metabolic errors, conjugation defects, breast milk syndrome,[533,605] hypothyroidism, intestinal obstruction, and hemotomas are all factors that may produce neonatal jaundice of the indirect-acting type.

In the children of diabetic mothers, the infants are usually large and hypotonic and have hypoglycemia. Infections that occur early, that is, during the first few days after birth or in the first 2 weeks of life, may be caused by any of many different organisms, though there has been a rise in the frequency of beta-hemolytic *Streptococcus* infections.[554,604] Rarely do the nonhemolytic indirect-acting hyperbilirubinemias require exchange transfusions.[589]

Direct-acting hyperbilirubinemia

Although any one of several diseases may cause an increase in direct-acting bilirubin,[542] such diseases may not become manifest until after the first week of life, for the liver is incapable of conjugating a large amount of bilirubin. Among the large number of diseases to be considered (Table 25-5),[534] three are most often responsible: biliary atresia, alpha$_1$-antitrypsin deficiency, and an idiopathic group collectively called neonatal hepatitis, though "hepatitis" may be a misnomer because evidence of infection is equivocal and inflammation is negligible. Other diseases, such as galactosemia, tyrosinemia, and fructosuria are far less common, though early diagnosis is imperative because of the irreversible changes that may occur in many organs if recognition and treatment are not prompt.

Biliary atresia

It is important to differentiate between neonatal hepatitis and biliary atresia because the later is often amenable to surgical treatment. Hepatic portoenterostomy (the Kasai operation),[575] a surgical procedure whereby a limb of jejunum is anastomosed to the hilum of the liver at the site of amputated sclerotic duct, has been successful at least for a short term in many cases.[557] Long-term defects may still develop in many if not all the successfully treated patients.

Many clinical, laboratory, and radiologic tests have been used to differentiate biliary atresia from other forms of intrahepatic cholestasis. Clinically in biliary atresia the earlier age at onset of acholic stools, a higher birth weight, and a large firm or hard liver are helpful clues in differentiating biliary atresia from neonatal "hepatitis" or alpha$_1$-antitrypsin deficiency.

Among the abnormal laboratory test results, the presence of glutamyl transpeptidase (GGT) above the level of 780 IU/liter is a sensitive test for the differentiation of biliary atresia from neonatal hepatitis and cholestatic diseases.[566] The use of N-substituted iminodiacetic acid (IDA) derivatives, especially diethyl IDA labeled with ^{99m}Tc, has proved helpful in the differential diagnosis of cholestatic disease.[600] In neonatal hepatitis after injection of diethyl IDA, the curve of hepatic-timed activities peaks early with a median of 1 minute and decays rapidly, whereas in biliary atresia the curves peak in 10 minutes and decay more slowly.[566] Because irreversible cirrhosis may be present within 3 months, surgical exploration is very important before this age in infants with biliary atresia.[565]

Grossly biliary atresia may involve a short segment or nearly all the extrahepatic duct system, including the gallbladder. The involved segments are reduced to cordlike structures. A Kasai operation is successful only when the right and left ducts are present and can be anastamosed to the bowel.

Both needle and excision biopsies are helpful in differentiating biliary atresia from neonatal hepatitis and other causes of intrahepatic cholestasis.[542] Portal fibrosis, ductular proliferation, and bile thrombi in the portal and periportal areas are the most constant findings in biliary atresia (Fig. 25-44). Giant cell transformation of a variable degree is common. Excision biopsy specimen of the extrahepatic ducts at surgery may show (1) fibrosis with complete absence of any glands or ductal structures, (2) one or more clusters of lumens lined with cuboid epithelium, seen peripherally, or (3) the presence of bile ducts at the center of concentrically

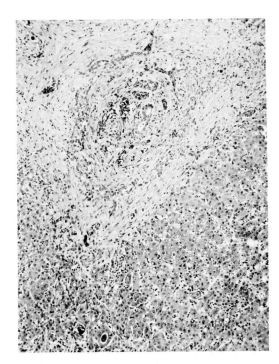

Fig. 25-44. Concentric bands of periportal connective tissue and bile stasis characteristic of biliary cirrhosis. Patient was 5-month-old infant with atresia of common bile duct.

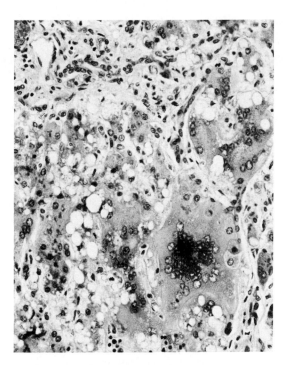

Fig. 25-45. Neonatal hepatitis (3-week-old male infant). Multinucleated giant cells compose most of parenchyma. Increased connective tissue can be seen along sinusoids and in periportal space. Intracanalicular bile stasis is at upper right and lower left.

arranged connective tissue. Surgical treatment is more successful in the last group. The Kasai operation, in which an anastomosis is made between the region of hepatic duct bifurcation and a loop of jejunum, relieves jaundice in some patients who have remained asymptomatic on follow-up studies. Other sequential biopsies indicate that fibrosis of the liver may continue and result in biliary cirrhosis with portal hypertension, even though bile flow is maintained.[530,561] Failure of establishment of a patent biliary tree produces severe perivenular cholestasis, bile duct proliferation, and periductal fibrosis that finally leads to biliary cirrhosis. At autopsy one third or more of the liver may be composed of fibrous tissue. However, there is considerable variation in severity not related to the duration of the obstruction. Children with unrelieved atresia who survive a few years may develop portal hypertension and die of bleeding esophageal varices.

Obstructive conditions other than extrahepatic biliary atresia, such as choledochal cysts and inspissated bile plugs,[556] may cause similar clinical findings. Hypoplasia of the extrahepatic bile ducts is a rare entity that has been diagnosed only with laparotomy and operative cholangiography.[583]

Neonatal "hepatitis" (NNH)

Neonatal hepatitis is a serious disorder of hepatocytes of unknown cause that may or may not be a true inflam-

matory disease. However, the term and its synonym, *giant cell hepatitis*, have been used for a long time in the pediatric literature.

NNH has about the same frequency as biliary atresia and much the same symptoms and laboratory findings. The disease is more prevalent in males with a birth weight less than those with biliary atresia. If all known cholangitic factors and relationships are excluded, about 85% of the patients recover; the other 15% die of chronic liver disease. Of those developing chronic liver disease, 60% have family histories of similar hepatic illnesses.[594] Microscopically, NNH is characterized by transformation of hepatocytes to gigantic multinucleated syncytial cells (Fig. 25-45), which may have eight to 40 nuclei. The hepatocytes are usually hydropic and contain bile pigment. With progression of the disease, the giant multinucleated cells become more numerous, bile stasis is more prominent, and often there are intralobular tubules filled with bile. Rather characteristic is the diffuse formation of intralobular connective tissue that tends to sharply surround the circumscribed giant cells. Excess hepatic hematopoiesis is nearly always present. A majority of patients have an increased amount of iron in the liver cells and usually excess iron in the spleen.[604] There is ordinarily some increase in connective tissue in the periportal spaces, but the bile ducts are usually not as prominent as they are in biliary atresia.

Alpha₁-antitrypsin deficiency

Sixteen percent to 20% of jaundice in neonates previously included in the catchall term *neonatal hepatitis* is related in some way to aberrations in the genetically controlled protease inhibitor (Pi) system. The principal Pi of the body is produced by the liver and known as alpha₁-antitrypsin. There are 26 Pi types or alleles, with new ones added yearly. Each allele is given an alphabetic designation that relates to its relative rate of electrophoretic migration on acid starch gel. There is one additional allele, called null, that in the homozygous state is associated with complete absence of protease inhibitor. About 90% of the population is homozygous for type M. The allele of recognized pathologic importance is Pi, type Z, which occurs in heterozygous form in 3% to 4% of the population and is associated with low serum levels of the Pi. It is the homozygous state of Pi Z that is related to liver disease in neonates, juveniles, and, rarely, adults. Not all patients homozygous for Pi Z have liver disease; some estimates have placed the association as low as 10%.[535] Clinically alpha₁-antitrypsin liver disease may cause jaundice at about 1 month of age. At this stage the liver biopsy usually shows only cholestasis, liver cell swelling, and often diminutive portal tracts (Fig. 25-46). Usually eosinophilic droplets in periportal hepatocytes can be found. The droplets are alpha₁-antitrypsin and can be specifically identified by immunoperoxidase or immunofluorescence methods. Alpha₁-antitrypsin is a glycoprotein and thus is readily demonstrated by periodic acid–Schiff stain after diastase digestion. However, only half the patients with Pi ZZ have the distinctive hepatocellular cytoplasmic droplets larger than 3 μm, a condition highly suggestive of the alpha₁-antitrypsin, and therefore serum phenotyping is essential.[545] Occasionally the bile ducts are greatly hyperplastic, and in some patients, considerable portal fibrosis develops during the first few months of life. In a few patients the disease progresses to cirrhosis within a year, but the majority of patients become asymptomatic before 6 months of age, only to develop signs of chronic liver disease, including varices and hepatic failure, during the late juvenile, adolescent, or young adult periods of life. The cirrhosis that develops is distinctly biliary in type. Parallel layers of collagen surround the cirrhotic nodules, interlobular bile ducts are absent (Fig. 25-47), and copper stains reveal copper-binding protein and copper content that rivals the amount seen in Wilson's disease or primary biliary cirrhosis. The eosinophilic droplets of alpha₁-antitrypsin are in periportal hepatocytes and range in size from barely discernible to an occasional globule that fills the entire cytoplasm.

Ultimately, patients who develop cirrhosis die of hepatic failure or gastrointestinal bleeding from varices. Undoubtedly, in the past, many of the juvenile cirrhotic patients with Pi ZZ were considered to have Wilson's disease. Liver transplantation has been performed successfully in several patients.[567,599] Some patients who have Pi ZZ develop cirrhosis at 50 to 60 years of age without having had an episode of neonatal jaun-

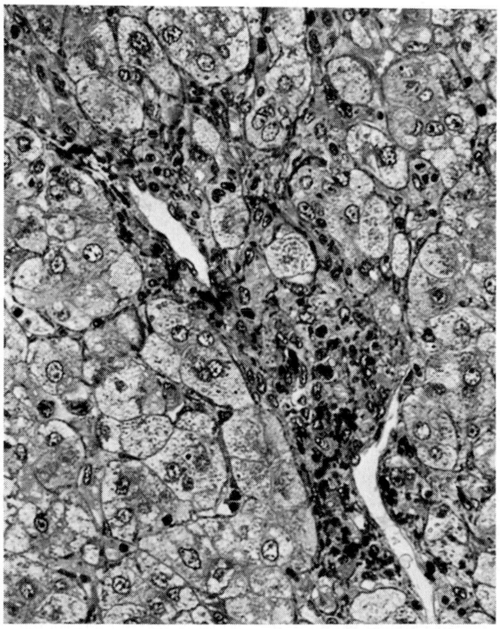

Fig. 25-46. Biliary dysgenesis associated with Pi ZZ phenotype. Notice poorly defined portal area with deficient duct structures.

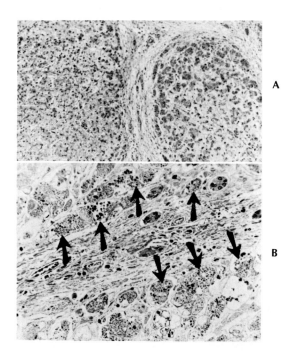

Fig. 25-47. Juvenile cirrhosis in alpha₁-antitrypsin deficiency (Pi ZZ). **A,** Lamellar fibrosis and duct deficiency. **B,** Periseptal hepatocytes filled with glycoprotein droplets *(arrows).*

dice,[618] and others are devoid of liver disease.

The importance of the heterozygous state in disease is unsettled. Many, probably most, patients with MZ do not develop liver disease, but there are numerous case reports of instances of cirrhosis with MZ phenotype and no other recognized basis for liver disease. There is disagreement about whether the coincidence of MZ and cirrhosis is greater than by chance. The number of reported cases of adult cirrhosis associated with heterozygosity of two abnormal Pi types, SZ, seems inordinately high.

Less common causes of jaundice

Among the less common causes of direct-acting hyperbilirubinemia in the first 3 months of life are infections, inborn errors of metabolism, and several other diseases.

In addition to bacterial infections that occur in the perinatal period, gram-negative infections caused by *E. coli*, involving particularly the urinary tract, may cause jaundice.[627] The same is true in hepatic abscesses that complicate sepsis, vessel cannulation, or abdominal surgery.[589] Coxsackie viremia may cause extensive necrosis of the liver and jaundice.[577] Massive necrosis may also occur after echovirus infection.[569]

Another group of infections is now known as the TORCH group, that is, toxoplasmosis, rubella, cytomegalovirus, and herpes.[591] These diseases are discussed in detail in Chapters 6 and 9. Congenital toxoplasmosis in its generalized form may cause hepatomegaly and jaundice.[612] In fatal cases the microscopic findings in the liver are usually nonspecific. Severe extramedullary hematopoiesis is common, as in bile stasis. Small foci of necrosis may be present. The disease may be difficult to diagnose with laboratory tests.[612] Severe hepatitis with cholestasis and giant cell change has been observed in the rubella syndrome.[603] Coagulative necrosis also has been reported.[613] In cytomegalic inclusion disease bile stasis is prominent.[535,592,593] Multinucleated giant cells may be seen, but necrosis of liver cells is variable. When present, the giant intranuclear inclusions in the bile duct epithelium are diagnostic (Fig. 25-48). The hepatic lesions may persist into infancy. As a rule the inclusions are more easily found in the kidney. Cytomegalovirus hepatitis may produce jaundice in the adult.[623]

Herpes simplex infection in the neonate usually occurs on the fourth to seventh days of life and results in high mortality. The disease is acquired during passage through the genital tract in women who are infected. The liver and adrenal gland are most often involved. In the liver there are coagulative necrosis and nuclear inclusions without inflammation.[609] There are two types of nuclear inclusions. One is an amphophilic, glassy body that occupies most of the nucleus. The second is

small, round, and surrounded by a halo. The first of these is the active infectious agent. Transplacental means of infection are rare.

Congenital syphilis still occurs, though in far lower incidence than 50 years ago. It may be manifested as heptosplenomegaly and either a conjugated or an unconjugated hyperbilirubinemia. Fibrosis, cellular injury, and cholestasis are the usual microscopic findings.[624] The presence of the organism and increase in fibrous tissue have been shown by electron microscopy.[541] It has been noted that results of serologic tests on the neonate who has congenital syphilis of the liver may be negative, whereas results of tests on the mother are positive.[606]

Acute viral hepatitis in the neonate as a cause of jaundice is uncommon, though there is a high incidence of transmission of the hepatitis B virus in the perinatal period. Usually the infant does not develop a clinical disorder.[607,608,617] However, there are examples of severe and even fatal cases of hepatitis in infants who have acquired the disease perinatally from infected mothers.[553]

Infants who do not acquire hepatitis from blood transfusions or an infected mother rarely develop hepatitis until they are in contact with many other children, as in nursery school. Hepatitis A acquired at this

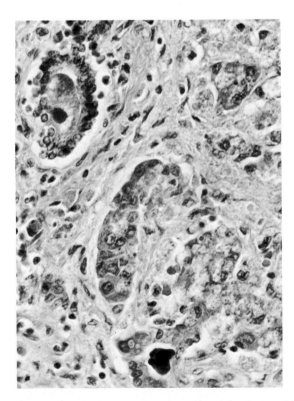

Fig. 25-48. Cytomegalic inclusion body in bile duct epithelial cell at upper left. Cholestasis and liver cell necrosis are evident. Patient had jaundice since birth and died at 2½ months of age.

time results in a mild illness or is asymptomatic. Hepatitis B may follow contact with blood or blood products, saliva, or other infected blood fluids. Infants and children who acquire hepatitis B are more likely to develop chronic active hepatitis B than adults are.

Metabolic defects

Three inborn errors of metabolism cause severe liver disease when left untreated. The first symptom of each is often jaundice. These diseases are galactosemia, fructosemia, and tyrosinemia. All are autosomal recessive disorders in which an important metabolic enzyme is absent. In galactosemia, galactose-1-phosphate uridyltransferase is deficient. This enzyme in normal persons catalyzes formation of uridine diphosphate (UDP)-galactose and glucose-1-phosphate from galactose-1-phosphate and UDP-glucose. The deficiency causes galactose-1-phosphate to accumulate in the lens, liver, brain, and kidneys of infants who receive galactose in their diet. In addition to hepatic disease, the toxic effects of galactose accumulation are noted in the eye, where lenticular opacities may develop quickly, and in the brain, where degeneration and mental retardation may result.[616] The diagnosis of this condition is highly important because the removal of galactose from the diet relieves the symptoms.[548] Recognition of the disease may be delayed for a few months, depending on the symptoms. Various screening methods have been used for its detection.[582,585]

The liver in galactosemia is enlarged and fatty and may become cirrhotic. Microscopically the lobules are large; a moderate to severe degree of fatty change is present, and bile stasis is the rule. The bile plugs are contained within large acini. Often numerous bile ducts entering the periphery of the lobules are likewise filled with bile (Fig. 25-49). An irregular increase in connective tissue widens and lengthens the periportal spaces, sometimes connecting adjacent ones, so that cirrhosis can be diagnosed. The combination of large liver lobules, fatty changes, and bile stasis seems to be characteristic of galactosemia. More rarely in galactosemia, the liver contains an excess of glycogen, with the cytoplasm of the cells being almost water-clear; delicate septa connect the periportal spaces, resulting in a different types of cirrhosis. In both of the foregoing morphologic patterns the terminal hepatic veins are visible and regenerative change seems to be minimal. In children with proved cirrhosis and ascites, proper treatment results in an apparent cessation of the disease process.

In hereditary fructose intolerance, a deficiency of the enzyme fructose-1-phosphate aldolase, which is responsible for catalyzing the hydrolysis of fructose-1-phosphate into glyceraldehyde and dihydroxyacetone phosphate,[555,626] fructose-1-phosphate accumulates in the liver and other organs. The disease becomes manifest

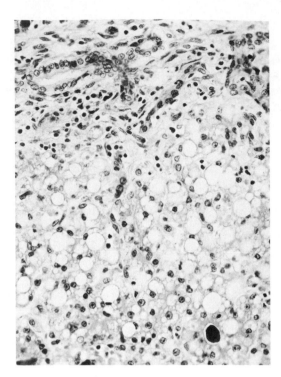

Fig. 25-49. Fatty change, intralobular bile stasis, and some increase of periportal connective tissue are characteristic of galactosemia. Patient was 3-week-old white male infant.

when the infant receives fruit or fruit juice. Vomiting, abdominal pain, excessive sweating, diarrhea, and even coma and convulsions may occur within 30 minutes after ingestion. Hypoglycemia, hypophosphatemia, hypermagnesemia, hyperuricemia, hyperfructosemia, and fructosuria are the most common laboratory findings. Aminoaciduria and other findings of the Fanconi syndrome may occur. All symptoms disappear on the fructose-free diet. Patients who continue to take fructose may develop fibrosis, fatty change, or even cirrhosis of the liver,[597] in addition to hyperbilirubinemia. Tyrosinemia type 1 is apparently caused by deficiency of the enzyme p-hydroxyphenylpyruvic acid oxidase, which converts p-hydroxyphenylpyruvic acid to homogentisic acid. Symptoms may begin during the first month of life, with death resulting from liver failure within 6 to 8 months.[588] More often the course is chronic, with later onset of jaundice, ascites, hypoglycemia, hypoprothrombinemia, and finally evidence of cirrhosis.[562,570] There are tyrosinemia,, multiple renal tubular defects, and increased urinary excretion of phenolic acids.[558] On microscopic examination, regeneration, fatty change, and fibrosis are noted. Liver cell carcinoma may arise in the course of the disease.[621] The management of tyrosinemia type 1 is difficult. In addition to the restriction of tyrosine and phenylalanine, the restriction of methionine has now been added.[588]

A group of familial intrahepatic cholestatic syndromes

has been identified based on clinical features, and as specific metabolic defects are identified for the syndrome, it is then separately classified, such as Zellweger's cerebrohepatorenal syndrome.[602] These syndromes are reported worldwide and may be given local names by country or population. As the reports increased in number over the years, it was recognized that different reports identified the same entity, and thus classification has been muddled. Several (but not all) major categories seem to be Alagille's syndrome (two types), Byler's syndrome, North American Indian cholestasis, and benign recurrent intrahepatic cholestasis (often not first recognized in childhood). Of this group, Alagille's syndrome may present with neonatal cholestasis; the others are discussed later. The syndromic form of Alagille's syndrome has typical facies, heart anomaly, pulmonary artery stenosis (peripheral), eye defects, vertebral body defects, and other organ malfunction. There is a similar hepatic form without extrahepatic changes (nonsyndromic type). Alagille's syndrome also called arteriohepatic dysplasia has as the classic hepatic change a "paucity of intrahepatic bile ducts," which is difficult to appreciate on needle biopsy, but difficulty in identifying well-developed open bile ducts and the presence of small distorted neoducts are hallmarks. The infants have pruritus and xanthomas at 3 to 6 months of age and then resolution of symptoms. A period of normal development followed by progressive hepatic disease, including hepatocellular carcinoma, may occur.

Parenteral nutrition (PN) in sick infants is often associated with development of severe cholestasis, especially in premature babies. Jaundice is noted, usually within 3 weeks after PN is initiated. Biopsy material discloses severe cholestasis accompanied by inflammation along the portal tracts, consisting of round cells, neutrophils, portal fibrosis, and bile duct proliferation. After cessation of PN the jaundice clears, but biopsies months later often disclose some residual fibrosis and cholestasis.[549] In infants who received total parenteral nutrition (TPN) for more than 300 days, severe hepatic fibrosis and fatal liver failure have been reported.[598] The effect of prolonged fasting as an etiologic factor in the production of hepatobiliary dysfunction has been suggested.[537]

Liver diseases of postneonatal infancy

The frequency of liver disease with onset in infants past 3 months of age, in children, and in juveniles is less than in the younger age group, though some of the diseases that start in the early months may continue as chronic liver disease and eventually develop into cirrhosis. These include the more common diseases already described. There are several acute or chronic diseases that begin or become manifest in the older pediatric group. Among these are certain metabolic disorders, anatomic abnormalities, intrahepatic cholestasis

of childhood (familial cholestasis), and a miscellaneous group.

Among the metabolic disorders, many of which are familial, are those caused by excess glycogen storage, Niemann-Pick and Gaucher's diseases, Wilson's disease, hemochromatosis, and gangliosidosis. Glycogenosis has been defined as any condition in which the glycogen concentration of a tissue is increased.[587] Normally the glycogen concentration in the liver should not exceed 6% of the net weight. Glycogen storage disease of the liver is now divided into types I to X, each with its specific enzyme defect. hepatic fibrous septa only have been observed in types III, VI, IX, and X, whereas type IV may progress to cirrhosis that is fatal, usually in childhood. In type IV, intracellular hyaline deposits may be present in the periportal areas and are difficult to distinguish from alpha₁-antitrypsin deficiency.[587] In type I the liver is enlarged and fatty, but chronic changes do not occur. A similar change is noted in type III. Clinical, laboratory, and morphologic studies are helpful, but the final diagnosis rests on quantitative biochemical analysis of the tissue.[587] The absence of glycogen synthase leads to inadequate glycogen formation and severe fatty change in the liver.

In Niemann-Pick disease there is an accumulation of sphingomyelin and other lipids in the body that particularly affects the liver and spleen and is accompanied by severe mental retardation. Five clinical categories have been recognized and are designated types A to E. Jaundice and severe liver changes, in both the hepatic reticuloendothelial system and the hepatocytes, have been noted. A perivenular distribution of Kupffer cell storage has also been described.[551]

Gaucher's disease is an inherited disorder in which there is a deficiency of the lysosomal enzyme, glucocerebrosidase.[562] Gaucher's cells are commonly present in the liver, but symptoms of liver disease are rare, though fibrosis associated with Gaucher's cells may lead to scarring and eventually to a nodular liver. Liver changes may be observed in some of the mucopolysaccharidoses.[562] In the Hurler-Hunter syndrome, fibrosis and cirrhosis may occur, usually in older children and adults. In Hurler's syndrome (gargoylism) there is an excess of dermatan sulfate and heparan sulfate in the urine and tissues, along with a decrease of alpha-galactosidase in the tissues. G_{M1} gangliosidosis is a genetically determined deficiency of alpha-galactosidase. Light and electron microscopy disclose many vacuoles in the hepatocytes and Kupffer cells. These have a characteristic ultrastructural appearance.[596] Wilson's disease and hemochromatosis are also inheritable disorders that may become manifest in childhood. These are discussed elsewhere in this chapter.

Two anatomic abnormalities, cystic fibrosis and congenital hepatic fibrosis, may become symptomatic or cause liver disease in infants and children. In cystic fibrosis the liver may contain focal areas of fibrosis associated with dilated bile ducts containing eosinophilic casts. Prolonged jaundice with cholestasis may be observed in neonates.[619] In more advanced states of liver disease a true cirrhosis may develop with formation of nodules of variable sizes. Portal venous hypertension may result.

Congenital hepatic fibrosis is a variant of polycystic disease[572]; microcysts are present in the dense fibrous tissue that surrounds the lobules. These are sometimes associated with tubular ectasia or polycystic disease of the kidney. The disease was first recognized in children[576] but may not become symptomatic until adulthood.[590] Although results of liver function tests are normal, portal hypertension is the predominating symptom. Portacaval shunts are usually successful, and hepatic encephalopathy does not develop.[531] Cholangitis may be a complication. The disease is characterized by an excessive amount of dense connective tissue that connects one portal tract with another and includes supernumerary small bile ducts.

The term *juvenile cirrhosis* is sometimes used for patients in this particular age group. With careful study, most of these cases can be put in one of the various etiologic types of cirrhosis already described, particularly alpha-1-antitrypsin deficiency, Wilson's disease, or chronic active hepatitis of unknown cause.

In addition to the intrahepatic cholestatic diseases, such as galactosemia and alpha$_1$-antitrypsin deficiency, there is a group of patients in whom the cause of liver disease is unknown. These include a broad spectrum of diseases that vary from benign recurrent jaundice to fatal familial cholestasis or Byler's disease. Fatal intrahepatic cholestasis may be familial or may occur sporadically. The familial form, known as Byler's disease, is named for the Byler family, whose seven children had the disease.[546] Usually the disease begins in the first few months of life and is characterized by jaundice, pruritus, and failure to thrive. The disease progresses rapidly or slowly over a period of months or years; ultimately, most of the patients die of a biliary type of cirrhosis. Biopsy specimens performed early in the disease disclose intense cholestasis. Bile acid studies show high serum levels and a very low content in the duodenum, but these are also noted in other forms of cholestasis. In the sporadic form several unusual features have been observed. Kayser-Fleischer–like rings may develop in the eyes.[571] Studies of copper metabolism show high plasma copper concentration and increased urinary copper excretion, in contrast to the finding in patients with Wilson's disease. The early age of onset, the predominantly cholestatic clinical picture, and familial history all aid in diagnosis.[552]

A severe familial cholestasis has been noted in a group of North American Indian children, 90% of whom developed cirrhosis. Neonatal hepatitis was documented in the majority of the cases. Electron microscopic studies disclosed evidence of microfilament dysfunction of the hepatocytes.[620] In yet another group of patients, familial or sporadic cirrhosis may occur that is not characterized by jaundice. No specific etiologic agent has been identified.[578] The prognosis in some of these patients is yet to be determined; however, biopsy findings have disclosed advanced cirrhosis of the postnecrotic type. In other familial types of cirrhosis, Kayser-Fleischer rings have been noted.[573]

Miscellaneous diseases

Indian childhood cirrhosis (ICC) is a poorly defined entity with many authors applying different criteria.[538] With the greater immigration of Indian people, the disease will likely be present in many areas of the world and not be restricted to India. Review of previous autopsy material indicates that ICC occurs in Caucasian children in the United States. True ICC is not cirrhosis as currently defined because regenerative nodules are not typical.[538] However, the disease is typical of young children (12 to 36 months of age), with hepatomegaly and even greater splenomegaly and death within 3 to 33 months. There is abundant orcein-positive deposits in hepatocytes, a moderate fatty change, and usually abundant alcoholic hyaline bodies. Whereas the histologic and clinical criteria of ICC are not uniformly adopted, identification of a cause has also been without agreement. However, the resemblance to alcoholic hepatitis is remarkable.

In the cerebrohepatorenal syndrome (Zellweger's syndrome) there are both a metabolic disorder and congenital anomalies. Jaundice with conjugated hyperbilirubinemia is often present in the first 2 weeks of life and is followed by progressive liver disease. Diffuse fibrosis of the lobules is characteristic of the early disease. With electron microscopy, mitochondrial defects that may be related to abnormal metabolism of the bile acids have been noted. Failure to oxidize the cholesterol side chain to form C-24 bile acids apparently leads to increased amounts of trihydroxycoprostanic acid, varanic acid, and dihydroxycoprostanic acid.[586]

In Reye's syndrome there is acute encephalopathy with fatty degeneration of the viscera, chiefly the liver.[601] The disease begins as an acute illness in a previously healthy infant or child and is characterized by vomiting that is usually followed within 24 hours by lethargy, stupor, convulsions, and coma. Death or recovery occurs within a few days. A wide range of laboratory findings may be present. Among these are hypoglycemia, hyperammonemia, hypertransaminasemia, and a prolonged prothrombin time. Liver biopsies performed within 48 hours usually disclose a fine foamy type of fatty change without nuclear displacement that is best seen in frozen sections stained for lipids. The hepatic lesion has been subdivided into three types, depending on the degree of glycogen deficiency: mild, type 1; moderate, type 2; and total, type 3.[540] The degree of depletion seems to correlate well with the occurrence of hypoglycemia, the severity of encephalopathy, and the mortality. The depletion of activity of several mitochondrial enzymes during the period of rapid lipid accumulation and low hepatic (manganese) content, coupled with the rarefied mitochondrial matrix and enlarged ameboid mitochondria seen on electron microscopy, is suggestive of a relationship that exists between transient mitochondrial dysfunction and the fatty change, glycogen depletion, hypoglycemia, and hyperammonemia.[540] Reye's syndrome has now been associated with some 16 groups of viruses, particularly influenza A and B,[584] and several other possible etiologic agents.[539,544,610,614] Aspirin may be involved in the etiology of Reye's syndrome. The patients are not jaundiced. At autopsy the liver is usually yellow, and there is cerebral edema. A dramatic decline in the number of patients with Reye's syndrome has occurred in the 1980s, and no definite reason has been advanced.[564]

Lastly, consideration must be given to a physical finding, hepatomegaly, and to a serious physiologic disorder, hypoglycemia. In the pediatric group symptomless hepatomegaly may be noted at any age. Often this solitary finding is caused by a neoplasm or cyst.

Hypoglycemia in the neonate, as well as in infants and children, deserves special consideration because its recognition and treatment may be lifesaving. Among the causes of hypoglycemia in the neonate are the hepatic enzyme deficiencies[595] such as glycogen-storage disease, fructose intolerance, galactosemia, glycogen synthase deficiency, and fructose 16-diphosphatase deficiency. Tyrosinemia and erythroblastosis may also be associated with hypoglycemia. In many of these diseases, jaundice is present. Neonatal cholestasis and hypoglycemia associated with endocrine disorders are possibly caused by cortisol deficiency.[579] Hypoglycemia must be defined relative to infant age. The following levels are considered to be hypoglycemic: (1) whole blood glucose concentrations less than 20 mg/dl (25 mg/dl of serum or plasma) in the preterm, low–birth weight infant; (2) whole blood glucose values less than 30 mg/dl (35 mg/dl of serum) from birth to 72 hours of age; and (3) whole blood levels less than 40 mg/dl (46 mg/dl of serum) in the full-sized or full-term infant after 72 hours of age. Prompt diagnosis and treatment are all important.

Hypoglycemia in infancy is comparatively rare but is caused by the same enzyme deficiencies just noted, and in addition, acquired liver diseases, such as hepatitis, cirrhosis, malnutrition with fatty liver,[622] and Reye's syndrome, must be considered.

LESS COMMON LIVER DISEASES
Wilson's disease (hepatolenticular degeneration)

Wilson's disease is a hereditary liver disease transmitted as an autosomal recessive trait. The gene responsible for Wilson's disease has been linked to the esterase D locus on chromosme 13.[657] Interestingly the gene for ceruloplasmin (a serum protein important in the diagnosis) appears to be on chromosome 3. Cirrhosis and neurologic defects first become apparent between late juvenile and young adult ages. In 7.5% of the cases the disease does not become apparent until the third decade, and rare cases have been reported that are not symptomatic until the fourth decade.[705] It is a disease associated with abnormalities in copper metabolism.

The homeostatic role of the liver in copper metabolism has been well established. Both a deficiency and an excess of this element may result in clinical disease. As in the case of iron, the liver is the chief storage organ. In the normal neonate the copper concentration is six to eight times the level in the adult. Within the first 6 months of life the hepatic copper level decreases to that seen in a normal adult, which is about 30 μg of copper per gram of dry tissue. Copper balance is achieved by an X-linked intestinal transport mechanism plus the regulation of copper stores by the liver. About 50% of the average daily intake, 2 to 5 mg, is absorbed into the blood and is loosely bound to albumin; this constitutes about 5% to 10% of the total copper circulating in the plasma. The absorbed copper is quickly cleared by the hepatocytes, in which two thiol-rich cytosol protein fractions are capable of storing the metal. One of these proteins has a higher molecular weight, 30,000 to 40,000 daltons, and has been termed "superoxide dismutase." The lower molecular weight proteins of about 10,000 daltons probably consist of both metallothioneine and nonmetallothioneine. These two protein fractions contain about 80% of the copper in the normal adult liver.[702] The remainder is incorporated into cytochrome c oxidase and ceruloplasmin or is present in lysosomes before being excreted in bile. The latter is the principal means of achieving copper balance, since about 1.5 mg of copper is excreted each day in the bile, bound to a carrier that prevents its reabsorption from the gut. A small portion of hepatic copper, approximately 0.5 to 1 mg daily, is incorporated into ceruloplasmin, a blue copper glycoprotein, and released into the blood.[702] Radioactive studies have shown that this incorporation occurs in the first few hours after absorption. The turnover rate of this copper in ceruloplasmin is high.

In Wilson's disease the patient is in positive copper balance, and excess quantities of copper are stored, first in the liver and eventually in other tissues, especially the brain, cornea, and kidney. The disease occurs in homozygotes who have inherited a pair of autosomal recessive genes, one from each parent. It is estimated that the frequency in heterozygotes is 1 in 200 and in homozygotes, 5 in 1 million,[702] though in one family the frequency was unusually high.[675] In the homozygote several abnormal physiologic phenomena occur, the exact mechanism of which is unclear. Foremost is the failure of the liver to excrete copper in the bile. Other changes measurable in the laboratory consist in an increased storage of copper in the dry liver tissue, about 50 μg/g; serum ceruloplasmin less than 20 μg/dl; and increased urinary copper greater than 50 μg/day. A prominent finding is the presence of Kayser-Fleischer rings. These are areas of brown pigmentation of Descemet's membrane at the limbus of the cornea. Once considered pathognomonic of Wilson's disease, it is now known that Kayser-Fleischer rings may be found on rare occasions in chronic cholestatic disorders, characterized by an excessive copper storage such as primary biliary cirrhosis.[652] See Plate 5, C.

The excess copper in the liver and later in the central nervous system, eyes, kidneys, and other organs leads to symptoms after 6 years of age; 50% of homozygotes have symptoms by 15 years of age.[702] These symptoms cover an extraordinarily wide range, most important being those caused by liver and basal ganglia involvement (Chapter 42). The liver disease may be manifested by symptoms of either acute or chronic liver disease and can be confused with acute viral hepatitis or chronic active hepatitis.[645,697] Occasionally cirrhosis may be diagnosed in an asymptomatic patient. Acute hemolytic anemia may occur during periods of acute accumulation of copper[644] and is an ominous sign. Various stages have been described in the progress of liver disease; however, the sequence probably varies from patient to patient. The earliest microscopic findings consist in fatty change, vacuolization of nuclei, and focal necrosis. In this stage the copper is present in the cytoplasm. In the next stage patients may have histologic changes indicative of chronic active hepatitis with peripheral necrosis. In these there may be stainable copper and atypical lipofuscin in the hepatocytes. Finally, cirrhosis of a nonspecific type, with either large nodules or both large and small nodules, is present, especially in patients dying of liver disease. In this latter stage, Mallory bodies may occur (Fig. 25-50). In the cirrhotic liver there may be sharp differences in the appearance of the hepatocytes from one pseudolobule to another or within the same lobule. This is noted particularly in regard to fatty change and the amount of lipochrome pigmentation. The septa in the cirrhosis of Wilson's disease vary greatly in thickness. Some are rather thin, whereas others are much thicker. These changes often give a nonuniform appearance to the cirrhosis of Wil-

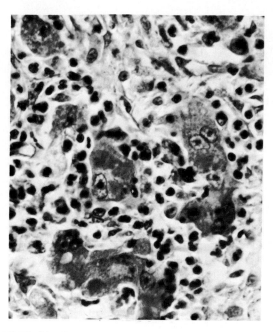

Fig. 25-50. Hyaline necrosis of hepatocytes in Wilson's disease. Abundant neutrophilic and round cell infiltrate in sinusoids.

son's disease. A copper stain is positive in about 90% of the cirrhotic livers, though in the early stage the regenerative nodules may not stain positive for copper. Electron microscopic studies have shown that early in the course of the disease the increase in hepatocytic copper is present in the cytoplasm,[659] where the copper ion is capable of causing episodes of necrosis. These may produce attacks of jaundice and a rise in the serum transaminase levels. Once cirrhosis has occurred, the copper is stored in lysosomes. Occasionally Wilson's disease may manifest biochemical and histologic characteristics that closely simulate those of active hepatitis. The diagnosis is even more difficult if Kayser-Fleischer rings are absent.[697] Prognosis of this pattern in Wilson's disease is frequently poor because it does not respond to D-penicillamine therapy. The use of radioactive copper may be helpful in differentiating the patient with Wilson's disease but who has low-normal ceruloplasmin levels and the histologic features of chronic active hepatitis from the nonwilsonian patient with chronic active hepatitis. It is also useful in distinguishing the homozygote with low-normal ceruloplasmin from the heterozygote. In Wilson's disease there is no positive slope for the labeled copper within 4 to 48 hours after oral administration.[703] These distinctions are of major importance because the homozygotes should be treated with D-penicillamine for the remainder of their life.

Increased storage of hepatic copper also occurs in patients with chronic cholestasis, such as primary biliary cirrhosis,[679] extrahepatic biliary obstruction,[642] intrahepatic cholestasis of childhood (IHCC),[651] cirrhosis of alpha$_1$-antitrypsin, and biliary atresia.[701] In IHCC the hepatic copper levels are equal to those in Wilson's disease. The serum copper level is abnormally elevated, whereas the urinary copper level is normal or very slightly elevated. An increase of hepatic copper may also occur in patients who do not have chronic cholestasis: excess copper has been noted in 30% of patients with alcoholic liver disease.[633] Excess copper has also been reported in livers of patients with chronic active hepatitis[701] and Indian childhood cirrhosis.[681,707] The Bedlington terrier has a copper storage disease that closely simulates Wilson's disease in the humans.[671]

Iron metabolism and liver disease

The liver is a major participant in the metabolism of iron because it stores the metal and also synthesizes transferrin, an iron-binding protein necessary for the transport of iron. Transferrin is responsible for the movement of iron from its absorption in the small bowel to storage in the liver and other tissues and to the most active metabolic area—in the bone marrow. An easily mobilized form of iron is stored as ferritin in the hepatocyte. Ferritin is a large protein molecule composed of 24 subunits that form a shell capable of storing some 4000 atoms of iron. Some 20 or so isoferritins have been identified; these vary from one tissue to another. Subunit analyses indicate that these isoferritins are derived from two or perhaps three subunit types.[647] The origin of serum ferritin is unknown. It does not bind as much iron as tissue ferritin does. In excess iron storage, ferritin apparently is degraded to hemosiderin and stored in lysosomes, known as siderosomes. Hemosiderin is rich in iron and poor in protein. The iron in hemosiderin is difficult to mobilize for transfer to bone marrow. Details of iron metabolism and storage are given in Chapter 1. Normally the body contains 4 to 5 g of iron, most of which is present in hemoglobin. Storage iron, present mostly in the liver, spleen, and bone marrow, has been estimated at some 800 mg in adult men and 300 mg in women in the reproductive age.[683]

Idiopathic hemochromatosis

Iron overload may occur by any one of several mechanisms: (1) inappropriate mucosal absorption of iron; (2) absorption related to chronic anemia, decreased gut iron binding, or increased dietary intake; and (3) parenteral administration of iron, in the form of either blood transfusions or therapeutic injections. In the first category there is an appropriate increase in iron absorption with parenchymal deposition of iron, eventual tissue damage, and functional insufficiency of the organs involved, especially the liver, pancreas, and heart.[683] This disease, known as idiopathic hemochromatosis

(IHC), is an inheritable disorder. Iron overload caused by parenteral administration or blood transfusions is deposited in the reticuloendothelial system and is known as hemosiderosis. However, in the latter, parenchymal cell deposition may eventually occur, and a secondary type of hemochromatosis is seen. It is still not clear whether the parenchymal iron deposition follows the parenteral administration of blood or results from the increased iron absorption from the gut, stimulated by the chronic anemia that was the reason for the transfusion therapy. Excessive dietary intake, as seen in the Bantu of South Africa, usually leads to reticuloendothelial system overload but can also cause hemochromatosis and cirrhosis.

Idiopathic hemochromatosis has been the subject of intense research in recent years. Family studies on the genetic abnormality have shown that IHC is inherited as an autosomal recessive trait. The abnormal homozygote with clinical manifestations of the disease carries two hemochromatosis alleles on chromosome 6 close to the HLA locus. The pattern of transmission of the predisposing alleles in a family has been traced by typing for the A and B alleles of the HLA complex.[632,637,710] In addition to the homozygotes with full expression of the disease, heterozygotes and normal persons have been identified in the pedigree studies.

In the homozygote with IHC there is an increase in iron absorption from early in life that is steady until about 60, at which time approximately 18 g of iron may be present in the liver of men but less in women because of menstrual loss. The mechanism for the unusual absorption is unknown. There is also an increase in hepatic uptake of iron, even when the serum iron is normal in patients with treated hemochromatosis. This occurs whether or not cirrhosis is present.[630] Actually, free iron may be absorbed into the portal vein blood and removed by the liver. The serum ferritin is increased in hemochromatosis, its levels increasing with the increase in iron stores. In normal persons and those with a modest iron overload, each microgram of serum ferritin per liter is equivalent to 8 mg of iron in storage.

The symptomatic homozygous state is usually diagnosed around 50 years of age. The laboratory findings most helpful in diagnosis[637] include an increased serum iron, usually 200 μg/dl (normal is 100 μg/dl); transferrin saturation above 80% (normal is less than 50%, average about 30%); and serum ferritin mean 2099 ng/ml in men and 301 ng/ml in women (normal is 93 in men and 48 in women). The hepatic iron in men with hemochromatosis averages 877 μg/100 mg of wet liver and 478 in women; in normal persons iron levels are less than 29 in men, 20 in women. A major iron load is defined as a transferrin saturation above 79% and hepatic iron concentration above 400 μg/100 mg of wet liver in men and above 250 µg/100 mg in women. A minor iron load is defined as a transferrin saturation greater than 50% or a hepatic iron concentration of 30 to 400 µg/100 mg of wet liver in men and of 20 to 250 µg/100 mg in women.

Early in IHC, there may be little dysfunction of the organs with a heavy iron overload. Recognizing this stage of disease in patients is important because phlebotomy may arrest the course of the disease. In untreated patients the liver becomes cirrhotic, and pancreatic deposition may result in diabetes. Other tissues that frequently have striking iron deposits and associated dysfunction include myocardial fibers, gastric mucosa, endocrine epithelium, and the testes. The classic clinical triad (seen after years of iron accumulation) is hepatomegaly, diabetes, and skin pigmentation. However, the mode of presentation varies greatly. The patient may complain of impotence, easy fatigability, or arthopathy and may have signs of heart failure. The arthropathy involves the second and third metacarpophalangeal joints of each hand.[690,695] Signs or symptoms of hepatic failure or portal hypertension are not the usual initial features. Despite the known diagnostic aids, a delay of several years often occurs before a correct diagnosis of IHC is made.[648] In one series of patients, the mean age at diagnosis of homozygous men was 52 years; for the homozygous woman the mean age was 44.8 years. In the heterozygotes there are no clinical manifestations of iron overload, but biochemical abnormalities may occur. The mean transferrin percentage saturation may reach 51% in men but much less in women.[637] Iron loading in the liver in the heterozygous men may increase sevenfold or eightfold over the normal. Some of these patients, though asymptomatic, have been subjected to phlebotomy until the iron reserves were depleted.

Early in IHC, hemosiderin is present microscopically in all the hepatocytes, but there is some predilection for the periportal areas. The intracytoplasmic iron is usually most prominent around the canaliculi. Kupffer cell iron is insignificant, and fibrosis is absent. With advancement of disease, a variable degree of fibrosis occurs along the portal tracts and within the lobules, leading to well-defined cirrhosis (Fig. 25-51).

Although there is usually some correlation between the amount of iron present and the severity of cirrhosis, occasionally some livers with advanced cirrhosis have less stainable iron than those with poorly developed septa. As the iron increases, the aggregates become larger and cellular detail may be obscured. Masses of hemosiderin are also seen within Kupffer cells, though this does not usually parallel the amount of hemosiderin within the hepatic cells. Focal areas of necrosis may occur, and after healing, such areas are characterized by closely packed macrophages whose cytoplasm contains dense accumulations of hemosiderin. After necrosis, regenerative nodules that have little or no stainable iron

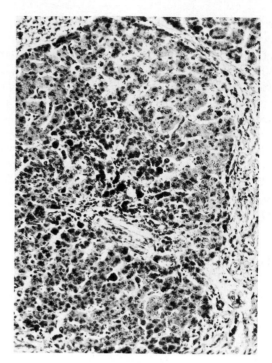

Fig. 25-51. Idiopathic hemochromatosis with pigmentary cirrhosis in 54-year-old white man who died of hepatocellular carcinoma of liver. Liver cells and Kupffer cells contain fine granules of hemosiderin. In area of recent necrosis near center, histiocytes are filled with hemosiderin.

within their cells develop. Fibrous septa connecting the portal spaces are similar to those in alcoholic cirrhosis except for iron-filled macrophages and, occasionally, iron-encrusted connective tissue fibers. An iron-free pigment, hemofuscin, may accumulate within both the fibrous tracts and the hepatic cells. Fatty change is seen in a small proportion of patients but is most prevalent in those who have diabetes mellitus. The latter, when present, is usually mild. The presence of increased iron in sweat glands or melanin in the skin may give the patient a blue-gray or bronzed appearance, hence the name *bronze diabetes* for this complication of hemochromatosis. In many patients with pigmentary cirrhosis there is a long course (10 years or more). Portal hypertension and ascites are not common complications, but primary carcinoma of the liver occurs more often than in most types of cirrhosis, to 25% of patients in some series.[684] Although, the life span of IHC patients has been prolonged by phlebotomy, heptocellular carcinoma still evolves and is the major cause of death.[677]

The question of whether iron produces fibrous scarring is unanswered. There is clinical evidence indicating that iron may be involved in the pathogenesis of the hemochromatosis.[682] In my experience there does not seem to be an association between the density of iron deposition and the degree of fibrosis in both liver and pancreas. The Bantu who stores large amounts of iron absorbed from his diet, however, develops a meager degree of fibrosis. Iron-loading experiments have usually failed to produce significant fibrosis, with notable exceptions.[669]

The mechanism by which iron may damage the liver and pancreas, producing necrosis and fibrosis, is not known. Studies with the electron microscope show that iron is deposited within the lysosomes of the liver cell and, to a lesser extent, in some of the mitochondria. The latter may then degenerate. It is likely that a point is reached at which some of the liver cells populating the lobules are unable to survive with so much of their cytoplasm occupied by iron.[708]

The presence of fibrosis preceding any evidence of cellular injury indicates that, by some mechanism, iron stimulates the synthesis of collagen.[663]

Few electron microscopic studies have been performed on liver biopsy material in idiopathic hemochromatosis.[651,678] In patients with thalassemia major, electron microscopic studies have shown that ferritin molecules are present in the cell sap and lysosomes.[663]

Neonatal hemochromatosis

Neonatal hemochromatosis is an uncommon hepatic condition with severe hepatic iron storage presumably occurring in utero and associated with failure to thrive with death at a few days to weeks of age.[634] Hepatic fibrosis with hepatocellular iron and iron storage in endocrine organs, heart, and renal tubules are the distinctive features.

Secondary hemochromatosis and siderosis

Hepatic iron stores may become greatly increased in certain other disorders. Quantitative analysis generally reveals that this deposition is much less in secondary hemochromatosis; liver iron usually is calculated to be less than 2 g/100 g dry weight of liver when the iron loading is the result of another disorder. Iron overload alone, without cirrhosis of the liver dysfunction, is usually called hemosiderosis of the liver. In addition to idiopathic hemochromatosis, excess iron is found in the following:

1. Any chronically anemic patient, except one having iron deficiency
2. Patients with multiple transfusions, especially more than 100 units (such patients are usually chronically anemic)
3. A small percentage of patients with any type of cirrhosis, especially alcoholic liver disease
4. A small percentage of patients who have undergone a portacaval shunt for portal hypertension
5. Most patients with porphyria cutanea tarda
6. Patients who have excessive dietary intake of iron salts, particularly if protein intake is low

Patients in the last group are principally South African Bantus, who ingest the large quantities of iron in food or drink prepared in iron utensils. This condition has been known as Bantu siderosis. It may lead to increased iron absorption and storage within the reticuloendothelial system and liver.[635] When the iron content of the liver is more than 2% of the dry weight, classical signs of hemochromatosis may develop. The effect of vitamin C deficiency on the deposition of iron in the Bantu is of interest because the excess iron is found in the reticuloendothelial cells of the spleen, liver, and pancreas; the heart and other endocrine glands are usually spared. The nearly normal serum iron level in the Bantus rises when they are given vitamin C. This may possibly have a deleterious effect.[678] In refractory anemias, especially those characterized by accelerated erythropoiesis and defects in normoblast maturation, secondary hemochromatosis and cirrhosis may eventually develop. Iron overload after multiple transfusions has now been studied in some detail.[692] Severe hemosiderosis and focal portal fibrosis are observed, along with a widespread subclinical organ dysfunction similar to that seen in idiopathic hemochromatosis. Total iron content in 100 transfusions is 20 g. In an autopsy series of patients who had thalassemia with and without transfusions, a definite relationship of fibrosis to quantity of iron and age of patient was observed.[687] After portacaval shunt for cirrhosis, increased hepatic iron stores may develop. Occasionally the classical picture of hemochromatosis develops.[680]

Distinction of alcoholic hemosiderosis from early asymptomatic idiopathic hemochromatosis (IHC) may be made by total hepatic iron content, in which case genetic hemochromatosis has greater than 22.3 mg of iron/gram dry weight.[629] Such a distinction is common because 25% of patients with IHC drink alcohol excessively.

Liver diseases in pregnancy

The frequency of jaundice in pregnancy is about 1 in 1500 patients. A few liver diseases occur almost exclusively in pregnancy, though other more common illnesses such as viral hepatitis, choledocholithiasis, and drug jaundice must also be considered. Viral hepatitis occurring during pregnancy seems to be no different from that seen in nonpregnant women. In our series of cases of fatal fulminant hepatitis from 1918 to 1981, two of the patients were pregnant, both in the first trimester, and another patient had recently given birth. This is in sharp contrast to a variety of non-A, non-B hepatitis with fecal-oral transmission, reported from Kashmir, in which both the incidence and the severity of disease were far greater in pregnant women.[667] Other reports of epidemics of hepatitis occurring in the Near East have similarly referred to the high fatality in pregnant women. Unfortunately, there has been little morphologic comparison with fulminant hepatitis seen in the United States. During the nineteenth century, "acute yellow atrophy" of the liver seemed more common in pregnant women; although some would probably now be called fatty liver of pregnancy (see the following), there may have been a disorder akin to that now seen in the Near East. Choledocholithiasis is a rare complication of pregnancy.

Among the disorders peculiar to pregnancy is obstetric cholestasis or recurrent jaundice of the third trimester. The condition is often familial and most often has its onset in the third trimester. It is accompanied by pruritus and tends to recur with succeeding pregnancies. Pruritus of pregnancy without jaundice is a variant. Recent investigations disclose a high perinatal mortality with low–birth weight babies and a higher frequency of postpartum hemorrhage.[665] Obstetric cholestasis is probably caused by an increased level of hormones in susceptible patients, especially since it has been shown that the same patients who develop recurrent jaundice of pregnancy may develop similar cholestasis and symptoms after the use of estrogens, progesterone, or both, as in oral contraceptives.[639,646] The possibility that intrahepatic cholestasis of pregnancy may represent an abnormal reaction to estrogen in predisposed persons is suggested.[685] A biopsy discloses perivenular cholestasis without necrosis. Laboratory findings include a serum bilirubin level of less than 10 mg/dl, a sharp elevation of serum alkaline phosphatase, and only a mild rise in AST levels. An associated rise in plasma bile acids is probably responsible for the pruritus.

Idiopathic fatty liver of pregnancy, initially described in 1940,[700] is a rare disorder that occurs in the third trimester. Although this is usually considered a highly fatal disease, a recent report indicates otherwise.[688] Many cases of fatty liver of pregnancy were reported during the early 1960s, but most of them occurred after the intravenous administration of tetracycline for the treatment of pyelonephritis.[668,688] It became apparent that tetracycline hepatotoxicity in pregnancy produced a fatty liver indistinguishable from the idiopathic type. Both are characterized by epigastric pain, vomiting, jaundice, and symptoms of hepatic and renal failure. The laboratory findings usually consist in hyperbilirubinemia, lactic acidosis, azotemia, hyperamylasemia, and depressed prothrombin activity. The transaminase levels are usually less than 500 units.[668] Those who survive an attack of idiopathic fatty liver of pregnancy may subsequently have an uncomplicated pregnancy.[672] At autopsy the liver is moderately decreased in size and is soft. Fatty change of a fine foamy type is present, the fat being most prominent on the sinusoidal border of the liver cell with the displacement of the granular portion of the cytoplasm to the pericanalicular area. Cholestasis is not prominent. Necrosis is slight, but syncytial change of hepatocytes is prominent in the perivenular zones. Pathologic changes also are seen in the renal tubules, pancreas, and brain. It is probable that tetracycline inhibits the synthesis of the proteins essential to the formation of lipoproteins, the principal form by which fat leaves the liver, thus leading to fatty liver.[668,676] The pathogenesis of the idiopathic fatty liver of pregnancy may be similar. Disseminated intravascular coagulation may complicate acute fatty liver of pregnancy.[636]

Eclampsia only rarely produces hepatic symptoms or clinical liver disease. Only one instance of fatal hepatic failure associated with the liver lesion of eclampsia was found at the Los Angeles County–University of Southern California medical complexes from 1918 to 1981. Jaundice in preeclampsia caused by disseminated intravascular coagulation has been reported.[670] However, hepatic fibrin deposition in preeclampsia that does not produce symptoms is common.[628] Despite the absence of hepatic symptoms, patients who die of eclampsia generally have a mottled discoloration of the liver, with hemorrhagic areas alternating with zones of pale, ischemic necrosis and intact liver (Fig. 25-52). The periportal regions often have fibrin in the sinusoids and are necrotic. The small branches of the portal vein may be thrombosed. Zones of infarction may cover several lobules. Occasionally, such hepatic alterations develop without the convulsions of eclampsia.[631,658] Rarely, dif-

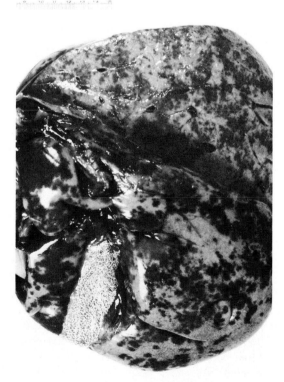

Fig. 25-52. Liver in eclampsia showing hemorrhagic appearance.

fuse coagulative necrosis occurs as a terminal event. Spontaneous rupture of the liver is a rare complication, usually in the third trimester of a multiparous woman who has toxemia, with or without eclampsia. The rupture most often occurs in the right lobe as a complication of subcapsular hematoma.[631,658,661] Rupture of the liver may occur in women taking contraceptive drugs.[656]

Liver disease during pregnancy is often difficult to evaluate because of alterations of laboratory values that are associated with pregnancy. The serum albumin level is ordinarily depressed to a range of 2.8 to 3.7 g/dl (normal is 3.5 to 4.8 g/dl), and the alkaline phosphatase activity often is elevated to as much as twice the upper limits of normal. Most chronic diseases of liver preclude pregnancy, though patients with chronic active viral hepatitis B apparently have no impairment in ability to become pregnant.[696] In nonviral chronic active hepatitis, fertility is apparently reduced, but those pregnancies that do occur may proceed without detriment to the mother provided prednisone treatment is maintained. Babies may be born prematurely, and a higher than normal fetal loss can be expected.[704]

Hepatic injuries

One of the various forms of hepatic injury constitutes the major indication for liver surgery in the United States. About 60% are caused by gunshot wounds, 20% by knife wounds, and 20% by blunt trauma. The mortality is high, between 10% and 20%, hemorrhage being the leading cause of death.[643,650] The liver, because of its size, weight, and soft consistency, is susceptible to blunt injury in high-speed vehicular accidents. The impact of the victim's body colliding with the steering wheel can be particularly harmful to the liver. Blunt injuries most often affect the right lobe, producing lacerations of variable configuration and severity

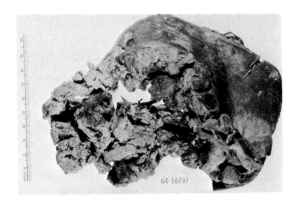

Fig. 25-53. Shattered right lobe of liver after bullet wound. Specimen was surgically resected.

that require surgery. Severe injury, without laceration of the capsule, may cause continued bleeding that results in a subcapsular hematoma and delayed rupture into the abdominal cavity 24 hours or more after the accident. A peritoneal tap may aid in the diagnosis of intrahepatic hemorrhage.[709] In some instances an intrahepatic hematoma ruptures into the biliary tract with resultant hemobilia,[686] in which the patient has gastrointestinal bleeding, often with hematemesis. Gunshot wounds may destroy much of the liver (Fig. 25-53).[674,709]

Liver injuries have been graded, based on the severity of the trauma, including whether bleeding is present.[643] Most traumatic lesions can be handled by simple surgical techniques; however, those with lobal destruction, central hematomas, and hepatic venous or retrohepatic vena caval injury require special techniques. Such severe injuries constitute only 10% of total cases of hepatic trauma. Extensive ligation of the hepatic artery and portal vein branches may be necessary to control hemorrhage. The highest mortality is from gunshot blasts and blunt trauma. Injury to other organs also increases the mortality. In traumatized liver removed at surgery there is a variable amount of hemorrhage and necrosis of the injured parenchyma, often with a neutrophilic exudate. On rare occasions an arteriovenous fistula has been known to occur after liver injury.[653] These are often present for many years before they are diagnosed. They are curable by surgery, but only if treated early. Left untreated, they lead to portal hypertension and ascites. Another rare complication of hepatic trauma is a biliary pleural fistula.[654]

Subcapsular hematomas of small or large size occur occasionally in newborn infants, especially those born prematurely, though they may require surgery or prove fatal. The frequency of unruptured hematomas as incidental findings in newborn premature infants makes it probable that many, or most, reabsorb without rupture. These hematomas may be caused by trauma during birth or may accompany blood dyscrasias, such as erythroblastosis fetalis.

Hereditary hyperbilirubinemia

Several syndromes that are caused by inborn errors in the metabolism of bilirubin have been described.[693,694] These may be divided into two groups. In Crigler-Najjar syndrome and Gilbert's syndrome, there are unconjugated hyperbilirubinemia and defects in the glucuronyl transferase system in the hepatocytes. In the second group, composed of Dubin-Johnson (Sprinz-Nelson) and Rotor's syndromes, conjugation of bilirubin occurs, but secretion is blocked. Some features of these disorders are given in Table 25-6. The Crigler-Najjar syndrome occurs in two forms: type 1 and type 2. In type 1 glucuronyl transferase is absent

Table 25-6. Hereditary hyperbilirubinemias

Syndrome	Age of onset of jaundice	Symptoms and course	Serum bilirubin Range (mg/dl)	Conjugated	Unconjugated	BSP excretion	Physiologic defect	Pathologic condition
Crigler-Najjar								
Type 1	Neonate	Jaundice at birth with or without kernicterus; death in first year of life	>20	—	Increased	Normal	Absence of glucuronyl transferase	Few bile thrombi
Type 2	Neonate	May live past 50 years	<20 mg	—	Increased	Normal	Partial deficiency of glucuronyl transferase	Few bile thrombi
Gilbert's	Birth to middle age (average 18 years)	Jaundice may be precipitated by fasting, fatigue, intermittent infections, alcohol, and stress	<5	Normal	Increased	Normal	Deficiency of glucuronyl transferase	Hypertrophy of smooth endoplasmic reticulum
Dubin-Johnson								
Classic	Most often 15 to 25 years	Pain over liver and hepatomegaly, especially during attacks of jaundice; dyspepsia; problem exists throughout life with fluctuations of jaundice	Normal to 6	Increased	Increased		Retention with late rise after 90 minutes	Pigment in liver, nature unknown
Variants in family members	Mild elevation of serum bilirubin after 10 years	None	>1 in 20% of family	Normal or increased	Normal or increased	Normal		Pigment in many but not related to increased bilirubin
Rotor's	Early life, usually before 20 years	Jaundice fluctuates	Normal to 6	Increased	Increased	Retention with no late rise		None

and hyperbilirubinemia is severe, usually greater than 20 mg/dl; the bile is almost completely colorless and contains only traces of unconjugated bilirubin (UCB). A similar disease occurs in the Gunn rat. In type 2 the patients have a partial deficiency of glucuronyl transferase, probably of the plasma membrane transglucuronidation enzyme. The hyperbilirubinemia is less severe, and the bile contains some bilirubin monoglucuronide. The conjugation defect in the first type is transmitted as an autosomal recessive trait and in the second type as an autosomal dominant characteristic. The jaundice appears in the neonate and persists with high concentrations of unconjugated bilirubin in the blood serum. Patients with type 1 often die in infancy, whereas those with type 2 have been known to survive past 50 years of age without neurologic disorders.[660] Administration of phenobarbital increases the hypertrophy of the smooth endoplasmic reticulum and lowers the serum UCB in type 2 patients only. As in Gilbert's disease, dietary restriction increases the UCB and a normal diet restores the former level. The intravenous administration of glucose after dietary restriction does not lower the UCB.[660]

Gilbert's syndrome (GS) is the most common of the hereditary hyperbilirubinemias.[693] Its frequency may total 2% to 6% of the population, as suggested by measurement of UCB. The frequency of jaundice, which usually begins after puberty, is much lower. The jaundice tends to be intermittent and may be precipitated by fasting. The most useful diagnostic test is the fasting test. Intravenous nicotinic acid is also used; either of these tests usually results in 100% rise in the serum bilirubin. All patients with GS have a defect in glucuronyl transferase, as shown on needle biopsy specimens. The defect has been postulated to be at the plasma membrane, since the bilirubin diglucuronide is decreased in the duodenal bile. However, two subpopulations of patients with GS have been recently reported. In one group endoplasmic reticulum is greatly increased, whereas the other group shows no increase. Patients with hypertrophy of the endoplasmic reticulum show a higher percentage of response to both caloric restriction and nicotinic acid injection.[640,641] No evidence of any defect is noted in the plasma membrane, either biochemically or by electron microscopy. In addition to the difficulty in the excretion of bilirubin that is attributable to the lack of glucuronyl transferase, there may also be a problem in bilirubin uptake in GS.[673]

Included in the second group of hereditary hyperbilirubinemia are the Dubin-Johnson (Sprinz-Nelson) and Rotor's syndromes. The Dubin-Johnson syndrome is characterized by a chronic or intermittent nonhemolytic type of jaundice in which there is an increase of both conjugated[666] and unconjugated bilirubin though mostly of the conjugated type. Glucuronide formation is presumed to be normal, but the hepatocytes have difficulty secreting bilirubin. Similarly the secretion of bromosulfophthalein and iopanoic acid is affected, and so there is BSP retention and the gallbladder cannot be viewed roentgenographically. Most helpful in diagnosis is the abnormal excretion of coproporphyrin isomers in the urine. Isomer I is increased and isomer III is decreased.[667a] The parenchymal cells, especially in the perivenular zone 3, contain large granules of lipochrome pigment (Fig. 25-54), often in such amounts that the liver is black. The electron spin resonance study of this pigment indicates that it is not melanin.[706] It is excreted in the urine in large amounts in patients with Dubin-Johnson syndrome who have acute viral hepatitis. During this time it disappears from the liver but reappears after recovery. The pigment is located within lysosomes.[698] A similar disease is seen in a Corriedale sheep mutant.[638] The disease in the human is inherited as an autosomal recessive trait with a high frequency of consanguinity of parents.[649] Improvement in the handling of bilirubin and bromosulfophthalein is noted in some patients after the use of phenobarbital, an enzyme inducer.[699]

In Rotor's syndrome there is likewise an increase in both conjugated and unconjugated serum bilirubin but no pigmentation of the liver cells. There is bromosul-

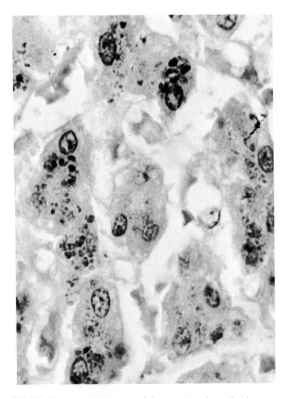

Fig. 25-54. Large masses of intracytoplasmic brown pigment in Dubin-Johnson syndrome.

fophthalein retention but a normal view of the gallbladder. It has been suggested that Rotor's syndrome is a variant of the Dubin-Johnson syndrome.

CIRCULATORY DISTURBANCES
Hypoxic necrosis

Any circulatory disorder that results in prolonged hypoxia may cause recognizable pathologic changes in the liver. The damage may be acute or chronic in nature, depending on the underlying disease responsible for the lack of oxygen. For example, the hypotension of shock may produce perivenular necrosis, whereas

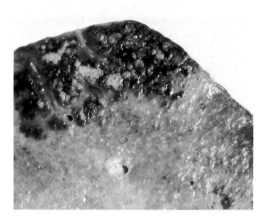

Fig. 25-55. Anoxic necrosis of liver in a patient with alcoholic cirrhosis and fatal hemorrhage from a duodenal ulcer.

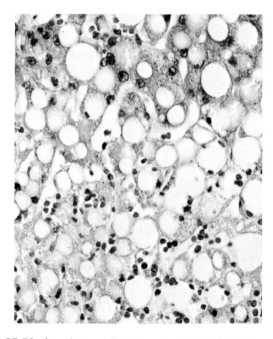

Fig. 25-56. Anoxic centrilobular necrosis in fatty liver of alcoholic patient who was in shock after variceal bleeding.

chronic heart failure often results in perivenular atrophy and occasionally fibrosis. The acute changes may be observed in a liver that was previously normal, or the changes may be superimposed on chronic passive congestion or cirrhosis. Trauma, hemorrhage, heart failure, and endotoxic shock resulting from septicemia are the most common causes.[715] Normally, endotoxins in portal blood are removed in the liver.[734] Shock lasting longer than 24 hours usually is associated with liver cell necrosis.[715] In a study of 1000 patients with cardiac dysfunction, perivenular necrosis was associated with shock and with other sequelae of arterial hypotension, including acute tubular necrosis of the kidney and corticomedullary junction necrosis of the adrenal.[712] Left-sided congestive heart failure apparently was not a factor. In the same study chronic passive congestion of the liver without necrosis was associated with right-sided heart failure and other conditions associated with elevated systemic venous pressure.[712] Other studies indicate that perivenular necrosis may complicate severe heart disease and cardiogenic shock resulting from heart failure, whether it is right sided, left sided, or both. Occasionally, hypoxic necrosis in the absence of any demonstrable hypotension may be seen. Jaundice is rare but does occur in endotoxic shock and in cardiac conditions. When anoxic necrosis is associated with a pronounced increase of transaminase, it may be confused with acute viral hepatitis.[719]

In noncirrhotic individuals hypoxic perivenular necrosis usually has a uniform distribution involving about one half the perivenular area. Grossly the areas of necrosis may or may not be recognized, but often the perivenular zones have a characteristic dull yellow to yellow-brown appearance. Microscopically coagulative necrosis is apparent with intensely acidophilic hepatocytes whose nuclei stain poorly or have disappeared. Neutrophils may be abundant, especially around the periphery of the necrotic zones. The degree of centrilobular hyperemia varies greatly; it may be so extreme that pools of blood fill the necrotic area. A distinctive perivenular hepatic lesion, characterized by hepatic cords filled with erythrocytes, has been described in patients with heart failure.[735] In some instances of hypoxic perivenular necrosis, a narrow rim of intact hepatocytes remains around the terminal venules. Although hypoxic necrosis is predominantly perivenular, the midzonal area is often affected. The necrotic cells slowly disappear, and in biopsy specimens taken in the healing stage, only dilated sinusoids and pigmented macrophages are seen, a histologic change difficult to distinguish from other types of healing centrilobular zonal necrosis.

The cirrhotic liver is particularly prone to hypoxic pseudolobular necrosis when there is bleeding from varices. The large pseudolobules of cirrhosis are rrobably poorly oxygenated as a result of an abnormal inflow and outflow pattern. Furthermore, much of the portal vein blood may be shunted around the liver, and so a fall in hepatic artery pressure during shock would lead rapidly to hypoxic necrosis. The areas of necrosis are often large and pale yellow-white and may be surrounded by a thin zone of hemorrhage (Fig. 25-55). Portions or entire pseudolobules may be involved by hypoxic necrosis (Fig. 25-56). It is likely that some of the depressed scars seen in the liver of cirrhotic patients who have bled from varices in the past may be of hypoxic origin.

Passive hyperemia and cardiac cirrhosis

Passive hyperemia of the liver is most often the result of cardiac disease with congestive failure, but also may result from compression and obstruction of the inferior vena cava or obstructions of the pulmonary circulation, leading to right-sided cardiac failure. Increased pressure in the venous system affects the liver severely because of the short distance between the point of entry of hepatic veins into the vena cava and the entry of the latter into the right auricle. Because the liver cells are particularly sensitive to hypoxia, the decreased oxygen content of the hepatic blood and the diminished flow in congestive failure are probably responsible for much of the histologic change that is observed.

In the early stages of passive congestion dilatation of only terminal hepatic veins and sinusoids is seen. Atrophy and disappearance of liver cells later lead to larger pools of blood in the dilated channels. Fragments of former sinusoid walls remain, but the normal architectural arrangement around the central vein tends to disappear. Often a correlation is lacking between the clinical course and severity of atrophy. When the perivenular one third to one half of the lobule has undergone atrophy, fatty change of the remaining liver cells near the margin is often present and is responsible for the gross "nutmeg" appearance (Fig. 25-57). However, in many instances the pale peripheral lobular zones do not contain fat vacuoles. The reason for their pallor is not apparent. An increase of fibrous tissue may ensue coincidentally with the perivenular atrophy.[756] Occasionally, especially in patients with tricuspid valvular disease, fibrosis links the perivenular areas together, and a diagnosis of cardiac cirrhosis may be made (Fig. 25-58). It has been suggested that perivenular fibrosis and cardiac cirrhosis may follow repeated acute attacks of hypoxic necrosis.[769] This remains to be proved by the use of repeated needle biopsies.

Portal fibrosis with communicating septa to the central fibrous areas is rare but does occur. Hyperplasia of the peripheral portions of the lobules is occasionally seen, sometimes with cardiac cirrhosis.

Grossly the liver in cardiac cirrhosis is of normal or

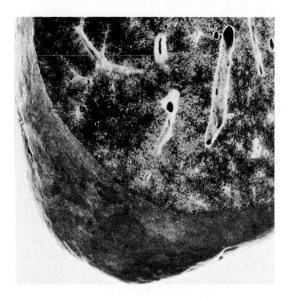

Fig. 25-57. "Nutmeg liver" in chronic passive congestion of liver.

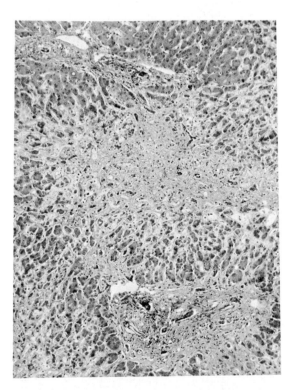

Fig. 25-58. Severe perivenular fibrosis (cardiac cirrhosis) in patient with tricuspid stenosis and chronic heart failure.

slightly reduced size, firm, and dark red-brown or purple-red. The surface is only slightly nodular, and the capsule is thickened. The cut surface shows a mottling of gray or yellow-gray areas separated by brown-red zones of variable size and shape. The hepatic veins are uniformly dilated, sometimes strikingly so, and their walls are thickened. Ill-defined nodules may be present in proximity to the portal tracts. Whether true cirrhosis of congestive origin exists is questionable. A small percentage of patients with long-standing congestive failure do have esophageal varices, but these rarely bleed.[739] In my experience the wedged hepatic vein pressure is not elevated in patients with congestive failure.

Vascular diseases—infarction

Several pathologic entities may affect the blood vessels of the liver, often producing clinical symptoms. Most of these diseases can be diagnosed by angiography. The diseases of the hepatic artery include arteriosclerosis, embolism, aneurysm, polyarteritis nodosa, and hepatoportal arteriovenous fistula.

Infarction of the liver is rare; most cases result from obstruction of the hepatic artery or some of its branches by arteriosclerosis or aneurysms, as well as by bland or septic emboli from the heart.[758] Obstruction of the proper hepatic artery beyond the gastroduodenal and right gastric arteries is most likely to result in infarction. Ligature proximal to the latter arteries is well tolerated because of retrograde flow of blood through the right gastric artery from its anastomoses. Ligature of the hepatic artery is sometimes accidental but also may be necessary in treating severe trauma to the liver. Polyarteritis nodosa is a rare cause of multiple infarcts (Fig. 25-59). Thickening of the walls of hepatic arteries

has been observed in women taking oral contraceptives[771] and in orthotopic transplants.

Hepatoportal arteriovenous fistulas may occur after trauma or biopsy.[750,767] Large fistulas necessitate obliteration either by surgical means or by embolization to prevent portal hypertension. Smaller fistulas may close spontaneously or do not require treatment. There are anastomoses between the arteries supplying hepatocellular carcinoma (HCC) and the branches of the portal veins in a high percentage of cases. These shunts especially occur because of the tendency of HCC to grow into branches of the portal vein carrying along its arterial supply.[711,746,750] Most hepatic artery aneurysms occur in the extrahepatic portion; however, mycotic aneurysms resulting from bacterial endocarditis or sepsis have been reported. Other causes include arteriosclerosis and trauma.[727]

Occlusion of the portal vein or one or more of its branches usually results from another disease (Fig. 25-60), such as cirrhosis of the liver, idiopathic portal hypertension, pancreatitis, hepatocellular carcinoma, carcinoma of the pancreas that grows into the intrahepatic portal veins, or pylephlebitis that follows abdominal suppuration or umbilical infection of the newborn infant. Among cirrhotic patients undergoing decompressive procedures for variceal bleeding, approximately 20% have portal vein thrombosis.[757] In these patients the mortality is higher because of rebleeding. Intrahepatic obstruction of the portal vein or one of the major branches usually causes only the atrophic red infarct of

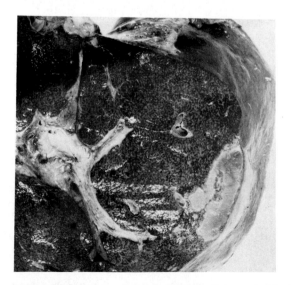

Fig. 25-59. Subcapsular infarct attributed to polyarteritis nodosa.

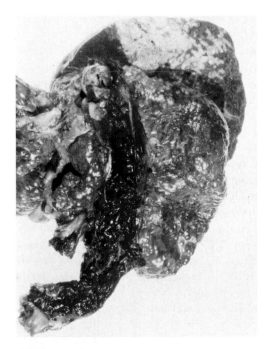

Fig. 25-60. Cirrhosis and thrombosis of portal vein. (Courtesy Dr. G. Lyman Duff.)

Zahn (Fig. 25-61), a discolored zone that does not show necrosis on microscopic examination. Occasionally thrombosis or neoplastic invasion of the trunk of the portal vein causes areas of necrosis in the liver. True infarcts may also follow thrombosis of both hepatic and portal veins.[725]

In an adult, gas in branches of the portal veins noted on x-ray examination is a sign of serious abdominal disease and necessitates surgery, except in patients with chronic ulcerative colitis.[738]

Idiopathic portal hypertension

Idiopathic portal hypertension is a term used for a syndrome first described by Banti.[728] The syndrome is characterized by esophageal varices, hypersplenism, and portal hypertension but no cirrhosis. The disease is more common in India[717] and Japan[733] than in the United States. In the United States most patients first seek medical care for bleeding esophageal varices, at which time splenomegaly and mild pancytopenia are noted. Hepatic function is normal, at least initially.

Grossly the liver surface is smooth, the edges are blunted, and the parenchyma is slightly firmer than normal. Microscopically the relationship between terminal hepatic venules and portal areas is inconstant. Two or more outflow venules are often found in a lobule. The portal area is widened within an intact limiting plate, and there are increased numbers of dilated, thin-walled angiomatous structures. The major intrahepatic portal veins have sclerotic walls (Fig. 25-62). As the dis-

ease progresses, collagen becomes more dense in the portal areas and may extend beyond the confines of the limiting plates to adjacent portal areas. The terminal portal vein radicles may become thickened. The end stage of idiopathic portal hypertension is a fibrotic, shrunken liver without regenerative nodules.

Both the pathogenesis and the cause of idiopathic portal hypertension are unknown. There is general agreement that increased portal vein flow from an enlarged spleen could not produce portal pressure levels equivalent to those found in this disorder. Small segments of occlusion or narrowing have been demonstrated in the intrahepatic portal vein radicals,[716,744] but similar portal vein lesions were also found in incidental autopsy findings in signficant numbers of patients who had no signs of portal hypertension.[768] Sclerosis and thickening of portal vein walls have also been described, but it is unclear whether thrombosis of diverse cause or phlebosclerosis is the pathogenic mechanism in such patients. The possibility of aberrant hepatic artery–portal vein communication has not been thoroughly explored. The histolic changes of idiopathic portal hypertension are similar to the changes in the livers of patients who have acquired an arterioportal fistula and consequent portal hypertension.[721] Abnormalities in hepatic veins that include unusual anastomoses by way of capsular veins to adjacent hepatic vein segments have been reported.[751]

Several etiologic factors and associations have been proposed, including induction of portal venular scle-

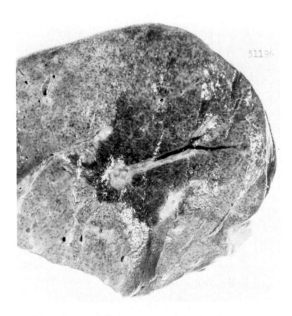

Fig. 25-61. Infarct of Zahn, area of dusky hyperemia attributed to thrombosis of branch of portal vein.

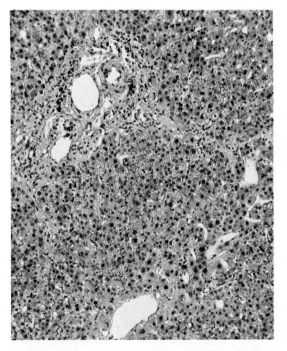

Fig. 25-62. Idiopathic portal hypertension with large vessels and increase of connective tissue in portal areas. Terminal hepatic veins are enlarged and prominent.

rosis by chronic inflammatory reaction or hepatitis, chronic arsenic exposure (a possible cause in India),[720] chronic exposure to vinyl chloride or polyvinylchloride,[752,766] and even cytomegalovirus infection.[722] The disease has also been reported after renal transplantation.[749]

Some patients with the foregoing findings have thrombotic or sclerotic occlusion of the extrahepatic portal vein. This occlusion is considered by many investigators to be the cause of extrahepatic portal hypertension, whereas others[742] have suggested that the portal vein occlusion occurs after idiopathic portal hypertension, just as it occasionally occurs after portal hypertension associated with cirrhosis.

Hepatic veins

The blood from the liver drains into the inferior vena cava via three large venous trunks—the right, middle, and left—plus some direct branches, chiefly from the caudata lobe.[748] Although trauma is the most common disorder affecting the veins, often necessitating surgery, there are two rather rare, intrinsic diseases that may involve the hepatic veins. One of these is hepatic vein thrombosis (HVT), which affects the larger trunks and is known clinically as the Budd-Chiari syndrome (BCS). The other, veno-occlusive disease (VOD), is a specific entity that affects the terminal hepatic and sublobular veins. This disorder most often follows the ingestion of one of the pyrrolizidine alkaloids[740] present in a wide variety of plants in many parts of the world.

Budd-Chiari syndrome

In the Budd-Chiari syndrome obstruction to the flow of blood usually occurs slowly and, over a period of weeks or months, ascites and a large tender liver become manifest. However, a few patients may have an acute onset with abdominal pain and a rapid accumulation of ascites. Portal hypertension, esophageal varices, and hematemesis commonly occur late in the course of the disease. When the vena cava is occluded, collateral veins may be noted along the anterio and posterior thorax.

Among the etiologic factors that have been implicated are polycythemia vera,[732] paroxysmal nocturnal hemoglobinuria (PNH),[737] oral contraceptives,[736] pregnancy,[764] neoplasms, chemotherapy,[713] graft-versus-host reaction,[714,760] radiation,[724] familial immune deficiency,[741] and membranes across or sclerosis of inferior vena cava near the mouths of the hepatic veins.[747] However, in approximately half of the patients with BCS, there is no recognizable etiologic factor. Polycythemia vera and PNH are among the most common causes of BCS when a cause can be identified. PNH is particularly likely to have an acute onset.[737] Although there are many reports of HVT after use of oral contraceptives, whether there is a real increase of the disease in women of childbearing age might be questioned.

In BCS two diagnostic tests have been found useful[737]: the liver scan showing the hepatic and splenic enlargement, along with an increased uptake in the caudate lobe,[729] and percutaneous hepatography that often shows the site and nature of the outflow block. The pathology in BCS depends on the duration of the disease and to a lesser extent on the cause. An early biopsy discloses severe perivenular congestion, a variable degree of necrosis, and fibrin thrombi in terminal hepatic venules. Erythrocytes are often present in the space of Disse and between the hepatocytes. In patients with MOVC (see below), perivenular congestion is absent in most of the biopsy specimens and if present may indicate fibrosis related to alcoholic injury.[754] Atrophy and fibrosis of the liver, along with closure of vessels, is evident later. In autopsy material there are both thrombosis and sclerosis of the larger venous trunks. Many become fibrotic, but recanalization is not prominent. Atrophy of the liver parenchyma may be extensive, but cholestasis is not noted. Since the blood from the caudate lobe is drained by several small veins directly into the inferior vena cava, this lobe is often uninvolved or less involved than the main right and left lobe. Thus as the remainder of the liver undergoes atrophy in BCS, the caudate lobe becomes enlarged because of hyperplasia. This may be sufficient to impinge on the inferior vena cava, causing venous collaterals to form.[745,765] The prognosis is poor in patients with hepatic venous thrombosis. More than 50% die within a few months. Side-to-side portacaval shunt has been used in the treatment of BCS.[753]

Membranous obstruction of the inferior vena cava (MOVC) may produce a second and different type of BCS that is associated with signs and symptoms of inferior vena cava hypertension. These membranes affect both the inferior vena cava and the hepatic veins in some 72% of the cases. In the remainder the obstruction may be only of the inferior vena cava or only of the hepatic veins.[747] Although the membrane may be thin, usually it is a sclerotic segment of vena cava just above the diaphragm. Symptoms usually develop slowly over a period of years, and surgery is often successful.[723] Since hepatic vein thrombosis may occur late in the disease, early diagnosis and treatment are important. The disease has been reported mostly from Japan, but the occurrence is far greater in blacks in South Africa and is associated with hepatocellular carcinoma in 47.5% of cases.[761] The diagnosis is made with cavogram.

Veno-occlusive disease

Veno-occlusive disease (VOD) occurs in widespread locations throughout the world and is caused by one or more of the pyrrolizidine alkaloids. The disease also produces fatalities among livestock. In the West Indies, both children and adults who have ingested "bush tea" made from boiling the leaves of foliage that includes *Crotolaria fulva* and *Senecio* plants may develop occlusive disease of the terminal hepatic and sublobular veins with resultant hepatomegaly, ascites, and often jaundice (Fig. 25-63).[718,759,763] The disease has also been reported in South America[726] and occasionally in Native Americans in the western United States.[763] The venous lesion is first characterized by edema and, later, by collagenization. The large hepatic veins usually are unaffected. The sinusoids are remarkably congested, and the perivenular hepatic cells atrophy. Later, in chronic cases a nonportal type of cirrhosis may develop. A similar disease apparently occurs after the use of flour contaminated with *Senecio* in Africa.[759] Egyptian children also suffer from a disease involving the hepatic veins.[730] A severe outbreak of VOD, caused by *Heliotropium* plant seeds contaminating wheat used for human consumption, occurred in 1972 in Afghanistan.

This involved several thousand patients and was usually fatal.[743] Another form of VOD with a high mortality has been noted after allogeneic bone marrow transplantation. Most of the patients who died had been treated for leukemia and had received chemoradiotherapy. In one report the VOD was most noticeable in patients who had received dimethyl busulfan.[760,770]

In symptomless disease of the hepatic veins sometimes seen at autopsy, small segments of the hepatic veins may be closed by thrombi or even by tumors that produce infarction. Primary carcinomas of the liver often grow into the hepatic veins but rarely fill the entire system.

Radiation injury

Heavy irradiation of the liver, 3000 to 5900 rad, produces perivenular necrosis, intense hyperemia, and damage to the small hepatic veins that taken together resemble VOD.[755] However, fibrin in the terminal hepatic veins and sinusoids has been observed in patients who had received fractionated radiation with total doses of 1850 to 4050 rad, or single doses of 1000 rad.[724]

The microscopic changes in a needle biopsy specimen taken in the acute stage of irradiation damage are most difficult to distinguish from idiopathic BCS. In the chronic stage, after several months, there is a shrunken, atrophied liver with lobular collapse and portal tract fibrosis. Vascular damage is still present. The presence of both acute and chronic changes may represent an intermediate stage of damage. The disease may be fatal and may be considered a form of VOD. Experimentally irradiation produces a fine structural change in the rough endoplasmic reticulum, characterized by the formation of dense membranes.[731]

CHRONIC INFECTIONS AND OTHER CHRONIC DISORDERS
Granulomatous hepatitis—chronic infections

Hapatic granulomas have been reported in 10% or less of all needle biopsy samples of the liver. In our patients in Los Angeles, the percentage has dropped over the years to 2.5% in 1981. The indications for biopsy in patients with proven granulomas include a fever of unknown origin, hepatomegaly, and a high serum alkaline phosphatase level. A small percentage of patients may have jaundice or a tender liver. The presence of granulomas in needle biopsy specimens may be a confirmatory finding for the clinicians, but in some patients granulomatous disease is unexpected. Extensive bacteriologic, viral, and radiologic studies; skin testing; and even biopsies of other tissues may be necessary to establish a diagnosis. Etiologic classification of granulomatous hepatitis includes infectious diseases, drug sensitivity, granulomas associated with neoplasms, foreign-body reaction, and a large and important group, includ-

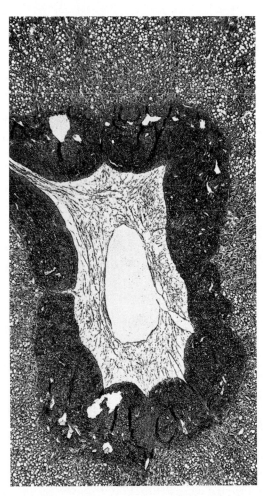

Fig. 25-63. Veno-occlusive disease of liver. (Courtesy Dr. G. Bras, Jamaica.)

ing sarcoidosis, the cause of which is not known.[782] Clinicopathologically, hepatic granulomas may be associated with (1) systemic granulomatosis, such as tuberculosis that involves one or more other organs; (2) another liver disease, such as primary biliary cirrhosis; and (3) a nonhepatic, nongranulomatous disease, such as abdominal cancer.[789] Most granulomas of the liver are nonnecrotizing and bear a certain similarity to one another, and in some instances very small aggregates of macrophages are difficult to categorize as granulomas. The definition of a granuloma as a "focal organized collection of mononuclear phagocytes"[772] seems applicable to the liver.

In our patients and probably in most large medical centers in the United States the major granulomatous diseases to be considered are sarcoidosis, tuberculosis, and granulomas associated with primary biliary cirrhosis and drug sensitivity. Other specific granulomas are rare, such as Q fever, but even after exhaustive studies, about 15% cannot be diagnosed. Tuberculous and sarcoid granulomas are the most frequently seen, and their differentiation is of practical importance. The lesion of sarcoidosis is composed of epithelioid cells with no particular arrangement. Caseation necrosis is not seen, and a few lymphocytes usually surround the granulomas (Fig. 25-64). Larger lesions are composed of multiple units, often with an occasional multinucleated giant cell. In some instances the noncaseating lesions of sar-

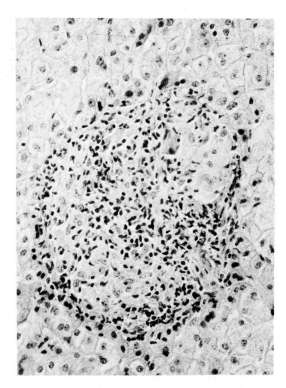

Fig. 25-64. Irregular arrangement of epithelioid cells and scanty lymphoid infiltrate in sarcoid granuloma of liver.

coidosis are observed in the walls of the terminal hepatic and sublobular veins. In healing, sarcoid granulomas usually become surrounded by concentric layers of connective tissue. Tubercles often have a caseous center, the epithelioid cells are arranged in a radial fashion at the periphery, and the exudate contains both lymphocytes and other mononuclear cells. Langhans' giant cells are frequent. Fibrin is often present, which helps to distinguish tuberculosis from sarcoidosis. In the small early lesions of tuberculosis, there may be no caseation, and the differentiation from sarcoidosis and leprosy is most difficult. An acid-fast stain should always be done on any granulomatous lesion that resembles tuberculosis. Occasionally the tubercles are concentrated along the portal tracts, and the bile ducts may be destroyed. In a patient so affected, jaundice may occur. More rarely, solitary or multiple tuberculomas have been observed. Tubercle bacilli may reach the liver from either an active pulmonary or an abdominal focus. After antituberculous chemotherapy, resolution of the granuloma and return to normal liver tissue is documented.[803]

In addition to tuberculosis, sarcoidosis must also be differentiated from PBC. The clinical and laboratory findings usually suffice, but occasionally the presence of granulomas on biopsy is the first indication of early PBC. These granulomas are usually along the portal tracts and may be in proximity to diseased bile ducts. They are also found within the lobules. These are usually solitary and do not have the complex structure of sarcoid. In the advanced stage of PBC, if extensive granulomas are present, the differentiation from sarcoidosis is difficult.[816] Also, on rare occasions sarcoidosis destroys branches of the intrahepatic bile ducts, producing chronic cholestasis and microscopic findings that are similar to PBC.[800]

Among the infectious granulomas, two are of major importance outside the United States. Schistosomiasis is a common cause of granulomas in which a specific diagnosis can be made by finding the larvae or the ova in the lesions. Liver involvement is also common in lepromatous leprosy and to a lesser extent in tuberculoid leprosy. The organisms are easily demonstrated with the Fite stain, especially in the foam cells. Leprosy involvement of the liver is usually symptomless; lesions are the result of bacteremia.[779]

Brucellosis infection causes a poorly defined granuloma or pseudogranuloma that consists of a jumblelike arrangement of epithelioid cells or round cells. They are located within the lobule and are associated with necrosis of hepatocytes.[799,814] Q fever produces rather characteristic lesions of variable size that often show a bright band of acidophilic material, apparently arising in the sinusoidal wall. These produce a doughnutlike lesion in the center of which is often a multinucleated giant cell.[762,767] The granulomas are present both in the triads and within the lobules and may at times form fairly large conglomerate lesions. Central vein involvement is noticed occasionally.

In visceral larva migrans the presence of the larvae of *Toxocara canis, T. cati,* or other parasites in the liver causes distinctive granulomas that may reach a diameter of several millimeters and are composed of a necrotic center surrounded by epithelioid cells having a radial arrangement, many eosinophils, and giant cells. The larvae may be identified on serial sectioning. The disease is seen in children, usually from 1½ to 6 years of age, who eat dirt (pica) and associate with dogs or cats. The syndrome is characterized by fever, hepatomegaly, eosinophilia, and hyperglobulinemia.[791] A reliable intradermal test using *Toxocara* antigen has been found useful.[818] *Toxoplasma gondii* occasionally causes a granuloma-like lesion of the liver.[776]

Where histoplasmosis is endemic, it is a fairly common cause of hepatic granulomas. In other parts of the United States, it is a rare cause.[798] In addition to granulomas, the organisms are commonly found in the Kupffer cells. Coccidioidal granulomas are of rare occurrence. Both histoplasmosis and coccidioidal organisms may be demonstrated with periodic acid–Schiff stains. Neonatal coccidioidomycosis with involvement of the liver has been observed.[813] Tularemia is discussed in Chapter 6.

The frequency of granulomas after drug use seems to be increasing. In one report nearly one third of patients with granulomatous hepatitis had acquired it after the use of drugs.[794] These granulomas are noncaseous and characterized by epithelioid cell reaction with giant cells and eosinophils. The presence of large numbers of the latter should make the pathologist suspect drug-induced or parasitic liver disease.[794] Among the more common drugs reported in association with granulomas are methyldopa,[796] hydralizine,[787] chlorpropamide,[808] quinidine,[777] allopurinol,[812,820] phenylbutazone,[774] and sulfonamides.

A rare disease characterized by granulomatous hepatitis, increased platelet aggregation, and hypercholesterolemia has been reported,[819] as has a single case of granulomatous disease of the small hepatic and portal veins.[801]

Numerous types of foreign material have been recognized as the cause of granulomas. Among these are copper, which has been noted in vineyard sprayers,[806] talcum crystals in narcotic addicts,[797] fluid silicone,[781] and silica in patients with advanced pulmonary silicosis.[778]

In the miscellaneous granuloma group associated with nonhepatic nongranulomatous disorders, there are abdominal neoplasms, Hodgkin's disease,[811] and Crohn's disease. Ileal bypass for obesity may also be complicated by nonnecrotizing granulomas in about one fourth of the patients. These granulomas do not seem to have clinical significance.[773]

Lastly, there are many cases (about 15% in our patients) in which no etiologic agent or association with another disease is ever demonstrated. The prognosis in these patients seems to be favorable.[807]

Syphilis of the liver

In congenital syphilis of the liver, now a rare entity, there is an overgrowth of mesenchymal tissue along the sinusoids that causes wide separation of the hepatic cells. Small gummas, or even large soft ones, occasionally are seen. Usually spirochetes are easily demonstrable. Syphilitic cirrhosis rarely occurs.

Secondary syphilis may rarely involve the liver, causing jaundice, a rise in the serum alkaline phosphatase, and mild rise in the AST.[792] The microscopic findings vary; usually there is portal tract inflammation, focal necrosis, disruption of the bile duct epithelium,[809] and occasional noncaseating granulomas. Spirochetes are difficult to demonstrate. Anal lesions are common.

Although common at one time, tertiary syphilis of the liver, complicating acquired syphilis, is now a rare disorder.[815] Gummas may be solitary or multiple and confluent, sometimes forming a large mass. On sectioning they have a dull gray-yellow area of central necrosis, an irregular outline, and a marginal zone of gray-white, glassy-appearing granulation tissue. They are often widespread, and, in healing, the scar tissue replacing them contracts to form deep scars that may incompletely divide the liver into masses of irregular size—hepar lobatum (Fig. 25-65). In other instances the crevices are not so deep, but stringy adhesions may bridge the indentations. More rarely, the liver is deformed by

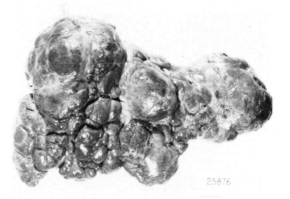

Fig. 25-65. Deeply scarred liver (hepar lobatum syphiliticum) that weighed only 710 g. Patient was 79-year-old white woman, known syphilitic, who had received some antisyphilitic therapy 3 years before death. Several large hyperplastic nodules are present. Stringy adhesions bridge some deep transverse fissures.

linear depressions. This occurs alone or in combination with the deeply scarred organ. Beneath these linear deformities are bands of connective tissue that do not have the appearance of healed gummas. In hepar lobatum syphiliticum, there may be little more than the normal amount of connective tissue or, on the contrary, the connective tissue may be diffusely increased.

The gross pattern of hepar lobatum may occur with submassive hepatic necrosis of viral hepatitis superimposed on chronic liver disease such as cirrhosis and others have noted the pattern after chemotherapy in breast cancer.[52]

Microscopically in the gummatous stage there are isolated areas of necrosis surrounded by granulation tissue relatively poor in fibroblasts and usually sparse in epitheloid cells (Fig. 25-66). The granulation tissue impinges on the liver parenchyma, and necrosis of the latter appears to occur at this junction. Lymphocytes and plasma cells are common, both around the areas of gummatous necrosis and along the portal tracts. Later, wide bands of scar tissue are irregularly distributed throughout the liver, sometimes in combination with unhealed gummas.

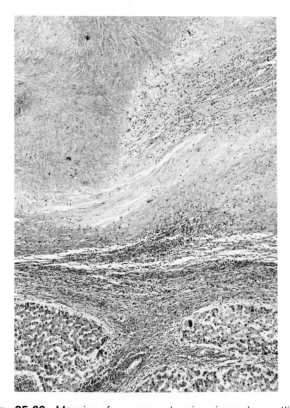

Fig. 25-66. Margin of gumma showing irregular outline, sparsity of epithelioid cells, and zone of granulation tissue. Patient was 41-year-old woman who died of massive gastrointestinal hemorrhage; syphilis was not diagnosed before death.

Amyloidosis

In systemic amyloidosis the liver is commonly involved. Usually, however, there is only symptomless hepatomegaly that may be accompanied by bromosulfophthalein retention and increase in serum alkaline phosphatase.[795,810] Rarely jaundice and even ascites may occur, both of which are poor prognostic signs. Amyloidosis occurs in about equal frequency in primary (immunocyte dyscrasia with amyloidosis) and secondary (reactive systemic amyloidosis).[785] Grossly the liver is large, firm, much lighter in color than normal, and waxy in appearance. Microscopically amyloid may be predominantly intralobular (reticular), portal (collagenous), or globular in form. Amyloidosis that produces symptoms is usually of the intralobular variety. The amyloid is deposited in Disse's space, and the hepatocytes are severely compressed or may nearly disappear.[805] Cholestasis is noted in the few patients who are jaundiced.[810] Portal amyloidosis involves the blood vessels and is symptomless, but the distribution pattern is that seen in patients with plasma cell dyscrasias. The third type of amyloidosis of the liver is the recently reported globular form that may be associated with systemic amyloid involvement, including adrenal glands and kidneys.[783,788] Globular amyloid has not been associated with dysproteinemia or myeloma; similarly, intralobular (reticular) amyloid seems unassociated with myeloma. An immense amount of research has been done on the biochemistry, fine structure, and classification of amyloidosis (see p. 38).[786]

Parasitic cirrhosis

Although many different species of parasites may cause infestation of the liver, *Schistosoma mansoni* and *S. japonicum* are most likely to cause chronic liver disease, even cirrhosis. It has been estimated that 100 million people have schistosomiasis and that portal hypertension with esophageal varices is probably present in several million patients.[817] The pathology of all parasitic diseases is described in Chapter 11. The pathology of schistosomiasis was first described in Egypt in 1904. The pipestem fibrosis of schistosomiasis causes a presinusoidal bloc in the absence of any noticeable changes in liver function tests.[793,817]

AIDS and the liver

Acquired immunodeficiency syndrome (AIDS) produces a wide spectrum of disseminated infectious disease and neoplasms that usually do not produce distinctive hepatic signs and symptoms.[784,802] Liver function tests may be abnormal and lead to biopsy, which allows recognition of hepatic involvement. At autopsy, hepatic involvement is noted for Kaposi sarcoma, *Mycobacterium avium-intracellulare* (MAI), cytomegalic inclusion virus (CMV), *Cryptococcus neoformans*, and other fungal agents. The immune deficiency allows a different histologic pattern for some of these agents because little or no lymphocytic reaction occurs and the "granuloma" of MAI is solely macrophages filled by light granular organisms, which are easily stained with Ziehl-Nielsen or periodic acid–Schiff stain and reveal a myriad of organisms. Chronic viral hepatitis occurs commonly in the male homosexual group as does AIDS but the course of chronic active hepatitis appears milder, probably because of the immune deficiency.[790]

LIVER DISEASE IN NONHEPATIC DISORDERS

Cirrhosis and other lesions may complicate the course of other serious diseases that are systemic or that primarily involve another organ or organ system in the body. Liver abnormalities are common in patients with inflammatory bowel disease.[823] Ulcerative colitis may be associated with fatty change, portal inflammation and fibrosis, chronic active hepatitis (which may follow transfusion), granulomas, amyloidosis, cirrhosis, bile duct carcinoma, pericholangitis (intrahepatic sclerosing cholangitis), and panductal sclerosing cholangitis.[829,830] The most common single laboratory finding is an elevated alkaline phosphatase level that is not associated with the cholestasis.[834] In patients with Crohn's disease the liver changes may be similar to those in ulcerative colitis but occur with much less frequency.[825] Pericholangitis and fibrosis may lead to protracted jaundice and, finally, a biliary type of cirrhosis. The liver in both ulcerative colitis and Crohn's disease may have an increased copper content.[832] The liver in both has occasionally been reported to improve after removal of the diseased bowel but in most instances seems unrelated to the course or the treatment of the colon disorder.

Fatty change, pericentric fibrosis, and even intracellular Mallory bodies may be observed in diabetes mellitus. Whether there is a progression from fatty change and a variable degree of fibrosis to cirrhosis is yet to be determined. An increased incidence of cirrhosis in diabetics has been suggested, but this is controversial.[826] It is well known that patients with alcoholic cirrhosis may secondarily become diabetic. Hepatic dysfunction in rheumatoid arthritis is common but usually asymptomatic. A rise in alkaline phosphatase, retention of bromosulfophthalein, and hepatomegaly are the more common findings.[827,828] In addition, infiltration of the portal tracts with round cells,[812] primary biliary cirrhosis, amyloidosis, and other findings have been recorded. Rarely the hepatic arteries are affected by rheumatoid arteritis.[828] The existence of liver disease in patients with systemic lupus erythematosus has been noted. A wide variety of changes occur, sometimes progressing to cirrhosis.[833] Regional enteritis, scleroderma,[822] rheumatic fever, hyperthyroidism,[821] and various bacterial infections occasionally may be complicated by cirrhosis. A mild degree of cirrhosis is not infrequently noted in the liver of elderly persons. This seems to be a slowly progressive disease that occurs in patients in whom there are no etiologically demonstrable factors, except possibly poor eating habits. In Boeck's sarcoidosis, the lesions in the liver may progress to cirrhosis.[831] Sickle cell anemia may be complicated by an unexplained type of micronodular cirrhosis. Presumably this follows vascular obstruction by the sickled cells, necrosis of hepatocytes, fibrosis, and regeneration.[804] A hemochromatotic type of cirrhosis may also occur. There is also the complication that non-A, non-B hepatitis followed by cirrhosis may develop in patients who receive many transfusions related to nonhepatic diseases. Thus one must be cautious not to ascribe cirrhosis or chronic active hepatitis too freely to some of the above-mentioned diseases. As an example, most cases of chronic active hepatitis associated with inflammatory bowel diseases are probably a result of posttransfusion chronic active hepatitis.

EXTRAHEPATIC EFFECTS OF HEPATIC DISEASES

Many other associations of extrahepatic diseases with hepatic disorders have been recognized: pulmonary hypertension and chronic active hepatitis have been reported to coexist[435] though the relationship is unclear, and Graves' disease has a deleterious effect on the course of acute viral hepatitis. Muscle degradation in hepatic failure has been shown to be increased in cirrhotic patients; it has been hypothesized that the increased breakdown is a result of the increase in glucagon levels that is attained because the normal hepatic catabolism of glucagon is defective in hepatic failure. Glucagon accentuates muscle degradation. Cardiomyopathy and pancreatitis occur in alcoholic patients and are not necessarily related to liver disease, but cardiomyopathy is also apparently associated with the accentuated protein degradation of cirrhosis.[464] Vasculitis and glomerulonephritis have been associated with chronic active hepatitis B.[443]

TUMORS AND TUMORLIKE LESIONS

The liver provides a suitable milieu for the growth of neoplastic cells, especially for metastatic tumor. In addition, the lymphomas, leukemias, and primary carcinoma all grow readily within this organ. Its size, anatomic location, dual blood supply, and the ready availability of nutritional material are factors that influence the deposition and growth of neoplasms. Between 40% and 50% of all primary cancers in the body are noted at death to have metastases within the liver.[855] Primary neoplasms and tumorlike lesions of liver occur much less frequently in the United States but nevertheless are important inasmuch as they may enter into the differential diagnosis of an enlarged liver noted clinically or observed at laparotomy. In Asia and Africa the most common malignant tumor is cancer originating in the liver. Hepatomegaly, often symptomless, is a common finding in neoplastic liver disease. Malignant tumors usually are associated with weight loss. Fever and jaundice are less common. Esophageal varices may occur as a complication of both primary and secondary tumors.[890] Laboratory findings often include an elevation of the serum alkaline phosphatase level and bromosulfophthalein retention. Angiograms, scintiscans, echograms, and computerized tomography are useful in determining the size, number, and anatomic location of hepatic neoplasms.

Percutaneous fine-needle aspiration biopsy of the liver, guided by radioisotope scintigrams and the fluoroscope, has proved to be highly successful in the diagnosis of malignant tumors of the liver.[868]

The classification of hepatic tumors is based on recognition of the cell of origin, though it is well recognized that considerable variation in morphologic and physiologic function may occur in neoplastic cells. Experimental hepatic tumors illustrate dramatic metaplastic change and challenge the principle of classification by cell of origin.[949] Tumors produced by injection of

Table 25-7. Classification of primary hepatic tumors

Benign hepatocellular tumors	Hepatocellular adenoma
	  Estrogen related
	  Spontaneous
	  Metabolic diseases
	  Anabolic steroid induced
	Multiple hepatocellular adenomas
	Nodular regenerative hyperplasia
	Macroregenerative nodule
	Focal nodular hyperplasia
	Mixed hamartoma

Benign bile duct tumors	Bile duct adenoma Bile duct cystadenoma
Benign mesodermal tumors	Cavernous hemangioma Infantile hemangioendothelioma Fibroma Lipoma and variants Mesenchymal hamartoma

Tumorlike lesions	Inflammatory myofibroblastic tumor
	Cysts
	  Traumatic
	  Parasitic
	  Solitary nonparasitic
	  Polycystic disease

Malignant hepatocellular tumors	Hepatocellular carcinoma (HCC)
	  Fibrolamellar HCC
	  Spindle cell HCC
	  Other variants (giant cell HCC)
	Combined HCC and cholangiocarcinoma

Malignant bile duct epithelial tumors	Cholangiocarcinoma
	  Hilar
	  Peripheral
	  Intraductal

Malignant mesodermal tumors	Angiosarcoma Epithelioid hemangioendothelioma Leiomyosarcoma Fibrosarcoma Malignant fibrous histiocytoma Embryonal sarcoma
Uncertain origin and rare tumors	Carcinoid tumors, primary Trophoblastic tumor Adrenal rest tumor Pheochromocytoma

Table 25-8. Incidence of primary hepatic tumors

Type	Number	Percent
Benign*	64	11.9%
Bile duct adenoma	16	3.0%
Hepatocellular adenoma	5	1.0%
Focal nodular hyperplasia	42	7.8%
Inflammatory pseudotumor	1	0.2%
Malignant epithelial	462	86.0%
Hepatocellular carcinoma	414	77.1%
Typical	388	72.3%
Sclerosing	15	2.8%
Fibrolamellar	5	1.0%
Giant cell	2	
Undifferentiated	3	
Spindle cell	1	
Hepatoblastoma	2	0.4%
Bile duct carcinoma	44	8.2%
Cholangiocarcinoma	44	8.2%
Hilar	14	2.6%
Peripheral	30	5.6%
Carcinoid	2	0.4%
Malignant mesenchymal	11	2.0%
Endothelial		
Angiosarcoma	2	
Epithelioid hemangioendothelioma	2	
Lymphoma	1	
Undifferentiated	5	1.0%
Embryonal sarcoma		
TOTAL	537	100%

From Los Angeles County–University of Southern California Medical Center and University of Southern California Liver Unit 96,625 autopsies from 1918 to 1982.
*Excluding benign hemangiomatous lesions.

single cell–derived clonal subpopulations reflected a wide variety of histologic patterns including epidermoid carcinoma, adenocarcinoma, mixed carcinoma and sarcoma, and tumors identical to hepatocellular carcinoma, cholangiocarcinoma, and hepatoblastoma.[949] Monoclonally derived tumors had both osteoid and chondroid stroma rather than only one type of differentiated stromal element. Nonetheless, it remains convenient to categorize hepatic tumors by the apparent cell of origin because most tumors appear fairly homogeneous and remain so during the course in a single patient, and prognosis correlates reasonably well. Primary tumors arise from hepatic cells (hepatocellular carcinoma), bile duct epithelium (cholangiocarcinoma), and mesodermal structures including smooth muscle (leiomyosarcoma), primitive mesenchymal stroma (such as mesenchymal sarcoma), endothelium (angiosarcoma, epithelioid hemangioendothelioma), and Glisson's capsule (fibroma and fibrosarcoma). Table 25-7 is a simplified classification based on cell of origin, and Table 25-8 indicates the relative numbers of various primary hepatic benign and malignant tumors seen in a large autopsy pathology practice over many years in a large teaching hospital. The commonest benign primary hepatic tumor, the hemangioma, has been omitted to simplify the table, and in the autopsy series of the same time period, approximately 900 hemangiomas were documented, a number twice that of all other tumors combined. Of the nonhemangiomatous tumors, the benign lesions were 12%; the malignant epithelial tumors were 86%; and the less common sarcomas were 2% of the total. Adequate tumor sampling is essential for classification. The small number of hepatoblastomas reflects the presence of a childrens' hospital referral center. Comparison of this table with current surgical pathology practice during a 2-year period, 1977 to 1978, revealed less benign lesions, which are commonly incidental findings.

Benign hepatocellular tumors

Hepatocellular adenoma (HCA) are derived from hepatocytes and usually are solitary large tumors that are readily seen from the external surface and have a bulging light-tan cut surface. About 10% are pedunculated, and they usually occur in the right lobe. HCAs tend to be large, with a fourth larger than 10 cm, and 3 were ruptured in our series. The larger tumors have hemorrhage, necrosis, and gelatinous areas secondary to previous infarction and hemorrhage (Fig. 25-67). The microscopic features are benign hepatocytes in cords of 1 to 2 cells, though large HCA have sheets of cells, and the HCA often has no fibrous capsule and blends into the adjacent liver (Fig. 25-67). The neoplastic hepatocytes are of four types, including (1) a common "neohepatocyte" with eosinophilic cytoplasm and appearing similar to the adjacent normal liver cell, (2) a "hydropic" type, (3) a pleomorphic cell with more cytoplasm and large nucleus and even giant cell formation, and (4) a clear cell type. Some HCAs contain fat, cholestasis, and alcoholic hyaline. The presence of numerous small vessels is a key feature and peliosis hepatis is common. HCAs were rare until the widespread use of oral contraceptives during the 1960s and have again become less frequent after a decreased estrogen content and less use of oral contraceptives. The risk for estrogen-induced HCA is increased with more than 5 years of use, and HCA occurring in pregnancy or postpartum are associated with rupture. Surgery is required if rupture is noted.[841] Regression usually occurs after cessation of oral contraceptives, and a new tumor occurs in 25% of women who take the medication again.[854,925] HCA may be classified by the underlying associated condition and thus we recognize (1) estrogen-related HCA, (2) spontaneous HCA (no drug related), (3) metabolic disease–associated HCA (tyrosinemia and glycogen storage disease type 1A), and (4) anabolic steroid–related HCA. This latter group often associated with oxymetholone and methyltestosterone treatment of Fanconi's anemia, chronic anemia of renal failure, aplastic anemia, cryptorchidism, and male impotence has striking resemblance to hepatocellular carcinoma. In the other forms of HCA, distinction from carcinoma is made because HCA lacks vascular invasion, lacks local invasion of sinusoids of adjacent normal liver, usually does not occur in cirrhosis, has characteristic neohepatocytes and degenerative changes of infarction and hemorrhage, and lacks a nodule in nodule growth pattern of carcinoma. The anabolic steroid–related HCAs have disturbing microscopic features of acini formation (which if not related to anabolic steroids is considered carcinoma on histologic grounds), large pleomorphic cells, and even invasion of major veins within the tumor.[911] Regression of HCA in glycogen storage disease occurs with dietary therapy.[912] The risk of carcinoma developing in HCA has prompted close follow-up study, and a small number of patients (less than 5%) may have carcinoma either develop or be present and misidentified as HCA. Hepatocellular carcinoma typically evolves from HCA in tyrosinemia.[954]

Multiple hepatocellular adenomatosis (MHCA) is a rare condition with numerous (more than four HCAs and often more than 100 HCAs diffusely scattered in both lobes of the liver.[792a] *Nodular regenerative hyperplasia* (NRH) differs because the lesions are smaller, being less than 1.5 cm in most cases and involving one lobule, whereas in MHCA the lesions vary considerably and are several centimeters in diameter. However, at the gross examination of the NRH liver, the numerous bulging nodules resemble metastatic carcinoma (see Fig. 25-68, *A*), and yet the microscopic features are bland and benign, and so the viewer is puzzled by the slide review wondering if the correct slide is examined. The nodules are single hepatocytes in cords growing in nodular fashion, with the adjacent nonnodular liver cords compressed. NRH is associated with portal hypertension and with numerous clinical diseases including rheumatoid arthritis, Felty's syndrome, multiple myeloma, macroglobulinemia, a variety of drugs,[941] diabetes mellitus, toxic oil syndrome,[935] and hemorrhagic telangiectasia.[953]

Focal nodular hyperplasia (FNH) occurs predominately in women 20 to 50 years of age and is usually a solitary circumscribed subcapsular firm tumor 1 to 8 cm in diameter (smaller average than HCA). The hallmark of the lesion is the central fibrous scar that has promoted the earlier name of focal cirrhosis, and the brown liver tissue bulges on cut surface. Occasionally FNH is pedunculated, and approximately 20% occur in childhood.[937] The presence of fibrous bands, the lack of true portal areas, the presence of numerous proliferat-

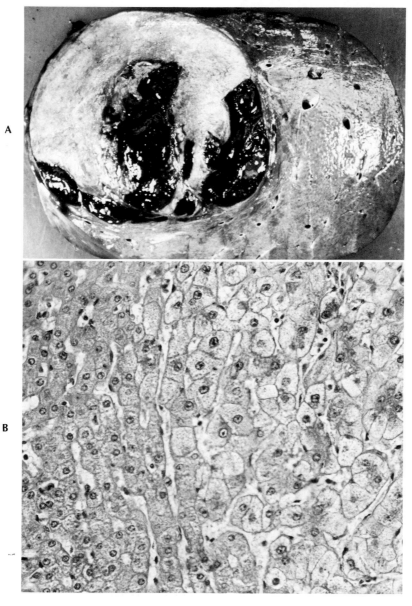

Fig. 25-67. Hepatic adenoma. **A,** Grossly mass is well defined with hemorrhage into tumor. **B,** Microscopically there is transition zone between adjacent liver and adenoma cells. Notice larger size of adenoma cells and more distinct cord arrangement around canaliculi.

ing small pseudoductules are the key microscopic features. The cause is unknown, but a vascular malformation is suspected.[952]

Macroregenerative nodule (MRN), or *adenomatous hyperplasia,* is a large (several centimeters) hyperplastic nodule of hepatocytes and portal areas that occurs after severe acute or chronic liver injury such as either submassive hepatic necrosis or cirrhosis. Such large nodules in the cirrhotic liver (see Fig. 25-68, *B*) resemble either tumor or with fibrous bands and indicate possible hepar lobatum. Following patients with cirrhosis caused by hepatitis B virus requires a careful search for developing carcinoma, and hyperplastic nodules are easily mistaken for malignant tumor, and MRN has been called cirrhotic pseudotumor.[905] Angiography may be useful in making the distinction.[921]

Mixed hamartoma (MH) is a rare solitary tumor composed of both hepatocytes and bile ducts including fibrous stroma.[923] These occur in young persons and may be large (more than 20 cm) and pedunculated.

Benign bile duct tumors

Bile duct adenoma (BDA) are usually solitary gray-white nodules less than 1 cm in diameter and located on Glisson's capsule. These nodules are easily mistaken for metastatic tumor, and light microscopy shows a mixture of benign bile ducts (round glands without mitosis or complex glandular formation) and a uniform fibrous stroma.[864]

Bile duct cystadenoma (BDCA), or hepatobiliary cystadenoma, are not proved to be of biliary origin and often have a distinctive mesenchymal stroma beneath a thin cuboid epithelial lining that is not seen in normal biliary structures.[955] BDCAs are multilocular cysts lined

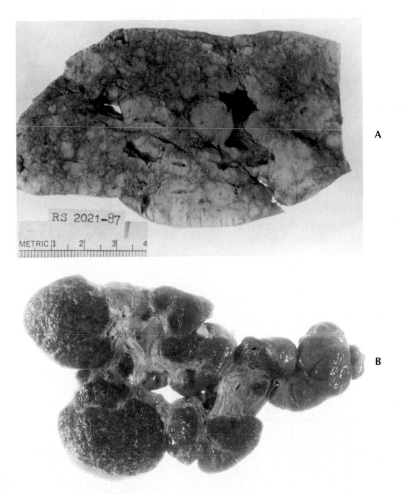

Fig. 25-68. A, Multiple bulging nodules up to 1 cm in diameter occur diffusely within the entire liver in an 85-year-old patient who died of gastrointestinal hemorrhage (nodular regenerated hyperplasia). **B,** Large macroregenerative nodules occur in both lobes of this patient dying from hepatitis (RA 52-87). Each large nodule contains numerous portal areas and surrounded by dense fibrous bands. (**A,** Courtesy Dr. Kenneth A. Frankel, Covina, Calif.)

by benign cuboid epithelium with a dense mesenchymal stroma and often hyalinized stroma. The age range is wide (19 to 67 years), and the size can be large up to 25 cm in diameter. The internal lining appears smooth with trabeculation, and a few have polypoid projections signifying malignant change (about an eighth). One variant of this tumor occurs as a large intraductal polyp, and removal of only the polyp may leave a substantial remnant that will regrow. BDCA in men differ by lacking the dense mesenchymal stroma, but numerous sections may be necessary to see the stroma in the female tumors.

Benign mesodermal tumors

Cavernous hemangioma (CH) is the most common tumor of the liver, is highly variable in size, and rarely has clinical significance unless very large and rupture may occur. Giant hemangioma is defined as one larger than 4 cm in diameter, and with special techniques such as computerized tomography scans more CH are discovered ante mortem and present clinical management problems.[836] The course of such tumors is highly variable, and the newborn may have a near replacement of the liver by diffuse CH and succumb to high output heart failure, whereas smaller lesions in the newborn usually spontaneously involute. In older age, CH seem more numerous, an indication that the tumor develops and grows in advancing years but follow-up study of these tumors has not been done in signficant numbers. Some CH have thrombosis and fibrosis with subsequent calcification that is apparent on roentgenograms. The typical CH has capillary angiomatous areas also, and the large blood-filled spaces are lined by thin endothelium placed on fibrous stalks (Fig. 25-69). A syndrome of systemic diffuse hemangiomatosis occurs with involvement of bone, lung, liver, and other organs.[883]

Infantile hemangioendothelioma (IHE) are congenital lesions noted at birth or during the first 6 months of life and are more common in girls. Abdominal enlargement, often cutaneous lesions, and heart failure are the major clinical signs. The lesions may be solitary or diffuse involving numerous portal areas. The portal veins are the major feeding vessels, and in time most of the vascular lesions undergo spontaneous involution. Microscopic classification into two types was outlined by Dehner, and type 1 is benign with an orderly proliferation of vessels lined by a single layer of endothelial cells. The center of the lesions may include cavernous areas and these correlate with the "puddling" noted by angiogram. Type 2 IHE have hyperchromatic endothelial cells with more pleomorphism and multilayered lining with budding and branching patterns. The type 2 IHE may be malignant, but separation into the two types is not easy. The abundance of small vessels in mesenchymal hamartoma may also indicate possible IHE.

Peliosis hepatis (PH) is a rare diffuse angiomatoid change of liver[958] that is seen more commonly with anabolic steroid use[904] and renal transplant patients and may occur outside the liver (as in the lung, spleen, and kidneys[874]). Peliosis hepatis is small blood-filled cavities with abundant or scant endothelial cells, and the lesion may be single or multiple and without preference for portal or perivenular location. Prominent portal vessels are a feature of *Osler-Weber-Rendu disease* (hereditary hemorrhagic telangiectasia).

Fibroma, a rare hepatic tumor, seems to arise from Glisson's capsule and may be pedunculated or grow internally forming a large mass. *Lipoma* may occur deep within the substance and must be distinguished from a pseudolipoma attributable to adhesion to the Glisson's capsule of an epiploica appendage of the colon.

Benign tumorlike lesions

Inflammatory pseudotumor (or inflammatory myofibroblastic tumor, IPT) occurs primarily in children and in the hilum of the liver with a mass of fibrous tissue containing acute and chronic inflammation producing jaundice by obstruction of the common bile ducts.[837]

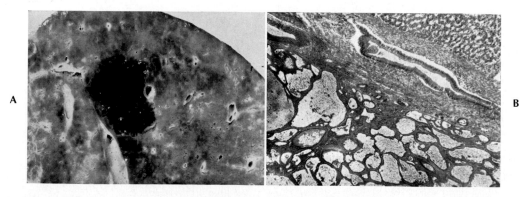

Fig. 25-69. A, Cavernous hemangioma of liver. **B,** Hepatic parenchyma at upper right.

Mesenchymal hamartoma (MH) is a large solitary tumor of childhood, composed of gelatinous myxoid stroma and cysts, and is recognized as a mass lesion. Males are more frequent in most series, and the age range is a few months to 10 years with the average age at diagnosis of 15 months.[940] MH is considered a hamartoma because of the normal "trapped" hepatic elements (bile ducts and hepatic cords) and the myxoid stroma, which appears to be benign but primitive hepatic mesenchyme that proliferates and grows into the adjacent liver tissue. The average size at diagnosis is 18 cm,[892] and resection is the usual treatment. Incomplete resection is not associated with adverse effects or malignant change.

Cysts of the liver include the solitary (nonparasitic cyst) that occurs more commonly in the male, and abdominal enlargement occurs. The cyst appears blue beneath Glisson's capsule and may be up to 15 or 20 cm in diameter.[865] *Echinococcus* cysts of the liver are discussed in Chapter 11. In North America, *E. granulosus* is most common, but hydatid disease of the liver is endemic in the Mediterranean and Baltic areas, South America, Australia, the Middle East, and northern Canada. Most patients have abdominal pain or tenderness and a single cyst in the right lobe. The cyst is composed of a fibrous wall (host derived) and a parasite-derived endocyst (Fig. 25-70). About half of the cysts communicate with the biliary tree or are infected, requiring external drainage.[894] Polycystic liver disease appears in two major forms: microcystic liver disease also called "congenital hepatic fibrosis," which has small cysts in contrast to the large cysts (1 to 4 cm in diameter), which may replace a large part of the liver and produce symptoms by hemorrhage into the multiple cysts. The two conditions are related because the portal regions of both contain von Meyenberg complexes in continuity with the cysts. Traumatic pseudocysts occur as infrequently as polycystic disease.

Primary hepatic carcinoma

Carcinoma primary in the liver occupies a unique position among neoplasms because of its propensity for arising in an organ that is already severely damaged by another disease—cirrhosis. Of the hepatocellular carcinomas studied in our liver unit, 77% arose in cirrhotic livers, 9% in what might be characterized as precirrhotic livers, and 14% in normal livers. Carcinomas most often are derived from hepatocytes, but a small percentage (less than 20%) are of bile duct origin. The preferred term for malignant tumors derived from hepatocytes is "hepatocellular carcinoma" (HCC), not "primary" hepatocellular carcinoma, a clearly redundant term, but one that with "hepatoma" and "liver cell carcinoma" continues to be used in the literature. There has been great interest in hepatic tumors over the past few decades but especially in recent years because of recognition of the part that hepatitis B virus plays in the etiology of HCC, particularly in the Orient and in Africa, where HCC is the leading malignant tumor. Hormones and environmental toxins may play additional roles. Incidence of HCC is reported to be between 0.2 per 100,000 population (about 0.1% of autopsies) in the British Isles[838] and about 173 per 100,000 in Taiwan.[840] Over a 60-year period in autopsies in Los Angeles, HCC has been found in 0.3% (0.15% in and before 1953; 0.88% by 1978); it comprises 1.8% of the malignant tumors studied at autopsy. In the Philippines, 4.5% of the deaths from malignancy are from HCC[898]; in Taiwan, 20% of all malignancies in both sexes combined are HCC.

The second major type of carcinoma primary in the liver arises from or resembles bile duct epithelium and is called cholangiocarcinoma. Cholangiocarcinomas may arise at any point in the biliary tree: those arising at or near the level of interlobular ducts are called peripheral cholangiocarcinomas (PCC); the rare instances of primary tumor in the major intrahepatic ducts are called cholangiocarcinoma of right or left hepatic duct; those at the bifurcation of the common hepatic duct are called hilar cholangiocarcinomas. The carcinomas arising in the remaining extrahepatic duct system are collectively called extrahepatic cholangiocarcinomas. A rare intrahepatic tumor that resembles the epithelium of the cholangiole throughout the tumor is called cholangilocellular carcinoma.

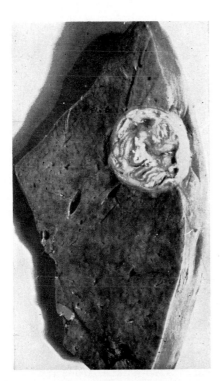

Fig. 25-70. *Echinococcus* cyst of liver. Notice convoluted membranous content.

Many hepatic carcinomas have tumor cells resembling hepatocytes with ductal elements also present; occasionally the ductal elements compose the major portion of the tumor. Many tumors with a continuum between hepatocyte and duct epithelium arise predominantly in the setting of hepatocellular carcinomas. Because the biologic activity of the tumor more closely resembles hepatocellular carcinoma, we at USC have considered such tumors to be HCC, reserving the term *combined* for cases in which there are separate HCC and peripheral cholangiocarcinomas in the same liver.

PCC is much less common than HCC, representing only 10% of liver cancers at our hospital but 16% in Japan. There is no apparent relationship between cholangiocarcinomas and hepatitis B virus.

Clinically HCC or PCC complicating cirrhosis is difficult to distinguish from cirrhosis alone. An enlarged abdominal mass, pain in the right upper quadrant (often severe), weight loss, rapidly accumulating ascites, and blood-stained ascitic fluid on paracentesis point toward a diagnosis of carcinoma of the liver. Jaundice is usually not severe and occurs in a third or less of patients. The liver is enlarged and is hard and tender in nearly every symptomatic patient. The tumor has often been present in the liver for years before symptoms develop. Usually symptoms occur when enough liver is replaced to produce some degree of hepatic failure, and symptoms develop earlier in cirrhotic patients than in noncirrhotic patients. Occasionally the tumor invades the portal vein or hepatic duct or metastasizes before a large tumor or liver replacement has developed. Such anomalous types of spread produce a different set of symptoms, earlier diagnosis, and usually earlier death with respect to tumor size. Exceptionally rapid rates of tumor growth seem to occur in the HCC developing in patients in parts of Africa, particularly Mozambique. Serum *alphafetoprotein* (AFP) is a helpful marker of HCC and also occurs in selected other nonhepatic tumors (germ cell endoplasms) and occasionally in metastatic adenocarcinoma to the liver (such as gastric adenocarcinoma). Fractionation of AFP may separate HCC from metastatic carcinoma.[877]

Hepatocellular carcinoma
Etiology

The most important feature in the etiology of HCC is cirrhosis or precirrhotic changes. There are clear differences in the propensity of different kinds of cirrhosis to give rise to HCC. Some types of cirrhosis (such as tyrosinemia) have a high incidence of development of HCC[954] but are rare entities; others (such as biliary atresia and familial cholestatic disorders) have a progression of the cirrhosis that is too rapid to allow sufficient survival time for the development of HCC. In another example, patients with alcoholic cirrhosis have a

far shorter life expectancy after development of cirrhosis than do patients with B viral cirrhosis, a factor that should be considered when the incidence of HCC in the two are considered. A third factor to be considered is that many types of chronic liver disease are labeled "cirrhosis" long before the development of nodular regeneration. Primary biliary cirrhosis (PBC) is an example: the time from the development of nodules to death is relatively short in PBC, even though the span of disease is well over a decade. Correspondingly, the percentage of patients with PBC who develop HCC is low though cases have been reported.

In all patients with cirrhosis the frequency of HCC is related to the causes of the particular types of cirrhosis. There are patients with certain very protracted types of cirrhosis who have a lower incidence of HCC than patients with other etiologic types of cirrhosis do. An example of long-term cirrhosis with low incidence of HCC occurs in Wilson's disease. With D-penicillamine therapy, patients may live 20 years or more with established cirrhosis. Only two HCCs arising in livers of patients with acceptably proved Wilson's disease have been reported.

Hepatitis B appears to be the most important etiologically related factor in hepatic carcinogenesis worldwide. In Taiwan, where about 80% of patients with HCC have a chronic form of hepatitis B,[945] the incidence of HCC in persons who are HBsAg positive is 1158:100,000, compared with 5:100,000 in HBsAg-negative patients.[840] Data from Hong Kong, Japan, the Philippines, and the United States indicate that between 40% and 45% of patients dying of B viral cirrhosis also have hepatocellular carcinoma,[855] whereas more precise data from Taiwan indicate that HCC develops in HBsAg carriers.[840] Thus it is unnecessary to hypothesize a cocarcinogen reacting with HBV infection in Asia or Africa to explain the high incidence of HCC in those countries. Differences in the incidence of HCC result from the difference in chronic HBsAg infection from one country to another. The high familial incidence of both HCC and chronic HBV infection in several countries[907,908,946] offers evidence for perinatal acquisition of HBV infection that is followed several decades later by development of HCC. Recent studies have detected hepatitis B viral DNA incorporated into the DNA of hepatocellular carcinoma.[901,919] Some patients with HCC but with no serologic evidence of past or current hepatitis B infection have been reported to have such B viral DNA incorporated into the tumor DNA.[844]

For purposes of comparison, since alcoholic cirrhosis is uncommon in Asia and Africa, if one excludes the patients with HCC arising in alcoholic cirrhosis in our series of patients with HCC from Los Angeles, more than 70% of the remaining patients with HCC arising in cirrhotic livers have chronic HBV infection.[916] Thus it appears that although chronic HBV infection is important in the etiology of HCC in the United States it occurs about 1% as often in the United States as in parts of Asia.

HCC is much less likely to develop in alcoholic cirrhotic patients than in patients with many other types of cirrhosis, but since alcoholic cirrhosis is much more common than other types of cirrhosis in the United States and Europe, it forms the basis for the greatest number of cases of HCC. Overall in the United States only about 4% of patients with alcoholic cirrhosis studied at autopsy have HCC. However, when HCC arises in the alcoholic cirrhotic liver, it does so only in the advanced cirrhotic liver, a stage reached by only a small percentage of alcoholic cirrhotic patients in the United States. In France and Italy, where average alcohol consumption is higher but less intense per alcoholic than in the United States, HCC is more likely to develop in the cirrhotic liver.[915] If the alcoholic cirrhotic patient discontinues alcohol consumption and thus prolongs survival, the chances of developing HCC increase.[896]

Aflatoxin, a product of *Aspergillus flavus*, may be involved in the etiology of liver cell carcinoma. This fungus has widespread distribution, growing on peanuts, soybeans, and cereals in humid parts of the world. Aflatoxin B_1, the most toxic of the aflatoxins, is highly carcinogenic for some animal species, particularly rats. As little as 15 μg/kg body weight/day produces cancer. The relationship of alfatoxin intake to primary carcinoma of the liver has been studied in Kenya,[930] Thailand,[913] and Mozambique. The last has the highest frequency of HCC in the world and also has the highest per capita intake of aflatoxins. It has been estimated that in Mozambique one male in each 40 households will die of HCC. There may be a short induction time after exposure to aflatoxins.[950] In studies of both biopsy and autopsy specimens in Bantus of Lourenço Marques, toxic changes that differed from viral hepatitis seen in the same population were observed. It has been suggested that these changes may be precancerous.[947] Yet on a case-by-case basis the relationship of HCC to high dietary aflatoxin intake has not been established. Because of the carcinogenic effect of single large doses of aflatoxins, an effect of these agents cannot readily be exluded, and many investigators propose a cocarcinogenic effect between hepatitis B and aflatoxins. This is difficult to prove, since the increased incidence of HCC in most Asian and African countries can probably be explained on the basis of increased incidence of chronic forms of hepatitis B alone.

Hemochromatosis is relatively uncommon in the United States and western Europe and therefore is not a major cause of HCC. However, HCC or cholangiocarcinoma develops in approximately 20% of patients with hemochromatosis. It is unclear whether treatment of hemochromatosis by iron removal reduces the incidence of development of HCC or allows longer survival and higher incidence of HCC.[843] Many cirrhotic livers have secondary increases in iron stores, ranging from only slightly more than normal quantities to amounts comparable to those in livers of patients with idiopathic hemochromatosis. Whether these increased stores contribute to carcinogenesis is unclear.

Hormones. A relationship between benign hepatocellular tumors and oral contraceptives has been discussed (see p. 1289); a much less frequent association of oral contraceptives and HCC has also been reported.[849,920] Although cases of HCC associated with oral contraceptives have been collected by various investigators from from a candidate population of approximately 12 to 15 million in the United States alone, there is little available information regarding the HCC incidence in the control population.

Anabolic steroids administered to young patients in treatment of aplastic anemia, particularly Fanconi's anemia, have been linked to occurrence of HCC. However, no definite metastatic HCC has been documented after anabolic steroid use, and histologic review of some of the reported tumors shows the typical acinar formation and dysplastic features associated with hepatocellular adenoma of the anabolic steroid type (so-called pseudocarcinoma appearance). Because these tumors regress off the medication and lack metastasis, I believe that they are not carcinoma despite their histologic appearance.

Cryptogenic cirrhosis. HCC arises in livers of about 10% of patients who have cirrhosis of unknown cause. Supposedly rare, there are reports of HCC rising in autoimmune cirrhosis.[845,880] Thirteen percent of the small series of lupoid cirrhotic patients studied at autopsy in our unit (8% of women with that disease and 50% of the men) have had HCC. However, nearly half of the patients with autoimmune liver disease died of submassive necrosis in a precirrhotic stage of chronic liver disease.

Non-A, non-B viral cirrhosis. The relationship between non-A, non-B viral hepatitis and cirrhosis is difficult to establish; undoubtedly many patients with so-called cryptogenic cirrhosis actually have chronic non-A, non-B viral infection. Although I have studied two patients who died of HCC arising in posttransfusion NAB cirrhosis, I have no solid information regarding the total number of cirrhotic patients in our hospital whose cirrhosis is NAB type.

Membranous obstruction of the vena cava. Membranous obstruction of the vena cava (MOVC) is a peculiar condition, rare in the United States[870] but frequently encountered in the Orient[886] and quite common in the black population in Pretoria, South Africa.[934] Of the Af-

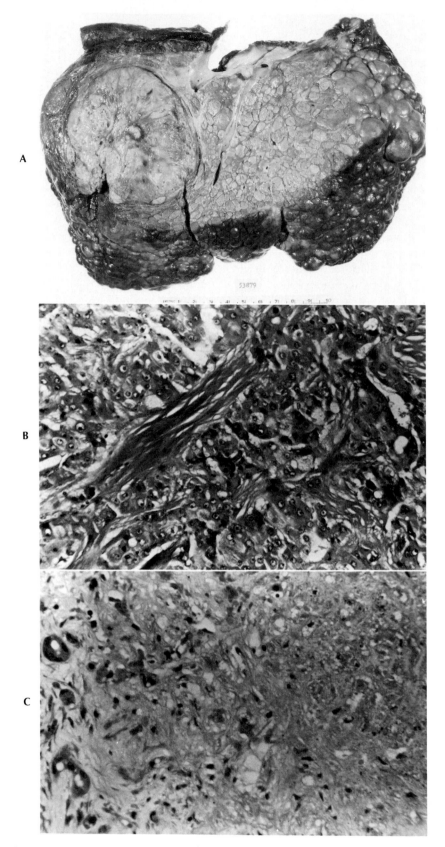

Fig. 25-71. A, Large, encapsulated, nodular liver cell fibrolamellar carcinoma of right lobe arising in liver of 38-year-old Oriental man. **B,** Fibrolamellar carcinoma with thin fibrous bands (lamellar) and polygonal pink carcinoma cells. **C,** Epithelioid hemangioendothelioma with abundant fibrous tissue in the central area containing scattered moderately large epithelioid cells.

rican patients who died of MOVC, 47.5% also had HCC. The weblike obstruction apparently has its origin in utero or during early extrauterine life and is usually not recognized until adulthood. Because of the chronicity, MOVC is not quite comparable to hepatic vein occlusion, but HCC has been reported in patients with chronic Budd-Chiari disease.[915]

Several rare diseases that do not contribute significantly to the total HCC incidence but have a significant coincidence with HCC include alpha$_1$-antitrypsin, aberrant Pi Z,[857,863] chronic immunodeficiency,[839,932] postradiation venous occlusion,[846,903] biliary atresia,[889] and tyrosinemia.[954]

Carcinoma of the liver may occur in infancy and childhood, especially in male infants before 2 years of age. Among adults the disease in Europe and the United States is most common in men between 40 and 50 years of age, whereas in Africa the average is nearer 30 years of age. When carcinoma arises in an otherwise completely normal liver, females are affected as often as males.

Pathologic anatomy

Hepatocellular carcinomas may be spreading, expanding, or multifocal. They usually arise as nodular or pseudolobular growths in the liver that is the seat of advanced cirrhosis.[853] A liver involved by HCC usually weighs between 2 and 3 kg but may be of normal size and weight. The right lobe is more frequently involved than the left in either the spreading or the expanding form. The cancer nodules often bulge beneath Glisson's capsule and are much softer to palpation than are areas of nodular regeneration. The nodules are rarely umbilicated.

In the expanding form of carcinoma the right lobe particularly may be largely replaced by well-circumscribed, soft, yellow-brown tumor (Fig. 25-71). Expanding type of tumor growth is more common in noncirrhotic livers. Small secondary nodules are sometimes present in other parts of the liver.

In the spreading type there is usually one mass that is larger, appears older, and is more circumscribed than any other lesion. Such a tumor may be regarded as the primary lesion (Fig. 25-72). Ordinarily nodules of smaller size are present throughout the remainder of the liver. Invasion of branches of the portal vein is usually demonstrable and is probably responsible for the rapid spread to all parts of the liver. Hemorrhage, necrosis, and bile staining may produce a wide variety of color changes within the nodules.

Hepatitis B virus in situ hybridization analysis of multiple HCC tumor nodules reveals that all nodules have the same pattern of integration and thus demonstrate that although there are many nodules of tumor the carcinoma is monoclonal in origin.[204]

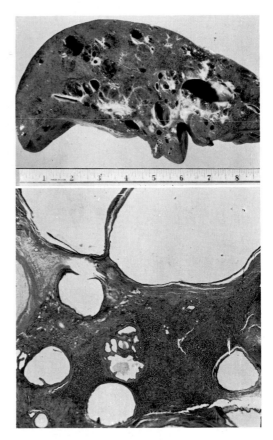

Fig. 25-72. Congenital cysts of liver.

The growth of carcinoma in the branches of the portal vein may lead to a tumor thrombus of the portal trunk and sudden increase of portal hypertension. Less often, the hepatic veins are invaded, and a tumor thrombus extends into the inferior vena cava. By this route the cancer may spread to the lungs and more distant structures.

Tumor cells of HCC stimulate normal liver cells, being characterized by large, round, hyperchromatic nuclei, prominent nucleoli, abundant granular eosinophilic cytoplasm, and a tendency toward arrangement in trabeculas that are usually two to eight cells wide (Fig. 25-73). They retain another feature indicative of their origin; the trabeculas (and liver cords) are covered by a thin connective tissue envelope having, external to this envelope, endothelial cells. This arrangement is particularly noted when the cancer grows into blood vessels. In the expanding carcinomas arising in previously normal liver, the trabecular pattern may not be so obvious. Regardless of variations in pattern, however, most HCCs are composed only of malignant cells and a capillary stroma. The excess connective tissue that characterizes most adenocarcinomas is usually absent. Some carcinomas form acini that may or may not contain bile. Many of the functions of normal liver cells

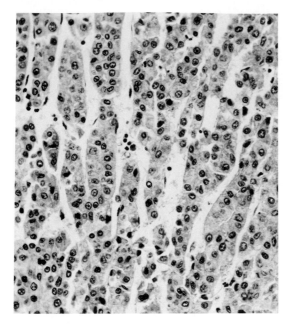

Fig. 25-73. Trabecular liver cell carcinoma with characteristic capillary pattern.

are retained in carcinomas, such as the ability to secrete bile and to store fat and glycogen. It has been suggested that the large amount of glycogen stored in a liver cell carcinoma is not available to form glucose, and this may result in hypoglycemia. Cytoplasmic hyaline inclusions, either globular or small Mallory bodies, are present in some neoplastic hepatocytes.

Several distinctive histologic variants of HCC have been identified. *Fibrolamellar HCC* occurs in young adults, often arises in the left lobe of a noncirrhotic liver, and has a better prognosis than HCC does and has a slow growth rate (Fig. 25-71, *B*). The histologic features are eosinophilic hepatocytes and fibrosis composed of lamellar strands.[847] Spindle cell HCC is distinctive also, with some cases having most of the tumor composed of either bland fibrous tumor or highly pleomorphic spindle cells.[882] In variants of HCC such as spindle cell and pleomorphic HCC, traceability to typical trabecular HCC is necessary to prove the origin.

Hepatocellular carcinomas in infants and children are large, multinodular lesions that, with rare exception, arise in noncirrhotic livers. Congenital defects have been noted in an abnormally high percentage of these patients.[858] Childhood tumors are classified as hepatoblastomas and hepatocarcinomas.[875] A fetal and embryonal cell is typical of hepatoblastoma and about half have osteoid. These tumors arise before 3 years of age (average age at diagnosis is 17 months), and surgical resection is successful in many.[891]

Cholangiocarcinoma

Cholangiocarcinomas may arise from bile ducts within the liver (peripheral cholangiocarcinoma) but originates most often from the large hilar ducts (hilar cholangiocarcinoma) or from the extrahepatic ducts. These are usually mucin-producing, well-differentiated, sclerosing adenocarcinomas that on histologic examination are difficult to distinguish from metastatic adenocarcinomas. In our patients in Los Angeles we have found that 25% of peripheral cholangiocarcinomas arise in cirrhotic livers.

Etiology

Cholangiocarcinoma is known to follow Thorotrast injection.[914,936] *Clonorchis sinensis* infestation,[862] hemochromatosis, polycystic disease, and duct ectasia disease,[869] and occasionally the tumor arises in patients with chronic ulcerative colitis.[922] In patients with the last the risk of cholangiocarcinoma is said to be tenfold higher than in normal persons. Peripheral cholangiocarcinoma is not as likely as HCC to grow within branches of the portal and hepatic veins, though it metastasizes just as widely to other organs but in a different pattern from that of HCC, favoring abdominal nodes, bones, and serosal structure.

Hilar cholangiocarcinoma

Hilar cholangiocarcinoma represents 25% of the total cholangiocarcinomas arising within the liver in our patients in Los Angeles. Reports from Japan indicate that in that country about 30%[942] to 50%[909] of the carcinomas are hilar in location. These carcinomas are characterized by slow growth; only about 15% have metastases at autopsy.[897] The predisposing factors are similar to those for PCC and include many of the same conditions, such as congenital cystic diseases of the duct system,[918] inflammatory bowel disease,[932] and *Clonorchis sinensis*.[862] Hilar cholangiocarcinoma, unlike peripheral cholangiocarcinoma, is characterized by pruritus and icterus at the onset. The course may be protracted, lasting more than 3 years on occasion.

Mesodermal tumors

Malignant tumors of mesodermal origin are rare. Hemangioendothelial sarcomas form bulky hemorrhagic masses and may metastasize to the lungs, portal lymph nodes, and spleen. It has been possible to remove some of these vascular sarcomas surgically.[835] Microscopically they are vasoformative tumors characterized by malignant endothelial lining cells. They may occur after ionizing radiation from Thorotrast[928] and after exposure to arsenic, both in vineyard workers and after the ingestion for therapeutic purposes,[893] as well as in vinyl chloride workers.[842,848] Nonmalignant lesions in vinyl chloride workers consist of portal fibrosis, sinusoidal dilatation, and atypical sinusoidal lining cells. The toxicity of vinyl chloride and polyvinylchloride has been the subject of a conference.[927] Hemochromatosis associated with hemangioendothelial sarcoma has been reported.

Malignant epithelioid hemangioendothelioma occurs as a primary hepatic sarcoma as well as primary tumor of lung and of soft tissue in which case it is less lethal than tumors arising in the liver. The tumor is slow growing and clinical symptoms are not specific. The age range is 19 to 86 years with females slightly more often affected than males.[876a] The gross features of the tumor are multiple nodules of densely fibrous tissue. Microscopic features are abundant fibrosis (even mimicking cirrhosis) in the central part of the tumor, with scattered vascular channels containing large "epithelioid" cells that stain for factor VIII by immunoperoxidase (Fig. 25-71, *C*). *Mesenchymal sarcoma* (also called embryonal sarcoma) occurs in the 6- to 10-year age group with equal sex incidence. Histologic features are a moderately cellular myxoid stroma with mitosis. Surgical resection is successful in less than a fifth.[867]

Although Kupffer cell sarcomas have been reported, this term should be restricted to vasoformative tumors in which the malignant cells are actively phagocytic. Some highly vascular sarcomas of the liver contain large stromal cells in variable quantity that appear to be myosarcomatous. A few cases of fibrosarcoma[948] and leiomyosarcoma have been reported.

Metastatic tumors

In metastatic cancer both lobes of the liver usually are involved, producing an enlarged nodular organ that is easily palpable in life. The cancer cells may reach the liver through the portal vein, hepatic artery, or hilar lymphatics or occasionally by direct extension. Once implanted, the cells may form small or large nodules or grow diffusely throughout the liver. Metastatic carcinoma often grows within sinusoids. The sinusoidal lining cells may be seen on biopsy around tiny metastatic growths (Fig. 25-74). In about 10% of the cases metastatic nodules are solitary. Characteristically, nodules of irregular size bulge beneath Glisson's capsule and are consistently depressed in their central portions (umbilicated) because of necrosis or fibrosis with contraction. Umbilication is practically never seen in HCC.

The pattern of growth of metastatic cancer appears to depend somewhat on the source; for example, carcinoma of the colon or stomach often produces large mucin-containing nodules that have a pebbled appearance on cut surface (Fig. 25-75). Breast cancer often forms smaller, discrete lesions, frequently oval in outline as seen beneath Glisson's capsule.

Metastatic carcinoma is usually gray to grayish white, but necrosis, hemorrhage, and mucus may add a variety

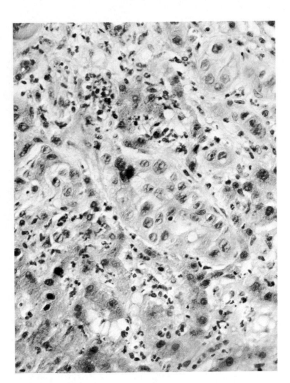

Fig. 25-74. Intrasinusoidal growth of metastatic carcinoma of liver.

of colors. Extensive hemorrhagic lesions are characteristic of choriocarcinoma and metastatic carcinoid. Malignant melanoma is black or brown but sometimes only faintly so.

Occasionally metastatic carcinoma may grow from the hilum outward along the portal tracts, causing them to be unusually prominent. Cancer from the gallbladder may grow directly into the liver, forming a solid mass along with smaller satellite deposits that decrease in size with increase in distance from their origin.

In 60% of the patients with metastatic carcinoma, the disease may be demonstrated by a needle biopsy of the liver. If possible, a biopsy should be performed on a palpable nodule.

Metastatic carcinoma usually grows rapidly in the liver, with patients rarely living more than a year after the diagnosis is made.[879] There are two notable exceptions: metastatic malignant carcinoid is not incompatible with survival of 5 to 25 years, and metastatic neuroblastoma of the adrenal gland in infancy may apparently be cured with radiotherapy. Metastasis to the liver occurs in 38% of all cancers (41% of lung cancers, 56% of colon cancers, 70% of pancreatic cancers, 53% of breast cancers, and 44% of gastric cancers).[855]

Surgical treatment of metastatic cancer is limited to palliative procedures, though occasionally a solitary metastasis may be resected. Hepatic dearterialization[900]

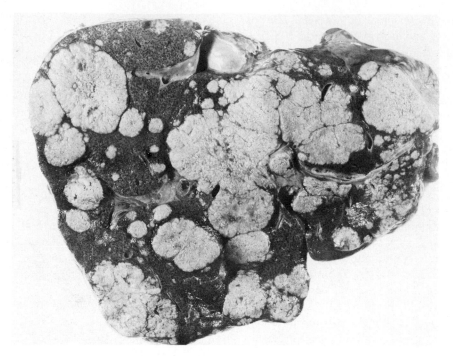

Fig. 25-75. Large metastatic nodules from primary carcinoma of stomach.

has been performed in some cases, since metastatic carcinoma, like HCC, derives its blood from the hepatic artery. These operations may prolong life somewhat and ameliorate symptoms in metastatic carcinoids.[902]

TRANSPLANTATION

Many orthotopic liver transplants have been performed worldwide, with a cumulative total of about 1000 patients by June 1984.[959] Current 1-year survival rates are greater than 50% at 1 year, with improved survival in children compared to adults and better survival with cyclosporin use compared to without the drug. Major diseases leading to transplantation in children include biliary atresia, cirrhosis, metabolic diseases including alpha$_1$-antitrypsin deficiency and in adults include primary biliary cirrhosis, sclerosing cholangitis, selected hepatic tumors (not hepatocellular carcinoma) such as epithelioid hemangioendothelioma and fibrolamellar carcinoma, and the Budd-Chiari syndrome. Transplantation of liver in alpha$_1$-antitrypsin deficiency results in donor-organ alpha$_1$-antitrypsin phenotype.[960] Liver biopsy of the transplanted liver may aid in evaluation of posttransplantation complications.[961] Rejection may be noted by biopsy by portal lymphocytic infiltration, portal PMNs, and bile duct lesions as well as hepatocellular cholestasis.

REFERENCES
General

1. Afroudakis, A., Liew, C.T., and Peters, R.L.: An immunoperoxidase technique for the demonstration of the hepatitis B surface antigen in human livers, Am. J. Clin. Pathol. **65:**533, 1976.
2. Ashare, A.B.: Radiocolloid liver scintigraphy: a choice and an echo, Radiol. Clin. North Am. **18:**315, 1980.
3. Bhathal, P.A., and Christie, G.W.: Fluorescence microscopy of terminal and subterminal portions of biliary tree, Lab. Invest. **20:**472, 1969.
4. Bloom, W.: The embryogenesis of human bile capillaries and ducts, Am. J. Anat. **36:**451, 1926.
5. Brensilver, H.L., and Kaplan, M.M.: Significance of elevated liver alkaline phosphatase in serum, Gastroenterology **68:**1556, 1975.
6. Reference withdrawn.
7. Contreras, P., Altieri, E., Liberman, C., Gac, A., Rojas, A., Ibarra, A., Ravanal, M., and Serón-Ferré, M.: Adrenal rest tumor of the liver causing Cushing's syndrome: treatment with ketoconazole preceding an apparent surgical cure, J. Clin. Endocrinol. Metab. **60:**21, 1985.
8. Corrigan, J.J., and Earnest, D.L.: Factor II antigen in liver disease and warfarin-induced vitamin K deficiency: correlation with coagulant activity using *Echis* venom, Am. J. Hematol. **8:**249, 1980.
9. Craig, J.R., Peters, R.L., and Edmondson, H.A.: Tumors of the liver and intrahepatic bile ducts, Armed Forces Institute of Pathology, ser. 2 fascicle, Washington, D.C. (In press.)
10. Crofton, R.W., Diesselhoff-den Dulk, M.M.C., and Van Furth, R.: Origin, kinetics and characteristics of Kupffer cells in the normal steady state, J. Exp. Med. **148:**1, 1978.
11. Dalan, M.F., and Janovski, N.A.: Adreno-hepatic union (adrenal dystopia), Arch. Pathol. **86:**22, 1968.
12. Edgington, T.S., and Ritt, D.J.: Intrahepatic expression of serum hepatitis virus–associated antigen, J. Exp. Med. **134:**871, 1971.

13. Enzan, H., and Hara, H., Yamashita, Y., Ohkita, T., and Yamane, T.: Fine structure of hepatic sinusoids and their development in human embryos and fetuses, Acta Pathol. Jpn. **33**:447, 1983.

14. Fraser, R., Day, W.A., and Fernando, S.: Review: the liver sinusoidal cells: their role in disorders of the liver, lipoprotein metabolism, and atherosclerosis, Pathology **18**:5, 1986.

15. French, S.W., and Davies, P.L.: Ultrastructural localization of actin-like filaments in rat hepatocytes, Gastroenterology **68**:765, 1975.

16. French, S.W., Kondo, I., Irie, T.J., Benson, N., and Munn, R.: Morphologic study of intermediate filaments in rat hepatocytes, Hepatology **2**:29, 1982.

17. Gabbiani, G., Ryan, G.B., Badonnel, M.C., Lamelin, J.P., Vassalli, P., and Majno, G.: Human smooth muscle autoantibody: its identification as antiactin antibody and a study of its binding to "non-muscular" cells, Am. J. Pathol. **72**:473, 1973.

18. Gerber, M.A., and Thung, S.: Histology of the liver, Am. J. Surg. Pathol. **11**:709, 1987.

19. Girolami, A., Patrassi, G., Cappellato, G., and Quaino, V.: An immunological study of prothrombin in liver cirrhosis, Blut **41**:61, 1980.

20. González-Crussi, F.: Extragonadal teratomas, Armed Forces Institute of Pathology, ser. 2, fasc. 18, p. 129, Washington, D.C., 1982.

21. Gudat, F., Bianchi, L., Sonnabend, W., Thiel, G., Aenishänslin, H.W., and Stalder, G.A.: Pattern of core and surface expression in liver tissue reflects state of specific immune response in hepatitis B, Lab. Invest. **32**:1, 1975.

22. Hadziyannis, S.T., Moussouros, A., Vissoulis, C., Afroudakis, A.: Cytoplasmic localization of Australia antigen in the liver, Lancet **1**:976, 1972.

23. Ham, J.M.: Partial and complete atrophy affecting hepatic segments and lobes, Br. J. Surg. **66**:333, 1979.

24. Hamlyn, A.N., and Berg, P.A.: Haemagglutinating anti-actin antibodies in acute and chronic liver disease, Gut **21**:311, 1980.

25. Hoofnagle, J.H.: Type B hepatitis: virology, serology and clinical course, Semin. Liver Dis. **1**:7, 1981.

26. Horn, T., Henriksen, J.H., and Christoffersen, P.: The sinusoidal lining cells in "normal" human liver: a scanning electron microscopic investigation, Liver **6**:98, 1986.

27. Horn, T., Lyon, H., and Christoffersen, P.: The blood hepatocytic barrier: a light microscopical transmission- and scanning electron microscopic study, Liver **6**:233-245, 1986.

28. Hoyes, A.D., Riches, D.J., and Martin, B.G.H.: The fine structure of haemopoiesis in human fetal liver. I. Haemopoietic precursor cells, J. Anat. **115**:99, 1973.

29. Huang, S.N.: Immunohistochemical demonstration of hepatitis B core and surface antigens in paraffin sections, Lab. Invest. **33**:88, 1975.

30. Johnstone, G.: Accessory lobe of liver presenting through a congenital deficiency of anterior abdominal wall, Arch. Dis. Child. **40**:541, 1965.

31. Jones, A.L., and Schmucker, D.L.: Current concepts of liver structure as related to function, Gastroenterology **73**:833, 1977.

32. Jones, E.A., and Summerfield, J.A.: Functional aspects of hepatic sinusoidal cells, Semin. Liver Dis. **5**:157, 1985.

33. Kaplan, M.A.: Akaline phosphatase, Gastroenterology **62**:452, 1972.

34. Kaneda, K., Kurioka, N., Seki, S., Wake, K., and Yamamoto, S.: Pit cell–hepatocyte contact in autoimmune hepatitis, Hepatology **4**:955, 1984.

35. Kent, G., Gay, S., Inouye, T., et al.: Vitamin A containing lipocytes and formation of type III collagen in liver injury, Proc. Natl. Acad. Sci. USA **73**:3719, 1976.

36. Klatskin, G., and Kantor, F.S.: Mitochondrial antibody in primary biliary cirrhosis and other diseases, Ann. Intern. Med. **77**:535, 1972.

37. Koga, A.: Morphogenesis of intrahepatic bile ducts of human fetus: light and electron microscopic study, Z. Anat. Entwicklungsgesch. **135**:156, 1971.

38. Lautt, W.W.: Hepatic vasculature: a conceptual review, Gastroenterology **73**:1163, 1977.

39. LeDouarin, N.M.: An experimental analysis of liver development, Med. Biol. **53**:427, 1975.

40. Ma, M.H., and Biempica, L.: Normal human liver cell: cytochemical and ultrastructural studies, Am. J. Pathol. **62**:353, 1971.

41. McLaren, D.S., Bitar, J.G., and Nassar, V.H.: Protein calorie malnutrition and the liver, Prog. Liver Dis. **4**:527, 1972.

42. Mendoza, A., Voland, J., Wolf, P., and Benirschke, K.: Supradiaphragmatic liver in the lung, Arch. Pathol. Lab. Med. **110**:1085, 1986.

43. Michels, N.A.: Variant blood supply and collateral circulation of liver, Am. J. Surg. **112**:337, 1966.

44. Mueller, A.F., and Leuthardt, F.: Conversion of glutamic acid to aspartic acid in liver mitochondria, Helv. Chir. Acta **33**:268, 1950.

45. Munro, C.J.: Computed tomography of the liver, Radiology **47**:73, 1981.

46. Nakanuma, Y., Nakamura, Y., Hoso, M., and Ohta, G.: Atrophy and ductopenia of the right hepatic lobe in a patient with choledocholithiasis, Acta Pathol. Jpn. **36**:1719, 1986.

47. Nakamura, S., and Tsuzuki, T.: Surgical anatomy of the hepatic veins and the inferior vena cava, Surg. Gynecol. Obstet. **156**:43, 1981.

48. Palmer, E.D.: Palpability of liver edge in healthy adults, U.S. Armed Forces Med. J. **9**:1685, 1958.

49. Pare, P., Hoefs, J.C., and Ashcavai, M.: Determinants of serum bile acids in chronic liver disease, Gastroenterology **81**:959, 1981.

49a. Peters, R.L., and Craig, J.R.: Liver pathology, New York, 1986, Churchill Livingstone.

50. Phillips, M.J., Poucell, S., Patterson, J., et al.: The liver: an atlas and text of ultrastructural pathology, New York, 1987, Raven Press.

51. Praaning-van Dalen, D.P., Brouwer, A., and Knook, D.L.: Clearance capacity of rat liver, Kupffer, endothelial and parenchymal cells, Gastroenterology **81**:1036, 1981.

52. Qizilbash, A., Kontozoglou, T., Sianos, J., and Scully, K.: Hepar lobatum associated with chemotherapy and metastatic breast cancer, Arch. Pathol. Lab. Med. **111**:58, 1987.

53. Rappaport, A.M.: Microcirculatory hepatic unit, Microvasc. Res. **6**:212, 1973.

54. Rohr, H.P., Luthy, J., Gudat, F., et al.: Stereology of liver biopsies from healthy volunteers, Virchows Arch. [A. Pathol. Anat.] **371**:251, 1976.

55. Rowsell, E.V.: Transaminations with L-glutamate and L-oxoglutarate, Biochem. J. **64**:235, 1956.

56. Rutenberg, A.M., Banks, B.M., Pineda, E.P., et al.: A comparison of serum aminopeptidase and alkaline phosphatase in the detection of hepatobiliary disease in anicteric patients, Ann. Intern. Med. **61**:50, 1964.

57. Severn, C.B.: Morphologic study of development of human liver. II. Establishment of liver parenchyma, extrahepatic ducts, and associated venous channels, Am. J. Anat. **133**:85, 1972.

58. Schiff, L., and Schiff, E.R.: Disease of the liver, ed 6, New York, 1987, J.B. Lippincott Co.

59. Shikata, T., Uzawa, T., Yoshiwara, N., et al.: Staining methods for Australia antigen in paraffin sections, Jpn. J. Exp. **44**:25, 1974.

60. Steiner, J.W., and Carruthers, J.A.: Structure of terminal branches of biliary tree: morphology of normal bile canaliculi, bile preductules, and bile ductules, Am. J. Pathol. **38**:639, 1961.

61. Tygstrup, N., Winkler, K., Mellemgaard, K., and Andreassen, M.: Hepatic arterial blood flow and oxygen supply during surgery, J. Clin. Invest. **41**:447, 1962.

62. Widrich, W.C., and Sequeria, S.R.: Interventional radiology of the liver and related structures, Radiol. Clin. North Am. **18**:297, 1980.

63. Wisse, E., DeZanger, R.B., Charels, K., van der Smissen, P., and McCuskey, R.S.: The liver sieve: considerations concern-

ing the structure and function of endothelial fenestrae, the sinusoidal wall and the space of Disse, Hepatology **5**:683, 1985.

64. Yamamoto, K., Fisher, M.M., and Phillips, M.J.: Hilar biliary plexus in human liver: a comparative study of the intrahepatic bile ducts in man and animals, Lab. Invest. **52**:103, 1985.

65. Yamamato, K., Sherman, I., Phillips, M.J., and Fisher, M.M.: Three-dimensional observations of the hepatic arterial terminations in rat, hamster, and human liver by scanning electron microscopy of microvascular casts, Hepatology **5**:452, 1985.

66. Yeh, H.C., and Rabinowitz, J.G.: Ultrasonography and computed tomography of the liver, Radiol. Clin. North Am. **18**:321, 1980.

67. Zamboni, L.: Hemopoietic activity of fetal liver, J. Ultrastruct. Res. **12**:525, 1965.

Basic hepatic histopathology

68. Adler, M., and Schaffner, F.: Fatty liver hepatitis and cirrhosis in obese patients, Am. J. Med. **67**:811, 1979.

69. Aikat, B.K., Bhattacharaya, T., and Walia, B.N.S.: Morphological features of Indian childhood cirrhosis: the spectrum of changes and their significance, Indian J. Med. Res. **62**:953, 1974.

70. Anthony, P.P., Ishak, K.G., Nayak, N.C., Poulsen, H.E., Schewer, P.J., and Sobin, L.H.: The morphology of cirrhosis, J. Clin. Pathol. **31**:395, 1978.

71. Bengmark, S., Engevik, L., and Rosengren, K.: Angiography of regenerating human liver after extensive resection, Surgery **65**:590, 1969.

72. Berk, P., and Javitt, N.B.: Hyperbilirubinemia and cholestasis, Am. J. Med. **64**:311, 1978.

73. Biava, C.: Electron microscopic studies on periodic acid–Schiff–positive nonglycogenic structures in human liver cells, Am. J. Pathol. **46**:435, 1965.

74. Blendis, L.M., Orrego, H., Crossley, I.R., Blake, J.E., Medline, A., and Israel, Y.: The role of hepatocytes enlargement in hepatic pressure in cirrhotic and noncirrhotic alcoholic liver disease, Hepatology **2**:539, 1982.

75. Brewer, D.B., and Heath, D.: Electron microscopy of anoxic vacuolization in the liver cell and its comparison with sucrose vacuolization, Pathol. Bacteriol. **90**:437, 1965.

76. Bruguera, M., Lamar, C., Bernet, M., and Rodés, J.: Hepatic disease associated with ground-glass inclusions in hepatocytes after cyanamide therapy, Arch. Pathol. Lab. Med. **110**:906, 1986.

77. Bucher, N.L.: Regeneration of mammalian liver, Int. Rev. Cytol. **15**:245, 1963.

78. Chedid, A., Jao, W., and Port, J.: Megamitochondria in hepatic and renal disease, Am. J. Gastroenterol. **73**:319, 1980.

79. Chedid, A., Mendenhall, C.L., Tosch, T., Chen, T., Rabin, L., García-Pont, P., Goldberg, S.J., Kiernan, T., Seeff, L.B., Serrell, M., et al.: Significance of megamitochondria in alcoholic liver disease, Gastroenterology **90**:1958, 1986.

80. Child, P., and Ruíz, A.: Acidophilic bodies, Arch. Pathol. **85**:45, 1968.

81. Ciba Foundation Symposium 55: Hepatotrophic factors, New York, 1978, Elsevier/North Holland, Inc.

82. Clement, B., Grimaud, J., Campion, J.P., Deugnier, Y., and Guillouzo, A.: Cell types involved in collagen and fibronectin production in normal and fibrotic human liver, Hepatology **6**:225, 1986.

83. Coward, W.A., and Lunn, P.G.: The biochemistry and physiology of kwashiorkor and marasmus, Br. Med. Bull. **37**:19, 1981.

84. Darlak, J.A., Moskowitz, M., and Kattan, K.R.: Calcifications in the liver, Radiol. Clin. North Am. **18**:209, 1980.

85. Davis, B.H., and Madri, J.A.: Hepatic fibrogenesis: an immunohistochemical and ELISA serum study in the CCl$_4$ rat model, Am. J. Pathol. **126**:137, 1987.

86. Denk, H., Franke, W.W., Eckerstorfer, R., Schmid, E., and Kerjaschki, D.: Formation and involution of Mallory bodies ("alcoholic hyalin") in murine and human liver revealed by immunofluorescence microscopy with antibodies to prekeratin, Proc. Nat. Acad. Sci. USA **76**:4112, 1979.

87. Essner, E., and Novikoff, A.B.: Human hepatocellular pigments and lysosomes, J. Ultrastructural Res. **3**:374, 1960.

88. Fauerholdt, L., Schlichting, P., Christensen, E., Poulsen, H., Tygstrup, N., and Juhl, E.: Conversion of micronodular cirrhosis into macronodular cirrhosis, Hepatology **3**:928, 1983.

89. Fausto, N.: New perspective on liver regeneration, Hepatology **6**:326, 1986.

90. Fletcher, G.F., and Galambos, J.T.: Phosphorus poisoning, Arch. Intern. Med. **112**:846, 1963.

91. French, S.W.: The Mallory body: structure, composition, and pathogenesis, Hepatology **1**:76, 1981.

92. French, S.W., Okanoue, T., Swierenga, S.H.H., and Marceau, N.: The cytoskeleton of hepatocytes in health and disease. In Farber, E., Phillips, M.J., and Kaufman, N., editors: Pathogenesis of liver diseases, Baltimore, 1987, Williams & Wilkins Co.

93. Galambos, M.R., Collins, D.C., and Galambos, J.T.: A radioimmunoassay procedure for type III procollagen: its use in the detection of hepatic fibrosis, Hepatology **5**:38, 1985.

94. Gärtner, U., Stockert, R.J., Morell, A.G., and Wolkoff, A.W.: Modulation of the transport of bilirubin and asialoorosomucoid during liver regeneration, Hepatology **1**:99, 1981.

95. Gerber, M.A., and Thung, S.N.: Hepatic oncocytes, Am. J. Clin. Pathol. **75**:498, 1981.

96. Gluud, C., Christoffersen, P., Eriksen, J., Wantzin, P., and Knudsen, B.B.: Influence of ethanol on development of hyperplastic nodules in alcoholic men with micronodular cirrhosis, Gastroenterology **93**:256, 1987.

97. Green, P.A., and Stephens, D.H.: Hepatic calcification in cancer of the large bowel, Am. J. Gastroenterol. **55**:466, 1970.

98. Hadziyannis, S., Gerber, M.A., Vissoulis, C., et al.: Cytoplasmic hepatitis B antigen in "ground-glass" hepatocytes of carriers, Arch. Pathol. Lab. Med. **96**:327, 1973.

99. Hall, P.M., Winkelman, E.I., Hawk, W.A., et al.: Calcification in the liver: an unusual feature of ductal cell hepatic carcinoma, Cleve. Clin. Q. **37**:93, 1970.

100. Hilden, M., Christoffersen, P., Juhl, E., and Dalgaard, J.B.: Liver histology in a "normal" population: examinations of 503 consecutive fatal traffic casualties, Scand. J. Gastroenterol. **12**:593, 1977.

101. Hruban, Z., Spargo, B., Swift, H., Wissler, R.W., and Kleinfeld, R.G.: Focal cytoplasmic degeneration, Am. J. Pathol. **42**:657, 1963.

102. International Association for Study of Diseases of the Liver and Biliary Tract: Standardization of nomenclature, diagnostic criteria and prognostic methodology, Fogarty International Proceedings no. 22, pub. no. 76-725, Washington, D.C., 1976, Department of Health, Education, and Welfare.

103. Itoh, S., Igarashi, M., and Tsukada, Y.: Nonalcoholic fatty liver with alcoholic hyalin after long-term glucocorticoid therapy, Acta Hepatogastroenterol. **24**:415, 1977.

104. Itoh, S., and Tsukada, Y.: Clinicopathological and electron microscopical studies on a coronary dilation agent 4,4′-diethylaminoethoxyhexestrol-induced injuries, Acta Hepatogastroenterol. **20**:204, 1973.

105. Kanel, G.C., Uchida, T., and Peters, R.L.: Globular hepatic amyloid: an unusual hepatic manifestation, Hepatology **1**:647, 1981.

106. Keeley, A.F., Iseri, O.A., and Gottlieb, L.S.: Ultrastructure of hyaline cytoplasmic inclusions in a human hepatoma: relationship to Mallory's alcoholic hyalin, Gastroenterology **62**:280, 1972.

107. Kerr, J.F.R.: Shrinkage necrosis: a distinct mode of cellular death, J. Pathol. **105**:13, 1971.

108. Kimura, H., Kako, M., Yo, K., and Oda, T.: Alcoholic hyalin (Mallory bodies) in a case of Weber-Christian disease: electron microscopic observations of liver involvement, Gastroenterology **78**:807, 1980.

109. LaBrecque, D.R., Steele, G., Fogerty, S., Wilson, M., and Barton, J.: Purification and physical-chemical characterization of hepatic stimulator substance, Hepatology **7**:100, 1987.

110. Leffert, H.L., and Koch, K.S.: Ionic events at the membrane initiate rat liver regeneration, Ann. NY Acad. Sci. **339**:201, 1980.

111. Lewis, C., Wainwright H.C., Kew, M.C., Zwi, S., and Isaacson, C.: Liver damage associated with perhexiline maleate, Gut **20**:186, 1979.
112. Ludwig, J., and Elveback, L.R.: Parenchyma weight changes in hepatic cirrhosis: a morphometric study and discussion of the method, Lab. Invest. **26**:338, 1978.
113. MacSween, R.N.M.: Mallory's (alcoholic) hyalin in primary biliary cirrhosis, J. Clin. Pathol. **26**:340, 1973.
114. MacSween, R.N.M., and Scott, A.R.: Hepatic cirrhosis: a clinico-pathological review of 520 cases, J. Clin. Pathol. **26**:936, 1973.
115. Mallory, F.B.: Cirrhosis of liver, N. Engl. J. Med. **205**:1231, 1932.
116. Martin, G.R., and Kleinman, H.K.: The extracellular matrix in development and in disease, Semin. Liver Dis. **5**:147, 1985.
117. McLaren, D.S., and Bitar, J.G., and Nassar, V.H.: Protein calorie malnutrition and the liver, Prog. Liver Dis. **4**:527, 1972.
118. Miller, M.W., and Shamoo, E.A.: Membrane toxicity, New York, 1977, Plenum Publishing Corp.
119. Minato, Y., Hasumura, Y., and Takeuchi, J.: The role of fat-storing cells in Disse space fibrogenesis in alcoholic liver disease, Hepatology **3**:559, 1983.
120. Monroe, S., French, S.W., and Zamboni, L.: Mallory bodies in a case of primary biliary cirrhosis: an ultrastructural and morphogenic study, Am. J. Clin. Pathol. **59**:254, 1973.
121. Morton, J.A., Bastin, J., Fleming, K.A., McMichael, A., Burns, J., and McGee, J.O.: Mallory bodies in alcoholic liver disease, Gut **22**:1, 1981.
122. Murata, K., Ochiai, Y., and Akashio, K.: Polydispersity of acidic glycosaminoglycan components in human and liver and the changes at different stages of liver cirrhosis, Gastroenterology **89**:1248, 1985.
123. Nagasue, N., Yukaya, H., Ogawa, Y., Kohno, H., and Nakamura, T.: Human liver regeneration after major hepatic resection, Ann. Surg. **206**:30, 1987.
124. Nishimura, R.N., Ishak, K.G., Reddick, R., Porter, R., James, S., and Barranger, J.A.: Lafora's disease: diagnosis by liver biopsy, Ann. Neurol. **8**:409, 1980.
125. Ouclea, P.R.: Anoxic changes of liver cells: electron microscopic study after injection of colloidal mercury, Lab. Invest. **12**:386, 1963.
126. Pariente, E.-A., Degott, C., Martin, J.P., Feldmann, G., Potet, F., and Benhamou, J.P.: Hepatocytic PAS-positive diastase-resistant inclusions in the absence of alpha-1-antitrypsin deficiency, Am. J. Clin. Pathol. **76**:299, 1981.
127. Partin, J.S., Partin, J.C., Schubert, W.K., et al.: Liver ultrastructure in abetalipoproteinemia: evolution of micronodular cirrhosis, Gastroenterology **67**:852, 1974.
128. Pérez-Tamayo, R.: Cirrhosis of the liver: a reversible disease? Pathol. Annu. **2**:183, 1979.
129. Peters, R.L.: Hepatic morphologic changes after jejunoileal bypass. In Popper, H., and Schaffner, F., editors: Progress in liver disease, vol. 6, New York, 1979, Grune & Stratton, Inc.
130. Peters, R.L., Gay, T., and Reynolds, T.B.: Postjejunal bypass hepatic disease: its similarity to alcoholic hepatic disease, Am. J. Clin. Pathol. **63**:318, 1975.
131. Petersen, P.: Alcoholic hyalin, microfilaments, and microtubules in alcoholic hepatitis, Acta Pathol. Microbiol. Scand. **85**:384, 1977.
132. Peura, D.A., Stromeyer, F.W., and Johnson, L.F.: Liver injury with alcoholic hyaline after intestinal resection, Gastroenterology **79**:128, 1980.
133. Phillips, M.J.: Mallory bodies and the liver, Lab. Invest. **47**:311, 1982. (Editorial.)
134. Phillips, M.J., Poucell, S., Patterson, J., and Valencia, P.: The liver: an atlas and text of ultrastructural pathology, New York, 1987, Raven Press.
135. Reference withdrawn.
136. Popper, H.: General pathology of the liver: light microscopic aspects serving diagnosis and interpretation, Semin. Liver Dis. **6**:175, 1986.
137. Porta, E.A., Koch, D.R., and Hartroft, W.S.: A new experimental approach in the study of chronic alcoholism, Lab. Invest. **20**:562, 1969.
138. Prockop, D.J., Kivirikko, K.I., Tuderman, L., and Guzman, N.A.: The biosynthesis of collagen and its disorders (in two parts), N. Engl. J. Med. **301**:13 and 77, 1979.
139. Pyke, K.W., and Gelfand, E.W.: Detection of T-precursor cells in human bone marrow and foetal liver, Differentiation **5**:189, 1976.
140. Rabes, H.M.: Kinetics of hepatocellular proliferation as a function of the microvascular structure and functional state of the liver. In Ciba Foundation Symposium 55: Hepatotrophic factors, New York, 1978, Elsevier/North Holland, Inc.
141. Rappaport, A.M., MacPhee, P.J., Fisher, M.M., and Phillips, M.J.: Review: The scarring of the liver acini (cirrhosis): tridimensional and microcirculatory considerations, Virchows Arch. [Pathol. Anat.] **402**:107, 1983.
142. Rojkind, M., and Dunn, M.A.: Hepatic fibrosis, Gastroenterology **76**:849, 1979.
143. Rojkind, M., Giambrone, M., and Biempica, L.: Collagen types in normal and cirrhotic liver, Gastroenterology **76**:710, 1979.
144. Ruebner, B.H.: Collagen formation and cirrhosis, Semin. Liver Dis. **6**:212, 1986.
145. Sakakibara, K., Ooshima, A., Igarashi, S., and Sakakibara, J.: Immunolocalization of type III collagen and procollagen in cirrhotic human liver using monoclonal antibodies, Virchows Arch. [Pathol. Anat.] **409**:37, 1986.
146. Salfeider, K., Seelkopf, C., and Inglessis, G.: Phosphorus poisoning, Zentralbl. Allg. Pathol. **108**:524, 1966.
147. Sato, S., Nouchi, T., Worner, T.M., and Lieber, C.S.: Liver fibrosis in alcoholics: detection by Fab radioimmunoassay of serum procollagen III peptides, JAMA **256**:1471, 1986.
148. Shibayama, Y., and Nakata, K.: Localization of increased hepatic vascular resistance in liver cirrhosis, Hepatology **5**:643, 1985.
149. Starzl, T.E., and Terblanche, J.: Hepatotrophic substances. In Popper, H., and Schaffner, F., editors: Progress in liver disease, vol. 6, New York, 1979, Grune & Stratton, Inc.
150. Sternberg, G.M.: Report on the etiology and prevention of yellow fever, U.S. Marine Hosp. Pub. Health Bull. **2**:151, 1890.
151. Stromeyer, F.W., and Ishak, K.G.: Histology of the liver in Wilson's disease, Am. J. Clin. Pathol. **73**:12, 1980.
152. Tamayo, R.P.: Is cirrhosis of the liver experimentally produced by CCl_4 an adequate model of human cirrhosis? Hepatology **3**:112, 1983.
153. Theron, J.A., and Liebenberg, N.: Fine cytology of parenchymal liver cells in kwashiorkor patients, J. Pathol. Bacteriol. **86**:109, 1963.
154. Uchida, T., et al.: Personal communication, Tokyo, 1986.
155. Uchida, T., and Peters, R.L.: The nature and origin of proliferated bile ductules in alcoholic liver disease, Am. J. Clin. Pathol. **79**:326, 1983.
156. Uchida, T., Kronberg, I., and Peters, R.L.: Giant mitochondria in the alcoholic liver diseases: their identification, frequency, and pathologic significance, Liver **4**:29, 1984.
157. Vasquez, J., and Pardo-Mindan, J.: Liver cell injury bodies similar to Lafora's in alcoholics treated with disulfiram (Antabuse), Histopathology **3**:377, 1979.
158. Webber, B.L., and Freiman, I.: The liver in kwashiorkor, Arch. Pathol. **98**:400, 1974.
159. Weinbren, K., Hadjis, N.S., and Blumgart, L.H.: Structural aspects of the liver in patients with biliary disease and portal hypertension, J. Clin. Pathol. **38**:1013, 1985.
160. Weiner, F.R., Czaja, M.J., Giambrone, M., Wu, C.H., Wu, G.Y., and Zern, M.A.: Development of molecular hybridization technology to evaluate albumin and procollagen mRNA content in baboons and man, Hepatology **7**:19S, 1987.
161. Whitcomb, F.F., Parikh, N.K., and Sedgwick, C.E.: Hydatid cyst disease, Am. J. Dig. Dis. **15**:711, 1970.
162. Wiggers, K.D., French, S.W., and Carr, B.N.: The ultrastructure of Mallory body filaments, Lab. Invest. **29**:652, 1973.
163. Yokoo, H., Minick, O.T., and Batti, F.: Morphologic variants of alcoholic hyalin, Am. J. Pathol. **69**:25, 1972.
164. Yokoo, H., Singh, S.K., and Hawasli, A.H.: Giant mitochondria in alcoholic liver disease, Arch. Pathol. Lab. Med. **102**:213, 1978.

165. Yunis, E.J., Agostini, R.M., and Glew, R.H.: Fine structural observations of the liver in alpha-1-antitrypsin deficiency, Am. J. Pathol. 82:265, 1976.

Infectious disorders

166. Afroudakis, A., Liew, C.T., and Peters, R.L.: An immunoperoxidase technic for the demonstration of the hepatitis B surface antigen in human livers, Am. J. Clin. Pathol. 65:533, 1976.
167. Afroudakis, A., Ashcavai, M., Peters, R.L., and Tong, M.J.: The immunohistochemical detection of HBsAg in liver function of serologically negative HBsAg patients, Am. J. Clin. Pathol. 66(suppl.):461, 1976. (Abstract.)
168. Aledort, L.M., Levine, P.H., Hilgartner, M., Blatt, P., Spero, J.A., Goldberg, J.D., Bianchi, L., Desmet, V., Scheuer, P., Popper, H., et al.: A study of liver biopsies and liver disease among hemophiliacs, Blood 66:367, 1985.
169. Alter, H.J., Hoofnagle, J.H.: Non-A, non-B: observations on the first decade. In Vyas, G.H., Dienstag, J.L., and Hoofnagle, J.H., editors: Viral hepatitis and liver disease, New York, 1984, Grune & Stratton, Inc.
170. Bechtelsheimer, H., Korb, G., and Gedigk, P.: The morphology and pathogenesis of "Marburg virus" hepatitis, Hum. Pathol. 3:255, 1972.
171. Bensabath, G., Hadler, S.C., Soares, M.C., Fields, H., Dias, L.B., Popper, H., and Maynard, J.E.: Hepatitis delta virus infection and Lábrea hepatitis, JAMA 258:479, 1987.
172. Berk, P.D., and Popper, H.: Fulminant hepatic failure: chairman's summary—a final evaluation, Am. J. Gastroenterol. 69:349, 1978.
173. Bernuau, J., Ruess, B., Clauvel, J.P., Degott, C., Terol, Y., and Benhamou, J.-P.: Non-inflammatory herpes simplex hepatitis in an adult with chronic neutropenia, Liver 1:244, 1981.
174. Biava, C., and Mukhlova-Montiel, M.: Electron microscopic observation on Councilman-like acidophilic bodies, Am. J. Pathol. 46:775, 1965.
175. Boeve, N.R., Winterscheid, L.C., and Merendino, K.A.: Fibrinogen-transmitted hepatitis in surgical patient, Ann. Surg. 170:833, 1969.
176. Bonino, F., Smedile, A., and Verme, G.: Hepatitis delta virus infection, Adv. Intern. Med. 32:345, 1987.
177. Bowen, E.T.W., Lloyd, G., Harris, U.J., et al.: Viral haemorrhagic fever in southern Sudan and northern Zaire, Lancet 1:571, 1977.
178. Boyer, J.L., and Klatskin, G.: Pattern of necrosis in acute viral hepatitis: prognostic value of bridging, N. Engl. J. Med. 283:1063, 1970.
179. Bradley, D.W., and Maynard, J.E.: Serodiagnosis of viral hepatitis A by radioimmunoassay, Lab. Management 16:29, 1978.
180. Bradley, D.W., Hornbeck, C.L., Cood, E.H., et al.: CsCl banding of hepatitis A associated virus-like particles, J. Infect. Dis. 131:304, 1975.
181. Brechot, C., Hadchouel, M., Scotto, J., Fonck, M., Potet, F., Vyas, G.N., and Tiollais, P.: State of hepatitis B virus DNA in hepatocytes of patients with hepatitis B surface antigen-positive and -negative liver diseases, Proc. Natl. Acad. Sci. USA 78:3906, 1981.
182. Brechot, C., Lugassy, C., and Dejean A.: Hepatitis B virus DNA in infected human tissues. In Vyas, G.M., Dienstag, J.L., and Hoffnagle, J.J., editors: Viral hepatitis and liver disease, New York, 1984, Grune & Stratton, Inc.
183. Brechot, C., Degos, F., Lugassy, C., Thiers, V., Zafrani, S., Franko, D., Bismuth, H., Trepo, C., Benhamou, J.P., Wands, J., et al.: Hepatitis B virus DNA in patients with chronic liver disease and negative tests for hepatitis B surface antigen, N. Engl. J. Med. 312:270, 1985.
184. Buitrago, B., Popper, H., Hadler, S.C., Thung, S.N., Gerberg, M.A., Purcell, R.H., and Maynard, J.E.: Specific histologic features of Santa Marta hepatitis: a severe form of hepatitis delta virus infection in northern South America, Hepatology 6:1285, 1986.
185. CDC Hepatitis Surveillance Report 1984, JAMA 257:911, 1987.

186. Chang, M.Y., and Campbell, W.G.: Fatal infectious mononucleosis: association with liver necrosis and herpes-like virus particles, Arch. Pathol. 99:186, 1975.
187. Chen, D., Lai, M., and Sung, J.: Delta agent infection in patients with chronic liver disease and hepatocellular carcinoma: an infrequent finding in Taiwan, Hepatology 4:502, 1984.
188. Child, P.L., and Ruíz, A.: Acidophilic bodies, Arch. Pathol. 85:45, 1968.
189. Chu, C., and Liaw, Y.: Intrahepatic distribution of hepatitis B surface and core antigen in chronic hepatitis B virus infection, Gastroenterology 92:220, 1987.
190. Combes, B.: The initial morphologic lesion in chronic hepatitis, important or unimportant? Hepatology 6:518, 1986.
191. Daemer, R.J., Feinstone, S.M., Gust, I.D., and Purcell, R.H.: Propagation of human hepatitis A virus in African green monkey kidney cell culture: primary isolation and serial passage, Infect. Immun. 32:388, 1981.
192. Darani, M., and Gerber, M.: Hepatitis B antigen in vaginal secretions, Lancet 2:1008, 1974.
193. Davis, G.L., Hoofnagel, J.H., and Waggoner, J.G.: Spontaneous reactivation of chronic hepatitis B virus infection, Gastroenterology 86:230, 1984.
194. DeBrito, T., Viera, W.T., and Dias, M.D.A.: Jaundice in typhoid hepatitis: light and electron microscopic study based on liver biopsies, Acta Hepatogastroenterol. 24:426, 1977.
194a. DeCock, K.M., Bradley, D.W., Sandford, N.L., Govindarajan, S., Maynard, J.E., and Redeker, A.G.: Epidemic non-A, non-B hepatitis in patients from Pakistan, Ann. Intern. Med. 106:227, 1987.
195. DeCock, K.M., Govindarajan, S., Chin, K.P., and Redeker, A.G.: Delta hepatitis in the Los Angeles area: a report of 126 cases, Ann. Intern. Med. 105:108, 1986.
196. DeCock, K.M., Govindarajan, S., Sanford, N., and Redeker, A.G.: Fatal reactivation of chronic hepatitis B, JAMA 256:1329, 1986.
197. DeCock, K.M., Govindarajan, S., Valinluck, B., and Redeker, A.G.: Hepatitis B virus DNA in fulminant hepatitis B, Ann. Intern. Med. 105:546, 1986.
198. Deinhardt, F., Holmes, A.W., Capps, R.B., et al.: Studies on the transmission of human viral hepatitis to marmoset monkeys. I. Transmission of disease, J. Exp. Med. 125:673, 1967.
199. Dienstag, J.L.: Hepatitis A virus: virologic, clinical, and epidemiologic studies, Hum. Pathol. 12:1097, 1981.
200. Dienstag, J.L.: Non-A, non-B hepatitis. I. Recognition, epidemiology, and clinical features, Gastroenterology 85:439, 1983.
201. Drew, R., Edington, G.M., and White, H.A.: The prognogy of Lassa fever, Trans. R. Soc. Trop. Med. Hyg. 66:381, 1972.
202. Eichberg, J.W., and Kalter, S.S.: Hepatitis A and B: serologic survey of human and non-human primate sera, Lab. Anim. Sci. 39:5411, 1980.
203. Elsner, B., Schwarz, E., Mando, O.G., et al.: Pathology of 12 fatal cases of Argentine hemorrhagic fever, Am. J. Trop. Med. Hyg. 22:229, 1973.
204. Esumi, M., Aritaka, T., Arii, M., Suzuki, K., Tanikawa, K., Mizuo, H., Mima, T., and Shikata, T.: Clonal origin of human hepatoma determined by integration of hepatitis B virus DNA, Cancer Res. 46:5767, 1986.
205. Fauerholdt, L., Asnaes, S., Ranek, L., Schiødt, T., and Tygstrup, N.: Significance of suspected chronic aggressive hepatitis and acute hepatitis, Gastroenterology 73:543, 1977.
206. Fawaz, K.A., and Matloff, D.S.: Viral hepatitis in homosexual men, Gastroenterology 81:537, 1981.
207. Flehmig, B., Ranke, M., Berthold, H., and Gerth, H.J.: Solid-phase radioimmunoassay for detection of IgM antibodies to hepatitis A virus, J. Infect. Dis. 140:169, 1979.
208. Gerber, M.A., and Thung, S.N.: Biology of disease: molecular and cellular pathology of hepatitis B, Lab. Invest. 52:572, 1985.
209. Gimson, A.E.S., O'Grady, J., Ede, R.J., Portmann, B., and Williams, R.: Late onset hepatic failure: clinical, serological and histological features, Hepatology 6:288, 1986.
210. Goodman, Z.D., Ishak, K.G., and Sesterhenn, I.A.: Herpes simplex hepatitis in apparently immunocompetent adults, Am. J. Clin. Pathol. 85:694, 1986.

211. Govindarajan, S., Uchida, T., and Peters, R.L.: Identification of T lymphocytes and subsets in liver biopsy cores of acute viral hepatitis, Liver 3:13, 1983.

212. Govindarajan, S., Chin, K., Redeker, A.G., and Peters, R.L.: Fulminant B viral hepatitis: role of delta agent, Gastroenterology 86:1417, 1984.

213. Govindarajan, S., DeCock, K.M., and Peters, R.L.: Morphologic and immunohistochemical features of fulminant delta hepatitis, Hum. Pathol. 16:262, 1985.

214. Govindarajan, S., DeCock, K.M., and Redeker, A.G.: Natural course of delta superinfection in chronic hepatitis B virus infected patients: histopathologic study with multiple liver biopsies, Hepatology 6:640, 1986.

215. Govindarajan, S., Valinluck, B., and Peters, R.L.: Relapse of acute B viral hepatitis: role of the delta agent, Gut 27:19, 1986.

216. Hadziyannis, S., Gerber, M.A., Vissoulis, C., et al.: Cytoplasmic hepatitis B antigen in "ground glass" hepatocytes of carriers, Arch. Pathol. 96:327, 1973.

217. Henigst, W.: Sexual transmission of infections associated with hepatitis B antigen, Lancet 2:1395, 1973.

218. Hilleman, M.R., Provost, P.J., Miller, W.J., et al.: Development and utilization of complement-fixation and immune adherence tests for hepatitis A virus and antibody, Am. J. Med. Sci. 270:93, 1975.

219. Hoofnagle, J.H.: Type B hepatitis: virology, serology and clinical course, Semin. Liver Dis. 1:7, 1981.

220. Hoofnagle, J., and Alter, H.J.: Chronic viral hepatitis. In Vyas, G.N., Dienstag, J.L., and Hoofnagle, J.H., editors: Viral hepatitis and liver disease, New York, 1984, Grune & Stratton, Inc.

221. Hoofnagle, J.H., Shafritz, D.A., and Popper, H.: Chronic type B hepatitis and the "healthy HBsAg carrier state, Hepatology 7:758, 1987.

222. Imazeki, F., Omata, M., Yokosuka, O., and Okudo, K.: Integration of hepatitis B virus DNA in hepatocellular carcinoma, Cancer 58:1055, 1986.

223. Immunocompromised homosexuals, Lancet 2:1325, 1981. (Editorial.)

224. Jackson, D., Tabor, E., and Gerety, R.J.: Acute non-A, non-B hepatitis: specific ultrastructural alterations in endoplasmic reticulum of infected hepatocytes, Lancet 1:1249, 1979.

225. Kanel, G.C., Govindarajan, S., and Peters, R.L.: Chronic delta infection and liver biopsy changes in chronic active hepatitis B, Ann. Intern. Med. 101:51, 1984.

226. Kao, H.W., Ashcavai, M., and Redeker, A.G.: The persistence of hepatitis A IgM antibody after acute clinical hepatitis A, Hepatology 4:933, 1984.

227. Karvountzis, G., Redeker, A.G., and Peters, R.L.: Long term follow-up studies of patients surviving fulminant viral hepatitis, Gastroenterology 67:870, 1974.

228. Katchaki, J.N., Siem, T.H., and Browser, R.: Serological evidence of presence of HBsAg undetectable by conventional radioimmunoassay, in anti-HBc positive donors, J. Clin. Pathol. 31:837, 1978.

229. Kiley, M.P., Regnery, R.L., and Johnson, K.M.: Ebola virus: identification of virion structural proteins, J. Gen. Virol. 49:333, 1980.

230. Kojima, M., Udo, K., Takahashi, Y., Yoshizawa, H., Tsuda, F., Itoh, Y., Miyakawa, Y., and Mayumi, M.: Correlation between titer of antibody to hepatitis B core antigen and presence of viral antigens in the liver, Gastroenterology 73:664, 1977.

231. Kojima, T., Callea, F., Desmyter, J., and Desmet, V.J.: Immune electron microscopy in hepatitis delta antigen in hepatocytes, Lab. Invest. 55:217, 1986.

232. Krugman, S., and Giles, J.P.: Viral hepatitis, type B (MS-2 strain): further observations on natural history and prevention, N. Engl. J. Med. 288:755, 1973.

233. Krugman, S., Giles, J.P., and Hammond, J.: Infectious hepatitis: evidence for two distinctive clinical, epidemiological and immunologic types of infection, JAMA 200:365, 1967.

234. Krugman, S., Giles, J.P., and Hammond, J.: Viral hepatitis type B (MS-2 strain) prevention with specific hepatitis B immune serum globulin, JAMA 218:1665, 1971.

235. Kryger, P., and Christoffersen, P.: Liver histopathology of the hepatitis A virus infection: a comparison with hepatitis type B and non-A, non-B, J. Clin. Pathol. 36:650, 1983.

236. Levine, R.A., and Payne, M.A.: Homologous serum hepatitis in youthful heroin users, Ann. Intern. Med. 53:164, 1960.

237. Lindsay, K.L., Redeker, A.G., and Ashcavai, M.: Delayed HBsAg clearance in chronic hepatitis B viral infection, Hepatology 1:586, 1981.

238. Lindsay, K., Nizze, J.A., Koretz, R., and Gitnick, G.: Diagnostic usefulness of testing for anti-HBc IgM in cute hepatitis B, Hepatology 6:1325, 1986.

239. MacGuarries, M.B., Forghani, B., and Wolochow, D.A.: Hepatitis B transmitted by a human bite, JAMA 230:723, 1974.

240. MacLachlan, M.J., Rodnan, G.P., Cooper, W.M., et al.: Chronic active ("lupoid") hepatitis, Ann. Intern. Med. 62:425, 1965.

241. Mathiesen, L.R., Drucker, J., Lorenz, D., Wagner, J.A., Gerety, R.J., and Purcell, R.H.: Localization of hepatitis A antigen in marmoset organs during acute infection with hepatitis A virus, J. Infect. Dis. 138:369, 1978.

242. Mathiesen, L.R., Fauerholdt, L., Møller, A.M., Aldershvile, J., Dietrichson, O., Hardt, F., Nielsen, J.O., and Skinhøj, P.: Immunoflourescence studies of hepatitis A virus and hepatitis B surface and core antigen in liver biopsies from patients with acute viral hepatitis, Gastroenterology 77:623, 1979.

243. Mathiesen, L.R., Skinrøj, P., Nielsen, J.O., Purcell, R.H., Wong, D., and Ranek, L.: Hepatitis type A, B, and non-A, non-B in fulminant hepatitis, Gut 21:72, 1980.

244. Matsaniotis, N., Kattamis, C., Laskari, S., Liapaki, K., Valassi-Adam, H., and Dionissopoulou, E.: Immune responses to hepatitis B vaccine, Lancet 1:210, 1981.

245. Michel, M., and Tiollais, P.: Structure and expression of the hepatitis B virus genome, Hepatology 7:61S, 1987.

246. Mirise, R.T., and Kitridou, R.C.: Arthritis and hepatitis, West. J. Med. 130:12, 1979.

247. Monath, T.P., Maher, M., Casals, J., et al.: Lassa fever in the Eastern province of Sierra Leone: 1970-1972. II. Clinical observations and virological studies, Am. J. Trop. Med. Hyg. 23:1140, 1974.

248. Mosley, J.W.: The epidemiology of viral hepatitis: an overview, Am. J. Med. Sci. 270:253, 1975.

249. Mosley, J.W., Edwards, V.M., Wapplehorst, B., et al: Hepatitis B virus subtypes ad and ay among blood donors in the Greater Los Angeles area, Transfusion 14:372, 1974.

250. Novick, D.M., Gelb, A.M., Stenger, R.J., Yancovitz, S.R., Adelsberg, B., Chateau, F., and Kreek, M.J.: Hepatitis B serologic studies on narcotic users with chronic liver disease, Am. J. Gastroenterol. 75:111, 1981.

251. Omata, M., Afroudakis, A., Liew, C.T., Ashcavai, M., and Peters, R.L.: Comparison of serum hepatitis B surface antigen (HBsAg) and serum anti-core with tissue HBsAg and hepatitis B antigen (HBcAg), Gastroenterology 75:1003, 1978.

252. Omata, M., Yokosuka, O., Imazeki, F., Ito, Y., Mori, J., Uchiumi, K., and Okuda, K.: Correlation of hepatitis B virus DNA and antigens in the liver, Gastroenterology 92:192-196, 1987.

252a. Perrillo, R.P., Regenstein, F.G., Peters, M.G., De Schryver-Kecskeméti, K., Bodicky, C.J., Campbell, C.R., and Kuhns, M.C.: Prednisone withdrawal followed by recombinant alpha interferon, in the treatment of chronic type B hepatitis, Ann. Intern. Med. 109:95, 1988.

253. Peters, R.L., Omata, M., Ashcavai, M., and Liew, C.T.: Protracted viral hepatitis. In Vyas, G.N., Cohen, S.N., and Schmid, R., editors: Viral hepatitis, Philadelphia, 1978, The Franklin Institute Press.

254. Plainos, R.C., Chloros, G., Tripatzi, I., Luciano, L., Kourepi-Logotheti, M., and Tsilivi, N.: Dane particles in homogenates of mosquitoes fed with HBs Ag-positive human blood, Lancet 1:1334, 1975.

255. Popper, H., and Schaffner, F.: The vocabulary of chronic hepatitis, N. Engl. M. Med. 284:1154, 1971.

256. Prince, A.M., Metselaar, D., Kafuko, G.W., Mukwaya, L.G., Ling, C.M., and Overby, L.R.: Hepatitis B antigen in wild-caught mosquitoes in Africa, Lancet 2:247, 1972.

257. Prince, A.M., Grady, G.F., Hazzi, C., Brotman, B., Kuhns, W.J., Levine, R.W., and Millian, S.J.: Long incubation post-transfusion hepatitis without serological evidence of exposure to hepatitis B virus, Lancet 2:241, 1974.

258. Provost, P.J., Wolanski, B.S., Miller, W.J., Ittensohn, O.L., McAleer, W.J., and Hilleman, M.R.: Physical chemical and morphologic dimensions of human hepatitis: a virus strain CR326 (38578), Proc. Soc. Exp. Biol. Med. 148:532, 1975.

259. Rakela, J.: Etiology and prognosis in fulminant hepatitis: acute hepatic failure study group represented by J. Rakela, Gastroenterology 77:A33, 1977. (Abstract.)

260. Rakela, J., and Redeker, A.G.: Chronic liver disease after acute non-A, non-B hepatitis, Gastroenterology 77:1200, 1979.

261. Redeker, A.G.: Viral hepatitis: clinical aspects, Am. J. Med. Sci. 270:9, 1975.

262. Redeker, A.G., Mosley, J.W., Gocke, D.J., McKee, A.P., and Pollack, W.: Hepatitis B immune globulin as a prophylactic measure for spouses exposed to acute type B hepatitis, N. Engl. J. Med. 293:1055, 1975.

263. Redeker, A.G., and Yamahiro, H.S.: Controlled trial of exchange transfusion therapy in fulminant hepatitis, Lancet 1:3, 1973.

264. Reiner, N.E., Judson, F.N., Bond, W.W., Francis, D.P., and Petersen, N.J.: Asymptomatic rectal mucosal lesions and hepatitis B surface antigen at sites of sexual contact in homosexual men with persistent hepatitis B virus infection, Ann. Intern. Med. 96:170, 1982.

265. Reynolds, T.B., Edmondson, H.A., Peters, R.L., and Redeker, A.: Lupoid hepatitis, Ann. Intern. Med. 61:650, 1964.

266. Rijntjes, R.J.M., Van Ditzhuijsen, T.J.M., Van Loon, A.M., Van Haelst, U.J., Bronkhorst, F.B., and Yap, S.H.: Hepatitis B virus DNA detected in formalin-fixed liver specimens and its relation to serologic markers and histopathologic features in chronic liver disease, Am. J. Pathol. 120:411, 1985.

267. Rizzetto, M., Canese, M.G., Purcell, R.H., London, W.T., Sly, L.D., and Gerin, J.L.: Experimental HBV and delta infections of chimpanzees: occurrence and significance of intrahepatic complexes of HBcAg and delta antigen, Hepatology 1:567, 1981.

268. Rizetto, M., Shih, J.W., Verme, G., and Gerin, J.L.: A radioimmunoassay for HBcAg in the sera of HBsAg carriers, Gastroenterology 80:1420, 1981.

269. Robinson, W.S., Miller, R.H., and Marion, P.L.: Hepadnaviruses and retroviruses share genome homology and features of replication, Hepatology 7:64S, 1987.

269a. Sanford, J.P.: Leptospirosis. In Schiff, L., and Schiff, E.R., editors: Diseases of the liver, ed. 6, Philadelphia, 1987, J.B. Lippincott Co.

270. Schweitzer, I.L., Dunn, A.E., Peters, R.L., et al.: Viral hepatitis B in neonates and infants, Am. J. Med. 55:762, 1973.

271. Scolnick, E.M., McLean, A.A., West, D.J., McAleer, W.J., Miller, W.J., and Buynak, E.B.: Clinical evaluation in healthy adults of a hepatitis B vaccine made by recombinant DNA, JAMA 251:2812, 1984.

272. Scott, R.M., Snitbhan, R., Bancroft, W.H., Alter, H.J., and Tingpalapong, M.: Experimental transmission of hepatitis B virus by semen and saliva, J. Infect. Dis. 142:67, 1980.

273. Seeff, L.B., Beebe, G.W., Hoofnagle, J.H., Norman, J.E., Buskell-Bales, Z., Waggoner, J.G., Kaplowitz, N., Koff, R.S., Petrini, J.L.J., Schiff, E.R., et al.: A serologic followup of the 1942 epidemic of post-vaccination hepatitis in the United States Army, N. Engl. J. Med. 316:965, 1987.

274. Sherlock, S., and Thomas, H.C.: Treatment of chronic hepatitis due to hepatitis B virus, Lancet 2:1343, 1985.

275. Shikata, T., Uzawa, T., Yoshiwara, N., et al.: Staining methods for Australia antigen in paraffin sections, Jpn. J. Exp. Med. 44:25, 1974.

276. Shimizu, Y.K., Mathiesen, L.R., Lorenz, D., Drucker, J., Feinstone, S.M., Wagner, J.A., and Purcell, R.H.: Localization of hepatitis A antigen in liver tissue by peroxidase-conjugated antibody method: light and electron microscopic studies, J. Immunol. 121:1671, 1978.

277. Shimizu, Y.K., Feinstone, S.M., Purcell, R.H., Alter, H.J., and London, W.T.: Non-A, and non-B hepatitis: ultrastructural evidence for two agents in experimentally infected chimpanzees, Science 205:197, 1979.

278. Smedile, A., Lavarini, C., Farci, P., Aricò, S., Marinucci, G., Dentico, P., Giuliani, G., Cargnel, A., Del Vecchio Blanco, C., and Rizzetto, M.: Epidemiologic patterns of infection with the hepatitis B virus–associated delta agent in Italy, Am. J. Epidemiol. 117:223, 1983.

278a. Shorey, J.: Does hepatitis B virus grow outside the liver? Gastroenterology 79:391, 1980.

279. Smith, D.H., Johnson, B.K., Isaacson, M., Swanapoel, R., Johnson, K.M., Killey, M., Bagshawe, A., Siongok, T., and Keruga, W.K.: Marburg-virus disease in Kenya, Lancet 1:816, 1982.

280. Snover, D.C., and Horwitz, C.A.: Liver disease in cytomegalovirus mononucleosis: a light microscopical and immunoperoxidase study of six cases, Hepatology 4:408, 1984.

281. Snyder, R.L., Tyler, G., and Summers, J.: Chronic hepatitis and hepatocellular carcinoma associated woodchuck hepatitis virus, Am. J. Pathol. 107:422, 1982.

282. Sternberg, G.M.: Report on the etiology and prevention of yellow fever, U.S. Marine Hosp. Pub. Health Bull. 2:151, 1890.

283. Sureau, C., Romet-Lemonne, J.-L., Mullins, J.I., and Essex, M.: Production of hepatitis B virus by a differentiated human hepatoma cell line after transfection with cloned circular HBV DNA, Cell 47:37, 1986.

284. Szmuness, W., Prince, A.M., Goodman, M., Ehrich, C., Pick, R., and Ansari, M.: Hepatitis B serum globulin in prevention of nonparenterally transmitted hepatitis B, N. Engl. J. Med. 290:701, 1974.

285. Szmuness, W., Dienstag, J.L., Purcell, R.H., Prince, A.M., Stevens, C.E., and Wong, D.C.: Distribution of antibody to hepatitis A antigen in urban adult population, N. Engl. J. Med. 295:755, 1976.

286. Szmuness, W., Dienstag, J.L., Purcell, R.H., Prince, A.M., Stevens, C.E., and Levine, R.W.: Hepatitis type A and hemodialysis: a seroepidemiologic study in 15 U.S. centers, Ann. Intern. Med. 87:8, 1977.

287. Szmuness, W., Dienstag, J.L., Purcell, R.H., Stevens, C.E., Wong, D.C., Ikram, H., Bar-Shany, S., Bensley, R.P., Desmyter, J., and Gaon, J.A.: The prevalence of antibody to hepatitis A antigen in various parts of the world: a pilot study, Am. J. Epidemiol. 106:392, 1977.

288. Szmuness, W., Stevens, C.E., Zang, E.A., Harley, E.J., and Kellner, A.: A controlled trial of the efficacy of the hepatitis B vaccine (Heptavax-B): a final report, Hepatology 1:377, 1981.

289. Szmuness, W., Stevens, C.E., Oleszko, W.R., and Goodman, A.: Passive-active immunization against hepatitis B: immunogenicity studies in adult Americans, Lancet 1:575, 1981.

290. Tassopoulos, N.C., Papaevangelou, G.J., Sjögren, M.H., Roumeliotou-Karayannis, A., Gerin, J.L., and Purcell, R.H.: Natural history of acute hepatitis B surface antigen–positive hepatitis in Greek adults, Gastroenterology 92:1844, 1987.

290a. Tavera, C.: Enterically transmitted non-A, non-B hepatitis—Mexico, JAMA 258(15):2036, 1987.

291. Teodori, U., Gentilini, P., and Surrenti, C.: Electron microscope observation of forms of viral hepatitis, Gastroenterologia (Basel) 108:105, 1967.

292. Thung, S.N., Gerber, M.A., Klion, F., and Gilbert, H.: Massive hepatic necrosis after chemotherapy withdrawal in a hepatitis B virus carrier, Arch. Intern. Med. 145:1313, 1985.

293. Uchida, T., Kronberg, I., and Peters, R.L.: Acute viral hepatitis: morphological and functional correlations in human livers, Hum. Pathol. 15:267, 1984.

294. Veeravahu, M.: Diagnosis of liver involvement in early syphilis: a critical review, Arch. Intern. Med. 145:132, 1985.

295. Vento, S., and Eddleston, W.F.: Immunological aspects of chronic active hepatitis, Clin. Exp. Immunol. 68:225, 1987.

296. Villarejos, V.M., Visona, K.A., Gutiérrez, A., et al.: Role of saliva, urine and feces in the transmission of type B hepatitis, N. Engl. J. Med. 291:1375, 1974.

297. Viral haemorrhagic fevers, Lancet **2**:1325, 1981. (Editorial.)

298. Wang, K.S., Choo, Q.-L., Weiner, A.J., Ou, J.H., Najarian, R.C., Thayer, R.M., Mullenbach, G.T., Denniston, K.J., Gerin, J.L., and Houghton, M.: Structure, sequence and expression of the hepatitis delta viral genome, Nature **233**:508, 1986.

299. Ware, A.J., Cuthbert, J.A., Shorey, J., Gurian, L.E., Eigenbrodt, E.H., Combes, B.: A prospective trial of steroid therapy in severe viral hepatitis, Gastroenterology **80**:219, 1981.

300. Weissberg, J.I., Andres, L.L., Smith, C.L., Weick, S., Nichols, J.E., Garcia, G., Robinson, W.S., Merigan, T.C., and Gregory, P.B.: Survival in chronic hepatitis B: an analysis of 379 patients, Ann. Intern. Med. **101**:613, 1984.

301. Whittingham, S., Irwin, J., Mackay, I.R., et al.: Smooth muscle autoantibody in "autoimmune" hepatitis, Gastroenterology **51**:490, 1966.

302. Winn, W.C., Jr., Monath, T.P., Murphy, F.A., et al.: Lassa virus hepatitis: observations on a fatal case from 1972 Sierra Leone epidemic, Arch. Pathol. **99**:599, 1975.

303. Yoshizawa, H., Akahane, Y., Itoh, Y., Iwakiri, S., Kitajima, K., Morita, M., Tanaka, A., Nojiri, T., Shimizu, M., Miyakawa, Y., and Mayumi, M.: Virus-like particles in a plasma fraction in the circulation of apparently healthy blood donors capable of inducing non-A, non-B hepatitis, Gastroenterology **79**:512, 1980.

304. Zimmerman, H.J., et al.: Jaundice due to bacterial infection, Gastroenterology **77**:362, 1979.

305. Zuckerman, A.J., and Simpson, D.I.H.: Exotic virus infections of the liver. In Popper, H., and Schaffner, F., editors: Progress in liver disease, vol. 6, New York, 1979, Grune & Stratton, Inc.

Chemical and drug injury

306. Al-Kawas, F.H., Seeff, L.B., Berendson, R.A., Zimmerman, H.J., and Ishak, K.G.: Allopurinol hepatoxicity: report of two cases and review of the literature, Ann. Intern. Med. **95**:588, 1981.

307. Arranto, A.J., and Sotaniemi, E.A.: Histologic follow-up of alpha-methyldopa–induced liver injury, Scand. J. Gastroenterol. **16**:864, 1981.

308. Arranto, A.J., and Sotaniemi, E.A.: Morphologic alterations in patients with alpha-methyldopa–induced liver damage after short- and long-term exposure, Scand. J. Gastroenterol. **16**:853, 1981.

309. Barker, J.D., deCarle, D.J., and Anuras, S.: Chronic excessive acetaminophen use and liver damage, Ann. Intern. Med. **87**:299, 1977.

310. Bassi, M.: Electron microscopy of rat liver after carbon tetrachloride, Exp. Cell Res. **20**:313, 1960.

311. Benjamin, S.B., Ishak, K.G., Zimmerman, H.J., and Grushka, A.: Phenyl-butazone liver injury: a clinical pathologic survey of 23 cases and review of literature, Hepatology **1**:255, 1981.

312. Benjamin, S.B., Goodman, A.D., Ishak, K.G., Zimmerman, H.J., and Irey, N.S.: The morphologic spectrum of halothane induced hepatic injury: analysis of 77 cases, Hepatology **5**:1163, 1985.

313. Black, M., Mitchell, J.R., Zimmerman, H.J., et al.: Isoniazid-associated hepatitis in 114 patients, Gastroenterology **69**:289, 1975.

314. Bonkowsky, H.L.: Chronic hepatic inflammation and fibrosis due to low doses of paracetamol, Lancet **1**:1016, 1978.

315. Breitenbucher, R., and Crowley, L.: Hepatorenal toxicity of tetracycline, Minn. Med. **53**:949, 1970.

316. Brown, B.R., and Sipes, I.G.: Biotransformation and hepatotoxicity of halothane, Biochem. Pharmacol. **26**:2091, 1977.

317. Burke, M.: Cytochrome P-450: a pharmacological necessity or a biochemical curiosity? Biochem. Pharmacol. **30**:181, 1981.

318. Chutlani, H.R.: Acute copper sulfate poisoning, Am. J. Med. **39**:849, 1965.

319. Deo, M.G., Roy, H., and Ramalingaswami, V.: Protein deficiency in carbon tetrachloride–induced hepatic lesions, Arch. Pathol. **99**:147, 1975.

320. Drill, A.: Benign cholestatic jaundice of pregnancy and benign cholestatic jaundice from oral contraceptives, Am. J. Obstet. Gynecol. **119**:165, 1974.

321. Emond, M., Erlinger, S., Berghelot, P., Benhamou, J., and Fauvert, R.: Effect of novobiocin on liver function, Can. Med. Assoc. J. **94**:900, 1966. (English abstract of French article.)

322. Ellard, G.A.: The hepatotoxicity of isoniazid among the three acetylator phenotypes, Am. Rev. Respir. Dis. **123**:568, 1981.

323. Erlinger, S.: Cholestasis: pump failure, microvilli defect or both, Lancet **1**:533, 1978.

324. Ferreyra, E.C. de, Castro, J.A., Díaz Gómez, M.I., Acosta, N.D., de Castro, C.R., and de Fenos, O.M.: Prevention and treatment of carbon tetrachloride hepatotoxicity by cysteine: studies about its mechanism, Toxicol. Appl. Pharmacol. **27**:558, 1974.

325. Hoft, R.H., Bunker, J.P., Goodman, H.I., and Gregory, P.B.: Halothane hepatitis in three pairs of closely related women, N. Engl. J. Med. **304**:1023, 1981.

326. Horváth, E., Saibil, F.G., Kovács, K., Kerényi, N.A., and Ross, R.C.: Fine structural changes in the liver of methotrexate-treated psoriatics, Digestion **17**:488, 1978.

326a. Kevat, S., Ahern, M., and Hall, P.: Hepatotoxicity of methotrexate in rheumatic diseases, Med. Toxicol. **3**:197, 1988.

327. Klatskin, G., and Kimberg, B.B.: Recurrent hepatitis attributable to halothane sensitization in an anesthetist, N. Engl. J. Med. **280**:515, 1969.

328. Klemola, H., Penttila, O., Runeberg, L., and Tallqvist, G.: Anicteric liver damage during nitrofurantoin medication, Scand. J. Gastroenterol. **10**:501, 1975.

329. Kline, M.A.: Enflurane-associated hepatitis, Gastroenterology **79**:126, 1980.

330. Knobler, H., Levij, I.S., Gavish, D., and Chajek-Shaul, T.: Quinidine-induced hepatitis, Arch. Intern. Med. **146**:526, 1986.

321. Lauterburg, B.H., and Mitchell, J.R.: Toxic doses of acetaminophen suppress hepatic glutathione synthesis in rats, Hepatology **2**:8, 1982.

332. Maddrey, W.C., and Boitnott, J.K.: Drug-induced chronic liver disease, Gastroenterology **72**:1348, 1977.

333. McCormick, D.J., Avbel, A.J., and Gibbons, R.B.: Nonlethal mushroom poisoning, Ann. Intern. Med. **90**:332, 1979.

334. Métreau, J.M., Dhumeaux, D., and Berthelot, P.: Oral contraceptives and the liver, Digestion **7**:313, 1972.

335. Mitchel, D.H.: Amanita mushroom poisoning, Annu. Rev. Med. **31**:51, 1980.

336. Mitchell, J.R., and Jollows, D.J.: Metabolic activation of drugs to toxic substances, Gastroenterology **68**:392, 1975.

337. Mitchell, J.R., Zimmerman, H.J., Ishak, K.G., Thorgeirsson, U.P., Timbrell, J.A., Snodgrass, W.R., and Nelson, S.D.: Isoniazid liver injury: clinical spectrum, pathology and probable pathogenesis, Ann. Intern. Med. **84**:181, 1976.

338. Mitchell, M.C., Schenker, S., Avant, G.R., and Speeg, K.V., Jr.: Cimetidine protects against acetaminophen hepatotoxicity in rats, Gastroenterology **81**:1052, 1981.

339. Mullick, F.G., and Ishak, K.G.: Hepatic injury associated with diphenylhydantoin therapy: a clinicopathologic study of 20 cases, Am. J. Clin. Pathol. **74**:442, 1980.

340. Nyfors, A., and Hopwood, D.: Liver ultrastructure in psoriatics related to methotrexate therapy, Acta Pathol. Microbiol. Scand. **85**:787, 1977.

341. Panner, B.J., and Hanss, R.J.: Hepatic injury in mushroom poisoning, Arch. Pathol. **87**:35, 1969.

342. Paracetamol hepatotoxicity, Lancet **2**:1189, 1975. (Editorial.)

343. Perrissoud, D., Auderset, G., Reymond, O., and Maignan, M.F.: The effect of carbon tetrachloride on isolated rat hepatocytes: early morphological alterations of the plasma membrane, Virchows Arch. [Cell Pathol.] **35**:83, 1981.

344. Peters, R.L., Edmondsen, H.A., Reynolds, T.B., Meister, J.C., and Curphey, T.J.: Hepatic necrosis associated with halothane anesthesia, Am. J. Med. **57**:748, 1969.

345. Phillips, M.J., Oda, M., and Kazuo, F.: Evidence for microfilament involvement in norethandrolone-induced intrahepatic cholestasis, Am. J. Pathol. **93**:729, 1978.

346. Portmann, B., Talbot, I.C., Day, D.W., et al.: Histopathological changes in the liver following a paracetamol overdose: correlation with clinical and biochemical parameters, J. Pathol. **117**:169, 1975.

347. Prescott, L.F., Ballantyne, A., and Park, J.: Treatment of parecetomal (acetaminophen) poisoning with *N*-acetylcysteine, Lancet **2**:432, 1977.

348. Prescott, L.F., Crome, P., Volans, G.N., Vale, J.A., Widdop, B., and Goulding, R.: Successful treatment of severe paracetamol (acetaminophen) overdose, Lancet **2**:829, 1976.

349. Recknagel, R.: Carbon tetrachloride hepatotoxicity, Pharmacol. Rev. **19**:145, 1967.

350. Recknagel, R.O., and Ghoshal, A.K.: Lipoperoxidation as vector in carbon tetrachloride hepatotoxicity, Lab. Invest. **15**:132, 1966.

351. Reynolds, T.B., Peters, R.L., and Yamada, S.: Chronic active and lupoid hepatitis caused by a laxative, oxyphenisatin, N. Engl. J. Med. **285**:813, 1971.

352. Rigas, B., Rosenfeld, L.E., Barwick, K.W., Enríquez, R., Helzberg, J., Batsford, W.P., Josephson, M.E., and Riely, C.A.: Amiodarone hepatotoxicity, Ann. Intern. Med. **104**:348, 1986.

353. Robertson, W.O.: Changing perspectives on acetaminophen, Am. J. Dis. Child. **132**:459, 1978.

354. Rubotham, J.L., Troxler, R.F., and Lietman, P.S.: Iron poisoning: another energy crisis, Lancet **2**:664, 1974.

355. Sato, C., Matsuda, Y., and Lieber, C.S.: Increased hepatotoxicity of acetaminophen after chronic ethanol consumption in the rat, Gastroenterology **80**:140, 1981.

356. Sherlock, S.: Halothane hepatitis, Lancet **2**:364, 1978.

357. Smith, R.L.: Biliary excretion and hepatotoxicity of contraceptive steroids, Acta Endocrinol. **185**:149, 1973.

358. Spechler, S.J., Sperber, H., and Doos, W.G.: Cholestasis and toxic epidermal necrolysis associated with phenytoin sodium ingestion: the role of bile duct injury, Ann. Intern. Med. **95**:455, 1981.

359. Stanko, R.T., Nathan, G., Mendelow, H., et al.: Development of hepatic cholestasis and fibrosis in patients with massive loss of intestine supported by prolonged parenteral nutrition, Gastroenterology **92**:197, 1987.

360. Stenger, R.J.: Organelle pathology of the liver—the endoplasmic reticulum, Gastroenterology **58**:554, 1970.

361. Storms, W.W.: Chloroform parties, JAMA **225**:160, 1973.

362. Tonder, M., Nordoy, A., and Elgio, K.: Sulfonamide-induced chronic liver disease, Scand. J. Gastroenterol. **9**:93, 1974.

363. Vergani, D., Mieli-Vergani, G., Alberti, A., Neuberger, J., Eddleston, A.L., Davis, M., and Williams, R.: Antibodies to the surface of halothane-altered rabbit hepatocytes in patients with severe halothane-associated hepatitis, N. Engl. J. Med. **303**:66, 1980.

364. Walker, C.O., and Combes, B.: Biliary cirrhosis induced by chlorpromazine, Gastroenterology **51**:631, 1966.

365. Weinstein, G., Roemigk, H., Maibach, H., Cosmides, J., Halprin, K., and Millard, M., et al.: Psoriasis-liver methotrexate interactions, Arch. Dermatol. **108**:36, 1973.

366. Wepler, W., and Opitz, K.: Histologic changes in the liver biopsy in *Amanita phalloides* intoxication, Hum. Pathol. **3**:249, 1972.

367. Wieland, T., and Faulstich, H.: Aflatoxins, phallotoxins, phallolysin, and antamanide: the biologically active components of poisonous *Amanita* mushrooms, CRC Crit. Rev. Biochem. **5**:185, 1978.

368. Zimmerman, H.J.: Classification of hepatotoxins and mechanisms of toxicity. In Zimmerman, H.J., editor: Hepatotoxicity, New York, 1978, Appleton-Century-Crofts.

369. Zimmerman, H.J.: Intrahepatic cholestasis, Arch. Intern. Med. **139**:1038, 1979.

370. Zimmerman, H.J.: Effects of aspirin and acetaminophen on the liver, Arch. Intern. Med. **141**:333, 1981.

Alcoholic liver disease

371. Baillie, M.: The morbid anatomy of some of the most important parts of the human body, vol. 28. In Rodin, A.E.: The influence of Matthew Baillie's morbid anatomy, Springfield, Ill., 1973, Charles C Thomas, Publisher.

372. Bell, H., and Nordhagen, R.: HLA antigens in alcoholics, with special reference to alcoholic cirrhosis, Scand. J. Gastroenterol. **15**:453, 1980.

373. Bruguera, M., Bordas, J.M., and Rodés, J.: Asymptomatic liver disease in alcoholics, Arch. Pathol. Lab. Med. **101**:644, 1977.

374. Burt, A.D., and MacSween, R.N.M.: Hepatic vein lesions in alcoholic liver disease: retrospective biopsy and necropsy study, J. Clin. Pathol. **39**:63, 1986.

375. Cederbaum, A.I.: Regulations of pathways of alcohol metabolism by the liver, Mt. Sinai J. Med. **47**:317, 1980.

376. Chedid, A., Jao, W., and Port, J.: Megamitochondria in hepatic and renal disease, Am. J. Gastroenterol. **73**:319, 1980.

377. Criteria Committee, National Council on Alcoholism: Criteria for the diagnosis of alcoholism, Ann. Intern. Med. **77**:249, 1972.

378. Deitrich, R.A., and McClearn, G.E.: Neurobiological and genetic aspects of the etiology of alcoholism, Fed. Proc. **40**:2051, 1981.

379. Edmondson, H.A.: Pathology of alcoholism, Am. J. Clin. Pathol. **74**:725, 1980.

380. Edmondson, H.A., Peters, R.L., Reynolds, T.B., and Kuzma, O.T.: Sclerosing hyaline necrosis of the liver in the chronic alcoholic: a recognizable clinical syndrome, Ann. Intern. Med. **59**:646, 1963.

381. Fleming, K.A., Morton, J.A., Barbatis, C., Burns, J., Canning, S., and McGee, J.O.: Mallory bodies in alcoholic and nonalcoholic liver disease contain a common antigenic determinant, Gut **22**:341, 1981.

382. French, S.W., Burbige, E.J., Tarder, G., Bourke, E., Harkin, C.G., and Denton, T.: Lymphocyte sequestration by the liver in alcoholic hepatitis, Arch. Pathol. Lab. Med. **103**:146, 1979.

383. Friedman, L.S., Dienstag, J.L., Watkins, E., Hinkle, C.A., Spiers, J.A., Rieder, S.V., and Huggins, C.E.: Evaluation of blood donors with elevated serum alanine aminotransferase levels, Ann. Intern. Med. **107**:137, 1987.

384. Gayre, G.R.: Wassail! In Mazers of mead, London, 1948, Phillimore & Co., Ltd.

385. Goodman, Z.D., and Ishak, K.G.: Occlusive venous lesions in alcoholic liver disease: a study of 200 cases, Gastroenterology **83**:786, 1982.

386. Hales, M.R., Allan, J.S., and Hall, E.M.: Injection corrosion studies of normal and cirrhotic livers, Am. J. Pathol. **35**:909, 1959.

387. Hultcrantz, R., Glaumann, H., Lindberg, G., and Nilsson, L.H.: Liver investigation in 149 asymptomatic patients with moderately elevated activities of serum aminotransferases, Scand. J. Gastroenterol. **21**:109, 1986.

388. International Group: Alcoholic liver disease: morphological manifestations, Lancet **1**:707, 1981.

389. Karasawa, T., Kushida, T., Shikata, T., and Kaneda, H.: Morphologic spectrum of liver diseases among chronic alcoholics, Acta Pathol. Jpn. **39**:505, 1980.

390. Kater, L., Jobsis, A.C., de la Faille-Kuyper, E.H., Vogten, A.J., and Grijm, R.: Alcoholic hepatic disease: specificity of IgA deposits in liver, Am. J. Clin. Pathol. **71**:51, 1979.

391. Keller, M.: A historical overview of alcohol and alcoholism, Cancer Res. **39**:2822, 1979.

392. Klatsky, A.L., Friedman, G.D., and Siegelaub, A.B.: Alcohol and mortality: a ten-year Kaiser-Permanente experience, Ann. Intern. Med. **95**:141, 1981.

393. Krebs, H.A., and Perkins, J.R.: The physiologic role of liver alcohol dehydrogenase, Biochem. J. **118**:635, 1970.

394. Kroyer, J.M., and Talbert, W.M.: Morphologic liver changes in intestinal bypass patients, Am. J. Surg. **139**:855, 1980.

395. Laënnec, R.T.H.: Traité de l'auscultation médiate, Paris, 1826, Chaude.

396. Levin, D.M., Baker, A.L., Riddell, R.H., Rochman, H., and Boyer, J.L.: Nonalcoholic liver disease: overlooked causes of liver injury in patients with heavy alcohol consumption, Am. J. Med. **66**:429, 1979.
397. Li, T.-K.: Human alcohol dehydrogenase isoenzyme (B), Alcoholism **5**:451, 1981.
398. Lieber, C.S.: Alcoholic and the liver: 1984 update, Hepatology **4**:1243, 1984.
399. Lieber, C.S., and de Carli, L.M.: Hepatic microsomal ethanol-oxidizing system: in vitro characteristics and adaptive properties in vivo, J. Biol. Chem. **245**:2505, 1970.
400. Lundquist, F., Tygstrup, N., Winkler, K., Mellemgaard, K., and Munck-Petersen, S.: Ethanol metabolism and production of free acetate in the human liver, J. Clin. Invest. **41**:955, 1962.
401. Mezey, D.: Alcoholic liver disease: roles of alcohol and malnutrition, Am. J. Clin. Nutr. **33**:2709, 1980.
402. Morgan, M.Y., Sherlock, S., and Scheuer, P.J.: Acute cholestasis, hepatic failure and fatty liver in the alcoholic, Scand. J. Gastroenterol. **13**:299, 1978.
403. Orrego, H., Blendis, L.M., Crossley, I.R., Medline, A., Macdonald, A., Ritchie, S., and Israel, Y.: Correlation of intrahepatic pressure with collagen in the Disse space and hepatomegaly in humans and in the rat, Gastroenterology **80**:546, 1981.
404. Orrego, H., Blake, J.E., Blendis, L.M., and Medline, A.: Prognosis of alcoholic cirrhosis in the presence and absence of alcoholic hepatitis, Gastroenterology **92**:208, 1987.
405. Parés, A., Caballería, J., Bruguera, M., Torres, M., and Rodés, J.: Histological course of alcoholic hepatitis, J. Hepatol. **2**:33, 1986.
406. Petersen, P.: Alcoholic hyalin, microfilaments, and microtubules in alcoholic hepatitis, Acta Pathol. Microbiol. Scand. **85**:384, 1977.
407. Popper, H., and Lieber, C.S.: Histogenesis of alcoholic fibrosis and cirrhosis in the baboon, Am. J. Pathol. **98**:695, 1980.
408. Randall, B.: Fatty liver and sudden death: a review, Hum. Pathol. **11**:147, 1980.
409. Reynolds, R.B., Aidemura, R., Michell, H., and Peters, R.: Portal hypertension without cirrhosis in alcoholic liver disease, Ann. Intern. Med. **70**:497, 1969.
410. Rubin, E., and Lieber, C.S.: Alcohol-induced hepatic injury in nonalcoholic volunteers, N. Engl. J. Med. **278**:869, 1968.
411. Schmid, W., and Popham, R.E.: The role of drinking and smoking in mortality from cancer and other causes in male alcoholics, Cancer **47**:1031, 1981.
412. Smith, M., Hopkinson, D.A., and Harris, H.: Developmental changes and polymorphism in human alcohol dehydrogenase, Ann. Hum. Genet. **34**:251, 1971.
413. Stanko, R.T., Mendelow, H., Shinozuka, H., and Adibi, S.A.: Prevention of alcohol-induced fatty liver by natural metabolites and riboflavin, J. Lab. Clin. Med. **91**:228, 1978.
414. Stanko, R.T., Nathan, G., Mendelow, H., and Adibi, S.A.: Development of hepatic cholestasis and fibrosis in patients with massive loss of intestine supported by prolonged parenteral nutrition, Gastroenterology **92**:197, 1987.
415. Swerdlow, M.A., and Chowdhury, L.N.: IgA deposition in liver in alcoholic liver disease, Arch. Pathol. Lab. Med. **108**:416, 1984.
416. Uchida, T., Kao, H., Quispe-Sjögren, M., and Peters, R.L.: Alcoholic foamy degeneration: a pattern of acute alcoholic injury of the liver, Gastroenterology **84**:683, 1983.
417. Uchida, T., Kronborg, I., and Peters, R.L.: Alcoholic hyalin-containing hepatocytes, Liver **4**:233, 1984.
418. van de Wiel, A., Delacroix, D.L., van Hattum, J., Schuurman, H.J., and Kater, L.: Characteristics of serum IgA and liver IgA deposits in alcoholic liver disease, Hepatology **7**:95, 1987.
419. Van Thiel, D.H., Lipsitz, H.D., Porter, L.E., Schade, R.R., Gottlieb, G.P., and Graham, T.O.: Gastrointestinal and hepatic manifestations of chronic alcoholism, Gastroenterology **81**:594, 1981.
420. Veech, R.L.: Metabolism of alcohol: enzymes, pathways, and metabolites (A), Alcoholism **5**:451, 1981.
421. Von Wartburg, J.P.: Alcohol metabolism and alcoholism: pharmacogenetic consideration, Acta Psychiatr. Scand. **62**(suppl. 286):179, 1980.
422. Yokoo, H., Singh, S.K., and Hawasli, A.H.: Giant mitochondria in alcoholic liver disease, Arch. Pathol. Lab. Med. **102**:213, 1978.

Pathophysiology of chronic liver disease

423. Bean, W.B.: Vascular "spiders" and palmar erythema, Am. Heart J. **25**:463, 1943.
424. Bennett, H.S., Baggenstoss, A.H., and Butt, H.R.: Testis, breast, and prostate of men who die of cirrhosis of liver, Am. J. Clin. Pathol. **20**:814, 1950.
425. Berenyi, M.R., Straus, B., and Avila, L.: T rosettes in alcoholic cirrhosis of the liver, JAMA **232**:44, 1975.
426. Berk, P.D., and Popper, H.: Fulminant hepatic failure: chairman's summary—a final evaluation, Am. J. Gastroenterol. **69**:349, 1978.
427. Berthelot, P., Walker, J.G., Sherlock, S., et al.: Arterial changes in the lungs in cirrhosis of the liver, N. Engl. J. Med. **274**:291, 1966.
428. Calabresi, P., and Abelmann, W.H.: Portopulmonary anastomoses, J. Clin. Invest. **36**:1257, 1957.
429. Cavanagh, J.B., and Kye, M.H.: The astrocyte in liver disease, Lancet **2**:1189, 1971.
430. Eisenmenger, W.J.: Ascites in patients with cirrhosis, Ann. Intern. Med. **37**:261, 1952.
431. Grahn, E., Dietz, A.A., Stefani, S.S., et al.: Burr cells, hemolytic anemia and cirrhosis, Am. J. Med. **45**:78, 1968.
432. Green, G., Poller, L., Thomson, J.M., and Dymock, I.W.: Association of abnormal fibrin polymerisation with severe liver disease, Gut **18**:909, 1977.
433. Herbert, V.: Hematopoietic factors in liver diseases, Prog. Liver Dis. **2**:57, 1965.
434. Kelty, R.H., Baggenstoss, A.H., and Butt, H.R.: Portal hypertension, Gastroenterology **15**:285, 1950.
435. Kissane, J.M.: Chronic active hepatitis and pulmonary hypertension. In Cryer, P.E., editor: Clinicopathologic conference, Am. J. Med. **63**:604, 1977.
436. Lieberman, F.L., Ito, S., and Reynolds, T.B.: Effective plasma volume in sclerosis of ascites, J. Clin. Invest. **48**:975, 1969.
437. Lieberman, F.L., and Peters, R.L.: Cirrhotic hydrothorax, Arch. Intern. Med. **125**:114, 1970.
438. Lieberman, F.L., Hidemura, R., Peters, R.L., et al.: Pathogenesis and treatment of hydrothorax complicating cirrhosis with ascites, Ann. Intern. Med. **64**:341, 1965.
439. Liebowitz, H.R.: Pathogenesis of ascites in cirrhosis of liver, NY J. Med. **69**:2012, 1969.
440. Liver disease and the renal prostaglandin system, Gastroenterology **77**:391, 1979. (Editorial.)
441. Maderazo, E.G., Ward, P.A., and Quintiliani, R.: Defective regulation of chemotaxis in cirrhosis, J. Lab. Clin. Med. **85**:621, 1975.
442. McDermott, W.V., Jr.: Surgery of the liver and portal circulation, Philadelphia, 1974, Lea & Febiger.
443. Michalak, T.: Immune complexes of hepatitis B surface antigen in the pathogenesis of periarteritis nodosa: a study of seven necropsy cases, Am. J. Pathol. **90**:619, 1978.
444. Mikkelsen, W.P., Edmundson, H.A., Peters, R.L., et al.: Extra- and intrahepatic portal hypertension without cirrhosis (hepato-portal sclerosis), Ann. Surg. **162**:602, 1965.
445. Mullane, J.F., and Gliedman, M.L.: Elevation of pressure in inferior vena cava, Surgery **59**:1135, 1966.
446. Nakashima, T.: Vascular changes and hemodynamics in hepatocellular carcinoma. In Okuda, K., and Peters, R.L., editors: Hepatocellular carcinoma, New York, 1976, John Wiley & Sons, Inc.
447. Norenberg, M.D., Lapham, L.W., Eastland, M.W., and May, A.G.: Division of protoplasmic astrocytes in acute experimental hepatic encephalopathy, Am. J. Pathol. **67**:403, 1972.
448. Olling, S., and Olsson, R.: Congenital absence of portal venous system in a 50-year-old woman, Acta Med. Scand. **196**:343, 1974.

449. Orloff, M.J., Ross, T.H., Baddeley, R.M., et al.: Experimental ascites, Surgery **56**:83, 1964.

450. Palmer, E.D.: Management of esophageal varices, Prog. Liver Dis. **1**:329, 1961.

451. Papper, S.: Role of kidney in Laënnec's cirrhosis, Medicine **37**:299, 1958.

452. Ramoff, O.D.: Hemostatic mechanisms in liver disease, Med. Clin. North Am. **47**:721, 1968.

453. Reynolds, T.B.: Portal hypertension. In Schiff, L., and Schiff, E.R., editors: Diseases of the liver, ed. 6, Philadelphia, 1987, J.B. Lippincott Co.

454. Reynolds, T.B., Hidemura, R., Michel, H., and Peters, R.: Portal hypertension without cirrhosis in alcoholic liver disease, Ann. Intern. Med. **70**:497, 1969.

455. Reynolds, T.B., Redeker, A.G., and Geller, H.M.: Wedged hepatic pressure, Am. J. Med. **22**:341, 1959.

456. Ring-Larsen, H., and Palazzo, U.: Renal failure in fulminant hepatic failure and terminal cirrhosis: a comparison between incidence, types, and prognosis, Gut **22**:585, 1981.

457. Schafer, D.F., and Jones, E.A.: Hepatic encephalopathy and the γ-aminobutyric-acid neurotransmitter system, Lancet **1**:18, 1982.

458. Silber, R., Amorosi, E., Lhowe, J., and Kayden, H.J.: Spur-shaped erythrocytes in Laënnec's cirrhosis, N. Engl. J. Med. **275**:639, 1966.

459. Soria, J., Soria, C., Ryckewaert, J.J., Samama, M., Thompson, J.M., and Poller, L.: Study of acquired dysfibrinogenaemia in liver disease, Thromb. Res. **19**:29, 1980.

460. Taylor, P., Schoene, W.C., Reid, W.A., Jr., and von Lichtenberg, F.: Quantitative changes in astrocytes after portacaval shunting in chimpanzees and in man, Arch. Pathol. Lab. Med. **103**:82, 1979.

461. Van Thiel, D.H., Lester, R., and Sherins, R.J.: Hypogonadism in alcoholic liver disease: evidence for a double defect, Gastroenterology **67**:1188, 1974.

462. Van Thiel, D.H., Gavaler, J.S., Spero, J.A., Egler, K.M., Wright, C., Sanghvi, A.T., Hasiba, U., and Lewis, J.H.: Patterns of hypothalamic-pituitary-gonadal dysfunction in men with liver disease due to differing etiologies, Hepatology **1**:39, 1981.

463. Wilkinson, S.P., Prytz, H., Jacob, A.I., Clemente, C., Tarao, K., Ringlarsen, H., and Fullen, W.D.: Kidney failure in liver disease, Br. Med. J. **1**:1375, 1978.

464. Wuhrmann, F.: Hepatogenic myocardosis, Scand. J. Gastroenterol. **7**(suppl.):97, 1970.

465. Zieve, L.: The mechanism of hepatic coma, Hepatology **1**:360, 1981.

Cholestatic disorders

466. Abul-Khair, M.H., Kenawi, M.M., Korashy, E.E., and Arafa, N.M.: Ultrasonography and amoebic liver abscesses, Ann. Surg. **193**:221, 1981.

467. Adson, M.A., and Wychulis, A.R.: Portal hypertension in secondary biliary cirrhosis, Arch. Surg. **96**:604, 1968.

468. Baggenstoss, A.H., Foulk, W.T., and Butt, H.R.: The pathology of primary biliary cirrhosis with emphasis on histogenesis, Am. J. Clin. Pathol. **42**:259, 1964.

469. Ball, T.J., Mutchnik, M.G., Cohen, G.M., et al.: Hemobilia following percutaneous liver biopsy, Gastroenterology **68**:1297, 1975.

470. Biava, C.G.: Fine structure of normal bile canaliculi, Lab. Invest. **13**:840, 1964.

471. Blackstone, M.O., and Nemchausky, B.A.: Cholangiographic abnormalities in ulcerative cholitis associated pericholangitis which resembles sclerosing cholangitis, Dig. Dis. Sci. **23**:579, 1978.

472. Bodenheimer, H.C., and Schaffner, F.: Primary biliary cirrhosis and the immune system, Am. J. Gastroenterol. **72**:285, 1979.

473. Boey, J.H., and Way, L.W.: Acute cholangitis, Ann. Surg. **191**:264, 1980.

474. Brandt, H., and Tamayo, R.P.: Pathology of human amebiasis, Hum. Pathol. **1**:351, 1970.

475. Chapman, R.W.G., Marborgh, B.A., Rhodes, J.M., Summerfield, J.A., Dick, R., Scheuer, P.J., and Sherlock, S.: Primary sclerosing cholangitis: a review of its clinical features, cholangiography, and hepatic history, Gut **21**:870, 1980.

476. Charcot, J.M.: Leçons sur les maladies du foie; des voies biliaires et des reins: recueillies et publiées par Bourneville et Sévestre, Paris, 1877, Progrès Médical.

477. Cheung, N.K., Malfitan, R.C., Najem, A.Z., and Rush, B.F., Jr.: Pyogenic liver abscess, Am. Surg. **44**:272, 1978.

478. Christensen, E., Crowe, J., and Doniach, D.: Clinical pattern and course of disease in primary biliary cirrhosis based on an analysis of 236 patients, Gastroenterology **78**:236, 1980.

479. Craig, J.R.: Recurrent pyogenic cholangiohepatitis. In Peters, R.L., and Craig, J.R., editors: Liver pathology, New York, 1986, Churchill Livingstone.

480. Crowe, J.P., Christensen, E., Butler, J., Wheeler, P., Doniach, D., Keenan, J., and Williams, R.: Primary biliary cirrhosis: the prevalence of hypothyroidism and its relationship to thyroid autoantibodies and sicca syndrome, Gastroenterology **78**:1437, 1980.

481. Dehner, L.P., and Kissane, J.M.: Pyogenic hepatic abscesses in infancy and childhood, J. Pediatr. **74**:763, 1969.

482. Delamarre, J., Capron, J.P., Remond, A., Dupas, J.L., and Verhaeg, P.: Traumatic hemobilia: a complication of Chiba needle transhepatic cholangiography, Gastroenterology **75**:771, 1978. (Letter.)

482a. Doppman, J.L., Dunnick, N.R., Girton, M., Fauci, A.S., and Popovsky, M.A.: Bile duct cysts secondary to liver infarcts: report of a case and experimental production by small vessel hepatic artery occlusion, Radiology **130**:1, 1979.

483. Fleming, C.R., Ludwig, J., and Dickson, E.R.: Asymptomatic primary biliary cirrhosis: presentation, histology, and results with D-penicillamine, Mayo Clin. Proc. **53**:587, 1978.

484. Fujiwara, Y., Ohizumi, T., Kakizaki, G., and Fujiwara, T.: Congenital dilatation of intrahepatic and common bile ducts with congenital hepatic fibrosis, J. Pediatr. Surg. **11**:273, 1976.

485. Gall, E.A., and Dobrogorski, O.: Obstructive jaundice, Am. J. Clin. Pathol. **70**:226, 1960.

486. Gallagher, P.J., Millis, P.R., and Mitchinson, M.J.: Congenital dilatation of the intrahepatic bile ducts with cholangiocarcinoma, J. Clin. Pathol. **25**:304, 1972.

487. Helzberg, J.H., Petersen, J.M., and Boyer, J.L.: Improved survival with primary sclerosing cholangitis, Gastroenterology **92**:1869, 1987.

488. Holt, J.M., and Spry, C.J.F.: Solitary pyogenic liver abscess in patients with diabetes mellitus, Lancet **2**:198, 1966.

489. Ishak, K.G., and Rogers, W.A.: Cryptogenic acute cholangitis: association with toxic shock syndrome, Am. J. Clin. Pathol. **76**:619, 1981.

490. Jaup, B.H., Lennart, S.W., and Zettergren, S.W.: Familial occurrence of primary biliary cirrhosis associated with hypergammaglobulinemia in descendants, Gastroenterology **78**:549, 1980.

491. Kanner, R., Weinfeld, A., and Tedesco, F.J.: Hepatic abscess: plain film findings as an early aid to diagnosis, Am. J. Gastroenterol. **71**:432, 1979.

492. Kaplan, M.M.: Primary biliary cirrhosis, N. Engl. J. Med. **316**:521, 1987.

493. Lawson, T.L.: Hepatic abscess: ultrasound as an aid to diagnosis, Dig. Dis. Sci. **22**:33, 1977.

494. Lefkowitch, J.H.: Primary sclerosing cholangitis, Arch. Intern. Med. **142**:1157, 1982.

495. Lin, C.S.: Suppurative pylephlebitis and liver abscess complicating colonic diverticulitis: report of two cases and review of literature, Mt. Sinai J. Med. NY **40**:48, 1973.

496. Lloyd, D.A.: Massive hepatobiliary ascariasis in childhood, Br. J. Surg. **68**:468, 1981.

497. Ludwig, L., Dickson, E.R., and McDonald, G.S.A.: Staging of chronic non-suppurative destructive cholangitis (syndrome of primary biliary cirrhosis), Virchows Arch. [Pathol. Anat.] **379**:103, 1978.

498. Ludwig, J., MacCarty, R.L., LaRusso, N.F., Krom, R.A., and Wiesner, R.H.: Intrahepatic cholangiectases and large-duct obliteration in primary sclerosing cholangitis, Hepatology 6:560, 1986.
499. Maher, J.A., Reynolds, T.B., and Yellin, A.E.: Successful medical treatment of pyogenic liver abscess, Gastroenterology 77:618, 1979.
500. Maingot, R.: Postoperative strictures of the bile ducts: causes, prevention, repair procedures, Br. J. Clin. Pract. 31:117, 1977.
501. Marx, W.J., and O'Connell, D.J.: Arthritis of primary biliary cirrhosis, Arch. Intern. Med. 139:213, 1979.
502. Meade, R.H., III: Primary hepatic actinomycosis, Gastroenterology 78:355, 1980.
503. Moss, T.J., and Pysher, T.J.: Hepatic abscess in neonates, Am. J. Dis. Child. 135:726, 1981.
504. Ochsner, A., DeBakey, M., and Murray, S.: Pyogenic abscess of the liver. II. An analysis of forty-seven cases with review of the literature, Am. J. Surg. 40:292, 1938.
505. Palmer, E.D.: The changing manifestations of pyogenic liver abscess, JAMA 231:192, 1975.
506. Perry, H.B., Boulanger, M., and Pennoyer, D.: Chronic granulomatous disease in an adult with recurrent abscesses, Arch. Surg. 115:200, 1980.
507. Peters, R.S., Gitlin, N., and Libdke, R.D.: Amebic liver abscesses, Annu. Rev. Med. 32:161, 1981.
508. Phillips, M.J., and Poucell, S.: Cholestasis: surgical pathology, mechanism, and new concepts. In Farber, E., Phillips, M.J., and Kaufman, N., editors: Pathogenesis of liver diseases, Baltimore, 1987, The Williams & Wilkins Co.
509. Piggott, J.A., and Hochholzer, L.: Human melioidosis, Arch. Pathol. 90:101, 1970.
510. Quispe-Sjögren, M., Uchida, T., and Peters, R.L.: Comparative clinico-histopathological study among PBC, PSC and liver disease, Gastroenterology 80:1354, 1981. (Abstract.)
511. Record, C.O., Shilkin, K.B., Eddleston, A.L., and Williams, R.: Intrahepatic sclerosing cholangitis associated with a familial immuno-deficiency syndrome, Lancet 2:18, 1973.
512. Reynolds, T.B., Denison, E.K., Frankl, H.D., Lieberman, F.L., and Peters, R.L.: Primary biliary cirrhosis with scleroderma, Raynaud's phenomenon and telangiectasia, Am. J. Med. 50:302, 1971.
513. Robenek, H., Herwig, J., and Themann, H.: The morphologic characteristics of intercellular junctions between normal human liver cells and cells from patients with extrahepatic cholestasis, Am. J. Pathol. 100:93, 1980.
514. Roll, J., Boyer, J.L., Barry, D., and Klatskin, G.: The prognostic importance of clinical and histologic features in asymptomatic and symptomatic primary biliary cirrhosis, N. Engl. J. Med. 308:1, 1983.
515. Rolleston, H.D.: Diseases of the liver, gallbladder, and bile ducts, Philadelphia, 1905, W.B. Saunders Co.
516. Rubin, R.H., Swartz, M.N., and Malt, R.: Hepatic abscess: changes in clinical, bacteriologic, and therapeutic aspects—a review, Ann. Intern. Med. 57:601, 1974.
517. Sabbaz, J., Sutter, V.L., and Finegold, S.M.: Anaerobic pyogenic liver abscess, Ann. Intern. Med. 77:629, 1972.
518. Sandblom, P.: Hemobilia (biliary tract hemorrhage): history, pathology, diagnosis, treatment, Springfield, Ill., 1972, Charles C Thomas, Publisher.
519. Schoenfield, L.J., Sjövall, J., and Perman, E.: Bile acids on skin of patients with pruritic hepatobiliary disease, Nature 212:93, 1967.
520. Sheehy, T.W., Parmley, L.F., Jr., Johnston, G.S., et al.: Resolution of an amebic liver abscess, Gastroenterology 55:26, 1968.
521. Sherlock, S., and Scheurer, P.J.: The presentation and diagnosis of 100 patients with primary biliary cirrhosis, N. Engl. J. Med. 289:674, 1973.
522. Silver, S., Weinstein, A., and Cooperman, A.: Changes in the pathogenesis of intrahepatic abscess, Am. J. Surg. 137:608, 1979.
523. Smith, N.D., and Boyer, J.L.: Are antimitochondrial antibodies of prognostic value in primary biliary cirrhosis? Hepatology 6:739, 1986.
524. Snape, W.J., Long, W.B., Trotman, B.W., et al.: Marked alkaline phosphatase elevation with partial common bile duct obstruction due to calcific pancreatitis, Gastroenterology 70:70, 1976.
525. Takada, T., Hanyu, F., Mikoshiba, Y., et al.: Severe choledochocholangitis causing numerous cystlike hepatic abscesses, Int. Surg. 59:180, 1974.
526. Thung, S.N., and Gerber, M.A.: Caroli's disease: a rarely recognized entity, Arch. Pathol. Lab. Med. 103:650, 1979.
527. Wiesner, R.H., and LaRusso, R.F.: Clinicopathologic features of the syndrome of primary sclerosing cholangitis, Gastroenterology 79:200, 1980.
528. Yadegar, J., Williams, R.A., Passaro, E., Jr., and Wilson, S.E.: Common duct stricture from chronic pancreatitis, Arch. Surg. 115:582, 1980.
529. Yellin, A.E., and Donovan, A.J.: Biliary lithiasis and helminthiasis, Am. J. Surg. 142:128, 1981.

Liver disease in infants and children

530. Altman, P.R., Chandra, R., and Lilly, J.R.: Ongoing cirrhosis after successful porticoenterostomy in infants with biliary atresia, J. Pediatr. Surg. 10:684, 1975.
531. Alvarez, F., Bernard, O., Brunelle, F., Hadchouel, M., Leblanc, A., Odièvre, M., and Alagille, D.: Congenital hepatic fibrosis in children, J. Pediatr. 99:370, 1981.
532. Amanullah, A.: Neonatal jaundice, Am. J. Dis. Child. 130:1274, 1976.
533. Arias, I.M., Gartner, L.M., Seifter, S., and Furman, M.: Prolonged neonatal unconjugated hyperbilirubinemia associated with breast feeding and a steroid, J. Clin. Invest. 43:2037, 1964.
534. Balistreri, W.F., and Schubert, W.L.: Liver disease in infancy and childhood. In Schiff, L., and Schiff, E.R., editors: Diseases of the liver, ed. 6, New York, 1987, J.P. Lippincott Co.
535. Bearn, A.G.: Alpha-1-antitrypsin deficiency: a biological enigma, Gut 19:470, 1978.
536. Becroft, D.M.O.: Prenatal cytomegalovirus infection. In Rosenberg, H.S., and Bernstein, J., editors: Perspectives in pediatric pathology, vol. 6, New York, 1981, Masson Publishing U.S.A., Inc.
537. Benjamin, D.R.: Hepatobiliary dysfunction in infants and children associated with long-term total parenteral nutrition: a clinico-pathologic study, Am. J. Clin. Pathol. 76:276, 1981.
538. Bhagwat, A.G., Walia, B.N.S., Koshy, A., et al.: Will the real Indian childhood cirrhosis please stand up? Cleve. Clin. Q. 50:323-337, 1983.
539. Bourgeois, C., Olson, L., Comer, D., Evans, H., Keschamras, N., Cotton, R., Grossman, R., and Smith, T.: Encephalopathy and fatty degeneration of the viscera: a clinicopathologic analysis of 40 cases, Am. J. Clin. Pathol. 56:558, 1971.
540. Bove, K.E., McAdams, A.J., Partin, J.C., Partin, J.S., Hug, G., and Schubert, W.K.: The hepatic lesion in Reye's syndrome, Gastroenterology 69:685, 1975.
541. Brooks, S., Hanchard, B., Terry, S., and Audretsch, J.J.: Hepatic ultrastructure in secondary syphillis, Arch. Pathol. Lab. Med. 103:451, 1979.
542. Brough, A.J., and Bernstein, J.: Conjugated hyperbilirubinemia in early infancy: a reassessment of liver biopsy, Hum. Pathol. 5:507, 1974.
543. Brown, A.K., and McDonagh, A.F.: Phototherapy for neonatal hyperbilirubinemia: efficacy, mechanism and toxicity, Adv. Pediatr. 27:341, 1980.
544. Chalhub, E.G., DeVivo, D.C., Kerting, J.P., Haymond, M.W., and Feigin, R.D.: Reye's syndrome complicated by a generalized herpes simplex virus type I infection, J. Pediatr. 98:73, 1981.
545. Clausen, P., Lindskov, J., Gad, I., Kreutzfeldt, M., Orholm, M., Reinicke, V., Larsen, H.R., and Strøm, P.: The diagnostic

value of alpha-1-antitrypsin globules in liver cells as a morphological marker of alpha-1-antitrypsin deficiency, Liver **4**:353, 1984.

546. Clayton, R.J., Iber, F.L., Ruebner, B.H., et al.: Byler disease—fatal familial intrahepatic cholestasis in an Amish kindred, Am. J. Dis. Child. **117**:112, 1969.

547. Committee on Infectious Disease: A special report: aspirin and Reye's syndrome, Pediatrics **69**:810, 1982.

548. Craig, J.M., Gellis, S.S., and Hsia, D.Y.: Cirrhosis of the liver in infants and children, Am. J. Dis. Child. **90**:299, 1956.

549. Dahms, B.B., and Halpin, T.C., Jr.: Serial liver biopsies in parenteral nutrition–associated cholestasis of early infancy, Gastroenterology **81**:136, 1981.

550. Dufour, D.R., and Monoghan, W.P.: ABO hemolytic diseases of the newborn, Am. J. Clin. Pathol. **73**:369, 1980.

551. Elleder, M., Smíd, F., Harzer, K., and Cihula, J.: Niemann-Pick disease: analysis of liver tissue in sphingomyelinase-deficient patients, Virchows Arch. [Pathol. Anat.] **385**:215, 1980.

552. Evans, J., Newman, S., and Sherlock, S.: Liver copper levels in intrahepatic cholestasis of childhood, Gastroenterology **75**:875, 1978.

553. Fawaz, K.A., Grady, G.F., Kaplan, M.M., et al.: Repetitive maternal-fetal transmission of fatal hepatitis B, N. Engl. J. Med. **293**:1357, 1975.

554. Freedman, R.M., Ingram, D.L., Gross, I., Ehrenkranz, R.A., Warshaw, J.B., and Baltimore, R.S.: A half century of neonatal sepsis at Yale, Am. J. Dis. Child. **135**:140, 1981.

555. Froesch, E.R.: Essential fructosuria, hereditary fructose intolerance, and fructose-1,6-diphosphatase deficiency. In Stanbury, J.B., et al., editors: Metabolic base of inherited disease, ed. 4, New York, 1978, McGraw-Hill Book Co.

556. Gates, G.F., Sinatra, F.R., and Thomas, D.: Cholestatic syndrome in infancy and childhood, Am. J. Pathol. **134**:1141, 1980.

557. Gautier, M., and Eliot, N.: Extrahepatic biliary atresia: morphological study of 98 biliary remnants, Arch. Pathol. Lab. Med. **105**:397, 1981.

558. Gentz, J., Jagenburg, R., Zetterström, R.: Tyrosinemia, J. Pediatr. **66**:670, 1965.

559. Gibbs, W.N., Gray, R., and Lowry, M.: Glucose-6-phosphate dehydrogenase deficiency and neonatal jaundice in Jamaica, Br. J. Haematol. **43**:263, 1979.

560. Goldstein, A.I., and Farrell, R.C.: Physiologic jaundice of the newborn: relation to maternal serum and amniotic fluid alpha-fetoprotein, Obstet. Gynecol. **51**:315, 1978.

561. Haas, J.E.: Bile duct and liver pathology in biliary atresia, World J. Surg. **2**:561, 1978.

562. Hardwick, D.F., and Dimmick, J.E.: Metabolic cirrhoses of infancy and childhood, Perspect. Pediatr. Pathol. **3**:103, 1976.

563. Hegyi, T., Polin, R.A., and Driscoll, J.M.: The pediatric corner: conjugated hyperbilirubinemia in infants with erythroblastosis fetalis, Am. J. Gastroenterol. **72**:297, 1979.

564. Heubi, J.E., Partin, J.C., Partin, J.S., and Schubert, W.K.: Reye's syndrome, Curr. Concepts Hepatol. **7**:155, 1987.

565. Hirsig, J., and Rickham, P.P.: Early differential diagnosis between neonatal hepatitis and biliary atresia, J. Pediatr. Surg. **15**:13, 1980.

566. Hitch, D.C., Leonard, J.C., Pysher, T.J., Manion, C.V., and Smith, E.I.: Differentiation of cholestatic jaundice in infants: utility of diethyl-IDA, Am. J. Surg. **142**:671, 1981.

567. Hood, J.M., Koep, L.J., Peters, R.L., Schröter, G.P., Weil, R., III, Redeker, A.G., and Starzl, T.E.: Liver transplantation for advanced liver disease with alpha-1-antitrypsin deficiency, N. Engl. J. Med. **302**:272, 1980.

568. Horiguchi, T., and Bauer, C.: Ethnic differences in neonatal jaundice: comparison of Japanese and Caucasian newborn infants, Am. J. Obstet. Gynecol. **121**:71, 1975.

569. Hughes, J.R., Wilfert, C.M., Moore, M., Benirschke, K., de Hoyos-Guevara, E.: Echovirus 14 infection associated with fatal neonatal hepatic necrosis, Am. J. Dis. Child. **123**:61, 1972.

570. Jagenburg, R., Landblad, B., DeMaré, J.M., and Rodjer, S.: Hereditary tyrosinemia: metabolic studies in a patient with partial *p*-hydroxyphenylpyruvate hydroxylase activity, J. Pediatr. **80**:994, 1972.

571. Jones, E.A., Rabin, L., Buckley, C.H., Webster, G.K., and Owens, D.: Progressive intrahepatic cholestasis of infancy and childhood: a clinicopathological study of a patient surviving to the age of 18 years, Gastroenterology **71**:675, 1976.

572. Jorgensen, M.: Stereological study of intrahepatic bile ducts: congenital hepatic fibrosis, Acta Pathol. Microbiol. Scand. **82**:21, 1974.

573. Kaplinsky, C., Sternlieb, I., Javitt, N., and Rotem, Y.: Familial cholestatic cirrhosis associated with Kayser-Fleischer rings, Pediatrics **65**:782, 1980.

574. Karp, W.B.: Biochemical alterations in neonatal hyperbilirubinemia and bilirubin encephalopathy: a review, Pediatrics **64**:361, 1979.

575. Kasai, M., Kimura, S., Asakura, Y., Suzuki, H., Taira, Y., and Ohashi, E.: Surgical treatment of biliary atresia, J. Pediatr. Surg. **3**:665, 1968.

576. Kerr, D.N.S., Harrison, C.V., Sherlock, S., and Walker, R.M.: Congenital hepatic fibrosis, Q. J. Med. **30**:91, 1961.

577. Kibrick, S., and Benirschke, K.: Severe generalized disease in newborn infant due to infection with coxsackievirus, group B, Pediatrics **22**:857, 1958.

578. Koçak, N., and Ozsoylu, S.: Familial cirrhosis, Am. J. Dis. Child. **133**:1160, 1979.

579. Leblanc, A., Odièvre, M., Hadchouel, M., Gendrel, D., Choussain, J.L., and Rappaport, R.: Neonatal cholestasis and hypoglycemia: possible role of cortisol deficiency, J. Pediatr. **99**:577, 1981.

580. Levi, A.J., Gatmaitan, Z., and Arias, I.M.: Deficiency of hepatic organic and anion-binding protein, impaired organic anion uptake and "physiologic" jaundice in newborn monkeys, N. Engl. J. Med. **283**:1136, 1970.

581. Levine, R.L.: Bilirubin, Pediatrics **64**:380, 1979.

582. Levy, H.L., and Hammersen, G.: Newborn screening for galactosemia and other galactose metabolic defects, J. Pediatr. **93**:871, 1978.

583. Longmire, W.P.: Congenital biliary hypoplasia, Ann. Surg. **159**:335, 1964.

584. Luscombe, F.A., Monto, A.S., and Baublis, J.V.: Mortality due to Reye's syndrome in Michigan: distribution and longitudinal trends, J. Infect. Dis. **142**:363, 1980.

585. Masters, P., Langton, S., Robertson, E., and Hill, G.: Galactosaemia: case for neonatal screening illustrated by recent Australian experience, Med. J. Aust. **2**:348, 1981.

586. Mathis, R.K., Watkins, J.B., Szczepanik-van Leeuween, P., and Lott, I.T.: Liver in the cerebro-hepato-renal syndrome: defective bile acid synthesis and abnormal mitochondria, Gastroenterology **29**:1311, 1980.

587. McAdams, A.J., Hug, G., and Bove, K.E.: Glycogen-storage disease, types I to X: criteria for morphologic diagnosis, Hum. Pathol. **5**:463, 1974.

588. Michals, K., Matalon, R., and Wong, P.W.K.: Dietary treatment of tyrosinemia type I, Research **73**:507, 1978.

589. Moss, T.J., and Pysher, T.J.: Hepatic abscess in neonates, Am. J. Dis. Child. **135**:726, 1981.

590. Murray-Lyon, I.M., Ockenden, B.G., and Williams, R.: Congenital hepatic fibrosis, is it a single clinical entity? Gastroenterology **64**:653, 1973.

591. Nahmias, A.J.: The TORCH complex, Hosp. Pract. **9**:65, 1974.

592. Nankervis, G.A., Cox, F.C., and Kumar, M.L.: Diseases produced by cytomegalovirus and its effect on the fetus, Pediatr. Res. **7**:148, 1973.

593. Nankervis, G.A., and Kumar, M.L.: Diseases produced by cytomegaloviruses, Med. Clin. North Am. **62**:1021, 1978.

594. Odièvre, M., Hadchouel, M., Landrieu, P., Alagille, D., and Eliot, N.: Long-term prognosis for infants with intrahepatic cholestasis and patent extrahepatic biliary tract, Arch. Dis. Child. **56**:373, 1981.

595. Pagliara, A.S., Karl, I.E., Haymond, M., and Kipnis, D.M.: Hypoglycemia in infancy and childhood, J. Pediatr. **82**:365, 1973.

596. Petrelli, M., and Blair, J.D.: Liver in GM₁ gangliosidosis types 1 and 2: light and electron microscopical study, Arch. Pathol. **99:**111, 1975.

597. Phillips, M.J., Little. J.A., and Ptak, T.W.: Subcellular pathology of hereditary fructose intolerance, Am. J. Med. **44:**910, 1968.

598. Postuma, R., and Trevenen, C.L.: Liver disease in infants receiving total parenteral nutrition, Pediatrics **63:**110, 1979.

599. Putman, C.W., Porter, K.A., Peters, R.L., Ashcavi, M., Redeker, A.G., and Starzl, T.E.: Liver replacement for alpha-1-antitrypsin deficiency, Surgery **81:**258, 1977.

600. Ram, P., and Poe, N.: Hepatobiliary imaging by radionuclide scintigraphy, West. J. Med. **134:**434, 1981.

601. Reyes, R.D.K., Morgan, G., and Baral, J.: Encephalopathy and fatty degeneration of the viscera, Lancet **2:**749, 1963.

602. Riely, C.A.: Familial intrahepatic cholestatic syndromes, Semin. Liver Dis. **7:**119, 1987.

603. Rosenberg, H.S., Openheimer, E.H., and Esterly, J.R.: Congenital rubella syndrome. In Rosenberg, H.S., and Bernstein, J., editors: Perspectives in pediatric pathology, vol. 6, New York, 1981, Masson Publishing U.S.A., Inc.

604. Ruebner, B.H., and Miyai, K.: Neonatal hepatitis and biliary atresia: hemopoiesis and hemosiderin deposition, Ann. NY Acad. Sci. **111:**375, 1963.

605. Saland, J., McNamara, H., and Cohen, M.I.: Navajo jaundice: a variant of neonatal hyperbilirubinemia associated with breast feeding, J. Pediatr. **85:**271, 1974.

606. Saxoni, F., Lapatsanis, P., and Pontelakis, S.N.: Congenital syphilis, Clin. Pediatr. **6:**687, 1967.

607. Schweitzer, I.L., Wing, A., McPeak, C., et al.: Hepatitis and hepatitis-associated antigen in 56 mother-infant pairs, JAMA **220:**1092, 1972.

608. Schweiter, I.L., Mosley, J.W., Ashcavai, M., et al.: Factors influencing neonatal infection by hepatitis B virus, Gastroenterology **65:**277, 1973.

609. Singer, D.B.: Pathology of neonatal herpes simplex virus infection. In Rosenberg, H.A., and Bernstein, J., editors: Perspectives in pediatric pathology, vol. 6, New York, 1981, Masson Publishing U.S.A., Inc.

610. Sinniah, D., and Baskaran, G.: Margosa oil poisoning as a cause of Reye's syndrome, Lancet **1:**487, 1981.

611. St. Geme, J.W., Jr.: Perinatal and neonatal infections, West. J. Med. **122:**359, 1975.

612. Stagno, S.: Congenital toxoplasmosis, Am. J. Dis. Child. **134:**1980.

613. Strauss, L., and Bernstein, J.: Neonatal hepatitis in congenital rubella, Arch. Pathol. **86:**317, 1968.

614. Tanaka, K.K., Kean, E.A., and Johnson, B.: Jamaican vomiting sickness, N. Engl. J. Med. **295:**461, 1976.

615. Thaler, M.M.: Jaundice in the newborn—algorithmic diagnosis of conjugated and unconjugated hyperbilirubinemia, JAMA **237:**56, 1977.

616. Tolstrup, N.: Clinical and biochemical aspects of galactosemia, Scand. J. Clin. Lab. Invest. **18**(suppl. 92):148, 1966.

617. Tong, M.J., Thursby, M., Rakela, J., McPeak, C., Edwards, V.M., and Mosley, J.W.: Studies on the maternal-infant transmission of the viruses which cause acute hepatitis, Gastroenterology **80:**999, 1981.

618. Triger, D.R., Millward-Sadler, G.H., Czaykowski, A.A., et al.: Alpha-1-antitrypsin deficiency and liver disease in adults, Q. J. Med. **45:**351, 1976.

619. Valman, H.B., France, N.E., and Wallis, P.G.: Prolonged neonatal jaundice in cystic fibrosis, Arch. Dis. Child. **46:**805, 1971.

620. Weber, A.M., Tuchweber, B., Yousef, I., Brochu, P., Turgeon, C., Gabbiani, G., Morin, C.L., and Roy, C.C.: Severe familial cholestasis in North American Indian children: a clinical model of microfilament dysfunction? Gastroenterology **81:**653, 1981.

621. Weinberg, A.G., Mize, C.E., and Worthen, H.G.: The occurrence of hepatoma in the chronic form of hereditary tyrosinemia, J. Pediatr. **88:**434, 1976.

622. Wharton, B.: Hypoglycemia in children with kwashiorkor, Lancet **1:**171, 1970.

623. Wills, E.J.: Electron microscopy of the liver in infectious mononucleosis/megalovirus hepatitis, Am. J. Dis. Child. **123:**301, 1972.

624. Wright, D.J.M., and Berry, C.L.: Liver involvement in congenital syphilis, Br. J. Vener. Dis. **50:**241, 1974.

625. Wysowski, D.K., Flynt, J.W., Jr., Goldberg, M.F., and Connell, F.A.: RH hemolytic disease, JAMA **242:**1376, 1979.

626. Yudokoff, M., Cohn, R.M., and Segal, S.: Errors of carbohydrate metabolism in infants and children, Clin. Pediatr. **17:**820, 1978.

627. Zimmerman, H.J.: Jaundice due to bacterial infection, Gastroenterology **77:**362, 1979.

Less common liver diseases

628. Arias, F., and Jiménez, R.M.: Hepatic fibrinogen deposits in preclampsia, N. Engl. J. Med. **295:**578, 1976.

629. Bassett, M.L., Halliday, J.W., and Powell, L.W.: Value of hepatic iron measurement in early hemochromatosis and determination of the critical iron level associated with fibrosis, Hepatology **6:**24, 1986.

630. Batey, R.G., Pettit, J.E., Nicholas, A.W., Sherlock, S., and Hoffbrand, A.V.: Liver physiology and disease: hepatic iron clearance from serum in treated hemochromatosis, Gastroenterology **75:**856, 1978.

631. Baumwol, M., and Park, W.: An acute abdomen: spontaneous rupture of liver during pregnancy, Br. J. Surg. **63:**718, 1976.

632. Beaumont, C., Simon, M., Fauchet, R., Hespel, J.P., Brissot, P., Genetet, B., and Bourel, M.: Serum ferritin as a possible marker of the hemochromatosis allele, N. Engl. J. Med. **301:**169, 1979.

633. Berresford, P.A., Sunter, J.P., Harrison, V., and Lesna, M.: Histological demonstration and frequency of intrahepatocytic copper in patients suffering from alcoholic liver disease, Histopathology **4:**637, 1980.

634. Blisard, K.S., and Bartow, S.A.: Neonatal hemochromatosis, Hum. Pathol. **17:**376, 1986.

635. Bothwell, T.H., and Isaacson, C.: Siderosis in Bantu, Br. Med. J. **1:**522, 1962.

636. Cano, R.I., Delman, M.R., Pitchumoni, C.S., Lev, R., and Rosenthal, W.S.: Acute fatty liver of pregnancy: complication by disseminated intravascular coagulation, JAMA **231:**159, 1975.

637. Cartwright, G.E., Edwards, C.Q., Kravitz, K., Skolnick, M., Amos, D.B., Johnson, A., and Buskjaer, L.: Hereditary hemochromatosis: phenotypic expression of the disease, N. Engl. J. Med. **304:**175, 1979.

638. Cornelius, C.E., Arias, I.M., and Osburn, B.: Syndrome in Corriedale sheep resembling Dubin-Johnson, J. Am. Vet. Med. Assoc. **146:**709, 1965.

639. Dalen, E., and Westerholm, B.: Occurrence of hepatic impairment in women jaundiced by oral contraceptives and in their mothers and sisters, Acta Med. Scand. **195:**459, 1974.

640. Dawson, J., Seymour, C.A., and Peters, T.J.: Gilbert's syndrome: analytical subcellular fractionation of liver biopsy specimens, Clin. Sci. **57:**491, 1979.

641. Dawson, J., Carr-Locke, D.L., Talbot, I.C., and Rosenthal, F.D.: Gilbert's syndrome: evidence of morphological heterogeneity, Gut **20:**848, 1979.

642. Derring, T.B., Dickson, E.R., Fleming, C.R., Geall, M.G., McCall, J.T., and Baggenstoss, A.H.: Effects of D-penicillamine on copper retention in patients with primary biliary cirrhosis, Gastroenterology **72:**1208, 1977.

643. Dickerman, R.M., and Dunn, E.L.: Splenic, pancreatic, and hepatic injury, Surg. Clin. North Am. **61:**3, 1981.

644. Diess, A., Lee, G.R., and Cartwright, G.E.: Hemolytic anemia in Wilson's disease, J. Intern. Med. **73:**413, 1970.

645. Don't forget Wilson's disease, Br. Med. J. **2:**1384, 1978. (Editorial.)

646. Drill, A.: Benign cholestatic jaundice of pregnancy and benign cholestatic jaundice from oral contraceptives, Am. J. Obstet. Gynecol. **119:**165, 1974.

647. Drysdale, J.W., Adelman, T.G., Arosio, P., Casareale, D., Fitzpatrick, P., Hazard J.T., and Yokota, M.: Human isoferritins in normal and disease states, Semin. Haematol. **14:**71, 1977.

648. Edwards, C.Q., Cartwright, G.E., Skolnick, M.H., and Amos, D.B.: Homozygosity for hemochromatosis: clinical manifestations, Ann. Intern. Med. **93:**519, 1980.

649. Edwards, R.H.: Inheritance of the Dubin-Johnson-Sprinz syndrome, Gastroenterology **68:**734, 1975.

650. Elerding, S.C., Aragon, G.E., and Moore, E.E.: Fatal hepatic hemorrhage after trauma, Am. J. Surg. **138:**883, 1979.

651. Evans, J., Newman, S., and Sherlock, S.: Liver copper levels in intrahepatic cholestasis of childhood, Gastroenterology **75:**875, 1978.

652. Fleming, D.R., Dickson, E.R., Hollenhorst, R.W., Goldstein, W.P., McCall, J.T., and Baggenstoss, A.H.: Pigmented corneal rings in a patient with primary biliary cirrhosis, Gastroenterology **69:**220, 1975.

653. Foley, W.J., Turcotte, J.G., Hoskins, P.A., et al.: Intrahepatic arteriovenous fistulas between the hepatic artery and portal veins, Ann. Surg. **174:**849, 1971.

654. Franklin, D.C., and Mathai, J.: Biliary pleural fistula: a complication of hepatic trauma, J. Trauma **20:**256, 1980.

655. No reference.

656. Frederick, W.C., Howard, R.G., and Spatola, S.: Spontaneous rupture of the liver in patient using contraceptive pills, Arch. Surg. **108:**93, 1974.

657. Frydman, M., Bonne-Tamir, B., Farrer, L.A., Conneally, P.M., Magazanik, A., Ashbel, S., and Goldwitch, Z.: Assignment of the gene for Wilson disease to chromosome 13: linkage to the esterase D locus, Proc. Natl. Acad. Sci. USA **82:**1819, 1985.

658. Golan, A., and White, R.G.: Spontaneous rupture of the liver associated with pregnancy, S. Afr. Med. J. **56:**133, 1979.

659. Goldfischer, S., and Sternlieb, I.: Changes in distribution of hepatic copper in relation to progression of Wilson's disease, Am. J. Pathol. **52:**883, 1968.

660. Gollan, J.L., Huang, S.N., Billing, B., and Sherlock, S.: Prolonged survival in three brothers with severe type 2 Crigler-Najjar syndrome: ultrastructural and metabolic studies, Gastroenterology **68:**1543, 1975.

661. Hibbard, L.T.: Spontaneous rupture of the liver in pregnancy: a report of 8 cases, Am. J. Obstet. Gynecol. **126:**334, 1976.

662. Reference withdrawn.

663. Iancu, T.C., Neustein, H.B., and Landing, B.H.: The liver in thalassemia major: ultrastructural observations. In Porter, R., and Fitzsimons, D.W.: Iron metabolism (Ciba Foundation symposium new series 51), New York, 1977, Elsevier/North-Holland, Inc.

664. Jacobs, A.: Iron overload: clinical and pathologic aspects, Semin. Hematol. **14:**89, 1977.

665. Johnston, W.G., and Baskett, T.F.: Obstetric cholestasis: a 14-year review, Am. J. Obstet. Gynecol. **133:**299, 1979.

666. Kawasaki, H., Kuchiba, K., Kondo, T., Kimura, N., and Hirayama, C.: Unconjugated bilirubin kinetics in Dubin-Johnson syndrome, Clin. Chim. Acta **92:**87, 1979.

667. Khuroo, M.S., Teli, M.R., Skidmore, S., Sofi, M.A., and Khuroo, M.I.: Incidence and severity of viral hepatitis in pregnancy, Am. J. Med. **70:**252, 1981.

667a. Koskelo, P., and Mustajoki, P.: Altered coproporphyrin-isomer excretion in patients with the Dubin-Johnson syndrome, Int. J. Biochem. **12:**975, 1979.

668. Kunelis, C.T., Peters, R.L., and Edmondson, H.A.: Fatty liver of pregnancy and its relationship to tetracycline therapy, Am. J. Med. **38:**359, 1965.

669. Lisboa, P.E.: Experimental hepatic cirrhosis in dogs caused by chronic massive iron overload, Gut **12:**363, 1971.

670. Long, R.G., Scheuer, P.J., and Sherlock, S.: Pre-eclampsia presenting with deep jaundice, J. Clin. Pathol. **30:**212, 1977.

671. Ludwig, J., Owen, C.A., Jr., Barham, S.S., McCall, J.T., and Hardy, R.M.: The liver in the inherited copper disease of Bedlington terriers, Lab. Invest. **43:**82, 1980.

672. MacKenna, J., Pupkin, M., Crenshaw, C., Jr., McLeod, M., and Parker, R.T.: Acute fatty metamorphosis of the liver: a report of two patients who survived, Am. J. Obstet. Gynecol. **127:**400, 1977.

673. Macklon, A.F., Savage, R.L., and Rawlins, M.D.: Research review: Gilbert's syndrome and drug metabolism, Clin. Pharmacokinet. **4:**223, 1979.

674. Madding, G.F., and Kennedy, P.A.: Trauma to the liver, ed. 2, Philadelphia, 1971, W.B. Saunders Co.

675. Melendez, M.G., Williams, D.M., Baty, B., and Cartwright, G.E.: Clinical studies of a large family with Wilson's disease, South. Med. J. **73:**607, 1980.

676. Mistilis, S.P.: Liver disease in pregnancy, Aust. Ann. Med. **17:**248, 1968.

677. Niederau, C., Fischer, R., Sonnenberg, A., Stremmel, W., Trampisch, H.J., and Strohmeyer, G.: Survival and causes of death in cirrhotic and in noncirrhotic patients with primary hemochromatoses, N. Engl. J. Med. **313:**1256, 1985.

678. Nienhuis, A.W.: Vitamin C and iron, N. Engl. J. Med. **304:**170, 1981.

679. Owen, C.A., Jr., Dickson, E.R., Goldstein, N.P., Baggenstoss, A.H., and McCall, J.T.: Hepatic sub-cellular distribution of copper in primary biliary cirrhosis: comparison with other hyperhepatocupric states, Mayo Clin. Proc. **52:**73, 1977.

680. Plumb, V., Ho, K.J., and Mihas, A.A.: Hemochromatosis associated with side-to-side portacaval shunt, South. Med. J. **70:**1369, 1977.

681. Popper, H., Goldfischer, S., Sternlieb, I., Nayak, N.C., and Madhavan, T.V.: Cytoplasmic copper and its toxic effects: studies in Indian childhood cirrhosis, Lancet **1:**1205, 1979.

682. Powell, L.W., Bassett, M.L., and Halliday, J.W.: Hemochromatosis: 1980 update, Gastroenterology **78:**374, 1980.

683. Powell, L.W., Halliday, J.W., and Bassett, M.L.: Recent advances in iron metabolism, Aust. NZ J. Med. **9:**578, 1979.

684. Powell, L.W., Mortimer, R., and Harris, O.D.: Cirrhosis of the liver: a comparative study of the four major etiological groups, Med. J. Aust. **1:**941, 1971.

685. Reyes, H., Ribalta, J., González, M.C., Segovia, N., and Oberhauser, E.: Sulfobromophthalein clearance tests before and after ethinyl estradiol administration, Gastroenterology **81:**226, 1981.

686. Richardson, R.E., Gumbert, J.L., and Gale, S.Q.: Traumatic intrahepatic hematoma, Arch. Surg. **95:**940, 1967.

687. Risdon, R.A., Barry, M., and Flynn, D.M.: Transfusional overload: the relationship between tissue iron concentration and hepatic fibrosis in the thalassemia, J. Pathol. **116:**83, 1975.

688. Rolfes, D.B., and Ishak, K.G.: Acute fatty liver of pregnancy: a clinicopathologic study of 35 cases, Hepatology **5:**1149, 1985.

689. Rolfes, D.B., and Ishak, D.G.: Liver disease in pregnancy, Histopathology **10:**555, 1986.

690. Rosen, I.A., Rosner, I.A., Askari, A.D., McLaren, G.D., and Muir, A.: Arthropathy, hypouricemia and normal serum iron studies in hereditary hemochromatosis, Am. J. Med. **70:**870, 1981.

691. Ross, C.E., Muir, W.A., Ng, A.B.P., Graham, R.C., and Kellermeyer, R.W.: Hemochromatosis: pathophysiologic and genetic considerations, Am. J. Clin. Pathol. **63:**179, 1975.

692. Schafer, A.I., Cheron, R.G., Dluhy, R., Cooper, B., Gleason, R.E., Soeldner, J.S., and Bunn, H.F.: Clinical consequences of acquired transfusional iron overload in adults, N. Engl. J. Med. **304:**319, 1981.

693. Scharschmidt, B.F., and Gollan, J.L.: Current concepts of bilirubin metabolism and hereditary hyperbilirubinemia. In Popper, H., and Schaffner, F., editors: Progress in liver disease, vol. 6, New York, 1979, Grune & Stratton, Inc.

694. Schmid, R., and McDonagh, A.F.: Hyperbilirubinemia. In Stanbury, J.B., Wyngaarden, J.B., and Fredrickson, D.S., editors: The metabolic basis of inherited disease, New York, 1978, McGraw-Hill Book Co.

695. Schumacher, H.R.: Hemochromatosis and arthritis, Arthritis Rheum. **7::**41, 1964.

696. Schweitzer, I.L., and Peters, R.L.: Pregnancy in hepatitis B antigen positive cirrhosis, Obstet. Gynecol. **48**(suppl.):53S, 1976.

697. Scott, J., Gollan, J.L., Samourian, S., and Sherlock, S.: Wilson's disease presenting as chronic active hepatitis, Gastroenterology **74**:645, 1978.

698. Seymour, C.A., Neale, G., and Peters, T.J.: Lysosomal changes in liver tissue from patients with the Dubin-Johnson-Sprinz syndrome, Clin. Sci. Mol. Med. **52**:241, 1977.

699. Shani, M., Seligsohn, U., and Ben-Ezzer, J.: Effect of phenobarbital on liver functions in patients with Dubin-Johnson syndrome, Gastroenterology **67**:303, 1974.

700. Sheehan, H.L.: Yellow atrophy: chloroform poisoning, J. Obstet. Gynecol. Br. Emp. **47**:49, 1940.

701. Smallwood, R.A.: Other liver diseases associated with increased liver copper concentration. In Powell, L.W., editor: Metals and the liver, New York, 1978, Marcel Dekker, Inc.

702. Sternlieb, I.: Copper and the liver, Gastroenterology **78**:1615, 1980.

703. Sternlieb, I., and Scheinberg, I.H.: The role of radiocopper in the diagnosis of Wilson's disease, Gastroenterology **77**:138, 1979.

704. Steven, M.M., Buckley, J.D., and Mackay, I.R.: Pregnancy in chronic active hepatitis, Q. J. Med. **48**(new ser.):519, 1979.

705. Strickland, G.T., and Leu, M.-L.: Wilson's disease: clinical and laboratory manifestations in 40 patients, Medicine **54**:113, 1975.

706. Swartz, H.M., Sarna, T., and Varma, R.: On the nature and excretion of the hepatic pigment in the Dubin-Johnson syndrome, Gastroenterology **76**:958, 1979.

707. Tanner, M.S., and Portmann, B.: Indian childhood cirrhosis, Arch. Dis. Child. **56**:4, 1981.

708. Theron, J.J., Hawtrey, A.O., Liebenberg, N., and Schirren, V.: Experimental dietary siderosis, Am. J. Pathol. **43**:73, 1963.

709. Trunkey, D.D, Shires, G.T., and McClelland, R.: Management of liver trauma in 811 consecutive patients, Ann. Surg. **179**:722, 1974.

710. Valberg, L.S., Lloyd, D.A., Ghent, C.N., Flanagan, P.R., Sinclair N.R., Stiller, C.R., and Chamberlain, M.J.: Clinical and biological expression of the genetic abnormality in idiopathic hemochromatosis, Gastroenterology **79**:884, 1980.

Circulatory disturbances

711. Adler, J., Goodgold, M., Mitty, H., Gordon, D., Kinkhabwala, M.: Ateriovenous shunts involving the liver, Radiology **129**:315, 1978.

712. Arcidi, M.M., Jr., Moore, G.W., and Hutchins, G.M.: Hepatic morphology in cardiac dysfunction: a clinicopathologic study of 1000 subjects at autopsy, Am. J. Pathol. **104**:159, 1981.

713. Asbury, R.F., Rosenthal, S.N., Descalzi, M.E., Ratcliffe, R.L., and Arseneau, J.C.: Hepatic veno-occlusive disease due to DTIC, Cancer **45**:2670, 1980.

713a. Banti, G.; see ref. 728.

714. Berk, P.D., Popper, H., Krueger, G.R., Decter, J., Herzig, G., and Graw, R.G., Jr.: Veno-occlusive disease of the liver after allogenic bone marrow transplantation, Ann. Intern. Med. **90**:158, 1979.

715. Birgens, H.S., Henriksen, J., Matzen, P., and Poulsen, H.: The shock liver: clinical and biochemical findings in patients with centrilobular liver necrosis following cardiogenic shock, Acta Med. Scand. **204**:417, 1978.

716. Boyer, J.L., Hales, M.R., and Klatskin, G.: "Idiopathic" portal hypertension due to occlusion of the intrahepatic portal veins by organized thrombi, Medicine **53**:77, 1974.

717. Boyer, J.L., Sen Gupta, K.P., Biswas, S.K., Pal, M.C., Basu Mallick, K.C., Iber, F.L., and Basu, A.K.: Idiopathic portal hypertension, Ann. Intern. Med. **66**:41, 1967.

718. Bras, G.: Veno-occlusive disease of liver with nonportal type of cirrhosis occurring in Jamaica, Arch. Pathol. **57**:285, 1954.

719. Cohen, J.A., and Kaplan, M.M.: Left-sided heart failure presenting as hepatitis, Gastroenterology **74**:583, 1978.

720. Datta, D.V., Mitra, S,K., Chhuttani, P.N., and Chakravarti, R.N.: Chronic oral arsenic intoxication as a possible aetiological factor in idiopathic portal hypertension (non-cirrhotic portal fibrosis) in India, Gut **20**:358, 1979.

721. Donovan, A.J., Reynolds, T.B., Mikkelsen, W.P., et al.: Systemic-portal arteriovenous fistulas: pathological and hemodynamic observations in two patients, Surgery **66**:474, 1969.

722. Dresler, S., and Linder, D.: Noncirrhotic portal fibrosis following neonatal cytomegalic inclusion disease, J. Pediatr. **93**:887, 1978.

723. España, P., Figuera, D., Fernández de Miguel, J.M., Anaya, A., Menéndez, J., and Durántez, A.: Membranous obstruction of the inferior vena cava and hepatic veins: Budd-Chiari syndrome? A treatable disease, Am. J. Gastroenterol. **73**:28, 1980.

724. Fajardo, L.F., and Colby, T.V.: Pathogenesis of veno-occlusive liver disease after radiation, Arch. Pathol. Lab. Med. **104**:584, 1980.

725. Ghandur-Mnaymneh, L.: Anemic infarction of the liver resulting from hepatic and portal vein thrombosis, Johns Hopkins Med. J. **139**:78, 1976.

726. Grases, P.J., and Beker, S.: Veno-occlusive disease of the liver: case from Venezuela, Am. J. Med. **53**:511, 1972.

727. Guida, P., and Moore, S.W.: Aneurysm of the hepatic artery, Surgery **60**:299, 1966.

728. Guido Banti: 1852-1925, JAMA **201**:693, 1967. (Editorial.)

729. Hartmann, R.C., Luther, A.B., Jenkins, D.E., Jr., Tenorio, L.E., and Saba, H.I.: Fulminant hepatic venous thrombosis (Budd-Chiari syndrome) in paroxysmal nocturnal hemoglobinuria, Johns Hopkins Med. J. **146**:247, 1980.

730. Hashem, M.: Etiology and pathology of types of liver cirrhosis in Egyptian children, J. Egypt Med. Assoc. **22**:319, 1939.

731. Hendee, W.R., Alders, M.A., and Garciga, C.E.: Development of ultrastructural radiation injury, Am. J. Roentgenol. **105**:147, 1969.

732. Hendrix, T.R., Kaufman, F.L., and Boitnott, J.K.: Clinical conferences at the Johns Hopkins Hospital; clinical-pathologic conference, Johns Hopkins Med. J. **147**:41, 1980.

733. Imanaga, H., Yamamoto, S., and Kuroyanagi, Y.: Surgical treatment of portal hypertension, Ann. Surg. **155**:42, 1962.

734. Jacob, A.I., Goldberg, P.K., Bloom, N., et al.: Endotoxin and bacteria in portal blood, Gastroenterology **72**:1268, 1977.

735. Kanel, G.C., Ucci, A.A., Kaplan, M.M., and Wolfe, H.J.: A distinctive perivenular hepatic lesion associated with heart failure, Am. J. Clin. Pathol. **73**:235, 1980.

736. Kent, D.R., Nissen, E., and Goldstein, A.I.: Oral contraceptives and hepatic vein thrombosis, J. Reprod. Med. **68**:113, 1981.

737. Leibowitz, A.I., and Hartmann, R.C.: Annotation: the Budd-Chiari syndrome and paroxysmal nocturnal haemoglobinuria, Br. J. Haematol. **48**:1, 1981.

738. Liebman, P.R., Patten, M.T., Manny, J., Benfield, J.R., and Hechtman, H.B.: Hepatic-portal venous gas in adults: etiology, pathophysiology and clinical significance, Ann. Surg. **187**:281, 1978.

739. Luna, A., Meister, H.P., and Szanto, P.: Esophageal varices in absence in cirrhosis, Am. J. Clin. Pathol. **49**:710, 1968.

740. McLean, E.K.: The toxic actions of pyrrolizidine (Senecio) alkaloids, Pharmacol. Rev. **22**:429, 1970.

741. Mellis, C., and Bale, P.M.: Familial hepatic venocclusive with probable immune deficiency, J. Pediatr. **88**:236, 1976.

742. Mikkelsen, W.P., Edmondson, H.A., Peters, R.L., et al.: Extra- and intrahepatic portal hypertension without cirrhosis (hepato-portal sclerosis), Ann. Surg. **162**:602, 1965.

743. Mohabbat, O., Younos, M.S., Merzad, A.A., Srivastava, R.N., Sedig, G.G., and Aram, G.N.: An outbreak of hepatic veno-occlusive disease in north-western Afghanistan, Lancet **2**:269, 1976.

744. Mukherjee, A.K., Ramalingaswami, V., and Nayak, N.C.: Hepatoportal sclerosis: its relationship to intrahepatic portal venous thrombosis, Indian J. Med. Res. **69**:152, 1979.

745. Mullane, J.F., and Gliedman, M.L.: Elevation of pressure in inferior vena cava, Surgery **59**:1135, 1966.

746. Nagasue, N., Inokuchi, K., Kobayashi, M., and Saku, M.: Hepatoportal arteriovenous fistula in primary carcinoma of the liver, Surg. Gynecol. Obstet. 145:504, 1977.

747. Nakamura, S., and Toshiharu, T.: Surgical anatomy of the hepatic veins and the inferior vena cava, Surg. Gynecol. Obstet. 152:43, 1981.

748. Nakamura, T., Nakamura, S., Aikawa, T., et al.: Obstruction of the inferior vena cava in the hepatic portion and the hepatic veins, Angiology 19:479, 1968.

749. Nataf, C., Feldmann, G., Lebrec, D., Degott, C., Descamps, J.M., Rueff, B., and Benhamou, J.P.: Idiopathic portal hypertension (perisinusoidal fibrosis) after renal transplantation, Gut 20:531, 1979.

750. Okuda, K., Musha, H., Nakajima, Y., Takayasu, K., Suzuki, Y., Morita, M., and Yamasaki, T.: Frequency of intrahepatic arteriovenous fistula as a sequela to percutaneous needle puncture of the liver, Gastroenterology 74:1204, 1978.

751. Okuda, K., Nakashima, T., Okudaira, M., Kage, M., Aida, Y., Omata, M., Musha, H., Futagawa, S., Sugiura, M., and Kameda, H.: Anatomical basis for hepatic venographic alterations in idiopathic portal hypertension, Liver 1:255, 1981.

752. Popper, H.: Alterations of liver and spleen among workers exposed to vinyl chloride, Ann. NY Acad. Sci. 246:172, 1975.

753. Prandi, D., Rueff, B., and Benhamou, J.P.: Side-to-side portacaval shunt in treatment of Budd-Chiari syndrome, Gastroenterology 68:137, 1975.

754. Rector, W.G., Jr., Xu, Y.H., Goldstein, L., Peters, R.L., and Reynolds, T.B.: Membranous obstruction of the inferior vena cava in the United States, Medicine 64:134, 1985.

755. Reed, G.B., Jr., and Cox, A.J., Jr.: Human liver after radiation injury, Am. J. Pathol. 48:597, 1966.

756. Safran, A.P., and Schaffner, F.: Chronic passive congestion of liver in man, Am. J. Pathol. 50:447, 1967.

757. Sarfeh, I.J.: Portal vein thrombosis associated with cirrhosis, Arch. Surg. 114:902, 1979.

758. Seeley, T.T., Blumenfeld, C.M., Ikeda, R., Knapp, W., and Ruebner, B.H.: Hepatic infarction, Hum. Pathol. 3:265, 1972.

759. Selzer, G., and Parker, R.G.F.: *Senecio* poisoning exhibiting as Chiari's syndrome: report on 12 cases, Am. J. Pathol. 27:885, 1951.

760. Shulman, H.M., McDonald, G.B., Matthews, D., Doney, K.C., Kopecky, K.J., Gauvreau, J.M., and Thomas, E.D.: An analysis of hepatic venocclusive disease and centrilobular hepatic degeneration following bone marrow transplantation, Gastroenterology 79:1178, 1980.

761. Simson, I.W.: Membranous obstruction of the inferior vena cava and hepatocellular carcinoma in South Africa, Gastroenterology 82:171, 1982.

762. Stillman, A.S., Huxtable, R., Consroe, P., Kohnen, P., and Smith, S.: Hepatic veno-occlusive disease due to pyrrolizidine (Senecio) poisoning in Arizona, Gastroenterology 73:349, 1977.

763. Stirling, G.A., Bras, G., and Urquhart, A.E.: Early lesion in veno-occlusive disease of liver, Arch. Dis. Child. 37:535, 1962.

764. Sultan, K.M., and Datta, D.V.: Budd-Chiari syndrome following pregnancy: report of 16 cases with roentgenologic, hemodynamic and histologic studies of the hepatic outflow tract, Am. J. Med. 68:113, 1980.

765. Tavill, A.S., Wood, E.J., Kreel, L., Jones, E.A., Gregory, M., and Sherlock, S.: Budd-Chiari syndrome: correlation between hepatic scintigraphy and the clerical, radiological, and pathological findings in hepatic venous flow obstruction, Gastroenterology 68:509, 1975.

766. Villeneuve, J.P., Huet, P.M., Joly, J.G., Marleau, D., Cote, J., Legare, A., Lafortune, M., Lavoie, P., and Viallet, A.: Idiopathic portal hypertension, Am. J. Med. 61:459, 1976.

767. Vujic, I., Meredith, H.C., and Ameriks, J.A.: Embolization for hepatoportal arteriovenous fistula, Am. Surg. 46:366, 1980.

768. Wanless, I.R., Bernier, V., and Seger, M.: Intrahepatic portal vein sclerosis in patients without a history of liver disease: an autopsy study, Am. J. Pathol. 106:63, 1982.

769. Ware, A.J.: The liver when the heart fails, Gastroenterology 74:62, 1978.

770. Woods, W.G., Dehner, L.P., Nesbit, M.E., Krivit, W., Coccia, P.F., Ramsay, N.K., Kim, T.H., and Kersey, J.H.: Fatal veno-occlusive disease of the liver following high dose chemotherapy, irradiation and bone marrow transplantation, Am. J. Med. 68:285, 1980.

771. Zafrani, E.S., Pinaudeau, Y., LeCudonnec, B., Julien, M., and Dhumeaux, D.: Focal necrosis of the liver: a clinicopathological entity possibly related to oral contraceptives, Gastroenterology 79:1295, 1980.

Chronic infections and other chronic disorders

772. Adams, D.O.: The granulomatous, inflammatory response, Am. J. Pathol. 84:164, 1976.

773. Banner, B.F., and Banner, A.S.: Hepatic granulomas following ileal bypass for obesity, Arch. Pathol. Lab. Med. 102:655, 1978.

774. Benjamin, S.B., Ishak, K.G., and Zimmerman, H.J.: Phenylbutazone liver injury: a clinical pathologic survey of 23 cases and review of the literature, Hepatology 1:255, 1981.

775. Bernstein, M., Edmondson, H.A., and Barbour, B.H.: The liver lesion in Q fever, Arch. Intern. Med. 74:198, 1965.

776. Bohm, W., and Willnow, U.: Granulomartige Hepatitis bei konnataler Toxoplasmose, Z. Kinderheilkd. 88:215, 1963.

777. Bramlet, D.A., Posalaky, Z., and Olson, R.: Granulomatous hepatitis as a manifestation of quinidine hypersensitivity, Arch. Intern. Med. 140:395, 1980.

778. Carmichael, G.P., Targoff, C., Pintar, K., and Lewin, K.J.: Hepatic silicosis, Am. J. Clin. Pathol. 73:720, 1980.

779. Chen, T.S.N., Drutz, D.J., and Whelan, G.E.: Hepatic granulomas in leprosy: their relation to bacteremia, Arch. Pathol. Lab. Med. 100:182, 1976.

780. Dupont, H.L., Hornick, R.B., Levin, H.S., Rapoport, M.I., and Woodward, T.E.: Q fever hepatitis, Ann. Intern. Med. 74:198, 1971.

781. Ellenbogen, R., and Rubin, L.: Injectable fluid silicone therapy, JAMA 234:308, 1975.

782. Fauci, A.S., and Wolff, S.M.: Granulomatous hepatitis. In Popper, H., and Schaffner, F., editors: Progress in liver disease, vol. 5, New York, 1976, Grune & Stratton, Inc.

783. French, S.W., Schloss, G.T., and Stillman, A.E.: Case reports: unusual amyloid bodies in human liver, Am. J. Clin. Pathol. 75:400, 1981.

784. Glasgow, B.J., Anders, K., Layfield, L.J., Steinsapir, K.D., Gitnick, G.L., and Lewin, K.J.: Clinical and pathologic findings of the liver in the acquired immune deficiency syndrome (AIDS), Am. J. Clin. Pathol. 83:582, 1985.

785. Glenner, G.G.: Amyloid deposits and amyloidosis: the beta-fibrilloses (in two parts), N. Engl. J. Med. 302:1283, 1333, 1980.

786. Husby, G.: A chemical classification of amyloid, Scand. J. Rheumatol. 9:60, 1980.

787. Jori, G.P., and Peschle, C.: Hydralizine disease associated with transient granulomas in the liver: a case report, Gastroenterology 64:1163, 1973.

788. Kanel, G.C, and Peters, R.L.: Globular amyloid: an unusual morphologic presentation, Hepatology 1:647, 1981.

789. Klatskin, G.: Hepatic granulomata: problems in interpretation, Mt. Sinai J. Med. 44:798, 1977.

790. Krogsgaard, K., Lindhardt, B.O., Nielsen, J.O., Anderson, P., Kryger, P., Aldershvile, J., Gerstoft, J., and Pedersen, C.: The influence of HTLV-III infection on the natural history of hepatitis B virus infection in male homosexual HBsAg carriers, Hepatology 7:37, 1987.

791. Kuzemko, J.A.: Toxocariasis in sibs, Arch. Dis. Child, 41:221, 1966.

792. Lee, F.I., Murray, S., and Norfolk, D.R.: Cholestatic jaundice in secondary syphilis, Br. J. Clin. Pract. 33:139, 1979.

792a. Lui, A.F.K., Hiratzka, L.F., and Hirose, F.M.: Multiple adenomas of the liver, Cancer 45:1001, 1980.

793. Marcial-Rojas, R.A.: Parasitic diseases of the liver. In Gall, A., and Mostofi, F.K., editors: The liver, Baltimore, 1973, The Williams & Wilkins Co.

794. McMaster, K.R., and Hennigar, G.R.: Drug-induced granulomatous hepatitis, Lab. Invest. **44**:61, 1981.

795. Melkebeke, P., Vandepitte, J., Hannon, R., and Fevery, J.: Huge hepatomegaly and portal hypertension due to amyloidosis of the liver, Digestion **20**:351, 1980.

796. Miller, A.C., and Reid, W.M.: Methyldopa-induced granulomatous hepatitis, JAMA **235**:2001, 1976.

797. Min, K.W., Györkey, F., and Cain, G.D.: Talc granulomata in liver disease in narcotic addicts, Arch. Pathol. **98**:331, 1974.

798. Mir-Madjlessi, S.H., Farmer, R.G., and Hawk, W.A.: Granulomatous hepatitis: a review of 50 cases, Am. J. Gastroenterol. **60**:122, 1973.

799. Nagalotimath, S.J., Darbar, R.D., and Jogalekar, M.D.: Granulomatous hepatitis in brucellosis, J. Ind. Med. Assoc. **72**:1, 1979.

800. Nakanuma, Y., Ohta, G., Yamazaki, Y., and Doishita, K.: Intrahepatic bile duct destruction in a patient with sarcoidosis and chronic intrahepatic cholestasis, Acta Pathol. Jpn. **20**:211, 1979.

801. Nakanuma, Y., Ohta, G., Doishita, K., and Maki, H.: Granulomatous liver disease in the small hepatic and portal veins, Arch. Pathol. Lab. Med. **104**:456, 1980.

802. Nakanuma, Y., Liew, C.T., Peters, R.L., and Govindarajan, S.: Pathologic features of the liver in acquired immune deficiency syndrome (AIDS), Liver **6**:158, 1986.

803. Okuda, K., Kimura, K., Takara, K., Ohta, M., Omata, M., and Lesmana, L.: Resolution of diffuse granulomatous fibrosis of the liver with antituberculous chemotherapy, Gastroenterology **91**:456, 1986.

804. Omata, M., Johnson, C.S., Tong, M., and Tatter, D.: Pathological spectrum of liver diseases in sickle cell disease, Dig. Dis. Sci. **31**:247, 1986.

805. Pfeifer, U., and Alterman, K.: Shedding of peripheral cytoplasm: a mechanism of liver cell atrophy in human amyloidosis, Virchows Arch. [Cell Pathol.] **29**:229, 1979.

806. Pimentel, J.C., and Meneges, A.P.: Liver granuloma containing copper in vineyard sprayer's lung, Am. Rev. Respir. Dis. **111**:189, 1975.

807. Reynolds, T.B., Campra, J.L., and Peters, R.L.: Hepatic granulomas. In Zakin, D., and Boyer, T., editors: Hepatology, a textbook of liver disease, Philadelphia, 1982, W.B. Saunders Co.

808. Rigberg, L.A., Robinson, M.J., and Espiritu, C.R.: Chlorpropamide-induced granulomas, JAMA **235**:409, 1976.

809. Romeu, J., Rubak, B., Dave, P., and Coven, R.: Spirochetal vasculitis and bile ductular damage in early hepatic syphilis, Am. J. Gastroenterol. **74**:352, 1980.

810. Rubinow, A., Koff, R.S., and Cohen, A.S.: Severe intrahepatic cholestasis in primary amyloidosis: a report of four cases and a review of the literature, Am. J. Med. **64**:937, 1978.

811. Sacks, E.L., Donaldson, S.S., Gordon, J., and Dorfman, R.F.: Epithelioid granulomas associated with Hodgkin's disease: clinical correlations in 55 previously untreated patients, Cancer **41**:562, 1978.

812. Simmons, F., Feldman, B., and Gerety, D.: Granulomatous hepatitis in a patient receiving allopurinol, Gastroenterology **62**:101, 1972.

813. Spark, R.P.: Does transplacental spread of coccidioidomycosis occur? Arch. Pathol Lab. Med. **105**:347, 1981.

814. Spink, W.W., Hoffbauer, F.W., Walker, W.W., and Green, R.A.: Histopathology of the liver in human brucellosis, J. Lab. Clin. Med. **34**:40, 1949.

815. Symmers, D., and Spain, D.M.: Hepar lobatum, Arch. Pathol. **42**:64, 1946.

816. Thomas, E., and Micci, D.: Chronic intrahepatic cholestasis with granulomas and biliary cirrhosis, JAMA **238**:337, 1977.

817. Warren, K.S.: Hepatosplenic schistosomiasis: a great neglected disease of the liver, Gut **19**:572, 1978.

818. Woodruff, A.W., and Thacker, C.K.: Infection with animal helminths, Br. Med. J. **1**:1001, 1964.

819. Yon, J.L., Anuras, S., Wu, K., and Forker, E.L.: Granulomatous hepatitis, increased platelet aggregation, and hypercholesterolemia, Ann. Intern. Med. **84**:148, 1976.

820. Young, J.L., Boswell, R.B., and Nies, A.S.: Severe allopurinol hypersensitivity: association with thiazides and prior renal compromise, Arch. Intern. Med. **134**:553, 1974.

Liver disease in nonhepatic disorders

821. Ashkar, F.S., Miller, R., Smoak, W.M., III, et al.: Liver disease in hyperthyroidism, South. Med. J. **64**:462, 1971.

822. Batholomew, L.G., Cain, J.C., Winkelmann, R.K., et al.: Liver disease in scleroderma, Am. J. Dig. Dis. **9**:43, 1964.

823. Dew, M.J., Thompson, H., and Allan, R.N.: The spectrum of hepatic dysfunction in inflammatory bowel disease, Q. J. Med. **48**:113, 1979.

824. Dietrichson, O., From, A., Christoffersen, P., and Juhl, E.: Morphological changes in liver biopsies from patients with rheumatoid arthritis, Scand. J. Rheumatol. **5**:65, 1976.

825. Eade, M.N., Cooke, W.T., Brooke, B.N., and Thompson, H.: Liver disease in Crohn's colitis: a study of 21 consecutive patients having colectomy, Ann. Intern. Med. **74**:518, 1971.

826. Falchuk, K.R., Fiske, S.C., Haggitt, R.C., Federman, M., and Trey, C.: Pericentral hepatic fibrosis and intracellular hyalin in diabetes mellitus, Gastroenterology **78**:535, 1980.

827. Fernandes, L., Sullivan, S., McFarlane, I.G., Wojcicka, B.M., Warnes, T.W., Eddleston, A.L., Hamilton, E.B., and Williams, R.: Studies on the frequency and pathogenesis of liver involvement in rheumatoid arthritis, Ann. Rheum. Dis. **38**:501, 1979.

828. Hocking, W.G., Lasser, K., Ungerer, R., Bersohn, M., Palos, M., and Spiegel, T.: Spontaneous hepatic rupture in rheumatoid arthritis, Arch. Intern. Med. **141**:792, 1981.

829. Kolmannskog, F., Aakhus, T., Fausa, O., Schrumpf, E., and Ritland, S., Gjone, E., and Elgjo, K.: Cholangiographic findings in ulcerative colitis, Acta Radiol. **22**:151, 1981.

830. Lupinetti, M., Mehigan, D., and Cameron, J.L.: Hepatobiliary complications of ulcerative colitis, Am. J. Surg. **139**:113, 1980.

831. Nelson, R.S., and Sears, M.E.: Massive sarcoidosis of liver, Am. J. Dig. Dis. **13**:95, 1968.

832. Ritland, S., Elgjo, K., Johansen, O., and Steinnes, E.: Liver copper content in patients with inflammatory bowel disease and associated liver disorders, Scand. J. Gastroenterol. **14**:711, 1979.

833. Runyon, B.A., LaBrecque, D.R., and Anuras, S.: The spectrum of liver disease in systemic lupus erythematosus: report of 33 histologically-proved cases and review of literature, Am. J. Med. **69**:187, 1980.

834. Samuelson, K., Aly, A., Johansson, C., and Norman, A.: Evaluation of fasting serum bile acid concentration in patients with liver and gastrointestinal disorders, Scand. J. Gastroenterol. **16**:225, 1981.

Tumors and tumorlike lesions

835. Adams, Y.B., Huvos, A.G., and Hajdu, S.I.: Malignant vascular tumors of liver, Ann. Surg. **175**:373, 1972.

836. Adams, Y.G., Huvos, A.G. and Fortner, J.G.: Giant hemangiomas of the liver, Ann. Surg. **172**:239, 1972.

837. Anthony, P.P., and Telesinghe, P.E.: Inflammatory pseudotumor of the liver, J. Clin. Pathol. **39**:761, 1986.

838. Aoki, K.: Cancer of the liver: international mortality trends, World Health Stat. Rep. **31**:28, 1978.

839. Arbus, G.C., and Hung, R.H.: Hepatocarcinoma and myocardial fibrosis in an 8¾-year-old renal transplant recipient, Can. Med. Assoc. J. **107**:431, 1972.

840. Beasley, R.P., Hwang, L.Y., Lin, C.C., and Chien, C.S.: Hepatocellular carcinoma and hepatitis B virus, Lancet **2**:1129, 1981.

840a. Berman, C.: Primary carcinoma of the liver in the Bantu races of South Africa, S. Afr. J. Med. Sci. **5**:54, 1940.

841. Bird, D., Voweles, K., and Anthony, P.P.: Spontaneous rupture of the liver cell adenoma after long term methyltestoster-

one: report of a case successfully treated by right hepatic lo-bectomy, Br. J. Surg. **66:**212, 1979.

842. Block, J.B.: Angiosarcoma of liver following vinyl chloride exposure, JAMA **29:**53, 1974.

843. Bomford, A., and Williams, R.: Long-term results of venous section therapy in idiopathic hemochromatosis, Q. J. Med. **45:**611, 1976.

844. Brechot, C., Nalpas, B., Couroucé, A.M., Duhamel, G., Callard, P., Carnot, F., Tiollais, P., and Berthelot, P.: Evidence that hepatitis B virus has a role in liver-cell carcinoma in alcoholic liver disease, N. Engl. J. Med. **306:**1384, 1982.

845. Burroughs, A.K., Bassendine, M.F., Thomas, H.C., and Sherlock, S.: Primary cancer in autoimmune chronic liver disease, Br. Med. J. **282:**273, 1981.

846. Chudecki, B.: Primary cancer of the liver following treatment of polycythemia vera with radioactive phosphorus, Br. J. Radiol. **45:**770, 1972.

847. Craig, J.R., Peters, R.L., Edmondson, H.A., and Omata, M.: Fibrolamellar carcinoma of the liver: a tumor of adolescents and young adults with distinctive clinico-pathologic features, Cancer **46:**372, 1980.

848. Creech, J.L., Jr., and Johnson, M.N.: Angiosarcoma of liver in manufacture of polyvinyl chloride, J. Occup. Med. **16:**150, 1974.

849. Davis, M., Portmann, B., Searle, M., Wright, R., and Williams, R.: Histological evidence of carcinoma in a hepatic tumour associated with oral contraceptives, Br. Med. J. **4:**496, 1975.

850. Dehner, L.P., and Ishak, K.G.: Vascular tumors of the liver in infants and children, Arch. Pathol. **92:**101, 1971.

851. Edmondson, H.A.: Differential diagnosis of tumors and tumor-like lesions of the liver in infancy and childhood, Am. J. Dis. Child. **91:**168, 1956.

852. Edmondson, H.A.: Tumors of the liver and intrahepatic bile ducts. In Atlas of tumor pathology, section 7, fascicle 25, Washington, D.C., 1958, Armed Forces Institute of Pathology.

853. Edmondson, H.A., and Steiner, P.E.: Primary carcinoma of the liver: a study of 100 cases among 48,900 necropsies, Cancer **7:**462, 1954.

854. Edmondson, H.A., Reynolds, T.B., Henderson, B., and Benton, B.: Regression of liver cell adenomas associated with oral contraceptives, Ann. Intern. Med. **86:**180, 1977.

855. Edmondson, H.A., and Craig, J.R.: Neoplasms of the liver. In Schiff, L., and Eugene R., editors: Diseases of the liver, ed. 6, Philadelphia, 1987, J.B. Lippincott Co.

856. Ein, S.H.: Malignant liver tumors in children, J. Pediatr. Surg. **9:**491, 1974.

857. Eriksson, S., and Hagerstrand, I.: Cirrhosis and malignant hepatoma in alpha-1-antitrypsin deficiency, Acta Med. Scand. **195:**451, 1974.

858. Fraumeni, J.F., Miller, R.W., and Hill, J.A.: Primary carcinoma of the liver in childhood: an epidemiologic study, J. Natl. Cancer Inst. **40:**1087, 1968.

859. Fraser, R., Day, W.A., Fernando, S.: Review: The liver sinusoidal cells: their role in disorders of the liver, lipoprotein metabolism, and atherosclerosis, Pathology **18:**5, 1986.

860. French, S.W., Kondo, I., Ihrig, T.J., et al.: Morphologic study of intermediate filaments in rat hepatocytes, Hepatology **2:**29, 1982.

861. Gerber, M.A., and Thung, S.: Histology of the liver, Am. J. Surg. Pathol. **11:**709, 1987.

862. Gibson, J.B., and Sun, T.: Clonorchiasis. In Marcial-Rojas, R.A., editor: Pathology of protozoal and helminthic disease, Baltimore, 1971, The Williams & Wilkins Co.

863. Govindarajan, S., Ashcavai, M., and Peters, R.L.: Alpha-1-antitrypsin phenotypes in hepatocellular carcinoma, Hepatology **1:**628, 1981. (Abstract.)

864. Govindarajan, S., and Peters, R.L.: The bile duct adenoma, Arch. Pathol. Lab. Med. **108:**922, 1984.

865. Hadad, A.R., Westbrook, K.C., Graham, G.G., Morris, W.D., and Campbell, G.S.: Symptomatic nonparasitic liver cysts, Am. J. Surg. **134:**739, 1977.

866. Harris, M.B., Shen, S., Weiner, M.A., et al.: Peliosis hepatis: An unusual case involving multiple organs, Acta Pathol. Jpn. **30:**109, 1980.

867. Harris, M.B., Shen, S., Weiner, M.A., Bruckner, H., Dasgupta, I., Bleicher, M., Fortner, J.G., Leleiko, N.S., Becker, N., Rose, J., et al.: Treatment of primary and undifferentiated sarcoma of the liver with surgery and chemotherapy, Cancer **54:**2859, 1984.

868. Ho, C.F., et al.: Guided percutaneous fine needle aspiration biopsy of the liver, Cancer **47:**1781, 1981.

869. Homer, L.W., White, H.J., and Read, R.C.: Neoplastic transformation of von Meyenburg complexes of the liver, J. Pathol. Bacteriol. **96:**499, 1968.

870. Horisawa, M., Yokoyama, T., Juttner, H., et al: Incomplete membranous obstruction of the inferior vena cava, Arch. Surg. **111:**599, 1976.

871. Horn, T., Henriksen, J.H., and Christoffersen, P.: The sinusoidal lining cells in "normal" human liver: a scanning electron microscopic investigation, Liver **6:**98, 1986.

872. Horn, T., Lyon, H., and Christoffersen, P.: The blood hepatocytic barrier: a light microscopical transmission and scanning electron microscopic study, Liver **6:**233, 1986.

873. Hoyes, A.D., Riches, D.G., and Martin, B.G.H.: The fine structure of haemopoiesis in human fetal liver. I. Haemopoietic precursor cells, J. Anat. **115:**99, 1973.

874. Ichijima, K., Korashi, Y., Yamabe, H., et al.: Peliosis hepatis: an unusual case involving multiple organs, Acta Pathol. Jpn. **30:**109, 1980.

875. Ishak, K.G., and Glunz, P.R.: Hepatoblastoma and hepatocarcinoma in infancy and childhood, Cancer **20:**396, 1967.

876. Ishak, K.G.: Hepatic lesions caused by anabolic and contraceptive steroids, Semin. Liver Dis. **1:**116, 1981.

876a. Ishak, K.G., Sesterhenn, I.A., Goodman, Z.D., Rabin, L., and Stromeyer, F.W.: Epithelioid hemangioendothelioma of the liver, Hum. Pathol. **15:**839, 1984.

877. Ishiguro, T., Sugitachi, I., Sakaguchi, H., Itani, S.: Serum alpha-fetoprotein subfractions in patients with primary hepatoma or hepatic metastasis of gastric cancer, Cancer **55:**156, 1985.

878. Jackson, C., Greene, H.L., O'Neill, J., and Kirchner, S.: Hepatic hemangioendothelioma: angiographic appearance and apparent prednisone responsiveness, Am. J. Dis. Child. **131:**74, 1977.

879. Jaffe, B.M., Donegan, W.L., and Watson, F.: Factors influencing survival in patients with untreated hepatic metastases, Surg. Gynecol. Obstet. **127:**1, 1968.

880. Jenkins, P.J., Melia, W.M., Portmann, B., Longworth Krafft, J.M., and Williams, R.: Hepatocellular carcinoma in HBsAg-negative chronic active hepatitis, Gut **22:**332, 1981.

881. Jones, E.A., and Summerfield, J.A.: Functional aspects of hepatic sinusoidal cells, Semin. Liver Dis. **5:**157, 1985.

882. Kakizoe, S., Kojiro, M., and Nakashima, T.: Hepatocellular carcinoma with sarcomatous change, Cancer **59:**310, 1987.

883. Kane, R.C., and Newman, A.B.: Diffuse skeletal hepatic hemangiomatosis, Calif. Med. **118:**41, 1973.

884. Kaneda, K., Kurioka, N., Seki, S., et al.: Pit cell–hepatocyte contact in autoimmune hepatitis, Hepatology **4:**955, 1984.

885. Kato, M., Sugarawara, I., Okada, A., et al.: Hemangioma of the liver, Am. J. Surg. **129:**698, 1975.

886. Kent, G., Gay, S., Inouye, T., Bahu, R., Minick, O.T., Popper, H.: Vitamin A containing lipocytes and formation of type III collagen in liver injury, Proc. Natl. Acad. Sci. USA **73:**3719, 1976.

887. Kimura, C., Matsuda, S., Koie, H., and Hirooka, M.: Membranous obstruction of the hepatic portions of the inferior vena cava: clinical study of nine cases, Surgery **72:**551, 1972.

888. Koga, A.: Morphogenesis of intrahepatic bile ducts of human fetus: light and electron microscopic study, Z. Anat. Entwicklungsgesch. **135:**156, 1971.

889. Kulkarni, P.B., and Beatty, E.C.: Cholangiocarcinoma associated with biliary cirrhosis due to congenital biliary atresia, Am. J. Dis. Child. **131:**442, 1977.

890. Kurtz, R.C., Sherlock, P., and Winawer, S.J.: Esophageal var-

ices: development secondary to primary and metastatic liver tumors, Arch. Intern. Med. **41**:221, 1966.

891. Lack, E.E., Neave, C., Vawter, G.F.: Hepatoblastoma: a clinical and pathologic study of 54 cases, Am. J. Surg. Pathol. **6**:693, 1982.
892. Lack, E.E.: Mesenchymal hamartoma of the liver: a clinical and pathological study of nine cases, Am. J. Pediatr. Hematol. Oncol. **8**:91, 1986.
893. Lander, J.J., Stanley, R.J., Sumner, H.W., Boswell, D.C., and Aach, R.D.: Angiosarcoma of liver associated with Fowler's solution (potassium arsenite), Gastroenterology **68**:1583, 1975.
894. Langer, J.C., Rose, D.B., Keystone, J.S., Taylor, B.R., and Langer, B.: Diagnosis and management of hydatid disease of the liver: a 15 year North American experience, Ann. Surg. **199**:412, 1984.
895. LeDouarin, N.M.: An experimental analysis of liver development, Med. Biol. **53**:427, 1975.
896. Lee, F.L.: Cirrhosis and hepatoma in alcoholics, Gut **7**:77, 1966.
897. Lees, C.D., Zapolanski, A., Cooperman, A.M., and Hermann, R.E.: Carcinoma of the bile ducts, Surg. Gynecol. Obstet. **151**:193, 1980.
898. Lingao, A.L., Domingo, E.O., and Nishioka, K.: Hepatitis B virus profile of hepatocellular carcinoma in the Philippines, Cancer **48**:1590, 1981.
898a. Liver Cancer Study Group: Primary liver cancer in Japan, sixth report, Cancer **60**:1400, 1987.
899. Ma, M.H., and Biempica, L.: The normal human liver cell, Am. J. Pathol. **62**:353, 1971.
900. Madding, G.F., and Kennedy, P.A.: Hepatic artery ligation, Surg. Clin. North Am. **52**:719, 1972.
901. Marion, P.L., Salazar, F.H., Alexander, J.J., and Robinson, W.S.: State of hepatitis B viral DNA in a human hepatoma cell line, J. Virol. **33**:795, 1980.
902. McDermott, W.V., Jr., and Hensle, T.W.: Metastatic carcinoid to the liver treated by hepatic dearterialization, Ann. Surg. **180**:305, 1974.
903. Moore, T.A., Ferrante, W.A., and Crowson, T.D.: Hepatoma occurring two decades after hepatic irradiation, Gastroenterology **71**:128, 1976.
904. Nadell, J., and Kosek, J.: Peliosis hepatis: 12 cases associated with oral androgen therapy, Arch. Pathol. Lab. Med. **101**:405, 1977.
905. Nagasue, N., Akamizu, H., Yukaya, H., et al: Hepatocellular pseudotumor in the cirrhotic liver: report of 3 cases, Cancer **54**:2487, 1984.
906. Nakamura, S., and Tsuzuki, T.: Surgical anatomy of the hepatic veins and the inferior vena cava, Surg. Gynecol. Obstet. **152**:43, 1981.
907. Ohbayashi, A.: Genetic and familial aspects of liver cirrhosis and hepatocellular carcinoma. In Okuda, K., and Peters, R.L., editors: Hepatocellular carcinoma, New York, 1976, John Wiley & Sons, Inc.
908. Ohbayashi, A., Okochi, K., and Mayumi, M.: Familial clustering of asymptomatic carriers of Australia antigen and patients with chronic liver disease or primary liver cancer, Gastroenterology **42**:618, 1972.
909. Okuda, K., and the Liver Cancer Study Group of Japan: Primary liver cancers in Japan, Cancer **45**:2663, 1980.
910. Okuda, K., Omata, M., Itoh, Y., Ikezaki, H., and Nakashima, T.: Peliosis hepatis as a late and fatal complication of Thorotrast liver disease: report of five cases, Liver **1**:110, 1981.
911. Paradinas, F.J., Bull, T.B., Westaby, D., and Murray-Lyon, I.M.: Hyperplasia and prolapse of hepatocytes into hepatic veins during long term methyltestosterone therapy, Histopathology **1**:225, 1977.
912. Parker, P., Burr, I., Slonim, A., Ghishan, F.K., and Greene, H.: Regression of hepatic adenomas in type Ia glycogen storage disease with dietary therapy, Gastroenterology **81**:534, 1981.
913. Peers, F.G., and Linsell, C.A.: Dietary aflatoxin and liver cancer: a population based study in Kenya, Br. J. Cancer **27**:473, 1973.

914. Person, D.A., Sargent, T., and Isaac, E.: Thorotrast-induced carcinoma of the liver, Arch. Surg. **88**:503, 1964.
915. Peters, R.L.: Pathology of hepatocellular carcinoma. In Okuda, K., and Peters, R.L., editors: Hepatocellular carcinoma, New York, 1976, John Wiley & Sons, Inc.
916. Peters, R.L., Afroudakis, A.P., and Tatter, D.: The changing incidence of association of hepatitis B with hepatocellular carcinoma in California, Am. J. Clin. Pathol. **68**:1, 1977.
917. Phillips, M.J., Poucell, S., Patterson, J., et al.: The liver: an atlas and text of ultrastructural pathology, New York, 1987, Raven Press.
918. Phinney, P.R., Austin, G.E., and Kadell, B.M.: Cholangiocarcinoma arising in Caroli's disease, Arch. Pathol. Lab. Med. **105**:194, 1981.
919. Popper, H., Shafritz, D.A., Hoofnagle, J.H.L.: Relation of the hepatitis B virus carrier state to hepatocellular carcinoma, Hepatology **7**:764, 1987.
920. Pryor, A.C., Cohen, R.J., and Goldman, R.L.: Hepatocellular carcinoma in a woman on long term oral contraceptives, Cancer **40**:884, 1977.
921. Rabinowitz, J.G., Kinkhabwala, M., and Ulreich, S.: Macroregenerating nodule in the cirrhotic liver: radiologic features and differential diagnosis, Am. J. Roentgenol. Radium Ther. Nucl. Med. **121**:401, 1974.
922. Rankin, J.G., Skyring, A.P., and Goulston, S.J.M.: Liver in ulcerative colitis: obstructive jaundice due to bile duct carcinoma, Gut **7**:433, 1966.
923. Rhodes, R.H., Marhildon, M.B., Luebke, D.C., Edmondson, H.A., and Mikity, V.G.: A mixed hamartoma of the liver: light and electron microscopy, Hum. Pathol. **9**:211, 1978.
924. Rohr, H.P., Luthy, J., and Gudat, F.: Stereology of liver biopsies from healthy volunteers, Virchows Arch. [A. Pathol. Anat.] **371**:251, 1976.
925. Rooks, J.B., Ory, H.W., Ishak, K.G., Strauss, L.T., Greenspan, J.R., Hill, A.P., and Tyler, C.W., Jr.: Epidemiology of hepatocellular adenoma, JAMA **242**:644, 1979.
926. Samelippo, P.M., Beahrs, O.H., and Weiland, L.H.: Cystic disease of liver, Ann. Surg. **179**:922, 1974.
927. Selikoff, I.J., and Hammond, E.C.: Toxicity of vinyl chloride–polyvinyl chloride, Ann. NY Acad. Sci. **246**:5, 1975.
928. Selinger, M., and Koff, R.S.: Thorotrast and the liver: a reminder, Gastroenterology **68**:799, 1975.
929. Severn, C.B.: Morphologic study of development of human liver. II. Establishment of liver parenchyma, extrahepatic ducts, and associated venous channels, Am. J. Anat. **133**:85, 1982.
930. Sewell, J.H., and Weiss, K.: Spontaneous ruptures of hemangioma of the liver, Arch. Surg. **83**:729, 1961.
931. Shank, R.C., Wogan, G.W., Gibson, J.B., and Nondasuta, A.: Dietary aflatoxins and human liver cancer. III. Field survey of rural Thai families for ingested aflatoxins, Food Cosmet. Toxicol. **10**:61, 1972.
932. Sherlock, S., and Scheuer, P.J.: The presentation and diagnosis of 100 patients with primary biliary cirrhosis, N. Engl. J. Med. **289**:674, 1973.
933. Simons, M.J., Yu, M., and Shanmugaratnam, K.: Immunodeficiency to hepatitis B virus infection and genetic susceptibility to development of hepatocellular carcinoma, Ann. NY Acad. Sci. **259**:181, 1975.
934. Simson, I.W.: Membranous obstruction of the inferior vena cava and hepatocellular carcinoma in South Africa, Gastroenterology **82**:171, 1982.
935. Slovis, T.L., Berdon, W.E., Haller, J.O., et al: Hemangiomas of the liver in infants: review of diagnosis, treatment and course, AJR **123**:791, 1975.
936. Smoron, G.L., and Battifora, H.A.: Thorotrast-induced hepatoma, Cancer **30**:1252, 1972.
937. Solís-Herruzo, J.A., Vidal, J.V., Colina, F., Santalla, F., and Castellano, G.: Nodular regenerative hyperplasia of the liver associated with the toxic oil syndrome: report of 5 cases, Hepatology **6**:687, 1986.

938. Stocker, J.T., and Ishak, K.G.: Undifferentiated (embryonal) sarcoma of the liver: report of 31 cases, Cancer **42**:336, 1978.

939. Stocker, J.T., and Ishak, K.G.: Focal nodular hyperplasia of the liver: a study of 21 pediatric cases, Cancer **48**:336, 1981.

940. Stocker, J.T., and Ishak, K.G.: Mesenchymal hamartoma of the liver: report of 30 cases and review of the literature, Pediatr. Pathol. **1**:245, 1983.

941. Stromeyer, F.W., and Ishak, K.G.: Nodular transformation (nodular "regenerative" hyperplasia) of the liver: a clinicopathologic study of 30 cases, Hum. Pathol. **12**:60, 1981.

942. Takasan, H., Kim, C.I., Arii, S., Takahashi, S., Uozumi, T., Tobe, T., and Honjo, I.: Clinicopathologic study of seventy patients with carcinoma of the biliary tract, Surg. Gynecol. Obstet. **150**:721, 1980.

943. Tao, L.C., Ho, C.S., McLoughlin, M.J., Evans, W.K., and Donat, E.E.: Cytologic diagnosis of hepatocellular carcinoma by fine needle aspiration biopsy, Cancer **53**:547, 1984.

944. Tesluk, H., and Lawrie, J.: Hepatocellular adenoma: its transformation to carcinoma in a user of oral contraceptives, Arch. Pathol. Lab. Med. **150**:296, 1981.

945. Tong, M.J., Sun, S.C., Schaeffer, B.T., Chang, N.K., Lok, J., and Petero, R.L.: Hepatitis associated antigen and hepatocellular carcinoma in Taiwan, Ann. Intern. Med. **75**:687, 1971.

946. Tong, M.J., Weiner, J.M., Ashcavai, M.W., and Vyas, G.N.: Evidence for clustering of hepatitis B virus infection in families of patients with primary hepatocellular carcinoma, Cancer **44**:2338, 1979.

947. Torres, F.O., Purchase, I.F.H., and Van der Watt, J.J.: Aetiology of primary liver cancer in the Bantu, J. Pathol. **102**:163, 1970.

948. Totzke, H.A., and Hutcheson, J.B.: Primary fibrosarcoma of the liver, South. Med. J. **58**:236, 1965.

949. Tsao, M., and Grisham, J.W.: Hepatocarcinomas, cholangiocarcinomas, and hepatoblastomas produced by chemically transformed cultured rat liver epithelial cells, Am. J. Pathol. **127**:168, 1987.

950. Van Rensburg, S.J., Van der Watt, J.J., Purchase, I.F., et al.: Primary liver cancer rate and aflatoxin intake in a high cancer area, S. Afr. Med. J. **48**:2506, 1974.

951. Wanless, I.R., Solt, L.C., Kortan, P., Deck, J.H., Gardiner, G.W., and Prokipchuk, E.J.: Nodular regenerative hyperplasia of the liver associated with macroglobulinemia, Am. J. Med. **70**:1203, 1981.

952. Wanless, I.R., Mawdsley, C., and Adams, R.: On the pathogenesis of focal nodular hyperplasia of the liver, Hepatology **5**:1194, 1985.

953. Wanless, I.R., and Gryfe, A.: Nodular transformation of the liver in hereditary hemorrhagic telangiectiasia, Arch. Pathol. Lab. Med. **110**:331, 1986.

954. Weinberg, A.G., Mize, C.E., and Worthen, H.G.: The occurrence of hepatoma in the chronic form of hereditary tyrosinemia, J. Pediatr. **88**:434, 1976.

955. Wheeler, D.A., and Edmondson, H.A.: Cystadenoma with mesenchymal stroma (CMS) in the liver and bile ducts, Cancer **56**:1434, 1985.

956. Wisse, E., DeZanger, R.B., Charels, K., Van der Smissen, P., and McCuskey, R.S.: The liver sieve: considerations concerning the structure and function of endothelial fenestrae, the sinusoidal wall and the space of Disse, Hepatology **5**:683, 1985.

957. Yamamoto, K., Sherman, I., Phillips, M.J., and Fisher, M.M.: Three dimensional observations of the hepatic arterial terminations in rat, hamster, and human liver by scanning electron microscopy of microvascular casts, Hepatology **5**:452, 1985.

958. Yanoff, M., and Rawson, A.J.: Peliosis hepatis, Arch. Pathol. **77**:159, 1964.

Transplantation

959. Busuttil, R.W., Goldstein, L.I., Danovitch, G.M., Ament, M.E., and Memsic, L.D.: Liver transplantation today, Ann. Intern. Med. **104**:377, 1986.

960. Porter, K.A.: Pathology of the orthotopic homograft and heterograft. In Starzl, T.E., editor: Experiments in hepatic transplantation, Philadelphia, 1969, W.B. Saunders Co.

961. Snover, D.C., Freese, D.K., Sharp, H.L., Bloomer, J.R., Najarian, J.S., and Ascher, N.L.: Liver allograft rejection: an analysis of the use of biopsy in determining outcome of rejection, Am. J. Surg. Pathol. **11**:1, 1987.

26 Gallbladder and Biliary Ducts

KATHERINE DE SCHRYVER-KECSKEMÉTI

ANATOMY

We owe our first records of gallbladder anatomy to the divination rites during the time of the Babylonians (3000 BC), including thorough observation and recording of the length of the bile duct and the presence of gallstones and swelling of the gallbladder in the various sacrificial animals.[3]

The gallbladder is a pear-shaped bag, 9 cm long, with a capacity of about 50 ml. The fundus is the broad end and is directed forward; this is the part palpated when the abdomen is examined. The body extends into a narrow neck, which continues into the cystic duct. The valves of Heister are spiral folds of mucous membrane in the wall of the cystic ducts and neck of the gallbladder. Hartmann's pouch, a sacculation at the neck of the gallbladder, is a common site for a gallstone to lodge.

The hepatic ducts emerge from the right and left lobes of the liver and unite in the porta hepatis to form the common hepatic duct. This is soon joined by the cystic duct from the gallbladder to form the common bile duct.

The common bile duct, measured at operation, is about 0.5 to 15 mm in diameter and runs between the layers of the lesser omentum, lying anterior to the portal vein and to the right of the hepatic artery. Numerous anatomic variants of this relationship are known to occur. Passing behind the first part of the duodenum the common duct enters it, usually joining the main pancreatic duct to form the ampulla of Vater. In about 30% of subjects the biliary and pancreatic ducts open separately into the duodenum. The duodenal portion of the common bile duct is surrounded by a thickening of both longitudinal and circular muscle fibers derived from the intestine, called the spincter of Oddi.

MORPHOLOGY

The biliary ducts, as well as the gallbladder, are lined by tall columnar epithelium. The normal epithelium functions as an absorptive surface and has little mucin-secreting activity. Acinar glands producing a mucinous secretion are present only in the neck of the gallbladder and are absent in its body and fundus. Beneath the epithelium a delicate lamina propria contains capillaries.

The mucosal surface of the gallbladder is immensely expanded by deep folds and ridges of varying heights. Microscopically the ridges are richly branching, and delicate connective tissue stalks are covered by tall columnar cells (Fig. 26-1). Under normal conditions there is no lymphoid tissue in the lamina propria.[1] External to the lamina propria is a fairly dense, fibrous connective tissue making up the wall of the extrahepatic biliary ducts. In the gallbladder, external to the lamina propria, are smooth muscle bundles arranged longitudinally and external to that obliquely or circularly. The muscular coat is surrounded by the perimuscular layer composed of a narrow zone of loose connective tissue, sometimes interspersed with adipose cells. Serosa covers the perimuscular layer over the peritoneal surface of the gallbladder. In the gallbladder fossa the connective tissue of the wall is continuous with the periportal spaces of the liver. On the surface, aberrant bile ducts (Luschka ducts) frequently occur.

PHYSIOLOGY

The function of the gallbladder is to concentrate hepatic bile and deliver it at intervals into the intestine to aid in the digestion and absorption of fat. Despite its limited capacity, the gallbladder concentrates and thus can accommodate up to half of the daily flow of hepatic bile and can sequester between meals the entire bile acid pool. The absorptive rate of the gallbladder, one of the highest among epithelia, is between 15% and 30% of intraluminal volume per hour, and the ionic profile of the residual concentrate is altered. Organic solutes comprise only 5% of human bile by weight and consist mainly of bile acid anions, phospholipids (mostly lecithin), and nonesterified cholesterol aggregated into mixed micelles.

The drive for bile secretion is predominantly attributable to the hepatic flow of bile acids having two components: bile acids that have been returned to the liver from the intestine and newly synthesized bile acids. Hence factors that modify intestinal bile acid absorption may alter hepatic bile acid secretion and also change its lipid composition throughout a 24-hour cycle.[2]

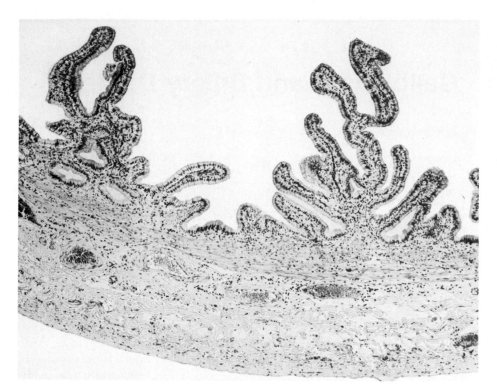

Fig. 26-1. Normal gallbladder in 33-year-old woman. In cross section of midportion, delicate connective tissue stalks are covered by tall columnar epithelium. Beneath tunica propria is muscular coat with smooth muscle bundles arranged longitudinally and then obliquely or circularly. External to muscular coat is perimuscular layer. (40×.)

The extent to which hepatic bile is normally "partitioned" into gallbladder before delivery into the intestine is estimated at 60% to 70% using cholescintigraphy.

Gallbladder motility, contraction, and choledochal relaxation are under the receptor-mediated control of a peptide hormone, cholecystokinin (CCK), which is released from the proximal intestine by partly digested proteins and fatty acids.

The extent of neural control of gallbladder motor function is uncertain. Adrenergic innervation of gallbladder muscle is sparse; most of the adrenergic fibers in the human gallbladder are distributed to blood vessels. The extent of vagal cholinergic innervation of gallbladder smooth muscle has yet to be defined; vagotomy is said to decrease nerve fibers in the wall of the gallbladder by 10%. Cholinergic agonists contact gallbladder smooth muscle, and beta-adrenergic agonists relax it.

Vasoactive intestinal peptide (VIP), immunoreactive nerve fibers, and cell bodies have recently been demonstrated in muscle and submucosal layers of the gallbladder in humans and other mammals and appear to reach the gallbladder via the vagus nerve.[5] VIP relaxes gallbladder muscle and antagonizes the contractile effect of CCK.[4] It seems reasonable to speculate that VIP and CCK function as the neural and hormonal limbs of a peptide system for the control of gallbladder motor activity. The control of gallbladder motility is probably far more complex. Indeed, a link has recently been demonstrated between intestinal migrating motor complex activity and gallbladder emptying, the mechanism of which is not understood.[6]

Certain substances, when injected intravenously or given by mouth, appear in the bile and reach the gallbladder. Some substances so administered accumulate in the gallbladder in concentrations not attained in the bile coming from the liver. Cholecystography, the visualization of the gallbladder roentgenographically, is based on this selective resorbing ability of the gallbladder. Radiopaque substances, after reaching the gallbladder, are resorbed more slowly than the bile, eventually attaining a concentration sufficient to cast a shadow on an x-ray film. Intraluminal lesions (stones or "polyps") appear as a radiolucent filling defect. Some antibiotics do also more selectively appear in bile, and so this property can be used in therapeutic decisions.

Congenital or developmental abnormalities

Many anomalous arrangements of the extrahepatic bile ducts and their arteries are usually asymptomatic and significant only for those involved in gallbladder surgery. Other abnormalities of the gallbladder include absence, duplication, and presence of heterotopic tissue. Agenesis may be associated with symptoms suggestive of inflammatory disease of the gallbladder. Exploration and T-tube cholangiography establish the diagnosis. The remainder of the biliary tract is usually normally developed in these cases.[10] Duplication and lobulation show histologically normal features.

Heterotopic tissue is nearly always accompanied by inflammation and lithiasis.[11] Gastric tissue is the most frequent finding,[8] but adrenal,[7] pancreas,[13] and thyroid[9] tissues have all been reported.

A group of conditions with a probably related pathogenesis, which are designated infantile obstructive cholangiopathy, includes biliary atresia, choledochal cyst, and neonatal hepatitis.[12] They are now believed to be part of an acquired progressive process that occurs postnatally. They are discussed in detail on p. 1262.

Acquired disorders
Cholelithiasis

Cholelithiasis results from the interplay of numerous factors. It is more frequent in women than in men. The incidence in the general population of the United States is 11% according to the Framingham Study.[16] The incidence increases with age, so that at the age of 60 years, about 25% of women have stones. In the Native American population the incidence is considerably greater.[24]

Gallstones contain cholesterol, calcium bilirubinate, and calcium carbonate either in pure form or in various combinations (Figs. 26-2 and 26-3). About 20% contain sufficient calcium to be radiopaque. Others appear as a filling defect in an opacified gallbladder. About half of patients with lithiasis have a gallbladder that cannot be visualized. Ultrasonography and computerized tomography are methods of choice for the investigation of symptoms referable to the gallbladder and common duct.[34] Ultrasonography has the advantage of being noninvasive, with no radiation exposure and modestly priced equipment, but it requires a high degree of interpretative skill.[30] Other procedures include percutaneous transhepatic cholangiography and endoscopic retrograde cholangiopancreatography (ERCP); these are invasive procedures and involve some radiation exposure but have high diagnostic accuracy.

Table 26-1 summarizes the appearance of various gallstones and the known factors in their formation. Intraluminal stones of different composition have different effects on the gallbladder mucosa. Gallbladders containing pure stones show little or no inflammatory reaction if the cystic duct is not obstructed. On the other hand, chronic cholecystitis is almost always present in gallbladders with mixed and combined gallstones, which represent the majority (90%) of cases of lithiasis (Fig. 26-4).

Numerous clinical and experimental studies have tried to elucidate the mechanism of stone formation in the gallbladder. It is increasingly evident that multiple factors are involved and that patients with cholelithiasis probably constitute a heterogeneous population. Some of the important factors identified in stone formation can be grouped according to three general categories[19,32]: (1) lithiasis resulting from abnormal composition of bile; (2) that resulting from abnormal contractility of the bladder; and (3) that resulting from abnormal epithelial secretion. However, in patients with lithiasis, the various factors exist synchronously, and their relative primary importance cannot be established independently. Supersaturation of bile in cholesterol is the major factor in gallstones associated with obesity and clofibrate therapy in coronary patients.[15] On the other hand, excessive bile salt loss is seen in lithiasis associated with intestinal bypass procedures in Crohn's disease.[22] Decreased bile acid secretion was identified in the lithogenic bile of the Native American women.

Cholelithiasis is rare in children.[29] A hemolytic disorder of one type or another is present in approximately 50% of afflicted children. These include congenital spherocytosis, sickle cell anemia (Fig. 26-5), and thalassemia. In one report of gallbladder disease in children, however, only 25 of 50 children had hemolytic disease. Two had acalculous cholecystitis, and three had cystic fibrosis. Importantly, the group without hemolytic disease had a long history of symptoms. Gallstones in children are rarely calcified and not seen on plain roentgenogram of the abdomen. Ultrasonography is clearly the method of choice for diagnosis.[26] In some of the other children there is a history of previous intra-abdominal sepsis. Both children and adults maintained on prolonged total parenteral nutrition (TPN) are at increased risk for gallstone formation (Fig. 26-6). Initially, there is formation of sludge, which is partially reversible.[23] The majority of gallstones developing under these circumstances consist of calcium bilirubinate.

Female sex hormones have long been suspected to be involved in gallbladder physiology and pathology. Estrogen and progesterone receptors of high affinity and specificity in both cytosol and nuclei were identified in gallbladder epithelium.[31] Some side effects on gallstone formation may result from altering respective bile constituents. The female preponderance and the association of gallbladder stones and parity are well known. Gallbladder function in the last trimester of pregnancy has been examined by real-time ultrasonography; an abnormal contractility and a large residual volume resulting in stasis were observed, whereas in patients taking contraceptive steroids, gallbladder kinetics were normal.[14] Interestingly, progesterone has been shown experimentally to impair gallbladder response to exogenous cholecystokinin. There is a significant association between gallstones, replacement estrogen therapy, and estrogen given for coronary artery

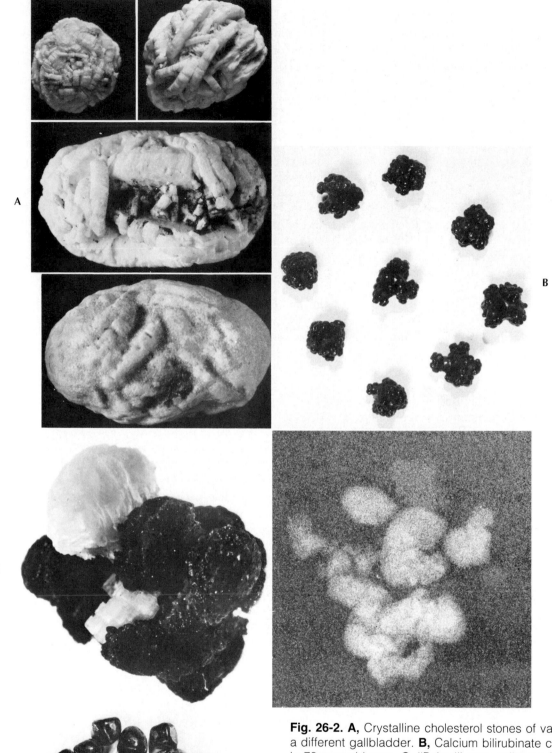

Fig. 26-2. A, Crystalline cholesterol stones of varying sizes, each from a different gallbladder. **B,** Calcium bilirubinate calculi from gallbladder in 78-year-old man. **C,** "Paired" pure gallstone from gallbladder in 41-year-old woman. Calculus is 0.9 cm in diameter. Attached to black calcium bilirubinate concretion are clusters of crystalline cholesterol. Calcium bilirubinate portion is radiopaque. **D,** Mixed gallstones from gallbladder in 68-year-old man. Calculi are of almost equal size with articulating faceted surfaces and are black with lighter black-brown centers. (**A,** 2×; **A** and **C,** courtesy Dr. Malcolm A. Hyman, New York.)

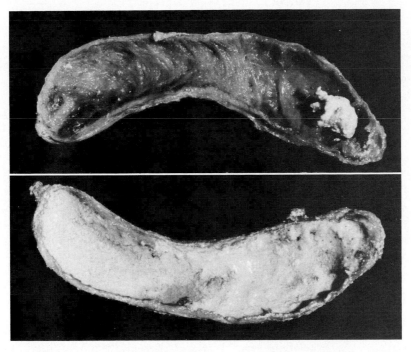

Fig. 26-3. Calcium carbonate stone and "lime paste" in gallbladder of 34-year-old man.

Table 26-1. Classification of gallstones

Type	Composition	Appearance	Factors in origin	Changes in gallbladder
Pure gallstones (10%)	Cholesterol (crystalline)	Solitary; crystalline surface	Increased cholesterol content in bile	Cholesterosis
	Calcium bilirubinate	Multiple; jet black; crystalline or amorphous	Increased pigment content in bile	No change
	Calcium carbonate	Grayish white; amorphous	Unknown	No change
Mixed gallstones (80%)	Cholesterol and calcium bilirubinate Cholesterol and calcium carbonate Calcium bilirubinate and calcium carbonate Cholesterol, calcium bilirubinate, and calcium carbonate	Multiple, faceted or lobulated, laminated, and crystalline on cut surfaces; hue depends on content: cholesterol, yellow; calcium bilirubinate, black; calcium carbonate, white	Chronic cholecystitis plus increased content in bile of cholesterol, calcium bilirubinate, or calcium carbonate	Chronic cholecystitis
Combined gallstone (10%)	Pure gallstone nucleus with mixed gallstone shell	Largest of gallstones when single; hue depends on composition of shell	As in pure gallstones, followed by chronic cholecystitis	Chronic cholecystitis
	Mixed gallstone nucleus with pure gallstone shell		As in mixed gallstones, followed by increased content in bile of cholesterol, calcium bilirubinate, or calcium carbonate	Chronic cholecystitis

disease in men. Interestingly, oral contraceptive usage is a risk factor only in women under 30 years of age. Over that age it actually decreases the risk of gallstones, as perhaps estrogens simply accelerate formation of gallstones in those predestined to get them through other risk factors.[28] The mechanism of this association is not determined but probably does not involve gallbladder motility itself. Vagotomy is said to predispose patients to lithiasis. In addition, in an elegant series of in vitro studies,[20] excess mucin secretion by the gallbladder epithelium has recently been identified as a critical nucleation factor for stone formation. And last, another iatrogenic factor predisposing to cholestasis and possibly gallstones is cyclosporin A, now widely used in all the organ-transplantation protocols.

Gallstones are formed in the gallbladder and may escape into the cystic duct or common duct. Approximately 15% of patients operated on for cholelithiasis also have concomitant choledocholithiasis.[34] In more than 1% of patients, symptoms of common duct lithiasis appear some time after cholecystectomy and are caused by stones overlooked at the time of operation.[17] The primary formation of stones in the extrahepatic ducts is so rare that common duct obstruction by stone is nearly always the result of gallbladder lithiasis. However, 20% of patients with agenesis of the gallbladder have had gallstones.[10] In rare cases, therefore, stones can and do form in the common duct. These so-called earthy stones are predominantly soft and dark in appearance. The common duct is invariably dilated.

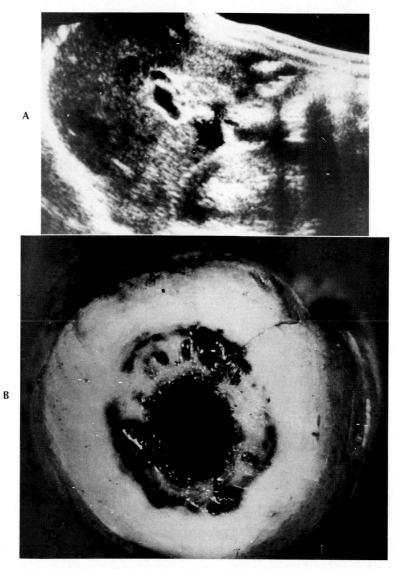

Fig. 26-4. Ultrasonogram, **A,** and transverse anatomic section of gallbladder, **B,** to show extent of thickening of wall in chronic cholecystitis. Appearance is grossly indistinguishable from that of sclerosing carcinoma.

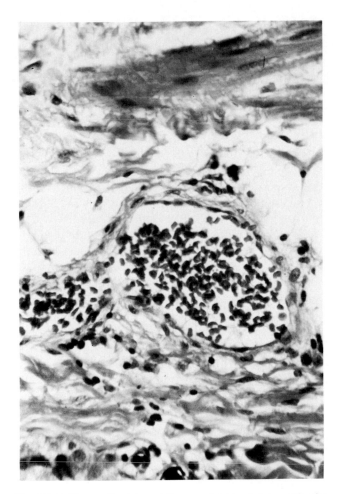

Fig. 26-5. The patient is a 12-year-old black boy with cholelithiasis. The cholecystectomy specimen revealed multiple brown calculi. Vessels of the submucosa and subserosa show numerous sickled red blood cells. (260×.)

Lithiasis, if untreated, has numerous complications.[21,33] Stones travel through the cystic duct to become impacted in the common duct or at the ampulla, causing intermittent jaundice and severe colicky pain. They are causes of obstruction with secondary acute cholecystitis. Gallstones may also lead to internal biliary fistulas, mostly between gallbladder and duodenum or gallbladder and colon. These result from inflammatory adhesions with subsequent perforation. Fistulas may be visualized on a plain film of the abdomen when an air column outlines the biliary tree. Gallstones are by far the commonest single cause of pancreatitis accounting for over half of documented cases. The rationale for removal of stones is thus the observed serious inflammatory and obstructive complications and not the possibility of associated cancer.[21,25,33]

Because there is substantial postoperative morbidity and mortality,[18] development of extracorporeal lithotripsy has become an area of major interest.[27]

ACUTE INFLAMMATION

Acute acalculous primary bacterial cholecystitis has been documented but is relatively rare in adults.[37] Strains of *Salmonella*, coliform bacteria, enterococci, and staphylococci have all been implicated in some cases. However, much more frequently, acute cholecystitis results from secondary bacterial infection caused by obstruction or impaction of a stone in the common duct. Thiazides have been incriminated in their ability to cause acute cholecystitis.[46] A temporary increase in bile salt content has also been shown experimentally to produce acute cholecystitis. Circulating bacterial toxins are also suspected to be able to damage gallbladder epithelium, as in the lesions of the toxic shock syndrome.[40]

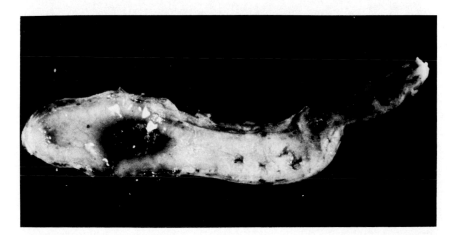

Fig. 26-6. The patient is an 18-month-old black girl with cholecystitis and no known hemolytic disorder. The cholecystectomy specimen measured 3.5 × 0.8 × 0.7 cm and contained a single stone, which occupied most of the gallbladder lumen. The patient was a severely premature baby on long-term total parenteral nutrition.

Whether acute cholecystitis occurring in the critically ill is a related phenomenon is not clear.[39] A review of 18 cases indicates that prolonged use of high-dose opiates in intensive care may cause constriction of the ampulla of Vater, causing bile stasis, and may play a role in the development of acute acalculous cholecystitis in this clinical setting.

In children, acute cholecystitis is more often the acalculous variety than in adults in up to 30% of gallbladder disease. Systemic infections such as scarlet fever, salmonellosis, and leptospirosis are considered significant factors in the etiology.[35] The exact mechanism by which acute inflammation of the gallbladder is initiated, however, is unknown.

More recently, in states of immunodeficiency, cytomegalovirus and *Cryptosporidium* have been identified in the gallbladder and in the intrahepatic biliary tree (Fig. 26-7).[41,42,45] Cytomegalovirus is also implicated in a primary sclerosing cholangitis-like presentation in patients with congenital or acquired immunodeficiency syndromes.[47]

In another report, cholecystectomy specimens of acute cholecystitis have been shown to actually contain the *Rickettsia rickettsii* organisms in two patients with Rocky Mountain spotted fever with attendant focal vascular thrombosis and hemorrhage.[48]

In acute cholecystitis the clinical symptoms and signs are those of an acute inflammation in the right upper quadrant of the abdomen. Grossly the gallbladder is enlarged and firm, with a thickened wall oozing serous or serosanguineous fluid. There is pronounced edema, and the outer surface is a dusky reddish brown. The mucosa is congested and grayish red. The mucosa may be intact or may show focal or extensive areas of ulceration. Microscopic examination show subserosal edema with all the layers spread apart, pronounced congestion, extravasation of red blood cells, and fresh thrombi within small veins. In distended capillaries, margination of white blood cells is conspicuous. A pronounced tissue reaction of polymorphonuclear cells is generally absent. Free perforation into the peritoneal cavity has become a rare complication. However, in an acutely distended gallbladder, bile may leak through the intact wall and cause bile peritonitis, which has a guarded prognosis. Hemorrhagic infarction of the gallbladder (gangrenous cholecystitis) may occur, often resulting from an impacted stone that interferes with the venous drainage of the gallbladder.

Occasionally a classic case of acute cholecystitis may show vasculitis with fibrinoid necrosis of the muscular arteries.[36,38,43] Some of these patients go on to full-blown multisystem disorders, whereas in others vasculitis-like changes are confined to the gallbladder. The incidence of gallstones is increased five- to tenfold in patients with Crohn's disease, but actual involvement of the gallbladder by Crohn's disease is rare.[44]

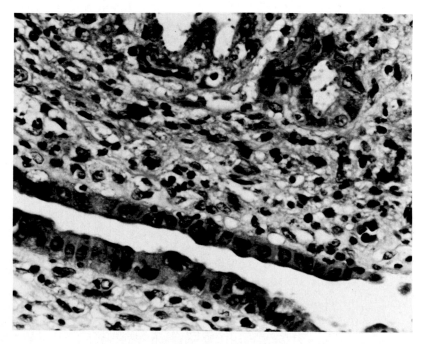

Fig. 26-7. Cytomegalovirus and *Cryptosporidium* cholecystitis. A cytomegalovirus inclusion–bearing cell is seen in an epithelial invagination. Two glandlike structures show cryptosporidial organisms attached to the luminal aspects of the cells. (490×; courtesy Dr. Jorge Albores-Saavedra, Miami, Fla.)

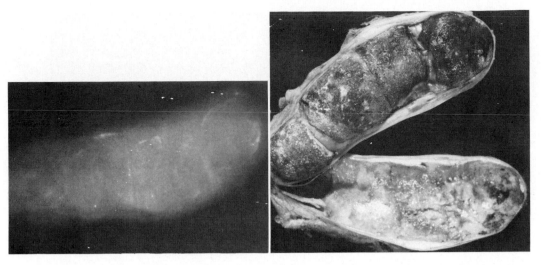

Fig. 26-8. Calcium impregnation of wall of gallbladder in 73-year-old man. Combined calculi with articulating faceted surfaces fill lumen. (Courtesy Dr. William R. Schmalhorst, Bakersfield, Calif.)

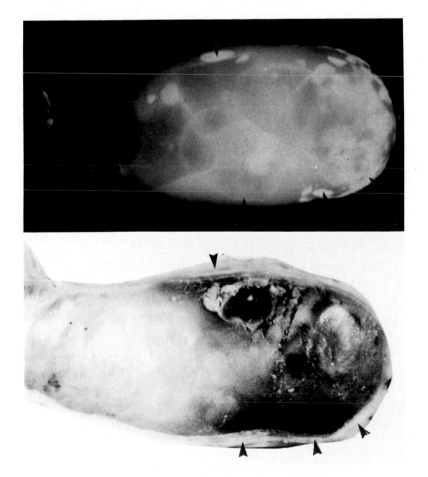

Fig. 26-9. Comparison of calcified material seen on the roentgenogram and the gross photograph in a so-called porcelain gallbladder, *arrows.*

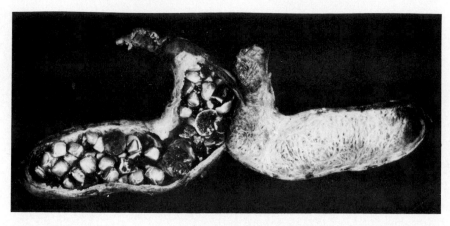

Fig. 26-10. Gallbladder with chronic cholecystitis containing mixed gallstones in 40-year-old man. There are noticeable trabeculations on mucosal surface. Calculi are faceted and yellow with brown centers.

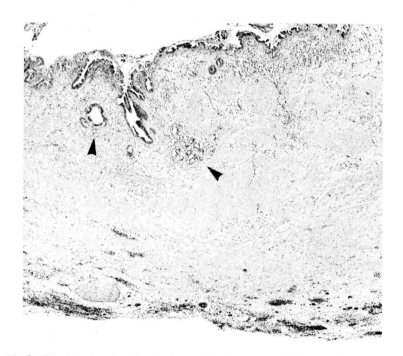

Fig. 26-11. Gallbladder in chronic cholecystitis. Compare thickness of wall to that in Fig. 26-1. Attenuation of mucosa and appearance of mucous cells *(arrows)* are characteristic. (Hematoxylin and eosin; 35×; WU 81-7968.)

CHRONIC INFLAMMATION

Chronic cholecystitis is rarely seen in the absence of lithiasis. The associated stones are of the mixed or combined type (Table 26-1). The gallbladder in chronic cholecystitis is characterized by prominent thickening and fibrosis of the wall, which may be grossly indistinguishable from sclerosing carcinoma (Fig. 26-4). Occasionally, diffuse calcification of the wall is also present (porcelain gallbladder, Figs. 26-8 and 26-9. The mucosal folds are coarse and may be completely obliterated. The surface may be trabeculated because of the muscular hyperplasia of the "fighting gallbladder" in the early phase of common duct obstruction (Fig. 26-10).

On microscopic examination the mucosa may be atrophic or show hyperplastic changes. The normal epithelium of the gallbladder secretes little mucin, but in chronic inflammation, newly formed mucous glands arise from the epithelium in the depths of the folds and may become complex (Fig. 26-11). The recently redefined crucial role of epithelial mucin in the pathogene-

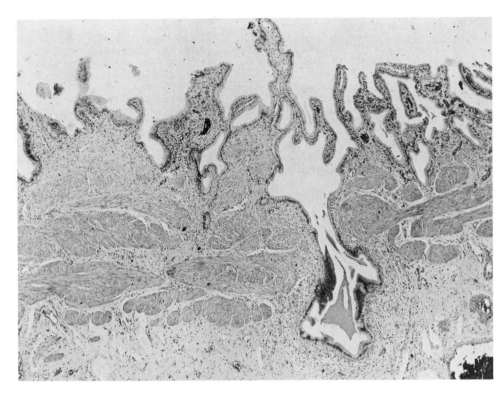

Fig. 26-12. Gallbladder with chronic cholecystitis that contained mixed gallstones in 57-year-old woman. In longitudinal section from body of viscus, folds of mucosa are coarse or delicate. Rokitansky-Aschoff sinus extends through entire thickness of greatly hypertrophied muscular coat. There is increase in connective tissue in tunica propria and between muscle bundles. Perimuscular layer is broad. In all layers there is slight infiltration with lymphocytes, plasma cells, large mononuclear cells, and some eosinophilic granulocytes. (Hematoxylin and eosin; 32×.)

sis of lithiasis is relevant.[20] Endocrine cells may be increased.[11] The muscle usually becomes hyperplastic with mucosal diverticula (Rokitansky-Aschoff sinuses) between its fascicles (Fig. 26-12). These normally occur at a site of existing weakness of the wall, along the path of penetrating blood vessels. According to Halpert, they result from inflammation and never occur in the normal gallbladder.[56] The perimuscular layer is fibrotic with coarse collagenous bundles. There is usually a moderate mixed inflammatory infiltrate involving all layers. Rarely, there is a prominence of lymphocytic infiltration with formation of lymph follicles and large germinal centers (chronic follicular cholecystitis).[54] These need to be differentiated from gallbladder involvement by malignant lymphoma.[49]

Numerous episodes of acute cholecystitis usually become superimposed on the chronic inflammatory process. Grossly the gallbladder appears acutely inflamed, red, and edematous with mucosal erosions and also contains stones (Fig. 26-13). Microscopically Rokitansky-Aschoff sinuses are numerous, and muscular hyperplasia and considerable fibrosis of the wall are present. In addition, a hemorrhagic fibrinopurulent exudate cov-

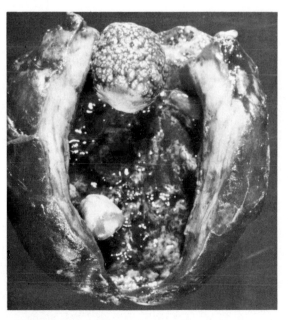

Fig. 26-13. Gross appearance of acute cholecystitis, superimposed on long-standing lithiasis. Hemorrhagic and fibrinopurulent deposits line gallbladder lumen, wall is greatly thickened, and stones are visible.

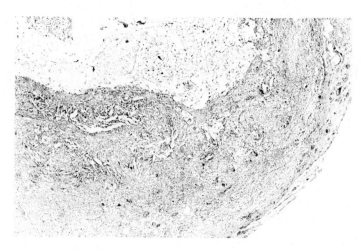

Fig. 26-14. Ulcerated gallbladder mucosa with underlying cholesterol granuloma that complicated long-standing lithiasis and chronic cholecystitis. (Hematoxylin and eosin; 35×; WU 81-7969.)

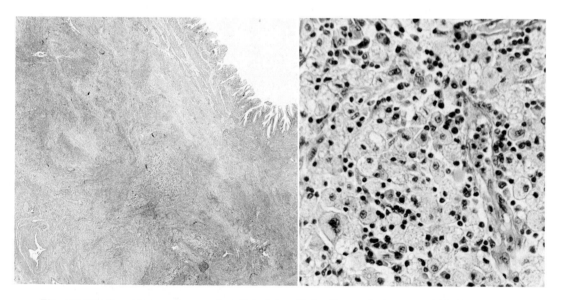

Fig. 26-15. Ceroid granuloma of gallbladder. Collections of pigmented histiocytes are seen deep in gallbladder wall, as is a chronic lymphoplasmacytic inflammatory infiltrate. (Hematoxylin and eosin; 10×; WU 81-10000; courtesy Dr. A.M. Wright, Penrose Hospital, Colorado Springs, Colo.)

ers extended areas of the mucosa, and the inflammatory infiltrate contains sheets of polymorphonuclear cells in the interstitium. This is the condition that most frequently necessitates cholecystectomy. Localized tissue reactions with cholesterol crystals may be seen within the thickened fibrous wall underlying an ulcer (Fig. 26-14). Ceroid granulomas have recently been described in the gallbladder[50] and probably represent a form of chronic cholecystitis. Bile is postulated to serve as the substrate for the ceroid pigment formation within his-

tiocytes (Fig. 26-15). What previously was called xanthogranulomatous cholecystitis probably represents the same entity.[8] Another previously unreported morphologic form of chronic cholestitis is malakoplakia with formation of Michaelis-Gutmann bodies[60a] (Fig. 26-16).

Strictures of the common duct usually result from operative trauma cased by inadvertent ligation.[57] The numerous anatomic variants of the extrahepatic duct and their vessels mentioned earlier are contributing factors in causing the error. Rarely the common duct may

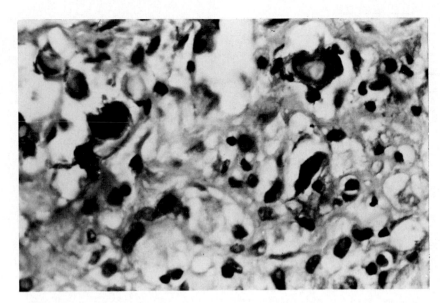

Fig. 26-16. A 27-year-old white woman had a 2-year history of occasional upper quadrant pain, with gallstones visible by ultrasound. The cholecystectomy specimen was not grossly remarkable except for seven round, soft, laminated, chalky yellow gallstones. Sections, however, showed collections of macrophages containing both clear foamy cytoplasm and granular PAS-positive cytoplasm underlying reactive and focally ulcerated epithelium. There are numerous Michaelis-Gutmann bodies, which stain positively with iron stains, consistent with malakoplakia. (540×.)

participate and get encased within a process of idiopathic retroperitoneal fibrosis.[61] Surgical repair in all these cases is extremely difficult. Extrinsic compression of the common duct by a calcified lymph node can occur.[52]

Primary sclerosing cholangitis, a rare disease of unknown cause, is characterized by fibrosis and diffuse thickening of the wall, predominantly affecting the common duct.[51,55] However, more extensive involvement of the entire system can occur, sometimes including the intrahepatic ducts, in which case the characteristic changes may be seen on liver biopsy. The diagnosis is based on examination of a section of the common duct, which shows the chronic inflammatory and fibrosing changes involving submucosa and subserosa, whereas the mucosa is relatively intact. Well-differentiated sclerosing adenocarcinoma, the principal element of the differential diagnosis, must be ruled out. The diagnosis of sclerosing cholangitis should be made only in patients who do not have gallstones and who had no previous operations on the biliary tract. The disease may be found with ulcerative colitis.[62] Rarely, it also affects children[53] and particularly children with immunodeficiency syndromes.[47,60] A sclerosing cholangitis–*like* clinical presentation can be seen after continuous hepatic artery infusion of fluorodeoxyuridine (FUDR) for the management of metastatic tumors to the liver. Eight of 46 (17.4%) patients developed strictures in one prospective study documented on ERCP.[58,59]

MISCELLANEOUS NONINFLAMMATORY CONDITIONS

Cholesterosis of the gallbladder has a characteristic morphologic pattern. Usually the lesion has no inflammatory component and the gallbladder mucosa is otherwise normal. Grossly the mucosa is congested and has yellow flecks of lipid in linear streaks. Cholesterol is increased in the bile but not in the blood. Microscopically collections of lipid-laden foamy cells are present in the lamina propria beneath a normal epithelium (Fig. 26-17).

Spontaneous perforation of the biliary tract occurs within the first year of life. It is usually solitary, and the most common site is the junction of the cystic duct and the common bile duct. The cause is unclear, but a preexisting malformation of the wall has been postulated.[64] It is an acute abdominal emergency, and the treatment is surgical.

Acute hydrops of the gallbladder is more often seen in children than in adults, and a precise cause had not been identified.[63] Right upper quadrant symptoms and often a mass are the clinical features. Grossly the gallbladder is distended without stones. The bile is pale, watery, or mucoid. The treatment is usually aspiration or cholecystotomy.

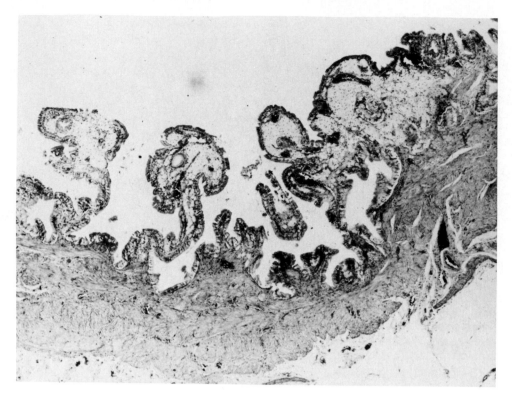

Fig. 26-17. Gallbladder with cholesterosis of mucosa in 46-year-old woman. Viscus contained crystalline cholesterol stone. In cross section from near neck, folds are enlarged and rounded. Connective tissue stalks contain many large mononuclear cells with light-stained cytoplasm and eccentric nuclei. These cells contain anisotropic lipoid substances that can be demonstrated by fat stains. (Hematoxylin and eosin; 60×.)

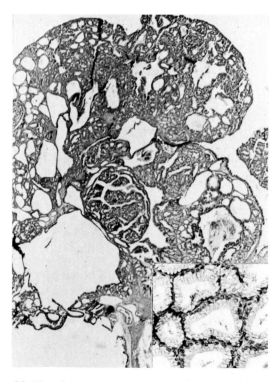

Fig. 26-18. Adenomatous polyp showing proliferated glands, some cystic, surrounded by scant connective tissue stroma. (Hematoxylin and eosin; 10×.)

TUMORS
Benign tumors and pseudotumors

Benign true neoplasms of the gallbladder and common duct are extremely rare.[8] They include adenomatous polyps (Fig. 26-18), villous adenomas, and cystadenomas.[69] Adenomatous polyps and villous adenomas represent a preneoplastic condition at this site as well as at all other sites of the gastrointestinal tract.[68,71,73] Distally in the common duct and at the ampulla of Vater and more rarely proximally these lesions can occur in Gardner's syndrome; therefore these sites must be part of the lifelong surveillance effort in these patients.[66,75] Granular cell myoblastomas have been reported in the biliary tract, and their morphology is similar to that at other sites seen by both light microscopy and electron microscopy.[77] Paragangliomas of the gallbladder have been reported,[72] as well as eosinophilic granuloma, which involved the common duct and occurred as a mass.[70]

More frequently, however, "masses" in the area of the gallbladder and extrahepatic system are "pseudotumors," including inflammatory polyps, cholesterol polyps, and reactive conditions. Cholesterol polyps are multilobular and yellow. Microscopically they consist of sheets of foamy histiocytes covered by an intact mucosa

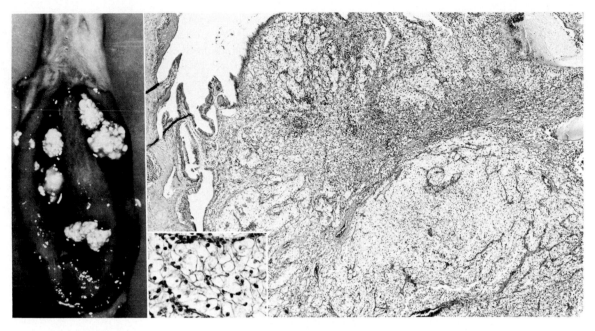

Fig. 26-19. Gross and microscopic appearances of pedunculated cholesterol polyps, consisting of sheets of foamy histiocytes lined by intact surface epithelium. (Hematoxylin and eosin; 35×; WU 81-7974.)

(Fig. 26-19). These may detach and become the nidus for stone formation.

Another condition, consisting of a complex system of tubular structures set within interlacing smooth muscle bundles, commonly involves the region of the fundus.[65] When sharply circumscribed, it appears grossly as a tumor (Fig. 26-20) and is called "adenomyoma." The condition may involve the gallbladder in a more diffuse manner and is then labeled "adenomyomatosis." It resembles cholecystitis glandularis and the various forms of gallbladder diverticuli. They probably all represent reactive conditions of the gallbladder mucosa possibly secondary to an abnormality of muscle contraction and may best be thought of as diverticular disease of the gallbladder.[76]

Amputation neuromas have been described at the junction of the common and cystic ducts; some are isolated, and some are seen in conjunction with intriguing and complex syndromes, such as soft-tissue tumors that secrete nerve growth factor.[74] Ganglioneuromatosis of the gallbladder has been described in the multiple endocrine neoplasia 2b syndromes.[67]

Malignant tumors
Etiology and pathogenesis

Primary carcinoma of the gallbladder and biliary tract is not a rare disease, being the fifth most common of the digestive tract.[85] There has been an apparent increase in incidence during the last 15 years.[112] Whether this is real or only a reflection of more accurate reporting remains to be determined. Although the causes of this disease are unknown, several possible factors have been suggested.

Gallstones have long been thought to play a role in the genesis of gallbladder carcinoma[29] as is apparent from the Western literature. In one study the percentage of patients with gallbladder carcinoma who were definitely stated not to have stones accompanying the carcinoma varied only from 3.4% to 17%. Another series reported 29 cases of carcinoma among 1488 cholecystectomies, whereas stones were detected in 4459 patients by roentgenologic examination[117]; thus in the presence of cholelithiasis, the incidence of documented carcinoma in that study appears to be only 0.66%. In yet another cumulative series, only 0.4% of 1419 patients with known untreated gallstones developed gallbladder carcinoma when followed for 10 years.[112] There is a high prevalence of gallbladder carcinoma in certain population groups, such as American Indians of the Southwest. In Native Americans the incidence of gallbladder carcinoma is six times that in whites.[90,96] The incidence of gallbladder cancer in the Hispanic population, which has a considerable Indian component in its gene pool, seems to be intermediate. However, chronic gallbladder diseases with lithiasis is also prevalent in these populations. The atypical epithelial lesions described in gallbladders of these populations, considered to be precursors to carcinoma, are invariably confined to the free surface epithelium and superficial epithelial invaginations.[78,90] These observations indicate that the mucosal atypia in these cases may be related to exposure to substances in the gallbladder lumen, presumably contained in bile or stones.

In Japan, on the other hand, there is a high incidence of carcinoma of the gallbladder associated with anoma-lous junctions of the pancreaticobiliary duct.[125] A study from Japan found that 16 out of 65 patients (24.6%) with an anomalous ductal union had a gallbladder cancer as opposed to 12 out of 635 healthy subjects (1.9%) and gallstones were present in only two of the 16.[103]

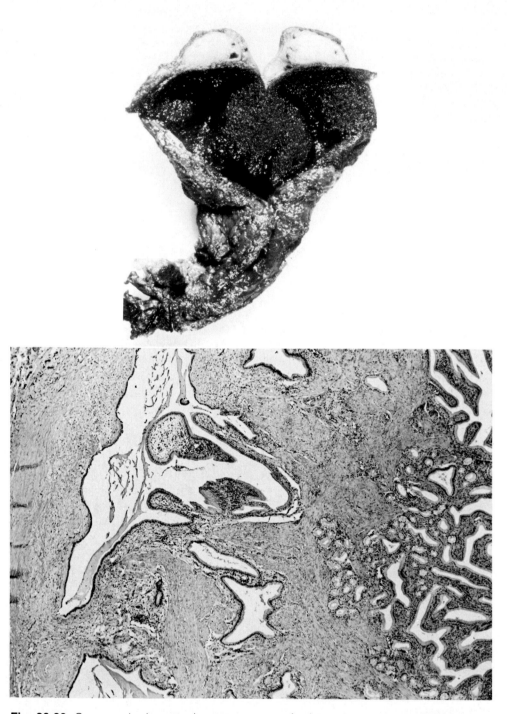

Fig. 26-20. Gross and microscopic appearances of adenomyoma of gallbladder that is localized to fundus. Sections show system of acinar tubular structures lined by cuboid or columnar cells in scanty connective tissue stroma. Interlacing smooth muscle bundles are also seen in stroma. (32×; courtesy Dr. Malcolm A. Hyman, New York.)

The role of chemical carcinogenesis in gallbladder cancer has also received considerable attention because of the structural similarity of some known carcinogens to the naturally occurring bile acids. Animal studies have implicated methylcholanthrene, *o*-aminoazotoluene, and various nitrosamines in the induction of gallbladder carcinoma.[88,112] Experimental animal studies, however, suffer from the problem of species differences in susceptibility and subsequent extrapolation of data from animals to humans. A higher incidence and earlier onset of cancer of the gallbladder have been reported in rubber industry workers.[107] Moreover, pesticides have been shown to be excreted in the bile. The therapeutic agent chenodeoxycholic acid, now available for the dissolution of cholesterol gallstones, may also have long-term effects that are not yet known.

A higher incidence of subsequent gallbladder carcinoma has also been reported in patients who had undergone previous operations on the biliary tract, usually a cholecystostomy. The association of chronic ulcerative colitis with carcinoma of the gallbladder had been reported[100] though the association with carcinoma of the bile ducts is more frequent.[91,92,109] Patients with ileal disease and those who have undergone bypass surgery are also at higher risk for gallbladder carcinoma. These same groups of patients, however, are also the ones with high incidence of gallbladder lithiasis.[99]

Liver fluke infections in the Orient are known promoters of bile duct carcinoma.[88] It is possible that the chronic inflammatory response they elicit potentiates the action of carcinomas in the bile. Similar conclusions have been drawn in experimental animals. There is an association of carcinoma with congenital cysts of the biliary tract, which may have a similar cause.[102] Caroli's disease is a congenital disorder of the intrahepatic biliary tree characterized by multiple segmental cystic dilatations of the bile ducts. Six of 138 cases have been complicated by cholangiocarcinoma.

In summary, chronic inflammation and fibrosis seem to be strongly associated with carcinoma of the biliary tract. It is interesting in this respect that patients with end-stage chronic cholecystitis, the calcified (porcelain) gallbladder, also have a very high incidence of malignancy[113] (Figs. 26-8 and 26-9). The exact nature of the relationship, however, has been elusive both in clinical and in experimental studies. Nevertheless, in the United States the incidence of gallbladder cancer has recently stabilized, or possibly even declined, concurrent with a rise in the number of cholecystectomies.[97] Two gallbladder carcinoma–derived cell lines have been shown to have epidermal growth factor receptor gene amplification, a finding consistent with an autocrine growth pattern of tumor growth in gallbladder carcinoma.[104]

Incidence and clinical presentation

The usual type of carcinoma of the gallbladder has a female preponderance (ratio of 4:1).[73] The mean age of 1728 patients was 65 years, with 0.1%, 1.5%, 8.9%, 19.6%, and 37% occurring in the third, fourth, fifth, sixth and seventh decades respectively.[71] In patients over 70 years of age who underwent operations on the biliary tract, 10% to 17% were found to have carcinoma. Gallbladder carcinoma that is associated with another condition than gallstones (ulcerative colitis, anomalous biliary tree, and so on) presents in a much younger age group.

In a few instances, cancer arises from the hepatic duct in the region of the porta hepatis in relatively young persons (Fig. 26-21).[105] Some of these tumors are extremely well differentiated, with relatively slow growth. The presence and location of tumor are best demonstrated by percutaneous transhepatic cholangiography.

Bile duct carcinoma appears to be less frequent than gallbladder carcinoma,[122] and there is no sex difference in its incidence. Carcinoma of the terminal portion of the common bile duct and that of intrahepatic ducts are discussed elsewhere.

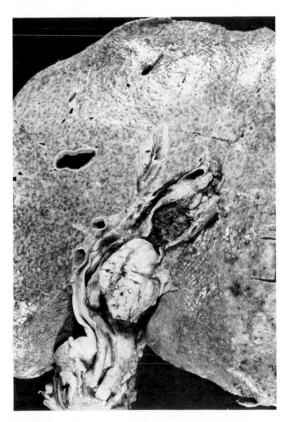

Fig. 26-21. Gross appearance of well-differentiated adenocarcinoma, "Klatskin tumor," arising in porta hepatis.

Clinically the lack of specific signs and symptoms prevents early detection of carcinoma of the gallbladder. The clinical presentation commonly mimics benign gallbladder disease, especially acute cholecystitis. Indeed, the most frequent symptoms are pain (75% of patients), obstructive jaundice, and weight loss. Jandice is the predominant symptom in up to 90% of patients, but although it is classically progressive, an intermittent character is present in about 8% of patients. This is sometimes attributable to tumor debris floating free within the bile duct. It was metastatic colon carcinoma in 3 of 6 cases reported.[116] As a result of the highly variable clinical presentation and the nonspecific physical, laboratory, and roentgenographic findings in gallbladder carcinoma, the mean correct preoperative rate of diagnosis is only 8.6%.[21] In diagnosed cases the tumor is advanced and usually inoperable. When the nature of the lesion becomes apparent to the surgeon at the time of exploration, the tumor is usually too advanced for cure. Results of a collective review of 993 patients revealed that 16% of patients underwent presumed complete resection of identified tumor and 72% underwent palliative procedures or biopsy alone. In a group of patients with a more favorable prognosis, however, "incidental" carcinoma was diagnosed only after microscopic examination of gallbladders that were removed for presumed benign disease.[87] In these cases

the difficulty of diagnosis lies in the gross similarity with inflammation fibrous tissue. Therefore microscopic examination of every excised gallbladder is mandatory.

Pathology, clinicopathologic correlation, and rationale for treatment

Tumors may occur in all parts of the gallbladder but are most frequent in the fundus.[123] The gross pattern of growth assumes either a papillary or an infiltrative character, which may be superimposed on preexisting deformities because of chronic inflammation or lithiasis. Infiltrative carcinoma grows diffusely, imparting a firm, leatherlike quality to the wall, with considerable thickening. Papillary carcinoma is a less common variant. It may be localized or diffusely involve the entire mucosa. The papillary fronds are prone to necrosis and hemorrhage. Obstructive symptoms and development of hydrops are encountered in tumors in the neck. Tumors arising in the fundus usually remain asymptomatic. Gallstones are found in 80% to 90% of the cases.

Most gallbladder cancers are adenocarcinomas that are well differentiated and secrete variable amounts of mucin (Fig. 26-22). This is mainly sialomucin in character, in contrast to the sulfomucin type secreted by the normal or inflamed gallbladder. Adenocarcinomas may exhibit varying degrees of squamous metaplasia. In less differentiated tumors the glandular pattern may be par-

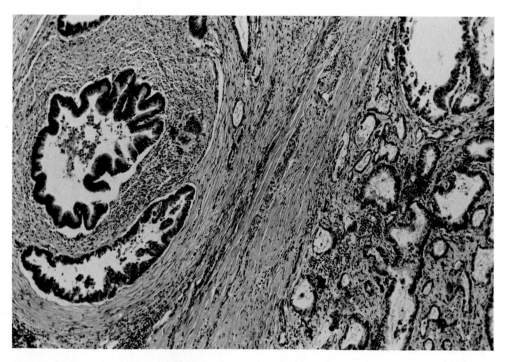

Fig. 26-22. Carcinoma of common bile duct in 83-year-old man. Neoplastic cuboid and columnar cells form acinar tubular structures or are mounted on delicate connective tissue stalks. Neoplastic cells are within sheath of nerve. There was complete obstruction of common bile duct but no involvement of regional lymph nodes and no distant metastasis. (Hematoxylin and eosin; 60×.)

tially or completely lost, and the tumor then grows in sheets (Fig. 26-23). Some cases represent poorly differentiated neuroendocrine carcinomas (Fig. 26-24). Carcinoid and composite tumors of the gallbladder have also been reported.[86,110,119] About half were metastatic at the time of diagnosis. Some of these malignant endocrine tumors produce "ectopic" hormones,[121] whereas others are detected because of the obstructive picture they produce.[101] Moreover, an endocrine component is not uncommonly present in the usual variety of gallbladder adenocarcinoma, with 7 of 42 (40%) and

surrounding metaplastic mucosa in 11 of 17 cases (64%).[79,80,95] Squamous cell carcinoma is rare (Fig. 26-24, C).

The precursor lesion of invasive gallbladder carcinoma has now been identified in a high-risk population for invasive carcinoma (Fig. 26-25).[82,89] It was concluded that a small number of hyperplasias of the gallbladder evolve toward atypical hyperplasia and that this in turn progresses to carcinoma in situ. The 10-year differences in the mean ages of patients with carcinoma in situ and those with invasive carcinoma gives additional

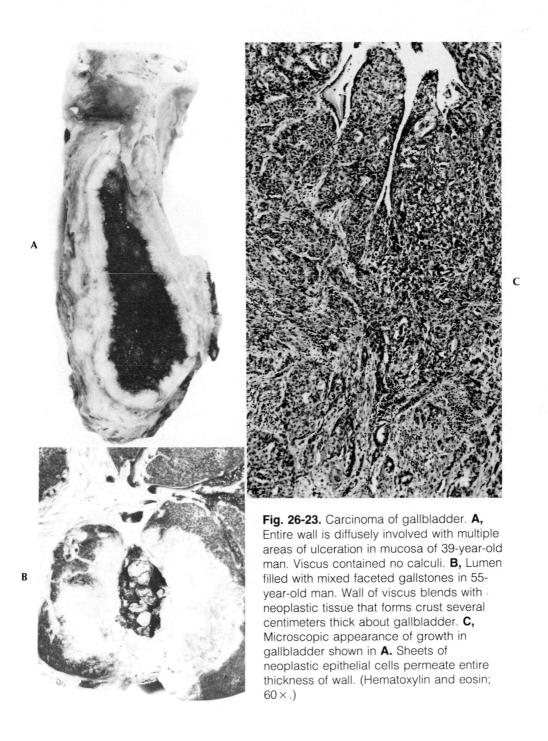

Fig. 26-23. Carcinoma of gallbladder. **A,** Entire wall is diffusely involved with multiple areas of ulceration in mucosa of 39-year-old man. Viscus contained no calculi. **B,** Lumen filled with mixed faceted gallstones in 55-year-old man. Wall of viscus blends with neoplastic tissue that forms crust several centimeters thick about gallbladder. **C,** Microscopic appearance of growth in gallbladder shown in **A.** Sheets of neoplastic epithelial cells permeate entire thickness of wall. (Hematoxylin and eosin; 60×.)

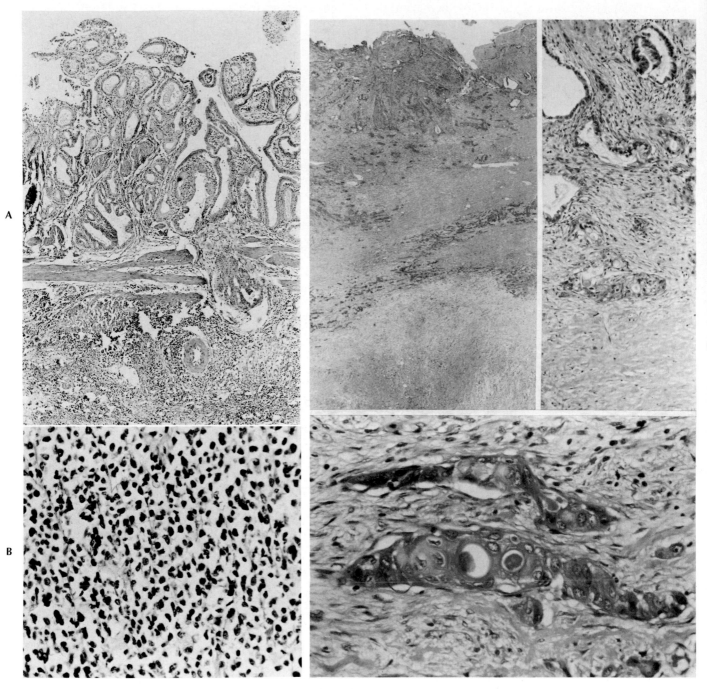

Fig. 26-24. A, Photomicrograph of gallbladder from a 76-year-old man who presented with jaundice, epigastric pain, abdominal distension, and diarrhea. A small-cell undifferentiated carcinoma infiltrating the mucosa and submucosa of the gallbladder was seen. **B,** The nesting pattern of tumor growth is suggestive of a neuroendocrine carcinoma. Tumor cells are positive for neuron-specific enolase and negative for leukocyte common antigen. The patient died of widespread metastatic disease 1 month after the cholecystectomy. **C,** White woman, 69 years of age, with "routine" cholecystectomy. At laparotomy there was gross transmural involvement of the gallbladder wall by tumor. Microscopically this was an ulcerating, moderately differentiated focally keratinizing squamous cell carcinoma. The patient died 3 months after surgery. (**A** and **C,** Hematoxylin and eosin; **A,** 60×; **B,** 400×; **C,** 30×, 280×, 490×; courtesy Dr. Timothy McDonnell, Washington University, St. Louis, Mo.)

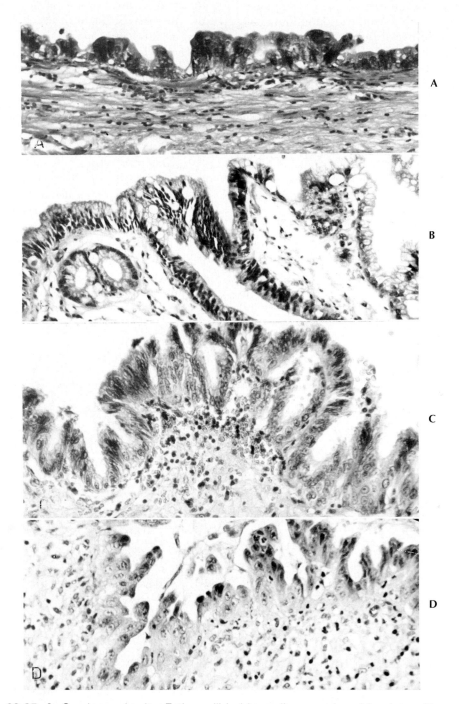

Fig. 26-25. A, Carcinoma in situ. Entire gallbladder wall was replaced by dense fibrous connective tissue, with no penetration of wall by cytologically malignant epithelium visible only on mucosal surface. Patient was free of disease at 4 years, one of the few survivors. **B,** Atypical hyperplasia indicated by variable enlargement of nuclei and crowding as seen especially in center of field. On right side is more normal epithelium for contrast. **C** and **D,** Similar microscopic changes in gallbladder mucosa at some distance from invasive adenocarcinomas. (Hematoxylin and eosin; 350×; courtesy Dr. William Black, University of New Mexico, Albuquerque; **C,** WU 81-10009; **D,** WU 81-10010.)

support to the idea of progression of a precursor lesion. Moreover, 18 cases of in situ carcinoma of the gallbladder are reported, with only microinvasion in four.[78]

Carcinomas of the proximal bile ducts are often extremely well differentiated and sclerotic, including the area of the porta hepatis (Fig. 26-21). The morphologic distinction between benign and malignant sclerosing processes in the area of the hepatic-duct junction can be difficult. Severe cytologic atypia and neural invasion are the two most important histologic criteria for malignancy in the interpretation of frozen sections from this area, including the upper third of the extrahepatic biliary tree.[114]

Nevin and associates[111] classified gallbladder carcinoma on the basis of staging and histologic grading and found a good correlation with survival. Patients with stage I (carcinoma in situ and intramucosal lesions) and stage II (invasion of submucosa) were generally cured by cholecystectomy alone. Local recurrence has, however, been reported. In stages III (involvement of all three layers) and IV (involvement of all three layers and

the cystic lymph node) the survival was 50%, whereas the stage V (involvement of the liver and other organs) the prognosis is hopeless. Well-differentiated papillary tumors also have a more favorable prognosis.

The biologic behavior of gallbladder carcinomas has been extensively studied by Fahim and co-workers.[98] The most common spread was shown to be lymphatic, vascular, neural, intraperitoneal, and intraductal, in decreasing order. Lymphatic drainage from the gallbladder is to lymph nodes along the cystic and common bile ducts and then via the pancreaticoduodenal nodes to the para-aortic chain. Venous drainage goes to the quadrate lobe of the liver. Vascular metastases to the liver are therefore localized near the gallbladder and are not in the whole liver as they are in other gastrointestinal carcinomas. Peritoneal seeding is rarely found.

Based on the knowledge that failure of treatment for gallbladder carcinoma results from local recurrence and not distant metastasis, radical cholecystectomy has been recommended as the treatment of choice.[112] More extensive resections have not yielded improvement in

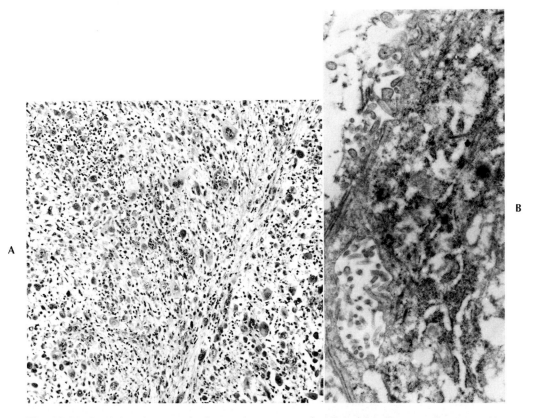

Fig. 26-26. A, Light micrograph of pseudosarcoma of gallbladder. Tumor cells grow without apparent cohesion, and multinucleated pleomorphic giant cells are numerous. **B,** By electron microscopy, however, intracellular lumens were present in tumor cells. Material was rescued from paraffin blocks. (**A,** Hematoxylin and eosin; 150×; WU 81-7976; **B,** uranyl acetate and lead citrate; 35,500×.)

prognosis. Since a substantial number of carcinomas are known to be incidental, especially in women over 70 years of age who have lithiasis, and since these cases are known to have a more favorable prognosis,[87] all gallbladders in these cases should be carefully examined at the time of operation. Frozen section examination elucidates the nature of suspicious lesions. Radiotherapy has recently been used in addition to surgery, with better results in bile duct carcinoma than in gallbladder carcinoma.[120]

Since depth of tumor invasion is the determining factor in survival, efforts should be directed toward early detection in populations at risk. Cytologic examination of specimens obtained at ERCP may prove to be one such method in the future. A cell line from a human gallbladder carcinoma has now been established and characterized. In vitro approaches may prove useful in learning more about the biologic behavior of the tumor, with possible therapeutic implications.[106]

In the patient population in which gallbladder malignancy usually occurs, totally anaplastic carcinomas are rare and include giant cell and spindle cell variants, which simulate sarcomas.[81,82] By electron microscopy,

one patient with pleomorphic spindle cell tumor of the gallbladder showed intracytoplasmic lumens with well-formed microvilli[83] (Fig. 26-26). Pure sarcomas have been reported in the literature, without ultrastructual proof of their nonepithelial derivation.[115,126] Many probably also represent carcinomas with a pseudosarcomatous pattern.

Embryonal rhabdomyosarcoma of the biliary tract is rare[93] but is the most common malignancy of extrahepatic ducts and gallbladder in children.[118] There is a slight female preponderance, and the mean age at diagnosis is between 3 and 4 years. Fever, malaise, and obstructive jaundice are the major symptoms. There is considerable dilatation of the common duct. Grossly the tumor is polypoid, and multiple mucoid glistening masses are attached to the mucosa. It has a deceptively benign soft polypoid appearance. Microscopically, loose myxoid tissue contains spindle-shaped tumor cells that are condensed beneath an intact ductal epithelium (Fig. 26-27). Some of these cases, when no ultrastructural studies are done, may well represent pleomorphic carcinomas as well (see preceding discussion). The prognosis is dismal because of local failure to control the disease.

Primary malignant melanomas have been documented,[12,41] but metastatic melanomas are more common.[108] Metastatic involvement of the gallbladder in melanoma is rare but constitutes the most common metastatic lesion involving this organ.

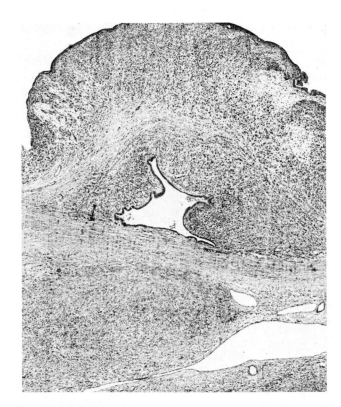

Fig. 26-27. Embryonal rhabdomyosarcoma of extrahepatic duct in child. There is condensation of spindle-shaped tumor cells under intact glandular and surface epithelium. (Hematoxylin and eosin; 33×; WU 81-10002; courtesy Dr. K.G. Ishak, Department of Hepatic Pathology, Armed Forces Institute of Pathology, Washington, D.C.)

REFERENCES
Normal morphology and brief overview of function

1. Albores-Saavedra, J., and Henson, D.E.: Tumors of the gallbladder and extrahepatic bile ducts. In AFIP: Atlas of tumor pathology, ed. 2, Washington, D.C., 1986, Armed Forces Institute of Pathology.
2. Carey, M.C., and Mazer, N.A.: Biliary lipid secretion in health and in cholesterol gallstone disease, Hepatology **4:**315, 1984.
3. Osler, W.: The evolution of modern medicine, New Haven, Conn., 1921, Yale University Press.
4. Ryan, J., and Cohen, S.: Effect of vasoactive intestinal peptide on basal and cholecystokinin-induced gallbladder pressure, Gastroenterology **73:**870, 1977.
5. Sundler, F., Alumets, J., Hakanson, R., Ingemansson, J., Fahrenkrug, J., Schaffalitzky de Muckadell, O.: VIP innervation of the gallbladder, Gastroenterology **72:**1375, 1977.
6. Toouli, J., Bushell, M., Stevenson, G., Dent, J., Wicherley, A., Iannos, J.: Gallbladder emptying in men related to fasting duodenal migrating motor contracting, Aust. NZ J. Surg. **56:**147, 1986.

Abnormalities believed to be congenital or developmental

7. Busuttil, A.: Ectopic adrenal within the gallbladder wall, J. Pathol. **113:**231, 1974.
8. Christensen, A.H., and Ishak, K.G.: Benign tumors and pseudotumors of the gallbladder: report of 180 cases, Arch. Pathol. **90:**423, 1970.
9. Curtis, L.E., and Sheahan, D.G.: Heterotopic tissues in the gallbladder, Arch. Pathol. **88:**677, 1969.
10. Gerwig, W.H., Jr., Countryman, L.K., and Gómez, A.C.: Congenital absence of the gallbladder and cystic duct: report of six cases, Ann. Surg. **153:**113, 1961.

11. Laitio, M.: Morphology and histochemistry of non-tumorous gallbladder epithelium: a series of 103 cases, Pathol. Res. Pract. **167**:335, 1980.
12. Landing, B.H.: Considerations of the pathogenesis of neonatal hepatitis, biliary atresia and choledochal cyst—the concept of infantile obstructive cholangiopathy, Prog. Pediatr. Surg. **6**:113, 1974.
13. Thorsness, E.T.: An aberrant pancreatic nodule arising on the neck of a human gallbladder from multiple outgrowths of the mucosa, Anat. Rec. **77**:319, 1940.

Acquired disorders
Lithiasis
14. Braverman, D.Z., Johnson, M.L., and Kern, F., Jr.: Effects of pregnancy and contraceptive steroids on gallbladder function, N. Engl. J. Med. **302**:362, 1980.
15. Corornary Drug Project Research Group: Gallbladder disease is a side effect of drugs influencing lipid metabolism. N. Engl. J. Med. **296**:1185, 1977.
16. Friedman, G.D., Kannel, W.B., and Dawber, T.R.: The epidemiology of gallbladder diseases: observations in the Framingham Study, J. Chron. Dis. **19**:273, 1966.
17. Glenn, F.: Retained calculi within the biliary ductal system, Ann. Surg. **179**:528, 1974.
18. Godfrey, P.J., Bates, T., Harrison, M., King, M.B., and Padley, N.R.: Gallstones and mortality: a study of all gallstone-related deaths in a single health district, Gut **25**:1029, 1984.
19. LaMorte, W.W., Schoetz, D.J., Jr., Birkett, D.H., and Williams, L.F., Jr.: The role of the gallbladder in the pathogenesis of cholesterol gallstones, Gastroenterology **77**:580, 1979.
20. Lee, S.P., Carey, M.C., and LaMont, J.T.: Aspirin prevention of cholesterol gallstone formation in prairie dogs, Science **211**:1429, 1981.
21. Lund, J.: Surgical indication in cholelithiasis: prophylactic cholecystectomy elucidated on the basis of long-term follow up on 526 nonoperated cases, Ann. Surg. **151**:153, 1960.
22. Marks, J.W., Conley, D.R., Capretta, T.L., Bonorris, G.G., Chung, A., Coyne, M.J., and Schoenfield, L.J.: Gallstone prevalence and biliary lipid composition in inflammatory bowel disease, J. Dig. Dis. **22**:1097, 1977.
23. Messing, B., Bories, C., Kunstlinger, F., and Bernier, J.-J.: Does total parenteral nutrition induce gallbladder sludge formation and lithiasis? Gastroenterology **84**:1012, 1983.
24. Morris, D.L., Buechley, R.W., Key, C.R., and Morgan, M.V.: Gallbladder disease and gallbladder cancer among American Indians in tricultural New Mexico, Cancer **42**:2472, 1978.
25. Perpetuo, M.D.C.M.O., Valdivieso, M., Heilbrun, L.K., Nelson, R.S., Connor, T., and Bodey, G.P.: Natural history study of gallbladder cancer: a review of 36 years experience at M.D. Anderson Hospital and Tumor Institute, Cancer **42**:330, 1978.
26. Pokorny, W.J., Saleem, M., O'Gorman, R.B., McGill, C.W., and Harberg, F.J.: Cholelithiasis and cholecystitis in childhood, Am. J. Surg. **148**:742, 1984.
27. Sackmann, M., Delius, M., Sauerbruch, T., Holl, J., Weber, W., Ippisch, E., Hagelauer, U., Wess, O., Hepp, W., Brendel, W., and Paumgartner, G.: Shock-wave lithotripsy of gallbladder stones: the first 175 patients, N. Engl. J. Med. **318**:393, 1988.
28. Scragg, R.K.R., Calvert, G.D., and Oliver, J.R.: Plasma lipids and insulin in gall stone disease: a case-control study, Br. J. Med. **289**:521, 1984.
29. Shrand, H., and Ackroyd, F.W.: Gallstones in children: case report, diagnostic clues and recent views on gallstone formation, Clin. Pediatr. **12**:191, 1973.
30. Simeone, J.F., and Ferrucci, J.T., Jr.: New trends in gallbladder imaging, JAMA **246**:380, 1981.
31. Singletary, B.K., Van Thiel, D.H., and Eagon, P.K.: Estrogen and progesterone receptors in human gallbladder, Hepatology **6**:574, 1986.
32. Smith, B.F., and Small, D.M.: The sequence of events in gallstone formation, Lab. Invest. **56**:125, 1987.
33. Wenckert, A., and Robertson, B.: The natural course of gallstone disease: eleven-year review of 781 nonoperated cases, Gastroenterology **50**:376, 1966.

34. Wilson, I.D., Delaney, J.P., Duane, W.C., Pries, J.M., Silvis, S.E., and Vennes, J.A.: Choledocholithiasis, Gastroenterology **75**:120, 1978.

Inflammation—acute
35. Barton, L.L., Escobedo, M.B., Keating, J.P., and Ternberg, J.L.: Leptospirosis with acalculous cholecystitis, Am. J. Dis. Child. **126**:350, 1973.
36. Bohrod, M.G., and Bodon, G.R.: Isolated polyarteritis nodosa of the gallbladder, Am. Surg. **36**:681, 1970.
37. Campbell, C.W., and Eckman, M.R.: Acute acalculous cholecystitis caused by *Salmonella indiana*, JAMA **233**:815, 1975.
38. Dillard, B.M., and Black, W.C.: Polyarteritis nodosa of the gallbladder and bile ducts, Am. Surg. **36**:423, 1970.
39. Flancbaum, L., Majerus, T.C., and Cox, E.F.: Acute post-traumatic acalculous cholecystitis, Am. J. Surg. **150**:252, 1985.
40. Ishak, K.G., and Rogers, W.A.: Cryptogenic acute cholangitis—association with toxic shock syndrome, Am. J. Clin. Pathol. **76**:619, 1981.
41. Kahn, D.G., Garfinkle, J.M., Klonoff, D.C., Pembrook, L.J., and Morrow, D.J.: Cryptosporidial and cytomegaloviral hepatitis and cholecystitis, Arch. Pathol. Lab. Med. **111**:879, 1987.
42. Kavin, H., Jonas, R.B., Chowdhury, L., and Kabins, S.: Acalculous cholecystitis and cytomegalovirus infection in the acquired immunodeficiency syndrome, Ann. Intern. Med. **104**:53, 1986.
43. LiVolsi, V.A., Perzin, K.H., and Porter, M.: Polyarteritis nodosa of the gallbladder, presenting as acute cholecystitis, Gastroenterology **65**:115, 1973.
44. McClure, J., Banerjee, S.S., and Schofield, P.S.: Crohn's disease of the gallbladder, J. Clin. Pathol. **37**:516, 1984.
45. Pitlik, S.D., Fainstein, V., Garza, D., Guarda, L., Bolívar, R., Rios, A., Hopfer, R.L., and Mansell, P.A.: Human cryptosporidiosis: spectrum of disease, Arch. Intern Med. **143**:2269, 1983.
46. Porter, J.B., Jick, H., and Dinan, B.J.: Acute cholecystitis and thiazides, N. Engl. J. Med. **304**:954, 1981.
47. Viteri, A.L., and Grune, J.F.: Bile duct abnormalities in the acquired immune deficiency syndrome, Gastroenterology **92**:2014, 1987.
48. Walker, D.H., Leseshe, H.R., Varma, V.A., and Thacker, W.C.: Rocky Mountain spotted fever mimicking acute cholecystitis, Arch. Intern. Med. **145**:2194, 1985.

Inflammation—chronic
49. Albores-Saavedra, J., personal communication, Miami, Fla., 1988.
50. Amazon, K., and Rywlin, A.M.: Ceroid granulomas of the gallbladder, Am. J. Clin. Pathol. **73**:123, 1980.
51. Chapman, R.W.G., Marborgh, B.A., Rhodes, J.M., Summerfield, J.A., Dick, R., Scheur, P.J., and Sherlock, S.: Primary sclerosing cholangitis: a review of its clinical features, cholangiography, and hepatic histology, Gut **21**:870, 1980.
52. Downey, R.S., Sicard, G.A., Lee, J.T., De Schryver-Kecskeméti, K., and Anderson, C.B.: Benign extrinsic compression of the common bile duct, Surgery **100**:113, 1986.
53. El-Shabrawi, M., Wilkinson, M.L., Portmann, B., Mieli-Vergani, G., Chong, S.K.F., Williams, R., and Mowat, A.P.: Primary sclerosing cholangitis in childhood, Gastroenterology **92**:1226, 1987.
54. Estrada, R.L., Brown, N.M., and James, C.E.: Chronic follicular cholecystitis: radiological, pathological and surgical aspects, Br. J. Surg. **48**:205, 1958.
55. Fee, H.J., Gewirtz, H., Schiller, J., and Longmire, W.D., Jr.: Sclerosing cholangitis and primary biliary cirrhosis—a disease spectrum? Ann. Surg. **186**:589, 1977.
56. Halpert, B.: Morphologic studies on the gallbladder. II. The "true Luschka ducts" and "Rokitansky-Aschoff sinuses" of human gallbladder, Bull. Johns Hopkins Hosp. **41**:77, 1927.
57. Kelley, C.J., Blumgart, L.H., and Benjamin, I.S.: Benign bile duct stricture following cholecystectomy, Br. J. Surg. **71**:836, 1984.

58. Kemeny, M.M., Battifora, H., Blayney, D.W., Cecchi, G., Goldberg, D.A., Leong, L.A., Margolin, K.A., and Terz, J.J.: Sclerosing cholangitis after continuous hepatic artery infusion of FUDR, Ann. Surg. **202:**176, 1985.

59. Laughlin, E.H.: Common duct stricture associated with hepatic artery infusion of FUDR, J. Surg. Oncol. **31:**56, 1986.

60. Naveh, Y., Mendelsohn, H., Spira, G., Auslaender, L., Mandel, H., and Berant, M.: Primary sclerosing cholangitis associated with immunodeficiency, Am. J. Dis. Child. **137:**114, 1983.

60a. Ranchod, M., and Kahn, L.B.: Malacoplakia of the gastrointestinal tract, Arch. Pathol. **94:**90, 1972.

61. Renner, I.G., Ponto, G.C., Savage, W.T., III, and Boswell, W.D.: Idiopathic retroperitoneal fibrosis producing common bile duct and pancreatic duct obstruction, Gastroenterology **79:**348, 1980.

62. Thorpe, M.E.C., Scheuer, E.P.J., and Sherlock, S.: Primary sclerosing cholangitis, the biliary tree, and ulcerative colitis, Gut **8:**435, 1967.

Miscellaneous noninflammatory conditions

63. Chamberlain, J.W., and Flight, D.W.: Acute hydrops of the gallbladder in childhood, Surgery **68:**899, 1970.

64. Prévot, J., and Babut, J.M.: Spontaneous perforations of the biliary tract in infancy, Prog. Pediatr. Surg. **1:**187, 1970.

Tumors
Benign neoplasms and pseudotumors

65. Beilby, J.O.: Diverticulosis of the gall bladder: the fundal adenoma, Br. J. Exp. Pathol. **48:**455, 1967.

66. Bombi, J.A., Rives, A., Astudillo, E., Pera, C., and Cardesa, A.: Polyposis coli associated with adenocarcinoma of the gallbladder: report of a case, Cancer **53:**2561, 1984.

67. Carney, J.A., Go, V.L., Sizemore, G.W., and Hayls, N.B.: Alimentary-tract ganglioneuromatosis: a major component of the syndrome of multiple endocrine neoplasia, type 2b, N. Engl. J. Med. **295:**1287, 1976.

68. Houdart, R., Palau, R., and Lavergne, A.: Should gallbladder polyps be removed? Does the adenoma-adenocarcinoma sequence exist? Gastroenterol. Clin. Biol. **10:**185, 1986.

69. Ishak, K.G., Willis, G.W., Cummins, S.D., and Bullock, A.A.: Biliary cystadenoma and cystadenocarcinoma: report of 14 cases and review of the literature, Cancer **38:**322, 1977.

70. Jones, M.B., Voet, R., Pagani, J., Lotysch, M., O'Connell, T., and Koretz, R.L.: Multifocal eosinophilic granuloma involving the common bile duct: histologic and cholangiographic findings, Gastroenterology **80:**384, 1981.

71. Majeski, J.A.: Polyps of the gallbladder, J. Surg. Oncol. **32:**16, 1986.

72. Miller, T.A., Weber, T.R., and Appelman, H.D.: Paraganglioma of the gallbladder, Arch. Surg. **105:**637, 1972.

73. Niv, Y., Kasakov, K., and Shcolnik B.: Fragile papilloma of the gallbladder, Gastroenterology **91:**999, 1986.

74. Waddell, W.R., Bradshaw, R.A., Goldstein, M.N., and Kirsch, W.M.: Production of human nerve-growth factor in a patient with a liposarcoma, Lancet **1:**1365, 1972.

75. Walsh, N., Qizilbash, A., Banerjee, R., and Waugh, G.A.: Biliary neoplasia in Gardner's syndrome, Arch. Pathol. Lab. Med. **111:**76, 1987.

76. Williams, I., Slavin, G., Cox, A., Simpson, P., and deLacey, G.: Diverticular disease (adenomyomatosis) of the gallbladder: a radiological-pathological survey, Br. J. Radiol. **59:**29, 1986.

77. Zvargulis, J.E., Keating, J.P., Askin, F.B., and Ternberg, J.L.: Granular cell myoblastoma: a cause of biliary obstruction, Am. J. Dis. Child. **132:**68, 1978.

Malignant tumors

78. Albores-Saavedra, J., Angeles-Angeles, A., Manrique, J.D., and Henson, D.E.: Carcinoma in situ of gallbladder, Am. J. Surg. Pathol. **8:**323, 1984.

79. Albores-Saavedra, J., and Henson, D.E.: Tumors of the gallbladder and extrahepatic bile ducts. In AFIP: Atlas of tumor pathology, ed. 2, Washington, D.C., 1986, Armed Forces Institute of Pathology.

80. Albores-Saavedra, J., Nadji, M., Henson, D.E., and Angeles-Angeles, A.: Entero-endocrine cell differentiation in carcinomas of the gallbladder and mucinous cystadenocarcinomas of the pancreas, Pathol. Res. Pract. **183:**169, 1988.

81. Albores-Saavedra, J., Cruz-Ortiz, H., Alcántara-Vázquez, A., and Henson, D.E.: Unusual types of gallbladder carcinoma: a report of 16 cases, Arch. Pathol. Lab. Med. **105:**287, 1981.

82. Albores-Saavedra, J., Alcántara-Vázquez, A., Cruz-Ortiz, H., Herrara-Goepfert, R.: The precursor lesions of invasive gallbladder carcinoma: hyperplasia, atypical hyperplasia and carcinoma in situ, Cancer **45:**919, 1980.

83. Alpers, C.E., and Smuckler, E.A.: Pleomorphic carcinoma of the gallbladder: case report and ultrastructural study, Ultrastruct. Pathol. **6:**29, 1984.

84. Appelman, H.D., and Coopersmith, N.: Pleomorphic spindle-cell carcinoma of the gallbladder, Cancer **23:**535, 1969.

85. Arminski, T.C.: Primary carcinoma of the gallbladder: a collective review with the addition of twenty-five cases from the Grace Hospital, Detroit, Michigan, Cancer **2:**379, 1949.

86. Bergdahl, L.: Carcinoid tumours of the biliary tract, Aust. NZ J. Surg. **46:**136, 1976.

87. Bergdahl, L.: Gallbladder carcinoma first diagnosed at microscopic examination of gallbladders removed for presumed benign disease, Ann. Surg. **191:**19, 1980.

88. Bismuth, H., and Malt, R.A.: Current concepts in cancer: carcinoma of the biliary tract, N. Engl. J. Med. **301:**704, 1979.

89. Black, W.C.: The morphogenesis of gallbladder carcinoma, Prog. Surg. Pathol. **2:**207, 1981.

90. Black, W.C., Key, C.R., Carmany, T.B., and Herman, D.: Carcinoma of the gallbladder in a population of southwestern American Indians, Cancer **39:**1267, 1977.

91. Case 29-1987: Case records of the Massachusetts General Hospital, N. Engl. J. Med. **317:**153, 1987.

92. Converse, C.F., Reagan, J.W., and DeCosse, J.J.: Ulcerative colitis and carcinoma of the bile ducts, Am. J. Surg. **121:**39, 1971.

93. Davis, G.L., Kissane, J.M., and Ishak, K.G.: Embryonal rhabdomyosarcoma (sarcoma botryoides) of the biliary tree: report of five cases and review of the literature, Cancer **24:**333, 1969.

94. Dayton, M.T., Longmire, W.P., Jr., and Tompkins, R.K.: Caroli's disease: a premalignant condition? Am. J. Surg. **145:**41, 1983.

95. De Schryver-Kecskeméti, K.: Neuroendocrine cells of the digestive tract. In Mendelsohn, G., editor: Diagnosis and pathology of endocrine diseases, Philadelphia, 1988, J.B. Lippincott Co.

96. Devor, E.J., and Buechley, R.W.: Gallbladder cancer in Hispanic New Mexicans. I. General population, 1957-1977, Cancer **45:**1705, 1980.

97. Diehl, A.K., and Beral, V.: Cholecystectomy and changing mortality from gallbladder cancer, Lancet **2:**187, 1981.

98. Fahim, R.B., McDonald, J.R., Richards, J.C., and Ferris, D.O.: Carcinoma of the gallbladder: a study of its modes of spread, Ann. Surg. **156:**114, 1962.

99. Hill, G.L., Mair, W.S.J., and Goligher, J.C.: Gallstones after ileostomy and ileal resection, Gut **16:**932, 1975.

100. Joffe, N., and Antonioli, D.A.: Primary carcinoma of the gallbladder associated with chronic inflammatory bowel disease, Clin. Radiol. **32:**319, 1981.

101. Judge, D.M., Dickman, P.S., and Trapukdi, B.S.: Nonfunctioning argyrophilic tumor (APUDoma) of the hepatic duct: simplified methods of detecting biogenic amines arising in tissue, Am. J. Clin. Pathol. **66:**40, 1976.

102. Kagawa, Y., Kashihara, S., Kuramoto, S., and Maetani, S.: Carcinoma arising in a congenitally dilated biliary tract: report of a case and review of the literature, Gastroenterology **74:**1286, 1978.

103. Kimura, K., Ohto, M., Saisho, H., Unozawa, T., Tsuchiya, Y., Morita, M., Ebara, M., Matsutani, S., and Okuda, K.: Association of gallbladder carcinoma and anomalous pancreaticobiliary ductal union, Gastroenterology **89:**1258, 1985.

104. King, C.R., Kraus, M.H., Williams, L.T., Merlino, G.T., Pastan, I.H., and Aaronson, S.A.: Human tumor cell lines with

EGF receptor gene amplification in the absence of aberrant sized mRNAs, Nucleic Acids Res. **13:**8477, 1985.

105. Klatskin, G.: Adenocarcinoma of the hepatic duct at its bifurcation within the porta hepatis: an unusual tumor with distinctive clinical and pathological features, Am. J. Med. **38:**241, 1965.

106. Koyama, S., Yoshioka, T., Mizushima, A., Kawakita, I., Yamagata, S., Fukutomi, H., Sakita, T., Kondo, I., and Kikuchi, M.: Establishment of a cell line (G-415) from a human gallbladder carcinoma, Gan **71:**574, 1980.

107. Mancuso, T.F., and Brennan, M.J.: Epidemiological considerations of cancer of the gallbladder, bile ducts and salivary glands in the rubber industry, J. Occupational Med. **12:**333, 1970.

108. McFadden, P.M., Krementz, E.T., McKinnon, W.M., Pararo, L.L., and Ryan, R.F.: Metastatic melanoma of the gallbladder, Cancer **44:**1802, 1979.

109. Morowitz, D.A., Glagov, S., Dordal, E., and Kirsner, J.B.: Carcinoma of the biliary tract complicating chronic ulcerative colitis, Cancer **27:**356, 1971.

110. Muto, Y., Okamoto, K., and Uchimura, M.: Composite tumors (ordinary adenocarcinoma, typical carcinoid and goblet cell adenocarcinoid) of the gallbladder, Am. J. Gastroenterol. **79:**645, 1984.

111. Nevin, J.E., Moran, J.J., Kay, S., et al.: Carcinoma of the gallbladder: staging, treatment and prognosis, Cancer **37:**141, 1976.

112. Piehler, J.M., and Greichlow, R.W.: Primary carcinoma of the gallbladder, Surg. Gynecol. Obstet. **147:**929, 1978.

113. Polk, H.C.: Carcinoma of the calcified gallbladder, Gastroenterology **50:**582, 1966.

114. Qualman, S.J., Haupt, H.M., Baver, T.W., and Taxy, J.B.: Adenocarcinoma of the hepatic duct junction: a reappraisal of the histologic criteria of malignancy, Cancer **53:**1545, 1984.

115. Rose, A.G.: Primary sarcoma of the gallbladder: a case report, S. Afr. Med. J. **53:**909, 1978.

116. Roslyn, J.J., Kuchenbecker, S., Longmire, P., Jr., and Tompkins, R.K.: Floating tumor debris: a cause of intermittent biliary obstruction, Arch. Surg. **119:**1312, 1984.

117. Russell, P.W., and Brown, C.H.: Primary carcinoma of the gallbladder, Ann. Surg. **132:**121, 1950.

118. Ruymann, F.B., Raney, R.B., Jr., Crist, W.M., Lawrence, W., Jr., Lindberg, R.D., and Soule, E.M.: Rhabdomyosarcoma of the biliary tree in childhood: a report from the Intergroup Rhabdomyosarcoma Study, Cancer **56:**575, 1985.

119. Shiffman, M.A., and Juler, G.: Carcinoid of the biliary tract, Arch. Surg. **89:**113, 1964.

120. Smoron, G.L.: Radiation therapy of carcinoma of gallbladder and biliary tract, Cancer **40:**1422, 1977.

121. Spence, R.W., and Burns-Cox, C.J.: ACTH-secreting "apudoma" of gall-bladder, Gut **16:**473, 1975.

122. Stewart, H.L., Loeber, M.M., and Morgan, D.R.: Carcinoma of the extrahepatic bile ducts, Arch. Surg. **41:**662, 1940.

123. Thorbjarnarson, B., and Glenn, F.: Carcinoma of the gallbladder, Cancer **12:**1009, 1959.

124. Verbanck, J.J., Rutgeerts, L.J., Van Aelst, F.J., Tytgat, J.H., Decoster, J.M., Noyez, D.N., Theunynck, P.J., and Gebdes, K.J.: Primary malignant melanoma of the gallbladder metastatic to the common bile duct, Gastroenterology **91:**214, 1986.

125. Yamauchi, S., Koga, A., Matsumoto, S., Tanaka, M., and Nakayama, F.: Anomalous junction of pancreaticobiliary duct without congenital choledochal cyst: a possible risk factor for gallbladder cancer, Am. J. Gastroenterol. **82:**20, 1987.

126. Yasuma, T., and Yanaka, M.: Primary sarcoma of the gallbladder: report of three cases, Acta Pathol. Jpn. **21:**285, 1971.

27 Pancreas and Diabetes Mellitus

JOHN M. KISSANE
PAUL E. LACY

NORMAL FORM AND DEVELOPMENT

The human pancreas is an elongated gland that extends from the concavity of the duodenal loop obliquely cephalad and to the left in the retroperitoneal space at the level of the junction between the first and second lumbar vertebrae, toward the hilum of the spleen. The adult gland is 12 to 15 cm long and weighs 60 to 100 g. The pancreas is subdivided into three topographic parts: (1) the head, dorsoventrally flattened, lying in the concavity of the duodenum with the uncinate (hooklike) process projecting ventramedially from the head of the pancreas to encompass the superior mesenteric artery and vein; (2) the body, the main portion of the gland; and (3) the thin, tapered tail extending toward the hilum of the spleen.

The pancreas is subdivided into rhomboid lobules by delicate connective tissue septa in which are found blood and lymphatic vessels, nerves, and ducts. The acini within the lobules are formed by pyramid-shaped acinar cells that contain numerous zymogen granules at their apices. Enzymes such as chymotrypsin, carboxypeptidase, and elastase have been demonstrated within individual zymogen granules by the fluorescent antibody technique. The basal portions of the acinar cells are basophilic and free of zymogen granules. Acini are intimately related to minute centroacinar ducts into which secretion products are discharged. Centroacinar ducts converge to form lobular ducts, which enter the major named pancreatic ducts. Islets possess no ductal system but release their secretory products—insulin, glucagon, gastrin, and perhaps others—directly into the circulation.

Ultrastructurally, zymogen granules appear as dense spherical structures encased within smooth membranous sacs. The basal portions of acinar cells are filled with a lamellar type of ergastoplasm with numerous ribonucleoprotein granules attached to the membranes. The ergastoplasm is responsible for the basophilic reaction of these cells. Electron microscopic and biochemical studies indicate that the zymogen granules are formed within the ergastoplasmic sacs, are subsequently transmitted to the Golgi zone where they apparently undergo further maturation, and finally move to the apical portion of the cell. After stimulation the zymogen granules with their encompassing sacs move to the apical surface of the cell; the membranous sacs fuse with the plasma membrane and rupture, and the zymogen granules are liberated into the lumans of the acini. The acinar and ductal cells are firmly attached by distinct desmosomes that prevent the enzymes within the zymogen granules from passing into the interstitial tissue.[5] The precise intracellular metabolic changes that initiate the migration and liberation of the zymogen granules are unknown.

Development. Among the several segmental diverticula of the foregut that appear in 3 to 4 mm embryos, two persist and give rise to the definitive pancreas. The larger dorsal pancreatic diverticulum arises from the foregut just cephalad to the hepatic diverticulum and elongates to the left in the retroperitoneal space. The smaller ventral pancreatic diverticulum arises in the angle between the hepatic diverticulum and foregut and, after more rapid growth of the hepatic diverticulum, comes to arise from that structure. Differential growth rotates the developing duodenum to the right and shifts the ventral pancreatic anlage into the dorsal mesentery, where it fuses with the dorsal anlage and contributes the uncinate process and most of the head to the definitive organ.[1]

Each pancreatic anlage possesses an axial duct. The distal end of the duct of the ventral pancreas ordinarily anastomoses with the duct of the dorsal pancreas and, as the duct of Wirsung, provides the major drainage for pancreatic secretions into the duodenum at the major duodenal papilla (of Vater). Distal to the point of anastomosis with the duct of Wirsung, the duct of the dorsal pancreas persists in about half of all individuals and, as the duct of Santorini, enters the duodenum at the minor duodenal papilla cephalad to the major papilla. In about 10% of individuals the duct of the ventral pancreas regresses, and the duct of Santorini provides the entire drainage into the duodenum.[2] These relationships are important in the pathogenesis of acute pancreatitis (see p. 1351).

Pancreatic acini appear initially as buds from the ducts and subsequently differentiate into acinar cells containing zymogen granules. Lumens of the acini retain communication with the centroacinar ducts that converge and form a passageway from exocrine secretions of the pancreas into the duodenum.[4] The islets of Langerhans also develop from the outer surfaces of the ultimate radicles of the pancreatic ducts. Solid masses of islet cells detach from the ducts and are vascularized by capillary sprouts. The first islets to be formed, primary islets, contain specific granules of beta cells as well as of delta cells. Insulin and several pancreatic enzymes have been identified very early in the primordial pancreas of rat embryos.[3] During the last 6 months of embryonic development, the primary islets undergo degeneration and a second generation of islet tissue originates from the ductal cells. Both primary and secondary islets arise from ductal tissue, not from acinar cells.[5]

ABNORMALITIES OF FORM AND DEVELOPMENT
Anular pancreas

Anular pancreas results from failure of rotation of the ventral pancreas. When the ventral pancreas fuses with the dorsal, it forms a ring of pancreatic tissue that envelops the second portion of the duodenum. Usually the encirclement is complete, but occasionally a gap may be found anteriorly. In children an anular pancreas may be associated with atresia or stenosis of the duodenum that results in intestinal obstruction.[7] In adults an anular pancreas usually produces no symptoms, though in some instances duodenal obstruction, peptic ulceration, and pancreatitis may be present. The relationship of anular pancreas to these symptoms is not clearly understood.

Ectopic pancreas

Pancreatic tissue may be found in the gastrointestinal tract in loci other than its normal anatomic area. The most common locations of ectopic pancreas are the duodenum, stomach, jejunum, and Meckel's diverticulum. Usually, nodules of ectopic pancreatic tissue are small, less than 1 cm in diameter, and located in the submucosa as circumscribed, mobile masses of firm yellow-white lobular tissue superficially suggestive of a neoplasm. Microscopically the masses consist of normal-appearing pancreatic tissue, often including islets of Langerhans. Usually pancreatic heterotopias are asymptomatic. Rarely such masses may produce pyloric or duodenal obstruction, lead to an intussusception, ulcerate and bleed, or serve as the site for an ectopic islet cell neoplasm.

Cystic fibrosis

Cystic fibrosis is a hereditary disorder characterized by increased viscosity of mucous secretions, including those of the pancreas, intestinal glands, tracheal and bronchial glands, and mucous salivary glands, and by increased concentrations of electrolytes, especially sodium and chloride, in secretions of other glands, notably eccrine sweat glands and also parotid salivary glands. The disease is transmitted as a mendelian recessive trait with clinical consequences only in homozygotes. Other genetic mechanisms have been considered.[18]

The frequency of heterozygous carriers in most white populations must range between 2% and 5%. Factors that contribute to maintaining this very high gene frequency despite the virtually lethal aspect of the homozygous state may include an as yet uncharacterized reproductive advantage in heterozygotes. Cystic fibrosis has been referred to as the most common hereditary disease in white populations.[21] The disease is very rare in blacks and almost unknown in Orientals. It is responsible for approximately 5% of all deaths in infants and children who are born alive. Meticulous clinical management has conspicuously improved the prognosis of the disease so that approximately half of affected persons reach adulthood.

The nature of the basic biologic defect in cystic fibrosis is unknown.[19,22] The initially attractive hypothesis that the essential disorder consists in increased viscosity of mucous secretions gave rise to the early designation "mucoviscidosis"[26] but could not be supported when more widespread disturbances, including those of eccrine sweat glands and serous glands such as parotid salivary glands, were discovered. In fact, the disease may represent the final pathophysiologic expression of several different basic abnormalities.

The traditional discussion of the disease among disorders of the pancreas is misleading on at least two counts; first, many organs other than the pancreas are involved and, second, the major clinical manifestations and chief threats to life result from pulmonary, not pancreatic, involvement. Lines of investigation of the basic defect in cystic fibrosis are currently directed in five, not necessarily exclusive, directions.

Biochemical composition of mucous secretions. Although results are not unanimous, the consensus is that mucous secretions of many origins from patients with cystic fibrosis are higher in the ratio of fucose to sialic acid than secretions of normal individuals are.[25] The subject of glycoproteins in cystic fibrosis has been reviewed.[13]

Autonomic function. Many of the deviations from normal in the eccrine secretions of patients with cystic fibrosis resemble those that result from exhaustive parasympathetic stimulation of normal secretory mechanisms. Such nonsecretory autonomic mechanisms as the speed of pupillary mydriasis in the dark appear to be impaired in patients with cystic fibrosis.[41]

Electrolyte-concentrating mechanism. In the normal formation of sweat, a solution with composition essentially that of an ultrafiltrate of plasma accumulates in the coiled portions of eccrine sweat glands. Preferential absorption of sodium chloride in excess of water from the duct results in the excretion of the normally hypotonic sweat. Micropuncture studies[35] suggest that primary secretion in the coil is normal in those with cystic fibrosis and that defective absorption of solute from the duct results in hypertonicity of the sweat. A defect in chloride transport into and out of cells may be involved, not in the transport mechanism itself but in the gate that opens and closes the channel. Recently, diminished resorption of sodium and chloride has been demonstrated in rat parotid glands perfused with sweat from patients with cystic fibrosis.[35] Sweat from normal children had no effect on the absorptive mechanism.

Effect on ciliary motility. Asynchronous and uncoordinated ciliary motility has been observed in cultured explants of rat tracheal mucosa exposed to serum from patients with cystic fibrosis. The factor responsible for this disturbance in ciliary motility is heat labile and nondialyzable. Similar effects were produced by sera from some parents of patients with cystic fibrosis.[44]

Metachromasia in cultured fibroblasts. Studies have demonstrated that cultured fibroblasts from patients with cystic fibrosis elaborate metachromatic material either as discrete cytoplasmic granules or as diffuse cytoplasmic metachromasia. Cultured fibroblasts from parents and other relatives of patients showed the same type of metachromasia.[21]

Clinical features

Clinical features of cystic fibrosis are highly variable, even among affected siblings. From 10% to 15% of affected newborns have intestinal, usually distal ileal, obstruction by chalky masses of inspissated intestinal contents, meconium ileus. The frequency of associated ileal atresia supports an acquired mechanism for intestinal atresia. Intestinal perforation in utero with production of sterile meconium peritonitis may occur. Acute or episodic intestinal obstruction beyond infancy is increasingly reported as "meconium ileus equivalent."

Failure to gain weight despite adequate appetite, nonspecific feeding problems, steatorrhea, or other manifestations of intestinal malabsorption characterize one fourth to one third of all patients with cystic fibrosis. Rectal prolapse occurs in as many as one sixth of all patients. Heat prostration may be an early manifestation. In older children, ascites, bleeding from esophageal varices, or unexplained splenomegaly may be the first symptoms of cystic fibrosis.

Beyond infancy, respiratory complications are by far the most common manifestations of cystic fibrosis and constitute its chief threat to life. Recurrent bouts of pneumonia, bronchiolitis, or bronchitis are usual but not invariable manifestations of the disease. Signs and symptoms of chronic respiratory insufficiency or of right ventricular failure occasionally may precede any indication of infection of the lower respiratory tract. The finding of inflammatory nasal polyps in the upper respiratory tract of a prepubertal child compels consideration of the diagnosis of cystic fibrosis.

Pathologic changes

Most pathologic changes in fibrocystic disease are interpretable as resulting from obstruction by abnormally viscid mucus in a variety of viscera.

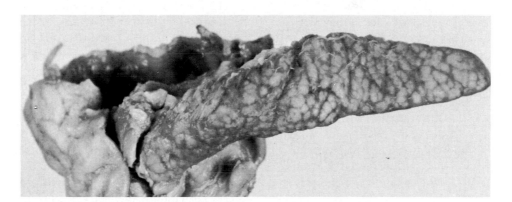

Fig. 27-1. Pancreas from child with cystic fibrosis showing accentuation of lobules but general preservation of size and contour of organ. (From Kissane, J.M., and Smith, M.G.: Pathology of infancy and childhood, ed. 2, St. Louis, 1975, The C.V. Mosby Co.)

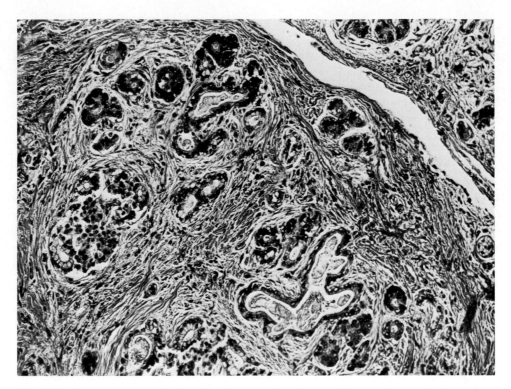

Fig. 27-2. Pancreas in cystic fibrosis showing dilated centrilobular ducts containing laminated concretions. Acini are almost totally replaced by fibrous tissue that still reflects lobular pattern of organ.

Pancreas. The pancreas is almost never normal in cystic fibrosis, though the degree of pancreatic involvement varies widely from case to case and correlates only crudely with age. Grossly, especially in infancy, the pancreas may appear deceptively normal (Fig. 27-1). Close examination even then, however, may disclose an almost too tidy demarcation of lobules and an increase in consistency. Later, pancreatic lobules come to assume an ovoid rather than a rhomboid or polyhedral contour and to bulge from the cut surface. Ultimately, the pancreas, still preserving relatively normal size and contour, represents gross fatty replacement of parenchyma. Fibrosis is rarely pronounced grossly, and macroscopic cysts are rarely discernible.

Microscopically, acinar atrophy and interlobular fibrosis are far out of proportion to the gross abnormality. Centroacinar ducts frequently contain laminated, eosinophilic concretions, and distal to these, acini are conspicuously atrophic, though stromal recapitulation of lobular architecture may be well preserved (Fig. 27-2). Islets persist until late in the evolution of the disease. Inflammation, fat necrosis, and pseudocyst formation are rarely prominent.

Intestine. In 12% to 15% of patients with cystic fibrosis, intestinal obstruction occurs in the newborn period. The obstructing lesion in meconium ileus is a plug of chalky, inspissated meconium in the distal ileum. Ileal atresia, volvulus, or perforation with the development of meconium peritonitis may occur secondarily, and total intestinal length usually is shortened. The occurrence of meconium ileus correlates more with dilation of intestinal glands by inspissated mucous secretions than with the extent of pancreatic lesions.

Attention has been called to the occurrence of peptic ulcers in patients with cystic fibrosis.[16] Above-normal frequency of peptic ulcer in parents of patients with cystic fibrosis has been claimed.

Respiratory tract. In a typical case the lungs show gross compensatory overexpansion anteriorly, alternating posteriorly with areas of atelectasis and overt consolidation. Bronchi are dilated and contain inspissated mucopurulent exudate. Dilated small bronchi containing similar material usually can be appreciated in the centers of consolidated pulmonary lobules. Microscopically the pulmonary lesion is a purulent bronchitis and bronchiolitis with resulting bronchiectasis and bronchiolectasis accompanied by a limited peribronchiolar pneumonia. Parenchymatous purulent necrosis with abscess formation is distinctly unusual (pp. 950 and 1348).

Larynx, trachea, and major bronchi show chronic inflammation, often with foci of squamous metaplasia. Submucous glands are distended with inspissated secretions. In the upper respiratory tract, inflammatory nasal polyps may be found.

Liver. The liver is usually of normal size. Significant fatty metamorphosis is not common. Focal stellate areas of portal fibrosis and ductular proliferation may be seen, occasionally sufficiently extensive to justify the designation *focal biliary cirrhosis.* The lesion may produce portal hypertension with its consequences—ascites, congestive splenomegaly, and gastroesophageal varices (see p. 1158 and also p. 788).

Sweat glands. In view of the constancy and diagnostic importance of hypersecretion of sodium and chloride in the sweat, microscopic alterations in sweat glands are disappointingly scanty. Munger and associates[36] described diminished vacuolation of mucoid cells.

Reproductive system. The frequent finding of azoospermia in postpubertal males with cystic fibrosis is attributable to discontinuity of the male sex ducts. Only 1% to 2% of postpubertal males with cystic fibrosis are fertile. There is no anatomic correlate for the high maternal mortality among pregnant women with cystic fibrosis.

Prenatal diagnosis. Prenatal diagnosis based upon diminished levels of certain microvillous enzymes in the amniotic fluid has an accuracy of about 95%.[37] Morphologic lesions have been described in aborted fetuses.[39]

PANCREATITIS

Inflammation of the pancreas constitutes a spectrum of disorders that ranges from acute hemorrhagic pancreatitis, a prostrating, catastrophic disease with a high mortality, to chronic relapsing pancreatitis, a disorder characterized by recurring episodes of upper abdominal pain and eventual pancreatic insufficiency. Elaborate clinical systems of classification reflect the tendency of the disorder to recur.

Acute hemorrhagic pancreatitis

Acute hemorrhagic pancreatitis is almost entirely a disease of adults between 40 and 70 years of age, slightly more common in women than in men. The onset is abrupt and calamitous, often occurring after a heavy meal or an alcoholic debauch. Severe epigastric pain, especially radiating to the back; nausea; vomiting; and shock are prominent clinical features. Peculiar ecchymotic mottling of the skin of the flanks, Grey-Turner spots, may be seen in severe cases. Early in the disease, pancreatic enzymes are liberated into the bloodstream, and increased levels of amylase and lipase in the serum are important in establishing the diagnosis. The mortality, even with vigorous supportive measures, is between 15% and 25%.

Pathologic changes

In the first few days the pancreas is swollen and edematous. After 1 or 2 days, friable foci of necrosis appear, followed by interstitial hemorrhage that varies

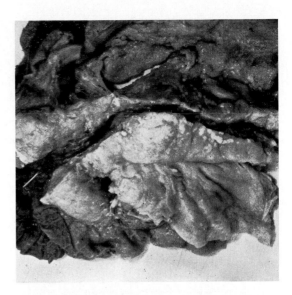

Fig. 27-3. Fat necrosis and acute pancreatitis. White opaque areas represent fat necrosis. Small white rod is in duct opening into duodenum.

from reddish reticulation between pancreatic lobules to obliteration of grossly recognizable pancreatic tissue in a massive retroperitoneal hematoma. Foci of fat necrosis in the peripancreatic tissue, mesentery, and omentum appear rapidly as small, ovoid, yellow-white nodules of pasty, gritty material (Fig. 27-3). The peritoneal cavity usually contains a moderate effusion of turbid rusty fluid with high amylase activity. Rarely, remote adipose tissues such as subcutaneous fat and fatty marrow may contain foci of necrosis attributable to lipolysis by enzymes borne in the plasma.

Very early in the disease the pancreas microscopically shows only interstitial edema. Later the pancreas contains patches of coagulative necrosis rimmed by infiltrates of polymorphonuclear leukocytes (Fig. 27-4). Still later, necrosis of arteries and arterioles is responsible for gross hemorrhages. Veins often are thrombosed. Eventually, as bacteria lodge in the necrotic pancreas, through either the ducts or the bloodstream, frank suppuration may occur.

A late complication of acute pancreatitis is the occasional development of a pseudocyst—an accumulation of enzyme-rich fluid, necrotic debris, and altered blood confined, not by an epithelial capsule, but by retroperitoneal connective tissue, adherent upper abdominal viscera, and the peritoneal components of the lesser omental sac. Pancreatic pseudocysts also may occur after blunt trauma to the abdomen.

Pathogenesis

The destructive changes that occur in the pancreas can be attributed to activation of proteolytic and lipo-

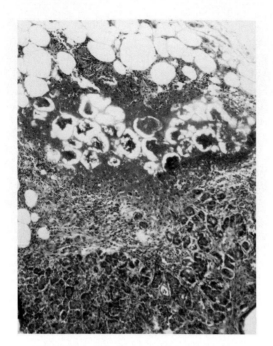

Fig. 27-4. Fat necrosis of pancreas.

lytic pancreatic enzymes and their liberation into the pancreatic interstitium. Normally the pancreas is protected from self-destruction by (1) synthesis and secretion of lytic enzymes as initially inactive proenzymes, which themselves require activation, often by trypsin; (2) elaborate compartmentalization of lytic systems within the cytoplasm of the acinar cell; and (3) the presence of trypsin inhibitors in acinar cells. Acinar cell injury by a variety of causes can disturb this relationship. When they gain access to the pancreatic interstitium,[58] active proteolytic enzymes such as trypsin and elastase produce necrosis of blood vessels, with resultant thrombosis and hemorrhage. Lipase liberated into the interstitial tissue causes necrosis of adipose tissue and the breakdown of triglycerides into fatty acids. Fatty acids combine with calcium in the interstitial tissue to form insoluble calcium soaps. This may produce a significant decrease in the level of serum calcium and lead to symptoms of hypocalcemia.

The pathogenesis of this sequence of events is not entirely clear. Experimentally, pancreatitis can be produced by injection of bile into the pancreatic duct at a pressure sufficient to rupture the ductal system. Opie's

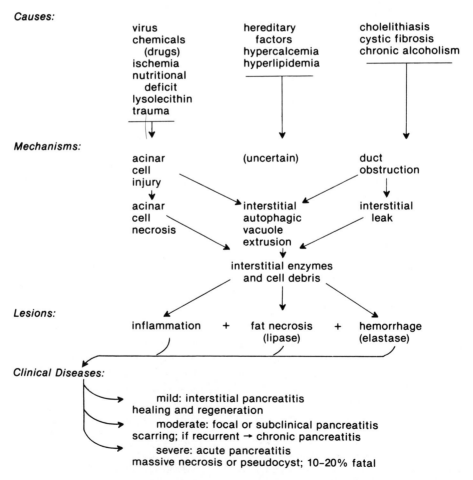

Fig. 27-5. Pathogenic mechanisms in pancreatitis. (From Longnecker, D.S.: Am. J. Pathol. **107**:103, 1982).

early report[60] of acute pancreatitis resulting from impaction of a gallstone in the ampulla of Vater directed perhaps undue attention toward the necessity for a "common channel" for biliary and pancreatic secretions to provide anatomically possible regurgitation of bile into the pancreatic duct. Detailed anatomic studies show that the configuration of the pancreatic ducts and common bile duct allows regurgitation of bile into the pancreatic duct in about 90% of specimens.[2]

Even in the presence of an anatomic common channel, measurements of pressures in the pancreatic duct and in the common bile duct indicate that the higher pressure in the pancreatic duct normally prevents the reflux of bile into the pancreatic duct. Increased intraductal pressure, whether from increased secretory pressure or as a result of duct obstruction, is, along with acinar cell injury, clearly a second general factor in the pathogenesis of pancreatitis.

The frequent association of chronic alcoholism indicates that alcohol may function not only by producing edema and partial obstruction of the sphincter of Oddi but also by stimulating pancreatic secretion. Pancreatic duct obstruction has been attributed to alcoholism.[64,65]

Ischemia has been implicated in the production of hemorrhagic pancreatitis, since it has been demonstrated experimentally that the pancreatic edema that occurs after ligation of the pancreatic duct in dogs can be transformed into acute hemorrhagic pancreatitis by the production of temporary ischemia in the pancreas. This factor alone is apparently not sufficient to produce the sequence of events, since vascular necroses in the pancreas in malignant hypertension are accompanied by only focal areas of necrosis, not a fulminating hemorrhagic pancreatitis.

Trauma also has been implicated as an etiologic factor. Acute pancreatitis is a recognized complication of closed abdominal trauma such as may result from "steering wheel" injuries to the abdomen. Acute pancreatitis also may complicate extensive surgery in the gastroduodenal area. On historical grounds, trauma can be excluded as a pathogenic mechanism in most cases.

Circulating antibodies to pancreatic tissue have been demonstrated in the bloodstream of patients with pancreatitis.[67] It is not clear whether these antibodies have an etiologic role in the production of pancreatitis or are simply immunologic by-products occurring after pancreatic necrosis in response to other factors. Fig. 27-5 summarizes current views as to pathogenic mechanisms.

Chronic pancreatitis

Chronic pancreatitis produces progressive destruction of the pancreas as the result of repeated episodes of necrosis of the parenchyma. Approximately one third of all patients who survive an episode of acute pancreatitis sustain subsequent acute episodes that ultimately progress to chronic pancreatitis. Some patients arrive at the stage of pancreatic insufficiency without sustaining a documented attack of acute pancreatitis. Chronic pancreatitis is a recognized manifestation of hyperparathyroidism and of a hereditary metabolic disorder usually, but not always, accompanied by aminoaciduria. The latter disorder accounts for only a small percentage of cases of chronic pancreatitis. Chronic relapsing pancreatitis occurs most frequently in the fourth or fifth decade. The disease is frequently associated with biliary tract disease or alcoholism.

Pathologic changes in the pancreas depend on the stage of development of the disease. In acute exacerbations, diffuse edema, local areas of necrosis, and peripancreatic inflammation may be present. After the acute attacks the pancreas will be firm and nodular, with areas of dense fibrosis, loss of acinar and islet tissue (Fig. 27-6), calcification in the interstitial tissue and pancreatic ducts, infiltration with plasma cells and lymphocytes, and formation of pseudocysts. The destruction of the pancreas eventually results in exocrine pancreatic insufficiency and, ultimately, diabetes mellitus.

Hereditary pancreatitis is a form of chronic pancreatitis that is transmitted as a mendelian dominant autosomal gene. In contrast to sporadic chronic pancreatitis, hereditary pancreatitis begins in childhood, and there is a relative infrequency of alcoholism and chronic biliary disease.[54]

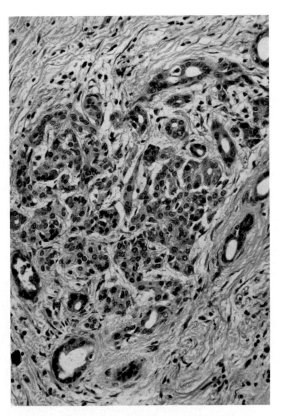

Fig. 27-6. Acinar atrophy occurring after pancreatic duct obstruction.

PANCREATIC LESIONS IN SYSTEMIC DISEASE

Dilatation of acini and ducts of the pancreas occurs in approximately 40% to 50% of patients with uremia. The dilated structures contain eosinophilic inspissated material. In some instances the individual lobules are separated by edematous tissue with a mild infiltrate of neutrophils.

Histologic changes in the acinar cells of the pancreatic lobules may be present in chronic congestive heart failure. Peripheral acinar cells in the pancreatic lobules appear atrophic, with diminished zymogen granules and decreased basophils of their cytoplasm, whereas cells adjacent to islets retain their normal appearance. These histologic changes are apparently related to increased venous pressure and vascular stasis within the pancreatic venous circulation.

NEOPLASMS OF EXOCRINE PANCREAS
Cystadenoma and cystadenocarcinoma

An uncommon but generally well-recognized pancreatic tumor is designated cystadenoma or mucinous cystadenoma. These lesions are more common in women than in men, are more common in the body or tail of the pancreas than in the head, and occur in middle-aged or elderly persons in whom a detectable mass is usually the only clinical manifestation.

Grossly cystadenomas are bulky neoplasms partially or totally circumscribed by a dense capsule that radiates, centrally compartmentalizing the lesion into locules (Fig. 27-7).

Microscopically, three variants are distinguishable.[72] A microcystic or spongiform type features cuboidal, non–mucin producing cells with clear cytoplasm lining small cystic spaces. The clear cytoplasm reflects accumulations of glycogen (hence "glycogen-rich cytoadenoma").[76] These lesions appear to be benign. The other variant (macrocystic) features tall, mucin-secreting cells that often fall into multilayered papillary folds about variable, mucin-filled cystic spaces. Distinction between benign and malignant variants may be impossible or even unjustified because metastases may occur many years after recognition of the lesion.[77]

A rare acinar cytadenoma has been described.[43]

Carcinoma

Carcinoma of the pancreas ranks fourth in frequency among fatal neoplastic diseases in the United States and is responsible for approximately 5% of all deaths caused by cancer. As a cause of death in the United States, carcinoma of the pancreas now exceeds such neoplastic diseases as carcinoma of the stomach, malignant lymphoma of all types, carcinoma of the prostate, and carcinoma of the cervix. Significantly increased risk of carcinoma of the pancreas has been attributed to and associated with disease of the gallbladder and extrahepatic biliary tree, cigarette smoking, high levels of consumption of fat, and high daily average total caloric intake.[111]

Association with alcohol consumption is not a prominent epidemiologic feature. At least in women, preexisting diabetes appears to be a risk factor. Data relating to previous episodes of pancreatitis are contradictory. Excess indulgence in coffee may be a factor. There is an increased risk of carcinoma of the pancreas among members of the American Chemical Society. Experi-

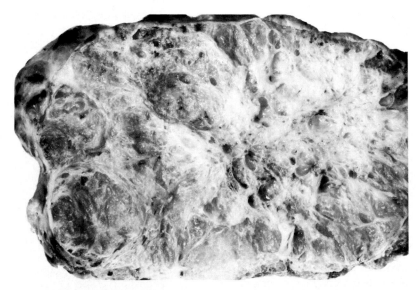

Fig. 27-7. Cystadenoma of pancreas. Coarse porous surface is typical. (From Rosai, J.: Ackerman's surgical pathology, ed. 7, St. Louis, 1989, The C.V. Mosby Co.)

mental models have been developed in animals.[85] Carcinoma of the pancreas is extremely rare before 40 years of age. Approximately two thirds of patients are over age 60. An uncommon, sluggishly malignant, histologically characteristic carcinoma of the pancreas has been described in children as "pancreatoblastoma"[82] (Fig. 27-8, *A*). Its cell of origin appears to be the acinar cell.

Clinical symptoms of carcinoma of the pancreas depend on the site of the origin of the tumor. If it arises in the head of the pancreas, obstruction of the common bile duct occurs early, producing obstructive jaundice (Fig. 27-9, *A*). Clinical recognition of carcinoma of the body and tail is difficult because of the paucity of distinctive signs and symptoms. Pain is the most common initial symptom of carcinoma of the pancreas, regardless of its location. Symptoms that appear later in the disease include anorexia, weight loss, cachexia, and weakness. The majority of patients with carcinoma of the pancreas are dead within a year after the onset of symptoms. The very high rate of failure of excisional surgery in the treatment of carcinoma of the pancreas has several possible explanations: initial symptoms are inconspicuous and nonspecific, and so early diagnosis is difficult; the organ lies deep in the retroperitoneum intimately related to vital structures, and so a conventional radical cancer operation is difficult; and multiple sites of origin within the pancreas have been described.[75]

Approximately one half of all deaths from carcinoma of the pancreas occur within 3 months of the onset of symptoms. Among selected patients with carcinoma of the pancreas who are subjected to radical pancreaticoduodenectomy, some 12% survive longer than 5 years.[108] This figure approaches 40% in cases of (usually well-differentiated) ampullary carcinoma, a lesion that should be distinguished from pancreatic carcinoma.

Approximately 70% of carcinomas of the pancreas occur in the head of the organ. The proximity of the neoplasm to the common bile duct results in neoplastic invasion of the wall of the duct, producing obstruction and dilatation. Obstruction of the common bile duct also occurs in cases of carcinoma of the body and tail of the pancreas. However, this is usually a late complication.

Carcinomas of the body and tail of the pancreas are,

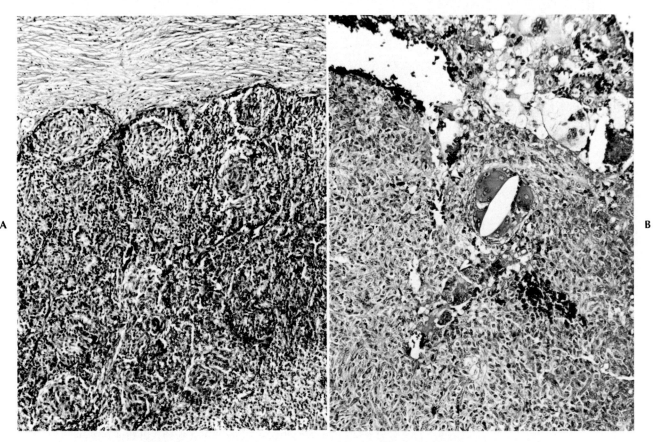

Fig. 27-8. A, Photomicrograph of a pancreatoblastoma showing a background of epithelial cells with vaguely tubular differentiation interspersed with globular areas of squamous cell–like differentiation. **B,** Solid and papillary epithelial tumor of the pancreas. Among the epithelial cells are foam cells in the stroma and characteristic lipid granulomas.

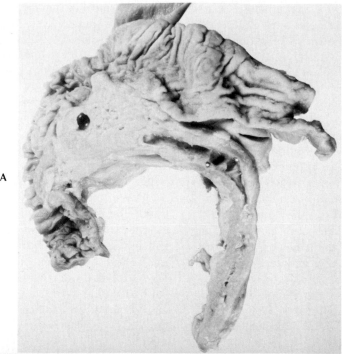

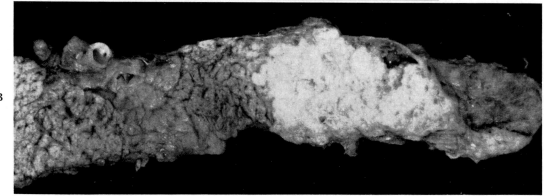

Fig. 27-9. Carcinoma of pancreas. **A,** Lesion of head of pancreas accompanied by atrophy of body and tail and dilatation of pancreatic duct. **B,** Lesion of body and tail of pancreas. (Courtesy Dr. Béla Halpert, Silver Spring, Md.)

on the average, larger than those of the head. Metastases occur most frequently in the regional lymph nodes, liver, lungs, peritoneum, and adrenal glands. The incidence of metastases is higher in cases of carcinoma of the body and tail than that of the head of the pancreas.

Grossly the neoplasm is an ill-defined, firm expansion of a portion of the pancreas, with no sharp line of demarcation between the neoplasm and the surrounding parenchyma (Fig. 27-9).

The following is a classification of epithelial malignancies of the pancreas*:

---

*From Kissane, J.M.: Cancer Treat. Res. 8:99, 1982.

A. Benign tumors
  1. Adenomas
    a. Clear cell adenoma
    b. Acinar cell adenoma
  2. Dermoid cyst
B. Malignant tumors
  1. Duct (ductular) cell origin
    a. Duct cell adenomcarcinoma
    b. Giant cell carcinoma
    c. Giant cell carcinoma (epulis with osteoid)
    d. Adenosquamous carcinoma
    e. Microadenocarcinoma
    f. Mucinous ("colloid") carcinoma
    g. Cystadenocarcinoma

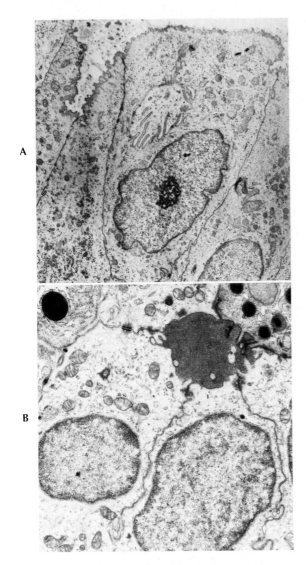

Fig. 27-10. Electron micrograph of pancreatic carcinoma compared with normal pancreatic ductule. **A,** Pancreatic adenocarcinoma. Cytoplasm of cell in center of field is traversed by canaliculus into which microvilli protrude. **B,** Normal pancreas shows a canaliculus with microvilli.

2. Acinar cell origin
    a. Acinar cell adenocarcinoma
3. Tumors of the inmature pancreas, pancreatoblastomas
    a. Pleomorphic type, acinar differentiation
    b. Solid and papillary type, ductal or ductular differentiation
4. Mixed type: acinar, duct, and islet-cell carcinoma
5. Unclassified
    a. Large cell
    b. Small cell
    c. Clear cell

Most carcinomas of the pancreas are moderately well-differentiated adenocarcinomas believed to arise from ductal epithelium (Fig. 27-10). These tumors recapitulate tubular and ductlike structures lined by one or several layers of neoplastic cells supported by dense fibrous stroma (Fig. 27-11, A). Although histochemical demonstration of mucin secretion by neoplastic cells can often be demonstrated, conspicuous extracellular production of mucin is uncommon. Occasional carcinomas of the pancreas present a peculiar histologic dimorphism between tubular and ductular structures and a sarcomatous stroma (Fig. 27-11, B).[84] The pancreas is one of the more common sites for the occurrence of adenosquamous carcinoma, a carcinoma with both squamous and glandular elements.[74] Pure epidermoid carcinoma occurs. Undifferentiated small cell carcinoma of the pancreas may closely resemble the similar neoplasms of the lung (Fig. 27-11, C).[78] Acinar carcinoma is a rare neoplasm that recaptibulates the pattern of acini in the normal pancreas. It may contain zymogen granules and manifest local features of lipolytic and proteolytic activity.[69,73] Peculiar giant cell tumors are rare.[106]

A mixed papillary and solid epithelial neoplasm with a definite predilection for girls and young women has been recognized[102] (Fig. 27-8, B). Many have been been detected incidentally, but these lesions are, at least sluggishly, malignant. Immunohistochemical studies suggest origin from a multipotent epithelial cell.[100]

Adenocarcinoma of the pancreas frequently invades the perineural lymphatics (Fig. 27-11, D). This invasion of the nerves accounts for the frequency of abdominal pain in these patients. Multiple venous thromboses may be associated with carcinoma of the pancreas and occur more frequently when the neoplasm is in the body or tail of the pancreas. The veins most frequently involved are the iliac and femoral. The mechanism of thrombosis is not clearly defined.

PERIAMPULLARY TUMORS
Carcinoma

Carcinoma of the periampullary region is a generic designation for a carcinoma that arises from any of four primary sites: (1) the true ampulla of Vater, the flask-shaped final channel of both biliary and pancreatic drainage; (2) the distal common bile duct; (3) the distal pancreatic duct (of Wirsung) or pancreatic ductules in its vicinity; or (4) the duodenal mucosa that invests the papilla of Vater. Often it is not possible from gross examination to assign a periampullary carcinoma to one or another of these sites of origin nor does conventional microscopy demonstrate differential features.

The unitary designation is appropriate because of the homogeneity of clinical features of these tumors. Jaundice, pain, and weight loss are common features. Peri-

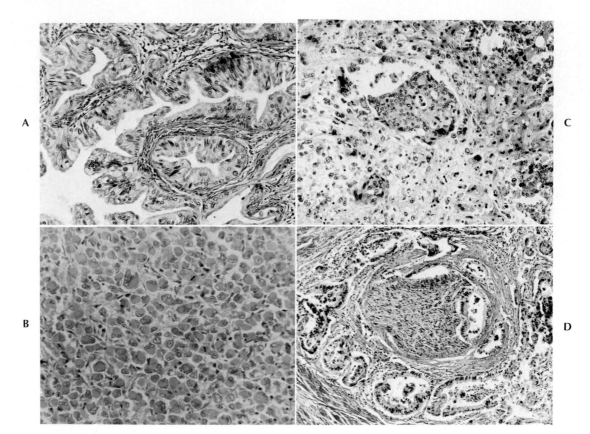

Fig. 27-11. Microscopic features of pancreatic carcinoma. **A,** Well-differentiated papillary adenocarcinoma. **B,** Adenosquamous carcinoma in which areas of epidermoid carcinoma occur in otherwise typical adenocarcinoma. **C,** Pleomorphic carcinoma, an anaplastic carcinoma consisting of large anaplastic cells in no particular architectural pattern. **D,** Invasion of nerve by pancreatic adenocarcinoma, a common microscopic feature.

ampullary carcinoma is considerably less common than carcinoma of the pancreas, but its recognition is important because its response to surgical treatment is much more favorable than that of pancreatic carcinoma.

Periampullary carcinoma presents with one or another of two gross appearances. Some of these tumors are distinctly papillary, but more commonly the lesion is seen as a knobby distorted enlargement of the papilla of Vater (Fig. 27-12). Microscopically these are usually moderately well-differentiated carcinomas as occur elsewhere in the pancreas or more commonly, the lung.

In a detailed study of 109 periampullary carcinomas, Yamaguchi and Enjoji promulgated a clinicopathologic staging system that correlates with survival after pancreatoduodenectomy.[113]

Adenoma. A few periampullary carcinomas have peripheral foci that resemble villous adenoma of the colon, suggestive of an origin of the carcinoma from a preexisting adenoma. Very rarely, exhaustive sectioning or a periampullary tumor discloses only a benign tumor, adenoma.

ENDOCRINE PANCREAS
Diabetes mellitus

Diabetes mellitus is a hereditary disease that affects approximately 2% to 4% of the population of the United States. The discovery of insulin and the use of this hormone in treatment have saved or prolonged the lives of diabetic patients but have not cured the disease. Today the major problems associated with diabetes are the complications that may affect the eye with resultant blindness, the kidney with resultant renal failure, the cardiovascular system with accelerated arteriosclerosis, and the peripheral nervous system with the development of neuropathy.

Clinically the disease has been divided into two major categories: type I and type II diabetes.[120] Type I corresponds to the older classification of juvenile onset diabetes and type II represents the previous classification of maturity onset diabetes. In type I diabetes, the disease usually begins abruptly, early in life, with a gradual loss of insulin reserve in the pancreas, and exogenous insulin is required for therapy. Type II diabe-

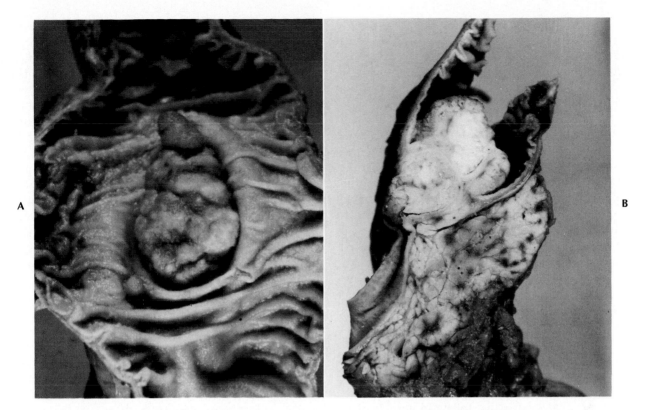

Fig. 27-12. A, Surface and, **B,** sectioned views of a papillary adenocarcinoma of the periampullary region. (From Rosai, J.: Ackerman's surgical pathology, ed. 7, St. Louis, 1989, The C.V. Mosby Co.)

tes occurs in older persons and has an insidious onset. The insulin reserve in the pancreas may be normal or moderately decreased, and exogenous insulin therapy is usually not required.

Etiology and pathogenesis

Type I diabetes. Type I diabetes is believed to be an autoimmune disease resulting from specific immune destruction of B-cells in the islets of Langerhans. The evidence supporting this concept is the presence of antibodies to islet cells at the time of onset of diabetes and for several years thereafter[126]; a higher frequency of HLA DR3 and DR4 histocompatibility antigens in type I diabetics as compared to the normal population[137]; and lymphocytic infiltration into the islets at the time of onset.[123,136] Immunosuppressive therapy with cyclosporin A started at the time of onset of diabetes has produced a remission of the disease in some patients with elimination of the need for insulin therapy and a rapid return to a diabetic state when immunotherapy is stopped. The most convincing evidence was the finding that B-cells were destroyed within a few weeks when a pancreas transplant was done between identical twins, and the diabetic recipient twin was not treated with immunosuppressive agents. The autoimmune state in the diabetic twin apparently recognized

and destroyed the B-cells bearing identical histocompatibility antigens on their surface.

Epidemiologic studies in identical twins have shown that if one twin has type I diabetes there is only a 50% chance that the second twin will also develop diabetes.[115,145] This finding indicates that a second environmental or endogenous factor is required for the initiation of the disease in addition to an immunologic susceptibility. Precipitating factors may be certain viruses or chemical agents. Experimentally, infection with encephalomyocarditis virus produces destruction of B-cells and diabetes in certain strains of mice.[119] Epidemiologic studies in humans have provided suggestive evidence of a greater incidence of coxsackievirus B infection in type I diabetes than in controls. A coxsackievirus B4 has been isolated from the pancreas of a diabetic child; however, in this instance an overwhelming infection with the virus was present. Streptozotocin and alloxan are two chemical agents that will produce specific destruction of B-cells in animals when administered in a single large dose. Repeated injections of a small amount of streptozotocin will induce immune destruction of B-cells in certain strains of mice.

Normal islet cells express only class I histocompatibility antigens on their surface; however, class II antigen expression has been demonstrated on B-cells at the time of onset of type I diabetes.[116] This finding has led to the suggestion that abnormal class II antigen expression on B-cells converts them to antigen-presenting cells, thus initiating an immune response that results in specific destruction of the B-cells. It is also possible that the induction of class II antigens on B-cells is secondary to the lymphocytic infiltration and release of lymphokines. Interferon-gamma and tumor necrosis factor will induce class II antigens on islet cells in vitro. Abnormal expression of class II antigens on B-cells in transgenic mice have been produced by the insertion of the genetic information for the insulin promoter coupled with the information for formation of class II histocompatibility antigens.[140] The B-cells in these transgenic animals expressed class II antigens and were destroyed; however, the mechanism of destruction is unknown, since a lymphocytic infiltration of the islets did not occur.

These fascinating, diverse findings indicate that environmental or endogenous factors may initiate damage to B-cells in susceptible individuals, which in turn leads to an autoimmune response and specific destruction of the B-cells. The specific mechanisms involved in these initiating events and the subsequent pathogenesis of the disease are unknown at the present time.

Type II diabetes. Epidemiologic studies on type II diabetes in identical twins have shown that if one of the twins develops type II diabetes the second twin has a 95% chance of developing the disease.[115,145] These findings clearly indicate that genetic factors play a definite role in the etiology of type II diabetes; however, there is no information available at the present time as to what these genetic factors may be. Clinical studies in type II diabetes have shown in some of these individuals an impaired initial responsiveness of the B-cells to glucose stimulation resulted in a delay in the release of insulin and resultant hyperglycemia.[117] These findings would indicate an impairment in the secretory mechanism of the B-cells with respect to insulin release. Obesity is a common finding in type II diabetes, and there is evidence of impaired sensitivity of peripheral tissues such as muscle and fat cells to insulin action in these individuals. Weight reduction of these obese patients produces a great improvement in the diabetic state. Thus it is not clear at present whether the primary genetic defect resides in the B-cells of type II diabetics or in the target cells for insulin action or a combination of these.

Normal structure and function of islet cells. The islets of Langerhans comprise about 1% to 3% of the weight of the pancreas, and the concentration of islets is greater in the tail than in the head or body of the pancreas. By use of immunohistochemical stains and electron microscopy, the islet cells of the human pancreas can be subclassified into A, B, D, F, and G cells (Fig. 27-13). Each cell type contains a specific hormone: A-cell, glucagon; B-cell, insulin; D-cell, somatostatin; F-cell, pancreatic polypeptide; G-cell, gastrin. Islets in the body and tail of the pancreas contain 60% to 70% B-cells and 20% to 30% A-cells; each of the remaining cell types comprises a small percentage of the islet population. In the head and uncinate process of the human pancreas are found islets that are composed of 95% F-cells with a few A- and D-cells. The secretory products from these different types of cells apparently modulate insulin secretion from B-cells. For example, purified B-cells have only a slight response to glucose stimulation, whereas, mixing A-cells with them with formation of pseudoislets results in a normal insulin secretory response to glucose stimulation. Presumably, somatostatin also in some way modulates the secretory activity of B-cells. The role of pancreatic polypeptide in affecting normal metabolic function in the body as well as within the confines of the islets is unknown. Thus the islets of Langerhans are in essence small organs containing different types of cells, releasing different hormones that modulate insulin secretion from B-cells.

Insulin synthesis and secretion. Stimulation of the B-cell with glucose results in the immediate release of stored insulin and also initiates a series of events that leads to new formation of insulin.[124,125,133,138,139,144] After glucose stimulation, proinsulin production is initiated in the endoplasmic reticulum. Human proinsulin is a single chain of 86 amino acids that consist of the A and B chains of insulin linked by a connecting peptide segment of 31 amino acids. This connecting segment is called the "C-peptide." Proinsulin is transferred by an energy-requiring mechanism to the Golgi complex, where the C-peptide is split off by a specific proteolytic enzyme. The insulin and C-peptide are packaged into secretory granules in the Golgi complex and then released into the cytoplasm after acquiring a membranous sac from the Golgi membranes, and the insulin is converted into a microcrystal of insulin that contains zinc.

Glucose stimulation of B-cells results in a biphasic pattern of insulin release with an immediate first phase of secretion lasting approximately 5 minutes followed by a slow second phase of release, which continues until the glucose level returns to normal limits. Glucose is the primary stimulus for insulin release in humans, and the mechanism of induction of insulin release by this hexose is still unknown. One concept is that glucose metabolism in the B-cells forms certain metabolites that initiate insulin release. Another concept is that glucose interacts with specific glucoreceptors in the B-cell resulting in insulin release. It is probable that both concepts are correct and that the first phase of insulin release may be attributable to an interaction of glucose

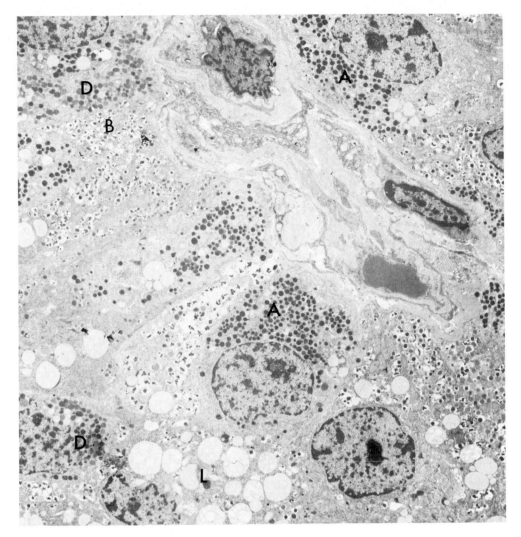

Fig. 27-13. Electron micrograph of islet cells of normal human pancreas. *A,* A-cell: *B,* B-cell; *D,* D-cell. Lipochrome pigment, *L,* is present in cells. (Courtesy Dr. Marie Greider, St. Louis, Mo.)

with a glucoreceptor whereas the second phase may be the result of glucose metabolism.

After glucose stimulation, the membranous sacs containing zinc-insulin crystals and C-peptide are conveyed to the plasma membrane of the B-cell by the microtubule-microfilament system. Cinephotomicrographic studies of living stimulated B-cells have demonstrated a saltatory motion of the beta granules along the microtubule-microfilament system. Intracellular calcium is required for insulin secretion; however, it is unknown how calcium and other factors activate the microtubule-microfilament system for movement of the granules to the cell surface. Studies with transmission and freeze-fracture electron microscopy have demonstrated that the final step in the secretion of insulin is by emiocytosis (Fig. 27-14). This is accomplished by fusion of the

membranous sacs surrounding the B-cell granules with the plasma membrane of the cell, resulting in the liberation of the granules and C-peptide into the extracellular space where insulin and C-peptide are then transported into the capillary system of the islets. The release of C-peptide with insulin makes it possible for one to assess the insulin reserve in the islets of diabetic patients by measuring C-peptide levels after stimulation of the B-cells.

A defect in any one of the steps in the secretory process could lead to an impairment or delay in the release of insulin by glucose stimulation. In type II diabetes, the B-cells in many of the patients do not respond immediately to glucose stimulation; thus a defect may exist in the putative glucoreceptor on the B-cells, intracellular calcium metabolism may be altered, the

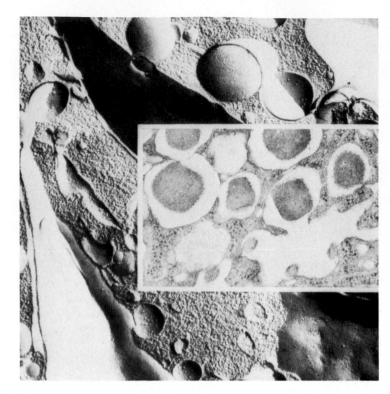

Fig. 27-14. Electron micrograph of freeze-fracture preparation of B-cell demonstrating emiocytosis. *Inset,* Electron micrograph of section of stimulated B-cell demonstrating release of B granule by emiocytosis. (Courtesy Dr. Lelio Orci, University of Geneva.)

microtubule-microfilament system may be defective, or the membranous fusion required for emiocytosis may be altered.

Pathologic changes in islets

The specific pathologic lesion or lesions of the islet cells that would explain the cause and pathogenesis of diabetes mellitus has not been elucidated. Despite this lack of specific knowledge, severel pathologic changes have been demonstrated in the islets in association with diabetes.

Type I diabetes. Leukocytic infiltration into the islets occurs at the time of onset of type I diabetes.[123,136,147] This lymphocytic insulitis does not affect all the islets at the same time, since a normal islet can be observed close to one involved with insulitis. The lymphocytic infiltrate is limited to islets and is apparently induced by the autoimmune process that has been initiated in these patients. In experimental animals a similar type of insulitis occurs in autoimmune diabetes in the BB rat and after the repeated administration of small amounts of streptozotocin to certain strains of mice (Fig. 27-15). This inflammatory response produces specific destruction of the B-cells either by the direct action of cytotoxic T-lymphocytes or by lymphokines released by this immune reaction or by a combination of these mechanisms. Interleukin-1 inhibits insulin release from iso-

lated islets and with tumor necrosis factor and interferon-gamma, the combined action of these lymphokines can result in destruction of B-cells. Over a period of months and years there is a gradual complete elimination of the B-cells leaving A, D, F, and G cells within the islets. One can demonstrate this loss of endogenous insulin reserve clinically by showing an absence of plasma C-peptide in these patients after a glucose tolerance test.

In the era before insulin therapy, the persistent hyperglycemia in these patients caused degranulation of the unaffected B-cells early in the course of diabetes and subsequently the deposition of massive quantities of glycogen in these cells.[146] Initially this lesion was called "hydropic degeneration of B-cells," since the cells appeared vacuolated and it was assumed that the vacuoles contained water. The use of special stains demonstrated that the vacuoles actually contained glycogen. Glycogenosis of B-cells also occurs in certain experimental animals with diabetes and sustained hyperglycemia (Fig. 27-16). The lesion rarely occurs now, since relatively few patients die in diabetic acidosis and severe hyperglycemia. Nevertheless, this lesion undoubtedly does occur during the life of diabetic subjects when there are periods of uncontrolled hyperglycemia.

Type II diabetes. In type II diabetes the B-cell mass and the degree of B-cell granulation may be normal or

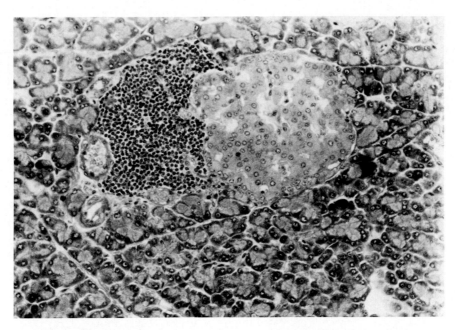

Fig. 27-15. Insulitis in an islet of a BB rat with autoimmune diabetes.

moderately reduced. The lesion that is found in the islets of some of the type II diabetics is amyloidosis of the islets.[121] By light microscopy, amyloid appears as an eosinophilic, amorphous material deposited around the capillaries of the islets, compressing and displacing the islet cells (Fig. 27-17). By electron microscopy, the amyloid has a fibrillar appearance, and it is deposited between the two basement membranes separating the islet cells from the capillaries.

Previously, this change was called "hyalinization of the islets of Langerhans" and was one of the earlier morphologic findings observed in diabetic patients. Amyloidosis does not involve all the islets within a single pancreas but has a patchy distribution. The lesion is not limited to diabetic patients but has been found to a minor degree in about 2% of nondiabetic persons over 40 years of age. It is unlikely that this pathologic change has a primary role in the cause of type II diabetes; however, it may play a role in delaying the release of insulin from affected islets in these persons.

Amyloidosis of the islets has been described in spontaneous diabetes in monkeys and cats. In cats, there have been reported occasional cases in which nearly all the islets were replaced with amyloid and, in some instances, calcification of the amyloid was present. In these instances with extensive involvement of the islets, it appears that amyloidosis is responsible for the diabetic state in these animals.

Newborn pancreas. Infiltration of eosinophils and some lymphocytes within and around the islets and in the interstitial tissue of the pancreas is observed in approximately 25% of infants who are born to diabetic

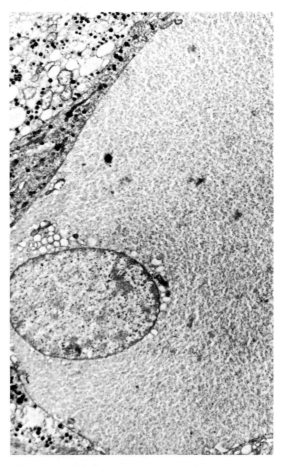

Fig. 27-16. Electron micrograph of B-cell containing massive accumulation of glycogen in diabetic hamster. Glycogen accumulation presents appearance of hydropic degeneration in ordinary microscopic preparations.

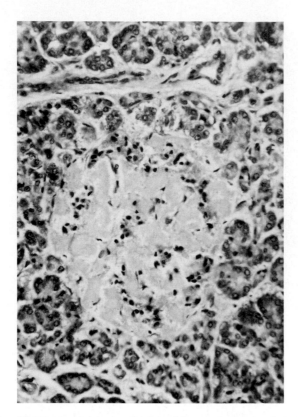

Fig. 27-17. Amyloidosis of islet of Langerhans in diabetic patient.

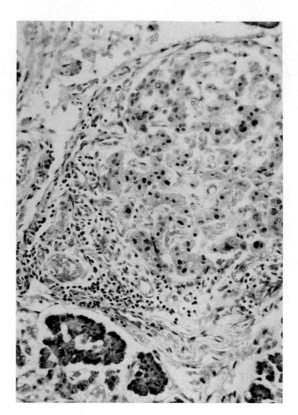

Fig. 27-18. Infiltration of eosinophils in peri-insular tissue of newborn infant of diabetic mother.

mothers and who die within 1 to 2 weeks after birth (Fig. 27-18). This eosinophil infiltration is invariably associated with hypertrophy and hyperplasia of the islets and is diagnostic of diabetes mellitus in the mother.[142] Experimentally a morphologic counterpart of this lesion has been produced by acute injections of anti-insulin serum into rats.[132] In these animals, a severe diabetic state is produced and an infiltration of eosinophils and lymphocytes is present in interstitial tissue and peri-insular areas of the pancreas. In monkeys with strepto-zotocin-induced diabetes, hyperplasia of the islets has been observed in the fetuses of the diabetic mothers; however, lymphocytic and eosinophil infiltration was not present. It appears that the hyperplasia and hypertrophy of the B-cells is attributable to the hyperglycemia; however, the lymphocytic and eosinophil infiltration may be caused by another factor involving an infectious agent or the transfer of specific antibodies to the fetus.

Diabetic microangiopathy

Pathologic changes in the small blood vessels and capillaries of the eye and kidney are responsible for the development of diabetic retinopathy and the Kimmel-stiel-Wilson syndrome in patients with diabetes mellitus. The cardinal pathologic change is the pronounced

accumulation of basement membrane–like material around the vessels. Ultrastructural studies have shown that this basement membrane change is not limited to only the eye and kidney but occurs also in capillaries of the muscle and skin of diabetic patients (Fig. 27-19). In nondiabetic persons, thickening of muscle capillary basement membranes occurs in a linear fashion in males with increasing age, whereas in females the basement membrane thickness increases until about 40 to 50 years of age, reaches a plateau, and increases again between 60 and 70 years of age.[127,148] In diabetics, the basement membrane is significantly thicker than in appropriate age- and sex-matched controls, and the thickening increases with the duration of the disease.

Both experimental and clinical evidence indicates that diabetic microangiopathy is a complication of the diabetic state and is not attributable to a separate genetic defect. It would appear that the changes are caused by the inability of maintaining the blood glucose within normal limits at all times with insulin therapy. These findings are of great importance, since they provide hope that if the diabetic state could be reverted to normal by new therapeutic means the early stages of the complications could be reversed and further progression of these lesions could be halted.

A unifying hypothesis for the pathogenesis of diabetic

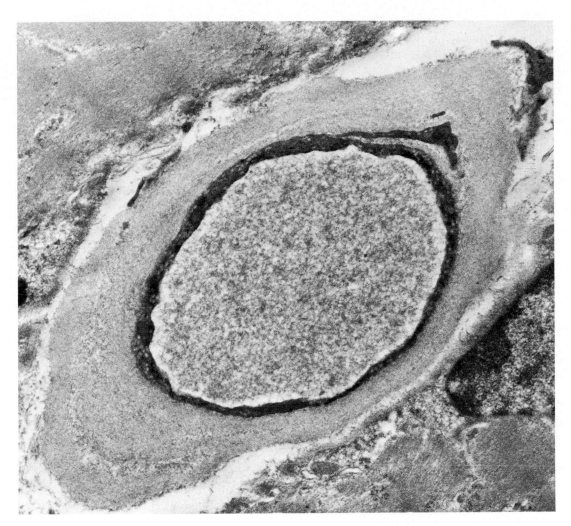

Fig. 27-19. Electron micrograph of capillary in skeletal muscle of diabetic patient. Basement membrane surrounding capillary tremendously thickened. (Courtesy Dr. Joseph R. Williamson, St. Louis, Mo.)

microangiopathy as well as for peripheral neuropathy, which occurs in diabetics, is that the recurrent hyperglycemia affects the structure and function of supporting cells. In capillaries, the supporting cells are embedded in the basement membrane and are called a pericyte in skeletal muscle, a mural cell in retinal capillaries, and a mesangial cell in the glomerulus of the kidney. In the same context, a Schwann cell would be considered a supporting cell for peripheral neves. A possible mechanism for alteration of these supporting cells by hyperglycemia could be the activation of the aldose reductase pathway of glucose metabolism resulting in the accumulation of sorbitol in the cells and depletion of *myo*-inositol in the plasma membranes. The aldose reductase enzyme has a low affinity for glucose and would therefore be activated only in the presence of hyperglycemia. Clinical studies are in progress to determine whether certain aldose reductase inhibitors will

affect the progression of these diabetic complications.

Recurrent hyperglycemia also produces glycosylation of hemoglobin and other proteins such as collagen and basement membrane material. Thus it has been suggested that these glycosylated products are altered and are unable to be removed, thus resulting in thickening of the basement membrane and alteration in the structure and function of capillaries and peripheral nerves.

Kidney in diabetes. The nodular lesions of the glomeruli described by Kimmelstiel and Wilson are characteristic pathologic changes found in the kidney in diabetes mellitus.[114,128] This lesion is the result of focal thickening of the basement membrane. Quantitative ultrastructural studies of the glomeruli in diabetic patients have demonstrated that the earliest change occurs in the mesangial area of the glomerulus. Initially there is a thickening of the basement membrane in this area and an increase in the number of mesangial cells.

Serial renal biopsies on these diabetic patients over a period of years have shown that the amount of basement membrane in the kidney gradually increases and results in the formation of the nodular lesions. These findings clearly indicate that the basement membrane changes result from the diabetic process. In experimentally induced diabetes in rats, an increase in the number of mesangial cells and the deposition of gamma globulin in the basement membrane occurs. Islet transplants into these diabetic animals have returned the diabetic state to normal and have completely reversed the pathologic changes in the glomeruli.[143]

Vacuolization of the pars recta of the proximal convoluted tubules at the corticomedullary junction may be observed in patients dying of uncontrolled diabetes and severe hyperglycemia. These vacuoles represent areas of glycogen deposition with the tubules that disappear when the hyperglycemia is maintained within normal limits. This condition is called the "Armanni-Ebstein lesion of the kidney."

Necrotizing renal papillitis is a rare but serious complication of diabetes mellitus. This condition is not limited to diabetic patients but also may occur in nondiabetic persons with obstructive lesions of the urinary tract. The condition is characterized clinically in the diabetic patient by the rapid onset of uremia and subsequent death caused by infarction and sloughing of the renal papillae.

Eye in diabetes. Diabetic retinopathy is now the first most common cause of blindness in the United States. The sequence of events in the development of this lesion is changes in the pattern of blood flow through the retina with resultant areas of ischemia, occurrence of microaneurysms in the retinal capillaries, new formation of capillaries within the retina, hemorrhage from these newly formed capillaries into the vitreous, and finally formation of granulation tissue. Development of these lesions requires many years with a varying degree of severity in individual patients and long periods of remission with no further impairment of vision.

The earliest anatomic change observed in the retina of diabetic patients is the loss of mural cells in the capillaries.[118] Ghostlike remnants of these cells persist for long periods of time. Presumably the loss of these cells affects the capillary tone and leads in some way to the changes in the pattern of blood flow through the retina and the subsequent development of microaneurysms of the retina.

The earliest clinical change in the eyes of diabetic patients is an increase in permeability of retinal capillaries, which can be demonstrated by quantitative measurements of fluorescein leakage into the anterior chamber and vitreous of the eye. This same change can be produced in rats with experimentally induced diabetes, and when the diabetic state is reversed to normal by islet transplantation, the abnormal leakage from the retinal capillaries is also reversed.[129]

Experimentally, microaneurysms and intraretinal hemorrhage have been observed in dogs with alloxan-induced diabetes. Tight control of these diabetic animals with insulin results in a sharp diminution in the number of microaneurysms, which adds further support to the concept that the vascular changes in the retina are associated with persistent recurrent hyperglycemia in these diabetic animals.

Peripheral nerves in diabetes. Peripheral neuropathy occurs in diabetic patients, with approximately 30% to 50% of the patients showing minor reflex changes, evanescent pains in the extremities, and delayed conduction times of the peripheral nerves.[122] The basic pathologic change in the peripheral nerves is a segmental demyelination. In experimental diabetes, greatly elevated levels of sorbitol and fructose are present in peripheral nerves of these animals. The elevated blood glucose in the diabetic state apparently activates the aldose reductase pathway for glucose metabolism resulting in the formation of sorbitol and fructose, which may in turn affect the structure and function of Schwann cells.

The autonomic nervous system may also be involved in diabetic patients with resultant development of severe diarrhea and abdominal pain as well as impaired catecholamine release. In experimental diabetes, degenerative changes have been demonstrated in autonomic nerve fibers of the mesenteric nerve supplying the intestine and were associated with the occurrence of megacolon in these animals. Control of the diabetic state by islet transplantation results in either prevention or disappearance of these degenerative lesions in the autonomic nerves.[141]

Arteriosclerosis and diabetes. Diabetes mellitus accelerates the development of arteriosclerosis with the resultant earlier onset of coronary arteriosclerosis and atherosclerosis in general. The arteriosclerotic process also involves vessels to the lower extremity with resultant production of gangrene of the toes and feet.

The precipitating causes of gangrene of the lower extremities are usually mechanical, thermal, or chemical trauma resulting in ulceration, infection, and subsequent gangrene. Comparison of the ultrastructure of dermal capillaries of the toes amputated from diabetic and nondiabetic persons indicates that thickening of basement membrane of the capillaries is limited to the diabetic group. Pronounced thickening in the basement membranes of the capillaries in diabetic patients may play some role in the inception and complication of the vascular insufficiency of the lower extremities, possibly by interference with nutrition and response of tissues to injury.

Islet transplantation in human diabetes. The devastating complications of diabetes involving the eye, kidney, cardiovascular system, and peripheral nervous system are apparently attributable to the inability of maintaining normoglycemia at all times in diabetic subjects using conventional insulin therapy. Thus the ideal approach for the treatment of diabetes would be to transplant islets into the patient early in the course of diabetes in order to maintain continuous normoglycemia and hopefully prevent these complications from occurring. Since these complications may require decades to occur, it would not be possible to transplant islets and prevent their rejection by continuous immunosuppression of the patient, since these drugs have serious toxic side effects. Thus methods were sought to try to prevent rejection of islet allografts in animals by pretreatment of the donor islets before transplantation. Studies in the last few years have clearly shown that it is possible to prevent rejection of islet allografts and even islet xenografts in rodents by use of procedures that alter or destroy lymphoid antigen-presenting cells in the donor islets before transplantation.[130,131,134,135] One of these methods is simply to culture the donor islets at low temperature (24° C) for 7 days before transplantation and provide a temporary immunosuppression of the recipient animals with either a single injection of antilymphocyte serum or three days of cyclosporin A therapy.

Since rejection of islet allografts could be prevented in animals without continuous immunosuppression, studies were initiated to resolve the next problem, which was mass isolation of human islets. This technical obstacle has been overcome, and procedures have been developed recently for the isolation of 400,000 to 600,000 islets from a single human pancreas. The human islets also survive with low-temperature culture similar to that of the rat islets, thus providing a means of attempting to alter immunogenicity of the donor islets before transplantation. Clinical trials are being initiated to determine whether the human islet transplants will maintain normoglycemia in diabetic patients with established kidney transplants, and if this is successful, trials will be initiated to determine whether alteration or destruction of antigen-presenting cells in the donor islets with temporary immunosuppression of the recipient will make it possible to accomplish islet transplants early in the course of diabetes without the need for continuous immunosuppressive therapy of the recipients.

As discussed earlier, type I diabetes is apparently an autoimmune disease. The approach that will be used to attempt to prevent recognition of the donor islets by the autoimmune process will be to mismatch histocompatibility antigens of the donor and recipient as far as possible. Studies in the autoimmune diabetes of BB rats have shown that transplants of islets from strains of rats entirely different from the BB rat will not be recognized by the autoimmune process, whereas transplants of islets from the same strain as the BB rat will permit immediate autoimmune recognition and destruction of the donor islet cells.[149] Thus there is available experimental evidence that this approach for prevention of recognition and destruction by the autoimmune process in type I diabetes might be avoided if the donor and recipient are mismatched. Obviously this can be answered only by clinical trials in human subjects in which the islets have been pretreated to decrease immunogenicity and the immunosuppressive agents have been withdrawn.

Neoplasms of pancreatic islets

Several different types of islet cell tumors occur in the pancreas and produce specific hormones.[150,152,156] These tumors cannot be differentiated on the basis of their morphologic appearance by use of hematoxylin and eosin preparations. To establish the specific identity of an islet cell tumor, immunohistochemical stains, electron microscopy, and immunoassay of the tumor for specific hormones are required. These procedures have revealed that islet tumors are composed of a predominant single type of islet cell and release a specific hormone but also contain minor elements of other types of islet cells and their hormones. It is mandatory that all the specialized techniques be used in the diagnosis of islet cell tumors to permit accurate identification of the tumor and appropriate therapy for the patients.

B-cell tumors (insulinomas). Functioning B-cell neoplasms retain the capacity to form, store, and release insulin into the bloodstream.[151,153-155] The neoplastic B-cells differ from normal in that they are no longer responsive to the normal control mechanisms affecting insulin release and thus release insulin at an uncontrolled rate, resulting in repeated attacks of hypoglycemia. Circulating levels of insulin are usually elevated in these patients during fasting and are increased during periods of hypoglycemia. Stimulation of insulin release from these neoplasms can usually be produced by the administration of either tolbutamide or arginine.

B-cell tumors are most commonly found in the body and tail of the pancreas. Grossly the tumors are usually encapsulated and well circumscribed, varying from 5 mm to 10 cm in diameter. Their homogeneous color and increased consistency make them easy to delineate from the surrounding normal pancreas.

Microscopically the tumors usually have a gyriform pattern with ribbons or cords of cells passing between vascular sinusoids (Fig. 27-20). It is extremely difficult to assess the degree of malignancy of these neoplasms based on the presence of anaplasia and hyperchromatism of the nuclei, since these changes may be present in a circumscribed adenoma or in one that has metas-

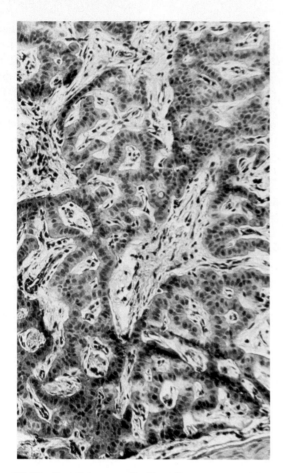

Fig. 27-20. B-cell tumor. Gyriform pattern resulting from anastomosing cords of B-cells. (Courtesy Dr. Marie Greider, St. Louis, Mo.)

tasized. The degree of granulation within the neoplasms may vary from a few scattered granules to an intense granulation similar to that in the normal B-cell. On electron microscopic examination the neoplastic cells contain the typical crystalline, rectangular granules that are present in normal B-cells, and the number of crystalline granules varies noticeably within different neoplasms. Amyloid frequently is observed between the two basement membranes separating the neoplastic cells from the capillaries, and in some instances calcification may be present in this area.

A-cell tumors (glucagonomas). A-cell tumors are rare neoplasms of the islet cells.[162,163] These tumors contain glucagon, and usually the level of circulating glucagon in the patient is greatly elevated. The clinical findings associated with high serum glucagon levels are a necrolytic migratory erythema, mild diabetes mellitus, and anemia. The skin rash is the main clinical diagnostic change that should arouse suspicion of hyperglucagonemia and the presence of an A-cell tumor in the pancreas. By light microscopy the neoplasms have a gyriform pattern similar to that of the B-cell tumors. Under electron microscopy the neoplastic cells have the ultrastructural appearance of normal A-cells and contain numerous secretory granules. The secretory granules of the tumors are round with an extremely dense core and have a diameter of 225 to 425 nm.

G-cell tumors (gastrinomas). Zollinger and Ellison[165] described a diagnostic triad that consists in a fulminating peptic ulcer diathesis persisting despite medical therapy or other radical procedures, gastric acid hypersecretion, and the presence of a non–B cell tumor in the pancreas. Approximately one third of the ulcers observed in these patients have been found in unusual locations, such as the esophageal, postbulbar, and jejunal areas. The tumors most frequently occur in the body and tail of the pancreas, and in a few instances the neoplasm has been found in the wall of the duodenum, apparently originating in heterotopic foci of pancreatic tissue. Multiple adenomas involving the pituitary, adrenal, and parathyroid glands and islets of Langerhans have been found in approximately one third of the patients.

With electron microscopy the tumors are shown to contain small, round granules similar to the secretory granules of gastrin-producing cells of the pyloric antrum. Gastrin can be demonstrated in extracts of the tumor by immunoassay and in the tumor cells by immunohistochemical techniques.[158,159,164]

D-cell tumors (somatostatinomas). Tumors of D-cells have been described recently.[161] Somatostatin has been isolated from the neoplasms and demonstrated in D-cells of the tumors by immunohistochemical techniques. Elevated circulatory levels of somatostatin have been found in these patients. The number of cases is small; however, the clinical findings associated with this neoplasm appear to be diabetes, achlorhydria, steatorrhea, and cholelithiasis. These clinical changes are consistent with the inhibitory action of somatostatin on the secretion of gastrin, insulin, glucagon, and pancreatic enzymes as well as on gallbladder contraction.

Pancreatic polypeptide has been demonstrated as a minor component of several different islet cell tumors. Information is lacking on the precise site of action of pancreatic polypeptide in normal metabolism. Further investigations should establish the normal function of this hormone and delineate clinical features associated with an F-cell tumor secreting predominantly pancreatic polypeptide.

Diarrheogenic tumors (vipomas). Verner and Morrison described a clinical syndrome associated with non–B cell tumors of the pancreas that was characterized by profuse diarrhea with hypokalemia and achlorhydria. The tumors usually occurred in the head and tail of the pancreas and were solitary or occasionally multiple in the pancreas.[157] Vasoactive intestinal polypeptide (VIP) has been isolated from the tumors. Administration of

VIP to experimental animals induces diarrhea and inhibits gastric acid secretion; thus VIP is apparently responsible for the clinical findings in patients with these neoplasms. VIP is present in autonomic nerve fibers, and it has been found that ganglioneuroblastomas may be associated with the clinical findings of diarrhea, hypokalemia, and achlorhydria. It is unknown at the present time whether VIP is produced by a specific type of islet cell.

Nesidioblastosis. Idiopathic hypoglycemia in infants is a syndrome encompassing several entities.[160] The majority of these infants suffer from ketotic hypoglycemia, show leucine hypersensitivity, or are infants of diabetic mothers. The hypoglycemia may be transitory, as occurs after birth from a diabetic mother, or may undergo remission when the diet of the infant is altered to prevent ketogenesis or to lower the leucine intake. In approximately one third of the infants with this syndrome the hypoglycemia is persistent, with inappropriate insulin secretion and a high insulin-to-glucose ratio in the blood. A common finding in the pancreas is a continued formation of islet cells from pancreatic duct epithelium. This pathologic change is called "nesidioblastosis." During normal embryologic development of the pancreas, islets form by budding from the ductular epithelium. In nesidioblastosis, new formation of islets continues after birth, and A, B, D, and F cells are present in these budding islets. Apparently abnormalities exist in the factors controlling the continued formation of islet cells after birth; however, it is unlikely that the hypoglycemia is simply the result of an increased mass of B-cells. Undoubtedly the B-cells are also defective, since the release of insulin is not controlled by the circulatory level of blood glucose and leucine stimulates insulin release in many of these patients.

REFERENCES
Normal form and development

1. Liu, H.M., and Potter, E.L.: Development of human pancreas, Arch. Pathol. **74**:439, 1962.
2. Milbourn, E.: On the excretory ducts of the pancreas in man with special reference to their relationships to each other, to the common bile duct, and to the duodenum, Acta Anat. **9**:1, 1950.
3. Rutter, W.J., et al: Epithelial-mesenchymal interactions, Baltimore, 1968, The Williams & Wilkins Co.
4. Wessels, N.K., and Cohen, J.H.: Early pancreas organogenesis: morphogenesis, tissue interactions, and mass effects, Dev. Biol. **15**:237, 1967.
5. Wessels, N.K., and Evans, J.: Ultrastructural studies of early morphogenesis and cytodifferentiation in the embryogenic mammalian pancreas, Dev. Biol. **17**:413, 1968.

Abnormalities of form and development

6. Barbosa, J.J. de C., Dockerty, M.B., and Waugh, J.M.: Pancreatic heterotopia: review of the literature and report of 41 authenticated surgical cases of which 25 were clinically significant, Surg. Gynecol. Obstet. **82**:527, 1946.
7. Elliott, G.B., Kliman, M.R., and Elliott, K.A.: Pancreatic annulus: a sign or cause of duodenal obstruction, Can. J. Surg. **11**:357, 1968.
8. Feldman, M., and Weinberg, T.: Aberrant pancreas: cause of duodenal syndrome, JAMA **148**:893, 1952.
9. Huebner, G.D., and Reed, P.A.: Annular pancreas, Am. J. Surg. **104**:869, 1962.
10. Lundquist, G.: Annular pancreas: pathogenesis, clinical features, and treatment with a report on two operation cases, Acta Chir. Scand. **117**:451, 1959.
11. Pearson, S.: Aberrant pancreas: review of literature and report of three cases, one of which produced common and pancreatic duct obstruction, Arch. Surg. **63**:168, 1951.
12. Van der Horst, L.F.: Annular pancreas, Arch. Surg. **83**:249, 1961.

Cystic fibrosis

13. Alhadeff, J.A.: Glycoproteins and cystic fibrosis: a review, Clin. Genet. **14**:89, 1978.
14. Anderson, D.H.: Cystic fibrosis of pancreas and its relation to celiac disease: clinical and pathologic study, Am. J. Dis. Child. **56**:344, 1938.
15. Anderson, D.H.: Pancreatic enzymes in duodenal juice in celiac syndrome, Am. J. Dis. Child. **63**:643, 1942.
16. Aterman, K.: Duodenal ulceration and fibrocystic pancreas disease, Am. J. Dis. Child. **101**:210, 1942.
17. Bodian, M.: Fibrocystic disease of the pancreas, New York, 1953, Grune & Stratton, Inc.
18. Bowman, B.H., and Mangos, J.A.: Current concepts in genetics: cystic fibrosis, N. Engl. J. Med. **294**:937, 1976.
19. Changus, H.C., and Pitot, H.C.: Cystic fibrosis: a dilemma in metabolic pathogenesis of genetic disease, Arch. Pathol. Lab. Med. **100**:7, 1976.
20. Clarke, J.T., Elian, E., and Shwachman, H.: Components of sweat in cystic fibrosis of the pancreas compared with controls, Am. J. Dis. Child. **101**:490, 1961.
21. Danes, B.S., and Bearn, A.G.: Cystic fibrosis of the pancreas: a study in cell culture, J. Exp. Med. **129**:775, 1969.
22. di Sant'Agnese, P.A., and Davis, P.B.: Research in cystic fibrosis (in three parts), N. Engl. J. Med. **295**:481, 534, 597, 1976.
23. di Sant'Agnese, P.A., and Lepore, M.J.: Involvement of abdominal organs in cystic fibrosis of the pancreas, Gastroenterology **40**:64, 1961.
24. di Sant'Agnese, P.A., and Talamo, R.C.: Pathogenesis and physiopathology of cystic fibrosis of the pancreas: fibrocystic disease of the pancreas (mucoviscidosis) (in three parts), N. Engl. J. Med. **277**:1287, 1344, 1399, 1967.
25. Dische, A., di Sant'Agnese, P., Pallavicina, C., and Youlous, J.: Composition of mucoprotein fractions from duodenal fluid of patients with cystic fibrosis of pancreas and from controls, Pediatrics **24**:74, 1959.
26. Farber, S.: Pancreatic function and disease in early life: pathologic changes associated with pancreatic insufficiency in early life, Arch. Pathol. **37**:238, 1944.
27. Farber, S.: Relation of pancreatic achylia to meconium ileus, J. Pediatr. **24**:387, 1944.
28. Frydman, M.I.: Epidemiology of cystic fibrosis: a review, J. Chronic. Dis. **32**:211, 1979.
29. Goodfellow, P.N.: Cystic fibrosis: classical and reverse genetics, Nature (London) **326**:824, 1987.
30. Gudjornsson, B.: Cancer of the pancreas 50 years of surgery, Cancer **60**:2284, 1987.
31. Kaplan, E., Shwachman, H., Perlmutter, A.D., Rule, A., Khaw, K.T. and Holsclaw, D.S.: Reproductive failure in males with cystic fibrosis, N. Engl. J. Med. **279**:65, 1968.
32. Kerlin, D.L., Frey, C.F., Bodai, B.I., Twomey, P.L., and Reubner, B.: Cystic neoplasms of the pancreas, Surg. Gynecol. Obstet. **165**:475, 1987.
33. Macdonald, J.A., and Trusler, G.A.: Meconium ileus: an eleven-year review at the Hospital for Sick Children, Toronto, Can. Med. Assoc. J. **83**:881, 1960.
34. Miettinen, M., Partanen, S., Fraki, O., and Kivilaakso, E.: Papillary cystic tumor of the pancreas: an analysis of cellular differentiation by electron microscopy and immunohistochemistry, Am. J. Surg. Pathol. **11**:855, 1987.

35. Mangos, J.A., and McSherry, N.R.: Sodium transport inhibitory factor in sweat of patients with cystic fibrosis, Science **158:**135, 1967.

36. Munger, B.L., Brusilow, S.W., and Cooke, R.E.: An electron microscopic study of eccrine sweat glands in patients with cystic fibrosis of the pancreas, J. Pediatr. **59:**497, 1961.

37. Newmark, P.: Testing for cystic fibrosis, Nature (London) **318:**309, 1987.

38. Oppenheimer, E.H., and Esterly, J.R.: Pathology of cystic fibrosis: review of the literature and comparison with 146 autopsied cases, Perspect. Pediatr. Pathol. **2:**241, 1975.

39. Ornoy, A., Arnon, J., Katznelson, D., Granat, M., Caspi, B., and Chemke, J.: Pathological confirmation of cystic fibrosis in the fetus following prenatal diagnosis, Am. J. Med. Genet. **18:**935, 1987.

40. Roberts, G.B.: Familial incidence of fibrocystic disease of the pancreas, Ann. Hum. Genet. **24:**127, 1960.

41. Rubin, L.S., Barbero, G.J., Chernick, W.S., et al.: Pupillary reactivity as a measure of autonomic balance in cystic fibrosis, J. Pediatr. **63:**1120, 1963.

42. Smoller, M., and Hsia, D.Y.: Studies on the genetic mechanism of cystic fibrosis of the pancreas, Am. J. Dis. Child. **98:**277, 1959.

43. Stamm, B., Burger, H., and Hollinger, A.: Acinar cell cystadenocarcinoma of the pancreas, Cancer **60:**2542, 1987.

44. Spock, A., Heick, H.M., Cress, H., et al.: In vitro studies of ciliary motility to detect individuals with active cystic fibrosis and carriers of disease, Mod. Probl. Paediatr. **10:**200, 1967.

45. Taussig, L.M., Lobeck, C.C., di Sant'Agnese, P.A., et al.: Fertility in males with cystic fibrosis, N. Engl. J. Med. **287:**586, 1972.

46. Welsh, M.J., and Fick, R.B.: Cystic fibrosis, J. Clin. Invest. **80:**1523, 1987.

Acquired diseases

47. Baggenstoss, A.H.: Pancreas in uremia, histopathologic study, Am. J. Pathol. **24:**1003, 1948.

48. Blumenthal, H.T., and Probstein, J.G.: Pancreatitis, Springfield, Ill., 1959, Charles C Thomas, Publisher.

49. Ciba Foundation Symposium: The exocrine pancreas, Boston, 1961, Little, Brown & Co.

50. Dreiling, D.A.: Pancreatic disease: a review, J. Mt. Sinai Hosp. NY **36:**388, 1969.

51. Edmonson, H.A., and Berne, C.J.: Calcium changes in acute pancreatic necrosis, J. Surg. Gynecol. Obstet. **79:**240, 1944.

52. Elliott, D.W., Williams, R.D., and Zollinger, R.M.: Alterations in the pancreatic resistance to bile in the pathogenesis of acute pancreatitis, Ann. Surg. **146:**669, 1957.

53. Gambill, E.E.: Pancreatitis, St. Louis, 1973, The C.V. Mosby Co.

54. Gross, J.B., and Comfort, M.W.: Chronic pancreatitis, Am. J. Med. **33:**358, 1962.

55. Gross, J.B., Gambill, E.E., and Ulrich, J.A.: Hereditary pancreatitis: description of a fifth kindred and summary of clinical features, Am. J. Med. **33:**358, 1962.

56. Hanna, W.A.: Rupture of pancreatic cysts: report of a case and review of the literature, Br. J. Surg. **47:**495, 1960.

57. Hranilovich, G.T., and Baggenstoss, A.H.: Lesions of the pancreas in malignant hypertension: review of 100 cases at necroscopy, Arch. Pathol. **55:**443, 1953.

58. Longnecker, D.S.: Pathology and pathogenesis of the diseases of the pancreas, Am. J. Pathol. **107:**103, 1982.

59. Murphy, R.F., and Hinkamp, J.F.: Pancreatic pseudocysts: report of 35 cases, Arch. Surg. **81:**564, 1960.

60. Opie, E.L.: The etiology of acute hemorrhagic pancreatitis, Bull. Johns Hopkins Hosp. **12:**182, 1901.

61. Ponka, J.L., Landrum, S.E., and Chaikof, L.: Acute pancreatitis in the postoperative patient, Arch. Surg. **83:**475, 1961.

62. Popper, H.L., Necheles, H., and Russell, K.C.: Transition of pancreatic edema into pancreatic necrosis, Surg. Gynecol. Obstet. **87:**79, 1948.

63. Rich, A.R., and Duff, G.L.: Experimental and pathologic studies on pathogenesis of acute hemorrhagic pancreatitis, Bull. Johns Hopkins Hosp. **58:**212, 1936.

64. Sarles, H.: Alcohol and the pancreas, Ann. NY Acad. Sci. **252:**187, 1975.

65. Sarles, H., and Tiscornia, D.: Ethanol and chronic calcifying pancreatitis, Med. Clin. North Am. **58:**1333, 1974.

66. Szymanski, F.J., and Bluefarb, S.M.: Nodular fat necrosis and pancreatic disease, Arch. Dermatol. **83:**224, 1961.

67. Thal, A.P.: The occurrence of pancreatic antibodies and the nature of the pancreatic antigen, Surg. Forum **11:**367, 1960.

68. Tumen, H.J.: Pathogenesis and classification of pancreatic disease, Am. J. Dig. Dis. **6:**435, 1961.

Tumors

69. Auger, C.: Acinous cell carcinoma of pancreas with extensive fat necrosis, Arch. Pathol. **43:**400, 1947.

70. Baczako, K., Büchler, M., Beger, H.G., Kirkpatrick, C.J., and Haferkamp, O.: Morphogenesis and possible precursor lesions of invasive carcinoma of the ampulla of Vater: epithelial dysplasia and adenoma, Hum. Pathol. **16:**305, 1985.

71. Bell, E.T.: Carcinoma of the pancreas, Am. J. Pathol. **33:**499, 1957.

72. Bogomoletz, W.W., Adnet, J.J., Widgren, S., Stavrou, M., and McLaughlin, J.E.: Cystadenoma of the pancreas a histologic, histochemical and ultrastructural study of seven cases, Histopathology **4:**309, 1980.

73. Burns, W.A., Matthews, M.J., Hamosh, M., et al.: Lipase-secreting acinar cell carcinoma of the pancreas with polyarthropathy: a light and electron microscopic, histochemical and biochemical study, Cancer **33:**1002, 1974.

74. Cihak, R.W., Kawashima, T., and Steer, A.: Adenoacanthoma (adenosquamous carcinoma) of the pancreas, Cancer **29:**1133, 1972.

75. Collins, J.J., Jr., Craighead, J.E., and Brooks, J.R.: Rationale for total pancreatectomy for carcinoma of the pancreatic head, N. Engl. J. Med. **274:**599, 1966.

76. Compagno, J., and Oertel, J.E.: Microcystic adenomas of the pancreas (glycogen-rich cystadenomas): a clinicopathologic study of 34 cases, Am. J. Clin. Pathol. **69:**289, 1978.

77. Compagno, J., and Oertel, J.E.: Mucinous cystic neoplasms of the pancreas with overt and latent malignancy (cystadenocarcinoma and cystadenoma): a clinicopathologic study of 41 cases, Am. J. Clin. Pathol. **69:**573, 1978.

78. Corrin, B., Gilby, E.D., Jones, N.F., and Patrick, J.: Oat cell carcinoma of the pancreas with ectopic ACTH secretion, Cancer **31:**1523, 1973.

79. Cubilla, A.L., and Fitzgerald, P.J.: Cancer of the pancreas (nonendocrine): a suggested morphologic classification, Semin. Oncol. **6:**285, 1979.

80. Cubilla, A.L., and Fitzgerald, P.J.: Morphological lesions associated with human primary invasive nonendocrine pancreas cancer, Cancer Res. **36:**2690, 1976.

81. Ehrenthal, D., Haeger, L., Griffin, T., and Compton, C.: Familial pancreatic adenocarcinoma in three generations: a case report and a review of the literature, Cancer **59:**1661, 1987.

82. Frable, W.J., Still, W.J.S., and Kay, S.: Carcinoma of the pancreas, infantile type: a light and electron microscopic study, Cancer **27:**667, 1971.

83. Frantz, V.K.: Tumors of the pancreas. In Atlas of tumor pathology, section VII, fascicles 27 and 28, Washington, D.C., 1959, Armed Forces Institute of Pathology.

84. Guillan, R.A., and McMahon, J.: Pleomorphic adenocarcinoma of the pancreas, Am. J. Gastroenterol. **60:**379, 1973.

85. Hayashi, Y., and Hasegawa, T.: Experimental pancreatic tumor in rats after intravenous injection of 4-hydroxyaminoquinoline 1-oxide, Gan **62:**329, 1971.

86. Hermreck, S., Thomas, C.Y., and Friesen, R.: Importance of pathologic staging in the surgical management of adenocarcinoma of the exocrine pancreas, Am. J. Surg. **127:**654, 1974.

87. Hodgkinson, D.J., and ReMine, W.H., and Weiland, L.H.:

Pancreatic cystadenoma: clinicopathologic study of 45 cases, Arch. Surg. **113**:512, 1978.

88. Kaplan, N., and Angrist, A.: Mechanism of jaundice in cancer of the pancreas, Surg. Gynecol. Obstet. **77**:199, 1943.

89. Kato, O., Kuno, N., Kasugai, T., and Matsuyama, M.: Pancreatic carcinoma difficult to differentiate from duodenal carcinoma, Am. J. Gastroenterol. **71**:74, 1979.

90. Kenney, W.E.: Association of carcinoma in body and tail of pancreas with multiple venous thrombi, Surgery **14**:600, 1943.

91. Kissane, J.M.: Carcinoma of the exocrine pancreas: pathologic aspects, J. Surg. Oncol. **7**:167, 1975.

92. Kissane, J.M.: Tumors of the exocrine pancreas in childhood, Cancer Treat. Res. **8**:99, 1982.

93. Lafler, C.J., and Hinerman, D.L.: A morphologic study of pancreatic carcinoma with reference to multiple thrombi, Cancer **14**:944, 1961.

94. MacMahon, B., Yen, S., Trichopoulos, D., Warren, K., and Nardi, G.: Coffee and cancer of the pancreas, N. Engl. J. Med. **304**:630, 1981.

95. Makipour, H., Cooperman, A., Danzi, J.T., and Farmer, R.G.: Carcinoma of the ampulla of Vater: review of 38 cases with emphasis on treatment and prognostic factors, Ann. Surg. **183**:341, 1976.

96. Malagelada, J.R.: Pancreatic cancer: an overview of epidemiology, clinical presentation, and diagnosis, Mayo Clin. Proc. **54**:459, 1979.

97. Mikal, S., and Campbell, A.J.A.: Carcinoma of the pancreas: diagnostic and operative criteria based on 100 consecutive autopsies, Surgery **28**:963, 1950.

98. Miller, J.R., Bagenstoss, A.H., and Comfort, M.W.: Carcinoma of the pancreas: effects of histological types and grade of malignancy on its behavior, Cancer **4**:233, 1951.

99. Mills, P.K., Beeson, W.L., Abbey, D.E., Fraser, G.E., and Phillips, L.P.: Dietary habits and past medical history as related to fatal pancreas cancer risk among adventists, Cancer **61**:2578, 1988.

100. Morohoshi, T., Kanda, M., Horie, A., Chott, A., Dryer, T., Klöppel, G., and Heitz, P.U.: Immunocytochemical markers of uncommon pancreatic tumors: acinar cell carcinoma, pancreatoblastoma, and solid cystic (papillary-cystic) tumor, Cancer **59**:739, 1987.

101. Neibling, H.A.: Primary sarcoma of the pancreas, Am. Surg. **34**:690, 1968.

102. Oertel, J.E., Mendelsohn, G., and Compagno, J.: Solid and papillary epithelial neoplasms of the pancreas, Cancer Treat. Res. **8**:167, 1982.

103. Pour, P., Mohr, U., Cardesa, A., et al.: Pancreatic neoplasms in an animal and model: morphological, biological, and comparative studies, Cancer **36**:379, 1975.

104. Probstein, J.B., and Blumenthal, H.T.: Progressive malignant degeneration of a cystadenoma of the pancreas, Arch. Surg. **81**:683, 1960.

105. Reyes, C.V., and Wang, T.: Undifferentiated small cell carcinoma of the pancreas: a report of five cases, Cancer **47**:2500, 1981.

106. Rosai, J.: Carcinoma of pancreas simulating giant cell tumor of bone: electron microscopic evidence of its acinar cell origin. Cancer **22**:333, 1968.

107. Salmon, P.A.: Carcinoma of the pancreas and extrahepatic biliary system, Surgery **60**:554, 1966.

108. Warren, K.W., Baasch, J.W., and Thum, C.W.: Carcinoma of the pancreas, Surg. Clin. North Am. **48**:601, 1968.

109. Weinstein, J.J.: Carcinoma of the head of the pancreas and periampullary area, Am. J. Gastroenterol. **37**:629, 1962.

110. Wise, L., Pizzimbono, C., and Dehner, L.P.: Periampullary cancer: a clinicopathologic study of sixty-two patients, Am. J. Surg. **131**:141, 1976.

111. Wynder, E.L., Mabuchi, K., Maruchi, N., and Fortner, J.G.: Epidemiology of cancer of the pancreas, J. Natl. Cancer Inst. **50**:645, 1973.

112. Wynder, E.L.: An epidemiological evaluation of the causes of cancer of the pancreas, Cancer Res. **35**:2228, 1975.

113. Yamaguchi, K., and Enjoji, M.: Carcinoma of the ampulla of Vater: a clinicopathologic study and pathologic staging of 109 cases of carcinoma and 5 cases of adenoma, Cancer **59**:506, 1987.

Diabetes mellitus

114. Allen, A.C.: So-called intercapillary glomerulosclerosis: a lesion associated with diabetes mellitus, Arch. Pathol. **32**:33, 1941.

115. Barnett, A.H., Eff, C., Leslie, R.D.G., and Pyke, D.A.: Diabetes in identical twins: a study of 200 pairs, Diabetologia **20**:87, 1981.

116. Bottazzo, G.F., Dean, B.M., McNally, J.M., MacKay, E.H., Swift, P.G.F., and Gamble, D.R.: In situ characterization of autoimmune phenomena and expression of HLA molecules in the pancreas in diabetic insulitis, N. Engl. J. Med. **313**:353, 1985.

117. Cerasi, E., and Luft, R.: The plasma insulin response to glucose infusion in healthy subjects and in diabetes mellitus, Acta Endocrinol. **55**:278, 1967.

118. Cogan, D.G., and Kuwabara, T.: Capillary shunts in the pathogenesis of diabetic retinopathy, Diabetes **12**:293, 1963.

119. Craighead, J.E., and Steinke, J.: Diabetes mellitus–like syndrome in mice infected with encephalomyocarditis virus, Am. J. Pathol. **63**:119, 1971.

120. Cudworth, A.G.: Type I diabetes mellitus, Diabetologia **14**:281, 1978.

121. Ehrlich, J.G., and Ratner, I.M.: Amyloidosis of the islets of Langerhans, Am. J. Pathol. **38**:49, 1961.

122. Ellenberg, M.: Current status of diabetes neuropathy, Metabolism **22**:657, 1973.

123. Foulis, A.K.: The pathogenesis of beta cell destruction in type I (insulin-dependent) diabetes mellitus, J. Pathol. **152**:141, 1987.

124. Howell, S.L., Kostianovsky, M., and Lacy, P.E.: Beta granule formation in isolated islets of Langerhans: a study by electron microscopic radioautography, J. Cell Biol. **42**:695, 1969.

125. Howell, S.L.: The mechanism of insulin secretion, Diabetologia **26**:319, 1984.

126. Irvine, W.J., McCallum, C.J., Gray, R.S., Campbell, C.J., Duncan, L.J.P., Farquhar, J.W., Vaughan, H., and Morris, P.J.: Pancreatic islet-cell antibodies in diabetes mellitus correlated with the duration and type of diabetes, coexistent autoimmune disease, and HLA type, Diabetes **26**:138, 1977.

127. Kilo, C., Vogler, N., and Williamson, J.R.: Muscle capillary basement membrane changes related to aging and to diabetes mellitus, Diabetes **21**:881, 1972.

128. Kimmelstiel, P., and Wilson, C.: Intercapillary lesions in the glomeruli of the kidney, Am. J. Pathol. **12**:83, 1936.

129. Krupin, T., Waltman, S.R., Scharp, D.W., Oestrich, C., Feldman, S.D., Becker, B., Ballinger, W.F., and Lacy, P.E.: Ocular fluorophotometry in streptozotocin diabetes mellitus in the rat: the effect of pancreatic islet isografts, Invest. Ophthalmol. Visual Sci. **18**:1185, 1979.

130. Lacy, P.E., Davie, J.M., and Finke, F.H.: Prolongation of islet allograft survival following *in vitro* culture (24° C) and a single injection of ALS, Science **204**:312, 1979.

131. Lacy, P.E., and Davie, J.M.: Transplantation of pancreatic islets, Annu. Rev. Immunol. **2**:183, 1984.

132. Lacy, P.E., and Wright, P.H.: Allergic interstitial pancreatitis in rats injected with guinea pig anti-insulin serum, Diabetes **14**:634, 1965.

133. Lacy, P.E.: Beta cell secretion—from the standpoint of a pathobiologist, Diabetes **19**:895, 1970.

134. Lacy, P.E.: Islet transplantation, Clin. Chem. **32**:B76, 1986.

135. Lafferty, K.J., Prowse, S.J., Simeonovic, C.J., and Warren, H.S.: Immunobiology of tissue transplantation: a return to the passenger leukocyte concept, Annu. Rev. Immunol. **1**:143, 1983.

136. Nagler, W., and Taylor, H.: Diabetic coma with acute inflammation of islets of Langerhans, JAMA **184**:723, 1963.

137. Nerup, J., Platz, P., Ryder, L.P., Thomsen, M., and Svejgaard, A.: HLA, islet cell antibodies, and types of diabetes mellitus, Diabetes **27**:247, 1978.

138. Orci, L.: A portrait of the pancreatic B cell, Diabetologia **10**:163, 1974.

139. Orci, L.: The insulin factory: a tour of the plant surroundings and a visit to the assembly line, Diabetologia **28**:528, 1985.

140. Sarvetnick, N., Liggitt, D., Pitts, S.L., Hansen, S.E., and Stewart, T.A.: Insulin-dependent diabetes mellitus induced in transgenic mice by ectopic expression of class III MHC and interferon-gamma, Cell **52**:773, 1988.

141. Schmidt, R.E., Plurad, S.B., Olack, B.J., and Scharp, D.W.: The effect of pancreatic islet transplantation and insulin therapy on experimental diabetic autonomic neuropathy, Diabetes **32**:532, 1983.

142. Silverman, J.L.: Eosinophile infiltration in the pancreas of infants of diabetic mothers, Diabetes **12**:528, 1963.

143. Steffes, M.W., Brown, D.M., Basgen, J.M., and Mauer, S.M.: Amelioration of mesangial volume and surface alterations following islet transplantation in diabetic rats, Diabetes **29**:509, 1980.

144. Steiner, D.F., Cunningham, D., Spigelman, L., and Aten, B.: Insulin biosynthesis: evidence for a precursor, Science **157**:697, 1967.

145. Tattersall, R.B., and Pyke, D.A.: Diabetes in identical twins, Lancet **2**:1120, 1972.

146. Toreson, W.E.: Glycogen infiltration (so-called hydropic degeneration) in the pancreas in human and experimental diabetes mellitus, Am. J. Pathol. **52**:1099, 1968.

147. Volk, B.W., and Arquilla, E.R.: The diabetic pancreas, ed. 2, New York, 1985, Plenum Medical Book Co.

148. Williamson, J.R., and Kilo, C.: Current status of capillary basement membrane disease in diabetes mellitus, Diabetes **26**:65, 1977.

149. Woehrle, M., Markmann, J.F., Silvers, W.K., Barker, C.F., and Naji, A.: Transplantation of cultured pancreatic islets to BB rats, Surgery **100**:334, 1986.

Neoplasms of pancreatic islets

150. Creutzfeldt, W.: Pancreatic endocrine tumors: the riddle of their origin and hormone secretion, Isr. J. Med. Sci. **11**:762, 1975.

151. Creutzfeldt, W., Arnold, R., Creutzfeldt, C., Deuticke, U., Frerichs, H., and Track, N.S.: Biochemical and morphological investigations of 30 human insulinomas, Diabetologia **9**:217, 1973.

152. Duff, G.L.: The pathology of islet cell tumors of the pancreas, Am. J. Med. Sci. **203**:437, 1942.

153. Frantz, V.K.: Tumors of islet cells with hyperinsulinism: benign, malignant, and questionable, Ann. Surg. **112**:161, 1940.

154. Howard, J.M., Moss, N.H., and Rhoads, J.E.: Hyperinsulinism and islet cell tumors of the pancreas, Int. Abstr. Surg. **90**:417, 1950.

155. Laidlaw, G.F.: Nesidioblastoma, the islet tumor of the pancreas, Am. J. Pathol. **14**:125, 1938.

156. Sieracki, J., Marshall, R.B., and Horn, R.C., Jr.: Tumors of the pancreatic islets, Cancer **13**:347, 1960

Glucagonomas, gastrinomas, vipomas, somatostatinomas, and diarrheogenic tumors

157. Bloom, S.R., and Polak, J.M.: Glucagonomas, VIPomas and somatostatinomas, Clin. Endocrinol. Metabol. **9**:285, 1980.

158. Greider, M.H., and McGuigan, J.E.: Cellular localization of gastrin in the human pancreas, Diabetes **20**:389, 1971.

159. Greider, M.H., Rosai, J., and McGuigan, J.E.: The human pancreatic islet cells and their tumors. II. Ulcerogenic and diarrheogenic tumors, Cancer **33**:1423, 1974.

160. Heitz, P.U., Klöppel, G., Häcki, W.H., Polak, J.M., and Pearse, A.G.E.: Nesidioblastosis: the pathologic basis of persistent hyperinsulinemia hypoglycemia in infants, Diabetes **26**:632, 1977.

161. Krejs, G.J., Orci, L., Conlon, J.M., Ravazzola, M., David, G.R., Raskin, P., Collins, S.M., McCarthy, D.M., Baetens, D., Rubenstein, A., Aldor, T.A., and Unger, R.H.: Somatostatinoma syndrome, N. Engl. J. Med. **301**:285, 1979.

162. Mallison, C.N., Bloom, S.R., Warin, A.P., Salmon, P.R., and Cox, B.: A glucagonoma syndrome, Lancet **2**:1, 1974.

163. McGavran, M.H., Unger, R.H., Recant, L., et al.: A glucagon-secreting A cell carcinoma of the pancreas, N. Engl. J. Med. **274**:1408, 1966.

164. McGuigan, J.E., and Trudeau, W.L.: Immunochemical measurement of elevated levels of gastrin in the serum of patients with pancreatic tumors of the Zollinger-Ellison variety, N. Engl. J. Med. **278**:1308, 1968.

165. Zollinger, R.M., and Ellison, E.H.: Primary peptic ulcerations of the jejunum associated with islet cell tumors of the pancreas, Ann. Surg. **142**:709, 1955.

28 Hematopoietic System: Bone Marrow and Blood, Spleen, and Lymph Nodes

ROGERS C. GRIFFITH
CHRISTINE G. JANNEY

The principal hematopoietic organs in the adult include the bone marrow and peripheral blood, the thymus gland, the spleen, and the lymph nodes. These organs are related in their development, structure, and function primarily through the production, sustenance, and circulation of blood cells (erythrocytes, granulocytes, and platelets) and cells of the immune system (lymphocytes and macrophages). The hematopoietic system is affected by congenital and acquired disorders and by neoplasia, which often affect the patient dramatically because of the generalized effects through a distributed organ system.

BONE MARROW AND BLOOD
Development, structure, and function

The earliest hematopoietic ('blood-forming') cells arise from the mesoderm of the embryonic yolk sac, where erythroblastic islands are detectable during the second week of gestation. Red blood cells that develop from the yolk sac are unique in that they contain embryonic hemoglobin, are quite large, and retain their nuclei throughout their life span. Yolk-sac hematopoiesis declines after the sixth week and ceases by the tenth week. The liver becomes the major blood-forming organ from the second to seventh month of gestation. Hepatic erythroblasts give rise to circulating anucleate, slightly macrocytic red blood cells. The predominant hemoglobin is fetal type (Hb F), though a small amount of adult type (Hb A) is detectable. The bone marrow assumes primary hematopoietic function during the third trimester, when granulocytes, megakaryocytes, and erythroid cells are produced. At birth, virtually all hematopoiesis takes place in the marrow. A switch from predominantly fetal to adult hemoglobin occurs in the immediate postnatal period, and the red blood cells produced are of normal size.[686]

At birth and for the first few years of life, virtually all possible marrow space contains hematopoietically active marrow. By 5 years of age, the rate of skeletal growth exceeds the requirement for blood-forming cells, and yellow, fatty marrow begins to replace the active, red marrow peripherally. At 20 years of age, hematopoietically active marrow is normally confined to the vertebrae, pelvis, proximal ends of long bones, sternum, ribs, and skull.[198] The total weight of red marrow in adults is estimated at 5% of body weight, nearly equal to that of the liver. By age 30, the red marrow contains equal parts of hematopoietic and adipose tissue, with a rate of myeloid cells to erythroid cells (M:E ratio) of about 2.5 to 1.

Structurally, marrow consists of blood-forming cells, fat cells, and a reticulin fiber network associated with arborizing blood vessels and stromal cells, and it fills the central and spongy portions of the bony skeleton.[120] The blood supply is derived from two sources: the central nutrient artery with its thin-walled arterial branches and the periosteal capillaries. These vessels communicate with a capillary-venous sinus network throughout the marrow, through which newly formed blood cells enter the circulation. The sinus endothelium is continuous and mediates this release by a transcellular passage rather than through intercellular spaces. Normally only mature erythrocytes, granulocytes, and platelets are discharged into the sinuses. Mechanisms regulating this release of mature cells while excluding immature cells are poorly understood. Megakaryocytes and erythroblastic islands lie adjacent to bone trabeculas, and lymphocytes and plasma cells next to the arterioles. Within the marrow space, hematopoietic cells lie in cords between the sinuses.[720] The sinus endothelia are capable of endocytosis, and closely associated monocytes provide additional phagocytic capacity.

Functionally, effective hematopoiesis depends on the integrity of the entire hematopoietic microenvironment, which includes the cellular and reticulin structural framework, and various growth, inhibitory, and other factors secreted by stromal cells, lymphocytes, and monocytes in the marrow.[20,169,815] Marrow, like other proliferating tissues, has cells capable of self-renewal and of differentiation, known as stem cells. All hematopoietic cells, including erythrocytes, granulo-cytes, mononuclear leukocytes (monocytes), mega-karyocytes, and lymphocytes, are derived from a common pluripotent stem cell. Under appropriate conditions, this cell gives rise to cells committed to lymphoid or to myeloid differentiation. These stem cells are morphologically indistinguishable and are detectable and classified on the basis of the type of cell colony that is produced in spleen or soft agar culture assays. Thus the myeloid stem cell may be called "CFU-S" or "CFU-GEMM" (colony forming unit—spleen, or colony forming unit—granulocyte, erythrocyte, macrophage, megakaryocyte) depending on the assay. Further differentiation is induced by specific colony-stimulating factors, including erythropoietin, other granulopoietins, thrombopoietin, and various leukokines, that results in stem-cell commitment to a single lineage and to morphologically recognizable red blood cell, granulocyte, and megakaryocyte precursors in the marrow.[271,304,578,664]

The morphologic stages of maturation in the different cell series are recognized by Romanowsky-stained (usually Wright's stain) marrow-aspirate smears and are thoroughly described and illustrated in atlases of hematology.[367,810] Although it is difficult to classify each cell in histologic section, assessment of the M:E ratio and general maturation can be done. In general, the youngest cells, myeloblasts and erythroblasts, have large nuclei with delicate chromatin and prominent nucleoli and a rim of dark-blue, ribosome-rich cytoplasm. As the cells mature, they develop their distinctive nuclear and cytoplasmic characteristics. In the red cell series, the round erythroblastic nucleus becomes smaller, darker, and progressively more pyknotic, and the cytoplasm becomes pinker, reflecting increasing hemoglobin content, until the normoblast stage is recognizable. Finally, the nucleus is extruded producing anuclear reticulocytes and mature red blood cells. In the myeloid line, the myeloblast enlarges and gains nonspecific azurophil granules to become a promyelocyte. Specific cytoplasmic granules in myelocytes distinguish granulocytic, eosinophilic, and basophilic precursors. Each then undergoes progressive changes in nuclear shape through the metamyelocyte and band forms, until the mature neutrophil, eosinophil, or basophil is formed. During megakaryocytic maturation, cells undergo cycles of DNA synthesis without cell division, producing polyploid mononuclear cells. Thus megakaryocytes are very large relative to other marrow cells because of their large, multilobed nuclei and abundant eosinophilic cytoplasm. Production of monocytes, lymphocytes, and mast cells also occurs in the marrow as well as in extramedullary tissues.

Other functions less obvious than blood cell formation are also performed by marrow elements. In addi-tion to its role in the release of blood cells into the circulation, an important function of sinus endothelium is the removal of intravascular particulate material by endocytosis. Marrow macrophages are important in phagocytosis of defective cells and extruded erythroblast nuclei, and they as well as T-lymphocytes are known to produce many growth, differentiation, and regulatory factors.[291,418,475,578,621]

Blood cells

Blood consists of plasma and mostly mature, nondividing cells, each type with specific functions and a finite life span. Maintenance of normal blood counts depends on the balance between rates of blood cell formation, release from the marrow, and survival in circulation. Normal blood cell counts and morphology imply normal marrow cellularity and function, and derangements of hematopoiesis are discussed at length later in this chapter. Measurements of cell release and survival are more difficult to obtain. A normal reticulocyte count, generally indicates normal release of mature red cells from the marrow. In hemolytic anemias, compensatory red cell production is effective, and the reticulocyte count is increased in response to the destruction of erythrocytes. A low reticulocyte count indicates erythrocytic hypoplasia or ineffective erythropoiesis, though other studies are necessary to distinguish the specific cause. Red cell survival averages 110 to 120 days and can be measured clinically by an in vivo radioisotopic chromium-labeling assay. Abnormal red cells often have shortened survival. Measures of similar parameters for neutrophils are not generally available. The life span of platelets is believed to be about 10 to 21 days, and white blood cells remain in the blood only a matter of hours before they enter the tissues. The measurement of neutrophils is difficult, since neutrophils may exit the circulation quickly into the tissues, or they may remain in one of two intravascular populations: a circulating population that is measured by the white blood cell count and a population that rests against blood vessel endothelium. Marginated white cells may be rapidly recruited into the circulation in response to the acute stress of infection, resulting in leukocytosis without, at least initially, an increase in granulopoiesis. Maintaining steady-state levels of blood cells is a dynamic and complex process and the blood does not always reflect what is occurring in the marrow.

Primary evaluation of bone marrow disorders

The marrow may be involved by a variety of pathologic conditions, not only hematologic disorders themselves, but also metastatic neoplasms, disseminated granulomatous infections, stromal reactions, metabolic bone disease, sarcoidosis, vasculitis, storage diseases, amyloidosis, and radiation effects. Thus there are numerous clinical indications for bone marrow examination, which includes among others the evaluation of cytopenias, myeloproliferative and lymphoproliferative states, hypercalcemia, and fevers of unknown origin, the assessment of chemotherapy effect and bone marrow transplantation, and staging of malignant neoplasms.

Two techniques are used to obtain marrow for study: aspiration and core biopsy.[35,52,73,460,613] Marrow may be aspirated through a large-bore needle, usually from the posterior iliac crest but also from the sternum in adults or the tibia in infants. Needle-core biopsy samples are usually obtained from the posterior iliac crest. Each type of specimen has certain advantages, and a combination of techniques yield the most information and is more frequently done in adults. Aspirated material is routinely used to prepare direct, particle smears, which when stained with a Romanowsky stain yields excellent cellular morphology. Aspirated marrow may also be processed for ancillary studies, such as cytochemistries, cell-marker studies, chromosome analysis, DNA-hybridization studies, electron microscopy, biochemical analysis, and microbiologic cultures. In contrast to smears, histologic sections of marrow biopsy specimens preserve the architecture of the tissue and the relationships between hematopoietic cells, stroma, blood vessels, and bone.[84,352] Biopsy is also more useful for the assessment of marrow cellularity and to demonstrate granulomas, fibrosis, vascular lesions, and focal involvement by neoplasms.[200,239,400] Biopsy should be performed when an aspiration yields no marrow tissue, which occurs as a result of fibrosis or pronounced hypercellularity. Lesions of bone can be evaluated only by a biopsy.

Aplasia, hypoplasia, and hyperplasia

Bone marrow cellularity is expressed as the percentage of the marrow area in section occupied by hematopoietic cells. Cellularity varies with age. At birth, the cellularity is 100%, adipose tissue can be identified in marrow particles at 2 weeks, and by 2 to 3 months of age the cellularity approaches 85% to 95%.[704] By 30 years of age and through most of adult life, the mean cellularity is 50% with a further decline after age 70.[308] In general, marrow that is less than 25% cellular is regarded as hypocellular or hypoplastic and that greater than 60% as hypercellular or hyperplastic. Aplasia refers to the virtual absence of hematopoietic cells in the marrow. Both hyperplasia and hypoplasia may be selective, affecting one or more cell lineages. Hypoplasia is reflected in blood by the reduction of affected circulating cells, that is, anemia, leukopenia, thrombocytopenia, or a combination of these. Generalized marrow hypoplasia results in pancytopenia, a reduced number of

all cell types. Similarly, marrow hyperplasia usually results in increasing the number of circulating cells of the hyperplastic lineage but not always. In some conditions, cytopenias are associated with hypercellular marrow, which may be attributable to accelerated destruction or consumption of cells in the circulation. In hemolytic anemias, for example, increased destruction of erythrocytes is accompanied by compensatory erythroid hyperplasia in the marrow; anemia results when the degree of hyperplasia is inadequate to compensate fully for the amount of hemolysis. Hypercellular marrow with cytopenias may also result from ineffective cell production, maturation defects, or defective cell release from the marrow. These mechanisms are believed to be important in the pathogenesis of megaloblastic anemias and in the myelodysplastic syndromes.

Disorders of erythrocytes

Red cell disorders may be classified in a variety of ways. In this section, we will consider selected erythrocyte disorders in terms of their effects on the rate and quality of erythropoiesis in various conditions. Pathologic conditions affecting red blood cells usually result in anemia, a reduction in red cell mass or concentration. Polycythemia, an increased red cell mass or concentration, is less common than anemia. Regardless of the cause of the anemia, the result is a decreased ability of the blood to oxygenate tissues. Signs and symptoms depend on severity and how quickly the drop in hematocrit (red cell concentration) occurred. Anemia of acute onset, as with sudden blood loss, is less well tolerated than a chronic anemia of similar severity is. General clinical findings include pallor, tachycardia, weakness, and fatigue. In an attempt to compensate for the diminished oxygen-carrying capacity of the blood, the cardiovascular system increases the cardiac output and shunts blood flow to organs most sensitive to hypoxemia. Dizziness, syncope, stroke, angina pectoris, and cardiac and renal failure may result from inadequate oxygenation of brain, heart, and kidneys.

Disorders with decreased red blood cell production

Aplastic anemia. Aplastic anemia is defined as at least two cytopenias, that is, anemia, leukopenia, or thrombocytopenia, associated with a marrow cellularity of less than 25% of normal. The marrow consists largely of adipose tissue with scattered, often perivascular, lymphocytes, and plasma cells (Fig. 28-1). Small clusters of hematopoietic elements are usually identified. Bone-marrow biopsy is necessary in patients with pancytopenia to exclude other causes, such as myelodysplasia, leukemia, malignant lymphoma, myelofibrosis, and metastatic carcinoma.

Aplastic anemia may be congenital, acquired, or id-

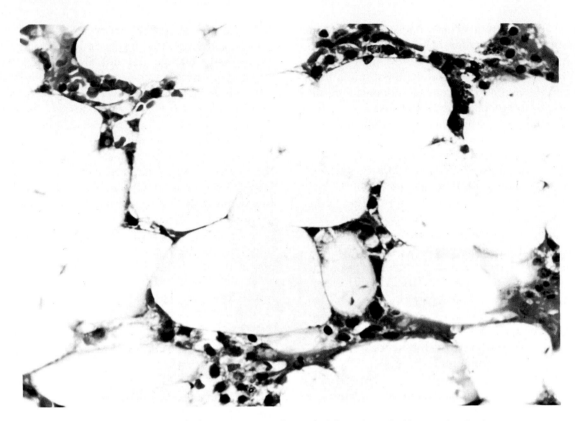

Fig. 28-1. Aplastic bone marrow after administration of chloramphenicol.

iopathic.[5,337] The disorder affects all ages and both sexes and may have an insidious, or less frequently, an abrupt onset. Exposure to chemicals or drugs is the most commonly known cause of aplastic anemia. When the offending agent is a predictable myelotoxin, such as benzene, alkylating agents, or arsenic, the marrow usually recovers when the agent is withdrawn. Aplasia from an idiosyncratic reaction to such drugs as phenylbutazone, streptomycin, chlorpromazine, or chloramphenicol is unpredictable and rare but may also be irreversible. Ionizing irradiation is a cause of aplastic anemia in persons receiving therapeutic irradiation, in radiologists, and in persons exposed to excessive radiation levels from nuclear explosions or accidents. Various infections, including infectious mononucleosis, hepatitis, and tuberculosis, dengue, and the multiple infections in AIDS, have been cited as causes of aplasia. However, since most infected patients are treated with drugs, the exact etiologic associations are uncertain in many cases. It is clear that a rare proportion of patients with infectious hepatitis of non-A, non-B type subsequently develop aplasia.[823] Congenital and familial aplastic anemia with or without congenital anomalies occur but are much less frequent than acquired forms of aplasia are. Fanconi's anemia is an autosomal recessive genetic disorder characterized by aplastic anemia, increased chromosomal breakage, and a variety of con-genital defects including hyperpigmentation, renal defects, and upper limb hypoplasias. An increased incidence of acute leukemias and possibly other tumors has been noted in this disorder.[642,643,712]

Despite the large number of possible causes of pancytopenia with hypocellular marrow, the cause remains unknown in almost two thirds of affected patients. In vitro studies of marrow growth from patients with aplastic anemia generally support the hypothesis that the disorder is most often attributable to stem cell injury or a defect.[111,208] Autoantibodies to stem cells or committed erythroid precursors have been documented in some patients with systemic lupus erythematosus and pure red cell aplasia.[296,824] Cell-mediated stem-cell cytolysis, defective colony-stimulating or colony-inhibiting factors, and an abnormal hematopoietic microenvironment in the marrow have been implicated in a few cases.[5,834]

Regardless of cause, aplastic anemia is a very serious disorder. A 5-year survival of 30% has been reported, with only 10% recovering full marrow function. Generally, younger persons in whom a known toxic chemical or drug can be withdrawn have the best prognosis. Recently, administration of antithymocyte globulin or colony-stimulating factors has benefited some patients.[452,564] Bone-marrow transplantation in selected patients offers the prospect of cure.[7,467]

Pure red blood cell aplasia. Pure red blood cell aplasia is a rare disorder characterized by severe anemia and the virtual absence of recognizable erythroid precursors in the marrow with sparing of the myeloid and megakaryocytic lineages.[5] The acquired or adult form of the disease is often associated with thymoma, though it also occurs with chronic lymphocytic leukemia, chronic myelocytic leukemia, systemic lupus erythematosus, and autoimmune thyroiditis and as an isolated disorder. Most cases of adult red cell aplasia appear to be mediated by IgG autoantibodies specific for erythroblasts or erythropoietin. In contrast, the less common congenital form of the disease, the Diamond-Blackfan syndrome, is usually attributed to T lymphocyte–mediated suppression of erythropoiesis. Evidence indicates that a defect in the marrow microenvironment, a primary erythroid stem cell defect, or autoantibodies to erythropoietin may be causative in some cases.[111,406] Transient aplastic crisis in sickle cell anemia represents a form of acquired pure red cell aplasia that is caused by human parvovirus infection with lysis of erythroid progenitor cells.[823] The role of viruses in other forms of aplasia is unclear. In addition to alleviating the primary disorder, red cell transfusions, plasmapheresis, and the administration of androgens, corticosteroids, and other immunomodulators may be effective therapy.[126,474] Bone marrow transplantation is an option in some patients.[799]

Megaloblastic anemia. Megaloblastic anemia is a group of disorders characterized by hematopoietic precursors that are larger than normal at all stages of differentiation with delayed nuclear maturation relative to that of the cytoplasm (referred to as nuclear-cytoplasmic asynchrony). The majority of megaloblastic anemias are caused by deficiency or impaired utilization of vitamin B_{12} or folate, which results in defective DNA synthesis.[119,310,316] The hematologic changes and morphology appear similar regardless of cause.

The marrow is hypercellular with a disturbed maturation that is most evident in the erythroid series but also affects the myeloid and megakaryocytic cells (Fig. 28-2). The megaloblastic change in erythroblasts consists in nuclear enlargement with fine, immature-appearing chromatin that fails to condense with cellular maturation. Many of the abnormal erythrocytes produced are destroyed before leaving the marrow. Characteristic macro-ovalocytes are released into the circulation and are hemolyzed at an accelerated rate. Nuclear-cytoplasmic asynchrony is also seen in the myeloid series as giant metamyelocytes, bands, and hypersegmented neutrophils and in the bizarre, hyperlobular megakaryocytes. Leukopenia, thrombocytopenia, or both frequently result. Other proliferating tissues, such as the gastrointestinal tract, are also affected by these vitamin deficiencies and show similar nuclear morphology.

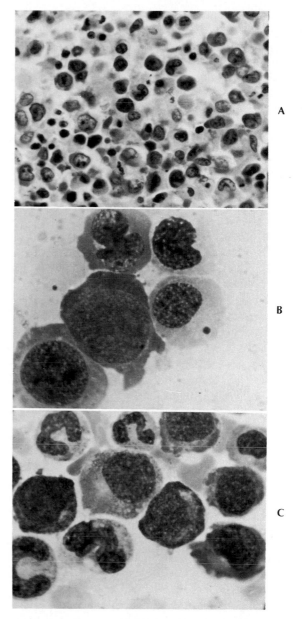

Fig. 28-2. Megaloblastic dyspoiesis in bone marrow. **A,** Histologic section. **B,** Smear. All cells are megaloblastic erythroid precursors. **C,** Smear. Notice giant neutrophilic metamyelocytes and band cells.

Megaloblastic anemia is diagnosed on the basis of blood and marrow examination. The specific cause can usually be determined by assays for serum vitamin B_{12} and serum and red cell folate levels. The distinction is important, for although there may be a hematologic response to folate administration, folate alone will not arrest the associated progressive neurologic disease that occurs in vitamin B_{12} deficiency known as "subacute combined degeneration of the spinal cord." Neurologic signs and symptoms include paresthesias, sensory loss, ataxia, impotence, and impairment of bladder and bowel control. Myelin and axonal degeneration affect the pyramidal tracts, initially in the lower cervical and upper thoracic cord. With time the degeneration may extend farther along the cord, and peripheral neuropathy may also result.

Vitamin B_{12} deficiency may occur because of a variety of causes and results in megaloblastic anemia. Malabsorption and inadequate dietary intake are the most important causes of vitamin B_{12} deficiency. Vitamin B_{12} is present in all foods of animal origin, including milk and eggs, and so dietary lack is virtually confined to strict vegetarians. Even in these persons, because the vitamin is conserved by an efficient enterohepatic circulation, it takes many years to deplete the body's stores. Much more common is impaired absorption by either deficiency of intrinsic factor or disease affecting the site of B_{12} absorption from the terminal ileum.

Pernicious anemia is vitamin B_{12} deficiency caused by inadequate production or function in intrinsic factor that is necessary for the intestinal absorption of B_{12}. Most patients with pernicious anemia are between 50 and 70 years of age, and the disease is rare before 30 years of age. Gastric atrophy with achlorhydria is characteristic. Autoantibodies against parietal cells, intrinsic factor, or intrinsic factor–B_{12} complexes are demonstrable in the majority of patients.[166] Other autoimmune disorders, such as Hashimoto's thyroiditis, Graves' disease, adrenal hypofunction, and rheumatoid arthritis, are more common in patients with pernicious anemia and their families, and there appears to be an increased risk of gastric carcinoma in patients with pernicious anemia.[320] Congenital absence of intrinsic factor production or deficiency in transcobalamin II, causing vitamin B_{12} deficiency, without autoantibodies or gastric atrophy is rare. Gastrectomy represents an acquired condition with absent intrinsic factor production. Disorders affecting the terminal ileum, such as Crohn's disease, sprue, or ileal resections may interfere with B_{12} absorption.[433] Abnormal bacterial flora in the upper gastrointestinal tract, especially with surgically constructed blind loops, diverticula, or other conditions causing stasis, may metabolize vitamin B_{12}, thus depleting the amount available for absorption. Fish tapeworms also compete with the body for vitamin B_{12} within the small intestine.

Folate deficiency causes a megaloblastic anemia indistinguishable from that attributable to vitamin B_{12} deficiency but is not associated with neurologic abnormalities.[697] Folates are present in most types of animal and vegetable foods but are heat labile and are largely destroyed in cooking. The absorption of folate from the upper small intestine is normally balanced by obligate losses in urine and sweat. Hepatic stores of folate may be depleted within months when the diet is folate de-

ficient or when an increased folate requirement is superimposed on marginal dietary intake. Inadequate dietary intake of folate is most common among the poor, alcoholics, and mentally impaired persons. Increased requirements occur in pregnancy, chronic hemolytic anemia, and malignancy.[260] Diseases affecting the upper small intestine, including Crohn's disease and tropical sprue, and certain drugs, such as phenytoin and oral contraceptives, may interfere with folate absorption.[433]

Megaloblastic anemias independent of vitamin B_{12} or folate deficiencies may be caused by drug-induced impairment of DNA synthesis.[646] Responsible agents include folate antagonists such as methotrexate, metabolic inhibitors of purine and pyrimidine synthesis, alkylating agents, and nitrous oxide. The majority of these drugs are used in the treatment of malignancies, and the mechanism of their antineoplastic effect, interference with DNA synthesis, also affects normal proliferating tissues, such as the marrow and gastrointestinal tract.

Iron-deficiency anemia. Iron deficiency is a very common cause of anemia, affecting an estimated 500 to 600 million persons worldwide.[141] The lack of iron results in deficient hemoglobin synthesis and ineffective erythropoiesis. As in other types of nutritional deficiencies, iron deficiency may be caused by inadequate dietary intake, intestinal malabsorption, or an increased requirement. The most common cause of iron deficiency in Western countries is chronic blood loss. In women whose total body iron stores are normally low because of menstruation, abnormal uterine bleeding because of dysfunctional bleeding or neoplasms may lead to severe iron deficiency. The gastrointestinal tract is the most common site of bleeding in men and postmenopausal women; varices, aspirin ingestion, peptic ulcer, diverticular disease, hemorrhoids, neoplasms, and a variety of other lesions may cause sufficient blood loss to deplete total body iron stores. Deficient dietary intake of iron by itself is uncommon as a cause of iron deficiency in adults in the United States but remains an important one in infants in developing countries. Increased requirement for iron accompanies rapid growth occurring during infancy, childhood, adolescence, and pregnancy and lactation. Iron stores may readily be depleted if ample amounts of iron are not obtained from the diet.[604] Intestinal malabsorption of iron occurs infrequently but may occur in association with sprue or after gastrectomy. Rarely, chronic hemoglobinuria results in iron deficiency.

Regardless of cause, the anemia of iron deficiency is a hypochromic, microcytic anemia. The red cells are abnormally small with pale cytoplasm related to insufficient hemoglobin content. The marrow is usually hypercellular predominantly because of erythroid hyperplasia of poorly hemoglobinized erythroid precursors.

An iron stain verifies that sideroblasts and hemosiderin normally present in the marrow are absent. Confirmatory laboratory values include decreased serum iron and ferritin levels, increased transferrin levels reflecting reduced iron stores in the marrow and liver, and increased red cell protoporphyrin levels because of deficient heme synthesis.[68,121]

Besides impaired hemoglobin production and resultant anemia, there is iron deficiency from a depletion of tissue iron that is required by iron-containing enzymes, causing dysfunction in nonhematologic organs. The gastrointestinal tract is particularly vulnerable, and atrophic glossitis, stomatitis, gastritis, and esophageal webs may result from chronic iron depletion. Less well characterized are the deleterious effects of iron deficiency on host defense mechanisms, including cell-mediated immunity and phagocytosis, and the impairment of neurologic function, especially cognitive function.[141,161]

Other causes of decreased erythropoiesis. Sideroblastic anemias are characterized by a defect in the utilization of iron, resulting in defective heme synthesis, increased tissue iron stores, and numerous pathologic ringed sideroblasts in the marrow.[63] Erythroid hyperplasia is present in the marrow, but erythropoiesis is ineffective with decreased numbers of hypochromic, microcytic red cells being produced. A dimorphic picture with macrocytic red cells is frequently seen in the acquired forms. Causes of sideroblastic anemias include pyridoxine deficiency, chronic exposure to some drugs or chemicals including lead, and chronic alcohol abuse.[312] Rarely a congenital form of the disease occurs. Acquired idiopathic sideroblastic anemia is considered a form of myelodysplasia, since as high as 10% of these patients subsequently develop leukemia.[6,125,425]

Many chronic diseases are associated with marrow failure of obscure cause that predominantly affect erythropoiesis producing mild to severe anemia.[107] These conditions include chronic liver disease, chronic renal failure, chronic inflammatory states, such as tuberculosis and rheumatoid arthritis, and certain endocrine deficiency disorders, especially hypothyroidism. The marrow findings are nonspecific. It may be normocellular or show erythroid hypoplasia or hyperplasia. The pathogenesis of the depressed erythropoiesis is unclear and possibly multifactorial, though in individual cases there is evidence to support several different mechanisms: low levels of erythropoietin, a defect in the utilization of iron, a circulating erythropoietic toxin or inhibitor, and a component of folate or iron deficiency.[598] Regardless of cause, control or treatment of the underlying disease often corrects the anemia.

Another important cause of marrow failure is myelophthisic anemia, which refers to failure because of massive infiltration of the marrow space and replacement of the normal hematopoietic cells by metastatic carcinoma, leukemia, lymphoma, myeloma, fibrous tissue, or granulomatous infiltrates. Marrow involvement that is extensive enough to cause marrow insufficiency implies advanced disease, and other signs and symptoms referable to the primary diseases are usually identifiable. Myelophthisic processes cause the early release of immature and misshapen red cells into the blood in association with mild anemia, thrombocytopenia, leukocytosis, and small numbers of myeloblasts and nucleated erythroid procursors, referred to as a leukoerythroblastic reaction.

Disorders with increased erythropoiesis

Blood-loss anemia. The most apparent initial effect of acute hemorrhage is the drop of blood volume, which, if massive, can result in shock or death. If the person survives, a series of cardiovascular and hematologic mechanisms are activated to compensate for the loss of blood volume. Immediately after significant hemorrhage, the hemoglobin and hematocrit are normal, since cells and plasma are lost in proportion. A mild transient leukocytosis and thrombocytosis may result as leukocytes and platelets are mobilized from the marginated intravascular pool. However within 72 hours, fluid and protein shifts into the intravascular compartment, effectively restoring the plasma volume, while reducing the hematocrit.[2,143] In response, the erythropoietin level rises, and the marrow responds appropriately with erythroid hyperplasia and production of red blood cells.[209] Reticulocytosis, an indicator of increased erythropoiesis, is evident within days and peaks at about 7 days, achieving levels of 10% to 15%. The rate of erythropoiesis then declines as normal steady-state levels of blood cells are reached.[192,767] With chronic blood loss, however, the body's stores of iron become depleted over time, impairing the effect of compensatory erythropoiesis and resulting in iron-deficiency anemia.

Hemolytic anemia. Hemolytic anemias are anemias that result from an accelerated destruction of erythrocytes and shortened red cell life span. Hemolysis occurs within the intravascular compartment and the spleen. The marrow in hemolytic anemia appears similar regardless of cause, exhibiting pronounced normoblastic erythroid hyperplasia (Fig. 28-3). Over time, there is also increased hemosiderin deposition in macrophages in the marrow and other organs.[568] In severely affected persons, the need for red cells may cause considerable expansion of hematopoietically active marrow, replacing fatty yellow marrow with active red marrow throughout the skeleton. This expansion of the marrow may cause widespread bony deformities and cortical thinning, predisposing the bones to fracture. Erythropoiesis may resume in extramedullary sites such as liver and spleen. Hemolysis causes increased production and excretion of

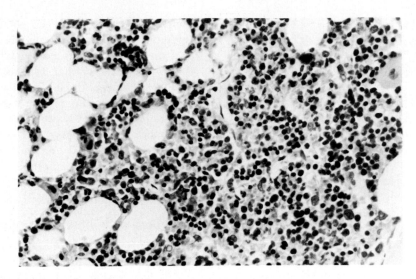

Fig. 28-3. Marrow section showing extensive erythroid hyperplasia in immune hemolytic anemia.

bilirubin, and the formation of pigment gallstones is common. Individuals with hemolytic anemias of diverse causes are susceptible to hypoplastic crises because of infections, especially with human parvovirus.[823] Typical laboratory findings in hemolytic states include reticulocytosis, low serum haptoglobin level, elevated serum, indirect bilirubin and hemoglobin concentration, and hemosiderin or hemoglobin in the urine.[730] Various abnormalities of red cells are present in the blood, depending on the cause of the hemolysis.

Numerous diverse causes of hemolytic anemia are recognized and are broadly divisible into intrinsic defects of the erythrocyte and extracorpuscular causes of hemolysis. With rare exceptions, intrinsic red cell abnormalities have a genetic basis, whereas extrinsic causes are acquired. Intrinsic red cell defects include erythrocyte membrane defects, abnormal hemoglobins, and enzyme deficiencies.

Hereditary spherocytosis, an autosomal dominant disorder, is the most common of the membrane disorders and is the most common hereditary hemolytic anemia among persons of northern European descent. The basic defect resides in the cytoskeleton and results in uniform and spherical but nondeformable and fragile erythrocytes. The expression of the disease is variable but, when severe, may cause pronounced anemia, jaundice, and splenomegaly. Splenectomy reduces the hemolysis allowing the spherocytosis to persist.

Paroxysmal nocturnal hemoglobinuria (PNH) is an acquired membrane defect of variable severity characterized by anemia with chronic intravascular hemolysis and a tendency to develop venous thromboses. Any age may be affected, though most patients are between 25 and 35 years of age. The hemolysis is paroxysmal and nocturnal in only about 25% of cases. In PNH, an increased susceptibility to complement-induced lysis can be demonstrated to affect not only erythrocytes but also granulocytes and platelets. The observation that granulocytes and platelets are also abnormal relates to the complications of frequent infections and the often fatal thrombosis of hepatic, portal, or cerebral veins seen in this disorder. PNH appears to be a stem cell disorder, occasionally transforming to aplastic anemia or acute leukemia.[225] The median survival is 10 years. Anticoagulants may benefit some patients, and bone marrow transplantations have been curative.

Disorders of hemoglobin synthesis includes the hemoglobinopathies, in which structurally abnormal hemoglobin molecules are synthesized, and the thalassemia syndromes, characterized by a reduced synthesis of one of the globin chains. These disorders are among the commonest of the single gene disorders, and the World Health Organization suggests that approximately 5% of the world population may be carriers of the more common ones.

Hundreds of structural variants of hemoglobin are known, but only a few are associated with significant disease. The most frequent molecular lesion is a point mutation, a single base substitution, in one of the globin genes; deletions and insertions are much less frequent. The red cells containing these hemoglobins may hemolyze because of denaturation or precipitation when deoxygenated (Hb S) or when exposed to certain drugs, or they may have an abnormal affinity for oxygen.

Sickle cell anemia and its variants are the most common of the hemoglobinopathies. In Hb S, there is a single base substitution in the sixth codon of the gene coding the beta-globin chain that results in the substitution of valine for glutamic acid. Although normally soluble when oxygenated, the mutant polymerizes when deoxygenated, causing the characteristic shape of the sickled erythrocyte, which results in abnormal flow characteristics of these cells. The prevalence of the abnormal gene is as high as 25% in parts of Africa and 10% in American blacks. The high prevalence in Africa relates to the advantageous resistance of heterozygous erythrocytes to parasitization by *Plasmodium falciparum* in areas of chronic endemic malaria.[777] The clinical manifestations of sickle cell disease are variable and are most severe in homozygous individuals and relatively benign in heterozygous carriers (sickle cell trait).[201] Intermediate severity may occur in individuals heterozygous for two abnormal globins, such as Hb S and Hb C. Jaundice, bilirubin gallstones, and splenomegaly are complications of chronic hemolysis. Autosplenectomy, or the chronic deterioration of splenic parenchyma and function because of recurring infarcts, occurs throughout childhood and contributes to increased susceptibility to serious infections such as pneumococcal sepsis (discussed later). Chronic leg ulcers may also be a problem. Crises caused by vaso-occlusion occur episodically and cause excruciating pain in the abdomen, chest, or extremities. Microinfarcts affecting kidneys, heart, lungs, and central nervous system may result in vascular insufficiency, organ failure, and death. Current therapy is supportive and consists in transfusions, hydration, prophylaxis, prompt treatment of infections, and analgesics. Experimental therapeutic approaches include inhibition of Hb S polymerization, induction of fetal hemoglobin synthesis, bone marrow transplantation, which has demonstrated early success, and replacement of the defective gene with a normal beta-globin gene.

The thalassemia syndromes are disorders of hemoglobin synthesis in which there is depression of the rate of synthesis of either alpha- or beta-globin chains, known as alpha-thalassemia and beta-thalassemia respectively. The molecular lesion in alpha-thalassemias is usually deletion of one or more of the four normal alpha-globin structural genes. In contrast, beta-thalassemia is rarely caused by simple gene deletion. More often there are mutations that affect the rate of transcription, produce nonfunctional mRNA, or cause abnormal mRNA splicing and processing.[686] Regardless of mechanism, the result is the same: an imbalance between alpha- and beta-chain synthesis. Thus each red cell contains reduced amounts of hemoglobin and an excess of globin chains, which may precipitate in the cytoplasm. The thalassemias have elements of both ineffective erythropoiesis and hemolysis of abnormal erythrocytes.

The clinical severity of the thalassemias is proportional to the degree of unbalanced synthesis of globin chains. Persons with alpha-thalassemia trait, in which one or two of the four genes is deleted or abnormal, are asymptomatic and usually exhibit subtle abnormalities in laboratory tests and a modestly shortened red cell life span. Hemoglobin H disease, in which three genes are deleted or abnormal, is associated with elevated Hb H, composed of four beta-chains, and chronic hemolytic anemia, which may be exacerbated by infection, drugs, or pregnancy. The absence of all four genes causes hydrops fetalis syndrome and is incompatible with extrauterine life. Most of the hemoglobin produced is Hb Barts, composed of four gamma-chains. Since the switch to beta-chain production occurs postnatally, no Hb A is produced. The beta-thalassemia syndromes also vary greatly in severity depending on whether the abnormal gene is associated with decreased or absent beta-chain synthesis. The beta-thalassemia disorders are most prevalent in Mediterranean countries, Southeast Asia, and parts of Africa. Heterozygotes with one normal beta-globin gene, known as beta-thalassemia minor, are usually asymptomatic but may exhibit mild hypochromic anemia. Beta-thalassemia major is the most severe form occurring in individuals homozygous for the beta-thalassemia gene. Severe anemia becomes apparent in the first year of life after the switch from fetal to adult hemoglobin occurs because of ineffective hematopoiesis and hemolysis. Untreated children develop pronounced deformities, hepatosplenolmegaly, and severe growth retardation, and die in infancy. Red cell transfusions help to compensate for the anemia and also reverse or suppress the exuberant erythropoiesis. However, over time, iron overload develops, and hemochromatosis can become a serious problem. Bone marrow transplantation has become an effective treatment, and the induction of fetal hemoglobin synthesis and gene-replacement therapy are current areas of investigation and experimental therapy for the severe forms of thalassemia.[149,287,542]

Deficiency of glucose-6-phosphate dehydrogenase (G6PD) is the most common of the red cell enzymatic defects.[749] The multiple variants of the disorder exhibit reduced G6PD activity, ranging from 20% to less than 5% of normal. Low levels of G6PD inhibit the pentose phosphate shunt, lowering levels of reduced glutathione and making the red cell susceptible to oxidative injury and subsequent hemolysis. An estimated 100 million persons are affected worldwide, including about 10% of American black men. Because the disease is X-linked, clinical manifestations are seen in hemizygous males and homozygous females. In the common, mild form (G6PDA), significant hemolysis is usually seen only during infectious illnesses or in association with several drugs, including sulfonamides, nitrofurantoin, phenacetin, and antimalarial drugs.

Acquired causes of hemolytic anemia include immunologic mechanisms, physical trauma, red cell infections such as malaria and babesiosis, oxidant chemicals and drugs, and hypersplenism. Immune hemolytic anemias may be mediated by preformed alloantibodies or by autoantibodies. Alloantibodies are specific for blood group antigens on the erythrocyte surface and are seen in transfusion reactions and erythroblastosis fetalis caused by maternal-fetal blood group incompatibility. Autoantibodies are specific for molecules in the red cell membrane itself and may be formed in association with underlying disease such as lymphoma, leukemia, systemic lupus erythematosus, and certain drugs and infections, or for reasons unknown. The direct and indirect Coombs' antiglobulin tests demonstrate the responsible antibodies on the patient's red cells or in the patient's serum.

Mechanical trauma to erythrocytes causes largely intravascular hemolysis with resultant hemoglobinuria and often fragmented erythrocytes in the blood and occurs with prosthetic heart valves, Teflon patches in the heart, valvular heart disease, large or multiple hemangiomas, or exceptionally severe, sustained athletic activity referred to as "march hemoglobinuria." Microangiopathic hemolytic anemia results from physical trauma to erythrocytes from fibrin deposition in the microvasculature, and characteristic abnormal red blood cells, a mixture of helmet cells and other fragmented forms, result. Disseminated intravascular coagulation, arteriovenous fistulas, malignant hypertension, purpura fulminans, thrombotic thrombocytopenic purpura, systemic lupus erythematosus, the Kasabach-Merritt and hemolytic-uremic syndromes, eclampsia, and metastatic mucinous adenocarcinoma are known causes.[810]

Infection by malarial parasites is the most common infectious cause of hemolytic anemia worldwide. Infection of blood and marrow cells results not only in parasitemia, which can range from 0.4 to 53 parasites per 1000 red blood cells, but also in a dyserythropoietic state that affects infected erythroblasts and simulates the nuclear changes of megaloblastic anemia.[394] The marrow responds to the shortened red cell life span with erythroid hyperplasia and increased red cell production. Thrombocytopenia, accompanied by megakaryocytic hyperplasia and minimal dysmyelopoiesis, may also be present. These abnormalities resolve after eradication of the parasite.

Drugs and toxins may cause direct intravascular lysis of erythrocytes or the formation of insoluble cytoplasmic precipitates of denatured hemoglobin (Heinz bodies), which may sufficiently deform or damage the red cells so that they are destroyed in the spleen.[554] Persons with G6PD deficiency and other red cell enzyme deficiencies are particularly susceptible to oxidative drug–induced hemolysis.

Polycythemia. The term "polycythemia" is commonly used as a synonym for erythrocytosis, or increased red blood cell and hemoglobin concentration in the blood. Polycythemia may be absolute and associated with increased red cell mass or relative. Relative polycythemia refers to the state in which increased red cell concentration is attributable to contracted plasma volume without an increase in erythropoiesis or red blood cell mass. It can result from dehydration caused by prolonged vomiting, diarrhea, sweating, decreased fluid intake, burns, or increased insensible fluid loss as in fever, hyperthyroidism, and diabetic ketoacidosis.

In absolute erythrocytosis, which can be primary or secondary, there is erythroid hyperplasia in the marrow with increased production of red blood cells that leads to an increase in the total circulating red cell mass and blood volume. Regardless of the cause, there occur certain signs and symptoms that are related to the increased blood volume and hyperviscosity.[265] The skin and mucous membranes become cyanotic, and the patient may complain of headaches, dizziness, tinnitus, and feeling of fullness in the head. The most serious effect is the real tendency to thrombosis and bleeding. Polycythemia vera (PV), primary polycythemia, is characterized by normal or low erythropoietin levels and trilineage marrow hyperplasia with erythrocytosis, leukocytosis, and thrombocytosis. PV is considered to be a myeloid stem cell malignancy and is discussed with the chronic myeloproliferative disorders.

In secondary erythrocytosis, the marrow hyperplasia is selective, affecting only erythroid elements.[403] There are many causes of secondary polycythemia, most of which are related to tissue hypoxia and elevated erythropoietin levels.[23] These causes include erythrocytosis caused by high altitude and low atmospheric oxygen pressure, chronic pulmonary disease, congenital heart disease with right to left shunts, and hypoventilation syndromes. Abnormal hemoglobins with an increased affinity for oxygen, which may be inherited or acquired because of drugs, toxins, or heavy smoking, cause impaired tissue oxygenation. Rarely, erythrocytosis may be caused by a variety of neoplasms, some of which have been shown to secrete erythropoietin, including renal cell carcinoma, hepatocellular carcinoma, cerebellar hemangioblastoma, and uterine smooth muscle neoplasms.[727] Benign renal lesions such as cystic renal disease and hydronephrosis also may cause aberrant erythropoietin elevations. Treatment of secondary polycythemia entails treating the primary condition, if possible, and periodic phlebotomy.

Disorders of white blood cells
Leukocytosis and leukopenia

In contrast to disorders of erythroid cells, most pathologic conditions affecting the white blood cells result in increased numbers of white cells in the blood or leukocytosis. These proliferations are often malignant, but numerous causes of benign, reactive leukocytosis occur as well. Most commonly, neutrophilia is an appropriate response to infection and results initially from the mobilization of marginated neutrophils from the reserve pool in blood and marrow and later from myeloid hyperplasia in marrow.[719] Causes of reactive neutrophilia include infection by pyogenic bacteria, some fungi and viruses, burns, infarcts, surgery, metabolic derangements, poisons, acute hemorrhage, hemolysis, malignant neoplasms, and corticosteroid administration.[596] Occasionally, leukocytosis may be severe and include a greater number of immature forms simulating leukemia, particularly chronic myelocytic leukemia. However, myelocytic hyperplasia usually appears in the marrow as patchy proliferations, localized around vessels and bony trabeculas and in the central marrow space in contrast to effacement of the marrow space in leukemia. However, when prolonged, the histology of so-called leukemoid reactions and leukemia may have a similar appearance in the marrow. The findings of normal or elevated leukocyte alkaline phosphatase, normal marrow chromosomes, and the lack of progression support a diagnosis of reactive granulocytosis.

Leukocytosis caused by increased numbers of other cell types occurs less frequently than neutrophilia. Lymphocytosis occurs in response to acute viral infection, chronic infections caused by tuberculosis, syphilis, brucellosis, and lymphoproliferative disorders and is physiologic in infants and children. Eosinophilia characteristically accompanies allergic reactions, parasitic infestations, drug reactions, and connective tissue diseases. Basophilia is usually associated with chronic myeloproliferative disorders, especially chronic myelocytic leukemia, but is also seen in myelodysplastic syndromes, acute leukemia, carcinoma, lymphoma, plasma cell myeloma, and iron-deficiency and aplastic anemias.[12] The degree of marrow hyperplasia generally parallels the degree of leukocytosis.

A large number of causes are known for leukopenia, which usually occurs in association with anemia and thrombocytopenia in aplastic anemia, infection, or nutritional deficiency. Isolated neutropenia does occur, however, with drug and immune reactions, rheumatoid arthritis, and unknown insults.[572,716] Regardless of cause, the degree of neutropenia should be graded, since the grade relates to the risk of infection: over 1000 granulocytes/dl is considered as slight, 500 to 1000 as moderate, and less than 500 as severe neutropenia, which has the highest risk of serious infection. Survival with severe neutropenia depends on prevention or controlling infection until the granulocyte count recovers.

Bone marrow biopsy is helpful in distinguishing the various causes of selective neutropenia. Drug-induced agranulocytosis is associated with the absence of iden-

tifiable myeloid cells from the marrow, whereas erythroid and megakaryocytic lineages are normal. Common offending drugs include phenothiazines, phenylbutazone, sulfonamides, antithyroid drugs, and chloramphenicol. Marrow recovery begins soon after withdrawal of the drug, and neutrophils reenter the circulation in about 1 to 2 weeks.

The pathogenic mechanisms responsible for immune neutropenia are analogous to those responsible for immune hemolytic anemia, isoimmunization, and autoimmunity. The first condition, the neutrophil equivalent of erythroblastosis fetalis, is attributable to the development of maternal antibodies directed against fetal neutrophilic antigens. The affected infants are normal at birth, but they develop infections and transient neutropenia in the first few weeks of life. However, recovery is the rule. Autoimmune neutropenia occurs in patients with systemic lupus erythematosus, rheumatoid arthritis, T cell–mediated neutropenia, and other disorders. In immune neutropenias, the marrow shows myeloid hyperplasia with immaturity. Since neutrophils are destroyed in the marrow and blood, they are present in relatively low numbers and can simulate the histologic condition seen in hypoplastic acute myeloid leukemia.

Felty's syndrome is the complex of rheumatoid arthritis, leukopenia, and splenomegaly that affects approximately 1% of patients with rheumatoid arthritis. Often, there is mild anemia and thrombocytopenia that accompanies the variably severe neutropenia; skin and pulmonary infections are frequent complications. Usually the marrow is hypercellular, and neutrophils may be present or virtually absent. The pathophysiology of the neutropenia is not understood, and there may be defective chemotactic and bactericidal properties as well as low numbers of neutrophils. Recovery of blood counts may occur after splenectomy.

Chronic idiopathic neutropenia is a rare form of selective granulocytopenia in which the neutrophil count remains low for many months or years with normal red cell and platelet counts and a normal spleen. The condition may be congenital, familial, or sporadic. Infections are not a problem until the absolute neutrophil count drops below 500/dl. This disorder appears to be an example of ineffective granulopoiesis, resulting in decreased production of neutrophils. There is a distinctive "maturation-arrest" abnormality in the marrow, characterized by normal or increased numbers of granulocyte precursors in the absence of more mature granulocytes. However, this is not a preleukemic condition, and occasional patients, usually children, may remit.

Several rare, usually congenital, neutrophil disorders have been reported in which functional abnormalities accompany the neutropenia leading to severe, morbid infections.[754] These disorders include the lazy leukocyte syndrome, with impaired migration from marrow into blood and defective chemotaxis; the Chediak-Higashi anomaly, characterized by chemotactic defects and giant nonfunctional lysosomal granules; and cyclic neutropenia, which probably represents a defect in granulopoietic control mechanisms. Similar disorders of monocytes with dysfunction in chemotaxis and phagocytosis occur as seen in the Wiskott-Aldrich syndrome.

Proliferative disorders of white blood cells

The leukemias, chronic myeloproliferative disorders, and myelodysplastic syndromes constitute the proliferative disorders of white cells. They represent a diverse but related group of stem cell disorders with many clinical features and pathogenic mechanisms in common. Traditional divisions into specific clinicopathologic entities, modified and refined by new information, retain their usefulness in guiding therapy and predicting outcome.

Leukemias are malignant clonal disorders characterized by the development of a neoplastic cell line within the marrow that coexists with normal hematopoietic stem cells. Leukemic cells exhibit aberrant growth and maturation resulting in an abnormal accumulation of cells at certain morphologic stages of differentiation. In contrast to most other malignancies, leukemias are systemic disorders at the time of diagnosis and most often involve the marrow diffusely.[292] The neoplastic cells have the propensity to circulate in the blood and to infiltrate a variety of tissues, either as diffuse infiltrates or by forming discrete tumor masses. However, the diagnosis of leukemia is usually not apparent clinically until there accumulates in the body a critical mass of leukemic cells, estimated at 10^{12} cells, that is usually accompanied by a leukocytosis of 15,000 to 20,000 cells/dl or more. Myelodysplasias and chronic myeloproliferative disorders are also clonal in origin and are apparently derived from a neoplastic stem cell, but they exhibit less severely deranged patterns of growth and maturation and retain a capability for producing differentiated cells.

The evidence for a clonal nature of these disorders is derived from several different kinds of studies.[292] A consistent and characteristic chromosome abnormality, the Philadelphia chromosome (Ph_1), was first identified in the leukemic cells of patients with chronic myelogenous leukemia (CML) in 1960.[528] Refined cytogenetic techniques now demonstrate clonal chromosomal abnormalities in the majority of leukemias and many of the myelodysplasias and myeloproliferative disorders, and many of these abnormalities, like the Ph_1, are characteristic of the subtype of leukemia.[633,825] In most acute lymphoblastic and chronic lymphocytic leukemias, the leukemic clone appears to be derived from a committed lymphoid precursor cell and does not in-volve other hematopoietic stem cells. This is not the case in the myeloproliferative disorders. In CML, clonal markers, such as the Ph_1, have been identified not only in granulocytes, erythroid cells, monocytes, and megakaryocytes, but in some cases B- or T-lymphocytes as well.[160,655] Recent studies of acute myeloblastic leukemia have also demonstrated clonal chromosome markers in nonmyeloid cells.[218,375] These findings indicate that the leukemic cell of origin may be a stem cell, often a multipotential myeloid stem cell, and sometimes a more primitive stem cell that is capable of myeloid and lymphoid differentiation. This hypothesis may partially explain the occurrence of lymphoid blast crisis of CML[59] and acute mixed-lineage (myeloid-lymphoid) leukemias. Other evidence of clonality in leukemia results from early studies of isoenzyme mosaicism in women heterozygous for the two forms of the X-linked enzyme glucose-6-phosphate dehydrogenase (G6PD). Because one X chromosome is randomly inactivated in each somatic cell, tissues have a mixture of two G6PD isoenzymes. In leukemic cell populations, however, only one isoenzyme is present, an indication of derivation from a single neoplastic precursor cell. The antigen receptors of lymphocytes, immunoglobulin of B-cells and the T-cell receptor of T-cells, usually demonstrate clonal expression of the receptor genes and their protein products in lymphoid leukemias and lymphomas. Studies of antigen-receptor clonality have become useful adjuncts in the evaluation of these neoplasms (discussed later).[13,765]

Epidemiology. Hematologic neoplasms are an important cause of mortality, accounting for an estimated 9% of all cancer deaths in the United States in 1988.[666] Leukemia is the leading cause of cancer death in children and in young men 15 to 34 years of age and is second only to breast cancer in young women. Males are more frequently afflicted at all ages than females are. Definite geographic variations in leukemia incidence are known. The distribution of leukemias in Western countries is estimated at 60% acute, with acute nonlymphoblastic leukemias (ANLL) being more common than acute lymphoblastic leukemias (ALL), 25% chronic lymphocytic leukemia (CLL), and 15% chronic myelocytic leukemia (CML).[292] In contrast, CLL is uncommon in Japan, comprising only about 2.5% of leukemia; this figure contributes to an overall incidence of leukemia in Japan of only half that in the United States.

Although any type of leukemia may occur at any age, characteristic age distributions are seen. Acute leukemias are more common than chronic leukemias at all ages with incidence peaks in children 3 to 4 years of age and in elderly persons 70 to 80 years of age. White children are affected more frequently than black children in the United States and children in Africa have the lowest incidence of leukemia. CML occurs rarely in childhood and becomes increasingly more common in older age groups, with a mean age of about 47 years. CLL is virtually unheard of in childhood and is rare before 35 years of age. It is the most frequent type of leukemia in elderly persons.

In the first half of this century, leukemia incidence and mortality were virtually identical; that is, leukemia was almost invariably fatal. In recent decades, chemotherapy and bone marrow transplantation have altered that outlook for some patients. Treatment successes with long-term survivals have been achieved largely in children with ALL, though some young adults with ANLL have also been cured. Allogenic bone marrow transplants are successful in some patients with ALL, ANLL, and CML, but the early mortality is still appreciable.[266] New information about the pathophysiologic and therapeutic responses of these disorders have led to altered approaches that offer hope for better control and eventual cure of these devastating diseases.

Etiology. The cause of leukemia and related disorders is unknown, but several factors may act singly or in combination to alter the incidence of leukemia. These etiologic factors include genetic and acquired diseases, myelodysplastic syndromes (preleukemia), exposure to ionizing radiation, benzene, alkylating agents, and viruses.

Some genetic disorders are associated with an increased incidence of leukemia and other neoplasms.[393,632] Numerically, the most important is Down's syndrome, trisomy 21, which exhibits up to a twentyfold increased risk of leukemia development, especially acute leukemia, in the first decade of life. Neonates with Down's syndrome occasionally have a transient myeloproliferative disorder that may be difficult to distinguish from leukemia but resolves spontaneously without therapy.[426,493] Patients with other constitutional chromosome abnormalities, especially sex-chromosome disorders such as Klinefelter's syndrome (XXY) have a slightly increased propensity to develop leukemia. The chromosomal breakage disorders are a group of rare inherited diseases that have in common increased spontaneous chromosomal breakage and fragility and an increased incidence of a variety of malignancies. Of these, persons with Fanconi's anemia, ataxia-telangiectasia, and Bloom's syndrome are particularly prone to the development of leukemia and lymphoma.[189,642] In addition to specific chromosomal defects, "leukemia families" are known in which multiple members of a family develop leukemia of the same type, usually CLL or ALL, or a complex of lymphoproliferative disorders, such as CLL and lymphoma. Acute leukemia may also develop in the course of certain acquired diseases that are often associated with chromosome abnormalities, including the chronic myeloproliferative disorders, myelodysplasias, and aplastic anemia.[55]

Ionizing radiation has long been known to be leukemogenic in experimental animals. A graphic demonstration of its potential role in human leukemogenesis is the observation that the survivors of atomic bombings of Hiroshima and Nagasaki developed leukemias at an increased rate.[662] Interestingly, CLL has not been reported to occur in any of the exposed persons and has remained rare in Japan. Other situations in which radiation clearly is associated with leukemia are radiotherapy administered for benign or malignant conditions and occupational exposure experienced by early radiologists.[565,745] Thus it appears that both single high doses and multiple small doses of radiation are capable of inducing leukemias. Overall, however, radiation exposure is a minor determinant of leukemia occurrence.

Some drugs and chemicals have been implicated in the causation of leukemia. Most of the putative leukemogens are known myelotoxins, and the relationship is most direct in individual instances where a "preleukemic phase" of myelodysplasia and blood abnormalities precedes the leukemia.[231] The resulting leukemia is ANLL. Benzene, other organic solvents, and alkylating agents are the most frequently cited compounds, though sulfonamides, nitrosoureas, chloramphenicol, phenylbutazone, and many others have also been implicated.[250,547,549,737] The precise mechanisms of chemical leukemogenesis are unknown, but these secondary leukemias often share characteristic, recurring chromosomal abnormalities, specifically complete or partial deletion of chromosomes 5 and 7.[412]

Viruses have long been known as etiologic agents in certain animal leukemias and other neoplasms, but very recently oncogenic retroviruses that contribute to the development of human leukemia have been isolated and characterized.[769] Human T-cell leukemia virus type I (HTLV-I) is associated with the adult T-cell leukemia-lymphoma syndrome, a leukemia that is endemic in parts of Japan and the Caribbean and has been reported in the United States. The incidence of HTLV-I seropositivity in endemic areas is much higher than that of the neoplasm is, an indication of a more complex etiologic relationship. A second human retrovirus, HTLV-II, has been implicated in the causation of the rare T-cell variant of hairy cell leukemia. Scattered reports of viral isolates from a few cases of other types of leukemia have appeared, but the associations seem tenuous at the present time.[252]

Much insight into leukemogenesis has been gained through the study of chromosome (chr) abnormalities identified in leukemias and other hematologic disorders.[781] The first consistent chromosomal abnormality identified in any neoplastic disease was the Ph₁ (Philadelphia) chromosome in CML, which was first believed

Table 28-1. Gene rearrangements and chromosomal abnormalities in hematologic diseases

Chromosomal abnormality	Associated genes	Gene alterations			Chromosomal localization	Diseases	References
		Translocation	Rearrangement	Deletion			
t(9;22)(q34;q11)	c-*abl*	+	+	−	9q34	CML, some	(190, 633)
	bcr	−	+	−	22q11	ALL	
t(8;14)(q24;q32)	c-*myc*	+	+	−	8q24	Burkitt's lym-	(148)
	heavy chain	−	+	−	14q32	phoma leukemia	
t(2;8)(p11;q24)	c-*myc*	−	+	−	8q24	Burkitt's lym-	(148)
	kappa chain	+	+	−	2p11	phoma leukemia	
t(8;22)(q24;q11)	c-*myc*	−	+	−	8q24	Burkitt's lym-	(148)
	lambda chain	+	+	−	22q11	phoma leukemia	
t(8;21)(q22;q22)	Hu-*ets*-2	+	+	−	21q22	ANLL-M2	(619)
	c-*mos*	−	−	−	8q22		
t(5;17)(q22;q21)	myeloperoxi-dase	+	−	−	17q22-24	ANLL-M3	(427)
	c-*erb* A	−	−	−	17q21-22		
t(9;11)(p22;q23)	Hu-*ets*-1	+	+	−	11q23-24	ANLL-M4 and	(174)
	alpha-interferon	−	?	−	9p22	M5	
t(4;11)(q21;q23)	Hu-*ets*-1	+	+	−	11q23-24	ALL, AUL	(619)
del 6 (q23)	c-*myb*	−	+	−	6q23	ALL, lymphoma	(25)
inv 14 (q11q32)	*tcl*-1	±	?	−	14q32	T-cell	(149)
or t(14;14) (q11;q32)	TCR	−	?	−	14q11	malignancies	
del 5 (q13q33)	c-*fms*, M-CSF	−	−	+	5q33-34	MDS, ANLL	(327, 522)
	GM-CSF, IL-3	−	−	+	5q23-31		

GM-CSF, Granulocyte macrophage–colony-stimulating factor; *M-CSF,* macrophage–colony-stimulating factor; *IL-3,* interleukin-3; *TCR,* T-cell receptor.
ALL, Acute lymphoblastic leukemia; *ANLL,* acute nonlymphoblastic leukemia; *AUL,* acute undifferentiated leukemia; *CML,* chronic myelocytic leukemia; *MDS,* myelodysplastic syndrome.

Table 28-2. French-American-British (FAB) classification of acute leukemias

FAB type	Characteristics of bone marrow
ACUTE NONLYMPHOBLASTIC (ANLL)	
M1: Myeloblastic, without maturation (AML)	>3% of blasts myeloperoxidase positive
M2: Myeloblastic, with maturation (AML)	Maturation to or beyond the promyelocyte stage, <20% monocytes
M3: Promyelocytic (APL)	Majority of cells are abnormal, hypergranular, promyelocytes
M4: Myelomonocytic (AMML)	Like M2, but with >20% monocytes (confirm with fluoride-inhibited esterase reaction)
M5: Monoblastic (AMoL)	Majority of cells monocytic, <20% granulocytic
M6: Erythroleukemia (EL)	>50% erythroblasts, or >30% if erythropoiesis is bizarre, must also have >30% myeloblasts and promyelocytes
M7: Megakaryoblastic (AMegL)	Blasts positive for platelet peroxidase reaction (by electron micros-copy) or antibodies against platelet glycoprotein Ib, IIb/IIIa, IIIa or factor VIII, fibrosis
ACUTE LYMPHOBLASTIC (ALL)	
L1: Predominantly small homogeneous cells with scant cytoplasm, dispersed nuclear chromatin, small nucleoli	
L2: Large, heterogeneous in size and chromatin pattern, irregular clefted and folded nuclei, variable large nucleoli	
L3: Large homogeneous cells, oval or round nuclei with finely stippled chromatin, usually several nucleoli; deeply baso-philic cytoplasm, often with prominent cytoplasmic vacuoles	

to represent a simple deletion of a G-group chromosome.[528] Only after the development of banding techniques could it be determined that the defect in CML represented a reciprocal translocation between chr 9 and chr 22. Subsequently, numerous nonrandom chromosomal changes have been identified in a variety of hematologic neoplasms (Table 28-1).[609,825] More importantly, these recurring abnormalities now provide specific diagnostic and prognostic information.[54,608,633]

Two major classes of cytogenetic abnormalities, numerical and structural, are identifiable. Hyperdiploidy refers to a chromosome number greater than the diploid number of 46 chromosomes; hypodiploidy, less than 46. The gain or loss of complete chromosomes are common in leukemias but are nonspecific abnormalities. Trisomy 8 (designated +8) and monosomy 7 (−7) are common in ANLL but may also occur in lymphomas and solid neoplasms. The most frequent type of structural abnormality in leukemia is a balanced reciprocal translocation involving a particular pair of chromosomes with very consistent breakpoints. Examples include the Ph_1, or t(9;22), translocation in CML, the t(8;21) translocation in AML, and the t(15;17) translocation in APL (Tables 28-1 and 28-2). Specific deletions of portions of chromosomes are more characteristic of certain solid neoplasms but also occur in hematologic malignancies, including deletion of the long arm of chr 7 (7q−) in ANLL and myelodysplasia, 5q− in myelodysplasia, and deletions of chr 5 and 7 in secondary ANLL. The third major type of structural cytogenetic abnormality includes extrachromosomal double minute chromosomes (DM) and abnormal homogeneously staining regions (HSR) integrated within chromosomes. DM were first identified in neuroblastomas in 1965, and HSR in 1976 after the development of banding techniques. Both abnormalities have been associated with hematologic disease only rarely. However, DM and HSR are important because they represent the cytogenetic manifestations of gene amplification, a correlation made during the study of mechanisms of drug resistance in cell lines.[639] The identity of amplified genes in DM and HSR in human neoplasms has proved in several instances to be cellular proto-oncogenes.[464] Similarly, several proto-oncogenes have been mapped to specific locations on human chromosomes, many of which are involved in characteristic rearrangements in specific hematologic diseases.[25,548,617] A more complete understanding of the pathogenesis of these diseases, particularly CML and Burkitt's lymphoma, has been gained through a combination of cytogenetic and molecular analytic techniques.[93,151,634,775]

Recently acquired knowledge of the genetics of cancer has led to a general hypothesis that the final common pathway for induced and spontaneous carcinogenesis is an alteration in proto-oncogene expression. Certainly involvement of these genes, so named because of close homology to oncogenic retroviral sequences, has been demonstrated in a variety of human neoplasms.[51,270,676] It was originally proposed that oncogenes represented endogenous viruses that had been incorporated into the host genome and could be activated by a variety of environmental conditions to cause tumors.[328] However, it is now clear that the identified proto-oncogenes are endogenous human genes that are controlled in a tissue-specific manner in fetal and adult organ systems. The observed pattern of expression of these genes seems to indicate that they have important roles in the regulation of normal cell growth and differentiation.[414,557,610] Recently, the definition of oncogene has been expanded to include any gene or gene product, even without viral homology, that is capable of initiating or maintaining the transformed state.[92]

Several mechanisms may potentially be responsible for activation of these genes to oncogenes. Except for the human T-cell leukemia virus, which has no apparent homology with human genes, retroviral insertion appears to have at most a minor role in oncogene activation in human leukemias.[313,457] Instead, somatic mutations, evidenced by chromosomal changes such as balanced translocations or deletions, may lead to expression of structurally altered genes that presumably confer a growth advantage (c-*abl*/*bcr* in CML)[93,98,190] or to altered transcriptional control of the normal genes (c-*myc* in Burkitt's lymphoma, discussed later).[317,762] Gene amplification through an increase in gene copy number is most graphically seen as DM and HSR (amplified N-*myc* in neuroblastoma). Less dramatic is an increase in gene dosage because of the presence of an extra chromosome (trisomy 8 in ANLL). Thus oncogene activation in most cases leads to the leukemic phenotype through aberrant production of oncogene products, such as growth factors or growth factor receptors, or by intracellular second messengers. Current evidence indicates that activation of a single oncogene may not be the only event in leukemogenesis.[118,219,407] Cytogenetic and molecular studies of hereditary cancer have identified mutant dominant cancer genes in xeroderma pigmentosum and Bloom's syndrome and mutant recessive cancer genes in retinoblastoma and Wilms' tumor that predispose individuals to the development of cancer.[393] A second mutational event appears necessary for the development of a neoplasm in these situations.[792] Similarly, specific deletions in hematologic disorders may unmask such genes, permitting development of the particular disorder.[804] Clearly, leukemogenesis is a complex, multifactorial, multistep process that is still not fully understood and is under intense investigation.

Classification of leukemia. Leukemia is classified as acute or chronic, and myeloid or lymphoid. Four major categories encompass most leukemias: acute nonlymphoblastic leukemia (ANLL), acute lymphoblastic leukemia (ALL), chronic myelocytic leukemia (CML), and chronic lymphocytic leukemia (CLL), though several other variants are also recognized. The diagnosis and classification of acute leukemia and myelodysplasia is based on the morphologic assessment of routinely prepared Romanowsky-stained bone marrow aspirate smears and supplemented by cytochemical reactions using criteria that were formulated by a group of hematologists from Europe and the United States in 1976 that has since been modified (Tables 28-2 and 28-3). This formulation is known as the French-American-British (FAB) classification.[36-38] Diagnosis and classification of chronic leukemias is usually straightforward, but 10% or more of acute leukemias are misclassified by Wright's stain alone. Accurate classification of leukemias is essential, since the selection of therapy and prognosis is directly related. Large series of newly diagnosed adult and childhood acute leukemias classified by the FAB classification and correlated with cell marker and cytogenetic studies indicate that the FAB classification is useful in delineating clinicopathologic entities of ANLL, but not ALL.[56,223,272,415,650] Cell marker and cytogenetic studies are necessary to define specific prognostic and therapeutic subgroups in ALL (Table 28-4).[223] Additional immunologic and karyotypic data for ANLL have tended to reinforce and expand the original FAB groupings (Tables 28-5 and 28-12).[498,650]

Pathophysiology of leukemia. Pathologic changes that affect cells and tissues of patients with leukemia result from the direct infiltration of tissues by leukemic cells, the decrease in hematopoietic cell production and function resulting in the frequent complications of infection and hemorrhage, the alterations of normal physiology including altered immune function, hemolysis, hyperviscosity, and metabolic derangements, and the adverse effects of therapy. Any tissue may be infiltrated by leukemic cells, and most are at the time of diagnosis. However, many organs show surprisingly little ill effects even with extensive infiltration. Some organs do show characteristic patterns of involvement and levels of dysfunction in certain types of leukemia. The marrow, of course, is extensively replaced by leukemic cells in almost every type of leukemia, and this results in anemia, neutropenia, and thrombocytopenia. Bone pain attributable to marrow expansion is characteristic of ALL. In addition to the physical displacement of hematopoietic cells by malignant cells, some leukemias elaborate substances that inhibit normal stem cell proliferation and contribute to the degree and frequency of complications attributable to cytopenias.[64,292] The morbidity and mortality from hemorrhage caused by thrombocytopenia has been decreased greatly by the use of platelet transfusions. Neutropenia is more difficult to manage and often leads to serious infectious complications and death. Cytopenias are particularly evident in hypoplastic ANLL, which usually occurs in elderly patients and in which the marrow is usually hypocellular. Treatment often results in profound, chronic marrow suppression and death from prolonged cytopenias. Supportive measures alone often produced longer than expected survival.[513] Leukemic infiltration of liver and spleen resulting in hepatosplenomegaly is most common in CML, prolymphocytic leukemia and hairy cell leukemia. In general, myeloid leukemias infiltrate the red pulp of the spleen, and the lymphoid leukemias infiltrate the white pulp, though extensive involvement by any type of leukemia usually completely effaces the splenic parenchyma. Splenic infarcts and rupture may occur as a consequence of acute leukemic infiltration. In contrast, hepatic enlargement usually causes no functional impairment. Acute and chronic lymphoid

Table 28-3. French-American-British (FAB) classification of myelodysplastic syndromes

Type	Blood findings	Marrow findings
Refractory anemia (RA)	Anemia, reticulocytopenia <1% blasts	<5% blasts, prominent erythroid hyperplasia with dyserythropoiesis
Refractory anemia with ringed sideroblasts (RARS)	Anemia, reticulocytopenia <1% blasts	>15% ringed sideroblasts, <5% blasts
Refractory anemia with excess of blasts (RAEB)	<5% blasts	Hypercellular, trilineage dyspoiesis, 5% to 20% blasts
Chronic myelomonocytic leukemia (CMML)	Monocytosis (>1 × 10⁹/L) <5% blasts	<20% blasts, increased promonocytes
Refractory anemia with excess blasts in transformation (RAEBIT)	>5% blasts or Auer rods present	20% to 30% blasts or Auer rods present

leukemias infiltrate and expand portal areas, whereas the myeloid leukemias preferentially infiltrate the hepatic sinusoids. Lymphadenopathy is characteristic of lymphoid leukemias and may cause pain or pressure symptoms related to compression of adjacent structures. Leukemic meningitis and brain parenchymal involvement are especially serious, life-threatening complications of ALL and may be encountered in ANLL and in blast crisis of CML. Chloromas, also called myeloblastomas or granulocytic sarcomas, are discrete, leukemic tumors composed of myeloblasts that may occur anywhere in the body but preferentially in bones of the skull and spine, dura, lymph nodes, and kidneys. Myeloblastomas usually appear during the course of known

Table 28-4. Morphologic, immunologic, and cytogenetic correlations in acute nonlymphoblastic leukemias

Morphology (FAB type)	Frequency of FAB type	Immunologic markers*	Karyotype	Karyotype frequency†
M1 (M2)‡	15%-30%	CD13/33 >25%	t(9;22)(q34;q11)	3%
M1 (M2, M4, M7) with thrombo-cytosis			inv (3)(q21q26)	1%
M2	25%-30%	CD15 >25% CD14 <25%	t(8;21)(q22;q22) often −X or −Y	10%-15%
M2, M4 with basophilia			t(6;9)(p21;q22) or del (6p)	<1%
M3	5%	AML 2.23 >25% DR, CD14 <25%	t(15;17)(q22;q34) variant t(17q)	10%
M4	30%-40%	CD14 25%-55%	t or del (11)(q23)	5%-10%
M4 with abnormal eosinophils			inv or del (16)(q22)	5%-10%
M5	5%-10%	CD14 >55%	t or del (11)(q23)	5%-10%
M6	10%	Glycophorin A >50% of blasts	Often abnormal, but no specific defects known	
M7	?5%-10%	Plt 1, factor VIII >25% of blasts	Often abnormal, but no specific defects known	

*Cell surface markers corresponding to myeloid differentiation antigens.
†Percentage of all acute nonlymphoblastic leukemia.
‡Less common karyotypic association in parentheses.
AML, Acute myeloblastic leukemia; *CD,* cluster of differentiation; *DR,* an HLA type; *Plt,* platelet.

Table 28-5. Morphologic, immunologic, and cytogenetic correlations in acute lymphoblastic leukemia

Morphology (FAB type)	Type (lineage)	Frequency	Immunologic markers	Common karyotype
L1 (L2)*	common (precursor B)	50%-60%	CD10, TdT, DR+	Modal number >50
L1 (L2)	pre-B	15%-20%	Cytoplasmic Ig + surface Ig −	t(1;19) t(9;22)
L2 (L1)	T-cell	15%-20%	pan T, CD2, TdT +	t(11;14), 6q −
L1, L2	Null	5%-10%	TdT +, Ig −, CD10 −	t(4;11), t(9;22)
L3	B-cell	1%	Surface Ig +	t(8;14), t(8;22), t(2;8), 6q −

*Less common FAB type in parentheses.

ANLL in a child or young adult,[798] but they may precede overt leukemia by months or even years[465] or herald the onset of blast crisis in chronic phase CML. Potential acute complications common to all leukemias include hyperuricemia with uric acid nephropathy, depressed immunity, and hyperviscosity with leukocytostasis, especially serious when the brain and lungs are affected. Antileukemic therapy, when effective, exacerbates suppression of marrow function during or after its administration and may lead to prolonged cytopenias in some cases. Delayed complications of infertility, central nervous system toxicity of mild intellectual impairment to severe demyelinating leukoencephalopathy, persistent immune depression, and secondary neoplasms are seen in long-term survivors of ALL.

Proliferative disorders of myeloid cells

Acute nonlymphoblastic leukemia, chronic myelocytic leukemia, the chronic myeloproliferative disorders, and the myelodysplastic syndromes are the principal groups of proliferative disorders that affect myeloid cells.

Myelodysplastic syndromes. Myelodysplastic syndromes (MDS) are a group of related disorders in which there is defective hematopoiesis that results in cytopenias, often monocytosis, and usually hypercellular marrow (Table 28-3). Variably these disorders may progress to ANLL and, for this reason, have sometimes been called "preleukemia."[436] However, this term is confusing and inadequate, since the incidence of leukemia is variable and even rare in some of these disorders. Other "preleukemic" disorders, such as paroxysmal nocturnal hemoglobinuria and aplastic anemia, differ from MDS and have not usually been classified as such.

Myelodysplastic syndromes may be primary without preexisting hematologic disease or secondary after chemotherapy, irradiation, or congenital and acquired hematologic stem cell disorders.[53,240,411] Most affected persons are over 50 years of age and are more often male than female. Blood findings include unexplained anemia with macro-ovalocytes, thrombocytopenia, or neutropenia with hyposegmentation and hypogranulation. The marrow is hypercellular or less frequently normocellular with evidence of ineffective hematopoiesis, pathologic ringed sideroblasts, and increased myeloblasts in some types.[240,618] The FAB classification is based on Romanowsky-stained marrow aspirate smears.[38] An elevated proportion of myeloblasts is unfavorable prognostically and is often associated with early leukemic transformation.[240,735] Symptoms are related to the type and degree of cytopenia. Although half or more of the patients with myelodysplasia ultimately develop ANLL, a significant number of patients die from marrow insufficiency because of infection or hemorrhage.[430,722] Secondary myelodysplasia after chemo-

therapy or radiotherapy may last months to several years before ANLL supervenes.[231] These ANLL are often difficult to classify and have a uniformly poor prognosis. Myelodysplasia rarely preceeds ANLL of FAB M2 or M3 type or Ph_1 chromosome–positive acute leukemia. Clonal chromosomal abnormalities are found in 40% to 80% of primary and nearly all secondary myelodysplasias and provide useful diagnostic and prognostic information.[61,343,829] Several specific cytogenetic abnormalities are seen in both myelodysplasia and ANLL, in particular trisomy 8 and monosomy 7 in primary disorders, and deletions of chr 5 and 7 in secondary disorders, but these abnormalities do not segregate with particular FAB types. The risk of leukemic transformation in MDS is higher in patients with chromosomal abnormalities. In patients with normal chromosomes, the dysplasia tends to remain stable for several years and survival is favorable, whereas patients with deletions of chr 5 and 7 or multiple complex chromosomal aberrations have a poor prognosis, with a median survival of 4 months.[829] Treatment of myelodysplasia has generally been supportive, and the role of chemotherapy has been controversial.[734] New therapeutic approaches include differentiation-inducing drugs and administration of recombinant colony-stimulating factors (CSF).[276,830]

A distinctive form of myelodysplasia is characterized by refractory macrocytic anemia and morphologically abnormal, often giant platelets in the blood and numerous macromegakaryocytes with small nonlobulated nuclei in the marrow. This form is referred to as the 5q− syndrome because of the consistent interstitial deletion of part of the long arm of chr 5 in the marrow cells of affected individuals.[751] Molecular studies have identified a cluster of genes involved in the regulation of hematopoiesis at the 5q site that are deleted in this syndrome, including CSF 1, granulocyte-macrophage CSF, the proto-oncogene c-*fms*, and interleukins 3 and 5.[327,710] The disorder primarily affects women 60 to 70 years of age, and symptoms related to anemia usually manifest the disorder. Because neutropenia is absent, infection is usually not a problem. When blood and marrow findings are indicative of this disorder, cytogenetic studies are warranted. Patients with the 5q− syndrome have been reported to develop acute leukemia, but the risk is relatively small, perhaps 5% to 10%, in comparison to other myelodysplasia syndromes when deletion of 5q− is the sole cytogenetic abnormality.[522]

Acute nonlymphoblastic leukemia. The acute nonlymphoblastic leukemias (ANLL) are the most common type of leukemia that affect middle-aged and elderly persons and infants less than 1 year of age. ANLL must be distinguished from acute lymphoblastic leukemia (ALL), since ANLL and ALL are treated and respond to therapy quite differently. Patients with ANLL present with the clinical findings of weakness, pallor, fever, bleeding, and infection, which are common to all acute leukemias, and certain subtypes exhibit characteristic findings. Acute promyelocytic leukemia (APL), a disease of young adults, is frequently associated with disseminated intravascular coagulation and hemorrhagic phenomena. APL is characterized by the unusually intense myeloperoxidase activity in the azurophilic granules of its cells. The myeloperoxidase gene, which has been mapped to chr 17, translocates specifically to chr 15 in APL.[427,780] This event provides a genetic marker for the continued study of the pathogenesis of this leukemia. Monoblastic leukemia has a greater tendency to involve the skin and gums than other ANLL. The diagnosis and subclassification of ANLL are made on the basis of characteristic blood and marrow findings in combination with cytochemical, karyotypic, and immunologic studies (Table 28-2). In histologic sections, the marrow space is usually fully replaced by an infiltrate of immature hematopoietic cells; often no adipose tissue and few normal hematopoietic cells remain (Fig. 28-4). The proportion of blasts varies from 30%, the minimum required to justify the diagnosis, to nearly 100% of the cells present. Sometimes reaction of the marrow stroma is quite striking, consisting in reticulin fibrosis, necrosis, or serous atrophy. Collagen fibrosis is a characteristic but nonspecific feature of acute megakaryoblastic leukemia, often thwarting the aspiration of leukemic cells.

The synthesis of clinical features, morphology, karyotype, and cell-marker findings are helpful in predicting how a given patient might respond to standard induction chemotherapy.[473,498,576,650] Overall, patients have a 65% to 85% chance of achieving a complete remission with standard therapy. Duration of remission ranges from 16 to 24 months in good-risk patients, and about 15% of these patients can expect to remain in remission for 3 years.[227] Infants and patients over 60 years of age as well as patients with very high white blood cell counts have a poor prognosis. Patients with APL often respond well to therapy with relatively good survival, whereas patients with AMML or AMoL have a relatively poor survival. In contrast, patients with acute myelomonocytic with abnormal eosinophils and inversion of chr 16 (FAB M4 Eo) have a relatively better survival. Most of the specific, nonrandom chromosome translocations and inversions confer an intemediate prognosis with 1- to 2-year median survival, whereas complex defects and monosomy 5 and 7 in secondary leukemia portend a survival of only a few months.[412,826,827] Cell-marker studies of differentiation antigens expressed by blasts yields independent prognostically useful information (see Tables 28-4 and 28-12). Expression of CD13 or CD14 is predictive of low response rate (55%), whereas patients with leukemias expressing neither antigen have a complete remission rate of 82%. The expression of class II human lymphocyte antigens (HLA-DR) by myeloblasts of patients who achieve remission is associated with a higher rate of relapse, 50% compared with 10% for DR-negative patients.[279]

Chronic myelocytic leukemia. Chronic myelocytic leukemia (CML), one of the chronic myeloproliferative disorders, is a neoplasm derived from a pluripotential

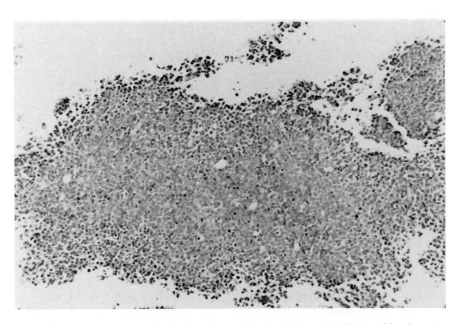

Fig. 28-4. Acute nonlymphoblastic leukemia. Marrow is hypercellular with almost complete replacement by myeloblasts. Notice monotonous appearance of cells.

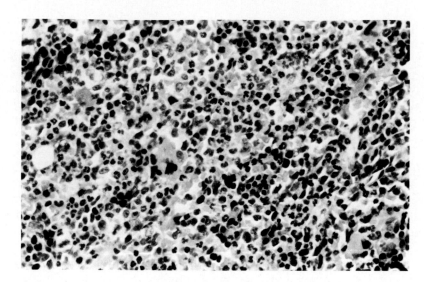

Fig. 28-5. Chronic myelocytic leukemia. Marrow section is hypercellular with virtually no adipose tissue present. Granulocytes, especially neutrophils, are greatly increased in number.

stem cell in which differentiated cells of the granulocytic series predominate in the blood and marrow.[268,489] CML occurs in all ages and both sexes but predominantly in middle-aged adults. Splenomegaly, often pronounced, is an invariable finding.[681] The blood shows granulocytosis, which is often greater than 100×10^9/L, anemia, and thrombocytosis that may approach 1000×10^9/L. In contrast to the lack of mature myeloid cells in acute leukemia, all stages of differentiation from myeloblasts to neutrophils are present, usually in normal proportions, and basophils are often increased. Morphologically, the myeloid cells appear relatively normal. However, leukemic neutrophils failing to differentiate normally is indicated by low or absent leukocyte alkaline phosphatase and inadequate phagocytic activity.[701]

The marrow in CML is greatly hypercellular, usually completely replacing the adipose tissue (Fig. 28-5). The granulocytic series is greatly hyperplastic with a myeloid-to-erythroid ratio of 5 to 20:1. The full maturation of the circulating cells reflects the marrow in which myeloblasts, promyelocytes, myelocytes, and neutrophils are in normal proportion. Eosinophils and basophils may be increased in number, whereas megakaryocytes may be normal, decreased, or increased but do not show significant dysplastic features. The red cell precursors are relatively scarce. Marrow fibrosis may be slight or pronounced, and increased fibrosis usually correlates with length of clinical disease. A progressive increase in the proportion of immature cells in the marrow occurs in some patients and characterizes the accelerated phase of CML.[366] The percentage increase

in blasts may make distinction from de novo Ph_1-positive acute leukemia difficult.

Most cases of CML, 85% to 90%, are Philadelphia chromosome positive, exhibiting either the typical t(9;22) translocation or a variant translocation (Fig. 28-6). The existence of Ph_1-negative CML has been questioned, since many of these cases are better classified as chronic myelomonocytic leukemia, one of the myelodysplastic syndromes.[732] Ph_1-negative CML generally progresses to acute leukemia more rapidly than Ph_1-positive CML.[624] However, with an increasing understanding of molecular events in CML, it has become apparent that the chimeric p210 protein product from the juxtaposition of the *bcr* gene from chr 22q11 and the *abl* gene from chr 9q34 are also detected in some cases of Ph_1-negative CML.[30,190,267]

Leukocytosis in CML is attributable to an abnormal accumulation rather than an accelerated proliferation of granulocytes. Thus conventional cytotoxic chemotherapy is ineffective in eradicating the neoplastic clone, and the Ph_1 chromosome will persist in apparent hematologic remission. The treatment rationale has been for control not cure of the disease, often with a single agent such as busulfan. Hematologic and cytogenetic remissions have been achieved with experimental alpha-interferon therapy.[718] Bone marrow transplantation may offer a cure in selected patients.[115,116]

Blast crisis develops in 80% to 100% of patients with CML after an average chronic phase of 3 to 4 years.[29] The appearance of myeloblastomas, pancytopenia, or drug resistance may herald its onset. Usually, the metamorphosis occurs gradually and is referred to more ap-

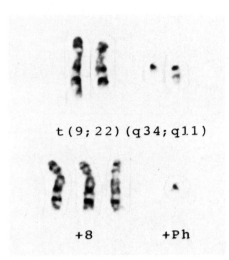

t(9;22)(q34;q11)

+8   +Ph

Fig. 28-6. Abnormal chromosomes in chronic myelocytic leukemia. *Above,* Giemsa-banded chromosomes showing the t(9;22) translocation. Extra chromosomal material on the long arm of chromosome 9 (first chromosome above) derived from chromosome 22 (third chromosome above), the Philadelphia chromosome. *Below,* Additional clonal abnormalities in blast crisis of chronic myelocytic leukemia, trisomy 8 (+8), and a second Philadelphia chromosome (+Ph).

propriately as the accelerated phase. Blast crisis presents abruptly in only 10% of patients, and it may present as de novo acute leukemia without a preceding chronic phase or after over 10 years of stable disease. The blasts of the blast crisis are myeloblastic in two thirds of the cases and lymphoblastic in one third and occasionally have features of both as in acute mixed-lineage leukemia.[314,566,630] Clonal chromosome abnormalities in addition to the t(9;22) translocation are often seen in blast phase and may include a second Ph_1 chr, trisomy 8 (Fig. 28-6) and isochromosome for the long arm of chr 17 (iso 17q).[112,622] The blast phase is usually fatal in less than 1 year.

Chronic myeloproliferative disorders. The chronic myeloproliferative disorders encompass four entities: polycythemia vera (PV), primary thrombocythemia (PT), primary myelofibrosis with myeloid metaplasia (PM), and chronic myelocytic leukemia. CML is the most common of these disorders, and the Philadelphia chromosome is diagnostic in the appropriate clinical context. Although each of these diseases represent clonal neoplasms of hematopoietic stem cells, the predominance of hemic cell types involved, whether granulocytic, erythroid, or megakaryocytic, the participation of stromal elements, the blood findings, and the clinical features differ in each disorder. When they are considered together, the disorder can usually be distinguished.[15,162]

In polycythemia vera, the erythroid lineage is predominantly affected, resulting in an absolute increase in red cell mass in the presence of normal or low erythropoietin serum levels.[227] Middle-aged males are affected predominantly. Patients experience plethora, headache, dizziness, and the tendency for hemorrhage and thrombosis because of severe polycythemia. The red cell, white cell, and platelet counts are usually increased, though sometimes the platelet count may be decreased and the white cell count may be normal. The marrow is usually hyperplastic, typically a cellularity of 80% to 90% with predominance of normoblastic erythroid hyperplasia and lesser degrees of megakaryocytic and myeloid hyperplasia.[195,196,403] Megakaryocytic dysplasia is often present. In established cases, some increase in reticulin may be present. An interstitial deletion of the long arm of chr 20 (20q−) was believed to be characteristic of polycythemia vera. However, it occurs in only a minority of patients, most of whom have had prior ^{32}P or chemotherapy, and it has been seen in other hematologic disorders.[42,713] PV usually has a chronic course and after an average of 10 years may eventuate in myelofibrosis or acute leukemia.[197,594] Evolution to acute leukemia occurs in 5% to 10% of cases. Treatment consists in phlebotomy and use of melphalan, hydroxyurea, or ^{32}P.

Essential, idiopathic, or primary thrombocythemia is characterized by persistently and greatly elevated platelet counts, in excess of $1000 \times 10^9/L$, accompanied by pronounced megakaryocytic hyperplasia in the marrow. The disorder is quite uncommon and affects middle-aged and elderly persons. The major clinical manifestations are hemorrhage, from the gastrointestinal or genitourinary tracts, and thrombosis of blood vessels in the leg, brain, or splenic vessels.[637] The marrow is variably cellular, ranging from 25% to 100%. The gross overabundance of megakaryocytes, often arranged in large clusters, show various degrees of dysplasia, including enlargement and nuclear-cytoplasmic dyssynchrony, and nuclear multilobulation is characteristic. As in other myeloproliferative disorders, other hemic cell lines proliferate to a variable but less degree. Neutrophilia may occur, but the leukocyte alkaline phosphatase is normal or increased, unlike in CML. Erythrocytosis, if present, is mild, but with chronic blood loss, iron deficiency may supervene. A therapeutic trial of iron usually distinguishes between PT and PV with superimposed iron deficiency: in PV, iron administration will result in a rapid rise in hemoglobin and hematocrit with the attendant risk of hemorrhage and thrombosis.[334] PT can usually be distinguished from the occasional case of CML with pronounced thrombocytosis on the basis of megakaryocyte morphology: in PT, the megakaryocytes are enlarged, with complex hyperlobulated nuclei, whereas in the variant CML, single,

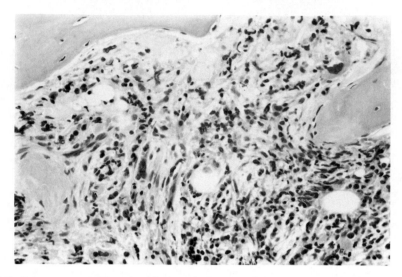

Fig. 28-7. Primary myelofibrosis. Marrow is hypercellular with dense fibrosis and little adipose tissue.

small, or bilobed micromegakaryocytes predominate. The leukocyte alkaline phosphatase and cytogenetic studies offer additional differential data; the chromosomes in PT are usually normal.[202] When fibrosis supervenes, the histologic appearance may be indistinguishable from primary myelofibrosis. Reactive thrombocytosis with marrow megakaryocytic hyperplasia may complicate hemorrhage, infectious and inflammatory diseases, and malignancies; however, the platelet count is usually only moderately increased in these disorders.

Primary idiopathic myelofibrosis, or agnogenic myeloid metaplasia, is characterized by marrow fibrosis and extramedullary hematopoiesis, most prominently affecting the spleen. It occurs as an apparently primary hematologic disease, and CML, PT, and PV may terminate in myelofibrosis, which is similar histologically.[344,410,770] The primary disorder affects middle-aged and elderly persons with the insidious onset of weakness, fatigue, and abdominal fullness and discomfort attributable to a greatly enlarged spleen. Moderate to severe anemia is the rule with characteristic morphologic abnormalities including teardrop forms, poikilocytes, and nucleated red cells. The white blood cell count may be normal, high, or low, and immature forms are usually present. Platelets are often large and function abnormally. Attempts at marrow aspiration are usually unsuccessful, though slight fibrosis may not thwart the procedure. The marrow may be hypercellular early in the course of the disease, but with time, progressive fibrotic replacement occurs (Fig. 28-7). Established fibrosis may also be present at diagnosis.[466] All hematopoietic cell lineages are represented, but megakaryocytes are especially predominant in the infiltrate and

are often encircled by coarse reticulin fibers (Fig. 28-8).[87] The cause of the marrow fibrosis is not clear, but it is not from a primary defect in fibroblasts, which are not neoplastic.[275] Rather, it is postulated that the fibrosis is caused by inappropriate release of platelet-derived growth factor and other platelet fibrogenic factors.[286] Chromosome abnormalities, when present, are usually of the nonspecific myeloproliferative type, that is, trisomy 8 or monosomy 7, but there have been suggestions that trisomy for the long arm or deletion of the short arm of chr 1 is more characteristic of PM.[103,109,484] The spleen in PM is enlarged and congested, weighing as much as 4 kg, and it becomes infarcted readily. Its size correlates with the duration of disease. Microscopically, there is diffuse extramedullary hematopoiesis including erythroid, granulocytic, and megakaryocytic precursors. Fibrosis and increased hemosiderin deposition are common. Extramedullary hematopoiesis may also involve the liver, lymph nodes, kidneys, adrenal glands, lungs, soft tissues, serous surfaces, and other sites, either diffusely or as discrete tumor masses. Relative prognosis can be predicted by the severity of systemic symptoms at presentation, and causes of death include infection, hemorrhage, thrombosis, cachexia, and congestive heart failure.[760,770] Acute myeloblastic or megakaryoblastic leukemia supervenes in 10% to 20% of cases.

Proliferative disorders of lymphoid cells

Lymphoproliferative disorders, like myeloproliferative disorders, have acute or chronic clinicopathologic forms. They represent the malignant clonal expansions of cells that mimic certain functional stages in normal lymphoid maturation (discussed later).[221] In contrast to

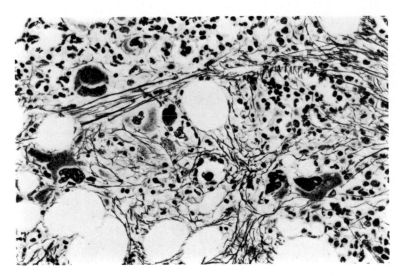

Fig. 28-8. Primary myelofibrosis. Coarse reticulin fibers in marrow space surrounding megakaryocytes (reticulin stain).

myeloid disorders, which almost always arise in the marrow, lymphoproliferative diseases originate in lymph nodes, spleen, thymus, other lymphoid tissues, and the marrow, or they may involve the marrow and other sites simultaneously. Lymphoid leukemias usually arise in the marrow.

Acute lymphoblastic leukemia. Acute lymphoblastic leukemia (ALL) is predominantly a disease of childhood, though it occurs in all ages. Signs and symptoms are similar to those of ANLL and include pallor, fever, weakness, bleeding, infection, and characteristically bone pain. The marrow is decidedly hypercellular and diffusely infiltrated by lymphoblasts, and normal myeloid, erythroid, and megakaryocytic cells are usually absent. Extensive marrow necrosis is seen occasionally in untreated ALL, and before more modern therapy, necrosis was indicative of poor prognosis.[401] Usually the blood is replete with lymphoblasts, and a marrow sample may not be essential for making the diagnosis in young children.

ALL may be classified in several ways. The FAB classification (Table 28-2), which is based on blast morphology alone, correlates with clinicopathologic groups in some degree.[37] Many childhood ALL have FAB L1 morphology, most adult ALL are FAB L2, and FAB-L3 includes many of the B-cell, Burkitt-like ALL. However, the immunologic classification of ALL defines prognostically relevant subgroups, and therapy is designed for the optimum management of low, intermediate, and high risk groups. In children, these groups are based upon immunophenotype, white blood cell count, age and sex, and other considerations including karyotype. Most ALL are CALLA (common ALL antigen), HLA-DR, and TdT (terminal deoxynucleotidyl

transferase) positive but negative for surface immunoglobulin (Ig) and T cell–associated antigens (discussed later), the phenotype of "common ALL" or non-T and non-B ALL (Tables 28-5 and 28-12). Recently, the demonstration of Ig gene rearrangement established in many cases indicates the precursor B-cell phenotype of common ALL. This group has a particularly favorable course in children in that remission is achieved in up to 90% with current therapy regimens with subsequent relapse rate of about 30% or less. Most of the long-term cures of patients with acute leukemia have been achieved in this group of patients; other immunologic types of ALL respond less well to standard therapy. Bone marrow transplantation holds some promise for some of these patients during first remission.

ALL of T-cell type accounts for about 15% of cases of ALL. Males are more frequently afflicted than females. The characteristic clinical presentation is that of a boy with a mediastinal mass, very high white blood cell count, often above 100×10^9/L, and meningeal infiltration. The presentation resembles that of lymphoblastic lymphoma in the same age group, except that blood and marrow involvement is lacking. The remission rate is lower and relapse rate higher than in common ALL, though prognosis is greatly improved with aggressive protocol therapy. ALL of B-cell type is rare and has morphologic, immunologic, and cytogenetic features of Burkitt's lymphoma. The response to conventional therapy is quite poor. Pre-B-cell and null-cell phenotypes are slightly more common that that of B-cell type and have an intermediate prognosis.

Nonrandom chromosomal abnormalities occur frequently in ALL, and they tend to segregate with phenotype and give additional prognostic information.[57,726,802] In general, hyperdiploidy greater than 50 chromosomes and the absence of translocations are prognostically favorable cytogenetic features. Both findings are characteristic of common ALL in childhood.[365] Translocations of any type, including t(9;22), t(4;11), and t(8;14), are associated with aggressive disease that is generally refractory to therapy.[801] The Philadelphia chromosome occurs in approximately 3% of childhood ALL and 25% of adult ALL. ALL patients with this translocation often have a poor prognosis. The molecular genetics of Ph_1-positive ALL is complex and as yet incompletely understood. At the cytogenetic banding level, the t(9;22) translocation in ALL and CML appears identical. However, two molecular lesions are known to occur in Ph_1-positive ALL. The first is associated with a chimeric c-abl/bcr gene and p210 tyrosine kinase product, as identified in CML. The second is an apparently unique rearrangement in ALL in which the breakpoint on chr 22 is outside the bcr region and results in the production of a p190 c-abl protein, which has not been demonstrated in CML.[130] The clinical significance of the two molecular forms is unknown.

Chronic lymphocytic leukemia. Chronic lymphocytic leukemia (CLL) is the most common leukemia in the elderly, with 90% of cases occurring after 50 years of age. It is twice as frequent in men as in women and is uncommon in Orientals. The onset of the disorder is insidious, and the diagnosis is often made in asymptomatic individuals being evaluated for persistent lymphocytosis. Patients with more advanced disease and correspondingly poorer prognosis exhibit mild but generalized lymphadenopathy, hepatosplenomegaly, anemia, and thrombocytopenia.[558,580,758] The absolute lymphocyte count at presentation is usually 27 × 10⁹/L

with a range of 8 to 1000 × 10⁹/L. The neoplastic small lymphocytes have characteristic clumped or "smudged" nuclear chromatin, and the vast majority of cases are of B-cell type. The cells express a low density of surface Ig with one light chain type indicative of a clonal population. Common chromosome abnormalities include trisomy 12 and 14q+; more complex changes usually indicate a clinically more aggressive leukemia and a poorer prognosis.[10,295,357-359,395,563]

Four patterns of marrow involvement in CLL have been described: interstitial, nodular, mixed, and diffuse.[440,611] In the interstitial type the lymphoid cells infiltrate and displace the hemic cells without a significant loss of adipose tissue. A minimum of 40% of cells should be small lymphocytes in a cellular marrow to support the clinical diagnosis of CLL. The nodular pattern is another pattern with focal involvement and limited replacement of adipose tissue (Fig. 28-9). Numerous lymphocytic nodules of slightly irregular size and shape, which tend to coalesce, are scattered throughout the marrow. The mixed type combines the nodular and interstitial patterns with increased cellularity and some loss of fatty tissue. In the diffuse type, sheets of small lymphocytes fill the marrow and almost completely replace the normal hemic cells and adipose tissue (Fig. 28-10). These patterns are prognostically important.[273,611] The nodular and interstitial patterns tend to occur in early, limited disease, and the mixed and diffuse types in advanced disease. The diffuse type is associated with cytopenias and organ infiltration and has the worst prognosis.[491]

Lymph node involvement in CLL can be histologically indistinguishable from small lymphocytic lymphoma (SL), though nodal capsule and trabeculas are

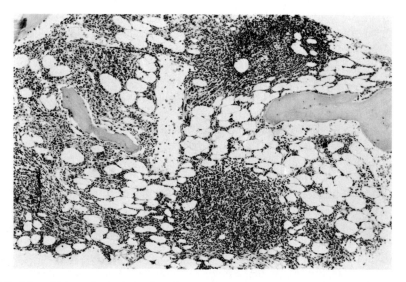

Fig. 28-9. Chronic lymphocytic leukemia, nodular type of infiltrate. The neoplastic small lymphocytic infiltrate is present focally in the marrow.

often infiltrated by leukemic cells.[179,540] However, any distinction is often arbitrary, since CLL and SL probably represent different manifestations of the same disease process. In contrast to SL, lymphadenopathy in CLL tends to be mild and symmetric without a dominant tumor mass initially. The spleen is enlarged because of expansion of the white pulp and infiltration of the red pulp. Discrete tumor nodules are usually not present. CLL involves the portal areas of the liver without gross tumor masses.

The clinical findings in CLL are related not only to direct tissue effects of leukemic cell accumulations but also to impaired humoral and cellular immunity and sometimes to autoimmune phenomena. Autoimmune hemolytic anemia, autoimmune thrombocytopenia, and pure red cell aplasia have been reported in CLL.[796] The course of CLL is often protracted and death usually results from unrelated causes. Treatment is usually instituted to control the white blood cell count or to treat anemia, thrombocytopenia, or bulky tissue infiltration in the later stages and not for curative intent. Acute leukemic termination occurs but is rare. More frequently, accelerated disease ensues as clonally related prolymphocytic transformation,[204] or diffuse large-cell non-Hodgkin's lymphoma (Richter's syndrome) develops in lymph nodes or in extranodal sites.[11,229,447]

Prolymphocytic leukemia. Prolymphocytic leukemia (PLL), like CLL, is a chronic lymphoid leukemia occurring exclusively in adults but is less common. It was originally described as a rare variant of CLL. However, sufficient differences have been shown to consider it as a separate clinicopathologic entity.[34,250] Most patients with PLL are elderly, with almost half of the cases diagnosed after age 70, and there is a male predominance. Clinically, there is pronounced splenomegaly and leukocytosis, with counts frequently above 1000×10^9 cells/L and sometimes above 2000×10^9/L. The marrow is greatly hypercellular, infiltrated by atypical lymphoid cells. The diagnosis rests on the identification of the prolymphocyte in the blood or marrow smears. The prolymphocyte is larger than a normal or malignant small lymphocyte and has a relatively condensed nuclear chromatin and a prominent, central nucleolus. Immunologic studies demonstrate B-cell lineage markers in approximately 80% of the cases. In contrast to CLL, surface immunoglobulin density in PLL is high. Almost 20% of PLL express T-cell lineage markers, compared to only 2% in CLL. Patients with PLL present with advanced disease and have short survivals. The median survival in stage IV PLL of T-cell type is 4 months compared to 9 months in PLL of B-cell and over 2 years in CLL of B-cell type.[796] Treatment of prolymphocytic leukemia may include aggressive chemotherapy, splenectomy, and leukopheresis. Unfortunately, patients are often refractory to treatment.

Hairy cell leukemia. Hairy cell leukemia (HCL), an unusual chronic lymphoid leukemia in which the involvement of marrow and spleen is predominant, is characterized by pancytopenia, splenomegaly, and the finding of a variable number of distinctive lymphoid cells in the blood.[82] Men are much more frequently affected than women, and the median age at diagnosis is

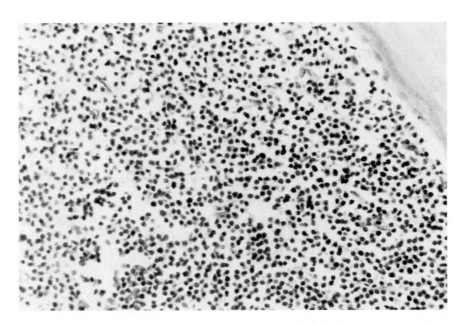

Fig. 28-10. Chronic lymphocytic leukemia, diffuse type of infiltrate. The marrow is replaced by a monotonous infiltrate of neoplastic small lymphocytes.

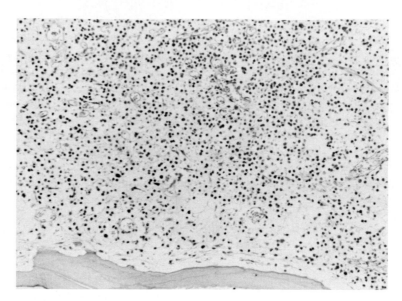

Fig. 28-11. Hairy cell leukemia. Marrow shows the characteristic loose infiltrate of separated neoplastic cells.

in the sixth decade. The neoplastic cells are somewhat larger than normal lymphocytes with more abundant amphophilic cytoplasm. The outline of the neoplastic cell appears ragged with numerous fine cytoplasmic processes projecting from the surface providing the illustrative name, hairy cell.[641] These processes are best visualized by phase microscopy. Characteristic hairy cells are usually detectable in the blood but may be found infrequently. Rodlike cytoplasmic inclusions may be identified by light microscopy that correspond to distinctive, ultrastructural ribosome-lamella complexes.[373] Cell-marker studies usually demonstrate B cell–associated antigens, clonal expression of Ig, clonal Ig gene rearrangements, and high-density interleukin-2 receptor expression.[110,577] The cells have monocyte-like features of phagocytosis and solid-phase adherence. Hairy cells express tartrate-resistant acid phosphatase (TRAP) in their cytoplasm, a reaction that is characteristic but not diagnostic of this leukemia.[501,516] Rarely, HCL may be of T-cell type. The marrow biopsy is diagnostic when marrow involvement is identified (Fig. 28-11).[79] In histologic sections, the neoplastic cells appear quite monotonous and bland, with round, oval, or indented nuclei surrounded by a wide margin of clear cytoplasm. Therefore the nuclei appear evenly and widely spaced and separated from one another. A diffuse, reticulin fibrosis characteristically encircles individual neoplastic cells. Because of this fibrosis, attempts at bone marrow aspiration are often unsuccessful. The diagnostic infiltrate may be extensive or patchy and relatively sparse.

The spleen in a HCL is greatly enlarged, both from leukemic infiltration of the red pulp and from conges-

tion. Pseudosinuses caused by the formation of ectatic spaces lined by neoplastic cells within splenic cords are a characteristic finding.[502] Similar lesions in the liver may produce the appearance of peliosis hepatis. Infiltration of other organs such as kidneys, lungs, and skin occurs but is less extensive and causes little functional impairment. HCL exhibits a highly variable clinical course and is compatible with a survival of many years. In patients with severe pancytopenia, which may be attributable to hypersplenism or extensive marrow infiltration, splenectomy may be helpful in preventing complications. Infections are potentially serious complications. Recently, alpha-2-interferon and 2-deoxycoformycin therapy have induced complete remission in a majority of patients and may be curative in some.[577]

Lymphoid hyperplasia and lymphoma. The normal number of interstitial lymphocytes, which are mostly B-cells, that is present in the marrow is higher in children than in adults. Lymphoid aggregates or nodules occur normally in the marrow of adults, and their frequency increases with age.[617] Histologically, these benign lymphoid nodules are sharply circumscribed and are usually delimited by adjacent adipose or hemic cells, creating a serrated edge. They are composed of cytologically normal-appearing small lymphocytes, plasma cells, and fewer large lymphoid cells. Occasionally germinal centers may be seen. Lymphoid hyperplasia (LH) is a subjective determination of an increase in the number of these lymphoid nodules beyond that expected for the age of the patient. LH may accompany a variety of disorders including pernicious anemia, hemolytic anemia, hyperthyroidism, chronic myeloproliferative disorders, inflammatory states, and autoimmune

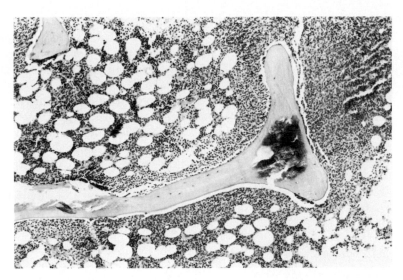

Fig. 28-12. Non-Hodgkin's lymphoma, paratrabecular pattern. Neoplastic lymphoid infiltrate is present adjacent to the bony trabeculas characteristically in lymphomas of follicular type.

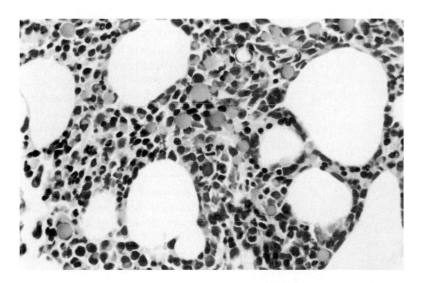

Fig. 28-13. Plasma cell myeloma, bone marrow, showing numerous Russell bodies.

conditions, such as rheumatoid arthritis. Distinguishing LH from neoplastic lymphoproliferative disorders may be difficult in certain cases requiring cell-marker studies of blood or marrow cells or biopsies of other tissues.

The reported incidence of marrow involvement by lymphoma is quite variable and depends on histologic type and method of sampling. Clearly, non-Hodgkin's lymphomas of small cleaved cell and small lymphocytic types more frequently involve the marrow than large cell lymphomas do, about 70% verses 10% (Fig. 28-12).[139,175,232] Bone marrow involvement by Hodgkin's disease is identified in only 10% of patients at presen-

tation and is virtually always accompanied by fibrosis.[529,778] Malignant lymphoid infiltrates in the marrow may be diffuse or focal, and central or paratrabecular. The diagnostic assessment of lymphoid infiltrates in the marrow requires correlation of the marrow aspirate and smears, the results of lymph node or tissue biopsy, and clinical findings.

Proliferative disorders of plasma cells

Plasma cells normally constitute less than 2% of marrow cells and are usually found adjacent to small blood vessels. Plasma cell hyperplasia in the marrow is seen

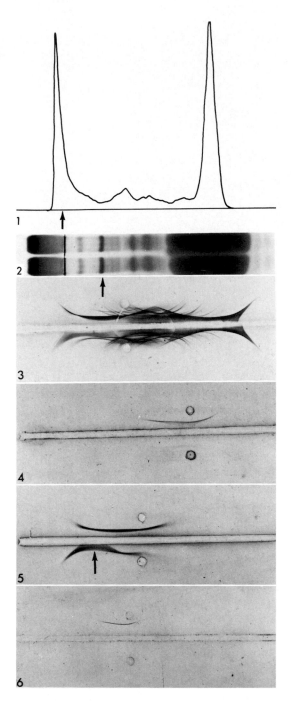

Fig. 28-14. Plasma cell myeloma. **1,** Electrophoretic pattern showing abnormal gamma peak *(arrow).* **2,** Starch gel electrophoresis showing abnormal gamma band *(arrow).* **3** to **6,** Immunoelectrophoresis: control subject *(top);* patient *(bottom).* **3,** Polyvalent antiserum showing abnormal gamma components. **4,** Anti-IgA serum showing reduction of IgA. **5,** Anti-IgG serum showing abnormal and increased IgG component *(arrow).* **6,** Anti-IgM serum showing decreased IgM. (From Miale, J.B.: Laboratory medicine—hematology, ed. 6, St. Louis, 1982, The C.V. Mosby Co.)

in a wide variety of conditions, including infection, carcinoma, Hodgkin's disease, metabolic disorders, cirrhosis, hemolytic, iron-deficiency, and megaloblastic anemias, and in hypoplastic or aplastic marrows.[332] The degree of hyperplasia is usually modest but may approach 50% of the cellularity in some processes. The morphology of the plasma cells may not aid in the distinction of benign from malignant proliferations. Intracytoplasmic immunoglobulin inclusions (or Russell bodies), intranuclear inclusions (or Dutcher bodies), nucleoli, and binucleate forms are common in both (Fig. 28-13). Biopsy is superior to the aspirate in assessment of the character, distribution, and extent of the plasma cells infiltrate. In hyperplasia it is usually heterogeneous, perivascular or interstitial, and minimal, whereas in neoplastic disorders it is usually homogeneous, focal or diffuse, and extensive.[88]

Plasma cell dyscrasias are clonal proliferations of Ig-secreting cells that are usually associated with elevated serum or urinary levels of monoclonal Ig or its components, light chains, or rarely heavy chains (Fig. 28-14). The excessive quantity of identical proteins forms a discrete, narrow band on serum protein electrophoresis, called an M-band or M-protein (monoclonal protein). This group of disorders, also called monoclonal gammopathies or paraproteinemias, include plasma cell myeloma, Waldenström's macroglobulinemia, primary amyloidosis, heavy-chain diseases, and monoclonal gammopathy of undetermined significance. All these conditions occur predominantly in middle-aged or elderly persons.

Plasma cell myeloma. Plasma cell myeloma, or multiple myeloma, is characterized by the proliferation and accumulation within the marrow of neoplastic cells that usually constitute greater than 20% of the marrow cells that morphologically resemble plasma cells (Fig. 28-15).[404] Usually the myeloma cells secrete Ig, light chains, or both; IgG and IgA are most frequent, IgD and IgE are rarely secreted, and nonsecretory myelomas occur in 1% of cases. Light chains (Bence Jones protein), which are not filtered by the glomeruli, may be demonstrated in the urine. Within the marrow, proliferations may be diffuse or form nodular masses. Radiographically, when the tumor burden is advanced, there is evidence of diffuse osteopenia or multiple, punched-out osteolytic lesions, thus multiple myeloma. Osteoclast-activating factors secreted by neoplastic cells has been demonstrated in myeloma and is postulated to cause the bone resorption. With rare exceptions, osteoblastic activity is not increased as demonstrated by a lack of radionuclide uptake in these cases. Lytic lesions most frequently involve the skull, vertebrae, ribs, and pelvis. Because of this central skeletal distribution, the diagnosis can usually be made by iliac crest biopsy.[103]

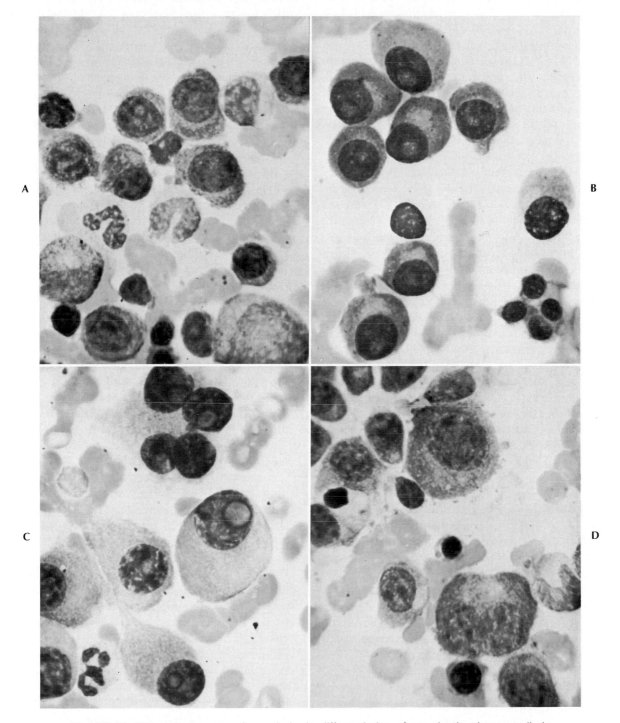

Fig. 28-15. Different degrees of morphologic differentiation of neoplastic plasma cells in myeloma. Marrow smears from most differentiated, **A,** to least, **D.** (From Miale, J.B.: Laboratory medicine—hematology, ed. 6, St. Louis, 1982, The C.V. Mosby Co.)

Occasionally at presentation, marrow involvement is patchy, and several biopsies may be required to allow detection of the infiltrate. Less commonly, solitary plasmacytomas occur in the upper respiratory tract including the paranasal sinuses, the lower respiratory tract, the gastrointestinal tract, soft tissues, various organs, and bone.[146,476,807] However, these lesions are most often nonsecretory and present as solitary, soft-tissue masses. In that plasmacytomas are occasionally cured with local treatment, a small proportion of these tumors are truly solitary at diagnosis, but disseminated myeloma will become evident ultimately in many patients.

The marrow in myeloma is infiltrated by plasma cells that may exhibit a range of cytologic appearances (Fig. 28-15). Most commonly, the tumor cells closely resemble mature plasma cells, forming extensive perivascular and paratrabecular infiltrates, scattered nodules, or confluent infiltrates.[99,103,456] Equivocal cases can be distinguished from plasma cell hyperplasia by the presence of a single type of light chain in the cytoplasm of myeloma cells[561]; reactive proliferations are polyclonal and express both kappa and lambda light chains. Poorly differentiated myeloma shows large cells with predominant central nuclei, prominent nucleoli, and multinucleation. Rarely, anaplastic tumors associated with a rapidly fatal course occur; demonstration of clonal Ig or light-chain and other plasma cell–associated antigens in the tumor cells may be necessary to establish the plasmacytic nature of the tumor.[242,698] Extraosseous plasma cell tumors occur quite frequently in myeloma, often as direct extensions into paraspinal tissue or extradural space causing spinal cord compression, or as infiltrates of orbital or cranial nerves. Dissemination also occurs, usually involving spleen, liver, and lymph nodes, but any visceral or cutaneous site may be affected. Plasma cell leukemia, defined as a neoplastic disorder with 20% plasma cells in the blood or an absolute plasmacytosis of 2×10^9 cells/L, occasionally complicates the terminal stage of disease in some patients or occurs as aggressive, fatal neoplasm usually in younger patients.[710]

The clinical manifestations of myeloma result from direct tissue effects of the neoplastic plasma cell infiltrate and from the effects of hypersecretion of Ig and light chains. Direct effects include anemia, hypercalcemia, and destructive, lytic bone lesions with bone pain and compression or pathologic fractures.[709] The hypersecretion of Ig may lead to blood hyperviscosity that impairs the circulation of red cells and results in neurologic manifestations, cardiac failure, and characteristic retinal lesions. Rouleau formation of red cells in the blood smear is attributable to hypergammaglobulinemia. Sometimes the paraprotein is a cryoglobulin, which can lead to tissue ischemia or necrosis after being precipitated in small peripheral vessels. Rarely, mono-

clonal Ig causes symptoms because of autoimmune activity, such as bleeding from anti–factor VIII activity. Humoral and cellular immunity is impaired in myeloma and results in infections, particularly with pneumococcus and herpes zoster. Chronic renal dysfunction is common in myeloma attributable to plasmacytic infiltration, amyloid, pyelonephritis, or "myeloma kidney." Myeloma kidney occurs in over 30% of patients, and its distinctive lesion is characterized by glassy or laminated tubular casts formed of precipitated Bence Jones protein that are surrounded by giant cells and accompanied by tubular atrophy, interstitial fibrosis, and glomerular lesions. Amyloidosis is a recognized complication of myeloma, occurring in approximately 10% of cases; amyloid deposits may be demonstrated in marrow as well as peripheral nerves, tongue, heart, synovium, and lungs, the same tissue distribution as in primary amyloidosis.[399] Amyloid appears as homogeneous, amorphous, eosinophilic material that may be directly associated with the plasma cells.

The treatment of myeloma includes corticosteroids, alkylating agents, combination chemotherapy, and local irradiation. Survival may be prolonged, but myeloma is currently incurable, with a median survival of 2 to 3 years.[26] Death occurs from infection, renal failure, progressive myeloma or immunoblastic transformation, myelodysplasia, or ANLL. The actuarial risk of developing ANLL is almost 20% within 5 years after treatment. ANLL may occur as part of the natural history of plasma cell neoplasms, since there is an increased risk of developing leukemia that is independent of treatment.[43]

Waldenström's macroglobulinemia. Waldenström's macroglobulinemia is an immunosecretory dyscrasia with features of both myeloma and lymphoma.[541] It is characterized by IgM monoclonal hypergammaglobulinemia (macroglobulinemia) with lymphadenopathy and hepatosplenomegaly. The marrow is almost always involved but usually without lytic bone lesions.[398,455] The marrow is focally or diffusely infiltrated by a mixture of neoplastic small lymphocytes, plasma cells, and plasmacytoid lymphocytes, which have a lymphocytic nucleus and plasma cell–like cytoplasm with a prominent Golgi region. Any of the cytoplasmic or nuclear inclusions found in plasma cell proliferations may be observed in Waldenström's macroglobulinemia.[615] Morphologic features suggestive of macroglobulinemia include plasmacytoid lymphocytes and PAS-positive material in blood vessel walls, in intravascular plasma, and in association with the lymphoid cell infiltrates (Fig. 28-16). The pattern and morphology of the infiltrate correlates with prognosis: patients with a predominance of small lymphocytes and focal disease replacing less than 20% of the marrow have a greater than 5-year median survival, whereas those with a polymorphous

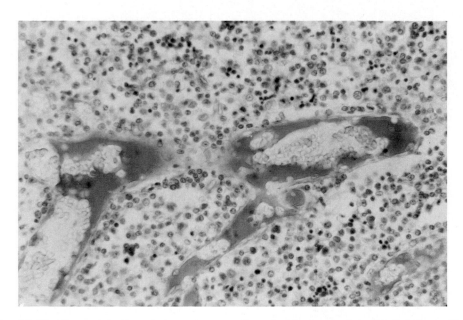

Fig. 28-16. Macroglobulinemia in marrow section showing periodic acid–Schiff–positive intravascular plasma. (PAS stain.)

infiltrate including immunoblasts and prolymphocytes replacing more than half of the marrow show rapid progression with death in a matter of months.[106] Common clinical manifestations of Waldenström's macroglobulinemia include weight loss, fatigue, anemia, bleeding tendency, the hyperviscosity syndrome, and enlargement of lymph nodes, spleen, and liver.[398] Bence Jones proteinuria and cryoglobulinemia are occasionally seen. Potential complications include amyloidosis, neuropathy, and infection as in myeloma; however, renal impairment is relatively infrequent.

Amyloidosis. Amyloidosis, characterized by extracellular tissue deposition of eosinophilic fibrillar material composed of light-chain protein may occur with or without an associated overt plasma cell dyscrasia. When associated with a plasma cell dyscrasia, the light chain class is more often lambda than kappa. The marrow in primary amyloidosis usually shows a modest plasmacytosis of 5% to 15%; amyloid deposits in blood vessels, sinuses, or interstice of the marrow may be present in up to 50% of cases.[399] The distribution of amyloid deposits in immunocyte-derived amyloidosis is characteristic and includes peripheral nerves, tongue, lungs, heart, gastrointestinal tract, and skin. In secondary amyloidosis, the kidneys, spleen, and liver are involved, and the amyloid is derived from non–Ig related A-protein. Histologic demonstration of amyloid deposits is necessary for the diagnosis of amyloidosis. Both primary and secondary types are characterized by congophilia with green birefringence under polarized light, nonbranching, 9 to 12 nm fibrils ultrastructurally, and fluorescence with thioflavin T. The two types can be

distinguished on the basis of resistance of light chain–derived amyloid to potassium permanganate oxidation and specific antisera.[757]

Monoclonal gammopathy of undetermined significance. Monoclonal gammopathy of undetermined significance, or benign monoclonal gammopathy, refers to the presence of a paraprotein of greater than 2 g/dl in the serum in the absence of any identifiable disease. Plasma cells in the marrow compose usually less than 10% of the cellularity, and cytologically atypical plasma cells may be present. Some persons have progressive disease, and over 25% will ultimately develop myeloma or a related disorder, sometimes after 20 years or more. The majority of patients, however, do not progress, and the paraprotein may even disappear. Stable paraprotein levels over time, normal serum albumin, absence of Bence Jones proteinuria, and normal blood T- to B-lymphocyte ratio have been suggested to indicate a low likelihood of progression.[684]

Proliferations of mast cells

Mast cell proliferations in the marrow occur in a variety of conditions, including myelodysplasia, acute leukemia, CLL, lymphoma, Waldenström's macroglobulinemia, and aplastic anemia as well as systemic mastocytosis.[574,821] Mast cells are easily identified in marrow smears because of their characteristic metachromatic cytoplasmic granules. In tissue sections, however, they exhibit a range of morphologic appearances. Often they contain round or oval nuclei and have abundant, slightly granular cytoplasm. The nucleus may be folded or lobular, resembling a histiocyte, and their

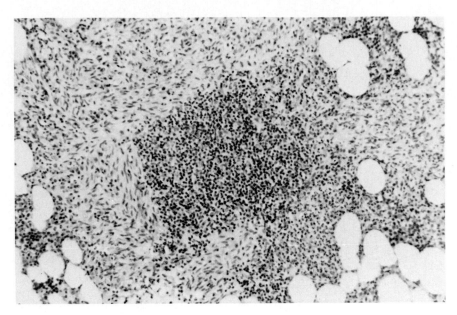

Fig. 28-17. Mastocytic eosinophilic fibrohistiocytic lesion. Lymphoid nodule is surrounded by mast cells characterized by regular, small, elongated nuclei. Eosinophils are not recognizable.

elongated, spindled cellular profile may be confused with a fibroblast. A clue to their presence is an increased number of eosinophils that are often associated with mast cell proliferations. Specific mast cell granules can be demonstrated by Giemsa, chloroacetate esterase, toluidine blue, or Ziehl-Neelsen acid-fast stains. Mast cell proliferations most frequently involve the skin as a localized lesion, a mastocytoma, or a generalized process, as in urticaria pigmentosa, which accounts for 99% of mastocytoses. Less frequently, there occurs systemic involvement or systemic mastocytosis in which the marrow, lymph nodes, spleen, and other organs are infiltrated by mast cells.[72,420,733]

Systemic mastocytosis, which accounts for about 10% of mastocytoses, affects middle-aged persons who usually have had long-standing urticaria pigmentosa.[779] Skin involvement is absent in about 10% of cases, however. Clinical manifestations include urticaria, pruritus, edema, flushing, hypotension, tachycardia, and diarrhea that is presumably related to histamine release. Generalized radiographic bone lesions and hepatosplenomegaly are caused by extensive infiltration by mast cells. The marrow in systemic mastocytosis contains aggregates or sheets of mast cells that displace normal hemic cells and results in cytopenias. Often, localized mast cell infiltrates are perivascular, paratrabecular, or associated with lymphoid follicles and are composed of prominently spindled, hypogranular mast cells intermixed with eosinophils.[812] Reticulin fibrosis may be increased, and osteopenia or osteosclerosis may be present.[212] The eosinophilic fibrohistiocytic lesion of bone, originally described as a likely result of drug hypersensitivity, probably represents part of the spectrum of systemic mast cell disease (Fig. 28-17).[616,721] The course of systemic mast cell disease is variable, and some reports distinguish between benign and malignant disease based on clinical and cytologic features.[420] When not associated with urticaria pigmentosa, it is more often a clinically progressive disease. Most deaths are attributable to disease progression or to mast cell leukemia, a very rare and particularly aggressive disorder, usually in the first 2 to 3 years after diagnosis. However, patients with systemic mastocytosis continue to be at risk for progression or the development of lymphoma or myeloid leukemia for many years.

Reactions and lesions of marrow stroma
Serous atrophy of marrow adipose tissue

Serous atrophy or gelatinous transformation of marrow fat may be seen in cachexia, disseminated carcinoma, chronic renal disease, tuberculosis, anorexia nervosa, and after chemotherapy for acute leukemia.[649,811] It is characterized histologically by the presence of homogeneous or slightly fibrillar faintly amphophilic extracellular material between fat cells (Fig. 28-18). The material consists of hyaluronic acid and fibrin. Fat cells may be normal in size or small and atrophic. The associated hemic cells are hypoplastic. It is important to distinguish serous atrophy from amyloid, necrosis, and generalized marrow aplasia.

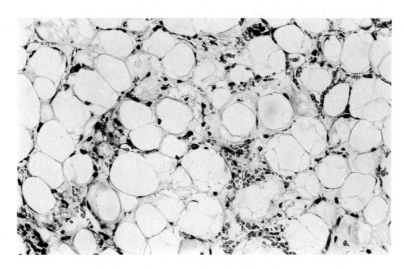

Fig. 28-18. Serous atrophy of fat present in marrow section. Homogeneous extracellular material separating variably sized fat cells.

Bone marrow necrosis

Necrosis of marrow is seen in association with hematopoietic or metastatic neoplasms, septicemia, sickle cell anemia, and caisson disease and in any disorder associated with disseminated intravascular coagulation.[69,140] The histology of marrow necrosis is similar to its appearance elsewhere: amorphous, granular, eosinophilic cytoplasm and pyknotic or fragmented nuclei. Necrosis may affect individual cells, small foci, or large confluent zones. With bone infarcts, the bony trabeculas are necrotic and acellular as well. Necrosis may be associated with bone pain, and rarely necrotic marrow embolizes to the lungs. The necrosis resolves by marrow regrowth, or the area, if extensive, may undergo fibrosis.[387]

Inflammatory reactions

Inflammatory lesions detectable in the marrow frequently are granulomatous, though acute and chronic inflammation attributable to localized or systemic infection also occurs. Granulomas, frequently encountered in marrow biopsy specimans, may be of an infectious or noninfectious origin. Lipid granulomas are the most frequent type, which is seen in nearly 10% of all marrow biopsy specimens.[614] The early lesion consists of variably sized fat vacuoles associated with macrophages, lymphocytes, plasma cells, and eosinophils, whereas mature lipid granulomas have more epithelioid or occasional giant cells. They resemble mineral oil–related granulomas of lymph nodes and spleen and appear to be a nonspecific inflammatory reaction unassociated with specific disease. Other nonspecific granulomas have been seen in association with infectious mononucleosis, viral hepatitis, Q fever, Whipple's disease, lymphomas, and other neoplasms.[321,533]

Specific granulomatous infections can be diagnosed by marrow biopsy when the infection is systemic. The etiologic agent can be demonstrated by appropriate histochemistry, immunohistochemistry, or microbiologic culture (Figs. 28-19 and 28-20).[58,546] Unusual organisms, including atypical mycobacteria, cytomegaloviruses, and *Pneumocystis carinii* have been encountered in patients with AIDS, organ transplants, or cancer.[311,499] The ability of these patient's marrow to develop typical inflammatory reactions to infection is often lacking, and routine histochemistry to exclude the presence of organisms is necessary. Noninfectious causes of marrow granulomas include sarcoidosis (Fig. 28-21), Hodgkin's and non-Hodgkin's lymphoma, myeloma, and drug hypersensitivity reactions.[546,812]

Marrow fibrosis

Fibrosis of the marrow occurs to a variable degree in a variety of conditions. Reticulin fibrosis refers to an increase in quantity, diameter, and distribution of stainable collagen fibers, which are normally fine and confined to perivascular and paratrabecular locations.[32] A variety of hematopoietic diseases, including myeloproliferative and lymphoproliferative disorders, hairy cell leukemia, and mast cell lesions, exhibit increased marrow reticulin.[87] Collagenous fibrosis, in which fibroblasts and extracellular collagen replace hemic cells, accompanies inflammatory disorders, metastatic carcinomas, renal osteodystrophy, Paget's disease, and numerous hematologic disorders.[466,763]

Vascular lesions

Systemic disorders involving blood vessels are detectable in marrow biopsy specimens, including fibrin-

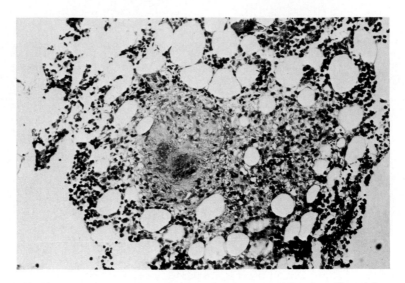

Fig. 28-19. Necrotizing granuloma present in marrow section in miliary tuberculosis.

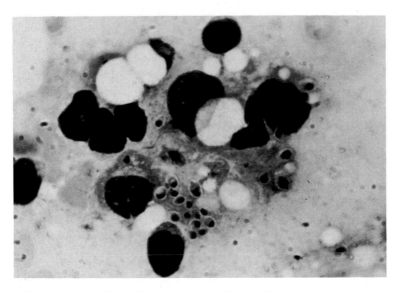

Fig. 28-20. Phagocytized *Histoplasma* sp. yeast forms *(lower center)* present in marrow smear (Wright's stain).

platelet thrombi in disseminated intravascular coagulation, thrombotic thrombocytopenia purpura, and most of the vasculitides. Atheroemboli originating from ulcerated atherosclerotic plaques can lodge in small vessels throughout the body, including the marrow as an incidental finding (Fig. 28-22). Widespread cholesterol emboli may be associated with multisystem microvascular occlusions, causing neurologic symptoms, ischemic digits, renal failure, anemia, and eosinophilia. Such lesions may be detected in the marrow during life or at autopsy.[555]

Metastatic neoplasms

The marrow is frequently involved by metastatic neoplasms. In almost 10% of marrow biopsy samples and 35% of marrow at autopsy in patients with cancer, metastatic carcinoma can be identified.[709] The most frequent primary sites in adults are the lung, breast, and prostate. Metastases may be found in the presence of radiographically detectable lesions but often are occult clinically.[674] Neuroblastoma, Ewing's sarcoma, and rhabdomyosarcoma are most common in children and may be difficult to distinguish from leukemia or lym-

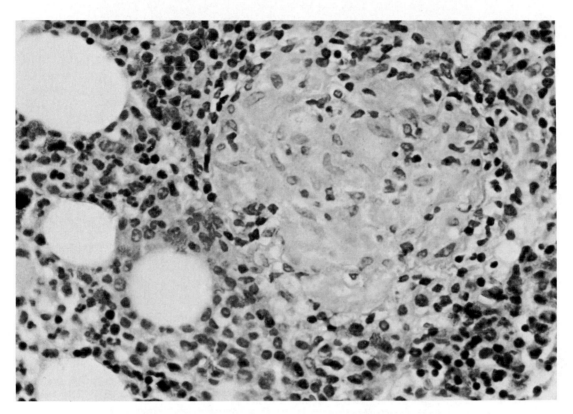

Fig. 28-21. Sarcoid granuloma present in bone marrow.

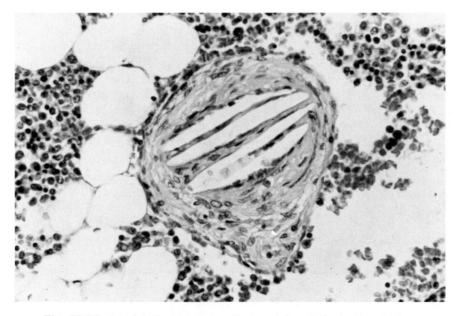

Fig. 28-22. Arteriole in marrow section contains cholesterol embolus.

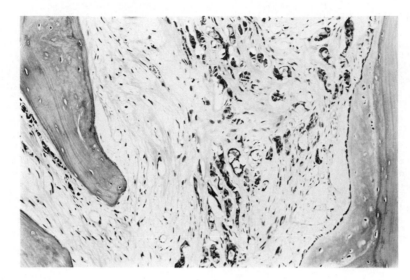

Fig. 28-23. Breast carcinoma metastatic to marrow with pronounced fibrosis accompanying the tumor cells.

phoma on the basis of the needle biopsy alone.[222] Generally, a combination of aspirate smears and needle biopsy has been shown to have the highest diagnostic yield.[8,253,636] Histologically, tumor may replace the normal hemic cells focally or extensively and is often associated with significant fibrosis (Fig. 28-23). Many metastatic tumors lead to bone resorption, which results in osteolytic lesions. Osteoblastic lesions with increased bone density are less common.[651] Often the pattern of tumor growth, its cytologic features, and associated stromal response are sufficiently distinctive, along with the patient's age and sex, to indicate the probable type and site of the primary tumor. Characteristic patterns include the linear infiltration and desmoplastic stroma in metastatic breast cancer, prominent osteoblastic reaction with prostatic adenocarcinoma, and rosettes and small, undifferentiated cells in a fibrillar background in metastatic neuroblastoma. In difficult cases, immunohistochemical studies demonstrating, for example, prostate-specific antigen or neuroendocrine antigens and electron microscopy can be helpful in classifying a given tumor.

SPLEEN
Structure and function

The spleen is the largest organized collection of lymphoreticular cells in the body. It lies within the abdomen in the upper left quadrant and is protected by the ninth, tenth, and eleventh ribs. The spleen performs as a complex filter within the bloodstream and obtains its blood supply from the splenic artery and empties into the portal venous system. Under normal conditions, the average weight of the spleen is about 135 g in the adult, with a range of 35 to 275 g.[496] It weighs less in young children and approaches adult values after 5 years of age. The spleen is contained by a thin capsule composed of dense fibrous and elastic connective tissue and smooth muscle and is covered by mesothelium. Connective tissue trabeculas extend into the pulp from the capsule and provide structure to the parenchyma and support to major vessels that enter and exit at the hilum. It is estimated that the spleen weighs 25% more in life because of the dynamic nature of its blood supply and its distensible structure. Macroscopically, the spleen consists of a homogeneous, soft, dark-red mass, called the "red pulp," that is interrupted by elongate, oval, gray-white islands, which measure 0.5 cm or less, collectively called the "white pulp." These individual malpighian bodies consist of functionally organized lymphoid tissue. Their white appearance is attributable to the refractile qualities of the densely arranged lymphocytes and accessory cells. The red pulp consists of an interlacing network of irregularly shaped, thin-walled blood vessels, called "venous sinuses," and adjacent, condensed blood spaces, called "cords of Billroth." The deep-red color of the red pulp is attributable to the abundance of the erythrocytes within the lumen of the sinuses and cords. Understanding the functional and pathologic complexities of the spleen begins with an understanding of the relationships of these structural compartments.[77,78,90]

These compartments are integrated by the splenic vascular system (Fig. 28-24). The splenic artery enters the hilum and divides into smaller arteries, which pass through the dense connective tissue of the trabeculas to enter the parenchyma as central arteries. A cylindric periarteriolar sheath of lymphoid tissue replaces the adventitia of the central artery, which in turn supplies the

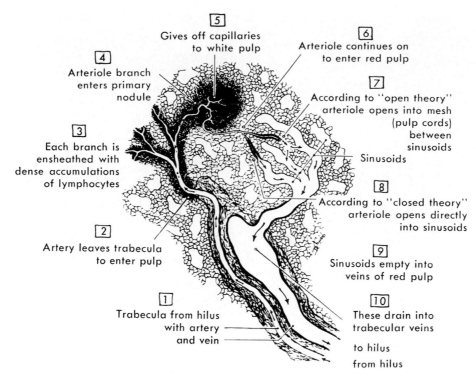

Fig. 5 Gives off capillaries to white pulp

Fig. 6 Arteriole continues on to enter red pulp

Fig. 4 Arteriole branch enters primary nodule

Fig. 7 According to "open theory" arteriole opens into mesh (pulp cords) between sinusoids

Fig. 3 Each branch is ensheathed with dense accumulations of lymphocytes

Sinusoids

Fig. 8 According to "closed theory" arteriole opens directly into sinusoids

Fig. 2 Artery leaves trabecula to enter pulp

Fig. 9 Sinusoids empty into veins of red pulp

Fig. 1 Trabecula from hilus with artery and vein

Fig. 10 These drain into trabecular veins

to hilus

from hilus

Fig. 28-24. Diagram of the splenic vascular system. (From Blaustein, A.: The spleen, New York, 1963, copyrighted by McGraw-Hill Book Co., used with permission.)

lymphoid tissue with capillaries. Further along the central artery, the lymphoid tissue widens asymmetrically to form a lymphoid follicle. The periarteriolar lymphoid tissue is organized into three functional areas: a T-cell area—the periarteriolar lymphoid sheath (PALS); a B-cell area—the germinal center and follicular cuff; and the marginal zone—a transitional area, which is unique to the spleen, located at the border of the malpighian body and the red pulp.[728] The central artery continues to branch and become smaller as the lymphoid sheath thins progressively to one or two layers of lymphocytes. At this point, it branches to form short penicillate arterioles, which enter the red pulp and further branch either into "sheathed" capillaries, which exhibit a characteristic thickening of their walls or into fewer numbers of simple capillaries. The thickening of the sheathed capillary consists of tall endothelia surrounded by reticulum cells, reticulum fibers, and macrophages. The sheathed capillary may function in the subtle regulation of blood flow. Both types of capillaries continue as simple capillaries. The pathway into the venous system is a functionally dynamic one through either the splenic cords or the splenic sinuses, but the structure of these pathways is unclear. The former pathway is explained by the "open-circulation" theory, and the latter by the "closed-circulation" theory. In reality, both pathways function and most probably simultaneously,

with the balance of blood flow depending on the prevailing hydrodynamic forces within the spleen.

The venous sinuses are wide, irregular vessels that permeate and occupy much of the volume of the red pulp. They are composed of fusiform epithelial cells that lie longitudinally along the axis of the sinus and perpendicularly to the encircling fenestrated architecture of the ring fibers of basal lamina material that supports them and into which they attach. The ring fibers are continuous with the reticulin fibers of the cordal spaces that are immediately adjacent, and they separate the sinusoid endothelial cells from the cordal reticulum cells and the large number of cordal macrophages. Whether within the sinuses or the cords, normal circulating blood cells may pass between the endothelia and the fenestrations of the basal lamina (Fig. 28-25). Abnormal cells, particularly erythrocytes and neoplastic cells, which are less compliant, remain entrapped within the cords (Fig. 28-26). The sinuses lead into the veins within the pulp, which leave through the trabeculas and hilum. Lymphatic vessels are sparsely distributed throughout the capsule and within the thickest trabeculas. Autonomic nerves are distributed along the arteries and arterioles as far as the central and penicillate arterioles.

The primary functions of the spleen are listed in Table 28-6. The spleen plays a major role in destroying

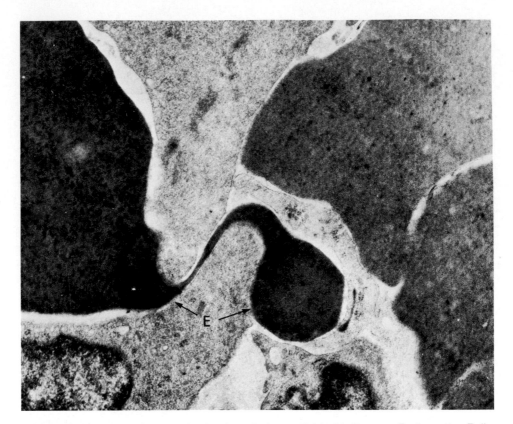

Fig. 28-25. Electron micrograph of spleen in hemoglobin H disease. Erythrocyte, *E,* lies partially within (smaller portion) and partially outside sinus. (From Wennberg, E., and Weiss, L.: Blood **31:**778, 1968; used with permission.)

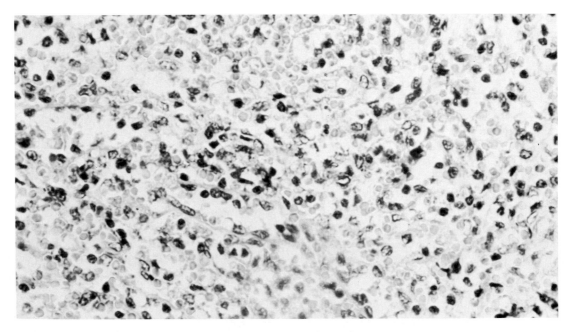

Fig. 28-26. Spleen in congenital spherocytosis. Notice congestion of the splenic cords.

Table 28-6. Primary functions of the normal spleen

Phagocytic functions	Removal of abnormal circulating cells and particulate debris from the blood
Immune functions	Production of immune responses to antigens circulating in the blood
Reservoir functions	Sequestration of normal platelets and storage of iron
Hematopoietic functions	Hematopoiesis during the development of the hematopoietic and immune systems and compensatory extramedullary hematopoiesis in states of relative marrow failure

defective or aged blood cells and platelets and in clearing the blood of foreign material. This filtering function depends on the abundant population of macrophages found in the splenic cords and is shared by similar, functional macrophages in the liver and marrow. Cordal macrophages, which are derived from the marrow, are a major component of the mononuclear-phagocytic system.[354] They compose only one of several phenotypically distinct subsets of macrophages that occupy distinct microanatomic niches within the spleen.[75] The cordal macrophage interrogates the blood cells as they pass through the interstices of the splenic cords, and they are particularly adept in this function and can excise cytoplasmic inclusions or small plasma membrane defects from erythrocytes and return them intact to the circulation. It is unclear exactly how the macrophage recognizes abnormal or effete blood cells, but it is believed that autoimmune antibodies play a role. Normal cells return freely to the circulation. During normal conditions, phagocytosis of intact cells by macrophages occurs exclusively, whereas in pathologic conditions, such as congenital spherocytosis, extracellular destruction, or erythroclasis, also occurs and results in the release of free hemoglobin and cell fragments into the circulation. The spleen also functions in early phases of iron and bilirubin metabolism through its phagocytic function. After phagocytosis of an aged erythrocyte, the heme moiety of hemoglobin is released intracellularly within the macrophage and degraded to bilirubin, which is released into the plasma where it binds to albumen for transport to the liver. The iron of hemoglobin is stored within the macrophage as ferritin and hemosiderin for transport to the marrow and other organs as needed.

Although the spleen acts as a reservoir of erythrocytes in some animal species, this function is vestigial in humans, though the human spleen does sequester reticulocytes temporarily until they mature. When the normal hematopoietic capacity of the marrow is compromised or overextended, the spleen, once a site of embryonic hematopoiesis, has the capacity to reinstate this function as extramedullary hematopoiesis. When extramedullary hematopoiesis occurs in association with primary myelofibrosis or other chronic myeloproliferative disorders, it is referred to as "myeloid metaplasia." Extramedullary hematopoiesis may also occur in the liver, another site of embryonic hematopoiesis. Hematopoiesis occurs in the splenic sinuses of the red pulp and can produce megakaryocytes, erythrocytes, or myelocytes or all three lineages, depending on the hemic deficit.

The spleen plays an important role in the systemic immune response to blood-borne antigens, such as bacteria and viruses. The spleen is an important source of certain antibodies, particularly anticarbohydrate antibodies. When exposed to antigen, the organized lymphoid tissue of the white pulp undergoes an immune response with a resultant proliferation of activated lymphocytes and the development of effector lymphocytes. This immune reaction results in lymphoid hyperplasia, seen as an expansion of the periarteriolar lymphoid sheath, germinal center formation, and differention of plasma cells in the marginal zones and within the cords. The temporal and functional relationships of immune responses in the spleen are similar to those in other lymphoid tissues.

Splenomegaly

Pathology in the spleen most often becomes known because of the enlargement of the spleen, a condition known as splenomegaly. Splenomegaly, which may occur in very many disorders, influences the activities of the functional compartments of the spleen. Some of the more frequent disorders that may be associated with splenomegaly are listed in Table 28-7. Quite often disorders associated with enlargement of the spleen are accompanied by the sequestration and destruction of significant numbers of blood cells, a condition referred to as hypersplenism (discussed below). Splenectomy may be the only means of diagnosis for some of these disorders and is definitive therapy for hypersplenism.

Asplenism, hyposplenism, and hypersplenism

Splenic pathology can be viewed in terms of how splenic function is altered by the various disorders that affect it. The functional alterations that affect the spleen range along a continuum from absence to excess and are termed asplenism, hyposplenism, and hypersplenism. Asplenism refers to a complete absence of splenic function, hyposplenism to functional deficiencies, and hypersplenism to functional excesses. The list below

Table 28-7. Disorders associated with splenomegaly

Circulatory disorders	Cirrhosis of the liver
	Portal or splenic vein thrombosis
	Cardiac failure
	Splenic infarcts
Infections	
Generalized infections	Acute splenic hyperplasia
	Bacterial endocarditis
	Typhoid fever
	Brucellosis
	Malaria
	Kala-azar
Granulomatous inflammation	Tuberculosis
	Histoplasmosis
	Sarcoidosis
Infections with atypical lymphocytosis	Infectious mononucleosis
	Cytomegalovirus
	Viral hepatitis
	Toxoplasmosis
	Pertussis
	Measles
	Mumps
Immunologic disorders	Rheumatoid arthritis and Felty's syndrome
	Systemic lupus erythematosus
	Drug reactions
	Autoimmune cytopenias
Infiltrative disorders	Sphingolipidoses
	Amyloidosis
Hematopoietic diseases	Hereditary hemolytic anemias
	Chronic myeloproliferative disorders
	Histiocytoses
	Leukemias
	Malignant lymphomas
	Systemic mast cell disease
Tumors and tumorlike conditions	Cysts
	Hamartomas
	Vascular neoplasms
	Metastatic neoplasms

shows some of the disorders and clinical syndromes that may alter splenic function. Although surgical absence of the spleen is encountered infrequently, congenital absence is very rare and is associated with cyanotic congenital heart disease and maldevelopment and malposition of the abdominal viscera.[814] All splenic functions are undoubtly absent in disorders of asplenism, whereas disorders that lead to hyposplenism reduce predominantly the functions of phagocytosis and immune responses. Those disorders that lead to hypersplenism increase primarily the functions of sequestra-

tion and phagocytosis. Other splenic functions are also altered, but the clinical consequences of these alterations are minimal and secondary.

Disorders that affect splenic function
  Asplenism and hyposplenism
    Asplenia syndrome
    Hypoplasia
    Atrophy
    Thrombosis of splenic vessels
    Splenectomy
  Hypersplenism
    Congestion
    Thrombosis of portal or hepatic veins
    Liver diseases
    Hereditary hemolytic anemias
    Autoimmune cytopenias
    Sphingolipidoses
    Histiocytoses
    Tumors and tumorlike lesions

In general, a disorder that causes the hyposplenic state results in a normal size or small spleen, which may go undetected. However, hyposplenism can be reliably detected through the examination of the routine blood smear by light microscopy by recognition of morphologic findings that indicate a deficiency in the spleen's phagocytic function. When the deficiency is severe, Howell-Jolly bodies are present. Howell-Jolly bodies are small cytoplasmic inclusions in erythrocytes that are normally extracted by the splenic macrophage.[155] In states of normal function, "cratered" erythrocytes can often be detected by phase microscopy. These erythrocytes appear "cratered" because they incur small pits in their plasma membranes after a successful encounter with a cordal macrophage in which an abnormality is excised. The number of cratered erythrocytes in the blood serves as a measure of relative splenic function. Asplenism usually permits the circulation of numerous abnormal cells, which are usually cleared from the blood. Hyposplenism also results in systemic infections caused by relative immune deficiencies.

In certain individuals, splenectomy can lead to overwhelming infections.[21,145,206,673] Serious infections usually occur within 12 to 24 months after splenectomy, and *Streptococcus pneumoniae* is the most frequent organism encountered regardless of the disease for which the spleen is removed. Antibody responses to pneumococcal capsular polysaccharide are impaired in postsplenectomy patients, and this impairment contributes to the propensity to infection.[178] Because other organs, such as the liver and marrow, contain appreciable amounts of lymphoreticular tissue, which is also exposed to circulating blood, the phagocytic and immune functions of the spleen are assumed gradually by these organs after splenectomy, but they never fully restore the splenic component. Hyposplenism, which results from the various congenital and acquired disorders, shares both the hematologic and immunologic features of the postsplenectomy state.

In contrast to hyposplenism, disorders that lead to a hypersplenism virtually always result in an enlarged spleen because of increased cell mass caused by increased sequestration and phagocytosis of blood cells and secondary hyperplasia of cordal macrophages and often the white pulp. Splenomegaly in association with cytopenias and a hypercellular marrow is indicative of the hypersplenic state. Splenectomy may be required to return the blood counts to normal when the specific disease is resistant to therapy.

Abnormalities of structure

Congenital anomalies of the spleen include several rare and profound developmental abnormalities: asplenia, polysplenia, and embryonic fusions with other organs. Asplenia is the congenital absence of the spleen, whereas polysplenia is the presence of multiple splenic tissue masses of essentially equal volume. Both asplenia and polysplenia occur in well-described syndromes that usually consist of partial or complete situs inversus in association with complex malformations of the heart and great vessels and other extensive developmental defects.[237,488,490,663] Hypoplasia of the spleen refers to a rare condition in which there is developmental hypoplasia primarily of the white pulp of the spleen.[380] The spleen usually weighs 1 g or less, and the lymphoid follicles appear diminished microscopically. Development of the thymus, lymph nodes, and other lymphoid tissue is unremarkable in this condition. Asplenia and hypoplasia of the spleen result in serious systemic infections, not unlike those seen in other hyposplenic states.

An accessory spleen should not be confused with polysplenia, since this condition refers to the presence of one or more small splenic masses in association with a normal spleen. In the majority of cases, accessory spleens are located at the splenic hilum, though they may be found within the tail of the pancreas, in the gastrosplenic and splenocolic ligaments, and in the omentum. The clinical importance of an accessory spleen lies in the recurrence of the splenic disease after therapeutic splenectomy should it not be recognized and excised. In addition, an accessory spleen may occasionally rupture, infarct, or simulate an abdominal neoplasm because of its mass.

During the second month of gestation, the spleen, which develops as a mesodermal proliferation from the left wall of the omental bursa, may merge with the developing nephrogenic mesoderm. This fusion occurs in an aberrant attempt of the dorsal mesogastrium to fuse with the posterior abdominal wall when forming the lienorenal ligament. Splenogonadal and more rarely splenorenal fusions result.[269] The most frequent fusion occurs between the spleen and the left testis.[472] Splenoovarian fusions have been described as well. Although the product of embryonic fusion is usually a contiguous organ mass, various degrees of discontinuity do occur, from splenic nodules within a connecting fibrous cord to a complete separation of the two organs, which results in the appearance of ectopic splenic tissue.

Degenerative changes

Atrophy of the spleen is more often related to pathologic disorders than to physiologic changes. Although age is an important factor in the involution of many organs, significant involution of the functional components of the spleen in the elderly has not been apparent in most large studies.[756] Splenic atrophy more frequently is associated with chronic hemolytic diseases, especially Hgb SS and SC diseases; a variety of intestinal malabsorption syndromes, particularly celiac disease and the chronic inflammatory bowel diseases; periarteriolar infiltrates in chronic myeloproliferative diseases, namely, chronic myelocytic leukemia and primary thrombocythemia; splenic vein thrombosis; and splenic vascular occlusions. The destructive changes, which lead to permanent atrophy, can be prevented by the successful treatment of the underlying disorder with a return to normal function. When left unabated, an otherwise transient loss of splenic function will eventually progress to a permanent loss by infarction, fibrosis, and scarring (Fig. 28-27). Atrophy with the complete loss of splenic function is referred to as autosplenectomy, a frequent occurrence in sickle cell anemia.

Amyloidosis, in its systemic form, involves the spleen more frequently than any other organ. The spleen may be normal in size or enlarged, and amyloid may involve the spleen in either a nodular or diffuse distribution. In the nodular pattern, amyloid is deposited in the walls of the central arteries and within the malpighian bodies. Macroscopically, the malpighian bodies appear exaggerated and translucent rather than gray-white. Rarely, clinical tumor nodules of amyloid form in the spleen as in other sites.[437] In the diffuse type, amyloid is deposited predominantly in the red pulp. Usually the spleen is enlarged and firm, and the cut surface is characteristically waxy in appearance. The functional loss encountered in either form is relative to the extent of amyloid deposition and the pace in which the amyloid is deposited.

Hyaline degeneration of the splenic arteries is common, occurs at all ages, and is accelerated in hypertensive cardiovascular disease. It is seen most prominently in the central arteries and arterioles of the malpighian bodies. Arterial hyaline degeneration has little func-

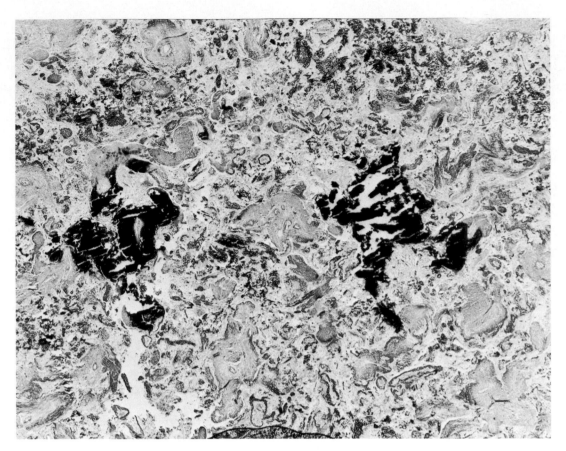

Fig. 28-27. Atrophy of spleen in long-standing sickle cell anemia. Notice complete loss of normal architecture and replacement by fibrous tissue, pigment, and calcium deposits.

tional significance. Arterial hyaline degeneration should not be confused with the characteristic periarterial lamellar lesions seen in systemic lupus erythematosus (SLE), which affect the central and the penicillate arterioles (Fig. 28-28). Although nondiagnostic, these lesions are characteristic of SLE and are of immunologic origin, since immunoglobulin, complement, and fibrinogen can be demonstrated within the lesion.

Rupture and autotransplantation

The most frequent cause of rupture or laceration of the spleen is trauma, which may or may not be associated with fractures of overlying ribs. Rupture is often a surgical emergency because of rapid blood loss and hemoperitoneum. Sometimes rupture is delayed for several days after the traumatic incident during which time a deep intrasplenic hematoma forms and expands with fluid before rupturing through the capsule. Should rupture not occur, a cystic hematoma results and eventually resolves to a splenic pseudocyst.

Splenosis is the autotransplantation of splenic tissue within the peritoneal cavity or sometimes in extraperi-

toneal sites and usually occurs after accidental rupture of the spleen.[226] Peritoneal splenic implants are usually quite numerous and appear as multiple, dark-red nodules on the surface of the peritoneum, mesentery, bowel wall, and omentum. The tissue remains functional, and unusual complications, such as infarction presenting as abdominal pain, or recurrent splenic disorders, such as hypersplenism, have been described.[731]

Pathologic or "spontaneous" rupture of the spleen is a rare clinical event that has been described as the most frequent complication of acute infectious mononucleosis. Pathologic rupture of the spleen is recorded as the most frequent cause of death in these patients. Spontaneous rupture has also been described as a complication of splenic abscess, sepsis, hepatitis, sarcoidosis, Gaucher's disease, amyloidosis, chronic myeloproliferative disorders, lymphoproliferative disorders, and metastatic carcinoma.[21,333,369] Trauma to the spleen almost certainly is the cause of splenic rupture in these conditions. In such cases, the trauma is unnoticed and may even occur as a result of palpation or abdominal straining.

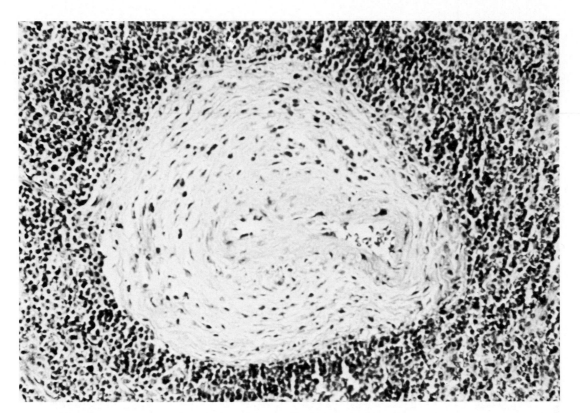

Fig. 28-28. Spleen in systemic lupus erythematosus. Notice the onion-skin appearance of arteriolar wall.

Circulatory disorders

Chronic passive congestion, or congestive spleno-megaly, is the most frequent cause of an enlarged spleen and results from a chronic increase in the hydro-dynamic pressure of the portal venous system. Portal hypertension results from an anatomic obstruction of the portal venous blood flow, which may be prehepatic, occurring in the portal or splenic veins or in the spleen itself; intrahepatic, occurring within the hepatic paren-chyma; and posthepatic, occurring in the systemic cir-culation distal to the liver. The two most frequent causes of palpable splenomegaly caused by chronic pas-sive congestion are cirrhosis of the liver and congestive heart failure. In congestive heart failure, the spleen is secondarily affected because of increased pressure with the hepatic venous system. The spleen may be moder-ately enlarged weighing more than 500 g. The spleen is firm because of slight fibrous thickening of the capsule and trabeculas, and the white pulp is reduced because of an increase in the red pulp mass. In long-standing cases, fibrosis of the red pulp occurs (Fig. 28-29), and the term "fibrocongestive splenomegaly" is appropriate.

Congestive splenomegaly attributable to portal hy-pertension causes enlargement of the spleen to 500 g and more. The splenic capsule is tense but not fibrotic,

and the cut surface is bulging and bloody obscuring the normal gross features of the spleen. Cirrhosis of the liver is the leading cause of portal hypertension, which occurs in 80% of cirrhotic livers attributable to the ob-struction of portal venous drainage into the hepatic venules. Portal hypertension may also occur because of extrahepatic obstruction to blood flow. Thromboses of the hepatic vein, the splenic vein, and the portal vein are well-described causes of prehepatic portal hyper-tension. Altered portal blood flow has also been de-scribed secondary to myeloid metaplasia in the spleen[602] and to altered circulation within the spleen itself.[551] A cause for portal hypertension may not always be demonstrable, and in such cases, portal hyperten-sion is considered to be idiopathic. Congestive spleno-megaly also occurs in moderate degree in high cardiac output states, such as thyrotoxicosis.

In long-standing portal hypertension, the spleen demonstrates all the histologic features of fibroconges-tive splenomegaly. The red pulp is expanded because of increased numbers of macrophages, fibrocytes, erythrocytes, and plasma cells. Fibrosis of the cordal space is always present to some degree, often with the formation of fibrotic fascicles. The sinuses may be open and dilated, or they may be narrowed in areas of dense

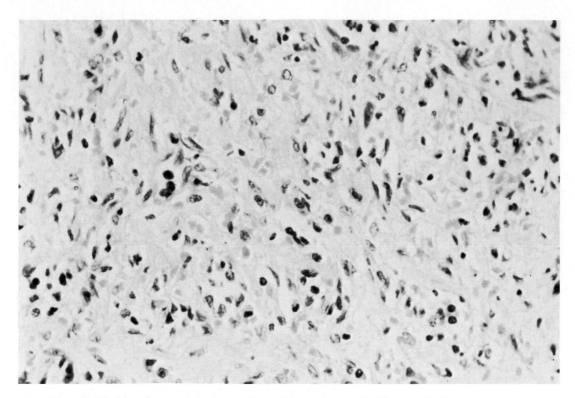

Fig. 28-29. Chronic passive congestion of the spleen with fibrosis. Notice pronounced fibrosis of red pulp.

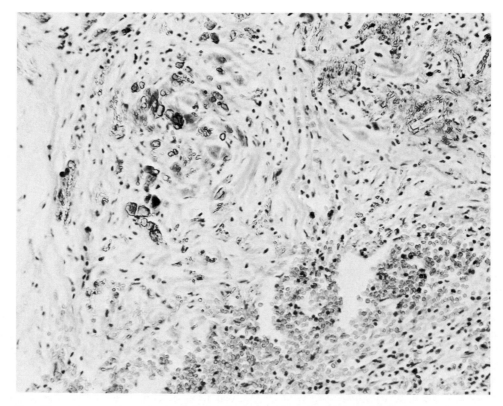

Fig. 28-30. Siderotic nodule or Gamna-Gandy body consisting of fibrous tissue, hemosiderin, hematoidin, and calcium in chronic passive congestion.

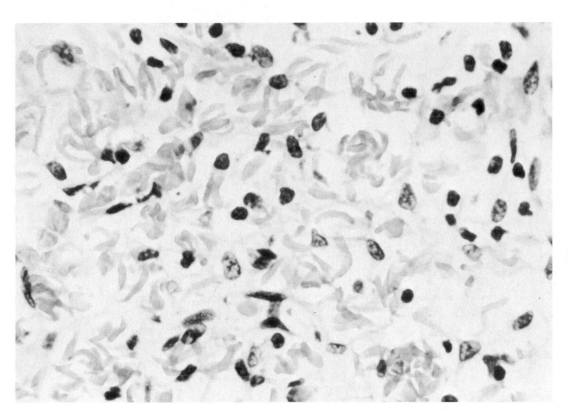

Fig. 28-31. Sickled erythocytes in the spleen in sickle cell anemia.

fibrosis. The malpighian bodies are atrophic because of pressure of the expanding red pulp, and perifollicular hemorrhage and fibrosis in the marginal zones are often present. When severe, the hemorrhages extend to the trabeculas and organize as siderotic nodules, called "Gamna-Gandy bodies" (Fig. 28-30). The association of fibrocongestive splenomegaly and hypersplenism is commonly referred to as "Banti's syndrome," though originally a more specific syndrome was described that was characterized by splenomegaly and anemia followed by gastrointestinal hemorrhage, hepatic cirrhosis, and ascites secondary to splenic vein thrombosis.[705]

Infarction

Infarcts of the spleen occur when the dependent arterial blood supply to a region is completely occluded by an embolus or thrombus. The majority of splenic infarcts occur secondarily to emboli, and most emboli to the spleen are attributable to thromboses associated with cardiovascular disease. Emboli may originate from mural thrombi within the chambers of the left side of the heart, or the aorta, and from the aortic or mitral valves. Septic emboli from bacterial vegetative endocarditis, especially of the cardiac valves, cause septic or less frequently bland infarcts in the spleen and other organs. Another frequent cause of splenic infarcts is sickle cell disease in which the microcirculation of the spleen becomes occluded by the nondeformable sickled erythrocytes (Fig. 28-31). Splenic infarcts also occur in patients with sickle cell trait when they are exposed to low atmospheric oxygen, such as at high altitudes. Involvement of the spleen by leukemias and lymphoproliferative disorders can result in neoplastic infiltrates in arterial vessels with secondary thrombi and infarcts on that basis. Infarcts also accompany massive splenomegaly because of myeloid metaplasia in patients with chronic myeloproliferative disorders, particularly in primary myelofibrosis. Splenic infarcts have also been described in vasculitides, in hypercoagulable states, and in association with amyloidosis.

Splenic infarcts are either ischemic, hemorrhagic, or suppurative. Macroscopically they are conical with their base at the capsular surface (Fig. 28-32). The cut surface appears irregular but well delineated from the adjacent, nonviable hyperemic parenchyma. Infarcts may appear pale, hemorrhagic, or necrotic depending on the time interval from the event and whether there is infection. Infarcts eventually heal by fibrosis, which contracts to produce a depressed scar in the overlying capsule.

Hemorrhagic infarction of part or all of the spleen may rarely result from acute torsion and occlusion of the splenic vessels.[168] Torsion occurs because of an increased mobility of the spleen attributable to developmental disturbances of the supporting ligaments and elongation of its vascular pedicle. Such a spleen is described as a "wandering" or "floating" spleen. Although the specific clinical diagnosis of splenic torsion is difficult, splenectomy results in a low mortality, if not delayed. Accessory spleens because of their inherent anatomic instability are particularly prone to torsion, and torsion has been described in some cases of splenosis.

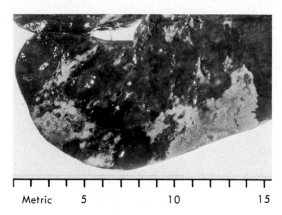

Fig. 28-32. Multiple infarcts of spleen. (From Rezek, P.R., and Millard, M.: Autopsy pathology, Springfield, Ill., 1963, Charles C Thomas, Publisher.)

Systemic infection

Splenomegaly of moderate degree, 250 to 350 g, is common in acute systemic infections and is referred to as "acute reactive hyperplasia," or "septic splenitis." Enlargement is caused both by reactive hyperplasia of the malpighian bodies and cordal macrophages and by active congestion of the cords attributable to increased cardiac output. The spleen is enlarged and soft, and the cut surface demonstrates an equal prominence of the red and white pulp. Lymphoid hyperplasia with germinal center formation is pronounced, and plasma cell hyperplasia is present in the marginal zone of the white pulp and in the cords. Histiocytic (cordal macrophage) hyperplasia is equally prominent. These reactive features are nonspecific and are present in most bacterial septicemias.

Infectious mononucleosis deserves mention because of the slight but real tendency to splenic rupture.[677] Infectious mononucleosis is a self-limited lymphoproliferative disorder that unlike most viremias is associated with splenomegaly that exceeds 500 g in 50% of cases. Cytomegalovirus infections may produce a similar clinical disorder in which the heterophil antibody test is negative.[355,651] Splenomegaly in infectious mononucleosis is attributable primarily to a massive influx of activated lymphocytes into the red pulp. These cells,

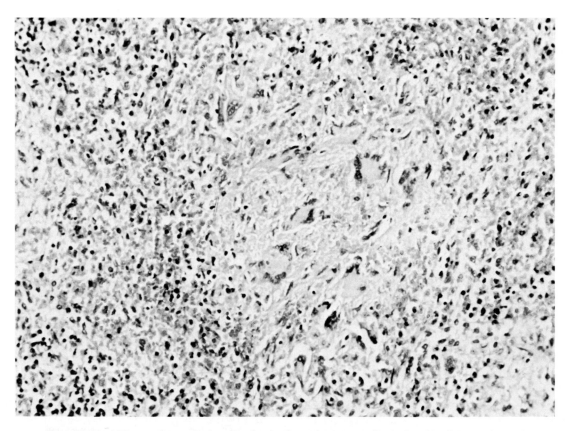

Fig. 28-33. Miliary tuberculosis of spleen. Granuloma consists of epithelioid cells and Langhan's giant cells without well-defined central necrosis.

which also circulate in the blood, are effector cytotoxic T-lymphocytes with specificity for the presence of Epstein-Barr virus–infected B-lymphocytes and are referred to as "atypical lymphocytes."[517] They infiltrate the cords and sinuses of the red pulp, the walls of splenic vessels, and the trabeculas and capsule of the spleen and promote its rupture in prolonged infections.

Abscesses in the spleen occur infrequently but most often in the spleens of young adults secondary to *Staphylococcus, Streptococcus,* or *Salmonella* infections.[129] The associated mortality may exceed 60% unless early diagnosis and prompt therapy is instituted. Hemoglobinopathies, such as sickle cell disease, nonpenetrating abdominal trauma, bacterial endocarditis, and gastrointestinal malignancies are predisposing causes of splenic abscess.

Granulomatous inflammation in the spleen occurs infrequently and is found in about 5% of surgical cases.[514] Granulomas are generally associated with splenic enlargement and often with generalized disease including hepatomegaly, fever, weight loss, and hypersplenism.[402] In some cases, the splenic weight exceeds 1000 g. The morphology of the granulomas ranges from sarcoidlike granulomas often associated with the malpighian bodies and the periarteriolar lymphoid sheath, to larger necrotizing granulomas, to confluent granulomatous masses. Sarcoidlike granulomas are found in a variety of disorders, both infectious and noninfectious: tularemia, brucellosis, histoplasmosis, leprosy, berylliosis, silica deposition, the sphingolipidoses, and Hodgkin's disease. Necrotizing granulomas (Fig. 28-33) are found in miliary tuberculosis and fungal diseases including histoplasmosis. Isolation of the causative microorganisms is rarely successful, and histochemistry results are generally negative in demonstrating the organism. Most splenic granulomas are noninfectious and are usually associated with Hodgkin's disease, sarcoidosis, chronic uremia, and the non-Hogkin's lymphomas. In those patients in which an associated disorder is not identified, the postsplenectomy course is uneventful and signs of hypersplenism disappear.

Sphingolipidoses

The sphingolipidoses are rare hereditary causes of histiocytic hyperplasia.[764] In these disorders, an enzymatic defect leads to an abnormal accumulation of an undegraded lipid in cells of the mononuclear phagocytic system and in the central nervous system. The accumulation of lipid-ladened histiocytes in the liver, spleen, lymph nodes, and marrow ultimately leads to enlargement and displacement of the normal parenchyma. Gaucher's disease, Niemann-Pick disease, and generalized gangliosidosis are associated with significant hepatosplenomegaly. The clinical features and functional deficits of each disorder depends on the specific enzyme defect and the extent to which normal organ function is disrupted (Table 28-8).

Gaucher's disease is caused by a deficiency of glucocerebrosidase, which results in a systemic hyperplasia of histiocytes that are filled with glucocerebroside (Fig. 28-34).[552] The disease presents in either an infantile form or an adult form and is most prevalent in Jews of Eastern European extraction. Because the clinical effects of this deficiency vary widely, some patients live relatively normal, symptom-free lives whereas others succumb to the disease in young adulthood.

The clinical features of Gaucher's disease are hepatosplenomegaly, cytopenias, erosive bone changes, and mental retardation in the infantile form. The spleen may be greatly enlarged, weighing more than 1000 g. Hypersplenism usually becomes the dominant clinical problem in this disorder and in other lipidoses and often required splenectomy. Histologically the sinuses and cords are filled by diffuse and patchy infiltrates of benign histiocytes (Fig. 28-35), referred to as Gaucher cells, whose cytoplasm appears striated and slightly vacuolated and stains faintly eosinophilic (Fig. 28-36). Similar histiocytes are also present in the sinuses of the liver and lymph nodes and within the medulla of the marrow. The histiocytic infiltrates may be so extensive in the marrow of long bones as to cause thinning of the cortex, which can be appreciated radiographically. The major precursor of the glucocerebroside that accumulates within the Gaucher cell is derived from senescent erythrocytes, white blood cells, and platelets. Gaucherlike cells can be found in states of rapid plasma membrane catabolism, such as chronic myelocytic leukemia or dyserythropoietic disorders.[419] Gaucher cells may be associated with a pronounced plasma cell hyperplasia in the marrow, and an increased incidence of monoclonal gammapathies including rare cases of plasma cell myeloma.[559,571] Amyloidosis resulting from hypergamma-

Table 28-8. Spinogolipidoses in which hepatosplenomegaly occurs

Disorder	Accumulated lipid	Enzyme defect	Clinical findings
Gaucher's	Glucocerebroside	Glucosidase	Bone changes, mental retardation
Niemann-Pick	Sphingomyelin	Sphingomyelinase	Mental retardation
Generalized	Ganglioside G_{M1}	Galactosidase	Mental retardation

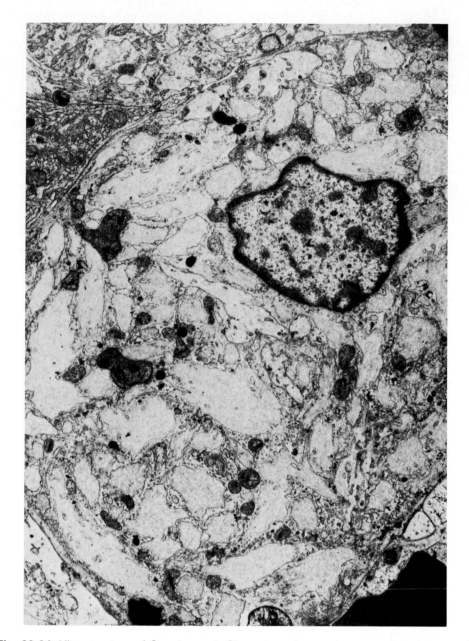

Fig. 28-34. Ultrastructure of Gaucher cell. Clear elongate membrane-enclosed spaces in cytoplasm contain lipid. (From Miale, J.B.: Laboratory medicine—hematology, ed. 6, St. Louis, 1982, The C.V. Mosby Co.)

globulinemia has been reported as a rare complication in Gaucher's disease.[297] Because some of the isolated Ig have shown a binding affinity for the glucocerebroside, it is believed that the glycolipid may induce a clonal expansion of plasma cells in some patients.

Niemann-Pick disease results from the deficiency of sphingomyelinase and is characterized by hepatosplenomegaly and mental retardation. The disease classically affects infants. The histiocytes accumulate sphingomyelin, which is derived from cell membranes and myelin sheaths. The histiocytes of Niemann-Pick dis-

ease appear foamy in microscopic section in contrast to the more distinctive appearance of the Gaucher cell, which appears striated. The sphingomyelin-containing histiocyte of Niemann-Pick disease also stains blue when stained with Giemsa stain, and this blue, granular, foamy-appearing histiocyte has been called the "sea-blue histiocyte."

The appearance of the sea-blue histiocyte is nonspecific, and similar histiocytes can be found in the spleen or marrow in many different hereditary and acquired conditions.[614] The staining qualities of this cell is char-

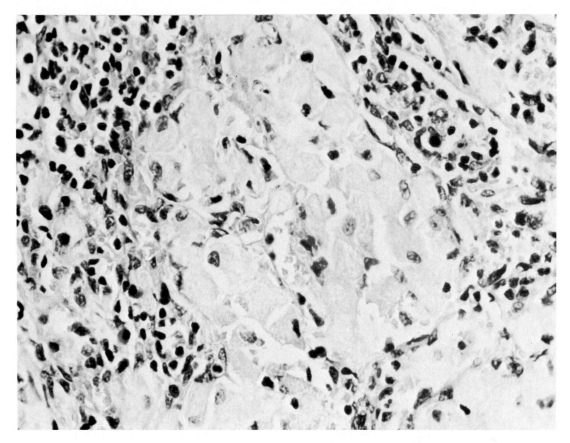

Fig. 28-35. Spleen in Gaucher's disease. Notice patchy infiltrate of Gaucher cells in splenic sinus.

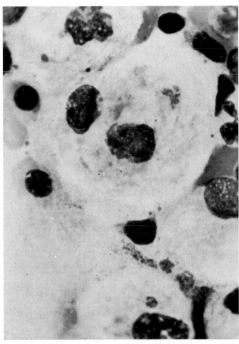

Fig. 28-36. Gaucher cell. (Spleen imprint; Wright's stain; 950×; from Miale, J.B.: Laboratory medicine—hematology, ed. 6, St. Louis, 1982, The C.V. Mosby Co.)

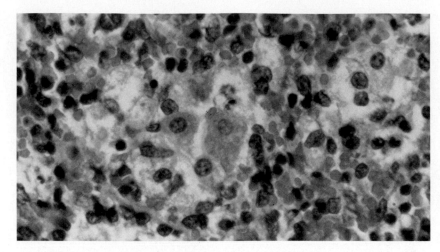

Fig. 28-37. Ceroid containing histiocytes in the spleen in hyperlipoproteinemia. Notice the large cells in the center with abundant granular cytoplasm.

acteristic of ceroid-containing histiocytes (Fig. 28-37). Ceroid, a form of lipofuchsin, results from the peroxidation and polymerization of unsaturated lipids[305] and is found in macrophages as a light, yellow or brown, autofluorescent pigment usually associated with lipid microvacuoles. The syndrome of splenomegaly of unknown cause with purpura secondary to hypersplenism manifested by severe thrombocytopenia has been referred to as the "sea-blue histiocyte syndrome" and is now recognized as ceroid histiocytosis.[669] Virtually all cases of "idiopathic ceroid histiocytosis" can be diagnosed specifically when thorough clinical and laboratory evaluations are done.

Histiocytoses

The generic term "histiocytoses" refers to a group of idiopathic clinicopathologic disorders in which there is a generalized proliferation of histiocytes.[263,284,517,519,581] Before this group of disorders can be considered as a possible diagnosis in a given circumstance, specific infections, immunologic-inflammatory disorders, and lipid storage diseases necessarily must be excluded as the primary cause.

Histiocytosis X (Langerhans' cell granulomatosis)

Histiocytosis X is a nosologic entity that represents a spectrum of described disorders that is characterized by the proliferation of cytologically benign-appearing histiocytes.[214,349,429] Historically this entity was divided into three clinical syndromes: eosinophilic granuloma, Hand-Schüller-Christian disease, and Letterer-Siwe disease.[581] There is still some discussion as to whether these named syndromes represent a spectrum of one or more disorders, but for pragmatic purposes, histiocytosis X is best divided into localized and disseminated forms: focal (monostotic and polyostotic eosinophilic granuloma) and disseminated (Letterer-Siwe disease).[159]

The term "eosinophilic granuloma" refers to a solitary lesion characterized by diffuse infiltrates of benign histiocytes accompanied by small lymphocytes, multinucleated histiocytes in varying numbers, and eosinophils, which may be quite numerous. There may also be focal necrosis including eosinophilic abscesses and fibrosis. The lesion occurs in all age groups but is more common in the first decade of life. The monostotic form most frequently involves the skull, femur, ribs, vertebrae, and pelvis, producing one or two radiographically well-circumscribed lytic lesions. Eosinophilic granulomas may also involve the lung,[31,135,682] lymph nodes,[132,588,803] skin,[483,816] and thymus[665] in isolation of any bony lesions. These lesions, like those of bone, may be the initial or only sign of disease. The prognosis of this form of histiocytosis X is excellent when the lesion is completely curetted or excised. The lesions have regressed spontaneously in some cases.

Polyostotic eosinophilic granuloma includes the syndrome of Hand-Schüller-Christian (HSC) disease and consists of multiple bony lesions that occur simultaneously or sequentially usually within the first 6 months of discovery of the initial lesion. Focal visceral infiltrates of the spleen, lung, and liver may be present as well. This form usually occurs in older children in contrast to the disseminated form. The classical triad of HSC disease (lytic lesions of the skull, exophthalmos, and diabetes insipidus) is frequently never fully expressed. The latter two sequelae result from lesions that occur in critical locations of the orbital and sphenoid bones and expand to infiltrate and destroy the hypothalamus. Again the prognosis is excellent in this lim-

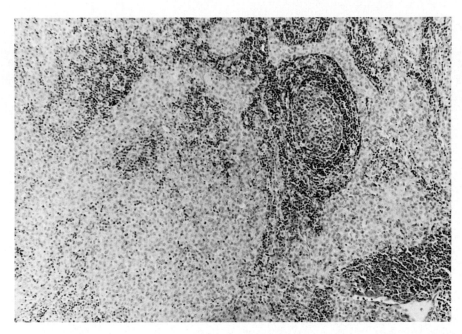

Fig. 28-38. Lymph node, eosinophilic granuloma. Subcapsular and cortical sinuses are filled by Langerhans histiocytes isolating a primary follicle.

ited form of disease when the severe symptoms of diabetes insipidus and exophthalmos are managed early and successfully. If not, patients may have a chronic course associated with diabetes insipidus, growth failure, mental retardation, blindness, or deafness.[480] Rare transitions have been described between monostotic and polyostotic eosinophilic granuloma eventuating in HSC disease.[431]

Disseminated differentiated histiocytosis (Letterer-Siwe disease) occurs in children less than 3 years of age. This form is an acute and progressive, systemic disease from the onset with infiltrates in the bone, liver, spleen, lymph nodes, lung, and skin. Primary immunodeficiency disorders, disseminated mycobacterial or fungal infections, and lymphoproliferative disorders resemble this clinical presentation and must be considered before this diagnosis is entertained. Malignant histiocytosis (discussed on p. 1425) may be especially difficult to distinguish from disseminated histiocytosis X in some patients.[335,774] The disseminated form is clinically the most serious and usually has an unfavorable outcome because of vital organ dysfunction.[521] Severe pancytopenia secondary to hypersplenism and infection, which may complicate the clinical course, can be ameliorated by splenectomy to improve survival. A rare congenital form of histiocytosis X, which is confined entirely to the skin, must be distinguished from the fatal disseminated form and treated conservatively, since spontaneous regression and recovery often occurs.[171,462]

The proliferative histiocytes of histiocytosis X are characteristic and can be recognized by light microscopy (Fig. 28-38). These differentiated histiocytes have abundant, pale eosinophilic cytoplasm, and vesicular nuclei with distinctive longitudinal, wavy grooves in the nuclear membrane. They infiltrate and expand the interstices of bone and lung and characteristically the sinuses of lymph nodes, spleen, and liver and lack the capacity of malignant histiocytes to infiltrate and destroy organ parenchyma. In chronic lesions, the histiocytes may become foamy because of the phagocytosis of endogenous lipids (Fig. 28-39). These foamy histiocytes cannot be distinguished from other ceroid-containing histiocytes. In the vast majority of cases that have been studied, the proliferating histiocyte shares morphologic and immunologic features with the Langerhans cell of the skin and other organs.[214] The Langerhans cell, a type of dendritic histiocyte, belongs to the mononuclear-phagocytic system and is characterized by the presence of ultrastructural Birbeck or X granules[48,294,480] and the expression of a specific antigenic profile.[349] It functions in the skin in antigen processing and presentation. Histiocytosis X is often referred to as "Langerhans cell histiocytosis or granulomatosis" in cases where the histologic features are typical of this cell type or when characteristic phenotypic features are present.[520] Localized Langerhans cell granulomatosis has also been reported in lymph nodes in association with malignant lymphomas, perhaps as a cellular reaction to the presence of the lymphoma.[85,389]

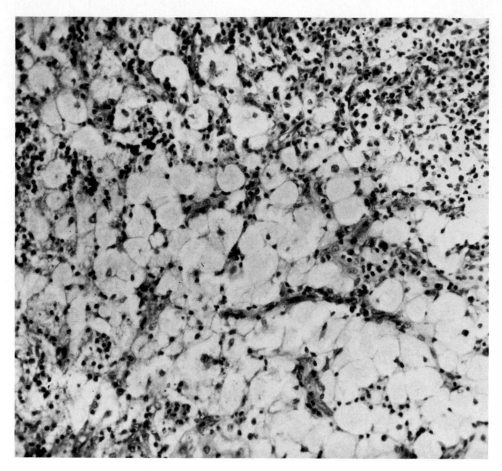

Fig. 28-39. Foamy histiocytes in spleen in histiocytosis X.

Familial histiocytic proliferative syndromes

Most cases of histiocytoses occur sporadically or as well-described clinicopathologic entities. However, rarely there are cases that are inherited and are easily and frequently confused clinically and pathologically with these entities (Table 28-9).[685] This confusion results because the tissues are infiltrated similarly by benign histiocytes preventing an accurate histologic separation of individual cases. Because these disorders tend to recur in families and are lethal, their recognition and categorization is necessary for appropriate genetic counseling.

Familial hemophagocytic lymphohistiocytosis is one of these syndromes that has been particularly well studied.[259,408,797] This disorder occurs in infants and in children as progressive hepatosplenomegaly accompanied by fever, jaundice, pancytopenia, hyperlipidemia, and coagulopathies. Infiltrates of benign histiocytes and lymphocytes are present throughout the tissues of the body but especially in the sinuses of the spleen and liver and in the marrow and central nervous system. Phagocytosis of erythrocytes and leukocytes is a particularly prominent feature of this disorder. The prolifer-

Table 28-9. Familial histiocytoses with inheritance patterns

Syndromes	Inheritance	Onset
Hemophagocytic lym-phohistiocytosis	R	I,C
Reticuloendotheliosis with eosinophilia	R	I
Chronic familial reticulosis	R	I
Histiocytic dermatoarthritis	D	C

C, Childhood; *D*, autosomal dominant; *I*, infancy; *R*, autosomal recessive.
Adapted from Spritz, R.A.: Pediatr. Pathol. **3**:43, 1985, and from others appearing in references 27, 213, 534, 567, 685, and 832.

ating histiocyte shares the phenotype of the sinusoid macrophage of the lymph node. Chromosome abnormalities usually associated with dysmyelopoietic and myeloproliferative disorders have been identified in one case.[392] Although there are reports of sporadic cases of this disorder and other hereditary histiocytoses, the incidence of this disorder in other family members is high. In familial hemophagocytic lymphohistiocytosis, the incidence approaches 75%.[353]

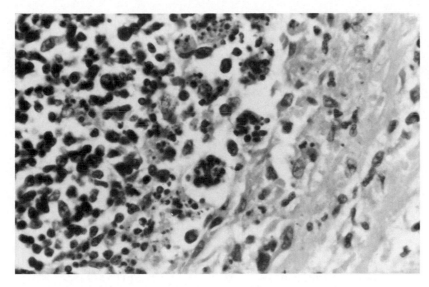

Fig. 28-40. Spleen in virus-associated hemophagocytic syndrome. Marginal zone of malpighian body with phagocytic histiocytes.

Virus-associated hemophagocytic syndrome

One of the morphologic hallmarks of many of the histiocytoses is the finding of erythrophagocytosis. However, this finding has proved to be nonspecific for any particular disorder and relates to the differentiation and functional integrity of the histiocytes. In certain clinical settings, hemophagocytosis has been associated with herpesvirus infections and a constellation of systemic signs and symptoms.[468] Patients with the virus-associated hemophagocytosis syndrome typically present with fever, hepatosplenomegaly, generalized lymphadenopathy, bilateral pulmonary infiltrates, skin rash, cytopenias, liver-function abnormalities, and coagulopathies. Histologically, there is depletion of lymphocytes in lymph nodes and the spleen. Organomegaly results from an extensive hyperplasia of actively phagocytic histiocytes (Fig. 28-40). Histologically the histiocytes appear benign without significant nuclear atypicality. Histiocytic hyperplasia in the marrow with prominent phagocytosis of erythrocytes and cellular debris is often apparent on marrow aspirate smears. Originally reported in renal transplant recipients and immunosuppressed patients, the syndrome has been observed in tuberculosis, brucellosis, and typhoid fever and as a complication of lymphoproliferative disorders and leukemia.[97,210,217,594,717,835] When the primary disorder is controllable, antiviral therapy is appropriate and usually effective in resolving the syndrome.

Malignant histiocytosis

Malignant histiocytosis is a progressive, systemic proliferation of neoplastic histiocytes and is an almost invariably fatal disease. Histologically it is recognized by the presence of abnormal histiocytes with varying degrees of nuclear atypicality and a proclivity to invade and destroy normal tissues.[95,581] These morphologic features separate malignant histiocytosis from the benign histiocytoses discussed before. In practice, this separation may be difficult in some cases.

First described as "histiocytic medullary reticulosis,"[647] malignant histiocytosis (MH) is characterized by fever, hepatosplenomegaly, jaundice, generalized lymphadenopathy, pulmonary infiltrates, skin lesions, and pancytopenia when the disease is fully developed. MH affects all age groups but occurs most frequently in the fourth decade. In the pediatric age group, the disease occurs more often after 3 years of age than before.

The spleen is usually massively enlarged and may be the first sign of disease in otherwise asymptomatic patients.[759] The white pulp is usually inconspicuous giving the organ a homogeneous, ruddy appearance on gross inspection. Discrete tumor masses are not apparent, which is in contrast to a recently recognized primary histiocytic neoplasm that forms a discrete mass.[234] Its natural history is unknown as yet. Microscopically, the neoplastic histiocytes of MH infiltrate the cords and eventually the sinuses of the spleen (Fig. 28-41). The neoplastic cells are characterized by their thick nuclear membranes, clumped chromatin, large irregular nucleoli, and mitotic activity. Pleomorphic tumor cells that resemble the Reed-Sternberg cell of Hodgkin's disease may be present occasionally or may predominate in some cases. Normal plasma cells are usually plentiful in the infiltrates. Phagocytosis of erythrocytes, leukocytes, and platelets by the neoplastic cells may or may not be evident in individual cases. Often the phagocy-

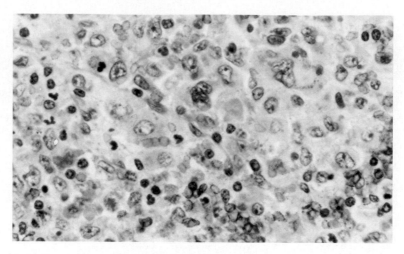

Fig. 28-41. Malignant histiocytosis in the spleen. Notice that the larger malignant histiocytes have atypical, occasionally pleomorphic nuclei and prominent nucleoli.

tizing cells appear better differentiated than the frankly malignant cells. The earliest infiltrates in the liver and lymph nodes are found in the sinuses. The malignant histiocytes ultimately infiltrate the adjacent parenchyma destroying its structure. In lymph nodes, this results in cortical and paracortical infiltrates, which isolate groups of lymphocytes and lymphoid follicles but tend to spare the capsule and perinodal tissues. In the skin, MH infiltrates the periadnexal structures of the deep dermis and the subcutaneous adipose tissue, producing palpable skin nodules. As MH disseminates, the marrow becomes involved compromising hematopoiesis. Marrow infiltrates are often identified in aspirated smears but ironically are difficult to appreciate in biopsy tissue unless extensive. Although biopsy specimens of the marrow and lymph nodes are usually the first tissues examined in patients with MH, splenectomy or liver biopsy is often required to establish the diagnosis.

In cases of MH in which cell-marker studies have been done, the neoplastic cells expressed antigens of phagocytic histiocytes and their precursors.[471,593,597] These studies have also identified many cases of non-Hodgkin's lymphoma of mature B- and T-lymphocyte phenotype in similar clinicopathologic situations.[342,346,362,790] MH has been described with increased frequency in association with other hematopoietic neoplasms: acute lymphoblastic leukemia, acute and chronic myeloproliferative disorders, and non-Hodgkin's lymphoma.[18,19,124,280,370] Before the use of combination chemotherapy, MH was almost a uniformly fatal disorder. Although most patients still succumb within a year of diagnosis, long-term complete remissions are being reported.[671]

Tumors and mass lesions
Nonhematopoietic tumors

Nonhematopoietic tumors of the spleen are rare causes of splenomegaly and include splenic cysts, hamartomas, inflammatory pseudotumors, vascular neoplasms, metastatic neoplasms, and less commonly sarcomas.[77,78,90,150,256,668] Splenic cysts present primarily in young people and are of two types: pseudocysts, which are without an epithelial lining, and true cysts, which are usually lined by epithelium. The majority of splenic cysts (80%) are in reality pseudocysts, and most of these occur because of trauma to the spleen. Most patients with splenic cysts present with abdominal pain or an abdominal mass. The wall of a pseudocyst consists of fibrous tissue with evidence of old hemorrhage, namely, hemosiderin pigment and cholesterol deposits, chronic inflammation, and dystrophic calcification. True cysts are referred to as "epidermoid cysts" and may be either nonparasitic, which are more frequent in the Western world, or parasitic, which are more frequent worldwide and are caused by *Echinococcus granulosus*. The nonparasitic, true cysts are lined by squamous epithelium or rarely by mucous cells or mesothelia and may be quite large, exceeding 1 kg.[50,581] Mucous glands and rarely sebaceous glands and hair follicles may be found in the epithelium. Splenectomy is the recommended treatment for all splenic cysts.

The splenic hamartoma is an infrequently encountered lesion of the spleen.[668] It is a well-demarcated nodular lesion that compresses the surrounding normal spleen and consists of plump, spindle cells that are inactive mitotically and disorganized. Occasional endothelium-lined spaces course through the lesion simulating a hemagioma or a sclerosing hemangioma. Whether

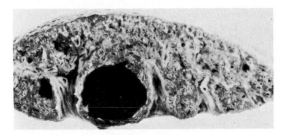

Fig. 28-42. Hemangioma of spleen with fibrosis.

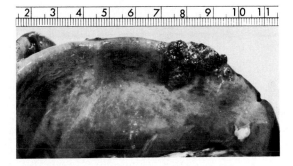

Fig. 28-43. Lymphangioma in capsule of spleen.

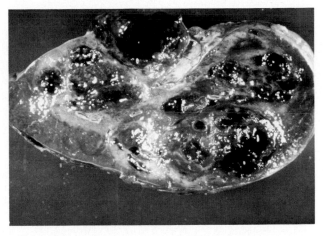

Fig. 28-44. Angiosarcoma of spleen. Notice bulging, rounded cystic areas filled by dark blood surrounded by solid, lighter areas of sarcomatous stroma.

the splenic hamartoma is developmental or acquired is unclear, but it is entirely benign. Another benign and rarely encountered solitary lesion is an inflammatory pseudotumor. Despite its alarming gross appearance that resembles a malignant neoplasm with areas of hemorrhage and necrosis, its microscopic appearance has the inflammatory and reparative features of inflammatory pseudotumors described in other sites, such as the lungs, gastrointestinal tract, and orbit.[150]

Hemangiomas, lymphangiomas, and angiosarcomas are rare primary neoplasms of the spleen.* Hemangiomas, benign neoplasms of blood vessels, are usually solitary and vary in size from minute to large cavernous lesions (Fig. 28-42). They may be located anywhere in the red pulp. Lymphangiomas arise from the splenic lymphatic vessels in the capsule or trabeculas and may be large and multicentric (Fig. 28-43). Histologically, lymphangiomas and hemangiomas are difficult to distinguish from one another. Occasionally these neoplasms may have a visceral distribution involving other organs, particularly the skeleton and the liver, in addition to the spleen.[14,158,256] Being vasoformative lesions, hemangiomas and lymphangiomas are prone to thrombosis

*References 117, 123, 144, 330, 667.

and infarction, and their clinical course may be complicated by consumptive coagulopathy and rupture, as with lymphangiomas.

Angiosarcomas represent the most frequently encountered nonhematopoietic malignant tumor of the spleen. Occasional examples of malignant fibrous histiocytomas, fibrosarcomas, and leiomyosarcomas have been described. Typically, angiosarcomas consist of solid areas of sarcomatous vascular stroma within the splenic pulp with centrally dilated, cystic spaces (Fig. 28-44). This tumor is highy lethal, with a median survival of less than a year. The clinical course may be complicated by rupture of the spleen, microangiopathic anemia, consumptive coagulopathy, and metastases to the liver and other organs. Splenic angiosarcoma has been described after long-term chemotherapy for low-grade non-Hodgkin's lymphomas.[836]

Metastatic neoplasms to the spleen occur late in the course of the disease and represent hematogenous dissemination of the malignant tumor and always occur in concert with metastases to other organs.[41] Splenic metastases may appear as discrete nodules or as aggregate tumor masses. The splenic weight in metastatic disease varies from nearly normal to over 1 kg. Lymphatic metastasis occurs rarely and only as retrograde growth of a tumor into the capsular and trabecular lymphatic vessels. When hematopoietic neoplasms are excluded, the incidence of splenic metastases is about 7% in autopsy series. The most frequent primary sites include the lung, breast, prostate, colon, and stomach in order of decreasing frequency. Direct extension from contiguous malignant neoplasms occurs with sarcomas, neuroblastomas, and renal neoplasms.

Hematopoietic neoplasms

In contrast to nonhematopoietic tumors, hematopoietic neoplasms frequently involve the spleen, are always malignant, and are rarely confined to the spleen. These tumors include acute and chronic leukemias, malignant histiocytosis, Hodgkin's disease, and non-Hodgkin's lymphomas. In some cases, non-Hodgkin's lymphomas and hairy cell leukemia may be confined to the spleen initially. A non-Hodgkin's lymphoma is the most likely cause of persistent splenomegaly without a detectable underlying disease in nontropical countries.[157,442] Lymphomas and leukemias characteristically infiltrate different anatomic areas of the spleen[77,78,90] and therefore create different macroscopic appearances.

Lymphomas most often involve the individual malpighian bodies and form nodular masses. The uniformity in the size, pattern, and distribution of the nodules relates to the specific histologic type of lymphoma. Hodgkin's disease and diffuse large-cell and mixed-cell non-Hodgkin's lymphomas as a group appear as discrete isolated nodules or as confluent nodules or tumor masses (Fig. 28-45). Localized reactive lymphoid hyperplasia, a benign proliferative process, has been reported to occur as a solitary, discrete nodule that closely resembles lymphoma or metastatic tumor grossly.[81] Most non-Hodgkin's lymphomas of follicular

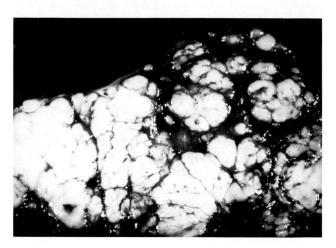

Fig. 28-45. Spleen involved by non-Hodgkin's lymphoma of diffuse large cell type. Notice the white, confluent, nodular tumor masses as well as the smaller nodules.

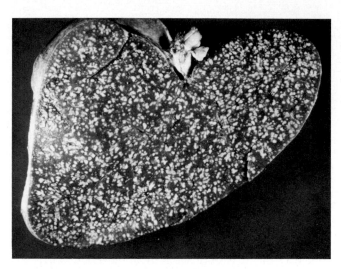

Fig. 28-46. Spleen involved by non-Hodgkin's lymphoma of follicular small cleaved cell type. Notice multiple, white tumor nodules, some of which are contiguous.

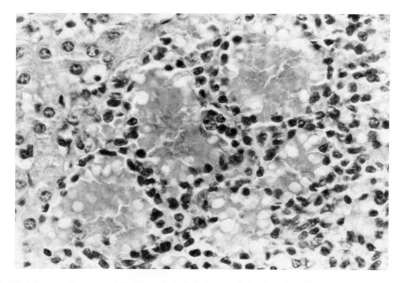

Fig. 28-47. Liver with portal infiltrates of hairy cell leukemia. Pseudosinusoid contains erythrocytes and is lined by neoplastic cells.

type appear as uniformly distributed expansions of the malpighian bodies (Fig. 28-46). Non-Hodgkin's lymphomas of small lymphocytic type and chronic lymphocytic leukemia also expand the white pulp but infiltrate the cords of the red pulp as well. The histology of lymphomas in the spleen are essentially the same as they are in lymph nodes. In some cases, diagnostic splenectomy may be curative in primary lymphomas presenting as splenomegaly.[696]

The leukemias create an entirely different macroscopic appearance in the spleen from that of most lymphomas because they infiltrate the splenic cords and eventually the sinuses and eventually efface the white pulp. This process gives the spleen a solid, ruddy appearance macroscopically. Tumor nodules are usually not formed. Chronic lymphoid leukemias, particularly chronic lymphocytic leukemia, infiltrate the red pulp and the malpighian bodies. Pseudosinuses may be seen in the cordal infiltrates of hairy cell leukemia[502] and may be seen grossly. These lesions represent blood lakes that are formed within the cord and lined by tumor cells. Similar lesions also occur in the sinuses of the liver (Fig. 28-47).[831] The spleen may weigh over 1500 g in chronic myelocytic leukemia, hairy cell leukemia, and prolymphocytic leukemia. Splenic infarcts occur frequently in spleens of this size. Spleens in chronic lymphocytic leukemia usually weigh between 500 and 1000 g, and those in acute leukemia weigh less than 500 g. Except for hairy cell leukemia, prolymphocytic leukemia, and some cases of chronic lymphocytic leukemia, it is unusual for the spleen to be involved

without evidence of leukemia in the marrow and blood. Malignant histiocytosis infiltrates the spleen in a manner similar to that of leukemia. Cell-marker studies may be helpful in determining the precise nature of the infiltrating neoplastic cells, when histology is indeterminant.

LYMPH NODES
Structure and function

Lymph nodes are small, encapsulated organs that are integral parts of the vast lymphatic network distributed throughout the body. The lymphatic vessels are unidirectional, valve-driven conduits that passively move lymph from hydrodynamically dependent areas of the body and its cavities. The structure of lymph nodes provides ready access for large numbers of macrophages and lymphocytes within the parenchyma to intercept, phagocytize, or react to microorganisms, particulate debris, and antigens within the lymph as it percolates through the node.

Lymph nodes therefore function as local centers of immune defense, a direct function of the constituent immune cells and their organization within the node. The ability of lymphocytes to react to antigen is reflected in the diverse morphology of reactive lymphoid tissue. When lymphocytes are stimulated by antigen or by nonspecific mitogens to proliferate and differentiate, their cytologic appearance is transformed as illustrated in the schematized Fig. 28-48. This transformation occurs in both B-lymphocytes within germinal centers and the medulla and T-lymphocytes within the paracor-

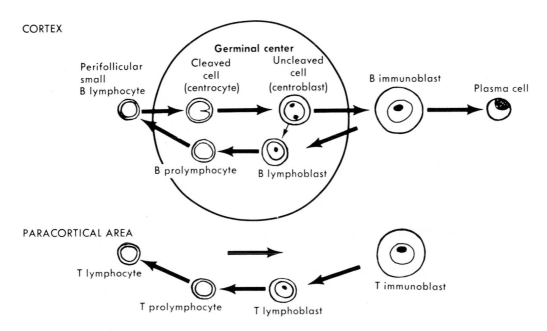

Fig. 28-48. Schema of transformation of B and T lymphocytes.

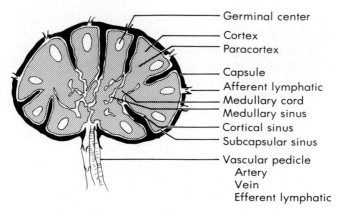

Germinal center
Cortex
Paracortex

Capsule
Afferent lymphatic
Medullary cord
Medullary sinus
Cortical sinus
Subcapsular sinus

Vascular pedicle
Artery
Vein
Efferent lymphatic

Fig. 28-49. Schema of a lymph node with its important anatomic structures.

tex. Small B-lymphocytes enter the germinal center from the perifollicular areas and are transformed into intermediate-sized cells, referred to as small cleaved and noncleaved follicular center cells, and finally into large cleaved and noncleaved follicular center cells. Morphometric studies indicate that the pathways of transformation of cleaved and noncleaved cells may be parallel rather than sequential.[164,623,738] The large cells migrate into the near paracortex as fully transformed B-lymphocytes, called "B-immunoblasts." B-immunoblasts may then differentiate into plasma cells or small memory cells. T-lymphocytes transform in a similar way within the paracortex and differentiate into effector or memory cells. Functionally different lymphocytes are not reliably distinguished by morphology. Lymphocytes circulate throughout the lymphatic and vascular systems, and certain long-lived, memory cells recirculate when stimulated by antigen. This mobility enhances the efficiency of immune surveillance and provides for functional as well as the pathologic interrelationships between regional and systemic, and central and peripheral lymphoid organs.

The lymph node consists of several component tissues that provide for its elaborate functional organization (Fig. 28-49): the fibrous capsule and trabeculas, the sinus system and blood vessels, the stationary reticulum cells and reticulin fibers, and the mobile immune cells—lymphocytes, macrophages, and mobile reticulum cells.[755] The fibrous capsule, trabeculas, and the sinuses and vessels together provide the structure and conduits to and from the nodal parenchyma for nutrients, antigens, and cells. Reticulin fibers produced by stationary reticulum cells provide the delicate substructure in which functional domains are organized.

The sinuses of the node consists of three interconnecting channels: the subcapsular, cortical, and medul-

lary sinuses. The afferent lymphatic vessels course through the capsule to enter the subcapsular sinuses directly. The space of the subcapsular sinus separates the capsule proper from the cortical parenchyma of the lymph node and is a useful landmark for the microscopic identification of a lymph node. Trabeculas bridge the sinus space to enter the parenchyma of the node. The intersecting reticulin and elastin fibers of the sinuses are invested by delicate cytoplasmic processes of endothelial cells that line the sinus. The subcapsular sinus leads into the cortical sinuses, which course through the cortex and deep paracortex to the medulla of the node and communicate with the efferent lymphatic vessels at the hilum. As the circuitous cortical sinuses continue into the medullary sinuses, they become larger and more tortuous and divide the parenchyma into the medullary cords. The predominant immune cells resident in the sinuses are the macrophages, which lie adherent to sinus endothelia. Lymphocytes are present but are less prevalent. Plasma cells are abundant within the medullary cords and in the sinuses. Blood vessels and nerves penetrate the lymph node at the hilum where the efferent lymphatic vessels exit. The large vascular trunks run within the trabeculas before branching into capillary plexuses in the cortex to surround the follicles and penetrate into the medulla. Some small vessels enter the trabeculas directly through the capsule rather than through the hilum. Capillaries give rise to venules except in the paracortex where specialized postcapillary venules arise before the simple venules. Nerve fibers are present in the capsule and trabeculas and accompany the small vessels into the parenchyma.

Three structurally and functionally integrated regions are identifiable within the lymph node: the outer cortex, the paracortex, and the medulla. Microscopically at low magnification, these regions are recognized by characteristic features. Lymphoid follicles identify the cortex of the normal lymph node. The lymphoid follicles have different appearances depending on whether they are antigenically stimulated. The primary follicle, which is unstimulated, and the secondary follicle or germinal center, which is stimulated, characteristically occur in the outer cortex beneath the subcapsular sinus. In highly stimulated nodes, germinal centers may be found throughout the nodal parenchyma and even beyond the capsule within the perinodal tissue. Primary follicles are structurally and kinetically simpler than the germinal centers are. The primary follicle is rounded with a small central area containing mostly reticulum cells and a few small and large lymphocytes surrounded by an ill-defined cuff of small lymphocytes. The germinal center, in comparison, is several times larger and usually oval in shape with the longitudinal axis perpendicular to the nearest sinus. The lymphocytic cuff is

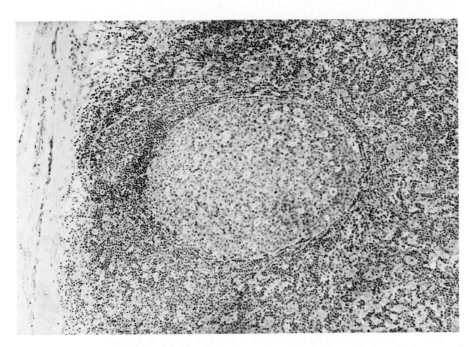

Fig. 28-50. Lymph node, germinal center. The lighter staining portion of the germinal center represents a higher density of the large lymphocytes and reticulum cells near the sinusoidal pole. The cuff is not well developed.

thinner toward the sinus and much thicker away. The germinal center consists of numerous mitotically active lymphocytes, referred to as follicular center cells, dendritic reticulum cells, and phagocytic reticulum cells, referred to as "starry-sky" macrophages, both of which are important antigen-processing cells.[527] Typically in the early stimulated germinal center, there is a size gradient of small to large follicular lymphocytes (Fig. 28-50) from the thick cap to the thinner cuff. With continued stimulation for several weeks, the germinal center enlarges, loses its gradient, assumes an irregular geographic appearance before resolving to a functionally exhausted, atretic state.

The paracortex is morphologically much simpler than the germinal center, but it is as complex functionally. Because of the morphologic simplicity, early pathologic changes in this area can be difficult to appreciate. This area is relatively less cellular and contains mostly small lymphocytes and fewer large lymphocytes. Interdigitating reticulum cells, homologous to the follicular dendritic reticulum cells, are present subtly in the background. Langerhans cells are also present in the paracortex. Of particular functional importance to this area are the postcapillary venules, which arise from the peripheral capillary plexuses and course through the inner cortex. They are identified by their specialized, high cuboid endothelium that is unsupported by a muscular layer. Molecules on the surface of these endothelia interact with receptors of lymphocytes to permit

their immigration into this area of the node.[249,350] Deep to the inner cortex is the medulla, which consists of freely anastomosing cords of vascular lymphoid tissue organized around medullary sinuses. The predominating cells of this area are the plasma cells.

The anatomy of the lymph node relates almost directly to its functional compartments: sinuses—macrophage activity; outer cortex and follicles—predominantly B-lymphocyte activity; paracortex—predominantly T-lymphocyte activity; and medulla—plasma cell maturation and Ig production and secretion. Immunohistochemistry studies have exquisitely documented the quantities and relationships of the various functional lymphocyte classes and subclasses that constitute the anatomic structures and functional compartments of normal resting and reactive lymph nodes.

Abnormalities of structure

Human lymph node development can be divided into early (eleventh to fourteenth gestational week) and late (fifteenth week and beyond) phases.[461] In general, mesenchymal elements differentiate within the early phase, and lymphoid development occurs later. Except for anatomic variations in distributions of regional lymph node groups, the early development is usually uneventful. Development within the late phase, however, depends on the quality of lymphopoiesis within the marrow and thymus. Whether the development of B- and T-lymphocyte functional domains in the peripheral

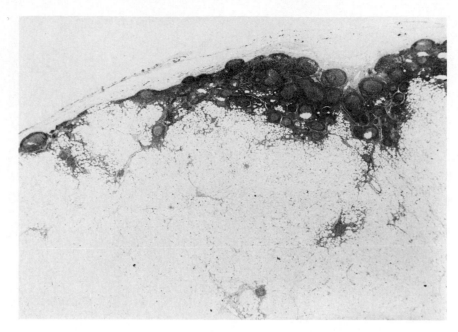

Fig. 28-51. Lymph node, axilla. Most of the nodal parenchyma has been replaced by adipose tissue.

lymphoid tissues is complete or incomplete depends on the integrity of these organs.

The morphology of a lymph node is related to age, location, and the relative amount of antigenic stimulation.[453] Gradual atrophy of nodal parenchyma occurs in aging individuals. The outer cortex and germinal center formation are more affected in this regard than the paracortex and medulla are. The peripherally located lymph nodes, where the tempo of antigenic stimulation declines with age, are more affected than the more centrally located lymph nodes are. Severe atrophy and replacement of lymphoid parenchyma by adipose tissue, fatty infiltration, is common in axillary, cubital, and popliteal nodes (Fig. 28-51). Fatty infiltration may be so extensive as to cause enlargement.[678]

Ectopic epithelial structures of various types are often found incidentally in lymph node biopsy samples and at autopsy.[193,371,605] Thyroid tissue has been described in cervical lymph nodes, epithelial glands in pelvic and paraortic nodes, and epithelial ducts, tubules, and cysts resembling breast epithelium in axillary nodes. Endometriosis involving endometrial glands, stroma, and decidua, and nerve cells has also been described. These inclusions are found most frequently within the nodal capsule or in the subcapsular sinus. Various theories have been entertained to explain the occurrence of ectopic epithelium in lymph nodes including implantation, metaplasia, and congenital rests, and each possibility may contribute in individual cases. The incidence of ectopic epithelium in lymph nodes varies widely from 0.3% to 40.8% and depends on the type of epithelium and the particular study. Dis-

tinguishing epithelial inclusions from metastatic carcinoma usually poses no difficulties in most cases.

Nevus cell aggregates are infrequently encountered nonepithelial ectopic structures found primarily in the capsule and perinodal tissue of the axillary, inguinal, and cervical lymph nodes.[592] The overall incidence of nevus cell aggregates is 0.3% to 6.2% in patients with axillary dissections for breast carcinoma. Blue-cell nevi have also been described in lymph nodes[17,205] and rarely in association with aggregates of nevus cells.[661] Migratory arrest of neural crest cells in mesenchyme during the early phase of lymph node development best explains this rare event.

Proteinaceous lymphadenopathy refers to an extensive replacement of nodal parenchyma by diffuse or focal deposits of acellular, amorphous, eosinophilic material.[518] The material may be solid and hyalinized or granular and fibrillary with small lymphocytes and plasma cells scattered in the less dense areas and at the periphery of the deposits (Fig. 28-52). Areas of hyalinized collagen may be associated. The proteinaceous material represents amyloid or other proteinaceous materials usually associated with chronic immune reactions within the node. Amyloidosis itself rarely presents as localized nodal enlargement but more frequently affects lymph nodes as part of a systemic process. Diagnostic morphologic features of amyloid include Congo red staining with green birefringence in polarized light, characteristic ultrastructural fibrils, and staining by amyloid-specific antisera. Focal nonamyloid proteinaceous deposits have been described in association with lymphoplasmacytic and non-Hodgkin's follicular lym-

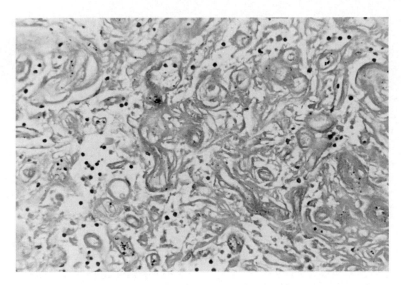

Fig. 28-52. Lymph node with proteinaceous lymphadenopathy. Notice concentric arrangement of hyaline material in this case.

phomas, Hodgkin's disease, angioimmunoblastic lymphadenopathy, carcinomas, and inflammatory conditions, such as sarcoidosis, and these deposits occur infrequently in apparent isolation of any disorder.[128,518] Immunoglobulin, other inflammatory-immune glycoproteins, and cell membrane material have been identified in these deposits, but amyloid has not.

Infarction or ischemic necrosis occurs in lymph nodes as in other organs because of vascular occlusion. However, because spontaneous infarcts occur infrequently in lymph nodes, other causes including iatrogenic ones should be considered first. Extensive necrosis is usually caused by the presence of a malignant neoplasm, either malignant lymphoma or metastatic neoplasm. Diagnostic efforts are often thwarted because of the extensive necrosis. In some cases, infarcts occur in uninvolved lymph nodes, signaling the presence of a malignancy in regional organs. The causes of focal infarcts of lymph nodes are many and include emboli, vasculitides including the mucocutaneous lymph node syndrome (Kawasaki's disease),[479] and many of the inflammatory-immune reactions of lymph nodes. Vascular transformation of sinuses may follow the unabated obstruction of hilar and perinodal veins. This reactive vasoproliferative lesion is a metamorphosis of the subcapsular and cortical sinuses into a vascular network that can extend into the perinodal soft tissues causing nodal enlargement. It is usually easily distinguishable from vascular, spindle-cell neoplasms, which may arise in or metastasize to lymph nodes.[293]

Inflammatory-immune reactions

Lymphoid tissue undergoes reactive changes to a wide variety of antigenic stimuli from infection by bacteria, fungi, and viruses, plant allergens, drugs, environmental pollutants, cellular debris from tissue injury, immune complex reactions, and neoplasia. The reaction within the node depends on the nature of the inflammatory stimulus encountered and the cellular response to it. Inflammatory and immune reactions are the most frequent causes of lymph node enlargement or lymphadenopathy and are self-limiting. Lymphadenopathy also occurs as a result of primary neoplasms of the lymph node itself and from metastases of malignant neoplasms from regional and distal organs.

Collectively the inflammatory-immune reactions that cause lymphadenopathy are called "reactive lymphoid hyperplasias." Lymph nodes are biopsied when the lymphadenopathy does not resolve after several weeks and a specific diagnosis has not been achieved by other means. Biopsies are done primarily for two purposes: pathologic diagnosis and microbiologic cultures. The probability of determining the cause of lymphadenopathy by biopsy can be as high as 60% when the biopsy is done under judicious, clinical restraint and when all clinical information is considered.[627,672] However, when infectious and neoplastic causes are excluded, histology leads to the specific cause of the adenopathy in less than 15% of cases. This low yield reflects the nonspecific histologic features that are seen in various reactive hyperplasias.

Reactive lymphoid hyperplasias are traditionally placed into one of two nosologic groups: the lymphadenitides, primarily inflammatory reactions, and the lymphadenopathies, primarily immune reactions (see the following list). These lists are not exhaustive but include the more frequently encountered conditions. Acute suppurative and necrotizing lesions are generally considered separately from reactive hyperplasias.

Lymphadenitides

Bacterial infections, others[338,688,715]

Cat-scratch disease[105,459,485,776]

Cytomegalovirus infection[629]

Fungal infections[338,688,715]

Herpes zoster lymphadenitis[544]

Infectious mononucleosis[127,323,469,629]

Lymphogranuloma venereum[768]

Mycobacterial infections[338,688,715]

Postvaccinial lymphadenitis[306]

Syphilis[264,307,363,740]

Toxoplasmosis[186,689]

Viral infections, others[338,688,715]

Lymphadenopathies

Angiofollicular lymph node hyperplasia[28,76,101,108,244,247,303,376,707]

Angioimmunoblastic lymphadenopathy[9,246,450,509,786]

Dermatopathic lymphadenopathy[83,142]

Phenytoin (Dilantin) lymphadenopathy[251,331,428,628]

Lymphangiographic lymphadenopathy[585]

Rheumatoid arthritis[101,526,800]

Sarcoidosis[351,601]

Sinus histiocytosis with massive lymphadenopathy[74,372,599,600,820]

Systemic lupus erythematosus[233]

Tumor reactions[338,688,715]

Inflammatory reactions

Acute inflammation. Some acute inflammatory reactions in lymph nodes can destroy the lymphoid parenchyma, if not abated. Acute suppurative lymphadenitis usually occurs in infections caused by pyogenic organisms like *Staphylococcus aureus*. The inflammatory process may involve the lymph node directly or secondarily through drainage of an abscess. When the node is not involved directly, the parenchyma is hyperemic, and neutrophils are present in the sinuses, around vessels, and within the parenchyma. The capsule may become fibrotic as the adjacent abscess resolves. When the node is involved directly, liquefactive necrosis and hemorrhage occur. If destruction of the parenchyma is extensive, healing occurs through fibrosis. Acute suppurative lymphadenitis may be seen less often in many other infections: cat-scratch disease, fungal infections, mycobacterial infections, listeriosis, lymphogranuloma venereum, and yersiniosis.

Acute necrotizing lymphadenitis may accompany the infections of many of the same pyogenic organisms, when suppuration does not occur. The histology of acute necrotizing lymphadenitis differs in that it may be partial or nearly complete, essentially acellular centrally, and conspicuously devoid of neutrophils. Necrotizing lymphadenitis is characteristic of bubonic plague and may also be seen in tularemia, tuberculosis, ty-

phoid fever, melioidosis, lymphogranuloma venereum, yersiniosis, and anthrax. Histologically, similar lesions may occur in noninfectious disorders: systemic lupus erythematosus, Wegener's granulomatosis, infarcts caused by nodal vessels thrombosis, vasculitides, and necrotizing neoplasms. Focal necrosis may be present at times in many of the reactive lymphoid hyperplasias and neoplasms of lymph nodes.

One form of necrotizing lymphadenitis maintains clinicopathologic specificity and has been referred to as histiocytic necrotizing lymphadenitis without granulocytic infiltration, Kikuchi's disease, or simply necrotizing lymphadenitis.[183,382,478,556,742,748] The disease primarily affects young women and generally involves cervical lymph nodes. Histologically, the necrosis is partial but extensive and characteristically is surrounded by histiocytes separating it from the surrounding viable nodal parenchyma. Most often the necrotizing process regresses spontaneously. Evidence of a *Yersinia* infection has been found in some cases.[215] Systemic lupus erythematosus should be included in the differential diagnosis in this group of patients.

Chronic inflammation. The concept of chronic inflammation in lymph nodes is not so clearly defined as it is in other tissues. Undoubtedly, reactive lymphoid hyperplasias, which are predominantly complex, immune reactions, qualify as chronic inflammation in the generic sense. Granulomatous inflammation of various causes and eosinophilic infiltrates associated with protozoan infections and drug reactions are also forms of chronic inflammation resulting from immune responses. Repair and healing of necrosis in lymph nodes as in other tissues usually evokes a chronic inflammatory response.

Granulomatous reactions in lymph nodes vary from fully developed granulomas to focal collections of histiocytes. The numbers of diseases, disorders, foreign substances, and neoplasms that can induce their formation is extraordinary. Some of the more frequently encountered conditions associated with granulomas in lymph nodes are listed in Table 28-10. Central necrosis occurs quite often in the granulomas of infection, especially tuberculosis (Fig. 28-53), histoplasmosis, cat-scratch disease, and tularemia. Occasionally, central necrosis may be present in sarcoid granulomas, which are usually void of necrosis (Fig. 28-54). Small granulomas and clusters of epithelioid histiocytes occasionally accompany the immune reactions of some reactive lymphoid hyperplasias, malignant lymphomas, and metastatic neoplasms.

Reactive lymphoid hyperplasia

Persistent antigenic stimuli will inevitably induce hyperplasia of the constituent cellular components of the lymph node resulting in its enlargement. As stated be-

Table 28-10. Conditions associated with granulomas in lymph nodes

Infectious diseases	Brucellosis
	Cat-scratch disease
	Fungal infections
	Infectious mononucleosis
	Mycobacterial infections
	Syphilis
	Toxoplasmosis
	Tularemia
Lymphoproliferative disorders and neoplasms	Angioimmunoblastic lymphadenopathy
	Hodgkin's disease
	Metastatic carcinomas
	Metastatic seminomas
	Non-Hodgkin's lymphomas
Immunologic disorders	Crohn's disease
	Immunodeficiency disorders
	Primary biliary cirrhosis
	Sarcoidosis
Foreign substances	Berylliosis
	Povidone deposits
	Silicosis
	Zirconiosis

fore, inflammatory reactions may accompany this process but are not the predominant reaction. The functional anatomic areas of the node are affected differently by the various stimuli that result in recurring morphologic patterns of hyperplasia. The causes of reactive lymphoid hyperplasia have been categorized into predominant groups based on these patterns (Table 28-11).[187] In practice, consideration of the histologic pattern in evaluation of the otherwise nonspecific histology of reactive hyperplasia reduces the number of possible causes in many cases and often leads to a more thorough clinical investigation. Clinical information and laboratory testing is necessary for the accurate diagnosis of the specific entities. Because malignant lymphomas and other neoplasms readily simulate these patterns, the observer's sensitivity to neoplastic disorders is enhanced through a familiarity with these reactive histologies.[89,187]

Follicular hyperplasias. Follicular hyperplasia is the most frequent pattern of reactive lymphoid hyperplasia encountered and occurs more frequently and more intensely in children than in adults. It represents an expansion of the B lymphocyte–dependent outer cortex and is characterized by an increase in the number of germinal centers. The extent of hyperplasia varies greatly depending on the intensity and chronicity of an-

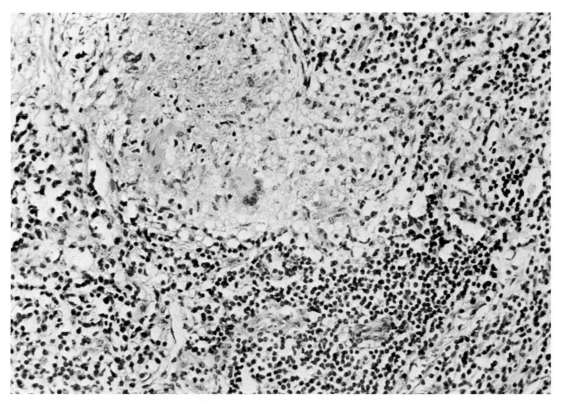

Fig. 28-53. Granuloma with central necrosis *(above center)* in tuberculosis involving a lymph node. Notice Langhans type of giant cell.

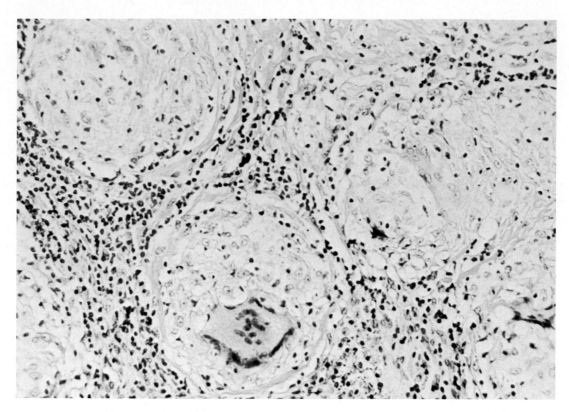

Fig. 28-54. Nonnecrotizing granulomas in sarcoidosis involving a lymph node.

Table 28-11. Patterns of reactive lymphoid hyperplasia

Pattern	Disorder found
Follicular	Nonspecific follicular hyperplasia
	Angiofollicular lymph node hyperplasia
	Rheumatoid disease
	Syphilis
Diffuse	Angioimmunoblastic lymphadenopathy
	Infectious mononucleosis
	Phenytoin (Dilantin) lymphadenopathy
	Dermatopathic lymphadenopathy
	Postvaccinial lymphadenitis
	Viral lymphadenitis
Sinus	Sinus histiocytosis
	Lymphangiographic lymphadenopathy
	Sinus histiocytosis with massive lymphadenopathy
Mixed	Cat-scratch disease
	Inflammatory pseudotumor
	Lymphogranuloma venereum
	Systemic lupus erythematosus
	Toxoplasmosis

tigenic stimulation. Germinal centers may proliferate to completely occupy the nodal area and perhaps extend beyond the capsule into perinodal tissues. Follicular hyperplasia to this extent is often referred to as florid follicular hyperplasia, which can be confused with follicular forms of non-Hodgkin's lymphoma.[511] In follicular hyperplasia, the germinal centers appear histologically as oval or irregularly expanded follicles and are composed of a mixture of normal, mitotically active, follicular center cells and interspersed phagocytic, dendritic reticulum cells (Fig. 28-55). The surrounding cuff of lymphocytes may be thinned or thickened and be asymmetric. The interfollicular areas are cellular with small and large lymphocytes and plasma cells, and vascular with prominent postcapillary venules. There may also be an associated medullary plasma cell hyperplasia and sinus histiocytosis. Follicular hyperplasia is frequently seen in primary and secondary syphilis in which plasma cell hyperplasia is pronounced in the interfollicular areas around vessels that are also affected by arteritis or endarteritis obliterans.[264,307,363,740] Follicular hyperplasia is also frequently seen in autoimmune disorders, such as rheumatoid arthritis, Felty's syndrome, Sjögren's syndrome, and related disorders.[24,526,800]

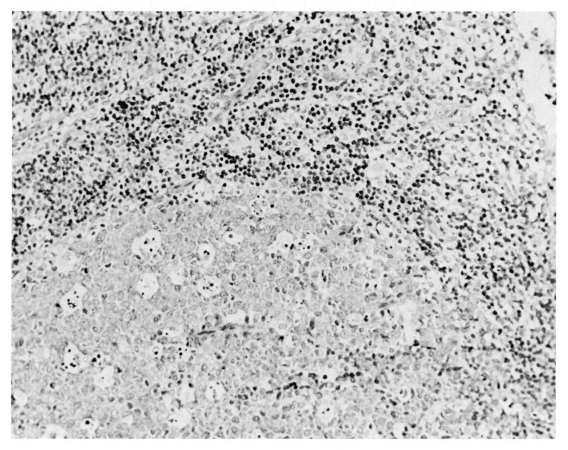

Fig. 28-55. Germinal center in reactive lymphoid hyperplasia of follicular type in a lymph node. Notice the phagocytic dendritic macrophages with clear cytoplasm containing debris.

Angiofollicular lymph node hyperplasia is a clinicopathologic variant of follicular hyperplasia in which solitary or multicentric lymphoid masses form.[76,108,244,303,376,784] Patients most often present with an incidental mediastinal mass, though many extramediastinal solitary lesions have been described in the lungs, abdomen, retroperitoneum, axillary and cervical regions, and various soft-tissues sites. All ages except infants and young children are affected. Two histologic forms are recognized: the hyaline-vascular type and the plasma-cell type. Cases in which histologic features of both types are present have also been reported. The hyaline-vascular type occurs in about 90% of cases and is more distinctive histologically. It is characterized by numerous small, round, lymphoid follicles that have concentrically arranged cuffs of small lymphocytes with distinct, hyalinized arterioles that course directly into the center of the follicle (Fig. 28-56). The immunophenotype of these follicular cells is similar to that of normal primary follicles.[101] The interfollicular areas are vascular with varying numbers of plasma cells, plasmablasts, small lymphocytes, and eosinophils.

The plasma cell form appears in less than 20% of cases and is characterized by germinal centers that are separated by abundant, vascular, interfollicular tissue in which there is a pronounced plasma cell hyperplasia. This form is more often accompanied by systemic manifestations of fever, anemia, and hyperglobulinemia. Hepatic dysfunction, nephrotic syndrome, thrombotic thrombocytopenic purpura, refractory anemia, peripheral neuropathies, and myasthenia gravis have also been described.[76,153,203,329] Excision or radiotherapy of the solitary mass effectively alleviates the syndrome in most cases. A clinicopathologic variant of the solitary plasma cell form, which is referred to as "multicentric angiofollicular lymph node hyperplasia," is also recognized. It presents with systemic manifestations very similar to those in the solitary plasma cell type and has similar histology. The hyperplasia, however, is manifest as generalized lymphadenopathy, hepatosplenomegaly, skin rash, and lymphoplasmacytic infiltrates in the marrow.[28,244,784] An association with Epstein-Barr virus and clonal rearrangement of antigen receptor genes have been demonstrated in some cases.[298] This syndrome

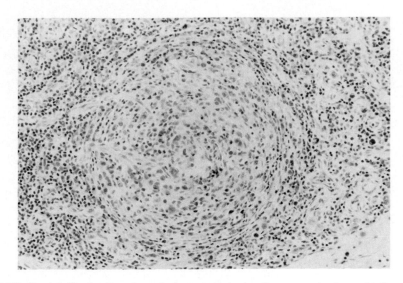

Fig. 28-56. Angiofollicular lymph node hyperplasia, hyaline-vascular type. Notice vessels entering lymphoid follicle with concentric layering of small lymphocytes *(left of center)* and hypervascularity of interfollicular tissue *(right).*

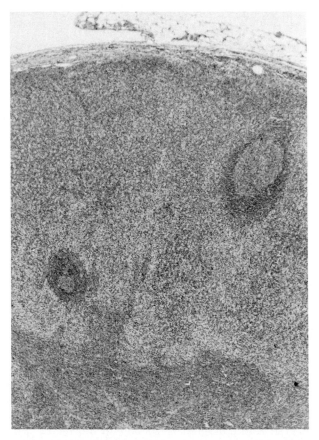

Fig. 28-57. Dermatopathic lymphadenopathy. Notice lighter staining, hyperplastic paracortex, which is expanded into the outer cortex and around germinal centers.

may be clinically aggressive and fatal and requires systemic management.

Paracortical and diffuse hyperplasias. Paracortical hyperplasia refers to hyperplasia of the T lymphocyte–dependent domain of the lymph node. Paracortical hyperplasia evolves to diffuse hyperplasia when cellular immunity dominates the immune response and the antigenic stimulus is prolonged. Dermatopathic lymphadenopathy (Figs. 28-57 and 28-58) and viral lymphadenitis (Fig. 28-59) are the prototypic causes of paracortical and diffuse hyperplasia, respectively. Paracortical hyperplasia is characterized histologically by expansion of the paracortex by increased numbers of immunoblasts and lymphocytes in varying stages of transformation, proliferation of interdigitating reticulum cells, and infiltrates of eosinophils and plasma cells in a vascular stroma. When the hyperplasia is predominantly paracortical, there arise immunoblasts from cells that migrate into the area from the blood through postcapillary venules and from the mitotic activity of the transformed cells in situ. This process may ultimately extend into and replace the outer cortex and medulla producing the diffuse pattern of reactive lymphoid hyperplasia. Germinal centers contribute to the number of paracortical immunoblasts in hyperplasias of mixed follicular and paracortical type. Since the paracortex is the site of early involvement of a lymph node by Hodgkin's disease and non-Hodgkin's lymphomas of T-cell derivation, cytologic atypicality in paracortical hyperplasia may be the first sign of an unexpected malignant lymphoma.

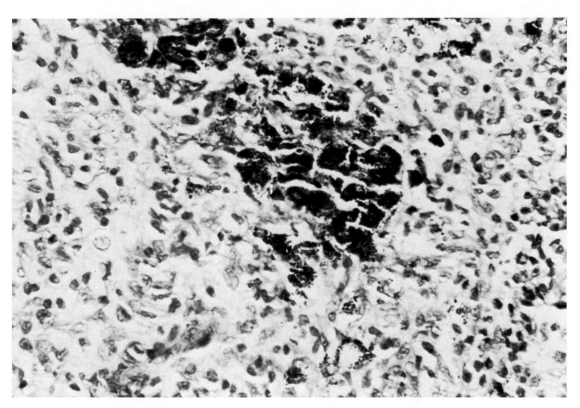

Fig. 28-58. Dermatopathic lymphadenopathy. Notice the dark melanin pigment within macrophages.

Angioimmunoblastic lymphadenopathy with dysproteinemia (AILD) describes a clinicopathologic entity in which diffuse hyperplasia occurs. AILD usually occurs in elderly patients and is characterized by generalized lymphadenopathy, hepatosplenomegaly, fever, hemolytic anemia, and hypergammaglobulinemia.[246,249] This syndrome shares many clinical features with that of multicentric angiofollicular lymph node hyperplasia discussed before. AILD has occurred after the use of various drugs, especially penicillin and other antibiotics. Phenytoin (Dilantin) lymphadenopathy may represent a variant form of AILD.[331,428,628] Histologically, AILD is characterized by the diffuse effacement of the nodal architecture, the great proliferation of small, arborizing blood vessels, a diffuse infiltrate of lymphocytes in varying states of immunoblastic transformation, small lymphocytes, eosinophils, and plasma cells, and the presence of an amorphous, eosinophilic, PAS-positive, interstitial material (Fig. 28-60). Lymphoid follicles, if present, are usually atretic, germinal centers. Pleomorphic immunoblasts resembling the Reed-Sternberg cell of Hodgkin's disease may be present occasionally. Similar infiltrates may also involve other organs, the skin, and the marrow. The histology of AILD has many features that are similar to those of experimental graft-

versus-host disease. An extreme form of immunoblastic proliferation, which probably represents a histologic subset of AILD in which follicles are not recognized, has been described as immunoblastic lymphadenopathy (IBL).[450] Immunoblastic lymphadenopathy may be confused histologically with some intense forms of diffuse, reactive hyperplasia, as in selected cases of acute infectious mononucleosis (Fig. 28-59).[127] Some cases of AILD and IBL may also be difficult to separate histologically from some types of diffuse non-Hodgkin's lymphoma.[509,786] The lack of cellular polymorphism in the infiltrate, the clustering of monomorphic immunoblasts, or a great degree of nuclear atypicality of the immunoblasts help to distinguish the lymphomas.

AILD presents a spectrum of disease severity both clinically and pathologically.[638] AILD is an aggressive systemic disorder with a median survival of only 30 months. Histologic transformation to lymphoma occurs in up to 18% of cases. Phenotypic and genotypic studies indicate that small clonal populations of T-lymphocytes may be present in the lymphadenopathy, which may progress to overt lymphoma in some cases.[773,786] Paradoxically, nearly 20% of patients undergo spontaneous complete remissions. Although prognostic factors have been identified in retrospective studies, it remains un-

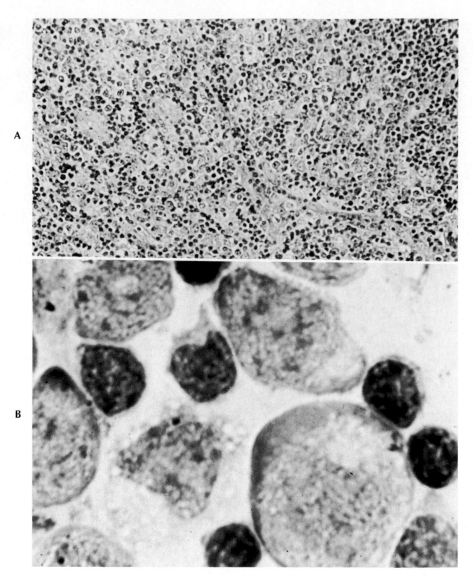

Fig. 28-59. A, Lymph node in infectious mononucleosis. **B,** Wright's stained imprint of **A** showing large immunoblasts. (Both courtesy Dr. Joseph Sieracki, Pittsburgh.)

clear in individual cases which patients will succumb to the disorder.[9,539] Chemotherapy, both single drug and combination regimens, has enjoyed only limited success in this disorder.[748]

Sinus hyperplasias. Sinus histiocytosis is a very frequent and nonspecific finding in lymph nodes. It may be seen in regional nodes draining inflammatory lesions or organs harboring carcinomas. Histologically the sinuses are expanded by a proliferation of constituent benign histiocytes that are characteristically large cells with pale, eosinophilic cytoplasm and small, oval nuclei containing inconspicuous nucleoli. The cells are phagocytic and may contain melanin or hemosiderin pigments, carbon, and other debris depending on the location of the node and the clinical situation. Lipophagic

phagocytosis by hyperplastic sinus histiocytes is seen in lymph nodes after lymphangiograms are taken. The radiopaque lipid material typically incites a foreign-body giant cell reaction by the histiocytes and an eosinophilic infiltrate.

Sinus histiocytosis with massive lymphadenopathy (SHML) is an extreme form of sinus histiocytosis that is associated with characteristic clinical features.[599,600] Although adults are occasionally affected, most patients are in the first and second decades of life and are often black and in previously good health. The disorder is characterized by painless, massive lymphadenopathy, which is most prominent in the cervical area. Extranodal involvement of the skin, orbit, nasopharynx, salivary gland, lung, gastrointestinal tract, gonads, bone,

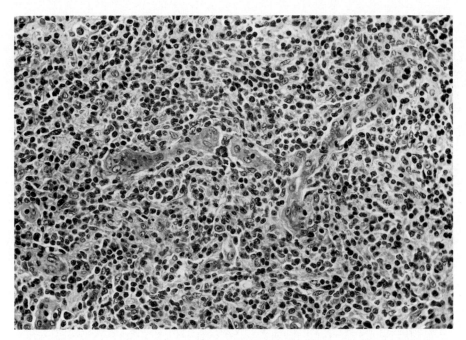

Fig. 28-60. Lymph node. Angioimmunoblastic lymphadenopathy. Arborizing vessels are prominent amid a polymorphic cellular infiltrate that includes immunoblasts, small lymphocytes, plasma cells, and eosinophils.

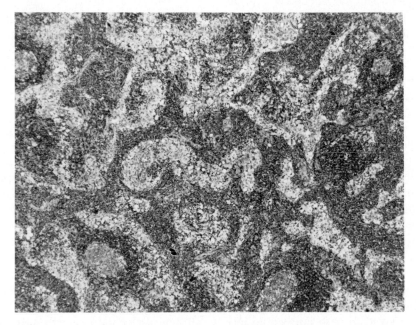

Fig. 28-61. Lymph node. Sinus histiocytosis with massive lymphadenopathy. The lymph node sinuses are expanded by a proliferation of benign histiocytes.

central nervous system, and soft tissues occurs in 25% of cases.[74,537,631,725,820] Fever, leukocytosis, and hyperglobulinemia are often associated findings, and the majority of patients show some evidence of immune dysfunction in the course of the disorder. Histologically the lymph node sinuses are greatly distended by benign histiocytes, small lymphocytes, and plasma cells (Fig. 28-61). The histiocytes are finely vacuolated and characteristically contain many small lymphocytes, which are mostly B-cells, within their cytoplasm as well as

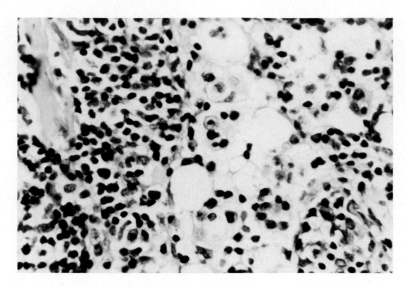

Fig. 28-62. Lymph node. Sinus histiocytosis with massive lymphadenopathy. Notice finely vacuolated histiocytes containing many small lymphocytes and plasma cells.

erythrocytes and plasma cells (Fig. 28-62).[372] The histiocytes maintain their sinusoid location, and plasma cell hyperplasia is present in the surrounding nodal parenchyma. The syndrome typically follows a protracted but benign clinical course with spontaneous resolution occurring within months to several years. Cytotoxic therapy is occasionally instituted in the treatment of severe complications.[706]

Mixed hyperplasias. Many nonspecific reactive lymphoid hyperplasias demonstrate a mixture of follicular and parafollicular hyperplasia and sinus histiocytosis histologically, but one feature usually predominates over the others. The mixed pattern of reactive hyperplasia refers to almost equal contributions of the aforementioned hyperplasias to the histology, which may be punctuated by focal necrosis or granulomatous inflammation. The lymphadenitis that accompanies acute, acquired toxoplasmosis best exemplifies the mixed form of reactive lymphoid hyperplasia. Histologically, prominent germinal centers are associated with small clusters of epithelioid histiocytes located in the interfollicular areas, within the germinal centers, and at the interface between them. Well-developed granulomas are not seen, and necrosis is usually absent. In addition to follicular hyperplasia associated with epithelioid histiocytes, the subcapsular and cortical sinuses are expanded by monocytoid cells, a reaction referred to as "immature sinus histiocytosis." Recently, these cells have been shown to be a proliferation of unusual-appearing B-lymphocytes rather than histiocytes and are now referred to as monocytoid B-cells.[167,481,659,691,752] The peculiar sinus infiltrate is most frequently associated with toxoplasmosis but may be seen in a variety of reactive and neoplastic lymph node disorders.[482,680] Malig-

nant lymphomas, which may represent the neoplastic phenotype of these cells, have been described.[523,658] Cysts of *Toxoplasma* may rarely be seen within the nodal parenchyma, but this finding is of itself non-diagnostic because of the high incidence of chronic infection by this protozoon. Even though the histologic appearance is characteristic of acute, acquired toxoplasmosis, this histologic reaction may be mimicked in the early development of many other disorders, both benign and neoplastic, and is not diagnostic. The definitive diagnosis requires confirmation by serologic studies such as the Sabin-Feldman or complement-fixation tests. *Toxoplasma* is proved causative in perhaps 85% of cases.

Cat-scratch disease is another characteristic form of the mixed type of reactive lymphoid hyperplasia. It is the most frequent cause of unilateral lymphadenitis involving axillary and cervical lymph nodes of young people, and in most cases there is a history of contact, scratch, or bite by a cat or other animal.[105,459] Typically, the lymph node shows paracortical and follicular hyperplasia early and the late appearance of star-shaped, central necrosis within large areas of paracortical granulomatous inflammation. The stellate necrosis characteristically contains some neutrophils and is surrounded by palisading rows of fibroblasts and histiocytes (Fig. 28-63).[524,809] Pleomorphic, gram-negative bacteria, which are positive with a modified Warthin-Starry stain, have been identified in several documented cases of cat-scratch disease.[485,776] Cat-scratch disease is usually self-limiting, requiring no therapy. Lymphogranuloma venereum lymphadenitis, caused by *Chlamydia trachomatis*, has similar centrally necrotic granulomas in a mixed hyperplastic pattern and should be distin-

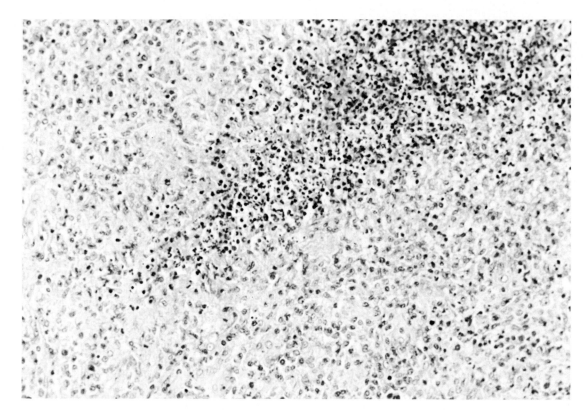

Fig. 28-63. Lymph node. Cat-scratch disease. Notice the elongate central necrosis surrounded by histiocytes and fibroblasts.

guished from cat-scratch disease. Its incidence is very low, and it usually involves inguinal lymph nodes, though it has been reported to involve supraclavicular lymph nodes simultaneously.[768] Tularemia, another common lymphadenitis that frequently affects axillary and epitrochlear lymph nodes unilaterally, can resemble cat-scratch disease histologically. Usually, the development of adenopathy follows the cleaning of wild rabbits or a tick bite and is accompanied by a prominent skin lesion at the organism's point of entry.[289]

Atypical lymphoid hyperplasia

Atypical lymphoid hyperplasia (ALH) is a diagnostic term that refers to lymphadenopathy that has unusual architectural or cytologic features unlike usual reactive lymphoid hyperplasia but is not diagnostic of malignant lymphoma. ALH does not refer to any particular clinical or pathologic entity. Inasmuch as the diagnosis of lymphoma is based on specific morphologic features that are not fully expressed by the lymphoid infiltrates in atypical lymphoid hyperplasia, ALH is a diagnosis of exclusion. However, the suspicion of lymphoma histologically and clinically in these cases is high. This diagnosis in one retrospective study from a large metropolitan hospital represented 3.1% of all lymph-node biopsies. The actual incidence will vary depending on

the demographic mix of patients, the surgical pathology laboratory, and the observer's experience and skill in the interpretation of lymph node pathology. In retrospective studies of ALH in which additional lymph node biopsy specimens were available for review, the diagnosis of a malignant lymphoproliferative disorder was made in 37% to 58% of patients.[627,644,672,714]

Malignant lymphoma
General considerations

Lymphomas are malignant neoplasms of lymphoreticular origin that are extremely heterogeneous both clinically and pathologically. As a group, they are the most studied of all human neoplasms, and some lymphomas are the most curable of all human cancers. These neoplasms are derived from the immune cells of lymphoid tissues, that is, from lymphocytes and mononuclear-phagocytic cells. Malignant lymphomas are divided into two clinicopathologic categories, which in most cases can be distinguished by routine histology: Hodgkin's disease (HD), which comprises about 25% of cases, and the non-Hodgkin's lymphomas (NHL). These two groups are further subdivided by various histopathologic classifications that distinguish distinct clinical groups of patients. Currently, the diagnoses and classification of these neoplasms depend entirely on histologic criteria. Within some of these histologic groups, relative biologic homogeneity has been demonstrated through immunologic, genetic, and molecular studies. About 34,000 new cases of lymphoma are reported each year. Males are more frequently affected than females are in a ratio of about 1.75:1. Hodgkin's disease patients, who average 32 years of age, are younger in general than patients with non-Hodgkin's lymphoma, who average 42 years. However, the age spectrum of most histologic categories of lymphoma is very broad.

Most lymphomas arise within lymph nodes, but they also develop in extranodal tissues and in all organs. Malignant lymphomas generally appear as a painless enlargement of one or more groups of lymph nodes that may be located superficially or deep in the body. The anatomic site of involvement often provides a clue to the type of lymphoma present. Hodgkin's disease generally presents in lymph node groups located above the diaphragm in the cervical or supraclavicular areas or in the mediastinum, though HD may occasionally present as retroperitoneal lymphadenopathy. HD rarely involves extranodal sites or the skin in the absence of nodal disease. Non-Hodgkin's lymphomas generally present in peripheral or abdominal lymph nodes. Some forms of NHL present as generalized, widespread disease, whereas others present as an extranodal tumor mass in soft tissue or in a nonlymphoid organ. Involvement of the spleen without the initial involvement of lymph nodes may occur in NHL.

Hodgkin's disease

Hodgkin's disease virtually always arises within lymph nodes and affects extranodal tissues secondarily. The diagnosis of HD is based on the identification of Reed-Sternberg (RS) cells in an appropriate histologic setting that appears inflammatory. The inflammatory infiltrate is polymorphous consisting of normal-appearing small lymphocytes, plasma cells, histiocytes, eosinophils, and stromal fibrosis in which RS cells are scattered as individual or clusters of cells. The frequency of diagnostic RS cells and the proportion of small lymphocytes and inflammatory cells in the tissue vary depending on the histologic subtype. Because of its inflammatory histologic appearance and the variable distribution of RS cells, HD usually lacks the histologic monotony that is characteristic of most non-Hodgkin's lymphomas and other neoplasms.

The classical, "diagnostic" Reed-Sternberg cell is a large cell that has a bilobular or multilobular nucleus with a thickened nuclear membrane and two or more prominent, eosinophilic, or amphophilic nucleoli often surrounded by a clear halo (Fig. 28-64). The identification of this cell is essential and necessary for the primary diagnosis of HD. RS cells are virtually always accompanied by the nondiagnostic Hodgkin's (H) cells, which are believed to be a kinetically more active and genetically more stable precursor of the RS cell. The H cell is characterized as a large, mononuclear cell with a central, prominent eosinophilic nucleolus and moder-

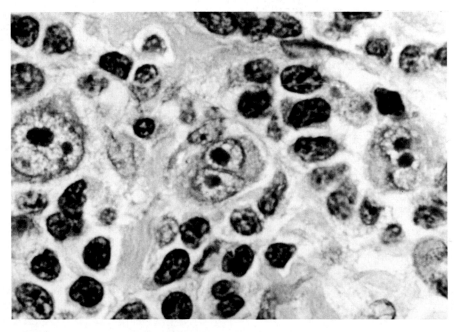

Fig. 28-64. Lymph node. Hodgkin's disease. Classical, diagnostic Reed-Sternberg cell *(center)*. Notice the nondiagnostic Hodgkin's cell to the left.

ate, amphophilic cytoplasm (Figs. 28-64 and 28-65). The cytologic appearance of the H cell resembles very closely that of the malignant immunoblast of NHL. Variant RS cells, which are cytologically abnormal but nondiagnostic cells, may be identified as well and aid in the subclassification and pathologic staging of the lymphoma.

Pathogenesis. The origin of the RS and H cells has not been clearly identified, though most lymphoreticular cells have been suggested as precursor cells. In most cases that have been studied immunologically, these cells lack specific markers of lymphocytes but do express a phenotype, which is restricted but not unique.* Cytogenetic studies of HD have demonstrated abnormalities that are common to both B and T cell–derived NHL, though ploidy characteristics are clearly different.[96] Cellular and molecular studies of small numbers of cases indicate that biologic heterogeneity may exist within the histologic types of Hodgkin's disease. In several cases of the Lukes' nodular form of lymphocytic predominance HD, the neoplastic cells appear to be derivatives of germinal-center B-lymphocytes,[421,560,692,729] which also give rise to follicular lymphomas, a predomi-

*References 188, 324, 325, 364, 562, 586, 690, and 695.

nant form of NHL. Clonal rearrangement of antigen receptor genes have been demonstrated in some cases of nodular sclerosis and mixed-cellularity HD, though it is still unclear whether the detected cell populations were neoplastic cells,[67,606,708,788] since Epstein-Barr virus genomic DNA was also identified in some of these cases, perhaps contributing to the development of the clonal lymphocyte populations.[787] In retrospective histologic studies, it is evident that a percentage of cases of mixed cellularity and lymphocytic depletion HD would be classified as NHL lymphoma if current criteria of NHL were applied.[723] It has been recognized for some time that cells morphologically similar if not identical to RS cells may be found in many malignant or benign disorders whose histologic appearance may differ or closely resemble that of HD.[703] In particular, NHL of peripheral T-cell type, which are often associated with HTLV-I infection, have pleomorphic histologic features that can be readily confused with mixed cellularity HD.[191] This new experience illustrates the dynamic quality of the present study of HD. There is no doubt that forthcoming observations will modify our concepts of HD until the histogenesis of the malignant cell is clarified and it can be reliably identified.

Classification. The diagnosis and classification of HD

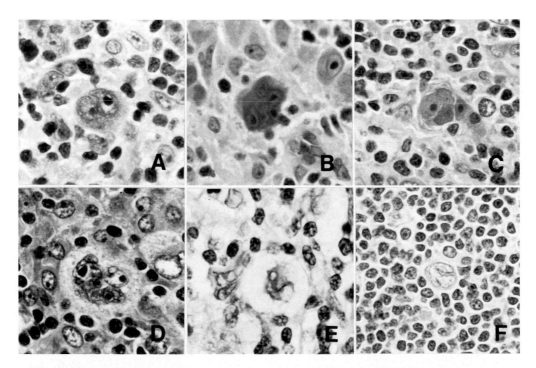

Fig. 28-65. Lymph node. Hodgkin's disease. Reed-Sternberg cells and RS variants. **A** to **C,** Bilobular and multilobular Reed-Sternberg cells. **D,** Multilobular Reed-Sternberg cell showing slight lacunar artifact. **E,** Lacunar RS variant cells. **F,** Lymphocytic and histiocytic variant RS cell.

is made solely by morphologic observations of routinely prepared microscopic slides. The current classification of HD was adopted at the Rye Conference in 1965 at Rye, N.Y., and is listed here.

Classification of Hodgkin's disease (Rye Conference, 1965)
  Lymphocytic predominance type (LP)
  Nodular sclerosis type (NS)
  Mixed cellularity type (MC)
  Lymphocytic depletion type (LD)

This list represents a clinicopathologic classification adapted from the histologic classification of Lukes, Butler, and Hicks,[94,448,451] as follows:

Lukes-Butler-Hicks classification of Hodgkin's disease
  Lymphocytic and histiocytic (L&H)
    Nodular
    Diffuse
  Nodular sclerosis
  Mixed
  Diffuse fibrosis
  Reticular

In the Rye classification, the two histologic forms of the lymphocytic and histiocytic type were condensed to the lymphocytic-predominance type, and the diffuse fibrosis and reticular types were combined as the lymphocytic-depletion type because of similar clinical features.

Nodular sclerosis is the most distinctive histologic type of HD and is characterized by bands of collagenous fibrosis that divide the neoplastic infiltrate within the node into lymphoid nodules (Fig. 28-66), thus the term "nodular sclerosis." Reed-Sternberg cells are present as well as lacunar cells (Fig. 28-67, *A*), variant RS cells that are characteristically plentiful in NS, in addition to an inflammatory infiltrate of normal-appearing small lymphocytes, eosinophils, histiocytes, and plasma cells. Reed-Sternberg cells are relatively rare in comparison to the large numbers of lacunar cells in the NS type. Lacunar cells (Fig. 28-67, *B*) are large cells that resemble RS cells in that their nuclei are polylobular. However, their nucleoli are generally less conspicuous and their cytoplasm is retracted from the peripheral plasma membrane toward the nucleus giving the cell its characteristic "lacunar" appearance in formalin-fixed tissue (Fig. 28-67, *B*). Lacunar cells are not restricted to NS necessarily and are found less frequently in both MC and LP types. They most probably represent an effete form of RS cell. Two variant histologic appearances of NS have been described, and they are infrequently encountered. The "cellular phase" of NS is characterized by similar clustered infiltrates of lacunar cells and relatively infrequent numbers of RS cells, but it lacks the circumferential fibrotic bands to fulfill the criteria for definitive subclassification.[136,702] Most often concurrent or subsequent lymph node biopsy specimens do show characteristic NS histology. The clinical significance of this variant is based on reports that patients who present initially with a cellular-phase NS histologic type may suffer a somewhat lower survival rate than patients with the typical NS histologic

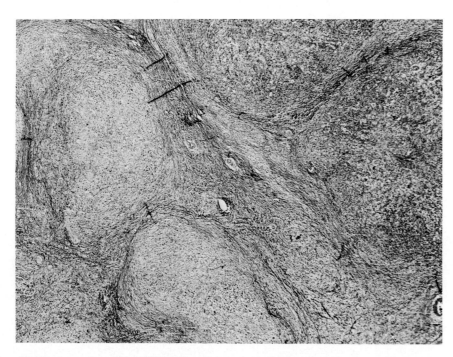

Fig. 28-66. Lymph node. Hodgkin's disease, nodular sclerosis type. Notice that the lymph node is divided into nodules by curvilinear bands of fibrosis.

type do.[138] Another variant histologic type is characterized by the partial effacement of the node by cohesive clusters or diffuse infiltrates of lacunar cells that may resemble NHL, metastatic neoplasms, or thymoma. Typical NS histologic appearance is usually present in other portions of the node. This histologic type has been referred to as the "syncytial variant" of NS and apparently has no clinical significance.[700]

The other types of HD, lymphocytic predominance, mixed cellularity, and lymphocytic depletion types, lack the sclerotic nodules that define the NS type. However, interstitial and capsular fibrosis is typically present. Each type demonstrates a characteristic frequency of RS cells and small lymphocytes, variant RS cells, and inflammatory cells including histiocytes, eosinophils, and plasma cells. In lymphocytic predominance, small lymphocytes are characteristically plentiful and diagnostic RS cells are rare, though variant RS cells, which are referred to as L&H cells (lymphocytes and histiocytes), are present (Figs. 28-68 and 28-69) and often plentiful. Variant L&H RS cells resemble reactive, pleomorphic immunoblasts with lobulated, twisted nuclei and small, often indistinct nucleoli (Fig. 28-65, F).

Inflammatory cells, except for histiocytes, are usually less numerous in LP than in the other types. Fine fibrosis is usually present interstitially in the nodal parenchyma and capsule. The Lukes classification recognizes two subgroups within the lymphocytic predominance type as defined by the Rye classification: the nodular subtype and the diffuse subtype. The nodular subtype (Fig. 28-69) resembles the progressively transformed germinal centers of aberrant follicular hyperplasia,[184] which may in some cases represent a precursor lesion of this subtype of LP Hodgkin's disease.[421,570] In the diffuse subtype, benign histiocytes are often numerous and arranged in small clusters intermixed with plentiful small lymphocytes. The diffuse subtype may be confused with the small lymphocytic type of NHL because of the diffuse pattern of tumor growth and the sparsity of diagnostic RS cells among numerous small lymphocytes. Cell-marker studies may be useful in distinguishing these forms of HD from NHL.[137]

In mixed cellularity HD, RS and H cells are numerous, and the inflammatory infiltrate includes many eosinophils, plasma cells, and histiocytes and relatively fewer small lymphocytes. Histiocytes may be plentiful

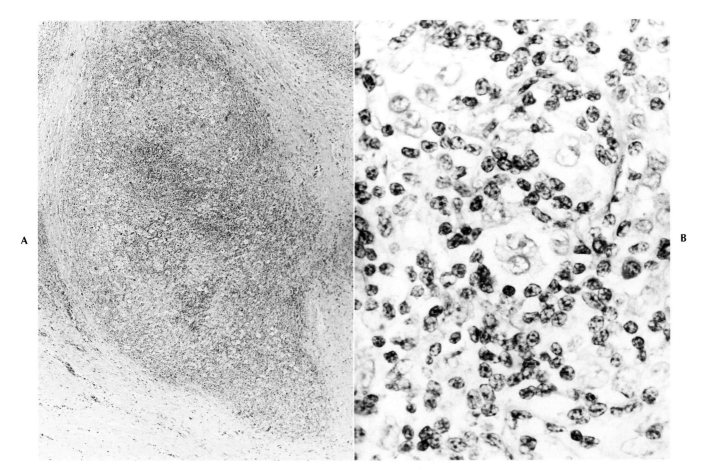

Fig. 28-67. Lymph node. Hodgkin's disease, nodular sclerosis type. Isolated sclerotic nodule in which the clear spaces denote clusters of lacunar cells. Lacunar cell in center surrounded by small lymphocytes.

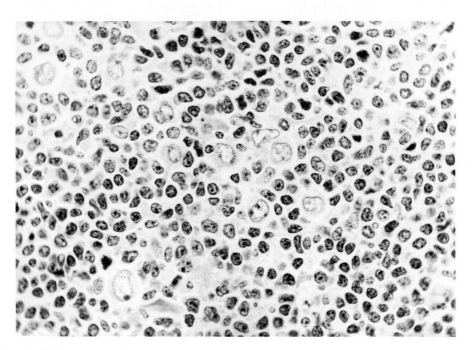

Fig. 28-68. Lymph node. Hodgkin's disease, lymphocytic predominance type. Several large leukocytic and histiocytic variant RS cells with lobular nuclei and indistinct nucleoli are surrounded by small lymphocytes.

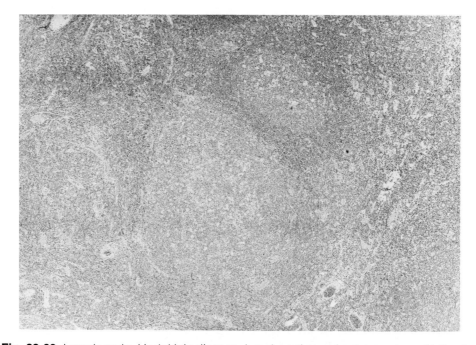

Fig. 28-69. Lymph node. Hodgkin's disease, lymphocytic predominance type. Notice two ill-defined nodules *(center)* representing the lymphocytic-histiocytic nodular form of Lukes.

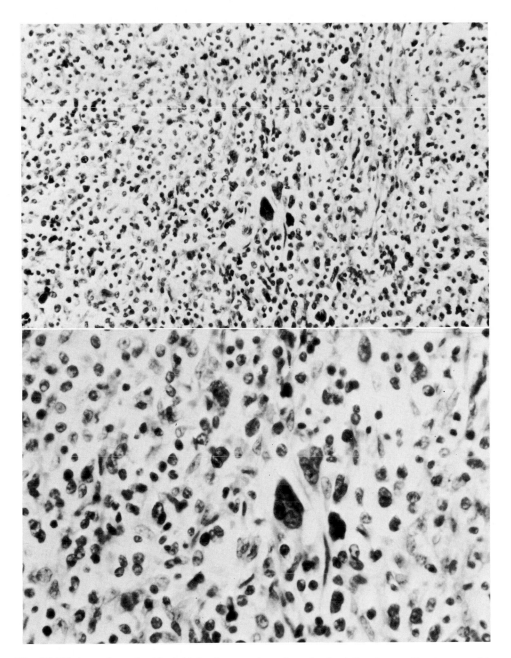

Fig. 28-70. Lymph node. Hodgkin's disease, lymphocyte depletion type with pleomorphic RS-variant cells.

and distributed in clusters resembling some forms of reactive hyperplasia. The RS cells are usually frequently pleomorphic with many nuclear lobules and exaggerated nucleoli. Lacunar cells may be present as well but are relatively less plentiful than RS cells are. Rarely, HD infiltrates of MC type may involve the paracortex without fully effacing the nodal parenchyma, a histologic type referred to as interfollicular HD.[179] Follicular hyperplasia is often prominent and may mask the presence of HD.

The lymphocytic depletion type as the name implies is relatively devoid of small lymphocytes in comparison to other types of HD. Two histologic varieties within

LD are recognized by the Lukes classification: the reticular type and the diffuse fibrosis type. These differ primarily in that the RS cells, which are characteristically very pleomorphic in LD (Fig. 28-70), are much more frequent in the reticular subtype than in the diffuse fibrosis type in which the fibrosis is a much greater. The benign inflammatory cell infiltrate, which is characteristically present in other types of HD, is less evident in LD. The lymphocytic depletion type can be confused histologically in some cases with malignant histiocytosis, some types of NHL, and metastatic, pleomorphic carcinomas and sarcomas.

In most cases, the histologic type of HD remains stable over the course of the disease, but transitions from one type to another do occur rarely. Most commonly, LP evolves to an MC and LD histologic type, or NS evolves to LD.[136,702] Prolonged therapy often affects the histologic appearance of HD such that it may closely resemble NHL of large cell, immunoblastic type when rebiopsied or at autopsy. Because of this observation, subclassification of posttherapy biopsy specimens in HD is not recommended.[138,181] When therapy is effective in eradicating the lymphoma, fibrosis may result at the site of disease forming a pseudotumor that clinically and radiographically mimics persistant HD.[122]

Staging. The extent to which a malignant neoplasm has spread in the body is the stage of the disease and is documented both clinically and pathologically. The stage provides a basis for selecting an appropriate therapeutic regimen for the patient. The staging system for HD was adopted at the Workshop on the Staging of Hodgkin's Disease, in Ann Arbor in 1971,[104] and has since been modified as follows[172,318]:

Staging classification for Hodgkin's disease (Ann Arbor, 1971)

Stage I   Involvement of single lymph node region, or I E

Stage II   Involvement of two or more lymph node regions on same side of diaphragm, or II E

Stage III Involvement of lymph node regions on both sides of diaphragm, or III E, S, or III ES.

Stage IV   Disseminated disease of one or more extralymphatic organs, including marrow and liver

A or B suffix, The respective absence, *A,* or presence, *B,* of constitutional symptoms: fever, night sweats, unexplained weight loss exceeding 10% of normal; *E,* extranodal organ or site; *S,* spleen.

The clinical stage differs from the pathologic stage in that the former determines the extent of the lymphoma by nonsurgical means: physical examination, laboratory tests, and radiologic imaging procedures including lymphangiogram, computerized axial tomography, and magnetic resonance imaging among others. The term "pathologic stage" is used after a second biopsy is done, which most often involves random bilateral bone marrow biopsy specimens from the posterior iliac pelvic crest. It has been recommended that staging include two marrow biopsies, since the yield of positive samples is higher than for a single biopsy or aspiration alone.[71] The higher yield has been attributed to the ability to evaluate densely cellular infiltrates involved by fibrosis and to detect focal disease by sampling a greater volume of marrow. When positive for HD, the lymphoma is considered to be distributed systemically, that is, pathologic stage IV, which mandates the use of a chemotherapeutic regimen. Complete pathologic staging includes a staging laparotomy in which splenectomy and biopsies of the liver and retroperitoneal, iliac, and mesenteric lymph nodes are done.[278] In women, oophoropexy may be done to preserve ovarian function when abdominal radiation therapy is anticipated. The histologic criteria to determine involvement of organs at staging or in subsequent biopsy specimens from patients with an established pathologic diagnosis of HD are not so stringent as are those required for the primary diagnostic biopsy.[386] The demonstration of H cells alone or cytologically atypical mononuclear cells in a histologic setting typical of HD without identification of RS cells is sufficient for staging purposes. A biopsy is only suggestive of involvement, when abnormal cells are not identified in the same setting.

The spleen is involved in about 40% of cases and is the most frequent abdominal site affected by HD.[172,185,361] Although most involved spleens weigh between 200 and 300 g or less, the weight may vary widely from 100 to 2500 g. Perhaps as many as 10% of palpable spleens are not involved by HD but are enlarged by granulomas, lymphoid hyperplasia, or hypersplenism. Splenic involvement occurs most frequently in MC and NS types. When involved, several tumor nodules are usually visible. Microscopically, early involvement begins in the T-lymphocyte zones of the malpighian bodies. Single nodules, which may be minute in size but still visible grossly, occur in about 10% of cases. Massive involvement with confluent tumor nodules occurs in about 5% of cases. The presence of more than four splenic tumor nodules has been shown to affect survival adversely because of the increased frequency of lower abdominal nodal involvement.[172,318] The location and number of abdominal sites involved may also significantly influence the survival rates. The liver is involved by HD in about 5% of cases and usually only in association with splenic involvement. HD infiltrates the portal tracts of the liver to form multiple tumor nodules. Involvement of other extranodal organs, such as the lungs or skin, occurs by extension from extensively involved regional lymph nodes or hematogenously in cases of high stage or histologic grade.

The overall incidence of marrow involvement at presentation is 15%, with a range of 5% to 30%.[39,495,529] However, the incidence rate in the LD type may approach 50%.[447] Most patients have clinical stage III disease with type B symptoms and cytopenias. The pattern of involvement of the marrow may be either focal or diffuse, and often the histology, especially the frequency of RS cells, is similar to that of nodal infiltrates with histiocytes, lymphocytes, plasma cells, eosinophils, and atypical mononuclear cells, H cells, and RS cells. Fibroblasts and fibrosis are always a component of the infiltrate that effectively effaces the normal hematopoietic cells and medullary adipose tissue. The uninvolved marrow in patients with HD is usually hyperplastic with increased numbers of eosinophils, plasma cells, and histiocytes scattered among the usual hemic cells.

Clinical and epidemiologic relationships. Because the

Rye classification is based on clinicopathologic considerations, the histologic types of HD often correlate with certain clinical patients groups and is helpful in predicting the extent or stage of a patient's disease. Nodular sclerosis more often presents asymptomatically in supradiaphragmatic lymph node groups and more frequently involves the mediastinum and lungs initially than other types do, and it is the most prevalent type of women, young people, and children of higher socioeconomic status.[662] NS usually has a predictable pattern of spread from one regional lymph node group to another, and this observation has been utilized in the development of effective radiotherapy.[368] The mixed cellularity type affects a broad population group and is prevalent in children of low socioeconomic means and in older populations. Hematogenous dissemination between noncontiguous nodal groups and to the spleen and marrow appears to have a greater role in the spread of the MC and LD types. Lymphocytic predominance and lymphocytic depletion types occur exclusively in adults. LP type affects men more than women and typically presents asymptomatically as disease limited to one or two nodal groups high in the cervical nodal chain

and axilla, though inguinal and femoral nodes may also be involved initially.[736] The Lukes nodular variant, which is often phenotypically different from other forms of HD, tends to relapse frequently when compared to the diffuse variant and other types of HD.[587] LD type occurs more frequently in the elderly population and frequently presents as retroperitoneal disease with fever and pancytopenia and with marrow involvement but without peripheral lymphadenopathy in some cases. As compared to other types of HD, the LD type usually follows an aggressive, clinical course, but significant complete remissions resulting in cures can be sustained when adequate therapy can be given.[33,277,515,679]

Essentially all patients with HD, even those in complete remission, have immunologic abnormalities related to cellular immunity. B-lymphocyte function is normal in patients before receiving therapy. The mechanism of impairment is unknown, but it may be related to prostaglandin E_2 production by the mononuclear cells. Radiation and chemotherapy alone or in combination act to diminish cellular immunity further through a slight but prolonged depletion of T-lymphocytes.

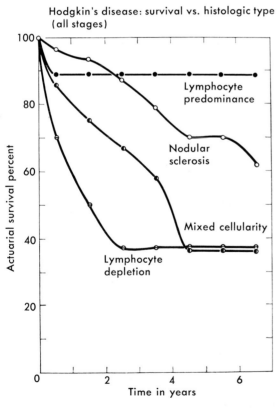

Fig. 28-71. Actuarial survival in 176 cases of Hodgkin's disease according to histologic types. Survival of nodular sclerosis and mixed cellularity groups at 5 years is significantly different ($p < 0.02$). (From Keller, A.R., et al.: Cancer **22:**487, 1968.)

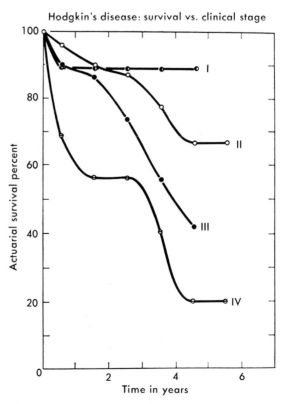

Fig. 28-72. Actuarial survival in Hodgkin's disease according to anatomic stages in 154 patients, all with lymphangiograms. Survival at 5 years of stages I and II, II and IV, and I and IV, are significantly different ($p < 0.02$). (From Keller, A.R., et al.: Cancer **22:**487, 1968.)

Survival and clinical relevance of histology. At the time of the Rye Conference, the prognostic significance of the histopathology of HD was clear (Fig. 28-71) and the contribution of pathologic stage to survival was appreciated (Fig. 28-72). The presence of certain histologic features within have been correlated with improved survival: mature collagenous fibrosis, numerous small lymphocytes, rarity of RS cells, and nonnecrotizing, sarcoidlike granulomas in uninvolved lymphoid organs.[136,530,620] Vascular invasion in the spleen and lymph nodes, poorly developed fibrosis, and numerous RS cells have been associated with a poorer prognosis.[388,497,583] However, the current therapy for HD is more successful than it was 20 years ago, and the overall cure rate is approaching 75% for a wide spectrum of patient prognostic groups. Only the stage of the disease, particularly marrow involvement, and the general health of the patient have independent prognostic significance today.[603] The Ann Arbor staging classification has become ineffective in separating significantly different prognostic groups, especially within the lower stage groupings. However, the histologic classification of HD remains important in that it promotes a reproducible recognition of its different pathologic forms. An accurate distinction of Hodgkin's disease from histopathologic conditions that mimic it, namely, some reactive lymphoid hyperplasias, non-Hodgkin's lymphomas, and other rarer neoplasms, is of prime importance because of the successful outlook of patients with Hodgkin's disease.

Unfortunately, severe complications of successful therapy regimens have become apparent as the number of long-term survivors of HD continues to increase. Sterility in young men and an earlier menopause in women, thyroid dysfunction, and an ominous number of secondary malignant neoplasms have been observed. A 17.6% cumulative risk of secondary cancers after 15 years is now reported.[739] This observation is particularly ominous for children because of their expected long survivals. Of most concern is ANLL, which evolves from myelodysplasia and is uniformly fatal. The risk of ANLL appears to reach a plateau of 3.3% at 10 years in patients who receive adjuvant chemotherapy or chemotherapy alone and differs with the dose of alkylating agents received. The risk of developing solid neoplasms, especially lung cancer, is 13.2%, and NHL is 1.6%, and both continue to rise. Newly designed, effective combination treatment regimens may ameliorate the high incidence of these complications.[100]

Non-Hodgkin's lymphomas

Non-Hodgkin's lymphomas (NHL) are a more heterogeneous group of neoplasms both clinically and pathologically than Hodgkin's disease appears to be. This heterogeneity has promoted the authorship of many classifications worldwide during the past two decades, each based upon shared or entirely different theoretic frameworks. This multiplicity of classifications has created confusion and controversy that is only now beginning to abate.

Classification. Three principal classifications that are currently in use illustrate the diversity of theory and terminology applied to NHL: the Rappaport classification, the Kiel classification, and the Lukes-Collins classification.[257,449,505] They are listed here:

Classification of non-Hodgkin's lymphomas

Modified Rappaport lymphomas
  Nodular
    Lymphocytic, poorly differentiated (WF 2)*
    Mixed lymphocytic-histiocytic (WF 2)
    Histiocytic (WF 4)
  Diffuse
    Lymphocytic, well differentiated (WF 1)
    Lymphocytic, intermediate differentiation
    Lymphocytic, poorly differentiated (WF 5)
    Mixed lymphocytic-histiocytic (WF 6)
    Histiocytic (WF 7, 8)
    Undifferentiated, Burkitt's and non-Burkitt's types (WF 21)
    Lymphoblastic (WF 9)
Kiel classification
  Low-grade malignancy
    Lymphocytic (WF 1)
    Lymphoplasmacytoid (WF 1, 6)
    Centrocytic (WF 5)
    Centroblastic-centrocytic
      Follicular (WF 2, 3, 4) or diffuse (WF 5, 6, 7), or both
  High-grade malignancy
    Centroblastic (WF 7)
    Immunoblastic (WF 8)
    Lymphoblastic
      Burkitt's type (WF 10)
      Convoluted cell type (WF 9)
      Unclassified (WF 9)
Lukes-Collins classification
  B-cell types
    Small lymphocytic (WF 1)
    Plasmacytoid lymphocytic (WF 1)
    Follicular center cell
      Small cleaved (WF 2, 3, 5, 6)
      Large cleaved (WF 3, 4, 6, 7)
      Small noncleaved (WF 10)
      Large noncleaved (WF 4, 6, 7)
    Immunoblastic sarcoma, B-cell (WF 8)
  T-cell types
    Small lymphocytic (WF 1)
    Mycosis fungoides/Sézary syndrome
    Convoluted lymphocytic (WF 9)
    Immunoblastic sarcoma, T-cell (WF 8)
  Histiocytic (WF 7, 8)
  Undefined cell types (WF 9)

---

*Equivalent categories within the working formulation (WF), p. 1453.

Before 1966, only three morphologic forms of NHL were recognized. Introduction of the Rappaport classification unmasked several clinicopathologic groups within these three forms, and it has since achieved broad, general clinical acceptance. It has been widely used in many clinicopathologic studies and remains an important classification today. The Rappaport classification is based on the precept that the cytology and growth pattern of a lymphoma is useful in predicting its natural history. Modifications of this classification since 1966 have maintained its clinical effectiveness. Despite these modifications, it still suffers from archaic nomenclature and biologic heterogeneity in several of its groups.

In contrast, the Lukes-Collins classification, which was introduced in 1974, is based on the morphologic recognition of the cell of origin of the lymphoma infiltrate, that is, whether derived from B-or T-lymphocytes, and discounts the prognostic value of the growth pattern. Its concepts were developed through immunologic-morphologic correlative studies. It too has become an important classification because it revealed several distinct entities that had been unrecognized within Rappaport groups, and it directed opinion toward the development of a functional classification of NHL. It suffers because immunologic heterogeneity has been demonstrated in some of its groups and because the complexities of lymphoma phenotypes and genotypes now far exceed a simple lymphocyte class distinction as first envisioned.

Theoretical middle ground is found in the Kiel classification, which was also published in 1974. This classification is based on the morphologic similarity of malignant lymphocytes to normal ones. Cytology rather than growth pattern of the malignant cells is emphasized in its criteria. However, even though its criteria are primarily morphologic, immunologic and cytochemical studies may augment the subclassification when available. Its nomenclature and criteria are complex, and until recently it has been unfamiliar to clinicians and pathologists outside the European medical community. It is still not widely used in the United States.

The nosologic turmoil surrounding the classification of NHL began to abate after the publication in 1982 of the NCI Working Formulation for Clinical Usage (WF), an extensive retrospective study of NHL classifications,[590] shown below:

National Cancer Institute Working Formulation for Clinical Usage

Low grade
1. Small lymphocytic
2. Follicular, predominantly small cleaved cell
3. Follicular, mixed, small cleaved and large cell

Intermediate grade
4. Follicular, predominantly large cell
5. Diffuse, small cleaved cell
6. Diffuse, mixed, small and large cell
7. Diffuse, large cell

High grade
8. Large cell, immunoblastic
9. Lymphoblastic
10. Small noncleaved cell

The study, which was sponsored by the National Cancer Institute of the United States, was a heroic effort to resolve the differences that existed among the principal classifications in use internationally. Through rigorous statistical analyses of clinical data from cases classified with each classification, the results indicated that each classification is usable and reproducible, that each separates patients into clinicopathologic prognostic groups, and that none was found to be superior to another in clinical relevance. Ten major clinicopathologic types of non-Hodgkin's lymphoma and some miscellaneous types were identified by the analysis, and these were sorted into favorable, intermediate, and unfavorable prognostic groups. Nosologic terms for each of the 10 WF types were identified in the six classifications analyzed. The WF was intended to be "a means of translation among the various systems and to facilitate clinical comparison of case reports and therapeutic trials" and "was not proposed as a new classification." However, it has been received by clinicians and pathologists in the United States as a classification of compromise with regard to Rappaport lymphoma types and Lukes-Collins terminology and concepts of large cell lymphomas. Transference between these two classifications through the WF, though not always entirely accurate, does appear straightforward. However, because biologic heterogeneity still exists within certain types of lymphoma and because some lymphoma types were not addressed by the WF, it is premature to expect that the WF and current classifications of NHL will not continue to require periodic revision as new observations dictate.[432,506]

Pathogenesis. Recent advances in several diverse fields of study have contributed extraordinarily to the present understanding of lymphomas and have brought into better focus certain intriguing observations that have been associated with these neoplasms for years. These include nonrandom chromosomal abnormalities and other clonal markers, associated endemic virus infections, and the prevalence of lymphomas in immunodeficiency states. It is becoming clear that these observations, once believed to relate only to a few specific lymphomas, have general significance in the origin of all lymphomas.

Malignant lymphomas are now rightly viewed as clonal proliferations of immune cells that recapitulate in aberrant ways the normal anatomic and functional organization of the immune system.[793] Collectively, about 65% of NHL are derivatives of B-lymphocytes, 35% of T-lymphocytes, and less than 2% of histiocytes. The cellular origin of Hodgkin's disease remains an enigma (discussed before), and recent studies have indicated some biologic heterogeneity in the histologic subtypes. In contrast to HD, the cytologic types of neoplastic cells in NHL have been related generally to hypothetical stages of lymphocyte development through immunologic studies, which are referred to as cell-marker studies (Table 28-12 and Figs. 28-73 and 28-74). In contrast to normal lymphocytes, malignant cells often do not express a normal phenotype fully and often express an array of differentiation antigens not anticipated in a normal cell. Recognizing these aberrancies enhance the diagnostic usefulness of these studies. Their use also provides a rapid means of distinguishing neoplasms of similar histology, that is, lymphoma from undifferen-

tiated carcinoma, sarcoma, and myeloblastoma; lymphoma from benign lymphoid infiltrates; and some specific histologic types of lymphoma, such as SNC, LB, and SL lymphomas (Table 28-13).[660] Despite their diagnostic importance, they have not as yet provided prognostic information that is independent of histologic classification.[645] Most of the experience with these studies has been with antibodies that are specific for antigenic epitopes that are denatured by routine tissue fixation. Therefore these studies have been limited to laboratories that are capable of analyzing unfixed tissue or cell suspensions. An ever-increasing number of antibodies are being developed that will be useful in analogous studies of routinely processed tissue.[165,434,525,699] Immunophenotyping of histologically well-defined lym-

Table 28-12. Selected list of antigens expressed by normal and neoplastic lymphoid cells

Antigen class	Designation	Name, specificity, and molecular weight
Non–lineage associated antigens	CD45	Leukocyte common antigen, gp200
	TdT	Terminal deoxynucleotidyltransferase
	DR	Class II MHC antigens
	CD10	CALLA; common ALL antigen; gp100
B cell–associated antigens	Ig	Immunoglobulin heavy and light polypeptide chains
	CD19	B cell–associated antigen; gp95
	CD20	B cell–specific antigen; gp30
	CD21	C3d; EBV receptor; gp140
	CD22	B cell–associated antigen; gp135
T cell–associated antigens	CD1	Common thymocyte; Langerhans cell–associated antigen; gp45
	CD2	Sheep erythrocyte ligand; gp50
	CD3	T cell receptor–associated antigen; gp 19–25
	CD4	Helper/inducer T cell subset–associated antigen; gp45
	CD5	T cell–associated antigen; B cell subset antigen; gp67
	CD7	T cell–associated antigen; gp41
	CD8	Cytotoxic/suppressor T cell subset–associated antigen; gp32
Myeloid cell–associated antigens	AML2.23	Myelocyte/monocyte-associated antigen
	CD11c	Monocyte-associated antigen
	CD13	Myeloid-associated antigen; MY7
	CD14	Myeloid-associated antigen; MY4
	CD15	Myeloid-associated antigen; Leul
	CD34	Blasts; PHCA1; MY10
	MPX/SBB	Myeloperoxidase/Sudan black B
	CAE	Chloroacetate esterase
Proliferative/activation antigens	CD25	IL-2 receptor; gp55
	CD30	Ki-1; B and T cell–associated activation antigen; gp90
	CD38	T cell–associated activation antigen; gp45
	Ki-67	Proliferation-associated antigen
	T9	Transferrin receptor

CD, Cluster of differentiation, assigned at the International Workshops on Leukocyte Differentiation Antigens to monoclonal antibodies that recognize cell surface molecules expressed by normal and neoplastic cells.

ALL, Acute lymphoblastic leukemia; *AML,* acute myeloblastic leukemia; *DR,* an HLA locus; *EBV,* Epstein-Barr virus; *gp,* glycoprotein; *Ig,* immunoglobulin; *IL,* interleukin; *Ki,* karyopyknotic index; *MHC,* major histocompatibility complex; *MY,* myeloid antigen; *PHCA,* progenitor hematopoietic ALL antigen.

phomas remain an active area of investigation; the results can be correlated with those from cell kinetic, molecular, and genetic studies.

Inherent in most of the classifications of NHL is the observation that higher tumor cell mitotic indices are associated with the histologic higher grades of lymphoma. Some studies using a variety of methods that measure the DNA content and synthesis by individual lymphoma cells have demonstrated directly the relationship of the proliferative capacity of a lymphoma to a histologic type and grade and to patient survival.[173,360,477,670] Flow cytometry permits a direct measurement of more than one property of the cell simultaneously and can be used to study antigen expression in relation to the cell cycle and DNA content of particular cell populations in the lymphoma as defined by specific arrays of cell antigens.[65] In one such study that correlated results with the NCI Working Formulation, the percentage of tumor cells in DNA-synthesis phase increased with increasing histologic grade and DNA aneuploidy, and significant positive correlations between the S-phase cell fraction, the presence of aneuploidy, and intermediate and high histologic grades were demonstrated.[360]

Investigations of the mechanisms by which lymphocytes generate the enormous diversity of the antigen receptor repertoire have progressed rapidly to address questions regarding the genetic basis of clonal development and the malignant phenotype.[49] Clonality of most lymphomas can be related to several specific, recurring chromosomal abnormalities that occur early in the expression of antigen receptors by tumor cells. The prototypic example is that of the 14q+ abnormalities of Burkitt's lymphoma, recognized in 1972. In some notable examples, certain proto-oncogenes that are involved in normal cell growth regulation are now known to become deregulated simultaneously and contribute to the neoplastic progression of the lymphoma. Growth factors and cytokines and their receptors are also implicated in promoting the growth and maintaining the malignant phenotype of the lymphoma.[654]

The lymphocyte antigen receptor is membrane-bound Ig in the B-lymphocyte and the T-cell receptor complex (TCR) in the T-lymphocyte. Ig consists of a pair of identical, covalently coupled heterodimers of heavy polypeptide chains and one of two light chains. The genes that encode these polypeptides are located on chr 14 for the heavy chain and on chr 2 and 22 for the kappa and lambda light chains respectively. The TCR consists of a complex of the nonpolymorphic, pentameric CD3 molecule and a noncovalent heterodimer of alpha and beta chains or gamma and delta chains de-

Table 28-13. Diagnostic applications of cell-marker studies

Cell marker	Application
Lymphoma versus nonlymphomatous neoplasms	
Cytokeratins	Epithelial neoplasms
Leukocyte common antigen	Hematopoietic neoplasms
Terminal deoxynucleotidyltransferase (TdT)	Lymphoblasts
Myeloperoxidase/Sudan black B	Myeloblasts
Chloroacetate esterase	Myeloid cells
Lymphoma versus reactive lymphoid hyperplasia	
Restricted expression of kappa versus lambda Ig light chains	B-cell neoplasms
Aberrant expression of antigens	T-cell neoplasms
Specific histologic types of lymphoma	
CD45, DR, CD19, CD5 +/−, IgM and K or L (low density)	Small lymphocytic lymphoma (98% B-cell phenotypes)
CD45, DR, CD19, CD21, IgH and K or L (high density)	Follicular lymphomas (100% B-cell phenotypes)
CD45, DR, CD19, IgM/G and K or L (high density)	Small noncleaved cell lymphomas (100% B-cell phenotypes)
TdT, CD1, CD3, CD4/CD8, and CD2 +/−, CD45 +/−	Lymphoblastic lymphomas (85% thymocyte phenotypes)
TdT, DR, CD19, CD10, Ig gene rearrangement	Lymphoblastic lymphomas (10% precursor B-cell phenotypes)
TdT +/−, DR, CD19, cytoplasmic IgM	Lymphoblastic lymphomas (5% pre-B-cell phenotypes)
CD15, CD30	Hodgkin's disease

CD, Cluster of differentiation.

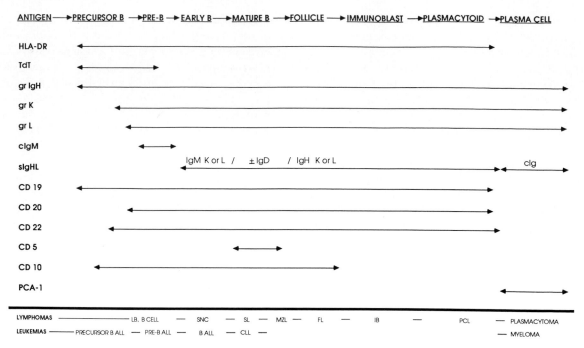

Fig. 28-73. Expression of antigens by normal and neoplastic B-lymphocytes in a hypothetical model of differentiation.

First column—antigens: *TdT*, terminal deoxynucleotidyl transferase; *gr*, gene rearrangement; *c*, cytoplasmic; *s*, surface membrane. *First line*—hypothetical stages of B cell differentiation; *last two lines*—acronyms of specific NHL and ALL relate vertically to normal stages of B-cell development and antigen expression: *LB*, lymphoblastic; *SNC*, small noncleaved cell; *SL*, small lymphocytic; *MZL*, mantle zone lymphoma; *FL*, follicular lymphoma; *IB*, immunoblastic; *PCL*, plasmacytoid lymphoma; *ALL*, acute lymphoblastic leukemia; *CLL*, chronic lymphocytic leukemia.

pending on the cell of expression.[62,66,309] The alpha and delta genes are located on chr 14, and the beta and gamma genes on chr 7. Expression of the receptor by the cell begins with the movement of gene-coding segments into juxtaposition to form a functional, structural gene before transcription occurs in a process called "gene rearrangement." Rearrangements, which occur in each polymorphic receptor protein gene, are hierarchically regulated and expressed.[397,635] Rearrangement results in the sequential movement and joining of single variable (V), joining (J), and constant (C) gene segments as illustrated in Fig. 28-75 for the kappa gene. The organization, structure, and number of gene segments differ for each of the various antigen receptor proteins. In the IgH gene, for example, diversity (D) segments, located between V and J regions, also become rearranged. Productive rearrangement results in a shortening of the gene with respect to DNA-restriction enzyme

sites for both alleles. The movement of the restriction enzyme sites during gene rearrangement provides a physical basis for discriminating nonrearranged or germline genes from rearranged genes.

DNA rearrangement is the earliest process known to occur when lymphocytes commit to differentiate into a functional lymphocyte subpopulation, and it results in the production of structural genes that are as unique to the individual cell as are its receptor proteins. When the progeny of a single cell proliferates to the extent of a clinical neoplasm, the quantity of the rearranged gene copies are more than sufficient to identify the rearrangement by DNA sizing and hybridization techniques using specific C-region gene probes (Fig. 28-75, *B* and *C*). The number of identically rearranged gene copies from cells in reactive, polyclonal proliferations usually cannot be detected in the same DNA hybridization assay. Molecular hybridization methods are specific and

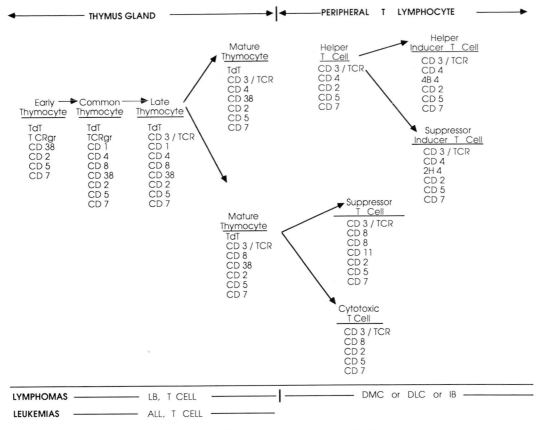

Fig. 28-74. Expression of antigens by normal and neoplastic T-lymphocytes in a hypothetical model of differentiation.
Last two lines—acronyms of specific NHL and ALL relate vertically to the normal stages of T-cell development and antigen expression: *LB*, lymphoblastic; *DMC*, diffuse small and large cell; *DLC*, diffuse large cell; *IB*, immunoblastic; *ALL*, acute lymphoblastic leukemia; *TdT*, terminal deoxynucleotidyl transferase; *TCR*, T-cell receptor; *gr*, gene rearrangement.

far more sensitive than other methods are for detecting clonal populations, in that 1 lymphoma cell in 1 million normal cells can be detected through gene-amplification methods.[13,154] These methods have proved useful in detection of residual lymphoma in patients in clinical remission.[154,416] However, several complex issues including the known occurrence of benign oligoclonal lymphoid proliferations in reactive and neoplastic disorders and the occurrence of life-threatening polyclonal lymphoid proliferations in certain immunodeficient patients preclude the use of this technology as an isolated, initial diagnostic test for lymphoma.[423]

Recurring cytogenetic abnormalities have long been identified with certain histologic types of lymphoma, notably chr 14q+ abnormalities in Burkitt's lymphoma (Table 28-14).[220] The t(8;14) translocation occurs in about 80% of Burkitt's lymphoma and involves the movement of the distal end of chr 8 to chr 14. Two

variant translocations involving the same portion of chr 8, t(8;22) and t(2;8), have since been described.[151] Recent studies of the complex translocations in Burkitt's lymphomas have discovered that these rearrangements involve the locus of the proto-oncogene c-*myc* on chr 8. A portion of the gene is translocated from its normal position to one of the three Ig gene loci. The breakpoint at 8q24 on chr 8 is the same for each translocation and is always located before the c-*myc* gene–coding regions. The aberrantly rearranged c-*myc* gene is believed by some to escape regulation associated with the normal growth state because its regulatory sequence is replaced with that of the respective, receptive Ig gene–altering transcriptional control.[113] Normally, c-*myc* gene products, two closely related normal cellular DNA-binding proteins, are present in cells that enter and maintain a proliferative state.[378] Cells that express this gene in tissue culture appear to have an unlimited

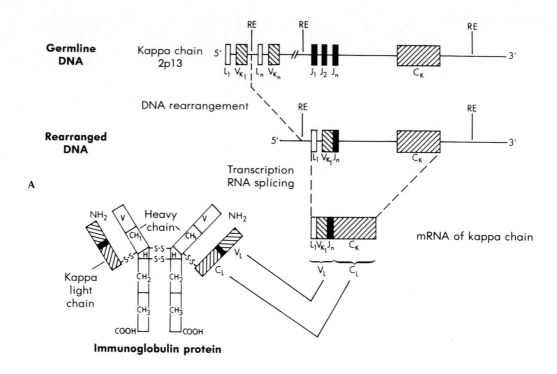

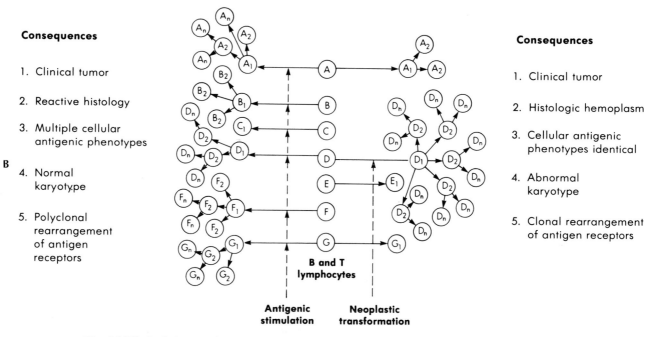

Fig. 28-75. A, Schema of rearrangement of the kappa Ig gene into a functional, structural gene from germline DNA and translation, transcription, and incorporation of the polypeptide chain into an Ig molecule. **B,** Schema of consequences of antigenic stimulation of lymphoid tissue *(left progression)* versus a neoplastic transformation event *(right progression)*. Equally dominant proliferations may produce multiclonal or oligoclonal populations that may persist during neoplastic progression.

Table 28-14. Correlations of specific karyotypic abnormalities and histologic types of non-Hodgkin's lymphoma

	SL	FSC	FM	FL	DSC	DM	DL	IB	SNC	LB
t(8;14)		+					+		+	
t(2;8)									+	
t(8;22)									+	
t(11;14)	+					+	+			+
t(14;18)	+	+	+	+	+	+	+	+	+	
Trisomy 12	+	+	+	+	+	+		+	+	
Trisomy 3	+		+		+	+		+		
14q11-13					+	+	+	+	+	

DL, Diffuse large-cell lymphoma; *DM,* diffuse mixed-cell lymphoma; *DSC,* diffuse small-cell lymphoma; *FL,* follicular large-cell lymphoma; *FM,* follicular mixed-cell lymphoma; *FSC,* follicular small-cell lymphoma; *IB,* immunoblastic lymphoma; *LB,* lymphoblast lymphoma; *SL,* small-lymphocyte lymphoma; *SNC,* small noncleaved-cell lymphoma.

proliferative capacity and are more responsive to exogenous growth factors.[409] In the Burkitt's cell, c-*myc* is dysregulated by a *cis*-acting influence, perhaps from the adjacent Ig gene, which modulates the constitutive c-*myc* mRNA and protein concentrations promoting fully the proliferative phenotype of Burkitt's lymphoma.[1,391] Similar mechanisms are believed to occur with other proposed proto-oncogenes, *bcl*-1 and *tcl*-1, which have been mapped to chr 11 and 14 respectively.[152,738] An-

other proto-oncogene, termed "*bcl*-2," which is located on chr 18, is frequently rearranged in a variety of B-cell lymphomas, especially follicular lymphomas.[3,417] Aberrant rearrangements of the IgH or TCR genes on chr 14 result in the t(14;18) abnormality, characteristic of most follicular lymphomas; the t(11;14) abnormality, seen in small-lymphocyte (SL) and diffuse lymphomas of B-cell type; and in the 14q11-13 abnormalities involving the alpha-chain locus of the TCR gene, found in many T-cell lymphomas. The products of these putative oncogenes have not as yet been identified, and it is unclear what effects, if any, these genes contribute to the phenotype of the neoplastic cells.

Recent studies indicate that additional chromosomal abnormalities other than the characteristic t(14;18)(q32;q21) abnormality occur in the course of some follicular lymphomas and undoubtedly contribute to the change in the clinicopathologic phenotype.[828] Lymphomas with divergent histology, particularly FM (follicular mixed-cell), FL (follicular large-cell), and DLC (diffuse large-cell), that develop in patients with otherwise indolent t(14;18)-positive FSC (follicular small-cell) lymphomas express an additional 6q deletion with partial or complete trisomy of chr 7 or 12 or both. Composite lymphomas of follicular and lymphoblastic histology in which t(14;18) and t(8;14) translocations were associated with activation of c-*myc* have been described.[170,549] Deletions of 13q32 have been found in FSC with t(14;18), and they develop significant lymphocytosis associated with acceleration of the clinical course. Trisomy 2 or 2p duplication often accompanies acceleration of the clinical disease and a poor therapeutic response in these lymphomas. These and other specific chromosomal abnormalities provide links to genetic mechanisms that are undoubtedly relevant to the development of clinical lymphoma phenotypes.

Two transforming viruses are now known to contribute to the development of certain malignant lympho-

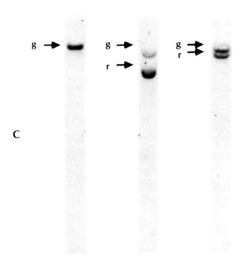

Fig. 28-75, cont'd. C, Clonal analysis of lymph node tissue by ^{32}P-labeled C$_k$/Hind III restriction enzyme digest in Southern blot hybridization that shows rearrangement of the kappa gene. *Lane I,* Control; *lane II,* lymphoma tissue; *g,* germline DNA; *r,* rearranged kappa alleles. (**C** courtesy Dr. Bratin K. Saha, St. Louis.)

mas. The Epstein-Barr virus (EBV), a DNA herpesvirus, has been extensively studied since it was isolated in 1964 from a Burkitt's lymphoma cell line. More recently, the human T-cell lymphotropic virus I (HTLV-I), an RNA retrovirus, has been associated with another form of non-Hodgkin's lymphoma, adult T-cell leukemia-lymphoma (ATL). The two viruses, though genetically distinct, have many biologic features in common. Both viruses are found in the general population and are capable of transforming normal lymphocytes in vitro. Lymphoma cells are infected by each virus, and the viral genomic DNA integrates at monoclonal sites that vary randomly between lymphomas of the same type. However, neither virus is known to produce the principal tumorigenic event in what is believed to be multistep progression to the malignant phenotype.

The pathophysiology of EBV infection is clearer than it is for HTLV-I. EBV infects B-lymphocytes by binding to the C3d receptor (CD21) and transforms the cells to a continuously proliferative state. In acute infectious mononucleosis, which is caused by EBV, the proliferation of B-lymphocytes is curtailed and controlled primarily by specific T cell–mediated immunity. In clinical settings of primary and secondary immunodeficiency, polyclonal B-cell proliferations driven by EBV may continue unabated because of suppressed T-cell function and can be recognized pathologically as polyclonal, multiclonal, oligoclonal, or monoclonal proliferations, as progression is sustained (Fig. 28-75, *B*).[133] In endemic Burkitt's lymphoma, it is believed that chronic recurring *Plasmodium falciparum* infection and high parasitemia in hyperendemic regions contribute to tumorigenesis by maintaining a milieu of polyclonal B-cell stimulation in relative T-cell deficiency. The unbridled proliferation results in a gradual expansion of EBV-transformed B-cell populations. It is in these predisposed B-cell populations that there occurs a rare tumorigenic Ig/c-*myc* translocation that ultimately produces a clonal malignancy.[441] Recently a new herpeslike human B-lymphotropic virus (HBLV), which is genetically distinct from EBV, has been isolated from patients with lymphoproliferative disorders, including AILD (angioimmunoblastic lymphadenopathy with dysproteinemia) and IB (immunoblastic) lymphoma, thus expanding the number of viruses implicated in lymphoma genesis.[625]

HTLV-I is associated with adult T-cell leukemia-lymphoma syndrome (ATL), an aggressive and usually rapidly fatal malignancy, which is characterized by generalized lymphadenopathy, polyclonal hypergamma-globulinemia, lytic bone lesions, lymphocytosis, and infiltration of the lungs, skin, and gastrointestinal tract.[743] The lymphoma cells express the phenotype of CD4-positive T-lymphocytes and are polymorphic with lobular nuclei that produce a variable histologic structure,

most frequently classified as IB lymphoma. ATL is endemic in Japan, Okinawa, Taiwan, and the Caribbean, and sporadic cases have been identified in Central and South America, the eastern United States, and Africa. The HTLV-I virus is not highly contagious, though many healthy adults in endemic areas are seropositive for it. The incidence of seropositivity increases with age. Fewer than 1% of infected persons ever develop ATL, usually after a latent period that may exceed 10 years. It is presently unknown exactly how HTLV-I contributes in the tumorigenesis. T-cells that are infected with the virus ultimately lose immunocompetence, and it is believed that this relative chronic T-cell immunodeficiency permits the emergence of malignantly transformed cells.[569]

These insights into the development of certain lymphomas has stimulated a rapid transfer of research technology into the clinical laboratory. Many of the methods have become important adjuncts in the diagnosis and monitoring of patients with lymphoma. Immunophenotyping, flow cytometric analysis of antigen expression and DNA content, and karyotypic and molecular genetic studies have become routine in medical centers involved in clinical research. Reference laboratories also provide these studies to general hospital laboratories, which do not provide their own. Information from these studies is useful clinically and, as emphasized before, is often relied upon to identify a clonal marker of the neoplasm or to support the subclassification of the lymphoma.[660] Even so, routine histology remains the essential method used to diagnose and classify malignant lymphomas. However, the histologic evaluation of lymphomas is anything but routine. Accurate interpretation of the suspect tissue requires that it be properly fixed at the time of biopsy. Tissue can be appropriated for the necessary ancillary studies at this time (Fig. 28-76). Obtaining the viable tissue quickly after biopsy requires an active dialog and coordination between the physician, surgeon, and pathologist in cases of suspected lymphoma.

Histopathology. The lymphomatous infiltrate of NHL most often enlarges the lymph node by completely effacing the normal architecture of the nodal parenchyma. The infiltrate may extend beyond the capsule to involve perinodal tissues. Partial involvement of the node may also occur with or without enlargement but less often. The infiltrate may appear as uniform nodules resembling germinal centers or as a diffuse infiltrate of cytologically abnormal cells. The infiltrate is composed of a mixture of one or more than one cytologic type of malignant lymphoid cell and is usually associated with normal cells. The "histologic types" of cells are believed to represent different states of transformation, activation, or differentiation.[274] Classification of the histologic type of NHL is achieved through the recognition of the

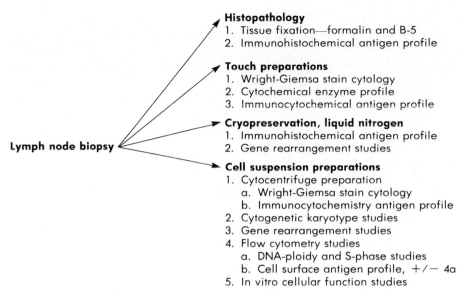

Fig. 28-76. Diagnostic and ancillary studies for lymphoma.

most prevalent or a mixture of the most prevalent abnormal cell types and their organizational pattern of growth as detailed by the particular classification used. As many as 20 different histologic types of NHL are recognized depending on the classification applied. Based upon this approach, broad clinicopathologic groups of NHL, which share similar natural histories, can be identified within each classification. The biologic heterogeneity within these groups can be identified by the application of ancillary diagnostic studies, that is, immunophenotypic, DNA-content analysis, and karyotypic and genotypic studies.

Lymphomas of follicular cells (FL). That certain non-Hodgkin's lymphomas grow in a nodular or follicular pattern is recognized by many classifications. Collectively, follicular lymphomas account for about 50% of cases of NHL. The cytologic features of these tumors consist of a mixture of malignant follicular center lymphocytes and are subclassified according to the predominant cell present: small cleaved-cell type (SCC), mixed small cleaved and large cell type (MC), and large cell type (LC). This subclassification is based upon a subjective estimate of the frequency of large noncleaved cells in the infiltrate.[163,458,512] The SCC type represents the most frequent type of follicular lymphomas, and the LC type the least frequent. The median age at presentation is between 40 and 50 years of age, and men and women are equally affected. Children very rarely develop follicular lymphomas.[243,808] Patients usually present with asymptomatic, generalized lymphadenopathy and widespread disease. Only 20% to 30% of cases are limited to stages I and II. These advanced stages are often attributable to marrow involvement, which occurs in 40% to 50% of cases. FL characteristically infiltrate the paratrabecular areas of the marrow, and the infiltrates are rarely extensive enough to affect hematopoiesis directly or influence survival.[230] Lymphomas of nonfollicular cells, in contrast, infiltrate the marrow in random sites. Lymphocytosis is common in FL, especially in the small cleaved cell type. The spleen and liver are also frequently involved by infiltrates that expand the malpighian bodies (Fig. 28-46) and the portal tracts.

Histologically, the malignant follicles are uniform in size and shape, are surrounded by cuffs or mantles of mostly small lymphocytes, and are closely arranged with little interfollicular tissue (Fig. 28-77). Malignant follicles must be distinguished from the germinal centers of reactive lymphoid hyperplasia. This task may be most difficult in cases of florid hyperplasia[511] and can require immunologic or genetic studies to support the diagnosis of lymphoma. In addition to their relative uniformity and high density within the tissue, malignant follicles have a cytologic monotony that reactive follicles lack: the cellular size gradient is absent, the number of phagocytic dendritic cells is decreased or absent, and reactive lymphocytes in varying states of antigenic activation are absent in lymphoma.

The cell types associated with follicular lymphoma include the small cleaved cell, the large cleaved cell, the large noncleaved cell, and less frequently the small noncleaved cell. Small cleaved cells are intermediate in size, that is, larger than malignant small lymphocytes but smaller than malignant large cells. They have an

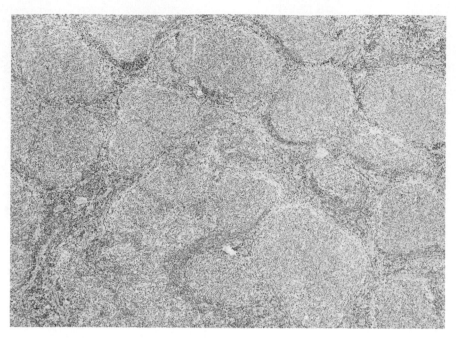

Fig. 28-77. Lymph node. Follicular lymphoma, small cleaved cell type.

elongated, folded nucleus with little discernible cytoplasm (Fig. 28-78), and the chromatin is more open than in the malignant small lymphocyte with indistinct nucleoli. The mitotic index is low. Malignant large cells are cells with nuclei that are similar in size or larger than those of endothelial cells or benign histiocytes in the same tissue section. Their nuclei may have an open chromatin pattern with several distinct nucleoli located at the edge of the nuclear membrane, in which case they are referred to as "large noncleaved cells" (Fig. 28-78), or they may have indistinct nucleoli with a slightly less open chromatin pattern, in which case they are referred to as "large cleaved cells" (Fig. 28-78). The cytoplasm of both cell types is minimal, and they are mitotically active. These malignant cells are derivatives of germinal center B-lymphocytes and are phenotypically similar to normal cells.[322,347] Benign B- and T-lymphocytes occupy the follicular cuffs along with infiltrating malignant cells. Benign T-lymphocytes are also present in the malignant follicles but are more prevalent in the interfollicular tissue. The t(14;18) chromosomal translocation is characteristic of FL and serves as a molecular marker for this group of lymphomas. It is most evident in the SCC type and is identified in about 85% of cases.[220,396,422]

In occasional cases, follicular lymphomas may display a diffuse growth pattern as well as the characteristic follicular pattern within the same lymph node.[771] This phenomenon of divergent histologic pattern is observed in 20% to 30% of NHL but occurs most frequently in FL. Composite lymphoma refers to a divergent histo-

logic pattern that occurs within the same lymph node region.[385] A divergent histologic pattern is most frequently recognized in sequential biopsy specimens during the course of disease, though it may also be recognized in biopsy specimens taken simultaneously. Progression of the histopathologic course of a lymphoma from a lower to a higher histologic grade is the common theme.[255] In most cases studied by immunologic or genetic methods, the observed changes reflect histologic derivatives of the same clonal neoplasm. Infrequently, two clonal neoplasms may arise within the same patients.[813,822] The prognosis in cases of histologic progression corresponds to that of the highest histologic grade of lymphoma identified.[326]

The median survival of patients with FL is greater than 7 years[590] and depends in part on the histologic type. In general, patients with FL enjoy longer survivals than those with diffuse lymphomas of the same cell type, and patients with the more prevalent SCC and MC types live longer than those with the LC type do.[693] It is uncertain whether diffuse areas within FL negatively influence survival, though this is most likely in the LC type.[694,771] Undoubtedly, the poorer survival of patients with diffuse lymphomas reported in many studies reflects the presence of biologic heterogeneity that is indiscernible histologically.[711]

Lymphomas of small lymphocytes (SL). Histologically the small lymphocytic lymphoma group of NHL is characterized by a diffuse infiltrate of malignant small lymphocytes (Fig. 28-79). In microscopic sections, the neoplastic cells are normal appearing but slightly enlarged

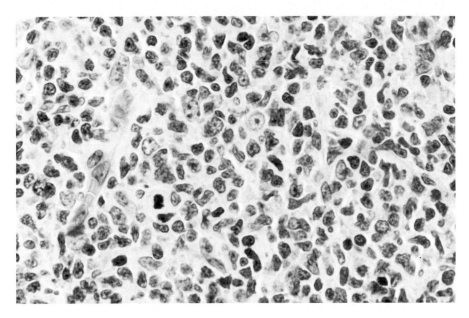

Fig. 28-78. Lymph node. Follicular lymphoma, mixed small cleaved and large cell type. Most of the cells are small cleaved cells. Fewer large cleaved and noncleaved cells are present.

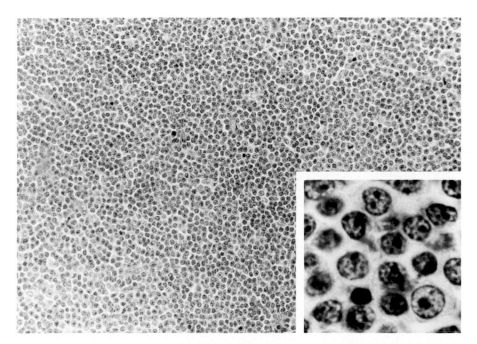

Fig. 28-79. Lymph node, small lymphocytic lymphoma. The malignant small lymphocyte is the predominant cell accompanied by fewer prolymphocytes. *Inset,* See cell descriptions in text.

lymphocytes with round nuclei and clumped chromatin. They appear identical to the cells of chronic lymphocytic leukemia. Mitoses are infrequent except in proliferation centers within the infiltrate. Proliferation centers are ill-defined concentrations of mitotically active prolymphocytes that sometimes give the diffuse infiltrate a pseudofollicular appearance. A true follicular pattern is never produced by SL. Prolymphocytes resemble the predominating small cells but are larger with single, central nucleoli and more open chromatin. Plasmacytoid features, that is, cells with nuclear features of a lymphocyte and cytoplasmic features of a plasma cell, may be exhibited by the small cells. Some classifications regard plasmacytic differentiation as a distinct variety of SL or as a more generalized phenomenon that may occur in other histologic types. Lymphomas with plasmacytoid features differ phenotypically from those without and often secrete measurable amounts of monoclonal Ig into the serum.[384] About 98% of SL are derivatives of B-lymphocytes, which phenotypically resemble the mature, antigen-naïve B-cell of the paracortex and are phenotypically very similar to those of chronic lymphocytic leukemia.[300,396,422,470] Cytogenic abnormalities, though identified in SL, are not characteristic.

Small lymphocytic lymphomas account for about 5% of NHL. The median age of onset is 55 to 60 years, and cases in patients under 40 years of age are rarely seen. These lymphomas are usually widespread at diagnosis with 70% to 80% in stage IV because of marrow involvement. Other SL present as isolated tumors particularly in extranodal sites, especially the lungs, perior-bital tissues, and gastrointestinal tract. SL, especially the nodal form, very often evolve into leukemia, indistinguishable from CLL. Even so, the prognosis for these patients is good with a median survival of more than 5 years.

Lymphomas of cuff or mantle zone cells (MZL). This group of lymphomas was identified by its unusual bimorphic population of lymphoma cells, an admixture of malignant small lymphocytes and small cleaved cells.[40] Most of these lymphomas grow in a diffuse pattern that effaces the nodal architecture, whereas a variant form is characterized by a vaguely nodular pattern attributable to the expansion of the cuff or mantle zone area by neoplastic cells around benign-appearing germinal centers (Fig. 28-80).[785] Cell-marker studies indicate that these cells may express the phenotype of B-lymphocytes of primary lymphoid follicles,[454,500,782] though some investigators suggest multiple derivations of MZL.[301,302] The original designation for this lymphoma, "lymphocytic lymphoma of intermediate differentiation," has been incorporated into the modified Rappaport classification. Most of these lymphomas classify as centrocytic type in the Kiel classification and are assigned to the category of diffuse, small cleaved cell type in the working formulation. The term "mantle zone lymphoma" has been proposed as an alternative, preferred name, which would avoid confusion with the generic designation of lymphomas of intermediate grade by the WF.[341,345,785]

Most patients with MZL are 50 years of age or older and present with generalized lymphadenopathy. About 85% of patients have stage IV disease initially, either because of marrow or liver involvement.[345,783] Lympho-

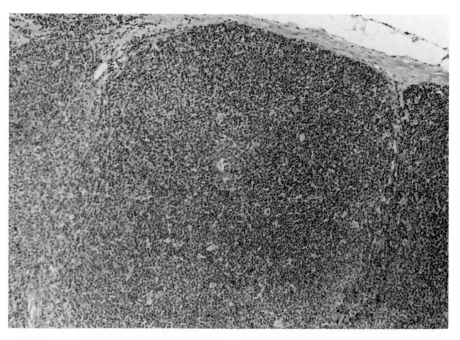

Fig. 28-80. Lymph node, mantle zone lymphoma. The lymphoma infiltrate expands the cuff around a small germinal center.

cytosis occurs in 20% of cases, and like in other indolent lymphomas, lymphocytosis usually does not affect overall survival. The reported median survival ranges from 3 to 7 years, and the range of survival may be quite broad from several months to over 10 years. Clinically aggressive forms of MZL do occur and appear to be different from typical cases only by a higher mitotic index.[199,783] In general, MZL, like other indolent lymphomas, do not appear to have a curative potential despite their long median survival.

Diffuse lymphomas of large cells (DL). Morphologically, there appears to be at least two major types of large cell lymphoma that proliferate in a diffuse pattern; lymphomas composed of large cells that resemble those of the follicular lymphomas and are specifically designated as large cell type (LC) and lymphomas composed of malignant immunoblasts and are designated as immunoblastic type (IB). About 70% of DL lymphomas are classified as the LC type. Although there is histologic overlap of the two subtypes, experienced pathologists can distinguish them about 85% of the time.[590] These histologic forms are biologically heterogeneous and do not have specific morphologic features that permit an objective distinction of cellular origin.[148,180,220,236,319,348,789]

The cytologic appearance of lymphomas of LC type is similar to that of large cell follicular lymphomas in that large cleaved cells and large noncleaved cells are recognized. Their prevalence within the infiltrates further defines two respective subtypes designated as large cleaved and large noncleaved subtypes. The large cleaved subtype should have less than 25% large noncleaved cells present. The lymphomas of IB type can be divided into three subtypes based upon the recognition of the variant cytologic appearance. The malignant IB is a large cell that has a uniform or pleomorphic nucleus with an open chromatin pattern and centrally located, prominent, usually singular nucleolus. The cells may have an eccentrically located nucleus with a moderate amount of amphophilic cytoplasm that creates a plasmacytoid appearance (Fig. 28-81, *A*), in which case the lymphoma is subclassified as plasmacytoid subtype, or the cytoplasm may be optically clear and the nucleoli less distinct (Fig. 28-81, *B*) and is subclassified as clear cell subtype. In the polymorphous subtype of IB, the nuclei are multilobulated and resemble the Reed-Sternberg cells of Hodgkin's disease. The mitotic index of these lymphomas is high.

Other variant histologic structures of DL, which are much less frequently encountered, have also been described and include multilobated NHL,[531,750] filiform large cell lymphoma,[46,536] and rare examples of lymphomas of dendritic and interdigitating reticulum cell derivation. The latter two forms require cell-marker studies to confirm their histocytic nature.[579] A rare, angiotrophic form of large cell lymphoma, which is called "malignant angioendotheliomatosis," or "intravascular malignant lymphomatosis," is characterized by the proliferation of large, pleomorphic neoplastic lymphoid cells within the lumen of small and medium-sized vessels.[795] This disorder, which is usually fatal, primarily involves cutaneous and central nervous system vessels as well as other organs, producing variable clinical findings. Extravascular DL lymphoma can be identified in lymphoid organs and in other sites in some patients. Clonal expression of Ig and Ig-gene rearrangements have been demonstrated in individual cases.[538]

The DL lymphomas comprise about 35% to 40% of NHL and about 30% of the NHL of childhood.[281,390,507,805] Most affected adults are between 50 and 60 years of age. These lymphomas usually appear clinically as localized tumors, and about one third arise in extranodal sites, such as bone, central nervous system, deep and subcutaneous soft tissues, nasopharynx, Waldeyer's throat ring, mediastinum, lung, thyroid, or testis. The marrow and central nervous system are involved initially in 10% of cases. In extranodal sites, their distinction from undifferentiated malignant neoplasms may be difficult by histology alone. Staging of these lymphomas usually requires only radiography and marrow biopsies, since tumor masses formed by these lymphomas are usually clinically and radiographically apparent. The disease characteristically progresses rapidly to involve other extranodal and nodal sites. Median survival is usually 1 to 2 years, but survival may exceed 5 years. Complete remissions with chemotherapy may occur in as many as 60% to 80% of patients, and long-term, disease-free survivals may be achieved in 30% to 60% of these patients.[224,675] Patients with large bulk disease, multicentric extranodal disease, and central nervous system involvement quite often do poorly.

The clinicopathologic features of the diffuse lymphomas of mixed small and large cell type (DM), which comprise 5% to 10% of NHL, as a group closely resemble those of the DL lymphomas. They are distinguished histologically from DL in that the frequency of large cells in the infiltrate is between 25% and 50% rather than 50% or more (Fig. 28-82). DM lymphomas, like the DL lymphomas, are also heterogeneous histologically. Diffuse lymphomas with cytologic structures and phenotypes similar to those of follicular lymphomas may be identified and comprise about 25% to 30% of this group. The survival characteristics of the DM lymphomas are generally better than for DL lymphomas. However, certain lymphomas within this group resemble histologically high-grade lymphomas in their clinical progression.[432,510]

Collectively, the DL and DM lymphomas have the greatest biologic heterogeneity of all NHL. Phenotypically, they are similar to differentiated, antigen-competent B- or T-lymphocytes of peripheral lymphoid tissues: about 65% of cases express B-cell phenotypes and

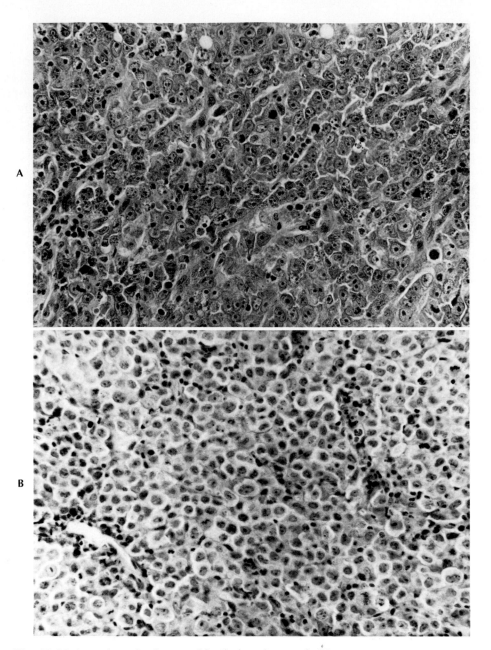

Fig. 28-81. Lymph node. Immunoblastic lymphoma. **A,** Plasmacytoid subtype. **B,** Clear cell subtype.

35% T-cell. The t(14;18) translocation, which is characteristic of follicular lymphomas, is also represented in this group of NHL.[220,828] T cell–associated antigens are expressed in about 70% of the DM and IB lymphomas. These diffuse, T cell–derived NHL are referred to as "peripheral T-cell lymphomas."[766] These lymphomas tend to have a polymorphous cellular infiltrate and to be associated with inflammatory infiltrates including histiocytes, epithelioid cell clusters or granulomas, eosinophils, and plasma cells, a tendency not exclusive of some B cell–derived lymphomas. Rare cells that are identical to Reed-Sternberg cells may also be present creating confusion with some forms of Hodgkin's disease. Many of these lymphomas occur as clinicopathologic entities of adult T-cell leukemia-lymphoma,[743,772] mycosis fungoides,[582] lymphoepithelioid cell (Lennert's) lymphoma,[80,216,543] and aggressive forms of lymphomatoid granulomatosis,[134,374,683] lethal midline granuloma,[257,439] polymorphic reticulosis,[28] and angioimmunoblastic lymphadenopathy.[773] Although there are no

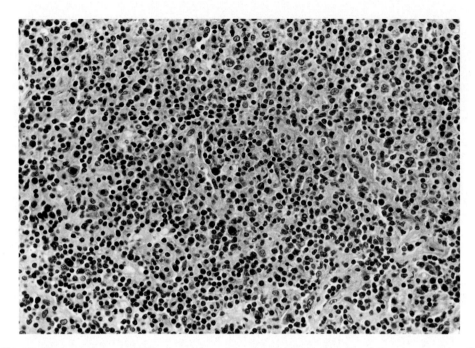

Fig. 28-82. Lymph node. Diffuse small and large cell lymphoma. The large lymphoid cells are intermixed with abnormal small cells. Mitotic figures are frequently identified in this lymphoma.

specific cytogenetic abnormalities within this group, certain abnormalities are prevalent within specific histologic types.[422]

Lymphomas of small noncleaved cells (SNC). The small noncleaved-cell lymphomas actually include three clinicopathologic entities: Burkitt's tumor (endemic or African Burkitt's lymphoma), Burkitt's type of lymphoma (sporadic Burkitt's) and non-Burkitt's lymphoma. The SNC lymphomas are grouped together because their histologic appearance is remarkably similar. Burkitt's tumor and Burkitt's type of lymphoma are identical histologically and are both referred to commonly as Burkitt's lymphoma. Burkitt's tumor is well-defined clinicopathologically, and its epidemiology has been extensively studied. It is endemic to Central Africa and New Guinea where it represents a significant proportion of non-Hodgkin's lymphoma. It has a predilection for involvement of the jaws and other extranodal sites of young children, whose mean age is 8 years. These children characteristically have an early exposure to Epstein-Barr virus (EBV) in the setting of chronic hyperendemic malaria, which is believed to contribute to an early susceptibility to the virus and the subsequent development of this lymphoma. EBV nuclear antigens, viral antigens expressed by infected cells, are identified in greater than 95% of the endemic tumors, whereas they are found in less than 15% of sporadic

Burkitt's type of lymphomas, implicating a tumorigenic role for EBV in Burkitt's tumor.

The small noncleaved cell is intermediate in size between the malignant small lymphocyte and malignant large cell and contains nuclei that may be more or less monotonously uniform with partially dispersed nuclear chromatin (Fig. 28-83). The nuclei contain one to five distinct nucleoli, which are usually located along the margin of the nuclear membrane. The cytoplasm is amphophilic and moderate in amount and in section abuts sharply against that of adjacent cells in a "squared-off" manner. Benign histiocytes with phagocytized cellular debris are characteristically isolated in the lymphoma infiltrate appearing as the stars in a starry sky. Other rapidly proliferating lymphomas, such as DLC, IB, and LB lymphomas, can also produce this effect. The malignant cells usually proliferate as a diffuse infiltrate, though germinal centers may be infiltrated or infrequently formed. The mitotic index of SNC lymphomas is the highest of NHL and of all human malignancies.[669] Histologically, non-Burkitt's lymphoma (NB) differs from Burkitt's lymphoma in that in NB there is a relatively greater cytologic polymorphism and fewer nucleoli.[377,545] Distinguishing between these two morphologic variants is highly subjective in practice and is poorly reproducible, even by experienced pathologists.[806]

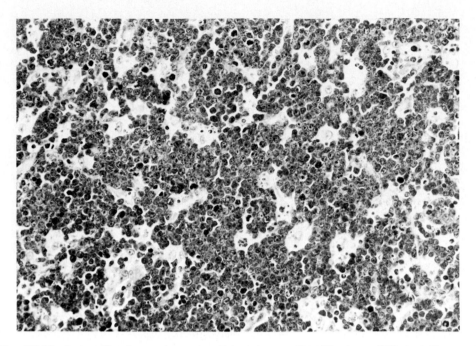

Fig. 28-83. Ileum. Small noncleaved cell lymphoma, Burkitt's type. Diffuse infiltrate of small noncleaved cells with benign, phagocytic histiocytes (larger cells with clear cytoplasm) interspersed.

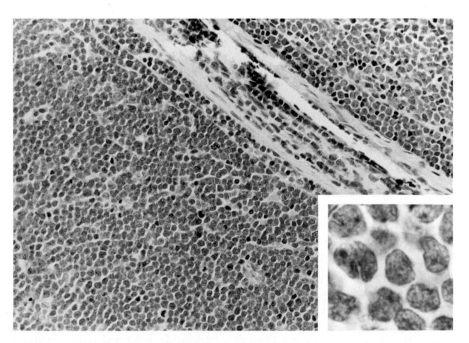

Fig. 28-84. Lymph node. Lymphoblastic lymphoma, convoluted type. Diffuse infiltrate of malignant lymphoblasts. Notice the lack of prominent nucleoli in nuclei and the high frequency of mitotic figures. *Inset,* An enlargement.

The incidence of Burkitt's type and non-Burkitt's lymphomas together is much lower than Burkitt's tumor in endemic areas, about 5% of NHL. As a group, however, SNC lymphomas represent about one third of childhood NHL.[281,377,390,805] Patients with Burkitt's type lymphomas are generally younger than those with non-Burkitt's lymphomas.[590] Lymphomas of Burkitt's type have a predilection for involving the ileocecal region of the gastrointestinal tract in children, whereas those of non-Burkitt's type have clinical characteristics that resemble those of the DLC lymphomas. Although the marrow is infrequently involved, almost 60% of patients have stage IV disease caused by involvement of the gastrointestinal tract or other extranodal sites. In most reported series, the response to treatment and survival rates of the SNC lymphomas are similar, though patients with Burkitt's type of lymphoma have been reported to fail in their response to chemotherapy more frequently.[806] The median survival of patients with SNC lymphomas is the poorest observed in NHL, but many patients do respond to therapy and may have remissions lasting many years.

Lymphomas of lymphoblasts (LB). Lymphoblastic lymphomas represent about 30% of the NHL of childhood[281,390,435,805] and about 5% of NHL in adults.[590] The malignant lymphoblast is a cell of intermediate size and is cytologically identical to lymphoblasts of acute lymphoblastic leukemia (ALL) (Fig. 28-84). The malignant lymphoblast has a nucleus with finely dispersed chromatin and inconspicuous nucleoli and has little discernible cytoplasm. In the majority of cases, the nuclear contour is conspicuously convoluted, whereas in others, nuclear convolutions are lacking. This observation is the basis for the morphologic subclassification into convoluted and nonconvoluted subtypes, which appear to be clinically indistinguishable. Mitoses are very frequent in these infiltrates, which always produce a diffuse growth pattern. The phenotype of about 85% of these lymphomas parallels those of developing thymocytes, and the remainder have precursor pre-B-cell and pre-B-cell phenotypes. LB lymphomas express phenotypes and genotypes that are seen in ALL, but the frequencies are inverted[44]; that is, the majority of LB phenotypes correspond to developmentally more mature cells than those in ALL. Cytogenetic findings are also similar to those in ALL.

The majority of the patients with LB lymphoma are adolescent males between 10 and 16 years of age who present with a large, anterior mediastinal mass. Mediastinal involvement may be so massive as to compromise respiratory function or induce the superior vena cava syndrome requiring immediate therapeutic intervention. However, LB lymphomas occur in other anatomic sites and in patients of all age groups.[508] These lymphomas often rapidly involve the marrow and typi-cally evolve to ALL usually within 6 months of presentation, when not controlled by therapy. Central nervous system involvement is frequent as is involvement of the skin, which may be the first sign of disease in some patients.[45,435] LB lymphomas respond better to therapy designed for ALL than to therapy that is effective for other high-grade lymphomas. Therefore it is imperative to distinguish between lymphoblastic and nonlymphoblastic lymphomas. This distinction is accomplished reliably by experienced observers[281,806] and can be supported by demonstrating a specific immunophenotype.[70,149,282,657] Nevertheless, the median survival and freedom from relapse is poor for this group of patients.

Lymphomas and lymphocytosis. Lymphoma cells may circulate in the peripheral blood and involve the marrow and other organs to some extent in every type of NHL.[486] Generally, lymphomas of low-grade (SL, SCC) are associated with lymphocytosis and marrow involvement more often than those of higher grades (DMC, DLC, IB, SNC, LB) except for LB lymphomas. In low-grade lymphomas, lymphocytosis indicates disseminated disease but does not have dire prognostic implications, whereas in lymphomas of high grade, it is indicative of widespread, clinically aggressive disease. In cases in which a B cell–derived lymphoma is suspected, clonality of the circulating cells can be inferred by demonstration of the predominant expression of a single light Ig chain by the circulating cells.[16] Lymphocytosis is also frequently associated with LB and SL lymphomas when the disease is widespread, and the clinical distinction of these lymphomas from ALL and CLL respectively is an arbitrary one. Two neoplastic T-cell lymphoproliferative disorders of adults have characteristic lymphocytosis: mycosis fungoides/Sézary's syndrome, a cutaneous T-cell lymphoma that may involve lymph nodes and other organs late in the clinical course, and adult T-cell leukemia-lymphoma, a clinicopathologic entity that is associated with HTLV-I infection and is endemic but not restricted to Japan and the Caribbean basin. The nuclei of the circulating cells are characteristically "cerebriform" in mycosis fungoides and "hyperconvoluted" in adult T-cell leukemia-lymphoma. The tissue structures of these infiltrates are variable but most frequently classify as DMC non-Hodgkin's lymphoma.

Monoclonal gammopathies in lymphoproliferative disorders. Monoclonal gammopathies occur in 3% to 9% of patients with diffuse NHL and 1% or less in patients with follicular lymphomas.[492] A monoclonal gammopathy is the appearance of a homogeneous Ig protein pattern in serum electrophoresis that presumably results from the secretion of monoclonal antibody by the clonal proliferation of B-lymphocytes. Usually these lymphomas consist of small lymphocytes, lymphoplasmacytoid lymphocytes, plasma cells, or less frequently small cleaved cells and would classify histologically as an NHL of low or intermediate grade. Similar lymphoplasmacytic infiltrates are found in Waldenström's macroglobulinemia, which characteristically is associated with high serum concentration of IgM. Rarely do lymphomas of large cell type secrete Ig in quantities detectable by usual laboratory methods. The amount of monoclonal Ig produced is often greater than 2 g/dl in a range of 0.6 to 4.6 g/dl and is proportional to the size of the neoplastic population of cells, the degree of plasma cell differentiation, and the effects of regulatory or therapeutic influences. Normal serum Ig levels are often reduced with monoclonal gammopathies. Occasionally, these antibodies have autoimmune specificity or unusual physical characteristics, such as cryoprecipitability, that produce paraneoplastic phenomena. Monoclonal gammopathies may also be detected in Hodgkin's disease and other malignancies and in a variety of nonneoplastic disorders.[463] The gammopathies in these disorders are considered to be reactive in nature, but their significance is unknown. Rarely a concomitant plasma cell neoplasm, non-Hodgkin's lymphoma, or chronic lymphocytic leukemia is discovered.

Heavy-chain diseases. Heavy-chain diseases (HCD) are uncommon lymphoplasmacytic malignancies characterized by the proliferation of neoplastic cells that synthesize and secrete truncated, defective Ig heavy chains that are not linked to light chains. Three types of HCD, which correspond to three of the five possible IgH isotypes, have been described: gamma HCD, alpha HCD, and mu HCD.[228,235,652] Molecular studies have been done in selective cases of gamma and mu HCD.[4,22,290] Extensive internal DNA deletions involve the variable and CH1 domains in gamma HCD, whereas in mu HCD, the defective heavy chain results from a transcriptional error of an effectively rearranged Ig gene that produces mRNA that lacks the variable, diversity, and joining segments. The secreted heavy chains in these disorders consist of intact Fc fragments and deletions of entire domains of the hinge region of the Fd fragments. It is unclear why light chains are not produced in gamma and alpha HCD. Kappa chains are produced in excess in mu HCD. The diagnosis of HCD depends on the recognition of the defective proteins and requires sophisticated immunoelectrophoresis and a competent immunochemist.

The clinical manifestations of gamma HCD usually include cervical or axillary lymphadenopathy, fever, and anemia and often hepatosplenomegaly or splenomegaly. Thrombocytopenia, leukopenia with atypical lymphocytosis, and plasmacytosis may also be present. Gamma HCD, or Franklin's disease, has been recognized in the United States, Canada, Europe, and Japan and affects mostly elderly patients though cases in young adults and children are reported. Survival in this disorder is variable, but it may be fatal within 1 year of diagnosis. The histology of gamma HCD is quite often nondiagnostic and resembles an inflammatory reactive hyperplasia. The neoplastic infiltrate consists of a mixture of small lymphocytes and lymphoplasmacytoid cells accompanied by histiocytes and eosinophils.

Mediterranean type of lymphoma (MTL) and alpha HCD are related lymphoproliferative diseases that are prevalent in Mediterranean and Middle Eastern countries.[381,424,504,584,626] Alpha HCD has been identified in an increasing number of patients with MTL. Both disorders have been included in the category of immunoproliferative small intestinal disease (IPSID) by the World Health Organization. These disorders are not restricted to the Mediterranean region and have been described in other parts of the world including Asia and South America. MTL and alpha HCD usually affect young patients who present with abdominal pain and intestinal malabsorption and are found to have disease in the proximal small bowel. IPSID is characterized by one of two forms histologically: a massive, diffuse infiltration of the lamina propria by plasma cells and lymphoplasmacytoid cells; or a diffuse, large cell infiltrate that is characteristic of immunoblastic lymphoma. In the plasma cell form, pleomorphic immunoblasts are frequently identified in the diffuse plasma cell infiltrate, and it is common to find distinct histologic transitions from the plasma cell form to the immunoblastic form in the same specimen. The chromosome abnormality, 14q+, is frequently identified as a clonal marker in these cases. Direct immunoblastic transformation from the low-grade plasma cell form has been demonstrated by immunologic studies and is well documented clinically. Survival is generally poor in MTL with an average survival of less than 3 years. Perforation of the bowel wall at sites of massive infiltration by lymphoma may occur after radiation or chemotherapy and can be avoided by prior surgical resection of massively infiltrated areas.

Mu HCD is the rarest form of this disorder, and clinically most patients appear to have chronic lymphocytic leukemia. However, patients with mu HCD differ in that they lack significant lymphadenopathy when hepatosplenomegaly is evident, abnormal vacuolated plasma cells are present in the marrow, and abundant free kappa light chains are excreted into the urine. Most patients are older than 40 years, and their prognosis is similar to that of patients with CLL.

Staging. The staging system that is most widely applied to NHL is the Ann Arbor system, which was developed for Hodgkin's disease (see p. 1450). Depending on the histologic type, the stage at diagnosis may have different implications for therapeutic strategy and prognosis, unlike in Hodgkin's disease. Pathologic staging

Table 28-15. Murphy staging system for childhood non-Hodgkin's lymphoma

Stage	Characteristics
I	A single (extranodal) tumor or single (nodal) area outside the mediastinum or abdomen
II	A single (extranodal) tumor with regional node involvement; two or more nodal areas on the same side of the diaphragm; two single (extranodal) tumors with or without involvement of associated mesenteric nodes only
III	Two single (extranodal) tumors on opposite sides of the diaphragm; two or more nodal areas above and below the diaphragm; all primary intrathoracic tumors
IV	Any of the above with initial central nervous system and bone marrow involvement

rarely includes laparotomy in NHL. Usually, only bone marrow biopsies are done to augment radiographic studies. As a staging system for lymphomas of low grade, the Ann Arbor system has been found to be deficient because involvement of stage IV sites, such as the marrow and liver, occur frequently, and usually it does not indicate a poor prognosis. Other staging systems, such as the Murphy system (Table 28-15), have been designed for assessing the stage of childhood NHL.[494] These systems account for many of the special modes of presentation and sites of involvement by NHL that affect children, that is, small bowel, mediastinum, and extranodal soft-tissue sites, and are now used in most children's cancer centers.

Malignant lymphomas in immunodeficiency states. The relationship of immunodeficiency states, whether primary (genetic) or secondary (acquired, iatrogenic), and cancer is unquestionable. The increased risk of developing a malignant neoplasm has been documented in cancer registries over the last 20 years. For patients with primary disorders, the risk is 4% or about 10,000 times greater than for normal persons.[379] A slightly higher risk is observed in organ-transplant recipients. A large variety of neoplasms has been described that include lymphomas, leukemias, and various carcinomas and sarcomas of the brain, liver, gonads, and soft tissues. Multiple neoplasms have been observed to occur in a small percentage of patients. The two most prevalent neoplasms observed by far are malignant lymphomas and nonmelanotic skin carcinomas. Within this decade, the acquired immunodeficiency syndrome and the expanded use of organ transplantation in medical care have confirmed the relationship of neoplasia and immunodeficiency and have increased the experience of

the general medical community with this often fatal complication.

Acquired immunodeficiency syndrome (AIDS). AIDS refers to the condition in which multiple, life-threatening, opportunistic infections, or Kaposi's sarcoma, or both, occur in patients without a history of primary or iatrogenic immunodeficiency. The syndrome results from infection by a retrovirus, the human immunodeficiency virus I (HIV-1), previously referred to as human T-cell lymphotropic virus type III (HTLV-III), lymphadenopathy-associated virus (LAV), or AIDS-related virus (ARV). HIV is related to the group of nontransforming, cytopathic lentiretroviruses, which include the visna virus and cause chronic neurodegenerative disorders in goats and sheep.[761] AIDS was first recognized in the Western world in 1981, or perhaps as early as 1978, and HIV was discovered in 1981. More recently, HIV-2, which has 60% homology with HIV-1, has been described as a cause of AIDS-like disease. HIV appears to exhibit unusual biologic variability.

Before February 1988, over 50,000 cases were diagnosed in the United States, and it has been estimated that the number of cases doubled every year since its recognition.[156,336] Almost 28,000 persons have died of the disease, 80% of whom died before 1985. The Centers for Disease Control (CDC) estimates that between 945,000 and 1,400,000 persons are infected by HIV as of 1988, and the Public Health Service has predicted that about 270,000 cases of AIDS will have development by 1991. Four population groups have been identified as being at high risk for developing AIDS in the United States and include homosexual or bisexual men (73%), intravenous drug users (17%), Haitians now living in the United States (4%), and hemophiliacs (1%). Recent observations in New York City, where seropositivity among drug addicts approaches 60%, indicate that AIDS is increasing faster among intravenous drug users and their offspring than among any other risk group. The CDC further estimates the average prevalence of seropositivity to be 20% to 25% for homosexuals, 25% to 60% for drug addicts, 63% for hemophiliacs before 1985, and 0.021% for heterosexuals without identified risks.[60] Two percent of AIDS cases have been associated with blood transfusions, most of which were received before 1985 and donor testing. The prevalence of HIV in blood donors has declined from 0.035% before 1985 to 0.015% in 1987. Heterosexual transmission is estimated to account for another 4% of cases, and 56% of these cases, in which 78% of the victims were women, were attributed to sexual contact with documented HIV-infected persons from one of the groups above. The remaining cases were among persons born in Haiti or central Africa where heterosexual contacts have been shown to be the major source of HIV infection.

The epidemiology of HIV infection resembles that of the hepatitis B virus, and the most prevalent routes of spread include communal intravenous drug use, intimate sexual contact with numerous partners especially receptive anal intercourse, congenital transmission, and blood-products transfusion. The risk of HIV transmission through casual, nonsexual contact, even if prolonged, or through insect vectors is essentially nonexistent.[238]

The virus infects at least two cells after entering the body, the CD4+ T-lymphocytes and mononuclear phagocytes, which also express the CD4 antigen and include the microglia of the central nervous system.[315] After binding to the CD4 molecule and entering the cell, the virus may have a cytotoxic effect either directly or indirectly upon activation of the cell by concomitant infection or allogeneic cells. This depletion of CD4+ T-cells, which are pivotal in many immune reactions, is paramount in causing the immunodeficient state.[211] The virus tends to accumulate within monocytes and remain insulated from antiviral immune responses. Monocytes appear to be important reservoirs for HIV within the body and may have a role as a vehicle in its transmission, since only a fraction of T-cells and as many as 15% of monocytes express viral protein, indicating infection. The demonstration of antibodies to HIV by ELISA assay is the basis of routine HIV screening. Antibodies are not usually demonstrable for 4 to 8 weeks in newly infected, infectious individuals. More than 90% of persons with AIDS and greater than 95% of asymptomatic carriers of HIV are antibody positive. Although almost 1.5 million persons are presently believed to be infected by HIV in the United States, the risk of developing AIDS once infected is estimated at 30% to 35%. The mean incubation period appears to be long and is estimated at 7.8 years for homosexual men and 8.2 years for transfusion-associated AIDS.[446] It is also estimated that 99% of infected homosexual men will eventually develop the syndrome. Once AIDS develops, the cumulative probability of survival for all groups appears to be about 49% at 1 year and 15% at 5 years.[607]

The clinical manifestations of HIV infection are protean and have been organized into a classification scheme by the CDC, which provides the basis for the definition of AIDS (Table 28-16).[131] Unexplained, generalized lymphadenopathy occurs in up to 30% of homosexual men who acquire AIDS. As many as 20% of those who sustain lymphadenopathy for 1 year will develop the syndrome. Therefore lymphadenopathy in HIV infection is regarded as a prodrome to AIDS, and it is referred to as the AIDS-related complex (ARC). However, the histopathologic findings, though sometimes described as progressive, are variable and nonspecific for HIV infection and do not appear to be predictive of the development of AIDS or lymphoma. The

Table 28-16. Abridged classification for human immunodeficiency virus (HIV) infection

Group	Characteristics
I	Acute infection
II	Asymptomatic infection
III	Persistent generalized lymphadenopathy
IV	Other disease
A	Constitutional disease
B	Neurologic disease
C	Secondary infectious disease
D	Secondary neoplasia
E	Other conditions

most frequent lymph-node histologic pattern identified in ARC is that of reactive follicular hyperplasia, which is sometimes florid.* Frequently the histologic appearance resembles that of acute, acquired toxoplasmosis in that hyperplasia is mixed with sinus monocytoid cell hyperplasia and epithelioid cell cluster formation with cuff effacement. Dermatopathic reaction in the deep paracortex is present frequently. Cellular lysis and hemorrhage within germinal centers also occurs. This finding appears to be nonspecific, even though HIV antigens and viruslike particles have been demonstrated in germinal centers,[47,724] an indication that the lymphoid follicles may be an important site of virus trapping and replication.[413] Florid follicular hyperplasia with a small number of neutrophils associated with paracortical sinus monocytoid cell hyperplasia is reported recently to be highly suggestive of HIV infection in patients with chronic lymphadenopathy at two or more noncontiguous, noninguinal sites.[91]

Alterations in the number and distribution of T-lymphocyte subpopulations have been described in lymph nodes of AIDS patients.[487,817,818] In some patients who have been followed with serial biopsies, hyperplastic follicles often involute with an increase in interfollicular tissue attributable to plasma cell hyperplasia, whereas others progress to lymphoid depletion either after follicle involution or directly. Some patients with ARC develop manifestations of autoimmunity described as immune thrombocytopenia, Sjögren's syndrome, various endocrinopathies, and allergic drug reactions.[182,744]

Malignant neoplasms occur in about 30% of AIDS patients of which Kaposi's sarcoma (20% to 30% incidence) and malignant lymphomas (4% incidence, which appears to be increasing) are the most prevalent. Approximately 30% of AIDS patients present with Kaposi's sarcoma (KS), a form of angiosarcoma, in association

---

*References 86, 288, 340, 532, 680, 687, 741.

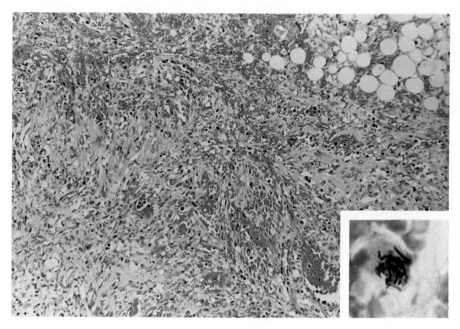

Fig. 28-85. Lymph node. Kaposi's sarcoma complicated by *Mycobacterium avium* and *M. intracellulare* infection (*inset,* intracellular mycobacteria). Notice the bland, spindle-shaped sarcoma cells and extravasated erythrocytes.

with one or more opportunistic infections. Unlike the classical form of Kaposi's sarcoma, which usually presents in cutaneous sites and follows an indolent course, that which occurs in AIDS is a multicentric, cutaneous, and visceral malignancy that frequently involves lymph nodes, gastrointestinal tract, and other organs. Histologically, Kaposi's sarcoma consists of a proliferation of spindle-shaped tumor cells with cleftlike spaces containing erythrocytes that extravasate with eventual hemosiderin pigment formation (Fig. 28-85). The endothelial nature of KS has been shown ultrastructurally and by immunohistochemistry.[612,648] In AIDS patients, KS may be identified in the same lymph node with an opportunistic infection or lymphoma (Fig. 28-85). Patients who present with KS generally have a less severe immune deficit than those who present with infection do. KS occurs far more frequently in homosexual than in nonhomosexual male patients with AIDS.[444] Homosexual patients with KS are infected with multiple strains of cytomegalovirus (CMV) and have been identified in tumor cells, suggestive of an etiologic relationship.[261,819]

Lymphomas that occur in AIDS patients are virtually all clinically aggressive neoplasms that affect a variety of different organs including sites, such as the brain, that are rarely involved by sporadic lymphoma. Hodgkin's disease, which represents about 10% to 15% of cases in most series, appears to have an altered natural history in AIDS in that many patients present in stage

IIIB or IVB and with unusual disease distributions, such as marrow involvement without splenic involvement.[445,573,640,746] Also, the histology of Hodgkin's disease in AIDS patients often appears atypical because of the depletion of lymphocytes, and the disease is generally more aggressive than in other patients. The incidence of non-Hodgkin's lymphoma reported in AIDS patients is much higher than in normal populations and resembles that seen in iatrogenically immunosuppressed organ transplant recipients.[299] The histologic appearance of most of the lymphomas described in AIDS patients has been either SNC, IB, or DLC.[177,339,833] Of the cases that have been studied and express cell antigens, most neoplasms appear to be clonal proliferations of B-lymphocytes, and the 14q+ chromosomal abnormalities have been identified in some cases, though rare cases of peripheral T-cell lymphomas have been documented.[114,194,503,794] Several lethal cases of polyclonal, B-cell lymphoproliferative disorders have also been reported.[256] In some cases, cell-marker studies in sequential biopsies have demonstrated progression of multiclonality to a clonal cell population, not unlike what has been observed in organ-transplant recipients.[285,438] Contributary roles for the Epstein-Barr virus and the proto-oncogene c-*myc* in these lymphoproliferative disorders have been proposed as they have been for endemic Burkitt's lymphoma, the X-linked lymphoproliferative syndrome, and organ-transplant recipients (discussed be-

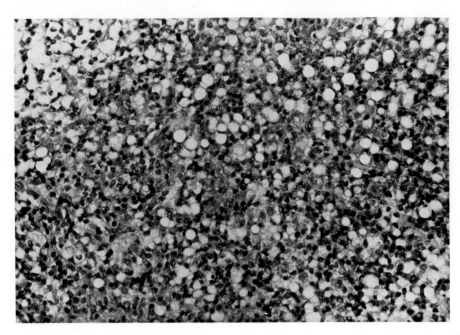

Fig. 28-86. Lymph node. Diffuse, small cleaved cell lymphoma, signet-ring variant. The round cytoplasmic vacuoles greatly distort the nuclei to crescent-shaped structures. Notice the relatively unperturbed neoplastic small lymphocytes to the right.

fore).[245,254,553,575,653,794] HTLV-I and other retroviruses may likewise participate in the development of some of these lymphomas.

Metastatic neoplasms

Enlarged lymph nodes are frequently the first sign of the presence of a malignant neoplasm. Usually metastases involve the regional lymph nodes before distant sites are involved. Generalized lymphadenopathy from metastases is infrequently encountered and always indicates the presentation of a highly malignant neoplasm or the late phase in a patient's clinical course with cancer. Extranodal organs are also involved in these circumstances. Carcinomas and malignant melanomas metastasize to lymph nodes more frequently than sarcomas do. In adults, lung, breast, and undifferentiated carcinomas from various other organs, cutaneous and extracutaneous malignant melanoma, and gonadal neoplasms are most frequently encountered, whereas in children, neuroblastoma and rhabdomyosarcoma predominate.

Metastatic neoplasms to lymph nodes usually demonstrate cellular or architectural features that permit their distinction from malignant lymphomas. Because some metastatic neoplasms are undifferentiated and frequently simulate the architectural patterns of lymphomas, the distinction in individual cases may be difficult. Metastatic undifferentiated carcinoma may show a sinusoid pattern that simulates lymphoma or malignant histiocytosis, and, alternatively, diffuse large cell NHL

may occur in a sinusoid pattern that mimics metastatic carcinoma.[535] Nonkeratinizing nasopharyngeal carcinoma metastatic to cervical lymph nodes is frequently confused with diffuse, large cell NHL. Metastatic seminoma to mediastinal lymph nodes are occasionally confused with Hodgkin's disease. A cytologic variant form of NHL, signet-ring lymphoma, may simulate metastatic poorly differentiated adenocarcinoma of signet-ring type from the gastrointestinal tract, pancreas, breast, prostate, and urinary bladder or malignant melanoma[283,383,589,656,753,791] (Fig. 28-86). Although signet-ring lymphoma was initially believed to be a variant of follicular lymphoma in which Ig could be demonstrated within the vacuoles, this variant has now been observed in various histologic types of NHL with both mature B- and T-cell phenotypes. Immunohistochemistry or ultrastructural studies can often resolve the differential diagnosis of lymphoma versus metastatic or another primary neoplasm when the possibility is considered.

REFERENCES

1. Adams, J.M., Harris, A.W., Pinkert, C.A., Corcoran, L.M., Alexander, W.S., Cory, S., Palmiter, R.D., and Brinster, R.L.: The c-*myc* oncogene driven by immunoglobulin enhancers induces lymphoid malignancy in transgenic mice, Nature **318**:533, 1985.
2. Adamson, J., and Hillman, R.S.: Blood volume and plasma protein replacement following acute blood loss in normal man, JAMA **205**:609, 1968.
3. Aisenberg, A.C., Wilkes, B.M., and Jacobson, T.O.: The bcl-2

gene is rearranged in many different B-cell lymphomas, Blood **71**:969, 1988.

4. Alexander, A., Steinmetz, M., Barritault, D., Frangione, B., Franklin, E.C., Hood, L., and Buxbaum, J.N.: γ Heavy chain disease in man: cDNA sequence supports partial gene deletion model, Proc. Natl. Acad. Sci. USA **79**:3260, 1982.

5. Alter, B.P., Potter, N.U., and Li, F.P.: Classification and aetiology of the aplastic anemias, Clin. Haematol. **7**:431, 1978.

6. Amenomori, T., Tomonaga, M., Jinnai, I., Soda, H., Nonaka, H., Matsuo, T., Yoshida, Y., Kuriyama, K., Ichimaru, M., and Suematsu, T.: Cytogenetic and cytochemical studies on progenitor cells of primary acquired sideroblastic anemia (PASA): involvement of multipotent myeloid stem cells in PASA clone and mosaicism with normal clone, Blood **70**:1367, 1987.

7. Anasetti, C., Doney, K.C., Storb, R., Meyers, J.D., Farewell, V.T., Buckner, C.D., Appelbaum, F.R., Sullivan, K.M., Clift, R.A., Deeg, H.J., et al.: Bone marrow transplantation for severe aplastic anemia: long-term outcome in fifty "untransfused" patients, Ann. Intern. Med. **104**:461, 1986.

8. Anner, R.M., and Drewinko, B.: Frequency and significance of bone marrow involvement by metastatic solid tumors, Cancer **39**:1337, 1977.

9. Archimbaud, E., Coiffier, B., Bryon, P.A., Vasselon, C., Brizard, C.P., and Viala, J.J.: Prognostic factors in angioimmunoblastic lymphadenopathy, Cancer **59**:208, 1987.

10. Arlin, Z.A., Friedland, M.L., and Mittelman, A.: Cytogenetic abnormalities in chronic lymphocytic leukemia, N. Engl. J. Med. **311**:123, 1984.

11. Armitage, J.O., Dick, F.R., and Corder, M.P.: Diffuse histiocytic lymphoma complicating chronic lymphocytic leukemia, Cancer **41**:422, 1978.

12. Arnalich, F., Lahoz, C., Larrocha, C., Zamorano, A.F., Jiménez, C., Gasalla, R., García-Puig, J., and Vázquez, J.J.: Incidence and clinical significance of peripheral and bone marrow basophilia, J. Med. **18**:293, 1987.

13. Arnold, A., Cossman, J., Bakhsi, A., Jaffe, E.S., Waldmann, T.A., and Korsmeyer, S.J.: Immunoglobulin-gene rearrangements as unique clonal markers in human lymphoid neoplasms, N. Engl. J. Med. **309**:1593, 1983.

14. Asch, M.J., Cohen, A.H., and Moore, T.C.: Hepatic and splenic lymphangiomatosis with skeletal involvement: report of a case and review of the literature, Surgery **76**:334, 1974.

15. Ash, R.C., Detrick, R.A., and Zanjani, E.D.: In vitro studies of human pluripotential hematopoietic progenitors in polycythemia vera: direct evidence of stem cell involvement, J. Clin. Invest. **69**:1112, 1982.

16. Ault, K.A.: Detection of small numbers of monoclonal B lymphocytes in the blood of patients with lymphoma, N. Engl. J. Med. **300**:1401, 1979.

17. Azzopardi, J.G., Ross, C.M.D., and Frizzera, G.: Blue naevi of lymph node capsule, Histopathology **1**:451, 1977.

18. Baer, M.R., Krantz, S.B., Cousar, J.B., Glick, A.D., and Collins, R.D.: Malignant histiocytoses developing in patients with B-cell lymphomas: report of two cases, Cancer **57**:2175, 1986.

19. Baer, M.R., Gleaton, J.H., Salhany, K.E., and Glick, A.D.: Malignant histiocytosis occurring with acute myelogenous leukemia in a patient with longstanding polycythemia vera, Cancer **59**:489, 1987.

20. Bagby, G.C.: Production of multilineage growth factors by hematopoietic stromal cells: an intercellular regulatory network involving mononuclear phagocytes and interleukin-1, Blood Cells **13**:147, 1987.

21. Baesl, T.J., and Filler, R.M.: Surgical diseases of the spleen, Surg. Clin. North Am. **65**:1269, 1985.

22. Bakhshi, A., Siebenlist, V., Guglielmi, P., Arnold, A., Ravetch, J., Leder, P., Waldmann, T.A., and Korsmeyer, S.J.: Molecular analysis of human mu heavy chain disease, Clin. Res. **32**:342A, 1984.

23. Balcerzak, S.P., and Bromberg, P.A.: Secondary polycythemia, Semin. Hematol. **12**:353, 1975.

24. Banks, P.M., Witrak, G.A., and Conn, D.L.: Lymphoid neoplasia following connective tissue disease, Mayo Clin. Proc. **54**:104, 1979.

25. Barletta, C., Pelicci, P.G., Kenyon, L.C., Smith, S.D., and Dalla-Favera, R.: Relationship between the c-myb locus and the 6q-chromosomal aberration in leukemias and lymphomas, Science **235**:1064, 1987.

26. Barlogie, B., and Alexian, R.L.: Biology and therapy of multiple myeloma, Acta Haematol. **78**:171, 1987.

27. Barth, R.F., Vergara, G.G., Khurana, S.K., et al.: Rapidly fatal familial histiocytosis associated with eosinophilia and primary immunological deficiency, Lancet **2**:503, 1972.

28. Bartoli, E., Massarelli, G., Soggia, G., and Tanda, F.: Multicentric giant lymph node hyperplasia: a hyperimmune syndrome with a rapidly progressive course, Am. J. Clin. Pathol. **73**:423, 1980.

29. Barton, J.C., and Conrad, M.E.: Current status of blastic transformation in chronic myelogenous leukemia, Am. J. Hematol. **4**:281, 1978.

30. Bartram, C.R., and Carbonell, F.: Bcr rearrangement in Ph-negative CML, Cancer Genet. Cytogenet. **21**:183, 1986.

31. Basset, F., Corrin, B., Spencer, H., Lacronique, J., Roth, C., Soler, P., Battesti, J.P., Georges, R., and Chrétien, J.: Pulmonary histiocytosis X, Am. Rev. Respir. Dis. **118**:811, 1978.

32. Bauermeister, D.E.: Quantitation of bone marrow reticulin: a normal range, Am. J. Clin. Pathol. **56**:24, 1971.

33. Bearman, R.M., Pangalis, G.A., and Rappaport, H.: Hodgkin's disease, lymphocyte depletion type: a clinicopathologic study of 39 patients, Cancer **41**:293, 1978.

34. Bearman, R.M., Pangalis, G.A., and Rappaport, H.: Prolymphocytic leukemia: clinical, histopathological, and cytochemical observations, Cancer **42**:2360, 1978.

35. Beckstead, J.H.: The bone marrow biopsy: a diagnostic strategy, Arch. Pathol. Lab. Med. **110**:175, 1986.

36. Bennett, J.M., Catovsky, D., Daniel, M.T., Flandrin, G., Galton, D.A., Gralnick, H.R., and Sultan, C.: Criteria for the diagnosis of acute leukemia of megakaryocytic lineage (M7), Ann. Intern. Med. **103**:460, 1985.

37. Bennett, J.M., Catovsky, D., Daniel, M.T., et al.: Proposals for the classification of the acute leukaemias, Br. J. Haematol. **33**:451, 1976.

38. Bennett, J.M., Catovsky, D., Daniel, M.T., Flandrin, G., Galton, D.A., Gralnick, H.R., and Sultan, C.: The Franco-American-British (FAB) Cooperative Group: proposals for the classification of the myelodysplastic syndromes, Br. J. Haematol. **51**:189, 1982.

39. Bennett, J.M., Gralnick, H.R., and DeVita, V.T.: Bone-marrow biopsy in Hodgkin's disease, N. Engl. J. Med. **278**:1179, 1968.

40. Berard, C.W., and Dorfman, R.F.: Histopathology of malignant lymphomas, Clin. Haematol. **3**:39, 1974.

41. Berge, T.: Splenic metastases: frequencies and patterns, Acta. Pathol. Microbiol. Scand. [Sect. A] **82**:499, 1974.

42. Berger, R., Bernheim, A., Le Coniat, M., Vecchione, D., Flandrin, G., Dresch, C., and Najean, Y.: Chromosome studies in polycythemia vera patients, Cancer Genet. Cytogenet. **12**:217, 1984.

43. Bergsagel, D.E.: Plasma cell neoplasms and acute leukaemia, Clin. Haematol. **11**:221, 1982.

44. Bernard, A., Boumsell, L., Reinherz, E.L., Nadler, L.M., Ritz, J., Coppin, H., Richard, Y., Valensi, F., Dausset, J., Flandrin, G., Lemerle, J., and Schlossman, S.F.: Cell surface characterization of malignant T cells from lymphoblastic lymphoma using monoclonal antibodies: evidence for phenotypic differences between malignant T cells from patients with acute lymphoblastic leukemia and lymphoblastic lymphoma, Blood **57**:1105, 1981.

45. Bernard, A., Murphy, S.B., Melvin, S., Bowman, W.P., Caillaud, J., Lemerle, J., and Boumsell, L.: Non-T, non-B lymphomas are rare in childhood and associated with cutaneous tumor, Blood **59**:549, 1982.

46. Bernier, V., and Azar, H.A.: Filiform large-cell lymphomas: an ultrastructural and immunohistochemical study, Am. J. Surg. Pathol. **11**:387, 1987.

47. Biberfeld, P., Chayt, K.J., Marselle, L.M., Biberfeld, G., Gallo, R.C., and Harper, M.E.: HTLV-III expression in infected lymph nodes and relevance to pathogenesis of lymphadenopathy, Am. J. Pathol. **125**:436, 1986.

48. Birbeck, M.D., Breathnach, A.J., and Everall, J.D.: An elec-

tron microscopic study of basal melanocytes and high level clear cells (Langerhans cells) in vitiligo, J. Invest. Dermatol. **37:**51, 1961.

49. Bishop, J.M.: The molecular genetics of cancer, Science **235:**305, 1987.
50. Blank, E., and Campbell, J.R.: Epidermoid cysts of the spleen, Pediatrics **51:**75, 1973.
51. Blick, M., Westin, E., and Gutterman, J.: Oncogene expression in human leukemia, Blood **64:**1234, 1984.
52. Block, M.: Bone marrow examination, Arch. Pathol. Lab. Med. **100:**454, 1976.
53. Bloomfield, C.D.: Chromosome abnormalities in secondary myelodysplastic syndrome, Scand. J. Haematol. **45**(suppl.):82, 1986.
54. Bloomfield, C.D., and Arthur, D.C.: Evaluation of leukemic cell chromosomes as a guide to therapy, Blood Cells **8:**501, 1982.
55. Bloomfield, C.D., and Brunning, R.D.: Acute leukemia as a terminal event in nonleukemic hematopoietic disorders, Semin. Oncol. **3:**297, 1976.
56. Bloomfield, C.D., and Brunning, R.D.: FAB M7 acute megakaryoblastic leukemia—beyond morphology, Ann. Intern. Med. **103:**450, 1985.
57. Bloomfield, C.D., Goldman, A.I., Alimena, G., Berger, R., Borgström, G.H., Brandt, L., Catovsky, D., de la Chapelle, A., Dewald, G.W., Garson, O.M., et al.: Chromosomal abnormalities identify high-risk and low-risk patients with acute lymphoblastic leukemia, Blood **67:**415, 1986.
58. Bodem, C.R., Hamory, B.H., Taylor, H.M., and Kleopfer, L.: Granulomatous bone marrow disease: a review of the literature and clinicopathologic analysis of 58 cases, Medicine **62:**372, 1983.
59. Boggs, D.R.: Hematopoietic stem cell theory in relation to possible lymphoblastic conversion of chronic myeloid leukemia, Blood **44:**449, 1974. (Editorial.)
60. Booth, W.: CDC paints a picture of HIV infection in U.S., Science **239:**253, 1988.
61. Borgström, G.H.: Cytogenetics of the myelodysplastic syndromes, Scand. J. Haematol. **45**(suppl.):74, 1986.
62. Borst, J., van de Griend, R.J., Van Oostveen, J.W., Ang, S.L., Melief, C.J., Seidman, J.G., and Bolhuis, R.L.: A T-cell receptor g/CD3 complex found on cloned functional lymphocytes, Nature **325:**683, 1987.
63. Bottomley, S.: Sideroblastic anaemia, Clin. Haematol. **11:**389, 1982.
64. Boyum, A., Løvhaug, D., Kolstø, A.B., Helgestad, J., and Melby, T.: Colony inhibiting factor in mature granulocytes from normal individuals and patients with chronic myeloid leukemia, Eur. J. Haematol. **38:**318, 1987.
65. Braylan, R.C., Benson, N.A., Nourse, V., and Kruth, H.S.: Correlated analysis of cellular DNA, membrane antigens and light scatter of human lymphoid cells, Cytometry **2:**337, 1982.
66. Brenner, M.B., McLean, J., Scheft, H., Riberdy, J., Ang, S.L., Seidman, J.G., Devlin, P., and Krangel, M.S.: Two forms of the T-cell receptor g protein found on peripheral blood cytotoxic T lymphocytes, Nature **325:**689, 1987.
67. Brinker, M.G., Poppema, S., Buys, C.H., Timens, W., Osinga, J., and Visser, L.: Clonal immunoglobulin gene rearrangements in tissues involved by Hodgkin's disease, Blood **70:**186, 1987.
68. Brittenham, G.M., Danish, E.H., and Harris, J.W.: Assessment of bone marrow and body iron stores: old techniques and new technologies, Semin. Hematol. **18:**194, 1981.
69. Brown, C.H.: Bone marrow necrosis: a study of seventy cases, Johns Hopkins Med. J. **131:**189, 1972.
70. Brownell, M.D., Sheibani, K., Battifora, H., Winberg, C.D., and Rappaport, H.: Distinction between undifferentiated (small noncleaved) and lymphoblastic lymphoma: an immunohistologic study on paraffin-embedded, fixed tissue sections, Am. J. Surg. Pathol. **11:**779, 1987.
71. Brunning, R.D., Bloomfield, C.D., McKenna, R.W., et al.: Bilateral trephine bone marrow biopsies in lymphoma and other neoplastic disease, Ann. Intern. Med. **82:**365, 1975.
72. Brunning, R.D., McKenna, R.W., Rosai, J., Parkin, J.L., and Risdall, R.: Systemic mastocytosis: extracutaneous manifestations, Am. J. Surg. Pathol. **7:**425, 1983.
73. Brynes, R.K., McKenna, R.W., and Sundberg, R.D.: Bone marrow aspiration and trephine biopsy: an approach to a thorough study, Am. J. Clin. Pathol. **70:**753, 1978.
74. Buchino, J.J., Byrd, R.P., and Kmetz, D.R.: Disseminated sinus histiocytosis with massive lymphadenopathy, Arch. Pathol. Lab. Med. **106:**13, 1982.
75. Buckley, P.J., Smith, M.R., Braverman, M.F., and Dickson, S.A.: Human spleen contains phenotypic subsets of macrophages and dendritic cells that occupy discrete microanatomic locations, Am. J. Pathol. **128:**505, 1987.
76. Burgert, E.O., Jr., Gilchrist, G.S., Fairbanks, V.F., et al.: Intra-abdominal, angiofollicular lymph node hyperplasia (plasmacell variant) with an antierythropoietic factor, Mayo Clin. Proc. **50:**542, 1975.
77. Burke, J.S.: Surgical pathology of the spleen: an approach to the differential diagnosis of splenic lymphomas and leukemias. Part I. Diseases of the white pulp, Am. J. Surg. Pathol. **5:**551, 1981.
78. Burke, J.S.: Surgical pathology of the spleen: an approach to the differential diagnosis of splenic lymphomas and leukemias. Part II. Diseases of the red pulp, Am. J. Surg. Pathol. **5:**681, 1981.
79. Burke, J.S.: The value of the bone-marrow biopsy in the diagnosis of hairy cell leukemia, Am. J. Clin. Pathol. **70:**876, 1978.
80. Burke, J.S., and Butler, J.J.: Malignant lymphoma with a high content of epithelioid histiocytes (Lennert's lymphoma), Clin. Pathol. **66:**1, 1976.
81. Burke, J.S., and Osborne, B.M.: Localized reactive lymphoid hyperplasia of the spleen simulating malignant lymphoma, Am. J. Surg. Pathol. **7:**373, 1983.
82. Burke, J.S., Byrne, G.S., Jr., and Rappaport, H.: Hairy cell leukemia (leukemic reticuloendotheliosis). I. A clinical pathologic study of 21 patients, Cancer **33:**1399, 1974.
83. Burke, J.S., Sheibani, K., and Rappaport, H.: Dermatopathic lymphadenopathy: an immunophenotypic comparison of cases associated and unassociated with mycosis fungoides, Am. J. Pathol. **123:**256, 1986.
84. Burkhardt, R.: Bone marrow histology. In Catovsky, D., editor: The leukemic cell, Edinburgh, 1981, Churchill Livingstone.
85. Burns, B.F., Colby, T.V., and Dorfman, R.F.: Langerhans' cell granulomatosis (histiocytosis X) associated with malignant lymphomas, Am. J. Surg. Pathol. **7:**529, 1983.
86. Burns, B.F., Wood, G.S., and Dorfman, R.F.: The varied histopathology of lymphadenopathy in the homosexual male, Am. J. Surg. Pathol. **9:**287, 1985.
87. Burston, J., and Pinniger, J.L.: The reticulin content of bone marrow in haematological disorders, Br. J. Haematol. **9:**172, 1963.
88. Buss, D.H., Prichard, R.W., Hartz, J.W., Cooper, M.R., and Feigin, G.A.: Initial bone marrow findings in multiple myeloma: significance of plasma cell nodules, Arch. Pathol. Lab. Med. **110:**30, 1986.
89. Butler, J.J.: Non-neoplastic lesions of lymph nodes of man to be differentiated from lymphomas, Nat. Cancer Inst. Monogr. **32:**233, 1969.
90. Butler, J.J.: Pathology of the spleen in benign and malignant conditions, Histopathology **7:**453, 1983.
91. Butler, J.J., and Osborne, B.M.: Lymph node enlargement in patients with unsuspected human immunodeficiency virus infections, Hum. Pathol. **19:**849, 1988.
92. Butturini, A., and Gale, R.P.: Oncogenes and human leukemias, Int. J. Cell Cloning **6:**2, 1988.
93. Butturini A., Sthivelman, E., Canaani, E., and Gale, R.P.: Oncogenes in human leukemias, Acta Haematol. **78**(suppl. 1):2, 1987.
94. Byrne, G.E., Jr.: Histopathologic diagnosis of Hodgkin's disease, Semin. Oncol. **7:**103, 1980.
95. Byrne, G.E., Jr., and Rappaport, H.: Malignant histiocytosis, GANN Monogr. Cancer Res. **15:**145, 1973.
96. Cabanillas, F., Pathak, S., Trujillo, J., Grant, G., Cork, A., Hagemeister, F.B., Velazquez, W.S., McLaughlin, P., Redman,

J., Katz, R., et al.: Cytogenetic features of Hodgkin's disease suggest possible origin from a lymphocyte, Blood **71:**1615, 1988.

97. Campo, E., Condom, E., Miro, M.J., Cid, M.C., and Romagosa, V.: Tuberculosis-associated hemophagocytic syndrome: a systemic process, Cancer **58:**2640, 1986.

98. Canaani, E., Gale, R.P., Steiner-Saltz, D., Berrebi, A., Aghai, E., and Januszewicz, E.: Altered transcription of an oncogene in chronic myeloid leukaemia, Lancet **1:**593, 1984.

99. Canale, D.D., and Collins, R.D.: Use of bone marrow particle sections in the diagnosis of multiple myeloma, Am. J. Clin. Pathol. **61:**382, 1974.

100. Canellos, G.P., Come, S.E., and Skarin, A.T.: Chemotherapy in the treatment of Hodgkin's disease, Semin. Hematol. **20:**1, 1983.

101. Carbone, A., Manconi, R., Volpe, R., Poletti, A., DePaoli, P., Tirelli, U., and Santini, G.: Immunohistochemical, enzyme histochemical, and immunologic features of giant lymph node hyperplasia of the hyaline-vascular type, Cancer **58:**908, 1986.

102. Carbone A., Manconi, R., Sulfaro, S., Vaccher, E., Zagonel, V., Poletti, A., Volpe, R., Tirelli, U., and Monfardini, S.: Practical importance of routine paraffin-embedded bone marrow biopsy in multiple myeloma, Tumori **73:**315, 1987.

103. Carbone, P., Barbata, G., Mirto, S., Marceno, R., Leone, S., and Granata, G.: Cytogenic studies in five patients with myelofibrosis and myeloid metaplasia, Cancer Genet. Cytogenet. **12:**209, 1984.

104. Carbone, P.P., Kaplan, H.S., Musshoff, K., et al.: Report of the Committee on Hodgkin's Disease Staging Classification, Cancer Res. **31:**1860, 1971.

105. Carithers, H.A., Carithers, C.M., and Edwards, R.O., Jr.: Cat-scratch disease: its natural history, JAMA **207:**312, 1969.

106. Carter, P., Koval, J.J., and Hobbs, J.R.: The relation of clinical and laboratory findings to the survival of patients with macroglobulinaemia, Clin. Exp. Immunol. **28:**241, 1977.

107. Cartwright, G.E., and Lee, G.R.: The anaemia of chronic disorders, Br. J. Haematol. **21:**147, 1971.

108. Castleman, B., Iverson, L., and Menéndez, V.P.: Localized mediastinal lymph-node hyperplasia resembling thymoma, Cancer **4:**822, 1956.

109. Castoldi, G., Cuneo, A., Tomasi, P., and Ferrari, L.: Chromosome abnormalities in myelofibrosis, Acta Haematol. **78:**104, 1987.

110. Catovsky, D., Pettit, J.E., Galetto, J., et al.: The B-lymphocyte nature of the hairy cell of leukaemic reticuloendotheliosis, Br. J. Haematol. **26:**29, 1974.

111. Cazzola, M., Bergamaschi, G., Huebers, H.A., and Finch, C.A.: Pathophysiological classification of the acquired bone marrow failure based on quantitative assessment of erythroid function, Eur. J. Haematol. **38:**426, 1987.

112. Cervantes, F., Ballesta, F., Mila, M., and Rozman, C.: Cytogenetic studies in blast crisis of Ph-positive chronic granulocytic leukemia: results and prognostic evaluation in 52 patients, Cancer Genet. Cytogenet. **21:**239, 1986.

113. Cesarman, E., Dalla-Favera, R., Bentley, D., and Groudine, M.: Mutations in the first exon are associated with altered transcription of c-*myc* in Burkitt lymphoma, Science **238:**1272, 1987.

114. Chaganti, R.S.K., Jhanwar, S.C., Koziner, B., Arlin, Z., Mertelsmann, R., and Clarkson, B.D.: Specific translocations characterize Burkitt's-like lymphoma of homosexual men with the acquired immunodeficiency syndrome, Blood **61:**1265, 1983.

115. Champlin, R.E., and Golde, D.W.: Chronic myelogenous leukemia: recent advances, Blood **65:**1039, 1985.

116. Champlin, R.E., Goldman, J.M., and Gale, R.P.: Bone marrow transplantation in chronic myelogenous leukemia, Semin. Hematol. **25:**74, 1988.

117. Chan, K.W., and Shaw, D.: Distinctive, multiple lymphangiomas of spleen, Pathology **131:**75, 1980.

118. Chan, T.W., and McGee, J.O'D.: Cellular oncogenes in neoplasia, J. Clin. Pathol. **40:**1055, 1987.

119. Chanarin, I.: Megaloblastic anaemia, cobalamin, and folate, J. Clin. Pathol. **40:**978, 1987.

120. Chanarin, I.: Structure and function of the bone marrow. In Irons, R.D., editor: Toxicology of the blood and bone marrow, New York, 1985, Raven Press.

121. Charache, S., Gittelsohn, A.M., Allen, H., Cox, C.W., Flanigan, V., Periasamy, V., LaFrance, N.D., and Perlstein, M.: Noninvasive assessment of tissue iron stores, Am. J. Clin. Pathol. **88:**33, 1987.

122. Chen, J.L., Osborne, B.M., and Butler, J.J.: Residual fibrous masses in treated Hodgkin's disease, Cancer **60:**407, 1987.

123. Chen, K.T.K., Bolles, J.C., and Gilbert, E.F.: Angiosarcoma of the spleen: a report of two cases and review of the literature, Arch. Pathol. Lab. Med. **103:**122, 1979.

124. Chen, T.K., Nesbit, M.E., McKenna, R., et al.: Leukemia of T cell origin, Am. J. Dis. Child. **130:**1262, 1976.

125. Cheng, D.S., Kushner, J.P., and Wintrobe, M.M.: Idiopathic refractory sideroblastic anemia: incidence and risk factors for leukemic transformation, Cancer **44:**724, 1979.

126. Chikkappa, G., Pasquale, D., Phillips, P.G., Mangan, K.F., and Tsan, M.F.: Cyclosporin-A for the treatment of pure red cell aplasia in a patient with chronic lymphocytic leukemia, Am. J. Hematol. **26:**179, 1987.

127. Childs, C.C., Parham, D.M., and Berard, C.W.: Infectious mononucleosis: the spectrum of morphologic changes simulating lymphoma in lymph nodes and tonsils, Am. J. Surg. Pathol. **11:**122, 1987.

128. Chittal, S.M., Caveriviere, P., Vaigt, J.J., Dumont, J., Benevent, B., Faure, P., Bordessoule, G.D., and Delsol, G.: Follicular lymphoma with abundant PAS-positive extracellular material: immunohistochemical and ultrastructural observations, Am. J. Surg. Pathol. **11:**618, 1987.

129. Chun, C.H., Raff, M.J., Contreras, L., Varghese, R., Waterman, N., Daffner, R., and Melo, J.C.: Splenic abscess, Medicine **59:**50, 1980.

130. Clark, S.S., McLaughlin, J., Crist, W.M., Champlin, R., and Witte, O.N.: Unique forms of the abl tyrosine kinase distinguish Ph-positive ALL, Science **235:**85, 1987.

131. Classification system for human T-lymphotropic virus type III/lymphadenopathy–associated virus infections, MMWR **35:**334, 1986.

132. Clayton, F.G., Mancini, A.E., and Frizzera, G.: Localized histiocytosis X of lymph nodes: a clinicopathologic report of six cases, Lab. Invest. **42:**106, 1980.

133. Cleary, M.L., and Sklar J.: Lymphoproliferative disorders in cardiac transplant recipients are multiclonal lymphomas, Lancet **2:**489, 1984.

134. Colby, T.V., and Carrington, C.B.: Pulmonary lymphomas: current concepts, Hum. Pathol. **14:**884, 1983.

135. Colby, T.V., and Lombard, C.: Histiocytosis X in the lung, Hum. Pathol. **14:**847, 1983.

136. Colby, T.V., and Warnke, R.A.: The histology of the initial relapse of Hodgkin's disease, Cancer **45:**289, 1980.

137. Colby, T.V., Warnke, R.A., Burke, J.S., and Dorfman, R.F.: Differentiation of chronic lymphocytic leukemia from Hodgkin's disease using immunologic marker studies, Am. J. Surg. Pathol. **5:**707, 1981.

138. Colby, T.V., Hoppe, R.T., and Warnke, R.A.: Hodgkin's disease at autopsy: 1972-1977, Cancer **47:**1852, 1981.

139. Coller, B.S., Chabner, B.A., and Gralnick, H.R.: Frequencies and patterns of bone marrow involvement in non-Hodgkin's lymphomas, Am. J. Hematol. **3:**105, 1977.

140. Conrad, M.E., and Carpenter, J.T.: Bone marrow necrosis, Am. J. Hematol. **7:**181, 1979.

141. Cook, J.D., and Lynch, S.R.: The liabilities of iron deficiency, Blood **68:**803, 1986.

142. Cooper, R.A., Dawson, P.J., and Rambo, O.M.: Dermatopathic lymphadenopathy: a clinicopathologic analysis of lymph node biopsy over a 15-year period, Calif. Med. **106:**170, 1967.

143. Cope, O., and Litwin, S.B.: Contribution of the lymphatic system to the replenishment of the plasma volume following a hemorrhage, Ann. Surg. **156:**655, 1962.

144. Cornaglia-Ferraris, P., Perlino, G.F., Barabino, A., Guarino, C., Oliva, L., Soave, F., and Massimo, L.: Cystic lymphangi-

oma of the spleen: report of CT scan findings, Pediatr. Radiol. **12**:94, 1982.

145. Corrigan, J.J., Van Wyck, D.B., and Crosby, W.H.: Clinical disorders of splenic function: the spectrum from asplenism to hypersplenism, Lymphology **16**:101, 1983.

146. Corwin, J., and Lindberg, R.D.: Solitary plasmacytoma of bone vs. extramedullary plasmacytoma and their relationship to multiple myeloma, Cancer **43**:1007, 1979.

147. Cossman, J., Chused, T.M., Fisher, R.I., Magrath, I., Bollum, F., and Jaffe, E.S.: Diversity of immunological phenotypes of lymphoblastic lymphoma, Cancer Res. **43**:4486, 1983.

148. Cossman, J., Jaffe, E.S., and Fisher, R.I.: Immunologic phenotypes of diffuse, aggressive, non-Hodgkin's lymphomas: correlation with clinical features, Cancer **54**:1310, 1984.

149. Costantini, F., Chada, K., and Magram, J.: Correction of murine β-thalassemia by gene transfer into the germ line, Science **233**:1192, 1986.

150. Cotelingam, J.D., and Jaffe, E.S.: Inflammatory pseudotumor of the spleen, Am. J. Surg. Pathol. **8**:375, 1984.

151. Croce, C.M., Tsujimoto, Y., Erikson, J., and Nowell, P.: Chromosome translocations and B cell neoplasia, Lab. Invest. **51**:258, 1984.

152. Croce, C.M., Isobe, M., Palumbo, A., Puck, J., Ming, J., Tweardy, D., Erikson, J., Davis, M., and Rovera, G.: Gene for alpha-chain of human T-cell receptor: location of chromosome 14 region involved in T-cell neoplasms, Science **227**:1044, 1985.

153. Couch, W.D.: Giant lymph node hyperplasia associated with thrombotic thrombocytopenic purpura, Am. J. Clin. Pathol. **74**:340, 1980.

154. Crescenzi, M., Seto, M., Herzig, G.P., Weiss, P.D., Griffith, R.C., and Korsmeyer, S.J.: Thermostable DNA polymerase chain amplification of t(14;18) chromosome breakpoints and the detection of minimal residual disease, Proc. Natl. Acad. Sci. USA **85**:4869, 1988.

155. Crosby, W.H.: Splenic remodeling of red cell surfaces, Blood **50**:643, 1977.

156. Curran, J.W., Jaffe, H.W., Hardy, A.M., Morgan, W.M., Selik, R.M., and Dondero, T.J.: Epidemiology of HIV infection and AIDS in the United States, Science **239**:610, 1988.

157. Dacie, J.V., Brain, M.C., Harrison, C.V., et al.: 'Non-tropical idiopathic splenomegaly' ('primary hypersplenism'): a review of ten cases and their relationship to malignant lymphomas, Br. J. Haematol. **17**:317, 1969.

158. Dadash-Zadeh, M., Czapek, E.E., and Schwartz, A.D.: Skeletal and splenic hemangiomatosis with consumption coagulopathy: response to splenectomy, Pediatrics **57**:803, 1976.

159. Daneshbod, K., and Kissane, J.M.: Idiopathic differentiated histiocytosis, Am. J. Clin. Pathol. **70**:381, 1978.

160. Dainiak, N., Liu, A., Dewey, M.C., Kulkarni, V.: Chromosome analysis of isolated colony erythroblasts in chronic myelogenous leukaemia, Br. J. Hematol. **56**:507, 1984.

161. Dallman, P.R.: Manifestations of iron deficiency, Semin. Hematol. **19**:19, 1982.

162. Dameshek, W.: Some speculations on the myeloproliferative syndromes, Blood **6**:372, 1951.

163. Dardick, I., and Caldwell, D.R.: Follicular center cell lymphoma: morphologic data relating to observer reproducibility, Cancer **58**:2477, 1986.

164. Dardick, I., Sinnott, N.M., Hall, R., Bajenko-Carr, T.A., and Setterfield, G.: Nuclear morphology and morphometry of B-lymphocyte transformation: implications for follicular center cell lymphomas, Am. J. Pathol. **111**:35, 1983.

165. Davey, F.R., Gatter, K.C., Ralfkiaer, E., Pulford, K.A., Krissansen, G.W., and Mason, D.Y.: Immunophenotyping of non-Hodgkin's lymphomas using a panel of antibodies on paraffin-embedded tissues, Am. J. Pathol. **129**:54, 1987.

166. DeAizpurua, H.J., Cosgrove, L.J., Ungar, B., and Toh, B.H.: Autoantibodies cytoxic to gastric parietal cells in serum of patients with pernicious anemia, N. Engl. J. Med. **309**:625, 1983.

167. DeAlmeida, P.C., Harris, N.L., and Bhan, A.K.: Characterization of immature sinus histiocytes (monocytoid cells) in reactive lymph nodes by use of monoclonal antibodies, Hum. Pathol. **15**:330, 1984.

168. DeBartolo, H.M., Jr., van Heerden, J.A., and Norris, D.G.: Torsion of the spleen: a case report, Mayo Clin. Proc. **48**:783, 1973.

169. DeBruyn, P.P.H.: Structural substrates of bone marrow function, Semin. Hematol. **18**:179, 1981.

170. DeJong, D., Voetdijk, B.M., Beverstock, G.C., van Ommen, G.J., Willemze, R., and Kluin, P.M.: Activation of the c-*myc* oncogene in a precursor-B-cell blast crisis of follicular lymphoma, presenting as composite lymphoma, N. Engl. J. Med. **318**:1373, 1988.

171. Dehner, L.P., Bamford, J.T., and McDonald, E.C.: Spontaneous regression of congenital cutaneous histiocytosis X: report of a case with discussion of nosology and pathogenesis, Pediatr. Radiol. **1**:99, 1983.

172. Desser, R.K., Golomb, H.M., Ultmann, J.E., et al.: Prognostic classification of Hodgkin's disease in pathologic stage III, based on anatomic consideration, Blood **49**:883, 1977.

173. Diamond, L.W., Nathwani, B.N., and Rappaport, H.: Flow cytometry in the diagnosis and classification of malignant lymphoma and leukemia, Cancer **50**:1122, 1982.

174. Diaz, M.O., LeBeau, M.M., Pitha, P., and Rowley, J.D.: Interferon and c-ets-1 genes in the translocation (9;11)(p22,q23) in human acute monocytic leukemia, Science **231**:265, 1985.

175. Dick, F., Bloomfield, C.D., and Brunning, R.D.: Incidence, cytology and histopathology of non-Hodgkin's lymphomas in the bone marrow, Cancer **33**:1382, 1974.

176. Dick, F.R., and Maca, R.D.: The lymph node in chronic lymphocytic leukemia, Cancer **41**:283, 1978.

177. DiCarlo, E.F., Amberson, J.B., Metroka, C.E., Ballard, P., Moore, A., and Mouradian, J.A.: Malignant lymphomas and the acquired immunodeficiency syndrome: evaluation of 30 cases using a Working Formulation, Arch. Pathol. Lab. Med. **110**:1012, 1986.

178. Di Padova, F., Dürig, M., Wadström, J., and Harder, F.: Role of spleen in immune response to polyvalent pneumococcal vaccine, Br. Med. J. **287**:1829, 1983.

179. Doggett, R.S., Colby, T.V., and Dorfman, R.F.: Interfollicular Hodgkin's disease, Am. J. Surg. Pathol. **7**:145, 1983.

180. Doggett, R.S., Wood, G.S., Horning, S., Levy, R., Dorfman, R.F., Bindl, J., and Warnke, R.A.: The immunologic characterization of 95 nodal and extranodal diffuse large cell lymphomas in 89 patients, Am. J. Pathol. **115**:245, 1984.

181. Dolginow, D., and Colby, T.V.: Recurrent Hodgkin's disease in treated sites, Cancer **48**:1124, 1981.

182. Doll, D.C., and List, A.F.: Burkitt's lymphoma in a homosexual, Lancet **1**:1026, 1982.

183. Dorfman, R.F.: Histiocytic necrotizing lymphadenitis of Kikuchi and Fujimoto, Arch. Pathol. Lab. Med. **111**:1026, 1987.

184. Dorfman, R.F.: Progressively transformation of germinal centers and lymphocyte predominant Hodgkin's disease: the Stanford experience, Am. J. Surg. Pathol. **11**:150, 1987.

185. Dorfman, R.F.: Relationship of histology to site in Hodgkin's disease, Cancer Res. **31**:1786, 1971.

186. Dorfman, R.F., and Remington, J.S.: Value of lymph-node biopsy in the diagnosis of acute acquired toxoplasmosis, N. Engl. J. Med. **289**:878, 1973.

187. Dorfman, R.F., and Warnke, R.: Lymphadenopathy simulating the malignant lymphomas, Hum. Pathol. **5**:519, 1974.

188. Dorfman, R.F., Gatter, K.C., Pulford, K.A., and Mason, D.Y.: An evaluation of the utility of anti-granulocyte and anti-leukocyte monoclonal antibodies in the diagnosis of Hodgkin's disease, Am. J. Pathol. **123**:508, 1986.

189. Dosik, H., Hsu, L.Y., Todaro, G.J., et al.: Leukemia in Fanconi's anemia: cytogenetic and tumor virus susceptibility studies, Blood **36**:341, 1970.

190. Dreazen, O., Canaani, E., and Gale, R.P.: Molecular biology of chronic myelogenous leukemia, Semin. Hematol. **25**:35, 1988.

191. Duggan, D.B., Ehrlich, G.D., Davey, F.P., Kwok, S., Sninsky, J., Goldberg, J., Baltrucki, L., and Polesz, B.J.: HTLV-I-induced lymphoma mimicking Hodgkin's disease: diagnosis by polymerase chain reaction amplification of specific HTLV-I sequences in tumor DNA, Blood **71**:1027, 1988.

192. Ebert, R.B., Stead, E.A., and Gibson, J.G.: Response of normal subjects to acute blood loss, Arch. Intern. Med. **68**:578, 1941.

193. Edlow, D.W., and Carter, D.: Heterotopic epithelium in axillary lymph nodes: report of a case and review of the literature, Am. J. Clin. Pathol. **59**:666, 1973.

194. Egerter, D.A., and Beckstead, J.H.: Malignant lymphomas in the acquired immunodeficiency syndrome: additional evidence for a B-cell origin, Arch. Pathol. Lab. Med. **112**:602, 1988.

195. Ellis, J.T., and Peterson, P.: The bone marrow in polycythemia vera, Pathol. Annu. **14**:383, 1979.

196. Ellis, J.T., Silver, R.T., Coleman, M., et al.: The bone marrow in polycythemia vera, Semin. Hematol. **12**:433, 1975.

197. Ellis, J.T., Peterson, P., Geller, S.A., and Rappaport, H.: Studies of the bone marrow in polycythemia vera and the evolution of myelofibrosis and second hematologic malignancies, Semin. Hematol. **23**:144, 1986.

198. Ellis, R.E.: The distribution of active bone marrow in the adult, Phys. Med. Biol. **5**:255, 1961.

199. Ellison, D.J., Turner, R.R., Van Antwerp, R., Martin, S.E., and Nathwani, B.N.: High-grade mantle zone lymphoma, Cancer **60**:2717, 1987.

200. Ellman, L.: Bone marrow biopsy in the evaluation of lymphoma, carcinoma and granulomatous disorders, Am. J. Med. **60**:1, 1976.

201. Embury, S.H.: The clinical pathophysiology of sickle cell disease, Annu. Rev. Med. **37**:361, 1986.

202. Emilia, G., Torelli, G., Sacchi, S., and Donelli, A.: Chromosomal abnormalities in essential thrombocythemia, Cancer Genet. Cytogenet. **18**:91, 1985.

203. Emson, H.E.: Extrathoracic angiofollicular lymphoid hyperplasia with coincidental myasthenia gravis, Cancer **31**:241, 1973.

204. Enno, A., Catovsky, D., O'Brien, M., Cherchi, M., Kumaran, T.O., and Galton, D.A.: "Prolymphocytoid" transformation of chronic lymphocytic leukemia, Br. J. Haematol. **41**:9, 1979.

205. Epstein, J.I., Erlandson, R.A., and Rosen, P.P.: Nodal blue nevi: a study of three cases, Am. J. Surg. Pathol. **8**:907, 1984.

206. Eraklis, A.J., and Filler, R.M.: Splenectomy in childhood: a review of 1413 cases, J. Pediatr. Surg. **7**:382, 1972.

207. Eridani, S., Sawyer, B., and Pearson, T.C.: Patterns of in vitro BFU-E proliferation in different forms of polycythaemia and in thrombocythaemia, Eur. J. Haematol. **38**:363, 1987.

208. Ershler, W.B., Ross, J., Finlay, J.L., and Shahidi, N.T.: Bone-marrow microenvironment defect in congenital hypoplastic anemia, N. Engl. J. Med. **302**:1321, 1980.

209. Ersley, A.G., and Caro, J.: Erythropoietin titers in response to anemia or hypoxia, Blood Cells **13**:207, 1987.

210. Ezdinli, E.Z., Kucuk, O., Chedid, A., Sinclair, T.F., Thomas, K., Singh, S., Sarpel, S., and Jovanovic, L.: Hypogammaglobulinemia and hemophagocytic syndrome associated with lymphoproliferative disorders, Cancer **57**:1024, 1986.

211. Fahey, J.L., Prince, H., Weaver, M., Groopman, J., Visscher, B., Schwartz, K., and Detels, R.: Quantitative changes in T helper or T suppressor/cytotoxic lymphocyte subsets that distinguish acquired immune deficiency syndrome from other immune subset disorders, Am. J. Med. **76**:95, 1984.

212. Fallon, M.D., Whyte, M.P., and Teitelbaum, S.L.: Systemic mastocytosis associated with generalized osteopenia: histopathological characterization of the skeletal lesion using undecalcified bone from two patients, Hum. Pathol. **12**:813, 1981.

213. Farquhar, J.W., and Claireaux, A.E.: Familial haemophagocytic reticulosis, Arch. Dis. Child. **27**:519, 1952.

214. Favara, B.E., McCarthy, R.C., and Mierau, G.W.: Histiocytosis X, Hum. Pathol. **14**:663, 1983.

215. Feller, A.C., Lennert, K., Stein, H., Bruhn, H.D., and Wuthe, H.H.: Immunohistology and aetiology of histiocytic necrotizing lymphadenitis: report of three instructive cases, Histopathology **7**:825, 1983.

216. Feller, A.C., Griesser, G.H., Mak, T.W., and Lennert, K.: Lymphoepithelioid lymphoma (Lennert's lymphoma) is a monoclonal proliferation of helper/inducer T cells, Blood **68**:663, 1986.

217. Fernándes-Costa, F., and Eintracht, I.: Histiocytic medullary reticulosis, Lancet **2**:204, 1979.

218. Fialkow, P.J., Singer, J.W., Adamson, J.W., Vaidya, K., Dow, L.W., Ochs, J., and Moohr, J.W.: Acute nonlymphocytic leukemia: heterogeneity of stem cell origin, Blood **57**:1068, 1981

219. Fialkow, P.J., Martin, P.J., Najfeld, V., Penfold, G.K., Jacobson, R.J., and Hansen, J.A.: Evidence for a multistep pathogenesis of chronic myelogenous leukemia, Blood **58**:158, 1981.

220. Fifth International Workshop on Chromosomes in Leukemia-Lymphoma: correlation of chromosome abnormalities with histologic and immunologic characteristics in non-Hodgkin's lymphoma and adult T cell leukemia-lymphoma, Blood **70**:1554, 1987.

221. Finger, L.R., Harvey, R.C., Moore, R.C., Showe, L.C., and Croce, C.M.: A common mechanism of chromosomal translocation in T- and B-cell neoplasia, Science **234**:982, 1986.

222. Finkelstein, J.Z., Skert, H., Isaacs, H., and Higgins, G.: Bone marrow metastases in children with solid tumors, Am. J. Dis. Child. **119**:49, 1976.

223. First MIC Cooperative Study Group: Morphologic, immunologic, and cytogenetic (MIC) working classification of acute lymphoblastic leukemias, Cancer Genet. Cytogenet. **23**:189, 1986.

224. Fisher, R.I., DeVita, V.T., Jr., Hubbard, S.M., Longo, D.L., Wesley, R., Chabner, B.R., and Young, R.C.: Diffuse aggressive lymphomas: increased survival after alternating flexible sequences of ProMACE and MOPP chemotherapy, Ann. Intern. Med. **98**:304, 1983.

225. Fleischmann, T., and Bodor, F.: Aneuploidy in paroxysmal nocturnal haemoglobinuria, Acta Haematol. **44**:251, 1970.

226. Fleming, C.R., Dickson, E.R., and Harrison, E.G., Jr.: Splenosis: autotransplantation of splenic tissue, Am. J. Med. **61**:414, 1976.

227. Foon, K.A., and Gale, R.P.: Controversies in therapy of acute myelogenous leukemia, Am. J. Med. **72**:963, 1982.

228. Forte, F.A., Prelli, F., Yount, W.J., et al.: Heavy chain disease of the μ (IgM) type: report of the first case, Blood **36**:137, 1970.

229. Foucar, K., and Rydell, R.E.: Richter's syndrome in chronic lymphocytic leukemia, Cancer **46**:118, 1980.

230. Foucar, K., McKenna, R.W., Frizzera, G., and Brunning, R.D.: Bone marrow and blood involvement by lymphoma in relationship to the Lukes-Collins classification, Cancer **49**:888, 1982.

231. Foucar, K., McKenna, R.W., Bloomfield, C.D., Bowers, T.K., and Brunning, R.D.: Therapy-related leukemia: a panmyelosis, Cancer **43**:1285, 1979.

232. Foucar, K., McKenna, R.W., and Frizzera, G.: Incidence and patterns of bone marrow and blood involvement by lymphoma in relationship to the Lukes-Collins classification, Blood **54**:1417, 1979.

233. Fox, R.A., and Rosahn, P.D.: The lymph nodes in disseminated lupus erythematosus, Am. J. Pathol. **19**:73, 1943.

234. Franchino, C., Reich, C., Distenfeld, A., Ubriaco, A., and Knowles, D.M.: A clinicopathologically distinctive primary splenic histiocytic neoplasm: demonstration of its histiocytic derivation by immunophenotypic and molecular genetic analysis, Am. J. Surg. Pathol. **12**:398, 1988.

235. Frangione, B., and Franklin, E.C.: Heavy chain diseases: clinical features and molecular significance of the disordered immunoglobin structure, Semin. Hematol. **10**:53, 1973.

236. Freedman, A.S., Boyd, A.W., Anderson, K.C., Fisher, D.C., Pinkus, G.S., Schlossman, S.F., and Nadler, L.M.: Immunologic heterogeneity of diffuse large cell lymphoma, Blood **65**:630, 1985.

237. Freedom, R.M.: The asplenia syndrome: a review of significant extracardiac structural abnormalities in 29 necropsied patients, J. Pediatr. **81**:1130, 1972.

238. Friedland, G.H., and Klein, R.S.: Transmission of the human immunodeficiency virus, N. Engl. J. Med. **317**:1125, 1987.

239. Frisch, B., and Bartl, R.: Bone marrow biopsy in clinical medicine: an overview, Haematologia **3**:245, 1982.

240. Frisch, B., and Bartl, R.: Bone marrow histology in myelodysplasia and secondary leukaemia, Scand. J. Haematol. **45**(suppl.):38, 1986.

241. Frisch, B., Bartl, R., and Chaichik, S.: Therapy-induced mye-

lodysplasia and secondary leukaemia, Scand. J. Haematol. 45(suppl.):38, 1986.

242. Fritz, E., Ludwig, H., and Kundi, M.: Prognostic revelance of cellular morphology in multiple myeloma, Blood 63:1072, 1984.

243. Frizzera, G., and Murphy, S.B.: Follicular (nodular) lymphoma in childhood: a rare clinical-pathological entity: report of eight cases from four cancer centers, Cancer 44:2218, 1979.

244. Frizzera, G., Banks, P.M., Massarelli, G., and Rosai, J.: A systemic lymphoproliferative disorder with morphologic features of Castleman's disease: pathological findings in 15 patients, Am. J. Surg. Pathol. 7:211, 1983.

245. Frizzera, G., Hanto, D.W., Gajl-Peczalska, K.J., Rosai, J., McKenna, R.W., Sibley, R.K., Holahan, K.P., and Lindquist, L.L.: Polymorphic diffuse B cell hyperplasias and lymphomas in renal transplant recipients, Cancer Res. 41:4262, 1981.

246. Frizzera, G., Moran, E.M., and Rappaport, H.: Angioimmunoblastic lymphadenopathy with dysproteinaemia, Lancet 1:1070, 1974.

247. Gaba, A.R., Stein, R.S., Sweet, D.L., and Variakojis, D.: Multicentric giant lymph node hyperplasia, Am. J. Clin. Pathol. 69:86, 1978.

248. Galasko, C.S.B.: Mechanisms of lytic and blastic metastatic disease of the bone, Clin. Orthop. Rel. Res. 169:20, 1982.

249. Gallatin, W.M., Weissman, I.L., and Butcher, E.C.: A cell surface molecule involved in organ specific homing of lymphocytes, Nature 303:30, 1983.

250. Galton, D.A.G., Goldman, J.M., and Wiltshaw, E.: Prolymphocytic leukemia, Br. J. Haematol. 27:7, 1974.

251. Gams, R.A., Neal, J.A., and Conrad, F.G.: Hydantoin-induced pseudo-pseudolymphoma, Ann. Intern. Med. 69:557, 1968.

252. Garfinkel, L.: Cancer clusters, CA 37:20, 1987.

253. Garrett, T.J., Gee, T.S., Lieberman, P.H., et al.: The role of bone marrow aspiration and biopsy in detecting marrow involvement by nonhematologic malignancies, Cancer 38:2401, 1976.

254. Gartner, J.G., Murphy, M.N., Diocee, M., de Sa, D.J., and McLain, K.L.: Demonstration of Epstein-Barr virus in immunoblastic sarcoma of B-cells arising in a child with primary immunodeficiency disease, Am. J. Surg. Pathol. 11:726, 1987.

255. Garvin, A.J., Simon, R.M., Osborne, C.K., Merrill, J., Young, R.C., and Berard, C.W.: An autopsy study of histologic progression in non-Hodgkin's lymphomas: 192 cases from the National Cancer Institute, Cancer 52:393, 1983.

256. Garvin, D.F., and King, F.M.: Cysts and nonlymphomatous tumors of the spleen, Pathol. Annu. 16:61, 1981.

257. Gaulard, P., Henni, T., Marolleau, J.P., Haioun, C., Henni, Z., Voisin, M.C., Divine, M., Goosens, M., Farcet, J.P., and Reyes, F.: Lethal midline granuloma (polymorphic reticulosis) and lymphomatoid granulomatosis: evidence for a monoclonal T-cell lymphoproliferative disorder, Cancer 62:705, 1988.

258. Gérard-Marchant, R., Hamlin, I., Lennert, K., Rilke, F., Stansfield, A.G., and van Unnik, J.A.M.: Classification of non-Hodgkin's lymphomas, Lancet 2:405, 1974.

259. Gilbert, E.F., Zu Rhein, G.M., Wester, S.M., Herrmann, J., Hong, R., and Opitz, J.M.: Familial hemophagocytic lymphohistiocytosis: report of four cases in two families and review of the literature, Pediatr. Pathol. 3:59, 1985.

260. Giles, C.: An account of 335 cases of megaloblastic anemia of pregnancy and puerperium, J. Clin. Pathol. 19:1, 1966.

261. Giraldo, G., Beth, E., Kourilsky, F.M., et al.: Antibody patterns to herpes-viruses in Kaposi's sarcoma with cytomegalovirus, Int. J. Cancer 15:839, 1975.

262. Glaser, S.L.: Regional variation in Hodgkin's disease incidence by histologic subtype in the US, Cancer 60:2841, 1987.

263. Glick, A.D., Bennett, B., and Collins, R.D.: Neoplasms of the mononuclear phagocyte system: criteria for diagnosis, Invest. Cell Pathol. 3:259, 1980.

264. Goffinet, D.R., Hoyt, C., and Eltringham, J.R.: Secondary syphilis misdiagnosed as lymphoma, Calif. Med. 112:22, 1970.

265. Golde, D.W., Hocking, W.G., Koeffler, H.P., and Adamson, J.W.: Polythemia: mechanisms and management, Ann. Intern. Med. 95:71, 1981.

266. Goldman, J.M.: Prospects for cure in leukemia, J. Clin. Pathol. 40:985, 1987.

267. Goldman, J.M.: The Philadelphia chromosome: from cytogenetics to oncogenes, Br. J. Haematol. 66:435, 1987.

268. Gómez, G.A., Sokal, J.E., and Walsh, D.: Prognostic features at the diagnosis of chronic myelocytic leukemia, Cancer 47:2470, 1981.

269. González-Crussi, F., Raibley, S., Ballantine, T.V., et al.: Splenorenal fusion: heterotopia simulating a primary renal neoplasm, Am. J. Dis. Child. 131:994, 1977.

270. Gordon, H.: Oncogenes, Mayo Clin. Proc. 60:697, 1985.

271. Graber, S.E., and Krantz, S.B.: Erythropoietin and the control of red cell production, Annu. Rev. Med. 29:51, 1978.

272. Gralnick, H.R., Galton, D.A.G., Catovsky, D., Sultan, C., and Bennett, J.M.: Classification of acute leukemia, Ann. Intern. Med. 87:740, 1977.

273. Gray, J.L., Jacobs, A., and Block, M.: Bone marrow and peripheral blood lymphocytosis in the prognosis of chronic lymphocytic leukemia, Cancer 33:1169, 1974.

274. Greaves, M.F.: Differentiation-linked leukemogenesis in lymphocytes, Science 234:697, 1986.

275. Greenberg, B.R., Woo, L., Veomett, I.C., Payne, C.M., and Ahmann, F.R.: Cytogenetics of bone marrow fibroblastic cells in idiopathic chronic myelofibrosis, Br. J. Haematol. 66:487, 1987.

276. Greenberg, P.L.: Biologic nature of myelodysplasic syndromes, Acta Hematol. 78:94, 1987.

277. Greer, J.P., Kinney, M.C., Cousar, J.B., Flexner, J.M., Dupont, W.D., Graber, S.E., Greco, F.A., Collins, R.D., and Stein, R.S.: Lymphocyte-depleted Hodgkin's disease: clinicopathologic review of 25 patients, Am. J. Med. 81:208, 1986.

278. Grieco, M.B., and Cady, B.: Staging laparotomy in Hodgkin's disease, Surg. Clin. North Am. 60:369, 1980.

279. Griffin, J.D., Davis, R., Nelson, D.A., Davey, F.R., Mayer, R.J., Schiffer, C., McIntyre, O.R., and Bloomfield, C.D.: Use of surface marker analysis to predict outcome of adult acute myeloblastic leukemia, Blood 68:1232, 1986.

280. Griffin, J.D., Ellman, L., Long, J.C., and Dvorak, A.M.: Development of a histiocytic medullary reticulosis-like syndrome during the course of acute lymphocytic leukemia, Am. J. Med. 64:851, 1978.

281. Griffith, R.C., Kelly, D.R., Nathwani, B.N., Shuster, J.J., Murphy, S.B., Hvizdala, E., Sullivan, M.P., and Berard, C.W.: A morphologic study of childhood lymphoma of the lymphoblastic type: the Pediatric Oncology Group experience, Cancer 59:1126, 1987.

282. Grogan, T., Spier, C., Wirt, D.P., Hicks, M.J., Paquin, M., Hutter, J., Miller, T., Rangel, C., Richter, L., and Jones, S.: Immunologic complexity of lymphoblastic lymphoma, Diagn. Immunol. 4:81, 1986.

283. Grogan, T.M., Richter, L.C., Payne, C.M., and Rangel, C.S.: Signet-ring cell lymphoma of T-cell origin: an immunocytochemical and ultrastructural study relating giant vacuole formation to cytoplasmic sequestration of surface membrane, Am. J. Surg. Pathol. 9:684, 1985.

284. Groopman, J.E., and Golde, D.W.: The histiocytic disorders: a pathophysiologic analysis, Ann. Intern. Med. 94:95, 1981.

285. Groopman, J.E., Sullivan, J.L., Mulder, C., Ginsburg, D., Orkin, S.H., O'Hara, C.J., Falchuk, K., Wong-Staal, F., and Gallo, R.C.: Pathogenesis of B cell lymphoma in a patient with AIDS, Blood 67:612, 1986.

286. Groopman, J.E.: The pathogenesis of myelofibrosis in myeloproliferative disorders, Ann. Intern. Med. 92:857, 1980.

287. Gruber, H.E., Finley, K.D., Hershberg, R.M., Katzman, S.S., Laikind, P.K., Seegmiller, J.E., Friedmann, T., Yee, J.K., and Jolly, D.J.: Retroviral vector-mediated gene transfer into hematopoietic progenitor cells, Science 230:1057, 1985.

288. Guarda, L.A., Butler, J.J., Mansell, P., Hersh, E.M., Reuben, J., and Newell, G.R.: Lymphadenopathy in homosexual men: morbid anatomy with clinical and immunologic correlations, Am. J. Clin. Pathol. 79:559, 1983.

289. Guerrant, R.L., Humphries, M.K., Butler, J.E., et al.: Tick-

borne oculoglandular tularemia: case report and review of seasonal and vectorial associations in 106 cases, Arch. Intern. Med. **136**:811, 1976.

290. Guglielmi, P., Bakhshi, A., Mihaesco, E., Broudet, J., Waldmann, T.A., and Korsmeyer, S.J.: DNA deletion in human gamma heavy chain disease, Clin. Res. **32**:348A, 1984.

291. Guigon, M., and Najman, A.: The inhibitors of hematopoiesis, Int. J. Cell Cloning **6**:69, 1988.

292. Gunz, F.W., and Henderson, E.S., editors: Leukemia, New York, 1983, Grune & Stratton, Inc.

293. Haferkamp, O., Rosenau, W., and Lennert, K.: Vascular transformation of lymph node sinuses due to venous obstruction, Arch. Pathol. **92**:81, 1971.

294. Hamoudi, A.B.: Significance of X granules in histiocytosis X: an ultrastructural study, Pediatr. Pathol. **3**:93, 1985.

295. Han, T., Ozer, H., Sadamori, N., Emrich, L., Gómez, G.A., Henderson, E.S., Bloom, M.L., and Sandberg, A.A.: Prognostic importance of cytogenetic abnormalities in patients with chronic lymphocytic leukemia, N. Engl. J. Med. **310**:288, 1984.

296. Hanada, T., Ehara, T., Nakahara, S., Suzuki, T., Nagasawa, T., and Takita, H.: Simultaneous transient erythroblastopenia and agranulocytosis: IgG-mediated inhibition of erythrogranulopoiesis, Eur. J. Haematol. **35**:10, 1985.

297. Hanash, S.M., Rucknagel, D.L., Heidelberger, K.P., and Radin, N.S.: Primary amyloidosis associated with Gaucher's disease, Ann. Intern. Med. **89**:639, 1978.

298. Hanson, C.A., Frizzera, G., Patton, D.F., Peterson, B.A., McClain, K.L., Gajl-Peczalska, K.J., and Kersey, J.H.: Clonal rearrangement for immunoglobulin and T-cell receptor genes in systemic Castleman's disease, Am. J. Pathol. **131**:84, 1988.

299. Hanto, D.W., Frizzera, G., Purtilo, D.T., Sakamoto, K., Sullivan, J.L., Saemundsen, A.K., Klein, G., Simmons, R.L., and Najarian, J.S.: Clinical spectrum of lymphoproliferative disorders in renal transplant recipients and evidence for the role of Epstein-Barr virus, Cancer Res. **41**:4353, 1981.

300. Harris, N.L., and Bhan, A.K.: B-7-cell neoplasms of the lymphocytic, lymphoplasmacytoid and plasma cell types: immunohistologic analysis and clinical correlation, Hum. Pathol. **16**:829, 1985.

301. Harris, N.L., and Bhan, A.K.: Mantle-zone lymphoma: a pattern produced by lymphomas of more than one cell type, Am. J. Surg. Pathol. **9**:872, 1985.

302. Harris, N.L., Nadler, L.M., and Bhan, A.K.: Immunohistologic characterization of two malignant lymphomas of germinal center type (centroblastic/centrocytic and centrocytic) with monoclonal antibodies: follicular and diffuse lymphomas of small-cleaved-cell type are related but distinct entities, Am. J. Pathol. **117**:262, 1984.

303. Harrison, E.G., and Bernatz, P.E.: Angiofollicular mediastinal lymph node hyperplasia resembling thymoma, Arch. Pathol. **75**:284, 1963.

304. Harrison, P.R.: Analysis of erythropoiesis at the molecular level, Nature (London) **262**:353, 1976. (Review article.)

305. Hartroft, W.S., and Porta, E.A.: Ceroid, Am. J. Med. Sci. **250**:324, 1965.

306. Hartsock, R.J.: Postvaccinial lymphadenitis: hyperplasia of lymphoid tissue that simulates malignant lymphomas, Cancer **21**:632, 1968.

307. Hartsock, R.J., Halling, L.W., and King, F.M.: Luetic lymphadenitis: a clinical and histologic study of 20 cases, Am. J. Clin. Pathol. **53**:304, 1970.

308. Hartsock, R.J., Smith, E.B., and Petty, C.S.: Normal variations with aging of the amount of hematopoietic tissue in bone marrow from the anterior iliac crest: a study made from 177 cases of sudden death examined by necropsy, Am. J. Clin. Pathol. **43**:326, 1965.

309. Hata, S., Brenner, M.B., and Krangel, M.S.: Identification of putative human T cell receptor d complementary DNA clones, Science **238**:678, 1987.

310. Herbert, V.: Megaloblastic anemias, Lab. Invest. **52**:3, 1985.

311. Heyman, M.R., and Rasmussen, P.: *Pneumocystis carinii* involvement of the bone marrow in acquired immunodeficiency syndrome, Am. J. Clin. Pathol. **87**:780, 1987.

312. Hillman, R.S.: Alcohol and hematopoiesis, Ann. NY Acad. Sci. **252**:297, 1975.

313. Hirai, H., Tanaka, S., Azuma, M., Anraku, Y., Kobayashi, Y., Fujisawa, M., Okabe, T., Urabe, A., and Takaku, F.: Transforming genes in human leukemia cells, Blood **6**:1371, 1985.

314. Hirsch-Ginsberg, C., Childs, C., Chang, K.S., Beran, M., Cork, A., Reuben, J., Freireich, E.J., Chang, L.C., Bollum, F.J., Trujillo, J., et al.: Phenotypic and molecular heterogeneity in Philadelphia chromosome–positive acute leukemia, Blood **71**:186, 1988.

315. Ho, D.D., Pomerantz, R.J., and Kaplan, J.C.: Pathogenesis of infection with human immunodeficiency virus, N. Engl. J. Med. **317**:278, 1987.

316. Hoffbrand, M.A.: Megaloblastic anemia, Clin. Haematol. **5**:1, 1976.

317. Holden, C.: Oncogene action probed, Science **237**:602, 1987.

318. Hoppe, R.T., Rosenberg, S.A., Kaplan, H.S., and Cox, R.S.: Prognostic factors in pathological stage IIIA Hodgkin's disease, Cancer **46**:1240, 1980.

319. Horning, S.J., Weiss, L.M., Crabtree, G.S., and Warnke, R.A.: Clinical and phenotypic diversity of T cell lymphomas, Blood **67**:1578, 1986.

320. Hoskins, L.C., Loux, H.A., and Britten, A.: Distribution of ABO blood groups in patients with pernicious anemia, gastric carcinoma and gastric carcinoma associated with pernicious anemia, N. Engl. J. Med. **273**:633, 1965.

321. Hovde, R.F., and Sundberg, R.D.: Granulomatous lesions in the bone marrow in infectious mononucleosis, Blood **5**:209, 1950.

322. Hsu, S., and Jaffe, E.S.: Phenotypic expression of B-lymphocytes. 2. Immunoglobulin expression of germinal center cells, Am. J. Pathol. **114**:396, 1984.

323. Hsu, S., and Zhao, X.: The H-RS-like cells in infectious mononucleosis are transformed interdigitating reticulum cells, Am. J. Pathol. **127**:403, 1987.

324. Hsu, S.M, Ho, Y.S., Li, P.J., Monheit, J., Ree, H.J., Sheibani, K., and Winberg, C.D.: L&H variants of Reed-Sternberg cells express sialylated Leu M1 antigen, Am. J. Pathol. **122**:199, 1986.

325. Hsu, S., Yang, K., and Jaffe, E.S.: Phenotypic expression of Hodgkin's and Reed-Sternberg cells in Hodgkin's disease, Am. J. Pathol. **118**:209, 1985.

326. Hubbard, S.M., Chabner, B.A., DeVita, V.T., Jr., Simon, R., Berard, C.W., Jones, R.B., Garvin, A.J., Canellos, G.P., Osborne, C.K., and Young, R.C.: Histologic progression in non-Hodgkin's lymphoma, Blood **59**:258, 1982.

327. Huebner, K., Isobe, M., Croce, C.M., Golde, D.W., Kaufman, S.E., and Gasson, J.C.: The human gene encoding GM-CSF is a 5q21-q32, the chromosome region deleted in the 5q − anomaly, Science **230**:1282, 1985.

328. Huebner, R.J., and Todaro, G.J.: Oncogenes of RNA tumor viruses as determinants of cancer, Proc. Natl. Acad. Sci. USA **64**:1087, 1969.

329. Humpherys, S.R., Holley, K.E., Smith, L.H., et al.: Mesenteric angiofollicular lymph node hyperplasia (lymphoid hamartoma) with nephrotic syndrome, Mayo Clin. Proc. **50**:317, 1975.

330. Husni, E.A.: The clinical course of splenic hemangioma, Arch. Surg. **83**:57, 1961.

331. Hyman, G.A., and Sommers, S.C.: The development of Hodgkin's disease and lymphoma during anticonvulsant therapy, Blood **28**:416, 1966.

332. Hyun, B.H., Kwa, D., Gabaldon, H., et al.: Reactive plasmacytic lesions of the bone marrow, Am. J. Clin. Pathol. **65**:921, 1976.

333. Hyun, B.H., Varga, C.F., and Rubin, R.J.: Spontaneous and pathologic rupture of the spleen, Arch. Surg. **104**:652, 1972.

334. Iland, H.J., Laszlo, J., Case, D.C., Jr., Murphy, S., Reichert, T.A., Tso, C.Y., and Wasserman, L.R.: Differentiation between essential thrombocythemia and polycythemia vera with marked thrombocytosis, Am. J. Hematol. **25**:191, 1987.

335. Imamura, M., Sakamoto, S., and Hanazono, H.: Malignant histiocytosis: a case of generalized histiocytosis with infiltration of Langerhans' granule-containing histiocytes, Cancer **28**:467, 1971.

336. Imrey, H.H., and Curran, J.W.: AIDS case definition, Science **240**:1263, 1988. (Letter.)

337. International Agranulocytosis and Aplastic Anemia Study: Incidence of aplastic anemia: the relevance of diagnostic criteria, Blood **70**:1718, 1987.

338. Ioachim, H.L.: Lymph node biopsy, Philadelphia, 1982, J.B. Lippincott Co.

339. Ioachim, H.L., Cooper, M.C., and Hellman, G.C.: Lymphomas in men at high risk for acquired immune deficiency syndrome (AIDS): a study of 21 cases, Cancer **56**:2831, 1985.

340. Ioachim, H.L., Lerner, C.W., and Tapper, M.L.: The lymphoid lesions associated with the acquired immunodeficiency syndrome, Am. J. Surg. Pathol. **7**:543, 1983.

341. Isaacson, P.G.: Lymphocytic lymphoma of intermediate differentiation, Hum. Pathol. **19**:492, 1988.

342. Ishii, E., Hara, T., Okamura, J., Suda, M., Takeuchi, T., Iida, K., and Ueda, K.: Malignant histiocytosis in infants: surface marker analysis of malignant cells in two cases, Med. Pediatr. Oncol. **15**:102, 1987.

343. Jacobs, R.H., Cornbleet, M.A., Vardiman, J.W., Larson, R.A., LeBeau, M.M., and Rowley, J.D.: Prognostic implications of morphology and karyotype in primary myelodysplastic syndromes, Blood **67**:1765, 1986.

344. Jacobson, R.J., Salo, A., and Fialkow, P.J.: Agnogenic myeloid metaplasia: a clonal proliferation of hematopoietic stem cells with secondary myelofibrosis, Blood **51**:189, 1978.

345. Jaffe, E.S., Bookman, M.A., and Longo, D.L.: Lymphocytic lymphoma of intermediate differentiation—mantle zone lymphoma: a distinct subtype of B-cell lymphoma, Hum. Pathol. **18**:877, 1987.

346. Jaffe, E.S., Costa, J., Fauci, A.S., Cossman, J., and Tsokos, M.: Malignant lymphoma and erythrophagocytosis simulating malignant histiocytosis, Am. J. Med. **75**:741, 1983.

347. Jaffe, E.S., Shevach, E.M., Frank, M.M., et al.: Nodular lymphoma: evidence for origin from follicular B lymphocytes, N. Engl. J. Med. **290**:813, 1974.

348. Jaffe, E.S., Strauchen, J.A., and Berard, C.W.: Predictability of immunologic phenotype of morphologic criteria in diffuse aggressive non-Hodgkin's lymphomas, Am. J. Clin. Pathol. **77**:46, 1982.

349. Jaffe, R.: Pathology of histiocytosis X, Perspect. Pediatr. Pathol. **9**:4, 1987.

350. Jalkanen, S., Reichert, R.A., Gallatin, W.M., Bargatze, R.F., Weissman, I.L., and Butcher, E.C.: Homing receptors and the control of lymphocyte migration, Immunol. Rev. **91**:39, 1986.

351. James, D.G., and Neville, E.: Pathobiology of sarcoidosis, Pathobiol. Annu. **7**:31, 1977.

352. Jamshidi, K., and Swain, W.R.: Bone marrow biopsy with unaltered architecture: a new biopsy device, J. Lab. Clin. Med. **77**:335, 1971.

353. Janka, G.E.: Familial hemophagocytic lymphohistiocytosis: review, Eur. J. Pediatr. **27**:931, 1961.

354. Johnston, R.B., Jr.: Monocytes and macrophages, N. Engl. J. Med. **318**:747, 1988.

355. Jordan, M.C., Rousseau, W., Stewart, J.A., et al.: Spontaneous cytomegalovirus mononucleosis, Ann. Intern. Med. **79**:153, 1973.

356. Joshi, V.V., Kauffman, S., Oleske, J.M., Fikria, S., Denny, T., Gadol, C., and Lee, E.: Polyclonal polymorphic B-cell lymphoproliferative disorder with prominent pulmonary involvement in children with acquired immune deficiency syndrome, Cancer **59**:1455, 1987.

357. Juliusson, G.: Immunologic and cytogenetic studies improve prognosis prediction in chronic B-lymphocytic leukemia: a multivariate analysis of 24 variables, Cancer **58**:688, 1986.

358. Juliusson, G., and Gahrton, G.: Poor age-corrected survival of chronic lymphocytic leukaemia patients with trisomy 12, Eur. J. Haematol. **38**:315, 1987.

359. Juliusson, G., Robèrt, K.H., Ost, A., Fribera, K., Biberfeld, P., Nilsson, B., Zech, L., and Gahrton, G.: Prognostic information from cytogenetic analysis in chronic B-lymphocytic leukemia and leukemic immunocytoma, Blood **65**:134, 1985.

360. Juneja, S.K., Cooper, I.A., Hodgson, G.S., Wolf, M.M., Ding, J.C., Ironside, P.N., Thomas, R.J., and Parkin, J.D.: DNA ploidy patterns and cytokinetics of non-Hodgkin's lymphoma, J. Clin. Pathol. **39**:987, 1986.

361. Kadin, M.E., Glatstein, E., and Dorfman, R.F.: Clinicopathologic studies of 117 untreated patients subjected to laparotomy for the Hodgkin's disease, Cancer **27**:1277, 1971.

362. Kadin, M.E., Kamoun, M., and Lamberg, J.: Erythrophagocytic Ig lymphoma: a clinicopathologic entity resembling malignant histiocytosis, N. Engl. J. Med. **304**:648, 1981.

363. Kahn, L.B., and Gordon, W.: Sarcoid-like granulomas in secondary syphilis, Arch. Pathol. **92**:334, 1971.

364. Kamesaki, H., Fukuhara, S., Tatsumi, E., Uchino, H., Yamabe, H., Miwa, H., Shirakawa, S., Hatanaka, M., and Honjo, T.: Cytochemical, immunologic, chromosomal, and molecular genetic analysis of a novel cell line derived from Hodgkin's disease, Blood **68**:285, 1986.

365. Kaneko, Y., Rowley, J.D., Variakojis, D., Chilcote, R.R., Check, I., and Sakurai, M.: Correlation of karyotype with clinical features in acute lymphoblastic leukemia, Cancer Res. **42**:2918, 1982.

366. Kantarjian, H.M., Dixon, D., Keating, M.J., Talpaz, M., Walters, R.S., McCredie, K.B., and Freireich, E.J.: Characteristics of accelerated disease in chronic myelogenous leukemia, Cancer **61**:1441, 1988.

367. Kapff, C.T., and Jandl, J.H.: Blood: atlas and sourcebook of hematology, Boston, 1981, Little Brown & Co.

368. Kaplan, H.S.: Hodgkin's disease, Cambridge, 1980, Harvard University Press.

369. Karakousis, C.P., and Elias, E.G.: Spontaneous (pathologic) rupture of spleen in malignancies, Surgery **76**:674, 1974.

370. Karcher, D.S., Head, D.R., and Mullins, J.D.: Malignant histiocytosis occurring in patients with acute lymphocytic leukemia, Cancer **41**:1967, 1978.

371. Karp, L.A., and Czernobilsky, B.: Glandular inclusions in pelvic and abdominal para-aortic lymph nodes: a study of autopsy and surgical material in males and females, Am. J. Clin. Pathol. **52**:212, 1969.

372. Karpas, A., Worman, C., Arno, J., and Nagington, J.: Sinus histiocytosis with massive lymphadenopathy: virological, immunological and morphological studies, Br. J. Haematol. **45**:195, 1980.

373. Katayama, I., Nagy, G.K., and Balogh, K., Jr.: Light microscopic identification of the ribosome-lamella complex in the "hairy cells" of leukemia reticuloendotheliosis, Cancer **32**:843, 1973.

374. Katzenstein, A., Carrington, C., and Liebow, A.: Lymphomatoid granulomatosis: a clinicopathologic study of 152 cases, Cancer **43**:360, 1979.

375. Keinänen, M., Griffin, J.D., Bloomfield, C.D., Machnicki, J., and de la Chapelle, A.: Clonal chromosomal abnormalities showing multiple-cell-lineage involvement in acute leukemia, N. Engl. J. Med. **318**:1153, 1988.

376. Keller, A.R., Hochholzer, L., and Castleman, B.: Hyaline-vascular and plasma-cell types of giant lymph node hyperplasia of mediastinum and other locations, Cancer **29**:670, 1972.

377. Kelly, D.R., Nathwani, B.N., Griffith, R.C., Shuster, J.J., Sullivan, M.P., Hvizdala, E., Murphy, S.B., and Berard, C.W.: A morphologic study of childhood lymphoma of the undifferentiated type: a pediatric oncology group study, Cancer **59**:1132, 1987.

378. Kelly, K., and Siebenlist, U.: The regulation and expression of c-myc in normal and malignant cells, Annu. Rev. Immunol. **4**:317, 1986.

379. Kersey, J.H., Spector, B.D., and Good, R.S.: Primary immunodeficiency diseases and cancer: the immunodeficiency-cancer registry, Int. J. Cancer **12**:333, 1973.

380. Kevy, S.V., Tefft, M., Vawier, G.F., et al.: Hereditary splenic hypoplasia, Pediatrics **42**:752, 1968.

381. Khojasteh, A., Haghshenass, M., and Haghighi, P.: Immunoproliferative small intestinal disease: a "third-world lesion," N. Engl. J. Med. **308**:1401, 1982.

382. Kikuchi, M., Yoshizumi, T., and Nakamura, H.: Necrotizing lymphadenitis: possible acute toxoplasmic infection, Virchows Arch. [Pathol. Anat.] **376**:247, 1977.

383. Kim, H., Dorfman, R.F., and Rappaport, H.: Signet ring cell lymphoma: a rare morphologic and functional expression of nodular (follicular) lymphoma, Am. J. Surg. Pathol. **2**:119, 1978.

384. Kim, H., Heller, P., and Rappaport, H.: Monoclonal gammopathies associated with lymphoproliferative disorders: a morphologic study, Am. J. Clin. Pathol. **59**:282, 1973.

385. Kim, H., Hendrickson, M.R., and Dorfman, R.F.: Composite lymphoma, Cancer **40**:959, 1977.

386. Kinney, M.C., Greer, J.P., Stein, R.S., Collins, R.D., and Cousar, J.B.: Lymphocyte-depletion Hodgkin's disease: histopathologic diagnosis of marrow involvement, Am. J. Surg. Pathol. **10**:219, 1986.

387. Kiraly, J.F., III, and Whelby, M.S.: Bone marrow necrosis, Am. J. Med. **60**:361, 1976.

388. Kirschner, R.H., Abt, A.B., O'Connell, M.J., et al.: Vascular invasion and hematogenous dissemination of Hodgkin's disease, Cancer **34**:1159, 1974.

389. Kjeldsberg, C.R., and Kim, H.: Eosinophilic granuloma as an incidental finding in malignant lymphoma, Arch. Pathol. Lab. Med. **104**:137, 1980.

390. Kjeldsberg, C.R., Wilson, J.F., and Berard, C.S.: Non-Hodgkin's lymphoma in children, Hum. Pathol. **14**:612, 1983.

391. Klein, G.: Constitutive activation of oncogenes by chromosomal translocations in B-cell derived tumors, AIDS Res. **2**(suppl.):167, 1986.

392. Kletzel, M., Gollin, S.M., Gloster, E.S., Jiménez, J.F., Golladay, E.S., and Berry, D.H.: Chromosome abnormalities in familial hemophagocytic lymphohistiocytosis, Cancer **57**:2153, 1986.

393. Knudson, A.G., Jr.: Genetics of human cancer, Annu. Rev. Genet. **20**:231, 1986.

394. Knuttgen, H.J.: The bone marrow of non-immune Europeans in acute malaria infection: a topical review, Ann. Trop. Med. Parasitol. **81**:567, 1987.

395. Knuutila, S., Elonen, E., Teerenhovi, L., Rossi, L., Leskinen, R., Bloomfield, C.D., and de la Chapelle, A.: Trisomy 12 in B cells of patients with B-cell chronic lymphocytic leukemia, N. Engl. J. Med. **314**:865, 1986.

396. Koduru, P.R.K., Filippa, D.A., Richardson, M.E., Jhanwar, S.C., Chaganti, S.R., Koziner, B., Clarkson, B.D., Lieberman, P.H., and Chaganti, R.S.: Cytogenetic and histologic correlations in malignant lymphoma, Blood **69**:97, 1987.

397. Korsmeyer, S.J., Arnold, A., Bakhshi, A., Ravetch, J.V., Siebenlist, U., Hieter, P.A., Sharrow, S.O., LeBien, T.W., Kersey, J.H., Poplack, D.G., Leder, P., and Waldmann, T.A.: Immunoglobulin gene rearrangement and cell surface antigen expression in acute lymphocytic leukemias of T cell and B cell precursor origins, J. Clin. Invest. **71**:301, 1983.

398. Krajny, M., and Pruzanski, W.: Waldenström's macroglobulinemia: review of 45 cases, Can. Med. Assoc. J. **114**:899, 1976.

399. Krause, J.R.: Value of bone marrow biopsy in the diagnosis of amyloidosis, South. Med. J. **70**:1072, 1977.

400. Krause, J.R.: An appraisal of the value of the bone marrow biopsy in the assessment of proliferative lesions of the bone marrow, Histopathology **7**:627, 1983.

401. Kundel, D.W., Brecher, G., Bodey, G.P., et al.: Reticulin fibrosis and bone infarction in acute leukemia: implications for prognosis, Blood **23**:526, 1964.

402. Kuo, T., and Rosai, J.: Granulomatous inflammation in splenectomy specimens, Arch. Pathol. **98**:261, 1974.

403. Kurnick, J.E., Ward, H.P., and Block, M.H.: Bone marrow sections in the differential diagnosis of polycythemia, Arch. Pathol. **94**:489, 1972.

404. Kyle, R.A.: Multiple myeloma: review of 869 cases, Mayo Clin. Proc. **50**:29, 1975.

405. Kyle, R.A.: Plasma cell leukemia, Ann. Intern. Med. **133**:813, 1974.

406. Lacombe, C., Casadevall, N., Muller, O., and Varet, B.: Erythroid progenitors in adult chronic pure red cell aplasia: relationship of in vitro erythroid colonies to therapeutic response, Blood **64**:71, 1984.

407. Land, H., Parada, L.F., and Weinberg, R.A.: Cellular oncogenes and multistep carcinogenesis, Science **222**:771, 1983.

408. Landing, B.H.: Lymphohistiocytosis in childhood: pathologic comparison with fatal Letterer-Siwe disease (disseminated visceral histiocytosis X), Perspect. Pediatr. Pathol. **9**:48, 1987.

409. Langdon, W.Y., Harris, A.W., Cory, S., and Adams, J.M.: The c-myc oncogene perturbs B lymphocyte development in Eu-myc transgenic mice, Cell **47**:11, 1986.

410. Laszlo, J.: Myeloproliferative disorders (MPD): myelofibrosis, myelosclerosis, extramedullary hematopoiesis, undifferentiated MPD, and hemorrhagic thrombocythemia, Semin. Hematol. **12**:409, 1975.

411. Layton, D.M., and Mufti, G.J.: Myelodysplastic syndromes: their history, evolution and relation to acute myeloid leukaemia, Blut **53**:423, 1986.

412. LeBeau, M.M., Albain, K.S., Larson, R.A., Vardiman, J.W., Davis, E.M., Blough, R.R., Golomb, H.M., and Rowley, J.D.: Clinical and cytogenetic correlations in 63 patients with therapy-related myelodysplastic syndromes and acute nonlymphocytic leukemia: further evidence for characteristic abnormalities of chromosome Nos. 5 and 7, J. Clin. Oncol. **4**:325, 1986.

413. LeTourneau, A., Audouin, J., Diebold, J., Marche, C., Tricottet, V., and Regnes, M.: LAV-like viral particles in lymph node germinal centers in patients with the persistent lymphadenopathy syndrome and the acquired immunodeficiency syndrome–related complex: an ultrastructural study of 30 cases, Hum. Pathol. **17**:1047, 1986.

414. Lebovitz, R.M.: Oncogenes as mediators of cell growth and differentiation, Lab. Invest. **55**:249, 1986.

415. Lee, E.J., Pollak, A., Leavitt, R.D., Testa, J.R., and Schiffer, C.A.: Minimally differentiated acute nonlymphocytic leukemia: a distinct entity, Blood **70**:1400, 1987.

416. Lee, M.S., Chang, K.S., Cabanillas, F., Freireich, E.J., Trujillo, J.M., and Stass, S.A.: Detection of minimal residual cells carrying the t(14;18) by DNA sequence amplification, Science **237**:175, 1987.

417. Lee, M.S., Blick, M.B., Pathak, S., Trujillo, J.M., Butler, J.J., Katz, R.L., McLaughlin, P., Hagemeister, F.B., Velasquez, W.S., Goodacre, A., et al.: The gene located at chromosome 18 band q21 is rearranged in uncultured diffuse lymphomas as well as follicular lymphomas, Blood **70**:90, 1987.

418. Lee, M., Segal, G.M., and Bagby, G.C.: Interleukin-1 induces human bone marrow–derived fibroblasts to produce multilineage hematopoietic growth factors, Exp. Hematol. **15**:983, 1987.

419. Lee, R.E., and Ellis, L.D.: The storage cells of chronic myelogenous leukemia, Lab. Invest. **24**:261, 1971.

420. Lennert, K., and Parwaresch, M.R.: Mast cells and mast cell neoplasia: a review, Histopathology **3**:349, 1979.

421. Lennert, K., and Hansmann, M.L.: Progressive transformation of germinal centers: clinical significance and lymphocytic predominance Hodgkin's disease—the Kiel experience, Am. J. Surg. Pathol. **11**:149, 1987.

422. Levine, E.G., Arthur, D.C., Frizzera, G., Peterson, B.A., Hurd, D.D., and Bloomfield, C.D.: There are differences in cytogenetic abnormalities among histologic subtypes of the non-Hodgkin's lymphomas, Blood **66**:1414, 1985.

423. Levy, N., Nelson, J., Meyer, P., Lukes, R.J., and Parker, J.W.: Reactive lymphoid hyperplasia with single class (monoclonal) surface immunoglobulin, Am. J. Clin. Pathol. **80**:300, 1983.

424. Lewin, K.J., Kahn, L.B., and Novis, B.H.: Primary intestinal lymphoma of "Western" and "Mediterranean" type, alpha chain disease and massive plasma cell infiltration: a comparative study of 37 cases, Cancer **38**:2511, 1976.

425. Lewy, R.I., Kansu, E., and Gazbuda, T.: Leukemia in patients with acquired idiopathic sideroblastic anemia: an evaluation of prognostic indicators, Am. J. Hematol. **6**:323, 1979.

426. Liang, D., Shen, E., and Chyou, S.: To early distinguish neonatal transient leukemoid proliferation from congenital leukemia by in vitro cell growth, Blut **53**:101, 1986.

427. Liang, J.C., Chang, K.S., Schroeder, W.T., Freireich, E.J., Stass, S.A., and Trujillo, J.M.: The myloperoxidase gene is translocated from chromosome 17 to 15 in a patient with acute promyelocytic leukemia, Cancer Genet. Cytogenet. **30**:103, 1988.

428. Li, F.P., Willard, D.R., Goodman, R., et al.: Malignant lymphoma after diphenylhydantoin (Dilantin) therapy, Cancer **36**:1359, 1975.

429. Lichtenstein, L.: Histiocytosis X: integration of eosinophilic granuloma of bone marrow, Letterer-Siwe disease and Schüller-Christian disease as related manifestations of a single nosologic entity, Arch. Pathol. **56**:84, 1953.

430. Lidbeck, J.: Studies on hemopoietic dysplasia (the preleukemic syndrome), Acta Med. Scand. **208**:459, 1980.

431. Lieberman, P.H., Jones, C.R., Dargeon, H.W., et al.: A reappraisal of eosinophilic granuloma of bone, Hand-Schüller-Christian syndrome and Letterer-Siwe syndrome, Medicine **48**:375, 1969.

432. Lieberman, P.H., Filippa, D.A., Straus, D.J., Thaler, H.T., Cirrincione, C., and Clarkson, B.D.: Evaluation of malignant lymphomas using three classifications and the Working Formulation: 482 cases with median follow-up of 11.9 years, Am. J. Med. **81**:365, 1986.

433. Lindenbaum, J.: Aspects of vitamin B_{12} and folate metabolism in malabsorption syndromes, Am. J. Med. **67**:1037, 1979.

434. Linder, J., Ye, Y.L., Harrington, D.S., Armitage, J.O., and Weisenburger, D.D.: Monoclonal antibodies marking T lymphocytes in paraffin-embedded tissue, Am. J. Pathol. **127**:1, 1987.

435. Link, M.P., Roper, M., Dorfman, R.F., Crist, W.M., Cooper, M.D., and Levy, R.: Cutaneous lymphoblastic lymphoma with pre-B markers, Blood **61**:838, 1983.

436. Linman, J.W., and Bagby, J.C.: The preleukemic syndrome (hemopoietic syndrome), Cancer **42**:854, 1978.

437. Lipper, S., and Kahn, L.B.: Amyloid tumor: a clinicopathologic study of four cases, Am. J. Surg. Pathol. **2**:141, 1978.

438. Lippman, S.M., Volk, J.R., Spier, C.M., and Grogan, T.M.: Clonal ambiguity of human immunodeficiency virus–associated lymphomas, Arch. Pathol. Lab. Med. **112**:128, 1988.

439. Lippman, S.M., Grogan, T.M., Spier, C.M., Koopmann, C.F., Jr., Gall, E.P., Shimm, D.S., and Durie, B.G.: Lethal midline granuloma with a novel T-cell phenotype as found in peripheral T-cell lymphoma, Cancer **59**:936, 1987.

440. Lipshutz, M.D., Mir, R., Rai, K.R., and Sawitsky, A.: Bone marrow biopsy and clinical staging in chronic lymphocytic leukemia, Cancer **46**:1422, 1980.

441. Lombardi, L., Newcomb, E.W., and Dalla-Favera, R.: Pathogenesis of Burkitt lymphoma: expression of an activated c-*myc* oncogene causes the tumorigenic conversion of EBV-infected human B lymphoblasts, Cell **49**:161, 1987.

442. Long, J.C., and Aisenberg, A.C.: Malignant lymphoma diagnosed at splenectomy and idiopathic splenomegaly: a clinicopathologic comparison, Cancer **33**:1054, 1974.

443. Long, J.C., and Aisenberg, A.C.: Richter's syndrome: a terminal complication of chronic lymphocytic leukemia with distinct clinicopathologic features, Am. J. Clin. Pathol. **63**:786, 1975.

444. Longo, D.L., Steis, R.G., Lane, H.C., Lotze, M.T., Rosenberg, S.A., Preble, O., Masur, H., Rook, A.H., Fauci, A.S., Jacob, J., et al.: Malignancies in the AIDS patient: natural history, treatment strategies and preliminary results, Ann. NY Acad. Sci. **437**:421, 1984.

445. Lowenthal, D.A., Straus, D.J., Campbell, S.W., Gold, J.W., Clarkson, B.D., and Koziner, B.: AIDS-related lymphoid neoplasia: the Memorial Hospital experience, Cancer **61**:2325, 1988.

446. Lui, K., Darrow, W.W., and Rutherford, G.W.: A model-based estimate of the mean incubation period for AIDS in homosexual men, Science **240**:1333, 1988.

447. Lukes, R.J.: Criteria for involvement of lymph node, bone marrow, spleen, and liver in Hodgkin's disease, Cancer Res. **31**:1755, 1971.

448. Lukes, R.J., and Butler, J.J.: The pathology and nomenclature of Hodgkin's disease, Cancer Res. **26**:1063, 1966.

449. Lukes, R.J., and Collins, R.D.: Immunological characterization of human malignant lymphomas, Cancer **34**:1488, 1974.

450. Lukes, R.J., and Tindle, B.H.: Immunoblastic lymphadenopathy: a hyperimmune entity resembling Hodgkin's disease, N. Engl. J. Med. **292**:1, 1975.

451. Lukes, R.J., Butler, J.J., and Hicks, E.B.: Natural history of Hodgkin's disease as related to its pathologic picture, Cancer **19**:317, 1966.

452. Lum, L.G., Seigneuret, M.C., Doney, K.C., and Storb, R.: In vitro immunoglobulin production, proliferation, and cell markers before and after antithymocyte globulin therapy in patients with aplastic anemia, Am. J. Hematol. **26**:1, 1987.

453. Luscieti, P., Hubschmid, T., Cottier, H., Hess, M.W., and Sobin, L.H.: Human lymph node morphology as a function of age and site, J. Clin. Pathol. **33**:454, 1980.

454. Manconi, R., Poletti, A., Volpe, R., Carbone, A., and de Paoli, P.: Mantle-zone lymphoma: additional arguments for its origin, Am. J. Surg. Pathol. **11**:333, 1987. (Letter.)

455. MacKenzie, M.R., and Fudenberg, H.H.: Macroglobulinemia: an analysis of forty patients, Blood **39**:874, 1972.

456. Mahmoud, L.A., Block, M.H., Franks, J.J., and Sayed, N.M.: Marrow biopsy and survival in multiple myeloma, Am. J. Clin. Pathol. **80**:363, 1983.

457. Mann, D.L., De Santis, P., Mark, G., Pfeifer, A., Newman, M., Gibbs, N., Popovic, M., Sarngadharan, M.G., Gallo, R.C., Clark, J., et al.: HTLV-1–associated B-cell CLL: indirect role for retrovirus in leukemogenesis, Science **236**:1103, 1987.

458. Mann, R.B., and Berard, C.W.: Criteria for the cytologic subclassification of follicular lymphomas: a proposed alternative method, Hematol. Oncol. **1**:187, 1982.

459. Margileth, A.M.: Cat scratch disease: nonbacterial regional lymphadenitis: the study of 145 patients and a review of the literature, Pediatrics **42**:803, 1968.

460. Mark, T., and Levin, A.: Histologic examination of the bone marrow: aspiration of trephine? South. Med. J. **74**:1447, 1981.

461. Markgraf, R., von Gaudecker, B., and Müller-Hermelink, H.K.: The development of the human lymph node, Cell Tissue Res. **225**:387, 1982.

462. Marsh, W.L., Jr., Lew, S.W., Heath, V.C., and Lightsey, A.L.: Congenital self-healing histiocytosis-X, Am. J. Pediatr. Hematol. Oncol. **5**:227, 1983.

463. Martin, N.H.: Macroglobulinaemia: a clinical and pathological study, Q. J. Med. **114**:179, 1960.

464. Marx, J.L.: Oncogenes amplified in cancer cells, Science **223**:40, 1984.

465. Mason, T.E., Demaree, R.S., Jr., and Margolis, C.I.: Granulocytic sarcoma (chloroma), two years preceding myelogenous leukemia, Cancer **31**:423, 1973.

466. McCarthy, D.M.: Fibrosis of the bone marrow: content and causes, Br. J. Hematol. **59**:1, 1985.

467. McGlave, P.B., Haake, R., Miller, W., Kim, T., Kersey, J., and Ramsay, N.K.: Therapy of severe aplastic anemia in young adults and children with allogeneic bone marrow transplantation, Blood **70**:1325, 1987.

468. McKenna, R.W., Risdall, R.J., and Brunning, R.D.: Virus associated hemophagocytic syndrome, Hum. Pathol. **12**:395, 1981.

469. McMahon, N.J., Gordon, H.W., and Rosen, R.B.: Reed-Sternberg cells in infectious mononucleosis, Am. J. Dis. Child. **120**:148, 1970.

470. Medeiros, L.J., Strickler, J.G., Picker, L.J., Gelb, A.B., Weiss, L.M., and Warnke, R.A.: "Well-differentiated" lymphocytic neoplasms: immunologic findings correlated with clinical presentation and morphologic features, Am. J. Pathol. **129**:523, 1987.

471. Mendelsohn, G., Eggleston, J.C., and Mann, R.B.: Relationship of lysozyme (muramidase) to histiocytic differentiation in malignant histiocytosis: an immunohistochemical study, Cancer **45**:273, 1980.

472. Mendez, R., and Morrow, J.W.: Ectopic spleen simulating testicular tumor, J. Urol. **102**:598, 1969.

473. Mertelsmann, R., Tzvi Thaler, H., To, L., Gee, T.S., McKenzie, S., Schaver, P., Friedman, A., Arlin, Z., Cirrincione, C., and Clarkson, B.: Morphological classification, response to therapy, and survival in 263 adult patients with acute nonlymphoblastic leukemia, Blood **56**:773, 1980.

474. Messner, H.A., Fauser, A.A., Curtis, J.E., and Dotten, D.:

Control of antibody-mediated pure red-cell aplasia by plasmapheresis, N. Engl. J. Med. **304:**1334, 1981.

475. Metcalf, D.: The molecular biology and functions of the granulocyte-macrophage colony-stimulating factors, Blood **67:**257, 1986.

476. Meyer, J.E., and Schulz, M.D.: "Solitary" myeloma of bone: a review of 12 cases, Cancer **34:**438, 1974.

477. Meyer, J.S., and Higa, E.: S-phase fractions of cells in lymph nodes and malignant lymphomas, Arch. Pathol. Lab. Med. **103:**93, 1979.

478. Michalek, H., and Henzan, E.: Necrotizing pseudolymphomatous lymphadenitis and rapidly fetal lymphoma in Okinawa, Histopathology **7:**209, 1983.

479. Michels, T.C.: Mucocutaneous lymph node syndrome in adults: differentiation from toxic shock syndrome, Am. J. Med. **80:**724, 1986.

480. Mierau, G.W., Favara, B.E., and Brenman, J.M.: Electron microscopy in histiocytosis X, Ultrastruct. Pathol. **3:**137, 1982.

481. Miettinen, M.: Histological differential diagnosis between lymph node toxoplasmosis and other benign lymph node hyperplasias, Histopathology **5:**205, 1981.

482. Miettinen, M., and Franssila, K.: Malignant lymphoma simulating lymph node toxoplasmosis, Histopathology **6:**129, 1982.

483. Mihm, M.C., Jr., Clark, W.H., and Reed, R.J.: The histocytic infiltrates of the skin, Hum. Pathol. **5:**45, 1974.

484. Miller, J.B., Testa, J.R., Lindgren, V., and Rowley, J.D.: The pattern and clinical significance of karyotypic abnormalities in patients with idiopathic and postpolycythemic myelofibrosis, Cancer **55:**582, 1985.

485. Miller-Catchpole, R., Variakojis, D., Vardiman, J.W., Loew, J.M., and Carter, J.: Cat scratch disease: identification of bacteria in seven cases of lymphadenitis, Am. J. Surg. Pathol. **10:**276, 1986.

486. Mintzer, D.M., and Hauptman, S.P.: Lymphosarcoma cell leukemia and other non-Hodgkin's lymphomas in leukemic phase, Am. J. Med. **75:**110, 1983.

487. Modlin, R.L., Meyer, P.R., Hofman, E.M., Mehlmauer, M., Levy, N.B., Lukes, R.J., Parker, J.W., Ammann, A.J., Conant, M.A., Rea, T.H., and Taylor, C.R.: T-lymphocyte subsets in lymph nodes from homosexual men, JAMA **250:**1302, 1983.

488. Moller, J.H., Nakib, A., Anderson, R.C., et al.: Congenital cardiac disease associated with polysplenia: a development complex of bilateral "left-sidedness," Circulation **36:**789, 1967.

489. Moloney, W.C.: Chronic myelogenous leukemia, Cancer **42:**865, 1978.

490. Monie, I.W.: The asplenia syndrome: an explanation for absence of the spleen, Teratology **25:**215, 1982.

491. Montserrat, E., and Rozman, C.: Bone marrow biopsy in chronic lymphocytic leukemia: a review of its prognostic importance, Blood Cells **12:**315, 1987.

492. Moore, D.F., Migliore, P.J., Schullenberger, C.C., et al.: Monoclonal macroglobulinemia in malignant lymphoma, Ann. Intern. Med. **72:**43, 1970.

493. Morgan, R., Hecht, F., Cleary, M.L., Sklar, J., and Link, M.P.: Leukemia with Down's syndrome: translocation between chromosomes 1 and 19 in acute myelomonocytic leukemia following transient congenital myeloproliferative syndrome, Blood **66:**1466, 1985.

494. Murphy, S.B.: Classification, staging and end results of treatment of childhood non-Hodgkin's lymphomas: dissimilarities from lymphomas in adults, Semin. Oncol. **7:**332, 1980.

495. Myers, C.E., Chabner, B.A., Devita, V.T., et al.: Bone marrow involvement in Hodgkin's disease: pathology and response to MOPP chemotherapy, Blood **44:**197, 1974.

496. Myers, J., and Segal, R.J.: Weight of the spleen. I. Range of normal in a nonhospital population, Arch. Pathol. **98:**33, 1974.

497. Naeim, F., Waisman, J., and Coulson, W.F.: Hodgkin's disease: the significance of vascular invasion, Cancer **34:**655, 1974.

498. Neame, P.B., Soamboosrup, P., Browman, G.P., Meyer, R.M., Benger, A., Wilson, W.E., Waker, I.R., Saeed, N., and McBride, J.A.: Classifying acute luekmia by immunophenotyping: a combined FAB-immunologic classification of AML, Blood **68:**1355, 1986.

499. Namiki, T.S., Boone, D.C., and Meyer, P.R.: A comparison of bone marrow findings in patients with acquired immunodeficiency syndrome (AIDS) and AIDS related conditions, Hematol. Oncol. **5:**99, 1987.

500. Nanba, K., Jaffe, E.S., Braylan, R.C., Soban, E.J., and Berard, C.W.: Alkaline phosphatase–positive malignant lymphoma: a subtype of B-cell lymphomas, Am. J. Clin. Pathol. **68:**535, 1977.

501. Nanba, K., Jaffe, E.S., Soban, E.J., et al.: Hairy cell leukemia: enzyme histochemical characterization, with special reference to splenic stromal changes, Cancer **39:**2323, 1977.

502. Nanba, K., Soban, E.J., Bowling, M.C., et al.: Splenic pseudosinuses and hepatic angiomatous lesions: distinctive features of hairy cell leukemia, Am. J. Clin. Pathol. **67:**415, 1977.

503. Nasr, S.A., Brynes, R.K., Garrison, C.P., and Chan, W.C.: Peripheral T-cell lymphoma in a patient with acquired immune deficiency syndrome, Cancer **61:**947, 1988.

504. Nassar, V.H., Salem, P.A., Shahid, M.J., Alami, S.Y., Balikian, J.B., Salem, A.A., and Nasrallah, S.M.: "Mediterranean abdominal lymphoma" or immunoproliferative small intestinal disease. Part II. Pathological aspects, Cancer **41:**1340, 1978.

505. Nathwani, B.N.: A critical analysis of the classifications of non-Hodgkin's lymphomas, Cancer **44:**347, 1979.

506. Nathwani, B.N.: Classifying non-Hodgkin's lymphomas. In Berard, C.W., Dorfman, R.F., and Kaufman, N., editors: Malignant lymphoma, Baltimore, 1987, The Williams & Wilkins Co.

507. Nathwani, B.N., Griffith, R.C., Kelly, D.R., Shuster, J.J., Hvizdala, E., Sullivan, M.P., Murphy, S.B., and Berard, C.W.: A morphologic study of childhood lymphoma of the diffuse "histiocytic" type: the Pediatric Oncology Group experience, Cancer **58:**1138, 1987.

508. Nathwani, B.N., Diamond, L.W., Winberg, C.D., Kim, H., Bearman, R.U., Glick, J.H., Jones, S.E., Gams, R.A., Nissen, N.I., and Rappaport, H.: Lymphoblastic lymphoma: a clinicopathologic study of 95 patients, Cancer **48:**2347, 1981.

509. Nathwani, B.N., Rappaport, H., Moran, E.M., Pangalis, G.A., and Kim, H.: Malignant lymphomas arising in angioimmunoblastic lymphadenopathy, Cancer **41:**578, 1978.

510. Nathwani, B.N., Metter, G.E., Gams, R.A., Bartolucci, A.A., Hartsock, R.J., Neiman, R.S., Bryne, G.E., Jr., Barcos, M., Kim, H., and Rappaport, H.: Malignant lymphoma, mixed cell type, diffuse, Blood **62:**200, 1983.

511. Nathwani, B.N., Winberg, C.D., Diamond, L.W., Bearman, R.M., and Kim, H.: Morphologic criteria for the differentiation of follicular lymphoma from florid reactive follicular hyperplasia: a study of 80 cases, Cancer **48:**1794, 1981.

512. Nathwani, B.N., Metter, G.E., Miller, T.P., Burke, J.S., Mann, R.B., Barcos, M., Kjeldsberg, C.R., Dixon, D.O., Winberg, C.D., Whitcomb, C.C., et al.: What should be the morphologic criteria for the subdivision of follicular lymphomas? Blood **68:**837, 1986.

513. Needleman, S.W., Burns, C.P., Dick, F.R., and Armitage, J.O.: Hypoplastic acute leukemia, Cancer **48:**1410, 1981.

514. Neiman, R.S.: Incidence and importance of splenic sarcoid-like granulomas, Arch. Pathol. Lab. Med. **101:**518, 1977.

515. Neiman, R.S., Rosen, P.J., and Lukes, R.J.: Lymphocyte-depletion Hodgkin's disease: a clinicopathologic entity, N. Engl. J. Med. **288:**751, 1973.

516. Neiman, R.S., Sullivan, A.L., and Jaffe, R.: Malignant lymphoma simulating leukemic reticuloendotheliosis: a clinicopathologic study of ten cases, Cancer **43:**329, 1979.

517. Nesbit, M.E., Jr., O'Leary, M., Dehner, L.P., and Ramsay, N.K.: Histiocytosis, continued: the immune system and the histiocytosis syndromes, Am. J. Pediatr. Hematol. Oncol. **3:**141, 1981.

518. Newland, J.R, Linke, R.P., and Lennert, K.: Amyloid deposits in lymph nodes: a morphologic and immunohistochemical study, Hum. Pathol. **17:**1245, 1986.

519. Nezelof, C., and Barbey, S.: Histiocytosis: nosology and pathobiology, Pediatr. Pathol. **3:**1, 1985.

520. Nezelof, C., Basset, F., and Rousseau, M.F.: Histiocytosis X: histogenetic arguments for a Langerhans' cell origin, Biomedicine **18:**365, 1973.

521. Nezelof, C., Frileux-Herbet, F., and Cronier-Sachot, J.: Dis-

seminated histiocytosis X: analysis of prognostic factors based on a retrospective study of 50 cases, Cancer **44**:1824, 1979.

522. Nimer, S.D., and Golde, D.W.: The 5q− abnormality, Blood **70**:1705, 1987.

523. Ng, C.S., and Chan, J.K.C.: Monocytoid B-cell lymphoma, Hum. Pathol. **18**:1069, 1987.

524. Niji, A.F., Carbonell, F., and Barker, H.T.: Cat scratch disease: a report of three new cases, review of the literature, and classification of the pathologic changes in the lymph nodes during various stages of the disease, Am. J. Clin. Pathol. **38**:513, 1962.

525. Norton, A.J., and Isaacson, P.G.: Detailed phenotypic analysis of B-cell lymphoma using a panel of antibodies reactive in routinely fixed wax-embedded tissue, Am. J. Pathol. **128**:225, 1987.

526. Nosanchuk, J.S., and Schnitzer, B.: Follicular hyperplasia in lymph nodes from patients with rheumatoid arthritis: a clinicopathologic study, Cancer **24**:343, 1969.

527. Nossal, G.J.V., Abbot, A., and Mitchell, J.: Antigens in immunity. XV. Ultrastructural features of antigen capture in primary and secondary lymphoid follicles, J. Exp. Med. **127**:277, 1968.

528. Nowell, P.C., and Hungerford, D.A.: A minute chromosome in human chronic granulocytic leukemia, Science **132**:1497, 1960.

529. O'Carroll, D.I., McKenna, R.W., and Brunning, R.: Bone marrow manifestations of Hodgkin's disease, Cancer **38**:1717, 1976.

530. O'Connell, M.J., Schimpff, S.C., Kirschner, R.H., et al.: Epithelioid granulomas in Hodgkin disease: a favorable prognostic sign? JAMA **233**:886, 1975.

531. O'Hara, C.J., Said, J.W., and Pinkus, G.S.: Non-Hodgkin's lymphoma, multilobated B-cell type: report of nine cases with immunohistochemical and immunoultrastructural evidence for a follicular center cell derivation, Hum. Pathol. **17**:593,1986.

532. O'Murchadha, M.T., Wolf, B.C., and Neiman, R.S.: The histologic features of hyperplastic lymphadenopathy in AIDS-related complex are nonspecific, Am. J. Surg. Pathol. **11**:94, 1987.

533. Okun, D.B., Sun, N.C.J., and Tanaka, K.R.: Bone marrow granulomas in Q fever, Am. J. Clin. Pathol. **71**:117, 1979.

534. Omenn, G.S.: Familial reticuloendotheliosis with eosinophilia, N. Engl. J. Med. **273**:427, 1965.

535. Osborne, B.M., Butler, J.J., and Mackay, B.: Sinusoidal large cell ("histiocytic") lymphoma, Cancer **46**:2484, 1980.

536. Osborne, B.M., MacKay, B., Butler, J.J., and Ordóñez, N.G.: Large cell lymphoma with microvillus-like projections: an ultrastructural study, Am. J. Clin. Pathol. **79**:443, 1983.

537. Osborne, B.M., Hagemeister, F.B., and Butler, J.J.: Extranodal gastrointestinal sinus histiocytosis with massive lymphadenopathy: clinically presenting as a malignant tumor, Am. J. Surg. Pathol. **5**:603, 1981.

538. Otrakji, C.L., Voight, W., Amador, A., Nadji, M., and Gregorios, J.B.: Malignant angioendotheliomatosis—a true lymphoma: a case of intravascular malignant lymphomatosis studied by Southern blot hybridization analysis, Hum. Pathol. **19**:475, 1988.

539. Pangalis, G.A., Moran, E.M., Nathwani, B.N., Zelman, R.J., Kim, H., and Rappaport, H.: Angioimmunoblastic lymphadenopathy: long-term follow-up study, Cancer **52**:318, 1983.

540. Pangalis, G.A., Roussou, P.A., Kittas, C., Mitsoulis-Mentzikoff, C., Matsouka-Alexandridis, P., Anagnostopoulos, N., Rombos, I., and Fessas, P.: Patterns of bone marrow involvement in chronic lymphocytic leukemia and small lymphocytic (well differentiated) non-Hodgkin's lymphoma: its clinical significance in relation to their differential diagnosis and prognosis, Cancer **54**:702, 1984.

541. Pangalis, G.A., Nathwani, B.N., and Rappaport, H.: Malignant lymphoma, well differentiated lymphocytic: its relationship with chronic lymphocytic leukemia and macroglobulinemia of Waldenström, Cancer **39**:999, 1977.

542. Parkman, R.: The application of bone marrow transplantation to the treatment of genetic diseases, Science **232**:1373, 1986.

543. Patsouris, E., Noel, H., and Lennert, K.: Histiological and immunohistological findings in lymphoepithelioid cell lymphoma (Lennert's lymphoma), Am. J. Surg. Pathol. **12**:341, 1988.

544. Patterson, S.D., Larson, E.B., and Corey, L.: Atypical generalized zoster with lymphadenitis mimicking lymphoma, N. Engl. J. Med. **302**:848, 1980.

545. Pavlova, Z., Parker, J.W., Taylor, C.R., Levine, A.M., Feinstein, D.I., and Lukes, R.J.: Small noncleaved follicular center cell lymphoma: Burkitt's and non-Burkitt's variants in the US. II. Pathologic and immunologic features, Cancer **59**:1892, 1987.

546. Pease, G.L.: Granulomatous lesions in bone marrow, Blood **11**:720, 1956.

547. Pedersen-Bjergaard, J., and Larsen, S.O.: Incidence of acute nonlymphocytic leukemia, preleukemia, and acute myeloproliferative syndrome up to 10 years after treatment of Hodgkin's disease, N. Engl. J. Med. **307**:965, 1982.

548. Pedersen-Bjergaard, J., Andersson, P., and Philip, P.: Possible pathogenetic significance of specific chromosome abnormalities and activated proto-oncogenes in malignant diseases of man, Scand. J. Haematol. **36**:127, 1986.

549. Pederson-Bjergaard, J., Osterlind, K., Hansen, M., Philip, P., Pedersen, A.G., and Hansen, H.H.: Acute nonlymphocytic leukemia, preleukemia and solid tumors following extensive chemotherapy of small cell carcinoma of the lung, Blood **66**:1393, 1985.

550. Pegoraro, L., Palumbo, A., Erikson, J., Falda, M., Giovanazzo, B., Emanuel, B.S., Rovera, G., Nowell, P.C., and Croce, C.M.: A 14;18 and an 8;14 chromosome translocation in a cell line derived from an acute B-cell leukemia, Proc. Natl. Acad. Sci. USA **81**:7166, 1984.

551. Pérez, M.A.: Portal hypertension of splenic origin, Am. J. Dig. Dis. **6**:780, 1961.

552. Peters, S.P., Lee, R.E., and Glew, R.H.: Gaucher's disease: a review, Medicine **56**:425, 1977.

553. Petersen, J.M., Tubbs, R.R., Savage, R.A., Calabrese, L.C., Proffitt, M.R., Manolova, Y., Manolova, G., Shumaker, A., Tatsumi, E., McClain, K., et al.: Small noncleaved B cell Burkitt-type lymphoma with chromosome t(8;14) translocation and carrying Epstein-Barr virus in a male homosexual with the acquired immune deficiency syndrome, Am. J. Med. **78**:141, 1985.

554. Petz, L.D.: Drug-induced immune hemolysis, N. Engl. J. Med. **313**:510, 1985.

555. Pierce, J.R., Jr., Wren, M.V., and Cousar, J.B., Jr.: Cholesterol embolism: diagnosis and antemortem by bone marrow biopsy, Ann. Intern. Med. **89**:937, 1978.

556. Pileri, S., Kikuchi, M., Helbron, D., and Lennert, K.: Histiocytic necrotizing lymphadenitis without granulocytic infiltration, Virchows Arch. [Pathol. Anat.] **395**:257, 1982.

557. Pimental, E.: Oncogenes and human cancer, Cancer Genet. Cytogenet. **14**:347, 1985.

558. Pines, A., Ben-Bassat, I., Modan, M., Blumstein, T., and Ramot, B.: Survival and prognostic factors in chronic lymphocytic leukaemia, Eur. J. Haematol. **38**:123, 1987.

559. Pinkhas, J., Djaldetti, M., and Yaron, M.: Coincidence of multiple myeloma with Gaucher's disease, Israel J. Med. Sci. **1**:537, 1965.

560. Pinkus, G.S., and Said, J.W.: Hodgkin's disease, lymphocyte predominance type, nodular—a distinct entity? Unique staining profile for L&H variants of Reed-Sternberg cells defined by monoclonal antibodies to leukocyte common antigen, granulocyte-specific antigen, and B-cell-specific antigen, Am. J. Pathol. **118**:1, 1985.

561. Pinkus, G.S., and Said, J.W.: Specific identification of intracellular immunoglobulin in paraffin sections of multiple myeloma and macroglobulinemia using an immunoperoxidase technique, Am. J. Pathol. **87**:47, 1977.

562. Pinkus, G.S., Thomas, P., and Said, J.W.: Leu-M1—a marker for Reed-Sternberg cells in Hodgkin's disease, Am. J. Pathol. **119**:244, 1985.

563. Pittman, S., and Catovsky, D.: Prognostic significance of chromosome abnormalities in chronic lymphocytic leukaemia, Br. J. Haematol. **58**:649, 1984.

564. Platanias, L., Gascon, P., Bielory, L., Griffith, P., Nienhaus, A., and Young, N.: Lymphocytic phenotype and lymphokines following anti-thymocyte globulin therapy in patients with aplastic anaemia, Br. J. Haematol. **66**:437, 1987.

565. Polhemus, D.W., and Koch, R.: Leukemia and medical radiation, Pediatrics **23**:453, 1959.

566. Polli, N., O'Brien, M., Tavares de Castro, J., Matutes, E., San

Miguel, J.F., and Catovsky, D.: Characterization of blast cells in chronic granulocytic leukaemia. I. Ultrastructural morphology and cytochemistry, Br. J. Haematol. **59**:277, 1985.

567. Polonovski, C., Seligmann, M., Zittoun, R., Navarro, J., and Saada, R.: Réticulose familiale chronique à forme hépatosplénoadénomégalique, Pédiatrie **23**:81, 1968.

568. Pootrakul, P., Kitcharoen, K., Yansakon, P., Wasi, P., Fucharoen, S., Charoenlarp, P., Brittenham, G., Pippard, M.J., and Finch, C.A.: The effect of erythroid hyperplasia on iron balance, Blood **71**:1124, 1988.

569. Popovic, M., Flomenberg, N., Volkman, D.J., Mann, D., Fauci, A.S., Dupont, B., and Gallo, R.C.: Alteration of T-cell functions by infection with HTLV-1 or HTLV-II, Science **226**:459, 1984.

570. Poppema, S., Kaiserling, E., and Lennert, K.: Hodgkin's disease with lymphocytic predominance, nodular type (nodular paragranuloma) and progressively transformed germinal centres: a cytohistological study, Histopathology **3**:295, 1979.

571. Pratt, P.W., Estren, S., and Kochwa, S.: Immunoglobulin abnormalities in Gaucher's disease: report of 16 cases, Blood **31**:633, 1968.

572. Price, T., and Dale, D.: The selective neutropenias, Clin. Haematol. **7**:501, 1978.

573. Prior, E., Goldberg, A.F., Conjalka, M.S., Chapman, W.E., Tay, S., and Ames, E.D.: Hodgkin's disease in homosexual men: an AIDS-related phenomenon? Am. J. Med. **81**:1085, 1986.

574. Prokocimer, M., and Polliack, A.: Increased bone marrow mast cells in preleukemic syndromes, acute leukemia, and lymphoproliferative disorders, Am. J. Clin. Pathol. **75**:34, 1981.

575. Purtilo, D.T., Sakamoto, K., Saemundsen, A.K., Sullivan, J.L., Synnerholm, A.C., Anret, M., Pritchard, J., Sloper, C., Sieff, C., Pincott, J., Pachman, L., Rich, K., Cruzi, F., Cornet, J.A., Collins, R., Barnes, N., Knight, J., Sandstedt, B., and Klein, G.: Documentation of Epstein-Barr virus infection in immunodeficient patients with life-threatening lymphoproliferative diseases by clinical, virological and immunopathological studies, Cancer Res. **41**:4226, 1981.

576. Quaglino, D., and DePasquale, A.: Relationships between different cytobiological aspects of myeloid leukaemias, Acta Haematol. **78**(suppl. 1):26, 1987.

577. Quesada, J.R., Gutterman, J.U., and Hersh, E.M.: Treatment of hairy cell leukemia with alpha interferons, Cancer **57**:1678, 1986.

578. Quesenberry, P.J., McNiece, I.K., Robinson, B.E., Woodward, T.A., Baber, G.B., McGerath, H.E., and Isakson, P.C.: Stromal cell regulation of lymphoid and myeloid differentiation, Blood Cells **13**:137, 1987.

579. Rabkin, M.S., Kjeldsberg, C.R., Hammond, M.E., Wittwer, C.T., and Nathwani, B.: Clinical, ultrastructural immunohistochemical and DNA content analysis of lymphomas having features of interdigitating reticulum cells, Cancer **61**:1594, 1988.

580. Rai, K.R., Sawitsky, A., Cronkite, E.P., et al.: Clinical staging of chronic lymphocytic leukemia, Blood **46**:219, 1975.

581. Rappaport, H.: Tumors of the hematopoietic system. In Atlas of tumor pathology, sect. III, fasc. 8, Washington, D.C., 1966, Armed Forces Institute of Pathology.

582. Rappaport, H., and Thomas, L.B.: Mycosis fungoides: the pathology of extracutaneous involvement, Cancer **34**:1198, 1974.

583. Rappaport, H., Strum, S.B., Hutchinson, G., et al.: Clinical and biological significance of vascular invasion in Hodgkin's disease, Cancer Res. **31**:1794, 1971.

584. Rappaport, H., Ramot, B., Hulu, N., et al.: The pathology of so-called Mediterranean abdominal lymphoma with malabsorption, Cancer **29**:1502, 1972.

585. Ravel, R.: Histopathology of lymph nodes after lymphagiography, Am. J. Clin. Pathol. **46**:335, 1966.

586. Ree, H.J., and Kadin, M.E.: Macrophage-histiocyte in Hodgkin's disease: the relation of peanut-agglutinin–binding macrophage-histiocytes to clinicopathologic presentation and course of disease, Cancer **56**:333, 1985.

587. Regula, D.P., Jr., Hoppe, R.T., and Weiss, L.M.: Nodular and diffuse types of lymphocyte predominance Hodgkin's disease, N. Engl. J. Med. **318**:214, 1988.

588. Reid, H., Fox, H., and Whittaker, J.S.: Eosinophilic granuloma of lymph nodes, Histopathology **1**:31, 1977.

589. Remmele, W., Weber, A., and Harding, P.: Primary signet-ring carcinoma of the prostate, Hum. Pathol. **19**:478, 1988.

590. Report of the Writing Committee: National Cancer Institute sponsored study of classifications on non-Hodgkin's lymphomas: summary and descriptions of a working formulation for clinical usage, Cancer **49**:2112, 1982.

591. Rickinson, A.B., Wallace, L.E., and Epstein, M.A.: HLA-restricted T-cell recognition of Epstein-Barr virus infected B cells, Nature **283**:865, 1980.

592. Ridolfi, R.L., Rosen, P.P., and Thaler, H.: Nevus cell aggregates associated with lymph nodes: estimated frequency and clinical significance, Cancer **39**:164, 1977.

593. Risdall, R.J., Brunning, R.D., Sibley, R.K., Dehner, L.P., and McKenna, R.W.: Malignant histiocytosis: a light- and electron-microscopic and histochemical study, Am. J. Surg. Pathol. **4**:439, 1980.

594. Risdall, R.J., McKenna, R.W., Nesbit, M.E., Krivit, W., Balfour, H.H., Jr., Simmons, R.L., and Brunning, R.D.: Virus-associated hemophagocytic syndrome: a benign histiocytic proliferation distinct from malignant histiocytosis, Cancer **44**:993, 1979.

595. Roberts, B.E., Miles, D.W., and Woods, C.G.: Polycythaemia vera and myelosclerosis: a bone marrow study, Br. J. Haematol. **16**:75, 1969.

596. Robinson, W.A.: Granulocytosis in neoplasia, Ann. NY Acad. Sci. **230**:212, 1974.

597. Roholl, P.J.M., Kleyne, J., Pijpers, H.W., and van Unnik, J.A.: Comparative immunohistochemical investigation of markers for malignant histiocytes, Hum. Pathol. **16**:763, 1985.

598. Roodman, G.D.: Mechanisms of erythroid suppression in the anemia of chronic disease, Blood Cells **13**:171, 1987.

599. Rosai, J., and Dorfman, R.F.: Sinus histiocytosis with massive lymphadenopathy: a newly recognized benign clinicopathologic entity, Arch. Pathol. **87**:63, 1969.

600. Rosai, J., and Dorfman, R.F.: Sinus histiocytosis with massive lymphadenopathy—a pseudolymphomatous benign disorder: analysis of 34 cases, Cancer **30**:1174, 1972.

601. Rosen, Y., Ambiavagar, P.C., Vuletin, J.C., and Macchia, R.J.: Sarcoidosis, from a pathologist's vantage point, Pathol. Annu. **14**:405, 1979.

602. Rosenbaum, D.L., Murphy, G.W., and Swisher, S.N.: Hemodynamic studies of the portal circulation in myeloid metaplasia, Am. J. Med. **41**:360, 1966.

603. Rosenberg, S.A.: Clinical relevance of morphologic studies in Hodgkin's disease, Am. J. Surg. Pathol. **11**:151, 1987.

604. Rosenmund, A., Gerber, S., Huebers, H., and Finch, C.: Regulation of iron absorption and storage iron turnover, Blood **56**:30, 1980.

605. Roth, L.M.: Inclusions of non-neoplastic thyroid tissue within cervical lymph nodes, Cancer **18**:105, 1965.

606. Roth, M.S., Schnitzer, B., Bingham, E.L., Harnden, C.E., Hyder, D.M., and Ginsberg, D.: Rearrangement of immunoglobulin and T-cell receptor genes in Hodgkin's disease, Am. J. Pathol. **131**:331, 1988.

607. Rothenberg, R., Woelfel, M., Stoneburner, R., Milberg, J., Parker, R., and Truman, B.: Survival with the acquired immunodeficiency syndrome: experience with 5833 cases in New York City, N. Engl. J. Med. **317**:1297, 1987.

608. Rowley, J.D.: Biological implications of consistent chromosome rearrangements in leukemia and lymphoma, Cancer Res. **44**:3159, 1984.

609. Rowley, J.D.: Do all leukemic cells have an abnormal karyotype? N. Engl. J. Med. **305**:164, 1981.

610. Rowley, P.T., and Skuse, G.R.: Oncogene expression in myelopoiesis, Int. J. Cell Cloning **5**:255, 1987.

611. Rozman, C., Montserrat, E., Rodríguez-Fernández, J.M., Ayats, R., Vallespí, T., Parody, R., Rios, A., Prados, D., Morey, M., Gomis, F., et al.: Bone marrow histologic pattern—the best

single prognostic parameter in chronic lymphocytic leukemia: a multivariate survival analysis of 329 cases, Blood **64**:642, 1984.

612. Rutgers, J.L., Wieczorek, R., Bonetti, F., Kaplan, K.L., Posnett, D.N., Friedman-Kien, A.E., and Knowles, D.M., II: The expression of endothelial cell surface antigens by AIDS-associated Kaposi's sarcoma: evidence for a vascular endothelial cell origin, Am. J. Pathol. **122**:493, 1986.

613. Rywlin, A.M.: The importance of bone marrow histology, Hum. Pathol. **6**:525, 1975.

614. Rywlin, A.M., and Ortega, R.S.: Lipid granulomas of the bone marrow, Am. J. Clin. Pathol. **57**:457, 1972.

615. Rywlin, A.M., Civantos, F., Ortega, R.S., et al.: Bone marrow histology in monoclonal macroglobulinemia, Am. J. Clin. Pathol. **63**:769, 1975.

616. Rywlin, A.M., Hoffman, E.P., and Ortega, R.S.: Eosinophilic fibrohistiocytic lesion of bone: a distinctive new morphologic finding probably related to drug hypersensitivity, Blood **40**:464, 1972.

617. Rywlin, A.M., Ortega, R.S., and Domínguez, C.J.: Lymphoid nodules of bone marrow: normal and abnormal, Blood **43**:389, 1974.

618. Saarni, M.I., and Linman, J.W.: Preleukemia: the hematologic syndrome preceding acute leukemia, Am. J. Med. **55**:38, 1973.

619. Sacchi, N., Watson, D.K., Guerts van Kessel, A.H., Hagemeijer, A., Kersey, J., Drabkin, H.D., Patterson, D., and Papas, T.S.: Hu-ets-1 and Hu-ets-2 genes are transposed in acute leukemias with (4;11) and (8;21) translocations, Science **231**:379, 1986.

620. Sacks, E.L., Donaldson, S.S., Gordon, J., and Dorfman, R.F.: Epithelioid granulomas associated with Hodgkin's disease: clinical correlations in 55 previously untreated patients, Cancer **41**:562, 1978.

621. Sachs, L.: The molecular control of blood cell development, Science **238**:1374, 1987.

622. Sadamori, N., Gómez, G.A., and Sandberg, A.A.: Chromosomes and causation of human cancer and leukemia. I. Therapeutic and prognostic value of chromosomal findings during acute phase in Ph₁-positive chronic myeloid leukemia, Hematol. Oncol. **1**:77, 1983.

623. Said, J.W., Sasson, A.F., Chien, K., Shintaku, I.P., and Pinkus, G.S.: Immunoultrastructural and morphometric analysis of B lymphocytes in human germinal cancers: evidence for alternate pathways of follicular transformation, Am. J. Pathol. **123**:390, 1986.

624. Sakurai, M., Hayata, I., and Sandberg, A.A.: Prognostic value of chromosomal findings in Ph₁-positive chronic myelocytic leukemia, Cancer Res. **36**:313, 1976.

625. Salahuddin, S.Z., Ablashi, D.V., Markham, P.D., Joseph, S.F., Sturzenegger, S., Kaplan, M., Halligan, G., Biberfeld, P., Wong-Staal, F., Kamarsky, B., et al.: Isolation of a new virus, HBLV, in patients with lymphoproliferative disorders, Science **234**:596, 1986.

626. Salem, P.A., Nassar, V.H., Shahid, M.J., Hajj, A.A., Alami, S.Y., Balikian, J.B., Salem, A.A., et al.: "Mediterranean abdominal lymphoma," or immunoproliferative small intestinal disease. Part I. clinical aspects, Cancer **40**:2941, 1977.

627. Saltzstein, S.L.: The fate of patients with nondiagnostic lymph node biopsies, Surgery **58**:659, 1965.

628. Saltzstein, S.L., and Ackerman, L.V.: Lymphadenopathy induced by anticonvulsant drugs and mimicking clinically and pathologically malignant lymphomas, Cancer **12**:164, 1959.

629. Salvador, A.H., Harrison, Jr., E.G., and Kyle, R.A.: Lymphadenopathy due to infectious mononucleosis: its confusion with malignant lymphoma, Cancer **27**:1029, 1971.

630. San Miguel, J.F., Tavares de Castro, J., Matutes, E., Rodríguez, B., Polli, N., Zola, H., McMichael, A.J., Bollum, F.J., Thompson, D.S., Goldman, J.M., et al.: Characterization of blast cells in chronic granulocytic leukaemia in transformation, acute myelofibrosis and undifferentiated leukaemia. II. Studies with monoclonal antibodies and terminal transferase, Br. J. Haematol. **59**:297, 1985.

631. Sánchez, R., Rosai, J., and Dorfman, R.F.: Sinus histiocytosis with massive lymphadenopathy: an analysis of 113 cases with special emphasis on its extranodal manifestations, Lab. Invest. **36**:349, 1977. (Abstract.)

632. Sandberg, A.A.: The chromosomes in human cancer and leukemia, New York, 1980, Elsevier Science Publishing Co., Inc.

633. Sandberg, A.A.: The chromosomes in human leukemia, Semin. Hematol. **23**:201, 1986.

634. Sandberg, A.A., Gemmill, R.M., Hecht, B.K., and Hecht, F.: The Philadelphia chromosome: a model of cancer and molecular cytogenetics, Cancer Genet. Cytogenet. **21**:129, 1986.

635. Sangster, R.N., Minowada, J., Suciu-Foca, N., Minden, M., and Mak, T.W.: Rearrangement and expression of the α, β, and γ chain T cell receptor genes in human thymic leukemia cells and functional T cells, J. Exp. Med. **163**:1491, 1986.

636. Savage, R.A., Hoffman, G.C., and Shaker, K.: Diagnostic problems involved in detection of metastatic neoplasms by bone-marrow aspirate compared with needle biopsy, Am. J. Clin. Pathol. **70**:623, 1978.

637. Schafer, A.I.: Bleeding and thrombosis in the myeloproliferative disorders, Blood **64**:1, 1984.

638. Schauer, P.K., Straus, D.J., Bagley, C.M., Jr., Rudolph, R.H., McCracken, J.D., Huff, J., Glucksburg, H., Bauermeister, D.E., and Clarkson, B.D.: Angioimmunoblastic lymphadenopathy: clinical spectrum of disease, Cancer **48**:2493, 1981.

639. Schimke, R.T.: Methotrexate resistance and gene amplification: mechanisms and implications, Cancer **57**:1912, 1986.

640. Schoeppel, S.L., Hoppe, R.T., Dorfman, R.F., Horning, S.J., Collier, A.C., Chew, T.G., and Weiss, L.M.: Hodgkin's disease in homosexual men with generalized lymphadenopathy, Ann. Intern. Med. **102**:68, 1985.

641. Schrek, R., and Donnelly, W.J.: "Hairy" cells in blood in lymphoreticular neoplastic disease and "flagellated" cells of normal lymph nodes, Blood **27**:199, 1966.

642. Schroeder, T.M., and Kurth, R.: Spontaneous chromosomal breakage and high incidence of leukemia in inherited disease, Blood **37**:96, 1971.

643. Schroeder, T.M., Drings, P., Beilner, P., et al.: Clinical and cytogenetic observations during a six-year period in an adult with Fanconi's anaemia, Blut **34**:119, 1976.

644. Schroer, K.R., and Franssila, K.O.: Atypical hyperplasia of lymph nodes: a follow-up study, Cancer **44**:1155, 1979.

645. Schuurman, H., Huppes, W., Verdonck, L.F., Baarlen, J.V., and van Unnik, J.A.M.: Immunophenotyping of non-Hodgkin's lymphoma: correlation with relapse-free survival, Am. J. Pathol. **131**:102, 1988.

646. Scott, J.M., and Weir, D.G.: Drug induced megaloblastic change, Clin. Haematol. **9**:587, 1980.

647. Scott, R.B., and Robb-Smith, A.H.T.: Histiocytic medullary reticulosis, Lancet **2**:194, 1939.

648. Scully, P.A., Steinman, H.K., Kennedy, C., Trueblood, K., Frisman, D.M., and Voland, J.R.: AIDS-related Kaposi's sarcoma displays differential expression of endothelial surface antigens, Am. J. Pathol. **130**:244, 1988.

649. Seaman, J.P., Kjeldsberg, C.R., and Linker, A.: Gelatinous transformation of the bone marrow, Hum. Pathol. **9**:685, 1978.

650. Second MIC Cooperative Study Group: Morphologic, immunologic, and cytogenetic (MIC) working classification of the acute myeloid leukemias, Cancer Genet. Cytogenet. **30**:1, 1988.

651. Seemeyer, T.A., Oligny, L.L., and Gartner, J.G.: The Epstein-Barr virus: historical, biologic, pathologic, and oncologic considerations, Perspect. Pediatr. Pathol. **6**:1, 1981.

652. Seligmann, M., Mihaesco, E., and Frangione, B.: Alpha chain disease, Ann. NY Acad. Sci. **190**:487, 1971.

653. Shapiro, R.S., McClain, K., Frizzera, G., Gajl-Peczalska, K.J., Kersey, J.H., Blazar, B.R., Arthur, D.C., Patton, D.F., Greenberg, J.S., Burke, B., et al.: Epstein-Barr virus associated B cell lymphoproliferative disorders following bone marrow transplantation, Blood **71**:1234, 1988.

654. Sharma, S., Mehta, S.R., and Ford, R.J.: Growth factor, viruses, and oncogenes in human lymphoid neoplasia, Lymphokine Res. **6**:245, 1987.

655. Shaw, M.T., Bottomley, R.H., Grozea, P.N., et al.: Heterogeneity of morphological, cytochemical, and cytogenetic features in the blastic phase of chronic granulocytic leukemia, Cancer **35**:199, 1975.

656. Sheibani, K., and Battifora, H.: Signet-ring cell melanoma: a rare morphologic variant of malignant melanoma, Am. J. Surg. Pathol. **12**:28, 1988.

657. Sheibani, K., Nathwani, B.N., Winberg, C.D., Burke, J.S., Swartz, W.G., Blayney, D., van de Velde, S., Hill, L.R., and Rappaport, H.: Antigenically defined subgroups of lymphoblastic lymphoma: relationship to clinical presentation and biologic behavior, Cancer **60**:183, 1987.

658. Sheibani, K., Sohn, C.C., Burke, J.S., Winberg, C.D., Wu, A.M., and Rappaport, H.: Monocytoid B-cell lymphoma: a novel B-cell lymphoma, Am. J. Pathol. **124**:310, 1986.

659. Sheibani, K., Fritz, R.M., Winberg, C.D., Burke, J.S., and Rappaport, H.: "Monocytoid" cells in reactive follicular hyperplasia with and without multifocal histiocytic reactions: an immunohistochemical study of 21 cases including suspected cases of toxoplasmic lymphadenitis, Am. J. Clin. Pathol. **81**:453, 1984.

660. Sheibani, K., Nathwani, B.N., Swartz, W.G., Ben-Ezra, J., Brownell, M.D., Burke, J.S., Kennedy, J.L., Koo, C.H., and Winberg, C.D.: Variability in interpretation of immunohistologic findings in lymphoproliferative disorders by hematopathologists: a comprehensive statistical analysis of interobserver performance, Cancer **62**:657, 1988.

661. Shenoy, B.V., Fort, L., and Benjamin, S.P.: Malignant melanoma primary in lymph node: the case of the missing link, Am. J. Surg. Pathol. **11**:140, 1987.

662. Shigematsu, I., and Kagan, A.: Cancer in atomic bomb survivors, Tokyo (and New York), 1986, Japan Scientific Societies Press (and Plenum Press, Inc.).

663. Shinohara, Y., Komiya, S., Nakashima, A., Nakashima, T., Takeuchi, S., Ono, E., Yukizane, S., Tanaka, C., Matsuishi, T., Koga, T., Hieda, Y., Nakashima, H., and Ichikawa, A.: Asplenia and polysplenia syndrome, Acta Pathol. Jpn. **32**:505, 1982.

664. Sieff, C.A., Emerson, S.G, Donahue, R.E., Nathan, D.G., Wang, E.A., Wong, G.G., and Clark, S.C.: Human recombinant granulocyte-macrophage colony-stimulating factor: a multilineage hematopoietin, Science **230**:1171, 1985.

665. Siegal, G.P., Dehner, L.P., and Rosai, J.: Histiocytosis X (Langerhans' cell granulomatosis) of the thymus: a clinicopathologic study of four childhood cases, Am. J. Surg. Pathol. **9**:117, 1985.

666. Silverberg, E., and Lubera, J.A.: Cancer statistics, 1988, CA **38**:5, 1988.

667. Silverman, M.L., Federman, M., and O'Hara, C.J.: Malignant hemangioendothelioma of the spleen: a case report with ultrastructural observations, Arch. Pathol. Lab. Med. **105**:300, 1981.

668. Silverman, M.L., and LiVolsi, V.A.: Splenic hamartoma, Am. J. Clin. Pathol. **70**:224, 1978.

669. Silverstein, M.N., Ellefson, R.D., and Ahern, E.J.: The syndrome of the sea-blue histiocyte, N. Engl. J. Med. **282**:1, 1970.

670. Silvestrini, R., Piazza, R., Riccardi, A., et al.: Correlation of cell kinetic findings with morphology of non-Hodgkin's malignant lymphoma, J. Natl. Cancer Inst. **58**:499, 1977.

671. Simon, J.H., Tebbi, C.K., Freeman, A.I., Green, D.M., Brecher, M.L., and Barcos, M.: Malignant histiocytosis: complete remission in two pediatric patients, Cancer **59**:1566, 1987.

672. Sinclair, S., Beckman, E., and Ellman, L.: Biopsy of enlarged superficial lymph nodes, JAMA **228**:602, 1974.

673. Singer, D.B.: Postsplenectomy sepsis. In Rosenberg, H.S., and Bolande, R.P., editors: Perspectives in pediatric pathology, vol. 1, Chicago, 1973, Year Book Medical Publishers.

674. Singh, G., Krause, J.R., and Breitfeld, V.: Bone marrow examination for metastatic tumor: aspirate and biopsy, Cancer **40**:2317, 1977.

675. Skarin, A.T., Canellos, G.P., Rosenthal, D.S., Case, D.C., Jr., MacIntyre, J.M., Pinkus, G.S., Moloney, W.C., and Frei, E., III: Improved prognosis of diffuse histiocytic and undifferentiated lymphoma by use of high dose methotrexate alternating with standard agents (M-BACOD), J. Clin. Oncol. **1**:91, 1983.

676. Slamon, D.J., de Kernion, J.B., Verma, I.M., and Cline, M.J.: Expression of cellular oncogenes in human malignancies, Science **224**:256, 1984.

677. Smith, E.B., and Custer, R.P.: Rupture of the spleen in infectious mononucleosis: a clinicopathologic report of seven cases, Blood **1**:317, 1946.

678. Smith T.: Fatty replacement of lymph nodes mimicking lymphoma relapse, Cancer **58**:2686, 1986.

679. Sobrinho-Simões, M., Paiva, M.E., Gonçalves, V., Saldanha, C., Vaz Saleiro, J., and Serrão, D.: Hodgkin's disease with predominant infradiaphragmatic involvement and massive invasion of the bone marrow: a necropsic study of nine cases, Cancer **52**:1927, 1983.

680. Sohn, C.C., Sheibani, K., Winberg, C.D., and Rappaport, H.: Monocytoid B lymphocytes: their relation to the patterns of the acquired immunodeficiency syndrome (AIDS) and AIDS-related lymphadenopathy, Hum. Pathol. **16**:979, 1985.

681. Sokal, J.E., Baccarani, M., Russo, D., and Tura, S.: Staging and prognosis in chronic myelogenous leukemia, Semin. Hematol. **25**:49, 1988.

682. Soler, P., Chollet, S., Jacque, C., Fukuda, Y., Ferrans, V.J., and Basset, F.: Immunocytochemical characterization of pulmonary histiocytosis X cells in lung biopsies, Am. J. Pathol. **118**:439, 1985.

683. Sordillo, P.P., Epremian, B., Koziner, B., Lacher, M., and Lieberman, P.: Lymphomatoid granulomatosis: an analysis of clinical and immunologic characteristics, Cancer **49**:2070, 1982.

684. Spira, A., Carter, A., Tatarsky, I., and Silvian, I.: Lymphocyte subpopulations in benign monoclonal gammopathy, Scand. J. Haematol. **31**:78, 1983.

685. Spritz, R.A.: The familial histiocytoses, Pediatr. Pathol. **3**:43, 1985.

686. Stamatoyannopoulos, G., Nienhuis, A.W., Leder, P., and Majerus, P.W.: The molecular basis of blood diseases, Philadelphia, 1987, W.B. Saunders Co.

687. Stanley, M.W., and Frizzera, G.: Diagnostic specificity of histologic features in lymph node biopsy specimens from patients at risk for the acquired immunodeficiency syndrome, Hum. Pathol. **17**:1239, 1986.

688. Stansfield, A.G.: Lymph node biopsy interpretation, Edinburgh, 1985, Churchill Livingstone.

689. Stansfield, A.G.: The histological diagnosis of toxoplasmic lymphadenitis, J. Clin. Pathol. **14**:565, 1961.

690. Stein, H.: Immunologic and tissue culture studies in Hodgkin's disease: investigation and diagnosis, Am. J. Surg. Pathol. **11**:148, 1987.

691. Stein, H., Lennert, K., Mason, D.Y., Liangru, S., and Ziegler, A.: Immature sinus histiocytes: their identification as a novel B-cell population, Am. J. Pathol. **117**:44, 1984.

692. Stein, H., Gatter, K., Falini, B., Delsol, G., Lemke, H., et al.: The expression of the Hodgkin's disease associated antigen Ki-1 in reactive and neoplastic lymphoid tissue: evidence that Reed-Sternberg cells and histocytic malignancies are derived from activated lymphoid cells, Blood **66**:848, 1985.

693. Stein, R.S., Cousar, J., Flexner, J.M., Graber, S.E., McKee, L.C., Krantz, S., and Collins, R.C.: Malignant lymphomas of follicular center cell origin in man. III. Prognostic features, Cancer **44**:2236, 1979.

694. Stein, R.S., Magee, M.J., Lenox, R.K., Cousar, J.B., Collins, R.D., Flexner, J.M., Ray, W., and Greer, J.P.: Malignant lymphomas of follicular center cell origin in man. IV. Large cleaved cell lymphoma, Cancer **60**:2704, 1987.

695. Strauchen, J., and Dimitriu-Bona, A.: Immunopathology of Hodgkin's disease: characterization of Reed-Sternberg cells with monoclonal antibodies, Am. J. Pathol. **123**:293, 1986.

696. Straus, D.J., Vance, Z.B., Kasdon, E.J., et al.: Atypical lymphoma with prolonged systemic remission after splenectomy: description of three cases, Am. J. Med. **56**:386, 1974.

697. Streiff, R.R.: Folic acid deficiency anemia, Semin. Hematol. **7**:23, 1970.

698. Strickler, J.G., Audeh, M.W., Copenhaver, C.M., and Warnke, R.A.: Immunophenotypic differences between plamacytoma/multiple myeloma and immunoblastic lymphoma, Cancer **61**:1782, 1988.

699. Strickler, J.G., Weis, L.M., Copenhaver, C.M., Bindl, J., McDaid, R., Buck, D., and Warnke, R.: Monoclonal antibodies reactive in routinely processed tissue sections of malignant lymphoma, with emphasis on T-cell lymphomas, Hum. Pathol. **18**:808, 1987.

700. Strickler, J.G., Michie, S.A., Warnke, R.A., and Dorfman, R.F.: The "syncytial variant" of nodular sclerosing Hodgkin's disease, Am. J. Surg. Pathol. **10**:470, 1986.

701. Strife A., and Clarkson, B.: Biology of chronic myelogenous leukemia: is discordant maturation the primary defect? Semin. Hematol. **25**:1, 1988.

702. Strum, S.B., and Rappaport, H.: Interrelations of the histologic types of Hodgkin's disease, Arch. Pathol. **91**:127, 1971.

703. Strum, S.B., Park, J.K., and Rappaport, H.: Observation of cells resembling Sternberg-Reed cells in conditions other than Hodgkin's disease, Cancer **28**:176, 1970.

704. Sturgeon, P.: Volumetric and microscopic pattern of bone marrow in normal infants and children. III. Histologic pattern, Pediatrics **7**:774, 1951.

705. Stutte, H.J.: Round table discussion: splenopathic inhibition of bone marrow and Banti's disease. In Lennert, K., and Harms, D., editors: The spleen, Berlin, 1970, Springer-Verlag.

706. Suárez, C.R., Zeller, W.P., Silberman, S., Rust, G., and Messmore, H.: Sinus histiocytosis with massive lymphadenopathy: remission with chemotherapy, Am. J. Pediatr. Hematol. Oncol. **5**:235, 1983.

707. Summerfield, G.P., Taylor, W., Bellingham, A.J., and Goldsmith, H.J.: Hyaline-vascular variant of angiofollicular lymph node hyperplasia with systemic manifestations and response to corticosteroids, J. Clin. Pathol. **36**:1005, 1983.

708. Sundeen, J., Lipford, E., Uppenkamp, M., Sussman, E., Wahl, L., Raffeld, M., and Cossman, J.: Rearranged antigen receptor genes in Hodgkin's disease, Blood **70**:96, 1987.

709. Suprun, H., and Rywlin, A.M.: Metastatic carcinoma in histologic sections of aspirated bone marrow: a comparative autopsy, South. Med. J. **69**:438, 1976.

710. Sutherland, G.R., Baker, E., Callen, D.F., Campbell, H.D., Young, I.G., Sanderson, C.J., Garson, O.M., Lopez, A.F., and Vadas, M.A.: Interleukin-5 is 5q31 and is deleted in the 5q− syndrome, Blood **71**:1150, 1988.

711. Swerdlow, S.H., Habeshaw, J.A., Murray, L.J., Dhaliwal, H.S., Lister, T.A., and Stansfield, A.G.: Centrocytic lymphoma: a distinct clinicopathologic and immunologic entity, Am. J. Pathol. **113**:181, 1983.

712. Swift, M.: Fanconi's anaemia in the genetics of neoplasia, Nature **230**:370, 1971.

713. Swolin, B., Weinfeld, A., and Westin, J.: Trisomy 1q in polycythemia vera and its relation to disease transition, Am. J. Hematol. **22**:155, 1986.

714. Symmers, W.S.C.: Survey of the eventual diagnosis in 600 cases referred for a second histological opinion after an initial biopsy diagnosis of Hodgkin's disease, Am. J. Clin. Pathol. **21**:650, 1968.

715. Symmers, W.S.C.: The lymphoreticular system. In Systemic pathology, Edinburgh, 1978, Churchill Livingstone.

716. Taetle, R.: Drug-induced agranulocytosis: in vitro evidence for immune suppression of granulopoiesis and a cross-reacting lymphocyte antibody, Blood **54**:501, 1979.

717. Takasaki, N., Kaneko, Y., Maseki, N., Sakurai, M., Shimamura, K., and Takayama, S.: Hemophagocytic syndrome complicating T-cell acute lymphoblastic leukemia with a novel t(11;14)(p15;q11) chromosome translocation, Cancer **59**:424, 1987.

718. Talpaz, M., Kantarjian, H.M., Kurzrock, R., and Gutterman, J.: Therapy of chronic myelogenous leukemia: chemotherapy and interferons, Semin. Hematol. **25**:62, 1988.

719. Tavassoli, M.: Structural alterations of marrow during inflammation, Blood Cells **13**:241, 1987.

720. Tavassoli, M., and Yaffey, J.M.: Bone marrow structure and function, New York, 1983, Alan R. Liss, Inc.

721. te Velde, J., Vismans, F.J., Leenheers-Binnendijk, L., Vos, C.J., Smeenk, D., and Bijvoet, O.L.: The eosinophilic fibrohistiocytic lesion of the bone marrow: a mastocellular lesion in bone disease, Virchows Arch. [Pathol. Anat.] **377**:277, 1978.

722. Teerenhovi, L., and Lintula, R.: Natural course of myelodys-

plastic syndromes: Helsinki experience, Scand. J. Haematol. **45**(suppl.):102, 1986.

723. Tejima, S., and Watanabe, S.: Hodgkin's disease in Japan: a reappraisal of 110 cases in National Cancer Center Hospital, Jpn. J. Res. **19**:347, 1980. [In Japanese.]

724. Tenner-Racz, K., Racz, P., Bofill, M., Schulz-Meyer, A., Dietrich, M., Kern, P., Weber, J., Pinching, A.J., Veronese-Dimarzo, F., Popovic, M., et al.: HTLV-III/LAV viral antigens in lymph nodes of homosexual men with persistent generalized lymphadenopathy and AIDS, Am. J. Pathol. **123**:9, 1986.

725. Thawerani, H., Sanchez, R.L., Rosai, J., and Dorfman, R.F.: The cutaneous manifestations of sinus histiocytosis with massive lymphadenopathy, Arch. Dermatol. **114**:191, 1978.

726. Third International Workshop on Chromosomes in Leukemia: Chromosomal abnormalities and their clinical significance in acute lymphoblastic leukemia, Cancer Res. **43**:868, 1983.

727. Thorling, E.B.: Paraneoplastic erythrocytosis and inappropriate erythropoietin production, Scand. J. Haematol. **17**(suppl. 17):1, 1972.

728. Timens, W., and Poppema, S.: Lymphocyte compartments in human spleen: an immunohistologic study in normal spleens and noninvolved spleens in Hodgkin's disease, Am. J. Pathol. **120**:443, 1985.

729. Timens, W., Visser, L., and Poppema, S.: Nodular lymphocyte predominance type of Hodgkin's disease is a germinal center lymphoma, Lab. Invest. **54**:457, 1986.

730. Todd, D.: Diagnosis of haemolytic states, Clin. Haematol. **4**:63, 1975.

731. Traub, A., Giebink, S., Smith, C., Kuni, C.C., Brekke, M.L., Edlund, D., and Perry, J.F.: Splenic reticuloendothelial function after splenectomy, spleen repair, and spleen autotransplantation, N. Engl. J. Med. **317**:1559, 1987.

732. Travis, L.B., Pierre, R.V., and DeWald, G.W.: Ph₁-negative chronic granulocytic leukemia: a nonentity, Am. J. Clin. Pathol. **85**:186, 1986.

733. Travis, W.D., and Li, C.Y.: Pathology of the lymph node and spleen in systemic mast cell disease, Mod. Pathol. **1**:4, 1988.

734. Tricot, G., Boogaerts, M.A., and Verwilghen, R.L.: Treatment of patients with myelodysplastic syndromes: a review, Scand. J. Haematol. **36**:121, 1986.

735. Tricot, G., Vlietinck, R., and Verwilghen, R.L.: Prognostic factors in the myelodysplastic syndromes: a review, Scand. J. Haematol. **45**(suppl.):107, 1986.

736. Trudel, M.A., Krikorian, J.G., and Neiman, R.S.: Lymphocyte predominance Hodgkin's disease: a clinicopathologic reassessment, Cancer **59**:99, 1987.

737. Tsongas, T.A.: Occupational factors in the epidemiology of chemically induced lymphoid and hemopoietic cancers. In Irons, R.D., editor: Toxicology of the blood and bone marrow, New York, 1985, Raven Press.

738. Tsujimoto, Y., Cossman, J., Jaffe, E., and Croce, C.M.: Involvement of the bcl-2 gene in human follicular lymphoma, Science **228**:1440, 1985.

739. Tucker, M.A., Coleman, C.N., Cox, R.S., Varghese, A., and Rosenberg, S.A.: Risk of second cancers after treatment for Hodgkin's disease, N. Engl. J. Med. **318**:76, 1988.

740. Turner, D.R., and Wright, K.J.M.: Lymphadenopathy in early syphilis, J. Pathol. **110**:305, 1973.

741. Turner, R.R., Levine, A.M., Gill, P.S., Parker, J.W., and Meyer, P.R.: Progressive histopathologic abnormalities in the persistent generalized lymphadenopathy syndrome, Am. J. Surg. Pathol. **11**:625, 1987.

742. Turner, R.R., Martin, J., and Dorfman, R.F.: Necrotizing lymphadenitis, Am. J. Surg. Pathol. **7**:115, 1983.

743. Uchiyama, T., Yodoi, J., Sagawa, K., et al.: Adult T cell leukemia, clinical and hematological features of sixteen cases, Blood **50**:481, 1977.

744. Ulirsch, R.C., and Jaffe, E.S.: Sjögren's syndrome–like illness associated with the acquired immunodeficiency syndrome–related complex, Hum. Pathol. **18**:1063, 1987.

745. Ulrich, H.: The incidence of leukemia in radiologists, N. Eng. J. Med. **234**:45, 1946.

746. Unger, P.D., and Strauchen, J.A.: Hodgkin's disease in AIDS complex patients: report of four cases and tissue immunologic marker studies, Cancer **58**:821, 1986.

747. Unger, P.D., Rappaport, K.M., and Strauchen, J.A.: Necrotizing lymphadenitis (Kikuchi's disease), Arch. Pathol. Lab. Med. **111**:1031, 1987.

748. Uphouse W.J., and Woods, J.C.: Angioimmunoblastic lymphadenopathy with dysproteinemia: complete remission with cisplatin-based chemotherapy, Cancer **60**:2161, 1987.

749. Valentine, W.N., and Paglia, D.E.: Erythrocyte enzymopathies, hemolytic anemia, and multisystem disease: an annotated review, Blood **64**:583, 1984.

750. Van Baarlen, J., Schuurman, H., and van Unnik, J.A.M.: Multilobated non-Hodgkin's lymphoma: a clinicopathologic entity, Cancer **61**:1371, 1988.

751. Van den Berghe, H.: The 5q− syndrome, Scand. J. Haematol. **45**(suppl.):78, 1986.

752. van den Oord, J.J., de Wolf-Peeters, C., De Vos, R., and Desmet, V.J.: Immature sinus histiocytosis: light- and electron-microscopic features, immunologic phenotype, and relationship with marginal zone lymphocytes, Am. J. Pathol. **118**:266, 1985.

753. van den Tweel, J.G., Taylor, C.R., Parker, J.W., and Lukes, R.J.: Immunoglobulin inclusions in non-Hodgkin's lymphomas, Am. J. Clin. Pathol. **69**:306, 1978.

754. van der Valk, P., and Herman, C.J.: Leukocyte functions, Lab. Invest. **57**:127, 1987.

755. van der Valk, P., and Meijer, C.J.L.M.: The histology of reactive lymph nodes, Am. J. Surg. Pathol. **11**:866, 1987.

756. van Krieken, J.H.J.M., te Velde, J., Hermans, J., Cornelisse, C.J., Welvaart, C., and Ferrari, M.: The amount of white pulp in the spleen: a morphometrical study done in methacrylate-embedded splenectomy specimens, Histopathology **7**:767, 1983.

757. van Rijswijk, M.H., and van Heusden, C.W.G.J.: The potassium permanganate method, Am. J. Pathol. **97**:43, 1979.

758. Van Scoy-Mosher, M.B., Bick, M., Capostagno, V., Walford, R.L., and Gatti, R.A.: A clinicopathologic analysis of chronic lymphocytic leukemia, Am. J. Hematol. **10**:9, 1981.

759. Vardiman, J.W., Byrne, G.E., and Rappaport, H.: Malignant histiocytosis with massive splenomegaly in asymptomatic patients: a possible chronic form of the disease, Cancer **36**:419, 1975.

760. Varki, A., Lottenberg, R., Griffith, R., annd Reinhard, E.: The syndrome of idiopathic myelofibrosis: a clinicopathologic review with emphasis on the prognostic variables predicting survival, Medicine **62**:353, 1983.

761. Varmus, H.: Retroviruses, Science **240**:1427, 1988.

762. Varmus, H.E.: Oncogenes and transcriptional control, Science **238**:1337, 1987.

763. Vigorita, V.J., Anand, V.S., and Einhorn, T.A.: Sampling error in diagnosing hyperparathyroid changes in bone in small needle biopsies, Am. J. Surg. Pathol. **10**:140, 1986.

764. Volk, B.W., Adachi, M., and Schneck, L.: The pathology of sphingolipidoses, Semin. Hematol. **9**:317, 1972.

765. Waldmann, T.A., Davis, M.M., Bongiovanni, K.F., and Korsmeyer, S.J.: Rearrangements of genes for the antigen receptor on T-cells as markers of lineage and clonality in human lymphoid neoplasms, N. Engl. J. Med. **313**:776, 1985.

766. Waldron, J.A., Leech, J.H., Glick, A.D., Flexner, J.M., and Collins, R.D.: Malignant lymphoma of peripheral T-lymphocytic origin: immunologic, pathologic, and clinical features in six patients, Cancer **40**:1604, 1977.

767. Walsh, R.J., and Sewell, A.K.: Some effects of blood loss on healthy males, Med. J. Aust. **1**:73, 1946.

768. Walzer, P.D., and Armstrong, D.: Lymphogranuloma venereum presenting as supraclavicular and inguinal lymphadenopathy, Sex. Transm. Dis. **4**:12, 1977.

769. Wantzin, G.L.: The isolation of human T-cell leukemia lymphoma virus I, Eur. J. Hematol. **38**:97, 1987.

770. Ward, H.P., and Block, M.H.: The natural history of agnogenic myeloid metaplasia (AMM) and a critical evaluation of its relationship with the myeloproliferative syndrome, Medicine **50**:357, 1971.

771. Warnke, R.A., Kim, H., Fuks, Z., and Dorfman, R.F.: The coexistence of nodular and diffuse patterns in nodular non-Hodgkin's lymphomas: significance and clinicopathologic correlation, Cancer **40**:1229, 1977.

772. Watanabe, S., Shimosato, Y., Shimoyama, M., Minato, K., Suzuki, M., Abe, M., and Nagatani, T.: Adult T cell lymphoma with hypergammaglobulinemia, Cancer **46**:2472, 1980.

773. Watanabe, S., Sato, Y., Shimoyama M., Manato, K., and Shimosato, Y.: Immunoblastic lymphadenopathy, angioimmunoblastic lymphadenopathy, and IBL-like T-cell lymphoma: a spectrum of T-cell neoplasia, Cancer **58**:2224, 1986.

774. Watanabe, S., Nakajima, T., Shimosato, Y., Sato, Y., and Shimizu, K.: Malignant histiocytosis and Letterer-Siwe disease: neoplasms of T-zone histiocyte with S100 protein, Cancer **51**:1412, 1983.

775. Watson, J.V.: Oncogenes, cancer and analytical cytology, Cytometry **7**:400, 1986.

776. Wear, D.J., Margileth, A.M., Hadfield, T.L., Fischer, G.W., Schlagel, C.J., and King, F.M.: Cat scratch disease: a bacterial infection, Science **221**:1403, 1983.

777. Weatherall, D.J.: Common genetic disorders of the red cell and the 'malaria hypothesis,' Ann Trop. Med. Parasitol. **81**:359, 1987.

778. Webb, D.I., Ubogy, G., and Silver, R.T.: Importance of bone marrow biopsy in the clinical staging of Hodgkin's disease, Cancer **26**:313, 1975.

779. Webb, T.I., Li, C.Y., and Yam, L.T.: Systemic mast cell disease: a clinical and hematopathologic study of 26 cases, Cancer **49**:927, 1982.

780. Weil, S.C., Rosner, G.L., Reid, M.S., Chisholm, R.L., Lemons, R.S., Swanson, M.S., Carrino, J.J., et al.: Translocation and rearrangement of myeloperoxidase gene in acute promyelocytic leukemia, Science **240**:790, 1988.

781. Weinberg, R.A.: The genetic origins of human cancer, Cancer **61**:1963, 1988.

782. Weisenburger, D.D., Sanger, W.G., Armitage J.O., and Purtilo, D.T.: Intermediate lymphocytic lymphoma: an immunohistologic study with comparison to other lymphocytic lymphomas, Hum. Pathol. **18**:781, 1987.

783. Weisenburger, D.D., Nathwani, B.M., Diamond, Z.W., Winberg, C.D., and Rappaport, H.: Malignant lymphoma, intermediate lymphocytic type: a clinicopathologic study of 42 cases, Cancer **48**:1415, 1981.

784. Weisenburger, D.D., Nathwani, B.N., Winberg, C.D., and Rappaport, H.: Multicentric angiofollicular lymph node hyperplasia: a clinicopathologic study of 16 cases, Hum. Pathol. **16**:162, 1985.

785. Weisenburger, D.D., Kim, H., and Rappaport, H.: Mantle-zone lymphoma: a follicular variant of intermediate lymphocytic lymphoma, Cancer **49**:1429, 1982.

786. Weiss, L.M., Strickler, J.G., Dorfman, R.F., Horning, S.J., Warnke, R.A., and Sklar, J.: Clonal T-cell populations in angioimmunoblastic lymphadenopathy and angioimmunoblastic lymphadenopathy-like lymphoma, Am. J. Pathol. **122**:392, 1986.

787. Weiss, L.M., Strickler, J.G., Warnke, R.A., Purtilo, D.T., and Sklar, J.: Epstein-Barr viral DNA in tissues of Hodgkin's disease, Am. J. Pathol. **129**:86, 1987.

788. Weiss L.M., Strickler, J.G., Hu, E., Warnke, R.A., and Sklar, J.: Immunoglobulin gene rearrangements in Hodgkin's disease, Hum. Pathol. **17**:1009, 1986.

789. Weiss, L.M., Crabtree, G.S., Rouse, R.V., and Warnke, R.A.: Morphologic and immunologic characterization of 50 peripheral T-cell lymphomas, Am. J. Pathol. **118**:316, 1985.

790. Weiss, L.M., Azzi, R., Dorfman, R.F., and Warnke, R.A.: Sinusoidal hematolymphoid malignancy ("malignant histiocytosis") presenting as typical sinusoidal proliferation: a study of nine cases, Cancer **58**:1681, 1986.

791. Weiss, L.M., Wood, G.S., and Dorfman, R.F.: T-cell signet-ring cell lymphoma: a histologic, ultrastructural, and immunohistochemical study of two cases, Am. J. Surg. Pathol. **9**:273, 1985.

792. Weissman, B.E., Saxon, P.J., Pasquale, S.R., Jones, G.R., Geiser, A.G., and Stanbridge, E.J.: Introduction of a normal human chromosome 11 into a Wilms' tumor cell line controls its tumorigenic expression, Science **236**:175, 1987.

793. Weissman, I.L., Warnke, R., Butcher, E.C., Rouse, R., and Levy, R.: The lymphoid system: its normal architecture and the potential for understanding the system through the study of lymphoproliferative diseases, Hum. Pathol. **9**:25, 1978.

794. Whang-Peng, J., Lee, E.C., Sieverts, H., and Magrath, I.T.: Burkitt's lymphoma in AIDS: cytogenetic study, Blood **63**:818, 1984.

795. Wick, M.R., Mills, S.E., Scheithauer, B.W., Cooper, P.H., Davitz, M.A., and Parkinson, K.: Reassessment of malignant "angioendotheliomatosis": evidence in favor of its reclassification as "intravascular lymphomatosis," Am. J. Surg. Pathol. **10**:112, 1986.

796. Wickramasinghe, S.N.: Blood and bone marrow, Edinburgh, 1986, Churchill Livingstone.

797. Wieczorek, R., Greco, M.A., McCarthy, K., Banetti, F., and Knowles, D.M., II: Familial erythrophagocytic lymphohistiocytosis: immunophenotypic, immunohistochemical, and ultrastructural demonstration of the relation to sinus histocytes, Hum. Pathol. **17**:55, 1986.

798. Wiernik, P.H., and Serpick, A.A.: Granulocytic sarcoma (chloroma), Blood **35**:361, 1970.

799. Wiktor-Jędrzejczak, W., Szczylik, C., Pojda, Z., Siekierzyński, M., Kansy, J., Klos, M., Ratajczak, M.Z., Pejcz, J., Jaskulski, D., and Gornas, P.: Success of bone marrow transplantation in congenital Diamond-Blackfan anaemia: a case report, Eur. J. Haematol. **38**:204, 1987.

800. Willkens, R.F., Roth, G.F., Husby, G., and Williams, R.C., Jr.: Immunocytological studies of lymph nodes in rheumatoid arthritis and malignant lymphoma, Ann. Rheum. Dis. **39**:147, 1980.

801. Williams, D.L., Harber, J., Murphy, S.B., Look, A.T., Kalwinsky, D.K., Rivera, G., Melvin, S.L., Stass, S., and Dahl, G.V.: Chromosomal translocataions play a unique role in influencing prognosis in childhood acute lymphoblastic leukemia, Blood **68**:205, 1986.

802. Williams, D.L., Raimondi, S., Rivera, G., George, S., Berardi, C.W., and Murphy, S.B.: Presence of clonal chromosome abnormalities in virtually all cases of acute lymphoblastic leukemia, N. Engl. J. Med. **313**:640, 1985.

803. Williams, J.W., and Dorfman, R.F.: Lymphadenopathy as the initial manifestation of histiocytosis X, Am. J. Surg. Pathol. **3**:405, 1979.

804. Willman, C.L., and Fenoglio-Preiser, C.M.: Oncogenes, suppressor genes, and carcinogenesis, Hum. Pathol. **18**:896, 1987.

805. Wilson, J.F., Jenkin, R.D., Anderson, J.R., Chilcote, R.R., Coccia, P., Exelby, P.R., Kersey, J., Kjeldsberg, C.R., Kushner, J., Meadows, A., et al.: Studies on the pathology of non-Hodgkin's lymphoma of childhood. I. The role of routine histopathology as a prognostic factor: a report from the Children's Cancer Study Group, Cancer **53**:1695, 1984.

806. Wilson, J.F., Kjeldsberg, C.R., Sposto, R., Jenkin, R.D., Chilcote, R.R., Coccia, P., Exelby, R.R., Kersey, J., Meadows, A., Siegel, S., et al.: The pathology of non-Hodgkin's lymphoma of childhood. II. Reproducibility and relevance of the histologic classification of "undifferentiated" lymphomas (Burkitt's versus non-Burkitt's), Hum. Pathol. **18**:1008, 1987.

807. Wiltshaw, E.: The natural history of extramedullary plasmacytoma and its relation to solitary myeloma of bone and myelomatosis, Medicine **55**:217, 1976.

808. Winberg, C.D., Nathwani, B.N., Bearman, R.M., and Rappaport, H.: Follicular (nodular) lymphoma during the first two decades of life: a clinicopathologic study of 12 patients, Cancer **48**:2223, 1981.

809. Winship, T.: Pathologic changes in so-called cat scratch fever: review of findings of 29 patients and cutaneous lesions of 2 patients, Am. J. Clin. Pathol. **23**:1012, 1953.

810. Wintrobe, M.M., Lee, G.R., Boggs, D.R., Bithell, T.C., Foerster, J., Athens, J.W., and Lukens, J.N.: Clinical hematology, Philadelphia, 1981, Lea & Febiger.

811. Wittels, B.: Bone marrow biopsy changes following chemotherapy for acute leukemia, Am. J. Surg. Pathol. **4**:135, 1980.

812. Wittels, B.: Surgical pathology of the bone marrow—core biopsy diagnosis. In Bennington, J.L. editor: Major problems in pathology, vol. 17, Philadelphia, 1985, W.B. Saunders Co.

813. Wolfe, J.A., and Borowitz, M.J.: Composite lymphoma: a unique case with two immunologically distinct B-cell neoplasms, Am. J. Clin. Pathol. **81**:526, 1984.

814. Wolfe, M.W., Vacek, J.L., Kinard, R.E., and Bailey, C.G.: Prolonged and functional survival with the asplenia syndrome, Am. J. Med. **81**:1089, 1986.

815. Wolff, N.S.: The haemopoietic microenvironment, Clin. Haematol. **8**:469, 1979.

816. Wolfson, S.L., Botero, F., Hurwitz, S., and Pearson, H.A.: "Pure" cutaneous histiocytosis-X, Cancer **48**:2236, 1981.

817. Wood, G.S., Burns, B.F., Dorfman, R.F., and Warnke, R.A.: In situ quantitation of lymph node helper, suppressor, and cytotoxic T cell subsets in AIDS, Blood **67**:596, 1986.

818. Wood, G.S., Burns, B.F., Dorfman, R.F., and Warnke, R.A.: The immunohistology of non-T cells in the acquired immunodeficiency syndrome, Am. J. Pathol. **120**:371, 1985.

819. Wormser, G.P.: Multiple opportunistic infections and neoplasms in the acquired immunodeficiency syndrome, JAMA **253**:3441, 1985.

820. Wright, D.H., and Richards, D.B.: Sinus histiocytes with massive lymphadenopathy (Rosai-Dorfman disease): report of a case with widespread nodal and extra nodal dissemination, Histopathology **5**:697, 1981.

821. Yoo, D., and Lessin, L.S.: Bone marrow mast cell content in preleukemic syndromes, Am. J. Med. **73**:539, 1982.

822. York, J.C., II, Cousar, J.B., Glick, A.D., Flexner, J.M., Stein, R., and Collins, R.D.: Morphologic and immunologic evidence of composite B- and T-cell lymphomas: a report of three cases developing in follicular center cell lymphomas, Am. J. Clin. Pathol. **84**:35, 1985.

823. Young, N., and Mortimer, P.: Viruses and bone marrow failure, Blood **63**:729, 1984.

824. Young, N.S., Leonard, E., and Platanias, L.: Lymphocytes and lymphokines in aplastic anemia: pathogenic role and implications for pathogenesis, Blood Cells **13**:87, 1987.

825. Yunis, J.J.: The chromosomal basis of human neoplasia, Science **221**:227, 1983.

826. Yunis, J.J.: Should refined chromosomal analysis be used routinely in acute leukemias and myelodysplastic syndromes? N. Engl. J. Med. **315**:322, 1986.

827. Yunis, J.J., Brunning, R.D., Howe, R.B., and Lobell, M.: High-resolution chromosomes as an independent prognostic indicator in adult acute nonlymphocytic leukemia, N. Engl. J. Med. **311**:812, 1984.

828. Yunis, J.J., Frizzera, G., Oken, M.M., McKenna, J., Theologides, A., and Arnesen, M.: Multiple recurrent genomic defects in follicular lymphoma: a possible model for cancer, N. Engl. J. Med. **316**:79, 1987.

829. Yunis, J.J., Rydell, R.E., Oken, M.M., Arnesen, M.A., Mayer, M.G., and Lobell, M.: Refined chromosome analysis as an independent prognostic indicator in de novo myelodysplasic syndromes, Blood **67**:1721, 1986.

830. Yuo, A., Kitagawa, S., Okabe, T., Urabe, A., Komatsu, Y., Itoh, S., and Takaku, F.: Recombinant human granulocyte colony-stimulating factor repairs the abnormalities of neutrophils in patients with myelodysplastic syndromes and chronic myelogenous leukemia, Blood **70**:404, 1987.

831. Zafrani, E.S., Degos, F., Guigui, B., Durand-Schneider, A.M., Martin, N., Flandrin, S., Benhamon, J.P., and Feldmann, G.: The hepatic sinusoid in hairy cell leukemia: an ultrastructural study in 12 cases, Hum. Pathol. **18**:801, 1987.

832. Zayid, I., and Farraj, S.: Familial histiocytic dermatoarthritis, Am. J. Med. **54**:793, 1973.

833. Ziegler, J.L., Beckstead, J.A., Volberding, P.A., Abrams, D.I., Levine, A.M., Lukes, R.J., Gill, P.S., Burkes, R.L., Meyer, P.R., Metroka, C.E., et al.: Non-Hodgkin's lymphoma in 90 homosexual men: relation to generalized lymphadenopathy and the acquired immunodeficiency syndrome, N. Engl. J. Med. **311**:565, 1984.

834. Zoumbos, N.C., Gascón, P., Djeu, J.Y., Trost, S.R., and Young, N.S.: Circulating activated suppressor T lymphocytes in aplastic anemia, N. Engl J. Med. **312**:257, 1985.

835. Zuazu, J.P., Duran, J.W., and Julia, A.F.: Hemophagocytosis in acute brucellosis, N. Engl. J. Med. **301**:1185, 1979.

836. Zwi, L.J., Evans, D.J., Wechsler, A.L., and Catovsky, D.: Splenic angiosarcoma following chemotherapy for follicular lymphoma, Hum. Pathol. **17**:528, 1986.

29 Thymus Gland

ROGERS C. GRIFFITH

DEVELOPMENT

The thymus gland is a complex, highly specialized lymphoreticular organ that has the central role in T-lymphocyte development.[114] It directs the development and ultimately the organization of the peripheral lymphoid tissues and the immune capabilities of the individual through its influence on T-cell development. The development of the human fetal thymus begins in the sixth gestational week when paired cellular proliferations emerge from the ectoderm of the third branchial cleft and from the endoderm of the ventral wing of the third pharyngeal pouch (Fig. 29-1). The inferior parathyroid glands arise similarly from the dorsal wing of the pharyngeal pouch. Both primordia separate from the pharyngeal wall and begin a caudal migration as the fetus grows. In this process the ectoderm of the third branchial cleft covers the endodermally derived epithelium.[30] The thymic primordium elongates caudally, trailing the incipient upper lobes of the thymus gland behind. During this migration, small fragments may separate from the primordium and persist postnatally along the migratory route. When the thymus gland ends its migration at the base of the heart, it lies anterior to the great vessels in the superior mediastinum with the upper poles of its two lobes extending laterally along the trachea to the base of the thyroid gland.

The complex, specialized stroma of the thymus is derived from at least three embryonic tissues: (1) the ectoderm of the third branchial cleft, which ultimately gives rise to the epithelium of the thymic cortex; (2) the endoderm of the third pharyngeal pouch, the anlage of the thymic medullary epithelium; and (3) mesenchymal stromal cells. Until the ninth gestational week, the embryonic thymus is composed entirely of these tissues when hematopoietic precursor cells from the fetal liver and bone marrow begin to colonize the thymus.[118] This influx of stem cells into the thymus occurs in successive waves[71,89] and is an active phenomenon[140] that depends on the maturational state of the thymic epithelium.[88] Lobulation occurs by the tenth week as the epithelial cells expand to surround mesenchymal septal ingrowths that communicate with the anlage through openings in

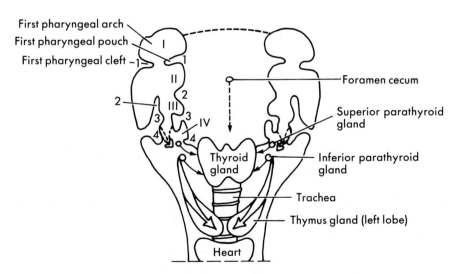

Fig. 29-1. Embryogenesis of thymus gland. In this schema of pharyngeal development, thymus gland originates from pouch and cleft of third pharyngeal structure.

the surrounding basal lamina. Inductive tissue interactions between the epithelial and mesenchymal components are necessary for this and further normal development to occur.[4] This development ultimately leads to significant structural and functional diversity among the epithelial cells.[54,109,196]

At this developmental stage, the epithelial cells at the periphery of the lobule develop a rounded contour, whereas those in the center appear more spindle shaped.[202] Adjacent epithelial cells are connected by well-developed desmosomes. Other large mesenchymal cells are present at this time in the septa and among the central epithelial cells, which lack intercellular junctions. These cells are related to interdigitating reticulum cells of thymus-dependent regions of peripheral lymphoid tissue in their bone marrow origin and function.[72,155] Macrophages colonize the thymus at the same stage as the lymphoid progenitors do. Precursors of both of these cell types invade the thymic stroma from the vasculature of the mesenchymal septa. Rare cells containing myofilaments, called "myoid cells," are present in the central anlage as early as the eighth week. Erythroblasts, residua from earlier hematopoiesis in the primordial gland, may also be found. However, by the twelfth gestational week most of the nonepithelial cells present are lymphoid cells.

The presumptive precursors of the characteristic Hassall's corpuscles of the postnatal thymus are present in the central region of the thymus by the twelfth week. They appear as electron-lucent epithelial cells that preferentially accumulate bundles of tonofilaments within their cytoplasm. Tubular structures often with microvilli projecting into a vestigial lumen have also been observed to contribute in their formation.[171] However, the histogenesis of Hassall's corpuscles is still uncertain. Arguments for direct derivation from senescent central epithelial cells,[15,106] for specific differentiation of central epithelial cells into keratinizing, stratified squamous epithelium[210] or for a separate embryonic origin distinct from the two epithelial primordia (anlagen)[30,171] have their proponents.

The development of the cortex and medulla is completed between the fourteenth and sixteenth gestational weeks, and any characteristic differences in the lymphocyte and epithelial cell populations of each region are apparent by this time. The mesenchymal septa extend to the corticomedullary junction and give rise to the vessels that enter the parenchyma of the gland. The cortex is filled with immature and maturing thymocytes, whereas the medulla contains very few lymphocytes but many compact epithelial cells and interdigitating reticulum cells at the border of the medulla and cortex. This contrasting cellularity creates the histologically distinct corticomedullary junction. The thymus at this stage of development resembles the postnatal thymus in all respects, except that it weighs only 0.2 g.

The thymus gland undergoes considerable growth before birth, when it attains its greatest weight in relation to body weight, weighing an average of 15 g. The thymus continues to increase in size until puberty, increasing in weight by another 50%. Afterward the natural process of involution begins, with a gradual replacement of parenchyma by adipose tissue. This process is never complete.[46] Individuals can display a considerable variation in thymic weight at all ages (Table 29-1).

STRUCTURE

The mature thymus gland maintains its fetal bilobed structure. Each lobe is separately encapsulated, and both lobes are invested in loose connective tissue that fuses into a continuous sheet anteriorly. The basic microscopic structure of each lobe is the lobule. The lobule structure is formed by the many primary and secondary invaginated mesenchymal septa (Figs. 29-2 and 29-3). The septa contain arterioles that enter the thymus at the corticomedullary junction and generate capillaries that ascend through the cortex to form an arcuate network. The capillaries descend from the outer cortex toward the medulla to form postcapillary venules at the boundary of the cortex and medulla and leave the thymus through the septa as interlobular veins. Lymphatic vessels are present in the septa but do not enter the parenchyma. Autonomic nerves are distributed along the arterioles.

The histologic pattern of the lobule and its distinct corticomedullary junction are the result of the rich thy-

Table 29-1. Weight of thymus

Age (yr)	Weight (g)		
	Minimum	Average	Maximum
Newborn	7.3	15.2	25.5
1-5	8.0	25.7	48.0
5-10	13.0	29.4	48.0
10-15	19.0	29.4	43.3
15-20	15.9	26.2	49.7
21-25	9.5	21.0	51.0
26-30	8.3	19.5	51.5
31-35	9.0	20.2	37.0
36-43	5.9	19.0	36.0
47-55	6.0	17.3	45.0
56-65	2.1	14.3	27.0
66-90	3.0	14.0	31.0

According to Hammar, J.A.: Die Menschenthymus in Gesundheit and Krankheit, Leipzig, 1926, Akademische Verlagsgesellschaft; from Fisher, E.R.: Pathology of the thymus and its relation to human disease. In Good, R.A., and Gabrielsen, A.E., editors: The thymus in immunobiology, New York, 1964, Paul B. Hoeber Medical Division, Harper & Row, Publishers, Inc.

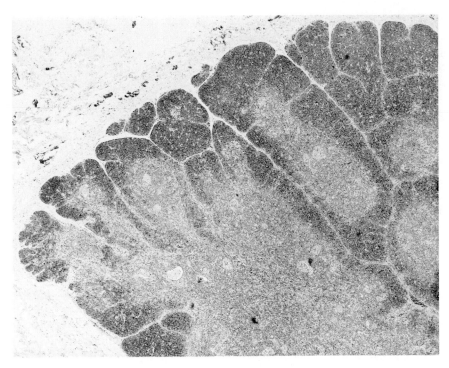

Fig. 29-2. Normal thymus gland from infant, showing lobulated structure, distinct corticomedullary junction, and prominent Hassall's corpuscles of medulla. (25×.)

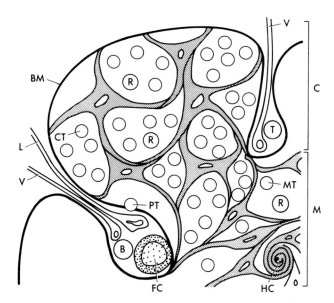

Fig. 29-3. Schema of structural organization of mature thymus gland. Epithelial cells *(elongated shaded cells)* providing primary structure are more densely associated in medulla *(M)* than in cortex *(C)*. Basal lamina *(BM)* circumscribes thymic parenchyma proper in which freely moving thymocytes develop. *B,* B-lymphocytes or plasma cells; *CT,* cortical thymocytes; *FC,* follicular center; *HC,* Hassall's corpuscle; *L,* lymphatic vessels; *MT,* medullary thymocytes; *PT,* prothymocyte; *R,* reticulum cells; *T,* T-lymphocytes; *V,* blood vessels.

mocyte population of the cortex. However, it is the stationary epithelial cells that provide the primary structure of the gland by means of their elongated interdigitating cytoplasmic processes. Microscopically the epithelial cells appear strikingly similar throughout the thymus gland. However, there are remarkable differences* that have profound functional importance in the ontogeny of the T-lymphocyte.[81,100,190,204,206] Obvious structural differences are that the cortical cells are less densely arranged and have very elongated cytoplasmic branches that form interstices, where the mobile thymocytes and macrophages are found. Similar attenuated cytoplasmic projections from subcortical epithelial cells line the inner surface of the capsule. Basal lamina material is present over the surface of these and other epithelial cells and circumscribes all the extrathymic areas in the mature gland, including the small blood vessels within the thymus.[12] An unusual subpopulation of epithelial cells, called "thymic nurse cells," are present in the middle to outer areas of the cortex, which contain the greatest concentration of thymocytes. These specialized cells have the unique quality of incorporating individual, actively dividing thymocytes within their cytoplasm completely surrounded by internal membranes. Medullary epithelial cells have blunted cytoplasmic projections and are more

---

*References 17, 34, 35, 55, 65, 68, 109, 120, 156, 196, 202, 203, 208.

densely associated than the cortical cells are. A consistent feature of these cells is the greater frequency of desmosomes and the dense tonofilaments in the cytoplasm that often insert into the desmosomes. These latter features are even better developed in those that abut on Hassall's corpuscles.

Hassall's corpuscles, the distinctive structures located within the medulla, are complex arrays composed of the epithelial interdigitations of concentrically arranged epithelial cells. Basal lamina material, numerous desmosomes, and dense tonofilaments are prominent ultrastructural features. Keratinization occurs in Hassall's corpuscles, and related keratinic and cytoplasmic antigens have been demonstrated in the thymus and the epidermis.[200] Their central areas can be either solid or cystic and often contain degenerative cellular debris. Lymphocytes, macrophages, and eosinophils may also be found within these structures.

The cortical epithelial cells express large amounts of class II (HLA-D) antigens and to a more variable extent class I (HLA-A, HLA-B, HLA-C) major histocompatibility complex (MHC) antigens at the plasma membrane surface. Thymic nurse cells also express both MHC class I and class II antigens. Epithelial cells of the medulla and subcapsular region are similar in that they express little if any MHC antigens, and they produce the thymic hormones thymopoietin and thymosin-α_1.[100,190] Thymosin-β_3 is an additional product of subcortical cells.

The thymic cortex is replete with thymocytes that en masse give the thymus gland its distinctive histologic appearance. Rapidly dividing prothymocytes comprise about 10% of the lymphoid cells and are found predominantly in the subcapsular portion of the outer cortex.[25] A gradient of smaller, less mitotically active cells occurs from the outer cortex to the deep cortex to the corticomedullary junction and into the medulla. In the cortex, intense lymphopoiesis, lympholysis, and active phagocytosis are indicative of the extensive amount of ineffective lymphopoiesis (probably 99% of thymocytes die in situ), now considered normal in an active thymus.[166]

Other cell types are found less frequently in the thymus. Macrophages are especially numerous in the cortex but are also found in the medulla. Interdigitating reticulum cells are very numerous in the medulla and at the corticomedullary junction. Both of these cells express class I and class II MHC antigens. Peripheral lymphocytes, plasma cells, mast cells, and eosinophils are frequently present in the extrathymic perivascular spaces of the septa. Lymphoid follicles with active germinal centers may also be found in otherwise normal thymuses, especially in children and adolescents.[112,199] These structures presumably arise within the perivascular space of the septa.[93] Myoid cells, cells with microscopic, ultrastructural, and immunohistochemical features of striated muscle, have been observed in the human thymic medulla of persons of all ages.[37,56,58,66] These cells are found clustered in the medulla and express acetylcholine receptors (AChR) on their surface.[73] Myoid cells are completely invested by epithelial cells, but evidence is lacking that these cells directly interact with epithelial cells or are derived from them. It is believed that they may provide an immunogenic form of the AChR and have a role in the pathogenesis of myasthenia gravis. Their histogenesis or function in the human thymus is not known.

FUNCTION

The thymus provides the essential microenvironment for the differentiation and expansion of T-lymphocyte subpopulations, which are necessary for the development of the complex network of immunoregulatory and cell-mediated effector functions attributable to mature, immunocompetent T-lymphocytes. Several functional subpopulations have been identified through their expression of cell surface molecules detected by monoclonal antibodies (Table 29-2). These cell functions,

Table 29-2. T-lymphocyte cell surface marker antigens

Marker antigen	Cellular expression	Molecular weight of glycoprotein (kilodaltons)	Function
T-cell receptor	Thymocyte, T-cell	40,43	ag receptor
CD1	Thymocyte, Langerhan's cell	43,45,49	
CD2	Thymocyte, T-cell	50	SRBC receptor
CD3	Thymocyte, T-cell	20,25	Associated with ag receptor
CD4	Thymocyte, T-cell	60	Helper/inducer
CD5	Thymocyte, T-cell, B-cell subpopulation	67	Activation
CD8	Thymocyte, T-cell	32	Suppressor/cytotoxic

From International Workshops on Human Leukocyte Differentiation Antigens.
ag, Antigen; *CD*, cluster of differentiation; *SRBC*, sheep red blood cells.

which may relate to more than one cell type, are outlined as follows:

1. Effector functions
   a. *Cell-mediated cytotoxicity* (CD8+ T-cells). Killing of foreign antigen-bearing cells (virus-infected, allogeneic, or tumor cells) within or outside the context of class I MHC antigens
   b. *Lymphokine production.* Production of nonimmunoglobulin mediators that induce, amplify, or regulate inflammation; specific and nonspecific immunity; B-lymphocytes and immunoglobulin production; and the activation and proliferation of nonlymphoid hemic cells
2. Regulatory functions
   a. *Helper* (CD4+ T-cells). Enhance or diminish B-lymphocyte responses to thymus-dependent antigens within the context of class II MHC antigens
   b. *Suppressor* (CD8+ T-cells). Diminish thymus-dependent B-lymphocyte responses and T-lymphocyte helper, cytotoxic functions, or delayed type of hypersensitivity

These functional subclasses of T-lymphocytes and their precursors develop as a consequence of intrathymic and postthymic events.[67,147,177,186,207] This process of differentiation begins after hematopoietic progenitor cells, prothymocytes, migrate from the bone marrow to the subcapsular area of the thymus and involves an intrathymic migration through theoretical cellular microenvironments from the cortex to the medulla within which interactions between the developing thymocytes and stromal thymic cells occur. Thymic nurse cell–thymocyte interaction is believed to be an early and important first step in this process.[35] At the end of this maturation gradient, thymocytes with essentially mature phenotypes exit through the thymus to the peripheral lymphoid compartment, where functional diversification is completed.[5,111,166] Antigen-activated, immunocompetent peripheral T-lymphocytes do immigrate to the thymic medulla where they may influence to some degree the final stages of clonal maturation of the thymocyte.[122]

The intrathymic portion of this process has been divided empirically into three stages of differentiation.[142] As the thymocytes encounter the various inductive, hormonal, and proliferative signals from various subpopulations of subcortical and cortical epithelial cells and interdigitating reticulum cells, genes are activated, and enzymes and surface receptor molecules, which identify these stages, are expressed (Table 29-3). Although the molecular events that are operative at this early stage of differentiation are not completely understood, it is now appreciated that genes that encode the T-cell antigen receptor complex and other important cell surface molecules of the thymocyte interact with epithelial MHC antigens.[68,156,217] The result of these interactions is a clonal selection for T-lymphocyte antigen receptors that distinguish self from nonself and recognize specific

Table 29-3. Stages of thymocyte differentiation

Stage	Thymocyte		Thymic epithelium	
I	**Prothymocytes**		**Subcortical cells**	
	CD2+		HLA-D ±	
	TdT+		Thymopoietin	
	γ-TCR gene		Thymosin-α_1 and -β_3	
			Thymic nurse cells	
II	**Common thymocytes**		**Cortical cells**	
	CD2+		HLA-D + + +	
	CD5+		HLA-A,B,C + + +	
	CD4+		Thymic nurse cells	
	CD8+			
	TdT+			
	γ- and β-TCR genes			
III	**Late thymocytes**			
	CD4+ T-cells	*CD8+ T-cells*	*Deep cortical and medullary cells*	
	CD4+	CD8+	HLA-D −	
	CD2+	CD2+	Thymopoietin	
	CD3+	CD3+	Thymosin α_1	
	Surface TCR	Surface TCR	*IDR cells*	
	α- and β-TCR genes	α-, β-, and γ-TCR genes	HLA-D + + +	
			HLA-A,B,C + + +	

TdT data from Ma, D.D.F., et al.: J. Immunol. **129**:1430, 1982. See reference 102.
CD, Cluster of differentiation; *IDR,* interdigitating reticulum cell; *TCR,* T-cell antigen receptor; *TdT,* terminal deoxynucleotidyltransferase.

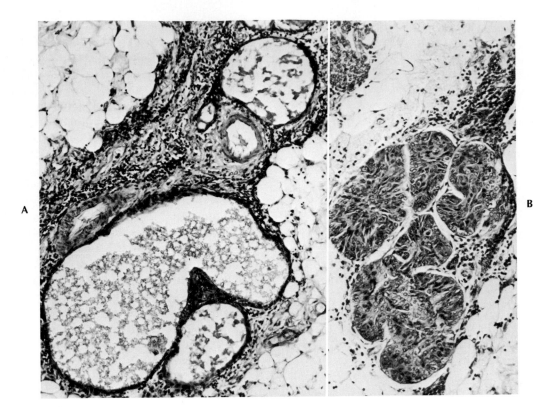

Fig. 29-4. Chronic involution of thymus. **A,** Cystic degeneration with epithelial cell atrophy and thymocyte depletion. **B,** Islets of spindle-shaped epithelial cells in abundant adipose tissue. (165×.)

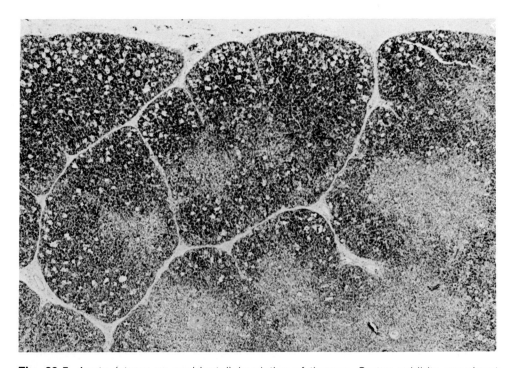

Fig. 29-5. Acute (stress or accidental) involution of thymus. Cortex exhibits prominent lympholysis and associated phagocytosis by macrophages—numerous "starry-sky" spaces. (55×.)

antigens in the context of class II MHC molecules,[220] and a clonal selection against those that cannot.[69,103,111] It is now believed that the complexing of cortical thymocytes within the environs of the thymic nurse cells may produce important ontologic niches in which thymocytes with restriction for self-MHC antigens are selected.[81] Only 1% or less of thymocytes that enter the thymus as prothymocytes or are produced as daughter cells ever mature to leave the thymus as immunocompetent cells—a very selective process indeed.

INVOLUTION

The thymus gland normally decreases in size and weight with advancing age resulting in the replacement of parenchyma by adipose tissue. This process of aging, called "age or physiologic involution," is accompanied by gradual changes in thymocyte populations relative to different rates of involution of the cortical and medullary epithelium[59,131,201] and a decline in the production of thymic hormones by thymic epithelium.[165,209] However, the thymus continues to serve as the site of T-cell differentiation and maturation throughout life.[183] In the young adult the parenchymal loss is primarily that of decreasing numbers of cortical thymocytes, with relative sparing of the epithelial architecture. With advancing age the epithelial component atrophies, and the gland consists of islands of spindle-shaped epithelial cells, with partially cystic, closely arranged Hassall's corpuscles and scattered small lymphocytes in abundant adipose tissue (Fig. 29-4). This gradual involution of the thymus is followed by a more gradual decrease in the volume of the peripheral T-lymphocyte compartment.[105]

The thymus gland with active lymphopoiesis responds dramatically to episodes of severe stress by a loss in size and weight, principally as a result of a loss of cortical thymocytes. A striking decrease in thymic size may be observed by roentgenogram within 24 hours of the onset of the illness. This process of accidental involution or stress-induced atrophy is mediated in part by the release of corticosteroids from the adrenal cortex, which results in rapid lympholysis of the cortical thymocytes. Microscopically a prominent karyorrhexis of thymocytes and phagocytosis of debris by numerous macrophages is seen in the early period (Fig. 29-5). If the stimulus continues, the extensive lympholysis results in a loss of corticomedullary distinction and an accentuation of the epithelial cells, cystic Hassall's corpuscles, and elongated epithelium-lined cystic spaces. With further loss of thymocytes, the lobular architecture progressively collapses and fibrosis ensues. Major stress, as from an extensive and severe thermal injury, results in immunosuppression, which may be clinically significant.[113]

CONGENITAL ANOMALIES

Faulty embryogenesis of the thymus gland can result in a failure of migration, an aberrant localization of thymic tissue, or a partial or complete failure of development, which is associated with one of the varieties of primary immunodeficiency disorders (discussed below). Failure of the thymic primordium to descend into the mediastinum can result in the development of one or both lobes in the neck. Symptoms of respiratory obstruction can result requiring surgical intervention.[3] A more common occurrence is the appearance of thymic tissue nodules in the lateral area of neck or within or adjacent to the thyroid or parathyroid glands. Likewise parathyroid glands may be observed within the thymus gland, reflecting their close developmental relationship. Cystic degenerative changes usually occur and lead to the discovery of the ectopic tissue. Such aberrant thymic nodules occur in perhaps 20% of the population[46] and may rarely be found outside the cervical migratory route.

PRIMARY IMMUNODEFICIENCY DISEASES

The primary immunodeficiency disorders are a heterogeneous group of genetic or acquired cellular defects that result in the faulty maturation, regulation, or function of antigen-specific lymphocytes. Concepts derived from the study of patients with these disorders as well as from experimental systems have expanded our knowledge of developmental immunobiology.[205] As our understanding of these disorders increases, more specific management of these patients will result.

Several classifications of immunodeficiency diseases have been proposed, but none of them are fully satisfactory. One of the current classifications of these disorders is based on criteria[43] that define altered functions of B- or T-lymphocytes or both. As a group, these disorders are rarely encountered in clinical medicine, since their fequency is less than 1 case per 50,000 to 100,000 persons.[188] Because of the rarity of these various disorders, only a few attempts have been made to correlate thymic morphology with clinical and immunologic information.[21,47,84] Specific immunodeficiency syndromes in which the thymus gland is morphologically abnormal are listed in Table 29-4.

Dysplasia of the thymus is the most frequently used term and the most thoroughly described histologic lesion used in describing the thymus glands in patients with cellular immune deficiency disorders. It is a constant feature in patients with severe combined immunodeficiency (SCID).[21,48] A fully dysplastic gland encompasses three invariant findings: (1) the loss of lymphoid cells, (2) the lack of a distinct corticomedullary junction, and (3) an embryonal appearance of the lobular structure. There are two exceptions among patients with SCID in whom the thymus gland may ap-

Table 29-4. Immunodeficiency disorders associated with an abnormal thymus gland

Syndrome	Inheritance	Associated findings
Congenital thymic hypoplasia (DiGeorge's syndrome)	S	HI variable Hypoparathyroidism Cardiovascular abnormalities Megaloblastic anemia
Severe combined immunodeficiencies (SCID)		
Reticular dysgenesis	AR	Neutropenia
Nezelof's syndrome	XL/AR	HI variable
Adenosine deaminase deficiencies	AR	Cartilage abnormalities
Purine nucleoside phosphorylase deficiency	AR	HI variable Hypoplastic anemia
MHC antigen deficiency	AR	Intestinal malabsorption
Ataxia telangiectasia	AR	Cerebellar ataxia Telangiectasia Chromosomal abnormalities Endocrine abnormalities
Wiskott-Aldrich syndrome	XL	Thrombocytopenia Eczema
Short-limbed dwarfism	AR	Cartilage and hair hypoplasia Neutropenia
Thymoma	S	Epithelial neoplasm Aplastic anemia Hypogammaglobulinemia
Immunodeficiency to Epstein-Barr virus (EBV)	XL/AR	Aplastic anemia Fatal infectious mononucleosis Lymphoproliferative disorders
Acquired immunodeficiency syndrome (AIDS)	S	Fatal opportunistic infections Kaposi's sarcoma Lymphoproliferative disorders

AR, Autosomal recessive; *HI,* humoral immunity; *MHC,* major histocompatibility complex; *S,* sporadic; *XL,* X-linked recessive.

pear normal or show mild atrophy as it does in pure immunoglobulin or B-lymphocyte deficiencies: (1) the disorders associated with specific enzymatic deficiencies in purine metabolism (adenosine deaminase deficiency and purine nucleoside phosphorylase deficiency), and (2) congenital thymic hypoplasia (DiGeorge's syndrome), in which the gland is completely absent or hypoplastic because of a variable failure in the embryogenesis of the pharyngeal pouches.

The thymus gland that is fully dysplastic is often small, weighing as little as 1 g, and it may not have completely descended into the mediastinum. It appears embryonal with small lobules that are composed of spindle-shaped epithelial cells and are essentially devoid of thymocytes, a condition that contributes to a pseudoglandular pattern (Fig. 29-6). Corticomedullary differentiation and Hassall's corpuscles are characteristically absent, though rudimentary development of these features may be present in some patients. However, the spectrum of histologic appearances of "dyspla-

sia" even in SCID cases is variable.[21,48] It ranges from a pseudoatrophic pattern, characterized by the continued presence of thymocytes and Hassall's corpuscles, through a morphologic continuum to a fully dysplastic gland. Greater variation in the histologic pattern is apparent in surgical biopsy specimens than in thymus glands examined at autopsy.[21,169] In surgical biopsies the epithelial cells may be larger and less atrophic, and larger numbers of thymocytes and macrophages may be present. Often the degree of immune function abnormality does not correlate directly with the degree of dysplasia observed histologically. This range of morphologic expression of thymic dysplasia may reflect (1) the heterogeneous nature of immunodeficiency, (2) the stage of progression of the disorder, or (3) the lack of involutional changes, which can simulate the histologic findings of dysplasia after a prolonged illness. The morphology of the thymus is also variable in patients with Wiscott-Aldrich syndrome, varying from simple atrophy to severe dysplasia-like changes.[126] The thymus from

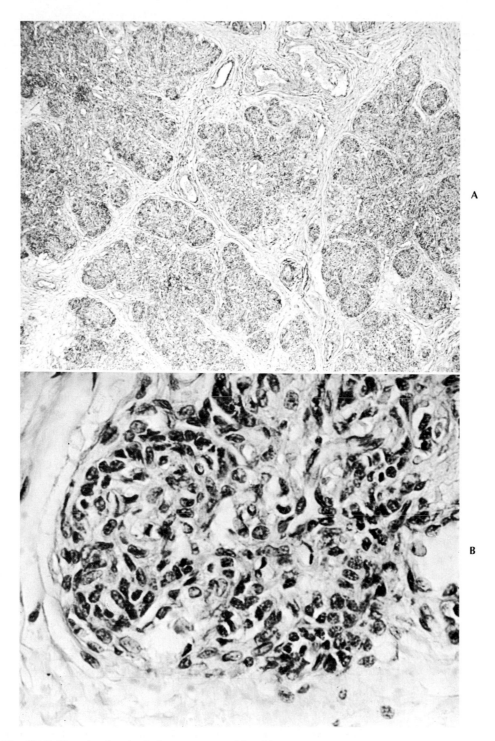

Fig. 29-6. Thymic dysplasia in severe combined immunodeficiency, thymic alymphoplasia. Poorly developed lobules are composed of spindle-shaped epithelial cells and are mostly devoid of thymocytes and Hassall's corpuscles. (**A,** 52×; **B,** 486×.)

patients with ataxia telangiectasia is most often simple hypoplasia.[126]

Histologic lesions similar to those of thymic dysplasia of primary immunodeficiency disease have been observed in patients with graft-versus-host disease (GVHD),[48,167] the acquired immunodeficiency syndrome (AIDS),[38,162,168] and fatal infectious mononucleosis (FIM) in the setting of immune deficiency to Epstein-Barr virus.[119] In these disorders, the thymus is devoid of thymocytes and Hassall's corpuscles, and definition of the corticomedullary junction is lost. In addition in GVHD, epithelial injury associated with a lymphocytic infiltrate is present as seen in other epithelial organs affected by GVHD. Although there may also be focal areas of epithelial necrosis indicative of epithelial injury in AIDS, a loss of epithelial antigens and hormones can be demonstrated with evidence of an immune response directed against the thymic epithelium itself. In FIM, some of the thymic lesions are dissimilar to the dysplasia in that Hassall's corpuscles are present.

It is recognized that infants with combined immunodeficiencies have an increased incidence of malignant lymphoproliferative disorders,[181] as do patients with other forms of profound primary or acquired immunodeficiencies. The fatal lymphomas in these patients have occurred after immunoreconstitution with cultured thymic epithelium grafts and spontaneously in untreated patients.[20,78] Appreciable numbers of both non-Hodgkin's lymphomas and Hodgkin's disease have now been described.[42] The frequency distribution among the various subclasses of lymphoma appears to be different from that the general population and predominantly of B-lymphocyte derivation. Both clonal and polyclonal tumors have been observed. The EBV nuclear antigen has been demonstrated within the neoplastic cell infiltrate of one polyclonal lymphoma after thymic epithelium engraftment.[141] This observation implicates one possible mechanism for the increased incidence of fatal lymphomas in these patients, that is, ineffective cellular immunity to a ubiquitous viral agent that is trophic for B-lymphocytes and vigorously stimulates their proliferation.[219]

THYMIC CYSTS

Cystic lesions of the thymus gland may be found anywhere along the lines of embryonic thymic descent, from the angle of the mandible to the body of the sternum. Thymic cysts are distinguished from other cysts by the presence of thymic tissue in their walls. These simple cysts are lined by epithelium, which may be flattened, columnar, squamous, or ciliated and are filled with accumulated serous fluid, cellular debris, or hemorrhagic extravation. Leakage of these contents into the surrounding tissues often stimulates the formation of granulomatous inflammation, which can resemble an

infectious process. The origin of some cysts is developmental from remnants of the third bronchial pouch. However, the origin of most thymic cysts, whether mediastinal or cervical in location, appears to be from degenerating Hassall's corpuscles or from other various foci within the mature thymus. One unusual intrathoracic thymic cyst that occurred in a 2-year-old girl contained not only thymic tissue in its walls but also parathyroid and salivary gland tissue, all tissues of pharyngeal origin.[23] Cystic lesions of other derivations arising in the thymus or in the same locations as thymic cysts include developmental cysts of respiratory, gastrointestinal, pericardial, and lymphatic tissues. Cystic degeneration of thymomas is common and may obscure the recognition of the neoplasm. Cyst formation can also occur after radiotherapy in patients with thymic involvement by Hodgkin's disease.[9]

THYMIC HYPERPLASIA

The concept of thymic hyperplasia embraces two morphologic forms.[96] The first form, massive or giant thymic hyperplasia,[62] is considered true thymic hyperplasia and is a dramatic enlargement of the gland through an increase in thymic tissue, which remains normally organized. Because of the wide weight variation of normal thymus glands throughout the population, the establishment of borderline hyperplasia is frequently problematic. Before standardized growth curves of the normal thymus were developed,[218] a proliferative lymphoid system and normally large thymus were frequently mininterpreted as a contributing cause of sudden respiratory death in infancy and led to the now archaic concept of "status thymolyphaticus." Thymus glands that are histologically unremarkable can weigh in excess of 200 g and are infrequently reported in infants[76,90,133] and children.[82] Massive thymic hyperplasia is unusual in infancy and is rarely encountered beyond 4 years of age. In older children thymic hyperplasia results in only mild respiratory symptoms because of compression of the airway. In infants hyperplasia can prevent the normal development of the lungs and results in pulmonary hypoplasia and secondary pulmonary hypertension. The pathogenesis and significance of thymic enlargement to massive proportions are unknown, and fortunately it rarely occurs. Recent evidence indicates that massive thymic hyperplasia may represent a maturation arrest in thymocyte development causing an accumulation of immature thymocytes and a reduction in the number of more mature cells.[127] Massive thymic hyperplasia has been reported in its pure form in patients without other associated diseases, in patients with Beckwith-Wiedemann syndrome (exomphalos, macroglossia, and gigantism,[6] and in patients who have recovered from acute stress involution. Lymphocytosis, presumably of antigen-responsive T-lymphocytes,[133] and an expansion of the thymus-dependent regions of lymph nodes often accompany thymic hyperplasia and resolve after thymectomy. Various cellular immunodeficiencies have been associated with massive thymic hyperplasia or have complicated the postoperative periods.[90]

The second form of thymic hyperplasia, lymphoid follicular hyperplasia,[63,134] is characterized by the presence of lymphoid follicles with germinal centers in the thymus gland, which may be either enlarged, atrophied, or involved by a neoplasm. (Fig. 29-7) The true incidence of this form of thymic hyperplasia is difficult to judge because of the wide range reported from the various populations studied. Based upon studies of thymus glands examined in victims of sudden accidental death or of those removed or biopsied during cardiac surgery,[112,174,199] the incidence in otherwise normal persons is 10% to 13%, with a slightly greater prevalence among young persons.

The presence of lymphoid follicles in the thymus gland is associated with a large number of diseases, most of which are believed to have an autoimmune basis, as follows: myasthenia gravis, primary hyperthyroidism, various endocrinopathies, systemic lupus erythematosus, rheumatoid arthritis, scleroderma, allergic vasculitides, aplastic anemia, some forms of chronic liver disease and chronic glomerulonephritis, and autoimmune skin disorders.[154] Myasthenia gravis is the disease most frequently associated with this form of hy-

perplasia, occurring in 85% of patients with myasthenia who have thymic abnormalities reported. Evidence up to now indicates that the thymus has a critical role in the pathogenesis of myasthenia gravis.[39] Although there appears to be an enhanced reactivity of patients with myasthenia gravis to autoantigens in general, T cell–dependent autoantibody production to the AChR appears to be the basic abnormality that reduces the number of available AChR at neuromuscular junctions ultimately causing the disease.[115,134,163] Formation of lymphoid follicles in the thymus glands of patients who develop myasthenia gravis may be pivotal in the early pathogenesis of this disease. Presumably in susceptible individuals, AChR antigen, perhaps originating within the thymus gland itself from epithelial cells or myoid stromal cells that are known to express AChR, is presented to and stimulates autoreactive thymocytes to proliferate, differentiate, and attract other T-lymphocytes and B-lymphocytes to formulate an immune response, which is directed against peripheral AChR.

The lymphoid follicles apparently arise in the thymus at the corticomedullary junction within the extrathymic, perivascular space of the septa and have been found to be structurally similar to those of peripheral lymphoid tissues.[93,182,192] In patients with myasthenia gravis, however, disruptions have been identified in the epithelial basal lamina at the borders of the germinal centers, which presumably allow communication of

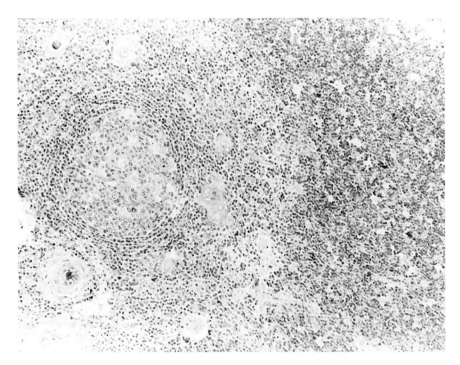

Fig. 29-7. Thymic hyperplasia. A germinal center immediately adjacent to Hassall's corpuscle, one form of thymic hyperplasia. (200×.)

lymphoid cells with the medullary epithelium.[19,29] Evidence of active lymphocyte–epithelial cell interaction in patients with myasthenia gravis includes structural evidence of epithelial damage to epithelial cells and epithelial cell hyperplasia, formation of high endothelial venules coincident with increased numbers of peripheral T-lymphocytes, and increased numbers of interdigitating reticulum cells and cortical thymocytes in the medulla.

Thymomas, often associated with intensive proliferations of the nonneoplastic thymocytic component of the neoplasm,[28] are associated with myasthenia gravis and many of these same autoimmune disorders. Numerous autoantigens, notably the AChR, various nuclear antigens, the carcinoembryonic antigen, and cytoplasmic antigens associated with cross-striations of skeletal muscle, have been detected in thymomatous cells.[32,214] Presumably then, all patients with thymomas are at risk for developing myasthenia gravis depending on the antigens expressed by the thymoma and the patient's immunogenetic potential. The true incidence of myasthenia gravis in thymoma patients is between 30% and 40%.[60,121,179] Myasthenia gravis has also been reported with thymolipomas,[132] an uncommon type of stromal tumor of the thymus, and after allogeneic bone marrow transplantation, in which lymphocytes from the donor graft were implicated as the contributing factor.[175]

As more becomes known about the aberrant immune regulation involved in myasthenia gravis, more specific and effective therapies or perhaps a cure for the disease will be devised. Current therapy consists in one or more methods: (1) pharmacologic, by enhancement of neuromuscular transmission through the use of anticholinesterase agents; (2) immunosuppressive, with steroids, cytotoxic agents, and cyclosporin A, or by exchanging plasma to deplete the patient's serum of anti-AChR autoantibodies; and (3) surgical, which has become more widely acceptable because of the possibility of long-term or permanent remissions.[2,36]

NEOPLASMS
Thymomas

The term "thymoma" refers to neoplasms of thymic epithelial cells.[151] Other primary tumors of the thymus gland are classified by their homologous identity to primary neoplasms in other locations, such as lymphomas, germ cell tumors, and neuroendocrine tumors. The prevalence of thymomas in a population increases with increasing age of individuals until after the fifth decade, when it begins to decline. The expected incidence in a large metropolitan population is about 1 per 10,000 to 20,000,[121] and the mean age of patients at diagnosis is about 48 years. Thymomas are rarely seen before 20 years of age, and both sexes and different ethnic groups are affected proportionally. Thymomas represent 9% to

17% of primary tumors of the mediastinum.[117] In over 50% of patients, thymomas are asymptomatic and are discovered by routine roentgenographic examination, which shows a lobated, anterior mediastinal mass. Linear calcifications may be observed at the tumor's periphery in some cases. In the remaining patients, symptoms bring attention to the tumor's presence. They may result from the physical presence of the tumor itself, such as cough, dyspnea, lassitude, dysphasia, chest pain, or superior vena cava compression, or from a systemic disease associated with the thymoma, namely, myasthenia gravis, hypogammaglobulinemia, or erythroid hypoplasia.[16,159] Superior vena cava syndrome or pain usually indicates invasion of adjacent anatomic structures by the tumor. Evidence of an associated systemic disease is discussed in 65% to 70% of all patients who present with symptoms.[121]

Typically thymomas occur in the anterior medastinum as well-encapsulated tumors that are easily removed surgically, though they may also arise in ectopic sites as in the neck along the route of embryonic migration.[145] In about 20% to 25% of cases the tumor is adherent to surrounding tissues, and most often tumor invasion of these tissues can be demonstrated microscopically.[108] Over half of the thymomas measure 5 to 10 cm in greatest diameter and weigh an average of 150 g.[151] Tumors that are not associated with myasthenia gravis often weigh more; however, rare thymomas of microscopic size or of gigantic proportions weighing more than 5 kg do occur.[176] The cut surface of the neoplasm usually reveals a thick fibrous capsule surrounding tumor lobules of varying sizes that are separated by prominent, fibrous trabeculas. Cystic degeneration of thymomas is common and can be so extensive as to obscure the presence of the neoplasm (Fig. 29-8).

Thymomas display a wide variation in their microscopic appearances, a fact that has frustrated the development of an acceptable classification. Because most thymomas maintain a constituency of nonneoplastic thymocytes (Fig. 29-9), they have been classified on the basis of the predominant cell type present—predominantly lymphocytic, predominantly epithelial, or mixed. Only rarely are thymomas purely epithelial. Thymomas have also been classified according to the cytology of the neoplastic epithelial cells—round, polygonal, spindle, or mixed, and as to their degree of cytologic differentiation.[117] Phenotyping of the epithelial cells by immunohistochemical methods has provided yet another means of classification.[27,116,146,197] These distinctions appear to be arbitrary, since there can be considerable variation of these features within the same tumor.

The neoplastic epithelial cells in thymomas are usually large, with a round or oval vesicular nucleus and indistinct, eosinophilic cytoplasm. The nucleus is usu-

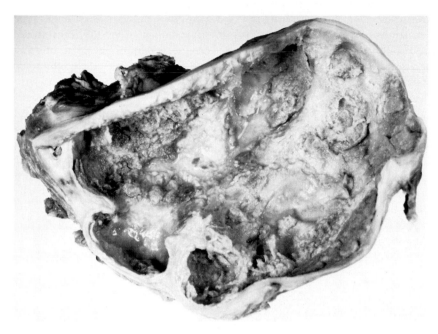

Fig. 29-8. Cystic degeneration of thymoma. Large central cyst was filled with necrotic, liquefied debris. Viable tumor was found microscopically in thick wall and in papillae that line cyst.

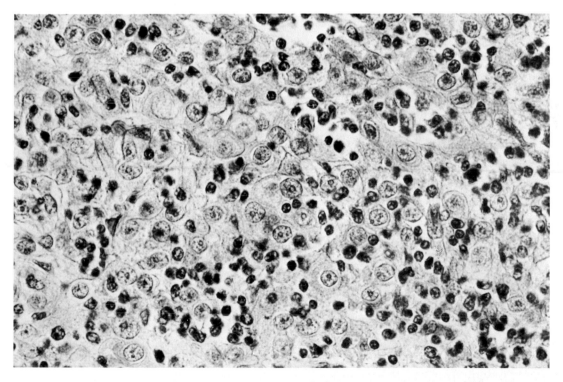

Fig. 29-9. Thymoma. Thymocytes are mixed with neoplastic epithelial cells. (585×.)

ally inconspicuous, though it may be prominent and centrally located within the nuclei in some tumors. Spindle-shaped cells are present in most thymomas, and when they predominate, the tumor is described as a spindle cell thymoma. This histologic patient is often seen in those tumors associated with hypoplastic anemia. Polygonal cells, which may be considered a transitional form between round cells and spindle cells, may also be present in any tumor, but they may also be the predominant cell type. Thymomas of this predominant cell type are often associated with myasthenia gravis. Rare thymomas showing differentiation toward both epithelial cells and myoid cells have also been observed.[41] The mitotic index in most thymomas is low, but it may be high in the thymocytic component and often accompanied by prominent lympholysis and a "starry-sky" pattern of phagocytosis of resulting cellular debris. Such cases can be misdiagnosed as non-Hodg-

kin's lymphoma if the arrangement and growth pattern of the epithelial component are not carefully observed. Immunohistochemistry and electron microscopy can be especially useful in establishing or excluding the diagnosis of thymoma in such cases by demonstrating the lymphoid or epithelial qualities of the neoplastic cells.[11,97,136]

The growth patterns of the neoplastic epithelial cells may be strikingly variable (Fig. 29-10). Some tumors grow in prominent whorled, storiform, or broad fascicular patterns. Others may show rosette-like or adenomatoid patterns or may resemble hemangiopericytomas.[151] Microcystic degeneration may be extensive in some tumors. Hassall's corpscles are found in about 15% of thymomas, which are considered well-differentiated neoplasms by some authors,[117] but may be entrapped in a small percentage of tumors. Quite often normal thymic tissue is found adjacent to thymomatous

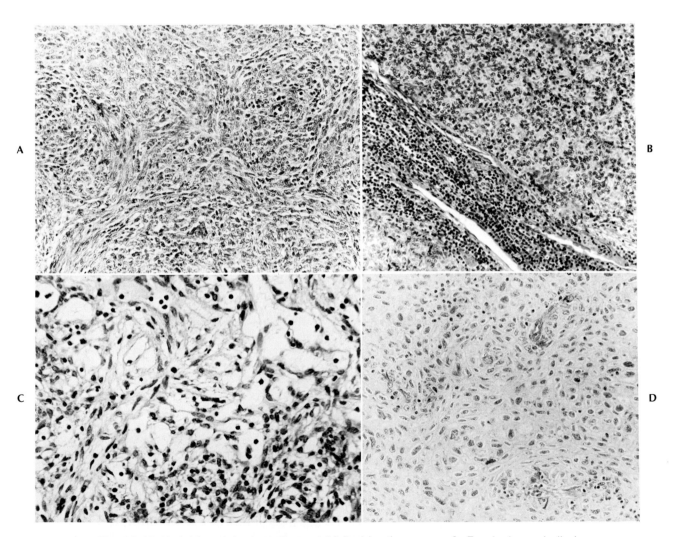

Fig. 29-10. Variable cytologic patterns exhibited by thymomas. **A,** Fascicular, spindled pattern. **B,** Rosettelike pattern. **C,** Microcystic pattern. **D,** Cytologically malignant pattern.

lobules. Thymic follicular hyperplasia may be observed in the adjacent tissue and rarely within the thymoma itself. This finding is common in cases associated with myasthenia gravis as discussed previously.

The lymphocytic component of thymomas is believed to be nonneoplastic, yet a close relationship appears to exist between lymphocytes and the tumor cells even in sites of metastases,[158,210] suggestive of the persistence of the functional properties of the epithelial cell. Most lymphocytes in thymomas express cellular antigens that are characteristic of the cortical thymocyte.[11,26,27,31,87,94,215] Thymomas of predominantly epithelial cell type and thymic carcinomas (to be discussed) contain many more mature T-lymphocytes and fewer thymocytes.[86,87,160] Although the epithelial cell microenvironment in thymomas is altered, cortical thymocyte differentiation appears to continue within some neoplasms.[161,191] T-cell lymphocytosis has also been observed in association with thymomas.[50,137]

Thymomas are slowly growing neoplasms that usually remain localized even to one lobe of the thymus gland for many years before invading adjacent anatomic structures. Invasion of an adjacent structure, such as lung or percardium, occurs in about 20% to 25% of the patients, 66% of whom have localizing symptoms.[16] Distant metastases rarely occur and most frequently involve the lung, thoracic lymph nodes, liver, axial skeleton, and central nervous system.[49,51] When thymomas are removed before local invasion has occurred, the prognosis is excellent, since tumor recurrence or death as result of a noninvasive tumor is a rare event.[40,85,91] Recurrences when they occur as localized mediastinal masses or pleural implants are amenable to secondary complete resection.[49] If resection by primary or secondary intent is not accomplished, death from cardiorespiratory complications of tumor invasion will result.

In assessing the short-term, malignant potential of a given thymoma, three characteristics of the tumor should be considered: (1) whether it is completely encapsulated and entirely excised, (2) whether it is considered invasive either macroscopically by the surgeon (this impression should be documented microscopically) or microscopically by the pathologist, and (3) whether it is benign or malignant histologically. For a given neoplasm, its history is the least powerful predictor of these three characteristics, since a thymoma with a benign history can be invasive and therefore malignant (these tumors are called "malignant thymomas") and a thymoma with a malignant history (called "thymic carcinomas") may not be invasive or metastatic and amenable to successful therapy. The malignant potential of thymomas therefore is more dependent on accurate clinicopathologic observations by the surgeon and pathologist. Most clinical staging systems for thymomas

Table 29-5. Clinical staging classification for thymomas

Stage	Clincopathologic characteristics
I	Encapsulated, noninvasive tumor, completely excised
II	Macroscopic invasion or microscopic capsular invasion
III	Macroscopic invasion into adjacent anatomic structures
IV	Mediastinal dissemination or distant metastases

Modified from Masaoka, A., et al.: Cancer **48:**2485, 1981.

incorporate these concepts[108,198,212] (Table 29-5). The 5-year survival rates for all patients with thymoma were 92.6% in stage I, 85.7% in stage II, 69.6% in stage III, and 50.0% in stage IV.[108] Nevertheless, strong statistical correlations have been made between tumor grade and the degree of invasiveness and prognosis in retrospective studies.[117,198]

Because some thymomas do display noticeable cytologic atypia in the neoplastic epithelial component, they are considered cytologically malignant (Fig. 29-10, *D*) and are referred to as "thymic carcinomas."[178] These true thymic carcinomas are more likely to be invasive and to metastasize.[107] Most of these carcinomas are either keratinizing or nonkeratinizing epidermoid carcinomas, though other morphologic variants do occur less frequently.[1,178] The finding that Epstein-Barr virus DNA has been detected in a case of nonkeratinizing thymic carcinoma raises the intriguing possibility of a causal role as in other morphologically similar carcinomas in tissues derived from embryonic pharyngeal epithelium.[79,98,157] A diagnosis of thymic carcinoma implies the exclusion of secondary involvement of the thymus gland by metastatic carcinoma, especially from the lung. Pleomorphic sarcomatous thymomas with morphologic features of the myoid cell have also been reported.[57]

Because of the improvement in management in systemic diseases, which are associated with thymomas, primarily myasthenia gravis, the long-term survival of patients with thymomas has improved.[104,198] More than 90% of patients with fully excised, noninvasive tumors are alive after 10 years regardless of whether they develop myasthenia gravis. Considering all patients with thymoma, the survival rate is 84% at 1 year, 77% at 3 years, and 57% at 10 years.[108] Thymomas in children, though uncommon, are much more aggressive than those in adults and have a considerably poorer prognosis.[22,33,44,110,159] Adjuvant radiotherapy and chemotherapy are indicated for patients after partial resection,[194] but the role of postoperative irradiation after total resection of a noninvasive tumor is controversial.[2,10,14,44] Recent reports indicate that postoperative radiotherapy may be advantageous in reducing local tumor recurrences.[104,108,129,194]

Thymomas in association with a large variety of systemic diseases have been described.[60,121,138,179] These include myasthenia gravis (10% to 15%), acquired hypogammaglobulinemia (12%),[138] erythroid hypoplasia (5%), and less frequently (1% or less) myositis, dermatomyositis, myocarditis, scleroderma, systemic lupus erythematosus, thyroiditis, Sjögren's syndrome, rheumatoid arthritis, pemphigus, and chronic mucocutaneous candidiasis. Occasionally more than one disorder is associated with thymomas.[45] Cushing's syndrome, previously reported in association with the thymomas, occurs in association with thymic carcinoid tumors.[149] Nonthymic malignancies, which include both lymphoreticular and nonlymphoreticular tumors, occurs in 20% of thymomatous patients.[180] Various mechanisms of autoimmunity are believed to function in each of these circumstances. What relationships exist between them is unclear. Differences are apparent between patients who do or do not have thymomas and are most distinctive in patients with myasthenia gravis. For example, as a group, myasthenia gravis patients with thymomas are older than myasthenic patients without tumors, but they are younger than nonmyasthenic patients with thymomas.[213] Thymomatous patients generally have a more severe form of myasthenia and higher mortality than myasthenic patients without thymomas.[121] The correlation of the histologic appearance of thymomas and the presence or absence of an associated syndrome has not been successful, except in myasthenia gravis in which spindle cell thymomas are rarely observed. In patients with myasthenia gravis, thymectomy has been ineffectual or has resulted in clinical improvement of remission in only some patients.[135] Paradoxically, myasthenia gravis has also followed the complete excision of thymomas in some patients.[45,121] Resection of thymomas in patients with other associated diseases have resulted in improvement in only a minority of patients.

Neuroendocrine (carcinoid) tumors

Before 1972 neoplasms arising from neuroendocrine cells of the thymus gland were confused with true thymomas of epithelial cell origin.[149] It was observed that these neoplasms had biological and morphologic features that were distinctly different from those of thymomas; that is, they were malignant neoplasms that were more often invasive and metastasized in about 30% of cases. These tumors, unlike thymomas, are associated with Cushing's syndrome in about one third of cases[96] but not with other endocrine aberrations. They do occur in association with multiple endocrine adenomatosis[150] and in association with bronchial and gastrointestinal carcinoid tumors.[149]

Morphologically these neoplasms most often resemble carcinoid tumors by their trabecular, rosette, or pseudoacinar pattern of growth of well-defined, uniform tumor cells. Like other carcinoid tumors of foregut derivation, the cells may stain by argyrophil techniques but not by argentaffin techniques, an indication of a lack of endogenous reducing capacity of the cell granules. Dense-core, membrane-bound neurosecretory granules (140 to 450 nm) can be demonstrated ultrastructurally. Peptide hormones can be identified immunohistochemically in 75% of cases.[211] In addition to adrenocortical hormone, somatostatin, calcitonin, and serotonin, neuron-specific enolase and chromogram have been demonstrated. Mitotic activity is often high, and necrosis with calcification may be present in areas of solid cell growth unlike typical carcinoid tumors found most often in other sites. Several rare morphologic variations of the tumor have been described: tumors resembling undifferentiated small cell carcinomas that are highly malignant and occur in other organs, especially the lung,[152] tumors that resemble spindle cell thymomas,[95] tumors that produce spindle cell thymomas,[95] tumors that produce melanin,[61,83] and tumors that produce melanin,[61,83] and tumors that resemble medullary thyroid carcinoma.[152] with abundant amyloid deposition (Fig. 29-11).

Germ cell tumors

Primary germ cell tumors, homologous to those in the gonads, arise in the thymus and include adult teratomas, seminomas, embryonal carcinomas, mixed germ cell tumors, teratocarcinomas, yolk sac tumors, and choriocarcinomas. It is generally accepted that these tumors have an origin similar to other midline extragonadal germ cell tumors—that is, an errant germ cell migration during embryogenesis[173]—but direct evidence of their cytogenesis is lacking. Mediastinal metastases primary germ cell tumors are rare but should always be considered as an alternative possibility. Most mediastinal germ cell tumors are benign adult teratomas. The malignant tumors have a predilection for men in the second and third decades of life, and as a group these tumors are highly malignant neoplasms that have poor prognosis.[64] However, seminomas are highly radiosensitive, and postoperative radiotherapy affords an excellent prognosis in most cases.[164,184] Combined chemotherapy can be effective therapy for nonseminomatous tumors.[52]

Microscopically, thymic germ cell neoplasms resemble their gonadal counterparts (Fig. 29-12). Thymic tissue can usually be found whithin these neoplasms or in the walls of their capsules, and it is often possible to

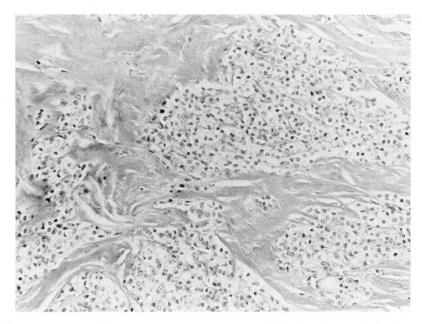

Fig. 29-11. Neuroendocrine (carcinoid) tumor. Tumor consists of solid areas of uniform cells with cleared cytoplasm arranged in abundant amyloid stroma. (900×.)

find teratoid elements in thymas. Primary thymic seminomas, though a distinct thymic neoplasm,[92] can be confused with thymomas and occasionally obscured by secondary granulomatous lesions, fibrosis, large cysts, and follicular lymphoid hyperplasia.[24] The prognosis of thymic seminomas is excellent when properly diagnosed and treated.

Malignant lymphomas

Malignant lymphomas most often involve the thymus gland secondarily in association with mediastinal or systemic disease. Lymphomas that do involve the thymus gland as a primary site include primarily Hodgkin's disease, lymphoblastic lymphomas, and large cell lymphomas. Other forms of lymphoma rarely involve the thymus as a primary event. Although clearly distinct pathologic entities, these tumors can provide diagnostic difficulties with thymoma. In contrast to thymomas, malignant lymphomas generally affect a younger patient population, demonstrate different patterns and more rapid rates of dissemination, and respond to nonsurgical therapeutic modalities (see Chapter 28).

Although Hodgkin's disease of the thymus gland has been distinguished from a histologic variant of thymoma and is recognized as a force of lymphoma, its histogenesis within the thymus remains as unclear as that of extrathymic, nodal Hodgkin's disease.[101,187] The nodular sclerosing subtype of Hodgkin's disease is by far the most common form that affects the thymus gland (Fig. 29-13). Hodgkin's disease in the thymus superfi-

cially resembles thymoma because of the interlacing bands of fibrosis and the inflammatory cell infiltrates that can be constituents of both neoplasms. Thymic epithelial cells can react with a peculiar hyperplastic response to the presence of the lymphoma and resemble the spindled cell proliferation of thymomas.[75] In Hodgkin's disease, however, the fibrous bands are rounded and not angulated as in thymomas; the epithelial cell hyperplasia is not pervasive throughout the tumor as in thymomas; and diagnostic Reed-Sternberg cells are identifiable, though occasionally with some difficulty.[128] Prognostic differences between thymic Hodgkin's disease and mediastinal Hodgkin's disease without thymic involvement are not apparent when differences in stage and histology are considered.[77] Thymic cyst formation after radiotherapy for thymic Hodgkin's disease has been described.[9] Synchronous cases of thymic Hodgkin's disease and thymoma,[144] thymolipoma,[139] myasthenia gravis,[130] and erythroid hypoplasia[143] have been reported.

Non-Hodgkin's lymphomas that involve the thymus gland as a first manifestation of disease are predominantly of two histologic types: lymphoblastic lymphoma and large cell lymphoma. Lymphoblastic lymphoma was first recognized in 1905 as lymphocytic sarcoma involving mediastinum that terminated in acute leukemia.[185] Characteristically the tumor is initially seen in adolescent males as a large mediastinal mass,[7,123] though this variety of lymphoma has been observed throughout the population and in many different pri-

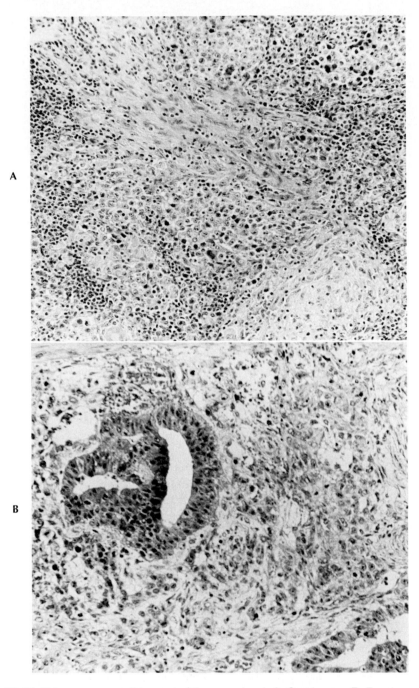

Fig. 29-12. Primary germ cell tumors of thymus gland. **A,** Seminoma. **B,** Teratocarcinoma. (900×.)

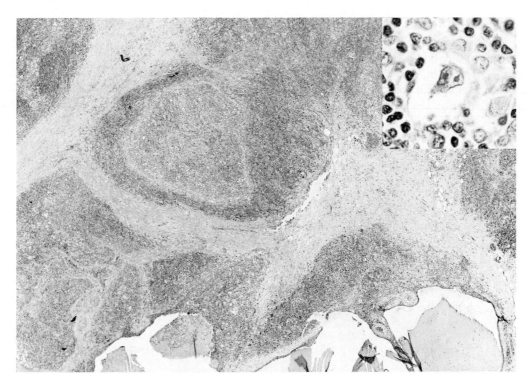

Fig. 29-13. Primary nodular sclerosing Hodgkin's disease of thymus gland. (80×.)

mary sites.[124,153] Mediastinal enlargement develops in a significant but lower frequency in adult patients, and when this occurs the thymus gland may not be directly involved.[125] But when the mediastinum is enlarged, early bone marrow involvement usually occurs and leukemia follows rapidly. The central nervous system and gonads are frequently involved in the course of the disease. Intense leukemic therapy for these patients is advocated from the time of diagnosis.[216] The neoplastic cells of this lymphoma resemble the cortical thymocytes in cytologic aspects, immunophenotype, and genotype.[170] The cells have a fine chromatin pattern and usually nuclear membrane convolutions. The mitotic index is high, and the tumor has a rapid growth phase. The rapidly proliferating cells expand the thymic lobules, surround persistent Hassall's corpuscles, infiltrate vessel walls, fibrous trabeculae, and the thymic capsule, and grow into the adjacent mediastinal adipose tissue. Observation of these histologic features usualy avoids diagnostic confusion with lymphocyte-predominant thymomas.

Large cell lymphomas may involve the mediastinum in adults and less frequently in children as primary disease localized to the thymus gland with or without accompanying lymph node involvement.[70] Thymic lymphoma of the large cell type virtually always has a diffuse growth pattern and is often of the immunoblastic subtype.[99] Nonimmunoblastic subtypes occurs less frequently, and true histiocytic lymphomas, which require cell-marker studies for their identification, have been described.[189] Large cell lymphoma in the thymus may occasionally be very difficult to distinguish from some thymomas, seminomas, or Hodgkin's disease, particularly when sclerosis is present.[136] Variable patterns of sclerosis may occur in over one third of cases, and pronounced fibrosis within a large cell lymphoma usually indicates a better prognosis. Since the optimal therapeutic approaches for these neoplasms are different, immunohistochemistry and electron microscopy may be necessary to distinguish them. Mediastinal large cell lymphomas may have a rapid onset and can be accompanied by symptoms of cardiorespiratory failure including dyspnea, heart failure, and superior vena cava syndrome. Because rapid systemic dissemination of these lymphomas usually occurs, they should be diagnosed and treated promptly with an effective chemotherapy regimen.[98]

Thymolipomas

Thymolipomas are rare, benign, encapsulated neoplasms of uncertain origin that arise in the thymus gland. They are usually found incidentally as asymptomatic mediastinal masses. They may attain a very large size, even greater than 16 kg, though most tumors weigh from 500 to 2000 g.[151] These tumors assume the configuration of the normal gland and are composed histologically of normal thymic tissue, which is excessive for age, and abundant mature adult adipose tissue.[18] One plausible explanation for this lesion is that it represents involution with compensatory fatty infiltration or previously unrecognized massive thymic hyperplasia. Thymolipomas may be associated with myasthenia gravis,[13] hypogammaglobulinemia,[148] hyperthyroidism,[13] red blood cell aplasia,[148] aplastic anemia,[8] and synchronous pharyngeal lipomas.[193]

Other proliferative lesions and neoplasms have been described as arising in the thymus gland,[148] and they include an inflammatory pseudotumor,[53] giant lymph node hyperplasia (Castleman's disease),[74,148] histiocytosis X,[172] granulocytic sarcoma,[80] malignant rhabdoid tumor,[148] liposarcoma,[148] and extraskeletal osteosarcoma.[195]

REFERENCES

1. Alguacil-García, A., and Halliday, W.C.: Thymic carcinoma with focal neuroblastoma differentiation, Am. J. Surg. Pathol. 11:474, 1987.
2. Alpert, L.I., Papatestas, A., Kark, A., et al.: A histologic reappraisal of the thymus in myasthenia gravis: a correlative study of thymic pathology and response to thymectomy, Arch. Pathol. 91:55, 1971.
3. Arnheim, E.E., and Gemson, B.L.: Persistent cervical thymus gland: thymectomy, Surgery 27:603, 1950.
4. Auerback, R.: Morphogenetic interactions in the development of the mouse thymus gland, Dev. Biol. 2:271, 1960.
5. Bach, J.F., and Popiernik, M.: Cellular and molecular signals in T cell differentiation. In Porter, R., and Whelan, J., editors: Microenvironments in haemopoietic and lymphoid differentiation (Ciba Foundation Symposium 84), London, 1981, Pitman Medical Publishing Co., Ltd.
6. Balcom, R.J., Hakanson, D.O., Werner A., and Gordon, L.P.: Massive thymic hyperplasia in an infant with Beckwith-Wiedemann syndrome, Arch. Pathol. Lab. Med. 109:153, 1985.
7. Barcos, M.P., and Lukes, R.J.: Malignant lymphoma of convoluted lymphocytes: a new entity of possible T-cell type. In Sinks, L.F., and Godden, J.O., editors: Conflicts in childhood cancer: an evaluation of current management, Prog. Clin. Biol. Res. 4:147, New York, 1975, Alan R. Liss, Inc.
8. Barnes, R.D.S., and O'Gorman, P.: Two cases of aplastic anemia associated with tumors of the thymus, J. Clin. Pathol. 15:485, 1976.
9. Baron, R.L., Sagal, S.S., and Baglan, R.J.: Thymic cyst following radiation therapy for Hodgkin's disease, Radiology 141:593, 1981.
10. Batata, M.A., Martini, N., Huvos, A.G., et al.: Thymomas: clinicopathologic features, therapy, and prognosis, Cancer 34:389, 1974.
11. Battifora, H., Sun, T.T., Baku, R.M., and Rao, S.: The use of antikeratin antiserum as a diagnostic tool: thymoma versus lymphoma, Hum. Pathol. 11:635, 1980.
12. Bearman, R.M., Bensch, K.G., and Levine, G.D.: The normal human thymic vasculature: an ultrastructural study, Anat. Rec. 183:485, 1976.
13. Benton, C., and Gerard, P.: Thymolipoma in a patient with Grave's disease: case report and review of the literature, J. Thorac. Cardiovasc. Surg. 51:428, 1966.
14. Bergh, N.P., Gatzinsky, P., Larson, S., Lundlin, P., and Ridell, B.: Tumors of the thymus and thymic region. I. Clinicopathological studies on thymomas, Ann. Thorac. Surg. 25:91, 1978.
15. Berman, R.M., Levine, G.D., and Bensch, K.G.: The ultrastructure of the normal human thymus: a study of 36 cases, Anat. Rec. 190:755, 1978.
16. Bernatz, P.E., Harrison, E.G., and Clagett, O.T.: Thymoma: a clinicopathologic study, J. Thorax. Cardiovasc. Surg. 42:424, 1961.
17. Bhan, A.K., Reinherz, E.L., Poppema, S., McCluskey, R.T., and Schlossman, S.F.: Location of T cell and major histocompatibility complex antigens in the human thymus, J. Exp. Med. 152:771, 1980.
18. Boetsch, C.H., Swoyer, G.B., Adams, A., and Walker, J.H.: Lipothymoma: report of two cases, Dis. Chest 50:539, 1966.
19. Bofill, M., Janossy, G., Willcox, N., Chilosi, M., Trejdosiewicz, L.K., and Newsom-Davis, J., et al.: Microenvironments in the normal thymus and the thymus in myasthenia gravis, Am. J. Pathol. 119: 462, 1985.
20. Borzy, M.S., Hong, R., Horowitz, S.D., Gilbert, E., Kaufman, D., DeMendonca, W., Oxelius, V.A., Dictor, M., and Pachman, L.: Fatal lymphoma after transplantion of cultured thymus in children with combined immunodeficiency disease, N. Engl. J. Med. 301:565, 1979.
21. Borzy, M.S., Schulte-Wissermann, H., Gilbert, E., Horowitz, S.D., Pellett, J., and Hong, R.: Thymic morphology in immunodeficiency diseases: results of thymic biopsies, Clin. Immunol. Immunopathol. 12:31, 1979.
22. Bowie, P.R., Teixeira, O.H.P., and Carpenter, B.: Malignant thymoma in a nine-year-old boy presenting with pleuropericardial effusion, J. Thorac. Cardiovasc. Surg. 77:777, 1979.
23. Breckler, I.A., and Johnston, D.G.: Choristoma of the thymus, Am. J. Dis. Child. 92:175, 1956.
24. Burns, B.F., and McCaughey, W.T.E.: Unusual thymic seminomas, Arch. Pathol. Lab. Med. 110:539, 1986.
25. Cantor, H., and Weissman, I.: Development and function of subpopulations of thymocytes and T lymphocytes, Prog. Allergy 20:1, 1976.
26. Chan, W.C., Zaatari, G.S., Tabei, S., Bibb, M., and Brynes, R.K.: Thymoma: an immunohistochemical study, Am. J. Clin. Pathol. 82:160, 1984.
27. Chilosi, M., Iannucci, A.M., Pizzolo, G., Menestrina, F., Fiore-Donati, L., and Janossy, G.: Immunohistochemical analysis of thymoma: evidence for medullary origin of epithelial cells, Am. J. Surg. Pathol. 8:309, 1984.
28. Chilosi, M., Iannucci, A., Menestrina, F., Lestani, M., Scarpa, A., Bonetti, F., Fiore-Donati, L., DiPasquale, B., Pizzolo, G., Palestro, G., et al: Immunohistochemical evidence of active thymocyte proliferation in thymoma: its possible role in the pathogenesis of autoimmune diseases, Am. J. Pathol. 128:464, 1987.
29. Chilosi, M., Iannucci, A., Fiore-Donati, L., Tridente, G., Pampanin, M., Pizzolo, G., Ritter, M., Bofill, M., and Janossy, G.: Myasthenia gravis: immunohistological heterogeneity in microenvironmental organization of hyperplastic and neoplastic thymuses suggesting different mechanisms of tolerance breakdown, J. Neuroimmunol. 11:191, 1986.
30. Cordier, A.C., and Haumont, S.M.: Development of the thymus, parathyroids and ultimo-brachial bodies in NMRI and nude mice. Am. J. Anat. 157:227, 1980.
31. Cossman, J., Deegan, M.J., and Schnitzer, B.: Thymoma: an immunologic and electron microscopic study, Cancer 41:2183, 1978.
32. Dardenne, M., Savino, W., and Bach, J.-F.: Thymomatous epithelial cells and skeletal muscle share a common epitope defined by a monoclonal antibody, Am. J. Pathol. 126:194, 1987.
33. Dehner, L.P., Martin, S.A., and Sumner, H.W.: Thymoma related tumors and tumor-like lesions in childhood with rapid clinical progression and death, Hum. Pathol. 8:53, 1977.
34. De Maagd, R.A., MacKenzie, W.A., Schuurman, H.J., Ritter, M.A., Price, K.M., Broekhuizen, R., and Kater, L.: The human thymus microenvironment: heterogeneity detected by monoclonal anti–epithelial cell antibodies, Immunology 54:745, 1985.
35. De Waal Malefijt, R., Leene, W., Roholl, P.J., Wormmeester, J., and Hoeben, K.A.: T cell differentiation within thymic nurse cells, Lab. Invest. 55:25, 1986.

36. Drachman, D.B.: Present and future treatment of myasthenia gravis, N. Engl. J. Med. 316:743, 1987.
37. Drenckhahn, D., von Gaudecker, B., Müller-Hermelink, H.K., Unsicker, K., and Gröschel-Stewart, U.: Myosin and actin containing cells in the human postnatal thymus: ultrastructural and immunohistochemical findings in normal thymus and in myasthenia gravis, Virchows Arch. [Cell Biol.] 32:33, 1979.
38. Elie, R., Laroche, A.C., Arnoux, E., Guérin, J.M., Pierre, G., Malebranche, R., Seemeyer, T.A., Dupuy, J.M., Russo, P., and Lapp, W.S.: Thymic dysplasia in acquired immunodeficiency syndrome, N. Engl. J. Med. 308:841, 1983.
39. Engel, A.G.: Myasthenia gravis and myasthenic syndromes, Ann. Neurol. 16:519, 1984.
40. Fechner, R.E.: Recurrence of noninvasive thymomas: report of four cases and review of literature, Cancer 23:1423, 1969.
41. Friedman, N.B.: Tumors of the thymus, J. Thorac. Cardiovasc. Surg. 52:163, 1967.
42. Frizzera, G., Rosai, J., Dehner, L.P., Spector, B.D., and Kersey, J.H.: Lymphoreticular disorders in primary immunodeficiencies: new findings based on an up-to-date histologic classification of 35 cases, Cancer 46:692, 1980.
43. Fudenberg, H., Good, R.A., Goodman, H.C., et al.: Primary immunodeficiencies: report of a World Health Organization committee, Pediatrics 47:927, 1971.
44. Fujimura, S., Kondo, T., Handa, M., Shiraishi, Y., Tamahashi, N., and Nakada, T.: Results of surgical treatment for thymoma based on 66 patients, J. Thorac. Cardiovasc. Surg. 93:708, 1987.
45. Fujimura, S., Kondo, T., Yamauchi, A., Handa, M., and Nakada, T.: Experience with surgery for thymoma associated with pure red blood cell aplasia: report of three cases, Chest 88:221, 1985.
46. Gilmour, J.R.: Some developmental abnormalities of the thymus and parathyroids, J. Pathol. Bacteriol. 52:213, 1941.
47. Gosseye, S., and Nezelof, C.: T-system immunodeficiencies in infancy and childhood, Pathol. Res. Pract. 171:142, 1981.
48. Gosseye, S., Diebold, N., Griscelli, C., and Nezelof, C.: Severe combined immunodeficiency disease: a pathological analysis of 26 cases, Clin. Immunol. Immunopathol. 29:58, 1983.
49. Gravanis, M.B.: Metastasizing thymoma: report of a case and review of the literature, Am. J. Clin. Pathol. 49:690, 1968.
50. Griffin, J.D., Aisenberg, A.C., and Long, J.C.: Lymphocytic thymoma associated with T-cell lymphocytosis, Am. J. Med. 64:1075, 1978.
51. Guillan, R.A., Zelman, S., Smalley, R.L., et al.: Malignant thymoma associated with myasthenia gravis, and evidence of extrathoracic metastases: an analysis of published cases and report of a case, Cancer 23:823, 1971.
52. Hainsworth, J.D., Einhorn, L.H., Williams, S.D., Stewart, M., and Greco, F.A.: Advanced extragonadal germ-cell tumors, Ann. Intern, med. 97:7, 1982.
53. Harpax, N., Gribetz, A.R., Krellenstein, D.J., and Marchevsky, A.M.: Inflammatory pseudotumor of the thymus, Ann. Thorac. Surg. 42:331, 1986.
54. Haynes, B.F.: The human thymic microenvironment, Adv. Immunol. 36:87, 1984.
55. Haynes, B.F., Scearce, R.M., Lobach, D.F., and Hensley, L.L.: Phenotypic characterization and ontogeny of mesodermal-derived and endocrine epithelial components of the human thymic microenvironment, J. Exp. Med. 159:1149, 1984.
56. Hayward, A.R.: Myoid cells in the human fetal thymus, J. Pathol. 106:45, 1972.
57. Henry, K.: An unusual thymic tumour with a striated muscle (myoid) component (with a brief review of the literature on myoid cells), Br. J. Dis. Chest 66:291, 1972.
58. Henry, K.: Mucin secretion and striated muscle in human thymus, Lancet 1:183, 1966.
59. Hirokawa, K.: Age-related changes of thymus: morphological and functional aspects, Acta Pathol. Jpn. 28:843, 1978.
60. Hirst, E., and Robertson, T.I.: The syndrome of thymoma and erythroblastopenic anemia: a review of 56 cases including 3 case reports, Medicine 46:225, 1967.
61. Ho, F.C.S., and Ho, J.C.I.: Pigmented carcinoid tumour of the thymus, Histopathology 1:363, 1977.
62. Hofmann, W.J., Möller, P., and Otto, H.F.: Thymic hyperplasia. I. True thymic hyperplasia: review of the literature, Klin. Wochenschr. 65:49, 1987.
63. Hofmann, W.J., Möller, P., and Otto, H.F.: Thymic hyperplasia. II. Lymphofollicular hyperplasia of the thymus: an immunohistologic study, Klin. Wochenschr. 65:53, 1987.
64. Hurt, R.D., Bruckman, J.E., Farrow, G.M., Bernatz, P.E., Hahn, R.G., and Earle, J.D.: Primary anterior mediastinal seminoma, Cancer 49:1658, 1982.
65. Hwang, W.S., Ho, T.Y., Luk, S.C., et al.: Ultrastructure of the rat thymus: a transmission, scanning electron microscope and morphometric study, Lab. Invest. 31:473, 1974.
66. Ito, T., Hoskino, T., and Abe, K.: The fine structure of myoid cells in the human thymus, Arch. Histol. Jpn. 30:207, 1969.
67. Janossy, G., Tidman, N., Papageorgiou, E.S., Kung, P.C., and Goldstein, G.: Distribution of T lymphocyte subsets in the human bone marrow and thymus: an analysis with monoclonal antibodies, J. Immunol. 126:1608, 1981.
68. Janossy, G., Thomas, J.A., Bollum, F.J., Granger, S., Pizzolo, G., Bradstock, K.F., Wong, L., McMichael, A., Ganeshaguru, K., and Hoffbrand, A.V.: The human thymic microenvironment: an immunohistologic study, J. Immunol. 125:202, 1980.
69. Jerne, N.K.L.: The somatic generation of immune recognition, Eur. J. Immunol. 1:1, 1971.
70. Jones, S.E., Fuks, Z., Bull, M., et al.: Non-Hodgkin's lymphomas. IV. Clinicopathologic correlation in 405 cases, Cancer 31:806, 1973.
71. Jotereau, F.V., Houssaint, E., and Le Douarin, N.M.: Lymphoid stem cell homing to the early thymic primordium of the avian embryo, Eur. J. Immunol. 10:620, 1980.
72. Kaiserling, E., Stein, H., and Müller-Hermelink, H.K.: Interdigitating reticulum cells in the human thymus, Cell Tissue Res. 155:47, 1974.
73. Kao, I., and Drachman, D.B.: Thymus muscle cells bear acetylcholine receptors: possible relation to myasthenia gravis, Science 195:74, 1977.
74. Karcher, D.S., Pearson, C.E., Butler, W.M., Hurwitz, M.A., and Cassell, P.F.: Giant lymph node hyperplasia involving the thymus with associated nephrotic syndrome and myelofibrosis, Am. J. Clin. Pathol. 77:100, 1982.
75. Katz, A., and Lattes, R.: Granulomatous thymoma or Hodgkin's disease of thymus: a clinical and histologic study and a reevaluation, Cancer 23:1, 1969.
76. Katz, S.M., Chatten, J., Bishop, H.C., and Rosenblum, H.: Massive thymic enlargement: report of a case of gross thymic hyperplasia in a child, Am. J. Clin. Pathol. 68:786, 1977.
77. Keller, A.R., and Castleman, B.: Hodgkin's disease of the thymus gland, Cancer 33:1615, 1974.
78. Kersey, J.H., et al.: Lymphoma after thymus transplantation, N. Engl. J. Med. 302:1615, 1974.
79. Klein, G.: The relationship of the virus to nasopharyngeal carcinoma. In Epstein, M.A., and Achong, B.G., editors: The Epstein-Barr virus, New York, 1979, Springer-Verlag.
80. Kubonishi, I., Ohtsuki, Y., Machida, K., Agatsuma, Y., Tokuoka, H., Iwata, K., and Miyoshi, I.: Granulocytic sarcoma presenting as a mediastinal tumor: report of a case and cytological and cytochemical studies of tumor cells in vivo and in vitro, Am. J. Clin. Pathol. 82:730, 1984.
81. Kyewski, B.A.: Thymic nurse cells: possible sites of T-cell selection, Immunol. Today 7:374, 1986.
82. Lack, E.E.: Thymic hyperplasia with massive enlargement: report of two cases with review of diagnostic criteria, J. Thorac. Cardiovasc. Surg. 81:741, 1981.
83. Lagrange, W., Dahm, H.H., Karstens, J., Feichtinger, J., and Mittermayer, C.: Melanocytic neuroendocrine carcinoma of the thymus, Cancer 59:484, 1987.
84. Landing, B.H., Yutue, I.L., and Swanson, V.L.: Clinicopathologic correlations in immunologic deficiency diseases of children with emphasis on thymic histologic patterns. In Kobayashi, N., editor: Immunodeficiency, its nature and etiological significance in human diseases, Baltimore, 1978, University Park Press.
85. Lattes, R.: Thymoma and other tumors of the thymus: an analysis of 107 cases, Cancer 15:1224, 1962.

86. Lauriola, L., Piantelli, M., Carbone, A., Dina, M.A., Scoppetta, C., and Musiani, P.: Subpopulations of lymphocytes in human thymomas, Clin. Exp. Immunol. **37**:502, 1979.

87. Lauriola, L., Maggiano, N., Marino, M., Carbone, A., Piantelli, M., and Musiane, P.: Human thymoma: immunologic characteristics of the lymphocytic component, Cancer **48**:1992, 1981.

88. Le Douarin, N.M., and Jotereau, F.V.: Homing of lymphoid stem cells to the thymus and the bursa of Fabricius studied in avian embryo chimeras. In Fourzereau, M., and Dausset, J., editors: Immunology 80, Prog. Immunol., vol. 4, London, 1980, Academic Press Inc., Ltd.

89. Le Douarin, N.M., and Jotereau, F.V.: Tracing of cells of the avian thymus through embryonic life in interspecific chimeras, J. Exp. Med. **142**:17, 1975.

90. Lee, Y., Moallem, S., and Lauss, R.H.: Massive hyperplastic thymus in a 22-month-old infant, Ann. Thorac. Surg. **27**:356, 1979.

91. Legg, M.A., and Brady, W.J.: Pathology and clinical behavior of thymomas: a review of 51 cases, Cancer **18**:1131, 1965.

92. Levine, G.D.: Primary thymic seminoma—a neoplasm ultrastructurally similar to testicular seminoma and distinct from epithelial thymoma, Cancer **31**:729, 1973.

93. Levine, G.D., and Bearman, R.: Electron microscopy of the thymus. In Johannessen, J.V., editor: Electron microscopy in human medicine, vol. 5, New York, 1980, McGraw-Hill Book Co.

94. Levine, G.D., and Polliack, A.: The T-cell nature of the lymphocytes in two human epithelial thymomas: a comparative immunologic, scanning and transmission electron microscopic study, Clin. Immunol. Immunopathol. **4**:199, 1975.

95. Levine, G.D., and Rosai, J: A spindle cell variant of thymic carcinoid tumor: a clinical, histologic, and fine structural study with emphasis on its distinction from spindle cell thymoma, Arch. Pathol. Lab. Med. **100**:293, 1976.

96. Levine, G.D., and Rosai, J.: Thymic hyperplasia and neoplasia: a review of current concepts, Hum. Pathol. **9**:495, 1978.

97. Levine, G.D., Rosai, J., Bearman, R.M., et al.: The fine structure of thymoma, with emphasis on its differential diagnosis: a study of ten cases, Am. J. Pathol. **81**:49, 1975.

98. Leyvraz, S., Henle, W., Chahinian, A.P., Perlmann, C., Klein, G., Gordon, R.E., Rosenblum, M., and Holland, J.F.: Association of Epstein-Barr virus with thymic carcinoma, N. Engl. J. Med. **312**:1296, 1985.

99. Lichtenstein, A.K., Levine, A., Taylor, C.R., Boswell, W., Rossman, S., Feinstein, D.I., and Lukes, R.J.: Primary mediastinal lymphoma in adults, Am. J. Med. **68**:509, 1980.

100. Low, T.L.K., and Goldstein, A.L.: Thymic hormones: an overview, Meth. Immunol. **116**:213, 1985.

101. Lowenhaupt, E., and Brown, R.: Carcinoma of the thymus of granulomatous type, Cancer **4**:1193, 1951.

102. Ma, D.D.F., Sylvestrowicz, T.A., Granger, S., Messaia, M., Franks, R., Janossy, G., and Hoffbrand, A.V.: Distribution of terminal deoxynucleotidyl transferase and purine degradative and synthetic enzymes in subpopulations of human thymocytes, J. Immunol. **129**:1430, 1982.

103. Ma, D.D.F., Sylvestrowicz, T.A., Tanossy, G., and Hoffbrand, A.V.: The role of purine metabolic enzymes and terminal deoxynucleotidyl transferase in intrathymic T cell differentiation, Immunol. Today **4**:65, 1983.

104. Maggi, G., Giaccone, G., Donadio, M., Ciufredda, L., Dalesio, O., Leria, G., Trifiletti, G., Casadio, C., Palestro, G., Mancuso, M., et al.: Thymomas: a review of 169 cases, with particular reference to results of surgical treatment, Cancer **58**:765, 1986.

105. Makinodan, T.: The thymus in aging. In Greenblatt, R.B., editor: Geratric endocrinology, vol. 5, Aging, New York, 1978, Raven Press.

106. Mandel, T.: The development and structure of Hassall's corpuscles in the guinea pig: a light and electron microscopic study, Z. Zellforsch. **89**:180, 1968.

107. Marino, M., and Müller-Hermelink, H.K.: Thymoma and thymic carcinoma: relation of thymoma epithelial cells to the cortical and medullary differentiation of thymus, Virchows Arch. [Pathol. Anat.] **407**:119, 1985.

108. Masaoka, A., Monden, Y., Nakahara, K., and Tanioka, T.: Follow-up study of thymomas with special reference to their clinical stages, Cancer **48**:2485, 1981.

109. McFarland, E.J., Scearce, R.M., and Haynes, B.F.: The human thymic microenvironment: cortical thymic epithelium is an antigenically distinct region of the thymic microenvironment, J. Immunol. **133**:1241, 1984.

110. McKenzie, F.N., and Youngson, G.G.: Malignant thymoma in childhood, J. Thorac. Cardiovasc. Surg. **79**:472, 1980.

111. McPhee, D., Pye, J., and Shortman, K.: The differentiation of T lymphocytes. V. Evidence for intrathymic death of most thymocytes, Thymus **1**:151, 1979.

112. Middleton, G.: The incidence of follicular structures in the human thymus at autopsy, Aust. J. Exp. Biol. Med. **556**:189, 1967.

113. Miller, C.L., and Claudy, B.J.: Suppressor T-cell activity induced as a result of thermal injury, Cell. Immunol. **44**:201, 1979.

114. Miller, J.F.A.P.: Immunological function of the thymus, Lancet **2**:748, 1961.

115. Mittag, T., Kornfeld, P., Tormay, A., et al.: Detection of antiacetylcholine receptor factors in serum and thymus from patients with myasthenia gravis, N. Engl. J. Med. **294**:691, 1976.

116. Mokhtar, N., Hsu, S.M., Lad, R.P., Haynes, B.F., and Jaffe, E.S.: Thymoma: lymphoid and epithelial components mirror the phenotype of normal thymus, Hum. Pathol. **15**:378, 1984.

117. Monden, Y., Tanioka, T., Maeda, M., Masaoka, A., Nakahara, K., Kawashima, Y., and Kitamura, H.: Malignancy and differentiation of neoplastic epithelial cells of thymoma, J. Surg. Oncol. **31**:130, 1986.

118. Moore, M.A.S., and Owen, J.J.T.: Chromosome marker studies on the development of the haematopoietic system in the chick embryo (in two parts), Nature **208**:966, 1965.

119. Mroczek, E.C., Seemayer, T.A., Grierson, H.L., Markin, R.S., Linder, J., Brichacek, B., and Purtilo, D.T.: Thymic lesions in fatal infectious mononucleosis, Clin. Immunol. Immunopathol. **43**:243, 1987.

120. Müller-Hermelink, H.K., Marino, M., and Palestro, G.: Pathology of thymic epithelial tumors. In Müller-Hermelink, H.K., editor: The human thymus: histophysiology and pathology, Curr. Top. Pathol. **75**:207, Berlin, 1986, Springer-Verlag.

121. Namba, T., Brunner, N.G., and Grob, D.: Myasthenia gravis in patients with thymoma, with particular reference to onset after thymectomy, Medicine **57**:411, 1978.

122. Naparstek, Y., Holoshitz, J., Eisenstein, S., Reshef, T., Rappaport, S., Chemke, J., Ben-Nun, A., and Cohen, I.R.: Effector T lymphocyte line cell migrate to the thymus and persist there, Nature **300**:262, 1982.

123. Nathwani, B.N., Kim, H., and Rappaport, H.: Malignant lymphoma, lymphoblastic, Cancer **38**:964, 1976.

124. Nathwani, B.N., Diamond, L.W., Winberg, C.D., Kim, H., Bearman, R.M., Glick, J.H., Jones, S.E., Gams, R.A., Nissen, N.I., and Rappaport, H.: Lymphoblastic lymphoma: a clinicopathologic study of 95 patients, Cancer **48**:2347, 1981.

125. Newcom, S.R., and Kadin, M.E.: T-cell leukemia with thymic involution, Cancer **43**:622, 1979.

126. Nezelof, C.: Pathology of the thymus in immunodeficiency states. In Müller-Hermelink, H.K., editor: The human thymus: histophysiology and pathology, Curr. Top. Pathol. **75**:151, Berlin, 1986, Springer-Verlag.

127. Nezelof, C., and Normand, C.: Tumor-like massive thymic hyperplasia in childhood: a possible defect of T-cell maturation, histological and cytoenzymatic studies of three cases, Thymus **8**:177, 1986.

128. Nickels, J., Franssila, K., and Hjelt, L: Thymoma and Hodgkin's disease of the thymus, Acta Pathol. Microbiol. Scand. **81**:1, 1973.

129. Nordstrom, D.G., Tewfik, H.H., and Latourette, H.B.: Thymoma: therapy and prognosis as related to operative staging, Radiat. Oncol. Biol. Phys. **5**:2059, 1979.

130. Null, J.A., LiVolsi, K.V.A., and Glenn, W.W.L.: Hodgkin's disease of the thymus (granulomatous thymoma) and myasthenia gravis: a unique association, Am. J. Clin. Pathol. **67**:521, 1977.

131. Oosterom, R., and Kater, L.: The thymus in the aging individual. II. Thymic epithelial function in vitro in aging and in thy-

mus pathology, Clin. Immunol. Immunopathol. **18**:195, 1981.

132. Otto, H.F., Löning, T., Lachenmayer, L., Janzen, R.W., Gürtler, K.F., and Fischer, K.: Thymolipoma in association with myasthenia gravis, Cancer **50**:1623, 1982.

133. O'Shea, P.A., Pansatiankul, B., and Farnes, P.: Giant thymic hyperplasia in infancy: immunologic histologic and ultrastructure observation, Lab. Invest. **39**:391, 1978.

134. Patrick, J., and Lindstrom, J.: Autoimmune response to acetylcholine receptor, Science **180**:871, 1973.

135. Papatestas, A.E., Alpert, L.I., Asserman, K.E., et al.: Studies in myasthenia gravis: effects of thymectomy: results on 185 patients with nonthymomatous and thymomatous myasthenia gravis, Am. J. Med. **50**:465, 1971.

136. Perrone, T., Frizzera, G., and Rosai, J.: Mediastinal diffuse large-cell lymphoma with sclerosis: a clinicopathologic study of 60 cases, Am. J. Surg. Pathol. **10**:176, 1986.

137. Pedraza, M.A.: Thymoma: immunological and ultrastructural characterization, Cancer **39**:1455, 1977.

138. Peterson, R.D.A., Cooper, M.D., and Good, R.A.: The pathogenesis of immunologic deficiency diseases, Am. J. Med. **38**:317, 1979.

139. Pillai, R., Yeoh, N., Addis, B., Peckham, M., and Goldstraw, P.: Thymolipoma in association with Hodgkin's disease, J. Thorac. Cardiovasc. Surg. **90**:306, 1985.

140. Pyke, L.W., and Bach, J.F.: The in vitro migration of murine fetal liver cells to thymic rudiments, Eur. J. Immunol. **9**:317, 1979.

141. Reese, E.R., Gartner, J.G., Seemayer, T.A., and Tongas, J.H.: Lymphoma after thymus transplantation, N. Engl. J. Med. **302**:302, 1980.

142. Reinherz, E.L., Kung, P.C., Goldstein, G., Levey, R.H., and Schlossman, S.F.: Discrete stages of human intrathymic differentiation: analysis of normal thymocytes and leukemic lymphoblasts of T-cell lineage, Proc. Natl. Acad. Sci. USA **77**:1588, 1980.

143. Remigio, P.A.: Granulomatous thymoma associated with erythroid hypoplasia, Am. J. Clin. Pathol. **55**:68, 1971.

144. Ridell, B., and Larsson, S.: Coexistence of a thymoma and Hodgkin's disease of the thymus, Acta Pathol. Microbiol. Scand. **88**:1, 1980.

145. Ridenhour, C.E., Henzel, J.H., DeWeese, M.S., et al.: Thymoma arising from undescended cervical thymus, Surgery **67**:614, 1970.

146. Ring, N.P., and Addis, B.J.: Thymoma: an integrated clinicopathological and immunohistochemical study, J. Pathol. **149**:327, 1986.

147. Romain, P.L., and Schlossman, S.F.: The T cell circuit: clinical and biological implications, Chicago, 1986, Year Book Medical Publishers, Inc.

148. Rosai, J.: The pathology of thymic neoplasia. In Berard, C.W., Dorfman, R.F., and Kaufman, N., editors: Malignant lymphoma, Monographs in pathology, Baltimore, 1987, Williams & Wilkins.

149. Rosai, J., and Higa, E.: Mediastinal endocrine neoplasm, of probably thymic origin, related to carcinoid tumor: clinicopathologic study of 8 cases, Cancer **29**:1061, 1972.

150. Rosai, J., Higa, E., and Davie, J.: Mediastinal endocrine neoplasm in patients with multiple endocrine adenomatosis: a previously unrecognized association, Cancer **29**:1075, 1972.

151. Rosai, J., and Levine, G.D.: Tumors of the thymus. In Firminger, H.I., editor: Atlas of tumor pathology, series 2, fascicle 13, Washington, D.C., 1976, Armed Forces Institute of Pathology.

152. Rosai, J., Levine, G., Weber, W.R., and Higa, E.: Carcinoid tumors and oat cell carcinomas of the thymus, Pathol. Annu. **11**:201, 1975.

153. Rosen, P.J., Feinstein, D.I., Pattengale, P.K., Tindle, B.H., Williams, A.H., Cain, M.J., Bonorris, J.B., Parker, J.W., and Lukes, R.J.: Convoluted lymphocytic lymphoma in adults: a clinicopathologic entity, Ann. Intern. Med. **89**:319, 1978.

154. Rosenow, E.C., and Hurley, B.T.: Disorders of the thymus: a review, Arch. Intern. Med. **144**:763, 1984.

155. Rouse, R.V. and Weissman, I.L.: Microanatomy of the thymus: its relationship to T cell differentiation. In Porter, R., and Whelan, J., editors: Microenvironments in haemopoietic and lymphoid differentiation (Ciba Foundation Symposium 84), London, 1981, Pitman Medical Publishing Co., Ltd.,

156. Rouse, R.V., van Ewyk, W., Jones, P.P., and Weissman, I.L.: Expression of MHC antigens by mouse thymic dendritic cells, J. Immunol. **122**:2508, 1979.

157. Saemundsen, A.K., Albeck, H., Hansen, J.P., Nielsen, N.H., Anvret, M., Henle, W., Henle, G., and Thomsen, K.A.: Epstein-Barr virus in nasopharyngeal and salivary gland carcinoma of Greenland Eskimoes, Br. J. Cancer **46**:721, 1982.

158. Salter, D.M., and Krajewski, A.S.: Metastatic thymoma: a case report and immunohistological analysis, J. Clin. Pathol. **39**:275, 1986.

159. Salyer, W.R., and Eggleston, J.C.: Thymoma: a clinical and pathological study of 65 cases, Cancer **37**:229, 1979.

160. Sato, Y., Watanabe, S., Mukai, K., Kodama, T., Upton, M.A., Goto, M., and Shimosato, Y.: An immunohistochemical study of thymic epithelial tumors. II. Lymphoid component, Am. J. Surg. Pathol. **10**:862, 1986.

161. Savino, W., Berrih, S., and Dardenne, M.: Thymic epithelial antigen, acquired during ontogeny and defined by the anti-p19 monoclonal antibody, is lost in thymomas, Lab. Invest. **51**:292, 1984.

162. Savino, W., Dardenne, M., Marche, C., Trophilme, D., Dupuy, J.M., Pekovic, D., Lapointe, N., and Bach, J.F.: Thymic epithelium in AIDS: an immunohistologic study, Am. J. Pathol. **122**:302, 1986.

163. Scadding, G.K., Vincent, A., Newsom-Davis, J., and Henry, K.: Acetylcholine receptor antibody synthesis by thymic lymphocytes: correlation with thymic histology, Neurology **31**:935, 1981.

164. Schantz, A., Sewall, W., and Castleman, B.: Mediastinal germinoma: a study of 21 cases with an excellent prognosis, Cancer **30**:1189, 1972.

165. Schuurman, H.J., Van de Wijngaert, F.P., Delvoye, L., Broekhuizen, R., McClure, J.E., Goldstein, A.L., and Kater, L.: Heterogeneity and age dependency of human thymus reticulo-endothelium in production of thymosin components, Thymus **7**:13, 1985.

166. Scollay, R.G., Butcher, E.C., and Weissman, I.L.: Thymus cell migration: quantitative aspects of cellular traffic from the thymus to the periphery in mice, Eur. J. Immunol. **10**:310, 1980.

167. Seemayer, T.A., and Bolande, R.P.: Thymus involution mimicking thymic dysplasia: a consequence of transfusion-induced graft versus host disease in a premature infant, Arch. Pathol. Lab. Med. **104**:252, 1980.

168. Seemayer, T.A., Laroche, A.C., Russo, P., Malebranche, R., Arnoux, E., Guérin, J.M., Pierre, G., Dupuy, J.M., Gartner, J.G., Lapp, W.S., et al.: Precocious thymic involution manifest by epithelial injury in the acquired immune deficiency syndrome, Hum. Pathol. **15**:469, 1984.

169. Shearer, W.T., Wedner, H.J., Strominger, D.B., Kissane, J., and Hong, R.: Successful transplantation of the thymus in Nezelof's syndrome, Pediatrics **61**:619, 1978.

170. Sheibani, K., Nathwani, B.N., Winberg, C.D., Burke, J.S., Swartz, W.G., Blayney, D., van de Velde, S., Hill, L.R., and Rappaport, H.: Antigenically defined subgroups of lymphoblastic lymphoma: relationship to clinical presentation and biologic behavior, Cancer **60**:183, 1987.

171. Shier, K.J.: The thymus according to Schambacher: medullary ducts and reticular epithelium of thymus and thymomas, Cancer **48**:1182, 1981.

172. Siegal, G.P., Dehner, L.P., and Rosai, J.: Histiocytosis X (Langerhans' cell granulomatosis) of the thymus: a clinicopathologic study of four childhood cases, Am. J. Surg. Pathol. **9**:117, 1985.

173. Simson, L.R., Lampe, I., and Abell, M.R.: Suprasellar germinomas, Cancer **22**:533, 1968.

174. Sloan, H.E.: The thymus in myasthenia gravis, Surgery **13**:154, 1943.

175. Smith, C.I.E., Aarli, J.A., Biberfeld, P., Bolme, P., Christenson, B., Gahrton, G., Hammarström, L., Lefvert, A.K., Löngqvist, B., Matell, G., et al.: Myasthenia gravis after bone-marrow transplantation: evidence for a donor origin, N. Engl. J. Med. **309**:1565, 1983.

176. Smith, W.F., DeWall, R.A., and Krumholz, R.A.: Giant thymoma, Chest **68**:383, 1970.

177. Snodgrass, H.R., Dembic, Z., Steinmetz, M., and von Boehmer, H.: Expression of the T-cell receptor genes during fetal development in the thymus, Nature (London) **315**:232, 1985.

178. Snover, D.C., Levine, G.D., and Rosai, J.: Thymic carcinoma: five distinctive histological variants, Am. J. Surg. Pathol. **6**:451, 1982.

179. Souadjian, J.V., Enríquez, P., Silverstein, M.N., et al.: The spectrum of diseases associated with thymoma: coincidence or syndrome? Arch. Intern. Med. **134**:374, 1974.

180. Souadjian, J.V., Silverstein, K.M.N., and Titus, J.L.: Thymoma and cancer, Cancer **22**:1221, 1968.

181. Spector, B.D., Perry, G.S., III, and Kersey, J.H.: Genetically determined immunodeficiency diseases (GDID) and malignancy: report from the Immunodeficiency-Cancer Registry, Clin. Immunol. Immunopathol. **11**:12, 1978.

182. Staber, F.G., Fink, U., and Sack, W.: B lymphocytes in the thymus of patients with myasthenia gravis, N. Engl. J. Med. **292**:1032, 1975.

183. Steinmann, G.G., and Müller-Hermelink, H.K.: Lymphocyte differentiation and its microenvironment in the human thymus during aging, Monogr. Dev. Biol. **17**:142, 1984.

184. Sterchi, M., and Cordell, A.R.: Seminoma of the anterior mediastinum, J. Thorac. Surg. **19**:371, 1975.

185. Sternberg, C.: Leukosarkomatose und Myeloblastenleukaemie, Beitr. Pathol. **61**:76, 1916.

186. Stutman, O.: Intrathymic and extrathymic T cell maturation, Immunol. Rev. **42**:138, 1978.

187. Suematsu, N., Watanabe, S., and Shimosato, Y.: A case of large "thymic granuloma": neoplasm of T-zone histiocyte, Cancer **54**:2480, 1984.

188. Summary report of a Medical Research Council working-party: Hypogammaglobulinemia in the United Kingdom, Lancet **1**:163, 1969.

189. Szporn, A.H., Dikman, S., and Jagirdar, J.: True histiocytic lymphoma of the thymus: report of a case and a study of the distribution of histiocytic cells in the fetal and adult thymus, Am. J. Clin. Pathol. **82**:734, 1984.

190. Sztein, M.B., and Goldstein, A.L.: Thymic hormones: a clinical update, Springer Semin. Immunopathol. **9**:1, 1986.

191. Takacs, L., Savino, W., Monostori, E., Ando, I., Bach, J.F., and Dardenne, M.: Cortical thymocyte differentiation in thymomas: an immunohistologic analysis of the pathologic microenvironment, J. Immunol. **138**:687, 1987.

192. Tamaoli, N., Habu, S., and Kameyu, T.: Thymic lymphoid follicles in autoimmune diseases. II. Histological, histochemical and electron microscopic studies, Keio J. Med. **20**:67, 1971.

193. Trites, A.E.W.: Thyrolipoma, thymolipoma, and pharyngeal lipoma: a syndrome, Can. Med. Assoc. J. **95**:1254, 1966.

194. Uematsu, M., and Kondo, M.: A proposal for treatment of invasive thymoma, Cancer **58**:1979, 1986.

195. Valderrama, E., Kahn, L.B., and Wind, E.: Extraskeletal osteosarcoma arising in an ectopic hamartomatous thymus, Cancer **51**:1132, 1983.

196. van de Wijngaert, F.P., Kendall, M.D., Schuurman, H.J., Rademakers, L.H., and Kater, L.: Heterogeneity of epithelial cells in the human thymus: an ultrastructural study, Cell Tissue Res. **237**:227, 1984.

197. van der Kwast, van Vliet, E., Cristen, E., van Ewijk, W., and van der Heul, R.O.: An immunohistologic study of the epithelial and lymphoid components of six thymomas, Hum. Pathol. **16**:1001, 1985.

198. Verley, J.M., and Hollmann, K.H.: Thymoma: a comparative study of clinical stages, histologic features, and survival in 200 cases, Cancer **55**:1074, 1985.

199. Vetters, J.M., and Barcley, R.S.: The incidence of germinal centers in thymus glands of patients with congenital heart disease, J. Clin. Pathol. **26**:683, 1973.

200. Viac, J., Schmitt, D., Staquet, M.J., and Thivolet, J.: Epidermis-thymus antigenic relations with special reference to Hassall's corpuscles, Thymus **1**:319, 1980.

201. von Gaudecker, B.: Ultrastructure of the age-involuted adult human thymus, Cell Tissue Res. **186**:507, 1978.

202. von Gaudecker, B., and Müller-Hermelink, H.K.: Ontogeny and organization of the stationary non-lymphoid cells in the human thymus, Cell Tissue Res. **207**:287, 1980.

203. von Gaudecker, B., and Schmale, E.M.: Similarities between Hassall's corpuscles of the human thymus and the epidermis: an investigation by electron microscopy and histochemistry, Cell Tissue Res. **151**:347, 1974.

204. von Gaudecker, B., Steinmann, G.G., Hansmann, M.L., Harpprecht, J., Milicevic, N.M., and Müller-Hermelink, H.K.: Immunohistochemical characterization of the thymic microenvironment: a light-microscopic and ultrastructural immunocytochemical study, Cell Tissue Res. **244**:403, 1986.

205. Waldmann, T.A., Strober, W., and Blaese, R.M.: T and B cell immunodeficiency diseases. In Parker, C., editor: Clinical immunology, Philadelphia, 1980, W.B. Saunders Co.

206. Weissman, I.L.: Nursing the thymus, Lab. Invest. **55**:1, 1986.

207. Weissman, I.L., Rouse, R.V., Kyewski, B.A., LePault, F., Butcher, E.C., Kaplan, H.S., and Scollay, R.G.: Thymic lymphocyte maturation in the thymic microenvironment, Behring Inst. Mitt. **70**:242, 1982.

208. Wekerle, H., Ketelsen, U., and Ernst, M.: Thymic nurse cells: lymphoepithelial cell complexes in murine thymuses: morphological and serological characterization, J. Exp. Med. **151**:925, 1980.

209. Weksler, M.E.: The immune system and the aging process in man, Proc. Soc. Exp. Biol. Med. **165**:200, 1980.

210. Wick, M.R., Nichols, W.C., Ingle, J.N., Bruckman, J.E., and Okazaki, H.: Malignant, predominantly lymphocytic thymoma with central and peripheral nervous system metastases, Cancer **47**:2036, 1981.

211. Wick, M.R., and Scheithauer, B.W.: Thymic carcinoid: a histologic, immunohistochemical, and ultrastructural study of 12 cases, Cancer **53**:475, 1984.

212. Wilkins, E.W., and Castleman, B.: Thymoma: a continuing survey at the Massachusetts General Hospital, Ann. Thorac. Surg. **28**:252, 1979.

213. Wilkins, E.W., Jr., Edmunds, L.H., Jr., and Castleman, B.: Cases of thymoma at the Massachusetts General Hospital, J. Thorac. Cardiovasc. Surg. **52**:322, 1966.

214. Willcox, N., Schluep, M., Ritter, M.A., Schuurman, H.J., Newsom-Davis, J., and Christensson, B.: Myasthenic and non-myasthenic thymoma: an expansion of a minor cortical epithelial cell subset? Am. J. Pathol. **127**:447, 1987.

215. Woda, B.A., Bain, K., and Salm, T.V.: The phenotype of lymphocytes in a thymoma as studied with monoclonal antibodies, Clin. Immunol. Immunopathol. **30**:197, 1984.

216. Wollner, N., Exelby, P.R., and Lieberman, P.R.: Non-Hodgkin's lymphoma in children: a progress report on the original patients treated with LSA2-L2 protocol, Cancer **44**:1990, 1979.

217. Yagüe, J., White, J., Coleclough, C., Kappler, J., Palmer, E., and Marrack, P.: The T cell receptor: the α and β chains define idiotype, and antigen and MHC specificity, Cell **42**:81, 1985.

218. Young, M., and Turnbull, H.M.: An analysis of the data collected by the Status Lymphaticus Investigation Committee, J. Pathol. Bacteriol. **34**:213, 1931.

219. Ziegler, J.L., Magrath, I.T., Gerber, P., et al.: Epstein-Barr virus and human malignancy, Ann. Intern. Med. **86**:323, 1977.

220. Zinkernagel, R.M.: Thymus and lymphohemopoietic cells: their role in T cell maturation in selection of T cell' H-2-restriction-specificity and in H-2 linked Ir gene control, Immunol. Rev. **42**:224, 1978.

30 Pituitary Gland

NANCY E. WARNER

EMBRYOLOGY

The pituitary gland arises from two quite separate primordia that meet and join early in embryonic life to form the definitive organ. The adenohypophysis, or anterior lobe, is an ectodermal derivative that arises from Rathke's pouch, a midline diverticulum of the roof of the stomodeum, or primitive buccal cavity. The pouch grows upward through the transient craniopharyngeal canal to fuse with the infundibulum, the downgrowth from the floor of the diencephalon that forms the neurohypophysis. By rupture of its attachment, Rathke's pouch loses its connection with the roof of the pharynx and comes to lie within the developing sphenoid bone. Cells of Rathke's pouch proliferate to form the adenohypophysis; thus the lumen of the pouch is reduced to a narrow cleft, which is eventually obliterated, though remnants may persist as small cysts. The anterior part of the pouch becomes the definitive pars distalis. An upward extension of the developing adenohypophysis forms a cuff that surrounds the pituitary stalk, known as the pars tuberalis. The portion of the pouch that lies in contact with the neurohypophysis becomes the pars intermedia, which thus is delimited by the cleft from the developing pars distalis. In humans the pars intermedia remains rudimentary. The developing neurohypophysis differentiates into the infundibulum, the infundibular stem (or stalk), and the infundibular process, or neural lobe. Whereas the adenohypophysis loses its connection with the pharynx as the craniopharyngeal canal closes, the neurohypophysis permanently retains direct connections with the brain by the infundibular stalk (Fig. 30-1). Rarely, the pituitary may occupy an ectopic suprasellar location.[8]

The adenohypophysis of the human fetus begins to produce hormones at 7 weeks of pregnancy, as demonstrated by immunocytochemical staining.[2] Hormones produced by the fetal hypophysis appear to have a crucial role in normal development of the thyroid and adrenal glands, since (1) congenital absence or hypoplasia of the human anterior lobe invariably leads to hypoplasia of thyroid and adrenals, and (2) experimental destruction of the fetal pituitary in the rat, mouse, and

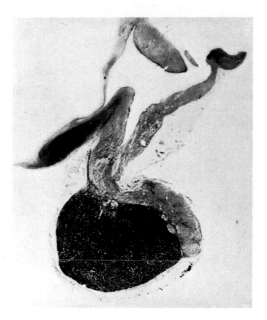

Fig. 30-1. Midsagittal section of pituitary gland to show neural attachments. (Hematoxylin and eosin; 4×; courtesy Drs. Dorothy S. Russell and A.R. Currie, Edinburgh.)

rabbit leads to reduction in size of the thyroid and adrenals, which can be avoided by injection of thyroid-stimulating hormone (TSH) or adrenocorticotropic hormone (ACTH) into the fetus.[13,20]

Remnants of Rathke's pouch regularly persist into postnatal life. The pharyngeal (caudal) end of the ruptured stalk of Rathke's pouch forms the pharyngeal pituitary.[5,12,14] The pharyngeal pituitary, which is present consistently in all age groups, is a small cylindrical body 5 to 6 mm in length, located in the midline in the roof of the nasopharynx, beneath the mucoperiosteum inferior to the vomerosphenoid junction (Fig. 30-2).[21] The extent of its function is uncertain.

Immunocytochemistry reveals the usual cell types.[6] Although the extent of its function is uncertain, the pharyngeal hypophysis may undergo hyperplasia in response to end-organ deficiency,[7] and hypertrophy after hypophysectomy has been reported. Other epithelial

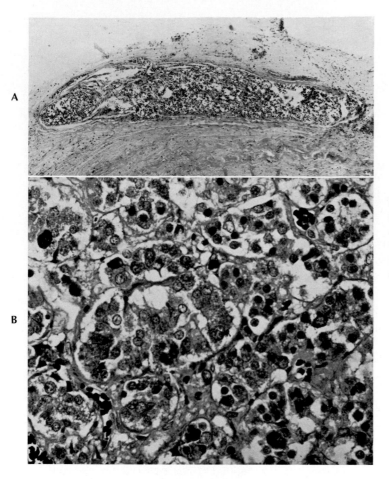

Fig. 30-2. A, Pharyngeal pituitary gland. **B,** Higher magnification showing typical configuration of adenohypophyseal cells in alveolar compartments. (**A,** Hematoxylin and eosin, 44×; **B,** acid fuchsin and aniline blue; 350×; courtesy Drs. Dorothy S. Russell and A.R. Currie, Edinburgh.)

remnants include parapituitary epithelial residua, persistent Rathke's cleft within the gland, and remains of the craniopharyngeal stalk within the sphenoid bone[21]; these elements may be the source of cysts or tumors (see p. 1536).

ANATOMY

The pituitary gland in the adult is a small, bean-shaped, bilaterally symmetric organ that weighs 500 to 900 mg.[17] The gland is usually heavier in women, and its weight may reach 1100 mg or more during pregnancy[10] when hyperplasia normally occurs. The gland has two major anatomic divisions, the reddish brown adenohypophysis and the pale gray neurohypophysis. The adenohypophysis consists of the pars distalis (or pars anterior), the pars intermedia, or zona intermedia,[9] and the pars tuberalis, which is an upward extension forming a cuff around the infundibular stem.

The pars anterior is divided into a median wedge and two lateral wings by a pair of fibrous trabeculas, which originate centrally at the junction of the zona intermedia and neurohypophysis and extend diagonally toward the anterior border of the gland to form a fibrous core.[11]

The neurohypophysis consists of the pars nervosa (also known as the neural lobe, or infundibular process), the infundibular stem, and the infundibulum proper. The gland is attached to the brain by the stalk, which contains the nerve tracts and blood vessels, vital links to the hypothalamus. The stalk in turn merges with the infundibulum, a cone-shaped projection of the tuber cinereum of the hypothalamus; this region is referred to as the median eminence.

The pituitary gland is located in the hypophyseal fossa of the sella turcica, a midline cavity in the sphenoid bone. In this position deep inside the head, the gland is unusually well protected, and surgical approach is difficult.

An extension of the dura mater lines the hypophyseal fossa, encapsulates the pituitary, and spreads out superiorly to form an incomplete covering for the sella, known as the diaphragma sellae.

An extension of the leptomeninges blends with the surface of the pituitary, and a subarachnoid space of variable size may be present.

Knowledge of the anatomic relationships of the pituitary to its environs is essential in understanding the symptoms caused by pituitary tumors, which often compress the vital structures adjacent to the pituitary gland. The optic chiasm, hypothalamus, and third ventricle lie directly above the gland. Just lateral to the pituitary on each side are the cavernous sinuses, each containing the internal carotid artery and cranial nerves III, IV, V, and VI. Minor anatomic variations of these relationships are common, a matter of great concern to the neurosurgeon who is operating for tumor or palliative ablation of the hypophysis.[4,15]

The arterial supply of the pituitary gland is derived from the internal carotid arteries by way of paired superior, middle, and inferior hypophyseal arteries.[3,11] The neurohypophysis is supplied by direct branches of these arteries.[22] The adenohypophysis also is supplied by direct branches of the same arteries,[11,19] which supply the capsular rete and each trabecular artery, but its major blood supply is derived from the hypophyseal portal system. The primary bed of this portal system consists of capillaries in the infundibulum and infundibular stem; the secondary bed is the network of capillaries in the adenohypophysis.[23] The primary capillary bed arises from small branches of the superior hypophyseal arteries, which terminate as specialized vascular structures known as gomitoli.[18] The capillaries in the infundibulum and upper region of the stem are drained by the long portal veins, which course to the adenohypophysis through the stalk. The capillaries of the lower part of the stem are drained by the short portal veins, which are contained within the body of the gland. Therefore transection of the stalk will destroy the long portal veins, but the short veins may remain intact unless the stalk is divided at its junction with the gland.[16] The portal veins deliver blood to the secondary capillary bed of the adenohypophysis, each group of vessels supplying a specific territory in the pars distalis.[1] The capillaries of both the pars distalis and the pars nervosa drain into the dural venous sinuses surrounding the pituitary.

The neural and vascular pathways that link the hypothalamus to the pituitary warrant special consideration, since they are crucial in the regulation of the secretion of hormones by both neurohypophysis and adenohypophysis. The pathway between the hypothalamus and the neurohypophysis is a direct neural connection, the hypothalamohypophyseal tract, which originates from neurons in the supraoptic and paraventricular nuclei, traverses the pituitary stalk, and terminates in the pars nervosa. The supraoptic and paraventricular nuclei secrete vasopressin and oxytocin, octapeptide hormones with antidiuretic and oxytocic effects. These hormones become attached to carrier substances, the neurophysins, and are transported down the axons of the hypothalamohypophyseal tract to the pars nervosa, where they are stored before release into the capillaries of the neural lobe. Whereas the neurohypophysis is connected directly to the hypothalamus by a single link, the hypothalamohypophyseal nerve

tract, the adenohypophysis is connected to the hypothalamus by a path consisting of two components, the tuberohypophyseal neural tract and the hypophyseal portal system. The tuberohypophyseal tract originates from neurons in the tuberal and other nuclei of the hypothalamus and terminates in the infundibulum, adjacent to the primary capillary beds of the hypophyseal portal system. Releasing and inhibiting factors synthesized in the cell bodies of tuberal nuclei pass down its axons and are deposited at the capillaries of the infundibulum, to be transported through the portal veins to the sinusoids of the adenohypophysis, where they control the release of hormones in the pars distalis.

HISTOLOGY AND FUNCTION
Adenohypophysis

The pars distalis is composed of cords and clumps of epithelial cells separated by a network of capillaries, the secondary plexus of the hypophyseal portal bed. The capillaries are surrounded by perivascular spaces (best shown by electron microscopy) into which the secretory granules are released from the epithelial cells by exocytosis. Some of these cells are arranged in follicles, with a small central lumen containing colloid.

With conventional stains, the epithelial cells can be separated into chromophils, which have cytoplasmic secretory granules with a strong affinity for dyes, and chromophobes, smaller cells with cytoplasm having no visible granules by light microscopy and a lesser affinity for dyes. In hematoxylin and eosin–stained sections, three types of epithelial cells can be distinguished: chromophil cells with acidophilic granules (about 40%), chromophil cells with basophilic granules (about 10%), and chromophobe cells with no visible granules (about 50%).

Acidophil cells are concentrated in the lateral wings, and basophil cells are mainly found in the median wedge. Efforts to subclassify the acidophils and basophils on the basis of special stains led to a succession of classifications[30,56] and resulted in chaos, principally for the reason that full understanding of functional cytology of the hypophysis was impossible without access to a broad range of techniques, some of which became available only recently. These techniques include histochemistry, enzyme immunohistochemistry (Fig. 30-3), electron microscopy of normal (Fig. 30-4) and abnormal hypophysis, ultrastructural analysis of cytoplasmic granules obtained by ultracentrifugation, autoradiography, and the histologic analysis of antigen-antibody reactions by immunofluorescence (Fig. 30-5). The functional classification, in which each cell was named according to its secretory activity,[60] was proposed by the International Committee for Nomenclature of the Adenohypophysis. This functional classification has been widely accepted, and a system of morphologic nomenclature has gradu-

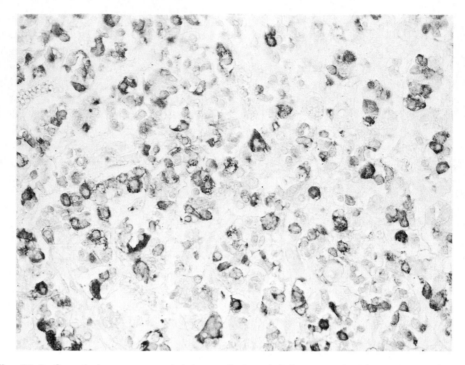

Fig. 30-3. Growth hormone–containing cells in adult human adenohypophysis. (Immunoperoxidase technique; 275×; courtesy Dr. Clive R. Taylor, Los Angeles.)

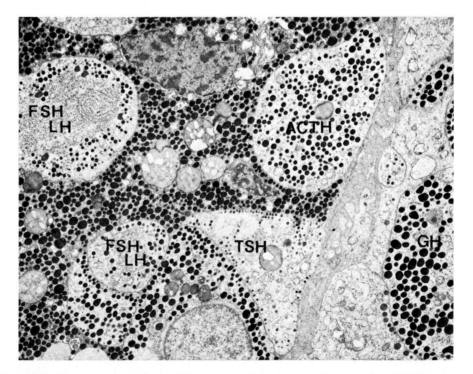

Fig. 30-4. Electron micrograph of normal pituitary removed transsphenoidally from 56-year-old woman with advanced mammary carcinoma. Smallest granules are in presumed thyrotroph (TSH) cell and largest granules are in presumed ACTH cell. Presumed FSH-LH cells have granules larger than TSH cell and smaller than ACTH cell. Mean granule sizes are TSH, 140 nm; FSH, 230 nm; ACTH, 330 nm; and GH, 470 nm. (4500×; courtesy Dr. I. Doniach, London.)

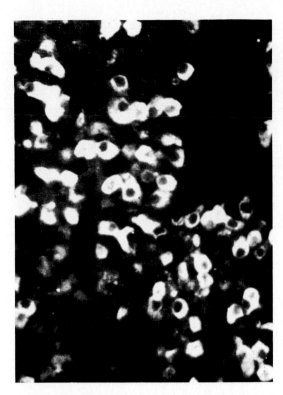

Fig. 30-5. Growth hormone–containing cells in adult human adenohypophysis. (Indirect immunofluorescence technique; 400×; from Porteous, I.B., Beck, J.S., and Currie, A.R.: J. Pathol. Bacteriol. **91**:539, 1966.)

ally emerged.[34,37] Previous classifications, recent developments, and relative percentages of cell types[37] are summarized in Table 30-1. McManus[41] first reported periodic acid–Schiff–positive granules in hypophyseal cells and Pearse[50] identified these cells as basophils (Fig. 30-6). These important discoveries marked the beginning of the histochemical studies that led ultimately to the demonstration of distinct classes of basophils.

The acidophils include somatotrophs and lactotrophs, which produce growth hormone (GH) and prolactin (PRL), respectively. Both hormones are simple proteins. In a horizontal section of the adenohypophysis, the acidophils are localized in the lateral wings.[34,49] Acidophils are readily identified by their affinity for eosin and other acidic dyes, such as orange G, erythrosin, and carmoisine.[26]

Differentiation of somatotrophs (GH cells) and lactotrophs (PRL cells) is based on immunostaining. By electron microscopy, somatotrophs and lactotrophs may be densely or sparsely granulated, with granules of various sizes.[37] Misplaced exocytosis, or release of secretory granules from cell surfaces not adjacent to perivascular spaces, is a characteristic feature of the lactotroph.[37] These cells also have concentric whorls of rough endoplasmic reticulum known as nebenkerns. In pregnancy, the lactotrophs are considerably enlarged and are known as pregnancy cells of Erdheim.[10] Cells containing both GH and PRL, known as mammosomatotrophic

Table 30-1. Functioning cells of adenohypophysis and corresponding hormones

Hormone	Hematoxylin and eosin	Periodic acid–Schiff–orange G	Herlant's tetrachrome[35]	PM-AT-PAS-orange G*[30,48]	Immunocytologic stains	Electron microscopy
Simple proteins 1. GH 2. PRL	*Acidophils*	*Acidophils* Orange G+	*Somatotrophs* Orange G+	*Acidophils* Orange G+	GH cell (50%)	Granules 250-700 nm[37]
			Lactotrophs Erythrosin+		PRL cell (15%-25%)	Granules 200-700 nm[37]; misplaced exocytosis
Glycoproteins 3. FSH 4. LH 5. TSH	*Basophils*	*Mucoid cells* PAS+	*Basophils*	*Gonadotrophs* PAS+ (magenta granules); cell contour round	FSH/LH cell (10%)	Granules 200-500 nm[37]; abundant rough endoplasmic reticulum
				Thyrotroph Thionine+ (blue purple granules); cell contour angular	TSH cell (5%)	Granules 100-300 nm[37]
Polypeptides 6. ACTH 7. MSH 8. LPH				*Corticomelanotrophs* PAS+ (red granules); cell contour oval	ACTH/MSH cell (15%-20%)	Granules 250-700 nm[37]; microfilaments, enigmatic bodies

*Permanganate–aldehyde thionine–periodic acid–Schiff–orange G.

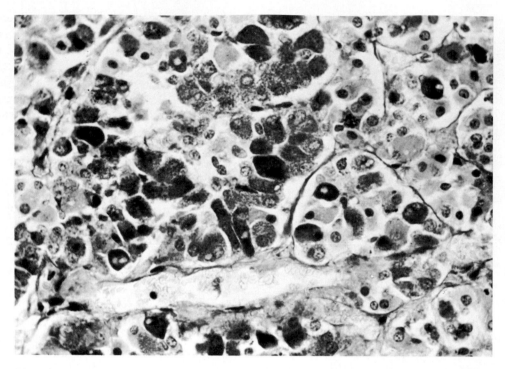

Fig. 30-6. Normal adult adenohypophysis showing groups of epithelial cells supported by connective tissue and sinusoids. Dark cells are basophils. (Periodic acid–Schiff–trichrome; 500×; courtesy Dr. A.R. Currie, Edinburgh.)

cells, also have been described in the human pituitary.[37,39]

The basophil cells include gonadotrophs, thyrotrophs, and corticotrophs. They are separated on the basis of immunostaining. The histochemistry of the adenohypophysis is summarized in Girod's comprehensive monograph.[32] Basophils contain polysaccharides and protein, and they are known collectively as mucoid cells.[50] Oxidation of the polysaccharide with periodic acid results in formation of free aldehyde groups, which form visible purple complexes with Schiff's reagent, the basis for the periodic acid–Schiff–positive reaction of the basophil cells.

Gonadotrophs are the source of FSH, and LH or interstitial cell–stimulating hormone (ICSH) and thyrotrophs are the source of TSH. FSH, LH, and TSH are glycoproteins. They are composed of two polypeptides known as alpha and beta subunits, plus a polysaccharide portion. The alpha subunit of the polypeptide is identical in all three hormones. The beta subunit is unique to each one, conferring on the hormone its special properties.

The corticotrophs produce ACTH, melanocyte-stimulating hormone (MSH, alpha and beta types), beta-lipotropin (LPH), and beta-endorphin.[27,37] ACTH, MSH, and LPH are simple peptides with a common

core and overlapping properties, derived from a common precursor, prepro-opiomelanocortin (prepropiocortin).[28,45] Corticotrophs also are known as ACTH/MSH cells, corticolipotropic cells, or melanocorticotropic cells.

The important characteristics of the three types of basophils may be summarized as follows. The gonadotrophs have a round or oval contour and an eccentric nucleus; in horizontal section they are most numerous in the posterior portion of the median wedge[34] but are also found in the lateral wings.[31] Phifer and associates[52] showed that antisera to FSH and LH reacted with the same cell types, indicating that FSH and LH may be secreted by the same cell, hence the designation FSH-LH cell. With electron microscopy, two populations of granules are described, measuring 200 to 300 nm and 300 to 500 nm.[37] The thyrotrophs are angular cells found in the median wedge, mainly in an anterior and subcapsular location.[34] By electron microscopy, the cells have an irregular shape and contain small granules 150 to 200 nm in diameter, which may have a peripheral distribution.[51] The corticotrophs are oval cells, concentrated in the anterior part of the median wedge and adjacent lateral wings. A separate group of corticotrophs is found consistently in the pars nervosa, at the junction with the pars distalis; these cells may be remnants of pars intermedia,[46,54] and they may have a function as yet unidentified.[42] Immunostaining demonstrates ACTH, MSH, beta-lipotropin and beta-endorphin in the corticotrophs.[28,47] Phifer and associates[53] showed that the corticotroph contains alpha-MSH as well as beta-MSH, though the latter is the principal form in humans. With the electron microscope, the ACTH cell contains granules 375 to 550 nm in diameter,[51] and typical filaments may be found in the cytoplasm.[29] Large lysosomal structures known as enigmatic bodies are frequent.[37]

With the advent of electron microscopy and immunostaining, the "chromophobes" in hematoxylin and eosin stain have proved to consist mainly of poorly granulated corticotrophs, thyrotrophs, or gonadotrophs. However, a subgroup of nonhormonal cells known as follicular, or folliculostellate, cells has been identified. These elongated stellate elements are scattered throughout the pars distalis, associated with follicles. Distinctive features include microvilli, cilia, and junctional complexes.[25] They are apparently derived from damaged adenohypophyseal cells.[37] Both S-100 protein and glial fibrillary acidic protein (GFAP) are present in the follicular cell.[44] Oncocytic cells also have been described in the human adenohypophysis.[37]

Immunostains have demonstrated other substances of interest in the cells of the adenohypophysis. These include cytokeratin,[43] chromogranin,[40] neuron-specific enolase,[24] gastrin,[38] renin,[57] and neurophysin.[36]

Neurohypophysis

The pars nervosa consists of interlacing nerve fibers and specialized glial elements known as pituicytes, with interspersed blood vessels. At its junction with the adenohypophysis, the neurohypophysis contains clusters of basophil cells,[54] referred to as basophil invasion of the pars nervosa. Granules of neurosecretory material, made up of the octapeptides vasopressin and oxytocin in association with carrier proteins termed "neurophysins," are present throughout the neurohypophysis. The neurophysins are a useful marker of neurosecretion, since they can be stained by the chrome alum–hematoxylin, the aldehyde fuchsin, or the performic acid–Alcian blue technique.[17] Vasopressin, or antidiuretic hormone (ADH), causes reabsorption of water from the renal tubules, and it is essential for maintaining osmolality of the plasma. Deficiency of ADH results in the condition known as diabetes insipidus, which is characterized by uncontrolled diuresis and polydipsia. Oxytocin is responsible for the ejection of milk from the lactating breast, by causing contraction of the mammary myoepithelium. It also stimulates contraction in the uterus at term.

The function of the pituicytes is unknown. Electron microscopy has revealed that pituicytes are closely apposed to neurosecretory fibers, and in lower animals a phagocytic function for disposal of neurophysins and membranes of granules has been suggested.

PITUITARY IN PREGNANCY

The hypophysis undergoes a striking enlargement during pregnancy and lactation, when it may reach 1100 mg or more. Although involution occurs subsequently, the gland remains heavier in multiparous women.[10] The basis for enlargement is the pronounced hypertrophy and hyperplasia of the lactotrophs. In the pituitary of nonpregnant, nonlactating adults, the lactotrophs are sparsely granulated and inconspicuous except with immunostains. However, during pregnancy and lactation the hypertrophic, hyperplastic lactotrophs can be recognized in hematoxylin and eosin–stained sections as enlarged acidophils, termed "pregnancy cells."[10] The lactotrophs also are selectively stained with erythrosin in the tetrachrome method of Herlant and Pasteels[35] or Brookes' carmoisine technique.[26]

PITUITARY IN DISORDERS OF OTHER ENDOCRINE GLANDS

Hypofunction of the thyroid, adrenals, or gonads generally produces morphologic changes in the thyrotrophs, corticotrophs, or gonadotrophs, respectively, ascribed to lack of negative feedback. Hyperfunction of the adrenal glands has profound effects on the corticotrophs, and hyperthyroidism produces alterations in the thyrotrophs.[75] Experimental evidence indicates that the changes occurring after hypofunction may be the result of stimulation of hypophyseal cells by hypothalamic-releasing hormones.[82]

Hypothyroidism

In untreated or inadequately treated myxedema caused by primary disease of the thyroid, hypertrophy and hyperplasia of the thyrotrophs lead to enlargement of the pituitary; weights up to 1.21 g have been recorded.[62] Historically such abnormal thyrotrophs have been designated thyroprival cells,[86] large chromophobes,[86] or hypertrophic amphophils.[63] With light microscopy the thyrotrophs can be recognized as large cells containing coarse vesicles, or droplets, in the cytoplasm; the typical basophil granules are lacking (Fig. 30-7). The droplets are periodic acid–Schiff and aldehyde thionine positive. In rats, high-resolution autoradiography has demonstrated that thyroidectomy cells originate from division of preexisting TSH cells.[84] After administration of ^{131}I to mice with hypothyroidism, the thyroidectomy cells by electron microscopy show ballooning of the ergastoplasmic cisternae, and secretory granules are decreased or absent, resulting in a chro-

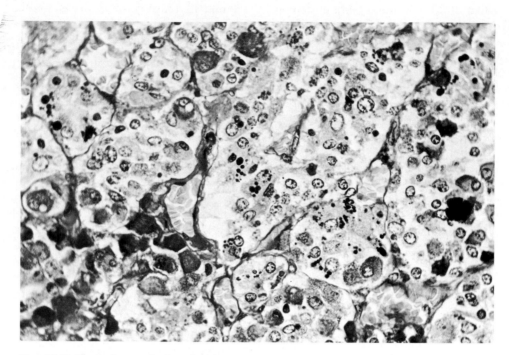

Fig. 30-7. Vesiculate cells in adenohypophysis of patient with myxedema. Notice variation in size of periodic acid–Schiff–positive granules. (Periodic acid–Schiff–trichrome; 500×; courtesy Dr. A.R. Currie, Edinburgh.)

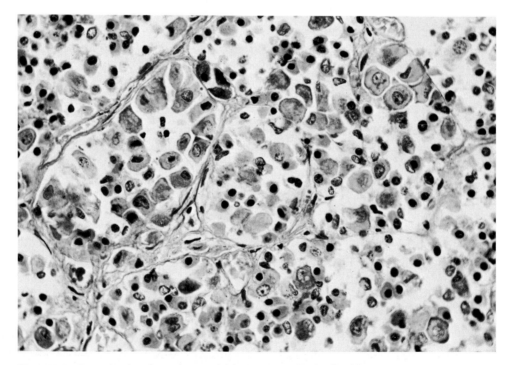

Fig. 30-8. Crooke's hyaline change in basophil cells in Cushing's syndrome. (Periodic acid–Schiff–trichrome; 500×; courtesy Dr. A.R. Currie, Edinburgh.)

mophobic appearance. In such animals, hyperplasia of thyrotrophs is followed by the appearance of microadenomas and then gross tumors.[68] In humans with untreated primary hypothyroidism, thyrotroph cell adenomas are well documented.[85]

Hyperthyroidism

Ezrin has described regression of thyrotrophs in patients who died of hyperthyroidism.[75] The regressed TSH cells have small nuclei, a thin rim of cytoplasm, and a few aldehyde thionine–positive droplets. These alterations in the TSH cells are reversible. In contrast to the characteristic findings in the adenohypophysis in myxedema, the abnormalities in hyperthyroidism are not considered diagnostic.[34]

Addison's disease

In Addison's disease, gross enlargement of the hypophysis has been recorded, with a weight of 1.2 g.[77] In Scheithauer's series of 19 cases, both diffuse and nodular hyperplasia were observed, and the extent of hyperplasia correlated with the duration of disease.[80] In two patients, microadenomas were present.

In patients with Addison's disease the number of thyrotrophs may be greatly increased.[30] This increase in thyrotrophs may be a reflection of the frequent association of idiopathic atrophy of the adrenal glands with atrophy of the thyroid, a condition known as Schmidt's syndrome, which has an autoimmune basis.[61,64,71]

Hyperadrenocorticism

A typical cytoplasmic alteration known as Crooke's hyaline change was first observed in the basophils in cases of Cushing's syndrome.[65] Subsequently the abnormality was found in other conditions characterized by excess circulating adrenocortical hormones, including therapy with exogenous glucocorticoids[73] and hypercorticism resulting from ectopic production of ACTH in lung cancer.[72] The basophils that are affected are the ACTH cells.[70] In Crooke's change the granules disappear and the cytoplasm gradually becomes periodic acid–Schiff negative.[70,81] In hematoxylin and eosin–stained section, the cytoplasm assumes a ground-glass, pale gray appearance. The nucleus and the cell body enlarge, and a few cytoplasmic vacuoles may be present (Fig. 30-8). By electron microscopy, the hyaline substance is made up of a dense feltwork of fine filaments,[29] which are cytokeratin positive.[76]

Hyperadrenocorticism also affects the population of thyrotrophs, or TSH cells. Halmi and McCormick[69] found that the thyrotrophs were scanty or undetectable at autopsy in patients with elevated levels of glucocorticoids, whether exogenous or endogenous. They postulated that the paucity of thyrotrophs was the morphologic basis for the tonic depression of TSH secretion that is observed clinically in sustained hyperadrenocorticism.

Deficiency of gonadal hormones

In rodents, ovariectomy removes the negative feedback exerted by ovarian steroids on the pituitary gonadotrophs. In such animals the degranulated, hyperactive gonadotrophs acquire large vacuoles, assume a signet-ring appearance, and are known as castration cells. By electron microscopy the signet-ring morphology results from fusion of distended elements of the endoplasmic reticulum and enlargement of individual cisternae.[67]

Although the same feedback action exists in humans, distinctive signet-ring castration cells such as those found in rodents do not occur. Nonetheless, changes are found in the gonadotrophs of patients with deficiency of gonadal hormones. Russfield[78] observed cellular hypertrophy and enlargement of the Golgi complex in the gonadotrophs of patients with gonadal deficiency; the changes were reversible by hormone therapy. In a man who underwent castration for carcinoma of the prostate, Russfield and Byrnes[79] found hyperplasia of sparsely granulated, periodic acid–Schiff–positive cells, but the staining method did not differentiate between the types of basophils. Phifer and associates[52] observed an increase in the size and number of gonadotrophs in a woman castrated 5 years previously. By light microscopy Ezrin[66] noted enlarged, vacuolated gonadotrophic basophils resembling chromophobes in patients with hypogonadism and in postmenopausal women. With the electron microscope, extreme dilatation of cisternae of the endoplasmic reticulum of these hypertrophied cells has been observed.[74]

HYPOPHYSECTOMY

Hypophysectomy has been shown to produce temporary remission of symptoms in about one third of women with disseminated mammary cancer.[88] Relief from bone pain is especially gratifying. In treatment of metastatic carcinoma, total ablation of adenohypophyseal function is the goal.

Several lines of evidence indicate that the pharyngeal hypophysis may be capable of active secretion of adenophypophyseal hormones in patients whose sellar hypophysis has been destroyed by tumor or hypophysectomy. In such patients Müller[92] reported "activation" of the cells of the pharyngeal pituitary, with typical acidophils and basophils, in contrast to the undifferentiated cells observed in the "inactive" state. McGrath[90] noted that acidophils predominated in the pharyngeal hypophysis after sellar hypophysectomy; basophils and chromophobes were also present. In extracts of pharyngeal hypophyses, McGrath[89] demonstrated PRL and

GH. McPhie and Beck[91] found GH in acidophils of pharyngeal pituitary in patients without endocrine disease. These findings strongly suggest that the pharyngeal hypophysis is capable of active secretion. However, the extent to which this organ can compensate for absence of the sellar hypophysis is uncertain.[87]

HYPOPITUITARISM

Hypopituitarism, or pituitary insufficiency, may involve the neurohypophysis, the adenohypophysis, or both. The pathology of the major causes of insufficiency is discussed in detail in the later sections; some of the clinical features are described briefly here.

Deficiency of the neurohypophysis results in the syndrome known as diabetes insipidus because of the loss of vasopressin. The condition is characterized by diuresis, polyuria, and uncontrollable thirst.

Deficiency of the adenohypophysis may involve one, several, or all of the trophic hormones. Deficiency of all hormones (panhypopituitarism) follows destruction of 70% or more of the adenohypophysis. Infarction and tumor are the most common causes. Isolated hormonal deficiency may be associated with incomplete adenohypophyseal destruction, but it may also occur in the absence of a recognizable pathologic lesion. In such cases a functional disorder of the hypothalamus has been postulated.

The classic clinical syndrome of panhypopituitarism in adults is known as Simmonds' disease. The advanced cachexia that characterized the cases observed by Simmonds is rarely observed now, probably because of the advances in medical care since then.[93] From this heterogeneous group of cases described by Simmonds, Sheehan[95] separated the clinicopathologic entity of postpartum necrosis of the adenohypophysis, and this syndrome now bears his name.

The effects of isolated hormone deficiency depend on the hormone involved and to some extent on the age of the patient. Deficiency of gonadotrophic hormones leads to hypogonadotrophic eunuchoidism in men and amenorrhea in women; before the age of puberty there are no clinical signs, but secondary sexual development fails to occur at adolescence.[94] Deficiency of corticotropin secretion leads to anorexia, weakness, weight loss, and hypoglycemia; in women axillary and pubic hair may be lost, and in girls it fails to appear. Isolated deficiency of thyrotropic hormone causes hypothyroidism in adults but has not been described in children. Isolated deficiency of growth hormone results in ateliotic dwarfism in children and microsplanchnia in adults.[66]

ANOMALIES
Agenesis

Agenesis of the pituitary is a rare anomaly that is almost always associated with cyclopia, a gross malformation involving the neural tube and axial skeleton. Even in this condition, agenesis is not universal, occurring in only about half the cases reported.[98] Agenesis of the anterior lobe has been described in a few normocephalic infants; in males the penis is unusually small, a finding that has been suggested as an external marker of this condition.[101] In such normocephalic infants, the sella turcica may appear normally formed but empty, or it may be smaller than normal with a persistent craniopharyngeal canal.[105] In all cases in which the anterior lobe of the pituitary is absent, the adrenal glands are hypoplastic and the thyroid gland is often similarly affected. The adrenal glands lack a fetal, or "X," zone, and the layers of the cortex are irregular and disordered. That the function of these abnormal adrenal glands is defective is supported by the observation of stable, low maternal urinary estriol levels in the last weeks of pregnancy.[101] The hypoplastic thyroid is small and may lack an isthmus. The testes may also be hypoplastic, and absence of interstitial cells of Leydig has been reported.[97] Several of these infants have survived a decade or more, exhibiting mental deficiency, dwarfism, failure of development, myxedema, hypoglycemic convulsions, and undeveloped genitalia.[104]

Agenesis of the anterior pituitary may occur without any anomaly of the posterior pituitary.

Hypoplasia

Hypoplasia of the pituitary is a constant finding in anencephaly. In this condition the sella turcica is flattened and the exposed base of the skull is covered by a mat of spongy, vascular tissue. The hypophysis usually cannot be recognized grossly, but it can be found by en bloc removal of the entire sella, decalcification, and vertical sectioning of the central portion.[96] The size and shape of the gland are quite variable. Whereas the pars anterior is nearly always present, the pars nervosa is often absent.

The adrenals in anencephaly are invariably hypoplastic, and the X zone, or fetal cortex, is greatly diminished or even absent, and so the glands are miniature replicas of those of older individuals,[102] with orderly cortical layers. The thyroid gland, gonads, and genitalia are unaffected.

Malposition

Malposition, or dystopia, of the hypophysis is a rare occurrence. Lennox and Russell[99] reviewed the literature and added two cases in which the pars nervosa lay between the infundibulum and the sella, being connected to the pars anterior by a stalk composed of pars tuberalis. No disorder of pituitary function was recognized. Another rare malposition occurs as a result of failure of contact between Rathke's pouch and the developing diencephalon, leading to displacement of pituitary tissue into a persistent craniopharyngeal duct.[92] In such cases, polypoid protrusion of pituitary anlage into the pharynx may occur. Adenomas may occur in ectopic pituitary tissue, and they have been reported in the nasal cavity, sphenoid sinus, sphenoidal wing, and temporal bone.[103] Ectopic pituitary adenoma with normal intrasellar pituitary also has been reported.[100]

EMPTY SELLA SYNDROME

Empty sella syndrome is characterized by an incomplete diaphragma sellae with extension of the subarachnoid space into the sella turcica. The sella may be enlarged and deformed, and the pituitary may be reduced to a flattened layer of tissue lining the floor of the sella.[110,111] Histologically the gland appears normal,[106,107] and endocrine function is not usually impaired. Hyperprolactinemia[109] and coexisting functional microadenoma have been reported in a few patients with empty sella syndrome.[108]

HEMORRHAGE

Severe skull trauma frequently injures the hypophysis, causing hemorrhage, laceration, and necrosis.[113] The patients who survive such injury may have diabetes insipidus as a result of damage to the neurohypophysis.[112,113] Hemorrhage in the posterior pituitary also occurs in patients who have cerebral hemorrhage, tumors of the brain, or "respirator brain" (deterioration of the brain that occurs as a complication of mechanical respirator therapy).[114]

PITUITARY APOPLEXY

Acute hemorrhage into a pituitary tumor is responsible for the condition known as pituitary apoplexy. It is characterized by sudden headache, ophthalmoplegia, meningismus, and signs of compression of the optic nerves or chiasm.[116] Sudden pituitary failure may result; impaction of the hypophysis by the expanding neoplasm has been cited as the mechanism. In some patients, pituitary apoplexy may be the first manifestation of hypophyseal tumor.[115]

ISCHEMIA

Foci of ischemic necrosis are occasionally observed post mortem, with an incidence of 1% to 3% in unselected autopsies.[122] These almost always involve the adenohypophysis. The associated conditions are varied[120] and include such diverse entities as obstetric shock,[124] elevated intracranial pressure, diabetes mellitus,[119,121] craniocerebral trauma, cerebrovascular accident, shock, mechanical respirator therapy ("respirator brain"),[114,118,125] transection of the hypophyseal stalk,[16,117] overwhelming sepsis, and carcinomatous permeation of local blood vessels.[17] The common denominator in most of these conditions appears to be inadequate perfusion of the adenohypophysis, resulting in ischemia and coagulative necrosis. The "life support" of the adenohypophysis is the hypophyseal portal system, and the direct arterial supply to the anterior pituitary is not sufficient to sustain the cells.[1,16] This arrangement renders the adenohypophysis more vulnerable to episodes of stasis and ischemia. The pathogenesis of the ischemia has been ascribed to such mechanisms as embolism, thrombosis, Shwartzman phenomenon, vascular spasm, and vascular compression.[121] In many patients with infarcts, the lesions occur as a terminal complication of a severe systemic illness; hence they are of little importance clinically whether large or small. Survivors with microinfarcts do not have symptoms of hypopituitarism because insufficiency is not apparent until 70% of the adenohypophysis is destroyed.[78] However, survivors of large infarcts do suffer from hypopituitarism.

The most important cause of pituitary insufficiency from massive infarction is obstetric shock, usually related to hemorrhage at the time of delivery. Postpartum necrosis of the pituitary is known as Sheehan's syndrome. In severe cases the extent of necrosis of the adenohypophysis approaches 99% (Fig. 30-9).[18] A narrow zone of tissue at the periphery may survive. The necrotic anterior lobe gradually shrivels and becomes replaced by a thin, semilunar collagenous scar (Fig. 30-9). The posterior lobe is unaffected. The degree of hypopituitarism depends on the extent of destruction. Failure of lactation may be the first sign, followed by amenorrhea and eventually by adrenocortical insufficiency and hypothyroidism.[123]

ACUTE INFLAMMATION

Acute purulent inflammation of the hypophysis may occur by direct extension of inflammation in an adjacent structure, by hematogenous dissemination during the course of overwhelming sepsis,[127] or as a complication of invasive pituitary adenoma.[128] Purulent meningitis causes acute hypophysitis by direct spread into the subarachnoid space surrounding the pituitary; inflammation in such a case may be limited to the surface of the gland. Rarely, the hypophysis is converted into a pus-filled sac.[126] Other causes include sinusitis, osteomyelitis of the sphenoid bone, thrombophlebitis of the cavernous sinus, and suppurative otitis media. In the case of hematogenous dissemination, microabscesses may form within the substance of the adenohypophysis or neurohypophysis.[127]

CHRONIC INFLAMMATION
Granuloma

Granulomatous diseases may involve the pituitary and cause destruction of both adenohypophysis and neurohypophysis. Symptoms of hypopituitarism are proportional to the extent of destruction and localiza-

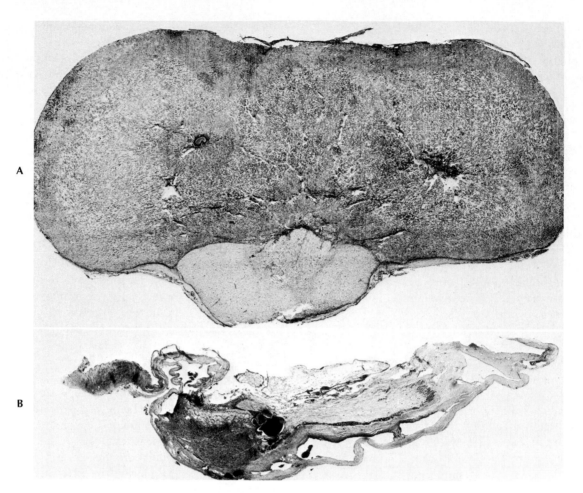

Fig. 30-9. Postpartum necrosis of pituitary gland. **A,** Most of anterior lobe affected. **B,** Gland shriveled and deformed. Patient survived for many years. (Hematoxylin and eosin; 10×; courtesy Prof. H.L. Sheehan, Liverpool, and Dr. A.R. Currie, Edinburgh.)

tion of the involvement. Tuberculosis occurs by hematogenous dissemination or by direct extension from tuberculous meningitis; miliary tubercles or areas of caseous necrosis are found at autopsy. Syphilis of the pituitary may be congenital or acquired; in the acquired cases the lesion may be a diffuse fibrosis or gummatous necrosis.[130] Boeck's sarcoid can affect the central nervous system, with involvement of the base of the brain, hypothalamus, and pituitary including both neurohypophysis and adenohypophysis.[131] Noncaseating tubercles composed of epithelioid cells, lymphocytes, and giant cells of Langhans' type, which may contain asteroid bodies and Schaumann bodies, characterize the lesions. No etiologic agent can be demonstrated, and special stains for acid-fast organisms and fungi are negative.

The entity known as giant cell granuloma of the pituitary presents a histologic picture similar to Boeck's sarcoid, but unlike sarcoidosis, giant cell granuloma is not a disease of multiple systems. This rare disorder affects the anterior pituitary, and the involvement may

progress to destruction of the adenohypophysis with consequent hypopituitarism and secondary atrophy of thyroid and adrenal glands. The hypophyseal lesions consist of noncaseating tubercles with Langhans' giant cells and associated chronic inflammatory cells. The condition occurs chiefly in middle-aged and elderly women.[132] The pathogenesis is obscure. In a few reported cases, similar granulomas were observed in the adrenals, and it has been suggested that giant cell granuloma may be an autoimmune or an infectious disorder.[129]

Lymphocytic hypophysitis

More recently, another variant of chronic inflammatory disease of the pituitary known as lymphocytic hypophysitis has been described.[134] The majority of patients have been postpartum women,[132,138] though a single case in a male has been reported.[135] In some patients the lesion presented as a pituitary tumor,[132,137] with transitory or permanent hypopituitarism involving

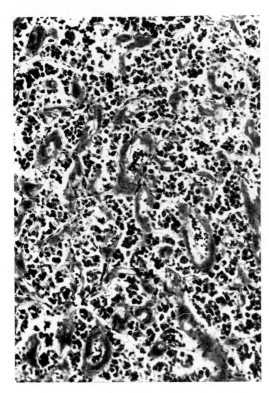

Fig. 30-10. Amyloid deposition in anterior lobe of pituitary gland. (Hematoxylin and eosin; 140×; courtesy Drs. Dorothy S. Russell and A.R. Currie, Edinburgh.)

deficiency of one or more hypophyseal hormones.[136,139] In some patients the lesion appeared as a pituitary tumor.[132,137] Microscopically the adenohypophysis is involved by extensive nodular or diffuse infiltration of lymphocytes, sometimes with fibrosis. Concomitant thyroiditis and adrenalitis have been observed, with lymphoid infiltration in these organs. An autoimmune basis has been postulated for this disorder.

INFILTRATIONS AND METABOLIC DISORDERS
Amyloidosis

Generalized secondary amyloidosis may involve the pituitary.[141] In this condition, amyloid is deposited in the walls of the blood vessels of the adenohypophysis (Fig. 30-10). Old age is associated with amyloid deposits in the pituitary and was found in 80% of patients over 90 years of age in the series of Voigt and co-workers.[146] Interstitial amyloid deposits may be found in pituitary adenomas,[147] and amyloid in the form of laminated concretions has been described in prolactinomas.[139,140,142-144]

Hand-Schüller-Christian disease

The posterior lobe, infundibular stem, and infundibulum are often involved by the xanthomatous deposits that characterize Hand-Schüller-Christian disease.[18] Usually the skull and dura mater adjacent to the hypophysis also are involved, with bony destruction. The infundibular lesions interfere with neurosecretion, and Hand-Schüller-Christian disease is an important cause of diabetes insipidus in children (see also p. 1422).

Hurler's syndrome (gargoylism)

The adenohypophyseal cells in Hurler's syndrome display a characteristic vacuolation with a foamy appearance, corresponding to the abnormal storage of mucopolysaccharides characteristic of this disorder. By electron microscopy the majority of the affected cells contain numerous membrane-bound vesicles. Lipid cytosomes with parallel-stacked or concentric osmiophilic lamellae known as "zebra bodies" also are present.[145]

Hyperplasia

Reversible hyperplasia secondary to endocrine imbalance and alteration in endocrine homeostasis is well known (see p. 1523). In contrast, primary hyperplasia of the pituitary has emerged as an established entity only recently.[37,148-151] Cushing's disease attributable to primary hyperplasia of corticotroph cells has been well documented. Two forms of primary hyperplasia are recognized, diffuse and nodular. Differentiation of nodular hyperplasia can be difficult or impossible if the entire gland is not available for study.

TUMORS

Formerly cited at about 6%, the occurrence of symptomatic tumors of the pituitary has risen sharply in the past two decades. This change is the result of the recognition of microadenomas (adenomas less than 10 mm) (Fig. 30-11) as a significant cause of the syndromes of pituitary hypersecretion. Although exact data are still lacking, it seems likely that their incidence may approach that of microadenomas at autopsy.[153] The early diagnosis of small intrasellar tumors has been greatly improved by advances in diagnostic radiology, clinical chemistry, and neurosurgery, the last enabling selective total adenomectomy without disturbing pituitary function. This turn of events has revolutionized the management of pituitary tumors.[155-157]

With improved clinical diagnosis of microadenomas and early surgical intervention, rapid intraoperative diagnosis by frozen section and smears has become essential.[37] In smears, the adenoma has a characteristic appearance, with discohesive, usually monomorphous cells.[154] For establishment of tumor margins, frozen sections stained with hematoxylin and orange G have been suggested.[152]

Tumors of the pituitary give rise to symptoms in two ways. Local effects result from expansion of the lesion, and distant effects are caused by hypersecretion or hy-

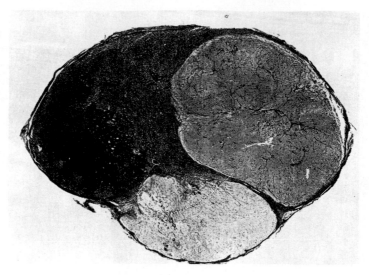

Fig. 30-11. Microadenoma of anterior lobe of pituitary gland. Clinically silent. (Acid fuchsin and aniline blue; 6×; courtesy Drs. Dorothy S. Russell and A.R. Currie, Edinburgh.)

Table 30-2. Classification of functioning tumors of adenohypophysis

| Hormone | Cell type | | Syndrome |
	Hematoxylin and eosin	Functional classification	
STH	Acidophil or chromophobe*	Somatotroph	Acromegaly
PRL		Lactotroph	Amenorrhea-galactorrhea
FSH-LH	Basophil or chromophobe*	Gonadotroph	—
TSH		Thyrotroph	Hyperthyroidism
ACTH-MSH		Corticomelanotroph	Cushing's syndrome, Nelson's syndrome

*Granules too small to be seen with light microscope.

posecretion of trophic hormones or hypothalamic principles. Unchecked local growth and expansion will ultimately erode and enlarge the sella turcica, and extension upward into the suprasellar region impinges on optic chiasm, optic nerves, neurohypophysis, and adjacent cranial nerves (Fig. 30-12). At the same time, uninvolved portions of the pituitary may become compressed and attenuated, with insufficiency of trophic hormones or diabetes insipidus caused by pressure on the adenohypophysis or neurohypophysis, respectively. Displacement of the hypothalamus may impair production and transport of releasing hormones and inhibitory factors, causing further endocrine imbalance and abnormality. In fact, analysis of the effect of tumors has given considerable insight into the function of the hypophysis and hypothalamus.

Adenomas

Adenomas are the most common of the pituitary tumors, and their incidence in unselected autopsies is about 25%.[164,166,193] The simple but inadequate classification of adenomas as acidophil, basophil, or chromophobe that was proposed by early workers has been expanded and clarified by the remarkable advances of the past two decades, resulting in the functional classification of adenohypophyseal cells summarized in Table 30-1.

In the light of ultrastructural and immunocytochemical data, it is clear that many neoplasms formerly designated "chromophobe adenomas" are in reality tumors with granules too small or too sparse to be seen with the light microscope, explaining the paradoxical occurrence of "chromophobe" tumors in patients with clear-

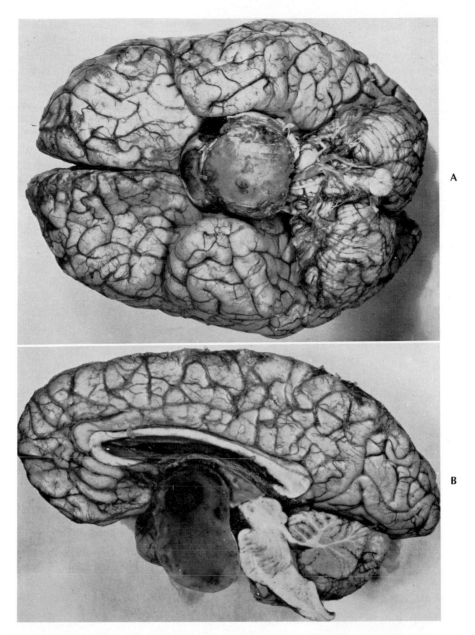

Fig. 30-12. A, Basal view of intrasellar part of large chromophobe adenoma. Notice distortion of optic chiasm. **B,** Midsagittal view of same specimen shown in **A.** (Courtesy Drs. Dorothy S. Russell and A.R. Currie, Edinburgh.)

cut syndromes of hyperpituitarism such as acromegaly, Cushing's disease, or hyperthyroidism.

In their excellent monograph on tumors of the pituitary, Kovacs and Horvath have integrated the functional and morphologic classifications and documented the recent advances in pathology of adenomas.[37] An abbreviated version of the modern classification of functioning pituitary adenomas is shown in Table 30-2. The screening of hematoxylin and eosin–stained sections in the analysis of a pituitary adenoma continues to be a point of departure for application of the advanced techniques required for functional classification and final diagnosis.

Although the cause is usually unknown, failure of a target organ is a causative factor in some patients. Constant stimulation of pituitary cells by hypothalamic releasing hormones in the absence of feedback inhibition has been suggested as the mechanism.[219] Thus primary hypothyroidism, hypogonadism, or hypoadrenalism can lead to formation of a pituitary tumor. TSH cell adenomas and the sequence of events in their pathogenesis after thyroid ablation are well known in animals.[168,171]

Basophil tumors also have been described in rats after gonadectomy.[174] The occurrence of thyrotroph cell adenoma associated with hypothyroidism in humans is well documented.[182] Pituitary tumors have also been reported in association with Addison's disease[80] and hypogonadism.[205]

Adenomas originate in the adenohypophysis and therefore arise in the hypophyseal fossa in the majority of cases. A few instances in which an adenoma originated outside the sella turcica, in an anomalous remnant of adenohypophysis, have been reported.[21,103]

Adenomas range from barely visible nodules (Fig. 30-11) to massive neoplasms with smooth or bosselated surfaces. Tumors less than 10 mm in diameter are termed microadenomas. Neurosurgeons have had the greatest experience in recognizing microadenomas; the consistency (soft, semisolid, or gelatinous) and color (creamy white, gray, or purple) of most microadenomas in contrast to the firm, yellow, "nonsuctionable" normal gland are regarded as diagnostic.[156,218] Externally, the adenohypophysis may appear normal, or symmetric and slightly enlarged. Microadenomas are typically discrete and well demarcated, but they lack a capsule. The larger tumors bulge upward from the sella turcica to encroach on the hypothalamus and third ventricle (Fig. 30-12). In such cases the tumor does not invade the brain, and it can be easily shelled from its bed in the compressed, invaginated cerebral tissue. Both large and small adenomas may be cystic, containing turbid or clear fluid. Also, infarction and hemorrhage may occur, producing the life-threatening syndrome of pituitary apoplexy in the case of larger tumors.[116]

With light microscopy, three patterns are observed: diffuse, sinusoidal, and papillary. The diffuse form is

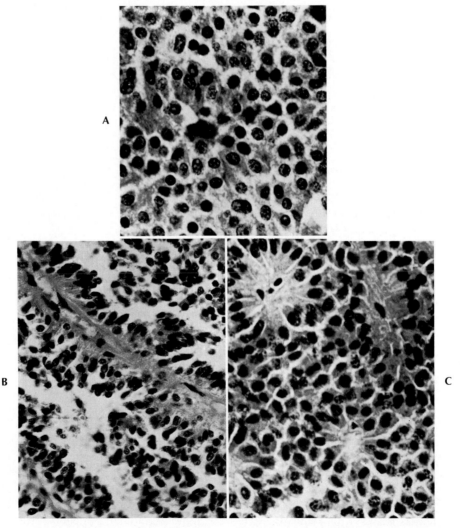

Fig. 30-13. Pituitary adenoma. **A,** Diffuse type. **B** and **C,** Perisinusoid type, with cells arranged about sinusoids. (**A** to **C,** Hematoxylin and eosin; **A,** 490×; **B,** 350×; **C,** 540×; courtesy Drs. Dorothy S. Russell and A.R. Currie, Edinburgh.)

composed of polygonal cells arranged in sheets, with inconspicuous stroma (Fig. 30-13). The sinusoidal form more or less resembles the structure of the normal adenohypophysis. The cells tend to be columnar or fusiform, and the stroma has fibrovascular septa with sinusoidal blood vessels to which the cells are oriented, creating a perisinusoidal arrangement (Fig. 30-13). In the papillary form, which is a variant of the sinusoidal pattern, cuboidal or columnar neoplastic cells are arranged radially about papillae with a vascular core. In all three types the cells are quite orderly and mitoses are rare. Microscopic criteria for diagnosis of microadenoma include uniformity of cells, a well-defined margin, absence of the reticular pattern of the normal gland, and evidence of compression of the adjacent pituitary.[153,161,165,181] Reticulin stain is a useful adjunct in identifying the extent of the neoplasm, since the reticular pattern of the normal gland is lacking in the tumor (Figs. 30-14).

Prolactin cell adenoma. In the past two decades, the lactotroph, or prolactin cell adenoma, has become the most commonly diagnosed pituitary tumor.[37] Functioning prolactin-cell adenomas are associated with infertility and amenorrhea in women[169,170] and impotence, oligospermia, and gynecomastia in men.[160,170,198,210] Galactorrhea may occur in either sex. Prolactinomas are densely or sparsely granulated,[37] and the cytoplasm is correspondingly acidophilic or chromophobic; the majority are sparsely granulated and chromophobic. By

electron microscopy the cells present a well-developed rough endoplasmic reticulum, nebenkerns, and a prominent Golgi apparatus. In the sparsely granulated tumors, the granules range from 125 to 300 nm; the densely granulated tumors have granules from 300 to 700 nm or more.[37,197] In both types, misplaced exocytosis is a characteristic feature.[37] Intra-adenomatous dystrophic calcification is a distinctive feature of prolactin-secreting adenomas[191]; ossification[194] and formation of pituitary "stone" also have been reported.[216]

Somatotroph cell adenoma. Functioning GH-cell adenoma, may produce gigantism or acromegaly, depending on the patient's age. GH-cell adenoma that occurs in a prepubertal patient whose epiphyses have not closed leads to proportionate growth of the body with gigantism. In the adult, epiphyses are closed, and abnormal growth is confined to the skull, jaw, hands, feet, and soft tissues, with enlargement of supraorbital ridges, the mandible, and phalanges, together with a characteristic coarsening of the features, thickening of heel pads, and enlargement of the viscera.

Somatotroph adenomas occur as densely or sparsely granulated forms, with acidophilic or chromophobic cytoplasm in hematoxylin and eosin stain. The densely granular form is associated with acromegaly.[43] The neoplastic GH-cell may closely resemble its normal counterpart. The granules range from 250 to 600 nm.[37] Filamentous aggregates known as fibrous bodies may be found in the sparsely granulated adenomas.[37,208]

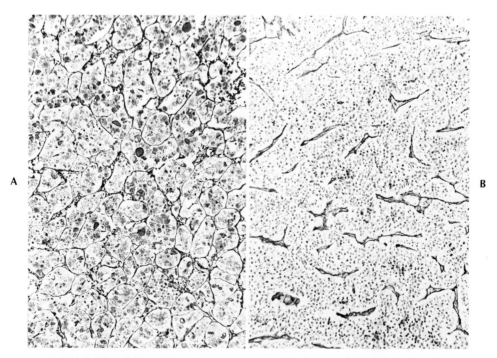

Fig. 30-14. Reticulin stain of, **A,** normal adenohypophysis and, **B,** pituitary adenoma. Normal alveolar pattern of reticulin is lost in tumor. (Gridley modification, silver impregnation method; 100×.)

Mixed somatotroph-prolactin (GH/PRL) adenomas.
Some 20% of acromegalics have hyperprolactinemia.[43]
Three types of tumors can be responsible. In the mixed
GH/PRL-producing tumor, the two hormones are produced by separate cell types in the same tumor.[181] In
the mammosomatotrophic adenoma, the hormones are
produced by a single type of neoplastic cell that can
make both.[180] The third type, known as the acidophil
stem cell tumor, also can produce both hormones in the
same cell; it is differentiated from the other two tumors
by its ultrastructural features (misplaced exocytosis, fibrous bodies).[37,177,179]

Corticotroph cell adenoma. Functioning corticotroph
cell tumors are associated with two distinctive clinical
disorders—Cushing's disease[167] and Nelson's syndrome.[195] In Cushing's disease the tumor causes hyperplasia of the adrenal cortex and overproduction of
adrenocortical hormones, thus producing the characteristic clinical findings that include truncal obesity,
moon face, purple striae, muscular wasting, hypertension, and abnormal glucose tolerance. Cushing's belief
that pituitary basophil adenomas were a significant
cause of adrenal hypersecretion recently has been substantiated.[163,203,215]

The second disorder associated with corticotroph cell
tumors is Nelson's syndrome—pituitary tumor and hyperpigmentation after bilateral adrenalectomy.[195] When
bilateral adrenalectomy is performed to control the
clinical manifestations of hypercorticism, about 10% of
patients develop cutaneous melanosis, signs and symptoms of a pituitary tumor, and elevated plasma ACTH.
Whether the tumor was present at the outset and was
the original cause of adrenal hyperplasia is not known
at present.

With light microscopy, neoplastic corticotroph cells
more or less resemble their normal counterparts. Typically the cytoplasm contains abundant basophilic granules, is periodic acid–Schiff positive, and contains
ACTH with immunoperoxidase technique. In addition,
corticotroph adenomas may contain other peptides derived from pro-opiomelanocortin, including beta-lipotropin (LPH), alpha- and beta-endorphins, and melanocyte-stimulating hormone (MSH).[28,37,196,201] The
extent of granularity in functioning adenomas is variable, and cells resembling chromophobes may be interspersed or may predominate. This variant has been
classified as sparsely granulated functioning corticotroph cell adenoma.[37]

By electron microscopy the secretory granules range
from 250 to 700 nm. Perinuclear accumulation of intermediate filaments 7 to 10 nm in diameter similar to
those seen in Crooke's cells is a characteristic feature in
adenomas with Cushing's disease.[37,200]

An important variant known as silent corticotroph adenoma contains immunoreactive ACTH and related
peptides but produces no clinical signs of Cushing's disease.[37,178] Progressive loss of vision is the usual presenting symptom, and infarction of the tumor is common.

Thyrotroph cell adenoma. Thyrotroph cell tumors
are rare; only a few dozen cases have been reported.[173,206] Clinically the tumor may be primary, arising autonomously in a previously euthyroid patient,[202,213] or it may be secondary to long-standing
hypothyroidism.[182,204] Pituitary tumors that cause hyperthyroidism secrete TSH, which in turn stimulates
the thyroid to produce excess hormones. Thus serum
levels of T_3, T_4, and TSH are simultaneously elevated.
The tumors that occur in association with hypothyroidism represent adenomatous transformation of thyrotroph cells in response to long-standing thyroid (end-
organ) failure.

Most thyrotroph tumors have grown to the size of
macroadenomas with suprasellar extension and visual
disturbances before they are diagnosed. Usually hypothyroidism is recognized and treated first, and only after an asymptomatic interval of months or years do
signs of intracranial tumor supervene.

Thyrotroph adenomas stain as chromophobe adenomas in hematoxylin and eosin–stained sections; the
cells are typically small, angular, and polyhedral, resembling normal thyrotrophs. Granules positive for periodic acid–Schiff and aldehyde thionine may be present. TSH immunoreactivity is variable and may be
negative. A significant proportion of TSH-cell adenomas
contain an admixture of cells producing a second hormone, usually PRL or GH.

By electron microscopy, the cells have long processes
and, in some tumors, may resemble normal thyrotrophs. The granules are small, varying in size and
number; they may localize along the cell membrane.[37,206]

Gonadotroph cell adenoma. Although uncommon,
the gonadotroph cell anenoma now is a firmly established entity.[37,206,214] The tumor may secrete FSH,
FSH and LH, or LH and alpha subunit.[37] Most patients
are middle-aged men with microadenomas and visual
problems but no gonadal hypofunction.[212] A few patients have had long-standing hypogonadism.[186,205]

Gonadotroph cell adenomas are chromophobe tumors
with a sinusoidal pattern in hematoxylin and eosin–
stained sections.[37] Periodic acid–Schiff stain may reveal
a few small positive granules. The tumor cells are small
and polyhedral or angular. FSH and LH are demonstrated by immunohistochemical staining but may be
lacking in some tumors.

Electron microscopy reveals two patterns.[37,176] In
women, the cells have long processes, uniform nuclei,
and Golgi apparatus resembling a honeycomb. In men
these features are lacking, and cytoplasmic organelles

are poorly developed. The secretory granules measure 350 nm or less.[176,214]

Alpha subunit adenoma. Alpha subunit adenoma, an uncommon variant of pituitary adenoma, is characterized by hypersecretion of alpha subunit of the glycoprotein hormones.[183,192,199] It has no recognized endocrine syndrome; rather, the symptoms and signs are those of an expanding lesion of the sella turcica. In hematoxylin and eosin sections, the cells are faintly acidophilic.[189] A small proportion of these adenomas have granular, acidophilic cytoplasm and prove to be oncocytomas by electron microscopy. The remainder have small sparse granules measuring 125 to 180 nm.[189]

Null cell adenoma. Null cell adenomas are endocrine inactive and have no morphologic or immunologic markers. Formerly known as chromophobe adenomas, these neoplasms constitute 20% to 30% of pituitary adenomas.[206] They are clinically silent until relatively far advanced, with headache and disturbed vision as the first symptoms.

Null cell tumors consist of small polyhedral or elongated cells with scanty agranular cytoplasm and small oval nuclei, forming diffuse, sinusoidal, or papillary patterns. The cytoplasm fails to stain with periodic acid–Schiff stain. Immunostains typically are negative; the occasional positive cell is interpreted as a sign of differentiation.[37] With electron microscopy, nuclei are irregular and the cytoplasm is poorly developed, having sparse granules less than 250 nm and abundant microtubules.[37,187]

Oncocytic adenoma. Oncocytic adenomas are hormonally inactive tumors composed of cells with granular, eosinophilic cytoplasm.[37,184,190] The diagnosis is reserved for nonfunctioning tumors, and hormonally active adenomas with oncocytic change should be excluded from this category.[37] The cytoplasm is densely packed with abnormal mitochondria, which is the basis for the acidophilia observed with the light microscope.[175] Thus positive identification of this tumor depends on electron microscopy and immunostains.

Multiple endocrine adenomatosis

Adenomas of the pituitary occur as an integral part of Wermer's syndrome, or multiple endocrine adenomatosis (MEA) type I.[162] This genetic disorder is inherited as an autosomal dominant, and familial involvement is the rule.[217] The disease is characterized by multiple adenomas involving pancreatic islets, parathyroids, and the pituitary. The endocrine involvement may be sequential rather than simultaneous. Clinically the patient usually has a combination of Zollinger-Ellison syndrome, hyperparathyroidism, and signs of pituitary tumor.

In the series of 40 patients with MEA type I reported by Scheithauer and associates,[207] three fourths of the

tumors were macroadenomas and 7 were invasive. Almost half were associated with production of growth hormone.

Carcinoma
Primary carcinoma

Identification of a primary tumor of the adenohypophysis with distant metastases as a carcinoma presents no problem.[220,224] However, the characteristic tendency of tumors of the adenohypophysis to erode bone and displace or compress soft tissues as the tumors expand, which already has been emphasized, has led to considerable debate on the criteria for malignancy of tumors without distant spread. It has been proposed that such tumors be designated "invasive adenomas." However, Kovacs and Horvath reserve the diagnosis of carcinoma for tumors with remote metastases.[37] It is clear that cytologic criteria are not absolute, since pleomorphism, hyperchromatism, and mitotic activity have been observed in tumors that are not infiltrative and tumors with none of these qualities have exhibited invasiveness.[221]

Metastatic carcinoma

Metastases to the pituitary gland occur in patients having widespread metastatic carcinoma. The usual primary site is the breast, and carcinoma of the lung is the second most common.[223,225] Most observers have found the pars nervosa to be involved more frequently than the pars distalis. Destruction of the posterior pituitary by metastatic carcinoma is a significant cause of diabetes insipidus in patients with carcinomatosis.[222]

Craniopharyngioma

Craniopharyngioma is a benign tumor believed to originate in remnants of Rathke's pouch that persist into postnatal life. An alternative explanation that the neoplasm arises by metaplasia of adenohypophyseal cells has been proposed. The onset of these tumors in childhood favors the origin from embryologic rests.[221] Whichever theory is correct, it is a fact that most craniopharyngiomas originate outside the sella turcica and are usually suprasellar in location. Occurrence within the sphenoid bone has also been reported.

Craniopharyngiomas make up 1% to 3% of intracranial tumors.[233,240,241] They are most common in children and young adults but may occur in older persons as well.

Grossly the tumor is encapsulated and firmly adherent to surrounding tissues, which suffer compression as the neoplasm slowly enlarges. Thus the structures involved are the brain above, the pituitary below, the optic chiasm anteriorly, and the circle of Willis at the periphery. The typical tumor is cystic, with intervening solid areas (Fig. 30-15). The content is fluid or semi-

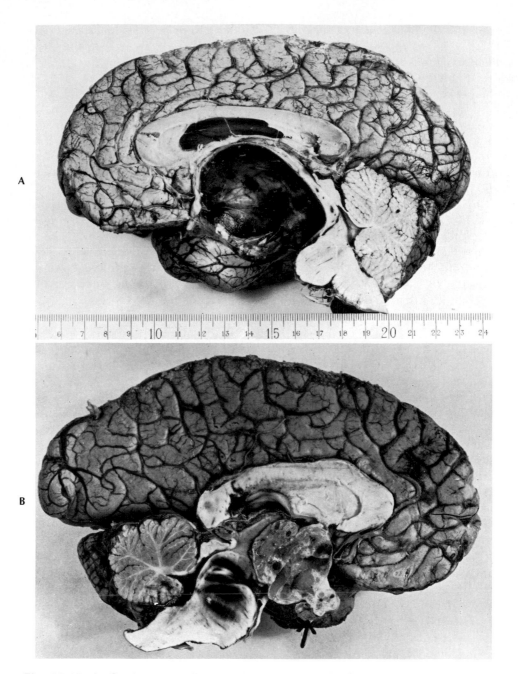

Fig. 30-15. A, Cystic suprasellar craniopharyngioma. **B,** Solid and cystic suprasellar craniopharyngioma. *Arrow,* Pituitary gland. (Courtesy Drs. Dorothy S. Russell and A.R. Currie, Edinburgh.)

solid, dark brown, greasy material containing cholesterol crystals, altered blood, and calcified debris.

Microscopically, the patterns are distinctive. The solid areas contain anastomosing cords of well-differentiated stratified squamous epithelium with a palisaded peripheral layer, set in a stroma of connective tissue (Fig. 30-16). Within the epithelium, areas composed of loosely arranged stellate cells may be found. Mitoses and cellular pleomorphism are uncommon. The cystic

regions may be lined by similar epithelial cords, with lipid histiocytes in the stroma and desquamated keratin in the cysts. The ultrastructure of craniopharyngioma has been described by Ghatak and associates.[229]

The histologic patterns may strikingly resemble those of ameloblastoma, an epithelial odontogenic tumor of the jaw.[236] Consequently, craniopharyngioma also is known as ameloblastoma. That a craniopharyngioma should resemble an ameloblastoma is not surprising,

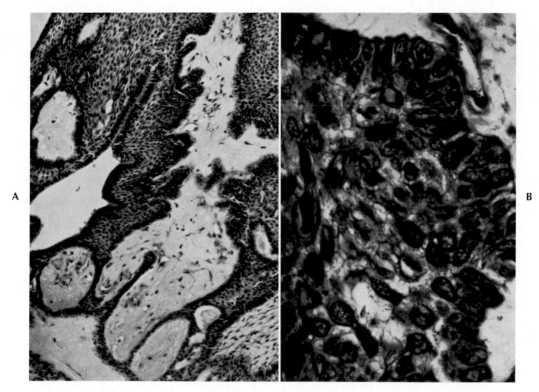

Fig. 30-16. Craniopharyngioma. **A,** Solid anastomosing trabeculas of cells. **B,** Surface cells of basal type and squamous cells. (**A,** Hematoxylin and eosin, 140×; **B,** phosphotungstic acid and hematoxylin, 850×; courtesy Drs. Dorothy S. Russell and A.R. Currie, Edinburgh.)

since the adenohypophysis itself arises in primitive buccal epithelium. It follows that neoplasms of its developmental remnants might be expected to reflect kinship with other buccal derivatives.

Although craniopharyngioma is histologically benign and grows slowly, ablation is difficult because of its location, and progressive enlargement is the rule.

Intrasellar cyst

Colloid-filled, epithelium-lined, asymptomatic benign cysts of microscopic size are commonly found at the junction of the pars distalis and the pars nervosa.[237] Such cysts are interpreted as remnants of Rathke's pouch. Rarely, larger benign cysts producing symptoms occur. They may be located entirely within the sella, or they may protrude above it, producing a dumbbell shape. The intrasellar cysts are usually lined by simple cuboidal epithelium, which may be ciliated.[143,237] The suprasellar portion of a dumbbell cyst may be lined by stratified squamous epithelium.[17] Kepes[230] has described a unique transitional epithelial tumor arising in the wall of a Rathke's cleft cyst.

Granular cell tumor (choristoma)

The granular cell tumor arises in the neurohypophysis, and it is the most common primary tumor of the posterior lobe. Nearly always asymptomatic, granular cell tumor is usually identified as an incidental finding at autopsy in persons past 30 years of age.[231] The incidence in Luse and Kernohan's series of autopsies was 6.4%.[231] Originally the name "choristoma" was proposed in the belief that the condition was a developmental anomaly. More recently, origin from Schwann cells[226] or pituicytes[232] has been suggested.

Grossly the lesion is generally too small to be seen. Microscopically it is composed of orderly, large polygonal cells with abundant granular pale pink cytoplasm and small, oval, eccentrically placed nuclei. The resemblance to the tumor known as granular myoblastoma found in extracranial locations is striking.

Rarely, granular cell tumor of the neurohypophysis may be large enough to produce symptoms. Such patients have signs and symptoms of a space-occupying intracranial lesion[238] or loss of vision as a result of compression of the optic chiasm.[235,239]

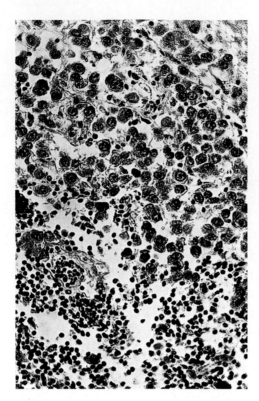

Fig. 30-17. Germinoma of pituitary stalk and posterior lobe of pituitary gland. (Hematoxylin and eosin; 260×; courtesy Drs. Dorothy S. Russell and A.R. Currie, Edinburgh.)

Germinal tumors

Tumors histologically identical to germinoma (seminoma) and teratoma of the gonads may occur within and adjacent to the sella turcica.[228,234] Because these tumors are more common in the pineal region, formerly they were designated "ectopic pinealoma" when they occurred in the hypothalamic region or the sella. However, the identity of the pinealoma with the germinoma (seminoma) of the testis was recognized by Friedman,[227] who emphasized their unmistakable morphologic congruity, and the term "germinoma" has become accepted.[234]

Grossly the germinoma is a fleshy, soft gray, diffusely infiltrating mass, frequently associated with hemorrhage. Microscopically the tumor is composed of large polygonal cells with abundant cytoplasm, a large vesicular nucleus, and one or more prominent nucleoli (Fig. 30-17). Mitoses are numerous. The cells are arranged in sheets or clusters separated by fibrovascular septa. Numerous small lymphocytes are usually present in the stroma. The resemblance to germinoma (seminoma) of the testis and dysgerminoma of the ovary is remarkable.

Teratomas also may occur in a suprasellar location. These neoplasms typically are cystic and are lined by ectodermal derivatives; bone and cartilage may be found in the wall.[234]

REFERENCES
Embryology and anatomy

1. Adams, J.H., Daniel, P.M., and Prichard, M.M.L.: Observations on the portal circulation of pituitary gland, Neuroendocrinology **1:**193, 1965-1966.
2. Baker, B.L., and Jaffe, R.B.: The genesis of cell types in the adenohypophysis of the human fetus as observed with immunocytochemistry, Am. J. Anat. **143:**137, 1975.
3. Bergland, R.M., and Page, R.B.: Can the pituitary secrete directly to the brain? (affirmative anatomical evidence), Endocrinology **102:**1325, 1978.
4. Bergland, R.M., Ray, B.S., and Torack, R.M.: Anatomical variations in the pituitary gland and adjacent structures in 225 human autopsy cases, J. Neurosurg. **28:**93, 1968.
5. Boyd, J.D.: Observations on the human pharyngeal hypophysis, J. Endocrinol. **14:**66, 1956.
6. Ciocca, D.R., Puy, L.A., and Stati, A.O.: Identification of seven hormone-producing cell types in the human pharyngeal hypophysis, J. Clin. Endocrinol. **60:**212, 1985.
7. Ciocca, D.R., Puy, L.A., and Stati, A.O.: Immunocytochemical evidence for the ability of the human pharyngeal hypophysis to respond to change in endocrine feedback, Virchows Arch. [Pathol. Anat.] **405:**497, 1985.
8. Colohan, A.R.T., Grady, M.S., Bonnin, J.M., Thorner, M.O., Kovacs, K., and Jane, J.A.: Ectopic pituitary gland simulating a suprasellar tumor, Neurosurgery **20:**43, 1987.
9. Doniach I.: Histopathology of the pituitary, Clin. Endocrinol. Metab. **14:**765, 1985.
10. Erdheim, J., and Stumme, F.: Über die Schwangerschaftsveränderungen bei der Hypophyse, Beitr. Pathol. Anat. **46:**1, 1909.
11. Gorczyca, W., and Hardy, J.: Arterial supply of the human anterior pituitary gland, Neurosurgery **20:**369, 1987.
12. Hinrichsen, K., Mestres, P., and Jacob, H.J.: Morphological aspects of the pharyngeal hypophysis in human embryos, Acta Morphol. Neerl.-Scand. **24:**235, 1986.
13. Jost, A.: Anterior pituitary function in foetal life. In Harris, G.W., and Donovan, B.T., editors: The pituitary gland, Berkeley, 1966, University of California Press.
14. Melchionna, R.H., and Moore, R.A.: The pharyngeal pituitary gland, Am. J. Pathol. **14:**763, 1938.
15. Renn, W.H., and Rhoton, A.L., Jr.: Microsurgical anatomy of the sellar region, Neurosurgery **43:**288, 1975.
16. Russell, D.S.: Effects of dividing the pituitary stalk in man, Lancet **1:**466, 1956.
17. Russell, D.S.: Pituitary gland (hypophysis). In Anderson, W.A.D., editor: Pathology, ed. 4, St. Louis, 1961, The C.V. Mosby Co.
18. Sheehan, H.L., and Kovacs, K.: Neurohypophysis and hypothalamus. In Bloodworth, J.M.B., Jr., editor: Endocrine pathology, ed. 2, Baltimore, 1982, The Williams & Wilkins Co.
19. Stanfield, J.P.: The blood supply of the human pituitary gland, J. Anat. **94:**257, 1960.
20. Wells, L.J., and Highby, D.N.: Experimental evidence of production of adrenotrophin by the fetal hypophysis, Proc. Soc. Exp. Biol. Med. **68:**487, 1948.
21. Willis, R.A.: The borderland of embryology and pathology, London, 1958, Butterworth & Co.
22. Xuereb, G.P., Prichard, M.M.L., and Daniel, P.M.: Arterial supply and venous drainage of human hypophysis cerebri, Q. J. Exp. Physiol. **39:**199, 1954.
23. Xuereb, G.P., Prichard, M.M.L., and Daniel, P.M.: The hypophysial portal system of vessels in man, Q. J. Exp. Physiol. **39:**219, 1954.

Histology and function

24. Asa, S.L., Ryan, N., Kovacs, K., Singer, W., and Marangos, P.J.: Immunohistochemical localization of neuron-specific enolase in the human hypophysis and pituitary adenomas, Arch. Pathol. Lab. Med. **108:**40, 1984.
25. Bergland, R.M., and Torack, R.M.: An ultrastructural study of follicular cells in the human anterior pituitary, Am. J. Pathol. **57:**293, 1969.

26. Brookes, L.D.: A stain for differentiating two types of acidophil cells in the rat pituitary, Stain Technol. **43**:41, 1968.
27. Celio, M.R.: Distribution of β-endorphin immunoreactive cells in human fetal and adult pituitaries and in pituitary adenomas, J. Histochem. Cytochem. **27**:1215, 1979.
28. Celio, M.R., Pasi, A., Bürgisser, E., Buetti, G., Höllt, V., and Gramsch, C.: 'Proopiocortin fragments' in normal human adult pituitary, Acta Endocrinol. **95**:27, 1980.
29. deCicco, F.A., Dekker, A., and Yunis, E.J.: Fine structure of Crooke's hyaline change in the human pituitary gland, Arch. Pathol. **94**:65, 1972.
30. Ezrin, C., and Murray, S.: The cells of the human adenohypophysis in pregnancy, thyroid disease and adrenal cortical disorders. In Benoit, J., and DeLage, C., editors: Cytologie de l'adénohypophyse, Paris, 1963, Centre National de la Recherche Scientifique.
31. Fowler, M.R., and McKeel, D.W., Jr.: Human adenohypophyseal quantitative histochemical cell classification, Arch. Pathol. Lab. Med. **103**:613, 1979.
32. Girod, C.: Histochemistry of the adenohypophysis. Handbuch der Histochemie, vol. 8, part 4, Stuttgart, 1976, Gustav Fischer Verlag.
33. Girod, C., Trouillas, J., and Dubois, M.P.: Immunocytochemical localization of S-100 protein in stellate cells (folliculo-stellate cells) of the anterior lobe of the normal human pituitary, Cell Tissue Res. **241**:505, 1985.
34. Halmi, N.S.: Current status of human pituitary cytophysiology, NZ Med. J. **80**:551, 1974.
35. Herlant, M., and Pasteels, J.L.: Histophysiology of human anterior pituitary, Methods Achiev. Exp. Pathol. **3**:250, 1967.
36. Kimura, N., Andoh, N., Sasano, N., et al.: Presence of neurophysins in the human pituitary corticotrophs, Cushing's adenomas, and growth hormone-producing adenomas detected by immunohistochemical study, Am. J. Pathol. **125**:269, 1986.
37. Kovacs, K., and Horvath, E.: Tumors of the pituitary gland. In Atlas of tumor pathology, series 2, fascicle 21, Washington, D.C., 1986, Armed Forces Institute of Pathology.
38. Larsson, L.I., and Rehfeld, J.F.: Pituitary gastrins occur in corticotrophs and melanotrophs, Science **213**:768, 1978.
39. Lloyd, R.V.: Analysis of mammosomatotropic cells in normal and neoplastic human pituitaries, Pathol. Res. Pract. **183**:577, 1988.
40. Lloyd, R.V., Wilson, B.S., Kovacs, K., et al.: Immunohistochemical localization of chromogranin in human hypophyses and pituitary adenomas, Arch. Pathol. Lab. Med. **109**:515, 1985.
41. McManus, J.F.A.: Histological demonstration of mucin after periodic acid, Nature **158**:202, 1946.
42. McNicol, A.M.: Patterns of corticotropic cells in the adult human pituitary in Cushing's disease, Diagn. Histopathol. **4**:335, 1981.
43. McNichol, A.M.: Pituitary adenomas, Histopathology **11**:995, 1987.
44. Morris, C.S., and Hitchcock, E.: Immunocytochemistry of folliculo-stellate cells of normal and neoplastic human pituitary gland, J. Clin. Pathol. **38**:481, 1985.
45. Nakanishi, S., Inoue, A., Kita, T., Nakamura, M., Chang, A., Cohen, S., and Numa, S.: Nucleotide sequence of cloned cDNA for bovine corticotrophin–β-lipoprotein precursor, Nature **278**:423, 1979.
46. Nieuwenhuijzen Kruseman, A.C., and Schröeder-van der Elst, J.P.: The immunolocalization of ACTH and α MSH in human and rat pituitaries, Virchows Arch. [Cell Pathol.] **22**:263, 1976.
47. Osamura, R.Y., Watanabe, K., Nakai, Y., and Imura, H.: Adrenocorticotropic hormone cells and immunoreactive β-endorphin cells in the human pituitary gland, Am. J. Pathol. **99**:105, 1980.
48. Paget, G.E., and Eccleston, E.: Simultaneous specific demonstrations of thyrotroph, gonadotroph, and acidophil cells in the anterior hypophysis, Stain Technol. **35**:119, 1960.
49. Paiz, C., and Hennigar, G.R.: Electron microscopy and histochemical correlation of human anterior pituitary cells, Am. J. Pathol. **59**:43, 1970.
50. Pearse, A.G.E.: Cytochemistry and cytology of the normal anterior hypophysis investigated by the trichrome–periodic acid–Schiff method, J. Pathol. Bacteriol. **64**:811, 1952.
51. Pelletier, G., Robert, F., and Hardy, J.: Identification of human anterior pituitary cells by immunoelectron microscopy, J. Clin. Endocrinol. **46**:534, 1978.
52. Phifer, R.F., Midgley, A.R., and Spicer, S.S.: Immunohistologic and histologic evidence that follicle-stimulating hormone and luteinizing hormone are present in the same cell type in the human pars distalis, J. Clin. Endocrinol. **36**:125, 1973.
53. Phifer, R.F., Orth, D.N., and Spicer, S.S.: Specific demonstration of human hypophyseal adrenocortico-melanotropic (ACTH/MSH) cell, J. Clin. Endocrinol. **39**:684, 1974.
54. Rasmussen, A.T.: Origin of the basophilic cells in the posterior lobe of the human hypophysis, Am. J. Anat. **46**:461, 1930.
55. Rehfeld, J.F., Hansen, H.F., Larsson, L.-I., et al.: Gastrin and cholecystokinin in pituitary neurons, Proc. Natl. Acad. Sci. USA **81**:1902, 1984.
56. Romeis, B.: Die mikroskopische Anatomie der Hypophyse. In von Möllendorff, W., editor: Handbuch der mikroskopischen Anatomie des Menschen, vol. 6, part 3, Berlin, 1940, Julius Springer Verlag.
57. Saint-André, J.-P., Rohmer, V., Alhenc-Gélas, F., Ménard, J., Bigorgne, J.C., and Corvol, P.: Presence of renin, angiotensinogen, and converting enzyme in human pituitary lactotroph cells and prolactin adenomas, J. Clin. Endocrinol. Metab. **63**:231, 1986.
58. van Oordt, P.G.W.J.: Nomenclature of the hormone-producing cells in the adenohypophysis: a report of the International Committee for Nomenclature of the Adenohypophysis, Gen. Comp. Endocrinol. **5**:131, 1965.
59. Velasco, M.E., Roessmann, U., and Gambetti, P.: The presence of glial fibrillary acidic protein in the human pituitary gland, J. Neuropathol. Exp. Neurol. **41**:150, 1982.
60. von Lawzewitsch, I., Dickmann, G.H., Amerzúa, L., et al.: Cytological and ultrastructural characterization of the human pituitary, Acta Anat. **81**:286, 1972.

Pituitary in endocrine disorders

61. Bloodworth, J.M.B., Jr., Kirkendall, W.M., and Carr, T.L.: Addison's disease associated with thyroid insufficiency and atrophy (Schmidt syndrome), J. Clin. Endocrinol. **14**:540, 1954.
62. Boyce, R., and Beadles, C.F.: Enlargement of the hypophysis cerebri in myxoedema; with remarks upon hypertrophy of the hypophysis, associated with changes in the thyroid body, J. Pathol. Bacteriol. **1**:224, 1893.
63. Burt, A.S., Landing, B.H., and Sommers, S.C.: Amphophil tumors of the hypophysis induced in mice by I[131], Cancer Res. **14**:497, 1954.
64. Carpenter, C.C.J., Solomon, N., Silverberg, S.G., et al.: Schmidt's syndrome (thyroid and adrenal insufficiency): a review of the literature and a report of fifteen new cases including ten instances of coexistent diabetes mellitus, Medicine **43**:153, 1964.
65. Crooke, A.D.: A change in the basophil cells of the pituitary gland common to conditions that exhibit the syndrome attributed to basophil adenoma, J. Pathol. Bacteriol. **41**:339, 1935.
66. Ezrin, C.: The adenohypophysis. In Ezrin, C., Godden, J.O., Volpé, R., and Wilson, R., editors: Systematic endocrinology, Hagerstown, Md., 1973, Harper & Row, Publishers, Inc.
67. Farquhar, M.G., and Rinehart, J.F.: Electron microscopic studies of the anterior pituitary gland of castrate rats, Endocrinology **54**:516, 1954.
68. Furth, J., and Clifton, K.H.: Experimental pituitary tumors. In Harris, G.W., and Donovan, B.T., editors: The pituitary gland, vol. 2, Berkeley, 1966, University of California Press.
69. Halmi, N.S., and McCormick, W.F.: Effects of hyperadrenocorticism on pituitary thyrotrophic cells in man, Arch. Pathol. **94**:471, 1972.
70. Halmi, N.S., McCormick, W.F., and Decker, D.A., Jr.: The natural history of hyalinization of ACTH/MSH cells in man, Arch. Pathol. **91**:318, 1971.
71. Irvine, W.J.: Autoimmunity in endocrine disease, Proc. R. Soc. Med. **67**:548, 1974.

72. Ketelbant-Balasse, P., Herlant, M., and Pasteels, J.L.: Modifications hypophysaires dans un cas d'hypercorticisme para-néoplastique, Ann. Endocrinol. **34**:743, 1973.
73. Kilby, R.A., Bennett, W.A., and Sprague, R.G.: Anterior pituitary gland in patients treated with cortisone and corticotropin, Am. J. Pathol. **33**:155, 1955.
74. Kovacs, K., and Horvath, E.: Gonadotrophs following removal of ovaries: a fine structural study of human pituitary glands, Endokrinologie **66**:1, 1975.
75. Murray, S., and Ezrin, C.: Effect of Graves' disease on the "thyrotroph" cell of the adenohypophysis, J. Clin. Endocrinol. **26**:287, 1966.
76. Neumann, P.E., Horoupian, D.S., Goldman, J.E., et al.: Cytoplasmic filaments of Crooke's hyaline change belong to the cytokeratin class, Am. J. Pathol. **116**:214, 1984.
77. Russfield, A.B.: The endocrine glands after bilateral adrenalectomy compared with those in spontaneous adrenal insufficiency, Cancer **8**:523, 1955.
78. Russfield, A.B.: Adenohypophysis. In Bloodworth, J.M.B., Jr., editor: Endocrine pathology, Baltimore, 1968, The Williams & Wilkins Co.
79. Russfield, A.B., and Byrnes, R.L.: Some effects of hormone therapy and castration on the hypophysis in men with carcinoma of the prostate, Cancer **11**:817, 1958.
80. Scheithauer, B.W., Kovacs, K., and Raymond, R.V.: The pituitary gland in untreated Addison's disease, Arch. Pathol. Lab. Med. **107**:484, 1983.
81. Schochet, S.S., Jr., Halmi, N.S., and McCormick, W.F.: PAS-positive hyalin change in ACTH/MSH cells of man, Arch. Pathol. **93**:457, 1972.
82. Shiino, M.: Morphological changes of pituitary gonadotrophs and thyrotrophs following treatment with LH-RH or TRH in vitro, Cell Tissue Res. **202**:399, 1979.
83. Siperstein, E.R., and Miller, K.J.: Hypertrophy of ACTH-producing cell following adrenalectomy: a quantitative electron microscopic study, Endocrinology **93**:1257, 1973.
84. Stratmann, I.E., Ezrin, C., Sellers, E.A., et al.: The origin of thyroidectomy cells as revealed by high resolution radioautography, Endocrinology **90**:728, 1972.
85. Takano, K., Kogawa, M., Tsushima, T., and Shizume, K.: A TSH secreting tumor accompanied by high stature: presentation of a case and review of the literature, Endocrinol. Jpn. **28**:215, 1981.
86. Thornton, K.R.: The cytology of the pituitary gland in myxoedema, J. Pathol. Bacteriol. **77**:249, 1959.

Hypophysectomy

87. Crome, L.: Underdevelopment of the pituitary, Dev. Med. Child. Neurol. **16**:222, 1974.
88. Manni, A., Pearson, O.H., Brodkey, J., and Marshall, J.S.: Transsphenoidal hypophysectomy in breast cancer, Cancer **44**:2330, 1979.
89. McGrath, P.: Prolactin activity and human growth hormone in pharyngeal hypophyses from embalmed cadavers, J. Endocrinol. **42**:205, 1968.
90. McGrath, P.: Extra-sellar post-hypophysectomy remnant, Br. J. Surg. **56**:64, 1969.
91. McPhie, J.L., and Beck, J.S.: Growth hormone in the normal human pharyngeal pituitary gland, Nature **219**:625, 1968.
92. Müller, W.: On the pharyngeal hypophysis. In Currie, A.R., and Illingworth, C.F.W., editors: Endocrine aspects of breast cancer, Edinburgh, 1958, E. & S. Livingstone, Ltd.

Hypopituitarism

93. Daughaday, W.H.: The adenohypophysis. In Williams, R.H., editor: Textbook of endocrinology, ed. 5, Philadelphia, 1975, W.B. Saunders Co.
94. Laron, Z.: The hypothalamus and the pituitary gland (hypophysis). In Hubble, D., editor: Paediatric endocrinology, Philadelphia, 1969, F.A. Davis Co.
95. Sheehan, H.L.: Post-partum necrosis of the anterior pituitary, J. Pathol. Bacteriol. **45**:189, 1937.

Anomalies

96. Angevine, D.M.: Pathologic anatomy of hypophysis and adrenals in anencephaly, Arch. Pathol. **26**:507, 1938.
97. Blizzard, R.M., and Alberts, M.: Hypopituitarism, hypoadrenalism, and hypogonadism in newborn infant, J. Pediatr. **48**:782, 1956.
98. Edmonds, H.W.: Pituitary, adrenal and thyroid in cyclopia, Arch. Pathol. **50**:727, 1950.
99. Lennox, B., and Russell, D.S.: Dystopia of the neurohypophysis: two cases, J. Pathol. Bacteriol. **63**:485, 1951.
100. Lloyd, R.V., Chandler, W.F., Kovacs, K., and Ryan, N.: Ectopic pituitary adenomas with normal anterior pituitary glands, Am. J. Surg. Pathol. **10**:546, 1986.
101. Moncrieff, M.W., Hill, D.S., Archer, J., et al.: Congenital absence of pituitary gland and adrenal hypoplasia, Arch. Dis. Child. **47**:136, 1972.
102. Potter, E.L., and Craig, J.M.: Pathology of the fetus and infant, ed. 3, Chicago, 1975, Year Book Medical Publishers, Inc.
103. Rasmussen, P., and Lindholm, J.: Ectopic pituitary adenomas, Clin. Endocrinol. **11**:69, 1979.
104. Steiner, M.W., and Boggs, J.D.: Absence of pituitary gland, hypothyroidism, hypoadrenalism and hypogonadism in a 17-year-old dwarf, J. Clin. Endocrinol. **25**:1591, 1965.
105. Willard, D., et al.: La dysgénésie antéhypophysaire primitive, Nouv. Presse Med. **1**:2237, 1972.

Empty sella syndrome

106. Bergeron, C., Kovacs, K., and Bilbao, J.M.: Primary empty sella: a histologic and immunocytologic study, Arch. Intern. Med. **139**:248, 1979.
107. Doniach, I.: Histopathology of the anterior pituitary, Clin. Endocrinol. Metab. **6**:21, 1977.
108. Ganguly, A., Stanchfield, J.B., Roberts, T.S., et al.: Cushing's syndrome in a patient with an empty sella turcica and a microadenoma of the adenohypophysis, Am. J. Med. **60**:306, 1976.
109. Jones, J.R., de Hempel, P.A., Kemmann, E., et al.: Galactorrhea and amenorrhea in a patient with an empty sella, Obstet. Gynecol. **49**(suppl. 1):9, 1977.
110. Kaufman, B.: The "empty" sella turcica—a manifestation of the intrasellar subarachnoid space, Radiology **90**:931, 1968.
111. Neelon, F.A., Goree, J.A., and Lebovitz, H.E.: The primary empty sella: clinical and radiographic characteristics and endocrine function, Medicine **52**:73, 1973.

Hemorrhage

112. Goldman, K.P., and Jacobs, A.: Anterior and posterior pituitary failure after head injury, Br. Med. J. **5217**:1924, 1960.
113. Kornblum, R.N., and Fisher, R.S.: Pituitary lesions in craniocerebral injuries, Arch. Pathol. **88**:242, 1969.
114. McCormick, W.F., and Halmi, N.S.: Hypophysis in patients with coma dépassé ("respirator brain"), Am. J. Clin. Pathol. **54**:374, 1970.

Pituitary apoplexy

115. Candrina, R., and Giustina, G.: Development of acromegaly after pituitary apoplexy, JAMA **256**:2998, 1986.
116. Wakai, S., Fukushima, T., Teramoto, A., and Sano, K.: Pituitary apoplexy: its incidence and clinical significance, J. Neurosurg. **55**:187, 1981.

Infarction and necrosis

117. Adams, J.H., et al.: The volume of the infarct in pars distalis of a human pituitary gland, 30 hr after transection of the pituitary stalk, J. Physiol. **166**:39P, 1963.
118. Daniel, P.M., Spicer, E.J.F., and Treip, C.S.: Pituitary necrosis in patients maintained on mechanical respirators, J. Pathol. **111**:135, 1973.
119. Frey, H.M.: Spontaneous pituitary destruction in diabetes mellitus, J. Clin. Endocrinol. **19**:1642, 1959.
120. Kovács, K.: Necrosis of anterior pituitary in humans, Neuroendocrinology **4**:170, 1969.
121. Kovács, K.: Pituitary necrosis in diabetes mellitus, Acta Diabetol. Lat. **9**:958, 1972.

122. Kovács, K.: Adenohypophysial necrosis in routine autopsies, Endokrinologie **60**:309, 1972.
123. Purnell, D.C., Randall, R.V., and Rynearson, E.H.: Postpartum pituitary insufficiency (Sheehan's syndrome): review of 18 cases, Mayo Clin. Proc. **39**:321, 1964.
124. Sheehan, H.L., and Davis, J.C.: Pituitary necrosis, Br. Med. Bull. **24**:59, 1968.
125. Towbin, A.: The respirator brain death syndrome, Hum. Pathol. **4**:583, 1973.

Acute inflammation

126. Domínguez, J.N., and Wilson, C.B.: Pituitary abscesses: report of seven cases and review of the literature, J. Neurosurg. **46**:601, 1977.
127. Simmonds, M.: Über embolische Prozesse in der Hypophyse, Virchows Arch. [Pathol. Anat. Physiol.] **217**:226, 1914.
128. Zorub, D.S., Martinez, A.J., Nelson, P.B., et al.: Invasive pituitary adenoma with abscess formation: case report, Neurosurgery **5**:718, 1979.

Granuloma

129. Doniach, I.: Histopathology of the anterior pituitary, Clin. Endocrinol. Metab. **6**:21, 1977.
130. Oelbaum, M.H.: Hypopituitarism in male subjects due to syphilis, Q. J. Med. **21**:249, 1952.
131. Plair, C.M., and Perry, S.: Hypothalamic-pituitary sarcoidosis, Arch. Pathol. **74**:527, 1962.

Lymphocytic hypophysitis

132. Asa, S.L., Bilbao, J.M., Kovacs, K., Josse, R.G., and Kreines, K.: Lymphocytic hypophysitis of pregnancy resulting in hypopituitarism: a distinct clinicopathologic entity, Ann. Intern. Med. **95**:166, 1981.
133. Cebelin, M.S., Velasco, M.E., de las Mulas, J.M., and Druet, R.L.: Galactorrhea associated with lymphocytic adenohypophysitis, Br. J. Obstet. Gynaecol. **88**:675, 1981.
134. Goudie, R.B., and Pinkerton, P.H.: Anterior hypophysitis and Hashimoto's disease in a young woman, J. Pathol. Bacteriol. **83**:584, 1962.
135. Guay, A.T., Agnello, V., Tronic, B.C., Gresham, D.G., and Freidberg, S.R.: Lymphocytic hypophysitis in a man, J. Clin. Endocrinol. Metab. **64**:631, 1987.
136. Jensen, M.D., Handwerger, B.S., Scheithauer, B.W., Carpenter, P.C., Mirakian, R., and Banks, P.M.: Lymphocytic hypophysitis with isolated corticotropin deficiency, Ann. Intern. Med. **105**:200, 1986.
137. Mayfield, R.K., Levine, J.H., Gordon, L., Powers, J., Galbraith, R.M., and Rowe, S.E.: Lymphoid adenohypophysitis presenting as a pituitary tumor, Am. J. Med. **69**:619, 1980.
138. McGrail, K.M., Beyerl, B.D., Black, P.M., Klibanski, A., and Zervas, N.T.: Lymphocytic adenohypophysitis of pregnancy with complete recovery, Neurosurgery **20**:791, 1987.

Infiltrations and metabolic disorders

139. Barr, R., and Lampert, P.: Intrasellar amyloid tumor, Acta Neuropathol. **21**:83, 1972.
140. Bilbao, J.M., Horvath, E., Hudson, A.R., et al.: Pituitary adenoma producing amyloid-like substance, Arch. Pathol. **99**:411, 1975.
141. Kraus, E.J.: Die Hypophyse. In Henke, F., and Lubarsch, O., editors: Handbuch der speziellen Anatomie und Histologie, vol. 8, Berlin, 1926, Julius Springer Verlag.
142. Kubota, T., Kuroda, E., Yamashima, R., et al.: Amyloid formation in prolactinoma, Arch. Pathol. Lab. Med. **110**:72, 1986.
143. Russell, D.S., and Rubinstein, L.J.: Pathology of tumours of the nervous system, ed. 4, Baltimore, 1977, The Williams & Wilkins Co.
144. Schober, R., and Nelson, D.: Fine structure and origin of amyloid deposits in pituitary adenoma, Arch. Pathol. **99**:403, 1975.
145. Schochet, S.S., Jr., McCormick, W.F., and Halmi, N.S.: Pituitary gland in patients with Hurler syndrome, Arch. Pathol. **97**:96, 1974.

146. Voigt, C., Saeger, W., Gerigk, C., et al.: Amyloid in pituitary adenomas, Pathol. Res. Pract. **183**:555, 1988.
147. Westermark, P., Grimelius, L., Polak, J.M., et al.: Amyloid in polypeptide hormone–producing tumors, Lab. Invest. **37**:212, 1977.

Hyperplasia

148. Horvath, E.: Pituitary hyperplasia, Pathol. Res. Pract. **183**:623, 1988.
149. McKeever, P.E., Koppelman, M.C., Metcalf, D., Quindlen, E., Kornblith, P.L., Strott, C.A., Howard, R., and Smith, B.H.: Refractory Cushing's disease caused by multinodular ACTH-cell hyperplasia, J. Neuropathol. Exp. Neurol. **41**:490, 1982.
150. Saeger, W., and Lüdecke, D.K.: Pituitary hyperplasia, Virchows Arch. [Pathol. Anat.] **399**:277, 1983.
151. Schnall, A.M., Kovacs, K., Brodkey, J.S., and Pearson, O.H.: Pituitary Cushing's disease without adenoma, Acta Endocrinol. **94**:297, 1980.

Tumors

152. Adelman, L.S., and Post, K.D.: Intra-operative technique for pituitary adenomas, Am. J. Surg. Pathol. **3**:173, 1979.
153. Burrow, G.N., Wortzman, G., Rewcastle, N.B., Holgate, R.C., and Kovacs, K.: Microadenomas of the pituitary and abnormal sellar tomograms in an unselected autopsy series, N. Engl. J. Med. **304**:156, 1981.
154. Franks, A.J.: Diagnostic manual of tumours of the central nervous system, Edinburgh, 1988, Churchill Livingstone.
155. Hardy, J.: Transsphenoidal surgery of hypersecreting pituitary tumors. In Kohler, P.O., and Ross, G.T., editors: Diagnosis and treatment of pituitary tumors, New York, 1973, American Elsevier Publishing Co.
156. Horvath, E., and Kovacs, K.: Pathology of the pituitary gland. In Ezrin, C., Horvath, E., Kaufman, B., Kovacs, K., and Weiss, M.H., editors: Pituitary diseases, Boca Raton, Fla., 1980, CRC Press, Inc.
157. Post, K.D.: General considerations in the surgical treatment of pituitary tumors. In Post, K.D., Jackson, I.M.D., and Reichlin, S., editors: The pituitary adenoma, New York, 1980, Plenum Publishing Corp.
158. Post, K.D., Biller, B.J., Adelman, L.S., Molitch, M.E., Wolpert, S.M., and Reichlin, S.: Selective transsphenoidal adenomectomy in women with galactorrhea-amenorrhea, JAMA **242**:158, 1979.
159. Wrightson, P.: The limitations of surgical treatment of pituitary microadenomas. In Faglia, G., Giovanelli, M.A., and MacLeod, R.M., editors: Pituitary microadenomas, Proceedings of the Serono Symposia, vol. 29, New York, 1980, Academic Press, Inc.

Adenomas

160. Abbassy, A.A., and Sakali, W.A.: Hyperprolactinemia and male infertility, Br. J. Urol. **54**:305, 1982.
161. Adelman, L.S.: The pathology of pituitary adenomas. In Post, K.D., Jackson, I.M.D., and Reichlin, S., editors: The pituitary adenoma, New York, 1980, Plenum Publishing Corp.
162. Ballard, H.S., Frame, B., and Hartsock, R.J.: Familial multiple endocrine adenoma–peptic ulcer complex, Medicine **43**:481, 1964.
163. Bigos, S.T., Somma, M., Rasio, E., Eastman, R.C., Lanthier, A., Johnston, H.H., and Hardy, J.: Cushing's disease: management by transsphenoidal pituitary microsurgery, J. Clin. Endocrinol. Metab. **50**:348, 1980.
164. Burrow, G.N., Wortzman, G., Rewcastle, N.B., Holgate, R.C., and Kovacs, K.: Microadenomas of the pituitary and abnormal sellar tomograms in an unselected autopsy series, N. Engl. J. Med. **304**:156, 1981.
165. Carmalt, M.H.B., Dalton, G.A., Fletcher, R.F., et al.: The treatment of Cushing's disease by transsphenoidal hypophysectomy, Q. J. Med. **46**:119, 1977.

166. Costello, R.T.: Subclinical adenoma of the pituitary gland, Am. J. Pathol. **12**:205, 1936.

167. Cushing, H.: The basophil adenomas of the pituitary body and their clinical manifestations (pituitary basophilism), Bull. Johns Hopkins Hosp. **50**:137, 1932.

168. Dingemans, K.P.: Development of TSH-producing pituitary tumors in mouse, Virchows Arch. [Cell Pathol.] **12**:338, 1973.

169. Forbes, A.P., et al.: Syndrome characterized by galactorrhea, amenorrhea and low urinary FSH: comparison with acromegaly and normal lactation, J. Clin. Endocrinol. **14**:265, 1954.

170. Frantz, A.G.: Prolactin, N. Engl. J. Med. **298**:201, 1978.

171. Furth, J., Moy, P., Hershman, J.M., et al.: Thyrotrophic tumor syndrome: a multiglandular disease induced by sustained deficiency of thyroid hormones, Arch. Pathol. **96**:217, 1973.

172. Gillespie, C.A., Walker, J.S., Burch, W.M., et al.: Cushing's syndrome secondary to ectopic pituitary adenoma in the sphenoid sinus, Otolaryngol. Head Neck Surg. **96**:569, 1986.

173. Girod, C., Trouillas, J., and Claustrat, B.: The human thyrotropic adenoma: pathologic diagnosis in five cases and critical review of the literature, Semin. Diagn. Pathol. **3**:58, 1986.

174. Griesbach, W.E., and Purves, H.D.: Basophil adenomata in the rat hypophysis after gonadectomy, Br. J. Cancer **14**:49, 1960.

175. Horvath, E., and Kovacs, K.: Pituitary chromophobe adenoma composed of oncocytes: a light and electron microscopic study, Arch. Pathol. **95**:235, 1973.

176. Horvath, E., and Kovacs, K.: Gonadotroph adenomas of the human pituitary: sex-related fine-structural dichotomy, Am. J. Pathol. **117**:429, 1984.

177. Horvath, E., Kovacs, K., Singer, W., Ezrin, C., and Kerényi, N.A.: Acidophil stem cell adenoma of the human pituitary, Arch Pathol. Lab. Med. **101**:594, 1977.

178. Horvath, E., Kovacs, K., Killinger, D.W., Smyth, H.S., Platts, M.E., and Singer, W.: Silent corticotrophic adenoma of the human pituitary gland: a histologic, immunocytologic, and ultrastructural study, Am. J. Pathol. **98**:617, 1980.

179. Horvath, E., Kovacs, K., Singer, W., Smyth, H.S., Killinger, D.W., Ezrin, C., and Weiss, M.H.: Acidophil stem cell adenoma of the human pituitary: clinicopathologic analysis of 15 cases, Cancer **47**:761, 1981.

180. Horvath, E., Kovacs, K., Killinger, D.W., Smyth, H.S., Weiss, M.H., and Ezrin, C.: Mammosomatotroph cell adenoma of the human pituitary: a morphologic entity, Virchows Arch. [Pathol. Anat.] **398**:277, 1983.

181. Kanie, N., Kageyama, N., Kuwayama, A., Nakane, T., Watanabe, M., and Kawaoi, A.: Pituitary adenomas in acromegalic patients: an immunohistochemical and endocrinological study with special reference to prolactin-secreting adenoma, J. Clin. Endocrinol. **57**:1093, 1983.

182. Katz, M.S., Gregerman, R.I., Horvath, E., Kovacs, K., and Ezrin, C.: Thyrotroph cell adenoma of the human pituitary gland associated with primary hypothyroidism: clinical and morphological features, Acta Endocrinol. **95**:41, 1980.

183. Klibanski, A., Ridgway, E.C., and Zervas, N.T.: Pure alpha subunit–secreting pituitary tumors, J. Neurosurg. **59**:585, 1983.

184. Kovacs, K., and Horvath, E.: Pituitary chromophobe adenoma composed of oncocytes: a light and electron microscopic study, Arch. Pathol. **95**:235, 1973.

185. Kovacs, K., Horvath, E., Van Loon, G.R., Rewcastle, N.B., Ezrin, C., and Rosenbloom, A.A.: Pituitary adenomas associated with elevated blood follicle–stimulating hormone levels: a histologic, immunocytologic and electron microscopic study of two cases, Fertil. Steril. **29**:622, 1978.

186. Kovacs, K., Horvath, E., Rewcastle, N.B., and Ezrin, C.: Gonadotroph cell adenoma of the pituitary in a woman with long-standing hypogonadism, Arch. Gynecol. **229**:57, 1980.

187. Kovacs, K., Horvath, E., Ryan, N., and Ezrin, C.: Null cell adenoma of the human pituitary, Virchows Arch. [Pathol. Anat.] **387**:165, 1980.

188. Landolt, A.M.: Biology of pituitary microadenomas. In Faglia, G., Giovanelli, M.A., and MacLeod, R.M., editors: Pituitary microadenomas, Proceedings of the Serono Symposia, vol. 29, New York, 1980, Academic Press, Inc.

189. Landolt, A.M., and Heitz, P.U.: Alpha-subunit–producing pituitary adenomas, Virchows Arch. [Pathol. Anat.] **409**:417, 1986.

190. Landolt, A.M., and Oswald, U.W.: Histology and ultrastructure of an oncocytic adenoma of human pituitary, Cancer **31**:1099, 1973.

191. Landolt, A.M., and Rothenbühler, V.: Pituitary adenoma calcification, Arch. Pathol. Lab. Med. **101**:22, 1977.

192. Macfarlane, I.A., Beardwell, C.G., Shalet, S.M., et al.: Glycoprotein hormone alpha subunit secretion by pituitary adenomas: influence of external irradiation, Clin. Endocrinol. **13**:215, 1986.

193. Mosca, L., Solcia, E., Capella, C., et al.: Pituitary adenomas: surgical versus post mortem findings today. In Faglia, G., Giovanelli, M.A., and MacLeod, R.M., editors: Pituitary microadenomas, vol. 29, New York, 1980, Academic Press, Inc.

194. Mukuda, K., Ohta, M., Uozumi, R., et al.: Ossified prolactinoma: case report, Neurosurgery **20**:473, 1987.

195. Nelson, D.H., Meakin, J., and Thorn, G.W.: ACTH-producing pituitary tumors following adrenalectomy for Cushing's syndrome, Ann. Intern. Med. **52**:560, 1960.

196. Osamura, R.Y., Watanabe, K., Seidah, N.G., Chan, J.S., and Chrétien, M.: Light and electron microscopic localization of the N-terminal fragment of human pro-opiomelanocortin in the human pituitary gland and in neoplasms, Virchows Arch. [Pathol. Anat.] **408**:281, 1985.

197. Peake, G.T., McKeel, D.W., Jarett, L., et al.: Ultrastructural, histologic and hormonal characterization of a prolactin-rich human pituitary tumor, J. Clin. Endocrinol. **29**:1383, 1969.

198. Racadot, J., Vila-Porcile, E., Peillon, F., et al.: Adénomes hypophysaires à cellules à prolactine: étude structural et ultrastructurale, corrélations anatomo-cliniques, Ann. Endocrinol. **32**:298, 1971.

199. Ridgway, E.C., Klibanski, A., Ladenson, P.W., Clemmons, D., Beitins, I.Z., McArthur, J.W., Martorana, M.A., and Zervas, N.T.: Pure alpha-secreting pituitary adenomas, N. Engl. J. Med. **304**:1254, 1981.

200. Robert, F., and Hardy, J.: Human corticotroph cell adenomas, Semin. Diagn. Pathol. **3**:34, 1986.

201. Robert, F., Pelletier, G., and Hardy, J.: Pituitary adenomas in Cushing's disease, Arch. Pathol. Lab. Med. **102**:448, 1978.

202. Saeger, W., and Lüdecke, D.K.: Pituitary adenomas with hyperfunction of TSH, Virchows Arch. [Pathol. Anat.] **394**:255, 1982.

203. Salassa, R.M., Laws, E.R., Jr., Carpenter, P.C., and Northcutt, R.C.: Transsphenoidal removal of a pituitary microadenoma in Cushing's disease, Mayo Clin. Proc. **53**:24, 1978.

204. Samaan, N.A., Osborne, B.M., Mackay, B., Leavens, M.E., Duello, T.M., and Halmi, N.S.: Endocrine and morphologic studies of pituitary adenomas secondary to primary hypothyroidism, J. Clin. Endocrinol. Metab. **45**:903, 1977.

205. Samaan, N.A., Stepanas, A.V., Danziger, J., and Trujillo, J.: Reactive pituitary abnormalities in patients with Klinefelter's and Turner's syndromes, Arch. Intern. Med. **139**:198, 1979.

206. Scheithauer, B.W.: Surgical pathology of the pituitary: the adenomas, Part I, Pathol. Annu. **19**(pt. 2):269, 1984.

207. Scheithauer, B.W., Laws, E.R., Jr., Kovacs, K., Horvath, E., Randall, R.V., and Carney, J.A.: Pituitary adenomas of the multiple endocrine neoplasia type I syndrome, Semin. Diagn. Pathol. **4**:205, 1987.

208. Schochet, S.S., McCormick, W.F., and Halmi, N.S.: Acidophil adenomas with intracytoplasmic filamentous aggregates: a light and EM study, Arch. Pathol. **94**:6, 1972.

209. Schteingart, D.E., Chandler, W.F., Lloyd, R.V., and Ibarra-Pérez, G.: Cushing's syndrome caused by an ectopic pituitary adenoma, Neurosurgery **21**:223, 1987.

210. Segal, S., Polishuk, W.Z., and Ben-David, M.: Hyperprolactinemic male infertility, Fertil. Steril. **27**:1425, 1976.

211. Shenker, Y., Lloyd, R.V., Weatherbee, L., Port, F.K., Grekin, R.J., and Barkan, A.L.: Ectopic prolactinoma in a patient with hyperparathyroidism and abnormal sellar radiography, J. Clin. Endocrinol. Metab. **62**:1065, 1986.

212. Snyder, P.J.: Gonadotroph cell pituitary adenomas, Endocrinol. Metab. Clin. **16:**755, 1987.
213. Tolis, G., Bird, C., Bertrand, G., McKenzie, J.M., and Ezrin, C.: Pituitary hyperthyroidism, Am. J. Med. **64:**177, 1978.
214. Trouillas, J., Girod, C., Sassolas, G., Claustrat, B., Lhéritier, M., Dubois, M.P., and Goutelle, A.: Human pituitary gonadotropic adenoma: histological, immunocytochemical, and ultrastructural and hormonal studies in eight cases, J. Pathol. **135:**315, 1981.
215. Tyrrell, J.B., Brooks, R.M., Fitzgerald, P.A., Cofoid, P.B., Forsham, P.H., and Wilson, C.B.: Cushing's disease: selective trans-sphenoidal resection of pituitary microadenomas, N. Engl. J. Med. **298:**753, 1978.
216. Von Westarp, C., Weir, B.K.A., and Shnitka, T.K.: Characterization of a pituitary stone, Am. J. Med. **68:**949, 1980.
217. Wermer, P.: Endocrine adenomatosis and peptic ulcer in a large kindred, Am. J. Med. **35:**205, 1963.
218. Wilson, C.B., and Dempsey, L.C.: Transsphenoidal microsurgical removal of 250 pituitary adenomas, J. Neurosurg. **48:**13, 1978.
219. Woolf, P.D., and Schenk, E.A.: An FSH-producing tumor in a patient with hypogonadism, J. Clin. Endocrinol. Metab. **38:**561, 1974.

Carcinoma

220. D'Abrera, V.S.E., Burke, W.J., Bleasel, K.F., et al.: Carcinoma of the pituitary gland, J. Pathol. **109:**335, 1973.
221. Evans, R.W.: Histological appearances of tumours, ed. 2, Edinburgh, 1966, E. & S. Livingstone, Ltd.
222. Houck, W.A., Olson, K.B., and Horton, J.: Clinical features of tumor metastasis to pituitary, Cancer **26:**656, 1970.
223. Kovacs, K.: Metastatic cancer of pituitary gland, Oncology **27:**533, 1973.
224. Queiroz, L. de S., Facure, N.O., Facure, J.J., et al.: Pituitary carcinoma with liver metastases and Cushing syndrome, Arch. Pathol. **99:**32, 1975.
225. Roessman, U., Kaufman, B., and Friede, R.L.: Metastatic lesions in the sella turcica and pituitary gland, Cancer **25:**478, 1970.

Other tumors

226. Fischer, E.R., and Wechsler, J.: Granular cell myoblastoma—a misnomer, Cancer **15:**936, 1962.
227. Friedman, N.B.: Germinoma of pineal—its identity with germinoma ("seminoma") of the testis, Cancer Res. **7:**363, 1947.
228. Ghatak, N.R., Hirano, A., and Zimmerman, H.M.: Intrasellar germinomas: a form of ectopic pinealoma, J. Neurosurg. **1:**670, 1969.
229. Ghatak, N.R., Hirano, A., and Zimmerman, H.M.: Ultrastructure of a craniopharyngioma, Cancer **27:**1465, 1971.
230. Kepes, J.J.: Transitional cell tumor of the pituitary gland developing from a Rathke's cleft cyst, Cancer **41:**337, 1978.
231. Luse, S.A., and Kernohan, J.W.: Granular-cell tumors of the stalk and posterior lobe of the pituitary gland, Cancer **8:**616, 1955.
232. Massie, A.P.: A granular-cell pituicytoma of the neurohypophysis, J. Pathol. **129:**53, 1979.
233. Petito, C.K., DeGirolami, U., and Earle, K.M.: Craniopharyngiomas: a clinical and pathological review, Cancer **37:**1944, 1976.
234. Rubinstein, L.J.: Tumors of the central nervous system. In Atlas of tumor pathology, series 2, fascicle 6, Washington, D.C., 1972, Armed Forces Institute of Pathology.
235. Satyamurti, S., and Huntington, H.W.: Granular cell myoblastoma of the pituitary: case report, J. Neurosurg. **37:**483, 1972.
236. Seemayer, T.A., Blundell, J.S., and Wiglesworth, F.W.: Pituitary craniopharyngioma with tooth formation, Cancer **29:**423, 1972.
237. Shuangshoti, S., Netsky, M.G., and Nashold, B.S., Jr.: Epithelial cysts related to sella turcica: proposed origin from neuroepithelium, Arch. Pathol. **90:**444, 1970.
238. Symon, L., Ganz, J.C., and Burston, J.: Granular cell myoblastoma of neurohypophysis: report of 2 cases, J. Neurosurg. **35:**82, 1971.
239. Waller, R.R., Riley, F.C., and Sundt, T.M., Jr.: A rare cause of the chiasmal syndrome, Arch. Ophthalmol. **88:**269, 1972.
240. Zimmerman, H.M.: Ten most common types of brain tumor, Semin. Roentgenol. **6:**48, 1971.
241. Zülch, K.J.: Brain tumors, their biology and pathology, ed. 2, New York, 1965, Springer Verlag.

31 Thyroid Gland

KAARLE O. FRANSSILA

DEVELOPMENT, STRUCTURE, AND FUNCTION

The thyroid gland arises from a midline invagination at the base of the tongue. The invagination grows downward to the normal position of the thyroid, and its lowest part proliferates to form the gland. The thyroglossal duct that initially connects the gland to the pharyngeal floor disappears by the sixth week of embryonic life. Its proximal end is represented in adults by the foramen cecum at the base of the tongue and its lowest part by the pyramidal lobe of the thyroid, which is present in about 40% of persons. The other epithelial component of the thyroid, the C-cells, are believed to have their origin in the neural crest.[6]

The thyroid in an adult weighs between 15 and 30 g, but this varies considerably in different areas of the world. The gland is composed of two lateral lobes connected by an isthmus that may have a pyramidal lobe that extends cranially. The cut surface of the thyroid is yellow-red and translucent.

The functional unit of the thyroid is a follicle, a spherical sac filled with acidophilic colloid and lined by cuboid epithelium with a thin basement membrane. The apical surface of the epithelial cells has numerous microvilli extending to the colloid,[5] which is composed of the glycoprotein thyroglobulin. The follicles are separated from each other by delicate fibrous tissue containing the blood vessels, nerves, and lymphatics. Between 20 and 40 follicles are surrounded by a thicker connective tissue sheath, forming a lobule.

Briefly, the synthesis of thyroid hormones is as follows. The epithelial cells absorb iodide from the blood, concentrate it more than twentyfold, and oxidize it to iodine. Iodine attaches to tyrosine residues of thyroglobulin to form monoiodotyrosine (MIT) and diiodotyrosine (DIT), which couple to form triiodothyronine (T_3) and tetraiodothyronine (T_4, or thyroxine). Both the oxidation of iodide and the coupling of tyrosines require the presence of proxidases. The release of thyroid hormones occurs through endocytosis of colloid and proteolysis of thyroglobulin by lysosomal enzymes. T_3 and T_4 are freed and discharged into blood, where they are bound to plasma proteins, mainly thyroxine-binding globulin. The synthesis and release of thyroid hormones are regulated by the hypophyseal thyroid-stimulating hormone (TSH).

C-cells, or parafollicular cells, are dispersed within the follicles, especially in the posterolateral parts of the lateral lobes. They make up about 0.1% of the epithelial mass.[7] These cells secrete a polypeptide hormone called calcitonin, which has a hypocalcemic effect. C-cells are almost impossible to identify by light microscopy without the use of special techniques such as sil-

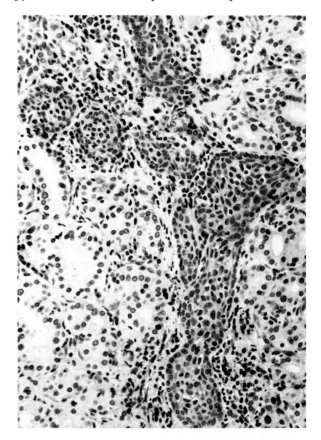

Fig. 31-1. Solid cell nest. Small cell groups resembling squamous epithelium and situated between the follicles. The follicular epithelium is hyperplastic because of Graves' disease. (240×.)

ver stains for argyrophil cells or immunohistochemical methods,[2] usually based on the calcitonin content of the cells.[7] Ultrastructurally C-cells contain secretory granules and occupy an intrafollicular position. They are separated from the interstitium by the follicular basement membrane and from the colloid by extensions of the follicular cell cytoplasm.[1] *Solid cell nests* are small cell groups that resemble squamous epithelium (Fig. 31-1) and are situated between the follicles, most often in the middle third of the lateral lobes.[8] They have been detected in up to 60% of cases in systematic autopsy studies[3] using semiserial sections and are believed to represent remnants of the ultimobranchial body.[4] There is usually a distinct increase of C-cells around them.[4] Solid cell nests should not be confused with papillary microcarcinomas or with C-cell hyperplasia.

FUNCTIONAL DISORDERS
Hypothyroidism

Hypothyroidism is defined as a clinical state resulting from inadequate production of thyroid hormones or, very rarely, from resistance of the peripheral tissues to the influence of thyroid hormones. Hypothyroidism may be congenital or may appear in children or adults. Adulthood hypothyroidism shows about a tenfold predominance among females and develops most often between 30 and 60 years of age.

The clinical features depend on the age at onset. Symptoms of overt adult hypothyroidism include lack of energy, cold intolerance, dryness of skin and hair, hoarseness of voice, and subcutaneous swelling that is most prominent around the eyes. Advanced hypothyroidism with subcutaneous swelling is called "myxedema." In mild hypothyroidism the symptoms are frequently minor or nonspecific. Serum T_4 concentrations are low in severe hypothyroidism but within the normal range in mild cases. Because of a negative feedback control, serum TSH values become elevated even before the patient has any symptoms (if the disease is not of hypophyseal origin). The causes of hypothyroidism can be grouped as follows:

A. Causes of congenital hypothyroidism
  1. Developmental anomalies
    a. Thyroid agenesis
    b. Ectopic thyroid
  2. Genetic defects in thyroid hormone synthesis (dyshormonogenesis)
    a. Iodide-transport defect (inability to concentrate iodide in the thyroid)
    b. Organification defect (inability to bind iodide to thyroglobulin, caused by deficiency in peroxidases)
    c. Coupling defect (inability to couple MIT and DIT to form T_3 and T_4)
    d. Dehalogenase defect (inability to deiodinate MIT and DIT, caused by deficiency in dehalogenase)
    e. Defects in thyroglobulin synthesis
  3. Endemic goiter and cretinism
  4. Fetal exposure to iodides, antithyroid agents, or radioactive iodine
  5. Transplacental passage of thyrotropin receptor–inhibiting antibodies in babies delivered by mothers with Hashimoto's thyroiditis.[16]
B. Causes of noncongenital hypothyroidism
  1. Lymphocytic (autoimmune) thyroiditis
    a. Hashimoto's thyroiditis
    b. Atrophic thyroiditis (spontaneous hypothyroidism)
  2. Ablation of thyroid by surgery or radiation
  3. Endemic and sporadic goiter
  4. Hypopituitarism
  5. Thyroid cancer destroying the gland
  6. Antithyroid drug administration
  7. Developmental anomalies and defects in thyroid hormone synthesis (mild cases, less than complete lack of thyroid hormone)

The most common cause of noncongenital hypothyroidism is autoimmune thyroiditis, especially its atrophic variant, and the next most common cause is ablation of the thyroid by radioactive iodine or surgery.[18]

Cretinism is the term given to congenital hypothyroidism if the lack of thyroid hormone is complete or almost complete and prolonged. Endemic cretinism occurs in the same areas as endemic goiter and is mainly caused by the lack of iodine. Sporadic cretinism, on the other hand, has many causes, the most common of which are developmental anomalies and genetic defects in thyroid hormone synthesis.[23] Because of iodination of salt, endemic cretinism is becoming very rare. In cretinism there is, in addition to hypothyroidism, an intellectual defect and growth retardation that are caused by thyroid hormone deficiency during fetal life. The early symptoms of cretinism, including decreased activity, feeding problems, enlarged tongue, and hoarse cry, appear during the neonatal period. The full clinical picture with physical and mental retardation develops slowly over several months.

Most endemic cretins have neurologic defects such as deaf-mutism or spastic diplegia, but they do not always have postnatal hypothyroidism, and sometimes they have no intellectual defect.[12] Although endemic cretins have lacked iodine and thyroid hormones during fetal life, their thyroids are usually capable of producing hormones postnatally if iodine is available.

Hypothyroidism that develops in children after the first year of life results in growth retardation but usually no intellectual defect.

Hyperthyroidism

Hyperthyroidism, also known as thyrotoxicosis, is defined as a hypermetabolic clinical state caused by increased production of thyroid hormones. It is characterized by emotional lability, nervousness, rapid pulse, weight loss, perspiration, heat intolerance, and fine tremor in the hands.

Hyperthyroidism may be caused by several diseases.[22] Graves' disease is the most common cause in areas where there is no endemic goiter, whereas in many endemic areas, toxic nodular goiter is the predominant cause.

Rarely, hyperthyroidism may be caused by hypersecretion of pituitary TSH because of a pituitary tumor, or by hypersecretion of thyrotropin-releasing hormone (TRH). Excessive secretion of chorionic gonadotropin by trophoblastic tumors, such as hydatidiform mole and choriocarcinoma, or by testicular tumors containing trophoblastic elements is another rare cause of hyperthyroidism. (Chorionic gonadotropin has a weak thyrotropic effect on the thyroid.) Hyperthyroidism may also be caused by excessive doses of thyroid hormones or iodine (jodbasedow), as well as by amiodarone, an iodine-containing drug used in the treatment of cardiac arrhythmias.[11,21] Congenital hyperthyroidism may develop when the mother has Graves' disease because the thyroid-stimulating immunoglobulins can cross the placental barrier. Painless thyroiditis begins with hyperthyroidism,[11] and in the initial phase of granulomatous thyroiditis there may be a transitional hyperthyroid phase. Rarely, hyperthyroidism may be caused by metastatic tumors in the thyroid[19] or by thyroid hormones secreted by a thyroid carcinoma or a struma ovarii (teratoma with thyroid components).

DEVELOPMENTAL ANOMALIES

Developmental anomalies of the thyroid result from disturbances in the descent of the thyroid anlage. Although rare, they are the most common cause of sporadic cretinism.

Thyroid agenesis

Complete failure of the thyroid anlage to develop results in total absence of thyroid tissue. Children with thyroid agenesis are born as cretins. In hemiagenesis only one of the thyroid lobes develops.

Ectopic thyroid

An ectopic thyroid may be located anywhere along the route of descent, usually between the normal position and the base of the tongue but sometimes caudally in the mediastinum.[13,14] The base of the tongue is the most common location. Such a lingual thyroid sometimes causes laryngeal or pharyngeal obstruction. Total absence of thyroid tissue from its normal location occurs in about two thirds of cases with an ectopic thyroid.[14]

In patients with an ectopic thyroid, the presence and severity of hypothyroidism depend on the quantity of residual thyroid tissue. Hypothyroidism may not develop until late in childhood or in adulthood.

"Lateral aberrant thyroid"

Lateral aberrant thyroid, a term denoting thyroid tissue occurring laterally in the neck, does not represent, at least in most cases, a developmental anomaly but may be a result of various disorders. It may represent a thyroid nodule connected to the gland by a very thin strand of tissue,[20] or nonneoplastic thyroid tissue implanted during a thyroid operation. Thyroid follicles occurring in the lymph nodes appear practically always to represent metastasis from a papillary thyroid carcinoma that is often occult,[17] though some authors have claimed that in rare cases they might represent nonneoplastic inclusions.[10] In metastatic papillary carcinoma at least some of the follicular cell nuclei usually but not always[17] have the ground-glass appearance and other nuclear features typical of this tumor (see p. 1557).

Thyroglossal cyst

Remnants of the thyroglossal duct may give rise to cysts or sinuses. Thyroglossal cysts occur in the midline, most commonly in the region of the hyoid bone. They are lined with columnar or squamous epithelium, though this may be lacking because of inflammation.[9] Follicles are sometimes present in the wall of the cyst. Cysts may communicate with the pharynx at the foramen cecum and form fistulas. If they are inflamed, they may rupture to the skin. Rarely, carcinoma may arise from a thyroglossal cyst. It is usually of the papillary type.[15]

GOITER (NODULAR GOITER AND DIFFUSE NONTOXIC GOITER)

The term "goiter" refers to thyroid enlargement that is caused by compensatory hyperplasia in response to thyroid hormone deficiency. Diffuse thyroid enlargement is called "diffuse nontoxic goiter," nodular enlargement is called "nodular or adenomatous goiter." Although the term "goiter" is sometimes used for all kinds of thyroid enlargement, here it does not include thyroid enlargement caused by other thyroid diseases such as neoplastic growth or inflammation.

Etiology

Goiter occurs in two epidemiologic forms: (1) endemic and (2) sporadic, or nonendemic. A goiter prevalence higher than 10% in an area indicates that the condition is endemic.[25] Endemic goiter is prevalent in several high mountainous areas or areas far from the sea, such as the Alps, the Himalayas, and the Andes, where iodine content of drinking water and food is low. Endemic goiter is a common disease; in 1960 it was estimated that 200 million people in the world had endemic goiter, but its prevalence is decreasing because of prophylactic iodination of salt. Most endemic goiter is caused by lack of iodine,[25] though in some cases goitrogens and genetic factors may be involved.

Sporadic goiter is also a common disease. A small proportion is caused by inborn errors in the synthesis of thyroid hormones. It has been suggested that this dyshormonogenic goiter is inherited according to simple mendelian rules.[23,24] The different types of this disorder are presented on p. 1545.

Goitrogens, substances that interfere with the production of thyroid hormones, are a rare cause of goiter. The most common goitrogens are drugs used for treatment of hyperthyroidism, but some other drugs and some foods (such as cabbage and cauliflower) are also goitrogenic. Goitrogens are able to cross the placental barrier and may cause congenital goiter.

In most cases of sporadic goiter the cause is unknown. On some occasions suboptimal iodine intake may predispose to goiter, especially during increased metabolic demand, as in puberty and pregnancy. Furthermore, genetic factors and undefinable dyshormonogenic defects may contribute to goiter development that is possibly multifactorial in origin. Recently, it has been suggested that growth-stimulating immunoglobulins might on some occasions be a factor in the development of goiter.[26]

Pathogenesis

Goiter is believed to be caused by long-term TSH stimulation during a period of suboptimal production of thyroid hormones. This stimulation leads to epithelial hyperplasia with development of new daughter follicles from the original ones.[28] Hyperplasia is often followed by involution. Both of these changes result in diffuse goiter. Nodular goiter is usually regarded as an end stage of diffuse goiter, caused by cyclic changes of hyperplasia and involution. This is supported by the finding that in endemic areas the goiter is hyperplastic in childhood, diffusely enlarged with colloid accumulation in adolescence, and nodular in adulthood.

Some patients with nodular goiter develop hyperthyroidism, a condition often called "toxic nodular goiter," or "Plummer's disease." It has been suggested that hyperthyroidism is attributable to an increased number of daughter follicles containing epithelial cells with high intrinsic iodine turnover ("hot" follicles in autoradiography with ^{131}I).[29] These hot follicles may be autonomous, and when occurring in clusters, they may appear as "hot nodules" in scintigrams.[29]

Clinical features

Goiter is more common in females than in males. Diffuse goiter often appears at puberty or in adolescence. It may regress, but if not, it often later turns nodular. Dyshormonogenic goiters are detected in early childhood or not until adulthood. The thyroid may be diffuse or nodular.[27]

Nodular goiter may produce compression symptoms, which may be severe if the goiter extends substernally. In endemic goiter hypothyroidism is rather common, varying in severity from clinical euthyroidism to cretinism. In sporadic goiter the patient usually remains euthyroid because of compensatory mechanisms, whereas patients with dyshormonogenic goiter are usually hypothyroid, with the most severe forms involving cretinism. In toxic nodular goiter the symptoms of hyperthyroidism usually develop more slowly than in Graves' disease.[29] Ophthalmopathy does not occur, but cardiac symptoms are common.

Morphology

In diffuse goiter, the thyroid is symmetrically and diffusely enlarged and may weigh several hundred grams. Histologically, the hyperplastic stage is characterized by epithelial hyperplasia with small follicles, high epithelium showing papillary infoldings, and scanty colloid. The involution stage, the stage usually seen in histologic specimens, is characterized by large follicles distended by colloid and lined by flattened follicular cells. On section the surface is gelatinous and colloidal at this stage (colloid goiter).

In nodular goiter the thyroid usually weighs 50 to 100 g but sometimes more than 500 g. The gland is usually asymmetric with nodules varying considerably in size (Fig. 31-2). Both macroscopically and histologically, it

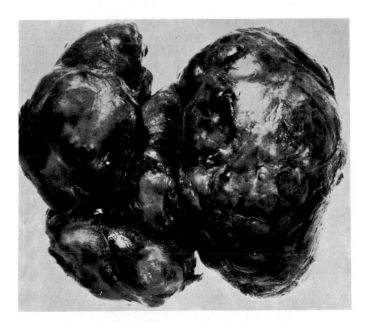

Fig. 31-2. Nodular goiter with areas of degeneration and hemorrhage. (From Anderson, W.A.D., and Scotti, T.M.: Synopsis of pathology, ed. 10, St. Louis, 1980, The C.V. Mosby Co.)

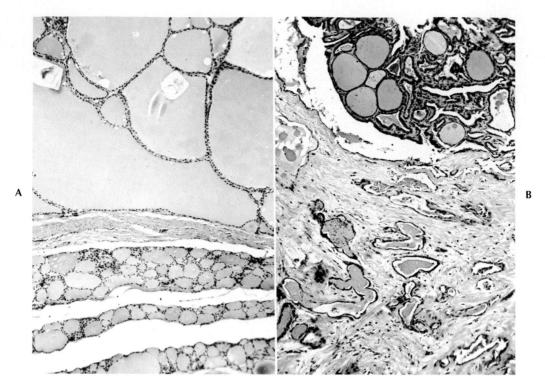

Fig. 31-3. Nodular goiter. **A,** Abundant colloid, flat epithelium, and fibrosis around upper nodule. **B,** Fibrosis and nodule with epithelial hyperplasia. (85×.)

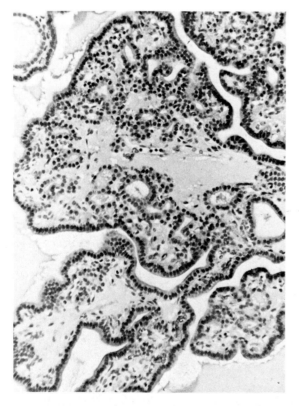

Fig. 31-4. Macropapillary structures in nodular goiter. Notice tall epithelium, dark nuclei against basement membrane, and follicles within papillae. (150×.)

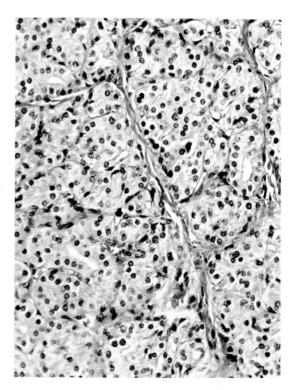

Fig. 31-5. Goiter from cretin with pale and notably hyperplastic epithelium. (240×.)

is characterized by considerable heterogeneity in structure. The nodules may be colloidal or show degenerative featues such as hemorrhages with hemosiderin deposits and cholesterol crystals, as well as calcifications, fibrous scarring, or cystic degeneration. The nodules are partially or occasionally completely encapsulated. The follicles may vary from small to large, and the epithelium from flat to high (Fig. 31-3). Some nodules may be composed of oxyphilic cells, often arranged in cords, and some are composed of so-called macropapillary structures (Fig. 31-4) that may be erroneously diagnosed as papillary carcinoma.

Dyshormonogenic goiters often show intense epithelial hyperplasia (Fig. 31-5), which may sometimes be difficult to differentiate from follicular carcinoma.[30]

It is not possible to evaluate thyroid function in nodular goiter morphologically because follicles composed of epithelial cells with a large iodine turnover are morphologically indistinguishable from follicles composed of cells with a small iodine turnover.[29] Therefore the diagnosis of toxic nodular goiter is not morphologic. Hyperplastic foci may occur in nodular goiter whether toxic or not.

GRAVES' DISEASE (DIFFUSE TOXIC GOITER)

Graves' disease, also known as Basedow's disease or primary hyperplasia, is characterized by hyperthyroidism, ophthalmopathy, and diffuse enlargement of the thyroid. In most countries it is the second most common thyroid disease, preceded only by nontoxic goiter. The disease occurs at all ages, most often during the third or fourth decade of life, and shows an approximately fivefold preponderance among females.

Almost all patients with Graves' disease exhibit what is known as a thyroid-stimulating antibody in their serum. There is strong evidence that this antibody stimulates thyroid function by binding to the antigen, the TSH receptor of the follicular cell surface.[35,50] It has been suggested that thyroid enlargement in Graves' disease is caused by another stimulator, the thyroid growth antibody that possibly also binds to the TSH receptor.[50] In addition, low levels of circulating autoantibodies against various thyroid constituents, mainly the microsomal antigen, occur in the serum of most patients with Graves' disease.

An aggregation of Graves' disease and Hashimoto's thyroiditis in the same families has been found, and it is assumed that these two diseases are immunologically closely related autoimmune disorders that occur in people with an inherited predisposition. In white populations Graves' disease is associated with HLA-DR3.[35] The cause of the autoimmune reactions in the two diseases has been suggested to be a genetically induced organ-specific defect in suppressor T-lymphocytes.[50]

The pathogenesis of Graves' ophthalmopathy has not been clarified, but it is probable that the damage to the eye muscles is attributable to an autoimmune process.[39,51] It is not certain either whether ophthalmopathy is a separate disease entity or is an integral part of Graves' disease.

Clinically, patients with Graves' disease have the typical features of hyperthyroidism (see p. 1546) and diffuse goiter. In addition, eye symptoms occur in about half the patients; the mildest and most common form is exophthalmos; in the most severe form there is limitation of eye movements and optic nerve damage. Rarely, patients may have pretibial myxedema or acropathy (peripheral soft-tissue swelling and periosteal changes).

The thyroid is usually moderately and symmetrically enlarged; its weight is in most cases less than 70 g. On section the surface is homogeneous and hyperemic, and the normal colloidal appearance is lacking. Histologically, considerable epithelial hyperplasia is seen; the follicles are small, and sometimes the epithelial cells form solid groups without any visible lumen. The follicular cells are tall, columnar, and often with papillary infoldings that project into the colloid (Fig. 31-6). The enlarged nuclei, which may show some variation in size, lie at the base of the cell. Occasional mitoses may be seen. The colloid is light staining and often finely vacuolated. Some follicles may appear quite empty. The stroma is vascular. In addition to epithelial hyperplasia, foci of lymphatic tissue, often with germinal centers, are seen in many cases. It has been proposed that the amount of lymphatic tissue may have a positive correlation with high microsomal antibody titers and with frequent occurrence of postoperative hypothyroidism.

Histologic differentiation of Graves' disease from papillary carcinoma (p. 1559) and from Hashimoto's thyroiditis (p. 1553) may occasionally be difficult.

Operative specimens do not often show the typical hyperplastic features of Graves' disease because nearly all patients receive preoperative medication. Iodine inhibits thyroid hormone synthesis and release, resulting in thyroid involution with accumulation of colloid in the follicles and decrease in vascularity and follicular cell height. The histologic picture may appear quite normal, though usually some hyperplastic foci persist.

Antithyroid drugs inhibit thyroid hormone synthesis, causing an increase in the level of TSH. As a result the thyroid may become even more hyperplastic, though the patient is often clinically euthyroid.

Exophthalmos is caused by an increase in the volume of extraocular muscles and other orbital tissues. Histologically, deposits of material rich in mucopolysaccharides (glycosaminoglycans) are seen, as are edema and mononuclear inflammatory cells, followed later by fibrosis.[46,48] In pretibial myxedema, metachromatic ma-

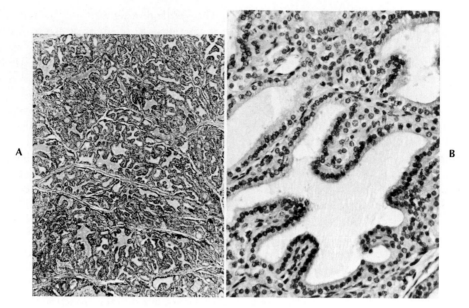

Fig. 31-6. Epithelial hyperplasia in Graves' disease. **A,** Notice preserved lobular structure. **B,** Papillary infoldings projecting into the follicle, high columnar epithelium, and pale staining colloid. (**A,** Low power; **B,** 300×.)

terial is seen in deeper layers of the dermis.[37] In Graves' disease, lymphatic hyperplasia may occur, not only in the thyroid, but also in the thymus, spleen, and lymph nodes.

THYROIDITIS
Infectious thyroiditis

Acute thyroiditis is a rare disease that usually develops as a complication of bacterial infection elsewhere in the body, often in the oropharynx or tonsils. Inflammation is usually suppurative, and the abscess may rupture to the skin, trachea, or esophagus. The thyroid is swollen and painful, and the patient usually has noticeable general symptoms such as fever and malaise.

Tuberculosis, syphilis, actinomycosis, and echinococcosis also occur in the thyroid but are very rare.[31,49]

Granulomatous thyroiditis

Granulomatous thyroiditis is synonymous with de Quervain's, subacute, and giant cell thyroiditis. Its cause is unknown, but a viral origin is supported by clinical features such as a prodromal phase, often a preceding respiratory infection, and usually a complete recovery. The disease is fairly common and occurs mainly in middle-aged and young women. The patient typically has fever and a painful and moderately enlarged thyroid. Manifestations of hyperthyroidism are common in the early phases of the disease and are probably caused by destruction of follicles and leakage of colloid.

Macroscopically, the thyroid is slightly or moderately enlarged and often asymmetric. The involvement is ir-

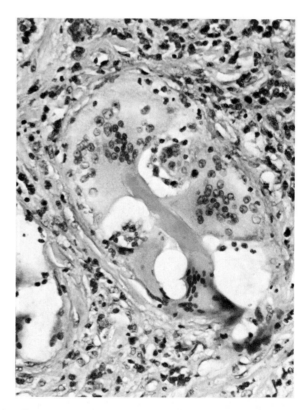

Fig. 31-7. Granulomatous (de Quervain's) thyroiditis. Multinucleated giant cells surround residual colloid in a follicle. Outside follicle are mononuclear inflammatory cells and fibrosis. (300×.)

regular but usually bilateral. The involved areas are whitish and firm. Slight adhesions may occur in the capsule, but the gland is easily separated from the surrounding structures.

The histologic findings vary according to the stage of the disease. The process appears to begin with destruction of follicular epithelium and infiltration of the disrupted follicles by neutrophils.[49] Neutrophils are replaced by histiocytes and multinucleated giant cells, which are situated inside the follicle and characteristically surround residual colloid (Fig. 31-7), producing a typical granulomatous appearance. The interstitium around the granulomas shows edema and an inflammatory infiltrate composed of lymphocytes and histiocytes. Later, fibroblastic proliferation and fibrosis are seen. The intensity of the process and its extent vary considerably, and there are often lesions at different stages of development in the same gland. The disease can be diagnosed with aspiration cytology; the diagnosis is based on the occurrence of giant cells, histiocytes, and lymphocytes.[54]

Granulomatous thyroiditis should be differentiated from so-called *palpation thyroiditis*, which has been described in patients with a thyroid disease and is believed to be attributable to mechanical injury caused by palpation of the thyroid.[32] In this disorder, there are scattered follicles containing foamy histocytes, lymphocytes, desquamated epithelial cells, and occasional multinucleated giant cells, but there is no continuous spectrum from granuloma to scar like that seen in granulomatous thyroiditis.

Lymphocytic (autoimmune) thyroiditis

Lymphocytic thyroiditis includes Hashimoto's thyroiditis, atrophic thyroiditis, and focal lymphocytic thyroiditis. These diseases have in common lymphocytic infiltrates in the gland and the occurrence of thyroid antibodies, but in many other respects they differ from each other both morphologically and clinically.

Hashimoto's thyroiditis

Hashimoto's thyroiditis (diffuse lymphocytic thyroiditis, goitrous autoimmune thyroiditis) is characterized by thyroid enlargement, lymphocytic infiltration of the gland, and occurrence of thyroid autoantibodies. The disease is fairly common, especially in women around menopause (sex ratio about 10:1). Certain variants of the disease are seen in childhood and adolescence and constitute about 40% of all cases of nontoxic thyroid enlargement occurring in childhood.[45]

Hashimoto's thyroiditis is an autoimmune disease that is immunologically closely related to Graves' disease and occurs often in the same families. The disease is associated with HLA-DR5.[51] Autoantibodies against different thyroid antigens, such as the microsomal component and thyroglobulin, are present in the sera of almost all patients,[33] whereas thyroid-stimulating antibody, common in Graves' disease, occurs infrequently in Hashimoto's thyroiditis. Tissue destruction in Hashimoto's thyroiditis is believed to be caused by cytotoxic antibodies and by cell-mediated immunity, mainly natural killer cells.[50] It has been suggested that, like Graves' disease, Hashimoto's thyroiditis might be attri-

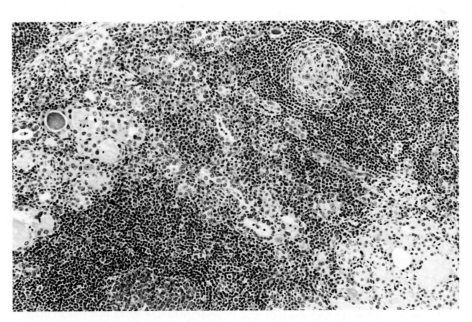

Fig. 31-8. Hashimoto's thyroiditis. Pronounced lymphocytic infiltration with germinal centers and destruction of follicles. (150×.)

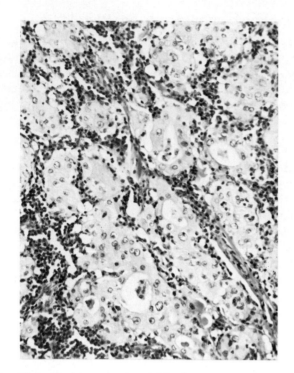

Fig. 31-9. Hashimoto's thyroiditis. Lymphocytic infiltration and oxyphilic cells with enlarged nuclei varying in size, and prominent nucleoli. (250×.)

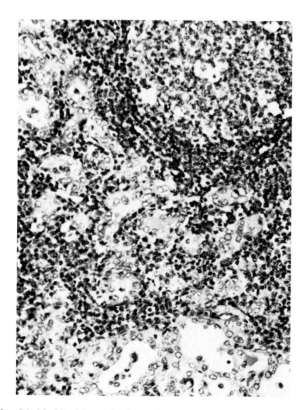

Fig. 31-10. Hashimoto's thyroiditis, juvenile variant. There is pronounced lymphatic hyperplasia with germinal centers. Cuboidal epithelium, no oxyphilic change. Some macrophages in follicular lumens. (250×.)

butable to a genetically induced organ-specific defect in suppressor T-cells.[50] Inadequate suppressor T-cell function would allow a randomly appearing "forbidden clone" of helper T-cells to help B-lymphocytes to produce self-reactive antibodies.[50]

Although the patient with classical Hashimoto's thyroiditis is clearly hypothyroid and has a large, rubbery hard goiter, most patients with this disease are either euthyroid or mildly hypothyroid and have only a slightly or moderately enlarged thyroid.[33]

The thyroid usually weighs around 40 to 60 g but sometimes as much as 300 g. Its consistency varies but is often firm or rubbery. Its surface is smooth or slightly bosselated, and the capsule is thin and unaltered. On section the surface is uniform, faintly lobulated, and opaque.

Histologically, the most prominent feature is noticeable diffuse lymphocytic infiltration, which usually contains lymphatic follicles with germinal centers (Fig. 31-8). Plasma cells are present in most cases. There is a decreased number of thyroid follicles, and the remaining follicles are generally small and often devoid of colloid. The epithelial cells usually have an abundant oxyphilic and faintly granular cytoplasm, an enlarged hyperchromatic nucleus, often varying in size, and a prominent nucleolus (Fig. 31-9). These oxyphil cells, also known as Askanazy or Hürthle cells, contain large numbers of mitochondria.[47] Slight fibrous thickening of the interlobular septa is common, giving the gland a typical lobulated appearance. In most cases only slight fibrosis occurs outside the septa.[56] The disease can be diagnosed by aspiration cytology, which reveals the oxyphil cells and lymphocytes.[54]

It is possible to distinguish within Hashimoto's thyroiditis histologic variants differing in their clinical features. In *juvenile thyroiditis* no or only a few oxyphil cells are seen, but the epithelium is cuboidal or sometimes columnar (Fig. 31-10) and often has papillary infoldings that give it a hyperplastic appearance. The follicular lumens often contain clusters of macrophages. Germinal centers are abundant, and fibrosis is slight or absent. This type of thyroiditis occurs mainly in children and young women. The patients are usually euthyroid and symptomless and exhibit low titers of thyroid antibodies, and their thyroids are only slightly enlarged.[45]

In about 10% of cases of Hashimoto's thyroiditis there is considerable fibrous replacement of thyroid parenchyma (Fig. 31-11), often accompanied by squamous metaplasia,[38] which may simulate neoplastic growth. Patients with this *fibrous variant of Hashimoto's thyroiditis* have a firm and enlarged thyroid, often with compression symptoms and high thyroid antibody titers, and frequently clinical hypothyroidism.[38]

Histologic differential diagnosis between Hashimoto's

thyroiditis and malignant lymphoma, follicular carcinoma, and Graves' disease may sometimes cause problems. In Graves' disease the lymphocytic infiltration is usually focal and mild, and there are no oxyphil epithelial cells. However, epithelial hyperplasia occurs, in addition to Graves' disease, sometimes also in Hashimoto's thyroiditis, especially in the juvenile variant. For the relation of Hashimoto's thyroiditis to malignant lymphoma, see p. 1565.

Atrophic thyroiditis

Atrophic thyroiditis corresponds to a clinical condition known as "spontaneous hypothyroidism." In atrophic thyroiditis the gland is not enlarged but is often decreased in size. Thyroid autoantibodies are present. Histologically, lymphocytic infiltration, atrophy of the follicles, and fibrosis are seen. It is believed that this condition is closely related to Hashimoto's thyroiditis except for the fact that the thyroid fails to regenerate; in Hashimoto's thyroiditis the thyroid enlargement is probably caused by regeneration of follicular epithelium induced by TSH.[50] It has been suggested that the lack of regeneration in atrophic thyroiditis might be caused by thyroid growth–blocking antibodies reported to occur in atrophic thyroiditis but not in Hashimoto's thyroiditis.[34]

Focal lymphocytic thyroiditis

In focal lymphocytic thyroiditis, focal aggregates of lymphocytes, often with germinal centers, are seen in the thyroid (Fig. 31-12). Especially in the more severe forms, the areas involved may show oxyphil epithelial cells, but most of the epithelium appears unaltered. This lesion has been reported to occur in up to 54% of women and 24% of men in systematic autopsy series[42] and to be twice as common in glands that have some other abnormality (nodular goiter, adenoma, papillary carcinoma) than in otherwise normal glands.[52] The patients often have low titers of thyroid antibodies, and the disease is usually classified under autoimmune thyroiditis. Its autoimmune origin is favored also by the presence of ultrastructural basement membrane changes, which are believed to represent immune-complex deposits both in focal lymphocytic and in Hashimoto's thyroiditis.[44] The disorder does not appear to be progressive or clinically important.[33]

Riedel's thyroiditis (invasive fibrous thyroiditis)

Riedel's thyroiditis is a rare disease; only 20 cases were found among 42,000 thyroidectomies at the Mayo Clinic.[55] The initial complaint of the patients is a stone-hard goiter that is densely adherent to adjacent struc-

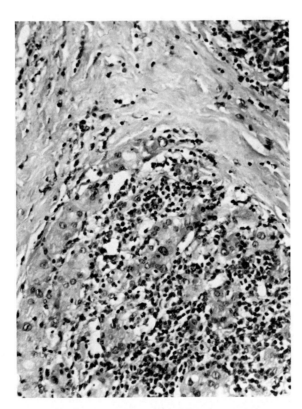

Fig. 31-11. Hashimoto's thyroiditis, fibrous variant. There is pronounced fibrous replacement of thyroid parenchyma, lymphocytic infiltration, follicle destruction with oxyphilic cytoplasmic change. (250×.)

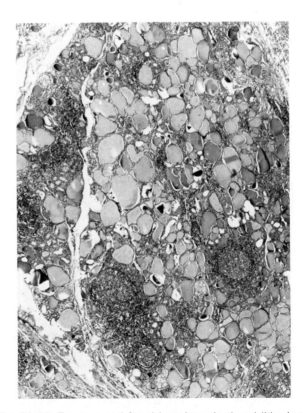

Fig. 31-12. Pronounced focal lymphocytic thyroiditis. Lymphocytic infiltrates have germinal centers. Follicles appear unaltered. (Low power.)

tures in the neck. Compression symptoms, such as dysphagia, may occur. Thus the clinical picture resembles that of cancer.

The cause is unknown, but it has been suggested that Riedel's thyroiditis belongs to a disease group collectively known as multifocal idiopathic fibrosclerosis, which also includes idiopathic retroperitoneal, mediastinal, and retro-orbital fibrosis, and sclerosing cholangitis. These disorders may occur simultaneously.[41,43]

The process involves the whole gland or a part of one lobe. In addition, contiguous structures, most often muscle, are involved, which contrasts with the findings in granulomatous thyroiditis and Hashimoto's thyroiditis. The involved areas are stone hard and whitish and show no lobulation on cross section. The thyroid capsule is not usually discernible. Histologically, fibrous tissue, accompanied by inflammatory cells, replaces normal thyroid structures and invades the adjacent muscle tissue.[40] The fibrous tissue may be extensively hyalinized. Usually neither germinal centers nor oxyphil cells are seen.

Painless thyroiditis

In the recently described disease painless thyroiditis, the patient has symptoms resembling those seen in granulomatous thyroiditis with one exception, the absence of pain. Typically the disease begins with rather abrupt onset of hyperthyroidism that resolves spontaneously.[40,53] Painless thyroiditis often occurs in the postpartum period. Originally the disease was believed to be related to granulomatous thyroiditis, but at present it is believed to be akin to autoimmune thyroiditis. The histologic features are not well known. Needle biopsy specimens during the hyperthyroid period have revealed features of lymphocytic thyroiditis.[36] However, oxyphil cells and fibrosis, characteristic of Hashimoto's thyroiditis, are not encountered.[42a]

RADIATION CHANGES

Ionizing radiation, whether external or from radioactive iodine, induces interstitial fibrosis, thickening of blood vessel walls, cytoplasmic oxyphilia, and nuclear atypia in the thyroid.[60] The nuclei are hyperchromatic and often bizarre and show considerable variation in size, with many giant forms. Considerable morphologic variation is seen between different follicles as well as within the same follicle; some of the nuclei appear morphologically normal, and some are hyperchromatic. The nuclear abnormalities appear some weeks after the radiation and persist for many years.[60] Late changes after low-dose irradiation have been reported to include nodule formation, oxyphil cells, and focal lymphocytic thyroiditis.[58,59] For the relation of radiation to carcinogenesis, see p. 1556.

AMYLOIDOSIS

The thyroid may be involved in systemic amyloidosis. Occasionally the infiltrates may be so massive that they replace most of the thyroid tissue. This kind of lesion has been called amyloid goiter.[57] In amyloid goiter, fat cells are usually seen between the amyloid masses (Fig. 31-13).

BENIGN TUMORS
Follicular adenoma

Follicular adenoma is an encapsulated noninvasive tumor arising from follicular cells and showing follicular cell differentiation.

Follicular adenoma is a common tumor that can occur at any age but mainly in young adults. It is about five times more common in females than in males. Clinically it usually presents as a solitary thyroid nodule that occasionally causes compression. Hemorrhage into an adenoma may cause pain and an acute increase in the size of the tumor.

Macroscopically adenomas are circumscribed and encapsulated spherical tumors that vary in size up to 10 cm in diameter. On section, the tumor is often less colloidal than the surrounding tissue, its color varies from white to red-brown, and its consistency from soft to

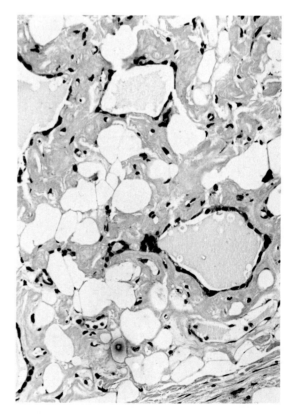

Fig. 31-13. Amyloid goiter. Masses of amyloid and some fat cells between few follicles. (150×.)

firm. Degenerative features such as a central scar or calcifications and hemorrhages are often seen.

Histologically the tumor is surrounded by a fibrous capsule that often contains wide vascular spaces. The tumor cells form follicles, usually of small size (Fig. 31-14), or occur in cords (trabeculas) or solid groups with little follicle formation (Fig. 31-15). These structures are separated by a hyalinized or edematous stroma or by thin fibrous septa, often containing abundant thin-walled vascular spaces (Fig. 31-16), which may give a sinusoid appearance. The nuclei of the tumor cells are often enlarged, and there may be some variation in their size and shape, but mitoses are infrequent.

Follicular adenomas are often divided according to their pattern into several subgroups such as trabecular and solid (old term "embryonal"), microfollicular ("fetal"), normofollicular ("simple"), and macrofollicular ("colloid") adenoma. Because adenomas are often composed of more than one type of structure and the subdivision does not show any clinical correlations, it can be regarded as unnecessary for practical purposes.

It may sometimes be difficult to distinguish follicular adenoma from follicular carcinoma (see p. 1561) and nodular goiter. Follicular adenoma has been said to differ from a nodule of nodular goiter in having a contin-uous capsule, a clear distinction in architecture between that inside and that outside of the capsule, a rather uniform histologic architecture inside the capsule, and compression of the surrounding thyroid tissue. Increased vascularity and small follicle size also point to adenoma. However, there are nodules in nodular goiter that fulfill these criteria. In practice, such nodules are usually called "adenomas" if they are single, and "nonneoplastic" if they are multiple.

Follicular adenoma of oxyphilic cell type (Hürthle cell adenoma) is composed of cells that have abundant oxyphil cytoplasm and usually a trabecular growth pattern (Fig. 31-16) but may also occur in solid groups or form follicles. The nuclei are clearly enlarged and often vary considerably in size. The nucleolus is usually prominent. Ultrastructurally the cytoplasm contains large numbers of mitochondria.[61] The tumor does not seem to differ from other follicular adenomas in clinical behavior.

Follicular adenoma of clear cell type is composed of cells with a clear cytoplasm. These cells contain distended and empty-looking mitochondria or large amounts of glycogen.[61] Differentiation between this tumor and metastatic renal cell carcinoma may sometimes be difficult.

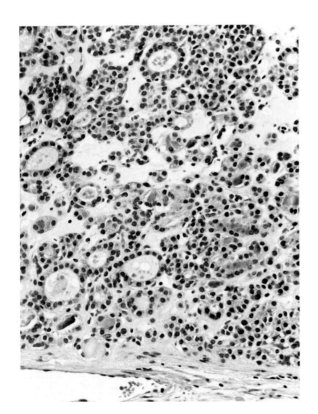

Fig. 31-14. Follicular adenoma. Encapsulated tumor is composed of follicles. Capsule contains wide vascular lumens. (250×.)

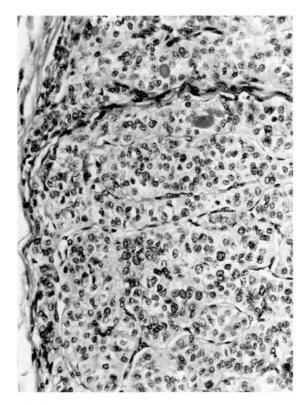

Fig. 31-15. Follicular adenoma. Trabecular growth pattern. Occasional colloid droplets are seen. (300×.)

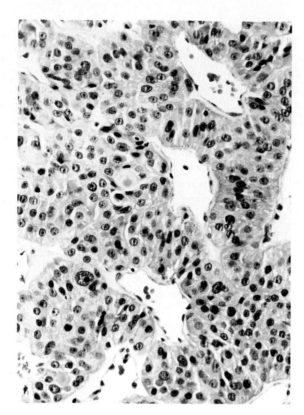

Fig. 31-16. Follicular adenoma of oxyphilic cell type. Trabecular structures composed of large cells with abundant eosinophilic cytoplasm, big nuclei, and prominent nucleoli as well as separation by wide vascular spaces. (300×.)

Atypical follicular adenoma is a term that has been given to adenomas showing features that can be regarded as indicative of malignancy, such as high cellularity, nuclear and architectural atypia, and increased number of mitoses.[65,67] This tumor does not show capsular penetration or invasion of blood vessels, which is characteristic of follicular carcinoma. To exclude malignancy, multiple sections of the capsular area should be examined. Flow cytometric analysis of nuclear DNA content does not help in differential diagnosis because adenomas are often aneuploid.[66]

Some follicular adenomas may contain *mucin-producing* or *signet-ring cells.*[64,68,69] A recently described *"hyalinizing trabecular adenoma"* may histologically mimic medullary or papillary carcinoma.[63]

Other benign tumors

Teratoma is a very rare tumor that occurs mainly in newborn infants.[70] Some teratomas may arise from the thyroid capsule, but others may originate from the adjoining structures. Teratomas are usually but not always[169] histologically and clinically benign, but they may grow large and cause compression of adjacent

structures. *Paragangliomas* have been rarely found within the thyroid gland.[62]

MALIGNANT TUMORS

Thyroid cancer is not a common disease; it makes up less than 1% of all cases of human cancer. Carcinoma is clearly the most common type, but sarcomas and primary lymphomas also occur. Usually thyroid carcinoma is divided into four principal histologic types: papillary, follicular, medullary, and undifferentiated (anaplastic).[75,76] Papillary and follicular carcinomas show follicular cell differentiation and stain positively for thyroglobin by immunohistochemical methods.[81] Medullary carcinoma shows C-cell differentiation and stains positively for calcitonin.[127]

Epidermoid,[153] mucoepidermoid,[143,148,149] mucinous,[141,150,154] and so-called columnar cell[142] carcinomas have also been reported to occur in the thyroid, but they are rare. Most tumors with epidermoid differentiation represent epidermoid metaplasia in papillary carcinoma.

There is a good correlation between histologic findings and prognosis in thyroid cancer.[71,73,80] In addition to prognosis, the histologic picture of the tumor correlates with other features of the natural history of the disease better than is true in malignant tumors of most other organs (Table 31-1).[72,78] For these reasons an accurate histologic classification of thyroid cancer is important.

Aspiration cytology is useful in the diagnosis of thyroid cancer.[77] However, follicular carcinoma and follicular adenoma cannot usually be cytologically differentiated because they differ from each other with respect to invasion but not essentially in cellular features.

Carcinoma

Papillary carcinoma. Papillary carcinoma is the most common type of thyroid carcinoma, comprising 45% to 70% of all cases.[71,72,80] It occurs at any age, including children, but the incidence rises with advancing age. The tumor is about three times more common in females than in males.[76]

It has been shown that people who have been exposed to irradiation in childhood have an increased risk of papillary carcinoma.[104,105] Radiation has been suggested to act as an initiating factor in thyroid carcinogenesis.[104] There appears to be a negative correlation between papillary carcinoma and endemic goiter; the incidence of the tumor is exceptionally high in Iceland, an iodine-rich area,[74,79] and the relative frequency of papillary carcinoma rose in Switzerland after administration of iodine in the diet.[96]

Papillary carcinoma is a slow-growing tumor that usually appears clinically as a solitary thyroid nodule. The primary tumor is in most cases limited to the gland, but

Table 31-1. Natural history in different types of thyroid carcinoma

	Papillary carcinoma	Follicular carcinoma	Medullary carcinoma	Undifferentiated carcinoma
Age	All ages	Middle and old age	Middle and old age (familial cases also in children)	Old age
Female-to-male ratio	About 3:1	About 2.5:1	About 1:1	About 1.5:1
Primary tumor	Usually within thyroid capsule	Usually within thyroid capsule	Usually within thyroid capsule	Usually large and invades contiguous structures
Regional metastases	Common	Very rare	Common	Common
Distant organ metastases	Rare	Common	Rare	Common
Ten-year survival	80% to 95%	50% to 70%	60% to 70%	5% to 10%, median survival about 2 months
Principal cause of death	Local invasion and distant metastases	Distant metastases	Distant metastases	Local invasion

especially in older people it may invade the surrounding structures, such as muscles, the esophagus, or the larynx. Regional lymph nodes in the neck are involved in almost half the cases at the time of diagnosis,[72,80] and this may be the only symptom of the disease. Lymph node involvement is most common at a young age.[72] Distant (organ) metastases occur mainly in the lungs but are rare; their frequency at diagnosis is less than 5%.[71,80,101]

The prognosis of papillary carcinoma is good, with a 10-year survival rate in the order of 80% to 95%.[73,80,101] Survival rate correlates with the extent of the primary tumor[110] and the presence of distant metastases but unexpectedly not with the presence of regional metastases.[73,80] Young age is associated with good prognosis.[73,83,102]

Macroscopically the tumor is usually a whitish, hard, scarlike, poorly limited area, but it may also be cystic. The primary tumor may be extremely small, only a few millimeters in diameter, though it may give rise to bulky regional metastases.

Histologically papillary carcinoma is composed of papillae, usually accompanied by follicles and sometimes by solid sheets of cells. The papillae are often long and slender and have a fibrovascular core that is usually thin but may be thick and hyalinized. The core is covered by one layer of tumor cells (Figs. 31-17 and 31-18). The follicles are usually well differentiated and often contain colloid (see Figs. 31-18 and 31-22). The solid growth pattern (Fig. 31-19) often occurs at the periphery of the tumor, and it is most often seen in tumors of young people. The nuclei of papillary carcinoma often overlap and have many typical features including a pale outlook

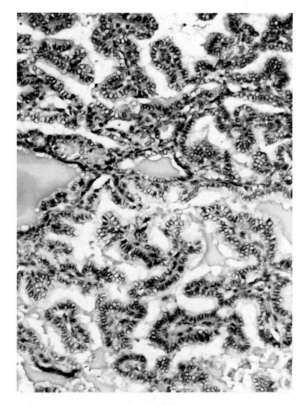

Fig. 31-17. Papillary carcinoma. Papillae have one layer of tumor cells with ground-glass nuclei. (150×.)

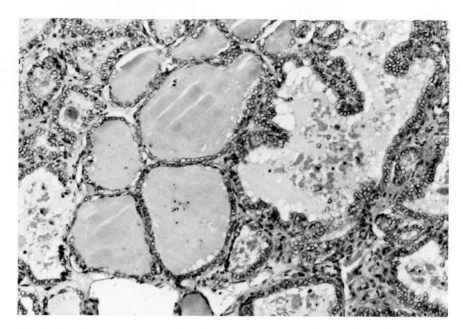

Fig. 31-18. Papillary carcinoma. Papillae are on right; follicles with colloid are on left. Notice ground-glass nuclei. (150×.)

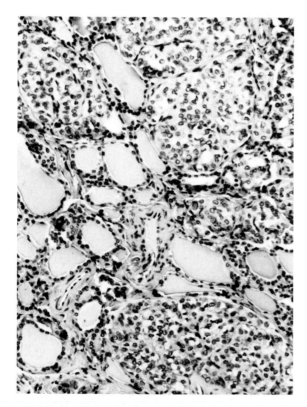

Fig. 31-19. Papillary carcinoma. Solid sheets of cells invade between normal follicles. In other parts of the tumor papillae and follicles were present. (100×.)

(ground-glass appearance), large size compared with normal follicular cells, irregular outline with deep grooves and cytoplasmic pseudoinclusions, rare mitoses, and an inconspicuous nucleolus.[86,94,111] All these nuclear features, which are regarded as important diagnostic criteria of papillary carcinoma, are not always seen in all tumor cells, but usually some of these features are present in most cells. These details may be difficult to discern in poorly fixed specimens, and, on the other hand, poor fixation of other types of lesions may yield a false ground-glass appearance. In frozen material, the nuclei often lose their ground-glass appearance, but they may show the nuclear grooves and pseudoinclusions. These features are better appreciated in alcohol-fixed cytologic smears made simultaneously with the frozen sections.

Follicles are often the predominant component of the tumor. It is generally agreed also that tumors composed solely of follicles and having the typical nuclear features of papillary carcinoma should be included under papillary carcinoma.[72,80,85] These tumors usually display the typical invasive growth pattern of papillary carcinoma. Their course resembles that of papillary carcinomas and differs from that of follicular carcinoma.[72] The smallest papillary carcinomas are often composed solely of follicles.

Papillary carcinoma is typically strongly invasive, and encapsulation is rare. Fibrosis and lymphocytic infiltration are often seen around the invading islands. Small foci of tumor tissue, which in most cases probably rep-

Table 31-2. Histologic differential diagnosis of papillary and follicular carcinomas

	Papillary carcinoma	Follicular carcinoma
Encapsulation	Rare	Common
Invasion	Strongly invasive, invades in small islands	Less invasive, invades in large islands with pushing border
Multiple tumor foci	Common	Rare
Blood vessel invasion	Rare	Common
Cellular pattern	Papillae, follicles, solid cell groups	Follicles, trabeculas, no papillae (pseudopapillary infoldings may occur)
Psammoma bodies	In about 50%	None (calcified colloid may occur)
Nuclei	"Ground-glass," grooves, pseudoinclusions, often overlapping	Normochromatic or hyperchromatic, no grooves, no overlap

resent intrathyroid lymphatic metastases, often occur far from the tumor proper, even as far as the other thyroid lobe. Blood vessel invasion is rare. Psammoma bodies, which are small, concentric, calcified spherules, are seen in almost one half of papillary carcinomas,[72] sometimes far from the tumor, and they have been regarded as diagnostic of the disease. They must, however, be distinguished from calcified colloid, which may occur in a variety of conditions, especially in follicular adenomas of oxyphilic cell type. Calcified colloid is located inside the follicles, whereas psammoma bodies are usually seen in the stroma. Epidermoid metaplasia,[100] which morphologically appears benign, may occur in papillary carcinoma and apparently does not have any prognostic importance.[72]

All papillary neoplasias are usually considered malignant, regardless of the presence or absence of encapsulation, but encapsulated papillary carcinomas have been reported to have a better prognosis than the invasive ones.[106]

Sometimes it may be difficult to distinguish papillary carcinoma from follicular (Table 31-2) and medullary carcinomas (p. 1563) and from epithelial hyperplasia and macropapillary structures in nodular goiter. In epithelial hyperplasia the nuclei may be large and pale, resembling those seen in papillary carcinoma, but there is no abrupt change in the nuclear morphology as that seen at the border of papillary carcinoma tissue. The papillary infoldings projecting into the follicles are short in epithelial hyperplasia, and the normal lobular struc-

ture is preserved (see Fig. 31-6), whereas it is distorted in papillary carcinoma. In macropapillary structures the typical nuclear features of papillary carcinoma are not seen, and the papillae are short and broad and often contain follicles (see Fig. 31-4), which is uncommon in papillary carcinoma.

Papillary microcarcinoma (occult papillary carcinoma, occult sclerosing carcinoma) is a term given to small papillary carcinoma (occult papillary carcinoma is defined as less than 1.5 cm,[80] and in the new WHO histologic classification of thyroid tumors, papillary microcarcinoma is less than 1.0 cm[75] in diameter) that may have a central fibrous scar.

Its prevalence is high, varying between 6% and 37%[92,94] in autopsy studies in which the thyroids were semiserially sectioned. Most of such incidentally found tumors are very small, under 1 mm in diameter.[94,103] Prevalence of this tumor appears to be rather constant after 20 years of age.[91]

The tumors may have regional lymph node metastases, though most tumors are detected as incidental findings in thyroids resected for another thyroid disease. Distant metastases or deaths from carcinoma are extremely rare in this tumor.[97] Irradiation seems to increase its prevalence.[104]

Papillary carcinoma is rarely composed of *oxyphil cells*.[88,109] These tumors show the usual growth pattern of papillary carcinoma but usually do not have the typical nuclear features. The nuclei in this type are similar to the nuclei of oxyphil cells in general (see p. 1555).

Diffuse sclerosing variant of papillary carcinoma is rare and occurs mainly in children. It is histologically characterized by diffuse invasion of the gland by small tumor islands with common epidermoid metaplasia, numerous psammoma bodies, and a strong lymphocytic reaction.[87,111] Its prognosis does not appear to be quite as good as that of other papillary carcinomas.[111]

Follicular carcinoma. Follicular carcinoma comprises about one fourth of all thyroid carcinomas. It is more common in females than in males[89] and is a disease of middle and old age. It has been claimed that there is a positive correlation between the risk of follicular carcinoma and endemic goiter,[79] but this is controversial.[74] The association between irradiation and follicular carcinoma is not clear.

The primary tumor in follicular carcinoma is in most cases confined within the thyroid capsule, but it may invade the surrounding structures. In contrast to papillary carcinoma, regional lymph node metastases are very rare, whereas distant metastases are common, occurring in as many as 25% of patients at diagnosis.[89] Their most common sites are the bones and the lungs. Symptoms caused by distant metastases, such as a pathologic fracture, may be the first symptoms of the disease. The prognosis of follicular carcinoma is be-

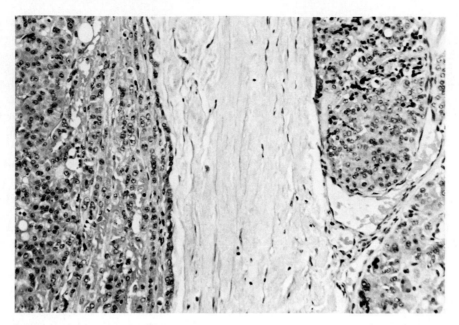

Fig. 31-20. Follicular carcinoma. Encapsulated tumor is composed of Hürthle cells with trabecular growth pattern. Tumor invades capsular vessel on right. Notice compact tumor thrombus surrounded by endothelium. (150×.)

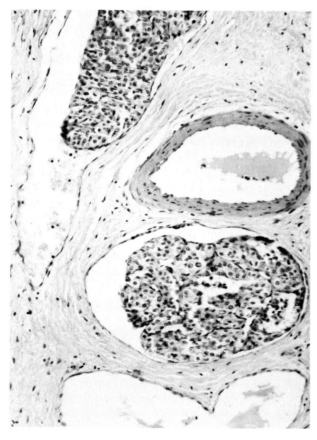

Fig. 31-21. Follicular carcinoma with blood vessel invasion. Tumor thrombi are compact and are surrounded by vascular endothelium. (80×.)

tween those of papillary and undifferentiated carcinomas.

Macroscopically, follicular carcinoma is usually circumscribed, resembling follicular adenoma. Histologically the tumor is often encapsulated. The capsule usually contains large, thin-walled blood vessels. Vascular invasion—often to these vessels—is common, a finding that explains the frequent occurrence of distant blood-borne metastases in follicular carcinoma (Figs. 31-20 and 31-21). When invasion to the surrounding thyroid or other tissues occurs, the invading islands are usually large and have a pushing border. Only tumors that show vascular or capsular invasion are considered malignant.[90,98]

Histologically, follicular carcinoma shows follicular differentiation but lacks the diagnostic features of papillary carcinoma.[75] Like follicular adenoma, follicular carcinoma is composed of follicular, trabecular, or solid structures.[84] The degree of follicular differentiation varies, but usually the follicles are smaller and less well differentiated than the follicles in papillary carcinoma. Between the trabeculas and groups of follicles are often abundant thin-walled blood vessels, which may form a sinusoid pattern. Neither papillary structures nor psammoma bodies occur; the nuclei are normochromatic or hyperchromatic (Fig. 31-22) and do not show the typical nuclear features of papillary carcinoma. The nuclear atypia varies but is usually not pronounced.

Metastatic follicular carcinomas are often extremely well differentiated and may be indistinguishable from

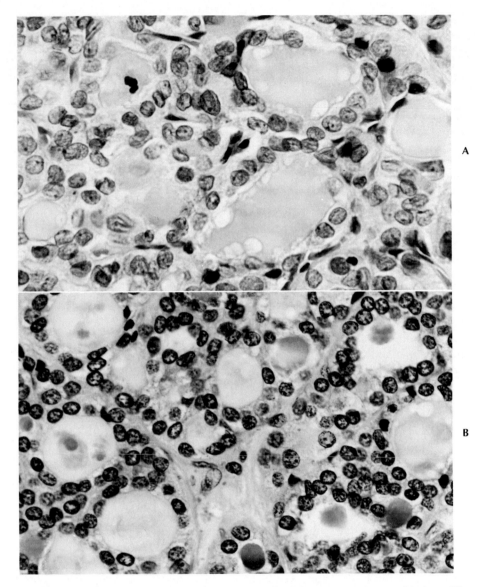

Fig. 31-22. A, Papillary carcinoma, follicular area. **B,** Follicular carcinoma. Notice difference in nuclear type. In papillary carcinoma the nuclei are overlapping and pale and grooved. (400×.)

nonneoplastic thyroid tissue. In such cases, the primary thyroid is almost invariably less well differentiated.

Follicular carcinoma is divided into two subtypes: *minimally invasive* (also called encapsulated) and *widely invasive*.[75] In the first subtype the tumor is encapsulated, and only minimal (difficult-to-find) vascular or capsular invasion is seen. In the second subtype the tumor is either nonencapsulated or encapsulated with considerable invasion. These two subtypes should be distinguished in prognosis[99] because the 10-year survival rate for the first type is 80% to 95% and for the second type 30% to 45%.[73,80,90]

Follicular carcinoma should be histologically distinguished from atypical follicular adenoma, atypical nodules of nodular goiter, papillary carcinoma (see Table 31-2), and thyroiditis. Follicular carcinoma differs from adenoma and atypical nodules in exhibiting capsular or vascular invasion. Capsular invasion can be regarded as having occurred if tumor tissue is seen outside the capsule; tumor tissue within the capsular wall may be caused by capsular infoldings. In vascular invasion, which is a more reliable criterion of malignancy than capsular invasion,[75] there is a compact tumor thrombus surrounded by vascular endothelium in a vessel within or outside the capsular wall (Figs. 31-20 and 31-21).[95] Loose tumor cells in vascular lumens should not be accepted as vascular invasion because in most cases they appear to be caused by manipulation of the tumor.[95] It is usually impossible to assess blood vessel invasion inside the tumor tissue because in most cases there is an intimate contact with the tumor cells and the vascular endothelium. In Hashimoto's thyroiditis, epithelial atypia may lead to an erroneous diagnosis of follicular carcinoma.

Follicular carcinoma of oxyphil cell type (Hürthle cell carcinoma). Carcinomas composed of oxyphilic cells usually have a follicular or trabecular growth pattern and are classified as follicular carcinomas (Fig. 31-20). The criteria of malignancy and the course of disease are the same as for other follicular carcinomas.[82,93]

Follicular carcinoma of clear cell type. Cells with a clear cytoplasm are seen fairly often in thyroid carcinomas. The clear appearance is caused by accumulation of glycogen or distended mitochondria.[108,145] Carcinomas composed solely of cells with a clear cytoplasm are rare. They usually form follicles and are then classified as follicular carcinomas. It may be difficult to distinguish them from metastatic renal cell carcinoma. Immunohistochemical methods based on the thyroglobulin content of most thyroid carcinomas with follicular cell differentiation may help in the differentiation.[81,107]

Undifferentiated (anaplastic) carcinoma. Undifferentiated carcinoma comprises 10% to 25% of all thyroid carcinomas.[72,80] The tumor is only slightly more common in women than in men and is a disease of old age. A differentiated component, either papillary or follicular carcinoma, is usually found in undifferentiated carcinomas studied with subserial sections,[151] and it has been assumed that the tumor arises from differentiated carcinoma.[138]

In contrast to differentiated carcinomas, the course of disease in undifferentiated carcinoma is characterized by invasion of adjacent soft tissues, trachea, and esophagus. That is why the first symptom is often dyspnea, hoarseness, dysphagia, or a rapidly growing tumor in the neck. Prognosis is poor; the 5-year survival rate is only in the order of 10%, and the median time of survival about 2 months.[73,138] Death is usually caused by local invasion of the tumor, though the tumor also metastasizes into both regional lymph nodes and distant organs, most often the lungs.

Macroscopically, undifferentiated carcinoma is usually large and firm and shows necrotic areas. Histologically the tumor is typically composed of polygonal, spindle (Fig. 31-23), and giant cells, which occur in varying proportions. This kind of tumor has been called spindle and giant cell type of undifferentiated carcinoma. Tumors that were previously called small cell undifferentiated carcinoma have often been found to represent either malignant lymphomas, small cell medullary carcinomas, or poorly differentiated follicular carcinomas.

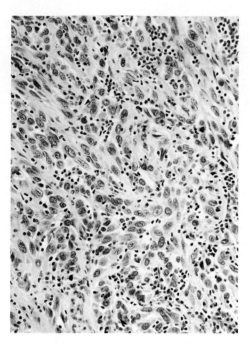

Fig. 31-23. Undifferentiated carcinoma composed of spindle cells. Some lymphocytes are seen between the tumor cells. (250×.)

Because the tumor is often composed of spindle cells, it may closely resemble sarcoma. However, areas that appear epithelial are usually also found. Some tumors may contain obvious sarcomatous foci; these include osteosarcoma, chondrosarcoma, and rhabdomyosarcoma.[75] If epithelial elements are found, either histologically or by using immunohistologic markers such as keratin,[139,151] the tumor is currently classified as undifferentiated carcinoma.[75] Occasional undifferentiated tumors do not show any signs of epithelial or definite sarcomatous differentiation. It has been suggested that such tumors should be included under undifferentiated carcinoma because they have a similar course.[75] Undifferentiated carcinoma does not generaly stain positively for thyroglobulin in immunohistology,[140,152] though the results are somewhat controversial.[137,144,146,147]

Tumors that are composed of both differentiated and undifferentiated carcinoma are classified as undifferentiated.[75] If the undifferentiated focus is small, the tumor generally carries a better prognosis than undifferentiated carcinoma in general. Undifferentiated carcinoma is sometimes difficult to distinguish from spindle-celled medullary carcinoma.

Medullary carcinoma. Basically, medullary carcinoma differs from other thyroid carcinomas in showing evidence of C-cell differentiation. Like normal C-cells, the tumor cells produce and secrete calcitonin. The tumor may also secrete prostaglandins,[121] histaminase,[121] and carcinoembryonic antigen (CEA),[130] and occasionally 5-hydroxytryptamine (5-HT) or adrenocorticotropic hormone (ACTH).[121]

Although most medullary carcinomas occur sporadically, about 10% have a genetic background.[113] The familial form has an autosomal dominant mode of inheritance and is often associated with pheochromocytoma and parathyroid hyperplasia or adenoma (multiple endocrine adenomatosis, MEN IIA)[113,132,133] or with pheochromocytoma and multiple mucosal neuromas (MEN IIB).[132] Although the sporadic carcinoma is generally unilateral, the familial tumor is usually bilateral and multicentric and often accompanied by C-cell hyperplasia, which precedes the development of medullary carcinoma.[1,134] Also, the associated pheochromocytoma is usually bilateral.[115]

C-cell hyperplasia is not diffusely distributed in the thyroid gland but is mainly found in the central parts of the lateral lobes.[112] In patients who also have medullary carcinoma, C-cell hyperplasia is usually seen in the thyroid tissue surrounding the tumor. The hyperplasia may be diffuse or nodular. Sometimes it may be difficult to differentiate between nodular hyperplasia and invasive islands of medullary carcinoma.

In autopsy studies, clusters of C-cells have been found in persons without hypercalcemia and without parathyroid or thyroid disease,[117] and around what are known as solid cell nests (see p. 1544), there are often many C-cells, which should not be confused with C-cell hyperplasia.[3,4] For demonstration of normal or hyperplastic C-cells, special techniques such as immunohistology (for the detection of calcitonin) should be used.

Medullary carcinoma is rather rare, comprising about 5% to 10% of all thyroid carcinomas. It is as common in men as in women and is usually detected at middle age. The most frequent finding is a solitary thyroid nodule, but sometimes enlarged cervical lymph nodes may be the first symptom. Regional lymph node metastases are common; they have been detected in about half the patients at the time of surgery.[120] Distant metastases also occur but less commonly. About one third of patients, mostly those with the most extensive disease, have diarrhea believed to be caused by calcitonin secretion.[114] Occasionally patients exhibit the carcinoid syndrome, and some have Cushing's syndrome.[121] The prognosis is moderate; the observed 10-year survival rate is in the order of 60% to 70%.[80] The familial form seems to have a better prognosis than the nonfamilial form. This may be attributable to earlier detection of these tumors brought about by screening of the families carrying the gene for medullary carcinoma.

Macroscopically the tumor is usually of hard consistency and rather well limited but not encapsulated. Histologically, it is composed of sheets of tumor cells that are usually divided into groups by fibrous septa. The cells may be polygonal, spindle shaped, or round (Fig. 31-24). Sometimes they are arranged in ribbonlike structures or small glands (Fig. 31-25).[119] In poorly fixed specimens, shrinkage may cause a pseudopapillary pattern, but very rarely true papillae are also seen.[112] The cytoplasm is eosinophilic and finely granular, and the nuclei are usually uniform in shape, though binucleate cells and occasional giant nuclei do occur. Mitoses are infrequent. There are often irregular calcifications in the stroma that may resemble psammoma bodies but do not show regular laminations. Irregular masses of amyloid are seen between the tumor cells, sometimes in their cytoplasm. The amyloid stains with the usual staining methods, such as Congo red, and is believed to be stored calcitonin in the form of prohormone. It is not always possible to find amyloid in medullary carcinoma. In such cases the diagnosis can be confirmed by use of silver stains for argyrophil cells[2] or immunohistochemical methods based on the calcitonin content of the tumor cells.[127,136] The tumor cells usually stain positively also for CEA[130] and sometimes for somatostatin, 5-HT, ACTH, and some other markers.[116,131,136] The cells are also positive for general neuroendocrine markers, like synaptophysin[118] and chromogranin.[129,130a] Medullary carcinoma has been reported to show focal mucin positivity in nearly half the cases.[135] The tumor may rarely be composed of clear cells[122] or contain melanin.[124]

Differentiation between medullary carcinoma and papillary carcinoma may cause problems if papillary structures are present. Medullary carcinoma with glandular structures may resemble poorly differentiated follicular carcinoma. It is important to distinguish medullary carcinoma with spindle cells from undifferentiated carcinoma. Problems may arise especially in those rare cases in which medullary carcinoma contains clusters of bizarre giant cells.[125,126]

Mixed medullary-follicular carcinoma[123,128] denotes a very rare tumor with morphologic features of medullary carcinoma with immunoreactive calcitonin, accompanied with morphologic features of follicular carcinoma with immunoreactive thyroglobulin. In such cases the possibility of entrapped normal follicles should be excluded as well as artifactual uptake of thyroglobulin from surrounding follicles. The histogenesis of this tumor is uncertain.

Malignant lymphoma

The thyroid is involved in about 20% of patients who die of generalized lymphoma. Also, primary lymphomas occur and comprise about 5% of all thyroid cancer. The tumor has a diffuse growth pattern; residual thyroid follicles are often seen within the tumor at the border

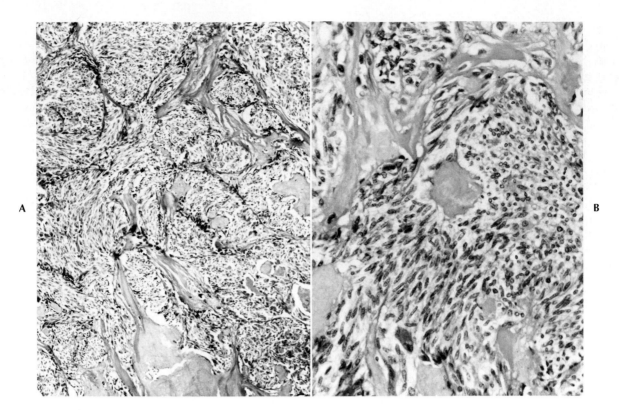

Fig. 31-24. Medullary carcinoma. **A,** Fibrous septa divide tumor cells into islands. **B,** Regular spindle-shaped tumor cells surround mass of amyloid. (**A,** 50×; **B,** 200×.)

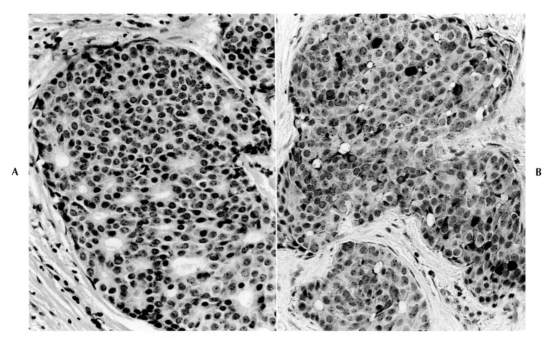

Fig. 31-25. A, Medullary carcinoma containing small glandular structures. **B,** Immuno-peroxidase staining of calcitonin, demonstrating positivity in some tumor cells, also at their luminal border. (**A,** 400×; **B,** 500×.)

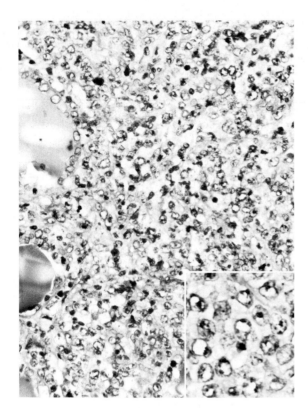

Fig. 31-26. Malignant lymphoma. Growth pattern is diffuse. Tumor cells invade between residual follicles on left. (200×.) *Inset,* Large vesicular nuclei and prominent nucleoli corresponding to large noncleaved cell lymphoma. (650×.)

(Fig. 31-26). Especially when the lymphoma is composed partly or solely of small cleaved cells (centrocytes), lymphoma cells are often seen in thyroid follicles, a finding that helps to differentiate between malignant lymphoma and chronic thyroiditis. In malignant lymphoma, the thyroid epithelium may show oxyphil cell change because of preexisting chronic thyroiditis.

Lymphomas are almost always of B-lymphocytic origin[160] and usually of follicle center cell origin,[155,157] the most common type being large noncleaved cell (centroblastic or centroblastic-centrocytic) lymphoma.[163] It has been suggested that thyroid lymphomas would represent neoplasms of mucosa-associated lymphoid tissue.[155,161] Hodgkin's disease probably does not involve the thyroid primarily. The prognosis in malignant lymphoma is better than in undifferentiated carcinoma; the 5-year survival rate is about 50%[158] and is higher in tumors confined within the thyroid capsule.[158,159] In most cases malignant lymphoma occurs together with lymphocytic thyroiditis,[159,162] an indication suggestive of evolution of the lymphoma from thyroiditis. Also plasmacytomas may occur in the thyroid.[156]

Other malignant tumors

Sarcomas, like fibrosarcomas[167] and malignant hemangioendotheliomas,[164,165] may occur in the thyroid, but they are extremely rare. The existence of the malignant hemangioendothelioma has been questioned.[164,170,171] In the past, sarcomas were rather common in studies from Central Europe, but most of these cases probably represented undifferentiated carcinomas.[167] A rare tumor composed of keratin-positive spindle cells and mucus-producing glandular structures[166] have been reported in the thyroid and called "spindle cell tumor with mucous cysts."

Metastatic tumors

Although clinically demonstrable metastases are uncommon[168] in the thyroid, in autopsies thyroid metastases have been detected in one fourth of patients who died of a metastasizing neoplasm.[172] The most common primary tumors are malignant melanoma and carcinomas of the kidney and bronchus. Metastatic renal cell carcinoma (hypernephroma) may cause a large tumor that may simulate primary thyroid neoplasm, mainly follicular carcinoma or adenoma.

REFERENCES
Development, structure, and function
 1. DeLellis, R.A., Nunnemacher, G., and Wolfe, H.J.: C-cell hyperplasia: an ultrastructural analysis, Lab. Invest. **36**:237, 1977.
 2. Grimelius, L., and Wilander, E.: Silver stains in the study of endocrine cells of the gut and pancreas, Invest. Cell Pathol. **3**:3, 1980.
 3. Harach, H.R.: Solid cell nests of the thyroid, J. Pathol. **155**:191, 1988.
 4. Janzer, R.C., Weber, E., and Hedinger, C.: The relation between solid cell nests and C cells of the thyroid gland, Cell Tissue Res. **197**:295, 1979.
 5. Klinck, G.H., Oertel, J.E., and Winship, T.: Ultrastructure of normal human thyroid, Lab. Invest. **22**:2, 1970.
 6. Pearse, A.G.E.: The APUD cell concept and its implications in pathology, Pathol. Annu. **9**:27, 1974.
 7. Wolfe, H.J., Voekel, E.F., and Tashijian, A.H., Jr.: Distribution of calcitonin-containing cells in the normal adult thyroid gland: a correlation of morphology with peptide content, J. Clin. Endocrinol. Metab. **38**:688, 1974.
 8. Yamaoka, Y.: Solid cell nests (SCN) of the human thyroid gland, Acta Pathol. Jpn. **23**:493, 1973.

Functional disorders: developmental anomalies
 9. Dalgaard, J.B., and Wetteland, P.: Thyroglossal anomalies: a follow-up study of 58 cases, Acta Chir. Scand. **111**:444, 1956.
10. Gerard-Marchant, R., and Caillou, B.: Thyroid inclusions in cervical lymph nodes, Clin. Endocrinol. Metab. **10**:337, 1981.
11. Himsworth, R.L.: Hyperthyroidism with a low iodine uptake, Clin. Endocrinol. Metab. **14**:397, 1985.
12. Ibbertson, H.K.: Endemic goitre and cretinism, Clin. Endocrinol. Metab. **8**:97, 1979.
13. Kantelip, B., Lusson, J.R., De Riberolles, C., Lamaison, D., and Bailly, P.: Intracardiac ectopic thyroid, Hum. Pathol. **17**:1293, 1986.
14. Larochelle, D., Arcand, P., Belzile, M., and Gagnon, N.B.: Ectopic thyroid tissue: a review of the literature, J. Otolaryngol. **8**:523, 1979.
15. LiVolsi, V.A., Perzin, K.H., and Savetsky, L.: Carcinoma arising in median ectopic thyroid (including thyroglossal duct tissue), Cancer **34**:1303, 1974.

16. McGregor, A.M., Hall, R., and Richards, C.: Autoimmune thyroid disease and pregnancy, Br. Med. J. **288**:1780, 1984.

17. Sampson, R.J., Oka, H., Key, C.R., et al.: Metastases from occult thyroid carcinoma: an autopsy study from Hiroshima and Nagasaki, Japan, Cancer **25**:803, 1970.

18. Sawin, C.T.: Hypothyroidism, Med. Clin. North Am. **69**:989, 1985.

19. Shimaoka, K.: Thyrotoxicosis due to metastatic involvement of the thyroid, Arch. Intern. Med. **140**:284, 1980.

20. Sisson, J.C., Schmidt, R.W., and Beierwaltes, W.H.: Sequestered nodular goiter, N. Engl. J. Med. **270**:927, 1964.

21. Smyrk, T.C., Goellner, J.R., Brennan, M.D., and Carney, J.A.: Pathology of the thyroid in amiodarone-associated thyrotoxicosis, Am. J. Surg. Pathol. **11**:197, 1987.

22. Spaulding, S.W., and Lippes, S.W.: Hyperthyroidism: causes, clinical features, and diagnosis, Med. Clin. North Am. **69**:937, 1985.

23. Stanbury, J.B.: Inborn errors of the thyroid, Prog. Med. Genet. **10**:55, 1974.

Goiter

24. Barsano, C.P., and DeGroot, L.J.: Dyshormonogenetic goitre, Clin. Endocrinol. Metab. **8**:145, 1979.

25. Clements, F.W.: Endemic goitre. In Beaton, G.H., and Bengea, J.M., editors: Nutrition in preventive medicine, World Health Organization Monogr., no. 62, Geneva, 1976, WHO, p. 83.

26. Doniach, D., Chiovato, L., Hanafusa, T., and Bottazzo, G.F.: The implications of "thyroid-growth-immunoglobulins" (TGI) for the understanding of sporadic nontoxic nodular goitre, Springer Semin. Immunopathol. **5**:433, 1982.

27. Kennedy, J.S.: The pathology of dyshormogenetic goiter, J. Pathol. **99**:251, 1969.

28. Ramelli, F., Studer, H., and Bruggisser, D.: Pathogenesis of thyroid nodules in multinodular goiter, Am. J. Pathol. **109**:215, 1982.

29. Studer, H., Peter, H.J., and Gerber, H.: Toxic nodular goitre, Clin. Endocrinol. Metab. **14**:351, 1985.

30. Vickery, A.L.: The diagnosis of malignancy of dyshormonogenetic goitre, Clin. Endocrinol. Metab. **10**:317, 1981.

Graves' disease; thyroiditis

31. Berger, S.A., Zonszein, J., Villamena, P., and Mittman, N.: Infectious diseases of the thyroid gland, Rev. Infect. Dis. **5**:108, 1983.

32. Carney, J.A., Moore, S.B., Northcutt, R.C., et al.: Palpation thyroiditis (multifocal granulomatous folliculitis), Am. J. Clin. Pathol. **64**:639, 1975.

33. Doniach, D., Bottazzo, G.F., and Russell, R.C.G.: Goitrous autoimmune thyroiditis (Hashimoto's disease), Clin. Endocrinol. Metab. **8**:63, 1979.

34. Drexhage, H.A., Bottazzo, G.F., Bitensky, L., Chayen, J., and Doniach, D.: Thyroid growth-blocking antibodies in primary myxoedema, Nature **289**:594, 1981.

35. Gossage, A.A.R., and Munro, D.S.: The pathogenesis of Graves' disease, Clin. Endocrinol. Metab. **14**:299, 1985.

36. Inada, M., Nishikawa, M., Naito, K., Ishii, H., Tanaka, K., and Imura, H.: Reversible changes of the histological abnormalities of the thyroid in patients with painless thyroiditis, J. Clin. Endocrinol. Metab. **52**:431, 1981.

37. Johnson, W.C., and Hellwig, E.B.: Cutaneous focal mucinosis: a clinicopathological and histochemical study, Arch. Dermatol. **93**:13, 1966.

38. Katz, S.M., and Vickery, A.L.: The fibrous variant of Hashimoto's thyroiditis, Hum. Pathol. **5**:161, 1974.

39. Kendall-Taylor, P.: The pathogenesis of Graves' ophthalmopathy, Clin. Endocrinol. Metab. **14**:331, 1985.

40. Levine, S.N.: Current concepts of thyroiditis, Arch. Intern. Med. **143**:1952, 1983.

41. Meyer, S., and Hausman, R.: Occlusive phlebitis in multifocal fibrosclerosis, Am. J. Clin. Pathol. **65**:274, 1976.

42. Mitchell, J.D., and Kirkham, N.: Focal lymphocytic thyroiditis in Southampton, J. Pathol. **144**:269, 1984.

42a. Mizukami, Y., Michigishi, T., Hashimoto, T., Tonami, N., Hisada, K., Matsubara, F., and Takazakura, E.: Silent thyroiditis: a histologic and immunohistochemical study, Hum. Pathol. **19**:423, 1988.

43. Nielsen, H.K.: Multifocal idiopathic fibrosclerosis: two cases with simultaneous occurrence of retroperitoneal fibrosis and Riedel's thyroiditis, Acta Med. Scand. **208**:119, 1980.

44. Pfaltz, M., and Hedinger, C.E.: Abnormal basement membrane structures in autoimmune thyroid disease, Lab. Invest. **55**:531, 1986.

45. Rallison, M.L., Dobyns, B.M., Keating, F.R., et al.: Occurrence and natural history of chronic lymphocytic thyroiditis in childhood, J. Pediatr. **86**:675, 1975.

46. Riley, F.C.: Orbital pathology in Graves' disease, Mayo Clin. Proc. **47**:975, 1972.

47. Shamsuddin, A.K.M., and Lane, R.A.: Ultrastructural pathology in Hashimoto's thyroiditis, Hum. Pathol. **12**:561, 1981.

48. Trokel, S.L., and Jakobiec, F.A.: Correlation of CT scanning and pathologic featues of ophthalmic Graves' disease, Ophthalmology **88**:553, 1981.

49. Volpé, R.: The pathology of thyroiditis, Hum. Pathol. **9**:429, 1978.

50. Volpé, R.: Autoimmune thyroid disease: a perspective, Mol. Biol. Med. **3**:25, 1986.

51. Wall, J.R., and Kuroki, T.: Immunologic factors in thyroid disease, Med. Clin. North Am. **69**:913, 1985.

52. Weaver, D.R., Deodhar, S.D., and Hazard, J.B.: A characterization of focal lymphocytic thyroiditis, Cleve. Clin. Q. **33**:59, 1966.

53. Woolf, P.D.: Thyroiditis, Med. Clin. North Am. **69**:1035, 1985.

54. Willems, J.-S., and Löwhagen, T.: Fine needle aspiration cytology in thyroid disease, Clin. Endocrinol. Metab. **10**:247, 1981.

55. Woolner, L.B., McConahey, W.M., and Beahrs, O.H.: Invasive fibrous thyroiditis (Riedel's struma), J. Clin. Endocrinol. Metab. **17**:201, 1957.

56. Woolner, L.B., McConahey, W.M., and Beahrs, O.H.: Struma lymphomatosa (Hashimoto's thyroiditis) and related thyroid disorders, J. Endocrinol. Metab. **19**:53, 1959.

Radiation changes; amyloidosis

57. James, P.D.: Amyloid goitre, J. Clin. Pathol. **25**:683, 1973.

58. Maxon, H.R.: Radiation-induced thyroid disease, Med. Clin. North Am. **69**:1049, 1985.

59. Spitalnik, P.F., and Straus, F.H.: Patterns of human thyroid parenchymal reaction following low-dose childhood irradiation, Cancer **41**:1098, 1978.

60. Vickery, A.L., Jr.: Thyroid alterations due to irradiation. In Hazard, J.B., and Smith, D.E., editors: The thyroid, International Academy of Pathology Monogr., no. 5, Baltimore, 1964, The Williams & Wilkins Co.

Benign tumors

61. Böcker, W., Dralle, H., Koch, G., de Heer, K., and Hagemann, J.: Immunohistochemical and electron-microscope analysis of adenomas of the thyroid gland. II. Adenomas with specific cytological differentiation, Virchows Arch. [Pathol. Anat.] **380**:205, 1978.

62. Buss, D.H., Marshall, R.B., Baird, F.G., and Myers, R.T.: Paraganglioma of the thyroid gland, Am. J. Surg. Pathol. **4**:589, 1980.

63. Carney, J.A., Ryan, J., and Goellner, J.R.: Hyalinizing trabecular adenoma of the thyroid gland, Am. J. Surg. Pathol. **11**:583, 1987.

64. Gherardi, G.: Signet ring "mucinous" thyroid adenoma: a follicle cell tumour with abnormal accumulation of thyroglobulin and a peculiar histochemical profile, Histopathology **11**:317, 1987.

65. Hazard, J.B., and Kenyon, R.: Atypical adenoma of the thyroid, Arch. Pathol. **58**:554, 1954.

66. Joensuu, H., Klemi, P., and Eerola, E.: DNA aneuploidy in follicular adenomas of the thyroid gland, Am. J. Pathol. **124**:373, 1986.

67. Lang, W., Georgii, A., Stauch, G., and Kienzle, E.: The differ-

entiation of atypical adenomas and encapsulated follicular carcinomas in the thyroid gland, Virchows Arch. [Pathol. Anat.] **385**:125, 1980.

68. Rigaud, C., Peltier, F., and Bogomoletz, M.V.: Mucin producing microfollicular adenoma of the thyroid, J. Clin. Pathol. **38**:277, 1985.
69. Schröder, S., and Böcker, W.: Signet-ring-cell thyroid tumors: follicle cell tumors with arrest in folliculogenesis, Am. J. Surg. Pathol. **9**:619, 1985.
70. Silberman, R., and Mendelson, I.R.: Teratoma of the neck: report of two cases and review of literature, Arch. Dis. Child. **35**:159, 1960.

Malignant tumors in general

71. Beaugié, J.M., Brown, C.L., Doniach, I., et al.: Primary malignant tumors of the thyroid: the relationship between histological classification and clinical behaviour, Br. J. Surg. **63**:173, 1976.
72. Franssila, K.: Value of histologic classification of thyroid cancer, Acta Pathol. Microbiol. Scand. [A] **225**(suppl).:1, 1971.
73. Franssila, K.O.: Prognosis in thyroid carcinoma, Cancer **36**:1138, 1975.
74. Franssila, K., Saxén, E., Teppo, L., Bjarnason, O., Tulinius, H., Normann, T., and Ringertz, N.: Incidence of different morphological types of thyroid cancer in the Nordic countries, Acta Pathol. Microbiol. Scand. [A] **89**:49, 1981.
75. Hedinger, C.E., Williams, E.D., and Sobin, L.H.: Histological typing of thyroid tumours, ed. 2, Berlin, 1988, Springer-Verlag.
76. Heitz, P., Moser, H., and Staub, J.J.: Thyroid cancer: a study of 573 thyroid tumors and 161 autopsy cases observed over a thirty-year period, Cancer **37**:2329, 1976.
77. Löwhagen, T., Willems, J.S., Lundell, G., Sundblad, R., and Granberg, P.O.: Aspiration biopsy cytology in diagnosis of thyroid cancer, World J. Surg. **5**:61, 1981.
78. Rosai, J., Carcangiu, M.L.: Pathology of thyroid tumors: some recent and old questions, Hum. Pathol. **15**:1008, 1984.
79. Williams, E.D., Doniach, I., Bjarnason, O., et al.: Thyroid cancer in an iodide-rich area, Cancer **39**:215, 1977.
80. Woolner, L.B., Beahrs, O.H., Black, B.M., McConahey, W.M., and Keating, F.R., Jr.: Classification and prognosis of thyroid carcinoma, Am. J. Surg. **102**:354, 1961.

Carcinoma
Papillary and follicular carcinomas

81. Böcker, W., Dralle, H., Hüsselmann, H., Bay, V., and Brassow, M.: Immunohistochemical analysis of thyroglobulin synthesis in thyroid carcinomas, Virchows Arch. [Pathol. Anat.] **385**:187, 1980.
82. Bondeson, L., Bondeson, A.G., Ljungberg, O., and Tibblin, S.: Oxyphil tumors of the thyroid: follow-up of 42 surgical cases, Ann. Surg. **194**:677, 1981.
83. Cady, B., Sedgwick, C.E., Meissner, W.A., et al.: Changing clinical, pathologic, therapeutic, and survival patterns in differentiated thyroid carcinoma, Ann. Surg. **184**:541, 1976.
84. Carcangiu, M.L., Zampi, G., Rosai, J.: Poorly differentiated ("insular") thyroid carcinoma: a reinterpretation of Langhans' "wucherende Struma," Am. J. Surg. Pathol. **8**:655, 1984.
85. Carcangiu, M.L., Zampi, G., Pupi, A., Castagnoli, A., and Rosai, J.: Papillary carcinoma of the thyroid: a clinicopathologic study of 241 cases treated at the University of Florence, Italy, Cancer **55**:805, 1985.
86. Chan, J.K.C., and Saw, D.: The grooved nucleus: a useful diagnostic criterion of papillary carcinoma of the thyroid, Am. J. Surg. Pathol. **10**:672, 1986.
87. Chan, J.K.C., Tsui, M.S., and Tse, C.H.: Diffuse sclerosing variant of papillary carcinoma of the thyroid: a histological and immunohistochemical study of three cases, Histopathology **11**:191, 1987.
88. Dickersin, G.R., Vickery, A.L., and Smith, S.B.: Papillary carcinoma of the thyroid, oxyphil cell type, "clear cell" variant: a light and electron-microscopic study, Am. J. Surg. Pathol. **4**:501, 1980.
89. Franssila, K.O.: Is the differentiation between papillary and follicular thyroid carcinoma valid? Cancer **32**:853, 1973.

90. Franssila, K.O., Ackerman, L.V., Brown, C.L., and Hedinger, C.E.: Session II: Follicular carcinoma, Semin. Diagn. Pathol. **2**:101, 1985.
91. Franssila, K.O., and Harach, H.R.: Occult papillary carcinoma of the thyroid in children and young adults: a systemic autopsy study in Finland, Cancer **58**:715, 1986.
92. Fukunaga, F.H., and Yatani, R.: Geographic pathology of occult thyroid carcinomas, Cancer **36**:1095, 1975.
93. Gonzáles-Cámpora, R., Herrero-Zapatero, A., Lerma, E., Sánchez, F., and Galera, H.: Hürthle cell and mitochondrion-rich cell tumors: a clinicopathologic study, Cancer **57**:1154, 1986.
94. Harach, H.R., Franssila, K.O., and Wasenius, V.-M.: Occult papillary carcinoma of the thyroid: a "normal" finding in Finland, a systematic autopsy study, Cancer **56**:531, 1985.
95. Hazard, J.B., and Kenyon, R.: Encapsulated angioinvasive carcinoma (angioinvasive adenoma) of thyroid gland, Am. J. Clin. Pathol. **24**:755, 1954.
96. Hofstädter, F.: Frequency and morphology of malignant tumours of the thyroid before and after the introduction of iodine-prophylaxis, Virchows Arch. [Pathol. Anat.] **385**:263, 1980.
97. Hubert, J.P., Jr., Kierman, P.D., Beahrs, O.H., McConahey, W.M., and Woolner, L.B.: Occult papillary carcinoma of the thyroid, Arch. Surg. **115**:394, 1980.
98. Kahn, N.F., and Perzin, K.H.: Follicular carcinoma of the thyroid: an evaluation of the histologic criteria used for diagnosis. In Sommers, S.C., and Rosen, P.P., editors: Pathol. Annu. **16**(pt.1):221, 1983.
99. Lang, W., Choritz, H., and Hundeshagen, H.: Risk factors in follicular thyroid carcinomas: a retrospective follow-up study covering a 14-year period with emphasis on morphological findings, Am. J. Surg. Pathol. **10**:246, 1986.
100. LiVolsi, L.A., and Merino, M.J.: Squamous cells in the human thyroid gland, Am. J. Surg. Pathol. **2**:133, 1978.
101. Mazzaferri, E.L., Young, R.L., Oertel, J.E., et al.: Papillary thyroid carcinoma: the impact of therapy in 576 patients, Medicine **56**:171, 1977.
102. McConahey, W.M., Hay, I.D., Woolner, L.B., van Heerden, J.A., and Taylor, W.F.: Papillary thyroid cancer treated at the Mayo Clinic, 1946 through 1970: initial manifestations, pathologic findings, therapy, and outcome, Mayo Clin. Proc. **61**:978, 1986.
103. Sampson, R.J., Key, C.R., Buncher, C.R., et al.: Smallest forms of papillary carcinoma of the thyroid, Arch. Pathol. **91**:334, 1971.
104. Sampson, R.J.: Prevalence and significance of occult thyroid cancer. In DeGroot, L.J., et al., editors: Radiation-associated thyroid carcinoma, New York, 1977, Grune & Stratton, Inc.
105. Schneider, A.B., Pinsky, S., Bekerman, C., and Ryo, U.Y.: Characteristics of 108 thyroid cancers detected by screening in a population with a history of head and neck irradiation, Cancer **46**:1218, 1980.
106. Schröder, S., Böcker, W., Dralle, H., Kortmann, K.B., and Stern, C.: The encapsulated papillary carcinoma of the thyroid: a morphologic subtype of the papillary thyroid carcinoma, Cancer **54**:90, 1984.
107. Schröder, S., and Böcker, W.: Clear-cell carcinomas of thyroid gland: a clinicopathological study of 13 cases, Histopathology **10**:75, 1986.
108. Sobrinho-Simões, M.A., Nesland, J.M., Holm, R., and Johannessen, J.V.: Transmission electron microscopy and immunocytochemistry in the diagnosis of thyroid tumors, Ultrastruct. Pathol. **9**:255, 1985.
109. Sobrinho-Simões, M.A., Nesland, J.M., Holm, R., Sambade, M.C., and Johannessen, J.V.: Hürthle cell and mitochondrin-rich papillary carcinomas of the thyroid gland: an ultrastructural and immunocytochemical study, Ultrastruct. Pathol. **8**:131, 1985.
110. Tscholl-Ducommun, J., and Hedinger, C.E.: Papillary thyroid carcinomas: morphology and prognosis, Virchows Arch. [A, Pathol. Anat.] **396**:19, 1982.
111. Vickery, A.L., Carcangiu, M.L., Johannessen, J.V., and Sobrinho-Simões, M.: Session I: Papillary carcinoma, Semin. Diagn. Pathol. **2**:90, 1985.

Medullary carcinoma

112. Albores-Saavedra, J., LiVolsi, V.A., and Williams, E.D.: Session IV: Medullary carcinoma, Semin. Diagn. Pathol. **2**:137, 1985.

113. Bigner, S.H.: Medullary carcinoma of the thyroid in the multiple endocrine neoplasia IIA syndrome, Am. J. Surg. Pathol. **5**:459, 1981.

114. Cox, T.M., Fagan, E.A., Hillyard, C.J., Allison, D.J., and Chadwick, V.S.: Rôle of calcitonin in diarrhoea associated with medullary carcinoma of the thyroid, Gut **20**:629, 1979.

115. DeLellis, R.A., Wolfe, H.J., Gagel, R.F., et al.: Adrenal medullary hyperplasia: a morphometric analysis of patients with familial medullary thyroid carcinoma, Am. J. Pathol. **83**:177, 1976.

116. Ghatei, M.A., Springall, D.R., Nicholl, C.G., Polak, J.M., and Bloom, S.R.: Gastrin-releasing peptide–like immunoreactivity in medullary thyroid carcinoma, Am. J. Clin. Pathol. **84**:581, 1985.

117. Gibson, W.C.H., Peng, T.-C., and Croker, B.P.: Age-associated C-cell hyperplasia in the thyroid, Am. J. Pathol. **106**:388, 1982.

118. Gould, V.E.: Synaptophysin: a new and promising pan-neuroendocrine marker, Arch. Pathol. Lab. Med. **111**:791, 1987.

119. Harach, H.R., and Williams, E.D.: Glandular (tubular and follicular) variants of medullary carcinoma of the thyroid, Histopathology **7**:83, 1983.

120. Hazard, J.B., Hawk, W.A., and Crile, G.: Medullary (solid) carcinoma of the thyroid: a clinicopathologic entity, J. Clin. Endocrinol. Metab. **19**:152, 1959.

121. Hazard, J.B.: The C cells (parafollicular cells) of the thyroid gland and medullary thyroid carcinoma: a review, Am. J. Pathol. **88**:214, 1977.

122. Landon, G., and Ordóñez, G.: Clear cell variant of medullary carcinoma of the thyroid, Hum. Pathol. **16**:844, 1985.

123. Ljungberg, O., Bondeson, L., and Bondeson, A.-G.: Differentiated thyroid carcinoma, intermediate type: a new tumor entity with features of follicular and parafollicular cell carcinoma, Hum. Pathol. **15**:218, 1984.

124. Marcus, J.M., Dice, C.A., and LiVolsi, V.A.: Melanin production in medullary thyroid carcinoma, Cancer **49**:2518, 1982.

125. Martinelli, G., Bazzocchi, F., Govoni, E., and Santini, D.: Anaplastic type of medullary thyroid carcinoma: an ultrastructural and immunohistochemical study, Virchows Arch. [Pathol. Anat.] **400**:61, 1983.

126. Mendelsohn, G., Baylin, S.B., Bigner, S.H., Wells, S.A., Jr., and Eggleston, J.C.: Anaplastic variants of medullary thyroid carcinoma: a light microscopic and immunohistochemical study, Am. J. Surg. Pathol. **4**:333, 1980.

127. Mendelsohn, G., Wells, S.A., and Baylin, S.A.: Relationship of tissue carcinoembryonic antigen and calcitonin to tumor virulence in medullary thyroid carcinoma, Cancer **54**:657, 1984.

128. Pfalz, M., Hedinger, C.E., and Muhlethaler, J.P.: Mixed medullary and follicular carcinoma of the thyroid, Virchows Arch. [A. Pathol. Anat.] **400**:53, 1983.

129. Schmid, K.W., Fischer-Colbrie, R., Hagn, C., Jasani, B., Williams, E.D., and Winkler, H.: Chromogranin A and B and secretogranin II in medullary carcinomas of the thyroid, Am. J. Surg. Pathol. **11**:551, 1987.

130. Schröder, S., and Klöppel, G.: Carcinoembryonic antigen and nonspecific cross-reacting antigen in thyroid cancer, Am. J. Surg. Pathol. **11**:100, 1987.

130a. Schröder, S., Böcker, W., Baisch, H., et al.: Prognostic factors in medullary thyroid carcinomas: survival in relation to age, sex, stage, histology, immunohistochemistry, and DNA content, Cancer **61**:806, 1988.

131. Sikri, K.L., Varndell, I.M., Hamid, Q.A., Wilson, B.S., Kameya, T., Ponder, B.A., Lloyd, R.V., Bloom, S.R., and Polak, J.M.: Medullary carcinoma of the thyroid: an immunocytochemical and histochemical study of 25 cases using eight separate markers, Cancer **56**:2481, 1985.

132. Sizemore, G.W., Heath, H., III, and Carney, J.A.: Multiple endocrine neoplasia type 2, Clin. Endocrinol. Metab. **9**:299, 1980.

133. Williams, E.D., Brown, C.L., and Doniach, I.: Pathological and clinical findings in a series of 67 cases of medullary carcinoma of the thyroid, J. Clin. Pathol. **19**:103, 1966.

134. Wolfe, H.J., Melvin, K.E., Cervi-Skinner, S.J., et al.: C-cell hyperplasia preceding medullary thyroid carcinoma, N. Engl. J. Med. **289**:437, 1973.

135. Zaatari, G.S., Saigo, P.E., and Huvos, A.G.: Mucin production in medullary carcinoma of the thyroid, Arch. Pathol. Lab. Med. **107**:70, 1983.

136. Zajac, J.D., Penschow, J., Mason, T., Tregear, G., Coghlan, J., and Martin, T.J.: Identification of calcitonin and calcitonin gene–related peptide messenger ribonucleic acid in medullary thyroid carcinomas by hybridization histochemistry, J. Clin. Endocrinol. Metab. **62**:1037, 1986.

Undifferentiated carcinoma; other carcinomas

137. Albores-Saavedra, J., Nadji, M., Civantos, F., and Morales, A.R.: Thyroglobulin in carcinoma of the thyroid: an immunohistochemical study, Hum. Pathol. **14**:62, 1983.

138. Aldinger, K.A., Samaan, N.A., Ibáñez, M., and Hill, C.S., Jr.: Anaplastic carcinoma of the thyroid: a review of 84 cases of spindle and giant cell carcinoma of the thyroid, Cancer **41**:2267, 1978.

139. Buley, I.D., Gatter, K.C., Heryet, A., and Mason, D.Y.: Expression of intermediate filament proteins in normal and diseased thyroid glands, J. Clin. Pathol. **40**:136, 1987.

140. Carcangiu, M.L., Steeper, T., Zampi, G., and Rosai, J.: Anaplastic thyroid carcinoma: a study of 70 cases, Am. J. Clin. Pathol. **83**:135, 1985.

141. Deligdisch, L., Subhani, Z., and Gordon, R.E.: Primary mucinous carcinoma of the thyroid gland, Cancer **45**:2564, 1980.

142. Evans, H.L.: Columnar-cell carcinoma of the thyroid: a report of two cases of an aggressive variant of thyroid carcinoma, Am. J. Clin. Pathol. **85**:77, 1986.

143. Franssila, K.O., Harach, R.H., and Wasenius, V.-M.: Mucoepidermoid carcinoma of the thyroid, Histopathology **8**:847, 1984.

144. Hurlimann, J., Gardiol, D., and Scazziga, B.: Immunohistology of anaplastic thyroid carcinoma: a study of 43 cases, Histopathology **11**:567, 1987.

145. Jao, W., and Gould, V.E.: Ultrastructure of anaplastic (spindle and giant cell) carcinoma of the thyroid, Cancer **35**:1280, 1975.

146. LiVolsi, V.A., Brooks, J.J., and Arendash-Durand B.: Anaplastic thyroid tumors: immunohistology, Am. J. Clin. Pathol. **87**:434, 1987.

147. deMicco, C., Ruf, J., Carayon, P., Chrestian, M.A., Henry, J.F., and Toga, M.: Immunohistochemical study of thyroglobulin in thyroid carcinomas with monoclonal antibodies, Cancer **59**:471, 1987.

148. Mizukami, Y., Matsubara, F., Hashimoto, T., Haratake, J., Terahata, S., Noguchi, M., and Hirose, K.: Primary mucoepidermoid carcinoma of the thyroid gland: a case report including an ultrastructural and biochemical study, Cancer **53**:1741, 1984.

149. Rhatigan, R.M., Roque, J.L., and Bucher, R.L.: Mucoepidermoid carcinoma of the thyroid gland, Cancer **39**:210, 1977.

150. Rigaud, C., and Bogomoletz, W.V.: "Mucin secreting" and "mucinous" primary thyroid carcinomas: pitfalls in mucin histo-

chemistry applied to thyroid tumours, J. Clin. Pathol. **40:**890, 1987.
151. Rosai, J., Saxén, E.A., and Woolner, L.: Session III: Undifferentiated and poorly differentiated carcinoma, Semin. Diagn. Pathol. **2:**123, 1985.
152. Ryff-de Lèche, A., Staub, J.J., Kohler-Faden, R., Müller-Brand, J., and Heitz, P.U.: Thyroglobulin production by malignant thyroid tumors: an immunocytochemical and radioimmunoassay study, Cancer **57:**1145, 1986.
153. Shimaoka, K., and Tsukada, Y.: Squamous cell carcinomas and adenosquamous carcinomas originating from the thyroid gland, Cancer **46:**1833, 1980.
154. Sobrinho-Simões, M., Stenwig, A.E., Nesland, J.M., Holm, R., and Johannessen, J.V.: A mucinous carcinoma of the thyroid, Pathol. Res. Pract. **181:**464, 1986.

Malignant lymphoma

155. Anscombe, A.M., and Wright, D.H.: Primary malignant lymphoma of the thyroid—a tumour of mucosa-associated lymphoid tissue: review of seventy-six cases, Histopathology **9:**81, 1985.
156. Aozasa, K., Inoue, A., Yoshimura, H., Miyauchi, A., Matsuzuka, F., and Kuma, K.: Plasmacytoma of the thyroid gland, Cancer **58:**105, 1986.
157. Aozasa, K., Inoue, A., Tajima, K., Miyauchi, A., Matsuzuka, F., and Kuma, K.: Malignant lymphomas of the thyroid gland: analysis of 79 patients with emphasis on histologic prognostic factors, Cancer **58:**100, 1986.
158. Burke, J.S., Butler, J.J., and Fuller, L.M.: Malignant lymphomas of the thyroid: a clinical pathologic study of 35 patients including ultrastructural observations, Cancer **39:**1587, 1977.
159. Compagno, J., and Oertel, J.E.: Malignant lymphoma and other lymphoproliferative disorders of the thyroid gland: a clinicopathologic study of 245 cases, Am. J. Pathol. **74:**1, 1980.
160. Heimann, R., Vannineuse, A., De Sloover, C., and Dor, P.: Malignant lymphomas and undifferentiated small cell carcinoma of the thyroid: a clinicopathologic review of the light of the Kiel classification for malignant lymphomas, Histopathology **2:**201, 1978.
161. Isaacson, P.G., and Spencer, J.: Malignant lymphoma of mucosa-associated lymphoid tissue, Histopathology **11:**445, 1987.
162. Maurer, R., Taylor, C.R., Terry, R., and Lukes, R.J.: Non-Hodgkin lymphomas of the thyroid: a clinico-pathological review of 29 cases applying the Lukes-Collins classification and an immunoperoxidase method, Virchows Arch. [Pathol. Anat.] **383:**293, 1979.
163. Schwarze, E.W., and Papadimitriou, C.S.: Non-Hodgkin lymphoma of the thyroid, Pathol. Res. Pract. **167:**346, 1980.

Other tumors; metastatic tumors

164. Eckert, F., Schmid, U., Gloor, F., and Hedinger, C.: Evidence of vascular differentiation in anaplastic tumours of the thyroid: an immunohistological study, Virchows Arch. [A, Pathol. Anat.] **410:**203, 1986.
165. Egloff, B.: The hemangioendothelioma of the thyroid, Virchows Arch. [A, Pathol. Anat.] **400:**119, 1983.
166. Harach, H.R., Saravia Day, E., and Franssila, K.O.: Thyroid spindle-cell tumor with mucous cysts—an intrathyroid thymoma? Am. J. Surg. Pathol. **9:**525, 1985.
167. Hedinger, C.E.: Sarcomas of the thyroid gland. In Hedinger, C.E., editor: Thyroid cancer, UICC Monogr., no. 12, Berlin, 1969, Springer-Verlag.
168. Ivy, H.K.: Cancer metastatic to the thyroid: a diagnostic problem, Mayo Clin. Proc. **59:**856, 1984.
169. Kimler, S.C., and Muth, W.E.: Primary malignant teratoma of the thyroid: case report and literature review of cervical teratomas in adults, Cancer **42:**311, 1978.
170. Krisch, K., Holzner, J.H., Kokoschka, R., Jakesz, R., Niederle, B., and Roka, R.: Hemangioendothelioma of the thyroid gland—true endothelioma or anaplastic carcinoma? Pathol. Res. Pract. **170:**230, 1980.
171. Mills, S.E., Stallings, R.G., and Austin, M.B.: Angiomatoid carcinoma of the thyroid gland: anaplastic carcinoma with follicular and medullary features mimicking angiosarcoma, Am. J. Clin. Pathol. **86:**674, 1986.
172. Silverberg, S.G., and Vidone, R.A.: Metastatic tumors in the thyroid, Pacif. Med. Surg. **74:**175, 1966.

32 Parathyroid Glands

JAMES E. OERTEL
JEFFREY M. OGORZALEK

The parathyroid glands are important regulators of the metabolism of calcium and phosphorus and act to maintain normal levels of these elements in the blood.

DEVELOPMENT AND STRUCTURE

The parathyroid glands, usually four in number, are developed from endoderm of the third and fourth branchial pouches, in intimate relation to portions of the thymus but quite independent of the thyroid gland.[1,5] The superior pair of glands is derived from the fourth pharyngeal pouches, whereas the inferior pair, derived from the third pouches, outdistances the superior pair and the thyroid gland in caudal migration and takes the lower position. Their close connection with the development of the thymus explains the occasional occurrence of one or more parathyroid glands near or even embedded in thymic tissue. This possibility should be borne in mind during a search for parathyroid tissue or a parathyroid adenoma by surgical procedures or at autopsy.[11,12]

Although four parathyroid glands are usually present, variations in number from two to 10 have been reported. The superior pair is nearly always situated on the medial part of the dorsal surface of each lobe of the thyroid gland, at about the junction of the middle and upper thirds, and lies close to ascending branches of the inferior thyroid artery. They often are embedded in thyroid substance but separated from it by a connective tissue capsule. The inferior parathyroid glands, more inconstant in position, are found usually on the dorsal surface of the lateral lobes of the thyroid gland, near the lower pole.

The parathyroid glands are brownish yellow, oval, somewhat flattened bodies that vary considerably in size in adults, reported as means of 35.2 mg each in whites, 47.5 mg each in blacks (95% upper limit: 73.1 mg and 91.6 mg respectively).[4] Also, the glands differ in size in each person. Each parathyroid gland possesses a capsule of connective tissue from which bands pass through the gland.

The parenchymal cells are arranged as solid masses or as irregular cords. Acinar or follicular structures occur, may contain colloid, and tend to increase in frequency with age. Interstitial adipose tissue is extremely variable in amount, is usually sparse or absent in children, and often is increased in adults, relating very approximately to body fat generally.

The parenchymal cells appear in three main forms: chief cells, water-clear cells, and oxyphil cells. Transitional forms occur.

The chief cell (6 to 8 μm in diameter) is the most numerous. Its cytoplasm is weakly acidophilic and may appear vacuolated by light microscopy. Electron microscopic studies have indicated that cyclic changes of secretory activity may occur in the cells, but some of these findings have been questioned as artifacts of fixation.

The water-clear cell is larger (10 to 15 μm), has abundant clear cytoplasm and a relatively small pyknotic nucleus, and has well-defined cell borders, a feature often evident in all varieties of parathyroid cells. This cell is rare in normal glands. Large membrane-limited cytoplasmic vacuoles are the most conspicuous aspect of its fine structure. Dense secretory granules are sparse.

The oxyphil cell is 8 to 14 μm in diameter. Its eosinophilic granular cytoplasm is packed with mitochondria, secretory granules are rare, and glycogen is present in moderate amounts. Before puberty, oxyphil cells are uncommon. They increase in number with age and in certain diseases, such as chronic renal failure.[57]

PARATHYROID HORMONE

Parathyroid hormone is a polypeptide that acts to elevate serum calcium and reduce serum phosphate. Reduction of serum ionized calcium promptly causes increased secretion of the hormone, whereas elevation of serum calcium results in decreased secretion. Elevation of magnesium ions in serum also causes decreased secretion of the hormone; magnesium depletion impairs the secretion of parathyroid hormone.

The opinions or assertions contained herein are the private views of the authors and are not to be construed as official or as reflecting the views of the Departments of the Army, Air Force, or Defense.

Parathyroid hormone acts on the tubular cells of the nephrons to inhibit reabsorption of phosphate and to promote absorption of calcium and magnesium, causes resorption of bone matrix and bone mineral, and increases renal production of 1,25-dihydroxycholecalciferol (which in turn promotes the absorption of calcium from the small intestine).

REGULATION OF CALCIUM METABOLISM

The regulation of calcium metabolism is a complex mechanism involving the effects of hormones and ions on bone, the absorption of calcium and phosphate from the small intestine, and the loss of calcium and phosphate in the urine and feces. Parathyroid hormone maintains the level of calcium in the blood and other extracellular fluids by the actions mentioned in the previous section. Calcitonin opposes parathyroid hormone partly by preventing resorption of bone and partly by enhancing renal excretion of sodium, calcium, and phosphate. It is released in response to elevations of serum calcium and probably also by certain hormones of the alimentary tract.

Vitamin D is required for absorption of calcium ions from the intestine and for adequate growth and mineralization of the skeleton. Its most active metabolite, 1,25-dihydroxycholecalciferol, is formed in the kidney; synthesis is enhanced by parathyroid hormone and by hypophosphatemia.

Calcium metabolism is also affected by the corticosteroids, by some of the hormones of the alimentary tract, and by thyroid hormone. Estrogens, androgens, and growth hormone also have long-term effects on the skeleton, but their short-term influence on divalent cation metabolism is unknown.

PATHOLOGIC CALCIFICATION

Pathologic calcification is the deposition of mineral salts, including calcium, in tissues not normally calcified as well as in excretory or secretory ducts. Mineral deposits are found quite regularly in some soft tissues (for instance, the pineal gland after puberty). Calcium phosphate (present most often as hydroxyapatite) mixed with small amounts of calcium carbonate is the most common form. Calcium oxalate deposits may also be present, especially in the urinary tract.

Pathologic calcification has been described under the categories of dystrophic calcification, metastatic calcification, calcification in tumors, calcinosis, and calciphylaxis.

Dystrophic calcification is the deposition of calcium salts in injured or dead tissue. The systemic chemical balance is normal, but the local environment is altered to favor precipitation of the salts. Metastatic calcification is the deposition of calcium salts in soft tissue as a result of a systemic disturbance in calcium and phos-

phate metabolism. Calcification in tumors is a form of dystrophic calcification in which a tumor contains calcium salts either as irregular masses in the tissue, often associated with regions of necrosis, or as psammoma bodies (concentrically laminated bodies formed of calcium apatite). Calcinosis is local or generalized calcification in or under the skin, sometimes including muscles, fasciae, nerves, and tendons, and occasionally is associated with a collagen vascular disease. Tumoral calcinosis refers to a localized, often cystic, calcific mass in the soft tissue, usually next to a large joint and usually solitary. In some persons there are disturbances in mineral metabolism; some cases are familial. Calciphylaxis is an experimental process in animals in which induced hypercalcemia is followed by injury to tissues by chemical or physical agents, and calcification of the damaged tissues results.

These categories of calcification of soft tissues are artificial because, regardless of whether there is an alteration in the levels of calcium and phosphate in the extracellular fluids or local injury to tissues, the mechanisms of calcification are similar. Current belief is that the avidity of mitochondria for calcium and their ability to store it lead to its accumulation within them. Elevated extracellular calcium and phosphate cannot be excluded by the cells (overloading the mitochondria), or an insult to the cells results in their inability to exclude extracellular calcium present in normal amounts (also overloading the mitochondria). Eventually the calcium salts interfere with mitochondrial metabolism, and the cell dies. Extracellular calcification apparently occurs on the membranes of matrix vesicles and on collagen fibrils.

Once the initial foci of calcium salts have been deposited, the growth of mineral crystals depends on the systemic chemical environment, local mechanisms for concentrating the ions, quantity and character of available matrix, and levels of inhibitors of calcification, such as pyrophosphate and proteoglycans. Major factors promoting calcification include elevation of the serum calcium-phosphate product (Ca × P in mg/100 ml) resulting from higher levels of calcium or phosphate or both, elevation of pH locally or systemically, and availability of a suitable matrix. The local elevation of pH in the eye and kidney (because the cells establish a hydrogen-ion gradient across their membranes) may enhance calcification.

HYPOPARATHYROIDISM

Diminution or absence of circulating parathyroid hormone causes a reduction of serum calcium (to as little as half the normal level) and an elevation of serum phosphate (to as much as three or four times normal levels). Little or no calcium appears in the urine. Tetany and other evidence of neuromuscular irritability are the most important clinical manifestations of hypoparathyroidism. If the disease is of long duration, the persons affected may have (in addition to tetany) skin disorders, abnormal nail growth, loss of hair, cataracts, a variety of disorders of the central nervous system, and roentgenographic evidence of increased bone density and calcification in the vessels of the basal ganglia of the brain. Convulsions, papilledema, and gastrointestinal disturbances may be present.

The most common cause of hypoparathyroidism is the removal of all or part of the parathyroid tissue during surgery on the neck, especially during thyroidectomy. If only part of the gland tissue is removed, or if the glands are partially injured by impairment of their blood supply or by postoperative edema, the hormonal deficiency will be temporary. Complete removal or more severe damage results in permanent impairment of function.

Temporary neonatal hypocalcemia may be a manifestation of the hypoparathyroidism that occurs normally in many infants for a brief period after birth. This state may persist in sick or injured infants and may become manifest as symptomatic hypocalcemia.[30,32,38]

So-called idiopathic hypoparathyroidism is a rare disease that is sporadic or familial and in some instances may be an autoimmune disorder. The glands either are replaced by fat or cannot be found.[33,36] Permanent idiopathic hypoparathyroidism developing during the first year of life may be associated with congenital hypoplasia or absence of the parathyroid glands and thymus, and the children usually die.[41] Another type of hypoparathyroidism that also occurs in childhood may be familial or sporadic and is associated with a variety of disorders, some of which are accompanied by autoimmune phenomena. These include idiopathic adrenocortical atrophy, lymphocytic thyroiditis, oophoritis, diabetes mellitus, gastric mucosal atrophy, hepatitis, alopecia totalis, and severe *Candida* infections.

PSEUDOHYPOPARATHYROIDISM

Pseudohypoparathyroidism is a group of disorders, also called Albright's hereditary osteodystrophy, with a female predominance, and characterized by clinical features suggestive of idiopathic hypoparathyroidism. Brachydactyly, short stature, and multiple foci of soft-tissue calcification and ossification are additional features. Defective responsiveness of hormone-sensitive adenylate cyclase and abnormalities of circulating parathyroid hormone have been found in some persons. Other pseudohypoparathyroid persons have normal or elevated levels of urinary cyclic adenosine monophosphate but nonetheless fail to exhibit the phosphaturic effects of parathyroid hormone. The parathyroid glands are normal or hyperplastic.

HYPERPARATHYROIDISM

Excessive production of parathyroid hormone results from several different disorders: from a disturbance of calcium and phosphorus metabolism originating elsewhere in the body (renal failure, vitamin D deficiency) and leading to secondary hyperplasia of parathyroid tissue, from primary hyperplasia of the parathyroid tissue, from benign and malignant tumors of the parathyroid glands, and from neoplasms not of parathyroid origin, such as carcinoma of the lung or of the kidney.

Hyperparathyroidism may occur at any age but is more likely after 30 years of age. It is more common in women, and there is evidence that primary hyperparathyroidism is especially likely to occur in women about the time of menopause.

In some patients incidental laboratory tests reveal the disorder. The most common symptoms in symptomatic patients are weakness and fatigability, followed in frequency by signs and symptoms of urinary calculi. Renal manifestations also include nephrocalcinosis and uremia. Less common are signs and symptoms of skeletal disease, such as pathologic fractures, bone pain, and generalized demineralization of the skeleton. Gastrointestinal disorders occur, including epigastric discomfort, constipation, and vague abdominal complaints. More important, peptic ulcers occur in 10% to 15% of hyperparathyroid patients, especially men. Central nervous system disturbances may constitute an important part of the clinical picture. These include depressive reactions, confusion, stupor, and personality changes. Additional manifestations of hypercalcemia include polydipsia and polyuria. The ophthalmologist may find band keratopathy, a corneal opacity extending across the cornea from within the limbus, and also may note crystals in the conjuctivae. Some patients have hypertension, often the result of renal damage, although in certain instances the relationship to kidney disease is unclear because impairment of renal function cannot be demonstrated.

Elevated levels of circulating parathyroid hormone cause increased urinary excretion of inorganic phosphate, decreased serum phosphate, and increased serum calcium. Intestinal absorption of calcium rises. If skeletal lesions are present, serum alkaline phosphatase is elevated, and the urinary excretion of hydroxyproline rises (see also p. 1575).

Hyperparathyroidism must be differentiated from other causes of hypercalcemia, such as hypervitaminosis A and D, hyperthyroidism, adrenocortical insufficiency, and milk-alkali syndrome (excessive ingestion of milk and absorbable alkalis, leading to hypercalcemia, alkalosis, and azotemia without hypophosphatemia), use of certain diuretics, sarcoidosis, tuberculosis, multiple myeloma, leukemia, lymphoma, and some other malignant neoplasms with and without metastatic foci in bone.[18] Idiopathic hypercalciuria with normal serum calcium and repeated formation of renal stones and the hypercalciuria present in renal tubular acidosis are conditions that also must be distinguished from hyperparathyroidism.

Secondary hyperplasia

Disturbances in calcium and phosphorus metabolism not primarily involving the parathyroid glands may in time cause changes in the glands as they respond to the metabolic abnormalities. Chronic renal glomerular insufficiency resulting in retention of phosphate and depression of intestinal absorption of calcium is the most common cause of compensatory parathyroid hyperfunction and hyperplasia. Very high levels of circulating parathyroid hormone may be present, but the glands are still responsive to changes in serum calcium. Hyperplasia may occur in rickets and osteomalacia caused by vitamin D deficiency, with intestinal malabsorption syndromes causing deficiencies of calcium and vitamin D, and in pseudohypoparathyroidism.

Hyperplastic glands range from normal size to strik-

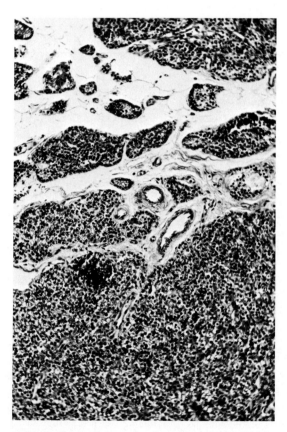

Fig. 32-1. Primary chief cell hyperplasia. Irregular involvement of gland can occur. Several small groups of cells appear to be normal.

ing enlargement. Variations in size of the individual glands in any one patient may be evident. As a rule the glands are not adherent to the surrounding tissue. The cut surfaces may be smooth or nodular. There is a decrease in or absence of stromal fat, and the glands are cellular, composed usually of pale and vacuolated chief cells (Fig. 32-1). Transitional oxyphil cells or transitional water-clear cells may predominate occasionally. The cells often are arranged in solid masses, but nests, cords, or acinar patterns may occur. Nuclei are normal sized or somewhat enlarged.

Adenoma and primary hyperplasia

Parathyroid adenoma (Fig. 32-2) and primary hyperplasia are the major primary proliferative disorders of the glands. Primary chief cell hyperplasia may affect all the glands uniformly, or there may be substantial differences in the size and apparent degree of involvement in the different glands. Also the process may be nodular, and a large nodule occupying much of a gland may be difficult or impossible to distinguish from an adenoma using routine measures. As a rule, normal parathyroid parenchyma contains evenly distributed cytoplasmic fat droplets, whereas adenomas do not contain such fat, and hyperplastic parenchyma has reduced or absent fat. These observations have been exploited to assist the surgeon in making intraoperative decisions regarding the extent of surgery.[42] Unfortunately, these fat droplets occasionally are numerous in adenomatous or hyperplastic tissue, and so results of fat stains may be misleading.[44] Ultrastructural studies have been recommended to assist in the distinction of normal glandular parenchyma from abnormal tissues, but obviously these procedures cannot be completed during the operation. Further complicating the problem of adenoma versus hyperplasia are the enzymatic studies,[65] which indicate that adenomas may be of multicellular origin, and the morphologic studies,[66] which indicate that "true" adenomas may be rare and most cases of primary hyperparathyroidism may be the result of hyperplasia. Because of these complexities, the pathologist's diagnostic evaluation must be cautious and developed in close collaboration with the surgeon's findings during exploration of the neck.

Fortunately, experience has demonstrated that removal of the largest gland often results in cure of the hyperparathyroidism, regardless of whether the subsequent pathologic study demonstrates a classic adenoma or indicates the possibility of uneven hyperplasia.

Primary hyperplasia occurs in the absence of any known primary metabolic disorder, may be familial, and may be a part of multiple endocrine adenopathies. If the parathyroid glands are all enlarged and have little or no stromal fat, hyperplasia is readily recognized by

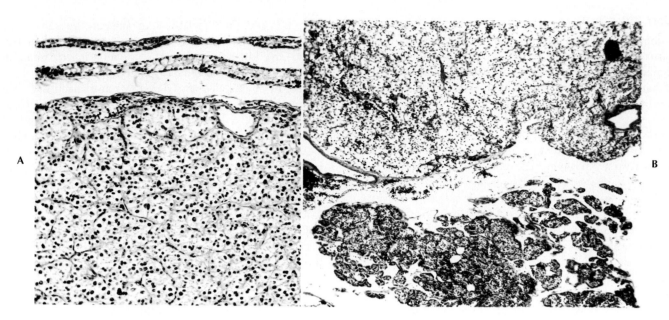

Fig. 32-2. A, Adenoma. Two delicate strands of remaining glandular tissue are above tumor. **B,** Remnant of normal tissue accompanies adenoma.

the surgeon and pathologist. Uneven involvement of the glands or a nodular proliferation is much more difficult to recognize as hyperplasia. The cells of hyperplastic glands vary from chief cells to transitional water-clear cells and transitional oxyphil cells. Scattered mitotic figures, focal degenerative changes, and fibrosis may occur.

A small number of patients undergoing surgery because of elevated serum ionized-calcium levels or other abnormalities suggestive of hyperparathyroidism have normal parathyroid glands by biopsy or have subtle abnormalities only suggestive of hyperplasia. Such instances may represent an early or mild form of hyperparathyroidism. Patients with familial hypocalciuric hypercalcemia have a modest degree of hyperplasia believed to be primary in type.[70]

Primary water-clear cell hyperplasia is very rare and is probably a variant of long-standing primary chief cell hyperplasia. The glands are enlarged, irregular, chocolate brown, nonadherent, and soft. They are composed of large water-clear cells that are 10 to 40 μm in diameter and have small dark-staining nuclei 4 to 8 μm in diameter.[69]

A single lesion designated as an adenoma causes primary hyperparathyroidism in about three fourths of patients with the disorder. Two adenomas are rare. Adenomas range in weight from less than 100 mg to several hundred grams (rarely), but most weigh only a few grams. The tumors are spherical to ovoid, soft, tan to reddish brown, occasionally gray, have a delicate capsule, and are usually not adherent to the surrounding tissues. The cut surface may be focally hemorrhagic

or cystic, and zones of fibrosis and calcification may be present. Deposits of brown pigment mark the sites of old hemorrhage.

The majority of adenomas are composed of chief cells, either normal or abnormal in appearance, but any cell type can predominate and any single tumor can contain a variety of cell types. Oxyphil cell tumors are often nonfunctional, but, except for these, there is no correlation between the degree of function and the cell type. Giant nuclei, bizarre nuclei, and multinucleated cells are fairly common. Mitoses are rare. The cells may be arranged as simply a solid mass, or they may form cords, nests, acini, or follicles resembling thyroid follicles. Nodules of single or mixed patterns may be evident. Rarely the tumor contains a large amount of adipose tissue.[64]

The remnant of a gland containing an adenoma often forms a rim of normal tissue outside the capsule of the adenoma, typically including some adipose tissue as part of its stroma and composed of small chief cells and sometimes oxyphil cells. Considerable neutral lipid is usually present within these glandular cells.

Tertiary hyperparathyroidism

Tertiary hyperparathyroidism is defined as persistent parathyroid hyperfunction that has developed from secondary hyperplasia after apparent removal of the cause of the secondary hyperplasia, such as restoration of renal function by dialysis or renal transplantation. The hyperplastic parathyroid tissue appears to persist, or a lesion recognizable as an adenoma or a carcinoma is found.

Carcinoma

Since nonfunctional parathyroid carcinomas are difficult to differentiate from thyroid carcinomas, most pathologists require the presence of hyperparathyroidism to make the diagnosis. Parathyroid hyperfunction is often pronounced. A moderate number of carcinomas are palpable on physical examination.

At surgery carcinoma is nearly always tightly adherent to surrounding tissue and is irregular in shape, but some resemble typical adenomas. The cut surface is gray, light tan, or brown and is firm, largely as a result of fibrous septa running through the tumor.

Typically carcinoma is surrounded by a thick capsule and is composed of solid masses of cells divided by irregular fibrous septa. The cells may be polygonal or elongated with clear, amphophilic, or eosinophilic cytoplasm. Nuclei are relatively large. The tumors may closely resemble adenomas, even on careful microscopic examination. Perivascular palisading and trabecular patterns are common. Mitotic figures are usually present.

The only certain criteria of malignancy are local invasion of adjacent tissues and distant metastatic lesions. Local recurrence may be a serious problem, even though distant metastases are rare.

Lesions associated with hyperparathyroidism

The hypercalcemia of hyperparathyroidism may lead to the deposition of calcium salts (known as metastatic calcification) in a variety of soft tissues. Renal calculi occur in at least half the patients with symptomatic hyperparathyrodism and often are the reason the patient seeks medical aid. A considerably smaller number of patients have osteoporotic lesions of the skeletal system, a condition that when fully developed is known as generalized osteitis fibrosa cystica.

Metastatic calcification

The kidneys and blood vessels are the most frequent sites of metastatic calcification, but some deposits, especially in acute hyperparathyroidism, may be found in the lungs, stomach, heart, eyes, and other tissues. Calcific deposits are particularly abundant when there is renal failure with phosphate retention.

In blood vessels the calcification is mainly in the media and particularly involves elastic tissue, and so the internal elastic lamella is often prominently calcified. The adjacent intima may be thickened by hyperplasia but is usually without calcification. Vascular calcification may be particularly severe in secondary renal hyperparathyroidism in which there is an increased level of blood phosphate. In some patients, ischemic muscle pains in the extremities and even gangrene have resulted.

Generalized osteitis fibrosa cystica

Osteitis fibrosa cystica (von Recklinghausen's disease) (Fig. 32-3) is essentially an osteoclastic resorption of bone and its replacement by connective tissue in which there are abortive attempts at new bone formation. The changes range from a slightly increased porosity of the bones, because of an increase in osteoclasts removing trabecular and cortical bone with minimal replacement of the marrow by fibrous stroma, to a pronounced dissecting osteitis of the trabeculas and large cutting cores in the bony cortex in advanced cases. Immature and poorly calcified bone develops in the connective tissue. The newly formed bone may undergo resorption. While endosteal resorption occurs, periosteal deposition of bone is taking place. Osteoclasts are abundant. Large fibrous scars develop in place of the original spongy bone. Brown tumors, usually in the jaws or long bones, are colored by blood pigment and consist of multinucleated giant cells, cellular fibrous stroma, macrophages filled with hemosiderin, and newly formed vessels. Cysts lined by connective tissue may result from degeneration or hemorrhage but are not always present. Characteristic early roentgenographic changes include subperiosteal resorption of bone, most frequently seen along the margins of the middle phalanges of the fingers. Plasma alkaline phosphatase is increased. Because skeletal collagen is resorbed, urinary hydroxyproline excretion is increased.

Renal lesions

The kidneys may be severely damaged in hyperparathyroidism as a result of the deposition of calcium salts (nephrocalcinosis) and the formation of renal stones. Excess parathyroid hormone apparently interferes with the ability of the tubules to concentrate urine. In acute hyperparathyroidism, some of the nephrons show calcification of tubular epithelial cells and tubular basement membranes. Calcific casts are formed.

In the milder chronic cases, patchy calcification usually involves the cells of the ascending limb of the loop of Henle, the distal convoluted tubule, and the collecting tubule.[53] Casts, usually calcific, are formed partly from desquamated cells and cellular debris and may cause obstruction of the nephron. Some interstitial calcification may occur. Foci of fibrosis with tubular and glomerular atrophy and infiltration by chronic inflammatory cells are common.

In advanced cases fibrosis, inflammation, and nephron destruction are extensive, and calcification of interstitial tissue may be striking. Both atrophy and cystic dilatation of the tubules proximal to obstructing calcific masses may be evident (Fig. 32-4).

Although hyperparathyroidism is an uncommon cause of renal calculi, its presence should be sought in every patient with renal stones. In some clinics, 4% of

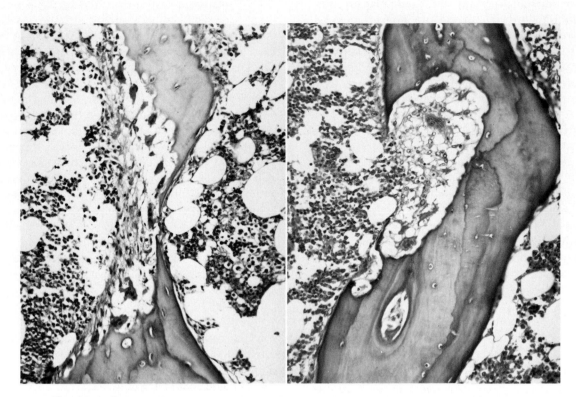

Fig. 32-3. Bone in hyperparathyroidism. Portions of trabeculas have been removed by osteoclasts, and small part of marrow has been replaced by fibroblasts.

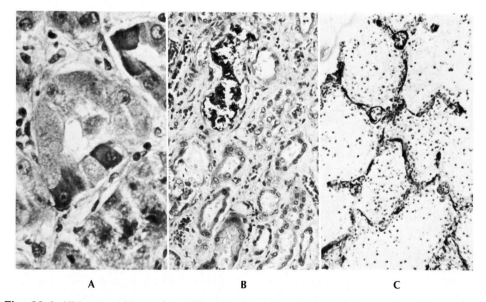

A   B   C

Fig. 32-4. Kidney and lung from 35-year-old man with large parathyroid adenoma. **A,** Several renal tubular cells have undergone calcification. **B,** Calcific material fills a renal tubule. **C,** Walls of alveoli and of blood vessels are calcified.

persons with renal stones have hyperparathyroidism. The calculi are predominantly calcium oxalate or calcium phosphate. Kidneys containing stones may have only minor tubular damage, or they may be extensively involved by calcific deposits and the associated parenchymal damage. Hydronephrosis may occur. Pyelonephritis is common in kidneys damaged by stones and by calcinosis.

Renal osteodystrophy and secondary hyperparathyroidism

The osteodystrophy occurring in chronic renal failure is characterized by varying degrees of osteitis fibrosa, osteomalacia, osteoporosis, and osteosclerosis.[80,81] The clinical and pathologic features in a single patient depend on the pathologic process that predominates during a particular time period. The pathologic processes, in turn, depend on which of the complex metabolic disturbances of uremia are most important in the person affected and how these disturbances are altered by therapeutic measures. Renal lesions of a type in which large amounts of renal parenchyma are lacking or destroyed and those that are stationary or very slowly progressive (renal insufficiency over a prolonged period) may result in these skeletal changes. Hemodialysis and renal transplantation prolong life and thereby have substantially increased the possibility that skeletal disease may develop.

One of the most important complications of the secondary hyperparathyroidism usually present in chronic renal disease is soft-tissue calcification. Sites commonly involved are the arteries, heart, kidneys, lungs, stomach, soft tissues around joints, eyes, and skin and subcutaneous tissues. Arterial, myocardial, and renal calcification may have grave clinical effects.

In children, remarkable skeletal deformities and growth disturbances (dwarfism) may result because bone growth is incomplete and the epiphyses are not united. The underlying renal lesion is most commonly a developmental malformation in the kidneys or urinary tract, such as congenital hypoplasia, congenital polycystic disease, strictures of the ureters, or congenital valves of the urethra. Infection (pyelonephritis) may be added to hydronephrotic atrophy in cases of obstruction in the lower urinary tract and may further decrease the functioning renal parenchyma.

The characteristic changes in the epiphyseal cartilages are probably the result of abnormal metabolism of vitamin D as well as of hyperparathyroidism. The epiphyseal cartilages are greatly increased in bulk but show degenerative changes, defects of calcium deposition, and distortion. The cartilage may be bent and twisted and displaced from its normal position at the end of the shaft. Extreme deformity often results. The skull may be greatly thickened, and the appearance of the calvaria closely resembles that in Paget's disease of bone.

The kidneys show less calcium deposition than in primary hyperparathyroidism, and renal calculi are less frequent.

OTHER ABNORMALITIES

Parathyroid cysts large enough to be clinically apparent are rare. They may occur within the thyroid gland and the mediastinum as well as in the lower neck near the thyroid gland. A few have been associated with hyperparathyroidism, perhaps because of the accumulation of the hormone within the cyst fluid. Such functional examples must be distinguished from cystic adenomas.

Inflammatory processes in parathyroid tissue are unusual and may be associated with different degrees of glandular function.[82] Sometimes inflammation in the thyroid gland extends into one or several glands. Rarely part of the gland tissue is replaced by amyloidosis or by secondary carcinoma, such as carcinomas of the lung and the thyroid gland.

REFERENCES
General; development and structure

1. Castleman, B., and Roth, S.I.: Tumors of the parathyroid glands. In Atlas of tumor pathology, ser. 2, fascicle 14, Washington, D.C., 1978, Armed Forces Institute of Pathology.
2. Dufour, D.R., and Wilkerson, S.Y.: The normal parathyroid revisited: percentage of stromal fat, Hum. Pathol. 13:717, 1982.
3. Dufour, D.R., and Wilkerson, S.Y.: Factors related to parathyroid weight in normal persons, Arch. Pathol. Lab. Med. 107:167, 1983.
4. Ghandur-Mnaymneh, L., Satterfield, S., and Block, N.L.: The parathyroid gland in health and disease, Am. J. Pathol. 125:292, 1986.
5. Gilmour, J.R.: The embryology of the parathyroid glands, the thymus, and certain associated rudiments, J. Pathol. Bacteriol. 45:507, 1937.
6. Gilmour, J.R.: The gross anatomy of the parathyroid glands, J. Pathol. Bacteriol. 46:133, 1938.
7. Gilmour, J.R.: The normal histology of the parathyroid glands, J. Pathol. Bacteriol. 48:187, 1939.
8. Nilsson, O.: Studies on the ultrastructure of the human parathyroid glands in various pathological conditions, Acta Pathol. Microbiol. Scand. [C] 263(suppl.):1, 1977.
9. Roth, S.I., and Capen, C.C.: Ultrastructural and functional correlations of the parathyroid gland, Int. Rev. Exp. Pathol. 13:161, 1974.
10. Thiele, J.: The human parathyroid chief cell—a model for a polypeptide hormone producing endocrine unit as revealed by various functional and pathological conditions: a thin section and freeze-fracture study, J. Submicrosc. Cytol. 18:205, 1986.
11. Thompson, N.W., Eckhauser, F.E., and Harness, J.K.: The anatomy of primary hyperparathyroidism, Surgery 92:814, 1982.
12. Wang, C.-A.: The anatomic basis of parathyroid surgery, Ann. Surg. 183:271, 1976.

Hormones; regulation of calcium metabolism

13. Audran, M., Gross, M., and Kumar, R.: The physiology of the vitamin D endocrine system, Semin. Nephrol. 6:4, 1986.
14. Carroll, P.R., and Clark, O.H.: Milk alkali syndrome. Does it exist and can it be differentiated from primary hyperparathyroidism? Ann. Surg. 197:427, 1983.

15. Chase, L.R., and Aurbach, G.D.: Renal adenyl cyclase: anatomically separate sites for parathyroid hormone and vasopressin, Science **159**:545, 1968.
16. Fisken, R.A., Heath, D.A., Somers, S., and Bold, A.M.: Hypercalcaemia in hospital patients; clinical and diagnostic aspects, Lancet **1**:202, 1981.
17. Forster, J., Querusio, L., Burchard, K.W., and Gann, D.S.: Hypercalcemia in critically ill surgical patients, Ann. Surg. **202**:512, 1985.
18. Strewler, G.J., Stern, P.H., Jacobs, J.W., Eveloff, J., Klein, R.F., Leung, S.C., Rosenblatt, M., and Nissenson, R.A.: Parathyroid hormone–like protein from human renal carcinoma cells: structural and functional homology with parathyroid hormone, J. Clin. Invest. **80**:1803, 1987.

Pathologic calcification

19. Anderson, H.C.: Calcification processes, Pathol. Annu. **15**(2):45, 1980.
20. Barr, D.P.: Pathological calcification, Physiol. Rev. **12**:593, 1932.
21. Dalinka, M.K., and Melchior, E.L.: Soft tissue calcifications in systemic disease, Bull. NY Acad. Med. **56**:539, 1980.
22. Lutz, J.F.: Calcinosis universalis, Ann. Intern. Med. **14**:1270, 1941.
23. Mortensen, J.D., and Baggenstoss, A.H.: Nephrocalcinosis: review, Am. J. Clin. Pathol. **24**:45, 1954.
24. Mulligan, R.M.: Metastatic calcification, Arch. Pathol. **43**:177, 1947.
25. Parfitt, A.M.: Soft-tissue calcification in uremia, Arch. Intern. Med. **124**:544, 1969.
26. Russell, R.G.G., Caswell, A.M., Hearn, P.R., and Sharrard, R.M.: Calcium in mineralized tissues and pathological calcification, Br. Med. Bull. **42**:435, 1986.
27. Selye, H.: Calciphylaxis, Chicago, 1962, University of Chicago Press.
28. Stewart, A.F., Horst, R., Deftos, L.J., Cadman, E.C., Lang, R., and Broadus, A.E.: Biochemical evaluation of patients with cancer-associated hypercalcemia: evidence for humoral and nonhumoral groups, N. Engl. J. Med. **303**:1377, 1980.
29. Veress, B., Malik, M.O.A., and El Hassan, A.M.: Tumoural lipocalcinosis: a clinicopathological study of 20 cases, J. Pathol. **119**:113, 1976.

Hypoparathyroidism; pseudohypoparathyroidism

30. Bainbridge, R., Mughal, Z., Mimouni, F., and Tsang, R.C.: Transient congenital hypoparathyroidism: how transient is it? J. Pediatr. **111**:866, 1987.
31. Chase, L.R., Melson, G.L., and Aurbach, G.D.: Pseudohypoparathyroidism: defective excretion of 3',5'-AMP in response to parathyroid hormone, J. Clin. Invest. **48**:1832, 1969.
32. David, L., and Anast, C.S.: Calcium metabolism in newborn infants: the interrelationship of parathyroid function and calcium, magnesium, and phosphorus metabolism in normal, "sick," and hypocalcemic newborns, J. Clin. Invest. **54**:287, 1974.
33. Drake, T.G., Albright, F., Bauer, W., and Castleman, B.: Chronic idiopathic hypoparathyroidism: report of six cases with autopsy findings in one, Ann. Intern. Med. **12**:1751, 1939.
34. Drezner, M., Neelon, F.A., and Lebovitz, H.E.: Pseudohypoparathyroidism type II: a possible defect in the reception of the cyclic AMP signal, N. Engl. J. Med. **289**:1056, 1973.
35. Farfel, Z., Brickman, A.S., Kaslow, H.R., Brothers, V.M., and Bourne, H.R.: Defect of receptor-cyclase coupling protein in pseudohypoparathyroidism, N. Engl. J. Med. **303**:237, 1980.
36. Mann, J.B., Alterman, S., and Hills, A.G.: Albright's hereditary osteodystrophy comprising pseudohypoparathyroidism and pseudo-pseudohypoparathyroidism, Ann. Intern. Med. **56**:315, 1962.
37. Mitchell, J., and Goltzman, D.: Examination of circulating parathyroid hormone in pseudohypoparathyroidism, J. Clin. Endocrinol. Metab. **61**:328, 1985.

38. Roberton, N.R.C., and Smith, M.A.: Early neonatal hypocalcaemia, Arch. Dis. Child. **50**:604, 1975.
39. Rodríguez, H.J., Villarreal, H., Jr., Klahr, S., et al.: Pseudohypoparathyroidism type II: restoration of normal renal responsiveness to parathyroid hormone by calcium administration, J. Clin. Endocrinol. Metab. **39**:693, 1974.
40. Spinner, M.W., Blizzard, R.M., and Childs, B.: Clinical and genetic heterogeneity in idiopathic Addison's disease and hypoparathyroidism, J. Clin. Endocrinol. Metab. **28**:795, 1968.
41. Taitz, L.S., Zarate-Salvador, C., and Schwartz, E.: Congenital absence of the parathyroid and thymus glands in an infant (3 and 4 pharyngeal pouch syndrome), Pediatrics **38**:412, 1966.

Hyperparathyroidism

42. Bondeson, A.-G., Bondeson, L., Ljungberg, O., and Tibblin, S.: Fat staining in parathyroid disease—diagnostic value and impact on surgical strategy: clinicopathologic analysis of 191 cases, Hum. Pathol. **16**:1255, 1985.
43. Castleman, B., and Mallory, T.B.: The pathology of the parathyroid gland in hyperparathyroidism: a study of 25 cases, Am. J. Pathol. **11**:1, 1935.
44. Chen, K.T.K.: Fat stain in hyperparathyroidism, Am. J. Surg. Pathol. **6**:191, 1982.
45. Corlew, D.S., Bryda, S.L., Bradley, E.L., III, and DiGirolamo, M.: Observations on the course of untreated primary hyperparathyroidism, Surgery **98**:1064, 1985.
46. Falko, J.M., Maeder, M.C., Conway, C., Mazzaferri, E.L., and Skillman, T.G.: Primary hyperparathyroidism: analysis of 220 patients with special emphasis on familial hypocalciuric hypercalcemia, Heart Lung **13**:124, 1984.
47. Heath, H., III, Hodgson, S.F., and Kennedy, M.A.: Primary hyperparathyroidism: incidence, morbidity, and potential economic impact in a community, N. Engl. J. Med. **302**:189, 1980.
48. Hellström, J., and Ivemark, B.I.: Primary hyperparathyroidism: clinical and structural findings in 138 cases, Acta Chir. Scand. **294**(suppl.):1, 1962.
49. Kelly, T.R.: Primary hyperparathyroidism: a personal experience with 242 cases, Am. J. Surg. **140**:632, 1980.
50. Larsson, L., Eneström, S., and Gillquist, J.: Biochemical and morphological findings in patients with increased serum ionized calcium, Acta Chir. Scand. **145**:435, 1979.
51. Lloyd, H.M.: Primary hyperparathyroidism: an analysis of the role of the parathyroid tumor, Medicine **47**:53, 1968.
52. Pugh, D.G.: Subperiosteal resorption of bone: a roentgenologic manifestation of primary hyperparathyroidism and renal osteodystrophy, Am. J. Roentgenol. **66**:577, 1951.
53. Pyrah, L.N., Hodgkinson, A., and Anderson, C.K.: Primary hyperparathyroidism, Br. J. Surg. **53**:245, 1966.
54. Rogers, H.M., Keating, F.R., Jr., Morlock, C.G., and Barker, N.W.: Primary hypertrophy and hyperplasia of the parathyroid glands associated with duodenal ulcer: report of an additional case, with special reference to metabolic, gastrointestinal, and vascular manifestations, Arch. Intern. Med. **79**:307, 1947.
55. Rudberg, C., Åkerström, G., Palmér, M., Ljunghall, S., Adami, H.O., Johansson, H., Grimelius, L., Thorén, L., and Bergström, R.: Late results of operation for primary hyperparathyroidism in 441 patients, Surgery **99**:643, 1986.
56. Salazar, J., Dembrow, V., and Egozi, I.: A review of 265 cases of parathyroid explorations, Am. Surg. **52**:174, 1986.

Secondary hyperplasia

57. Åkerström, G., Malmaeus, J., Grimelius, L., Ljunghall, S., and Bergström, R.: Histological changes in parathyroid glands in subclinical and clinical renal disease: an autopsy investigation, Scand. J. Urol. Nephrol. **18**:75, 1984.
58. Åkerström, G., Rudberg, C., Grimelius, L., Bergström, R., Johansson, H., Ljunghall, S., and Rastad, J.: Histologic parathyroid abnormalities in an autopsy series, Hum. Pathol. **17**:520, 1986.
59. Castleman, B., and Mallory, T.B.: Parathyroid hyperplasia in chronic renal insufficiency, Am. J. Pathol. **13**:553, 1937.

Primary hyperplasia and adenoma

60. Albright, F., Bloomberg, E., Castleman, B., and Churchill, E.D.: Hyperparathyroidism due to diffuse hyperplasia of all parathyroid glands rather than adenoma of one: clinical studies on three such cases, Arch. Intern. Med. **54:**315, 1934.
61. Arnold, B.M.: Kovacs, K., Horvath, E., Murray, T.M., and Higgins, H.P.: Functioning oxyphil cell adenoma of the parathyroid gland: evidence for parathyroid secretory activity of oxyphil cells, J. Clin. Endocrinol. Metab. **38:**458, 1974.
62. Badder, E.M., Graham, W.P., and Harrison, T.S.: Functional insignificance of microscopic parathyroid hyperplasia, Surg. Gynecol. Obstet. **145:**863, 1977.
63. Castleman, B., Schantz, A., and Roth, S.I.: Parathyroid hyperplasia in primary hyperparathyroidism: a review of 85 cases, Cancer **38:**1668, 1976.
64. Ducatman, B.S., Wilkerson, S.Y., and Brown, J.A.: Functioning parathyroid lipoadenoma: report of a case diagnosed by intraoperative touch preparations, Arch. Pathol. Lab. Med. **110:**645, 1986.
65. Fialkow, P.J., Jackson, C.E., Block, M.A., et al.: Multicellular origin of parathyroid "adenomas," N. Engl. J. Med. **297:**696, 1977.
66. Ghandur-Mnaymneh, L., and Kimura, N.: The parathyroid adenoma: a histopathologic definition with a study of 172 cases of primary hyperparathyroidism, Am. J. Pathol. **115:**70, 1984.
67. Golden, A., Canary, J.J., and Kerwin, D.M.: Concurrence of hyperplasia and neoplasia of the parathyroid glands, Am. J. Med. **38:**562, 1965.
68. Liechty, R.D., Teter, A., and Suba, E.J.: The tiny parathyroid adenoma, Surgery **100:**1048, 1986.
69. Stout, L.C., Jr.: Water-clear-cell hyperplasia mimicking parathyroid adenoma, Hum. Pathol. **16:**1075, 1985.
70. Thorgeirsson, U., Costa, J., and Marx, S.J.: The parathyroid glands in familial hypocalciuric hypercalcemia, Hum. Pathol. **12:**229, 1981.

Tertiary hyperparathyroidism

71. Krause, M.W., and Hedinger, C.E.: Pathologic study of parathyroid glands in tertiary hyperparathyroidism, Hum. Pathol. **16:**772, 1985.

Carcinoma

72. Cohn, K., Silverman, M., Corrado, J., and Sedgewick, C.: Parathyroid carcinoma: the Lahey Clinic experience, Surgery **98:**1095, 1985.
73. Schantz, A., and Castleman, B.: Parathyroid carcinoma: a study of 70 cases, Cancer **31:**600, 1973.
74. Smith, J.F., and Coombs, R.R.H.: Histological diagnosis of carcinoma of the parathyroid gland, J. Clin. Pathol. **37:**1370, 1984.

Lesions associated with hyperparathyroidism

75. Andersen, D.H., and Schlesinger, E.R.: Renal hyperparathyroidism with calcification of the arteries in infancy, Am. J. Dis. Child. **63:**102, 1942.
76. Anderson, W.A.D.: Hyperparathyroidism and renal disease, Arch. Pathol. **27:**753, 1939.
77. Follis, R.H., Jr., and Jackson, D.A.: Renal osteomalacia and osteitis fibrosa in adults, Bull. Johns Hopkins Hosp. **72:**232, 1943.
78. Herbert, F.K., Miller, H.G., and Richardson, G.O.: Chronic renal disease, secondary parathyroid hyperplasia, decalcification of bone and metastatic calcification, J. Pathol. Bacteriol. **53:**161, 1941.
79. Mehls, O., Ritz, E., Kreusser, W., and Krempien, B.: Renal osteodystrophy in uraemic children, Clin. Endocrinol. Metab. **9:**151, 1980.
80. Sherrard, D.J.: Renal osteodystrophy, Semin. Nephrol. **6:**56, 1986.
81. Slatopolsky, E.: The interaction of parathyroid hormone and aluminum in renal osteodystrophy, Kidney Int. **31:**842, 1987.

Other abnormalities

82. Bondeson, A.-G., Bondeson, L., and Ljungberg, O.: Chronic parathyroiditis associated with parathyroid hyperplasia and hyperparathyroidism, Am. J. Surg. Pathol. **8:**211, 1984.
83. Ramos-Gabatin, A., Mallette, L.E., Bringhurst, F.R., and Draper, M.W.: Functional mediastinal parathyroid cyst: dynamics of parathyroid hormone secretion during cyst aspirations and surgery, Am. J. Med. **79:**633, 1985.
84. Rosenberg, J., Orlando, R., III, Ludwig, M., and Pyrtek, L.J.: Parathyroid cysts, Am. J. Surg. **143:**473, 1982.

33 The Adrenal Glands

JOHN G. GRUHN
VICTOR E. GOULD

The adrenal consists of two anatomically and physiologically distinct components that also differ in embryologic origin and development—the cortex and the medulla.[1-8]

Eustachius[3] first depicted the adrenals in 1552. In 1611, Bartholinus the Elder[1] called them "atrabiliary capsules" and suggested that they were detoxifying organs. In 1629, Riolan[6] coined the term "suprarenal capsules," which Addison later used. By 1805, Cuvier[2] distinguished the cortex from the medulla.

The adrenal cortex is an endocrine organ that produces hormones essential for life. Cortical disorders are relatively rare. Clinical signs and symptoms suggestive of adrenocortical disorders are highly prevalent but are nonspecific; hence selective laboratory testing is needed to discriminate genuine adrenal disorders from their mimics. Adrenocortical disorders may produce spectacular clinical syndromes; thus they fascinate clinicians. Morphologic changes in the cortex often cannot and usually should not be interpreted without a context of clinical, biochemical, and functional data.

STRUCTURE

The right adrenal tends to be pyramidal, the left crescentic. The right adrenal sits closely adjacent to the inferior vena cava. Modern diagnostic imaging techniques permit accurate clinical evaluation of the gross anatomy of the adrenal; CT technology permits identification of more than 99% of normal adrenal glands and can allow detection of masses of the order of 1 cm.[38-45]

The adult human adrenal consists of a head, body, and tail. Medullary tissue is concentrated in the body and head. On section, the outer cortex is yellow, whereas the inner cortex is brown and the medulla is gray. The normal cortex measures 1 to 2 mm in width.

The average weight of normal adrenal glands removed surgically (as from patients with breast cancer) or from "normal nonhospitalized adults" who died suddenly from trauma has been stated to be from 4.16 to 4.6 g per adrenal.[24,28,30] To attain an accurate weight, all fat must be removed from the adrenal. Adrenal weight is important in the evaluation of hyperplasia or atrophy.

The adrenal cortex consists of three zones—the glomerulosa, the fasciculata, and the reticularis. The glomerulosa of man does not usually form an outer layer of uniform thickness. It may be focally discontinuous and sometimes extends into the fasciculata as triangular wedges. The glomerulosa consists of ovoid pockets of cuboid cells with relatively clear cytoplasm. It makes up approximately 10% of the cortex. The fasciculata consists of parallel cords of light or clear cells that make up approximately 70% of the cortex. The reticularis consists of interconnecting cords of more compact eosinophilic staining cells; it makes up the remainder of the cortex.[9-12,14,16-18,20-21,23,25-27,29,31,33-34]

Ultrastructurally, steroid-producing adrenocortical cells have a rich smooth endoplasmic reticulum and prominent mitochondria with tubular cristae.[13,35]

Three adrenal arteries supply each gland—the superior adrenal artery arising from the inferior phrenic artery, the middle adrenal artery arising from the aorta, and the inferior adrenal artery arising from the renal artery.[17,40] The left adrenal vein joins the inferior phrenic vein and enters the left renal vein. On the right, three venous trunks form a common vein that joins the posterior aspect of the inferior vena cava directly in 90% of cases; in 10% of cases, it enters the vena cava through a hepatic vein.[17]

EARLY DEVELOPMENT

The cortex and medulla arise from separate primordia. In some lower species the cortex and medulla are topographically separate organs.[19,46-52]

In 1861, Kölliker[48] demonstrated that the cortex forms during fetal development from the mesodermal urogenital ridge and that neural elements subsequently enter to form the medulla.

During the perinatal period, the adrenal gland is quite large in relation to the kidney; the fetal adrenal gland is about 20 times its relative size in the adult and may reach a weight of 2 to 4 g each at birth. In the neonate, the adrenal is about one third the weight of the kidney (Fig. 33-1).[50,51]

During the last two trimesters of pregnancy, the normal adrenal cortex greatly increases in width; it consists of two zones, an outer cortex, which will persist, and an inner fetal cortex, which may occupy 75% of the cortex, which involutes later.

The fetal cortex lacks enzymes such as 3β-hydroxydehydrogenase; hence it cannot make cortisol, corticosterone, or aldosterone, but it converts pregnenolone sulfate formed in the placenta to dehydroepiandrosterone, which is hydroxylated by the fetal liver to 16α-hydroxy-dehydroepiandrosterone,[52] which in turn is converted to estriol in the placenta. The fetal cortex involutes rapidly after birth.

Characteristically, anencephalic fetuses have either no pituitary or a very hypoplastic pituitary.[50,52,78] It is not surprising that anencephalics have hypoplastic adrenals lacking a fetal cortex. The adrenals may be absent in some anencephalics. The fetal zone is usually normal in anencephalics until the early second trimester, but it degenerates during the latter period of pregnancy. Urinary excretion rates of estrogens are reduced in mothers bearing an anencephalic fetus.

One or both adrenals may be absent. Bilateral absence is incompatible within life. Approximately 10% of babies with unilateral renal agenesis lack the corresponding adrenal.

Heterotopic adrenal tissue may be found at many sites related embryologically to the urogenital ridge; these include the retroperitoneal space, the root of the mesentery, the region of coeliac plexus, the spermatic cord, the hilum of the testis and ovary, the site beneath the renal or hepatic capsules, and so on.[49] Rarely the adrenals may be fused. Most of these heterotopic tissues are of no clinical relevance but may provide sites for the origin of the adrenocortical type of neoplasms.

The commonest variant is the presence of small, rounded collections of adrenal tissue just outside the capsule that have been designated as capsular extrusions. They are usually less than 2 mm in diameter and should not be misconstrued as nodules or adenomas. They have no functional significance but may be conspicuous in cases of adrenal hyperplasia.

FUNCTION

Cortical function is controlled by two major tropic hormone systems: (1) ACTH for the synthesis of cortisol and androgens, and (2) angiotensin for the synthesis of aldosterone. The fasciculata and reticularis are under the control of the pituitary (ACTH); they produce the glucocorticoids (cortisone) and "sex steroids." The role of hypothalamic corticotropin-releasing factor (CRH) is now well established. The zona glomerulosa functions relatively independent of the pituitary; it produces the hormones regulating electrolyte balance (aldosterone).

The adrenal cortex produces more than 50 steroids in three principal groups.* Aldosterone, a mineralocorticoid, is manufactured principally in the glomerulosa. Glucocorticoids (cortisol) are manufactured in the fasciculata and reticularis as are "sex steroids." Glucocorticoids and mineralocorticoids are 21-carbon compounds essential for life. The "sex steroids" are 18- or 19-carbon compounds. Normally, dehydroisoandrosterone (also called dehydroepiandrosterone), a weak androgen, is the "sex steroid" produced in the largest quantity.

Normally at least nine enzymes (Fig. 33-2) are involved in the major biosynthetic pathway. Pregnenolone is produced from precursor cholesterol. Normally enzymatic transformations from pregnenolone to the end products (cortisol, aldosterone, and DHEA) occur rapidly without the accumulation of significant amounts of biosynthetic intermediates, which would be of pathophysiologic import. Adrenal steroids are *not* stored in the cortex. The amounts present are not sufficient to maintain normal rates of secretion for more than a few minutes without continuing biosynthesis. The major biosynthetic pathways are illustrated in Fig. 33-2.

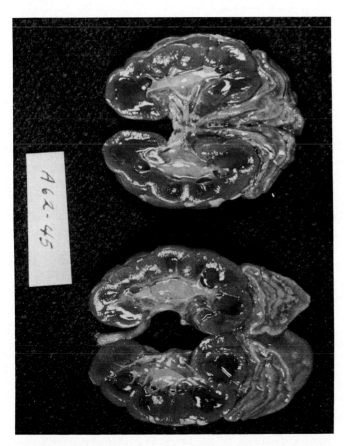

Fig. 33-1. Large adrenals in the normal newborn.

---

*References 10, 14, 15, 18, 23, 25, 27, 36.

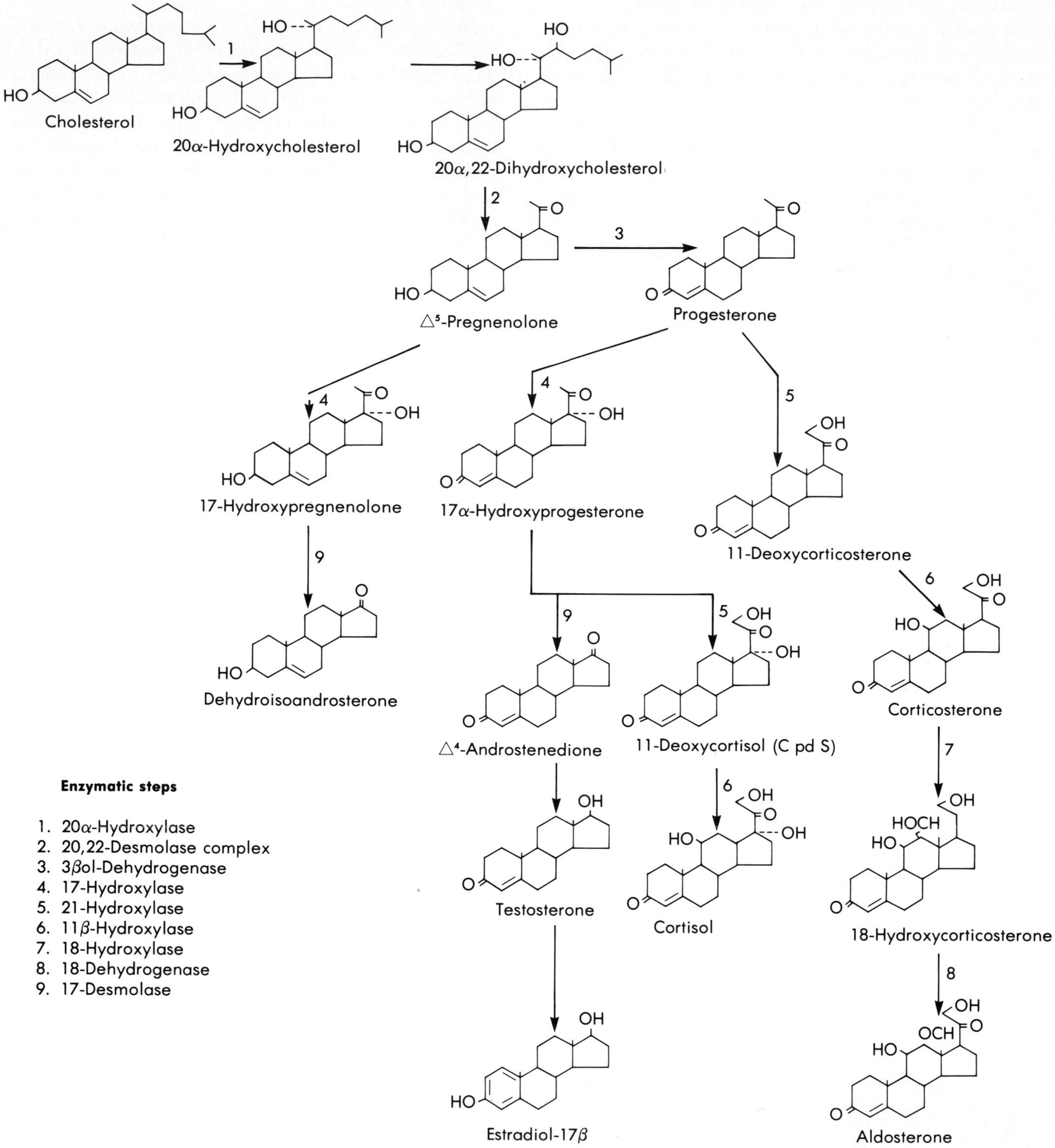
Cholesterol
20α-Hydroxycholesterol
20α,22-Dihydroxycholesterol
Δ⁵-Pregnenolone
Progesterone
17-Hydroxypregnenolone
17α-Hydroxyprogesterone
11-Deoxycorticosterone
Dehydroisoandrosterone
Δ⁴-Androstenedione
11-Deoxycortisol (C pd S)
Corticosterone
Testosterone
Cortisol
18-Hydroxycorticosterone
Estradiol-17β
Aldosterone
Enzymatic steps
1. 20α-Hydroxylase
2. 20,22-Desmolase complex
3. 3βol-Dehydrogenase
4. 17-Hydroxylase
5. 21-Hydroxylase
6. 11β-Hydroxylase
7. 18-Hydroxylase
8. 18-Dehydrogenase
9. 17-Desmolase

Fig. 33-2. Major biosynthetic pathways for adrenal steroids. The enzymatic steps are from *1* to *9*.

Since the steroids are not stored, the rates of synthesis are approximately the rates of secretion. Throughout the day the mean plasma concentration of a given steroid equals the rates of the secretion rate divided by the metabolic clearance rate of the steroid. Urinary excretion rates are measured routinely just as plasma levels of hormones are.

One must be familiar with the tests of adrenal function to correlate structure with function.[10,14,22-23,32,36-37] Current technology permits reasonably precise diagnostic evaluation of adrenocortical function and the hypothalamic-pituitary-adrenal axis.

DISORDERS OF INFANCY AND CHILDHOOD
Adrenal hypoplasia

Several types of adrenal hypoplasia may occur in infants and children, the principal ones being hypoplasia associated with anencephaly, hypoplasia associated with pituitary aplasia or hypoplasia, hypoplasia associated with hypothalamic malformations, idiopathic hypoplasia, adrenal cytomegaly in the newborn, and precocious involution. Adrenal hypoplasia associated with anencephaly has already been discussed. Those associated with pituitary aplasia or hypoplasia or with hypothalamic malformations are virtually identical to those associated with anencephaly.

Idiopathic hypoplasia. There are several forms of idiopathic hypoplasia.[59,61-63,66,71,76-77] The pituitary and hypothalamus are morphologically unremarkable in these cases.

Criteria that have been sited include the following:
1. Each gland is less than 1 g and is less than one twelfth the weight of the corresponding kidney.
2. The adrenal weight is less than one eight-hundredth the body weight for a premature baby or less than one seven-hundredth for a mature infant.

At least three different histologic patterns of adrenal morphology have been reported:
1. In one type, the adrenals resemble those associated with a primary pituitary disorder though the pituitary is normal.
2. Another group is associated with adrenal cytomegaly, which is subsequently discussed.
3. A third form reported by Larroche[65] manifests a miniature of the normal adrenal.

Several different modes of genetic inheritance including autosomal recessive and sex-linked modes have been reported.[70,88] No definite correlation between morphologic pattern and mode of inheritance has yet been established.

Idiopathic hypoplasia may be congenital, more common in males, and familial. A familial variant in females is said to be resistant to ACTH.

The diagnosis of adrenal hypoplasia is seldom made clinically.

Adrenal cytomegaly in the newborn. Cytomegaly is usually an incidental finding in adrenals of normal weight in newborns, but it may be associated with hypoplasia.[53,64,68] Adrenal cytomegaly is a morphologic phenomenon that may occur in from 1% to 3% of newborns, prematures, or stillborn infants. No known clinical abnormality is usually associated with these morphologic changes. Fetal cortical cells may reach 100 μm in diameter; their cytoplasm is brightly eosinophilic. Vacuoles may be present in the cytoplasm, and cytoplasmic evaginations into the nuclei may mimic nuclear inclusions. No cellular inflammatory reaction is usually present. This condition should not be confused with cytomegalovirus inclusions. These lesions are more common in Beckwith's syndrome. Neither the cause nor the significance of this lesion is currently known.

Precocious involution. Precocious involution of the fetal cortex may occur in postmature infants or in various newborn illnesses.

Adrenal leukodystrophy

The concurrence of diffuse demyelination of cerebral white matter and the adrenal atrophy has been known since 1923. Adrenal leukodystrophy is now known to be the result of a basic metabolic defect involving very long chain fatty acids; culture of skin fibroblasts from these patients reveals excessive synthesis of hexacosanoic and other long-chain fatty acids.[72-74] Inheritance is based on an X-linked recessive transmission, affecting males almost exclusively. Four clinical forms have been described.

The cerebral disorder is a diffuse sudanophilic demyelinating process.

Ultrastructurally, the earliest adrenal lesion is the appearance of intracytoplasmic striations in cortical cells that appear as lipid-lamellar profiles with trilaminar structure because of the formation of abnormal long-chain fatty acids (Fig. 33-3). This interferes with normal steroidogenesis, produces decreased cortisol levels, and induces ACTH overproduction.

The adrenal cortices may become severely atrophic, the medulla is unaffected, and the glomerulosa may be spared while the inner fasciculata and reticularis are most severely affected. These zones may have ballooned cells containing inclusions, which may stain metachromatically with periodic acid–Schiff stain. The ballooning and vacuolation may be a consequence of ACTH stimulation. There is also striation of the cytoplasm. Adrenolysis tends to outstrip regeneration, leading to severe atrophy. There may also be lymphocytic infiltration, but usually inflammatory reaction is not a feature.

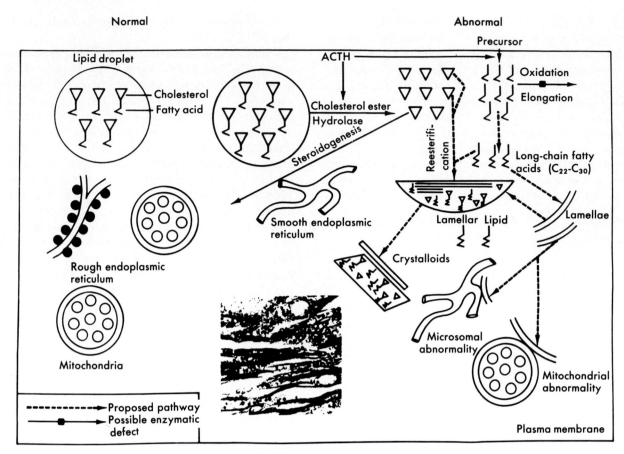

Fig. 33-3. Schema of adrenal leukodystrophy. Intracellular lesion in adrenoleukodystrophy involves formation of abnormal long-chain fatty acids that interfere with steroidogenesis and produce cytoplasmic lamellar lipid striations shown in inset. (22,000×; modified from Powers, J.M., et al.: Invest. Cell Pathol. **3:**353, 1980.)

Electron microscopic studies by Martin and co-workers have also demonstrated curved or rectilinear clefts in Schwann cells from skin and conjunctiva.[58]

Congenital adrenal hyperplasia

All forms of congenital adrenal hyperplasia are the result of diminution or absence of enzymes essential for steroid biosynthesis.[54-58,67,69,82-87,89] The biochemical common denominator is reduction in the production of cortisol followed by a compensatory increase in ACTH secretion. Precursor steroids proximal to the block may accumulate and may be shunted to other metabolic pathways involving androgen biosynthesis or excess mineralocorticoid synthesis, or both.

Currently recognized enzymatic defects, their frequency, and the ensuing clinical syndromes have been summarized by White and co workers[82]; the clinical features are naturally related to the site of the enzyme block. Since it is now possible to diagnose and treat these syndromes, gross and microscopic sections of

adrenal glands are no longer usually available for pathologic study. Distinctive gross and microscopic patterns have been described for some of these syndromes. In most of these syndromes, the adrenals are enlarged; sometimes the weight of both glands together reached 20 g. Most of these disorders cannot be differentiated from one another solely by histologic criteria.

Molecular genetic techniques have provided significant new data that may influence prenatal diagnosis and therapy.[82] For example, 20-hydroxylase deficiency is now known to be inherited as a monogenic autosomal recessive trait closely related to the HLA major histocompatibility complex on the short arm of chromosome 6. It has been suggested that the locus for 21-hydroxylase deficiency is located between HLA-B and HLA-DR near the class III genes. The various forms of this particular deficiency are inherited as alleles at a single locus.

Several recent monographs provide detailed discussions of congenital adrenal hyperplasia.[67,69]

Other neonatal hyperplasias

At least three other conditions with adrenal hyperplasia in the newborn infant have been reported.[31] Infants of diabetic mothers may have increased urinary corticoids as part of an edematous, pseudoerythroblastosis syndrome, sometimes with an apparent increase of fetal cortical width. In infants dying of erythroblastosis fetalis or α-thalassemia, the fetal cortex may be thick and excessively vacuolated; an accompanying thymic atrophy is suggestive of adrenal hyperfunction, possibly because of chronic intrauterine hypoxia. Antenatal infection is also reported to be associated with adrenocortical hyperplasia in the newborn.

Acquired disorders in infants and children

Hemorrhage. Clinically significant hemorrhage is relatively uncommon. Hemorrhage is more common in premature and postmature infants. Some hemorrhage may occur in 10% of newborns. In adults, anticoagulant therapy is the most common cause of adrenal hemorrhage. Hemorrhage usually occurs at the junction of the provisional and definitive cortex. There are several reports of massive hemorrhage that were treated surgically. Very rarely hemorrhage may be associated with adrenal insufficiency.[33,104]

Waterhouse-Friderichsen syndrome. In 1911, Waterhouse[81] described "a case of suprarenal apoplexy," and in 1918, Friderichsen[60] described adrenal apoplexy in small children. They described fulminant meningococcemia manifested by profound irreversible peripheral circulatory collapse, cutaneous petechiae, and massive bilateral adrenal hemorrhage. Since fibrin microthrombi are frequently found in the capillaries of the adrenals and other organs, disseminated intravascular coagulation (DIC) is a significant pathologic feature of this syndrome. Pathogenetically, this syndrome is an endotoxemia; it represents a clinical instance of the generalized Shwartzman reaction whereby activation of the coagulation mechanisms induces DIC resulting in ischemic hemorrhagic necrosis. Endotoxemia attributable to other gram-negative bacteria, especially Enterobacteriaceae and *Pseudomonas*, may also induce the Waterhouse-Friderichsen syndrome, which is attributable to endotoxemia not to microthrombi. Injection of purified endotoxin into animals produces a shock syndrome identical to that occurring in gram-negative bacteremia. Antibodies against endotoxin can greatly reduce the occurrence of shock in gram-negative bacteremia. Neither the fibrin microthrombi nor the adrenal hemorrhage are responsible for the shock syndrome that is attributable to endotoxemia. Patients may die rapidly before cortisol levels are significantly reduced. There is still clinical controversy regarding the role of acute adrenal insufficiency in the mortality associated with adrenal hemorrhage and regarding the role of cortisol therapy.

Infections in neonates. The adrenal cortex is relatively resistant to common bacterial infections, but staphylococcal sepsis may be associated with adrenal abscesses.

Before the availability of modern antibiotics, tuberculosis accounted for almost 90% of granulomatous destruction that produced Addison's disease in children. Histoplasmosis is now more common in childhood than tuberculosis is. Mycotic infections such as candidiasis and aspergillosis are not rare in terminal childhood leukemias at autopsy.

In about half the autopsied cases of infantile toxoplasmosis, adrenal granulomas with or without recognizable organisms are found. In generalized histoplasmosis, coccidioidomycosis, and brucellosis, there occur epithelioid, caseous, or partly calcified adrenal granulomas, sometimes extensive enough to cause death from adrenocortical insufficiency. Congenital syphilis may show subcapsular adrenal fibrosis and abundant treponemes. Tuberculous Addison's disease of children is similar to the adult condition. Listeriosis may also produce granulomas.

Infections producing necrosis. Hepatoadrenal necrosis is another usually fatal lesion, especially in premature infants with systemic herpes simplex infection acquired at birth, probably by transmission from maternal herpes vaginitis.[75,79-80] Both the adrenocortical and hepatic cells are extensively destroyed. Some contain intranuclear Cowdry type A inclusion bodies. Cytomegalic inclusion disease is accompanied by typical, large, intranuclear viral inclusions, and cortical necrosis is about one third of generalized cytomegalovirus infections. Comparable adrenal involvement may occur in adults as a complication of immunosuppression associated with lymphoma or leukemia. Systemic *Pneumocystis* or *Cryptococcus* infections may localize in the adrenal glands. Varicella and herpes zoster of the adrenal glands produce medullary intranuclear inclusions.

Cushing's syndrome in childhood

About 20% of cases of Cushing's syndrome develop before puberty. Guinn and Albert reported a 3-month-old infant who developed Cushing's syndrome because of an adrenocortical carcinoma. During childhood, Cushing's syndrome is usually attributable to a functioning, hormone-producing adrenocortical carcinoma rather than to pituitary-induced cortical hyperplasia. The disorder tends to progress rapidly and has a poor prognosis. Two thirds of the patients are females. With functioning tumors, ACTH is suppressed and the opposite and contiguous adrenal becomes atrophic.

Hyperaldosteronism in children

In children, hyperaldosteronism is more likely to be attributable to cortical hyperplasia than cortical adenoma, the reverse of what occurs in adults.

Neoplasms in children

Most cortical neoplasms in children produce overt endocrinologic changes, and a majority have been regarded as malignant.[58] Recently Cagle and coworkers[141] suggested that histologic criteria for adult neoplasms may lead to overdiagnosis of pediatric tumors.

HYPOCORTISOLISM—ADRENAL INSUFFICIENCY (ADDISON'S SYNDROME)

Thomas Addison[90] originally reported in 1849 the disorder that now bears his name. He was the first to relate a clinical syndrome to a specific endocrine organ.

Pathophysiologic mechanisms

It is now recognized that the basic pathophysiology of Addison's syndrome is hypocortisolism, which may be attributable to any of the mechanisms included in following outline:*

I. Primary adrenal disorder—destruction or cell loss
  A. Adults
    1. Addison's disease
      a. Idiopathic (autoimmune; approximately 80% of cases)
      b. Infectious or granulomatous
        (1) Tuberculosis (approximately 10% of cases)
        (2) Fungal
        (3) Other
      c. Amyloidosis
      d. Metastatic carcinoma
      e. Lymphoma
      f. Miscellaneous, including sarcoidosis and hemochromatosis
    2. Massive hemorrhage
  B. Congenital lesions (usually in children)
    1. Congenital adrenal hypoplasia—cytomegalic or karyomegalic type
    2. Congenital adrenal hyperplasia (adrenogenital syndrome)
    3. Congenital lipoid hyperplasia
    4. Adrenal cyst
II. Primary hypothalamic or pituitary disorder (secondary adrenocortical insufficiency caused by lack of ACTH)
  A. Adults
    1. Pituitary tumors
    2. Pituitary infarction
      a. Sheehan's syndrome
      b. Simmond's disease
    3. Hypophysectomy
    4. Pituitary destruction caused by
      a. Irradiation
      b. Metastases
      c. Infections
    5. Isolated ACTH deficiency
    6. Abrupt withdrawal after prolonged cortisol administration
  B. Children
    1. Disorder caused by anencephaly, etc.
    2. Disorder consequent to congenital adrenal hypoplasia—anencephalic type

Clinical syndrome

The clinical signs and symptoms of primary adrenocortical dysfunction reflect the low corticoid levels, low sodium levels, and depletion of blood volume together with the effects of increased melanin-stimulating hormone in the pituitary.[10,14,18,23,26] The latter effect does not occur in primary hypothalamic or pituitary disorders. The clinical phenomena include fatigue, muscular weakness, weight loss, skin and mucous membrane hyperpigmentation, hypotension, anorexia, nausea, and vomiting and may include salt craving.

Laboratory diagnosis

Common abnormal findings commonly noted on routine laboratory tests include hyponatremia (88%), hyperkalemia (64%), azotemia, anemia, eosinophilia, lymphocytosis, hypoglycemia, and hypercalcemia.

Specific laboratory studies of patients suspected to have adrenocortical deficiency usually include rapid ACTH stimulation tests, plasma ACTH, and other determinations to establish the existence of adrenocortical deficiency and determine whether there is primary or secondary adrenocortical disease.[10,14,18,23,26,32,37]

The pathologic processes

Idiopathic or autoimmune disease. Currently in developed countries an autoimmune disorder is responsible for approximately 80% of primary adrenocortical insufficiency. This process has also been designated as idiopathic atrophy, cytotoxic atrophy, or lymphocytic adrenalitis.

From 51% to 74% of patients with idiopathic Addison's disease have adrenal antibodies.* Autoimmune Addison's disease may occur alone or in combination with other autoimmune disorders and may be associated with the presence of several autoantibodies to adrenal, thyroid, gastric parietal, gonadal, and other

---

*References 10-12, 14, 18, 21, 23, 25, 26, 33, 97, 99, 101, 105, 106, 113.

*References 91-94, 96, 98, 102, 107, 108, 112.

cells. Addison's disease may be associated with thyrotoxicosis, Hashimoto's thyroiditis, goiter, pernicious anemia, diabetes, hypoparathyroidism, gonadal failure, and vitiligo. Concurrent Addison's disease and Hashimoto's disease have been dubbed "Schmidt's syndrome."[94,111] Recent studies of histocompatibility antigens (HLA groups) indicate that genes controlling immune responses may be closely linked and may eventually prove to be the common denominator for these processes.[96,110]

Grossly the adrenals in autoimmune (idiopathic) Addison's disease are small and contracted; they have been described as leaflike. Average combined weights range from about 2 to 3 g. It may be difficult to recognize the adrenals at autopsy in advanced cases. Histologically the medulla is preserved, but the cortex is disorganized, and there is loss of cortical cells. The cortex is infiltrated with lymphocytes and plasma cells in early stages and becomes fibrotic in later stages. In end-stage disease, there may be a few mononucleated cells, and residual antibodies may no longer be detected (Fig. 33-4).[12,26-27,30-31,34]

Granulomatous diseases

Tuberculosis. In the decade 1928 to 1938, tuberculosis still accounted for 79% of cases of Addison's disease. Currently, it accounts for approximately 10% in developed countries.[109] Patients with widespread disseminated tuberculosis do not usually manifest Addison's disease, and patients with extensive adrenocortical tuberculosis often manifest little evidence of widespread tuberculosis. In contrast with the autoimmune process, the medulla is virtually always destroyed along with the cortex. Anatomically the adrenals are usually enlarged (Fig. 33-5). Histologically, caseous necrosis predominates.[12,26,27,30,31,33] The granulomatous reaction tends to be suppressed. It is generally considered that high local cortisol concentration initially diminishes the local inflammatory reaction. More than 90% of the cortex must be destroyed to produce Addison's disease.

Others. Granulomatous disease may also be attributable to histoplasmosis, candidiasis, coccidioidomycosis, blastomycosis, paracoccidioidomycosis, and leprosy. Since the tissue reactions may be similar, diagnosis depends on identification of the causal organism.*

Amyloidosis. Amyloidosis accounts for fewer than 1% of cases of Addison's disease.[30,31,33,99,100] Primary amyloidosis is usually confined to the walls of arterioles but

---

*References 12, 26, 27, 30, 31, 33, 95, 103.

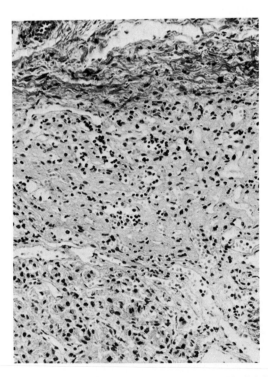

Fig. 33-4. Idiopathic adrenocortical atrophy with Addison's disease. Cortical cells have practically disappeared and stroma is collapsed. Adrenal medulla and central veins can be seen below. (120×.)

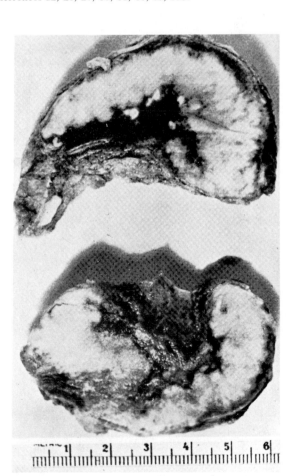

Fig. 33-5. Tuberculosis of adrenal glands in Addison's disease.

may rarely produce Addison's disease. More commonly, secondary amyloidosis, associated with processes such as rheumatoid arthritis, caused amyloid deposition in the cortex. Deposition massive enough to cause Addison's disease is very rare. When amyloidosis causes Addison's disease, the adrenals may be enlarged to a combined weight of 30 to 40 g and may be firm, gray, and translucent.

Miscellaneous processes. Addison's disease attributable to metastatic neoplasms is rare. Adrenal leukodystrophy, familial cytomegalic adrenocortical hypoplasia, and hemorrhage are other rare causes.

Secondary Addison's disease caused by primary pituitary disorders. Destruction of the pituitary (Simmond's disease, Sheehan's syndrome, neoplasia, infection, or hypophysectomy) will result in a great reduction of ACTH, which contrasts with the high level of ACTH noted in primary adrenal insufficiency. This produces a simple atrophy manifested by low adrenal weight and thinned cortices consisting of cells resembling fasciculata without an inflammatory cellular infiltrate.

Iatrogenic adrenal insufficiency. Cortisol therapy also

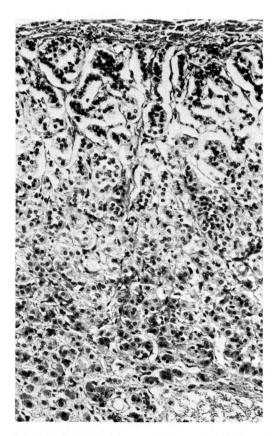

Fig. 33-6. Poststeroid atrophy. After prolonged cortisone therapy, zona fasciculata cells become shrunken and cortical thickness is reduced to 0.5 mm, half the normal width. Zona glomerulosa and zona reticularis are unaffected and appear prominent. (120×.)

suppresses ACTH and leads to iatrogenic adrenal atrophy, which was often observed by surgical pathologists during the period when patients with metastatic breast cancer were treated with steroids and bilateral adrenalectomy. The morphology of the adrenals simulates the pattern seen in primary pituitary disorders, reflecting the lack of ACTH. A similar pattern is also seen in the nontumorous adrenal tissue of patients whose Cushing's syndrome is attributable to a functioning adenoma or carcinoma of the adrenal that suppresses ACTH (Fig. 33-6).

Survival

Current therapy usually achieves a virtually normal life span for what had formerly been a disorder with a high mortality.[10,14,25]

BASIC DEFINITIONS OF SELECTED PATHOLOGIC LESIONS
Nodules

Neville and O'Hare[27] noted that "nodules . . . represent one of the principal remaining enigmas of adrenal pathology." Distinction between a nodule and an adenoma may be arbitrary. Dobbie concluded that nodular hyperplasia and so-called large adenomas represent different degrees of the same proliferated cell process.[147] There is no absolute criterion to distinguish a small solitary nodule from a small, nonfunctional, nonencapsulated adenoma. Symington noted that tiny adenomas may not be big enough to produce enough hormone to alter the plasma level or induce an endocrine syndrome.[33,34]

Although most nodules are minute, some may exceed 2 cm. Nodules commonly vary in size and shape; they are not sharply circumscribed or encapsulated. Cellular pleomorphism or nuclear enlargement is unusual. The remaining intervening adrenal cells are usually neither compressed, atrophic, nor hypertrophic. Nodules are not associated with alteration of the nonnodular cortex; by contrast, adenomas that induce hypercortisolism usually cause atrophy of the remainder of the adrenal cortex (Fig. 33-7). Small, nonfunctional nodules are of no known clinical relevance. The incidence of nodules has been reported to increase with increasing age, whereas the incidence of adenomas is reported not to increase with age. Approximately half the population over 50 years of age have multiple, small, rounded nodules of the zona fasciculata.[33,171,173]

Nodules are present with increased frequency in hypertension, Cushing's syndrome, primary aldosteronism, cirrhosis, and cancer.[31]

Multinodular adrenals

Multinodular adrenals are common at autopsy.[33,173] Although the glands may reach four times the size and weight of a normal gland, they produce no evidence of

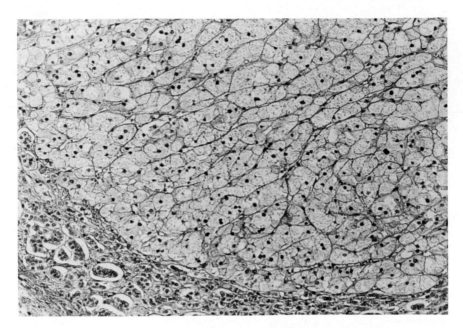

Fig. 33-7. Cortical nodule. Notice lack of encapsulation and bland cytologic features.

clinical hyperfunction and are of no known clinical significance. They usually consist of lipid-rich cells. The number and size of the nodules tends to increase with increasing age. In contrast with nodular lesions of functional significance, the remainder of the cortex manifests no evidence of hyperplasia or hyperactivity. Nodules are almost always multiple. They are not encapsulated. Lesions are almost always bilateral, but the sides often differ in size and weight.

The largest masses in multinodular adrenals represent dominant nodules not adenomas. Multinodular adrenals should be distinguished from multinodular adrenal hyperplasia and the microadenomatous adrenal, which are subsequently described.

The adrenals in patients with multiple endocrine neoplasia syndrome may also have multiple nodules, but most glands in this syndrome are neither increased in weight nor enlarged and none has been reported to manifest autonomous function.

Adrenocortical hyperplasia

Hyperplasia is an absolute increase in the number of cells per unit of tissue or organ. Criteria for adrenal hyperplasia include gland weight exceeding the top 5% of normal weight, gland weight above twice the standard deviation from the mean, and cortices exceeding 2 mm in thickness.[12,30,31,33,34,173] Fox suggested that "in . . . Cushing's disease . . . a single adrenal is abnormal if its weight is more than 6 g at operation or 9 g at autopsy."[30]

The best understood adrenal hyperplasia is the one that accompanies Cushing's disease and is caused by increased ACTH production by the pituitary. Plasma ACTH may be increased by many mechanisms. Pituitary microadenomas and adenomas now designated as corticotropic rather than basophilic are the commonest causal pituitary lesions. The normal pituitary secretes excess ACTH as a result of stress or hypoglycemia. Stress is the commonest cause of adrenal hyperplasia observed at autopsy. Ectopic ACTH secretion by nonadrenal tumors is the commonest cause of adrenal hyperplasia in elderly hospitalized males, half of whom have a small-cell neuroendocrine lung carcinoma. Exogenous ACTH administration also causes adrenal hypertrophy.

The cortex usually has a stereotypic response to ACTH. The characteristic reaction is that the clear cells of the inner two thirds of the fasciculata lose much of their stainable lipid, become compact like the reticularis, and leave a narrow rim of clear fasciculata cells on the surface. Usually the cortex increases in thickness. Fig. 33-8 illustrates Symington's extensive experimental studies of this reaction.

According to Symington,[33] the histologic features of the cortex differ in Cushing's syndrome, Conn's syndrome, adrenogenital hyperplasia and ectopic ACTH syndrome. A sketch of the first three of these conditions is presented in Fig. 33-9. The microscopic appearance of the adrenal cortex in the ectopic ACTH syndrome may be so typical that the diagnosis can be suggested from the histologic section. The cortex tends to be greatly thickened. It consists of elongated columns of large compact cells that reach to the capsule of the cortex. Most commonly, isolated islands of clear cells are found scattered amidst compact cells. There are no distinctive changes of the zona glomerulosa.

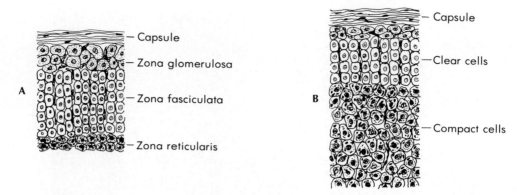

Fig. 33-8. Effect of ACTH on the adrenal cortex. **A,** Normal adrenal cortex. **B,** Effect of 30 to 50 units/mg of purified ACTH. (Modified from Symington, T.: Functional pathology of human adrenal gland, Edinburgh, 1969, E. & S. Livingstone, Ltd.)

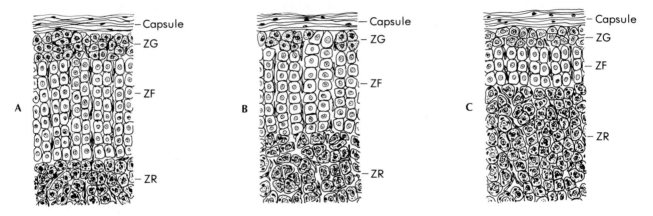

Fig. 33-9. Adrenal cortex in, **A,** Conn's syndrome, **B,** Cushing's syndrome, and, **C,** adrenogenital syndrome. *ZF,* Zona fascicularis; *ZG,* zona glomerulosa; *ZR,* zona reticularis. (Modified from Symington, T.: Functional pathology of human adrenal gland, Edinburgh, 1969, E. & S. Livingstone, Ltd.)

Ultrastructural studies of diffuse adrenal hyperplasia associated with Cushing's syndrome demonstrate that mitochondria are increased in size and complexity and smooth endoplasmic reticulum is increased and dilated. Basal laminal reduplication has also been noted.[13,35]

Nonspecific adrenocortical hyperplasia occurs with acromegaly, in thyrotoxicosis (about 40%), hypertension associated with arteriosclerosis and arteriolosclerosis (about 16%), cancer, and diabetes (3.4%). Adrenal weights are usually increased in patients who die in congestive heart failure.

Some instances of hyperplasia are not clearly explicable.[173,183]

Diffuse hyperplasia

Endocrine pathologists tend to reserve the term "diffuse hyperplasia" for glands for which there is supporting evidence for increased function.[33,125,173,183] There is

a generalized, symmetric, diffuse increase in cortical cells that usually results in an increase in size and weight of the glands (Fig. 33-10). This pattern is most commonly associated with Cushing's syndrome because of an increase in ACTH because of pituitary hypersecretion, but similar patterns can result because of ectopic ACTH secretion, administration of ACTH, or congenital adrenal hyperplasia. In Cushing's disease, the glands usually weigh between 6 and 8 g. Rarely adrenals in Cushing's disease are not increased in weight. When the glands reach 12 g, they almost always become focally nodular as well. With the ectopic ACTH syndrome, the glands usually weigh approximately 12 to 20 g each and may reach 30 g. Incidentally, such glands may also harbor metastatic deposits from the neoplasm causing the syndrome. About 20% of patients with hyperaldosteronism have a diffuse adrenal hyperplasia with a microscopically prominent glomerulosa.

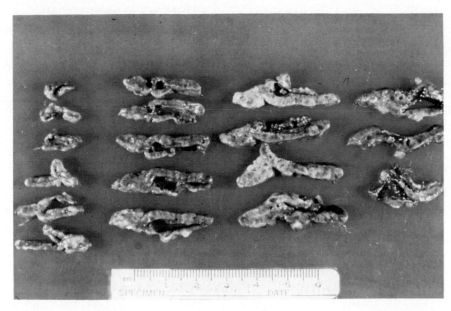

Fig. 33-10. Diffuse adrenal cortical hyperplasia. Notice uniform increased thickness of cortex.

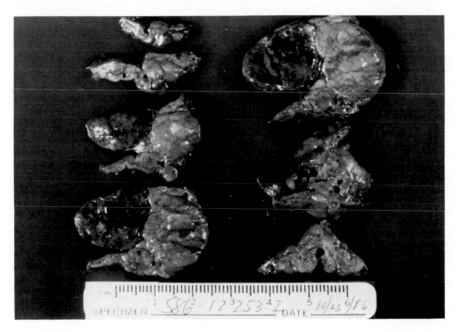

Fig. 33-11. Nodular hyperplasia of adrenal cortex.

Diffuse and nodular hyperplasia

Some hyperfunctional states are associated with enlarged adrenals in which diffuse hyperplasia is accompanied by nodular hyperplasia (Fig. 33-11). Nodules vary from microscopic size to about 2.5 cm but may reach 5 cm. Glands weighing more than 12 g almost regularly manifest nodular as well as diffuse hyperplasia. Most such cases are associated with Cushing's syndrome. Diffuse and multinodular hyperplasia should not be confused with multinodular adrenals, multino-dular adrenal hyperplasia, or microadenomatous hyperplasia.

Multinodular hyperplasia and hypercortisolism

The term "multinodular hyperplasia and hypercorti-solism" has recently been introduced to define an uncommon entity associated with Cushing's syndrome that differs from the variants of the spectrum of diffuse and nodular hyperplasia and multinodular adrenals previously described.[173] In this uncommon condition, the glands each weigh 30 to 50 g but may reach 100 g. Prominent, irregularly distributed nodules varying from about 0.3 to 3 cm are present throughout the gland in such profusion that identifying the intervening cortex is difficult. This entity appears to manifest autonomous function in that it is not suppressed by high-dose dexamethasone. This lesion has also been described as pseudoadenomatous hyperplasia.

Microadenomatous adrenal with hypercortisolism (microadenomatous hyperplasia)

In this relatively rare entity, the adrenals are usually of normal size and weight but contain multiple, evenly distributed, 1 to 5 mm–sized nodules consisting of large cells with eosinophilic cytoplasm containing pigment similar to that seen in black adenomas.[121,127,130,131,162] Nodularity may not be obvious grossly. The intervening cortical cells are small and inactive. This lesion is most common in children and young adults. Functionally, this lesion behaves and responds to test procedures as an autonomous adrenal neoplasm. There is usually a moderate elevation of cortisol levels with low ACTH levels. Cortisol is not suppressed by high-dose dexamethasone. ACTH stimulation gives equivocal results. The condition may be familial.

The term "microadenomatous hyperplasia" is a misnomer. This disorder was probably originally reported in 1952 by Rose and co-workers[130] as a distinctive type of hyperplasia. Meador and associates[127] reported that entity as primary adrenocortical nodular dysplasia in 1967. In 1986, Grant and associates[121] reported seven patients from the Mayo Clinic as primary pigmented nodular adrenocortical disease. They stressed the importance of preoperative diagnosis, since this disorder should be treated by adrenalectomy. Pituitary surgery is contraindicated.

CUSHING'S SYNDROME
From Cushing to the evolution of current concepts

In 1932, Harvey Cushing delineated this syndrome in a classic paper.[120] In his book, *The Pituitary Body and Its Disorders*, published in 1912,[119] he included a case of a "polyglandular syndrome" and suggested the possibility of pituitary or adrenal origin. He noted that "we may, per chance, be on the way toward recognition of consequences of hyperadrenalism." By 1934, Walters, Wilder, and Kepler[134] recognized that an identical clinical syndrome could occur in patients with adrenal adenomas or carcinomas. Soon thereafter, Anderson, Haymaker, and Joseph[115] suggested that the common denominator for Cushing's syndrome was an excess of adrenal hormone. Within the next few years, methods became available to measure adrenal hormones, and the concept of a common denominator of hypercortisolism was established. After potent synthetic glucocorticoids became available, iatrogenic Cushing's syndrome became more common than the classic disorder.

The current status of the pituitary in Cushing's syndrome is detailed in the chapter on the pituitary.

Although the term "ectopic ACTH syndrome" was only established in the 1960s, Gabcke[18a,25] had described a case in his dissertation in 1896. Brown's paper[116] in 1928 has long been regarded as the first description of the ectopic hormonal effect of a tumor; he described a woman with an "oat cell" lung carcinoma who became diabetic and developed a dark beard. The first very well-documented case of severe Cushing's syndrome caused by a corticotropin-secreting oat cell carcinoma of lung was reported by Meador and co-workers in 1961. In 1962, Liddle, Island, and Meador noted that Cushing's syndrome caused by ectopic ACTH was a distinct clinicopathologic entity.[23] In 1965,

Table 33-1. Pathophysiologic classification of Cushing's syndrome

ACTH dependent	Hypothalamic-pituitary dependent
	With or without overt pituitary basophilic microadenomas or other lesions
	Caused by ectopic secretion of ACTH by other tumors
	Caused by prolonged use of ACTH
ACTH independent	Caused by adrenal adenoma
	Caused by adrenal carcinoma
	Caused by prolonged use of glucocorticoids

Table 33-2. Pathologic lesions in Cushing's disorder in adults

Lesion	Frequency (current estimate)
Pituitary based	80%
With diffuse hyperplasia	
With nodular hyperplasia	
Primary adenoma	5%-10%
Primary cancer	5%
Multinodular adrenal hyperplasia	Uncommon
Microadenomatous hyperplasia	Uncommon
Ectopic ACTH production	10%-15%

Liddle and co-workers used the term "ectopic ACTH secretion" in their report on ACTH-like activity in tissue from patients who had elevated levels of ACTH clinically, though their pituitary glands at autopsy had decreased ACTH.[23] Ectopic ACTH production is now known to be one of the common ectopic hormonal syndromes.[10,25,118,122] About 50% of patients with the syndrome have a neuroendocrine carcinoma of the lung. Among patients with neuroendocrine lung carcinoma, about 2.8% have findings of ectopic ACTH syndrome; approximately one half of these patients do not have overt clinical Cushing's syndrome but do have elevated cortisol levels not suppressed by high-dose dexamethasone. At present, a clinical example of Cushing's syndrome in a hospitalized male is more likely to be caused by ectopic ACTH secretion by a lung cancer rather than a primary endocrine organ disorder.

Clinical patterns

Review of the effects of glucocorticoids facilitates understanding of the phenomena associated with clinical hypercortisolism.[10,114,117,123,124,126,128,132]

The diagnosis of classic Cushing's syndrome may be strongly suggested by the characteristic appearance of the patient. Patients with the ectopic ACTH syndrome often fail to manifest obesity or other characteristic signs and symptoms. Comprehensive laboratory verification is always mandatory to validate the diagnosis.

Current classification

It is common clinical practice to use the term "Cushing's syndrome" to include the clinical effects of glucocorticoid excess without regard to cause. The term "Cushing's disease" implies that the disorder is attributable to pituitary hypersecretion of ACTH. A pathophysiologic classification of Cushing's syndrome is presented in Table 33-1.

Pathologic substrata and laboratory differential diagnosis

The pathologic lesions that may be responsible for hypercortisolism are summarized in Table 33-2 and illustrated in Figs. 33-12 to 33-16.

Frequency of incidence of adrenal lesions in adults and children

It has been estimated that the prevalence of Cushing's syndrome approximates 6 per 1 million persons in the United States. The frequency of incidence of adrenal lesions in Cushing's syndrome differs considerably in adults and children. Table 33-2 presents a current estimate of the pathologic substrata for adults.

Ectopic ACTH secretion

The tumors commonly associated with ectopic ACTH production are listed in Table 33-3.

HYPERALDOSTERONISM

Conn first described primary hyperaldosteronism in 1955.[144] The essential pathophysiology is an increased production of aldosterone, which induces hypertension, potassium depletion, metabolic alkalosis, and suppresses plasma renin activity.[143-145]

Probably less than 1% of hypertension is attributable to hyperaldosteronism, but as many as one fourth of hypertensives have low renin activity levels. The clinical findings usually mandate laboratory screening for hyperaldosteronism. The pathologic lesions associated with hyperaldosteronism[135,136,143,173,178,179] are listed in Table 33-4 and illustrated in Figs. 33-17 to 33-20.

Adrenal adenomas causing Conn's syndrome are sometimes difficult to localize preoperatively because of their relatively small size. The classic features of an aldosteroma are cited in the tabular summary on adenomas. Most patients with adenomas are cured by sur-

Table 33-3. Tumors associated with ectopic ACTH production

Tumor	Frequency (%)
Small-cell neuroendocrine lung carcinoma	50
Thymic neuroendocrine tumors	10
Islet cell carcinoma of pancreas	10
Medullary carcinoma of thyroid	5
Pheochromocytoma, neuroblastoma	5
Others (parotid, breast, gallbladder, colon, testis, ovary, prostate uterus, kidney, liver, esophagus, trachea, gut carcinoid, cervix, argentaffinoma)	15

Table 33-4. Pathologic substrata of primary hyperaldosteronism

	Conn (1960)*	Page et al. (1986)†
Single adenomas	70%	~80%
Multiple adenomas	15%	
Bilateral hyperplasia	9%	20%
Carcinoma	None	About 20 documented cases
Normal adrenals	6%	—

*From Conn, J.W.: JAMA **172:**1650, 1960.[143]
†From Page, D.L., et al.: In Atlas of tumor pathology, ser. 2, fasc. 23, p. 52, Washington, D.C., 1986, Armed Forces Institute of Pathology.

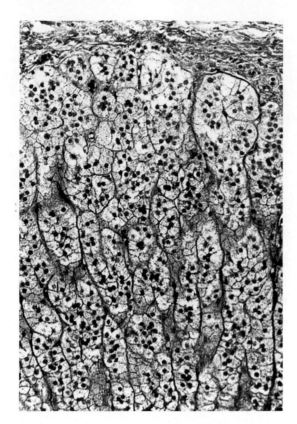

Fig. 33-12. Cushing's syndrome with diffuse adrenocortical hyperplasia. Outer zona fasciculata cells are typically enlarged to form club-shaped cords. (120×.)

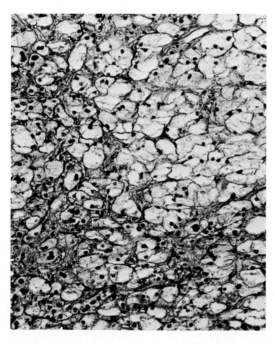

Fig. 33-13. Nodular hyperplasia of zona fasciculata with Cushing's syndrome associated with irregular cellular enlargement and locally increased lipid in adrenocortical cells. (120×.)

gery. Hyperaldosteronism associated with bilateral cortical hyperplasia without adenomas tends to respond poorly to adrenalectomy.

VIRILIZATION AND FEMINIZATION

Virilization and feminization may be attributable to gonadal or adrenal disorders.* Extra-adrenal causes of these manifestations are beyond the scope of this chapter.

Virilization is the appearance of adult masculine characteristics in prepubertal males or in females of any age. In females, virilization usually results in genital abnormalities ranging from clitoromegaly to pseudohermaphroditism. In children, virilization is usually attri-

*References 10, 14, 18, 25, 33, 58, 89, 149, 151, 166, 168, 173, 183.

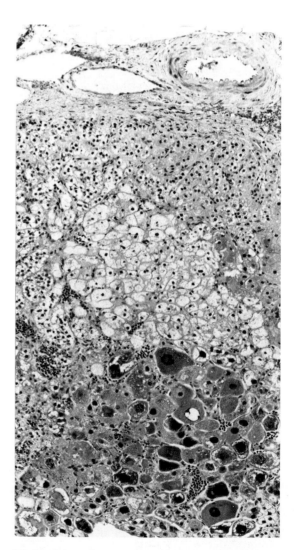

Fig. 33-14. Adrenalectomy specimen of normal-sized gland in adolescent with Cushing's syndrome showing notable nodularity and cytologic atypia of cells in deeper nodules. (100×.)

butable to congenital adrenal hyperplasia. In adults, adenomas and carcinomas may induce virilization. The majority of virilizing adrenal neoplasms in adults are malignant. Usually, but not invariably, there is also defeminization of adult women, with cessation of menses, loss of feminine body contour, and breast atrophy. Very rarely, patients with a virilizing tumor have become pregnant. Two common symptoms of virilization are hirsutism and clitoromegaly.

Feminization caused by an adrenocortical neoplasm may occur in children and postmenopausal women but more commonly occurs in men between 25 and 50 years of age. Clinical changes include gynecomastia, reduced or lost libido, feminizing hair changes, and testicular atrophy with azoospermia. Tumor size has ranged from 10 to 2000 g, but most are large and many were clinically palpable. Feminization may rarely be attributable to an adrenal adenoma but, as a rule, is usually attributable to a carcinoma. Modern imaging technology usually permits localization of such lesions. In contrast with the subtle morphologic clues for malignancy in some adrenal cancers, the morphologic evidence for malignancy is usually overt in cancers causing feminization.

ADRENOCORTICAL ADENOMA

An adenoma is defined as a benign neoplasm whose cells resemble normal adrenal cells morphologically (Fig. 33-21) but that usually manifests functional autonomy. An adenoma is usually a spherical, discrete, well-localized lesion that is usually encapsulated. Most but

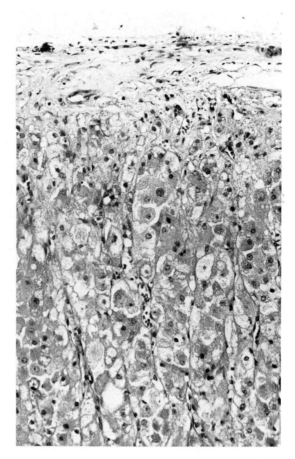

Fig. 33-15. Enlargement and lipid depletion of maximally stimulated outer zona fasciculata cells produced by ectopic ACTH. (120×.)

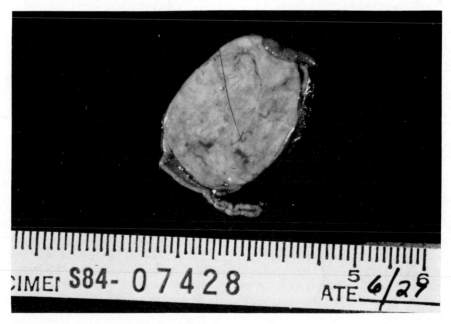

Fig. 33-16. Adenoma associated with Cushing's syndrome. Uninvolved cortex is atrophic.

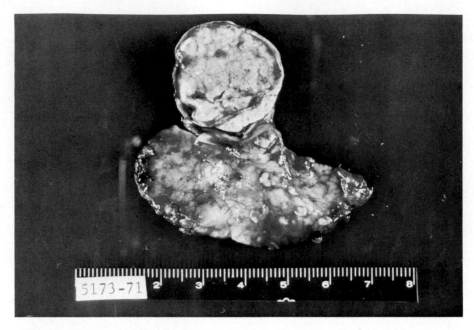

Fig. 33-17. Sectioned rounded mass above adrenal gland is cortical adenoma responsible for primary aldosteronism.

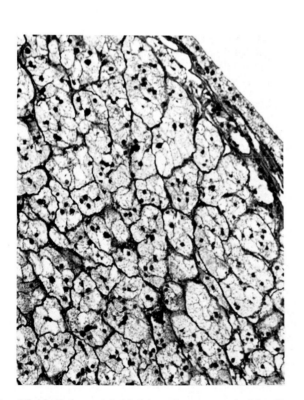

Fig. 33-18. Enlarged lipid-rich cells surrounded by fibrous capsule characterize adrenocortical adenomas, in this instance aldosteronoma. (120×.)

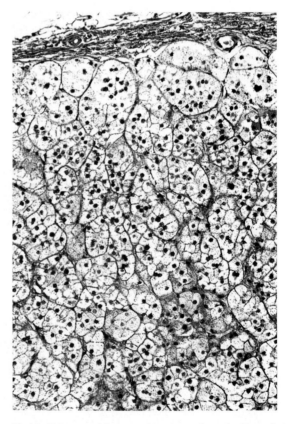

Fig. 33-19. Primary aldosteronism associated with unilateral adrenocortical hyperplasia. Zona glomerulosa cells are enlarged and finely granular. (120×.)

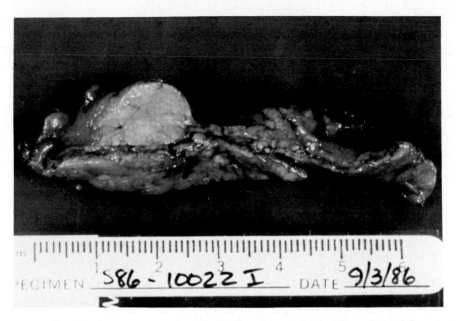

Fig. 33-20. Small adenoma associated with Conn's syndrome. Remainder of cortex is normal.

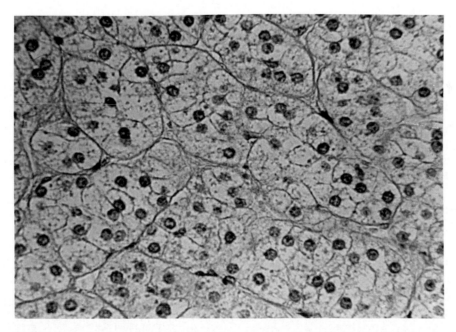

Fig. 33-21. Microphotograph of a typical benign adenoma. Notice the uniformity of cytoplastic and nuclear features.

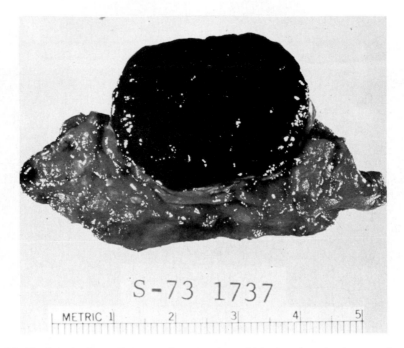

Fig. 33-22. Black adenoma. Intense pigmentation of black adrenal adenoma is caused by lipochromes. (Courtesy Dr. Mary B. King, Chicago.)

Table 33-5. Adenomas

Clinical state	Percentage attributable to adenoma	Classic gross features	Usual microscopic features	Status of adjacent gland uninvolved by adenoma
Hyperaldosteronism	80% of cases attributable to adenoma; usually solitary	Small; difficult to localize; average 1.5 cm; bright yellow	Hybrid and clear cells	Normal or hyperplastic glomerulosa
Hypercortisolism	5%-10% attributable to adenoma	Average 4 cm; yellow-brown; may be black	Compact and clear cells	Atrophy especially reticularis; glomerulosa normal
Virilization	Majority in adult are cancer; some adenomas in childhood	Large; average 5 cm or more	Compact cells	Normal
Feminization	Virtually always cancer in adults; diagnose adenoma warily	Same as above	Same as above	Normal

Modified from Page, D.L., et al.: In Atlas of tumor pathology, ser. 2, fasc. 23, Washington, D.C., 1986, Armed Forces Institute of Pathology.

not all exceed 2 cm and are usually larger than nodules. Most adenomas are solitary.*

Most but not all adenomas are hyperfunctional and produce clinical syndromes because of overproduction of hormones. Adenomas usually produce either aldosterone or cortisol and only rarely produce androgens. Lesions that cause feminization almost always behave as cancer. Carcinomas usually secrete a variety of steroids. The color and cellular composition of adenomas are usually related to the functional status as outlined in Table 33-5. The status of the nonadenomatous residual adrenal is also related to the functional status of the adenoma as outlined in Table 33-5. It is not possible to reliably characterize function from the histologic features of the tumor alone. Adenomas conventionally regarded as nonfunctional may produce biologically inactive steroid products.

Adenomas located centrally in the adrenal may be difficult to distinguish from a pheochromocytoma without marker studies. Ultrastructural studies for neurosecretory granules or immunohistochemical analysis for

*References 12, 27, 30, 31, 33, 58, 137, 139-141, 143, 153, 156, 163, 173, 175, 176, 181, 183, 186.

neuroendocrine and cytoskeletal components should establish the difference.

"Black adenomas"

In the original fascicle on adrenal tumors in 1950, Karsner[163] stated that the "black adenoma" is rare (Fig. 33-22). Subsequent studies have demonstrated that black nodules are relatively frequent at autopsy. Robinson and co-workers[174] found an incidence of 10.4% in a retrospective review of 1000 autopsies in which only random sections had been made. Their prospective review of 100 autopsies, in which 3 mm sections of adrenal were evaluated, demonstrated 37% of adrenals had pigmented nodules. Currently it is recognized that "black adenomas" are indeed rare, but black-pigmented nodules, often misclassified as "black adenomas," are relatively frequent. Black nodules can be differentiated from melanoma, myelolipoma, hemangioma, and hematoma by microscopic examination.

Typically, pigmented nodules are black or brown, are circumscribed but not encapsulated, arise at the corticomedullary junction, and extend into the cortex. The pigment has been considered to be lipofuscin based on the histochemical staining reactions and because ultrastructurally the pigmented masses consist of membrane-bound structures containing osmiophilic droplets, dense granular conglomerates, and a pale matrix. Tabular summaries or cytochemistry of lipofuscin and neuromelanin have been provided by Damron[146] and by Robinson.[174]

Most pigmented nodules are incidental findings at autopsy; they are usually not associated with endocrine abnormalities, hormonal disorders, electrolyte disorders, or hypertension.[138,174] Black nodules discovered incidentally at autopsy are commonly single, unilateral, and black or dark brown, whereas pigmented lesions associated with Cushing's syndrome are likely to be multiple, bilateral, and less pigmented. Atrophy of the remaining cortex is associated with Cushing's syndrome but not with incidental lesions. Black-pigmented adenomas have been associated with Cushing's syndrome with or without virilism and rarely with hyperaldosteronism. "Black adenomas" may cause any of the common syndromes of adrenal hyperfunction.

Pigmented nodules and adenomas should be distinguished from the microadenomatous adrenal associated with Cushing's syndrome. This latter lesion, described previously, has also been designated as primary pigmented nodular adrenocortical disease and by several other terms.

Spironolactone bodies

Spironolactone is an aldosterone antagonist. Spironolactone administration may induce the formation of "spironolactone bodies" in the cells of the glomerulosa and outer fasciculata, but these bodies may occur with-

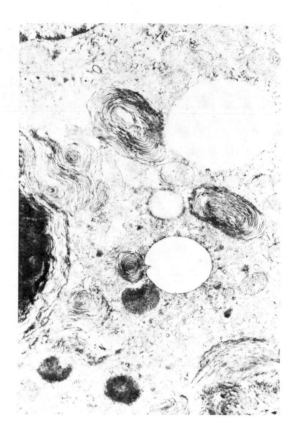

Fig. 33-23. Spironolactone bodies are complex whorled membranous structures in adrenal zona glomerulosa. (12,000×; from Bloodworth, J.M.B., Jr., Horvath, E., and Kovacs, K.: Fine structural pathology of the endocrine system. In Trump, B.F., and Jones, R.T., editors: Diagnostic electron microscopy, vol. 3, New York, 1980, John Wiley & Sons, Inc.)

out such therapy. With hematoxylin and eosin stains, these bodies tend to be round, palely eosinophilic, intracytoplasmic masses about 2 to 25 μm in diameter. They vary considerably in size and shape. Since they are phospholipid, they stain well with Sudan black. Ultrastructurally they consist of laminated osmiophilic structures consisting of layers of membranelike material believed to be compressed arrays of smooth endoplasmic reticulum (Fig. 33-23).

PRIMARY ADRENOCORTICAL CARCINOMA
Incidence and prevalence

It is difficult to obtain accurate data on the incidence and prevalence of adrenal carcinoma.[140,142,152,164,170] Based on SEER (the National Cancer Institute's Surveillance, Epidemiology and End Results program) data for 1973-1977, approximately 132 new cases occur in the United States annually or approximately 0.5 new cases per 1 million persons. The prevalence has been estimated at 2 per 1 million persons in the United States. Clearly, adrenal carcinoma is relatively uncom-

Table 33-6. Summary of functional status of adrenal carcinomas

Syndrome	Number of cases per institution (date of report)			Summary of tallies	
	M.D. Anderson (1975*)†	Mayo (1983)‡	Memorial (1986)§	Number of cases	Percentage of 141 cases
Cushing's alone	7	15	9	31	22%
Cushing's with virilization	4	12	7	23	16.3%
Cushing's with aldosteronism	0	0	1	1	0.7%
SUM OF CANCERS WITH CUSHINGOID FEATURES	(11)	(27)	(17)	(55)	(39%)
Virilization alone	4	3	5	12	8.5%
Feminization	0	1	3	4	2.8%
Aldosteronism	—	4	1	5	3.5%
SUM OF FUNCTIONAL CANCERS	15	35	26	76	53.9%
TOTAL CANCERS	32	62	47	141	100.0%

*The M.D. Anderson Report of 77 cases in 1983 does not tabulate their functional status (Nader, S., et al.: Cancer **52**:707, 1983[170]).
†Haffar, R.A., et al.: Cancer **35**:549, 1975.[152]
‡Henley, D.J., et al.: Surgery **94**:926, 1983.[155]
§Cohn, K., et al.: Surgery **100**:1170, 1986.[142]

mon; it has been estimated to comprise from 0.02% to 0.2% of all malignancies.

Functional status

Adrenal carcinomas may or may not be functional. Early estimates were that only 10% were nonfunctional, but current estimates were that almost 50% may not produce clinically overt hormonal syndromes. Patients with functioning carcinomas most commonly present with cushingoid features, but often they may concurrently manifest virilism and mineralocorticoid excess. Pure endocrine syndromes are less common. Tumors that cause feminization are usually malignant. Tumors that produce mixed endocrine syndromes are more likely to be malignant than those that produce Cushing's syndrome alone. A few cases of hyperaldosteronism have been attributed to an adrenal carcinoma.* A summary of the functional status of 141 cortical carcinomas from three major centers is presented in Table 33-6.

Adrenocortical cancers are usually considered nonfunctional if there is no *clinical* evidence of a hormone imbalance and *conventional* test procedures do not reveal evidence of physiologically detectable hormones. Tumors, however, may produce biologically inactive steroidal products. Moreover, they may not produce excess amounts of cortisol, aldosterone, or sex steroids, but may secrete pregnenolone whose metabolites may be detected in urine. These tumors are unable to carry out further steroid biosynthesis for reasons not yet elucidated, possibly because of enzymatic defects. In this

sense, the tumors are biologically inactive rather than truly nonfunctional. Copeland[38] regarded the distinction between functional and nonfunctional as relative and dependent on the thoroughness of search for appropriate metabolites and clinical clues.

Neville and O'Hare[172] and Page and co-workers[173] note that histology correlates poorly with function of tumors. There are no reliable histologic criteria to permit determination of functional status of the tumor itself. However, the status of residual or contralateral nonneoplastic adrenal may provide useful data. The associated gland is "normal" with nonfunctioning tumors, is atrophic with cortisol producers, and may show a prominent zona glomerulosa in association with hyperaldosteronism. It may be possible to study such patients by studying the precursor metabolites rather than studying the standard hormonal products.

The evaluation of the steroid content of tumor tissue may not reflect the rate of secretion. Carcinomas of the cortex are inefficient producers of hormones; hence functioning tumors also tend to be large at the time of diagnosis. In general, functioning adrenal carcinomas do not have a better prognosis than their nonfunctioning counterparts.

Age and sex incidence

Cortical carcinoma may occur at any age, but most childhood cancers occur before 5 years of age, and most adults are afflicted during late midlife. Functional tumors are somewhat more common in women, whereas nonfunctional tumors are more common in men. Neoplasms of young children are more likely to be malignant than tumors of adults.

---

*References 135, 136, 142, 155, 156, 173, 178.

Gross examination

The typical adrenal carcinoma is large and may weigh considerably more than 100 g (Fig. 33-24).* It is likely to be soft, focally hemorrhagic, and necrotic. Invasion and fixation to adjacent structures is common; 70% of the Memorial Hospital (New York) surgical cases extended outside the gland.[142] Gross invasion of vessels occurs rarely.

It may not be possible to find normal adrenal tissue on the affected side. Approximately 25% of the Memorial Hospital cases presented with obvious metastases.[142]

Most cancers weigh several hundred grams, but a few documented carcinomas weigh less than 50 g. Some carcinomas may be completely encapsulated and may not show gross necrosis or hemorrhage. Gross examination alone may not permit a seasoned examiner to differentiate a borderline cancer from an adenoma. Rarely a large metastasis to the adrenal may grossly mimic a primary carcinoma.

Localizing techniques

Modern imaging techniques especially CAT scan, now widely available and of great clinical utility, reflect the gross anatomy of a tumor.[38-41] Several representative illustrations are provided (Figs. 33-25 to 33-27).

---

*References 31, 33, 142, 152, 155, 156, 158, 159, 161, 170, 173, 181, 183.

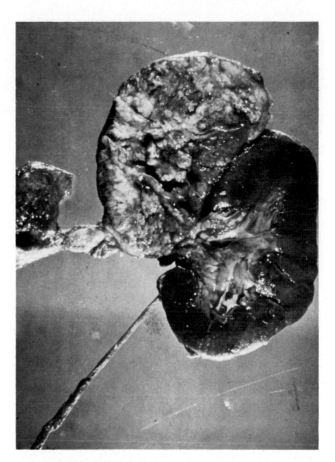

Fig. 33-24. Large adrenal carcinoma.

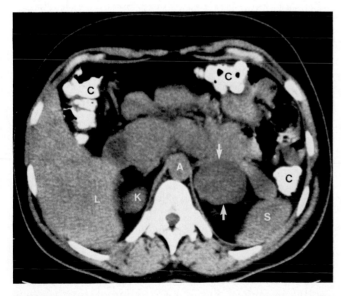

Fig. 33-25. Adrenal adenoma. A noncontrast CT scan of the upper abdomen demonstrates a 3.3 × 4 cm left adrenal mass, *arrows*. Unopacified bowel is seen anterior to the mass. *A,* Aorta; *C,* contrast-filled colon; *K,* top of right kidney; *L,* liver; *S,* spleen.

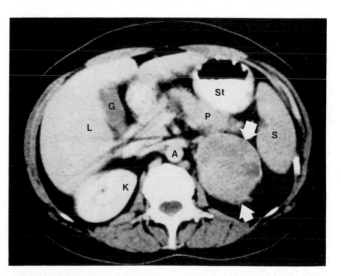

Fig. 33-26. Adrenal carcinoma. Scan after contrast material was given and obtained through the upper abdomen demonstrates a 6 cm soft-tissue mass, *arrows*, in the left adrenal gland. Notice several regions of low attenuation along the lateral and anterior margins of the tumor. These probably represent areas of necrosis. *A,* Aorta; *G,* gallbladder; *K,* right kidney; *L,* liver; *P,* pancreatic tail; *S,* spleen; *St,* stomach filled with orally administered contrast material.

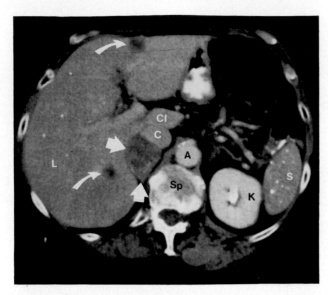

Fig. 33-27. Adrenal metastasis from adenocarcinoma of the lung. This contrast material–enhanced CT scan demonstrates a 4.4 × 3.4 cm in homogeneous right adrenal mass, *straight arrows.* Two low-attenuation regions, *curved arrows,* are seen in the liver, *L,* and represent metastases as well. *A,* Aorta; *C,* inferior vena cava; *CL,* caudate lobe of liver; *K,* kidney; *S,* spleen; *Sp,* spine.

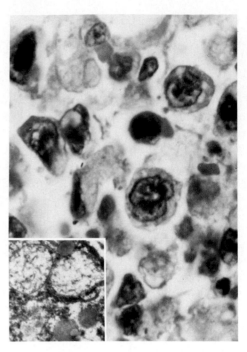

Fig. 33-28. Carcinoma of adrenal cortex. Tumor cells show considerable variation in size, shape, and intensity of staining. (900×.) *Inset,* Cytoplasmic lipid droplets and mitochondria of adrenocortical type. (5080×.)

Significant advances are being reported with magnetic resonance imaging (MRI).[42-45] Glazer has claimed that the technique permits differentiation between a primary carcinoma and a functional or nonfunctional adenoma and between a primary and a metastatic carcinoma. Doppman[42-44] has reported that nonfunctioning carcinomas are easy to differentiate from adenomas by MRI because they have a high T_2-weighted image signal.

Histopathology

Adrenal carcinomas may manifest a broad spectrum of histologic findings ranging from obviously pleomorphic patterns that are clearly malignant to borderline tumors with subtle histologic evidence for malignancy.*

Experienced histopathologists have acknowledged that histologic distinction between benign and malignant tumors may be difficult. In 1978, Waisman[181] stated that microscopic findings did not provide a reliable index of survival; occasionally the clinical course provides the final proof of its nature.

Most carcinomas feature a diffuse sheetlike growth of cells that are not well organized into trabecular or alveolar patterns. The cells manifest varying degrees of

pleomorphism that is sometimes extreme. By itself, moderate cellular pleomorphism is not a reliable criterion of malignancy. Usually there is a predominance of granular cells.

Typically there are foci of necrosis and hemorrhage, but the observer should be aware that benign lesions may become infarcted and necrotic and that surgical manipulation may induce hemorrhage.

A mitotic rate greater than five mitoses per 50 high-power microscopic fields or atypical mitoses or venous invasion is virtually diagnostic for carcinoma, but these factors are not invariably present (Figs. 33-28 and 33-29).

Benign adenomas may show some pleomorphism and a rare mitosis, whereas occasional small cortical carcinomas may be completely encapsulated, manifest sparse mitoses, and may lack capsular and vascular involvement.

Recently, several authors have evaluated histologic criteria on groups of tumors based on whether or not recurrences or metastases occurred during a defined follow-up period.[156,173,184] Generally, it has not been possible to achieve absolute separation of tumors based on any single histologic criterion or parameter. Several authors have proposed the utilization of clusters of histologic and nonhistologic criteria sometimes expressed as numerical indices to reach a definitive diagnosis.

Weiss[184] proposed evaluation of nine histologic fea-

---

*References 30, 31, 33, 58, 137, 150, 152, 156-161, 163, 164, 170, 173, 181, 183, 184, 186.

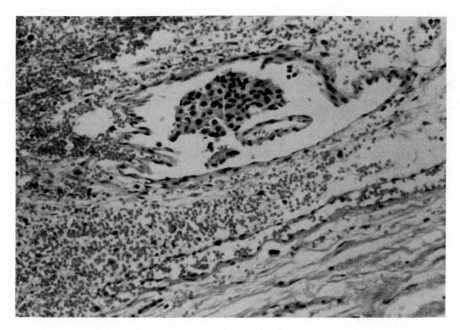

Fig. 33-29. Intravascular tumor in adrenal carcinoma.

Table 33-7. Histologic assessment of adrenal neoplasms by criteria of Weiss

Criterion	Definition
Nuclear grade	Types III and IV according to criteria of Fuhrman et al.*
Mitotic rate	Greater than 5 mitoses per 50 high-power fields†
Atypical mitoses	Abnormal distribution of chromosomes or excessive number of mitotic spindles
Cytoplasm	Clear cells comprise 25% or less of tumor
Architecture of tumor	Diffuse if over a third of tumor is composed of patternless sheets of cells
Necrosis	Present if occurs in at least confluent nests of cells
Invasion of venous structures	Unequivocal invasion of endothelial vessel with smooth muscle as component of the wall
Invasion of sinusoid structures	Unequivocal invasion of endothelium-lined vessel without supporting tissues
Invasion of capsule of tumor	Present if nests or cords of tumor extended into or through capsule with corresponding stromal reaction

From Weiss, L.M.: Am. J. Surg. Pathol. **8:**163, 1984.[184]
*From Fuhrman, S.A., et al.: Am. J. Surg. Pathol. **6:**655, 1982.[148]
†The observer counts at least 50 high-power fields and records the total number of mitoses. It is *not* adequate to state 1 mitosis per 10 high-power fields because that is average.

tures listed in Table 33-7. In Weiss's cases, no tumor that manifested two or fewer criteria recurred or metastasized whereas all but 1 of 19 cases that manifested four or more of these criteria did recur or metastasize.

Page, DeLellis, and Hough[173] have emphasized that certain nonhistologic findings such as extensive tumor necrosis, tumor weight over 100 g, and a feminizing syndrome indicate that a given neoplasm may be a carcinoma. The presence of mixed endocrine syndromes (that is, mixed Cushing's syndrome and virilism) or no endocrine syndrome also indicates probable carcinoma.

Only a rare lesion is likely to remain (un)classified as a borderline or indeterminate tumor after the pathologist correlates a study of multiple blocks from a tumor with the gross, clinical, radiologic, and biochemical/endocrinologic data. Electron microscopy and flow cytometry have not provided unequivocal differential diagnostic criteria.

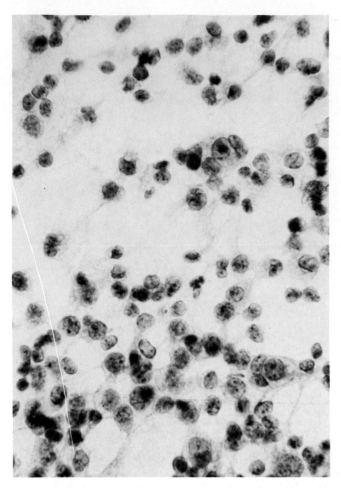

Fig. 33-30. Cytologic appearance: multinucleated cells with macronucleoli.

Cytologic criteria

Cytologic criteria that we currently utilize for adrenocortical carcinoma include the following:

Mononuclear cells with macronucleoli (Levin[188]) (Fig. 33-30)

Mononuclear cells with clear cytoplasm mimicking renal adenocarcinoma (Zajicek[189])

Mononuclear cells with dense cytoplasm, fine chromatin, small nucleoli, and irregularity of the nuclear envelope (Levin[188])

Clusters of cells attached to capillaries (Zajicek[189])

Cardozo also provided criteria in his atlas in 1975.[187]

Immunohistochemistry

Early histochemical studies were concerned with evaluation of the sites of steroid reactions and tumor diagnosis. Studies prior to 1969 were reviewed by Symington.[33] Some of the early studies, with the Ashbel-Seligman reaction,[177] which was believed to stain ketosteroids, and the Vine fuchsinophil stain, which was believed to stain androgens, led to erroneous conclusions, since the stains are not specific for ketosteroids or androgens.

Immunohistochemical studies on well-preserved tumor samples utilizing well-characterized antibodies reveal that adrenocortical carcinomas express cytokeratin polypeptides that may be coexpressed with vimentin. Thus the cytoskeletal intermediate filament complement of these carcinomas does not differ from that expressed by renal cortical carcinomas, whereas it does differ from that of pheochromocytomas, which express neurofilament proteins.[118,169,185]

Ultrastructure

Ultrastructurally, adrenocortical carcinoma may show partial or complete disappearance of the cellular basement membrane, increased numbers of large and normal-sized mitochondria, increased smooth endoplasmic reticulum, herniation of cytoplasm into nuclei, and increased collagen in the intercellular spaces. Detailed presentations of ultrastructural changes in adrenal cancer and adenoma are available elsewhere.[13,33,35] Ultrastructural study is rarely useful in differentiating adrenal adenoma from carcinoma but may provide definitive distinction between a primary and metastatic adrenal carcinoma.

Tissue culture

Neville and O'Hare[27] claimed that tissue culture demonstrates a significant difference between malignant and benign neoplasms. Functioning malignant tumors produce an abnormal amount of androgens and 11-deoxysteroids and manifest a blunted reaction to ACTH.

Flow cytometry

In 1983, Hedley and co-workers[192] reported a method for the analysis of cellular DNA content of tissue from paraffin blocks using flow cytometry. Essentially this technology permits an investigator to distinguish diploid from aneuploid cells. Representative DNA histograms from Amberson and co-workers[190] illustrate how this distinction is determined.

Ploidy has not yet been shown to be an absolute discriminant for carcinoma.[190-191,194] Although Klein and co-workers[193] reported that two adenomas were diploid and four carcinomas were aneuploid, Amberson and co-workers[190] that in a study of 48 adrenocortical neoplasms and 23 nonneoplastic adrenals reported that diploid DNA content did not assure a benign clinical course, and they considered that the size of the tumor was as useful as ploidy in predicting the outcome.

Metastases from adrenocortical carcinoma

Adrenocortical carcinoma is usually a highly malignant tumor that extends and metastasizes widely and rapidly.[173] A majority of adrenal carcinomas extend outside the adrenal. Approximately 25% have already metastasized by the time the diagnosis is established. Most other patients develop metastases within 2 years after diagnosis.

Surveys of the incidence at autopsy of metastases from primary adrenocortical carcinoma reveal that approximately 50% spread locally or to lungs or liver. Approximately 10% to 15% spread to nodes, peritoneum, or bone. Less commonly, in about 2% to 7%, tumor spreads to the contralateral kidney or adrenal or to the brain or skin. The presence of metastases automatically assigns a patient to stage IV by the staging criteria of Sullivan.

Ectopic adrenal carcinoma

There are rare reports of adrenal carcinoma arising in a site of ectopic adrenal tissue.[173] Ectopic adrenal carcinoma is likely to be mistaken as a metastatic carcinoma on initial evaluation. Both functional and nonfunctional variants have been reported. Such rare cases are likely to pose diagnostic difficulties that may not be resolved until complete autopsy study. Proof of such a diagnosis requires unequivocal evidence that the tumor is of cortical type and may require ultrastructural studies to exclude other primary lesions, especially from liver and kidney. If the adrenals are involved by metastases, it would be difficult to exclude an adrenal primary. Only a single case with a large extra-adrenal tumor has been claimed to be an extra-adrenal cortical carcinoma with metastases to both adrenals. Various gonadal lipid cell tumors may also mimic extra-adrenal cortical carcinoma.

Staging

The American Joint Committee on Cancer has not formally adopted staging criteria for adrenal cortical carcinoma, but the criteria proposed by Macfarlane in 1958 as modified by Sullivan and associates in 1978 have been utilized to stage patients at the time of diagnosis at the Mayo Clinic and Memorial–Sloan-Kettering Cancer Center.[142]

METASTASES TO THE ADRENAL

Metastatic carcinoma is frequently encountered in the adrenals at autopsy.[195-207] It has been reported that as many as 58% of breast cancers, 50% of melanomas, 42% of lung cancers, and 16% of gastric cancers metastasize to the adrenals. Although metastases to the adrenal are common, they are believed to account for less than 0.5% of cases of adrenal insufficiency. However, clinical problems referable to adrenal metastases may be obscured because weakness, asthenia, lassitude, weight loss, nausea, and even electrolyte imbalance may be regarded as nonspecific effects of widespread neoplastic disease. In the past, discovery of adrenal metastases was usually made at autopsy by the pathologist.

Currently, computerized tomographic (CT) scans commonly detect enlarged adrenal glands. Functional studies of cortisol after ACTH administration can establish the existence of Addison's disease and percutaneous needle aspiration or biopsy can confirm the diagnosis of metastases. It has recently been claimed that Addison's disease attributable to metastatic carcinoma may be underdiagnosed and that it is not as rare as previously supposed. Seidenwurm and co-workers[205] claimed that 20% of patients with metastatic cancer who had enlarged adrenals demonstrable by CT eventually developed clinical adrenal insufficiency.

Addison's disease has been reported as a consequence of destruction of the adrenal cortex because of metastases from breast cancer, lung cancer, gastric and colorectal cancer, esophageal, uterine, and renal cancer, seminoma, lymphoma, and Hodgkin's disease. Lymphoma limited to the adrenals with adrenal insufficiency has been reported; Carey and co-workers[196] reported the first known example of reversal of Addison's disease after antineoplastic therapy for lymphomatous adrenal infiltration.

MISCELLANEOUS TUMORS
Myelolipoma

The name "myelolipoma" was suggested by Oberling in 1929,[210] but the entity had been initially described by Gierke in 1905.[209] The myelolipoma is a relatively rare, tumorlike mass of fatty and myeloid tissue that usually presents as a small incidental lesion found at autopsy without associated clinical symptoms; incidence at autopsy has been reported from 0.08% to 0.2%. Currently, myelolipomas are increasingly being found incidentally on CAT scans performed for unrelated reasons.

Myelolipomas have not been noted before puberty, are most common in middle age, have no sex predilection, and bear no relationship to hematopoietic disease, compensatory hematopoiesis, or anemia. No endocrine dysfunction has been associated with most myelolipomas, but a few cases of endocrine dysfunction and association with Cushing's disease have been cited.

Most myelolipomas are small, ranging from microscopic foci to 8 cm, but rare examples have reached 25 cm and 1250 g. Microscopically, lesions run a broad gamut from almost all fatty tissue to almost all myeloid tissue (Fig. 33-31). Plaut[211] provided a meticulously detailed review of the morphology of the largest series studied by an expert observer.

Rarely lesions that produce vague abdominal discomfort or manifest hemorrhage may necessitate operative removal. The first report of surgical removal of a mylolipoma was published in 1957.[208] By 1979, the surgical removal of 12 cases had been reported. The diagnostic features of a myelolipoma include biochemical nonfunction, radiolucency on routine x-ray film, a solid mass by ultrasonography, no neovascularity on angiography, and

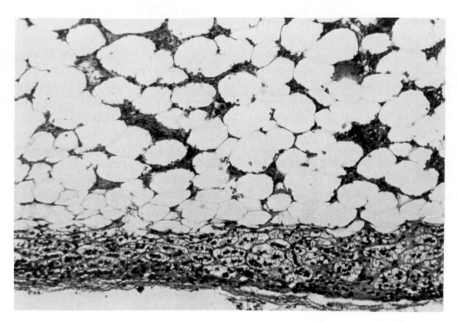

Fig. 33-31. Microphotograph of myelolipoma showing hematopoietic elements amidst fatty tissue.

typical patterns on CAT and MRI.

Multiple theories have been proposed for the cause and pathogenesis. Currently, the concept of metaplasia is most widely supported.

At least two examples of a myelolipoma in a heterotopic adrenal have been reported.[207a]

Others

Other adrenal neoplasms are usually small, benign, connective tissue tumors, including neurilemoma, neurofibroma, lipoma, leiomyoma, osteoma, and angioma, as well as mixed mesenchymoma.[31]

Primary malignant melanoma has been rarely diagnosed. Usually, multiple metastases are present elsewhere. The pigment must be identified as melanin, and one must exclude other possible primary sites, such as adrenal tumors capable of producing melanin, including pheochromocytomas, neuroblastomas, and malignant schwannomas.[31]

Rare examples of leiomyosarcoma, plasmacytoma, and lymphoma have also been reported.[31]

CYSTS

Cystic lesions of the adrenal are relatively rare. By 1979, approximately 250 cystic lesions have been reported.[213] Before 1956, the diagnosis of adrenal cyst had been made preoperatively in only 19 patients. Most cysts are asymptomatic lesions discovered post mortem. Abeshouse and others[212] first called attention to a "clinical triad" of (1) flank discomfort, (2) palpable mass, and (3) downward displacement of the adjacent kidney on x-

ray film. Obviously this clinical triad is seen only with large cysts. In 1961, Barron and Emanuel[212a] proposed a classification into epithelial, endothelial, parasitic, and pseudocysts, which included many previously proposed classifications. Symington in 1969 regarded the simple classification of true and pseudocysts proposed by Hodges and Ellis in 1958 as adequate for practice purposes.[33] Most cysts are pseudocysts. It is often difficult to determine the causal factor. Hemorrhage has been noted in newborns and during pregnancy and has been associated with cysts. Cystic changes within adenomas or carcinomas are secondary degenerative changes. Echinococcal cysts of the adrenal have been reported but are quite rare. The glandular cyst lined by ciliated cells reported by Sick[214b] in 1903 may be the only known example of an epithelial cyst. In 1938, Rabson and Zimmerman[214a] reported that lymphangiomatous cysts, usually small, either single or multiple, occurred as incidental autopsy findings. In 1979, Incze and co-workers[213] studied two such cases by light and electron microscopy. They suggested that some fibrous tissue–lined pseudocysts may have originated as endothelial cysts. Cystic angiomas have exceeded 20 cm. Modern imaging technology may increase the number of cysts detected clinically. Kearney described functioning cysts.[214]

MISCELLANEOUS PHENOMENA
Adrenal hemorrhage in the adult

Massive bilateral adrenal hemorrhage can destroy hormone-secreting adrenal tissue. Anticoagulant therapy is the commonest single cause of adrenal hemorrhage in adults; it accounts for approximately one third of cases.

Massive adrenal hemorrhage may be associated with severe infections and septicemia, trauma, malignant hypertension, heart disease including infarction and congestive failure, pulmonary emboli, toxemia of pregnancy, burns, coagulation disorders, leukemias, lymphomas, venous thrombi, disseminated intravascular coagulation, and metastatic tumor. Meningococcemia and *Pseudomonas* septicemia are more likely to cause adrenal hemorrhage in children than in adults.

At autopsy, massive hemorrhage may produce greatly enlarged glands that are virtually destroyed. There are a few documented cases of adrenal insufficiency after fulminant meningococcemia and anticoagulant therapy in which the patient survived without permanent adrenal damage.

Adrenal and regulation of blood pressure

Addison[90] called attention to hypotension in 1855, and Fränkel[216] observed hypertension with a pheochromocytoma in 1866.

Soon after the basic biochemistry of steroids was clarified, Selye[219] and others experimentally produced hypertension in animals with deoxycorticosterone. Selye focused attention on the adrenal cortex during the 1940s with his extensive studies of the "alarm reaction" and "general adaptation syndrome."[219]

It is now well known that hypertension occurs in primary aldosteronism, Cushing's syndrome, two forms of congenital adrenal hyperplasia (those associated with deficiency of C-11 hydroxylase and C-17 hydroxylase); it also occurs associated with pheochromocytoma (see the discussion of the adrenal medulla in the next column; the lesions associated with each of these disorders have already been described).[215,218,220,221] Since some adrenal causes of hypertension are potentially curable surgically, hypertensive patients may require screening for evaluation of adrenal abnormalities. Currently, less than 1% of hypertensive patients suffer from primary adrenal disorders. An early study by Gifford of almost 5000 hypertensive patients evaluated at the Cleveland Clinic during 1966 and 1967 led him to estimate that primary aldosteronism might account for as much as 0.5% of hypertension, Cushing's for 0.2%, and pheochromocytoma for 0.2%.[217] These figures appear high. By contrast, a study of 26,589 hypertensive patients at the Mayo Clinic included resection for aldosteroma in 0.01% and resection for pheochromocytoma in 0.04%.[221] Older pathologic literature includes many reports of increased weight or increased nodulation of the adrenals of hypertensive patients.[31] Heinivaara[154] and Dobbie[147] were able to document increased muscle wall thickness of the adrenal vein in hypertensives. The clinical relevance of most of these morphologic studies is obscure.

Calcification

Calcification of the adrenals is relatively uncommon.[222-229] Ball and others[222] reported an occurrence rate of one per 300 in a review of abdominal roentgenograms. Seligman and others[228] reported adrenal calcification in four per 1185 autopsies. Calcification of the adrenals is common in Addison's disease because of tuberculosis but does not occur invariably.[227] Jarvis and others[224] reported that calcifications can be demonstrated by roentgenograms in about 24% of cases of adrenal tuberculosis. It has been reported that calcification of the adrenals occurs less frequently if the extent of glandular destruction does not produce adrenal insufficiency. It has also been documented that the frequency of radiologically evident calcification has declined significantly as the frequency of tuberculous Addison's disease has declined. Calcification may occur in association with cystic adenoma, cortical carcinoma, choristoma, and pheochromocytoma. In children, neuroblastomas may calcify. Calcifications may be a radiologic finding of diagnostic significance. Adrenal hemorrhage may be followed by calcification. Snelling and Erb[229] have reported adrenal calcification after severe birth trauma and intercurrent infection. Jarvis and Seaman[225] reported "idiopathic calcification" in healthy children, but most of their cases had a history of birth trauma or prolonged anoxia.

AIDS and the adrenal cortex

Guenthner and co-workers[231] reported the first case of primary Addison's disease in an AIDS patient in 1984. Early in 1987, a review[230] of 38 autopsied patients with AIDS from the Chicago area disclosed unequivocal morphologic evidence of cytomeglovirus (CMV) infection of the adrenal in 14 patients (36.8%).

Irradiation

The effect of irradiation on the adrenal has rarely been described.[232]

ADRENAL MEDULLA

The bulk of the adrenal medullary tissue resides in the head of the glands toward the vertebral column; thus sections from the more lateral and caudal portions of the glands may not include medullary tissue.[237] As stated previously, the anatomic and functional integrity of the adrenal cortices is essential for life. This does not hold true for the adrenal medullas that are important components of the dispersed neuroendocrine system (DNS) but whose secretory functions are either nonessential or can be taken over by other paraganglia and possibly other neuroendocrine cells.

Adrenal medullary cells produce epinephrine and norepinephrine; in children the latter predominates over the former, whereas in adults the opposite is the case. In addition to neuroamines, neuropeptides such as calcitonin, somatostatin, and VIP (vasoactive intestinal polypeptide)[255,256] may be demonstrated. Adrenal medullary cells are readily immunostained with antibodies to chromogranin A,[261] NSE (neuron-specific enolase),[266] and synaptophysin.[244,245,273] Their intermediate filament cytoskeleton is composed of neurofilament proteins (NFP)[257]; thus adrenal medullary cells display "neural" cytoskeletal features differing from the "epithelial" features characteristic of most peripheral components of the DNS that express cytokeratin polypeptides and desmosomal plaque proteins (desmoplakins). Many structural, functional, and immunohistochemical characteristics of the paraganglia are similar to those of the adrenal medulla; notable particularly in the paraganglia is the presence of "sustentacular" cells around parenchymal cell clusters. These elongated elements are surrounded by basal lamina and display many features reminiscent of Schwann cells; not surprisingly, they are immunostained with antibodies to vimentin and S-100 protein.[263]

Neoplasms are the most frequent and clinically significant abnormalities occurring in the adrenal medulla; they include neuroblastomas particularly in infants and pheochromocytomas in children and adults.

Vascular lesions and hyperplasias

Vascular disturbances involving the adrenal medulla are uncommon but may attain clinical significance because venous thrombosis and hemorrhages may result in necrosis of both cortex and medulla. As the inner layer of the fetal adrenal cortex normally involutes in the early postnatal period, focal hemorrhages may be noted, but these do not result in adrenal failure.[242] Hemorrhages occurring as a result of birth trauma have been described, but only in rare cases where both glands are compromised will clinically significant problems ensue. As clinical entities, acute or chronic inflammation of the adrenal medullas only are practically unknown. In cases of severe chronic pyelonephritis, aggregates of lymphocytes and plasma cells may be found surrounding the adrenal medullas. This phenomenon is believed to be a component of the perirenal phlebitis that may be associated with pyelonephritis and is usually an autopsy finding of questionable clinical significance.[242]

Hyperplasia of the adrenal medulla is rare. A convincing diagnosis of medullary hyperplasia requires not merely gross and microscopic examination but also morphometric confirmation.[237,270] In cases of hyperplasia, medullary tissue may be found in the body and tail of the glands.

Adrenal medullary hyperplasia may be found in as-sociation with multiple endocrine neoplasia syndromes types II and III involving patients known to suffer the condition as well as clinically unaffected family members. In these persons, adrenal medullary hyperplasia may represent the contralateral manifestation of a pheochromocytoma or its forerunner.[263]

Adrenal medullary hyperplasia may occur in patients with neurofibromatosis and angiomatosis; in these cases it may also represent an early phase in the development of pheochromocytomas. Adrenal medullary hyperplasia has also been described in association with the sudden infant death syndrome[242]; the notion has been advanced that in these cases hyperplasia is the result of chronic hypoxemia. Extremely rare cases of "solitary" adrenal medullary hyperplasia have been diagnosed and are apparently unassociated with any of the aforementioned syndromes.[265,270]

Neoplasms

Pheochromocytoma is the most frequent and generally but not invariably benign tumor of the adrenal medulla and paraganglia[242]; it is at times also referred to as chromaffin paraganglioma. The term "pheochromocytoma" was introduced to describe an adrenal medullary tumor that takes on a dark brown color upon exposure to chromate-containing fixatives. That reaction is referred to as chromaffin, and it relates to the presence of substantial amounts of epinephrine. However, a good number of morphologically and functionally indistinguishable tumors of the adrenal medulla and paraganglia do not show that reaction. Thus, terms as chromaffin versus nonchromaffin paraganglioma were proposed; this in turn has resulted in much confusion, which can be corrected as our understanding of these tumors has improved. Since chromaffinity has no diagnostic, clinical, or therapeutic significance, the current approach is simply to apply the term "pheochromocytoma" when the tumor arises in the adrenal medulla but to apply the designation "paraganglioma" when one is referring to the counterparts arising in extra-adrenal paraganglia.[241,242,263] Indeed, the very notion of determining the chromaffinity of these tumors has been virtually abandoned.

The sex distribution of pheochromocytomas is approximately equal though some studies indicated a slight female predominance. "Sporadic" pheochromocytomas arise predominantly in the third to fifth decades of life. Pheochromocytomas are part of the MEN II (multiple endocrine neoplasia, type II, or Sipple) syndome. In the type IIa variant, pheochromocytomas are associated with medullary thyroid carcinoma and parathyroid adenomas or hyperplasia. In the type IIb, they are associated with mucosal neuromas, particularly of the lips and tongue, whereas parathyroid abnormalities are less frequent. Pheochromocytomas as part of MEN syndromes tend to develop in children, adolescents, and young adults. Occasional examples of congenital pheochromocytomas have been reported. In nonfamilial pheochromocytomas, the right adrenal is more often involved than the left.[242,263]

The overwhelming majority of pheochromocytomas are associated with clinically detectable hormonal syndromes that can be very dramatic as well as life threatening. Most pheochromocytomas produce epinephrine and norepinephrine; the former predominates in patients with MEN, whereas the latter is dominant in the sporadic cases. Determinations of urinary vanillylmandelic acid and metanephrines are diagnostic in 80% to 90% of cases; measurement of plasma catecholamines is even more sensitive. Most but not all signs and symptoms can be explained by the overproduction of catecholamines.[235,242,263]

Paroxysmal or sustained hypertension is almost the rule, and patients with constant hypertension may still experience paroxysmal episodes. Headaches are also almost the rule, and they may be accompanied by nausea and vomiting. Less frequent but still significant manifestations include diaphoresis, palpitations with and without tachycardia, tremors, anxiety, chest and abdominal pain, and visual disturbances. Elevated fasting blood glucose levels may be found. Serious and occasionally fatal complications of untreated pheochromocytomas include myocardial arrhythmias and infarction, cerebral hemorrhages, nephrosclerosis, and retinopathies.[235,242,263]

Catecholamine overproduction may result in a type of cardiomyopathy characterized by focal degeneration and leukocytic infiltration leading subsequently to fibrosis and scarring. This type of injury has been reproduced in experimental animals, and it may also be observed in patients treated with norepinephrine for hypotension.[233,263]

Occasionally pheochromocytomas may overproduce other hormones pertaining to the dispersed neuroendocrine system and present with other syndromes; cases of ACTH production resulting in Cushing's syndrome and VIP (vasoactive intestinal polypeptide) overproduction with associated watery diarrhea syndrome have been reported.[234,238,251,254,256,267] Poorly understood clinical problems associated with pheochromocytomas including abdominal cramps and hypercalcemia may be the direct or indirect result of the production of the aforementioned or other substances. Rarely, pheochromocytomas do not present clinical hormonal syndromes. Possible explanations include small tumor size or low level of hormonal production, impaired release mechanism, enzymatic inactivation of the hormones within the tumor, increased tolerance by the pertinent receptors, and possible antagonism by other materials produced by the tumors.

The majority of pheochromocytomas may be diagnosed preoperatively by modern methods including selective angiography and CAT scans. Most pheochromocytomas appear as 3 to 5 cm in diameter, round, apparently encapsulated masses weighing in the range of 100 g. Tumors weighing over 3 kg have been re-

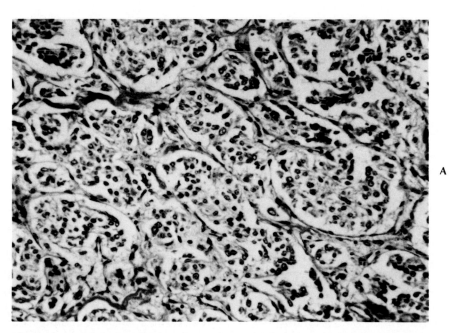

Fig. 33-32. A, Pheochromocytoma associated with paroxysmal hypertension and elevated levels of norepinephrine. Notice solid cell nests separated by delicate fibrovascular strands. Pleomorphism is mild.   *Continued.*

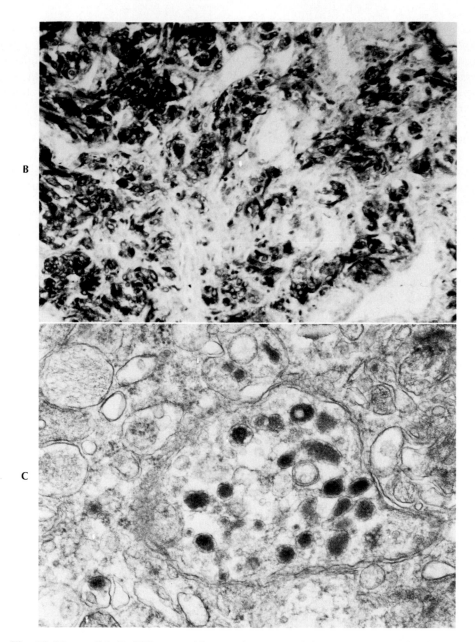

Fig. 33-32, cont'd. B, Diffuse and intense immunostaining with synaptophysin antibody. **C,** Electron micrograph depicts cytoplasmic process and adjacent segments of cytoplasm. Notice aggregate of comparatively small neurosecretory granules suggestive of neuropeptide storage. **(A,** Hematoxylin and eosin, 450×; **B,** avidin-biotin-complex method, 450×; **C,** 16,500×.)

ported. Freshly cut surfaces range from gray to pink with occasional tan areas; a rim of bright yellow adrenal cortex may be noted in the periphery. Hemorrhages, myxoid changes, necrosis, and cyst formation are frequent. As tumors grow larger, areas of calcification may be noted. Necrosis may also follow arteriography.[242,263]

The characteristic microscopic pattern of pheochromocytomas is one of solid, round cell aggregates *(Zellballen)*, cords, ribbons or trabeculas separated by a rich fibrovascular stroma (Fig. 33-32, *A*). Around the clusters, elongated "sustentacular" type of cells may be noted. Several patterns may be seen in the same tumor. Pheochromocytomas comprise polyhedral cells reminiscent of but larger than those of the adrenal medulla. After formalin or Bouin's fixation, the cytoplasm is eosinophilic and may be granular and, less frequently, vacuolated. Nuclear pleomorphism and atypism may be considerable; neither of these features is diagnostic for malignancy, and focal vascular invasion or rare mitoses are also not diagnostic. Some nuclei may show inclusions representing cytoplasmic evaginations. Occasional tumors may display conspicuous vascular pools that may result in mistaken diagnoses of vascular tumors.[242,253] Amyloid deposition in the stroma has been reported.

By electron microscopy, abundant neurosecretory granules are noted (Fig. 33-32, C). Most granules range from 250 to 400 nm. Granules with eccentric cores and crescent-shaped halos indicating norepinephrine storage tend to predominate; granules with large, centrally located cores are suggestive of epinephrine. Most if not all pheochromocytomas also have smaller granules of variable size, shape, and density consistent with the storage of other materials. Junctions rarely suggestive of true desmosomes, Schwann-like cells and basal lamina in the periphery of the clusters, arrays of microtubules, and so on may be noted.[240,242,252]

Given adequate tissue preservation, pheochromocytomas are invariably immunostained with antibodies to neuron-specific enolase, chromogranin A, and synaptophysin (Fig. 33-32, B).[244,245,247,261,264,266,273] Neuropeptides including calcitonin, VIP, bombesin, and somatostatin as well as serotonin may also be shown regardless of clinical manifestations.[234,238,245,251,254,256] The intermediate filament complement of pheochromocytoma consists of neurofilament proteins.[245,246,248,257] Coexpression of cytokeratin and desmoplakins has been shown in the PC12 rat pheochromocytoma in culture.[239] The Schwann-like sustentacular cells express vimentin and S-100 protein.[246]

Recurrences, distant metastases, and development of pheochromocytoma in the remaining adrenal are more frequent in children and in patients with a family history of this or related tumors. In sporadic cases, malignancy is more likely to be associated with a large tumor size than with capsular invasion or pleomorphism. Helpful but not absolute criteria include extensive necrosis, small tumor cell size, and abundant mitoses.[242,249,258,263] In cases of MEN syndrome, when metastatic pheochromocytoma may have to be differentiated from metastatic medullary thyroid carcinoma, the most helpful immunohistochemical probes pertain to the complement of intermediate filaments, such as cytokeratin, with or without neurofilaments and vimentin in medullary carcinomas versus neurofilaments only in pheochromocytomas.[245,248,257,273]

Neuroblastoma is a comparatively frequent childhood neoplasm; indeed, it is the most frequent extracranial solid tumor—as distinct from leukemias—of infancy and childhood. The incidence is higher if the so-called in situ neuroblastomas are added; the latter, however, are as a rule incidental autopsy findings in neonates that presumably progress toward maturity. About two thirds of clinically diagnosed neuroblastomas develop in children under 5 years of age; nevertheless, they are also found in adolescents and young adults.[242,263]

The most frequent primary site for neuroblastomas is the adrenal medulla and related retroperitoneal neural structures, but they also develop in the posterior mediastinum, neck, and olfactory mucosa[268]; rarely they may arise in the cerebrum. Malignant small cell tumors similar to neuroblastomas may arise in peripheral soft tissues and even bone. Many of these tumors are designated as peripheral neuroblastomas or neuroepitheliomas. Similar neoplasms arise in the chest wall, presumably from intercostal nerves (Askin tumor). Some investigators have grouped these tumors under the generic description of primitive neuroectodermal tumors (PNET) (for marker studies see p. 1612).[236,250,260]

The majority of neuroblastomas in infants present initially as an abdominal mass; fever, pain, and irritability are also significant signs. Other significant presentation signs include paraplegia, enlarged lymph nodes, proptosis, nasal obstruction, and hemorrhages. Angiographic studies are important for the diagnosis of neuroblastomas; in the case of abdominal tumors, pyelography is also important, given that tumor growth often results in the displacement of the renal calyceal system. Conventional radiography and CT scanning of the retroperitoneum, chest, and skeletal system are also important for assessment of the extent of the disease and metastases. Foci of calcification may be noted in neuroblastomas and may constitute radiologically important diagnostic signs.[242,263]

Neuroblastomas of the adrenal medulla range from microscopic foci (in situ neuroblastomas) to large masses that occupy most of the abdominal cavity. Most neuroblastomas appear as nodular masses, several centimeters in diameter. They may appear deceptively circumscribed and surrounded by a bright yellow rim of preserved adrenal cortex; more frequently, however, invasion of the capsule and extension beyond the site of origin are evident. Cut surfaces of well-preserved tumors are pink-gray; however, well-preserved tumors are exceptional since neuroblastomas are exceedingly friable with pronounced tendency to necrosis, hemorrhage, and cystic degeneration. Neuroblastomas primarily in the adrenal and retroperitoneum readily engulf or displace the major vessels, kidneys, and ureters. They may also directly invade neighboring viscera including kidney, liver, pancreas as well as the spinal cord via the vertebral foramina.[242,263]

Microscopically, neuroblastomas consist of small, round, and fusiform cells, often only slightly larger than lymphocytes. They are arranged in irregular sheets separated by fibrovascular strands. In well-preserved areas, round aggregates of tumor cells may be noted (Fig. 33-33). Classical neuroblastomas show Homer-

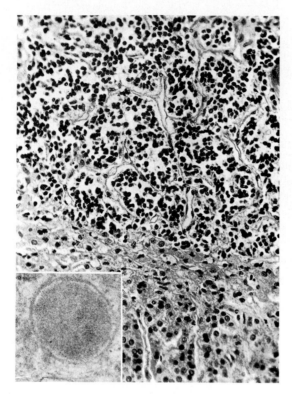

Fig. 33-33. Adrenomedullary neuroblastoma in newborn infant. (200×.) *Inset,* Membrane-enclosed catecholamine granule. (50,000×.)

Wright rosettes defined by a circle of dark tumor cells polarized toward a pale center, which is eosinophilic and faintly fibrillar; these structures, however, are found in only about one third of cases. The nuclei are deeply basophilic, and nucleoli are not prominent; the mitotic activity is variable but often brisk. The cytoplasm is scanty and poorly defined. Often one notices a loose and faintly eosinophilic fibrillar matrix or background, which corresponds to tangles of nerve fibrils. Given the gross description, necrosis, hemorrhage, and cystic changes may dominate the picture; calcification may also be noted. Invasion of lymphatics and veins is often found.[242,263]

"Maturing" neuroblastomas are characterized by the presence of increasingly large tumor cells with vesicular nuclei and nucleoli, increasing amounts of cytoplasm, increasing numbers of cell processes and rosettes, and recognizable ganglion cells.[242,263]

By electron microscopy, the fibrillar matrix consists of tangles of cell processes showing predominantly arrays of microtubules and some mitochondria; occasional aggregates of small neurosecretory granules may be noted. Cells and processes may be linked by nondesmosomal junctions. Neuroblastoma rosettes lack a basal lamina, a feature that differentiates them readily from the tubules in Wilms' tumor.[240,248,252]

By immunocytochemistry, given well-preserved material, neuroblastomas can be shown to express neuron-specific enolase[248,262] and synaptophysin.[244,245,273] Their intermediate filament complement consists exclusively of neurofilament proteins.[244-246,257,262] The related but distinct peripheral neuroectodermal tumors may express similar neural and neuroendocrine markers, such as neuron-specific enolase and synaptophysin, and neurofilament proteins respectively; however, peripheral neuroectodermal tumors have a different and more complex complement of intermediate filament proteins because they express predominantly vimentin and may variably coexpress neurofilament proteins, cytokeratins, and glial filament proteins.[246] Additional differential diagnoses include Ewing's sarcoma whose intermediate filament complement is composed very predominantly of vimentin with subpopulations that may express cytokeratins and neurofilament proteins.[259] By electron microscopy Ewing's sarcoma displays characteristic glycogen pools. Lymphomas may also pose differential diagnostic problems; in this case, the demonstration of characteristic lymphoma markers and the fact that lymphomas express vimentin only should prove helpful.[248]

Metastases of neuroblastomas are frequent and travel through lymphatic and venous systems. Characteristically, metastases develop in regional lymph nodes, bones, and liver. The development of extensive osseous neuroblastoma metastases involving particularly the skull is referred to as "Hutchinson's syndrome," whereas the development of massive liver metastases with resulting hepatomegaly is referred to as "Pepper's syndrome." Metastases in long bones may elicit a multilayered subperiosteal bone formation reflected in roentgenograms by an "onion-skin" pattern.[242,263]

Neuroblastomas seldom present with a clinical hormonal syndrome but nevertheless produce variable amounts of dopamine and catecholamines. In most cases, catecholamines or some of their metabolites may be determined in the urine. Particularly helpful in the diagnosis, in the monitoring of neuroblastoma response to therapy and the appearance of metastases, are the determinations of vanillylmandelic acid (VMA) and homovanillic acid (HVA). Rare neuroblastomas may present with hormonal syndromes related to the secretion of peptide hormones, such as VIP oversecretion with resulting watery diarrhea syndrome. Presumably typical "neuroblastoma antigens" as well as carcinoembryonic antigen (CEA) and certain still poorly understood immune complexes have been reported in neuroblastomas. It has also been noted that immune mechanisms may play a significant role in the rare but well-documented cases of total regression of untreated neuroblastomas.[242,263,269]

Neuroblastomas are malignant neoplasms; nevertheless, their aggressiveness varies considerably. In very young infants they are distinctly less malignant. Also notable is their occasional evolution or "maturation" to less malignant, indeed benign tumors, such as ganglioneuromas, which may occur with and without intervening therapy. Intermediate tumor types, such as ganglioneuroblastomas, also occur. Still, the majority of neuroblastomas diagnosed beyond 1 year of age have already metastasized at presentation.[242,263]

Paraganglioma is the preferred designation for pheochromocytoma arising in various sites, including viscera and particularly in paraganglia other than the adrenal medulla.[241,242,263] The organ of Zuckerkandl consists of a cluster of retroperitoneal paraganglia at the bifurcation of the aorta; these are comparatively prominent during infancy but involute subsequently. This organ as well as the posterior mediastinum are not uncommon primary sites of paragangliomas. Other sites are the retroperitoneum in general, the base of the skull, the neck, and vagal and aortic bodies, in addition there are well-defined paraganglia such as the carotid and jugular bodies and other named and unnamed clusters of paraganglionic cells. The larynx and small intestine and particularly the urinary bladder are visceral sites of paraganglioma. Urinary bladder paragangliomas occasionally present with a dramatic syndrome of headaches and hypertensive crises upon urination.[241,242,263]

The "carotid body tumor" is a classic paraganglioma. It may present as a palpable neck mass encompassing the carotid artery. These tumors tend to be soft; their cut surfaces are pale gray-pink or yellow; large tumors may be partly necrotic and cystic. By light and electron microscopy as well as by immunocytochemistry, paragangliomas are indistinguishable from pheochromocytomas. Also similar to pheochromocytomas, the presence of cellular atypism in paragangliomas is not tantamount to malignancy. Most paragangliomas do not metastasize. Nevertheless, it should be noted that, as a group, paragangliomas are more likely to develop metastases than pheochromocytomas; paragangliomas may also recur and spread locally and develop metastases more readily than their counterparts of the adrenal medulla. The potential of paragangliomas to develop metastases should not be excluded by the conventional 5-year, disease-free interval, since paraganglioma metastases presenting 10 to 30 years after removal of the primary have been recorded.[242,243,253,271,272]

Paraganglioma cells have an abundant complement of typical and generally large neurosecretory granules*; occasionally paragangliomas may produce sufficient amounts of catecholamines to cause hypertension. By immunocytochemistry, neuropeptides are readily demonstrable in most paragangliomas.[253,271,272] Nevertheless, hormonal syndromes associated with such materials are rare; such syndromes include watery diarrhea syndrome associated with the overproduction of VIP. With regard to intermediate filament proteins, paraganglioma cells express only neurofilament proteins,[245,248] but associated Schwann-like cells express vimentin.[246]

Ganglioneuromas are benign tumors appearing grossly as well-demarcated, encapsulated masses with distinctly myxoid cut surfaces; they arise in the same sites as pheochromocytomas, paragangliomas, and neuroblastomas but are most frequent in the posterior mediastinum and retroperitoneum. Microscopically, they consist of prominent, well-differentiated ganglion cells that are readily recognized as such with their large nuclei and typically prominent nucleoli.[242,263] Ganglioneuromas also include neural processes and an abundant and loose stroma and may also have some Schwann-like cells. By electron microscopy, neurosecretory granules are noted particularly in the cell processes.[240,242,252] By immunohistochemistry, ganglioneuromas can be shown to express neuron-specific enolase and synaptophysin; neuropeptide hormones such as calcitonin, somatostatin, and VIP may be demonstrable irrespective of the fact that most ganglioneuromas are not associated with clinical hormonal syndromes.[245] Their intermediate filament complement consists exclusively of neurofilament proteins,[245,273] though if Schwann-like cells are present, the Schwann-like cells will express vimentin.[246]

Ganglioneuromas, pheochromocytoma-paragangliomas, and neuroblastomas of all sites are regarded as a spectrum of neoplasms that are structurally, functionally, and embryogenetically closely related. They all arise in organs or sites that include cells that are part of the dispersed neuroendocrine system (DNS). Not surprisingly, all these tumors have the capability to produce biologically active neuroamine and neuropeptide hormones; but, although this capability is invariably demonstrable immunohistochemically or biochemically, the frequency of clinical hormonal syndromes is, as outlined, very variable.[248]

REFERENCES
Historical background

1. Bartholinus, T.: Anatomica ex Caspari Bartholini Parentis Institutionibus, Lugdini Batavorum: apud Franciseum Hackium, 1651; London, 1668, John Streater.
2. Cuvier, G.: Leçons d'anatomie comparée, Paris, 1805.
3. Eustachius, B.: Tabulae anatomicae (edited by Lancisius), Amsterdam, 1722.
4. Gaunt, R.: History of the adrenal cortex. In Greep, R.O., and Astwood, E.B., editors: Handbook of physiology; sect. 7, Endocrinology; vol. VI, Adrenal gland, Washington, D.C., 1975, American Physiological Society.
5. Medvei, V.C.: A history of endocrinology, Hingham, Mass. (Lancaster, Eng.), 1982, MTP Press.
6. Riolan, J.: Les œuvres anatomiques, Paris, 1629.
7. Rolleston, H.D.: The endocrine organs in health and disease with an historical review, London, 1936, Oxford University Press.

---

*References 240, 242, 253, 271, 272.

8. Thorn, G.W.: The adrenal cortex. 1. Historical aspects, Johns Hopkins Med. J. **123:**49-77, 1968.

Structure and function

9. Arnold, J.: Ein Beitrag zu der feineren Structur und dem Chemismus der Nebennieren, Arch. Pathol. Anat. Physiol. Klin. Med. **35:**64-107, 1866.
10. Baxter, J.D., and Tyrrell, J.B.: The adrenal cortex. In Felig, P., Baxter, J.D., Broadus, A.E., and Frohman, L.A., editors: Endocrinology and metabolism, ed. 2, New York, 1987, McGraw-Hill Book Co.
11. Bethune, J.E.: The adrenal cortex, Kalamazoo, Mich., 1974, Upjohn Co.
12. Bloodworth, J.M.B., Jr.: The adrenal. In Sommers, S.C., editor: Endocrine pathology decennial 1966-1975, New York, 1975, Appleton-Century-Crofts.
13. Bloodworth, J.M.B., Jr., Horvath, E., and Kovacs, K.: Fine structural pathology of the endocrine system. In Trump, B.F., and Jones, R.T., editors: Diagnostic electron microscopy, vol. 3, New York, 1980, John Wiley & Sons, Inc.
14. Bondy, P.K.: Disorders of the adrenal cortex. In Wilson, J.D., and Foster, D.W., editors: Williams textbook of endocrinology, Philadelphia, 1985, W.B. Saunders Co.
15. Brooks, R.V.: Biosynthesis and metabolism of adrenal cortical steroids. In James, V.T., editors: The adrenal gland, New York, 1979, Raven Press.
16. del Regato, J.A., and Spjut, H.J.: Lymphatics of the suprarenal glands, p. 697 in del Regato, J.A., and Spjut, H.J., editors: Ackerman and del Regato's cancer, ed. 5, St. Louis, 1977, The C.V. Mosby Co.
17. Dobbie, J.W., and Symington, T.: The human adrenal gland with special reference to the vasculature, J. Endocrinol. **34:**479-489, 1966.
18. Forsham, P.H., and Melmon, K.L.: The adrenals. In Williams, R.H., editor: Textbook of endocrinology, ed. 4, Philadelphia, 1968, W.B. Saunders Co.
18a. Gabcke, C.E.: Ueber einen Fall vom primären Spindelzellensarkom des Thymus, inaugural dissertation, Kiel, 1896, P. Peters; quoted by Leyton, D., Turnbull, H.M., and Bratton, A.B.: Primary cancer of thymus with pluriglandular disturbance, J. Pathol. Bacteriol. **34:**635, 1931.
19. Gottschau, M.: Struktur und embryonale Entwicklung der Nebennieren bei Säugetieren, Arch. Anat. Physiol. (Leipzig), pp. 412-458, 1883.
20. Idelman, S.: The structure of the mammalian adrenal cortex. In Jones, I.C., and Henderson, I.W., editors: General, comparative and clinical endocrinology of the adrenal cortex, vol. 2, London, 1976, Academic Press.
21. James, V.H.T.: Comprehensive endocrinology: the adrenal gland, New York, 1979, Raven Press.
22. Liddle, G.W.: Tests of pituitary-adrenal suppressibility in the diagnosis of Cushing's syndrome, J. Clin. Endocrinol. Metab. **20:**1539-1560, 1960.
23. Liddle, G.W.: The adrenals. In Williams, R.H., editor: Textbook of endocrinology, Philadelphia, 1981, W.B. Saunders Co.
24. Ludwig, J.: Current methods of autopsy practice, ed. 2, pp. 661-663, Philadelphia, 1979, W.B. Saunders Co.
25. Mulrow, P.J., editor: The adrenal gland, New York, 1986, Elsevier Science Publishing Co; quoting from ref. 18a.
26. Netter, F.H.: The CIBA collection of medical illustrations, vol. 4: Endocrine system and selected metabolic diseases, New York, 1965, CIBA.
27. Neville, A.M., and O'Hare, M.J.: Aspects of structure, function and pathology. In James, V.H.T., editor: The adrenal gland, New York, 1979, Raven Press.
28. Schulz, D.M., Giordano, D.A., and Schulz, D.H.: Weights of organs of fetuses and infants, Arch. Pathol. **74:**244-250, 1962.
29. Selye, H.: The adrenals. In Textbook of endocrinology, Montreal, 1947, Acta Endocrinologica.
30. Sloper, J.C., and Fox, B.: The adrenal glands. In Symmers, W.St.C., editor: Systemic pathology, ed. 2, vol. 4, Edinburgh, 1978, Churchill Livingstone.

31. Sommers, S.C.: Adrenal glands. In Kissane, j.M., editor: Anderson's pathology, ed. 8, St. Louis, 1985, The C.V. Mosby Co.
32. Sunderman, F.W., and Boerner, F.: Normal values in clinical medicine, Philadelphia, 1949, W.B. Saunders Co.
33. Symington, T.: Functional pathology of the human adrenal gland, Edinburgh, 1969, E&S Livingstone Ltd.
34. Symington, T.: The adrenal cortex. In Bloodworth, J.M.B., editor: Endocrine pathology, ed. 2, Baltimore, 1982, The Williams & Wilkins Co.
35. Tannenbaum, M.: Ultrastructural pathology of the adrenal cortex, Pathol. Annu. **8:**109-156, 1973.
36. Temple, T.E., and Liddle, G.W.: Inhibitors of adrenal steroid biosynthesis, Annu. Rev. Pharmacol. **10:**199-218, 1970.
37. Watts, N.B., and Keffer, J.H.: Practical endocrine diagnosis, ed. 3, Philadelphia, 1982, Lea & Febiger.

Imaging

38. Copeland, P.M.: The incidentally discovered adrenal mass, Ann. Intern. Med. **98:**940-945, 1983.
39. Hussain, S., Belldegrun, A., Seltzer, S.E., Richie, J.P., Gittes, R.F., and Abrams, H.L.: Differentiation of malignant from benign adrenal masses: predictive indices on computed tomography, AJR **144:**61-65, 1985.
40. Kenney, P.J., Kenney, P.J., Berlow, M.E., and Ellis, D.A.: Current imaging of adrenal masses, RadioGraphics **4(5):**743-783, Sept. 1984.
41. Mitty, H.A., and Yeh, H.-C.: Radiology of the adrenals with sonography and CT, Philadelphia, 1982, W.B. Saunders Co.
42. Reinig, J.W., Doppman, J.L., Dwyer, A.J., Johnson, A.R., and Knop, R.H.: Adrenal masses differentiated by MR, Radiology **158:**81-84, 1986.
43. Reinig, J.W., Doppman, J.L., Dwyer, A.J., Johnson, A.R., and Knop, R.H.: Distinction between adrenal adenomas and metastases using MR imaging, J. Comput. Assist. Tomogr. **9(5):**898-901, 1985.
44. Reinig, J.W., Doppman, J.L., Dwyer, A.J., and Frank, J.: MRI of indeterminate adrenal masses, AJR **147:**493-496, 1986.
45. Schultz, C.L., Haaga, J.R., Fletcher, B.D., Alfidi, R.J., and Schultz, M.A.: Magnetic resonance imaging of the adrenal glands: a comparison with computed tomography, AJR **143:**1235-1240, 1984.

Embryology and fetal development

46. Arey, L.B.: Developmental anatomy, ed. 4, Philadelphia, 1940, W.B. Saunders Co.
47. Graham, L.S.: Celiac accessory adrenal glands, Cancer **6:**149-152, 1952.
48. Kölliker, A.: Entwickelungsgeschichte des Menschen und höheren Thiere, Leipzig, 1861, W. Engelmann.
49. Nelson, A.A.: Accessory adrenal cortical tissue, Arch. Pathol. **27:**955-965, 1939.
50. Potter, E.L., and Craig, J.M.: Adrenal glands. In Pathology of the fetus and the infant, ed. 3, Chicago, 1975, Year Book Medical Publishers.
51. Vales-Dapena, M.A.: The adrenal gland. In Histology of the fetus and newborn, Phladelphia, 1979, W.B. Saunders Co.
52. Wigglesworth, J.S.: Perinatal pathology, Philadelphia, 1984, W.B. Saunders Co.

Disorders of infancy and childhood

53. Aterman, K., Kerenyi, N., and Lee, M.: Adrenal cytomegaly, Virchows Arch. [A, Pathol. Anat.] **355:**105-122, 1972.
54. Bartter, F.C.: Adrenogenital syndromes from physiology to chemistry (1950-1975). In Lee, P.A., Plotnick, L.P., Kowarski, A.A., and Migeon, C.J., editors: Congenital adrenal hyperplasia, Baltimore, 1977, University Park Press.
55. Bartter, F.C., Albright, F., Forbes, A., Leaf, A., Dempsey, E., and Carroll, E.: The effects of adrenocorticotropic hormone and cortisone in the adrenogenital syndrome associated with congenital adrenal hyperplasia: an attempt to explain and correct its disordered hormonal pattern, J. Clin. Invest. **30:**237-251, 1951.
56. Bartter, F.C., Henkin, R.I., and Bryan, G.T.: Aldosterone hy-

persecretion in "non-salt-losing" congenital adrenal hyperplasia, J. Clin. Invest. **47:**1742-1752, 1968.

57. Bullock, W., and Sequiera, J.H.: On the relation of the suprarenal capsules to the sex organs, Trans. Pathol. Soc. Lond. **56:**189-208, 1905.

58. Dehner, L.P.: Pediatric surgical pathology, ed. 2, Baltimore, 1987, The Williams & Wilkins Co.; quoting from ref. 68a.

59. Favara, B.E., Franciosi, R.A., and Miles, V.: Idiopathic adrenal hypoplasia in children, Am. J. Clin. Pathol. **57:**287-296, 1972.

60. Friderichsen, C.: Nebennierenapoplexie bei kleinen Kindern, Jahrbuch Kinderheilkd. **87:**109-125, 1918.

61. Golden, M.P., Lippe, B.M., and Kaplan, S.A.: Congenital adrenal hypoplasia and hypogonadotropic hypogonadism, Am. J. Dis. Child. **131:**1117-1118, 1977.

62. Göksu, N., Cağlar, M., Tunçer, M., and Senocak, M.E.: A case of congenital adrenal hypoplasia and review of the literature, Turk. J. Pediatr. **24:**103-108, 1982.

63. Gutai, J.P., and Migeon, C.J.: Adrenal insufficiency during the neonatal period, Clin. Perinatol. **2:**163-186, 1975.

64. Hay, I.D., Smail, P.J., and Forsyth, C.C.: Familial cytomegalic adrenocortical hypoplasia: an X-linked syndrome of pubertal failure, Arch. Dis. Child. **56:**15, 1981.

65. Larroche, J.C.: Developmental pathology of the neonate, Amsterdam, 1977, Excerpta Medica.

66. Laverty, C.R.A., Fortune, D.W, and Belscher, N.A.: Congenital idiopathic adrenal hypoplasia, Obstet. Gynecol. **41:**655-664, 1973.

67. Lee, P.A., Plotnick, L.P., Kowarski, A.A., and Migeon, C.J., editors: Congenital adrenal hyperplasia, Baltimore, 1975, University Park Press.

68. Marsden, H.B., and Zakhour, H.D.: Cytomegalic adrenal hypoplasia with pituitary cytomegaly, Virchows Arch. [A, Pathol. Anat.] **378:**105-110, 1978.

68a. Martin, J.J., Ceuterick, C., and Libert, J.: Skin and conjunctival nerve biopsies in adrenoleukodystrophy and its variants, Ann. Neurol. **8:**291, 1980.

69. New, M.I., and Levine, L.S.: Congenital adrenal hyperplasia, Berlin, 1984, Springer-Verlag.

70. Peterson, K.E., Bille, T., and Jacobsen, B.B.: X-linked congenital adrenal hypoplasia: a study of five generations of a Greenlandic family, Acta Paediatr. Scand. **71:**947-951, 1982.

71. Peterson, K.E., Tygstrup, I., and Thamdrup, E.: Familial adrenocortical hypoplasia with early clinical and biochemical signs of mineralocorticoid deficiency (hypoaldosteronism), Acta Endocrinol. **84:**605-619, 1977.

72. Powers, J.M., and Schaumburg, H.H.: Adreno-leukodystrophy (sex-linked Schilder's disease), Am. J. Pathol. **76:**481-492, 1974.

73. Powers, J.M., Schaumburg, H.H., Johnson, A.B., and Raine, C.S.: A correlative study of the adrenal cortex in adrenoleukodystrophy: evidence for a fatal intoxication with very long chain saturated fatty acids, Invest. Cell Pathol. **3:**353-376, 1980.

74. Powers, J.M.: Adreno-leukodystrophy (adreno-testiculo-leukomyeloneuropathic complex), Clin. Neuropathol. **4:**181-199, 1985.

75. Ruiz-Palacios, G., Pickering, L.K., vanEys, J., and Conklin, R.: Disseminated herpes simplex with hepatoadrenal necrosis in a child with acute leukemia, J. Pediatr. **91:**757-759, 1977.

76. Russell, M.A., Opitz, J.M., Viseskul, C., et al.: Sudden infant death due to congenital adrenal hypoplasia, Arch. Pathol. Lab. Med. **101:**168-169, 1977.

77. Sperling, M.A., Wolfsen, A.R., and Fisher, D.A.: Congenital adrenal hypoplasia: an isolated defect in organogenesis, J. Pediatr. **82:**444-449, 1973.

78. Sucheston, M.E., and Cannon, M.S.: Microscopic comparison of the normal and anencephalic human adrenal gland with emphasis on the transient zone, Obstet. Gynecol. **35:**544-553, 1970.

79. Templeton, A.C.: Generalized herpes simplex in malnourished children, J. Clin. Pathol. **23:**24-30, 1970.

80. Tucker, E.S., III, and Scofield, G.F.: Hepatoadrenal necrosis, Arch. Pathol. **71:**538-547, 1961.

81. Waterhouse, R.: A case of suprarenal apoplexy, Lancet **1:**577-578, 1911.

82. White, P.C., New, M.I., and Dupont, B.: Medical progress: congenital adrenal hyperplasia, N. Engl. J. Med. **316:**1519-1524, 1580-1586, 1987.

83. Wilkins, L., Blizzard, R.M., and Migeon, C.J.: The diagnosis and treatment of endocrine disorders in childhood and adolescence, ed. 3, Springfield, Ill., 1965, Charles C Thomas, Publisher.

84. Wilkins, L., and Cara, J.: Further studies on the treatment of congenital adrenal hyperplasia and cortisone. Part V. Effects of cortisone therapy on testicular development, J. Clin. Endocrinol. Metab. **14:**287-296, 1954.

85. Wilkins, L., Crigler, J.F., Silverman, S.H., Gardner, L.I., and Migeon, C.J.: Further studies on the treatment of congenital adrenal hyperplasia with cortisone. Part II. The effects of cortisone on sexual and somatic development with a hypothesis concerning the mechanism of feminization, J. Clin. Endocrinol. Metab. **12:**277-295, 1952.

86. Wilkins, L., Fleischmann, W., and Howard, J.E.: Macrogenitosomia precox associated with hyperplasia of the androgenic tissue of the adrenal and death from corticoadrenal insufficiency, Endocrinology **26:**385-395, 1940.

87. Wilkins, L., Lewis, R.A., Klein, R., and Rosemberg, E.: The suppression of androgen secretion by cortisone in a case of congenital adrenal hyperplasia, Bull. Johns Hopkins Hosp. **86:**249-255, 1950.

88. Wittenberg, D.F.: Familial X-linked adrenocortical hypoplasia association with androgenic precocity, Arch. Dis. Child. **56:**633-639, 1981.

89. Young, H.H.: Genital abnormalities, hermaphroditism, and related adrenal diseases, Baltimore, 1937, The Williams & Wilkins Co.

Addison's disease

90. Addison, T.: On the constitutional and local effects of diseases of the supra-renal capsules, London, 1855, Samuel Highley; reprinted by Classics of Medicine Library, Birmingham, Alabama, 1980.

91. Anderson, J.R., Goudie, R.B., Gray, K.G., and Timbury, G.C.: Autoantibodies in Addison's disease, Lancet **1:**1123-1124, 1957.

92. Blizzard, R.M., Chee, D., and Davis, W.: The incidence of adrenal and other antibodies in the sera of patients with idiopathic adrenal insufficiency (Addison's disease), Clin. Exp. Immunol. **2:**19-30, 1967.

93. Blizzard, R.M., and Kyle, M.: Studies of the adrenal antigens and antibodies in Addison's disease, J. Clin. Invest. **42:**1653-1660, 1963.

94. Carpenter, C.J., Soloman, N., Silverberg, S.G., et al.: Schmidt's syndrome (thyroid and adrenal insufficiency): a review of the literature and a report of 15 new cases including 10 instances of co-existent diabetes mellitus, Medicine **43:**153-180, 1964.

95. Crispell, E.R., Parson, W., Hamlin, J., et al.: Addison's disease associated with histoplasmosis: report of four cases and review of the literature, Am. J. Med. **20:**23-29, 1956.

96. Doniach, D., Cudworth, A.G., Khoury, E.L., and Bottazzo, G.F.: Autoimmunity and the HLA-system in endocrine disease. In O'Riordan, J.L.H., editor: Recent advances in endocrinology and metabolism, London, 1982, Churchill Livingstone.

97. Frawley, T.F.: Adrenal cortical insufficiency. In Eisenstein, A.B., editor: The adrenal cortex, Boston, 1967, Little, Brown & Co.

98. Goudie, R.B., McDonald, E., Anderson, J.R., and Gray, K.: Immunological features of idiopathic Addison's disease: characterization of the adrenocortical antigens, Clin. Exp. Immunol. **3:**119-131, 1968.

99. Guttman, P.H.: Addison's disease: a statistical analysis of 566 new cases and a study of the pathology, Arch. Pathol. (Chicago) **10:**742-785, 895-935, 1930.

100. Heller, E.L., and Camarata, S.I.: Addison's disease from amyloidosis of adrenal glands, Arch. Pathol. **49:**601-604, 1950.

101. Irvine, W.J., and Barnes, E.W.: Adrenocortical insufficiency, Clin. Endocrinol. Metab. **1:**549-594, 1972.

102. Irvine, W.J., Chan, M.M.W., and Scarth, L.: The further characterization of auto-antibodies reactive with extra-renal steroid-producing cells in patients with adrenal disorders, Clin. Exp. Immunol. 4:489-503, 1969.

103. Maloney, P.J., Addison's disease due to chronic disseminated coccidioidomycosis, Arch. Intern. Med. 90:869-878, 1952.

104. Margaretten, W., Hisayo, N., and Landing, B.H.: Septicemic adrenal hemorrhage, Am. J. Dis. Child. 105:346-351, 1963.

105. Nelson, D.H.: Addison's disease (primary adrenal insufficiency). In Nelson, D.H., editor: The adrenal cortex: physiological function and disease, major problems in internal medicine, vol. 18, Philadelphia, 1980, W.B. Saunders Co.

106. Nerup, J.: Addison's disease: clinical studies: a report of 108 cases, Acta Endocrinol. 76:127-141, 1974.

107. Nerup, J., and Bendixen, G.: Antiadrenal cellular hypersensitivity in Addison's disease. II. Correlation with clinical and serological findings, Clin. Exp. Immunol. 5:341-353, 1969.

108. Nerup, J., and Bendixen, G.: Antiadrenal cellular hypersensitivity in Addison's disease. III. Species-specificity and subcellular localization of the antigen, Clin. Exp. Immunol. 5:355-364, 1969.

109. O'Donnell, W.M.: Changing pathogenesis of Addison's disease, with special reference to amyloidosis, Arch. Intern. Med. 86:266-279, 1950.

110. Platz, P., Ryder, L., Nielsen, L.S., et al.: HL-A and idiopathic Addison's disease, Lancet 2:289, 1974.

111. Schmidt, M.B.: Eine biglanduläre Erkrankung (Nebennieren und Schilddruse) bei morbus Addisonii, Verh. Dtsch. Ges. Pathol. 21:212-220, 1926.

112. Spinner, M.W., Blizzard, R.M., Gibbs, J., et al.: Familial distributions of organ-specific antibodies in the blood of patients with Addison's disease and hypoparathyroidism and their relatives, Clin. Exp. Immunol. 5:461, 1969.

113. Thorn, G.W.: The diagnosis and treatment of adrenal insufficiency, Springfield, Ill., 1951, Charles C Thomas, Publisher.

Cushing's syndrome

114. Albright F., Parson, W., and Bloomberg, E.: Therapy in Cushing's syndrome, J. Clin. Endocrinol. 1:375-384, 1941.

115. Anderson, E., Haymaker, W., and Joseph, M.: Hormonal and electrolyte studies of patients with hyperadrenocortical syndrome (Cushing's syndrome), Endocrinology 23:398-402, 1938.

116. Brown, W.H.: A case of pluriglandular syndrome: "diabetes of bearded women," Lancet 2:1022-1023, 1928.

117. Carpenter, P.C.: Cushing's syndrome: update of diagnosis and management, Mayo Clin. Proc. 61:49-58, 1986.

118. Coates, P.J., Doniach, I., Howlett, T.A., Rees, L.N., and Besser, G.M.: Immunocytochemical study of 18 tumours causing ectopic Cushing's syndrome, J. Clin. Pathol. 39:955-960, 1986.

119. Cushing, H.: The pituitary body and its disorders, Philadelphia, 1912, W.B. Saunders Co.; reprinted by Classics of Medicine Library, Birmingham, Alabama, 1980.

120. Cushing, H.: The basophil adenomas of the pituitary body and their clinical manifestations (pituitary basophilism), Bull. Johns Hopkins Hosp. 50:137-195, 1932.

121. Grant, C.S., Carney, J.A., Carpenter, P.C., and van Heerden, J.A.: Primary pigmented nodular adrenocortical disease: diagnosis and management, Surgery 100:1178-1182, 1986.

122. Howlett, T.A., Drury, P.L., Perry, L., Doniach, I., Rees, L.H., and Besser, G.M.: Diagnosis and management of ACTH-dependent Cushing's syndrome: comparison of the features in ectopic and pituitary ACTH production, Clin. Endocrinol. (Oxf.) 24:699-713, 1986.

123. Krieger, D.T.: Cushing's syndrome, Berlin, 1982, Springer-Verlag.

124. Larsen, J.L., Cathey, W.J., and Odell, W.D.: Primary adrenocortical nodular dysplasia, a distinct subtype of Cushing's syndrome: case report and review of the literature, Am. J. Med. 80:976-984, 1986.

125. Marshall, R.B.: Adrenal cortical hyperplasia in Cushing's disease, Anatomic Pathology Check Sample AP-43, Chicago, 1977, American Society of Clinical Pathologists.

126. McArthur, R.G., Cloutier, M.D., Hayles, A.B., et al.: Cushing's disease in children, Mayo Clin. Proc. 47:318-326, 1972.

127. Meador, C.K., Bowdoin, B., Owen, W.C., Jr., et al.: Primary adrenocortical nodular dysplasia: a rare cause of Cushing's syndrome, J. Clin. Endocrinol. Metab. 27:1255-1263, 1967.

128. Orth, D.N., and Liddle, G.W.: Results of treatment in 108 patients with Cushing's syndrome, N. Engl. J. Med. 285:243-247, 1971.

129. Plotz, C.M., Knowlton, A.I., and Ragan, C.: The natural history of Cushing's syndrome, Am. J. Med. 13:597-616, 1952.

130. Rose, E.K., Enterline, H.T., Rhoads, J.E., and Rose, E.: Adrenal cortical hyperfunction in childhood, Pediatrics 9:475-484, 1952.

131. Ruder, H.J., Loriaux, D.L., and Lipsett, M.B.: Severe osteopenia in young adults associated with Cushing's syndrome due to micronodular adrenal disease, J. Clin. Endocrinol. Metab. 39:1138-1147, 1974.

132. Scott, H.W., Jr., Foster, J.H., Liddle, G., and Davidson, E.T.: Cushing's syndrome due to adrenocortical tumor, Ann. Surg. 162:505-516, 1965.

133. Soffer, L.J., Iannaccone, A., and Gabrilove, J.L.: Cushing's syndrome, Am. J. Med. 30:129-146, 1961.

134. Walters, W., Wilder, R.M., and Kepler, E.J.: The suprarenal cortical syndrome with presentation of ten cases, Ann. Surg. 100:670-688, 1934.

Nodules, adenoma, carcinoma, aldosteronism

135. Aberg, H., Johansson, H., Mörlin, C., and El-Sherief, A.: Malignant aldosteronoma, Acta Chir. Scand. 147:735-737, 1981.

136. Arteaga, E., Biglieri, E.G., Kater, C.E., López, J.M., and Schambelan, M.: Aldosterone-producing adrenocortical carcinoma, Ann. Intern. Med. 101:316-321, 1984.

137. Ashley, D.J.B.: Evans' histological appearances of tumours, ed. 3, vol. 1, Edinburgh, 1978, Churchill Livingstone.

138. Bahu, R.M., Battifora, H., and Shambaugh, G., III: Functional black adenoma of the adrenal gland, Arch. Pathol. 98:139-142, 1974.

139. Birke, G., Franksson, C., Gemzell, C.-A., Moberger, G., and Plantin, L.O.: Adrenal cortical tumors, Acta Chir. Scand. 117:233-246, 1959.

140. Brennan, M.F., and Macdonald, J.S.: Cancer of the endocrine system: the adrenal gland. In DeVita, V.T., Hellman, S., and Rosenberg, S.A., editors: Cancer: principles and practice of oncology, ed. 2, Philadelphia, 1985, J.B. Lippincott Co.

141. Cagle, P.T., Hough, A.J., Pysher, T.J., Page, D.L., Johnson, E.H., Kirkland, R.T., Holcombe, J.H., and Hawkins, E.P.: Comparison of adrenal cortical tumors in children and adults, Cancer 57:2235-2237, 1986.

142. Cohn, K., Gottesman, L., and Brennan, M.: Adrenocortical carcinoma, Surgery 100:1170-1176, 1986.

143. Conn, J.W.: Evolution of primary aldosteronism as a highly specific clinical entity, JAMA 172:1650-1653, 1960.

144. Conn, J.W.: Primary aldosteronism, new clinical syndrome, J. Lab. Clin. Med. 45:6-17, 1955.

145. Conn, J.W., and Louis, L.H.: Primary aldosteronism, new clinical entity, Ann. Intern. Med. 44:1-15, 1956.

146. Damron, T.A., Schelper, R.L., and Sorensen, L.: Cytochemical demonstration of neuromelanin in black pigmented adrenal nodules, Am. J. Clin. Pathol. 87:334-341, 1987.

147. Dobbie, J.W.: Adrenocortical nodular hyperplasia: the aging adrenal, J. Pathol. 99:1-18, 1969.

148. Fuhrman, S.A., Tasky, L.C., and Limas, C.: Prognostic significance of morphologic parameters in renal cell carcinoma, Am. J. Surg. Pathol. 6:655-663, 1982.

149. Gabrilove, J.L., Sharma, D.C., Wotiz, H.H., et al.: Feminizing adrenocortical tumors in the male, Medicine 44:37-79, 1965.

150. Gandour, M.J., and Grizzle, W.E.: A small adrenocortical carcinoma with aggressive behaviour, Arch. Pathol. Lab. Med. 110:1076-1079, 1986.

151. Grizzle, W.E., Tolbert, L., Pittman, C.S., et al.: Corticotropin production by tumors of the autonomic nervous system, Arch. Pathol. Lab. Med. 108:545-550, 1984.

152. Hajjar, R.A., Hickey, R.C., and Samaan, N.A.: Adrenal cortical carcinoma, Cancer **35**:549-554, 1975.
153. Hartmann, W.H., Warner, N.E., and Oertel, J.E.: Proceedings of the 43rd Annual Anatomic Pathology Slide Seminar, Chicago, 1977, American Society of Clinical Pathologists.
154. Heinivaara, O.: On the structure of the human suprarenal vein, Ann. Med. Int. Fenn. **43**(suppl. 19):1-65, 1954.
155. Henley, D.J., van Heerden, J.A., Grant, C.S., Carney, J.A., and Carpenter, P.C.: Adrenal cortical carcinoma: a continuing challenge, Surgery **94**:926-931, 1983.
156. Hough, A.J., Hollifield, J.W., Page, D.L., and Hartmann, W.H.: Prognostic factors in adrenal cortical tumors, Am. J. Clin. Pathol. **72**:390-399, 1979.
157. Humphrey, G.B., Pysher, T., Holcombe, J., et al.: Overview on the management of adrenocortical carcinoma (ACC). In Humphrey, G.B., Grindey, F.B., Dehner, L.P., et al., editors: Adrenal and endocrine tumors in children, Boston, 1984, Martinus Nijhoff Publishers.
158. Hutter, A.M., Jr., and Kayhoe, D.E.: Adrenal cortical carcinoma, Am. J. Med. **41**:572-580, 1966.
159. Huvos, A.G., Hajdu, S.I., Brasfield, R.D., et al.: Adrenal cortical carcinoma, Cancer **25**:354-361, 1970.
160. Ibáñez, M.L.: The pathology of adrenal cortical carcinoma: study of 22 cases. In (M.D. Anderson Hospital:) Endocrine and nonendocrine hormone-producing tumors, Chicago, 1971, Year Book Medical Publishers.
161. Javadpour, N., Woltering, E.A., and Brennan, M.F.: Adrenal neoplasms, Curr. Probl. Surg. **17**:3-52, 1980.
162. Kaplowitz, P.B., Carpenter, R., Newsome, H.H., Jr., et al.: Cushing's syndrome resulting from primary pigmented nodular adrenocortical disease, Am. J. Dis. Child. **140**:1072-1075, 1986.
163. Karsner, H.T.: Tumors of the adrenal. In Atlas of tumor pathology, sect. 8, fascicle 29, Washington, D.C., 1950, Armed Forces Institute of Pathology.
164. King, D.R., and Lack, E.E.: Adrenal cortical carcinoma, Cancer **44**:239, 1979.
165. Kovacs, K., Horvath, E., and Singer, W.: Fine structure and morphogenesis of spironolactone bodies in the zona glomerulosa of the human adrenal cortex. J. Clin. Pathol. **26**:949, 1973.
166. Lewinsky, B.S., Grigor, K.M., Symington, T., et al.: The clinical and pathologic features of "non-hormonal" adrenocortical tumors: report of twenty new cases and review of the literature, Cancer **23**:778-790, 1974.
167. Lipsett, M.B., Hertz, R., and Ross, G.T.: Clinical and pathophysiological aspects of adrenocortical carcinoma, Am. J. Med. **35**:374, 1963.
168. McKenna, T.T., Miller, R.B., and Liddle, G.W.: Plasma pregnenolone and 17-OH-pregnenolone in patients with adrenal tumors, ACTH excess, or idiopathic hirsutism, J. Clin. Endocrinol. Metab. **44**:231-236, 1977.
169. Miettinen, M., Lehto, V.P., and Virtanen, I.: Immunofluorescence microscopic evaluation of the intermediate filament expression of the adrenal cortex and medulla and their tumors, Am. J. Pathol. **118**:360-366, 1985.
170. Nader, S., Hickey, R.C., Sellin, R.V., and Samaan, N.A.: Adrenal cortical carcinoma: a study of 77 cases, Cancer **52**:707-711, 1983.
171. Neville, A.M.: The nodular adrenal, Invest. Cell Pathol. **1**:99-111, 1978.
172. O'Hare, M.J., Monaghan, P., and Neville, A.M.: The pathology of adrenocortical neoplasia: a correlated structural and functional approach to the diagnosis of malignant disease, Hum. Pathol. **10**:137-154, 1979.
173. Page, D.L., DeLellis, R.A., and Hough, A.: Tumors of the adrenal. In Atlas of tumor pathology, ser. 2, fascicle 23, Washington, D.C., 1986, Armed Forces Institute of Pathology.
174. Robinson, M.J., Pardo, V., and Rywlin, A.M.: Pigmented nodules (black adenomas) of the adrenal: an autopsy study of incidence, morphology, and function, Hum. Pathol. **3**:317-325, 1972.
175. Schteingart, D.E., Oberman, H.A., Friedman, B.A., et al.: Adrenal cortical neoplasms producing Cushing's syndrome, Cancer **22**:1005-1013, 1968.
176. Scott, H.H., Abumrad, N.N., and Orth, D.N.: Tumors of the adrenal cortex and Cushing's syndrome, Ann. Surg. **201**:586-594, 1985.
177. Seligman, A.M., and Ashbel, R.: Histochemical demonstration of ketosteroids in virilizing tumors of the adrenal cortex, Endocrinology **49**(1):110-126, 1951.
178. Slee, P.H.T.J., Schaberg, A., and VanBrummelen, P.: Carcinoma of the adrenal cortex causing primary hyperaldosteronism, Cancer **51**:2341-2345, 1983.
179. Sommers, S.C., and Terzakis, J.A.: Ultrastructural study of aldosterone-secreting cells of the adrenal cortex, Am. J. Clin. Pathol. **54**:303, 1970.
180. Tang, C.K., and Gray, G.F.: Adrenocortical neoplasms: prognosis and morphology, Urology **5**:691-695, 1975.
181. Waisman, J.: The adrenal glands. In Coulson, W.F., editor: Surgical pathology, Philadelphia, 1978, J.B. Lippincott Co.
182. Warner, N.E.: Basic endocrine pathology, Chicago, 1971, Year Book Medical Publishers.
183. Warner, N.E., and Strauss, F.H.: The adrenal. In Silverberg, S.G., editor: Principles and practice of surgical pathology, vol. 2, New York, 1983, John Wiley & Sons.
184. Weiss, L.M.: Comparative histologic study of 43 metastasizing and nonmetastasizing adrenocortical tumors, Am. J. Surg. Pathol. **8**:163-169, 1984.
185. Wick, M.R., Cherwitz, D.L., McGlennen, R.C., and Dehner, L.P.: Adrenocortical carcinoma: an immunohistochemical comparison with renal cell carcinoma, Am. J. Pathol. **122**:343-352, 1986.
186. Williams, E.D., Siebenmann, R.E., and Sobin, L.H.: Histological typing of endocrine tumors, International histological classification of tumours, no. 23, Geneva, 1980, World Health Organization.

Adrenocortical carcinoma
Cytologic criteria

187. Cardozo, P.L.: Atlas of clinical cytology, Leyden, The Netherlands, 1975, Targa b.v.'s–Hertogenbosch (privately printed).
188. Levin, N.P.: Fine needle aspiration and histology of adrenal cortical carcinoma: a case report, Acta Cytol. **25**:421-424, 1981.
189. Zajicek, J.: Aspiration biopsy cytology. Part 2. Cytology of infradiaphragmatic organs, Basel, 1979, S. Karger, AG.

Flow cytometry

190. Amberson, J.B., Vaughan, E.D., Jr., Gray, G.F., and Naus, G.J.: Flow cytometric analysis of nuclear DNA from adrenocortical neoplasms: a retrospective study using paraffin-embedded tissue, Cancer **59**:2091-2095, 1987.
191. Bowlby, L.S., DeBault, L.E., and Abraham, S.R.: Flow cytometric analysis of adrenal cortical tumor DNA: relationship between cellular DNA and histopathologic classification, Cancer **58**:1499-1505, 1986.
192. Hedley, D.W., Friedlander, M.L., Taylor, I.W., Rugg, C.A., and Musgrove, E.A.: Method for analysis of cellular DNA content of paraffin-embedded pathological material using flow cytometry, J. Histochem. Cytochem. **31**:1333-1335, 1983.
193. Klein, F.A., Kay, S., Ratliff, J.E., White, F.K., and Newsome, H.H.: Flow cytometric determinations of ploidy and proliferation patterns of adrenal neoplasms: an adjunct to histological classification, J. Urol. **134**:933-935, 1985.
194. Taylor, S.R., Roederer, M., and Murphy, R.F.: Flow cytometric DNA analysis of adrenocortical tumors in children, Cancer **59**:2059-2063, 1987.

Metastases to the adrenal

195. Black, R.M., Daniels, G.H., Coggins, C.H., Mueller, P.R., Data, R.E., and Lichtenstein, N.: Adrenal insufficiency from metastatic colonic carcinoma masquerading as isolated aldosterone deficiency, Acta Endocrinol. (Copenh.) **98**:586-591, 1981.
196. Carey, R.W., Harris, N., and Kliman, B.: Addison's disease secondary to lymphomatous infiltration of the adrenal glands: recovery of adrenocortical function after chemotherapy, Cancer **59**:1087-1090, 1987.
197. Cedermark, B.J., Blumenson, L.E., Pickren, J.W., et al.: The

significance of metastasis to the adrenal gland from carcinoma of the stomach and esophagus, Surg. Gynecol. Obstet. **145**:41-48, 1977.

198. Cedermark, B.J., and Olsen, H.: Computed tomography in the diagnosis of metastasis of the adrenal glands, Surg. Gynecol. Obstet. **152**:13-16, 1981.

199. Cedermark, B.J., and Sjöberg, H.E.: The clinical significance of metastasis to the adrenal glands, Surg. Gynecol. Obstet. **152**:607-610, 1981.

200. Glomset, D.A.: The incidence of metastases of malignant tumors to the adrenals, Am. J. Cancer **32**:57-61, 1938.

201. Gupta, D.T., and Brasfield, R.: Metastatic melanoma, Cancer **17**:1323-1339, 1964.

202. Kliman, B., and Carey, R.W.: Recovery of adrenocortical function after chemotherapy in a case of Addison's disease caused by malignant infiltration of the adrenal glands (Abstr. 348), Presented at the Sixth International Congress on Hormonal Steroids, Jerusalem, Israel, Sept. 5, 1982.

203. Mackenzie, D.H.: Fatal suprarenal hemorrhage in an adult due to a metastasis from a bronchial carcinoma, J. Pathol. Bacteriol. **49**:333-335, 1955.

204. Redman, B.G., Pazdur, R., Zingas, A.P., and Loredo, R.: Prospective evaluation of adrenal insufficiency in patients with adrenal metastasis, Cancer **60**:103-107, 1987.

205. Seidenwurm, D.J., Elmer, E.B., Kaplan, L.M., Williams, E.K., Morris, D.G., and Hoffman, A.F.: Metastases to the adrenal glands and the development of Addison's disease, Cancer **54**:552-557, 1984.

206. Shea, T.C., Spark, R., Kane, B., and Lange, R.F.: Non-Hodgkin's lymphoma limited to the adrenal glands with adrenal insufficiency, Am. J. Med. **78**:711-714, 1985.

207. Willis, R.A.: Pathology of tumours, St. Louis, 1953, The C.V. Mosby Co.

Myelolipoma

207a. Damjanov, I., Moriber Katz, S., Catalano, E., Mason, D., and Schwartz, A.: Myelolipoma in a heterotopic adrenal gland, Cancer **44**:1350-1356, 1979.

208. Desai, S.B., Dourmashkin, L., Kabakow, B.R., and Leiter, E.: Myelolipoma of the adrenal gland: case report, literature review and analysis of diagnostic features, Mt. Sinai J. Med. **46**(2):155-158, 1979.

209. Gierke, E.: Ueber Knochenmarksgewebe in der Nebenniere, Beitr. Pathol. Anat. (suppl. 7):311-325, 1905.

210. Oberling, C.: Les formations myélo-lipomateuses, Bull. Assoc. Franç. Cancer **18**:234-246, 1929.

211. Plaut, A.: Myelolipoma in the adrenal cortex (myeloadipose structures), Am. J. Pathol. **34**(3):487-515, 1958.

Cysts

212. Abeshouse, G.A., Goldstein, R.B., and Abeshouse, B.S.: Adrenal cysts: review of the literature and report of three cases, J. Urol. **81**:711-719, 1959.

212a. Barron, S.H., and Emanuel, B.: Adrenal cysts: a case report and review of the pediatric literature, J. Pediatr. **59**:592-599, 1961.

213. Incze, J.S., Lui, P.S., Merriam, J.C., Austen, G., Widrich, W.C., and Gerzof, S.G.: Morphology and pathogenesis of adrenal cysts, Am. J. Pathol. **95**:423-432, 1979.

214. Kearney, G.P., Mahoney, E.M., Maher, E., et al.: Functioning and nonfunctioning cysts of the adrenal cortex and medulla, Am. J. Surg. **134**:363-368, 1977.

214a. Rabson, S.M., and Zimmerman, E.F.: Cystic lymphangiectasia of the adrenal, Arch. Pathol. **26**:869-872, 1938.

214b. Sick, K.: Film der Epithelicyten in der Nebennierenkapsel und in einer Becken-Lymphdruse, Virchows Arch. [Pathol. Anat.] **172**:445-459, 1903.

Miscellaneous phenomena
Adrenal and regulation of blood pressure

215. Baxter, J.D., Perloff, D., Hsueh, W., et al.: The endocrinology of hypertension. In Felig, P., Baxter, J.D., Broadus, A.E., and Frohman, L.A., editors: Endocrinology and metabolism, ed. 2, New York, 1987, McGraw-Hill Book Co.

216. Fränkel, F.: Ein Fall von doppelseitigem, vollig latent verlaufenen Nebennierentumor und gleichzeitiger Nephritis mit Veränderungen am Circulations-apparat und Retinitis, Virchows Arch. [Pathol. Anat. Physiol.] **103**:244-263, 1886.

217. Gifford, R.W.: Evaluation of the hypertensive patient with emphasis on detecting curable causes, Milbank Mem. Fund Q. **47**(3, pt. 2):170-218, 1969.

218. Kaplan, N.M.: Clinical hypertension, ed. 4, Baltimore, 1986, The Williams & Wilkins Co.

219. Selye, H.: The general-adaptation syndrome and the diseases of adaptation. In Textbook of endocrinology, Montreal, 1947, Acta Endocrinologica.

220. Sherwin, R.P.: Present status of the pathology of the adrenal gland in hypertension, Am. J. Surg. **107**:136-143, 1964.

221. Tucker, R.M., and Labarthe, D.R.: Frequency of surgical treatment for hypertension in adults at the Mayo Clinic from 1973 through 1975, Mayo Clin. Proc. **52**:549-556, 1977.

Calcification

222. Ball, R.G., Greene, C.H., Camp, J.D., and Rowentree, L.G.: Calcification in tuberculosis of the suprarenal glands: roentgenographic study in Addison's disease, JAMA **98**:954-961, 1932.

223. Cohen, K.L., Harris, S., and Keohane, M.: Upper abdominal calcification in a young man, JAMA **240**:1639-1640, 1978.

224. Jarvis, J.L., Jenkins, D., Sosman, M.C., and Thorn, G.W.: Roentgenologic observations in Addison's disease: a review of 120 cases, Radiology **62**:16-29, 1954.

225. Jarvis, J.L., and Seaman, W.B.: Idiopathic adrenal calcification in infants and children, Am. J. Roentgenol. **82**:510-520, 1959.

226. Martin, J.F.: Suprarenal calcification, Radiol. Clin. North Am. **3**:129-138, 1965.

227. Nerup, J.: Addison's disease—clinical studies: a report of 108 cases, Acta Endocrinol. **76**:127-141, 1974.

228. Seligman, B.: Calcification of the suprarenal gland, Am. J. Pathol. **4**:457-462, 1928.

229. Snelling, C.E., and Erb, I.H.: Hemorrhage and subsequent calcification of the suprarenal, J. Pediatr. **6**:22-41, 1935.

AIDS and the adrenal cortex

230. Miller-Catchpole, R., Variakojis, D., Anastasi, J., and Abrahams, C.: A cooperative autopsy study of "AIDS" in the Chicago area, Proc. Inst. Med. Chicago **40**:2-3, 1987.

231. Guenthner, E.E., Rabinowe, S.L., VanNiel, A., Naftilan, A., and Dluhy, R.G.: Primary Addison's disease in a patient with the acquired immunodeficiency syndrome, Ann. Intern. Med. **100**:847-848, 1984.

Irradiation

232. Sommers, S.C., and Carter, M.: Adrenocortical postirradiation fibrosis, Arch. Pathol. **99**:421-423, 1975.

Adrenal medulla

233. Alpert, L.I., Pai, S.H., Zak, F.G., et al.: Cardiomyopathy associated with a pheochromocytoma, Arch. Pathol. Lab. Med. **93**:544-548, 1972.

234. Berenyi, M.R., Singh, G., Gloster, E.S, et al.: ACTH-producing pheochromocytoma, Arch. Pathol. Lab. Med. **101**:31-35, 1977.

235. Bravo, E.L., and Gifford, R.W.: Pheochromocytoma: diagnosis, localization and management, N. Engl. J. Med. **311**:1298-1303, 1984.

236. Dehner, L.P., Abenoza, P., and Sibley, R.K.: Primary cerebral neuroectodermal tumors: neuroblastoma, differentiated neuroblastoma and composite neuroectodermal tumor, Ultrastruct. Pathol. 12:479-494, 1988.

237. DeLellis, R.A., Wolfe, H.J., Gagel, R.F., et al.: Adrenal medullary hyperplasia, Am. J. Pathol. 83:177-196, 1976.

238. DeLellis, R.A., Tischler, A.S., Lee, A.K., Blount, M., and Wolfe, H.J.: Leu-enkephalin-immunoreactivity in proliferative lesions of the adrenal medulla and extra-adrenal paraganglia, Am. J. Surg. Pathol. 7:29-37, 1983.

239. Franke, W.W., Grund, C., and Achstaetter, T.: Coexpression of cytokeratins and neurofilament proteins in a permanent cell line: cultured rat PC12 cells combine neuronal and epithelial features, J. Cell Biol. 103:1942-1943, 1986.

240. Ghadially, F.: Diagnostic electron microscopy of tumors, London, 1980, Butterworth, & Co., Inc.

241. Glenner, G.G., and Grimley, P.M.: Tumors of the extra-adrenal paraganglion system (including chemoreceptors). In Atlas of tumor pathology, ser. 2, fascicle 9, Washington, D.C., 1974, Armed Forces Institute of Pathology.

242. Gould, V.E., and Sommers, S.C.: Adrenal medulla and paraganglia. In Bloodworth, J.M.B., Jr., editor: Endocrine pathology, ed. 2, Baltimore, 1982, The Williams & Wilkins Co.

243. Gould, V.E., Warren, W.H., and Memoli, V.A.: Metastatic paraganglioma in lung, Ultrastruct. Pathol. 5:299-306, 1983.

244. Gould, V.E., Lee, I., Wiedenmann, B., Moll, R., Chejfec, G., and Franke, W.W.: Synaptophysin: a novel marker for neurons, certain neuroendocrine cells and their neoplasms, Hum. Pathol. 17:979-983, 1986.

245. Gould, V.E., Wiedenmann, B., Lee, I., Schwechheimer, K., Dockhorn-Dworniczak, B., Radosevich, J.A., Moll, R., and Franke, W.W.: Synaptophysin expression in neuroendocrine neoplasms as determined by immunocytochemistry, Am. J. Pathol. 126:243-257, 1987.

246. Gould, V.E., and Jansson, D.: Neuroendocrine and nerve sheath neoplasms. In Osborn, M., and Weber, K., editors: Cytoskeletal proteins in tumor diagnosis, Current Communications in Molecular Biology, Cold Spring Harbor, New York, 1989, Cold Spring Harbor Laboratory.

247. Haimoto, H., Takahashi, Y., Koshikawa, T., Nagura, H., and Kato, K.: Immunohistochemical localization of gamma-enolase in normal tissues other than nervous and neuroendocrine tissues, Lab. Invest. 52:257-263, 1985.

248. Hammar, S., and Gould, V.E.: Neuroendocrine neoplasms. In Azar, H., editor: Pathology of human neoplasms, New York, 1988, Raven Press.

249. Harrison, T.S., Feier, D.T., and Cohen, E.L.: Recurrent pheochromocytoma, Arch. Surg. 108:1027-1032, 1978.

250. Hashimoto, H., Enjoji, M., Nakajima, T., Kiryu, H., and Daimaru, Y.: Malignant neuroepithelioma (peripheral neuroblastoma), Am. J. Surg. Pathol. 7:309-318, 1983.

251. Heath, H., III, and Edis, A.J.: Pheochromocytoma associated with hypercalcemia and ectopic secretion of calcitonin, Ann. Intern. Med. 91:208-210, 1979.

252. Henderson, D.W., Papadimitriou, J.M., and Coleman, M.: Ultrastructural appearances of tumors: a diagnostic atlas, ed. 2, Edinburgh, 1986, Churchill Livingstone.

253. Jao, W., Warren, W.H., Chejfec, G., et al.: Late development of pulmonary and systemic metastases from a retroperitoneal paraganglioma, Ultrastruct. Pathol. 6:83-88, 1984.

254. Lamovec, J., Memoli, V.A., Terzakis, J.A., Sommers, S.C., and Gould, V.E.: Pheochromocytoma producing ACTH with Cushing's syndrome, Ultrastruct. Pathol. 7:41-48, 1984.

255. Linnoila, R.I., DiAugustine, R.P., Hervonen, A., and Miller, R.J.: Distribution of [Met5]- and [Leu5]-enkephalin-, vasoactive intestinal polypeptide- and substance P-like immunoreactivity in human adrenal glands, Neuroscience 5:2247-2259, 1980.

256. Lundberg, J.M., Hamberger, B., Schultzberg, M., Hökfelt, T., Granberg, P.O., Efendic, S., Terenius, L., Goldstein, M., and Luft, R.: Enkephalin- and somatostatin-like immunoreactivities in human adrenal medulla and pheochromocytoma, Proc. Natl. Acad. Sci. USA 76:4079-4083, 1979.

257. Miettinen, M., Lehto, V.-P., and Virtanen, I.: Immunofluorescence microscopic evaluation of the intermediate filament expression of the adrenal cortex and medulla and their tumors, Am. J. Pathol. 118:360-366, 1985.

258. Miettinen, M., and Saari, A.: Pheochromocytoma combined with malignant schwannoma: unusual neoplasm of the adrenal medulla, Ultrastruct. Pathol. 12:513-527, 1988.

259. Moll, R., Lee, I., Gould, V.E., Berndt, R., Roessner, A., and Franke, W.W.: Immunocytochemical analysis of Ewing's tumors: patterns of expression of intermediate filaments and desmosomal proteins indicate cell type heterogeneity and pluripotential differentiation, Am. J. Pathol. 127:288-304, 1987.

260. Nesbitt, K.A., and Vidone, R.A.: Primitive neuroectodermal tumor (neuroblastoma) arising in sciatic nerve of a child, Cancer 37:1562-1570, 1976.

261. O'Connor, D.T., Burton, D., and Deftos, L.J.: Chromogranin A: immunohistology reveals its universal occurrence in normal polypeptide hormone producing endocrine glands, Life Sci. 33:1657-1663, 1983.

262. Osborn, M., Dirk, T., Kaeser, H., Weber, K., and Altmannsberger, M.: Immunohistochemical localization of neurofilaments and neuron-specific enolase in 29 cases of neuroblastoma, Am. J. Pathol. 122:433-442, 1986.

263. Page, D.L., DeLellis, R.A., and Hough, A.J., Jr.: Tumors of the adrenal. In Atlas of tumor pathology, ser. 2, fascicle 23, Washington, D.C., 1986, Armed Forces Institute of Pathology.

264. Pahlmann, S., Esscher, T., and Nilsson, K.: Expression of gamma subunit of enolase in human non-neuroendocrine tumors and derived cell lines, Lab. Invest. 54:554-560, 1986.

265. Rudy, F.R., Bates, R.D., Cimorelli, A.J., Hill, GS., and Engelman, K.: Adrenal medullary hyperplasia: a clinicopathologic study of 4 cases, Hum. Pathol. 11:650-657, 1980.

266. Schmechel, D., Marangos, P.J., and Brightman, M.: Neuron-specific enolase in a molecular marker for peripheral and central neuroendocrine cells, Nature 276:834-836, 1978.

267. Spark, R.K., Connolly, P.B., Gluckin, D.S., White, R., Sacks, B., and Lansberg, L.: ACTH secretion from a functioning pheochromocytoma, N. Engl. J. Med. 301:416-418, 1979.

268. Taxy, J.B., Bharani, N.K., Mills, S.E., Frierson, H.F., Jr., and Gould, V.E.: The spectrum of olfactory neural tumors, Am. J. Surg. Pathol. 10:687-695, 1986.

269. Tischler, A.S., Slayton, V.W., Costopoulos, D., Leape, L.L., DeLellis, R.A., and Wolfe, H.J.: Nerve growth factor as a survival factor in human neuroblastoma, Cancer 54:1344-1347, 1984.

270. Visser, J.W., and Axt, R.: Bilateral adrenal medullary hyperplasia: a clinicopathology entity, J. Clin. Pathol. 28:298-304, 1975.

271. Warren, W.H., Caldarelli,D.D., Javid, H., Lee, I., and Gould, V.E.: Neuroendocrine markers in paragangliomas of the head and neck, Ann. Otol. Rhinol. Laryngol. 94:555-566, 1985.

272. Warren, W.H., Lee, I., Gould, V.E., Memoli, V.A., and Jao, W.: Paragangliomas of the head and neck: immunohistochemical and ultrastructural analysis, Ultrastruct. Pathol. 8:333-343, 1985.

273. Wiedenmann, B., Franke, W.W., Kuhn, C., Moll, R., and Gould, V.E.: Synaptophysin: a marker protein for neuroendocrine cells and neoplasms, Proc. Natl. Acad. Sci. USA 83:3500-3505, 1986.

34 Female Genitalia

FREDERICK T. KRAUS

Abnormalities and diseases of the female genitalia have been the object of fascination for centuries and the basis for one of the oldest medical specialties. An abnormal external physical appearance may provide clues to significant underlying malformations, some of which are life threatening. The genital tract is the portal of entry for infectious diseases of remarkable variety with far-reaching effects on the patient and sometimes in her progeny. Neoplasms of the female genitalia are unsurpassed for bizarre appearance and variety of systemic effects and size; they also represent the second most common source of fatal cancer in women. Many insights into the biology of infections and neoplasms are afforded by a study of these conditions; the correct application of principles of prevention and treatment of these diseases may offer a greater prospect for relief of suffering and extension of life than is possible in any other area of the body.

EMBRYOLOGY OF FEMALE GENITAL TRACT

Knowledge of the anatomic changes in the early development of the female genitalia is helpful in understanding various pathologic conditions. Some malformations become recognizable as a failure in the completion of a developmental sequence. There is a close relationship between primitive urinary and genital structures, so that malformations often affect both systems, sometimes in predictable ways. For instance, recognition of ambiguous sexual differentiation of the vulva may be the first evidence of the potentially fatal, but curable, adrenogenital syndrome. Finally, the histologic similarities in neoplasms are understandable in terms of the embryologic relationships that form the basis of their classification. A brief summary of female genital tract embryology is supplied as a basis for such an understanding; for more detailed descriptions see standard texts.[10]

Genital ridges and müllerian ducts

With the exception of the germ cells, the internal genitalia arise from the mesoderm (celomic epithelium and adjacent mesenchyme) of the posterior body wall. Bilateral urogenital ridges are formed parallel to the body axis. In a 6 mm embryo (about 5 weeks old) each of these has become segregated longitudinally into a lateral mesonephric ridge and a medial genital ridge (Fig. 34-1).

By the end of the sixth week the primitive gonad is represented by proliferating surface epithelial cells and an inner blastema of loose mesenchymal cells. A lateral groove forms in the surface epithelium of each urogenital ridge, rolls inward, and closes to form the müllerian (paramesonephric) duct on each side. The cranial ends remain open and eventually become the fimbriated open ends of the uterine tubes. The caudal ends burrow medially in front of the mesonephric ducts and farther caudad toward the urogenital sinus. The point at which they end in the dorsomedial aspect of the urogenital sinus is transiently marked by a swelling, Müller's tubercle. The distal ends of the müllerian ducts fuse to become the uterus, cervix, and upper vagina. The myometrium and endometrial stroma differentiate from the surrounding mesenchyma (Fig. 34-2).

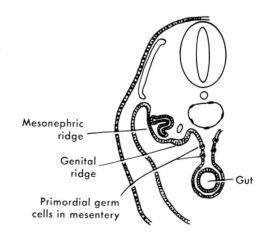

Fig. 34-1. Diagrammatic cross section of 6 mm embryo showing migrating germ cells, genital ridge, and mesonephros. (From Kraus, F.T.: Gynecologic pathology, St. Louis, 1967, The C.V. Mosby Co.)

In a 60 mm embryo the ovary is suspended by its mesovarium from the ventral surface of the mesonephros, which is still prominent (Fig. 34-3). The mesonephric ducts are functional at this time and pass into the urogenital sinus through the lateral walls of the developing myometrium.

Differentiation of ovary

Each ovarian blastema is covered by a surface layer of celomic epithelium, closely related but not identical to the cells that form the müllerian ducts. Perhaps because of this close relationship in early development, the adenocarcinomas that arise from ovarian surface epithelium closely resemble typical adenocarcinomas of the tube, endometrium, cervix, and vagina. As a result of this similarity of patterns, it has become customary to regard the common ovarian epithelial neoplasms as

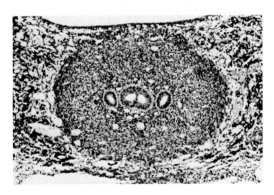

Fig. 34-2. Cross section of uterine anlage of 60 mm embryo. Müllerian ducts have nearly fused at center. Mesonephric ducts are situated on each side. Peritoneum of cul-de-sac is at top. (150×; from Kraus, F.T.: Gynecologic pathology, St. Louis, 1967, The C.V. Mosby Co.)

müllerian, even though the ovary does not actually form from the müllerian duct. The advantage of conceptual understanding overshadows the sacrifice of conformity to rigid embryologic fact. Pelvic mesothelium and underlying mesenchyme also maintain the capacity to generate, rarely, primary epithelial and stromal neoplasms identical to those of the uterus, tubes, and ovaries.[32]

The germ cells originate in the yolk sac endoderm near the hindgut, move through the primitive hindgut mesentery, and finally settle in the blastemas of the primitive ovaries.[21] The segregation of an occasional straggler along the way may explain some retroperitoneal germ cell tumors and the development of heterotopic ovarian tissue along the trail of this migration. This migration is completed by the tenth week. The germ cells begin to proliferate by mitosis on arrival, notably after the eighth week; by the twelfth week some begin the first meiotic division. At birth, germ cell mitosis has ceased, and most ova, at this time called oogonia, are in the dictyotene stage of meiosis. The adjacent stromal cells differentiate into a single layer of flattened granulosa cells, forming a primary follicle. The granulosa cells proliferate; a cavity, the antrum, appears, forming a graafian follicle; follicles may be numerous and some are large at birth. The ovaries descend into the pelvis attached to connective tissue strands, the gubernacula, which will become the medial ovarian ligaments and the round ligaments, extending from the uterine horns to the labia majora.

Differentiation of müllerian ducts

The separate proximal portions of the müllerian ducts develop into the uterine (fallopian) tubes. The fused middle and distal portions complete their merger by the twelfth week, forming the uterus and upper part of

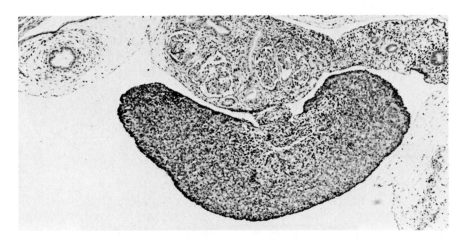

Fig. 34-3. Transverse section of ovary and adjacent mesonephros. Mesonephric glomeruli persist at this 60 mm stage. (90×; from Kraus, F.T.: Gynecologic pathology, St. Louis, 1967, The C.V. Mosby Co.)

Table 34-1. Correlation of age, size, and sequence of development of female urogenital organs

Age (approximately*)	Crown-rump length (mm)	Developmental levels in female urogenital tract
23-25 days	2.5	Limb buds appear
25 days		Pronephros formed; pronephric duct grow caudad as blind tubes; cloaca and cloacal membrane present; embryo has 14 somites
25-28 days	5	Closure of neural tube
32 days		Pronephros degenerated; mesonephric tubules forming; pronephric (now mesonephric) ducts reach cloaca; metanephric bud forms at distal end of mesonephric duct
30-35 days	8	Retinal pigment appears
35 days		Genital ridge bulges; ureteric and renal pelvic primordia formed
35-36 days	13	Finger plate appears
40 days		Urorectal septum begins to subdivide cloaca; genital tubercle and labioscrotal swellings evident; müllerian duct begins to form
37-45 days	22	Elbow appears
40-46 days		Knee appears
7 weeks		Urogenital membrane dissovles; cloaca separated into urogenital sinus and rectum; glans of phallus is evident
8 weeks	30	Testis and ovary become recognizable as such; müllerian ducts approach urogenital sinus and begin to fuse (distal portion) to become uterovaginal primordium
10 weeks	46	Mesonephric ducts atrophy; glands of urogenital sinus (vulvourethral and vestibular glands) appear
12 weeks	56	Uterine horns absorbed; muscular walls appear in uterus, vagina, and fallopian tubes; distinction of sex from external genitalia becomes possible
16 weeks	112	Uterus and vagina become distinctive structures
5 months	150	Primary ovarian follicles are found; vagina develops lumen; urogenital sinus becomes shallow vestible
7 months	230	Uterine glands appear

*There is no accurate way of determining embryonic age from the length; the figures given represent a composite or average and are based on the stages described by Hamilton, W.J., Boyd, J.D., and Mossman, H.W.: Human embryology, Baltimore, 1962, The Williams & Wilkins Co.; by Van Wagenen, G., and Simpson, M.E.: Embryology of the ovary and testis, New Haven, 1965, Yale University Press; and by Kalousek, D.K., and Poland, B.J.: Embryonic and fetal pathology of abortion, Chapter 2 in Perrin, V.D.K., editor: Pathology of the placenta, New York, 1984, Churchill Livingstone.

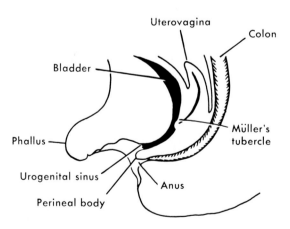

Fig. 34-4. Diagrammatic sagittal section showing relationship between urinary bladder, urogenital sinus, and Müller's tubercle. Age is approximately 10 weeks. (Redrawn from Arey, L.B.: Developmental anatomy, ed. 6, Philadelphia, 1954, W.B. Saunders Co.)

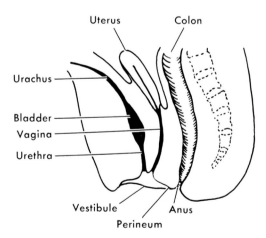

Fig. 34-5. Caudad growth of perineum and urovaginal septum separates bladder and vagina and enlarges separation between vulvar vestibule and anus. (Redrawn from Arey, L.B.: Developmental anatomy, ed. 6, Philadelphia, 1954, W.B. Saunders Co.)

the vagina, respectively. The myometrium differentiates from the surrounding mesenchyme, enveloping the adjacent segments of the withering mesonephric ducts.

Between the eighth and eleventh weeks the primitive vagina is a solid cord of epithelial cells ending distally in the urogenital sinus at Müller's tubercle. Evaginations of the urogenital sinus on either side of Müller's tubercle enlarge, fuse, and merge to form the hymen and distal vaginal wall. The lining of the vagina is formed by proliferation of epithelial cells from the dorsum of the urogenital sinus, extending craniad toward the cervix, which is lined by simple columnar epithelium. This process occurs between the twelfth and eighteenth weeks, which is a crucial period for female infants exposed in utero to the drug diethylstilbestrol and its derivatives.

Differentiation of vulva

The primitive hindgut, urinary ducts, and genital ducts all empty into a common chamber, the cloaca. By the sixth week the urorectal septum has formed as a transverse ridge separating the urogenital sinus and rectum. Müller's tubercle moves progressively caudad. The urinary bladder forms from the allantois, so that the müllerian and urinary orifices empty as separate orifices into the shallow remains of the urogenital sinus, now the vestibule of the vulva (Figs. 34-4 and 34-5).

The development of the vulva begins at a sexually indeterminate stage.[29] At about 36 days (9 mm) the external structures are represented by a genital tubercle (a conic anterior midline protuberance) and the labioscrotal swellings (two broad lateral elevations located just caudad to the genital tubercle on either side of the cloacal groove) (Fig. 34-6). The cloacal groove at first is closed by the cloacal membrane. After the urorectal

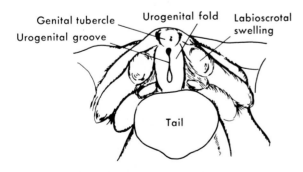

Fig. 34-6. External genitalia at about 7 weeks are sexually indeterminate. (Redrawn from Arey, L.B.: Developmental anatomy, ed. 6, Philadelphia, 1954, W.B. Saunders Co.)

septum grows down to meet it, the cloacal membrane becomes divided into an anterior urogenital groove, closed by the urogenital membrane, and a posterior anal membrane. The urogenital membrane disintegrates at about 42 days; a glans becomes evident on the genital tubercle in the 46-day-old (19 mm embryo). The urogenital groove extends anteriorly on the caudal aspect of the phallus thus formed. A sexual distinction is made evident by the urethral groove, which extends onto the phallus from the urogenital groove; the urethral groove extends distally onto the glans in the male but not in the female. This distinction is probably not a reliable indicator of sex until after the eleventh week (50 mm). The urethral folds lateral to the urethral groove fuse to form the male penile urethra; they persist as separate structures, the labia minora, in the female. The labioscrotal swellings enlarge to form the labia majora; they fuse posteriorly at the posterior commissure at about 50 mm. In the 4-month-old (100 mm) embryo the prepuce forms around the glans of the clitoris.

The most significant events in the embryology of the female genital tract are summarized in Table 34-1. This timetable of development is useful in relating malformations to possible teratogenic events such as maternal infection with a virus or exposure to a teratogenic drug.

Sexual differentiation: male and female

Female genital developmental anomalies often involve some degree of substitution of male-directed organogenesis. Therefore genital development in the male is basic to any understanding of the anatomy and physiology of intersex states in children or adults reared as females. The specific genes that determine testicular differentiation—hence "maleness"—are located on the Y chromosome and are expressed on the surface membrane of all male cells as a weak, sex-specific histocompatibility antigen, the H-Y antigen.[35] In the absence of a Y chromosome and H-Y antigen the embryo develops (at least transiently) ovaries, müllerian ducts and their derivatives, vagina, vulva, and a basically female phenotype. Full expression of all female secondary sexual characteristics and development of a functional ovary require a second X chromosome.

The gonadal blastemas begin similarly in both sexes and at first are morphologically indistinguishable from one another. The definitive ovary and testis have been identified by Van Wagenen and Simpson[34] in 23 mm embryos after the age of 42 days. In the female the müllerian ducts and vulva develop appropriately, but this progression is *not* dependent on the presence of one or both ovaries. In males, however, the persistence and development of the mesonephric (wolffian) ductal system, together with atrophy of the müllerian ducts and the structures that form from them, are dependent on two factors: a local-acting müllerian inhibitory factor (MIF) and circulating testosterone, both produced by the testis.[15]

Testosterone induces the formation of epididymis, vas deferens, and seminal vesicle from the mesonephric duct. Dihydrotestosterone, produced from testosterone by the action of 5-alpha-reductase within the cells of the perineal tissues, stimulates fusion of labioscrotal folds and growth of the glans and shaft of the penis, enclosed penile urethra, and scrotum. Male structures fail to develop when the somatic cells of a fetus are unresponsive to testosterone, which occurs in androgen-insensitivity (resistance) syndromes.

Because MIF acts locally, it must be produced in adequate amounts by both testes to prevent completely the development of both tubes, uterus, and upper vagina. Therefore an individual with a testis on one side and a streak (no gonad), an ovary, or ovotestis on the other usually will have a uterus and upper vagina and possibly a tube on the side opposite the testis.

In the strongly estrogenic maternal environment, genital development is female independent of the presence of a fetal ovary. Therefore at birth a fetus with no gonadal tissue on either side (bilateral streaks or bilateral agenesis) will have a uterus, vagina, tubes, and the female pattern of external genitalia. Individuals with abnormal (dysgenetic) testes, which may not produce either MIF or testosterone in adequate amounts, will have some degree of müllerian tract development and either female external genitalia or incompletely formed male external genitalia. A single testis might be expected to inhibit müllerian development on the same side but not to inhibit that on the opposite side or the entire uterus; however, it could generate enough dihydrotestosterone to masculinize the external genitalia.

Genital anomalies

Because of the importance of sex in social development, genital anomalies have a devastating impact. Any classification of female genital tract anomalies must reflect the incomplete knowledge of genetics and of teratogenic factors such as viruses and toxic chemicals or drugs. At present it is convenient to divide genital malformations into two broad groups: (1) those related to intersex states, in which a genetic abnormality of a sex chromosome is demonstrable or suspected, and (2) those more simply structural and localized developmental abnormalities in which one of the processes of the growth, fusion, canalization, or separation of developing tubular structures is incomplete. A detailed classification in relation to biochemical and cytogenetic anomalies has been prepared by Park, Aimakhu, and Jones.[20]

Intersex states and cytogenetic abnormalities

Normal sexual development is determined first of all by the presence in the zygote of a normal set of sex chromosomes. XX for a female and XY for a male. The initial factor in many genital anomalies is the contribution of abnormal or deficient genetic material by one of the gametes. Alternatively, during the first division of the zygote some genetic material may be lost or unevenly distributed in the daughter cells (nondisjunction), resulting in a mixture (mosaic) of two or more types of cells as the organism develops further. Although the loss, severe alteration, or duplication of an autosome is usually lethal, most sex chromosomal abnormalities exert their most notable effects in the form of altered genital structure and function.

A significant chromosomal abnormality can be detected in about 50% of spontaneous abortions when the fetus is either absent or morphologically abnormal,[27] and 5% of perinatal deaths or stillbirths involve chromosomal anomaly.[16] Among 50 women who failed to begin to menstruate (primary amenorrhea), Sarto[23] found chromosomal anomalies in 19.

A bewildering array of intersex states has been described, together with associated cytogenetic analyses and deranged endocrine physiology. Extensive clinical descriptions and genetic studies are available in monographs such as those by Smith[28] and Mittwoch.[18] This discussion is limited to a summary of the usual findings in a few of the more common intersex syndromes, with Table 34-2 for comparison. This table is a generalization. There is no perfect correspondence between phenotype, karyotype, and other features of these syndromes at the present state of the art: many patients will not fit the chart.

Certain commonly used terms require definition, as follows.

hermaphrodite An inexact term indicating that an individual has some kind of mixture of both male and female gonads, external genitalia, and sexual characteristics. A true hermaphrodite has both ovarian and testicular tissue, either or both of which may be functional.

pseudohermaphrodite An inexact, confusing, and often unnecessary general term for an individual with gonads and genotype of one sex and external genitalia more consistent with the opposite sex. A male pseudohermaphrodite has testes but otherwise appears to be female (typically represented by the androgen-insensitivity syndrome). A female pseudohermaphrodite has ovaries, but the external genitalia are masculinized (typically represented by congenital adrenal hyperplasia). It is nearly always possible, desirable, and sufficient to name the specific condition or syndrome.

genotype An expression of the genetic characteristics of an individual cell as determined by analysis of the number and morphologic characteristics of the chromosomes examined at metaphase; for example, 46XX indicates that the individ-

Table 34-2. Intersex syndromes affecting females, apparent females, or female genitalia

Syndrome	Gonads	Karyotype (genotype)	Inheritance	Internal genitalia	External genitalia	Habitus (phenotype)	Comment
Pure gonadal dysgenesis with abnormal karyotype	Bilateral streaks	XX/XO; XO/XY	No	Vagina, uterus, and tubes		Female	
Pure gonadal dysgenesis with normal karyotype	Streaks	XX	Autosomal recessive	Female	Female	Female	Some with nerve deafness
Pure gonadal dysgenesis with male karyotype (Swyer syndrome)	Bilateral streaks	XY	X-linked recessive or autosomal dominant	Vagina, uterus, and tubes	Female	Female	Gonadal neoplasms; virilization
Turner's syndrome	Bilateral streaks	XO, mosaics	No	Vagina, uterus, and tubes	Female	Female	Multiple malformations
Gonadal agenesis	Absent	XY	Uncertain	Rudimentary tubular structures; no uterus or vagina	Ambiguous or female	Female	Minor malformations in some cases
Mixed gonadal dysgenesis	Streak and dysgenetic testis	XO/XY	No	May be uterus and tubes	Variable male-female	Female	Gonadal neoplasms; virilization at puberty
True hermaphrodite	Ovary and testis	Majority XX Some XY	No	Usually vagina, uterus, and tubes	Ambiguous, variable	Variable male-female	
	Ovotestis Ovotestis with ovary or testis	Many mosaics					
Female pseudohermaphrodite (chiefly adrenogenital syndrome)	Ovaries	XX	Autosomal recessive	Vagina, uterus, and tubes	Ambiguous	Female	Some infants virilized by iatrogenic androgens
47XXX syndromes	Ovaries	XXX, XXXX, and a variety of mosaics	No	Uterus, vagina, and tubes	Female	Female	Some have been mentally retarded
Male XX	Testes	XX	No	Male	Male		Similar to Klinefelter's syndrome (see Chapter 19)
Male pseudohermaphrodite with normal karyotype							
1. Defect in testosterone synthesis	Testes	XY	Autosomal recessive	Male—may be rudimentary	Variable	Variable	
2. Defect in testosterone synthesis	Testes	XY	Autosomal recessive	Male	Ambiguous	Female	Virilization at puberty
3. Müllerian inhibitory factor (MIF) failure	Testes	XY	?	Female—no male structures	Male	Male	
4. Testicular feminization syndrome	Testes	XY	?	Male	Female	Female	

Courtesy Dr. Robert H. Shikes, Denver.

ual has 44 normal autosomes and two normal X chromosomes, the genotype of a normal female; 46XY is the normal male genotype; and 45XO indicates 44 autosomes, one X, and deletion of the second sex chromosome, as seen in Turner's syndrome.

phenotype The external habitus and general appearance of the individual. In intersex states, it refers more specifically to the appearance of the external genitalia (male or female). In the postpubertal individual it generally also includes secondary sexual characteristics such as hair distribution, wide or narrow hips, laryngeal enlargement.

dysgenetic gonad An ovary or testis that has been abnormal from the beginning, usually as the result of the absence or other abnormality of a sex chromosome complement of the cells. The streak gonad (as in Turner's syndrome) can be regarded as a dysgenetic ovary. Neoplasms, especially gonadoblastoma, are likely to occur in dysgenetic gonads.[26]

gonadal dysgenesis The gonads are streaks composed of fibrous ovarian stroma with no follicles and no ova (Fig. 34-7). The phenotype is female, and fallopian tubes, uterus, and vagina are present. Patients with associated short stature, webbing of the neck, widely spaced nipples, and, less frequently, coarctation of the aorta and red-green color blindness are said to have Turner's syndrome. Those with the gonadal lesion only are classified as having pure gonadal dysgenesis. The cytogenetic lesion is some kind of abnormality—usually absence—of the second sex chromosome in at least some of the cells—typically 45XO.

Hilum cells, mesonephric duct remnants, and a fibrous stroma reminiscent of ovarian stroma usually are identifiable. The presence of a few ova suggests that the patient is a mosaic; the XO karyotype has been leavened with a few XX (or other karyotype with a second X) cells. Cordlike structures similar to an immature testis support the existence of at least a few Y chromosomes.[17]

mixed gonadal dysgenesis One gonad is a fibrous streak, as in Turner's syndrome, and the other is a testis, usually an immature or rudimentary testis, but occasionally the dysgenetic gonad opposite the streak is replaced by a tumor. The internal genitalia include a uterus, upper vagina, and, despite the influence of the testis, usually two fallopian tubes. The phenotype varies considerably, from normal male to normal female with variable degrees of ambiguity in many instances; a few have the appearance of those with Turner's syndrome. The chromosomal lesion varies but commonly includes mosaicism with both XO and XY stem lines.

gonadal agenesis Gonads and internal genitalia are completely absent. Phenotype is female; genotype is XY. This is an extremely rare condition; the absence of müllerian duct derivatives is unexplained.

True hermaphroditism. Recognizable ovarian and testicular tissues are both present, together in the same gonad (an ovotestis), on opposite sides, or in combinations such as ovotestis on one side with ovary or testis on the other. There is nearly always a uterus. The side with a testis has a vas deferens; the side with an ovary has a tube. A wide variety of internal genitalia combinations occurs and the phenotypes and external genitalia are also extremely variable. Most patients have a 46XX karyotype, but 46XY and a variety of mosaics have been reported. Some testes (but not ovotestes) have produced spermatozoa; there have been rare pregnancies.[31]

Androgen-insensitivity (resistance) syndromes and other male pseudohermaphroditism. Androgen-insensitivity syndromes are the most common cause of male pseudohermaphroditism; there are three groups, all with XY genotypes and testes.[9] In the first group, absence of the intracellular enzyme 5-alpha-reductase blocks formation of dihydrotestosterone, on which development of external genitalia depends: the external genitalia appear to be female. At puberty testicular androgens induce masculine habitus and phallus enlargement. The second category, testicular feminization, is a generalized insensitivity to all androgens; not only are the external genitalia female, but also at puberty the breasts enlarge and a typical general female body habi-

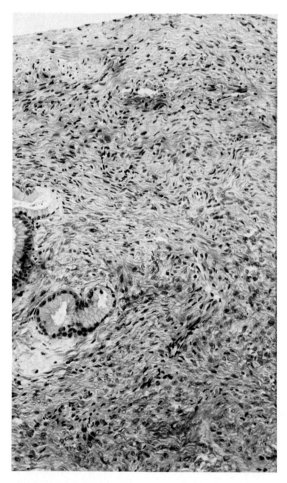

Fig. 34-7. Streak gonad from patient with Turner's syndrome. Tiny müllerian cysts *(lower left)* and hilar Leydig cells are occasionally evident, but germ cells and follicles are absent after birth. (150×.)

tus with normal female self-image develops. The vagina is short and ends blindly. A comparable syndrome exists in rats.[3] The third, somewhat variable group may be lumped together as Reifenstein's syndrome. The predominant phenotype is male, and external genitalia appear male but with defects, notably hypospadias. Gynecomastia occurs at puberty. The testes are small and immature, spermatogenesis is defective, and infertility is the rule. Rare instances of deficient testosterone synthesis result in incomplete development of wolffian duct derivatives and female or ambiguous external genitalia. Finally, ineffective müllerian inhibitory factor results in a phenotypic male with testes (often cryptorchid), male internal and external genitalia, and uterus and fallopian tubes.

Congenital adrenal hyperplasia and other hormonally induced causes of female pseudohermaphroditism. Congenital adrenal hyperplasia is fundamentally an adrenal abnormality in which defective hydrocortisone synthesis leads to androgen excess (see p. 1589). The gonads are normal ovaries; the uterus and tubes are likewise normal. The morphologic genital defect involves the external genitalia only and is the result of excessive androgen production by hyperplastic adrenal glands. This is the most common cause of ambiguous genitalia; it is also the most effectively treatable so that fertility and all other aspects of a normal sex role can usuallly be achieved. Because of the hydrocortisone deficiency, it is also likely to be fatal if unrecognized and is therefore the most important abnormality of sexual development to recognize at birth.

Rarely a similar masculinization of the external genitalia has been caused by the androgenic effect of progestogens administered to pregnant women in the hope of preventing abortion.

Other chromosomal syndromes. Other cytogenetic abnormalities affecting the sex chromosomes are less likely to be seen as malformations of female genitalia. The female with one or more extra X chromosomes (such as 47XXX) is phenotypically normal; some have mental retardation. Klinefelter's syndrome (usually 47XXY) involves a malformation of the male genitalia.

Localized developmental anomalies

Ovary. An ovary may be absent. The tube and uterine horn on the same side usually are also absent, and, of great clinical significance, the kidney and ureter on the affected side may be absent as well. Supernumerary ovaries and accessory ovarian tissue are most commonly found adjacent to a normally situated ovary and should be distinguished from lobulation of a single ovary. In rare instances ovarian tissue has been identified in the retroperitoneum, posterior bladder wall, and omentum and sigmoid mesentery.[22,36] Occasionally a cystic teratoma has arisen at such a site; the rare finding of other neoplasms of ovarian type that seem to have arisen in the pelvic retroperitoneum may in some instances be explained on a similar basis.

Fallopian tube. Duplication and atresia of the fallopian tubes occur rarely. Occasionally tiny accessory ostia, like miniature representatives of the fimbriated end, sprout from the side of the fallopian tube, especially the distal half.[38] Small patches of mucinous and endometrial epithelium may occur, especially when there is inflammation or endometriosis, so that it may not be clear whether this change in the tubal lining is congenital or acquired by metaplasia.

Unilateral absence of a tube is uncommon and is associated with ureteral and renal abnormalities, including absence of ipsilateral kidney and ureter.

Uterus, vagina, and vulva. The most common anomaly of the uterus, vagina, and vulva is the result of failure of fusion of some or all of the lower müllerian ducts. All gradations may occur, from complete separation causing the development of two complete genital tracts, to minimum failure with an incomplete sagittal septum at the uterine fundus. In the presence of a complete double vagina a double cervix and uterus are usual, but duplication of a distal structure such as the cervix does not invariably indicate that the uterine corpus is duplicated. Pregnancy may occur in either side or both. Both elements of a duplicated structure may not be of equal size. Development of one side may be discontinuous; a semidetached uterine horn may form a muscular walled cyst connected to the cervix by a fibrous cord.

Anomalies involving failure of fusion or establishment of patency in the lower müllerian system are often associated with urinary tract anomalies, including unilateral renal agenesis and misplaced ureters that discharge into the bladder at an abnormal site such as the uterus or vagina.

Transverse septa and atresias in the vagina probably result from the failure to canalize the distal end of the müllerian duct. Retention of fluid (hydrocolpos or hematocolpos) is usually caused by a transverse septum situated proximal to a patent hymen.

Nearly all patients with congenital absence of the vagina have no uterus; however, when the vagina is apparently absent and accumulated menstrual blood forms a bulging cystic mass, the obstruction is almost always below the cervical level.

An extreme degree of hypoplasia of the cervix—or apparent absence or atresia of the cervix—occasionally also causes a cystic accumulation of menstrual blood in the normally formed uterine corpus; successful term pregnancy is possible after surgical reconstruction.[6]

Associated with internal duplications, there may be even more rarely a duplication of the external genitalia, including both labia, the clitoris, and the urethra. Congenital fistulas between the anus or rectum and vestibule, anterior displacement of the anus, and vestibular location of the anus have been described in detail by Stephens.[30] These anomalies depend chiefly on the extent of the contribution by the uroanal septum to the formation of the perineum.

Double vulva is consistently associated with duplication in the lower gastrointestinal tract and urinary bladder, but other anomalies, especially congenital heart disease, are also common and represent the most important cause of morbidity and mortality.[5]

VULVA
Anatomy

The vulva is composed of the labia majora, labia minora, mons veneris, clitoris, vestibule, hymen, Bartholin's glands, and minor vestibular glands. The mons veneris and labia majora are covered externally by skin with hair follicles, sebaceous glands, and sweat glands, including apocrine sweat glands. The inner surfaces of the labia majora, labia minora, and vestibule have sebaceous glands but no hair and are covered by a less keratinized epidermis. The vulva is profusely permeated by lymphatics that cross the midline extensively so that a lesion on one side is very likely to affect the lymph nodes on the opposite side. Lymph from the labia flows to the superficial inguinal nodes; lymph from the vestibule and clitoris may flow directly to the deep femoral nodes. An inconspicuous layer of specific stroma similar to that beneath the epithelium of the vagina and cervix also extends beneath the vulvar epithelium.

The vulvar epithelium is subject to all the dermatoses that affect the body skin generally, as well as specific dystrophic conditions that may also affect the perineum and perianal skin. Reactive changes expressed as atrophy and inflammation with pruritus that occur in women with diabetes mellitus and pernicious anemia are relieved by control of the primary disease.

Inflammation

The vulva represents the portal of entry and the site of destructive results of most venereal infections. Many inflammatory lesions are ulcerated and painful or pruritic. The most common cause in a large series of women with vulvar ulcers was herpes simplex.[127] The inflammatory patterns vary considerably; although none is entirely specific, the pathologic changes are often sufficiently distinctive to indicate the agent responsible. Confirmation by culture or serologic techniques usually is possible.

The specific pathologic features of venereal diseases and other specific infectious diseases of the vulva are described in the chapters devoted to bacterial diseases (Chapter 6), viral diseases (Chapter 9), and fungal diseases (Chapter 10). Crohn's disease of the intestinal tract (p. 1163) may produce destructive vulvar granulomas and abscesses.[55] Amebiasis may simulate carcinoma grossly and microscopically.[97]

Bartholin's gland cyst and abscess

Bartholin's glands may be invaded by any bacterial agent; the ducts may become dilated behind an obstruction, so that an abscess, which may be acutely swollen and painful, is produced. A less severe chronic bacterial infection may evolve more slowly into a fluid-filled cyst. The most common cause of Bartholin's gland abscesses and cysts is gonorrhea, but other pathogenic bacteria can cause the same reactions. The mass must be distinguished from a neoplasm, and therefore a biopsy at the time of drainage is desirable, especially in the absence of any prior symptoms of acute inflammation.

Herpes simplex

Herpes simplex infection of the vulva deserves special attention. There has been a remarkable increase in the incidence of genital herpes. A distinctly specific strain of virus (herpesvirus, type 2) that is indigenous to the genital tract has emerged.[86]

Vulvar herpetic lesions begin as painful vesicles, ulcerate, and heal in about 2 weeks (Fig. 34-8). The lesions are more numerous and slightly larger in primary infections. Herpes simplex virus has been implicated by epidemiologic data as an initiator (among others, such as smoking) of genital cancers,[85] but the dominant factors appear to be certain strains of human papillomavi-

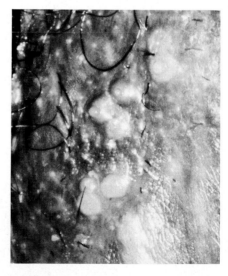

Fig. 34-8. Herpes simplex of vulva. Ulcers have yellow shaggy necrotic base and surrounding erythema. (Courtesy Dr. Ernst R. Friedrich, St. Louis, Mo.)

rus.[128] Active vulvar herpes infections are especially threatening during pregnancy because transmission to the newborn at parturition is usually fatal.[42]

Cells with viral inclusions are easily identifiable in degenerating squamous cells at the margins of vulvar vesicles or ulcers and in vaginocervical smears (see p. 1638).

Dystrophies, keratoses, and atrophy
Terminology

The vulvar epithelium is subject to a group of chronic conditions of unknown origin, chiefly affecting older women. The skin appears white, mottled red and white, or, less commonly, red. There are variable degrees of atrophy of the subcutaneous tissue so that at an advanced stage the labia are obliterated and the introitus is stenotic. Pruritus is common and may be severe and unremitting. The perineum and perianal skin may also be affected.

The term "leukoplakia" often is used by clinicians to describe the patchy areas of whitened skin. Similarly, the term "kraurosis" indicates that the atrophy and shrinkage are advanced. As the result of extremely varied usage in the past, both terms have no specific pathologic diagnostic meaning at this time. Their use by a pathologist now is undesirable.

Many benign conditions and some developmental forms of carcinoma have the clinical appearances described above, but in some women similar vulvar lesions represent a complication of a systemic disease, notably diabetes mellitus and pernicious anemia. It is necessary to identify the nature of all vulvar lesions by biopsy and conduct appropriate screening for specific metabolic abnormalities. Specific dermatoses such as psoriasis and lichen planus occasionally affect the vulva, usually as a part of a more generalized process on other cutaneous surfaces.

Lesions characterized as "dystrophies" in the vulva by gynecologists have many synonyms in the lexicons of dermatologists and other medical specialists. The term listed first in the following discussion are those proposed for general use by the International Society of Gynecologic Pathologists and the International Society for the Study of Vulvar Disease.[124]

Squamous hyperplasia (hyperkeratosis, hyperplastic dystrophy, lichen simplex chronica)

The combination of a thick layer of surface keratin, hyperplastic but cytologically benign squamous epithelium, and a mixture of chronic inflammatory cells distributed through the underlying dermis (Fig. 34-9) causes the vulva to appear thickened and white and usually to itch unremittingly. Scratching adds trauma and chronic inflammation and thereby probably reinforces the pruritus. Areas where the keratin layer is lacking appear red. The epidermis is usually hyperplastic; elongation of rete ridges in obliquely oriented microscopic sections may falsely indicate an invasive lesion. Either hyperkeratosis or parakeratosis may occur at the surface. The pattern is often indistinguishable from the condition known to dermatologists as "lichen simplex chronica" at other cutaneous locations.

The cause is unknown. Symptomatic relief has resulted from use of topical creams containing hydrocortisone or other corticoid hormone preparations. Lesions that include cells with atypical or dysplastic cytologic abnormalities are classified as dysplasia or vulvar intraepithelial neoplasia, as discussed on pp. 1632 and 1633.

Lichen sclerosus (lichen sclerosus et atrophicus)

Lichen sclerosus et atrophicus is not confined to the vulva and may affect both sexes at any age. However, the majority of patients who consult a gynecologist about this are postmenopausal women whose lesion and symptoms are either confined to the vulva or associated with perianal and perineal involvement.

The lesions appear first as small coalescent macules, which may have central pits resulting from follicular plugging. There is progressive shrinkage of the vulvar connective tissues so that the skin becomes smooth, shiny, and thin. Eventually the atrophic connective tissue changes obliterate the labia and produce stenosis of the introitus. Although usually white and opaque, the skin may appear mottled red and white.

The microscopic appearance is specific and character-

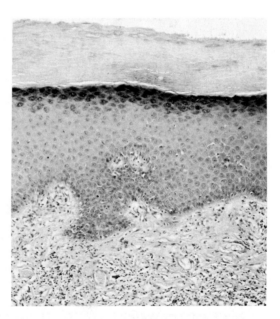

Fig. 34-9. Squamous hyperplasia (hyperkeratosis). Notice dense keratin layer at surface and fibrosis and chronic inflammation in underlying dermis. Cytologic pattern is benign. (85×.)

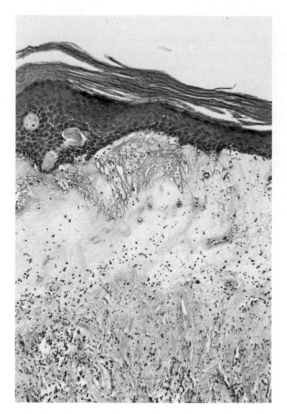

Fig. 34-10. Lichen sclerosus. Epidermis is thin and atrophic; underlying dermal collagen is hyalinized and edematous. Beneath this area of degenerative change is moderate chronic inflammation. There is surface hyperkeratosis. (85×.)

istic: the epidermis in cross section is a thin atrophic band without rete ridges. The surface layer is hyperkeratotic. The most distinctive feature is the amorphous homogeneous degenerative change in the dermal collagen, usually in a wide band beneath the epidermis. Elastic fibers are absent; the collagen that remains may stain densely or faintly and is relatively acellular, except for scattered lymphocytes. A band of lymphocytes with a few plasma cells lies beneath, in the middermis. There is often separation at the epidermal-dermal junction, at least in focal areas (Fig. 34-10).

Ultrastructurally, anchoring fibrils degenerate and disappear, elastic fibers become clumped, amorphous, and reduced in number.[88] An excessive elastase activity may explain the altered elastic tissue components.[66] Many patients respond to topical testosterone applications, an indication of abnormal androgen metabolism in the vulva.[63]

Clinicopathologic correlation

Lichen sclerosus and hyperplastic dystrophy may occur together, and other more threatening lesions may also be present. Multiple biopsies are necessary for evaluation of an extensive lesion, especially if its appearance varies from place to place.

The frequency of subsequent malignant change has been much debated. In the few large series of patients whose original lesion was a benign dystrophy, subsequent malignant change has been uncommon, in the range of 1% to 3%[81] even after follow-up periods of many years. Detailed pathologic studies have failed to show any evidence that lichen sclerosus et atrophicus predisposes vulvar epithelium to the development of cancer.[73]

It is important to emphasize that vulvectomy for a chronic vulvar dystrophy is not likely to relieve the symptoms, remedy the disease, or change the small possibility of subsequent cancer.[81] The best results up to now have occurred after topical treatment with corticosteroids for hyperplastic dystrophy and androgens for lichen sclerosus et atrophicus. Both lesions recur in grafted skin.

Neoplasms
Benign tumors and tumorlike conditions

Hidradenoma (hidradenoma papilliferum). Hidradenoma is a small papillary neoplasm that forms a nodule in the subcutaneous tissue of the vulva. The papillary fronds are covered by a double layer of epithelial cells, supported by a delicate fibrovascular stalk, an arrangement that resembles papilloma of the breast (Fig. 34-11). As in the breast, clusters of pink apocrine cells may form a part of the pattern. Most are located in the labia; about one fifth of the cases reported[100] occurred in the perianal region.

Granular cell tumor. Although it is more commonly found in other sites such as tongue, breast, and respiratory tract, granular cell tumor occasionally produces a poorly circumscribed indurated gray or yellow solid mass in the subcutaneous tissue of the vulva. The tumor cells are large, with abundant pink granular cytoplasm and benign, uniform, round nuclei. Ultrastructural studies show a varied appearance suggestive of a cell full of secondary lysosomes. Some of the cells contain larger granular structures, called angulate bodies, that are packed with fibrillar material and are sometimes lipid.

The ultrastructural features are like those occurring in Schwann cells during wallerian degeneration. Immunocytochemical reactions indicate the presence of S-100 protein and myelin basic protein.[94] Infiltration at margins and in nearby nerves should not be taken as evidence of malignant behavior but may explain an occasional recurrence.[94] The malignant counterpart exists but is rare.[112]

Fibroadenoma. The vulva is at the caudal end of the embryonic milk line, and nodular masses of breast tissue measuring as much as 10 cm in diameter have been

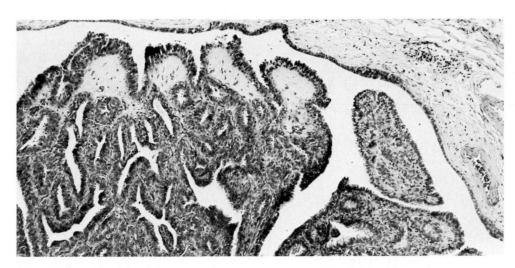

Fig. 34-11. Hidradenoma papilliferum. All the papillary processes have a delicate fibrovascular support, and there is a double layer of epithelial cells covering each of the papillary processes. (90×.)

reported. Sometimes the lesion first becomes evident during lactation as the result of rapid and alarming enlargement. The various patterns associated with chronic cystic disease of the breast also occur in vulvar breast tissue. Fibroadenomas in the vulva resemble breast fibroadenomas. A primary adenocarcinoma of the vulva with the patterns of breast adenocarcinoma has actually occurred[71] but is most unusual; the finding of such a lesion in the vulva is strongly suggestive of metastatic and disseminated breast adenocarcinoma.[54]

Stromal polyps. Cutaneous polyps are invested externally by an orderly epidermis that covers a loose fibrous connective tissue stroma with a variable component of adipose tissue and vessels; most polyps of the vulva have this pattern.

Rarely a stroma polyp may include scattered large giant cells of the type encountered more commonly in the vagina (see p. 1640). The specific subepithelial stroma of the cervix and vagina also extends beneath the epithelium of the vulva.

Condyloma acumination. Condyloma acuminatum is a papillary lesion of squamous epithelium that occurs chiefly as multiple soft warty masses. They may be large or small and can be distributed about the anus, perineum, vaginal wall, and cervix, as well as the vulva (Fig. 34-12). The infectious nature and apparent relationship to sexual behavior have apparently been recognized for centuries.[89] Virologic studies confirm a high rate of transmission between sexual partners even in the absence of clinically obvious condylomas. Furthermore, it appears that juvenile laryngeal papillomatosis is often transmitted to infants from maternal condylomas, presumably at parturition.[98] In the United States the incidence of patients seeking treatment rose by

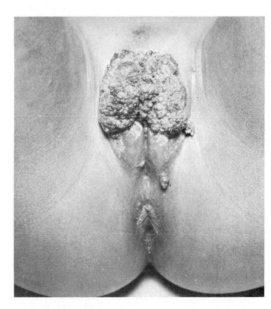

Fig. 34-12. Condyloma acuminatum. Exuberant keratotic papillary processes may cover and obliterate large areas of vulva.

over 400% between 1966 and 1981; two thirds of the patients were between 15 and 29 years of age.

The squamous epithelium that covers the papillary fronds is histologically benign and is supported by a uniformly distributed fibrovascular stroma that ramifies into all the papillary projections (Fig. 34-13). Perinuclear vacuolation, called "koilocytosis," is common and characteristic. Scattered cells may have enlarged, darkly stained nuclei related to polyploidy and arrested mitoses.

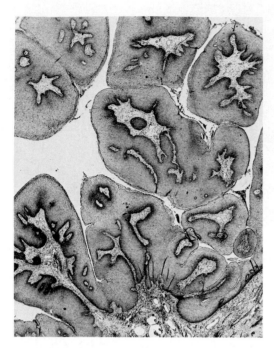

Fig. 34-13. Condyloma acuminatum. Papillary processes are covered by orderly squamous epithelium, each supported by a fibrovascular connective tissue stalk. (20×.)

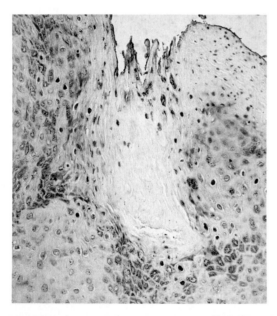

Fig. 34-14. Human papilloma virus demonstrated in infected cells at the surface of condyloma acuminatum. Immunoperoxidase stain, anti–human papilloma virus antiserum, with hematoxylin counterstain. Virus is localized in the blackened nuclei. Latent virus is not detected by this method. (150×.)

The etiologic agent is a papovavirus closely related to the virus of the ordinary cutaneous wart. Most lesions respond to podophyllin, cautery, excision, or freezing. The surprising effectiveness of an autogenous vaccine in eradicating large or resistance condylomas is at present unexplained.[107]

Over 50 strains of human papillomavirus (HPV) have been identified,[128] and the numbers continue to increase. Types 6 and 11 have been recovered from most condylomas. In contrast, similar-appearing lesions with dysplastic nuclear changes and many carcinomas (in situ and invasive) are associated with distinctly different strains of the virus (types 16, 18, and 31). Latent virus may be present in normal-appearing skin adjacent to a condyloma, which may account for the high frequency of local recurrence after treatment.[58] Lesions are often multicentric and the same patient may be infected by more than one viral subtype. Variations in histologic pattern, size, and location indicate that host response can vary and that the appearance of a lesion may represent focal breakdown of host resistance within a larger field of latent papillomaviral infection.[110] HPV is identifiable in tissue sections by immunocytochemical methods (Fig. 34-14) and by in situ hybridization.[49]

Miscellaneous benign neoplasms. Benign mucinous cysts lined by a single layer of columnar cells are more common than is generally appreciated. Most have appeared in the vicinity of the vestibule. The tissue of origin is the urogenital sinus vestiges.[64]

A collection of 34 benign vulvar neoplasms studied by Lovelady, McDonald, and Waugh[95] included 16 fibromas, seven lipomas, five hemangiomas, two neurofibromas, two leiomyomas, one ganglioneuroma, and one lymphangioma. Infiltrating margins and numerous mitoses are the most reliable indicators of aggressive behavior of smooth muscle tumors.[118] Collected reviews[94,101] include examples of pleomorphic adenoma, various sweat gland adenomas, and mesenchymal tumors. Aggressive angiomyxoma,[117] characterized by a loose myxoid matrix traversed by numerous vessels of variable size, is important to recognize because margins are indistinct and some lesions recur locally. Cutaneous lesions such as pyogenic granuloma, seborrheic keratosis, nevi of various types, and single squamous papillomas have no distinctive features when encountered in the vulva and are discussed in Chapter 36. Despite persistent statements to the contrary, vulvar nevi are no more dysplastic or "premalignant" than those at other cutaneous locations.[47]

Endometriosis occurs in the vulva usually as the result of implantation of endometrial tissue in minor operative wounds, notably episiotomy scars.

Dysplasia, intraepithelial neoplasia, and carcinoma in situ. The occurrence of cancerlike changes (dysplasia, atypia) in some cells of the skin and squamous mucosa

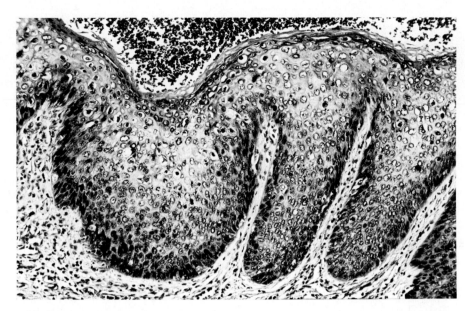

Fig. 34-15. Vulvar intraepithelial neoplasia (VIN). Cytologic atypia of many cells scattered through all layers of epidermis. Prominent clear spaces around nuclei of many cells is a human papilloma virus–associated change called "koilocytosis." This lesion would be graded as moderate dysplasia or VIN-II. (150×.)

of the vulva is distinguished by separate terminology in recognition of its neoplastic potential. The affected areas may be white, red, or brown, forming indistinct patches or well-defined papules. The characteristic changes include nuclear hyperchromasia, cellular pleomorphism, crowding, abnormal mitoses, dyskeratotic cells, perinuclear clear spaces (koilocytosis), hyperkeratosis, parakeratosis, and loss of epithelial cell maturation (Fig. 34-15). Because the numbers and distribution of the cytologically abnormal cells vary considerably, a convention to grade the severity of the process, as seen in histologic sections, has been developed.

These lesions, termed "vulvar intraepithelial neoplasia" (VIN), or "vulvar dysplasia," have been subclassified by the Nomenclature Committees of the International Society of Gynecologic Pathologists and the International Society for the Study of Vulvar Disease[124] as follows:

Mild dysplasia (VIN I). The above-noted abnormalities occupy the lower one third of the epithelium.

Moderate dysplasia (VIN II). The above-noted abnormalities occupy the lower two thirds of the epithelium.

Severe dysplasia (VIN III) and carcinoma in situ: The above-noted abnormalities occupy more than two thirds, nearly the full thickness of the epithelium (surface keratization may or may not be present).

Further discussion is on p. 1635.

The expression "bowenoid papulosis" is a descriptive clinical term applied when the lesion appears as elevated brown papules, usually multiple, in the vulvar,

perineal, or perianal skin and squamous mucosal surfaces; it is not a defined histopathologic entity. Bowen's disease, erythroplasia of Queyrat, and carcinoma simplex are additional vaguely synonymous terms.

The above-mentioned conditions are generally believed to be "precancerous." They have become increasingly common, especially in young women and even in children. Actual transition to invasive carcinoma occurs but has thus far been observed infrequently in young women, and some lesions regress spontaneously. Untreated lesions in middle-aged and elderly women are more likely to become invasive in periods of 2 to 5 years.[83] Association with the more carcinogenic strains of human papillomavirus has been demonstrated repeatedly.[49]

Malignant tumors

The predominant malignant tumor of the vulva is epidermoid carcinoma (at least 96%). Malignant melanomas make up another 2%, and the rest are a mixture of rare adenocarcinomas, soft-tissue sarcomas, and an occasional basal cell carcinoma. Vulvar carcinomas comprise less than 1% of all cancers and 5% of genital tract cancers in women.

Epidermoid carcinoma. Invasive epidermoid carcinoma is chiefly a disease of postmenopausal women. Smaller lesions are usually elevated and superficial with an irregular granular, nodular, or ulcerated surface. Larger lesions tend to protrude as an outward-growing warty mass with a weeping ulcerated surface and a mottled red-gray or yellow surface (Fig. 34-16). More ag-

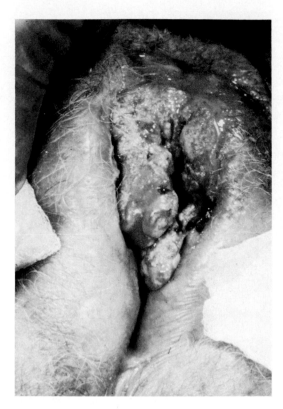

Fig. 34-16. Carcinoma of vulva. Tumor forms nodular erythematous mass with ulceration and erythema. Adjacent labia are edematous.

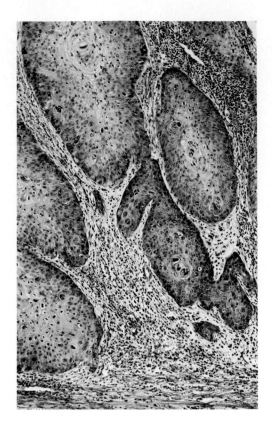

Fig. 34-17. Epidermoid carcinoma of vulva. Irregular rounded masses of well-differentiated keratinizing epidermoid carcinoma with well-circumscribed margin and associated inflammatory changes. (80×.)

gressive, poorly differentiated, infiltrating tumors have ulcerated surfaces with elevated, undermined margins.

Associated carcinoma in situ or dystrophic changes in the adjacent skin are commonly present. Women with vulvar carcinoma are likely to have diabetes mellitus, obesity, hypertension, early menopause, and other neoplasms.[68] The usual location is the labia majora, especially the inner aspect, and most carcinomas begin on the anterior two thirds of the vulva.

Most vulvar epidermoid carcinomas are well differentiated, produce keratin, and have well-circumscribed margins (Fig. 34-17). Lesions with this pattern are more likely to remain localized and have a better prognosis. Poorly differentiated carcinomas have a more diffusely infiltrating pattern, invade nerve sheaths and lymphatics, grow in narrow strands, and have a more aggressive natural history. The loose fibroblastic stroma in such cases is usually relatively abundant, and the tumor margin is indistinct.

It is important to emphasize that a physical examination is an unreliable indicator of metastatic spread; even an experienced examiner is likely to miss metastases or overdiagnose their presence in about 40% of patients.[122] The presence of a hyperkeratotic dysplastic

lesion in the adjacent skin is associated with a significantly better prognosis.[67]

The size of the primary tumor is not a reliable indicator of metastasis; in the experience of Green, Ulfelder, and Meigs[69,70] one third of the lesions 1 cm in maximum diameter or smaller and half of the well-differentiated grade I epidermoid carcinomas were associated with lymph node metastases.

A large collaborative study by the Gynecologic Oncology Group found that the most significant predictors of node metastases were tumor thickness, palpable nodes, lymphatic space invasion, midline location, and poorly differentiated histologic pattern. Predictive value in an individual case is enhanced when one considers all the above factors together.[115] The complex topography of the vulva and its cancers make measurements of depth of "microinvasive" lesions extremely difficult to reproduce. Careful orientation of the specimen and thorough pathologic study are necessary to identify the "early" lesions[113] that can be safely treated without lymph node dissection. Wilkinson has reviewed the pathologic approaches to this problem, which remains unsettled.[123] Measurements must be made with an ocular micrometer. Thickness is the distance between the surface of the cancer and its maximum depth; depth is the distance between the epithelialstromal junction of the most superficial adjacent dermal papilla and the deepest point of invasion. Lymph node metastases commonly appear in the opposite side of the vulva, and so bilateral inguinal lymph node dissections are necessary. Lesions located anteriorly or on the clitoris are more likely to spread to deeper (pelvic, iliac) lymph nodes.

There is a distant association with other areas of carcinoma of the lower genital tract, notably the cervix[40,53] and upper vagina, as well as the anus and perineum.

Earlier diagnosis has resulted in increased effectiveness of surgical treatment, fewer women with lymph node metastases, and improved survival.[68]

Verrucous carcinoma. Verrucous carcinoma is an extremely well-differentiated form of epidermoid carcinoma first described by Ackerman as a lesion occurring primarily in the oral cavity. It may become quite large and expands inexorably into adjacent tissues. The vulva is the most common site of genital verrucous carcinoma, but it also occurs in the vagina and cervix.[77]

Although the histologic and cytologic pattern appears benign, it is possible to distinguish verrucous carcinoma from condyloma acuminatum by the uneven distribution of the fibrovascular stromal support in the former.

Lymph node metastases occur only rarely, but any tissue, including lymph nodes and nerve sheaths, may be involved by direct extension. A satisfactory response to radiotherapy is unusual.[91]

Epidermoid carcinoma in situ. Epidermoid carcinomas in situ are white or mottled red and white patches that often form plaquelike elevations. Some lesions have a brown papillomatous appearance (called "bowenoid papulosis"). Pruritus is common. Distinction between benign dystrophy and carcinoma in situ is impossible without biopsy.

Before 1970 the typical patient was a postmenopausal woman, and the condition was uncommon. In a more recent series 40% of the women were under 40 years of age.[45] Many had prior or concomitant condyloma acuminatum,[84,120] and even more common was a history of vulvar herpes simplex infection.[86] The presence of virus-specific markers was demonstrated in the lesions of many women by both immunocytochemistry[86] and in situ hybridization,[48] strongly suggestive of herpes simplex virus being an important etiologic factor. The relative importance of these two common viral infections individually or in concert is not established, but both viruses seem to be strongly associated with the increasing incidence of vulvar neoplasms in young women.

The affected epithelium is composed almost entirely of small, relatively uniform dysplastic or anaplastic squamous epithelial cells that lie typically beneath a keratotic surface of variable thickness (Fig. 34-18). It is

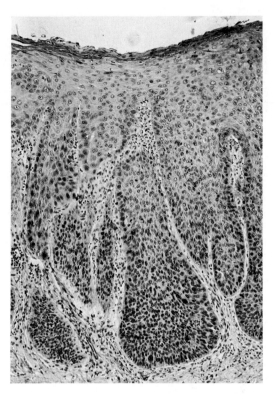

Fig. 34-18. Vulvar carcinoma in situ. Notice hyperchromatic dysplastic nuclei, mitoses, and disorderly pattern in comparison with hyperkeratosis. (140×.)

important to identify invasion if it is present.

A variant, more pleomorphic pattern called "Bowen's disease" now occurs with increasing frequency in young women. The lesions are brown papules, usually multiple, and often extend to involve the anus (Fig. 34-19, *A*). The histologic pattern is heterogeneous with a scattering of large bizarre cells, dyskeratotic cells, and bizarre mitoses distributed through a background of smaller uniform dysplastic cells (Fig. 34-19, *B*). Ulbright and colleagues[121] found a lesser risk of invasive cancer among younger women whose lesions were more uniform and did not involve the pilosebaceous apparatus. The histologic pattern sometimes includes koilocytosis and other features of condyloma acuminatum.[49] Although the same type of lesion may recur in an adjacent area, invasive carcinoma has not developed in most young women with this condition, prompting a consensus in favor of conservative treatment and close follow-up study when possible.[45,49,78,84,121] Lesions that appear during pregnancy may regress spontaneously in the postpartum period.[60,116]

Extramammary Paget's disease. Vulvar Paget's disease begins as an intraepidermal, noninvasive adenocarcinoma. The affected skin is mottled red and white, scaly, elevated, and slightly indurated. Characteristically there are small, white, keratotic patches separated

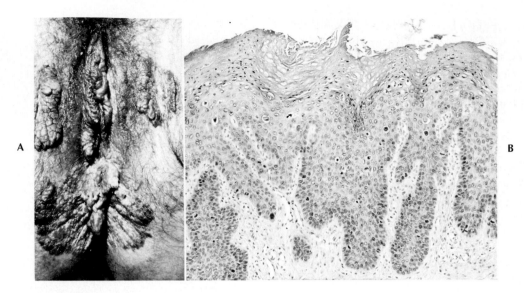

Fig. 34-19. A, Vulva with carcinoma in situ, Bowen's disease type. Elevated red-brown plaques composed of warty, sometimes papillary, anaplastic epithelium. There was no invasion in this extensive lesion. **B,** Vulva with carcinoma in situ, Bowen's disease type. Large, multinucleated, anaplastic cells and isolated dyskeratonic cells are distinguishing histologic features of this variant pattern of carcinoma in situ. Perinuclear vacuolation (koilocytosis) indicates possible condyloma virus infection, (150×.)

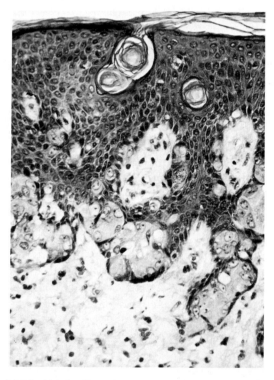

Fig. 34-20. Vulvar Paget's disease. Neoplastic cells infiltrate epidermis individually and in small clumps. Squamous cells of epidermis itself are histologically benign and compressed by tumor. There is no infiltration of underlying dermis. (260×.)

by red fissures of irregular bands from which the superficial epidermis has exfoliated. Extensive lesions may eventually spread onto the pubic area, thighs, or sacral region.

The epidermis is infiltrated by large pale adenocarcinoma cells, scattered between compressed but normal-appearing squamous epithelial cells (Fig. 34-20). The epithelium of hair follicles and apocrine sweat glands is characteristically involved. Many of the Paget cells contain stainable epithelial mucin. In ultrastructural studies various patterns of cytologic differentiation, resembling eccrine, apocrine, and squamous cell patterns, have been described. Immunocytochemical stains consistently identify epithelial membrane antigen, casein, and carcinoembryonic antigen, and fibrocystic disease fluid protein is identifiable in most cases.[101] The latter appears to be a reliable marker for apocrine epithelium.[99]

If there is no invasion, the prognosis is good. Margins are difficult to see, and local recurrence is therefore common. The colposcope may refine the planning of surgical margins.

Approximately one patient in three has an underlying tumor mass composed of infiltrating adenocarcinoma, usually poorly differentiated; foci of squamous differentiation are commonly present. In the presence of invasion, metastases are likely, and the prognosis is very poor.

Adenocarcinoma and Bartholin's gland carcinoma. Adenocarcinomas of the vulva are uncommon; they may arise in Bartholin's gland or the minor vestibular glands. The initial appearance is a subcutaneous lump. The microscopic pattern may be that of an adenoid cystic adenocarcinoma, papillary adenocarcinoma, mucoepidermoid carcinoma, or mucinous adenocarcinoma. About one third of Bartholin's gland carcinomas are epidermoid carcinomas.

The principles of treatment are the same as those for other vulvar carcinomas. Many patients are premenopausal: half of the lesions studied by Chamlian and Taylor[46] were originally underestimated as Bartholin's gland cysts. Adenoid cystic adenocarcinomas characteristically do not metastasize to lymph nodes but invade widely along nerve sheaths.

Malignant melanoma. Most malignant melanomas are located anteriorly near the midline. Local recurrence is usually at vaginal and urethral margins where the impulse to temporize is greatest.

Lesions of the squamous mucosa are usually of the mucosal membrane type of acral lentiginous melanoma with junctional clusters of spindle cells, whereas lesions of vulvar skin have the pagetoid intracutaneous pattern of superficial spreading melanomas.[46] The customary treatment is radical surgery with lymph node dissection,[102,103] though the generally poor results have caused some writers to question its effectiveness[51] because very thin (less than 1.49 mm) lesions usually have no nodal metastases and patients with larger lesions have a high frequency of local recurrence and poor survival.

Metastatic carcinoma. Metastatic carcinoma was the third most common malignant tumor encountered in a study by Dehner,[54] comprising 22 of 262 primary malignant neoplasms (8%). The most common primary sources are cervix and endometrium. Metastatic cancers from the colon, breast, and ovary also are found in the vulva and should not be mistaken for primary vulvar cancer.

Rare malignant neoplasms. Malignant fibrous histiocytoma, epithelioid sarcoma,[52] leiomyosarcoma, rhabdomyosarcoma, and malignant lymphoma may occur in the soft tissues of the vulva.[52] Basal cell carcinomas of the vulvar skin[50] resemble those occurring in more common cutaneous locations (see Chapter 36).

VAGINA
Anatomy and physiology

The vagina is a collapsed cylinder situated between the vestibule externally and the cervix internally. It has an inner lining of nonkeratinized squamous epithelium surrounded by a layer of connective tissue stroma, all supported by a double layer of smooth muscle. There are no named glands, but small glandular remnants of the mesonephric ducts occasionally persist and may form cysts.

The histologic and cytologic features of the squamous epithelium are affected by hormonal stimuli. During the reproductive years estrogens increase the thickness of the epithelium and the amount of cytoplasmic glycogen. The epithelium is thin in childhood and atrophic after menopause, when estrogen stimulation is minimal.

Cytologic patterns, as seen in the vaginal smear, vary with age and undergo cyclic changes with the menstrual cycle. During the first 14 days of the menstrual cycle, a period of estrogen predominance, the exfoliated cells,

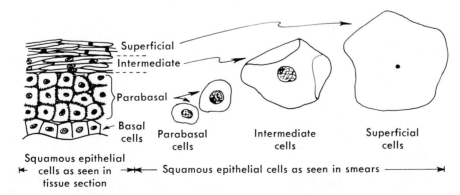

Fig. 34-21. Diagram of relationship between squamous mucosa of vagina and ectocervix, and parabasal, intermediate, and superficial cells exfoliated and seen in smears. Superficial cells predominate in estrogenic smears of first 2 weeks of menstrual cycle, and intermediate cells predominate in second 2 weeks after ovulation under influence of progesterone. (Redrawn from Frost, J.K.: Concepts basic to general cytopathology, Baltimore, Md., 1972, The Johns Hopkins Press.)

called superficial cells, are large and flattened and have pyknotic nuclei. After ovulation, under the superimposed influence of progesterone, the nuclei are larger and vesicular, and the cell margins are folded; these are called intermediate cells (Fig. 34-21). The amount of cytoplasmic glycogen is greatly increased, and cytoplasmic margins are dense and accentuated in pregnancy. In childhood, after menopause, and after childbirth the mucosa is atrophic and the predominant exfoliated cells are small, round or oval, parabasal cells that have little glycogen. Small amounts of estrogen administered at these times induce maturation to the estrogenic pattern of superficial cell predominance.

Knowledge of the normal cytologic variations is important in the identification of neoplastic cells and other pathologic states.

Cytologic manifestations of pathologic states
Endocrine disturbances

The vaginal cell population in precocious puberty shows pronounced maturation with superficial cell predominance as the result of estrogen stimulation. Exposure to any estrogenic drug, including estrogen-containing face creams, will have a similar effect. Digitalis is said to have an estrogenic effect on the vaginal smear of some postmenopausal women. Death of a fetus with inevitable abortion results in a reversion of the pregnancy pattern to the superficial cell smear of estrogen predominance.

Women taking artificial progestogens cyclically (the contraceptive pill) may have increased numbers of large parabasal cells or intermediate cells with large but cytologically benign nuclei. Syndromes of ovarian dysfunction such as the Stein-Leventhal syndrome are associated with continuous exfoliation of intermediate cells, without any sort of cyclic change.

Vaginal inflammation

The vaginal smears of women with active gonorrhea contain the typical intracellular diplococci of *Neisseria gonorrhoeae* located in the cytoplasm of polymorphonuclear leukocytes. Streptococci, staphylococci, and *Escherichia coli*, as well as several other bacteria, may cause vulvovaginitis. Vaginitis caused by *Gardnerella vaginalis* is associated with malodorous leukorrhea. It is likely that multiple organisms interact together to produce the syndrome of nonspecific vaginitis, which is now more properly designated "bacterial vaginosis."

The most common causes of symptomatic vaginitis are a fungus, *Candida albicans*, and a protozoon, *Trichomonas vaginalis*. Hyphae of *Candida* species and trichomonads are easily identified in smears (Fig. 34-22). In *Trichomonas* infections the vagina has a red punctate appearance with abundant frothy discharge. Candidiasis is associated in typical cases with white patches of mycelia attached to an inflamed mucosa and is more common in pregnant and diabetic women.[142] The vulva and cervix are usually involved simultaneously.

The least common, but much more serious, are the shallow ulcers that result from the use of vaginal tam-

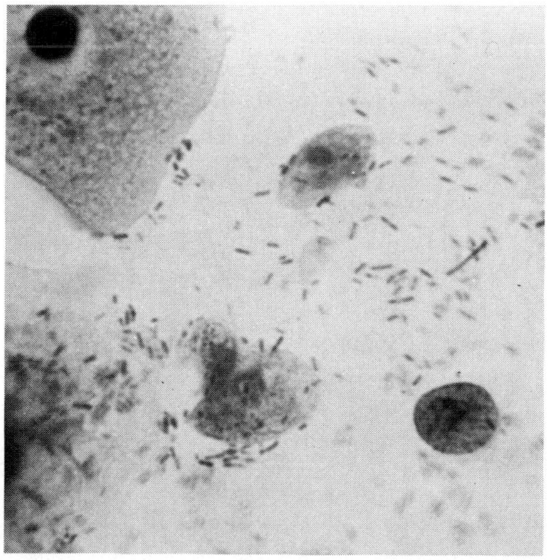

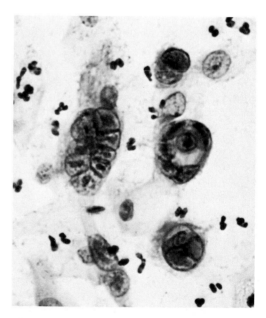

Fig. 34-22. *Trichomonas* organisms in cervicovaginal smear. Organisms are above and below the center. Portion of superficial squamous cell is present at top left, indicating relative size. (1000×.)

Fig. 34-23. Vaginal smears showing epithelial cells containing typical herpes simplex viral inclusions. Notice syncytial clustering of nuclei. (600×.)

pons when they occur in association with a specific form of staphylococcal infection. Absorption of enterotoxin F and exotoxin C produced by *Staphylococcus aureus* of phage group 1 results in the toxic shock syndrome, characterized by fever, erythematous rash, and shock, attended by a mortality of nearly 6%.[174]

The most important viral disease identifiable by vaginal cytology is herpes simplex. The infected epithelial cells form a multinucleated syncytium, like a cluster of bubbles. Ng, Reagan, and Lindner[155] have described two types of intranuclear inclusions and have found that one type with a homogeneous ground-glass appearance is more common in primary infections, whereas the typical eosinophilic inclusions surrounded by a clear zone are seen more frequently in secondary or recurrent infections (Fig. 34-23).

Cysts and nonneoplastic growths
Subepithelial cysts

Vaginitis emphysematosa is a remarkable process characterized by the presence of numerous subepithelial gas-filled cysts, which may pop audibly when traumatized (Fig. 34-24). They are essentially stromal bubbles with no epithelial lining, associated with a slight inflammatory response, including scattered giant cells. Many patients are pregnant, and a significant association with *Trichomonas* infection has been suggested.[141]

Epithelial cysts

Gartner's duct cysts of the lateral vaginal wall are lined with cuboid glandular epithelium without cyto-

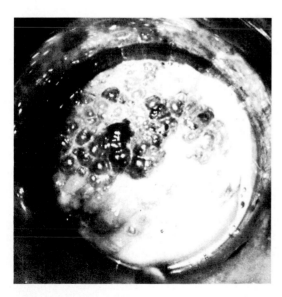

Fig. 34-24. Vaginitis emphysematosa. Vesicles and vaginal discharge as photographed through a cylindrical speculum. (From Close, J.M., and Jesurun, H.M.: Obstet. Gynecol. **19**:513, 1962.)

plasmic mucin; they are considered to arise from dilated vestiges of the mesonephric ducts.

Given the uncertainty surrounding the origins of all parts of the vagina, it is probably better to classify vaginal cysts according to the type of epithelium that predominates, such as mucinous, squamous, and endometrial.[108] Mucinous cysts, considered to be of urogenital sinus origin, seem to be more commonly situated near the vestibule[139] and are actually more common.[136] An occasional paramesonephric cyst contains ciliated cells.

Squamous epithelial inclusion cysts, lined by squamous epithelium and filled with keratin, occur in the vaginal mucosa, as they do in the skin. Endometriosis of the vagina forms multiple blue mucosal cysts, which may rupture and bleed during menses. The usual cause is implantation of endometrium in an incision, especially an episiotomy.

Adenosis, clear cell carcinoma, and in utero diethylstilbestrol exposure

Adenosis in the context of vaginal pathologic conditions refers to the presence of histologically benign mucinous epithelium of typical endocervical pattern in an area that is normally covered by stratified squamous vaginal mucosa. The extent ranges from tiny foci 1 or 2 mm in greatest diameter to a virtual conversion of the entire vaginal lining to a surface of columnar mucous epithelium.

The affected mucosa has a reddened, velvety appearance, in contrast to the more opaque pale pink of the normal squamous mucosa (Fig. 34-25, A). Focal lesions require a colposcope for identification; larger patches are visible in ordinary physical examination.

The epithelium in areas of adenomas is composed of a single layer of mucinous columnar epithelial cells, but glandular crypts and slight papillary in some areas (Fig. 34-25, B). Occasional patches of epithelium are composed of ciliated columnar cells without mucin vacuoles, resembling tubal mucosa.[164] Some degree of squamous metaplasia is often present, beginning as a proliferation of reserve cells beneath the gland cell layer, as in the cervix; a complete conversion to a squamous epithelial lining probably occurs eventually in most cases.

Adenosis in adolescent girls received considerable notoriety after the demonstration of a causal relationship with exposure in utero to diethylstilbestrol ingested by the mother. It has been shown that the crucial period of exposure is before the eighteenth week of gestation. After this time formation of the vagina is completed, and susceptibility to the effects of diethylstilbestrol is apparently lost. Diethylstilbestrol-induced adenosis may also occur in the mucosa of the portio vaginalis of the cervix. About one third of the patients have an anomalous ridge or "hood" of muscular connec-

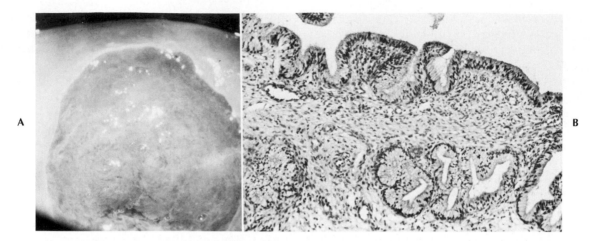

Fig. 34-25. Vaginal adenosis. **A,** Glandular mucosa covers ectocervix and adjacent vaginal mucosa in place of normal squamous epithelium. **B,** Photomicrograph of abnormal epithelium shown in **A.** Epithelial surface is covered by columnar mucinous epithelium, thrown into tiny clefts and folds. (**B,** 150×; **A** and **B,** courtesy Dr. James G. Blythe, St. Louis, Mo.)

tive tissue surrounding the cervix. This and other upper genital tract changes have adverse effects on pregnancy.[150] Many of the structural anomalies occurring in humans exposed to diethylstilbestrol have been reproduced in animal models[168] and provided insights into the normal embryology of the vagina.

The incidence of adenosis in diethylstilbestrol-exposed infants is probably very high, if minute areas are searched for carefully with a colposcope. A much more significant but fortunately less common association is clear cell adenocarcinoma of the vagina and cervix.[146,147] Both the mucinous epithelium of adenosis and the clear cell adenocarcinomas are probably of müllerian duct origin.

Neoplasms
Benign tumors

Fibroepithelial polyp (stroma polyp). The subepithelial connective tissue of the vagina may form single or multiple polypoid masses, covered by orderly vaginal squamous mucosa. This stroma characteristically has a loose myxoid appearance, interspersed with giant cells (Fig. 34-26). Benign polyps lack the subepithelial crowded zone of proliferating immature cells found in sarcoma botryoides, and they occur in young women, especially during pregnancy.[137,157] Rarely there is a component of mucinous epithelial glands intermixed with the stroma. Bleeding and awareness of a mass are the common initial symptoms.[133]

Leiomyoma. The most common benign connective tumor of the vagina is leiomyoma, and even these are rare. The morphologic features are like those of more common uterine leiomyomas. Tavassoli and Norris[169] found that recurrence and metastasis occurred in large

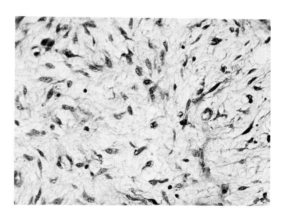

Fig. 34-26. Connective tissue of stromal polyp of vagina has loose myxoid appearance. Cells are spindle shaped or stellate and may be multinucleated. (260×.)

tumors, with more than five mitoses per 10 high-power microscopic fields and infiltrating margins. Only five of 60 smooth muscle tumors recurred; only one metastasized.

Other benign tumors. Other benign tumors include neurofibroma and neurilemoma. Kurman and Prabha[152] identified ectopic parathyroid and thyroid tissue in vaginal nodule and reviewed six reported cases of vaginal teratoma. Rare benign mixed tumors are composed of islands of squamous or mucinous epithelium scattered through a stroma of spindle cells that resemble endometrial stroma.[166] Ulbright and I[171] have encountered endometrial type of stromal nodules in the perivaginal connective tissue. A glandular papilloma of the vaginal wall of a child studied ultrastructurally had morphologic features suggestive of müllerian origin.[170] A benign rhabdomyoma has also been reported.[143,194]

Occasionally after a hysterectomy the tubal fimbria may herniate into the vaginal apex, simulating a neoplasm.[165] Granulation tissue, which may contain rapidly proliferating blood vessel sprouts, can produce sizable lumps at the vaginal apex after surgery.

Malignant tumors

Most cancers encountered in the vaginal wall are metastatic. According to the definition adopted by the International Federation of Gynecology and Obstetrics, a lesion that extends to the cervical os is classified as a cancer of the cervix, and a lesion that extends to the vulva is a vulvar carcinoma. The remaining true primary vaginal carcinomas compose slightly less than 1% of female genital cancers.

Over 95% of vaginal cancers are epidermoid carcinomas; of these, 10% have not invaded the vaginal wall and are called in situ carcinomas. The remaining 5% are adenocarcinomas, malignant melanomas, and sarcomas.

Epidermoid carcinoma in situ. It is uncommon to first find a carcinoma in situ in the vagina. In most instances there has been a prior or concurrent, in situ or invasive carcinoma in the cervix or vulva.

The histologic and colposcopic features are identical to those of an epidermoid carcinoma of the cervix. If there is no invasion, local excision of involved areas is adequate treatment; the use of a colposcope is a valuable and important way to identify all areas of involvement and their margins. An associated carcinoma of the vulva, cervix, or both is highly probable and must be excluded before therapy is planned.

Vaginal carcinoma in situ may appear 10 or more years after treatment of a carcinoma in situ of the cervix or vulva. The prognosis for in situ lesions is good even if superficial invasion is present, which emphasizes the importance of continued cytologic follow-up study of women treated for carcinoma of the cervix or vulva.

Invasive epidermoid carcinoma. Most invasive vaginal epidermoid carcinomas are indurated, ulcerated nodules; a few are elevated, soft, and papillary. The histologic pattern is commonly (about 50%) moderately differentiated, without keratinization. Well- and moderately differentiated carcinomas with keratinization account for about 15% each, and the rest are poorly differentiated without keratinization. Moderately differentiated keratinizing lesions with large anaplastic nuclei seemed to be more aggressive in the series studied by Perez and associates.[158] Most patients are elderly postmenopausal women; the usual location is the upper posterior vaginal wall. Significant etiologic factors have not been identified. Lesions of the distal aspect of the vagina may metastasize to inguinal lymph nodes.

For evaluating the prognosis and comparing the results of treatment, the extent of spread is classified by stages according to criteria agreed on by the International Federation of Gynecology and Obstetrics, as follows:

Stage 0   Carcinoma in situ
Stage I   Limited to vaginal wall
Stage II   Involving subvaginal tissue without extension to pelvic wall
Stage III   Extension to pelvic wall
Stage IV   Extension beyond true pelvis or to mucosa of bladder or rectum
    a. Spread to adjacent organs
    b. Spread to distant organs

Radiotherapy has been selected for most patients; about 75% of those with stage I disease survive for 5 years. Unfortunately, less than one third of the patients have stage I lesions; overall, less than half the patients survive for 5 years.

Metastatic cancer. The most frequent primary source of metastatic carcinoma in the vagina is the uterine cervix, often by direct extension. Carcinomas of the urinary bladder, rectum, vulva, urethra, or anus may infiltrate directly into the vagina. Embolic metastases from the endometrium, ovary, kidney, breast, or intestinal tract occur less frequently. The first evidence of a choriocarcinoma may be a vaginal metastasis.

Adenocarcinoma. Adenocarcinomas of the vagina are rare. Clear cell adenocarcinoma associated with adenosis in adolescent girls (as discussed previously) is currently the most frequently encountered pattern. The occurrence of an adenocarcinoma is estimated to be between 0.14 and 1.4 per 1000 diethylstilbestrol-exposed women through 24 years of age; the incidence appears to have peaked in 1975.[148] Similar tumors also occur rarely in older women not exposed to diethylstilbestrol. The tumors are usually superficial and either papillary or nodular (Fig. 34-27). Most have been located in the upper or middle third of the vagina, primarily on the anterior wall.

The histologic pattern, like that of clear cell carcinomas found elsewhere in the female genitalia, consists of tubules or small cysts with inconspicuous stroma (Fig. 34-28). Tumors with a tubulocystic pattern are attended by better survival at 5 years (90%) as compared to papillary tumors or those composed of solid masses of clear cells. The tumor cells are large with variable degrees of nuclear anaplasia. There is abundant clear cytoplasm, containing much glycogen and no mucin; there may be some intraluminal mucin. The nuclei of cells lining cystic spaces may protrude into the lumens; the cells are separated and produce a pattern that is said to resemble hobnails in a boot.

Vaginal adenosis has been found in almost all patients with adenocarcinoma. Factors associated with recur-

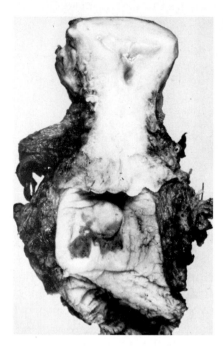

Fig. 34-27. Vagina with clear cell adenocarcinoma subsequent to in utero exposure to diethylstilbestrol. Carcinoma forms elevated nodule in vagina just below cervix (center). Dark patches of adenosis are contiguous, just below tumor.

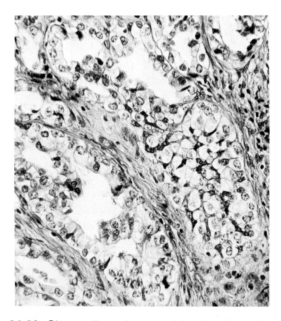

Fig. 34-28. Clear cell carcinoma arising in adenosis of vagina of young woman exposed to diethylstilbestrol in utero. Tumor cells contain glycogen but not mucin. (300×; courtesy Dr. Robert E. Scully, Boston, Mass.)

rence and poor prognosis are large size, proximity to resection margins, and penetration more than 3 mm into the wall of the vagina. Girls under 15 years of age have a less favorable prognosis than those over 19. The use of oral contraceptives does not seem to influence tumor behavior.[148] The entire subject of diethylstilbestrol-associated lesions has been reviewed extensively.[130]

Mucinous adenocarcinomas also occur in the vagina. Although usually well differentiated, they are characteristically aggressive and may metastasize widely. Some tumors of this type have been associated with adenosis[163]; these lesions occurred in older women whose birth dates precluded any possibility of diethylstilbestrol exposure in utero.

Embryonal rhabdomyosarcoma (sarcoma botryoides). Embryonal rhabdomyosarcoma is a malignant tumor of undifferentiated muscle cells. It tends to produce ovoid masses that protrude into the vagina, covered by normal epithelium (Fig. 34-29). There is a cambium zone of immature round or spindle cells crowded beneath the epithelium; this contrasts with the looser, more myxoid pattern of the central core. The cambium layer is seen best in smaller polyps.

Most of the patients are infants; 90% are under 5 years of age. After puberty there is an overwhelming probability that a polypoid lesion with myxoid-appearing stroma is a benign stromal polyp (p. 1640). Embryonal rhabdomyosarcoma has a predilection for the anterior vaginal wall and tends to invade extensively in the pelvis and metastasize to regional lymph nodes and distant sites such as lung and liver.[149] Most instances of successful treatment have resulted from early diagnosis and radical surgery. As with other forms of rhabdomyosarcoma, chemotherapy may offer some benefit.[134] Similar tumors may arise also in the orbit, urinary bladder, external auditory canal, and biliary tract. There is probably no relationship to malignant mixed müllerian tumor; glandular components have been absent in nearly all cases reported.[149]

Distinctive adenocarcinoma of infant vagina (endodermal sinus tumor). Distinctive vaginal adenocarcinoma in infants arises as multiple polypoid masses, resembling the botryoid gross appearance of embryonal rhabdomyosarcoma. The histologic pattern is identical to that of a type of germ cell carcinoma that has been called the endodermal sinus tumor, arising in the ovary (see Fig. 34-79) or infants testis.[156] The tumor cells produce alpha-fetoprotein, which circulates in the blood and serves as a tumor marker to monitor therapy. The prognosis has been poor, though promising results have been reported with chemotherapy.[129]

Other neoplasms. Rare instances of leiomyosarcoma[169] and malignant melanoma[131] have been reported. The pathologic features do not differ significantly from those of similar lesions in more common locations.

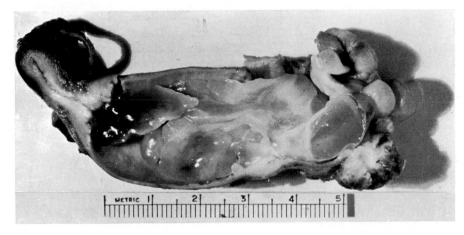

Fig. 34-29. Embryonal rhabdomyosarcoma of vagina (sarcoma botryoides) in sagittal section. Tumor arose in and filled vagina of 16-month-old infant and invaded adjacent pelvic tissues including base of urinary bladder. (Courtesy Dr. Sidney Farber, Boston, Mass.)

CERVIX
Anatomy and physiology

The distal third of the adult uterus is channeled by a central endocervical canal that communicates superiorly with the endometrial canal that communicates superiorly with the endometrial cavity at an ill-defined internal os and inferiorly with the vagina through an equally ill-defined external os. The endocervical canal is lined by a single layer of tall columnar mucin-producing cells. The endocervical mucosa is thrown into redundant, longitudinally oriented folds, separated by clefts. Opposing walls of clefts tend to fuse irregularly to form irregular tunnels that may reenter the endocervical canal or end blindly. These grooves and tunnels may produce an intricate pattern on cross section and commonly are referred to as glands; in fact, they represent extensions of the endocervical mucosa.

The physical properties of the cervical mucus vary during the menstrual cycle. After menses the mucus is at first viscous and sticky; under the influence of estrogen it becomes thin, glossy, and permeable to spermatozoa; when it dries on a glass slide, the sodium chloride crystallizes in delicate arborizing patterns (fern test). After ovulation and in pregnancy, when progesterone predominates, this crystallization is inhibited.

The portio vaginalis is part of the cervical mucosa exposed to the vagina; these surfaces are covered by stratified squamous epithelium, which is resistant to infection. Variable areas of exposed cervical mucosa may be covered with glandular endocervical mucosa at birth (congenital erosion). Of greater significance is the fact that cervical reconstitution and healing after parturition leave variable areas of endocervical glandular surfaces everted into the vagina and exposed to its contents. Such areas of eversion appear red and have been called "erosions." This expression is misleading because the mucosal layer is actually intact; glandular mucosa is transparent, and the visible underlying vessels give a red color.

The exposed glandular surfaces are less resistant to infections of all kinds; a discharge is common, and the subepithelial layers are infiltrated by chronic inflammatory cells. The resulting chronic cervicitis is the invariable morphologic finding in the cervix of women with a normal reproductive life.

Squamous metaplasia (squamous prosoplasia)

The normal response to eversion is the gradual conversion of exposed glandular epithelium to squamous epithelium. Local factors such as pH and estrogen[217] stimulate the proliferation of an underlying layer of reserve cells that eventually forms a multilayered covering serveral cells thick (Fig. 34-30). The surface gland cells slough away to leave mature stratified squamous epithelium. The area involved in these changes is called the transition zone.

Hyperkeratosis

The squamous epithelium of the portio vaginalis may develop a thick surface layer of keratin, especially in patients with uterine prolapse. Biopsy is important, especially if the process is patchy, since some well-differentiated carcinomas may have a similar appearance. The keratotic process is itself benign, as in the vulva.

Microglandular hyperplasia

A very characteristic pattern of gland cell hyperplasia occurs in young women taking oral contraceptives.[236,283] The larger lesions are polypoid. They are formed of masses of small endocervical gland cells intermixed with reserve cells in an early stage of squamous metaplasia, producing an intricate but recognizable pattern

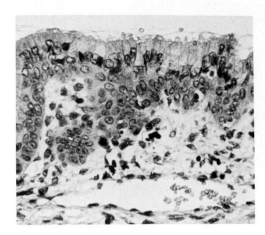

Fig. 34-30. Squamous metaplasia of cervix begins by proliferation of reserve cells beneath columnar epithelium. This new layer thickens, keratinizes, and will become a squamous mucosal surface when surface gland cells ultimately are sloughed away. (300×.)

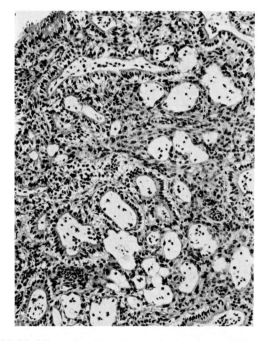

Fig. 34-31. Microglandular hyperplasia of cervix has complicated pattern produced by many small glandular spaces surrounded by immature proliferating reserve cells and squamous epithelial cells intermixed with inflammatory cells and strands of fibrous stroma. This pattern should not be confused with a neoplasm. (150×.)

(Fig. 34-31) that should never be confused with carcinoma. Similar changes occur in pregnancy. Less commonly, gland cells with large, dark, but cytologically benign polyploid nuclei may be found. This change is analogous to the secretory gestational hyperplasia described in the endometrium by Arias-Stella[297] (see p. 1654). There is no evidence that birth control pills have any direct carcinogenic effect on the cervix.[290]

The mesenchymal cells of the subepithelial stroma are often multinucleated and occasionally have a prominent appearance, which should not be mistaken for a neoplasm.[200] They resemble similar cells in a fibrous papule of the nose and, in polyps, have occasionally contained inclusions like those of infantile digital fibroma.[193] The function of these cells is unknown; they have not been implicated in any significant morbid condition.

Vestigial and heterotopic structures

Vestiges of the mesonephric ducts commonly persist in the lateral walls of the cervix and occasionally produce sizable collections. These are distinguished from well-differentiated cervical adenocarcinoma by the absence of cytoplasmic mucin and benign cytologic pattern. A few mesonephric cysts have been large enough to produce a mass.[271]

Roth and Taylor[264] described heterotopic hyaline cartilage in the cervix. Benign stromal polyps containing well-differentiated skeletal muscle, like those in the vagina,[194] also occur on the cervix. In most instances it is possible to show that apparent heterotopic tissues are the result of implantation of aborted fetal tissues.[184,202] Endometriosis of the cervix may appear as one or more blue hemorrhagic nodules or blisters on the portio vaginalis.

The startling occurrence of sebaceous glands, hair, and sweat glands[289] is harder to explain in this mesodermal organ. Lesions with a similar appearance, called Fordyce's spots, occurred simultaneously in the mouth of the patient described by Watson and Cochran.[285]

Inflammation

Acute cervicitis may be associated with an acute gonococcal infection or puerperal sepsis. Caustic substances used as abortifacients, such as potassium permanganate, produce extensive ulceration and hemorrhage. Occasionally biopsy of a primary chancre will be performed to exclude carcinoma. Acute cervicitis occurs also with herpes simplex infection; the characteristic multinucleated cells and intranuclear viral inclusions are demonstrated infrequently. Ulcerated lesions may resemble cancer on visual inspection. The clinical and pathologic features have been well illustrated by Kaufman and associates[225] and Naib and associates.[247] The relationship between herpes simplex infections and cervical cancer is discussed on p. 1647.

Cervical infection caused by *Chlamydia trachomatis* has been identified with increasing frequency as cultural techniques become more widely available. Although not all infected women are symptomatic, approximately 45% have extensive inflammation in the transitional zone, as seen with the colposcope, and severe histologic changes, including intraepithelial microabscesses, epithelial necrosis, and ulceration.[253] The presence of chlamydial organisms in infected cells can be demonstrated by immunocytochemical techniques, with gland cells being most commonly affected.[203] Some also have had cervical dysplasia, a possible relationship that deserves further study.

"Chronic cervicitis" is so common in sexually active women that the term is essentially useless as an informative pathologic diagnosis. Characteristically the everted endocervical mucosa may have a slightly papillary appearance, and the stroma is infiltrated by lymphocytes and plasma cells. The epithelium is intact, and usually some degree of squamous metaplasia is in progress, at least focally.

Exotic inflammatory lesions

Amebiasis may cause painful ulcerative lesions in the cervix and vagina.[201] Schistosomiasis is common in some parts of Africa[187]; the finding of calcified ova in the stroma is characteristic. The tiny vessels in which they are lodged may be difficult to identify in most histologic preparations.

Polyps and papillomas

Endocervical polyps represent the growth of redundant folds of endocervical mucosa, including both stroma and epithelium. There is often squamous metaplasia of the epithelium, especially at the tip. Much of the substance of the polyp may be the result of cystic dilatation of endocervical glands. Stroma polyps of the cervix resemble those in the vagina, described on p. 1631.

Condyloma acuminatum may occur as a typical papilloma in the cervix, but flattened keratotic papules with cytologic features of condyloma are more common and have been recognized with increasing frequency.[261] The cytologic hallmark in cervical scrapings or histologic sections is koilocytic atypia: nuclei are enlarged, appear wrinkled, stain densely but evenly, and are surrounded by a clear halo. This pattern probably is frequently misinterpreted as dysplasia.[243] Particles resembling human papillomavirus organisms appear in affected cells studied by electron microscopic, immunohistochemical, and in situ hybridization[219] techniques. Coxcomb polyp, a rare lesion of pregnancy, and true papilloma, with more dysplastic-looking epithelium, are difficult to distinguish from condyloma acuminatum.[258]

The application of recombinant DNA techniques to genital neoplasms has resulted in the identification of more than 50 subtypes of the virus,[128] many of which have distinctive morphologic features. The usual condyloma acuminatum is type 6 or 11, whereas most carcinomas are types 16, 18, or 31.[204] Virus subtypes can be identified by hybridization with labeled DNA probes. Southern blot hybridization applied to tissue homogenates is more sensitive, whereas the technique applied to microscopic sections or smears (in situ hybridization) is less sensitive but has the advantage of localizing viral DNA within the cells.[205]

Neoplasms
Benign tumors

Leiomyomas of the cervix resemble those in the myometrium, described later. They may cause cervical stenosis with secondary pyometra or hematometra. The occasional polypoid smooth muscle mass with an admixture of endocervical or endometrial glands and stroma is an adenomyoma.

Rarely a glandular papilloma, said to be of mesonephric duct origin, has been described in children.[223] The stroma is inconspicuous, and the epithelial component is cytologically benign. Hemangiomas include the cervix in their ubiquitous distribution; the cervix itself is very vascular, and many reported "hemangiomas" are nothing more than a conspicuous demonstration of local vascularity.

Dysplasia, carcinoma in situ, cervical intraepithelial neoplasia, microinvasion, and pathogenesis of epidermoid carcinoma of cervix

In some women the sequence of repair by squamous metaplasia in the transition zone does not proceed in an orderly manner to form mature stratified squamous epithelium. Instead the proliferating epithelial surface contains many cells that resemble carcinoma cells. These abnormal cells are confined to the surface epithelium and do not invade the stroma. The progressively more anaplastic-appearing lesions that result seem to evolve from dysplasia, which can be graded as slight, moderate, or severe, into carcinoma in situ. An alternative classification widely used to represent the same basic concept is cervical intraepithelial neoplasia (CIN), which is similarly graded from I to III. According to this scheme, CIN I is the equivalent of slight dysplasia, and CIN III is equivalent to carcinoma in situ.[213] Currently there is a consensus that carcinoma in situ (CIN III) is an important stage in the development of invasive epidermoid carcinoma of the cervix. An estimated 40,000 women with carcinoma in situ are treated annually in the United States.[274]

Definitions. The term "dysplasia" (CIN I and II) indicates that many but not all the cells of an epithelial surface resemble cancer cells; it is possible to recognize a sequence of maturation from basal layer to surface,

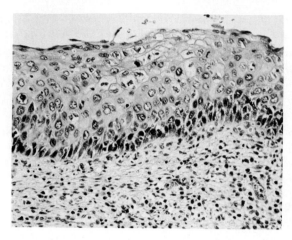

Fig. 34-32. Dysplasia (CIN II) of cervix. Abnormal squamous epithelial cells appear anaplastic, but they vary considerably in size and shape and have a relative abundance of cytoplasm. Sequence of maturation is evident as the surface is approached. (150×.)

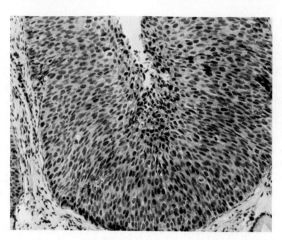

Fig. 34-33. Carcinoma in situ (CIN III) of cervix. Abnormal cells have a more uniform size and shape and relatively scant cytoplasm, and sequence of maturation is lost. (130×.)

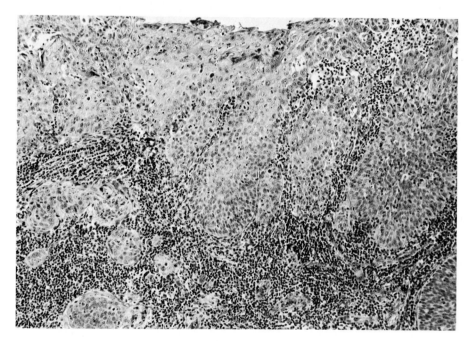

Fig. 34-34. Carcinoma in situ (CIN III) with microinvasion. Early invasive clumps have a more differentiated appearance with more abundant cytoplasm. Prominent inflammatory infiltrate in adjacent stroma is characteristic. (130×.)

though it may be disorderly (Fig. 34-32).

The term "carcinoma in situ" indicates that all the cells in the affected area from basement membrane to surface resemble cancer cells (Fig. 34-33), and they tend to resemble one another. Both dysplasia and carcinoma in situ occur within endocervical glandular crypts; such a locus may represent a separate focus of involvement but is not evidence of invasion or that the process is more aggressive.

Although there is general agreement about the definitions of dysplasia and carcinoma in situ,[216] the histologic distinctions are necessarily subjective. Complete agreement among a group of pathologists will occur in about 65% of the cases they examine.[207]

A microinvasive carcinoma is a small carcinoma that has invaded the cervical stroma to a limited extent. The maximum allowable depth of penetration and how to measure it are debated; a majority of reports favor a limit of 3 mm.[210] Measurement from the surface of the lesion to the point of maximum penetration gives the most reproducible figure in most cases.

The earliest invasive changes have the appearance of tiny irregular sprouts of neoplastic epithelial cells projecting into the cervical stroma, usually beneath an area of carcinoma in situ (Fig. 34-34). The cells at the interface between infiltrating epithelium and stroma appear more differentiated, have more cytoplasm, and are often degenerated. The adjacent stroma is infiltrated by lymphocytes and plasma cells. No metastases or deaths from such lesions have been reliably documented. These early changes, including the stromal reaction and cytologic features at the stromal interface, were described and discussed in an interesting early account by Stoddard[282] in 1952.

Small confluent growths composed of nests of invasive epidermoid carcinoma cells in the cervical stroma are classified as occult invasive carcinomas, if they are more than 3 mm in diameter, because metastases to lymph nodes have been demonstrated, rarely with a fatal outcome.[210] The presence of histologically apparent involvement of lymphatic spaces did not correlate with demonstrable lymph node metastases in 30 cases of microinvasive carcinoma studied by Roche and Norris.[263] It is rare to find lymph node metastases in radical hysterectomy specimens that include nodes, and long-term follow-up study after simple hysterectomy has shown favorable results in over 98% of women with microinvasive carcinoma.

Pathogenesis. Studies of epidemiology, viral culture, cytogenetics, marker enzymes, and tumor-specific immune response have added many dimensions to the understanding of the biology of carcinoma in situ and its relationship to invasive carcinoma of the cervix.

Cytogenetic studies have shown that dysplastic cells not only look different but also have profoundly altered chromosomes. A relatively small proportion of cells from dysplasia of the cervix show this change.[228] Both the number of chromosomes and their appearance vary widely among the abnormal cells; there is no consistent pattern in the genetic derangement.

In contrast, many or most of the cells from an area of carcinoma in situ are cytogenetically abnormal, and furthermore, the abnormal genetic patterns, though not identical, tend to be similar in a sizable proportion of the cells. Apparently an aggressive strain of cells (modal group) has emerged and managed to proliferate more rapidly than other cell types do.

One or more modal groups are characteristically present in carcinoma in situ; in microinvasive carcinoma there is usually a single modal group. Marker chromosomes having a distinctive and recognizable shape are also often present in early invasive lesions.[279] This suggests that all the affected cells are closely related, possibly members of a clone originating from a single cell.

Radioautographic studies of epithelium incubated with tritiated thymidine confirm increased DNA replication in large numbers of cells scattered throughout the epithelium.[268] Replication normally occurs only in the parabasal cells in the nonneoplastic cervical epithelium. The most striking increases in DNA replication occur in early "budding" areas of microinvasion.[266]

The ultrastructure of the cells of dysplasia and carcinoma in situ is similar. Mitochondria remain numerous even in surface layers, there are many free ribosomes, and the glycogen accumulation normally found in surface cells does not occur. These changes together reflect increased metabolic activities in the individual cells and decreased organization and surface maturation of the epithelium as a whole.[272]

Epidemiologic analyses of large populations of women with carcinoma of the cervix indicate that a considerable increase in risk is associated with early sexual activity, especially with multiple partners.[186,265] This observation prompted a search for a venereally transmissible etiologic factor. A variety of possible pathogenic agents have been investigated, including spermatozoa, mycoplasma, and various other organisms.[179] An interesting study of the potential role of the male as a carrier found that the subsequent wives of men whose first spouse had cervical carcinoma are themselves at greater risk of developing cervical carcinoma.[226]

Virologic and immunologic studies of women with in situ and invasive cervical cancer first implicated herpesvirus 2 as a promising etiologic agent. Antibodies to herpesvirus 2 are present in the sera of women with cervical carcinoma more often than in control subjects; furthermore, the titers are higher, and the high titers appear at an earlier age.[260] Membrane antigens extracted from cervical carcinoma cells seem to be specific markers for the presence of the virus genome in the tumor cells.[222] Latent virus can be unmasked from cultured cervical cancer cells, and 90% of patients with cervical cancer have antibody to a virus-specific antigen (AG-4) that is not found in control subjects or in successfully treated patients; many other virus-associated proteins have been identified in tumor cells and patient sera.[183] Tumor cells also contain messenger RNA with sequences corresponding to those of viral RNA.[241] Even inactivated herpesvirus is carcinogenic in mice.[235]

More recently a dominant role has been ascribed to the human papillomavirus (HPV), implicating a specific set of HPV types (most commonly 16, 18, and sometimes 30) as opposed to the types usually found in condylomas (types 6 and 11).[128] *Viral localization studies consistently identify HPV in many but not all cervical dysplasias and squamous carcinomas.*[204,205,219,234] Patterns of sexual transmission are well established.[110] The consistent finding of specific strains of virus in cancers (as opposed to condylomas) strengthens the concept of a central role for HPV. On the other hand, the subject cannot be regarded as settled because some patients and even individual lesions are colonized by multiple types of virus. Virus can be recovered from morphologically normal squamous epithelium, and all patients with viral lesions do not develop carcinoma. It would appear that HPV may be an important initiator and that other factors such as herpesvirus, age, oncogenes, and toxic exposure (smoking) may serve as promoters or co-carcinogens.

Recombinant DNA analysis of human papillomavirus (HPV) interactions. Integrated transcripts of HPV DNA 16 or 18 occur in virtually all primary cervical cancers and in immortalized cell lines cultured from cervical cancers. Sequencing of cDNA clones of HPV 18 transcripts in three cancer cell lines show a small intron introduced into the E6 open reading frame (ORF). As a result the second E6 exon is read in a different ORF, now encoding for a new protein with some features similar to epidermal growth factor. The same splice donor and acceptor sites exist for HPV 16 and 33 (other "malignant" strains of HPV) but not in HPV 6 or 11 (which are "benign" HPV strains associated with condylomas but not with carcinoma).[291a]

Normal human cervical keratinocytes can be "immortalized" (that is, continue to grow and divide in tissue cultures for many generations beyond the usual survival time of normal cells in vitro) by insertion of HPV 16 and 18 DNA. These cells are not tumorigenic when injected into nude mice; it appears therefore that HPV 16 and 18 may not be carcinogenic without some assistance.[289a] Other studies have indicated some potential cofactors. One study used a cell line already immortalized by transfection with herpes simplex virus type 2 (HSV-2); further transfection with HPV 16 and 18 produced cell lines that were fully tumorigenic in nude mice. This result indicates a possible initiator role for HSV-2 and a promotor role for HPV 16 and 18. Of great interest is the fact that persistence of the integrated viral sequences in tumor cell DNA does not appear necessary once oncogenic transformation is complete.[221a] Furthermore, the E6 and E7 ORFs, which seem to be the active viral component in carcinogenesis, can cooperate with the *ras* oncogene to transform primary rat cells.[185a] Another interesting observation is that the E7 protein can complex and thereby probably inactivate the protein encoded by the retinoblastoma (Rb) gene in vitro.[208a] The Rb gene and the protein encoded by it appear to be "tumor-suppressor" factors

that are absent in some cancer cells. In a well-studied model, inactivation of Rb protein by adenovirus early region 1A protein (E1A protein) is tumorigenic. The first 37 amino acids encoded by HPV 16 E7 are like adenovirus E1A, an indication that HPV and adenovirus may have similar oncogenic mechanisms.

Some interesting diagnostic applications arise from recombinant DNA techniques. Monoclonal antibodies to an HPV E6 peptide have been developed; these can be used to demonstrate the E7 protein in human cervical cancer tissue as well as in cultured cervical cancer cell lines.[268a] The E6 DNA itself can be demonstrated directly by use of the *polymerase chain reaction* (PCR), capable of remarkable sensitivity, detecting less than one virus genome per cell. Target DNA sequences are selectively amplified by repeated cycles of denaturation, annealing with oligomer primers complimentary to flanking regions of target DNA sequence, and primer extension with DNA polymerase-I. Final reaction products are detected by dot blot using a ^{32}P-labeled probe.[271a] The potential of these techniques for detecting cells that have escaped intracellular control mechanisms show promise in helping solve the current enigma of separating dysplasias that can or will progress to cancers from those that cannot, thus allowing identification of the patients at greatest risk.

Immunopathology. Epidermoid carcinoma of the cervix, like other cancers, produces circulating tumor-specific antigens, and patients form antibodies to them. Circulating antigens appear before invasion occurs. Cell-mediated immune response is unimpaired,[196] and lymphocytes of patients with cervical carcinoma are sensitized to epidermoid carcinoma cells and can destroy them in vitro.[208] Using a specific erythrocyte absorption test, Davidsohn and associates[206] have shown that A, B, and H blood group surface antigens normally also found in squamous epithelium are lost or masked

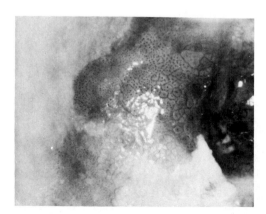

Fig. 34-35. Colposcopic photograph of carcinoma in situ of cervix. This mosaic pattern and accentuated punctate vessels emphasized against a background of opaque whitened epithelium are characteristic. (Courtesy Dr. James G. Blythe, St. Louis, Mo.)

in invasive and metastatic epidermoid carcinomas.

Colposcopy. The use of a magnifying instrument, the colposcope, has remarkably improved the accuracy of physical diagnosis of lesions of the cervix.[202,231] Based chiefly on differences in vascular pattern, distinctions can be made between squamous metaplasia, dysplasia, carcinoma in situ, and early invasive carcinoma (Figs. 34-35 and 34-36). Used with cytologic studies, biopsy, and conization, the colposcope has significantly improved the accuracy of diagnosis and the effectiveness of local treatment.[195,202,285]

Clinical significance of dysplasia and carcinoma in situ of cervix. Opinions about the significance of carcinoma in situ of the cervix vary widely. The name implies a threat of death, poised, yet momentarily held in check. Accepted forms of treatment include local excision (conization) designed to excise most of the transformation zone, some form of cautery (laser, freezing), and hysterectomy. The results are remarkably similar.

Dysplasia, left undisturbed, may progress to carcinoma in situ.[262] If there is no intervention of any sort, the observed conversion of dysplasia and carcinoma in situ to invasive carcinoma is nearly constant: 21% in 5 years, 28% in 10 years, 33% in 15 years, and 38% in 20 years.[227,278] However, local treatment in the form of conization or cautery effectively interrupts the process

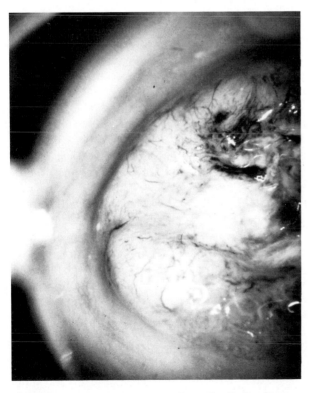

Fig. 34-36. Invasive carcinoma of cervix. Protruding mass and irregular tortuous blood vessels running over surface of lesion are features of invasive process. (Courtesy Dr. James G. Blythe, St. Louis, Mo.)

in a high percentage of patients.[195,218,234,284] Residual in situ carcinoma has been identified in as much as one third of hysterectomy specimens obtained after cervical conization.[270] Those patients who require more extensive treatment can be identified by colposcopy and cytologic studies, if one assumes that meticulous follow-up examinations will be carried out. Prospective studies designed to show the best form of treatment have not been carried out.[229] Ignoring cytologic evidence of carcinoma carries an unacceptably high risk of invasive carcinoma and death.[227] In a carefully conducted long-term study of 1121 women with carcinomma in situ, subsequent invasive carcinoma was found in 2.1% of those treated by hysterectomy and in 0.9% of those treated only by conization.[230] The popularity of hysterectomy may be related to the fact that it solves other problems.

The screening of large populations of women has identified hundreds of women with carcinoma in situ, as well as early invasive carcinomas. Treatment of the lesion at this stage has considerably reduced the number of women with advanced cervical cancer, for which treatment is much less effective, and has improved survival. The desirability of annual mass screening of women has been debated.[239] Success has been notable only in programs that include groups at greatest risk.[189,199] Various factors influence the frequency of false-negative and false-positive interpretation of smears. One of the most important and least defensible is the high frequency (88.2%) of failure of cytologists to identify and report technically inadequate specimens, as documented in surveys conducted by the College of American Pathologists.[207] Persistence of the cervical lesion as shown by cytologic or colposcopic abnormalities is very significant regardless of the treatment selected. In a group of 949 women attended closely for 5 to 28 years, 86% had consistently normal cytologic features and among these 12 (1.5%) ultimately developed invasive carcinoma. By comparison, of the 131 who continued to have abnormal cytology, 29 (22%) developed invasive carcinoma; the carcinomas occurred with approximately the same frequency whether the patients were initially treated by conization or by hysterectomy.[242]

There is a definite but apparently small group of invasive cervical carcinomas that originate from the basal layer of histologically normal squamous epithelium. There may be no detectable surface abnormality at any point in the cervix, until (presumably) the lesion ulcerates, sloughing the surface and exposing the cancer beneath.[248] Approximately 10% of cervical carcinomas may arise in this manner.[175]

Adenocarcinoma in situ. Adenocarcinoma in situ is a rare lesion characterized by replacement of the gland cells of endocervical mucosa and its crypts by cytologically malignant gland cells. The columnar pattern is usually retained, but the basal polarity of the nuclei is lost, the cytoplasmic mucin is replaced by amphophilic cytoplasm, and the nuclei have malignant cytologic features. If involved, gland-space outlines resemble those lined by normal epithelium in the same cervix, and if only part of the gland-space lining is affected, it is reasonable to conclude that stroma invasion has not occurred. Associated epidermoid carcinoma in situ is often present. The histologic pattern has been extensively illustrated by Burghardt.[192] In nearly every case the lesion is discovered when malignant gland cells are found in the cervical cytologic smear.[258]

Christopherson, Nealon, and Gray[197] concluded that adenocarcinoma in situ is a precursor to invasive adenocarcinoma because it was invariably found with very small (microinvasive) adenocarcinomas. Adenocarcinoma in situ is also located higher in the endocervix; a residual lesion remains in the resected uterus after conization in 66% of cases, which implies that conization for this lesion is probably an inadequate treatment.

Invasive carcinoma of cervix

In contrast to the remarkable increase in the numbers of women treated for carcinoma in situ of the cervix, it was estimated that the number of patients with invasive cervical carcinoma had decreased to 12,900 in 1988 from 19,000 in 1975 and 20,000 in 1970.[273] After several decades as the most common gynecologic cancer, cervical carcinoma is now encountered less often than endometrial carcinoma, which has increased to first place in many institutions in the United States.

Gross appearance. Cervical carcinomas large enough to be visible and palpable have one of three growth patterns, sometimes in combination. The ulcerating type has an infiltrative pattern of growth and eventually becomes necrotic in the center and sloughs, leaving a cavity surrounded by invasive cancer. The exophytic type is often papillary and may form a bulky mass of considerable size while still confined to the superficial portions of the cervix. The nodular type originates typically in the endocervix, forming multiple firm masses that expand the cervix and isthmus. The mass may be large, and when it is distributed circumferentially, it has been called the barrel-shaped cervix. The gross relationships are important clinically because they affect the placement of radioactive sources used in treatment.

Clinical stages. The extent of involvement of the cervix and pelvic tissues is determined by physical examinations. The clinical staging of the extent of disease must be determined before treatment is begun. It is in part the basis of selection of the best treatment for the patient and forms the standard for comparing the results of treatment of large groups of patients.

Definitions of the different clinical stages in carci-

noma of the cervix uteri, as established by the Cancer Committee of the International Federation of Gynecology and Obstetrics, are as follows:

0	Preinvasive carcinoma (intraepithelial carcinoma, carcinoma in situ).
I	Carcinoma strictly confined to the cervix (extension to the corpus should be disregarded).
Ia	Preclinical carcinomas of the cervix, that is, diagnosed only by microscopy.
Ia1	Minimal microscopically evident stroma invasion.
Ia2	Lesions detected microscopically that can be measured. The upper limits of the measurement should not show a depth of invasion of more than 5 mm taken from the base of the epithelium, either surface or glandular, from which it originates; and a second dimension, the horizontal spread, must not exceed 7 mm. Larger lesions should be staged as Ib.
Ib	Lesions of greater dimensions than stage Ia2, whether seen clinically or not. Preformed space involvement should not alter the staging but should be recorded specifically to determine whether it should affect treatment decisions in the future.
II	Invasive carcinoma that extends beyond the cervix but has not reached either lateral pelvic wall; involvement of the vagina is limited to the upper two thirds.
III	Invasive carcinoma that extends to either lateral pelvic wall and/or the lower third of the vagina.
IV	Invasive carcinoma that involves urinary bladder and/or rectum or extends beyond the true pelvis.

Microscopic appearance. The majority of invasive cervical carcinomas, about 80%, are epidermoid carcinomas; adenocarcinomas comprise about 10%, and the remainder is a variety of unusual adenocarcinoma patterns or mixtures.[175]

Epidermoid carcinoma. A moderately differentiated, nonkeratinizing, large cell epidermoid carcinoma is the most common pattern (70%) and in some series, at least, has the best prognosis (Fig. 34-37). Well-differentiated keratinizing epidermoid carcinoma occurs less frequently (25%); small cell undifferentiated carcinoma is uncommon (about 5%) and has a distinctly poor prognosis.[250]

Adenocarcinoma. Although they are much less common than epidermoid carcinomas, the proportion of cervical carcinomas arising from gland cells doubled in the decade from 1960 to 1970.[175,176] The patterns vary from a well-differentiated mucinous adenocarcinoma (Fig. 34-38), sometimes papillary, to a clear cell pattern containing glycogen but no mucin. Many resemble endometrial adenocarcinoma. A mixed adenosquamous carcinoma apparently arises from subcolumnar reserve cells capable of both squamous and gland cell differentiation.

Spread of carcinoma of cervix. It is important to recognize simultaneous involvement of the cervix and endometrium because this distribution affects principles

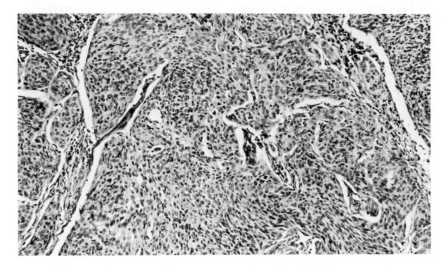

Fig. 34-37. Epidermoid carcinoma of cervix. This poorly differentiated, nonkeratinizing pattern is most common histologic type. (150×.)

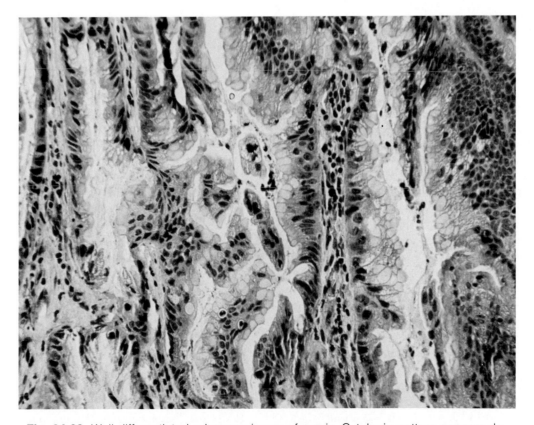

Fig. 34-38. Well-differentiated adenocarcinoma of cervix. Cytologic pattern appears deceptively benign, but bridges formed by epithelial cells without stromal support identify lesion as a carcinoma. (275×.)

of treatment; the prognosis is not so good as that for carcinoma limited to the cervix. Hysterectomy with radiotherapy improves the results, probably because the more extensive distribution of some lesions interferes with the spatial arrangement of intrauterine radiation sources.

Carcinoma of the cervix spreads by direct extension into contiguous tissues, through lymphatics to regional lymph nodes, and less often by blood vessel invasion to embolize throughout the body. Because of their close anatomic relationship to the cervix, the ureters may be obstructed; secondary hydronephrosis, pyelonephritis, and renal failure remain the most common causes of death.[185] Distant metastases to lungs and liver are found in about 25% of fatal cases at autopsy. In patients dying of cancer of the cervix, central pelvic recurrences are more common after surgery, and distant metastases are more common after radiotherapy.[185] Less than 2% of patients with stage I or IIa carcinoma of the cervix treated by megavoltage radiotherapy with adequate dosage and distribution of the radiation will have a central pelvic recurrence.[254]

Local recurrence occurs in 5% of patients with stage IIb disease, 7.5% with stage IIIa, and 17% with stage IIIb. Over half the distant metastases become evident within the first year after treatment, and 95% appear by the end of the fifth year after treatment. Because most of the patients without evidence of cancer 5 years after treatment die of unrelated causes, this follow-up period is customarily used in evaluating the effectiveness of therapy.

Rare tumors. Verrucous carcinoma, an extremely well-differentiated form of epidermoid carcinoma, resembles and behaves like the same lesion in the vulva. Clear cell adenocarcinomas identical to those in the vagina (p. 1641) also occur occasionally in the cervix after in utero exposure to diethylstilbestrol. This pattern of adenocarcinoma also has been called "mesonephroma"; in fact, origin from mesonephric remnants is rarely if ever demonstrable. Rarely a cervical adenocarcinoma may have a histologic pattern similar to that of adenoid cystic carcinoma, which is highly specific and more common in the salivary gland. This lesion in the cervix is highly aggressive, occurs in older women, and nearly always is associated with a more conventional epidermoid carcinoma or adenosquamous carcinoma pattern.[245] As seen in the cervix, adenoid cystic carcinoma is clearly different from the similar-appearing tumor of the salivary gland; it should be distinguished also from adenoid basal cell carcinoma, which has a much better prognosis.[211]

An extremely well-differentiated mucinous adenocarcinoma may be difficult to recognize because the epithelial pattern closely resembles that of benign endocervical epithelium, even in metastases. With adequate treatment the prognosis is probably the same as that of any adenocarcinoma at the same stage.[276] In our experience[244] these tumors have distinctive histologic features and produce cytoplasmic carcinoembryonic antigen, which may be diagnostically helpful.

Malignant mixed müllerian tumors, carcinosarcomas, and leiomyosarcomas of the cervix resemble those occurring in the endometrium (p. 1662) and share the same unfavorable prognosis.[177] Carcinoid tumors occur in the cervix as distinctly aggressive neoplasms. Like other tumors of the diffuse endocrine (APUD) system, they contain argyrophil and neurosecretory granules.[178] The less-differentiated cases resemble oat cell carcinoma in the lung; one cervical carcinoma of this type produced ACTH, causing Cushing's syndrome.[224] Melanin is rarely evident in basal cells of the cervix. Blue nevi and primary malignant melanomas are rare; Hall and associates[220] have reported a dramatic example that produced fatal metastases. Botryoid sarcoma in the cervix resembles the vaginal lesion described above but tends to occur at a somewhat older age and may have a better prognosis, especially with chemotherapy.[190]

Metastatic adenocarcinoma in the cervix is not common, but one should not mistake it for a primary lesion, thereby exposing the patient to a lengthy, painful, and expensive treatment that would be inappropriate. A cervical metastasis is usually the harbinger of rapid dissemination and death. The most common primary sites have been the ovary, colon, and breast.[237]

ENDOMETRIUM

The function of the normal endometrium is to produce a satisfactory substrate in which a healthy blastocyst may implant and flourish. Many of the pathologic changes that occur in the endometrium reflect its responsiveness to either hormonal stimulation or the lack of it.

Normal cyclic changes

The endometrial cycle starts with a phase of proliferation for about 14 days under the influence of estrogen. If ovulation occurs, the endometrium then undergoes prominent secretory changes for the next 7 days, in time for implantation if the ovum has been fertilized. If not, the secretion wanes slowly during the following 7 days, after which the endometrium sloughs away, and the whole cycle begins anew.

The histologic, ultrastructural, and histochemical changes of the endometrial cycle have been reviewed in detail by Noyes,[364] Ferenczy and Richart,[326] and Boutselis,[307] respectively. By convention, the first day of a cycle begins with the onset of menstrual flow, which results from ischemic necrosis of the inner layer of the endometrial stroma. The denuded surface heals after about 4 days. Under the influence of estrogen the stromal cells and endometrial gland cells proliferate rapidly (Fig. 34-39, *A*). The associated histochemical

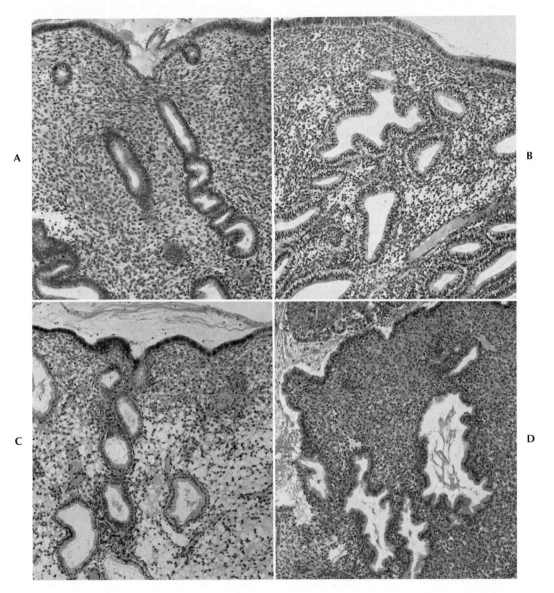

Fig. 34-39. A, Late proliferative endometrium at or about time of ovulation. Tortuous, pseudostratified glands with many mitoses are characteristic. Stroma, without predecidual reaction, may have variable degree of edema. **B,** Sixteen-day secretory endometrium. This early postovulatory endometrium is characterized by tortuous growing glands with irregular vacuolization caused by accumulation of glycogen in cytoplasm beneath nuclei. **C,** Twenty-two-day secretory endometrium. Significant features of this stage are massive stromal edema, tortuosity of glands nearing secretory exhaustion, thin-walled blood vessels, and absence of predecidua. This coincides with peak of corpus luteum activity during which time ovum is in process of implanting. **D,** Premenstrual endometrium. This phase is characterized by nearly complete predecidual transformation of stroma, secretory exhaustion of glands (which have serrated pattern), and inspissation of secretion. There is also leukocytic infiltration—both polymorphonuclear and monocytic. (150×; from Noyes, R.W., Hertig, A.T., and Rock, J.: Fertil. Steril. **1:**3, 1950.)

events are related chiefly to protein synthesis; RNA, glucose-6-phosphatase, alkaline phosphatase, beta-glucuronidase, and nonspecific esterase are especially abundant.

After ovulation, under the influence of progesterone, there is a rise in enzymes related to carbohydrate synthesis. Lactic dehydrogenase, glucose-6-phosphate dehydrogenase, and isocitric, succinic, and malic dehydrogenases are active as increasing amounts of glycogen become evident in the gland cells.

The morphologic changes related to secretion follow a distinctive sequence. Thirty-six hours after ovulation, prominent basal vacuolation appears in the glandular epithelial cells, representing an accumulation of glycogen (Fig. 34-29, B). Ultrastructural studies have related the appearance of a unique and specific nucleolar channel system to ovulation. It is seen in endometrium on the sixteenth day and for several days thereafter.[326,385] Giant mitochondria with tubular cristae also appear and increase in numbers in step with the secretory process.[300] During the next 3 days secretion increases, occupying the entire cytoplasmic mass. Coincident with the time of implantation (day 20 or 21) abundant edema is present in the stroma (Fig. 34-39, C). If implantation does not occur, there follows a progressive decrease in secretion and stromal edema, as the activity of the corpus luteum wanes. During the 2 or 3 days before menses, cytoplasmic secretion is exhausted, and stromal cells undergo a predecidual reaction, that is, become progressively plump and prominent, especially around the spiral arterioles and beneath the surface epithelium (Fig. 34-39, D). On the twenty-eighth day of a typical cycle the spiral arterioles contract, the stroma crumbles, and menstrual bleeding and expulsion of the functional endometrial lining occur.

If implantation occurs, the presence of gestation is reflected in the endometrial pattern of the twenty-fifth day, 3 days before the next period of bleeding is expected to begin. Hertig[337] has shown that this early gestational hyperplastic pattern is a highly characteristic combination of recrudescence of glandular secretion and accentuation of stromal edema, together with normal predecidual reaction and increased vascular prominence. A distinctive pattern of gestational glandular hyperplasia, emphasized by Arias-Stella,[297] especially in ectopic pregnancy and in abortions, is formed by masses of enlarged gland cells with abundant clear cytoplasm and large bizarre nuclei; there is no decidual reaction in the intervening stroma.

The importance of relative proportions of estrogen to progesterone in producing the normal sequence of menstrual patterns has been shown by Good and Moyer[330] in a study of endometrial biopsies in *Macaca mulatta* monkeys.

Pathologists vary in their willingness to ascribe a specific day in the cycle to an endometrial biopsy; physicians vary in their request for and acceptance of a specific date supplied by a pathologist.[375] In the course of infertility investigations, endometrial biopsy may be used to confirm that ovulation has occurred and that the morphologic development of the endometrium is sufficiently normal to support implantation. In general, a pathologic process such as atrophy or hyperplasia indicates that the prospects for pregnancy are poor.[382] Some patients who are unable to develop an adequate secretory response may be helped by hormonal therapy.[322]

Effects of hormones

Physicians treat women with estrogens or progestogens or both, most frequently to alleviate the symptoms of estrogen deficiency (especially after menopause) and to control conception. The morphologic changes that result in the endometrium vary with the dosage and the sequence with which different combined preparations are used.

Estrogens

The characteristic changes of the proliferative phase are produced by estrogen. The estradiol produced by the ovarian follicle and synthetic estrogens have similar effects. Unremitting estrogen stimulation may occur with approximately physiologic estrogen concentrations at the time of menopause, in postmenopausal women treated with estrogen, or in younger women after multiple anovulatory cycles, as in the Stein-Leventhal syndrome. In such cases proliferative activity continues, producing a characteristic anovulatory pattern with intraglandular protrusions of redundant epithelium and a compact stroma (Fig. 34-40). After longer periods or with higher degrees of estrogen stimulation the endometrium may become hyperplastic. The pattern in some cases may resemble atypical hyperplasia. High doses of estrogen in animal experiments actually cause endometrial atrophy.

Progestogens

The therapeutic addition of progesterone or artificial progestogens causes estrogen-primed endometrial gland cells to differentiate into a secretory pattern, and further growth is inhibited. This effect is produced if the endometrium has become hyperplastic, even in the case of atypical hyperplasia or carcinoma in situ.[348] The secretory changes induced are followed by regression, gland cell atrophy, and a decidua-like reaction in the stroma.

Estrogens and progestogens

If dosages and sequences are regulated carefully, it is possible to reproduce physiologically normal cycles

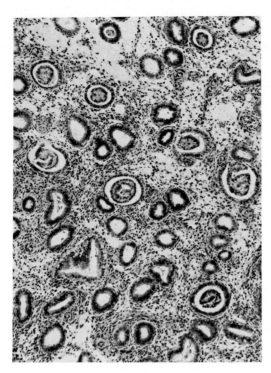

Fig. 34-40. Anovulatory endometrium. Irregular gland outlines are frequently found after anovulatory cycles, especially at time of menopause. The intraluminal protrusions of epithelium are believed to be an ar ifact caused by the dilatation and curettage procedure. (85×.)

with a normal morphologic sequence in the endometrium. This fact has had some application in treatment of functional bleeding, dysmenorrhea, endometriosis, menopausal symptoms, infertility, and some intersex states.

Unquestionably the most common application of hormonal therapy in gynecology is in conception control. Estrogen-progestogen combination regimens produce secretion at an early point in the cycle, arresting the proliferative stimulus of estrogen at an incompletely developed state. Continuation of the same stimulus leads to further gland atrophy, with a relatively pronounced decidua-like stroma reaction at the end of the cycle. Estrogen-progestogen sequential regimens operate in a different manner. The estrogen stimulus is carried past the time of ovulation and implantation so that secretion is delayed until about the twenty-fifth day and does not exceed the early secretory pattern of endometrium of the eighteenth day. Predecidual stromal changes do not appear.

After several months of cyclic therapy with combination agents the endometrial lining becomes thin and atrophic. Stromal cells are plump, with abundant cytoplasm. Vessels are small. The glands are generally small and lined with small, low columnar cells with traces of cytoplasmic secretion. (Fig. 34-41).

The atrophy is less pronounced after long-term exposure to sequential agents. Perhaps because of the stimulative effects of estrogen, hyperplasia and even carcinoma have developed in occasional patients at a

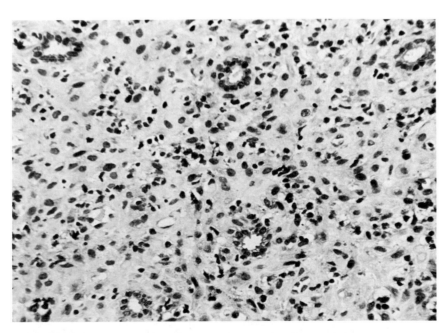

Fig. 34-41. Secretory atrophic pattern after long-term exposure to combination type of contraceptive hormonal preparation. Stromal cells are large and decidua like; glands are small and atrophic with faint traces of secretion. (350×.)

relatively young age after long-term exposure to sequential agents,[379] which are no longer used or produced for this reason.

Luteal phase defect

Infrequently, perhaps in 3% of infertile women, the endometrium fails to produce a fully developed secretory reaction, apparently because an inadequate corpus luteum fails to produce enough progesterone.[296,341] Early abortion has also been attributed to this condition. In a large proportion of women the basic disorder may be pituitary overproduction of prolactin, which in excess seems to diminish progesterone production. Rarely the endometrium lacks progesterone receptors. The diagnosis is customarily based on endometrial biopsy, which shows a lag in development of more than 2 days according to the dating scheme described previously. The syndrome is ill defined, appears to have many causes, and responds variably to progesterone replacement.

Metaplasia

Squamous metaplasia occasionally appears in the endometrium much the same as in the endocervix. Small clusters of cells proliferate beneath the glandular epithelium and eventually replace it. Actual keratinization is unusual. Chronic inflammation from various causes has been the most common associated factor; squamous metaplasia may occur after long-term estrogen therapy and in patients with hyperplasia. The rounded masses, or morules,[323] usually are easily recognized. Extensive squamous metaplasia produces a more complicated pattern that has been confused with carcinoma because the confluent masses of metaplastic cells resemble the epithelial bridging of carcinoma.[318] Most patients are obese young women with the polycystic ovary syndrome. The cytologic pattern confirms the benign prognosis. Other, less common eithelial metaplasias include mucinous patterns (like those in the endocervix), ciliated cells (like those in the fallopian tube), eosinophilic cells, and papillary metaplasia, all extensively illustrated by Hendrickson and Kempson.[335]

More exotic tissues such as cartilage,[372] bone,[328] and glial tissue[398] probably also arise as metaplastic foci sometimes, but implanted aborted fetal tissue may be the most common cause. It is also possible that the endometrial stroma may react to organizing substances produced by an aborted embryo.

Hysterectomy and normal uterus

The uterus is one of the most commonly resected organs in any institution in which major surgical procedures are performed on women. There is surprisingly little objectve data or discussion on the measurements, appearance, and significance of the "normal" uterus, which accounts for some pointless disagreement in hospital tissue committees.

Langlois[354] has reviewed sizes and weights of a series of 461 uteri considered to have normal gross appearance in that there was no detectable lesion known to have an effect on uterine size. The principal factor determining uterine weight in this population was parity. In general, it was found that the weight above which a uterus is *probably* abnormal was 130 g for the nulliparous woman, 210 g for parity of one to three, and 250 g for parity of four and more.

As a practical matter, objective pathologic data about the uterus frequently have little relevance to the reason for hysterectomy. Nearly half the "normal" uteri in the series reported by Langlois[354] were resected for relief of symptoms related to prolapse or abnormal bleeding. Assuming that the associated symptoms and abnormal physical findings are truthfully reported, hysterectomy is an extremely valuable means of providing relief for these patients. The uterus itself, however, usually shows no morphologic changes commensurate with the degree of preoperative symptoms. Review of the pathologists' reports alone in these circumstances does not provide the data required to audit the desirability of the surgical procedure. The endometrium examined by prior curettage either is normal, especially in the case of prolapse, or has one of the types of benign anovulatory or mixed patterns discussed subsequently.

A more controversial basis for hysterectomy is that it is undeniably an effective form of contraception. In certain ethnic and religious groups it may actually be the only available approach to contraception, though other diagnoses and symptoms are necessarily and even sincerely offered and believed by both patient and physician.

The estimated hysterectomy rate for women 15 to 44 years of age in the United States between 1970 and 1975 rose from 7.2 to 9.1 per 1000 women.[311] Estimated costs, potential benefits, and ultimate reasons for hysterectomy are perceived differently and are still debated.[308]

Dysfunctional uterine bleeding

Uterine bleeding that occurs at irregular intervals in excessive or scant amounts, especially when prolonged, is said to be dysfunctional when there is no easily assignable cause such as hyperplasia, neoplasm, polyps, trauma, blood dyscrasia, pregnancy, or hormone administration.

The morphologic findings are variable. The presence of a mixed proliferative and secretory pattern (irregular shedding) is believed to be the result of continued progesterone secretion from a corpus luteum that fails to involute. Another common pattern is irregular nonsecretory glands with intraluminal protrusions of epithe-

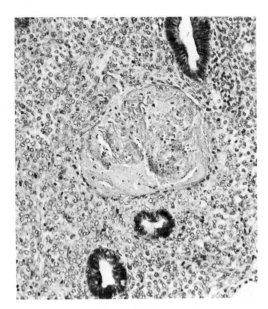

Fig. 34-42. This large fibrin thrombus distending a thin-walled vessel, with irregular proliferative phase gland outlines, indicates anovulatory endometrial bleeding. (150×.)

lial folds, a somewhat disorganized proliferative pattern that is common after a series of anovulatory cycles. Pathologic findings that confirm the history of bleeding include fragmentation of the stroma into compact ball-like masses, stromal fibrin accumulations, hemosiderin, and scattered tiny fragments of nuclear material sometimes called nuclear dust (Fig. 34-42). The histologic abnormality can be readily identified in currettings and is best classified as "anovulatory bleeding pattern."

A majority of the patients are in the perimenopausal period, have elevated follicle-stimulating hormone levels, and tend to have anovulatory cycles. A second group is young perimenarcheal women with the Stein-Leventhal syndrome, obesity, stress, or ovarian anomalies; most have abnormal luteinizing hormone levels, either elevated or prolonged.[294] A detailed classification has been presented by Arronet and Arrata.[301]

Inflammation
Chronic endometritis

The finding of an infiltrate of plasma cells in the endometrial stroma is the pathologic basis for the diagnosis of chronic endometritis. Most patients have menstrual disturbances, and about half may have pelvic pain or tenderness. The most common etiologic factors are recent abortion or recent delivery, coexisting pelvic inflammatory disease, and the presence of an intrauterine contraceptive device (IUD).[309]

The finding of hyalinized thick-walled stromal vessels and stellate glands with moderate secretory changes is sufficiently characteristic to identify a recent abortion as

the most likely cause, even in the absence of villi.[366] Although the endometrium seems to be sterile in the presence of most IUDs, serious infections do occur, some of which have been fatal.[342]

Tuberculous endometritis is rare in the United States in comparison with other countries; the disparity so far is unexplained by factors such as variations in sophistication of treatment or public health control.[343] Granulomas are usually small, sparse, and without caseation. Patients are usually sterile; tubal infection typically occurs first.

Organisms implicated as possible causes of endometritis that deserve more study include *Mycoplasma*[321] and *Listeria*[296] species, especially with respect to chronic endometrial infection and infertility or repeated abortion. Rare causes of endometritis have been reviewed by Dallenbach-Hellweg.[320]

Acute endometritis

The most significant form of acute endometritis is postpartum bacterial sepsis originating in the endometrium. The pathologic lesion is an acute invasive suppurative infection with progressive infiltration of the endometrium, myometrium, and parametrium by polymorphonuclear leukocytes. The portal of entry is the vagina. The classic agent is the streptococcus, but anaerobic bacteria, notably *Bacteroides* species, have more recently been implicated.[306] The precise role of anaerobes is controversial. Because of the prevalence of these organisms in the lower genital tract, the significance of a positive culture may be difficult to interpret.

Hyperplasia

Abnormally prolonged, profuse, and irregular uterine bleeding in the menopausal or postmenopausal woman is commonly associated with proliferative glandular and stromal patterns called "hyperplasia." Hyperplastic endometrial patterns vary, and the diagnostic terms used are confusing because their usage by different writers has varied widely. The following terminology is recommended by the World Health Organization[368] and employed in widely used textbooks of gynecologic pathology.[331]

Cystic hyperplasia is characterized by large dilated gland spaces with rounded profiles lined by relatively atrophic epithelium, separated by edematous, sparsely cellular stroma. Cystic atrophy would be a more apt designation.

Adenomatous hyperplasia is represented by a more distinctly proliferative pattern; the glands are lined by tall columnar epithelial cells with large nuclei often distributed at different levels, but basal polarity of nuclei is generally maintained. The gland outlines are irregular because of outpouchings and papillary infoldings of glandular epithelium. The stroma is dense, cellular,

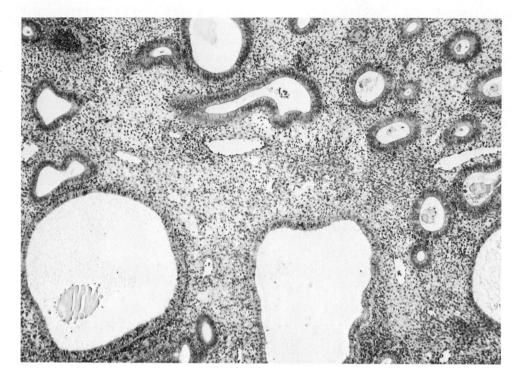

Fig. 34-43. Adenomatous hyperplasia. Dilated glands with irregular outlines and abundant stroma. (150×; from Kraus, F.T.: Gynecologic pathology, St. Louis, 1967, The C.V. Mosby Co.)

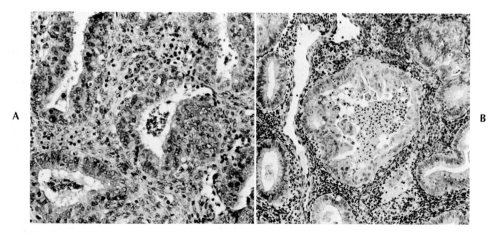

Fig. 34-44. Atypical hyperplasia. **A,** Epithelium two or three cells thick, loss of polarity, and atypical cytologic pattern (not evident at this magnification, 175×). **B,** Piled-up masses of large cells with abundant dense pink cytoplasm, small round nuclei, and loss of polarity. (75×.)

and compact. There are numerous mitoses in both glands and stroma (Fig. 34-43).

Atypical hyperplasia is more controversial as a concept and in terms of the histologic pattern it represents. There is general agreement that the cytologic features—large cells and large irregular nuclei and nucleoli—are more like those of adenocarcinoma. The cells that line the glands lose columnar orientation, and cytoplasm often has a dense eosinophilic staining character (Fig. 34-44). As reported by Tavassoli and Kraus,[383] leukocytes may or may not be present. The terms *anaplasia* and *carcinoma in situ* are frequently used as synonyms. In the original description[338] carcinoma in situ designated glands lined by enlarged irregularly heaped cells with abundant homogeneous eosinophilic cytoplasm, pale nuclei, and, notably, an absence of leukocytes. Two benign conditions with large eosinophilic cells and consistent leukocytic infiltrate—but no neoplastic connotations—are eosinophilic metaplasia and some postabortal gestational endometrial glands, which also often have large polyploid nuclei.

In 1988 the Nomenclature Committee of the International Society of Gynecologic Pathologists adopted the following modifications of terms for endometrial hyperplasia:

Simple hyperplasia

Complex hyperplasia (adenomatous hyperplasia without atypia)

Atypical hyperplasia (adenomatous hyperplasia with atypia)

These designations correspond in general to the three terms described above. By far the most significant morphologic characteristic for identifying lesions that have the potential to be or become malignant is cytologic atypia.[352]

Small foci of well-differentiated adenocarcinoma can be identified in about one fourth of uteri resected as treatment for atypical hyperplasia.[383] The significance of this observation is uncertain; carcinoma seldom develops in women with atypical hyperplasia whose uteri are not resected, if they are treated with progestogens. The minimal criteria for diagnosis of adenocarcinoma developing in endometrial hyperplasia are not as clear or settled as most textbooks imply.[337]

The etiology and significance of hyperplastic lesions is debated, and the varied use of terms has not clarified understanding of the subject. Unquestionably, estrogen administration produces hyperplasia.[349] Prolonged periods of anovulation with steady estrogen secretion that omit the periodic differentiating stimulus of progesterone have a similar effect, even in young women.[313,331,389] Atypical hyperplastic patterns may occur after prolonged anovulation in the Stein-Leventhal syndrome and will regress after therapeutic induction of ovulation.[344]

Actual progression of hyperplastic lesions to carcinomas has been observed, as reviewed by Gore and Hertig[332] and by Vellios,[389] but not frequently; most patients have been treated with progestogens or by hysterectomy, usually to control bleeding within a few months or years of the diagnosis of hyperplasia. The lesions classified here as atypical hyperplasia and carcinoma in situ apparently respond completely to the differentiating effect of progestogens.[348] For this reason the term "carcinoma in situ" as applied to the endometrium may be semantically confusing. Despite reversal of the morphologic lesion, abnormal bleeding often resumes and eventually is the basis for hysterectomy in many women treated for endometrial hyperplasia.

Those lesions that do not respond to treatment (progestogens, discontinued estrogen therapy, and dilatation and curettage) are most likely to occur in women with polycystic ovary syndrome, pronounced obesity, or both.[352] The carcinomas that develop in this clinical setting are usually well differentiated, confined to the uterus, and associated with hyperplasia; they have an excellent prognosis.[352]

Benign polyploid lesions

Endometrial polyps are composed of a mixture of endometrial glands and stroma organized into a circumscribed mass that protrudes into the endometrial cavity. The histologic pattern usually resembles that of so-called cystic hyperplasia, as described previously. There may be variable degrees of stromal fibrosis, traces of smooth muscle are commonly present, and stromal vessels are disproportionately large. When smooth muscle is abundant, the lesion is classified as a pedunculated adenomyoma. Squamous metaplasia in an atypical *polypoid adenomyoma* produces a complex pattern that is easily confused with cancer.[357] Follow-up data currently indicate a benign course.

Endometrial polyps may be a source of abnormal uterine bleeding. An isolated carcinoma arising in an endometrial polyp is rare; the patients who had a focal carcinoma in a polyp, described by Salm,[374] also had a focal carcinoma elsewhere in the endometrium. Armenia[298] found that 17 of 482 women with endometrial polyps subsequently were shown to have carcinoma of the endometrium. This is a greater incidence than expected in all women of the same age, but such an association is not commonly demonstrable.

Neoplasms
Adenocarcinoma

Carcinoma of the endometrium is primarily a disease of menopausal and postmenopausal women. The patients are more commonly nulliparous and as a group are more likely to be obese, diabetic, and hypertensive than a comparable group of women with a normal endometrium. Although endometrial carcinoma occurred with one tenth the frequency of cervical carcinoma 40 years ago, it has become increasingly common and has finally surpassed the incidence of cervical carcinoma.[360]

The cause is unknown, but long-continued noncyclic endometrial stimulation by estrogen, even at normally occurring concentrations, seems to be an important factor, especially when unopposed by the periodic differentiating stimulus provided by progestogen.

Estrone appears to be the most significant estrogenic hormone in this postulated relationship to cancer. Estrone is produced by conversion from adrenal (or ovarian) androstenedione in women who are menopausal, have polycystic ovary syndrome, or are obese. Conversion apparently occurs in peripheral adipose tissue. Statistical studies indicate that endometrial carcinoma is four to eight times more likely to develop in the postmenopausal woman who takes estrogens than in a group of matched control subjects,[381] especially with estrogens composed principally of estrone. The carcinomas identified in estrogen users differ from those occurring without estrogen use; they are well differentiated, superficial, and identified at a younger age and appear to behave less aggressively.[369,380] Also, in contrast to less-differentiated cancers in women who did not take estrogens, there is often an associated hyperplasia in adjacent endometrium. The addition of a progestogen on a cyclic dosage schedule seems to eliminate the risk of cancer among women taking estrogens in the perimenopausal period.[333,386] This is fortunate because estrogens are effective in delaying osteoporosis and the consequent debilitating fractures that may occur in postmenopausal women.[391]

Hyperstimulation by high levels of estrogen may produce an extremely hyperplastic pattern that may be difficult to distinguish from that of a well-differentiated carcinoma. Such a pattern also has been produced by exogenous estrogens and by endogenous estrogen from ovarian neoplasms, especially granuloma cell–theca cell tumors. Lesions of this type seem to be estrogen dependent, since they may regress when the stimulus is removed, and there are few documented reports of death or metastases. More recently a relationship between the use of the sequential type of contraceptive hormone preparation and endometrial cancer has been suggested. The relatively extended exposure to estrogen may be responsible. Some kind of constitutional predisposition may also be necessary; few cases have been identified.[379]

Gross appearance. Endometrial adenocarcinoma forms large irregular masses of friable, granular, gray-tan tissue that protrude into the endometrial cavity. Extension into the muscular wall of the uterus is identified in cut sections by the presence of softer bulging masses of lighter gray granular tissue that replaces the myometrium.

Microscopic appearance. Most endometrial adenocarcinomas are well differentiated and composed of fes-

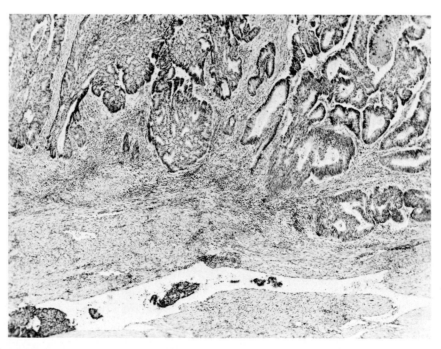

Fig. 34-45. Endometrial adenocarcinoma, moderately differentiated, invading myometrium and dilated lymphatic. (46×; AFIP 264087-2.)

toons and ribbons of columnar epithelium, forming multiglandular masses. The gland spaces are typically bridged by strands of epithelium that lack stroma support (Fig. 34-45). Nuclei are large and have irregular outlines, clumped chromatin, and prominent nucleoli. Focal histologically benign squamous metaplasia is common especially in well-differentiated tumors, a pattern that is designated "adenoacanthoma" (Fig. 34-46). Ng and associates[360] recommended that the term "adenosquamous carcinoma" be used to identify mixed carcinomas in which the squamous and glandular elements both are malignant. Rarely an endometrial carcinoma is composed of large clear cells that produce abundant glycogen; these clear cell adenocarcinomas resemble the endometrial hypersecretory pattern seen during pregnancy. Ultrastructural studies indicate a müllerian histogenesis; there is no evidence for a relationship to mesonephric structures.[378]

Many endometrial carcinomas include a few cells that produce vacuoles of mucin, and occasionally adenocarcinomas limited to the fundus may be composed chiefly of typical mucinous epithelium of the cervical type. For this reason histochemical stains for mucin are of little use in identifying the precise location of an adenocarcinoma; one must examine tissue from the endocervix and endometrium specifically and separately to localize the extent of an adenocarcinoma of the uterus. There are occasional reports of endometrial epidermoid carcinoma.[344] A highly aggressive form of papillary endo-

metrial carcinoma closely resembles ovarian serous carcinoma; psammoma bodies may present, the tumor cells are highly anaplastic, lymphatic invasion may be extensive, and multifocal disease in the peritoneal cavity is common.[312]

Factors affecting prognosis. Nearly 90% of women with endometrial cancer limited to the endometrium survive 5 years. As invasion extends to the inner half of the myometrium, survival falls to 70%, and with cancer spread outside the uterus, survival is less than 15%. Endometrial carcinomas that involve the cervix are more likely to metastasize to pelvic lymph nodes, with a similar distribution to that of cervical carcinoma. For this reason cervical involvement must be determined before treatment can be planned on a rational basis. Survival is good (85%) when the cancer is well differentiated and bad (30%) when it is poorly differentiated.[359] Well-differentiated adenocarcinomas with a well-differentiated or benign-appearing squamous component have a good prognosis; adenocarcinomas with a poorly differentiated squamous component generally have a poorly differentiated glandular component also, occur in older women, and have a poor prognosis.[396]

Endometrial stromal neoplasms

Benign endometrial stroma nodules form single, well-circumscribed masses that can often be distinguished grossly from leiomyomas by their yellow color and softer consistency. Most are in the myometrium, but some protrude into the endometrial cavity. The histologic appearance closely resembles that of normal endometrial stroma, with numerous evenly distributed small vessels forming a distinctive part of the pattern. Stromal lesions of similar origin that have a distinct trabecular pattern have also been called "plexiform tumorlets."[365] The endometrial stroma can form a variety of glandlike structures, some of which mimic ovarian stromal tumor patterns, including sex cords and Call-Exner bodies.[358] The epithelial elements appear benign; they may occur in stromal nodules as well as low-grade and high-grade stromal sarcomas, including those with prominent intravascular components.[316] Low-grade endometrial stromal sarcomas occur as grossly circumscribed nodules with or without extensive intravascular extensions (endolymphatic stromal myosis). The microscopic pattern resembles stromal nodule, but margins may infiltrate adjacent myometrium and mitotic figures are common and may be numerous.[346]

Endolymphatic stromal myosis is a distinctive subgroup of low-grade stromal sarcoma that forms multiple bulging masses of variable size, though there is often a single dominant endometrial mass. The most dramatic and characteristic feature is the presence of numerous wormlike masses of stromal tissue that extrude from vascular channels when the uterine wall is

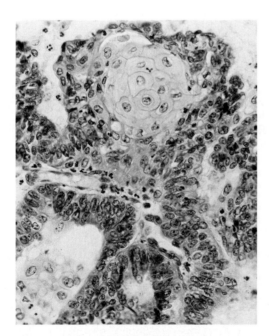

Fig. 34-46. Adenocarcinoma with squamous metaplasia (adenoacanthoma). Benign squamous epithelial pattern distinguishes this from adenosquamous carcinoma in which squamous component is malignant. (235×; AFIP 264048-1.)

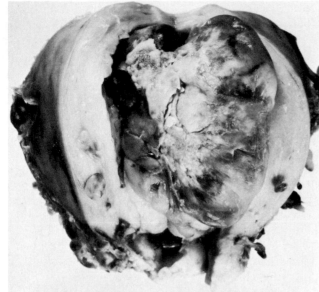

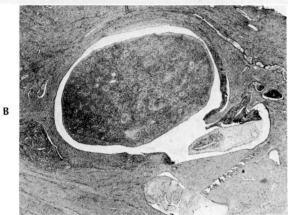

Fig. 34-47. Endolymphatic stromal myosis. **A,** Large, soft, polypoid mass distends endometrial cavity; extensions of mass protrude wormlike from dilated vascular spaces in sectioned uterine wall. **B,** Photomicrograph of neoplastic stroma extending through vascular space in uterine wall. Myometrium is not infiltrated.

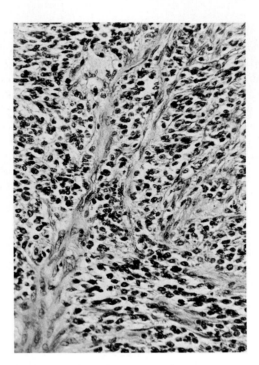

Fig. 34-48. Endometrial stromal sarcoma. Myometrial fibers are separated by infiltrating anaplastic endometrial stromal cells. (150×.)

cut (Fig. 34-47). Margins of stromal growths are well circumscribed; mitoses are infrequent. The clinical course is usually benign, but incompletely resected lesions may recur slowly in the pelvis, and in an occasional patient a pulmonary metastasis has developed. One of the 19 patients reported by Norris and Taylor[363] died of the tumor 12 years after the initial resection. Some metastatic lesions have regressed after progestogen therapy.[351] Similar stromal lesions may arise in the pelvic retroperitoneum.[388]

High-grade endometrial stromal sarcoma is a malignant tumor that characteristically forms one or more polypoid endometrial masses. Margins are indistinct as the result of diffuse infiltration of the myometrium by

poorly differentiated small cells (Fig. 34-48). Mitoses are numerous; more than 10 per 10 high-power microscopic fields indicate a poor prognosis.[363]

Malignant mixed müllerian tumor (carcinosarcoma, mixed mesodermal tumor), and other lesions with mixed epithelial and stromal elements

An uncommon and highly malignant group of endometrial cancers is composed of a mixture of carcinoma and sarcoma patterns. The patients are usually elderly and postmenopausal. A surprisingly large proportion have had prior radiotherapy.[362]

Abnormal bleeding is the most common symptom; the tumor may appear as a polyp protruding through the cervical canal. The carcinoma component includes the full range of patterns seen in endometrial carcinoma. Poorly differentiated endometrial adenocarcinoma is usually predominant. Focal components of clear cell adenocarcinoma, epidermoid carcinoma, and even papillary serous adenocarcinoma like that in the ovary also are common, and occasional embryonic-appearing gland structures are characteristic. If the stroma component is an undifferentiated sarcoma, the tumor is said to be homologous mixed müllerian tumor or carcinosarcoma (Fig. 34-49). Heterologous mixed müllerian tumors are those that also contain chondrosarcoma, osteosarcoma, or rhabdomyosarcoma.

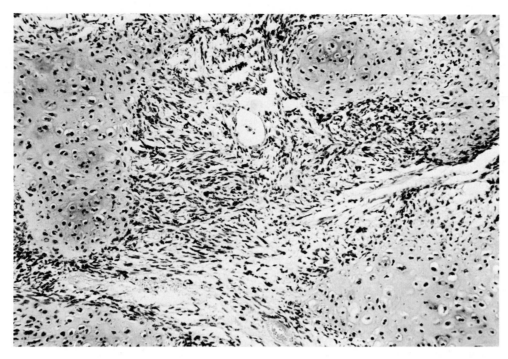

Fig. 34-49. Malignant mixed müllerian tumor. Sarcoma pattern, undifferentiated at center, with chondrosarcoma at margins. (150×; from Kraus, F.T.: Gynecologic pathology, St. Louis, 1967, The C.V. Mosby Co.)

The prognosis is extremely poor. Metastases occur early. The few survivors have had small lesions confined to the uterus, but even with such limited involvement the tumor often may disseminate widely, rapidly, and fatally.[303] The presence or absence of heterologous elements has not affected the prognosis significantly in most series. Radiotherapy may control localized lesions.[365] My experience and some reports[304] indicate improved results with chemotherapy.

An uncommon variant with a benign epithelial component mixed with a sarcomatous stroma has been called adenosarcoma by Clement and Scully.[316] Mitoses among the stromal cells exceed 4 per 10 high-powered microscopic fields; the most aggressive lesions are those that invade the uterine wall.[397]

Adenofibroma, the benign extreme in the spectrum of mixed müllerian tumors of the uterus, is distinguished by its circumscribed growth pattern and fewer than 4 mitoses per 10 high-power microscopic fields among the stromal cells. The histologic pattern resembles that of the more common ovarian adenofibroma.[397] Other rare lesions with mixed components, including carcinofibroma and adenomyoma are discussed in a comprehensive review by Clement and Scully.[316]

Metastatic carcinoma

Carcinoma metastatic from distant primary sites is rare in the endometrium. The most common origin noted is usually breast cancer identified at autopsy.[350] Gastrointestinal cancer has also been reported and may be identified in endometrial curettage. The simultaneous finding of areas of neoplastic change in the endometrium together with cancer of the tube, cervix, or ovary occasionally may represent a metastasis, but in most instances it probably has a multifocal origin.[394]

Primary malignant lymphomas originating in the cervix and body of the uterus have a relatively good prognosis when confined to the uterus.[314] Harris and Scully found that the cervix was the most common point of origin.[334] Nodular lymphomas and diffuse lymphomas with a preponderance of large cleaved cells were more often localized and had the best prognosis.

MYOMETRIUM

The myometrium provides a tough envelope for the developing fetus and propels it into independent life at parturition. It is painful when ischemic, as in the case of prolonged contraction and perhaps with infarction of a smooth muscle neoplasm.

Adenomyosis

The abnormal distribution of nests of histologically benign endometrial tissue within the myometrium is adenomyosis. It may be focal or diffuse. The involved portions of myometrial smooth muscle are hypertrophied.

The typical uterus is enlarged and globular, often with lateral humps at the horns. The posterior wall is most commonly affected and is more extensively involved when the process is diffuse. The cut surface of areas of adenomyosis bulges and has ill-defined margins and a coarse trabecular appearance. The scattered foci of endometrial tissue appear depressed, soft, and occasionally hemorrhagic (Fig. 34-50).

The islands of ectopic endometrium appear normal on histologic examination, except that orientation of glands is lacking. Both glands and stroma are present. Recent hemorrhage and hemosiderin in macrophages, indicating past hemorrhage, are usually found only in occasional areas. Both glands and stroma may respond to hormonal stimulation but not in all cases or in all parts of the same lesion.

The minimum criteria for diagnosis are vague. Most texts refer to the depth of more than 1 low-power microscopic field as the borderline beyond which endometrium qualifies for the diagnosis of adenomyosis. Microscopes vary. It is probable that the occasional superficial foci of endometrial growth that retain cystic accumulation of old blood are symptomatic and significant even if they do not qualify as adenomyosis by this criterion. The presence of associated muscle hypertrophy, as detected by bulges on the fresh-cut surface, also probably indicates a pathologic process. The common extensions of endometrium that retain continuity with the surface but reach a depth of 1 to 2 mm are probably not significant. Some judgment is required in the evaluation of the possibility that a superficial process may have been the cause of symptoms; rigid criteria of measurement alone probably will never enable one to classify all cases reliably.

The symptoms ascribed to adenomyosis are pain, especially with menstrual periods, cramps, and abnormally prolonged and profuse menstrual bleeding. Correlation of the degree of symptoms with the extent of the pathologic process is frequently poor. Occasionally a uterus is found to be extensively involved, with no history of menstrual difficulty. Just as often, an enlarged uterus is removed for all the appropriate reasons, but no adenomyosis can be demonstrated by the pathologist to justify the symptoms or the hysterectomy.[405]

The pathogenesis is unexplained. Adenomyosis is not seen in children and is much less common in young women, a finding indicating that it is unlikely to be a congenital malformation. The most popular concept is that the endometrium extends into the myometrium; a metaplasia of the myometrium is equally tenable. Estrogen stimulation may be an important etiologic factor. Adenomyosis is not usually associated with endometriosis, even when the endometriosis is extensive. It does seem to occur more frequently in women with endometrial hyperplasia or endometrial carcinoma.[413] In such cases the foci of adenomyosis may occasionally also appear hyperplastic or neoplastic, in step with the endometrial lesion.

Neoplasms of smooth muscle
Leiomyoma

The most common lesion of the myometrium is a benign neoplasm composed of smooth muscle with a variable fibrous tissue component. Leiomyomas are well-circumscribed, rounded, firm or hard rubbery masses of gray-white tissue with a characteristic whorled appearance on cut surface. They are often multiple and vary considerably in size (Fig. 34-51). Most occur during the years of active reproductive life; growth may be stimulated by pregnancy or hormonal therapy.

Symptoms vary with location. Subserosal leiomyomas may impinge on the bladder or the sacral plexus, for example, causing urinary frequency or pain. Submucous leiomyomas that protrude into the endometrial cavity cause abnormal bleeding. Rarely very large leiomyomas have been associated with polycythemia[417,421]; whether the leiomyoma secretes an erythropoietic factor itself or stimulates the kidney to do so remains to

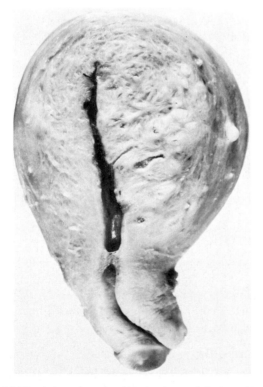

Fig. 34-50. Adenomyosis. Uterus has globular shape. In sagittal section, myometrial mass is poorly circumscribed. Soft depressions are composed of heterotopic endometrium; some are hemorrhagic.

be shown. Leiomyomas undergoing infarction or hemorrhage may be painful. Hysterography may amplify physical findings in establishing the diagnosis and sites of involvement with considerable accuracy.[420]

The histologic pattern is familiar, with streaming masses of smooth muscle separated by strands or masses of collagen (Fig. 34-52). Some remarkable variations occur, with pronounced edema or massive calcification or hyalinization. Leiomyomas that have a sizable adipose tissue component have been called lipoleiomyomas.[411]

Cellular leiomyomas have a threatening histologic appearance because of the absence of fibrotic areas and the large size of the individual cells and their nuclei. They are distinguished from leiomyosarcoma by the absence of mitoses.[403]

Bizarre leiomyomas have an even more frightening microscopic appearance because of the many large giant cells with very large, cytologically malignant-looking nuclei, which may be multiple. These lesions also lack the mitoses that characterize leiomyosarcoma and have proved to be benign after many years of follow-up study.[403] Fechner[406] has described bizarre leiomyomas in a few younger women who were using oral contraceptives. A direct relationship has not been established; the prognosis has been good.

Clear cell leiomyomas (leiomyoblastomas) are rare uterine counterparts of a similar tumor found in the stomach,[428] characterized histologically by abundant clear cytoplasm. Nearly all are benign; the few aggressive lesions have had more numerous mitoses.

Borderline smooth muscle lesions

Rarely proliferating masses of smooth muscle may behave in an aggressive manner that belies their benign microscopic appearance. Kempson and Hendrickson have provided a comprehensive review of the distinctive features of these unusual lesions.[346]

Peritoneal leiomyomatosis. Peritoneal leiomyomatosis refers to the extensive spread of histologically benign masses of smooth muscle about the peritoneal surfaces but limited to the peritoneal cavity. There seems to be a close relationship to pregnancy; it is probable that the origin is metaplastic rather than metastatic from the uterus.[418,429] Regression occurs in most cases after the stimulatory hormonal factors have been withdrawn.[346]

Metastasizing leiomyoma. Rarely a histologically benign leiomyoma may seem to be the source of lymph

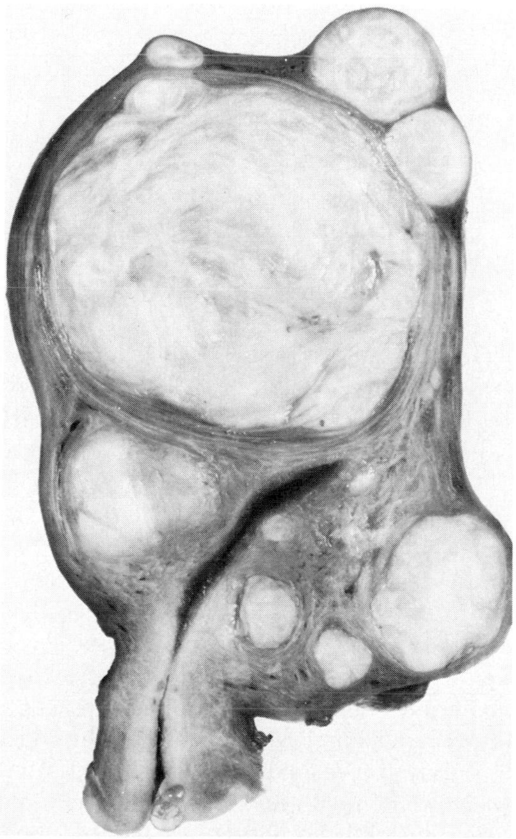

Fig. 34-51. Multiple leiomyomas in sagittal section. Typical, well-circumscribed, solid, light gray nodules distort uterus.

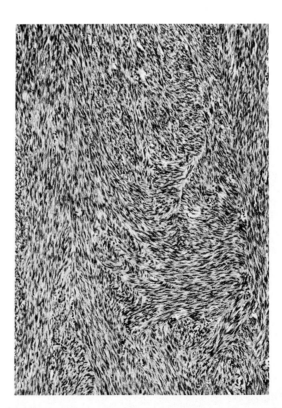

Fig. 34-52. Leiomyoma. Typical interlacing pattern. (140×; from Kraus, F.T.: Gynecologic pathology, St. Louis, 1967, The C.V. Mosby Co.)

nodal or pulmonary metastases.[410] Mitoses are not seen. In some cases progression seems related to hormonal factors, including pregnancy.[402] Intravenous extensions of the uterine tumor are absent.

Cramer and associates[404] identified estrogen receptors in an aggressive metastasizing leiomyoma and noted regression after termination of pregnancy. Other smooth muscle lesions (pulmonary lymphangiomyomatosis) have appeared to respond to endocrine manipulation.[399] Wolff, Silva, and Kaye[393] argue cogently that most or all "multiple pulmonary fibroleiomyomas" are actually metastatic uterine smooth muscle tumors, despite admixed (entrapped) glandular components.

Intravenous leiomyomatosis. Intravenous leiomyomatosis is a benign smooth muscle neoplasm that produces fleshy outgrowths of histologically benign smooth muscle into pelvic veins. Mitoses are absent. The prognosis is good even if all the intravenous extensions cannot be resected.[416,425] The changes are dramatic when extensive; less obvious cases are probably often overlooked.

Histologically benign leiomyoma with numerous mitoses. Occasionally one or more leiomyomas are excised from the uterus of a young woman. The finding of numerous mitoses in an otherwise benign-looking leiomyoma in these circumstances usually causes great consternation. A consideration of the peculiar smooth muscle tumors just described justifies acceptance of the possibility that any leiomyoma may rarely behave in an unexpected aggressive manner. However, all young women with histologically benign leiomyomas with numerous (5 to 15 mitoses per 10 high-power microscopic fields) normal-appearing mitoses that I have seen or heard about[346,419] have had a benign clinical course thereafter, with or without hysterectomy. It is unfortunate that so many have been overtreated.

Leiomyosarcoma

Leiomyosarcoma, the most common of uterine sarcomas, arises from the muscular wall of the uterus; although origin from a leiomyoma is possible and associated leiomyomas are present in a minority of cases, it is unusual to be able to prove such an occurrence.[345,403,416,426] The incidence is approximately 0.6 per 100,000 women over 20 years.[405,423] The mean age of patients at the time of diagnosis in most series is over 50, with a range of 40 to 80 years. Nonspecific symptoms related to uterine enlargement and abnormal uterine bleeding form the usual basis for exploration; only occasionally does tissue obtained by curettage establish a preoperative diagnosis.

Most leiomyosarcomas are large and soft; the yellow or tan color, lack of a trabeculated pattern, at least in some areas, and poorly circumscribed margins may indicate the diagnosis on gross inspection.

The histologic pattern nearly always includes areas

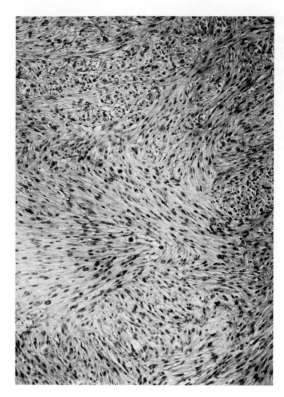

Fig. 34-53. Leiomyosarcoma, well differentiated. Tumor cells are only moderately pleomorphic, but mitoses are numerous. (150×; from Kraus, F.T.: Gynecologic pathology, St. Louis, 1967, The C.V. Mosby Co.)

with typical swirling masses of spindle-shaped smooth muscle cells containing identifiable myofibrils (Fig. 34-53). Nuclei are large and hyperchromatic with irregularly clumped chromatin. Most leiomyosarcomas include a few areas with large pleomorphic or anaplastic tumor cells. The most significant indicator of malignant behavior is the number of mitoses found in microscopic sections. Lesions that contain areas with more than 10 mitoses per 10 high-power fields are classified as sarcomas.[403,431] Lesions with less than 5 mitoses per 10 high-power fields have been associated with a good prognosis.[345,403,423,426] Those lesions in which the numbers of mitoses lie between 5 and 10 per 10 high-power fields constitute a borderline group; most of these patients will survive, at least for 5 years, but several reports have recorded a few deaths in this category. The most significant clinical prognostic factor is age. Over half the premenopausal patients studied by Vardi and Tovell[432] survived 5 years; in contrast, only 1 of 18 postmenopausal women with leiomyosarcoma survived.

Extension beyond the uterus is associated uniformly with a fatal prognosis. Chemotherapy with doxorubicin (Adriamycin) has seemed to produce a transient antitumor effect in a few patients.[400]

Other neoplasms

Lipomas, composed entirely of adipose tissue, are rare and probably result from metaplasia in smooth muscle or stromal cells.[424] Adenomatoid tumor is an uncommon benign nodular mass that resembles a leiomyoma grossly but microscopically has a microcystic honeycomb appearance caused by numerous small spaces lined by vacuolated cells.[433] Similar lesions occur in the fallopian tube. Ultrastructural and histochemical studies support a mesothelial origin.[407,430]

Uterine hemangiopericytoma is another rare benign nodular tumor. It resembles an endometrial stromal nodule grossly and microscopically; the photomicrographs of many reported cases appear more consistent with a stromal nodule. Reticulin stains accentuate the pericapillary growth of plump, spindle-shaped pericytes that make up the tumor. This histogenetic concept is supported by ultrastructural study.[427]

FALLOPIAN TUBE
Anatomy and physiology

The paired fallopian tubes are divided into specific regions, each of which has somewhat different functions. The interstitial portion is a narrow channel through the cornual wall of the uterine fundus. The isthmic portion, about 2 to 3 cm long, is immediately distal to the tubouterine junction. The muscular wall, both longitudinal and circular, is especially prominent in this portion and probably functions as a sphincter. The ampullary portion, about 5 to 8 cm long, has a much wider lumen and an extensive mucosa as the result of the complex folds, or plicae, which greatly increase its surface and secretory capacity. The infundibulum is the trumpetlike distal portion that terminates in the tubal fimbriae. The infundibular muscle also has the capacity to act as a sphincter.

The tubal mucosa is composed of three types of cells. The ciliated cells have an obvious function in transport through the tube. The secretory cells are columnar; they become especially tall and actively secreting during the secretory half of the menstrual cycle. Also present are narrow, dark intercalated cells, which apparently represent secretory cells at an inactive or exhausted stage. Both scanning and transmission electron microscopy have contributed considerably to current concepts of tubal mucosal morphology.[437]

The outer serosal covering is a mesothelial structure; tiny nodular masses of mesothelial proliferation may glisten like dewdrops on the outer surface of the tube; these so-called Walthard's cell rests should not be confused with tumor implants. The ultrastructural pattern is similar to that of urinary transitional epithelium, apparently involving a metaplastic change in mesothelial cells.

The fallopian tubes are complex structures that represent considerably more than conduits from ovary to endometrial cavity. The fringelike fimbriae are actively approximated to the ovary at ovulation by a fold of smooth muscle.

Coordination of muscular activity, epithelial proliferation, ciliary activity, and mucosal secretion is under endocrine control and varies with the phases of the menstrual cycle. Muscular activity also is probably affected by coitus. Mitochondria are greatly increased in both ciliated and secretory cells during the secretory half of the menstrual cycle; granular endoplasmic reticulum and secretion granules appear in the secretory cells at this time.

The circular smooth muscle layer can have a peristaltic effect under appropriate stimulation; spermatozoa are conveyed to the ampullary portion of the tube, where fertilization takes place faster than can be achieved with their unaided locomotive powers. The secretions of the tubal epithelium provide factors that result in capacitation of both spermatozoa and ova, without which fertilization cannot take place. The transport of the zygote cannot be unduly accelerated or retarded if the blastocyst is to develop and implant properly. In vitro fertilization techniques must take these relationships into account.

Inflammation
Acute salpingitis and pelvic inflammatory disease

Acute inflammation of the fallopian tube originates chiefly as a complication of venereally transmitted infections of the lower genital tract. Puerperal or postabortal salpingitis occurs especially after intrauterine instrumentation. Intra-abdominal infections such as appendicitis with peritonitis may secondarily affect the tube. Hematogenous spread is important in the pathogenesis of tuberculosis of the tube and some cases of pneumococcal salpingitis occurring in children.

The most common infectious organism at this time is *Chlamydia trachomatis*,[462] followed closely by the still very significant *Neisseria gonorrhoeae*. The frequency with which salpingitis and pelvic inflammatory disease occur after exposure is probably 50%,[450] much higher than the 10% figure[451] commonly accepted in the past. Subsequently, with the formation of more extensive pelvic tubo-ovarian abscess, numerous other organisms, notably anaerobes, have been cultured. IUDs may increase the potential for salpingitis and more extended pelvic infection after lower genital tract infections, including gonorrhea.[464] The significance of sperm and possibly *Trichomonas* organisms as motile vectors for the upward spread of both organisms has been generally disregarded, but it seems clear that sperm, especially, is directly implicated.[440,443]

Meticulous culture techniques are important because the most common anaerobes identified have been *Bac-*

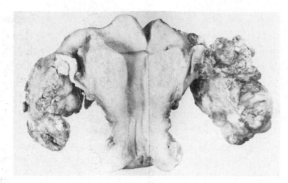

Fig. 34-54. Notice bilateral retort-shaped, swollen, sealed tubes and adhesions of ovaries, typical of salpingitis.

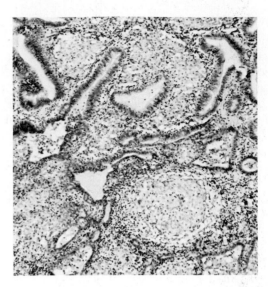

Fig. 34-55. Tuberculous salpingitis. Severe chronic inflammation, inconspicuous granulomas, and exuberant glandular epithelial proliferation. (90×.)

teroides species, which are not sensitive to penicillin[458] and pose a considerable threat to the patient if inadequately controlled. Mycoplasmas also represent important organisms that will not be cultured by "routine" bacteriologic cultural techniques in most laboratories unless the possibility is specifically stressed by the physician performing the culture.[446] *Chlamydia trachomatis* infections require specialized cultural techniques utilizing cultured cells. Laparoscopic examinations are especially effective in establishing an accurate diagnosis.[441]

The fallopian tubes are nearly always affected bilaterally. The fimbriated ends are sealed by organizing inflammatory exudate, and the lumens are dilated, especially the ampullary portion, producing a retort-shaped deformation (Fig. 34-54). The serosa is red and covered with purulent exudate, which extends to the ovaries and pelvic wall. Loculated pockets of pus may accumulate, producing a tubo-ovarian abscess, with the tube, uterus, broad ligament, and ovary forming parts of the surrounding abscess wall.

Microscopically the lumen of the tube is filled with polymorphonuclear leukocytes, which also extensively infiltrate the tubal mucosa and wall. The mucosal epithelium may be focally ulcerated but generally remains intact.

Chronic salpingitis

After approximately 10 days plasma cells, macrophages, and lymphocytes begin to dominate the inflammatory cell pattern. Fibrosis becomes progressively more apparent as the exudate organizes. The tubal plicae form adhesions in many areas, sometimes producing a complicated multiglandular pattern. As the inflammatory process finally resolves, this arrangement persists. The epithelium lining the spaces thus formed by inflammatory entrapment produces secretions, eventually forming small cysts, which in aggregate form a multicystic structure sometimes termed "follicular salpingitis."

It must be emphasized that active inflammation is not a self-perpetuating process, and the expression "sterile pus" is a fallacy. The causative organisms, often anaerobes, may be difficult to culture, but they are there and can be identified and treated effectively.[459] Anaerobes are especially likely to be present in the most serious and life-threatening pelvic infections.

Granulomatous salpingitis

Granulomatous salpingitis is most commonly caused by *Mycobacterium tuberculosis*. The tube is dilated, with a thickened wall. The exudate within the lumen usually appears purulent rather than caseous. Typical caseating granulomas are identified in microscopic sections, however. The glandlike pattern produced by the combination of adhesions of plicae and epithelial hyperplasia may be remarkably proliferative and has been mistaken for adenocarcinoma (Fig. 34-55). In a very large clinicopathologic study researchers[448] found that tubal tuberculosis was invariably present when any part of the female genital tract was affected; two thirds of the women were between 25 and 35 years of age, and the most common initial complaint was infertility (94%).

Foreign-body granulomas in the tube may occur after instillation of oily contrast media used in hysterosalpingography, and talc granulomas have occurred after laparotomy. Rare instances of sarcoidosis, actinomycosis, and schistosomiasis have been reported.[463]

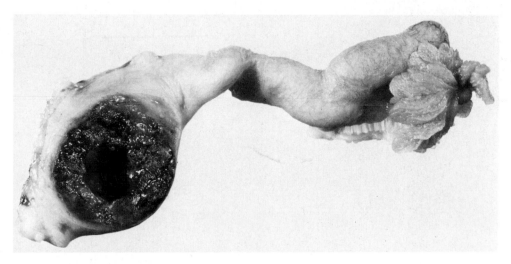

Fig. 34-56. Tubal ectopic pregnancy. Placental villi and trophoblast have infiltrated muscular wall, forming a hemorrhagic mass.

Endometriosis

Ectopic growth of endometrial glands and stroma can occur in all parts of the tube. Serosal implants appear as small red or red-brown patches or nodules with hemorrhage and fibrous adhesions. They are most common as a part of more generalized pelvic endometriosis. Involvement of the muscular wall stimulates muscle proliferation, and a nodular enlargement results. In about 10% of cases the tubal mucosa is replaced by endometrial glandular epithelium and stroma.[453]

In pregnancy focal decidual reaction may involve the serosa or mucosal stroma, especially in the plicae of the ampullary portion of the tube. The cells are large with refractile borders and closely resemble endometrial decidual cells; they must not be confused with granulomas or metastatic carcinoma.

Salpingitis isthmica nodosa

The characteristically bilateral nodular enlargements of salpingitis isthmica nodosa are located in the tubal isthmus and may be multiple. They vary from a few millimeters to a few centimeters in diameter, are firm, and appear gray, yellow, or brown on the cut surface.

Microscopically the nodules are composed of channels or spaces, lined by benign tubal epithelium separated by bundles of smooth muscle, which forms the major component of the mass. Inflammatory changes are inconspicuous or absent. The glandular channels communicate with the tubal lumen and therefore can be demonstrated by hysterosalpingography.[460]

The lesions apparently are acquired, but the pathogenesis is unknown. Benjamin and Beaver[435] considered inflammation to be an unlikely cause and suggested that the process is analogous to that of adenomyosis. Most patients are sterile.

Ectopic pregnancy

Implantation of a fertilized ovum may occur in the tube, especially when tubal structure or function has been altered or impaired by inflammation. The muscular wall is weakened by trophoblastic infiltration and attenuated because the lumen is distended by hemorrhage (Fig. 34-56). Vascular invasion by trophoblast is invariably present.

The diagnosis is not always easy because only a minority of the patients report the typical clinical picture of amenorrhea, pain, and vaginal bleeding, and at least half will have negative pregnancy test results.[463] Salpingectomy is done to control the massive hemorrhage that often results from rupture of the tube. Repeat tubal pregnancy occurs in about 10% of patients.

Attempts to enhance future fertility by excision of the ectopic gestation by means of a linear salpingostomy may be successful,[456] but this procedure is attended by a high rate of repeated ectopic pregnancy.[461] This risk is worth consideration when future pregnancy is desired because the expectation of an intrauterine pregnancy is about 50%. Occasionally the residual trophoblast may persist, requiring reoperation.[452]

Benign tumors and cysts

Hydatids of Morgagni are unilocular, thin-walled cysts that hang from the tubal fimbriae. Ferenczy and Richart[437] have shown that the epithelium is like that of the tube and undergoes cyclic changes in step with tubal epithelium; these are true tubal cysts.

Mesonephric (paratubal or parovarian) cysts are also unilocular thin-walled cysts filled with clear straw-colored fluid. The epithelium of these cysts resembles that of the mesonephric duct remnants of the mesovarium and does not undergo cyclic changes as tubal epithe-

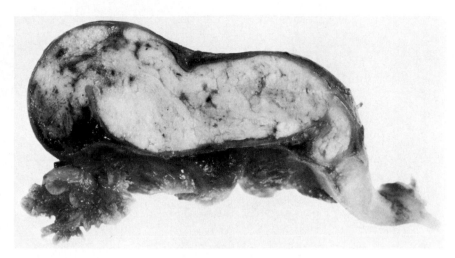

Fig. 34-57. Adenocarcinoma of fallopian tube, distending tubal lumen with soft gray tissue.

lium does.[437] The larger cysts spread to the mesovarium and mesosalpinx, and so the tube often is compressed and attenuated into a longer structure.

Adenomatoid tumors of the tube are histologically identical to those in the uterine wall (p. 1667). In the tube they form a small nodular mass that compresses the tubal lumen to one side. It is important to recognize the pseudoglandular pattern to avoid a mistaken diagnosis of adenocarcinoma.[465]

Rare instances of papillary proliferation composed of large polygonal cells with vesicular nuclei and abundant acidophilic cytoplasm have been reported under the name of "metaplastic papillary tumor."[442] The clinical course is benign, and the pathogenesis is uncertain but is believed to be the consequence of a reactive change found in postpartum women at the time of tubal ligation. Leiomyomas of the tube are surprisingly rare in view of their common occurrence in the adjacent uterus and the smooth muscle origin of both organs. Of the 60 or 80 cases reported, a few have been remarkably large.[463]

Teratomas in rare instances have originated from within the tube.[447] Most have been intraluminal and cystic and have resembled ovarian cystic teratomas (dermoid cysts). A few have been solid. A single instance of malignant teratoma is recorded.[457]

The histogenesis of these lesions is much debated. I have seen one instance of ovarian tissue, including ova and typical ovarian stroma, within tubal mucosa. The patient had been subjected to pelvic surgery, but the wall of the tube appeared to be intact. Such a finding also may explain the unique report of a Sertoli-Leydig cell tumor of the tube,[436] but a satisfactory explanation for the ovarian tissue itself at this location is still lacking.

Malignant tumors
Adenocarcinoma

Adenocarcinoma, the least common of female genital tract carcinomas, is also one of the most aggressive. The symptoms of pain and vaginal discharge are more characteristic of tubal inflammation, which commonly is also present. The inflammatory changes usually affect only the tube containing the neoplasm, a finding indicating that the neoplasm appears first; primary inflammation of the tube usually affects both sides at the same time. The often mentioned symptom of sudden copious watery discharge accompanied by relief of pain, dignified by the Latin term *hydrops tubae profluens*, is not commonly encountered. In about one patient in five, both tubes are affected.

Because of the nonspecific symptoms, the diagnosis is rarely made before laparotomy. Cancer cells were found in the vaginal smears of 24 of the 40 patients by Sedlis,[455] but a lower incidence is found in most series.

The affected tube resembles a distorted sausage and tends to feel firm instead of fluctuant (Fig. 34-57). The appearance of the tumor in the opened tube is usually papillary but may be soft or solid. Simultaneous involvement of tube and ovary may occur, in which case the lesion is considered by convention to be of ovarian origin.

The histologic appearance closely resembles the various patterns of papillary serous adenocarcinoma of the ovary (Fig. 34-58). Better-differentiated lesions may contain psammoma bodies. It is common to see invasion of the tubal stroma and muscle.

The prognosis is poor; about one patient in five lives for 5 years after the diagnosis is established. The few survivors have tended to have well-differentiated le-

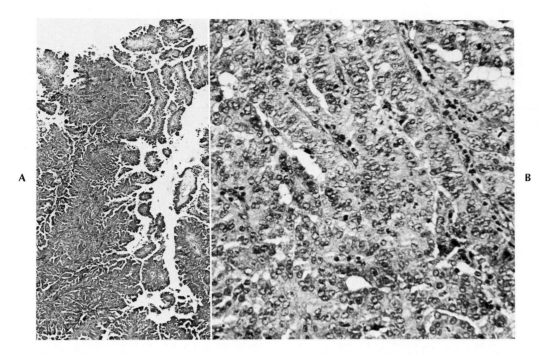

Fig. 34-58. Adenocarcinoma of fallopian tube. **A,** Typical papillary pattern. **B,** Higher magnification showing poorly differentiated adenocarcinoma. (**A,** 40×; **B,** 350×; from Kraus, F.T.: Gynecologic pathology, St. Louis, 1967, The C.V. Mosby Co.)

sions confined to the tubal mucosa, situated within a sealed tube.

Malignant mixed müllerian tumor of the tube is extremely rare. It has no gross distinguishing features. The histologic patterns and clinical correlations are similar to those described for carcinosarcoma and malignant mixed müllerian tumors of the endometrium.[436] The prognosis is very poor.

Metastatic carcinoma involving the tube is more common than primary carcinoma. The most frequent primary site is from one of the more common female genital tract carcinomas, but breast and gastric adenocarcinoma are also encountered. The conspicuous lymphatic involvement and lack of neoplastic change in the tubal epithelium easily distinguish metastatic from primary carcinomas in most instances.

OVARY

The ovary has a complex structure and operates on a multiphasic schedule. Its function is to produce eggs to implant after fertilization in the endometrium, whose preparation is coordinated afresh each time by the ovarian hormones. To do this, the ovary must react appropriately to a set of trophic substances (hormones, prostaglandins) whose stimulation schedules these activities.

The disarray of body structure and function that can occur when the ovarian hormonal stimuli appear inappropriately is often devastating and in many cases still incompletely explained. The bizarre collection of neoplasms and their fascinating effects on the patient rival the repertory of any other organ.

Both the disorders of physiology and the tumors are more easily understood when the morphology and activities of the cellular components of the ovary have been explained. For a more extended description of ovarian histology with physiologic correlations see the review by Clement.[487]

Anatomy and physiology

The two bean-shaped ovaries hang from either tube posterior to the broad ligament, attached to the tube by a mesentery, the mesovarium. The blood vessels and lymphatics enter and leave through the lateral suspensory ligaments and thence through long channels to terminate at the level of the kidneys. The first order of lymph nodes that drain the ovaries is therefore in the aortic chain at the level of the kidneys, which must be remembered when the possible extent of an ovarian neoplasm is being investigated.

Cells of ovary

Germ cells. At birth the germ cells are represented by oocytes, in a resting stage of the first meiotic division, a process that will not be completed until ovulation occurs and fertilization is in process. Ultrastructural features of these events have been compiled by

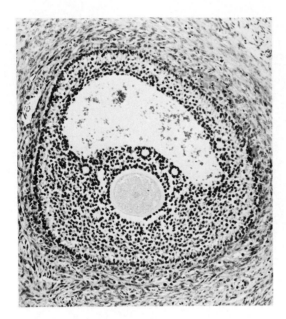

Fig. 34-59. Ovarian follicle. Large ovum is surrounded by mass of granulosa cells in which four Call-Exner bodies can be seen. Concentrically arranged plump spindle cells surrounding the follicle margin compose theca externa. (150×.)

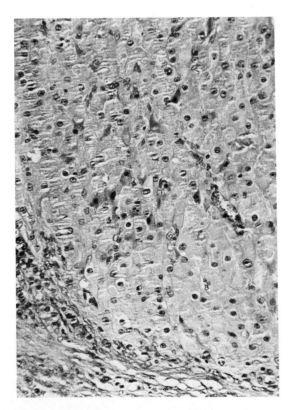

Fig. 34-60. Corpus luteum late in menstrual cycle. Luteinized granulosa cells are large and pale. Luteinized theca cells are smaller, intermixed with stromal cells at peripheral margin *(lower left)*. (275×.)

Ferenczy and Richart.[437] Germ cells have the potential for reproducing tissues of all germ layers and are considered to be the cell of origin of teratomas. They do not themselves produce ovarian hormones but organize the cells that do; adjacent ovarian stromal cells are induced to specialize and form the granulosa and theca cells that produce estrogens and progestogens.

Specialized gonadal stroma cells

Granulosa cells. In the primary follicle of an infant the granulosa cells lie in a single layer around the oocyte. Under the influence of follicle-stimulating hormone they proliferate, forming a fluid that contains the precursor of the zona pellucida, a dense capsule that surrounds the maturing oocyte. Cytoplasmic projections of granulosa cells extend through the zona pellucida and abut on the oocyte cell membrane. As the graafian follicle enlarges, a fluid-filled space, the antrum, forms. The oocyte, surrounded by a hillock of granulosa cells, lies eccentrically near the wall of the follicle (Fig. 34-59). Small round masses of dense pink material surrounded by a rosette of granulosa cells are usually evident in sections; these Call-Exner bodies are a specific product of granulosa cells, normal and neoplastic. The granulosa layer is avascular until ovulation.

Granulosa cells can synthesize estrogen (estrone) and various intermediates, including dehydroepiandrosterone.[574] At the time of ovulation they enlarge and form the corpus luteum, described subsequently.

Theca cells. As the maturing graafian follicle enlarges, the immediately surrounding stromal cells also enlarge and become rounded and plump. This change in an ovarian stromal cell is called "luteinization." The luteinized theca layer becomes noticeably more vascular than the adjacent stroma. Follicle-associated theca cells thus activated produce estrogen (both estrone and estradiol) and are considered to be the primary source of estrogen in the preovulatory stage of the menstrual cycle.

Corpus luteum. In response to the midcycle peak of pituitary luteinizing hormone (and with local help from prostaglandins[480]), the graafian follicle ruptures, expels the oocyte, and rapidly becomes a corpus luteum. The granulosa layer becomes vascularized, and the granulosa cells enlarge to accommodate a massive accumulation of cytoplasm; they are then said to be luteinized (Fig. 34-60). This transformation probably results from luteinizing hormone stimulation alone.[527] Electron micrographs show abundant cytoplasmic agranular reticulum and mitochondria with tubular cristae typical of steroid hormone–producing cells. The corpus luteum is the principal source of progesterone (which stimulates the secretory endometrial pattern) and estrone and estradiol as well. If a pregnancy does not occur, the corpus luteum rapidly regresses. The morphologic changes attending the growth and decline of the corpus luteum have been extensively discussed by Adams and Hertig.[468] The roles of gonadotropins in the rise, and prostaglandins in the fall, of the corpus luteum have been reviewed by Hammerstein.[515]

A corpus luteum of pregnancy should be recognized by the larger cell size, enlarged polyploid nuclei, dense eosinophilic cytoplasm, and small eosinophilic hyaline bodies scattered between the cells. The progesterone output of this organ is indispensable until after the sixth or seventh week of pregnancy; relaxin, a major peptide hormone that inhibits uterine contractions and promotes cervical softening and distensibility, is the other major endocrine product.

Unspecialized ovarian stroma. The unspecialized ovarian stroma is a deceptively innocent-appearing mass of spindle-shaped cells. They produce collagen and also are capable of responding to gonadotropic stimuli to become luteinized producers of steroid hormones. They are considered to be the cells of origin from which hyperplastic and stromal tumors (such as granulosa-theca cell and Sertoli-Leydig cell) arise. The ovarian stroma also contains smooth muscle fibers, which respond to prostaglandins, cholinergic agents, and oxytocin; contractile responses to drugs vary with the stage of the menstrual cycle.[495]

Surface mesothelium. The ovary is invested with a mesothelial covering, like other organs of the abdominal cavity (Fig. 34-61). It is the mesothelium of the urogenital ridge from which the müllerian ducts arise; the surface covering of the ovary seems to share or retain some specialized potential for differentiation with the related müllerian cells that form the lining of tube, endometrium, cervix, and upper part of the vagina. This relationship seems to be the basis for the close similarity between the epithelial cell types found in hyperplastic, metaplastic, and neoplastic growths that occur in or on the ovary.

Focal decidual reaction is regularly present on the surface of the ovaries in pregnancy and may be extensive on peritoneal surfaces generally. These areas look like tiny pink patches of serosal thickening. Rarely a similar change is seen in postmenopausal women[553] (Fig. 34-62).

Hilum cells (hilar Leydig cells). Clusters of large cells with abundant pink cytoplasm commonly are associated with nonmyelinated nerve fibers in the hilum of the ovary at the insertion of the mesovarium. Hilum cells regularly contain proteinaceous crystalloids of Reinke, a feature shared with testicular Leydig (interstitial) cells but not with luteinized stromal cells in the ovary. The physiologic significance of hilum cells in the ovary has not been demonstrated; they are increased in the newborn in association with pregnancy complications such as toxemia, diabetes, and multiple pregnancy, perhaps as a response to increased amounts of placental chorionic gonadotropin.[611]

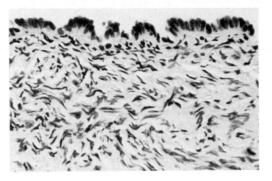

Fig. 34-61. Ovarian surface, covered by low columnar or cuboid coelomic epithelium; cortical stroma immediately below has fibrotic appearance. (300×.)

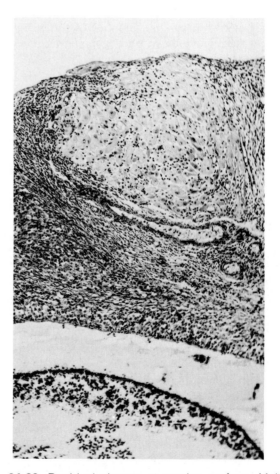

Fig. 34-62. Decidual change at ovarian surface. Multiple foci are found in ovaries of all pregnant women and rarely in postmenopausal women. (100×; AFIP 294919-17074.)

Vestigial structures. Traces of the mesonephros persist as isolated small ducts in the mesovarium; a more plexiform glandular structure, the rete ovarii, is situated at the margin of the ovarian-hilar junction. It is homologous with the rete testis; confusion with focal neoplastic change is to be avoided.

Tiny nodules of heterotopic adrenocortical tissue occur in the ovarian suspensory ligament, broad ligament, and mesovarium. They are common if carefully sought, especially in children.[500] Although there is some potential for neoplastic change in any cell, no important type of neoplasm has been consistently related to either mesonephric or adrenal rests.

Ovarian senescence, failure, and atrophy

The ovary at birth contains about a half million oocytes.[483] Between 300 and 400 oocytes may mature as potential gametes. Some of the rest form small follicles, which undergo atresia, but the majority lyse and disappear without a trace.

As the age of menopause approaches, the number of oocytes diminishes and the number of anovulatory cycles increases. The follicles undergoing atresia leave behind a thin convoluted skein of hyalinized tissue. A few residual oocytes can be identified during the sixth decade in about 25% of ovaries studied; functional corpora lutea with secretory endometrial changes are present in about 10%.[552]

The postmenopausal ovary is composed chiefly of stroma, which remains biochemically active and may be slightly or moderately hyperplastic. It produces chiefly the androgenic steroids dehydroepiandrosterone, androstenedione, and testosterone; it does not aromatize androgens to estrogen.[543]

Menopausal changes may occur prematurely in young women from 15 to 25 years of age. The ovaries are small and atrophic and usually contain no follicles. A few or no oocytes are present.[590] Gonadotropin titers are characteristically elevated, and the ovaries do not respond to gonadotropin therapy.

The basis of premature ovarian atrophy has not been explained by morphologic study, except in some instances of autoimmune ovarian failure. Thus far the patients with autoimmune ovarian destruction have had other well-recognized forms of autoimmune disease, notably Addison's disease and Hashimoto's thyroiditis.[494] At an active stage of the antiovarian immune response, the follicles are infiltrated by lymphocytes and plasma cells.

A form of ovarian atrophy that usually is reversible is caused by prolonged use of contraceptive progestogen-estrogen drugs. The ovaries are small and contain essentially no graafian follicles, but numerous oocytes persist.[542]

Nonneoplastic cysts and hyperplasia
Surface inclusion cysts

The ovary gradually develops a convoluted surface, perhaps as the result of contraction after ovulation, when the stigma of rupture heals, leaving a crevice with buried epithelium and delicate surface adhesions.[604] The buried epithelium may proliferate and often undergoes metaplastic changes, typically to a tubal epithelial pattern.[408] With accumulation of fluid, small cysts result. The resulting surface-inclusion cysts usually remain tiny; an occasional large unilocular cyst may also originate in this fashion.

Follicle cyst, corpus luteum cyst

Follicles and corpora lutea generally do not exceed 2 cm in diameter; when either exceeds a diameter of 3 cm, it may be regarded as cystic, that is, larger than usual. Symptoms that can be related to such a cyst usually do not occur, though menstrual irregularities have been attributed to corpus luteum cysts in some reports.[559] Rarely a large follicle cyst may be a source of excessive estrogen secretion; such a lesion in a child has been reported as a cause of sexual precocity.[591] Severe hemorrhage may originate from the site of rupture in an early corpus luteum.[466]

Luteoma of pregnancy and other luteinized cysts and nodules

Luteoma of pregnancy. Nodular masses of theca-lutein hyperplasia have been discovered chiefly as incidental findings during cesarean section.[592] They are solid and orange-brown and may be bilateral or multiple within the same ovary.

The cells are large and uniform, about half the diameter of a luteinized granulosa cell, and form solid masses or, less commonly, microcystic follicle-like structures. Mitoses may be numerous (Fig. 34-63).

A minority of women and a few female infants have been virilized; testosterone levels may be elevated.[560] Luteomas of pregnancy regress when the pregnancy terminates.

Theca-lutein cysts. Hyperplasia of luteinized theca cells regularly occurs in pregnancy, usually without significant disturbance in the gross morphologic traits of the ovary. Occasionally the process is greatly accentuated, producing multiple large cysts with prominent luteinization of theca cells but not of granulosa cells. This change, sometimes called hyperreactio luteinalis, is seen in association with hydatidiform mole, multiple pregnancy, erythroblastosis fetalis, and conditions in which chorionic gonadotropin titers are increased.[510] Occasional cases have been associated with otherwise uncomplicated pregnancy.[493] A remarkable degree of theca-lutein cystic hyperplasia can be produced when

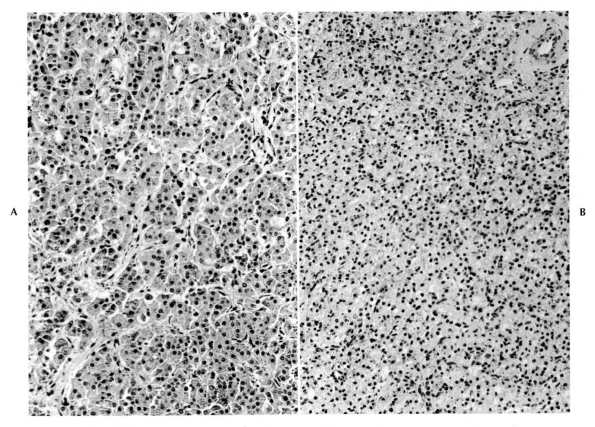

Fig. 34-63. A, Pregnancy luteoma composed of large luteinized stromal cells occurred as multiple red-brown nodules, identified at cesarean section. Female infant was temporarily masculinized. **B,** Section from ill-defined yellow area in opposite ovary 2 months later. (Courtesy Drs. L.R. Malmak and George V. Miller.)

clomiphene or gonadotropin is administered to stimulate ovulation.[576]

Stromal luteoma. Scully[577] has described nodular theca-lutein proliferation of the ovarian stroma, chiefly in postmenopausal women. Associated endometrial changes indicated probable estrogen or progesterone production. In view of the somewhat elevated gonadotropin secretion at this age, the pathogenesis may be analogous to that of pregnancy luteoma; the original lesions were considered to be neoplastic. The lesions reported have been small and benign.

Polycystic ovary (Stein-Leventhal) syndrome

The syndrome described by Stein and Leventhal[590] in 1935 included infertility, secondary amenorrhea, hirsutism, and obesity in a group of young women whose only notable endocrine lesion was enlarged, pale, cystic ovaries. Actual masculinization with clitoral hypertrophy, frontal balding, a deep voice, and changes of body habitus does *not* occur. Since that time a great many facts have been accumulated, but a fully satisfactory explanation remains to be found. In any series there is a general similarity in the endocrine problems, but only a minority of patients have all the criteria just listed. The condition is sometimes hereditary.[490]

The ovarian lesion is not specific; it is almost certainly just a reactive change like the other features of the syndrome. The appearance is essentially that of an anovulatory ovary. Numerous follicles are present; typically they form a layer beneath the thickened white cortex. The medullary stroma that forms the central core is solid, gray, and somewhat edematous (Fig. 34-64). Microscopically the follicles and atretic follicles are all surrounded by a relatively prominent luteinized theca cell layer. The stromal cells themselves may be focally luteinized. Except in rare cases there is no corpus luteum. The ovaries usually are enlarged, sometimes more than 6 cm in diameter, but may be of normal size.

Unquestionably more than one basic physiologic defect triggers the entire symptom complex and physical changes, including those in the ovary. For instance, an-

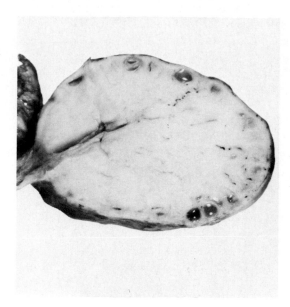

Fig. 34-64. Enlarged ovary from young woman with polycystic ovary (Stein-Leventhal) syndrome. Notice abundant central stroma and peripheral subcapsular follicles.

drogens from adrenal hyperplasia or neoplasm can do it; a similar syndrome has resulted from use of contraceptive steroids.[471,601] A common thread seems to be consistently elevated secretion of androgen, especially testosterone. It is necessary to identify the concentration of the protein-bound testosterone component, as well as the total, because only the unbound component reacts biologically; women with the polycystic ovary syndrome have low levels of testosterone-binding protein, which rises as they respond to treatment.[598]

Greenblatt and Mahesh[513] note that the pituitary follicle-stimulating hormone is inhibited to low levels by testosterone, but luteinizing hormone is not always so affected. The levels of luteinizing hormone are sufficient to stimulate the ovarian theca and stromal cells to luteinize[506]; they may then secrete androgens inappropriately because of the abnormal pattern of initial gonadotropin stimulation, perpetuating the abnormal anovulatory state.

Any intervention that elicits a surge of follicle-stimulating hormone sufficient to stimulate maturation of a follicle and ovulation will correct this abnormal state, at least temporarily. This has been done by direct injection of gonadotropins, by stimulation of their production with hypothalamic follicle-stimulating and luteinizing hormone–releasing factors,[491,596,610] and by reduction of ovarian steroid feedback effect through ovarian injury (chiefly wedge resection), clomiphene,[572] or suppression with corticoids. One review presents current concepts of pathogenesis and treatment selection in the context of the contrasting needs of different patients.[519]

Hyperthecosis and stromal hyperplasia

The amount of ovarian stroma varies, and it may be abundant even at menopause and thereafter. When stromal proliferation is excessive, it is said to be hyperplastic.

In some young women stromal hyperplasia is sufficiently pronounced to cause enlargement or displacement of follicles and other structures. Variable degrees of stromal luteinization may occur. The abnormal stromal cells produce androgens, especially testosterone; in some patients masculinization may be severe. The ovaries may be solid or partly cystic. The clinical and pathologic features tend to overlap with those of the polycystic ovary syndrome, except that hyperthecosis produces masculinization. This condition is harder to treat than the polycystic ovary syndrome. Some patients have responded to oophorectomy.[478]

Massive edema

Massive edema is a rare form of ovarian enlargement that usually occurs in young women who are initially seen either with severe abdominal pain or with severe masculinization. The ovarian enlargement may be unilateral or bilateral. There often seems to be some degree of torsion, especially in patients who have pain. The masculinizing lesions have histologic evidence of stromal luteinization that resembles hyperthecosis. Both types of ovaries are massively edematous, and so the water leaks copiously from the cut surface. The pathogenesis is unknown; it has been suggested that torsion is responsible.[569] Total ovariectomy is probably unnecessary for this benign condition; resection to a normal-sized remnant has been recommended.[580]

Endometriosis

Ectopic endometrium in the ovary is troublesome because it forms fibrous adhesions and hemorrhagic cysts, which are painful and a cause of infertility. Accumulated hemorrhage results from stromal breakdown at the time of menstrual bleeding. Cysts may become large and typically are filled with semisolid, dark brown, altered blood. Endometrial tissue usually can be found somewhere in the fibrous wall, but a search may be necessary. Smaller foci of hemorrhage organize and contract, leaving a characteristic puckered scar tinged yellow-brown with hemosiderin (Fig. 34-65).

The pathogenesis has been debated. Implants from a reflux of menstrual blood have been shown to occur, and implants have been observed growing from such material. Serosal metaplasia is another possibility and almost certainly has been the cause in some cases. In a

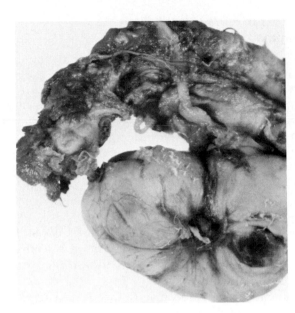

Fig. 34-65. Ovarian endometriosis forming characteristic puckered hemorrhagic scar and extensive tubal adhesions.

given case it is usually impossible to demonstrate the origin of the lesion.

Heterotopic ovarian tissue

Misplaced ovarian tissue is rare. The usual sites lie near the migratory route of the germ cells, in the pelvic retroperitoneum and mesosigmoid[604]; unquestionable nodules of ovarian stroma with oocytes have been encountered beneath the uterine serosa.[469] Heterotopic ovarian tissue has been the site of neoplasm (see discussion of fallopian tubes) and a source of unexpected ovarian function after bilateral ovariectomy.[531]

Neoplasms
Classification

Because of their remarkable diversity, ovarian tumors may be bewildering. Natural history and response to treatment vary considerably from one group of tumors to another. Especially in the area of chemotherapy and radiotherapy, the best therapeutic approach may be highly specific for a single type of neoplasm; accordingly, accurate histologic diagnosis is often a critical factor in achieving an optimum treatment response. It is extremely important therefore that the pathologist responsible for diagnosis and the physician responsible for therapy communicate clearly. Similarly, the classification used in any discussion of new therapeutic techniques must be understandable, or the pathologist's report is useless.

Neoplasms arise from and tend to resemble any of the normally occurring cellular components of the ovary described at the beginning of this section. This classification is based on histogenesis: the cell or tissue of origin. It is essentially the classification presented by the World Health Organization[583] with minor abridgments in the interest of clarity for this introduction to the subject.

  I. Tumors of surface epithelium

    A. Serous tumors

      1. Benign cystadenoma, cystadenofibroma, and papillary cystadenoma

      2. Borderline serous tumors

      3. Malignant serous cystadenocarcinomas, papillary carcinomas

    B. Mucinous tumors

      1. Benign mucinous cystadenoma

      2. Borderline mucinous tumors

      3. Malignant mucinous carcinomas

    C. Endometrioid tumors

      1. Benign (cystic endometriosis?)

      2. Borderline; rare lesions resembling atypical endometrial hyperplasia

      3. Malignant

        a. Adenocarcinomas, well differentiated and poorly differentiated, and adenosquamous carcinoma

        b. Endometrioid stromal sarcoma

        c. Malignant mixed müllerian tumor

    D. Clear cell tumors

      1. Benign clear cell tumor (chiefly cystadenofibroma)

      2. Borderline clear cell tumors

      3. Malignant clear cell adenocarcinoma

    E. Brenner tumor

      1. Benign

      2. Borderline (proliferating Brenner tumor)

      3. Malignant

    F. Mixed (such as serous and mucinous)

    G. Undifferentiated carcinoma (always malignant)

  II. Sex cord stromal tumors

    A. Granulosa-theca cell tumors

      1. Granulosa cell tumor

      2. Thecoma

      3. Fibroma

      4. Mixed and indeterminate types

    B. Sertoli-Leydig cell tumors (androblastomas,"arrhenoblastomas")

      1. Well differentiated; tubular and Leydig cell types

      2. Intermediate differentiation

      3. Poorly differentiated (sarcomatoid)

    C. Gynandroblastoma

  III. Lipid cell tumors (such as hilum cell tumor, "adrenal rest" tumor)

IV. Germ cell tumors
    A. Dysgerminoma
    B. Endodermal sinus tumor
    C. Embryonal carcinoma, polyembryoma
    D. Choriocarcinoma
    E. Teratomas
        1. Mature: chiefly benign cystic teratoma (dermoid cyst)
        2. Immature (malignant teratoma)
        3. Specialized (such as struma, carcinoid)
    F. Mixed forms
V. Gonadoblastoma

It was estimated that about 19,000 women in the United States would be found to have ovarian cancer in 1988, and that in the same year about 12,000 would die of ovarian cancer.[272] The yearly death rate from ovarian cancer remained about 8.5 per 100,000 women from 1950 to 1975.[274]

The relative frequency with which different types of ovarian neoplasms occur is summarized in Table 34-3. The proportions indicated are approximate and represent a synthesis of numerous reports. This is necessary because older studies use uncertain criteria for malignancy and do not distinguish important tumor categories, especially endometrioid carcinoma. More recent reports from cancer treatment centers do not reflect the true incidence of common benign neoplasms, which are usually treated in less specialized institutions.

Table 34-3. General classification of primary ovarian neoplasms

Cell of origin (representative tumor types)	Relative proportion of all ovarian neoplasms (%)*	Relative proportion of malignant neoplasms only (%)
Surface epithelium (serous, mucinous, endometrioid, clear cell, etc.)	65	95
Germ cells (immature ova) (cystic teratoma, solid teratoma, dysgerminoma, etc.)	20	1
Stromal cells (sex cords) (granulosa-theca cells, Sertoli-Leydig cells, lipid cells, fibroma, etc.)	12	2
Tumors in dysgenetic gonads (gonadoblastoma)	1	—
Unclassified (chiefly undifferentiated carcinoma)	2	2

*The relative proportion of figures noted here represents an approximation.

Tumors of surface epithelium (common epithelial tumors)

Tumors of the surface epithelium form the most common group of ovarian neoplasms and include the majority of ovarian carcinomas (Table 34-3). The tissue of origin is considered to be the surface celomic mesothelium that covers the ovary (Fig. 34-66); it seems to retain, in neoplasms, the capacity to recapitulate tumor patterns that resemble the epithelial components of the müllerian ducts. For example, the epithelium of serous tumors resembles that lining the tube; the cells that line mucinous cystadenomas resemble endocervical mucosa. These neoplasms usually have a prominent cystic component with single or multiple loculations, often a variable amount of fibrous stroma, and an epithelial lining that often is thrown into papillary tufts.

It is necessary to recognize a spectrum of aggressiveness that is divided into benign, malignant, and borderline or low malignant potential (LMP) categories. Clearly benign cystic tumors are lined by a single layer of well-oriented columnar epithelial cells; papillary projections, if present, are supported by fibrovascular stromal stalks and covered by the same type of epithelium. Obviously malignant tumors have an anaplastic epithelial component that invades the stroma of the tumor or other structures, in addition to forming the epithelial lining. The epithelial cells are often several layers thick and have anaplastic nuclei, with a loss of polarity. The prognosis is very poor; about 15% of patients survive for 5 years, regardless of treatment.

The important intermediate, or borderline (LMP), group is identified chiefly by the absence of invasion in an otherwise highly proliferative neoplasm. A complex papillary pattern is often present, and the epithelium may be two or three cells thick. The epithelial cells generally appear only moderately dysplastic and maintain some degree of columnar orientation in most areas. Even proliferative epithelial masses with an anaplastic cytologic pattern do not signify a carcinoma in the absence of stromal invasion; the clinical behavior is still that of a borderline (LMP) tumor.[525]

Although the behavior of borderline tumors is unpredictable in individual cases, as a group they have a much better prognosis than malignant tumors of the ovary do. More than 90% of patients survive 5 years, and 70% survive 15 years, even in the presence of implants on peritoneal surfaces.[562] Recurrences typically appear after several years, if at all; the minority of tumors that have a malignant course tend to progress slowly.

Survival varies with extent (stages) of disease at the time of diagnosis. Patients with lesions limited to one or both ovaries have survival rates approaching 100%. Persistent or recurrent tumor sufficient to cause symp-

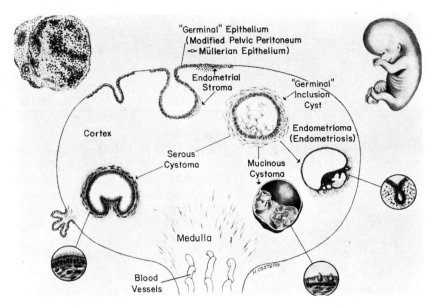

Fig. 34-66. Semidiagrammatic drawing of ovary to illustrate origin and types of cystomas derived from "germinal" epithelium. Notice papillary growth on surface and various types of cystic tumors derived from infolding of this type of epithelium. Embryonic ovary and müllerian duct *(top left)* are drawn from 35 mm embryo *(top right)* and illustrate embryonic similarity of müllerian duct to germinal epithelium. The three types of cystomas (and their malignant counterparts) derived from "germinal" inclusion cysts are serous, endometrial, and mucinous—all recapitulating müllerian system, to which germinal epithelium is embryologically closely related. Low- and high-power drawings are from actual specimens. (From Hertig, A.T., and Gore, H.M.: Rocky Mountain Med. J. **55:**47, 1958.)

toms occurs in 30% to 60% of women who have extraovarian involvement in the pelvis, omentum, or other peritoneal surfaces[518,561]; radiation therapy may prolong symptom-free survival in some of these women.[518]

Borderline (low malignant potential) tumors occasionally present as a unilateral ovarian mass in a young woman who has much to benefit from conservation of her uterus and opposite ovary. The risk that another tumor will develop in a normal-appearing ovary in these circumstances is about 15% in a 5- to 7-year period.[597] Most significantly, the tumors that do recur consistently maintain their borderline (LMP) clinical and pathologic characteristics, including an excellent prognosis.

Various tumor-associated antigens may circulate in the blood of women with borderline and malignant tumors of common epithelial type. CA-125 antigen is most commonly associated with serous and endometrioid tumors; mucinous tumors often produce carcinoembryonic antigen (CEA), as colon cancers do. Monitoring the appropriate antigen titers is very useful in identification of occult metastases,[503] monitoring of therapeutic response,[536] and detection of asymptomatic recurrence at an early stage. Evaluation of tumor cell DNA (ploidy) by flow cytometry shows promise as an independent

prognostic factor in evaluation of the aggressive potential of ovarian cancers.[566]

Serous tumors. Benign serous cysts and cystadenomas may form single or multiple loculations, lined by low columnar epithelium, which is sometimes ciliated, often distinctly resembling tubal epithelium (Fig. 34-67). The cyst fluid is watery or viscous and clear and contains a variety of mucins; however, the epithelial cells that secrete the fluid do not have the characteristic vacuolated pattern of mucinous epithelium. Papillary processes are common and may be numerous and complicated. The epithelial component of serous tumors, unlike other neoplasms of surface epithelium, may appear on the external surfaces; occasional lesions are composed entirely of a surface papillary growth with no cystic component. It is common to find tiny round laminated calcific concretions called "psammoma bodies" in the stroma of the papillary processes.

A relatively prominent or abundant fibrous tissue stroma produces plump papillae and large solid fibrous masses, as well as cysts. The resulting growths are papillary adenofibromas and cystadenofibromas.

Borderline serous tumors are often multilocular (Fig. 34-68) and have a more complex papillary pattern; fine papillae, closely packed, may resemble solid epithelial proliferation. Variable degrees of dysplastic nuclear change and mitotic activity are present (Fig. 34-69).

The presence of stromal invasion is the basis for identifying a serous tumor as a serous carcinoma[526] (Fig. 34-70). Bilateral ovarian involvement occurs in about two thirds of both borderline and malignant serous tumors and in one third of tumors that have not spread beyond the uterus, tubes, and ovaries. Microscopic foci of cancer may lurk in an apparently normal ovary when serous carcinoma is present on the opposite side.

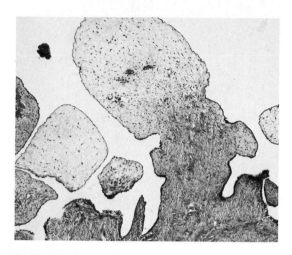

Fig. 34-67. Benign papillary serous tumor, with abundant fibrous stroma covered by single layer of small flattened epithelial cells. (85×.)

Mucinous tumors. Mucinous tumors are also typically unilocular or multilocular cystic masses. The epithelium that lines the cysts is composed of tall columnar goblet cells with basal nuclei and prominent mucin vacuoles; it resembles endocervical mucosa (Fig. 34-71). In some instances the pattern appears even more like intestinal epithelium, including argentaffin cells and even Paneth's cells.[579] Rarely a mucinous tumor has produced enough gastrin to cause Zollinger-Ellison syndrome.[491] Since about 5% of mucinous tumors are associated with cystic teratomas, it has been suggested that some, at least, originate from germ cells; an intestinal metaplasia of these exotic cell types seems more likely, despite the apparent production of endodermal derivatives by mesodermal cells.[502] A larger number, however, may have endometrioid or serous elements, which supports their classification with surface epithelial tumors. Since the biologic activity of mucinous tumors is more like the biologic activity of other surface epithelial tumors, their inclusion in this section has a solid practical basis, which outweighs the potential quibble over histogenesis.

The presence of strands or clusters of cytologically malignant cells infiltrating the stroma, with or without associated pools of mucin is unquestionably the most significant histologic attribute of an aggressive mucinous carcinoma.[485] Such neoplasms are usually at a higher stage, with extraovarian spread at the time of diagnosis. Hart and Norris[516] have noted that a multilayered epithelial proliferation more than three cells

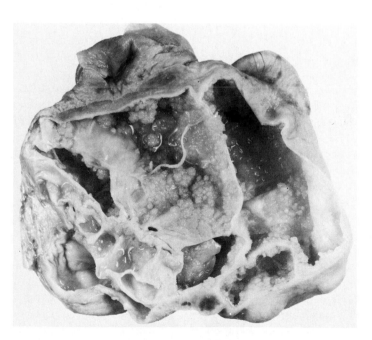

Fig. 34-68. Borderline serous tumor of ovary, a multilocular cystic mass with spaces lined by papillary epithelial masses.

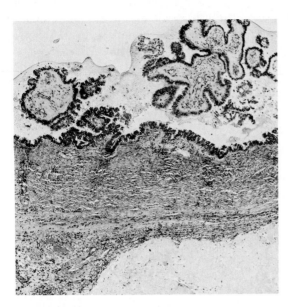

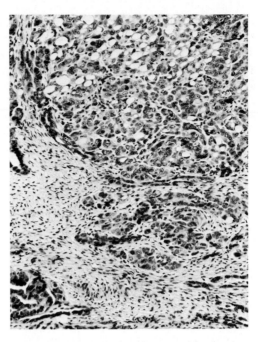

Fig. 34-69. Borderline serous cystadenoma of ovary without invasion. Epithelium is pleomorphic and forms small papillary processes. (46×; AFIP 264082-1.)

Fig. 34-70. Serous carcinoma of ovary showing invasion of stroma by strands and small clusters of adenocarcinoma cells. (100×.)

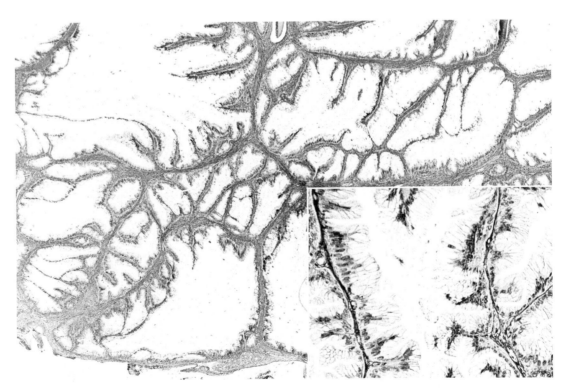

Fig. 34-71. Mucinous cystadenoma of ovary. Gland spaces are lined with tall columnar cells with basal nuclei and large apical mucin vacuoles. Notice resemblance to cervical mucosa. (40×; *inset,* 300×.)

thick also correlates well with malignant behavior. Borderline mucinous tumors, then, are defined as mucinous tumors in which there is no stromal invasion, and the epithelial proliferation, though sometimes cytologically atypical, remains no more than two or three cells thick.[516] In cases selected by these criteria, more than 90% of women with borderline tumors survived for 10 years; in the same report 59% of patients with mucinous carcinoma (all stage I) survived for 10 years. Survival at 10 years in mucinous carcinoma (all stages) is 34%.[575]

Bilateral ovarian involvement occurs in about one fifth of both borderline and malignant mucinous tumors but in only 10% of cases in which there is no spread beyond the uterus, tubes, and ovaries. Kottmeier[530] found no instance of microscopic involvement of an apparently normal ovary on the side opposite a mucinous carcinoma.

Borderline mucinous tumors with a pure endocervical type of pattern have a distinctly better prognosis than the more common mucinous tumors of intestinal type, even in the presence of extraovarian spread.[573]

Mucinous ascites (pseudomyxoma peritonei) occasionally occurs in association with a well-differentiated borderline mucinous tumor. The ovarian tumor characteristically contains mucin-filled cystic spaces that dissect the ovarian stroma. The neoplastic epithelium in the ovary and in the peritoneal lesion is sparse and well differentiated.[516] Chemotherapy with alkylating agents has provided symptomatic improvement and prolonged survival in some patients.[539]

Endometrioid tumors. Endometrioid carcinomas are so named because the histologic pattern closely resembles that of uterine endometrial adenocarcinoma. The distinction is most easily made in well-differentiated carcinomas (Fig. 34-72). Less-differentiated lesions may have a typical endometrioid pattern only in focal areas or a few patches of squamous metaplasia as the only clues to their identity, which accounts for some of the variation in the frequency with which they are reported. They probably comprise between 15% and 20% of ovarian cancers.

The benign counterpart is probably represented by some cases of cystic endometriosis of the ovary. A clearly defined concept of the borderline endometrioid tumor is lacking; certainly such lesions are rare.

Endometrioid carcinomas are often partly cystic, frequently with prominent solid areas; the cyst fluid is often brown or bloody. The cyst lining has a velvety or papillary appearance. Association with endometriosis is demonstrable in about one third of cases,[575] but the presence of endometriosis is not the basis for inclusion of a tumor within this group. Endometriosis is a common lesion of the ovary and occurs with other ovarian neoplasms, especially clear cell tumors.

The prognosis for well-differentiated carcinomas is good; about 60% of patients survive for 5 years, compared with 23% survival for poorly differentiated carcinomas.[575]

In about one third of the patients there is a coexistent adenocarcinoma of the endometrium. It is generally accepted that both lesions are separate primary cancers

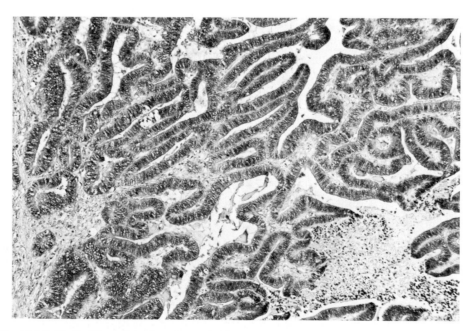

Fig. 34-72. Well-differentiated endometrioid adenocarcinoma of ovary. Pattern is identical to that of uterine endometrial adenocarcinoma. (150×.)

because the survival rate in the presence of endometrial involvement is not appreciably lower.[498] Furthermore, the two lesions commonly occur together without evidence of any other metastatic lesion; the common presence of multiple foci of dysplastic endometrial change is further evidence of a multifocal process. In contrast, simultaneous uterine and ovarian involvement by common epithelial carcinomas of other types such as serous or clear cell carcinomas is usually attended by a poor prognosis.[498]

Other endometrioid neoplasms such as stromal sarcoma, malignant mixed müllerian tumor, and adenosarcoma have been reported rarely as primary tumors of the ovary. The histologic features and prognosis (poor) do not differ significantly from those of similar lesions occurring in the endometrium.

Clear cell tumors. The gross appearance of clear cell tumors is often a combination of solid and cystic components much like that of endometrioid carcinoma. The cyst is usually unilocular; the fluid is commonly brown, and the solid areas form nodular masses that protrude into the lumen.

The histologic pattern is characterized by masses of large epithelial cells with abundant clear cytoplasm, supported by delicate fibrous trabeculas (Fig. 34-73). The cytoplasm contains abundant glycogen. A variation in this pattern is the presence of small cystic spaces lined by a single layer of large cuboid cells that are somewhat separated from one another; the nuclei may be oriented toward the cyst lumen rather than the basal area, producing a hobnail pattern.

Less than 10% are bilateral. Benign and borderline varieties occur, chiefly in the form of clear cell adenofibroma with an abundant fibrous stroma, but the malignant variety is much more common. Association with endometriosis is six times as great as with ovarian carcinoma in general.[579]

Because the clear cell histologic pattern resembles that of renal adenocarcinoma and because of the proximity of adjacent mesonephric structures, the term *mesonephroma* has also been used to designate this type of neoplasm. There is no convincing evidence to support the concept of mesonephric origin.[581] On the other hand, ovarian clear cell carcinomas and identical neoplasms of the endometrium, cervix, and vagina seem to be related to tumors of müllerian epithelial type, especially endometrioid tumors. Endometrioid and clear cell patterns occur together in ovarian and endometrial carcinomas, and clear cell tumors have been shown to arise in patients with endometriosis.[581] Clear cell carcinoma patterns also occur in many malignant mixed müllerian tumors. Survival rates are in an intermediate range; 37% survive 5 years.

Brenner tumor. Brenner tumors are solid gray or yellow-gray masses of fibrous tissue; occasionally it is possible to find scattered tiny cysts on cut section. The external serosal surface is smooth and shiny.

The microscopic appearance of scattered epithelial masses on a field of fibrous stroma is distinctive (Fig. 34-74). The epithelial component is composed of ovoid cells with clear cytoplasm, vesicular nuclei, and a characteristic nuclear groove. Mucinous epithelial cells form tiny cysts in the epithelial masses in about one third of the tumors, and one fifth have a conspicuous cystic mucinous component.

In the borderline variety of Brenner tumor (called proliferating Brenner tumor) the epithelial masses form

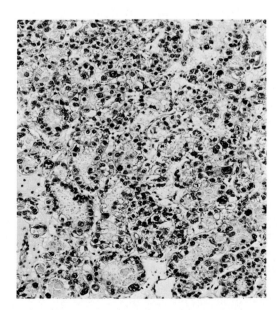

Fig. 34-73. Clear cell adenocarcinoma. There is abundant cytoplasmic glycogen; mucin is found only in extracellular secretions. (100×.)

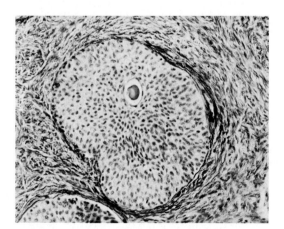

Fig. 34-74. Brenner tumor. Typical sharply circumscribed nest of uniform cytologically benign cells surrounded by dense fibrous stroma. (140×; AFIP 305334-1-4-2.)

larger cysts with a redundant, sometimes papillary lining of cells that look identical to transitional cell papilloma of the urinary bladder. Malignant Brenner tumors have an anaplastic epithelial component that resembles poorly differentiated transitional cell carcinoma or epidermoid carcinoma and invades the stroma of the tumor. Borderline and malignant Brenner tumors are both extremely rare; one needs to identify a well-differentiated Brenner tumor pattern in some part of the lesion to establish the diagnosis. Basing themselves on the similarity of histologic patterns, Austin and Norris[475] have identified a specific group of transitional cell carcinomas of the ovary that resemble both the malignant component of malignant Brenner tumor and urinary transitional cell carcinoma. Most of these have progressed to an advanced stage at the time of diagnosis, and the prognosis is poor.

Arey's wax model reconstructions[470] have shown that the epithelial islands are actually anastomosing cords of epithelial cells, in continuity with the covering serosal epithelium of the ovary. The ultrastructural appearance of Brenner epithelial cells resembles that of urinary bladder transitional epithelium and the Walthard's cell nests of the tubal serosa. On the basis of these studies it is generally accepted that Brenner tumors probably represent a neoplastic proliferation of ovarian surface epithelial cells that further differentiate into urinary transitional epithelium.[492,567,586]

Less than 10% are bilateral. The stromal component is not always inert. In occasional cases the stromal cells appear luteinized and contain birefringent lipid; associated endometrial hyperplasia has indicated secretion of estrogen by the tumor.[497]

Mixed forms. Surface epithelial tumors often include a combination of the foregoing types. Unless two or more patterns form a distinct and prominent component, the neoplasm is usually and most reasonably classified after the predominant cell type represented.

Cystadenofibromas combine any of the cystic epithelial patterns described previously with a prominent solid fibrous tissue component. Epithelial atypia, even when pronounced, has not been associated with aggressive behavior in the few instances described by Kao and Norris.[524] Malignant mixed müllerian tumor, histologically identical to its uterine counterpart (see p. 1662), occurs rarely as a highly aggressive ovarian primary neoplasm.[479]

Undifferentiated carcinoma. Nearly all adenocarcinomas too undifferentiated for subclassification probably belong to the group of tumors originating from surface epithelium. About 54% are bilateral; they comprise about 4% of ovarian carcinomas. The prognosis is extremely poor. Many are composed of small cells of nearly uniform size. Mitoses are numerous; nuclei are anaplastic. It is a mistake to classify such lesions as granulosa cell carcinomas. Confusion of this highly malignant group of neoplasms with granulosa cell tumors only blurs the distinct clinical correlation associated with these two different neoplastic diseases.

Sarcomas. Malignant mixed müllerian tumors and stromal sarcomas like those found more typically in the endometrium also occur rarely as primary ovarian neoplasms. Metastases occur early and the prognosis is poor.[584]

Extragenital tumors with müllerian histologic patterns. The peritoneal and retroperitoneal tissues of the female pelvis occasionally generate primary neoplasms resembling any of the foregoing tumor types without necessarily involving any part of the uterus, tubes, or ovaries. Thus serous tumors with psammoma bodies,[505] mucinous tumors,[570] adenosarcomas,[488] and even endometrial stromal tumors[388] may be found on or beneath the peritoneal surface of any part of the pelvis. Various metaplastic changes also occur; Lauchlan[535] refers to this versatile tissue as the "secondary müllerian system."

Sex cord stromal tumors (sex cord–mesenchyme tumors)

The sex cord stromal tumors arise from specialized ovarian stromal cells. The general designation of sex cord–mesenchyme tumors is favored by Scully[579] because the assumption that the embryonic sex cords and their derivatives are mesenchymal or stromal derivatives (rather than celomic epithelium) remains unproved. It is the specialized stromal cells that produce ovarian steroid hormones. The tumors that arise from them produce the full range of the ovarian and testicular steroid hormonal repertory, including intermediates, and occasionally adrenal steroids as well.

Granulosa-theca cell tumors. About half the granulosa-theca cell tumors are thecomas, a fourth are composed only of granulosa cells, and the remaining fourth are a mixture of both.

Granulosa cell tumors are often partly cystic, and multiple areas of hemorrhage are common. Solid areas are yellow-brown. Thecomas are solid, firm, and yellow or yellow-white with dense streaks and patches of hyalinized white tissue. Mixed granulosa-theca tumors are made firm and solid by the fibrotic thecal component.

Granulosa cells have uniform, small, oval or rounded nuclei, with a fold or cleft in the nuclear membrane. The cells are distributed in masses with little intervening stroma. Ultrastructural studies support and extend the resemblance to normal granulosa cells.[557] Characteristic rosettelike structures, or Call-Exner bodies, are nearly always present; they are rounded masses of pink inspissated material surrounded by a circular row of typical granulosa cells and resemble structures found in the normal graafian follicle (Fig. 34-75). Unlike acini,

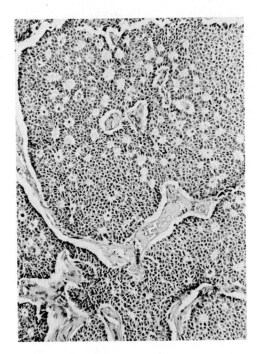

Fig. 34-75. Granulosa cell tumor. Many rounded spaces (Call-Exner bodies) containing amorphous eosinophilic material are scattered among uniform small cells with compressed-appearing nuclei. Compare with Fig. 34-59. Strands of hyalinized stroma are characteristic feature. (70×.)

with which they are often confused, the central cytoplasmic margins are indistinct, there is no stainable mucin, and the nuclei tend to lie adjacent to the inner rim of the space.

A variety of microscopic patterns occur; microfollicular and macrofollicular tumors resemble clusters of small or large graafian follicles. The descriptive terms *trabecular, insular, gyriform, solid tubular,* and *diffuse* are often applied, without significant clinical correlations. Paradoxically the cystic macrofollicular tumors produce androgenic effects.[550] The so-called sarcomatoid variety, in which large masses of granulosa cells tend to form swirling patterns of somewhat spindle-shaped cells, may have a more aggressive natural history.[538] Scully[580] has identified a distinctive juvenile pattern, chiefly prepubertal, in which both granulosa and thecal components are strikingly luteinized.

The most consistent indicator of aggressive behavior has been the presence of metastases or invasion of structures outside the ovary at the time of diagnosis.[481,499,504,549] Also unfavorable but less significant factors are large tumor size, increasing age, abdominal symptoms, and tumor rupture. Frequent mitoses correlate poorly with prognosis in my experience and that reported by Norris and Taylor.[549]

Thecomas are solid fibrotic masses in which some of

the spindle-shaped cells that form the tumor are plump and rounded and contain abundant cytoplasm that reacts with lipid stains. Another characteristic feature is the presence of hyaline plaques.

Granulosa-theca cell tumors characteristically produce estrogenic hormones, but they are occasionally androgenic. Using immunohistochemical techniques Kurman, Goebelsmann, and Taylor[532] found that granulosa and theca cells both produce a wide range of steroid hormones, but the chief product of granulosa cells is estradiol, and luteinized theca cells make progesterone.

The most common symptom is uterine bleeding. Women with estrogen-secreting granulosa-theca cell tumors often have endometrial hyperplasia. Well-differentiated endometrial adenocarcinoma occurs in 9%[549] to 24%[541] of cases in postmenopausal women. Although the morphologic features of these adenocarcinomas meet the criteria of a well-differentiated adenocarcinoma, they have a remarkably good prognosis; reports of death or metastasis related to these cancers are very difficult to find. It is possible that some of these endometrial carcinomas are highly estrogen dependent and therefore fail to progress when the source of estrogen is withdrawn.

Less than 5% of granulosa cell tumors are bilateral. Over 90% of the patients studied by Norris and Taylor[549] survived for 10 years, and some had residual tumor. Recurrences continued to appear as late as 25 years after original treatment. Studies that report a less favorable prognosis[481,504] include a larger proportion of poorly differentiated tumors with a high mitotic rate than I have encountered. It is reasonable to conserve the opposite ovary and uterus of a young woman with a small tumor confined to one ovary. Thecomas can be regarded as invariably benign.

Fibroma. Large fibrous tumors of the ovary without clinical or morphologic evidence of endocrine activity are relatively common, forming about 5% of all ovarian tumors in most large series. Densely collagenized fibrous tissue forms a monotonous histologic pattern, broken by areas of calcification in some cases. Occasionally there may be an associated benign ascites and pleural effusion, which disappear when the tumor is resected (Meigs' syndrome).

Fibrosarcoma is extremely rare.

Sertoli-Leydig cell tumors (arrhenoblastoma, androblastoma). Although Sertoli-Leydig cell tumors often produce androgens and masculinize the patient, many are hormonally inert, and some even have estrogenic effects.[544] Testosterone and a variety of androgenic precursors may be secreted in variable proportions. In an immunohistochemical study Kurman and associates[534] demonstrated both testosterone and estradiol in Sertoli cells, in Leydig cells, and also in less-differentiated stromal cells. Although their histologic patterns resemble those of developing male gonadal structures, Sertoli-Leydig cell tumors arise from the same female sex cord stromal cells as granulosa-theca cell tumors and consistently contain female sex chromatin.[554] Some ultrastructural studies confirm a closer relationship to ovarian stroma than to the testis[520,526]; however, the finding of cilia and other structures[522] leaves the subject unsettled.

Three histologic types are distinguishable. Well-differentiated tumors form tubular structures composed of Sertoli cells, separated by a fibrous stroma, intermixed with large round Leydig cells in poorly circumscribed clumps (Fig. 34-76). Tumors of intermediate differentiation have a biphasic pattern in which large pink Leydig cells are prominent, separated by a spindly stroma in which the abortive tubule formation resembles early sex cords of the embryonic testis (Fig. 34-77). A few tumors contain unexpected heterologous elements such as neoplastic mucinous glands, cartilage, and rhabdomyoblasts.[580]

Least differentiated is the sarcomatoid variety, composed of spindle cells that condense focally into a vague trabecular arrangement, separated by a looser myxoid component composed of the same type of cell. Leydig cells may or may not be present.

About half the well-differentiated tumors, three fourths of intermediate tumors, and all sarcomatoid tumors are androgenic. Pure Sertoli cell tumors occur in younger women and children; most cause hyperestrinism, including isosexual precocious puberty in children, but few have caused virilization.[594]

Nearly all Sertoli-Leydig cell tumors are benign, despite reports indicating malignant behavior in more than 20%; it has been suggested that the higher figures resulted from inclusion of other kinds of adenocarcinoma, primary and metastatic, with functioning stroma.[554]

Pathologic features that correlate with poor prognosis and rupture with or without extraovarian spread at the time of diagnosis, poor differentiation, and heterologous mesenchymal elements.[607,608] Malignant behavior takes the form of intraabdominal implantation, ordinarily without distant metastases.

Gynandroblastoma. Rarely, a sex cord stromal tumor may include both granulosa-theca cell and Sertoli-Leydig cell patterns.[551] Most have been benign. Those with hormonal function have produced androgens. Authentic examples are extremely rare.

Lipid cell tumors

Lipid cell tumors are a distinctive group of neoplasms that occur in the form of soft yellow or yellow-brown nodules. Examples are hilum cell tumors, "adrenal rest" tumors, and luteomas. The cells that compose them may be relatively small and rounded with dense

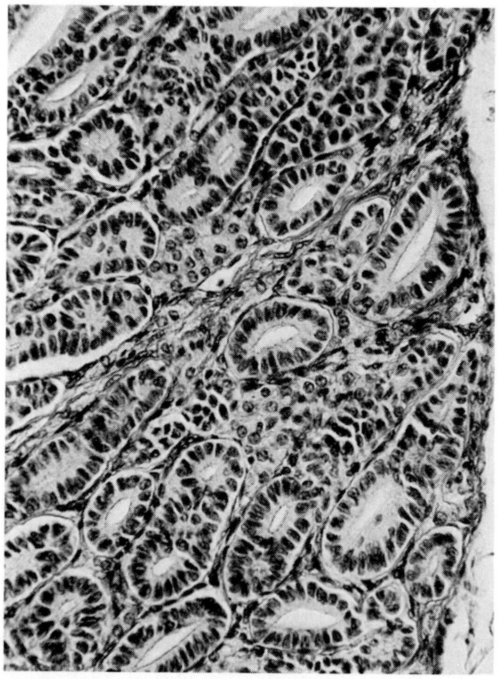

Fig. 34-76. Well-differentiated Sertoli-Leydig cell tumor, forming small tubules composed of Sertoli cells. Leydig cells are scattered through stroma *(center)*. (250×.)

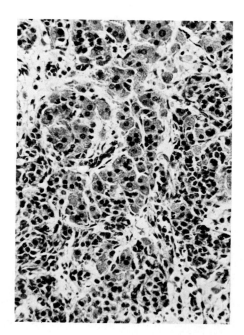

Fig. 34-77. Moderately differentiated intermediate type of Sertoli-Leydig cell tumor. Large, dense, eosinophilic Leydig cells are intermixed with cordlike strands of smaller Sertoli cells in a loose, sparsely cellular stroma. (275×.)

Table 34-4. Status of contralateral ovary in patients with stage I germ cell tumors of ovary

Tumor	Number of patients		Number of stage Ia patients with microscopic involvement of opposite ovary	
	Stage Ia	Stage Ib	Number examined microscopically	Number positive
Dysgerminoma	71	7	21	4
Endodermal sinus tumor	51	0	24	0
Immature teratoma	40	0	6	0
Embryonal carcinoma	9	0	0	0
Mixed germ cell tumor	20	0	5	1

Courtesy Drs. Robert J. Kurman and Henry J. Norris, Washington, D.C.

pink cytoplasm or larger with foamy or clear cytoplasm. Occasionally the smaller cells may contain crystalloids of Reinke, as in testicular Leydig cells and ovarian hilum cells. Both types of cells may occur in the same tumor. The ultrastructure is consistent with ovarian stromal origin; the cytoplasmic organelles resemble those of steroid-secreting cells,[526] such as the cells of the adrenal cortex. Crystalloids of Reinke must be identified to support classification as hilar Leydig cell or hilum cell tumor.

Most are benign. The few that behave aggressively are likely to be larger and to invade contiguous structures and may have atypical cytologic features.[595] The

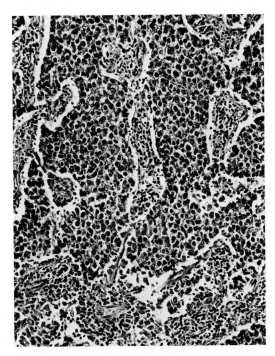

Fig. 34-78. Dysgerminoma. Masses of large uniform germ cells are separated by fibrous trabeculas that are infiltrated by lymphocytes. (130×.)

most common endocrine abnormality is virilization; a few have caused Cushing's syndrome.

Germ cell tumors

Ovarian germ cells are those that produce the female gametes—ova. They retain the capacity to produce an extremely diverse group of tissues in tumors. Most are benign cystic teratomas and occur chiefly in the young; malignant teratomas nearly always occur in children and young women. Optimum therapy depends on accurate identification and knowledge of the natural history of each type of neoplasm; various combinations of the different types are likely to occur.

Dysgerminoma. Dysgerminomas are large, solid, encapsulated masses of soft, gray-white tissue, often with foci of hemorrhage and necrosis. They are composed of large vesicular cells indistinguishable from the primordial germ cells of the embryonic gonad, distributed in large clumps and masses separated by fibrous trabeculas (Fig. 34-78). The fibrous stroma is almost always infiltrated by lymphocytes and may contain sarcoidosis-like granulomas. This pattern is indistinguishable from that of testicular seminoma. About 10% are bilateral.[472] The opposite ovary may contain microscopic foci of dysgerminoma even when it appears grossly normal (Table 34-4); if it is to be preserved, biopsy with frozen-section examination is desirable.

Dysgerminoma is extremely radiosensitive and curable with radiotherapy even in the presence of metastases. Thus, since most patients are young, unilateral oophorectomy is desirable and sufficient when the opposite ovary is normal. The 5-year survival rate is between 70% and 90%. For pure dysgerminoma limited to one ovary, the 5-year survival rate in one large series[512] was 94% for patients whose treatment was limited to resection of the affected ovary. The occasional dysgerminoma that contains syncytiotrophoblastic giant cells looks worse but does not behave more aggressively.[609] These tumors may produce human chorionic gonadotropin (HCG); all patients should be tested for it by radioimmunoassay of serum or urine, since HCG can serve as a tumor marker for early detection of recurrence.

Endodermal sinus tumor. Teilum[598] has established endodermal sinus tumor as a morphologically distinct entity. The most specific feature of this rare neoplasm is the presence of isolated papillary projections with a central blood vessel and peripheral sleeve of malignant embryonic epithelial cells (Fig. 34-79). Cross sections of this structure once were erroneously compared with immature glomeruli. In fact, they closely resemble invaginations of yolk sac endoderm, as seen best in the rat placenta, forming the endodermal sinuses of Duval.[598] Another distinctive feature is the presence of periodic acid–Schiff–positive, diastase-resistant hyaline globules partly composed of alpha-fetoprotein.[599] Some tumors contain multiple gland spaces with an hourglass constriction resembling yolk sac vesicles, a pattern that Teilum has designated polyvesicular vitelline tumor.

The gross appearance is much like that of dysgerminoma except for the more extensive yellow and red areas of hemorrhage and necrosis and the often present cystic areas. Endodermal sinus tumors consistently produce alpha-fetoprotein, which can be demonstrated in tissue sections by immunohistochemical techniques[599] and in the patient's serum.[476] This substance is produced in the yolk sac of the developing embryo and may serve as a tumor marker in evaluating the course of the patient after treatment. All the patients have been children or young adults. The prognosis is very poor; remissions have occurred in some patients treated postoperatively with multiple chemotherapeutic agents. Bilateral involvement in stage I is unlikely (Table 34-4).

Embryonal carcinoma. Embryonal carcinoma is an uncommon germ cell tumor that has been confused with endodermal sinus tumor, which it resembles. The patients are young, have an abdominal mass, and consistently have positive pregnancy test results because the tumors produce HCG. Premenarchal girls undergo precocious puberty. The histologic pattern resembles that of testicular embryonal carcinoma: large primitive anaplastic cells form solid masses interspersed with glandlike clefts and scattered giant cells. The multinucleated giant cells of syncytiotrophoblastic types are common, and immunohistochemical studies have shown that they contain HCG.[523] Similarly, mononuclear embryonal cells contain alpha-fetoprotein. Both substances can and should be used as tumor markers to evaluate therapeutic response and detect recurrence early.

Although these tumors are highly malignant, chemotherapy has resulted in some long-term survivors. There is little to gain from resecting a normal-appearing opposite ovary (tested by biopsy), since most tumors are unilateral, and occult metastases probably lie elsewhere.

Polyembryoma. Some germ cell tumors contain large numbers of embryoid bodies that closely resemble an early embryo, typically distributed in a primitive mesenchymal stroma.

Choriocarcinoma. Nongestational primary choriocarcinoma of the ovary is rare and malignant. The histologic pattern and clinical correlations are similar to those of gestational choriocarcinoma (p. 1709), except that the remarkable response to chemotherapy usually does not occur. There have been occasional survivors.[517]

Teratomas. Teratomas are composed of recognizable

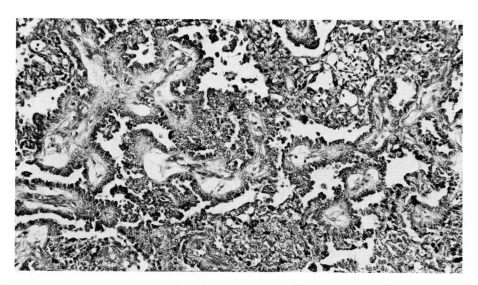

Fig. 34-79. Endodermal sinus tumor. There is a tangle of papillary processes with central blood vessel, usually covered by single layer of anaplastic germ cells; stroma is inconspicuous. (150×.)

tissues of ectodermal, mesodermal, and endodermal origin, in any combination. They are common and usually benign and inert but rarely produce remarkably bizarre and varied syndromes, reflecting the diverse potentials of the germ cell.

Benign cystic teratoma (dermoid cyst). Cystic teratomas are composed of mature somatic tissues of almost every description. Most cysts are unilocular, and the tissue that forms the lining is usually skin (Fig. 34-80). The desquamated keratin and secretions, notably from sebaceous glands, accumulate with masses of hair to fill the lumen of the cyst. This disagreeable mixture is liquid at body temperature but solidifies when chilled. Other common components are salivary gland; bronchus; fat; smooth muscle; cartilage; bone; neural tissue, including ganglia, glia, and choroid plexus; retina; pancreas; thyroid; and teeth. Characteristically a protuberance from the inner surface is the locus of growth of most of the hair and the richest depository of odd tissues. Uncommon tissues are skeletal and cardiac muscle, kidney, and liver.

In collected series bilateral teratomas occurred in 8% to 15% of cases. Cystic teratomas comprise 20% of all ovarian tumors in adults and 50% of all ovarian tumors in children. Most patients are between 20 and 40 years, but the tumors occur at all ages. Roentgenograms often are diagnostic, especially when teeth or bone is present. Most patients are operated on because a mass was discovered during a physical examination.

The pathogenesis of teratomas has always excited speculation because of their exotic composition; Blackwell and associates[482] have made an interesting historical review of this subject. Analysis of more recent cytogenetic studies using chromosome-banding techniques indicates that ovarian teratomas are parthenogenetic tumors that must originate from a single germ cell after its first meiotic division.[537]

Malignant change in a cystic teratoma is certainly less frequent than the 1.8% of cases reported[558] because most benign teratomas are not reported. Almost any component may become malignant; epidermoid carcinoma is most common, but sweat gland carcinoma, thyroid carcinoma, malignant melanoma, and various sarcomas, including osteosarcoma, occur rarely.

Solid teratomas (teratomas with abundant solid tissue and relatively small cysts) are nearly all malignant (as discussed subsequently), but a few benign solid teratomas have been reported.[600] All the tissue components of a benign solid teratoma are as mature as the other tissues of the patient in whom they occur.

Immature teratoma (malignant teratoma). Malignant teratoma is a unilateral solid mass with a heterogeneous appearance on cut surface. The histologic pattern is also extremely variable; many tissues have an embryonic appearance, with numerous mitoses. Islands of immature cartilage, bone, and glandular structures are distributed through a poorly differentiated stroma of actively growing spindle-shaped myxoid or undifferentiated sarcoma cells (Fig. 34-81). Bilateral involvement in patients with stage I malignant teratoma is rare (Table 34-4).

Relatively mature (grade I) malignant teratomas have a good prognosis, whereas immature teratomas (grade III) have an extremely poor prognosis.[533,563] The relative amount of primitive neuroepithelial tissue is an important factor in grading and determining the prognosis.[533] Areas of endodermal sinus tumor, embryonal carcinoma, and choriocarcinoma are extremely unfavorable. Tumors that lack these structures but have an abundant neural component—resembling ganglioneuroblastoma—are more unpredictable; nearly half these patients survive for 2 years. The neural component, even in peritoneal implants, may mature, leaving well-differentiated glial vestiges on the peritoneal surfaces. Although they may persist for many years, mature glial implants are innocuous and not a basis for radical treatment.[563] Therefore the grading of metastases, once they have occurred, is also prognostically important.[533] In contrast to the dismal results obtained by surgery or radiation in the past, combination chemotherapy had produced remarkable results resulting in over 70% survival.[508]

Specialized teratomas. Rare teratomas composed solely of thyroid tissue are usually benign but may function and even cause thyrotoxicosis.[546] Carcinoid tumors with the insular pattern typical of midgut derivatives[562] and trabecular carcinoids of the foregut and hindgut type also occur as primary ovarian tumors. The latter type may be mixed with thyroid tissue. Both are nearly always unilateral and benign; insular carcinoids, especially if large, may cause the carcinoid syndrome. On

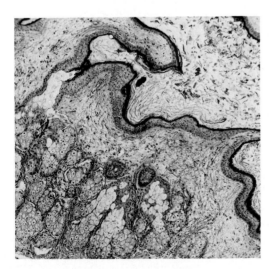

Fig. 34-80. Lining of typical benign cystic teratoma (dermoid cyst) is composed chiefly of skin with sebaceous glands, hair follicles, and sweat glands. (75×; AFIP 510588-07023.)

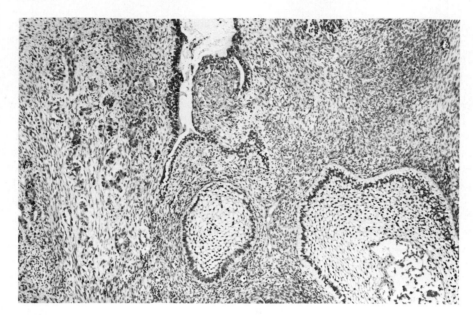

Fig. 34-81. Malignant teratoma. In addition to differentiated structures, there is an embryonic stroma resembling sarcoma *(upper right)*. (80×.)

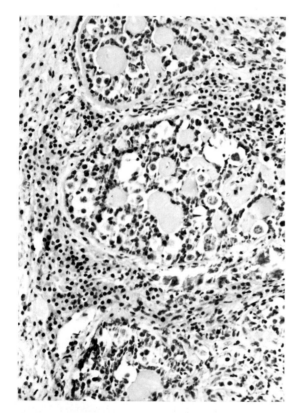

Fig. 34-82. Gonadoblastoma. Large germ cells and hyaline globules are intermixed with smaller granulosa cells, forming islands or nests. Clumps of Leydig cells are scattered through intervening stroma. (160×; courtesy Dr. Jerzy Teter, Warsaw, Poland; from Scully, R.E.: Androgenic lesions of the ovary. In Grady, H.G., and Smith, D.E., editors: The ovary, Baltimore, 1963, The Williams & Wilkins Co.)

the other hand, intestinal carcinoids metastatic to the ovary are usually bilateral and have a poor prognosis. It is especially important to distinguish them from granulosa cell tumors and Sertoli-Leydig cell tumors, as well as from primary ovarian carcinoids.[562]

Mixed forms. Germ cell tumors occur in various combinations. Solid areas in the wall of a cystic teratoma deserve careful study, since they may represent a locus of endodermal sinus tumor or other malignant category with a greatly different prognosis and implications for further treatment.

Malignant mixed germ cell tumors (stage I) have a poor prognosis if more than one third of the tumor consists of endodermal sinus tumor, choriocarcinoma, or stage III teratoma. Tumors that contain less than one third of these components or contain combinations of dysgerminoma, embryonal carcinoma, or stage I or II teratoma have a good prognosis. Patients with tumors less than 10 cm in diameter are more likely to survive regardless of tumor composition.[533]

Gonadoblastoma. Gonadoblastoma is a rare tumor that may arise in a dysgenetic gonad. The patients are usually phenotypic females, but nearly all are genotypic males (that is, have a Y chromosome). The tumor contains both immature germ cells and sex cord–stromal cells, which resemble granulosa or Sertoli cells, growing in small islands, intermixed with rounded pink hyaline bodies. Leydig cells or lutein cells are distributed through the intervening stroma in about two thirds of the cases (Fig. 34-82). Small calcifications may be extensive and have a distinctive roentgenographic pat-

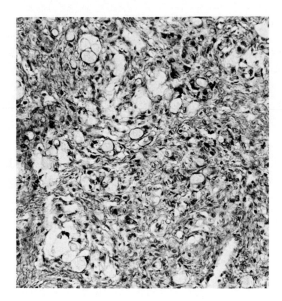

Fig. 34-83. Metastatic adenocarcinoma to ovary from stomach. Signet-ring cells and small acini are present. Stromal cells are hyperplastic. (150×.)

tern. Most are benign, but dysgerminomas and other malignant germ cell tumors develop occasionally.[578]

Metastatic carcinoma

Metastatic carcinomas represent 6% of ovarian cancers encountered in the course of surgical exploration of the abdomen. The primary site in most instances is the colon, stomach, or breast; it may be small and difficult to locate, even when the ovarian metastases are large.

The characteristic pattern of growth is diffuse infiltration of the ovarian stroma by strands and small nests of poorly differentiated carcinoma cells, forming a solid mass. The external surface is knobby and smooth. The eponymic designation of "Krukenberg's tumor" is usually reserved for this typical presentation when the tumor cells have large eccentric mucin vacuoles (signet-ring cells) and the primary site is the stomach (Fig. 34-83). The same pattern rarely occurs in a lesion that seems to be primary in the ovary after a thorough search for extraovarian primary carcinoma.[521] Because of wide variation in the use of this name, it is essentially useless; since Krukenberg's original paper erroneously concluded that the tumors were primary in the ovary, there is little point in clamoring for a rigorous use of this term for metastatic carcinoma. Colon cancers metastatic to the ovary may secrete enough mucin to produce cystic cavities; distinction in these cases from primary mucinous carcinoma of the ovary may be difficult. The dense cytoplasmic eosinophilia, sharp apical margins of the cells that line gland spaces, and lack of a

component to mucinous epithelial cells are helpful markers to suggest a colonic primary.[602]

The most important clinical correlation is the surprising fact that the ovarian metastases are often the only metastases apparent, and if they and the primary lesion are resected, the patient may live without symptoms for several years. For this reason ovarian metastases should generally be resected.

The basis for the selective enhancement of growth of certain adenocarcinoma cells in the ovary is unexplained. It is of interest that most of the patients are premenopausal, about a decade younger than those with primary ovarian adenocarcinoma; the phenomenon may be hormone dependent.

The ovarian stroma may be stimulated to secrete both androgenic and estrogenic hormones in the presence of metastatic carcinoma, especially colon carcinoma.

Malignant lymphoma

Like any other tissue, the ovaries may be involved by leukemic and lymphomatous infiltrate in patients with systemic disease. They rarely represent the primary locus of lymphoma, especially the poorly differentiated lymphocytic form of non-Hodgkin's lymphoma.[486] The ovaries, like the facial bones and orbital tissue, are preferential sites of involvement in Burkitt's lymphoma, including the American variety. An occasional instance of granulocytic leukemia has initially appeared as an ovarian tumor (so-called granulocytic sarcoma).[477]

The cells of diffuse lymphomas are often distributed in single-file rows, producing a histologic pattern easily confused with metastatic breast carcinoma of infiltrating lobular type.[555] Lymphomas limited to one ovary and those with a follicular (nodular) pattern have a better prognosis.[555]

Pathologic factors affecting prognosis

The foregoing discussion has emphasized that each different type of ovarian neoplasm is in fact a separate disease. There are other general characteristics that also affect the outcome of treatment.

Clinical stage. The extent of disease at the time of diagnosis is an important determinant of the outcome of therapy and must be stated in any comparison of effectiveness of different therapeutic techniques. The following internationally recognized criteria for staging primary ovarian carcinoma have been established by the International Federation of Gynecology and Obstetrics, based on findings at clinical examination and surgical exploration. The histology is to be considered in the staging, as is cytology as far as effusions are concerned.

Staging (FIGO)*: carcinoma of ovary

Stage I: Growth limited to the ovaries.

Stage Ia: Growth limited to one ovary; no ascites. No tumor on the external surface; capsule intact.

Stage Ib: Growth limited to both ovaries; no ascites. No tumor on the external surface; capsules intact.

Stage Ic: Tumor either stage Ia or stage Ib but with tumor on the surface of one or both ovaries; or with capsule ruptured; or with ascites present containing malignant cells; or with positive peritoneal washings.

Stage II: Growth involving one or both ovaries with pelvic extension

Stage IIa: Extension and/or metastases to the uterus and/or tubes.

Stage IIb: Extension to other pelvic tissues.

Stage IIc: Tumor either stage IIa or IIb but with tumor on the surface of one or both ovaries; or with capsule or capsules ruptured; or with ascites present containing malignant cells; or with positive peritoneal washings.

Stage III: Tumor involving one or both ovaries, with peritoneal implants outside the pelvis and/or positive retroperitoneal or inguinal nodes. Superficial liver metastasis qualifies as Stage III.

Stage IIIa: Tumor grossly limited to true pelvis, with negative nodes but with histologically confirmed microscopic seeding of abdominal peritoneal surfaces.

Stage IIIb: Tumor of one or both ovaries with histologically confirmed implants of abdominal peritoneal surfaces, none exceeding 2 cm in diameter. Nodes are negative.

Stage IIIc: Abdominal implants greater than 2 cm in diameter and/or positive retroperitoneal or inguinal nodes.

Stage IV: Growth involving one or both ovaries with distant metastases. If pleural effusion is present, there must be positive cytologic findings to allot a case to stage IV. Parenchymal liver metastases equals stage IV.

Special category: Unexplored cases that are believed to be ovarian carcinoma.

Stage is based on findings at *clinical examination* and surgical exploration. The final histology after surgery is to be considered in the staging, as well as cytology as far as effusions are concerned.

Ascites is peritoneal effusion that, in the opinion of the surgeon, is pathologic and/or clearly exceeds normal amounts.

---

*Cancer Committee of the International Federation of Gynecology and Obstetrics (FIGO), 1985, Obstet. Gynecol. **69:**138, 1987.

Implants. The significance of implants depends on the nature of the primary lesion. The prognosis is good, even in the presence of omental or other peritoneal implants, if the primary tumor is borderline.[579] It is extremely important to examine the undersurface of the diaphragm for distant metastases in establishing the stage of an ovarian cancer because this may be the only area with grossly evident metastases.[501]

Ascites. The significance of effusions depends on the nature of the primary lesion. Effusions associated with fibromas or Brenner tumors (Meigs' syndrome) are benign and do not recur after the tumor has been resected. Effusions that contain cancer cells, originating from an invasive ovarian cancer, indicate an average survival of 7.2 months.[529]

Rupture. The significance of rupture depends on the nature of the neoplasm. It has no demonstrable effect in the case of benign or borderline tumors. The prognosis of an invasive carcinoma, which is poor in any case, may be adversely affected, but it is difficult to demonstrate such a change convincingly.[514]

Metastases. The lymphatic drainage of the ovaries is directly to the aortic lymph nodes at the level of the renal veins. Biopsies inferior to this site are generally useless. From a study of aortic lymph node biopsy specimens it is clear that many ovarian cancers believed to be confined to the ovaries have actually produced lymph node metastases at the time of diagnosis.[528]

Role of pathologic study in management of apparently normal opposite ovary in young women. Preservation of an apparently normal ovary is extremely important in young women. A comparison of the results of ovarian conservation in the presence of apparently unilateral invasive carcinoma with a similar group of patients treated by bilateral ovariectomy shows no significant difference in survival.[545,565] On the other hand, Kottmeier[530] found that invasive serous carcinomas produced microscopic metastases that were grossly undetectable in a third of the patients in his series of 71 cases and recommended bilateral oophorectomy for this specific neoplasm in all cases.

PLACENTA*
Examination of placenta

The placenta is best examined fresh. The decisions to prepare for electron microscopy and to culture viruses,

---

*Although this entire chapter on pathology of the female genitalia derives heavily from the towering work of Arthur T. Hertig, the debt is nowhere as immense and obvious as in this section on the placenta. These illustrations and the words to describe them will be recognized by anyone who has so much as glanced at the subject, since they are unique and have been published necessarily by every writer who sets out to review the morphology of the early conceptus. The best and only completely original review of the subject is the monograph in which Hertig[674] summarizes earlier work done by himself and in collaboration with others.

bacteria, or tissues for cytogenetic study must be made immediately after delivery, based on historical data, physical examination of mother and infant, and gross inspection of the placenta itself. Subsequent examination of the placenta by a pathologist is not impeded seriously by refrigeration for a few hours.

The first step is to reconstruct the relationships of the membranous sac, with the width of the narrowest margin between the site of rupture and the placental margin being noted. Any margin at all excludes placenta previa.

After an inspection the membranes are cut away from the placental margin, rolled into a sausage-shaped structure, and held thus by transfixation with a pin; after fixation a cross section of this roll is submitted for microscopic study.

The cord is next examined and measured; the number of vessels is recorded. The cord is separated by a cut near the placenta, and the placenta is weighed. Placental weight when correlated with length of gestation and fetal weight provides highly significant information about growth, development, and neonatal prognosis.[705] Low placental weight associated with accelerated villous development indicates reduced uteroplacental blood flow and impaired development in childhood. Increased weight with villous edema indicates prenatal hypoxia with resulting neurologic abnormalities, respiratory distress syndrome, and death.[705] The surfaces are inspected for disruption or exudate. A whole mount of the amnion may be examined immediately for the presence of bacteria or sex chromatin. The placenta is then sliced in cross section like a loaf of bread, and representative blocks are cut for microscopic study. In order to evaluate the functional status of the placenta at the time of delivery, it is especially important to include *at least one section of normal-appearing placenta*. Infarcts and other grossly obvious abnormalities should be sampled, but these areas do not reflect overall placental development. A detailed protocol prepared for the National Institutes of Health collaboration study has been described with further comments about more specialized techniques.[674]

Development: anatomy and physiology

Significant stages in the formation of the placenta are as follows:

1. Implantation of the 6- to 7-day blastocyst occurs, with formation of solid trophoblast from its wall at the point of contact with the endometrium (Fig. 34-84, *A*).
2. Gradual peripheral orientation of the syncytiotrophoblast, in which vacuoles appear and then coalesce to form the intervillous space, occurs, with central orientation of the cytotrophoblast, which proliferates as isolated masses, forerunners of the primordial villi; these changes occur from the ninth to thirteenth day of development (Fig. 34-84, *B*).
3. Conversion of the cytotrophoblastic masses covered by syncytiotrophoblast to primordial villi occurs from the fourteenth to seventeenth day (Figs. 34-84, *C*, and 34-85, *D*).
4. Branching of primordial villi occurs from the eighteenth day through the first trimester; each primordial villus with its derivatives constitutes a cotyledon of the mature placenta (Fig. 34-85).
5. Gradual enlargement of the entire ovum occurs from the twentieth day to the twentieth week, resulting in the following.
   a. Obliteration of the entire uterine cavity by fusion of decidua capsularis and decidua vera
   b. Progressive thinning of the abembryonic chorion to become the chorion laeve
   c. Progressive growth of the amnion with gradual obliteration of the chorion cavity by fusion of chorionic and amniotic fibrous tissue
   d. Progressive growth of the chorion frondosum, forming eight to 15 cotyledons, constituting the placenta (Fig. 34-86)

Amnion

Significant phases in the formation of the amnion are as follows:

1. Its in situ delamination from the adjacent cytotrophoblast of the implanting ovum during the seventh to ninth day of development
2. Resulting formation of a veil-like membrane over and attached to the periphery of the circular concave germ disc during the ninth to thirteenth day of development (Fig. 34-84, *B*)
3. Gradual transformation of this membrane to amniotic epithelium during the fourteenth to twenty-fifth day of development (Fig. 34-84, *C*)
4. Simultaneous accumulation of a second mesoblastic layer
5. Progressive distension of the amniotic cavity, growth of the embryo, and its prolapse into the amniotic cavity
6. Gradual obliteration of the chorionic cavity by fusion of connective tissue of amnion and chorion

Umbilical cord

Significant stages in the formation of the umbilical cord are as follows:

1. Its origin as a mass of chorionically derived mesoblast at the caudal end of the embryonic disc when the latter develops its longitudinal axis during the fourteenth to sixteenth day (Fig. 34-85, *C*)
2. Gradual shifting of the caudally located body stalk to a more ventrally situated umbilical cord as the embryo grows caudally
3. Gradual prolapse of the embryo accompanied by

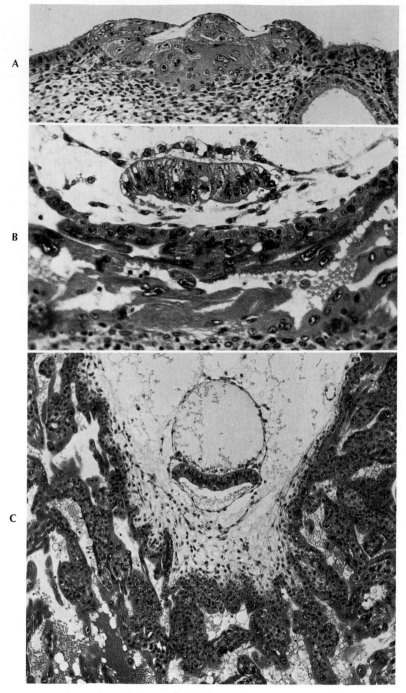

Fig. 34-84. A, Human 7½-day ovum superficially implanted for 36 hours on edematous 22-day secretory endometrium. Notice solid trophoblast, derived from blastocyst wall at its contact with endometrium and composed of pale cytotrophoblast and darker syncytiotrophoblast. **B,** Human 12½-day ovum showing embryonic disc *(above)* and adjacent trophoblast in contact *(below)* with predecidual stroma of 26-day secretory endometrium. Notice inner cytotrophoblast, beginning to form primordial chorionic villi, and outer syncytiotrophoblast, whose lacunar spaces contain maternal blood, beginning of uteroplacental circulation. **C,** Human 14-day ovum showing embryo *(upper center)* surrounded by early chorion frondosum. Notice simple unbranched primordial villi composed largely of central cytotrophoblastic core, beginning to form mesenchymal core and surrounded by syncytium, which lines intervillous space. (**A,** 150×; **B,** 250×; **C,** 100×; **A** to **C,** courtesy Department of Embryology, Carnegie Institution of Washington; **A** and **C,** Carnegie No. 7801; from Heuser, C.H., Rock, J., and Hertig, A.T.: Contrib. Embryol. **31:**85, 1945; **B,** Carnegie No. 7700; from Hertig, A.T., and Rock, J.: Contrib. Embryol. **29:**127, 1941.)

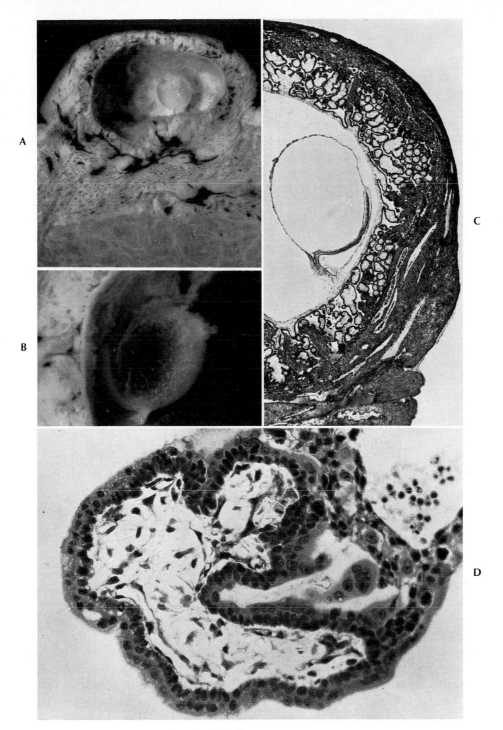

Fig. 34-85. Gross and microscopic aspects of chorionic, embryonic, and body stalk development at developmental age of 19 days (menstrual age of 33 days). **A,** Ovisac and implantation site bisected to show embryo, chorionic cavity, and chorionic villi around entire circumference. Thin decidua capsularis above, decidua vera laterally, and decidua basalis below, but above myometrium. For gross details of embryo viewed at right angles, see **B. B,** Embryo showing yolk sac with blood islands *(right),* curved germ disc *(left),* and crescent-shaped amniotic cavity between chorionic membrane *(extreme left)* and body stalk *(below).* For microscopic details (in mirror image), see **C. C,** Midsagittal section of embryo, body stalk, and adjacent chorion, the last representing one half of chorion and including both chorion laeve *(top)* and chorion frondosum *(bottom).* **D,** Detail of chorionic villus from pregnancy comparable to that shown in **A** to **C.** Notice immature stroma containing developing blood vessels. Trophoblast consists of outer syncytium and inner Langhans' epithelium. Between streamers of solid trophoblast *(upper right)* are maternal blood cells within intervillous space. (**A,** 4×; **B** and **C,** 12×; **D,** 300×. **A** to **D,** Courtesy Department of Embryology, Carnegie Institution of Washington; Carnegie Numbers: **A,** 8671, seq. 2; **B,** 8671, seq. 6; **C,** 8671, sect. 10-4-2; **D,** 5960, sect. 5-2-1; **D,** from Hertig, A.T.: Contrib. Embryol. **25:**37, 1935.)

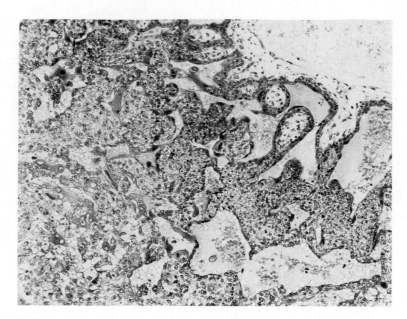

Fig. 34-86. Primordial chorionic villi from normal human placenta of approximately 15 days' gestation. These villi *(upper right)* are comparable to that shown in Fig. 34-85, *D,* and are continuous with cytotrophoblast of cell column and placental floor. The latter is contiguous with decidual basalis *(left margin).* Remnants of peripheral syncytiotrophoblast appear as giant cells *(center)* from which placental site giant cells will be derived. (150×.)

its cord into the amniotic cavity and simultaneous covering of the cord by amniotic epithelium

Chorionic villi

The immature villi are covered by an outer layer of syncytiotrophoblast and an inner layer of cytotrophoblast cells (Fig. 34-85, *D*). The latter divide, mature, and become incorporated into the growing syncytiotrophoblast layer, a process that is virtually completed by the sixteenth week. Only syncytiotrophoblast is evident thereafter. The capillary vessels are very small. The stromal core contains fibroblasts, collagen, and Hofbauer cells, which are macrophages with very large vacuoles that apparently result from the imbibition of large amounts of water.[656] In mature placental villi the cytotrophoblast cells have disappeared, the stroma is scant, capillaries are multiple with thin walls, and the immensely active syncytiotrophoblast layer is thin, except where nuclei accumulate into clusters or knots. The morphology of placental anatomy and development has been described in detail in the beautifully illustrated monographs by Hertig[674] and Boyd and Hamilton.[631]

The syncytiotrophoblast cells of the villi are responsible for sorting and distributing nutrients to the fetus and fetal metabolic by-products back to the mother and for synthesizing a remarkable variety of hormones. Placental functions are so numerous and placental products so varied that a completely satisfactory clinical test of placental function remains to be elaborated. The steroid hormones include estrogens, progesterone, androgens, adrenocorticosteroids, and aldosterone. The placental peptide hormones include HCG, chorionic somatomammotropin (HCS), also called human placental lactogen (HPL), chorionic thyrotropin, and adrenocorticotropic hormone. These placental activities have been summarized in monographs by Jaffe[684] and Gruenwald.[667] An additional group of placental peptides for which definite functions have not been established are pregnancy-specific beta$_1$-glycoprotein (SP1), pregnancy-associated plasma protein-A (PAPP-A), and others.[691] When the exact cell origin of substances identified in the mother during gestation involves fetal and placental tissues together, the metabolic products are considered to define the functional status of the fetoplacental unit; for example, the amount of estriol in maternal urine is dependent on fetal adrenal glands and liver, as well as the placenta, and a decline indicates a threat to survival of the fetus, though the site of the lesion responsible may not have been determined.

HCG alters the maternal immune response and is probably an important factor in the survival of the placental allograft. Trophoblast is antigenic.[627,681] Circulating HCG levels throughout pregnancy are not so high as those required for complete in vitro inhibition of lymphocyte transformation[613] or mixed lymphocyte culture reaction. However, local concentrations in the syn-

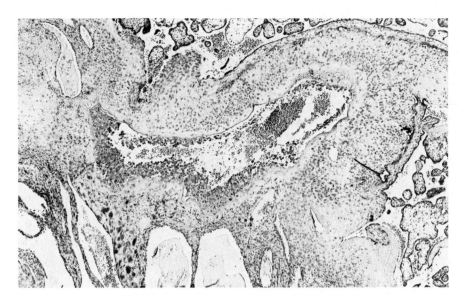

Fig. 34-87. Decidual spiral arteriole *(center)* during fifth month, showing dilatation, replacement of endothelium by intermediate trophoblast, and hyalinization of vessel wall. Decidua is infiltrated by intermediate trophoblast cells at lower left. Placental villi are at top, and dilated decidual glands are at bottom center. (40×.)

cytiotrophoblast layer are very high in comparison with those in other tissues.[647,651] There seems to be an important electronegative barrier of sialic acid (an HCG moiety) at the syncytiotrophoblast surface.[710] This surface is the interface between maternal and fetal tissues and ultimately the locus at which accommodation between the two must be settled. Of great interest is the apparent paradox that maternal sensitization to trophoblast, which must be blocked for the placenta to survive, actually enhances implantation and subsequent fetal growth.[623]

One postulated protective factor active soon after implantation is uteroglobin, a protein activated locally in the uterus by transglutaminase. Uteroglobin appears to cross-link with embryonic transplantation antigens, masking them from maternal immune response. In addition, an immunologic blocking antibody, present in maternal serum, is necessary for successful pregnancy; women without it abort repeatedly.[668,727] It is actually genetic compatibility between parents that seems to mediate this cause of habitual abortion.

One important line of cancer research is based on the similarity between cancer cells and trophoblast: cancers produce HCG and other placental hormones[745]; they also recapitulate the placental capacity for immunologic hiding.[664]

The dynamics of placental circulation are unique. Maternal blood from the uterine arteries works its way through the uterine wall into the spiral arterioles of the maternal endometrium (now decidua vera) and empties in spurts into the intervillous space of the placenta. The

openings of the spiral arterioles are distributed about the placental floor; between them are the openings of the decidual veins, through which blood from the intervillous space returns into the maternal venous system.

In the early weeks of pregnancy an extremely important sequence of changes enlarges the flow capacity of the decidual spiral arteries. The trophoblast cells of the outer margin of the conceptus invade opened ends of these small arteries, replace the endothelium, and infiltrate the muscular walls; the muscular layer and elastic tissue are destroyed (Fig. 35-87). By the middle of the second trimester this change has extended to involve the myometrial segments of the spiral arteries. The result is a group of 100 to 150 tortuous, greatly widened, funnel-shaped arterial channels—the true uteroplacental arteries—with walls composed of fibrinoid material and a lining of trophoblast. Thus the placenta must structure its vascular supply line.

Kurman and others[692] have emphasized the functional importance of a third group of trophoblast cells, which they have called "intermediate trophoblast," as contrasted with the syncytiotrophoblast and cytotrophoblast of the villi. These placental site trophoblast cells invade the maternal decidua as well as the spiral arteries and have distinctive and different activities as shown by their immunocytochemical properties.

The fetal circulation begins with the umbilical arteries, which come to the placenta through the umbilical cord. The umbilical arteries divide and redivide in the placenta, ultimately into small capillaries of the villi, and return through tributaries of the umbilical vein into the umbilical cord.

The intervillous space is a single vast pool of maternal blood in which the placental villi dangle, rootlike, with margins sealed by tight contact between decidua and placental membranes. There is no "marginal sinus" in the sense of an anatomic walled structure to collect maternal blood before its return to the uterus. A premature separation at this margin may allow maternal blood to leak out rapidly, an alarming event that is still called "marginal sinus tear."

Anomalies
Abnormal shapes

The umbilical cord usually inserts near the center of the placenta, but in about 10% of cases it may insert at the placental margin (battledore placenta). Less frequent (1%) but of greater potential importance is velamentous insertion, in which the cord runs for variable distances through the membranes before reaching the placenta. This fixes the location of the cord and may result in compression or even rupture if the area involved passes over the cervical outlet.

A placenta divided into two parts is bipartite; a small accessory succenturiate lobe is important as a cause of bleeding if left behind, an event that can be detected because the vessels that extend to it end abruptly at a tear in the membranes.

Single umbilical artery

In a series of 39,773 white and black single births, 0.9% of umbilical cords contained a single umbilical artery.[660] Fourteen percent of the infants so affected were stillborn or died in the neonatal period; of those on whom autopsies were performed, half were found to have significant congenital anomalies, chiefly affecting the cardiovascular or genitourinary system. Although the presence of a single umbilical artery implies a 10- to 20-fold increase in serious congenital malformations,

affected infants who survive the perinatal period have normal prospects, except for a 1 in 20 chance of developing an inguinal hernia.

Abnormalities of cord length are very important. Normal cords vary from 55 to 61 cm in total length. Segments removed for blood gas analysis must be taken into account. Short cords indicate probable reduced fetal movements and correlate with chronic neurologic abnormalities as well as cord rupture, uterine inversion, abruptions, and other problems during labor.[704] Long cords may prolapse or encircle fetal parts resulting in fatal cord compression or localized injuries.

Placenta membranacea

Persistence of villi surrounding the entire conceptus is called "placenta membranacea;" the situation is comparable to placenta previa, including the threat of severe hemorrhage.[659] Arteriographic studies may be misleading.[645]

Amnion nodosum

Amnion nodosum occurs with any condition resulting in extreme oligohydramnios, such as renal agenesis. Clusters of squamous cells, fibrin, and other amorphous debris become inspissated and form loosely attached plaques on the amnionic surfaces.[629] It should be distinguished from focal squamous metaplasia of the amnion, which is common around the insertion of the cord and has no known significance.

Multiple gestation

The question of genetic relationship in multiple pregnancy has increased importance because of the potential need for organ transplantation and because of the threatening implications of circulatory connections in monochorionic placentas. The relationships of the membranes are diagrammed in Fig. 34-88.

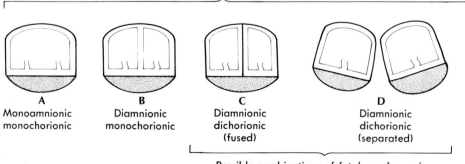

Possible combinations of fetal membranes in monozygous twin placenta (identical twins)

A	B	C	D
Monoamnionic monochorionic	Diamnionic monochorionic	Diamnionic dichorionic (fused)	Diamnionic dichorionic (separated)

Possible combinations of fetal membrane in dizygous twin placenta (fraternal twins)

Fig. 34-88. Diagram of common morphologic variations in twin placentation. Types **A** and **B** occur only in identical twins; types **C** and **D** are common to both. (From Kraus, F.T.: Gynecologic pathology, St. Louis, 1967, The C.V. Mosby Co.)

Dichorionic diamnionic twin placenta

If two separate zygotes implant concurrently, the placentas may fuse; the twins in this case are fraternal (not identical). Separate placentas (chorions) also result if a single zygote divides and the two daughter cells separate completely and implant; each will mature, producing identical twins. The fused placentas will be recognizable by a persistent ridge of chorion at the base of the septum between the two amnions after the amniotic membranes are stripped away. Histologic section of the septum shows two amnions and an intervening layer of chorion. It appears that about 20% of twins with this type of placenta are monozygotic (identical), and 80% are dizygotic (fraternal).[625]

Monochorionic diamnionic twin placentas

If two germ discs form after implantation of a single zygote, the twins (always identical) will share a single placenta. Vascular connections are large and easily demonstrated, and no chorionic ridge is present when the amnions are stripped away.[630] There is no layer of chorion (trophoblast) between the two amnions that fuse to form the septum between the amnionic cavities.

Monochorionic monoamnionic twin placentas

When there is no intervening septum, the twins (always identical) share the same amnionic cavity. The prospects for entanglement are great, and mortality is high.

Clinicopathologic correlation

In a series of 250 twin placentas carefully correlated by all possible factors to confirm zygosity (fraternal versus identical), 56% of placentas were dizygotic and 44% were monozygotic. Thirty percent of the monozygotic twins had dichorionic placentas, and 70% had monochorionic placentas; 3% of the latter had monochorionic monoamnionic placentas. Eighty percent of twins with dichorionic placentas are dizygotic. Thus, by examination of a twin placenta, one can conclude that the twins are definitely identical in the case of a monochorionic placenta and probably fraternal (four chances in five) in the case of a dichorionic placenta.[625]

Twins are exposed to greater risks of many kinds; both morbidity and mortality are increased. Malformations are more common than in single births; monozygotic twins sharing the same circulation both may be injured by unequal distribution, and prematurity is much more common. The abnormal relationships, causes, and pathologic physiology of multiple gestations have been comprehensively presented by Benirschke and Kim.[626]

Higher orders of multiple pregnancy

The same criteria of zygosity may be applied by examination of the septal membranes between adjacent amnionic cavities.

Abnormal implantation
Extrachorial implantation

In about 18% of deliveries the margins of the placenta lie submerged beneath the decidua. If the amnionic membrane extends to the placental rim and is reflected back toward the center, it is called a "circumvallate placenta" (Fig. 34-89). The amnion of a marginate placenta does not follow the placental rim beneath the decidua but continues out over the decidual surface. Scott[731] found no significant risk to mother or infant attributable to this relationship; there may be a slight increase in vaginal bleeding.

Placenta accreta

Placental separation at parturition occurs by cleavage through the decidua. If there is no intervening decidua,

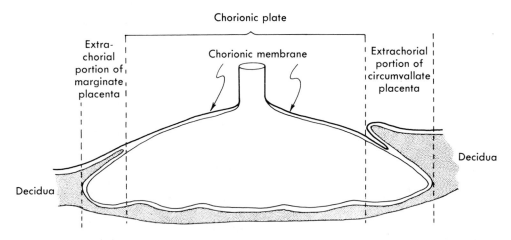

Fig. 34-89. Diagrams of placenta-uterus relationships in extrachorial placenta. (Modified from Scott, J.S.: J. Obstet. Gynaecol. Br. Cwlth. **67:**904, 1960.)

the villi become attached to the myometrium and will not separate. The condition may be complete over the entire base of the placenta or, more commonly, only partial; the villi may extend into the myometrium (placenta increta) or entirely through it, resulting in rupture (placenta percreta).[634] In all cases the placenta cannot be delivered, the uterus cannot contract, and hemorrhage is usually brisk. In most cases hysterectomy is necessary to control bleeding.

Ectopic pregnancy

Implantation may occur outside the uterine cavity. The most common site is the uterine tube. Less frequent sites include the interstitial part of the tube, the cervix, the ovary, and the intra-abdominal peritoneal surface.[633]

Tubal ectopic pregnancy usually occurs in a tube altered by prior inflammation, which apparently interferes with transport of the ovum. Fetal abnormalities also probably contribute to ectopic gestation; Poland, Dill, and Styblo[719] found embryos with gross abnormalities, apparently genetically induced, in about one fourth of a series of carefully examined ectopic pregnancies. In all sites there is a threat of rupture attended by severe hemorrhage. Maternal death, sudden, unexpected, and always a calamity, continues to challenge obstetricians and threaten their patients.[633,731]

The endometrium may or may not show gestational histologic changes, depending on the extent to which the gestation has progressed and the length of time between fetal death and onset of bleeding. It is important to note that no morphologic changes in the endometrium, including the presence of villi, will exclude an ectopic gestation; simultaneous intrauterine and ectopic gestations are uncommon but have been described with increasing frequency, mainly in women who were treated with gonadotropins in the management of infertility.[695] An occasional abdominal pregnancy is successfully terminated by cesarean section, but the fetal mortality exceeds 90%[622]; attempts at placental removal at delivery (laparotomy) may lead to serious hemorrhage.[680]

Placenta previa

After low implantation of a normal ovum the enlarging placenta may come to lie over the internal os of the cervix. Even before onset of labor the exposed maternal surface may be a source of bleeding, and with the onset of labor the certainty of massive hemorrhage necessitates cesarean section. Variable degrees of placenta accreta often accompany placenta previa, probably because of the generally deficient endometrium in the lower uterine segment.[674]

Spontaneous abortion (miscarriage)

The termination of a pregnancy, regardless of the mechanism, before the fetus can survive (if it is present) is called an abortion. Spontaneous abortion is usually the result of a pathologic ovum, infection, or maternal disease. Missed abortion is retention of a dead fetus longer than 2 months.

By far the most common abnormality leading to spontaneous abortion is a genetic defect of the conceptus. In about half of all spontaneous abortions the fetus is either absent or grossly malformed. Hertig[674] has written a detailed description and classification of various gross abnormalities. Cytogenetic studies have shown a chromosomal abnormality in about a third of the cases,[640] but the incidence was nearly 60% in a small series using more refined chromosome-banding techniques.[699] The most common chromosomal anomalies demonstrated have been triploidy, 45XO karyotype, and single autosomal trisomy.[624]

The decidua associated with spontaneous abortion shows hemorrhage, necrosis, and leukocytic infiltration. The endometrium away from the implantation site often shows the pattern of secretory gestational hyperplasia described by Arias-Stella.[297]

The chorionic villi may appear nearly normal or be surrounded by dense deposits of intervillous fibrin clot. In a majority of the cases in which the embryo is absent, the villous stroma is swollen and hydropic as the result of fluid accumulation. This is the hallmark of a "blighted" ovum and probably a result of continued trophoblast function in the absence of a vascular transport to carry the accumulated fluid, since there is no fetus. Hydropic villi have no direct significance for the mother and especially should not be confused with hydatidiform mole.

Philippe[716] has correlated cytogenetic studies of spontaneous abortions with histologic patterns. Invagination of the surface trophoblast into the core of the villus was found chiefly in instances of triploidy (Fig. 34-90). The pronounced hydropic change in the villi of triploid abortions has prompted the designation of "partial hydatidiform mole"[740]; it is important to recognize that hydatidiform mole is clinically, grossly, microscopically, and cytogenetically very different (as discussed later). Choriocarcinoma as a complication of a triploid abortion remains a remote possibility that has never been convincingly demonstrated.[624] Cases with autosomal trisomy show migration of occasional large cytotrophoblast cells into the villous stroma. Detailed examination of the embryo or fetus provides extremely important correlations with abnormal karyotypes including indications for genetic counseling and sometimes for parental karyotyping. Some combinations of facial clefts, abnormal digits, neural tube defects, impaired limb bud development, and others may correlate

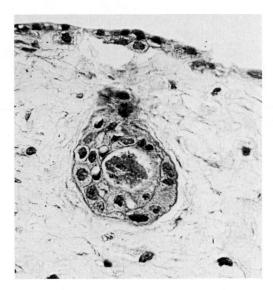

Fig. 34-90. Trophoblastic invagination in villus, shown in cross section. Chromosomal analysis of cultured cells showed a 69XXX triploid karyotype, which correlates consistently with this morphologic abnormality. (Courtesy Dr. Emile Philippe, Strasbourg, France.)

with specific abnormal karyotypes.[619] Occasional abortuses with large edematous winglike projections from the posterior area of the neck suggestive of hygromas have been shown to have a 45XO karyotype.[717]

Maternal factors in abortion include induced abortion and its complications, often related to infection. Infectious diseases generally have been considered to be an uncommon primary cause of spontaneous abortion. With the increased use of sophisticated microbiologic techniques, infections have been detected in increasing numbers; their role in abortion and fetal loss will have to be reevaluated. The organisms that have been implicated include herpesvirus,[661,708] cytomegalic inclusion virus,[646,703] virus of rubella,[712] *Listeria monocytogenes*,[720] *Toxoplasma gondii*,[617,649] and mycoplasmas.[670,679] Anaerobic bacteria are especially important in the pathogenesis of septic abortion and its maternal complications.[615] When compared with the pain and vast expense incurred by disabled living children injured by intrauterine infection, abortion may be one of the least problematic outcomes.

Toxemia of pregnancy (eclampsia and preeclampsia)

Toward the end of pregnancy, salt retention, edema, albuminuria, and hypertension develop in about 6% of women. This syndrome is called toxemia of pregnancy or preeclampsia. The most severe manifestation, eclampsia, is accompanied by convulsions; there is extensive intravascular coagulation with fibrin thrombi and focal necrosis in the liver, kidneys, and brain.

The pathogenesis of toxemia of pregnancy has been extensively studied but remains unexplained; theories are numerous.[712] The most significant pathologic lesion seems to be in the uterine spiral arteries. As described originally by Hertig,[673] there is fibrinoid necrosis of the walls of the terminal ends of the spiral arteries in the decidua. The myometrial segments of the uteroplacental arteries of the placental bed and the basal arteries that supply the decidua are also affected. In addition, there is an accumulation of foamy lipophages in the necrotic vessel walls and an infiltrate of small mononuclear cells in and around the vessels. These changes, called acute atherosis, begin with lipid accumulation in smooth muscle cells, necrosis of smooth muscle, exudation of fibrin into the vessel wall, and infiltration of the vessel wall by phagocytic macrophages that become swollen with accumulated lipid. They are often accompanied by thrombosis.[725]

Brosens, Dixon, and Robertson[636] have found that the physiologic trophoblastic invasion of placental bed spiral arteries (see p. 1697) does not extend into the myometrial segments of these vessels. These segments cannot expand and therefore represent a constriction between the proximal radial arteries and the distended distal segments in the decidua. It is in these areas that acute atherosis occurs. The similarity between acute atherosis and vascular changes in rejected renal allografts indicates that this placental vascular lesion may be the result of a local immunologic attack, which ordinarily is blocked by the physiologic invasion of trophoblast. Immunofluorescence studies provide some support for this.[690]

Complement-fixing immune complexes in maternal serum ultimately deposit in uterine spiral arteries and interfere with the necessary activities of the intermediate trophoblast; the resulting problems include preeclampsia and idiopathic intrauterine growth retardation.[694] Similar lesions occur in some women with diabetes mellitus, systemic lupus erythematosus, thrombocytopenia purpura, and chronic hypertension. Atherosis appears to be the basic lesion ultimately causing reduced blood flow to the placenta and impaired fetal development.[694]

Regardless of how they are produced, the lesions of acute atherosis impair blood flow to the placenta and to the decidua itself. In this ischemic background, placental infarction, retroplacental hematoma, premature placental separation, fetal distress, and the small fetus appear. The morphologic features of reduced uteroplacental blood flow upon the placenta itself are on p. 1703.

In experimental models of eclampsia McKay[701] has emphasized the similar features of the generalized Shwartzman reaction and the degenerative changes in the placental trophoblast. The placental lesions are not specific, but the ischemia and accentuation of degener-

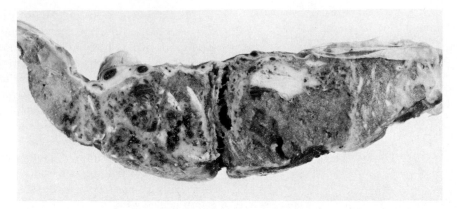

Fig. 34-91. Placental infarcts. Notice granular cut surface, mottled white and red of old and recent lesions, and irregular margins. The mother had severe toxemia.

ative changes produce a very abnormal pattern. Syncytiotrophoblast nuclei form tight clusters. Some are necrotic. The cytoplasm of the syncytiotrophoblast becomes vacuolated. The amount of intervillous fibrin material—always present at term—is increased. Infarcts are common and may be extensive.

Circulatory lesions

In addition to the changes more clearly related to toxemia, there are other disturbances in the vascular supply of the placenta and its decidual support. These include infarcts, hematomas, and vascular lesions resulting from systemic maternal disease and unrelated to pregnancy.

Infarcts

The blood supply that supports the placenta comes from the maternal circulation. Impaired maternal circulation in local areas produces placental infarcts; impaired fetal circulation results in avascular fibrotic villi, often in clusters.

The lesion responsible may be thrombosis of a group of decidual spiral arteries or atherosclerotic changes in branches of the uterine artery. A recent infarct appears red and granular. As the blood pigment is broken down and carried away, the infarct becomes progressively lighter, eventually achieving a pale yellow color (Fig. 34-91).

Small infarcts (less than 1 cm) in full-term placentas have no clinical significance, but they indicate low uteroplacental blood flow in preterm placentas; infarcts larger than 3 cm are all abnormal and are associated with increased perinatal mortality.[704] *Maternal floor infarcts* are characterized by extensive deposits of fibrin in the decidua basalis that extend to engulf the adjacent villi. The maternal surface of the placenta is indurated and has a convoluted "brainlike" appearance. Adjacent decidua may be focally necrotic and infiltrated by in-

flammatory cells.[706] Uteroplacental blood flow is reduced, mortality is high, and there may be an increased association with chorioamnionitis.

Intraplacental hematoma

Clots that develop in the intervillous space have a characteristic laminated pattern. They are red if recent and pale yellow if old. Since the villi are pushed aside as the hematoma forms, there are no villi in it, and the granularity of an infarct is not seen. The blood is of maternal origin.

A specific type of placental hematoma forms in the subchorionic area, producing a large tuberous mass. It usually but not always is associated with missed abortion and is called a "Breus mole"; there is no relationship to hydatidiform mole.[734]

Premature separation

The normally implanted placenta may become detached before the onset of labor. The bland decidual necrosis that disrupts the normal attachment may be the result of vascular disease, such as toxemia, or possibly poor nutrition, especially folic acid deficiency.[677]

The placenta is compressed by the clot that forms behind it (Fig. 34-92). As the result of consumption of clotting factors in this large hematoma, the circulating blood is depleted; thus there is a severe bleeding diathesis in at least one fifth of the patients. The uterine bleeding often leads to shock. The subsequent disseminated intravascular coagulation may be associated with bilateral renocortical necrosis and pituitary infarction. Any delay in delivery of the fetus results in prolonged anoxia and fetal death; the perinatal mortality is high.

Premature separation carries an increased risk of amniotic fluid embolism, a grave complication with a high mortality found also in women of high parity, with intrauterine fetal death or hypertonic labor, or with symptoms such as sudden onset of dyspnea, shock, or

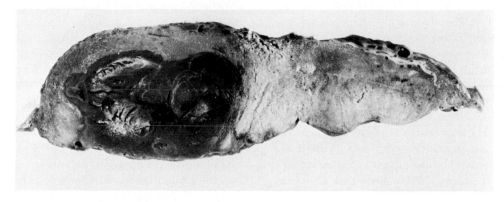

Fig. 34-92. Premature separation (abruptio placentae) with large hematoma that compresses overlying placenta.

disseminated intravascular coagulation.[715] The presence of amniotic fluid is not always easily identified at autopsy with standard histologic sections but is readily demonstrated with the colloidal iron stain for acid mucopolysaccharide.[726]

Reduced uteroplacental blood flow

An impaired vascular supply retards placental growth and fetal growth and is the major cause of fetal growth retardation, antenatal hypoxia, and stillbirth at delivery. The placenta is usually small for gestational duration, hence the importance of accurate recording of weight.[705] The placental villi under these circumstances are disproportionately small, trophoblastic knots are increased, and cytotrophoblast cells proliferate, a combination that is called "accelerated placental maturation."[704] The distribution of this lesion is uneven and patchy because some spiral arteries are affected more than others and villi at a distance from the source of supply are more severely affected. Because the placental margins generally are less well supplied, histologic sections from this area do not reflect the true state of overall placental blood supply. Obviously, more than one section of placenta is required to evaluate accelerated maturation; areas of infarct must be avoided for this purpose.

Prolonged gestation and the hypermature placenta

The threat of perinatal mortality increases in gestations that last longer than 42 weeks. One explanation is based upon recognition that fetal growth continues rapidly while placental growth slows down and at some point the placenta fails to support the rapidly growing fetus. Morphologic markers of functional inadequacy in this situation are uncertain. No specific changes have been identified. Kaufman and co-workers have noted "abnormal knoblike twisted and branched terminal

villi" in scanning electron micrographs.[687] It is probable that a variety of changes including increased intervillous fibrin deposits, meconium staining, and obliteration of fetal vessels sometimes resulting in fibrosis and villous edema all combine to impair adequate function of the post-term placenta.[748] Detailed correlation between gestational dates, clinical problems at delivery, fetal and placental weights, and multiple histologic sections are required to evaluate this problem adequately. Morphologic features of low uteroplacental blood flow are not evident.[704] The fetus continues to elongate at the expense of body fat stores, which become progressively depleted.

Villous edema

A major cause of hypoxia in preterm infants is villous edema.[704] The pathogenesis is unknown, but it is a common complicating factor in chorioamnionitis. It is most common between the twenty-fifth and thirty-second weeks and is uncommon in term placentas. According to Naeye it peaks shortly after the onset of a fetal stress event and then slowly recedes even though the basic problem continues; it is believed that compression of fetal vessels reduces blood flow and gas exchange, thus producing fetal anoxia.[704] It is a common indicator of fetal brain damage and usually signifies that a problem was well established before onset of delivery.

Atherosclerosis: essential hypertension and diabetes mellitus

Young women with essential hypertension who also happen to become pregnant have hyperplastic intimal atherosclerotic lesions affecting the myometrial segments of the spiral arteries of the placental bed. The lesions here are often disproportionately severe in comparison with similar vessels elsewhere in the body. If the arterial physiologic changes of pregnancy (p. 1697) progress normally, the prognosis for the fetus is good.[725] Decidual arterioles in diabetes mellitus may be thick walled with hyalinized media.[625] Either situation may be further complicated by lesions of atherosis if toxemia develops; the consequences are usually severe.

Haust[671] has illustrated in great detail the morphologic changes in the placenta and implantation site of diabetic mothers. The placentas are often large, and the edematous cords have increased diameter. The villi are large and appear immature with abundant stroma, increased numbers of Hofbauer cells, and prominent, sometimes continuous cytotrophoblast cells. Arterioles of the implantation site may have thickened walls and hyalinized media.

Infectious diseases

Intrauterine infection may be transplacental or may ascend from the vagina. Unquestionably infection is an underestimated cause of spontaneous abortion. Many birth defects once considered to be "acts of God" are now reliably ascribed to a specific infectious organism, notably viruses. The extent to which the cytogenetic alterations described in the section on abortions might be virus induced is essentially unexplored. Midtrimester abortion is especially likely to be the result of chorioamnionitis.[614] About one fourth of placentas of small-for-gestational-age infants show nonspecific villitis; the mortality for this group is 16%.[615]

Bacterial infections

Rupture of the fetal membranes before the onset of labor provides a path for ascending bacterial infection. If the infection is well developed by the time of delivery, purulent exudate may be obvious on gross inspection of the fetal surfaces of the placenta and membranes, and similar advanced infection may be presumed to exist in the infant's lungs. Microscopically a dense infiltrate of neutrophils obliterates the amniotic epithelium; bacterial colonies may or may not be present. In many instances an infiltrate of leukocytes and fibrin in the subchorionic plate of the placenta is the only histologic evidence of infection. The most common species of organisms are those that inhabit the vagina in pregnancy, including *Escherichia coli* and *Streptococcus*, *Proteus*, and *Pseudomonas* species and highly virulent anaerobes such as *Bacteroides* and *Peptostreptococcus* species. Colonization of the upper endocervix by bacteria that release proteolytic enzymes may represent the initiating factor that predisposes to membrane rupture. Many of the organisms involved also produce phospholipase A_2, which initiates prostaglandin synthesis and thereby stimulates the onset of labor.

Placental tuberculosis occurs rarely as a combination of miliary spread in the mother. Syphilis may cause villitis and fetal endovasculitis, but none of the gross or microscopic changes is specific for *Treponema pallidum*

infection. Group B streptococcus, which is rarely a human pathogen, colonizes the vagina of 3% to 25% of pregnant women. Transmission to the fetus, which can cause pneumonia and meningitis, takes place only if maternal antibodies fail to develop. Vaginal colonization is detected by culture, since the women are asymptomatic; antibiotic coverage may not be necessary in the presence of adequate antibody response.[618]

The morphologic lesion in the placenta produced by bacterial growth in the amniotic fluid is *acute chorioamnionitis*. The earliest reliable evidence in the placenta is accumulation of maternal neutrophils at the underside of the chorionic plate, followed by migration into the connective tissues of the chorionic plate and finally to the amnion itself. The earliest changes will be recognized best where the chorionic plate is thin. In our experience bacterial pathogens are most reliably identified, and one can exclude contaminants by sampling the subchorionic plate area rather than swabbing the amnionic surface; the severity and extent of the inflammatory reaction correlated positively with the presence of fetal and maternal morbidity.[757] In addition to organisms recovered by conventional bacteriologic study, *Chlamydia trachomatis* has become recognized as another major pathogen.[739] Premature labor and fetal infections occurring in these circumstances are a major cause of perinatal mortality in developed as well as underdeveloped countries.[706] Villous edema associated with chorioamnionitis correlates most significantly with perinatal death[704] when hypoxia is added to the other injurious effects of infection. Term infants of well-nourished mothers are less likely to be affected and may show little morbidity from chorioamnionitis.

Listeria monocytogenes produces a severe placentitis characterized by miliary abscesses and is one of the less recognized causes of septic abortion, especially repeated abortion.[721] The histologic appearance of the abscesses is a characteristic collection of polymorphonuclear leukocytes and mononuclear cells at the tip of a villus, enveloped by an attenuated layer of trophoblast (Fig. 34-93). The organism is better known as a cause of fetal wastage in animals, especially cattle; the basis for its selective pathogenicity in pregnancy is unknown.[625] The newborn is also susceptible, developing a distinctive disseminated infection called granulomatosis infantiseptica, in which the liver, lungs, spleen, and adrenal glands are riddled with miliary abscesses; the cause of death in the few born alive is acute meningitis.[702] The organism is a small gram-positive rod, which must not be hastily classified as a diphtheroid. Maternal endometrial infection may be chronic and should be treated even though it is asymptomatic.

Chronic villitis occurs as a focal process and in most instances has little significance in term infants. An etiologic factor is usually not identified, but villitis is the

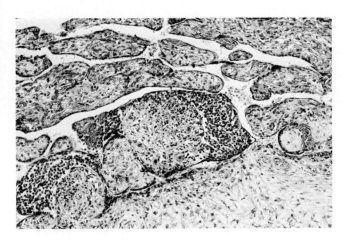

Fig. 34-93. Placental villitis associated with *Listeria monocytogenes* infection. Inflammatory cells expand villus, but thin envelope of attenuated trophoblast persists. (130×.)

type of lesion caused by most viruses and protozoa. Recurrent villitis in sequential pregnancies may have an autoimmune basis and is associated with high perinatal mortality.[722]

Viral infections

Transmission of viruses to the fetus may be hematogenous and transplacental or by contact at the time of delivery. Smallpox, varicella, herpes simplex, and cytomegalic inclusion virus[703] cause necrotizing villitis with typical intranuclear inclusions. Herpes simplex cultures in the absence of clinically evident maternal lesions have no predictive value, whereas active vulvar lesions pose a threat of intrapartum or postpartum transmission to the fetus.[663] Placental lesions in congenital rubella infection include acute necrotizing villitis, older fibrotic areas, and cytoplasmic viral inclusions. Ornoy and associates[711] found a close correlation between severe fetal anomalies and placental inflammation (including cytoplasmic inclusions) in pregnancies complicated by rubella infection. They suggested that evaluation of placental biopsy specimens would aid in the decision of whether to continue a pregnancy in the face of maternal rubella exposure or infection.

Perinatal infection with cytomegalovirus in term infants born alive is usually transmitted by contact with recently contracted active cervical infection in the mother.[724] First and second trimester abortion caused by necrotizing villitis and deciduitis has also been reported, but its numerical significance is uncertain. Primary infection of the mother during pregnancy poses a significant (30% to 40%) risk of intrauterine transmission and severe central nervous system injury when infection occurs in the first half of the gestation.[737] The immature nervous system is most susceptible to intra-

uterine infection. Mental retardation, deafness, impaired vision, low birth weight, and microcephaly are the more devastating disabilities that follow. The social costs are incalculable. The total cost for 5000 infants affected annually by cytomegalovirus certainly is comparable to the $161,000 direct cost estimated for each rubella-affected child; cytomegalovirus is clearly a billion dollar problem.

Protozoal infections

Toxoplasmosis is transmitted to the infant through the placenta. Mothers who have antibodies before pregnancy do not have infected infants. The most serious fetal lesions are produced when maternal exposure occurs during the first two trimesters of pregnancy. The encysted organisms can be demonstrated histologically, but often with difficulty; more consistent identification is obtained by intraperitoneal injection in mice.[649] The placental lesion is focal necrosis and villitis, with a mononuclear infiltrate. Cysts without inflammation may be found in the placentas of neonates who develop severe disease months later.[629] The injuries are not rare and include deafness, blindness, and mental retardation.[752] The accumulated direct costs from each year's total of 3300 disabled infants exceed $200 million in the United States alone.[751] The toll in misery and frustration is impossible to calculate. Effective control in the form of simple hygienic measures should be available to everyone.[751]

When infection is severe, fetal hydrops occurs, and the placental appearance mimics erythroblastosis grossly and microscopically.[617]

Malarial parasites have been identified in maternal erythrocytes in the intervillous space.

Fungous infections

The most common fungous infection of the placenta is that caused by *Candida* organisms that invade transvaginally after premature rupture of the membranes. Associated bacterial infection is common. Fungal hyphae may infiltrate the umbilical cord. Instances of *Coccidioides* infection have been reported.[625]

Mycoplasma infection

Mycoplasma organisms have been implicated in infertility[679] and abortion,[702] and organisms have been cultured in cases of chorioamnionitis. The lesions resemble those produced by bacteria, with a polymorphonuclear leukocytic infiltrate. Correlation between placental lesions caused by T mycoplasmas and any sort of fetal disease seems to be poor.[737]

Hemorrhagic endovasculitis

Sander[729] has described a distinctive form of focal intravillous hemorrhage; fragmented and intact erythrocytes are scattered through the vessel walls and villous stroma. Stillbirth and intrauterine growth retardation are common. There is a high incidence of central nervous system injury among liveborn children evaluated at 5 years of age. No etiologic agent has been identified.

Erythroblastosis fetalis

The placenta in erythroblastosis fetalis is greatly enlarged, from two to four times the normal size and weight. The fetal membranes are pale gray when associated with fetal hydrops. The cut surface is pale, spongy, and granular. The microscopic appearance represents a recapitulation of the immature state, with prominent cytotrophoblast cells, abundant villous stroma, and many Hofbauer cells.[672] Nucleated red blood cells in clusters may fill and distend capillary spaces.

Trophoblastic hyperplasia and neoplasia

The aggressive overgrowth of trophoblast, benign or malignant, is an unusual but always dramatic complication of pregnancy. All the lesions described subse-

quently are frequently discussed together as forms of "trophoblastic disease."

Hydatidiform mole

Hydatidiform mole is a form of pathologic pregnancy that is uncommon in the United States (about 1 per 2000 pregnancies) but for reasons still unknown occurs with about 10 times that frequency in various parts of Asia and Central America.[711] There is a rapid increase in uterine size, often with symptoms of toxemia and vaginal bleeding. Ultrasonography can be used to confirm the absence of the fetus. By the middle of the second trimester the uterus may approach the size of a uterus at term; bleeding begins at this time, if not before.

A hydatidiform mole itself is actually a placenta composed entirely or almost entirely of immensely swollen villi. The volume varies from about 1 to 3 liters (Fig. 34-94). There is usually an abundance of hyperplastic trophoblast covering some or all of the villi and infiltrating the decidua at the implantation site. It is possible but rare to find a fetus (Fig. 34-95). In the presence of a fetus, or in smaller abortions composed of a mixture

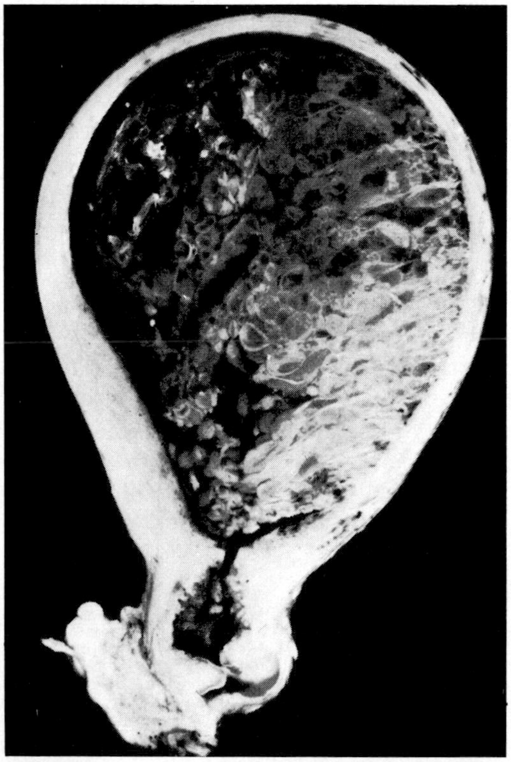

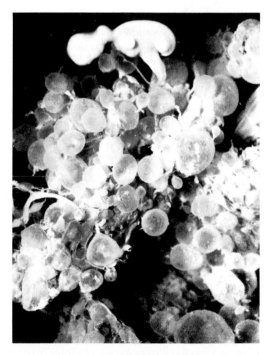

Fig. 34-94. Midsagittal section of typical molar uterus approaching term size though of gestational age of only about 20 weeks. Uterine cavity is greatly distended, but small, oval, centrally located chorionic sac may still be identified. (Courtesy Dr. H. Sheehan, Armed Forces Institute of Pathology, Washington, D.C.)

Fig. 34-95. Grapelike vesicles of varying size constituting hydatidiform mole. Stunted, macerated fetus at menstrual age of approximately 6 weeks was within intact chorionic sac (not shown here) when mole was delivered at hysterectomy. This is unusual, since chorionic sac is usually empty. (2×; Carnegie No. 8723, seq. 1; from Hertig, A.T.: Hydatidiform mole and chorionepithelioma. In Meigs, J.V., and Sturgis, S.H., editors: Progress in gynecology, vol. 2, New York, 1963, Grune & Stratton, Inc.; by permission.)

of normal and hydropic villi, subsequent choriocarcinoma is extremely unlikely. The term "hydatidiform mole" should be avoided in such cases, which are usually triploid abortions, as described previously.[740]

The pathogenesis is unknown. The considerably higher incidence in the lowest socioeconomic populations is suggestive of a nutritional factor that remains undefined. The cytogenetics of hydatidiform mole are startling. The karyotype is consistently 46XX and occasionally 46XY; in either case *both* sets of chromosomes are paternally derived.[686] The mechanism is not certain; it appears, however, that the female nucleus is expelled, and the genetic complement of a single sperm usually replicates by endoreduplication. The XY molar karyotype is dispermic. Follow-up studies of 61 women with hydatidiform moles showed a much greater tendency for aggressive behavior among those with dispermic moles.[749]

The histologic pattern of the villous core varies little; the jellylike edematous stroma is nearly clear and trav-

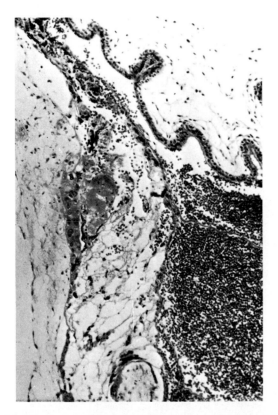

Fig. 34-96. Group II mole (probably benign). Despite benign appearance, clinically invasive mole (chorioadenoma destruens) developed 5 weeks after evacuation of mole. These portions of two villi show normal double-layered trophoblast on upper right and pleomorphism of Langhans' epithelium and vacuolization of syncytiotrophoblast on other villus. (110×; from Hertig, A.T., and Sheldon, W.H.: Am. J. Obstet. Gynecol. **53:**1, 1947.)

ersed by thin strands of connective tissue, most of which are ruptured (Fig. 34-96). Capillary structures are not apparent in ordinary microscopic examination but can be demonstrated by electron microscopy. The most significant component is the trophoblast that covers the villi and infiltrates the implantation site. There is considerable variation, from thin layers of atrophic degenerated attenuated syncytiotrophoblast cells with pyknotic nuclei to piled-up hyperplastic masses of syncytiotrophoblast, cytotrophoblast, or both. Large anaplastic-looking nuclei often have the appearance of a malignant neoplasm (Fig. 34-97, A). In fact, the manner in which cytotrophoblast and syncytiotrophoblast remain segregated is characteristic and resembles the trophoblast pattern in the area of the cytotrophoblast shell of a 10- to 12-day implantation.

Extreme degrees of dysplastic and anaplastic nuclear change undeniably have an ominous appearance when present. As a practical matter, the presence of the villi, even hydropic villi, serves to classify the lesion in question as benign. Grading of moles on the basis of degrees of anaplastic change in the trophoblast has little prognostic significance in an individual case.[625,674,713]

The most important factor in the decision to treat the patient is the demonstration of a rise in HCG titers after the fall attending the removal of the mole. Since it is extremely important to detect this rise early, a suitably sensitive assay is absolutely necessary. The radioimmunoassay of serum or urine samples for the presence of the beta subunit of HCG is specific and sufficiently sensitive to detect minute amounts and capable of showing changes in ranges at which the ordinary immunoassay of standard pregnancy tests will not react.[745]

Invasive mole (destructive mole). In addition to the threat that attends severe bleeding and the possibility of infection, hydatidiform mole may invade the wall of the uterus (Fig. 34-98), and molar tissue may be deported to other sites. Invasion of the uterine wall is a source of hemorrhage after the mole has been passed or removed. Molar trophoblast cells, like normal trophoblast,[616] are constantly embolizing the general circulation. Molar tissue may be deported to the lungs[620] or vaginal wall and produce local nodular lesions, which are usually hemorrhagic because of the vascular destructiveness of trophoblasts. Such a lesion is regarded as benign in the sense that it is not a malignant neoplasm, but the potential for hemorrhage is a strong inducement for treatment. Before the availability of chemotherapy it was generally recognized that such lesions regressed and could usually be managed conservatively.

The most devastating complication of hydatidiform mole is the subsequent occurrence of choriocarcinoma (as discussed later) in about 2.5% of patients. The mor-

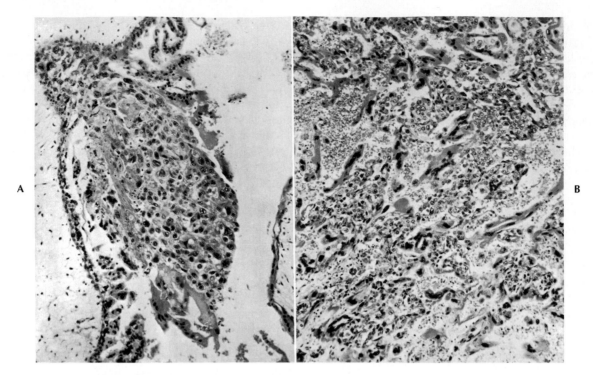

Fig. 34-97. A, Mass of molar trophoblast with pronounced anaplasia attached to villus while remainder of trophoblast is not unusually active. Although mole gave rise to choriocarcinoma, this trophoblast does not resemble that of tumor shown in **B. B,** Renal metastasis of typical choriocarcinoma in patient whose original mole is shown in **A.** Patient died 16 months after delivery of hydatidiform mole. (110×; courtesy Rhode Island Hospital, Providence; AFIP 218754-562 and 218754-563.)

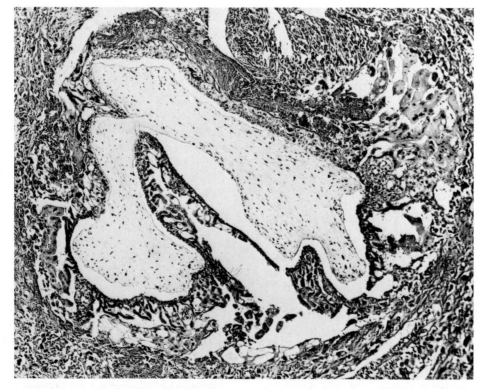

Fig. 34-98. Single hydatidiform villus invading myometrium, pathognomonic of invasive mole. (48×; AFIP 298593-2.)

phologic findings are not so important a factor in the decision to treat the patient as continued HCG production. Demonstration of a rising HCG titer after delivery of the mole is the basis for starting chemotherapy, regardless of the presence of a demonstrable lesion. The production of HCG is a constant and consistent property of trophoblast and is generally proportional to the amount of trophoblast present in a given patient. Rising titers mean growing trophoblast. If the location of proliferating trophoblast is uncertain or inaccessible, it is not necessary or desirable to identify it morphologically before instituting chemotherapy. A detailed plan for the follow-up care of patients after passage of a mole is obviously important; the protocols at the regional centers for treatment of trophoblastic disease are similar.[666,669] The drugs used successfully have been methotrexate and actinomycin D.

Having emphasized the overriding significance of HCG in management of clinical problems, we should give attention to some interesting morphologic correlations. Hydatidiform mole in the presence of a fetus is often associated with unusually severe toxemia and hypertension; subsequent choriocarcinoma is most unlikely.[714] Transitional (partial) moles (abortions of small size with a high proportion of vesicular villi) are followed rarely if ever by choriocarcinoma. Women who have had one mole are somewhat more likely to have another than are women who have not. The trophoblast cells of the molar implantation site occasionally persist for several months, with slowly *declining* HCG titers, and may be a source of bleeding. The histologic pattern is not that of choriocarcinoma, and demonstration of trophoblast cells at the implantation site of a mole does not mean that the patient has or ever will have a choriocarcinoma, but it is a reasonable basis for extending the period of follow-up study.

Placental-site trophoblastic tumor

The intermediate trophoblast cells that normally infiltrate the implantation site on rare occasions may proliferate to form a tumor mass. Small, circumscribed, often partly hyalinized nodules, usually discovered as an incidental finding in a hysterectomy specimen, are called "placental-site nodules."[756] All have been benign and appear to be asymptomatic.

Placental-site trophoblastic tumor is larger and clinically significant. The patients usually have noted amenorrhea for several months, the uterus is enlarged, and about one third have a positive pregnancy test. The tumors may be polypoid or intramural, and a few have perforated the uterus causing peritoneal hemorrhage. The tumor mass may be circumscribed or have ill-defined margins and are generally soft and yellow or tan, without the hemorrhagic appearance of choriocarcinoma. Microscopically the myometrial fibers are separated by large pale, trophoblast cells, mostly mononuclear, interspersed with occasional multinucleated giant cells. Although the giant cells stain deeply with anti-HCG antisera, the predominant mononuclear intermediate trophoblast cells usually do not. The mononuclear cells do stain particularly well with antisera to human placental lactogen (HPL) as intermediate trophoblast cells normally do.[758] Rare instances of placental-site trophoblastic tumor have caused fatal metastases. These lesions are monomorphic and stain more intensely with antisera to HCG but not HPL, in this respect resembling the staining qualities of choriocarcinoma.[758]

Choriocarcinoma

Gestational choriocarcinoma is a malignant neoplasm of trophoblast; it may occur after hydatidiform mole (50%), spontaneous abortion (25%), normal pregnancy (22.5%), and even rarely an ectopic pregnancy (Fig. 34-99).

Intravascular metastases occur early and disseminate widely. They are found chiefly in the lung (60%), vagina (40%), brain (12%), liver (16%), and kidney (13%), but virtually any site perfused by blood vessels is possible. The uterine lesion may be small, and often no uterine lesion can be identified.

The tumor masses are soft, necrotic, and hemorrhagic wherever they are found. The bulk of a nodular lesion is often a blood clot, and the trophoblastic tissue is occasionally difficult to find.

The histologic pattern varies only slightly. Plexiform masses of syncytiotrophoblast and cytotrophoblast are intimately intermixed, forming a distinctive biphasic pattern (Fig. 34-97, *B*). Nuclei of both cell types may be bizarre and anaplastic; mitoses occur in the cytotrophoblast cells. Unlike other malignant neoplasms of all types, choriocarcinoma has no stroma and no vascular supply of its own. In a study of treated patients, Mazur, Lurain, and Brewer[698] found an unexpected change in histologic pattern among four women whose tumors were resistant to treatment after multiple courses of chemotherapy. Instead of the typical biphasic pattern, these tumors were characterized by a significant predominance of cytotrophoblast growing in masses and infiltrating strands producing a histologic pattern that is more like that of a conventional carcinoma.

Choriocarcinoma is the best example of a malignant tumor that responds to chemotherapy. Nearly always fatal in the past, it has now become nearly always curable; many of the patients go on to have children. The drugs used most successfully have been actinomycin D and methotrexate. It is important to monitor therapy with serial HCG determinations. The drugs themselves can be dangerous, and the protocol for treatment can be extremely complicated. The results in the regional centers for treatment of trophoblastic disease have been

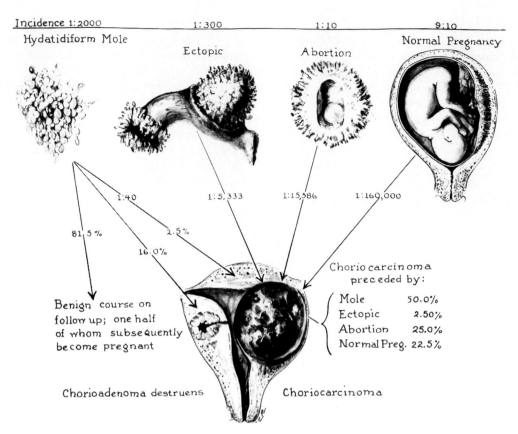

Fig. 34-99. Schema of relationship between various types of pregnancy and chorioadenoma destruens and choriocarcinoma. (Adapted from Hertig, A.T.: Hydatidiform mole and chorionepithelioma. In Meigs, J.V., and Sturgis, S.H., editors: Progress in gynecology, vol. 2, New York, 1963, Grune & Stratton, Inc.; by permission.)

excellent.[666,669] Their consultation and support are generally available on request and should be sought, since the results without highly specialized clinical and laboratory facilities can be disastrous.

The prognosis for the patient with cerebral or liver metastases is poor. Very high HCG titers are also an unfavorable finding; the inhibition of the immune response by large amounts of HCG could be the responsible factor. It would be interesting to know if its removal, for example, by plasmapheresis, would help in these grave circumstances. Gestational choriocarcinoma after an otherwise normal pregnancy has an unfavorable prognosis, probably because the diagnosis is delayed. In rare instances it has been possible to identify a small focus of choriocarcinoma in such a placenta.[635] In each case the patient was seen first with evidence of metastases while carrying a normally developing fetus. The primary tumors were inconspicuous, often requiring an extensive search.

Other neoplasms

Chorioangioma is a small and insignificant hemangioma that has been reported in 0.5% to 7% of placentas. Large lesions may be associated with hydramnios, toxemia, prematurity, and even a hydrops fetalis syndrome unrelated to Rh sensitization. Metastatic malignant tumors of maternal origin, notably breast and malignant melanoma, occur occasionally but usually do not cross the placental barrier to the fetus.[723] Rarely, malignant lesions of the fetus affect the placenta (leukemia, neuroblastoma), and instances of congenital giant nevus with placental metastasis have occurred.[648]

ACKNOWLEDGMENT

The continued use of Figs. 24, 29, 39, 45, 46, 62, 63, 66, 69, 74, 80, 82, 84, 85, and 94 to 99 in this chapter, originally prepared by Dr. Arthur T. Hertig, is gratefully acknowledged.

REFERENCES
Embryology and congenital malformations

1. Bernstein, R.: The Y chromosome and primary sexual differentiation, JAMA **245**:1953, 1981.
2. Boczkowski, K.: Abnormal sex determination and differentiation in man, Obstet. Gynecol. **41**:310, 1973.
3. Bullock, L.P., and Bardin, C.W.: *In vivo* and *in vitro* testosterone metabolism by the androgen insensitive rat, J. Steroid Biochem. **4**:139, 1973.
4. Dewhurst, C.J.: Congenital malformations of the genital tract in childhood, J. Obstet. Gynaecol. Br. Cwlth. **75**:377, 1968.
5. Fanning, J.: Double vulva: a case report, J. Reprod. Med. **32**:297, 1987.
6. Farber, M., and Marchant, D.J.: Congenital absence of the uterine cervix, Am. J. Obstet. Gynecol. **121**:414, 1975.
7. Forsberg, J.G.: Origin of vaginal epithelium, Obstet. Gynecol. **25**:687, 1965.
8. Green, L.K., and Harris, R.E.: Uterine anomalies: frequency of diagnosis and associated obstetric complications, Obstet. Gynecol. **47**:427, 1976.
9. Griffin, J.E.: The syndromes of androgen resistance, N. Engl. J. Med. **302**:198, 1980.
10. Hamilton, W.J., Boyd, J.D., and Mossman, H.W.: Human embryology, ed. 4, Baltimore, 1972, The Williams & Wilkins Co.
11. Holmes, L.B.: Current concepts in congenital malformations, N. Engl. J. Med. **295**:204, 1976.
12. Jacobs, P.A., Melville, M., and Ratcliffe, S.: A cytogenetic survey of 11,680 newborn infants, Ann. Hum. Genet. **37**:359, 1974.
13. Jost, A.: Problems of fetal endocrinology, Recent Prog. Horm. Res. **8**:379, 1953.
14. Jost, A.: Hormonal factors in the development of the fetus, Cold Spring Harbor Symp. Quant. Biol. **19**:167, 1954.
15. Jost, A., Vigier, B., Prépin, J., and Perchellet, Y.P.: Studies on sex differentiation in mammals, Recent Prog. Horm. Res. **29**:1, 1973.
16. Machin, G.A.: Chromosome abnormality and perinatal death, Lancet, **1**:549, 1974.
17. Márquez-Monter, H., Armendares, S., Buentello, L., and Villegas, J.: Histopathologic study with cytologic correlation in 20 cases of gonadal dysgenesis, Am. J. Clin. Pathol. **57**:449, 1972.
18. Mittwoch, U.: The genetics of sexual differentiation, New York, 1973, Academic Press, Inc.
19. Naftolin, F., and Judd, H.L.: Testicular feminization, Obstet. Gynecol. Annu. **2**:25, 1973.
20. Park, I.J., Aimakhu, V.E., and Jones, H.W., Jr.: An etiologic and pathogenic classification of male hermaphroditism, Am. J. Obstet. Gynecol. **123**:505, 1975.
21. Pinkerton, J.H., McKay, D.G., Adams, E.C., and Hertig, A.T.: Development of the human ovary—a study using histochemical techniques, Obstet. Gynecol. **18**:152, 1961.
22. Prinz, J.L., Choate, J.W., Townes, P.L., and Harper, R.C.: The embryology of supernumerary ovaries, Obstet. Gynecol. **41**:246, 1973.
23. Sarto, G.E.: Cytogenetics of 50 patients with primary amenorrhea, Am. J. Obstet. Gynecol. **119**:14, 1974.
24. Sarto, G.E., and Opitz, J.M.: The XY gonadal agenesis syndrome, J. Med. Genet. **10**:288, 1973.
25. Schellhas, H.F.: Malignant potential of the dysgenetic gonad, Obstet. Gynecol. **44**:298, 1974.
26. Scully, R.E.: Gonadoblastoma: a review of 74 cases, Cancer **25**:1340, 1970.
27. Singh, R.P., and Carr, D.H.: Anatomic findings in human abortions of known chromosomal constitution, Obstet. Gynecol. **29**:806, 1967.
28. Smith, D.W.: Recognizable patterns of human malformation, ed. 3, Philadelphia, 1982, W.B. Saunders Co.
29. Spaulding, M.H.: The development of the external genitalia in the human embryo, Contrib. Embryol. **13**:67, 1921.
30. Stephens, F.D.: The female anus, perineum, and vestibule: embryogenesis and deformities, Aust. NZ J. Obstet. Gynaecol. **8**:55, 1968.
31. Tegenkamp, T.R., Brazzell, J.W., Tegenkamp, I., and Labidi, F.: Pregnancy without benefit of surgery in a bisexually active true hermaphrodite, Am. J. Obstet. Gynecol. **135**:427, 1979.
32. Ulbright, T.M., and Kraus, F.T.: Endometrial stromal tumors of the extra-uterine tissue, Am. J. Clin. Pathol. **76**:371, 1981.
33. Van Niekerk, W.A.: True hermaphroditism: an analytic review with a report of three cases, Am. J. Obstet. Gynecol. **126**:890, 1976.
34. Van Wagenen, G., and Simpson, M.E.: Embryology of the ovary and testis: *Homo sapiens* and *Macaca mulatta*, New Haven, Conn., 1965, Yale University Press.
35. Wachtel, S.S.: H-Y antigen and the biology of sex determination, New York, 1983, Grune & Stratton Co.
36. Wharton, L.R.: Two cases of supernumerary ovary and one of accessory ovary, with an analysis of previously reported cases, Am. J. Obstet. Gynecol. **78**:1101, 1959.
37. Wilson, J.D., Harrod, M.J., Goldstein, J.L., Hemsell, D.L., and MacDonald, P.C.: Familial incomplete male pseudohermaphroditism, type I: evidence for androgen resistance and variable clinical manifestations in a family with the Reifenstein syndrome, N. Engl. J. Med. **290**:1097, 1974.
38. Woodruff, J.D., and Pauerstein, C.J.: The fallopian tubes, structure, function, pathology, and management, Baltimore, 1969, The Williams & Wilkins Co.
39. Woolf, R.M., and Allen, W.M.: Concomitant malformations: the frequent, simultaneous occurrence of congenital malformations of the reproductive and urinary tracts, Obstet. Gynecol. **2**:236, 1953.

Vulva

40. Abell, M.R.: Adenocystic (pseudoadenomatous) basal cell carcinoma of the vestibular glands of the vulva, Am. J. Obstet. Gynecol. **86**:470, 1963.
41. Abell, M.R., and Gosling, J.R.G.: Intraepithelial and infiltrative carcinoma of vulva: Bowen's type, Cancer **14**:318, 1961.
42. Amstey, M.S., Monif, G.R., Nahmias, A.J., and Josey, W.E.: Cesarean section and genital herpes infection, Obstet. Gynecol. **53**:641, 1979.
43. Benda, J.A., Platz, C.E., and Anderson, B.: Malignant melanoma of the vulva: a clinicopathologic review of 16 cases, Int. J. Gynecol. Pathol. **5**:202, 1986.
44. Burger, R.A., and Marcuse, P.M.: Fibroadenoma of the vulva, Am. J. Clin. Pathol. **24**:965, 1954.
45. Buscema, J., Woodruff, J.D., Parmley, T.H., and Genadry, R.: Carcinoma in situ of the vulva, Obstet. Gynecol. **55**:225, 1980.
46. Chamlian, D.L., and Taylor, H.B.: Primary carcinoma of Bartholin's gland: a report of 24 patients, Obstet. Gynecol. **39**:489, 1972.
47. Christensen, W.N., Friedman, K.J., Woodruff, J.D., and Hood, A.F.: Histologic characteristics of vulvar nevocellular nevi, J. Cutan. Pathol. **14**:87, 1987.
48. Crum, C.P., Braun, L.A., Shah, K.V., Fu, Y.S., Levine, R.U., Fenoglio, C.M., Richart, R.M., and Townshend, D.E.: Intraepithelial neoplasia of the vulva and vagina: an analysis for herpes simplex-2 by *in-situ* hybridization techniques, Lab. Invest. **44**:13A, 1981. (Abstract.)
49. Crum, C.P.: Vulvar intraepithelial neoplasia: histology and viral changes. In Wilkinson, E.J., editor: Pathology of the vulva and vagina, New York, 1987, Churchill Livingstone.
50. Cruz-Jiménez, P.R., and Abell, M.R.: Cutaneous basal cell carcinoma of the vulva, Cancer **36**:1860, 1975.
51. Davidson, T., Kissance, M., and Westbury, G.: Vulvo-vaginal melanoma. Should radical surgery be abandoned? Br. J. Obstet. Gynaecol. **94**:473, 1987.
52. Davos, I., and Abell, M.R.: Soft tissue sarcomas of vulva, Gynecol. Oncol. **4**:70, 1976.
53. Dean, R.E., Taylor, E.S., Weisbrod, D.M., and Martin, J.W.: The treatment of premalignant and malignant lesions of the vulva, Am. J. Obstet. Gynecol. **119**:59, 1974.
54. Dehner, L.C.: Metastatic and secondary tumors of the vulva, Obstet. Gynecol. **42**:47, 1973.

55. Devroede, G., Schlaeder, G., Sánchez, G., and Haddad, H.: Crohn's disease of the vulva, Am. J. Clin. Pathol. **63**:348, 1975.
56. Dgani, R., Czernobilsky, B., Borenstein, R., and Lancet, M.: Granular cell myoblastoma of the vulva: report of four cases, Acta Obstet. Gynecol. Scand. **57**:385, 1978.
57. Edsmyr, F.: Carcinoma of the vulva: an analysis of 560 patients with histologically verified squamous cell carcinoma, Acta Radiol. **217**(suppl.):1, 1963.
58. Ferenczy, A., Mitao, M., Nagai, N., Silverstein, S.J., and Crum, C.P.: Latent papillomavirus and recurring genital warts, N. Engl. J. Med. **313**:784, 1985.
59. Franklin, E.W., and Rutledge, F.D.: Epidemiology of epidermoid carcinoma of the vulva, Obstet. Gynecol. **39**:165, 1972.
60. Friedrich, E.G.: Reversible vulvar atypia, Obstet. Gynecol. **39**:173, 1972.
61. Friedrich, E.G.: Vulvar disease, Philadelphia, 1976, W.B. Saunders Co.
62. Friedrich, E.G., Cole, W., and Middlekamp, J.N.: Herpes simplex, Am. J. Obstet. Gynecol. **104**:758, 1969.
63. Friedrich, E.G., Jr., and Kalra, P.S.: Serum levels of sex hormones in vulvar lichen sclerosus, and the effect of topical testosterone, N. Engl. J. Med. **310**:488, 1984.
64. Friedrich, E.G., and Wilkinson, E.J.: Mucous cysts of the vulvar vestibule, Obstet. Gynecol. **42**:407, 1973.
65. Gardner, H.L., and Kaufman, R.H.: Benign diseases of the vulva and vagina, St. Louis, 1969, The C.V. Mosby Co.
66. Godeau, C., Frances, C., Hornebeck, D., Brechemier, D., and Robert, L.: Isolation and partial characterization of an elastase-type protease in human vulva fiberblasts: its possible involvement in vulvar elastic tissue destruction of patients with lichen sclerosus et atrophicus, J. Invest. Dermatol. **78**:270, 1982.
67. Gosling, J.R., Abell, M.R., Drolette, B.M., and Loughrin, T.D.: Infiltrative squamous cell (epidermoid) carcinoma of the vulva, Cancer **14**:330, 1961.
68. Green, T.H.: Carcinoma of the vulva: a reassessment, Obstet. Gynecol. **52**:462, 1978.
69. Green, T.H., Ulfelder, H., and Meigs, J.V.: Epidermoid carcinoma of the vulva: analysis of 238 cases. I. Etiology and diagnosis, Am. J. Obstet. Gynecol. **75**:834, 1958.
70. Green, T.H., Ulfelder, H., and Meigs, J.V.: Epidermoid carcinoma of the vulva: analysis of 238 cases. II. Therapy and end results, Am. J. Obstet. Gynecol. **75**:848, 1958.
71. Guerry, R.L., and Pratt-Thomas, H.R.: Carcinoma of supernumerary breast of vulva with bilateral mammary cancer, Cancer **38**:2570, 1976.
72. Hart, W.R.: Paramesonephric mucinous cysts of the vulva, Am. J. Obstet. Gynecol. **107**:1079, 1970.
73. Hart, W.R., Norris, H.J., and Helwig, E.B.: Relationship of lichen sclerosus et atrophicus of the vulva to development of carcinoma, Obstet. Gynecol. **45**:369, 1975.
74. Hassim, A.M.: Bilateral fibroadenoma in supernumerary breasts of the vulva, J. Obstet. Gynaecol. Br. Cwlth. **76**:275, 1969.
75. Helwig, E.B., and Graham, J.H.: Anogenital (extramammary) Paget's disease: a clinicopathological study, Cancer **16**:387, 1963.
76. Hertig, A.T., and Gore, H.: Tumors of the female sex organs. II. Tumors of the vulva, vagina, and uterus. In Atlas of tumor pathology, section IX, fascicle 33, Washington, D.C., 1970, Armed Forces Institute of Pathology.
77. Isaacs, J.H.: Verrucous carcinoma of the female genital tract, Gynecol. Oncol. **4**:259, 1976.
78. Iverson, T., Abeler, V., and Kolstad, P.: Squamous cell carcinoma in situ of the vulva: a clinical and histopathological study, Gynecol. Oncol. **11**:224, 1982.
79. Janovski, N.A., and Ames, S.: Lichen sclerosus et atrophicus of the vulva: a poorly understood disease entity, Obstet. Gynecol. **22**:2697, 1963.
80. Japaze, H., Garcia-Bunuel, R., and Woodruff, J.D.: Primary vulvar neoplasia: a review of *in situ* and invasive carcinoma 1935-1972, Obstet. Gynecol. **49**:404, 1977.
81. Jeffcoate, T.N.A.: Chronic vulval dystrophies, Am. J. Obstet. Gynecol. **95**:61, 1966.
82. Jimerson, G.K., and Merrill, J.A.: Multicentric squamous malignancy involving both cervix and vulva, Cancer **26**:150, 1970.
83. Jones, R.W., and McLean, M.R.: Carcinoma in situ of the vulva: a review of 31 treated and 5 untreated cases. Obstet. Gynecol. **68**:499, 1986.
84. Kaplan, A.L., Kaufman, R.H., Birken, R.A., and Simkin, S.: Intraepithelial carcinoma of the vulva with extension to the anal canal, Obstet. Gynecol. **58**:368, 1981.
85. Kaufman, R.H., and Faro, S.: Infectious diseases of the vulva and vagina. In Wilkinson, E.J., editor: Pathology of the vulva and vagina, New York, 1987, Churchill Livingstone.
86. Kaufman, R.H., Dreesman, G.R., Burek, J., Korhonen, M.O., Matson, D.O., Melnick, J.L., Powell, K.L., Purifoy, D.J., Courtney, R.J., and Adam, E.: Herpes-induced antigens in squamous cell carcinoma in situ of the vulva, N. Engl. J. Med. **305**:483, 1981.
87. Kelly, J.: Malignant disease of the vulva, J. Obstet. Gynaecol. Br. Cwlth. **79**:265, 1972.
88. Kint, A., and Geerts, M.L.: Lichen sclerosus et atrophicus: an electron microscopic study, J. Cutan. Pathol. **2**:30, 1975.
89. Kluzak, T.R., and Kraus, F.T.: Condylomata, papillomas, and verrucous carcinomas of the vulva and vagina. In Wilkinson, E.J., editor: Pathology of the vulva and vagina, New York, 1987, Churchill Livingstone.
90. Kolstad. P., and Stafl, A.: Atlas of colposcopy, Baltimore, 1972, University Park Press.
91. Kraus, F.T., and Pérez-Mesa, C.: Verrucous carcinoma: a clinical and pathologic study of 105 cases involving oral cavity, larynx, and genitalia, Cancer **19**:26, 1966.
92. Kurman, R.J., Shah, K.H., Lancaster, W.D., and Jenson, A.B.: Immunoperoxidase localization of papillomavirus antigens in cervical dysplasia and vulvar condylomas, Am. J. Obstet. Gynecol. **140**:931, 1981.
93. Lee, S.C., Roth, L.M., Ehrlich, C., et al.: Extramammary Paget's disease of the vulva: a clinicopathologic study of 13 cases, Cancer **39**:2540, 1977.
94. LiVolsi, V.A., and Brooks, J.J.: Soft tissue tumors of the vulva. In Wilkinson, E.J., editor: Pathology of the vulva and vagina, New York, 1987, Churchill Livingstone.
95. Lovelady, S.B., McDonald, J.R., and Waugh, J.M.: Benign tumors of the vulva, Am. J. Obstet. Gynecol. **42**:309, 1941.
96. Lukas, W.F., Benirschke, K., and Lebherz, T.B.: Verrucous carcinoma of the female genital tract, Am. J. Obstet. Gynecol. **119**:435, 1974.
97. Majmudar, B., Chaikeu, M.L., and Lee, K.U.: Amebiasis of clitoris mimicking carcinoma, JAMA **236**:1145, 1976.
98. Majmudar, B., and Hallden, C.: Juvenile laryngeal papillomatosis and maternal condyloma, Lab. Invest. **52**:40A, 1985.
99. Mazoujian, G., Pinkus, G.S., and Haagensen, D.E., Jr.: Extramammary Paget's disease: evidence for apocrine origin, Am. J. Surg. Pathol. **8**:43, 1984.
100. Meeker, J.H., Neubecker, R.D., and Helwig, E.B.: Hidradenoma papilliferum, Am. J. Clin. Pathol. **37**:182, 1962.
101. Michael, H., and Roth, L.M.: Congenital and acquired cysts, benign and malignant skin adnexal tumors, and Paget's disease of the vulva. In Wilkinson, E.J., editor: Pathology of the vulva and vagina, New York, 1987, Churchill Livingstone.
102. Morrow, C.P., and DiSaia, P.S.: Malignant melanoma of the female genitalia: a clinical analysis, Obstet. Gynecol. Surv. **31**:233, 1976.
103. Morrow, C.P., and Rutledge, F.N.: Melanoma of the vulva, Obstet. Gynecol. **39**:745, 1972.
104. Neilson, D., and Woodruff, J.D.: Electron microscopy of in situ and invasive vulvar Paget's disease, Am. J. Obstet. Gynecol. **113**:719, 1972.
105. Ng, A.B.P., Reagan, J.W., and Lindner, E.: The cellular manifestations of primary and recurrent herpes genitalis, Acta Cytol. **14**:124, 1970.
106. Palladino, V.S., Duffy, J.L., and Bures, G.J.: Basal cell carcinoma of the vulva, Cancer **24**:460, 1969.
107. Powell, L.C., Jr.: Condyloma acuminatum, Clin. Obstet. Gynecol. **15**:948, 1972.

108. Pradham, S., and Tobon, H.: Vaginal cysts: a clinicopathological study of 41 cases, Int. J. Gynecol. Pathol. **5**:35, 1986.
109. Ragni, M.V., and Tobon, H.: Primary malignant melanoma of the vagina and vulva, Obstet. Gynecol. **43**:658, 1974.
110. Reid, R., Greenberg, M., Jenson, A.B., Husain, M., Willett, J., Daoud, Y., Temple, G., Stanhope, C.R., Sherman, A.I., Phibbs, G.D., and Lorincz, A.T.: Sexually transmitted papillomaviral infections, Am. J. Obstet. Gynecol. **156**:212, 1987.
111. Robboy, S.J., Ross, J.S., Prat, J., Keh, P.C., and Welch, W.R.: Urogenital sinus origin of mucinous and ciliated cysts of the vulva, Obstet. Gynecol. **51**:3447, 1978.
112. Robertson, A.J., McIntosh, W., Lamont, P., and Guthrie, W.: Malignant granular cell tumor (myoblastoma) of the vulva, Histopathology **5**:69, 1987.
113. Ross, M.J., and Ehrmann, R.L.: Histologic prognosticators in stage I squamous cell carcinoma of the vulva, Obstet. Gynecol. **70**:774, 1987.
114. Roth, L.M., Lee, S.C., and Erlich, C.E.: Paget's disease of the vulva: a histogenetic study of five cases including ultrastructural observations and a review of the literature, Am. J. Surg. Pathol. **1**:193, 1977.
115. Sedlis, A., Homesley, H., Bundy, B.N., Marshall, R., Yorden, E., Hocker, N., Lee, J.H., and Whitney, C.: Positive groin nodes in superficial squamous cell vulvar cancer, Am. J. Obstet. Gynecol. **156**:1159, 1987.
116. Skinner, M.S., Sternberg, W.H., Ichinose, H., and Collins, J.: Spontaneous regression of Bowenoid atypia of the vulva, Obstet. Gynecol. **42**:40, 1973.
117. Steeper, T., and Rosai, J.: Aggressive angiomyxoma of the female pelvis and perineum, Am. J. Surg. Pathol. **7**:43, 1983.
118. Tavassoli, F.A., and Norris, H.J.: Smooth muscle tumors of the vulva, Obstet. Gynecol. **53**:213, 1979.
119. Tsukada, Y., López, R.G., Pickren, J.W., Piver, M.S., and Barlow, J.J.: Paget's disease of the vulva: clinicopathologic study of eight cases, Obstet. Gynecol. **45**:78, 1975.
120. Tuthill, R.J., and Wheeler, J.E.: Simple condylomata acuminata of vulva with focal squamous carcinoma, Lab. Invest. **44**:69A, 1981. (Abstract.)
121. Ulbright, T.M., Stehman, F.B., Roth, L.M., Ehrlich, C.E., and Ransburg, R.G.: Bowenoid dysplasia of the vulva, Cancer **50**:2910, 1982.
122. Way, S., and Benedet, J.L.: Involvement of inguinal lymph nodes in carcinoma of the vulva: a comparison of clinical assessment with histological examination, Gynecol. Oncol. **1**:119, 1973.
123. Wilkinson, E.J.: Superficially invasive carcinoma of the vulva. In Wilkinson, E.J., editor: Pathology of the vulva and vagina, New York, 1987, Churchill Livingstone.
124. Wilkinson, E.J., Kneale, B., and Lynch, P.J.: Report of the ISSVD Terminology Committee, J. Reprod. Med. **31**:973, 1986.
125. Woodworth, H.J., Dockerty, M.B., Wilson, R.B., and Pratt, J.H.: Papillary hidradenoma of the vulva: clinicopathologic study of 69 cases, Am. J. Obstet. Gynecol. **110**:501, 1971.
126. Yackel, D.B., Symmonds, R.E., and Kempers, R.D.: Melanoma of the vulva, Obstet. Gynecol. **35**:625, 1970.
127. Young, A.W., Tovell, H.M.M., and Sadri, K.: Erosions and ulcers of the vulva: diagnosis, incidence, and management, Obstet. Gynecol. **50**:35, 1977.
128. zur Hausen, H.: Papillomaviruses in human cancer, Cancer **59**:1692, 1987.

Vagina

129. Allyn, D.L., Silverberg, S.G., and Salzberg, A.M.: Endodermal sinus tumor of the vagina: report of a case with 7-year survival and literature review of so-called "mesonephromas," Cancer **17**:1231, 1971.
130. Antonioli, D.A.: Vaginal adenosis, clear cell adenocarcinoma and congenital and acquired cysts of the vagina and vulvar vestibule. In Wilkinson, E.J., editor: Pathology of the vulva and vagina, New York, 1987, Churchill Livingstone.
131. Berman, M.C., Tobon, H., and Surti, U.: Primary malignant melanoma of the vagina, Am. J. Obstet. Gynecol. **139**:963, 1981.
132. Berry, A.: A cytopathological and histopathological study of bilharziasis of the female genital tract, J. Pathol. Bacteriol. **91**:325, 1966.
133. Chirayil, S.J., and Tobon, H.: Polyps of the vagina: a clinicopathologic study of 18 cases, Cancer **47**:290, 1981.
134. Copeland, L.J., Gershenson, D.M., Saul, P.B., Sneige, N., Stringer, C.A., and Edwards, C.L.: Sarcoma botryoides of the female genital tract, Obstet. Gynecol. **66**:262, 1985.
135. Davos, I., and Abell, M.R.: Sarcomas of the vagina, Obstet. Gynecol. **47**:342, 1976.
136. Deppisch, L.M.: Cysts of the vagina: classification and clinical correlations, Obstet. Gynecol. **45**:632, 1975.
137. Elliot, G.B., and Elliot, J.D.A.: Superficial stromal reactions of lower genital tract, Arch. Pathol. **95**:100, 1973.
138. Fentanes de Torres, E., and Benítez-Bribiesca, L.: Cytologic detection of vaginal parasitosis, Acta Cytol. **17**:252, 1973.
139. Friedrich, E.G., and Wilkinson, E.J.: Mucous cysts of the vulvar vestibule, Obstet. Gynecol. **42**:407, 1973.
140. Frost, J.K.: Concepts basic to general cytopathology, Baltimore, 1972, Johns Hopkins University Press.
141. Gardner, H.L., and Fernet, P.: Etiology of vaginitis emphysematosa, Am. J. Obstet. Gynecol. **88**:680, 1964.
142. Gardner, H.L., and Kaufman, R.H.: Benign diseases of the vulva and vagina, St. Louis, 1969, The C.V. Mosby Co.
143. Gold, J.M., and Bosseu, E.H.: Benign vaginal rhabdomyoma, Cancer **37**:2283, 1976.
144. Gray, L.A., and Christopherson, W.W.: In-situ and early invasive carcinoma of the vagina, Obstet. Gynecol. **34**:226, 1969.
145. Hart, W.R.: Paramesonephric mucinous cysts of the vulva, Am. J. Obstet. Gynecol. **107**:1079, 1970.
146. Herbst, A.L., Green, T.H., Jr., and Ulfelder, H.: Primary carcinoma of the vagina: an analysis of 68 cases, Am. J. Obstet. Gynecol. **106**:210, 1970.
147. Herbst, A.L., Robboy, S.J., Scully, R.E., and Poskanzer, D.C.: Clear cell adenocarcinoma of the vagina and cervix in girls: analysis of 170 registry cases, Am. J. Obstet. Gynecol. **119**:713, 1974.
148. Herbst, A.L., Cole, P., Norusis, M.J., Welch, W.R., and Scully, R.E.: Epidemiologic aspects and factors related to survival in 384 registry cases of clear-cell adenocarcinoma of the vagina and cervix, Am. J. Obstet. Gynecol. **135**:876, 1979.
149. Hilgers, R.D., Malkasian, G.D., Jr., and Soule, E.H.: Embryonal rhabdomyosarcoma (botryoid type) of the vagina: a clinicopathologic review, Am. J. Obstet. Gynecol. **107**:484, 1970.
150. Kaufman, R.H., Adam, E., Binder, G.L., and Gerthoffer, E.: Upper genital tract changes and pregnancy outcome in offspring exposed in utero to diethylstilbestrol, Am. J. Obstet. Gynecol. **137**:299, 1980.
151. Koss, L.G.: Diagnostic cytology and its histopathologic bases, ed. 2, Philadelphia, 1968, J.B. Lippincott Co.
152. Kurman, R.J., and Prabha, A.C.: Thyroid and parathyroid glands in the vaginal wall: report of a case, Am. J. Clin. Pathol. **59**:503, 1973.
153. Malkasian, G.D., Welch, J.S., and Soule, E.H.: Primary leiomyosarcoma of the vagina: report of eight cases, Am. J. Obstet. Gynecol. **86**:730, 1963.
154. McIndoe, W.A., and Green, G.H.: Vaginal carcinoma in situ following hysterectomy, Acta Cytol. **13**:158, 1969.
155. Ng, A.B.P., Reagan, J.W., and Lindner, E.: The cellular manifestations of primary and recurrent herpes genitalis, Acta Cytol. **14**:124, 1970.
156. Norris, H.J., Bagley, G.P., and Taylor, H.B.: Carcinoma of the infant vagina: a distinctive tumor, Arch. Pathol. **90**:473, 1970.
157. Norris, H.J., and Taylor, H.B.: Polyps of the vagina: a benign lesion resembling sarcoma botryoides, Cancer **19**:227, 1966.
158. Perez, C.A., Zivnuska, F., Askin, F., et al.: Prognostic significance of endometrial extension from primary carcinoma of the uterine cervix, Cancer **35**:1493, 1975.
159. Prempree, T., Thavinsakdi, V., Slawson, R.G., Wizenberg, M.J., and Cuccia, C.A.: Radiation management in primary carcinoma of the vagina, Cancer **40**:109, 1977.
160. Pride, G.L., Schultz, A.E., Chuprevich, T.W., and Buchler,

D.A.: Primary invasive squamous carcinoma of the vagina, Obstet. Gynecol. **53**:218, 1979.

161. Robboy, S.J., Herbst, A.L., and Scully, R.E.: Clear cell adenocarcinoma of the vagina and cervix in young females: analysis of 37 tumors that persisted or recurred after primary therapy, Cancer **34**:606, 1974.

162. Robboy, S.J., Scully, R.E., Welch, W.R., and Herbst, A.L.: Intrauterine diethylstilbestrol exposure and its consequences, Arch. Pathol. Lab. Med. **101**:1, 1977.

163. Sandberg, E.C., Danielson, R.W., Cauwet, R.W., and Bonar, B.E.: Adenosis vaginae, Am. J. Obstet. Gynecol. **93**:209, 1965.

164. Scully, R.E., Robboy, S.J., and Herbst, A.L.: Vaginal and cervical abnormalities, including clear cell adenocarcinoma, related to prenatal exposure to diethylstilbestrol, Am. Clin. Lab. Sci. **4**:222, 1974.

165. Silverberg, S.G., and Frable, W.J.: Prolapse of fallopian tube into vaginal vault after hysterectomy, Arch. Pathol. **97**:100, 1974.

166. Sirota, R.L., Dickersin, G.R., and Scully, R.E.: Mixed tumors of the vagina: a clinicopathological analysis of eight cases, Am. J. Surg. Pathol. **5**:413, 1981.

167. Stabler, F.: The treatment of adenosis (adenomatosis) vaginae, J. Obstet. Gynecol. Br. Cwlth. **74**:493,1967.

168. Taguchi, O., Cunha, G.R., and Robboy, S.J.: Experimental study of the effect of diethylstilbestrol (DES) on the development of the human female reproductive tract, Biol. Res. Pregnancy Perinatol. **4**:56, 1983.

169. Tavassoli, F.A., and Norris, H.J.: Smooth muscle tumors of the vagina, Obstet. Gynecol. **53**:689, 1979.

170. Ulbright, T.M., Alexander, R.W., and Kraus, F.T.: Intramural papilloma of the vagina: evidence of Müllerian histogenesis, Cancer **48**:2260, 1981.

171. Ulbright, T.M., and Kraus, F.T.: Endometrial stromal tumors of extrauterine tissue, Am. J. Clin. Pathol. **76**:371, 1981.

172. Underwood, P.B., Jr., and Smith, R.: Carcinoma of the vagina, JAMA **217**:46, 1971.

173. Vooijs, P.G., Ng, A.B.P., and Wentz, W.B.: The detection of vaginal adenosis and clear cell carcinoma, Acta Cytol. **17**:59, 1973.

174. Wagner, J.P.: Toxic shock syndrome: a review, Am. J. Obstet. Gynecol. **146**:93, 1983.

Cervix

175. Abell, M.R.: Invasive carcinomas of the cervix. In Norris, H.J., Hertig, A.T., and Abell, M.R., editors: The uterus, Baltimore, 1973, The Williams & Wilkins Co.

176. Abell, M.R., and Gosling, J.R.G.: Gland cell carcinoma (adenocarcinoma) of the uterine cervix, Am. J. Obstet. Gynecol. **83**:729, 1962.

177. Abell, M.R., and Ramírez, J.A.: Sarcomas and carcinosarcomas of the uterine cervix, Cancer **31**:1176, 1973.

178. Albores-Saavedra, J., Larrazo, O., Poucell, S., and Martínez, H.A.R.: Carcinoid of the uterine cervix, Cancer **38**:2328, 1976.

179. Alexander, E.R.: Possible etiologies of cancer of the cervix other than herpesvirus, Cancer Res. **33**:1485, 1973.

180. Ashley, D.J.B.: The biologic status of carcinoma in situ of the uterine cervix, J. Obstet. Gynaecol. Br. Cwlth. **73**:372, 1966.

181. Aurelian, L.: Virions and antigens of herpes virus type 2 in cervical carcinoma, Cancer Res. **33**:1539, 1973.

182. Aurelian, L., Schumann, B., Marcus, R.L., et al.: Antibody to HSV-2 induced tumor specific antigens in serums from patients with cervical carcinoma, Science **181**:161, 1973.

183. Aurelian, L., Kessler, I.I., Rosenshein, N.B., and Barbour, G.: Viruses and gynecologic cancers: herpesvirus protein (ICP 10/AG-4), a cervical tumor antigen that fulfills the criteria for a marker of carcinogenicity, Cancer **48**:455, 1981.

184. Ayers, L.R., Drosman, S., and Saltzstein, S.L.: Iatrogenic paracervical implantation of fetal tissue during therapeutic abortion: a case report, Obstet. Gynecol. **37**:755, 1971.

185. Badib, A.O., Kurohara, S.S., Webster, J.H., and Pickren, J.W.: Metastasis to organs in carcinoma of the uterine cervix, Cancer **21**:434, 1968.

185a. Banks, L., and Crawford, L.: Analysis of human Papillomavirus type 16 polypeptides in transformed primary cells, Virology **165**:326, 1988.

186. Beral, V.: Cancer of the cervix: a sexually transmitted infection? Lancet **1**:1037, 1974.

187. Berry, A.: A cytopathological and histopathological study of bilharziasis of the female genital tract, J. Pathol. Bacteriol. **91**:325, 1966.

188. Boyes, D.A.: The value of a pap smear program and suggestions for its implementation, Cancer **48**:613, 1981.

189. Boyes, D.A., Worth, A.J., and Fidler, H.K.: The results of treatment of 4389 cases of pre-clinical cervical squamous carcinoma, J. Obstet. Gynaecol. Br. Cwlth. **77**:769, 1970.

190. Brand, E., Berek, J.S., Nieberg, R.K., and Hacker, N.F.: Rhabdomyosarcoma of the cervix: sarcoma botryoides, Cancer **60**:1552, 1987.

191. Brudnell, J.M., Cox, B., and Taylor, C.: The Royal College of Obstetricians and Gynaecologists' carcinoma situ survey, J. Obstet. Gynaecol. Br. Cwlth. **80**:673, 1973.

192. Burghardt, E.: Early histological diagnosis of cervical cancer, Philadelphia, 1973, W.B. Saunders Co.

193. Cachaza, J.A., Caballero, J.J.L., Fernández, J.A., and Salido, E.: Endocervical polyp with pseudosarcomatous pattern and cytoplasmic inclusions: an electron microscopic study, Am. J. Clin. Pathol. **85**:633, 1986.

194. Ceremsak, R.J.: Benign rhabdomyoma of the vagina, Am. J. Clin. Pathol. **52**:604, 1969.

195. Chanen, W., and Hollyock, V.E.: Colposcopy and the conservative management of cervical dysplasia and carcinoma in situ, Obstet. Gynecol. **43**:527, 1974.

196. Chen, S.S., Koffler, D., and Cohen, C.J.: Cellular hypersensitivity in patients with squamous cell carcinoma of the cervix, Am. J. Obstet. Gynecol. **121**:91, 1975.

197. Christopherson, W.M., Nealon, N., and Gray, L.A., Sr.: Noninvasive precursor lesions of adenocarcinoma and mixed adenosquamous carcinoma of the cervix uteri, Cancer **44**:975, 1979.

198. Christopherson, W.M., and Parker, J.E.: Control of cervix cancer in women in low income in a community, Cancer **24**:64, 1969.

199. Christopherson, W.M., and Scott, M.A.: Trends in mortality from uterine cancer in relation to mass screening, Acta Cytol. **21**:5, 1977.

200. Clement, P.B.: Multinucleated stromal giant cells of the uterine cervix, Arch. Pathol. Lab. Med. **109**:200, 1985.

201. Cohen, C.: Three cases of amoebiasis of the cervix uteri, J. Obstet. Gynaecol. Br. Cwlth. **80**:476, 1973.

202. Coppleson, M., Pixley, E., and Reid, B.: Colposcopy: a scientific and practical approach to the cervix in health and disease, Springfield, Ill., 1971, Charles C Thomas, Publisher.

203. Crum, C.P., Mitao, M., Winkler, B., Reumann, W., Boon, M.E., and Richart, R.M.: Localizing chlamydial infection in cervical biopsies with the immunoperoxidase technique, Int. J. Gynecol. Pathol. **3**:191, 1984.

204. Crum, C.P., Mitao, M., Levine, R.U., and Silverstein, S.: Cervical papillomaviruses segregate within morphologically distinct precancerous lesions, J. Virol. **54**:675, 1985.

205. Crum, C.P., Nagi, N., Levine, R.U., and Silverstein, S.: In situ hybridization analysis of HPV 16 DNA sequences in early cervical neoplasia, Am. J. Pathol. **123**:174, 1986.

206. Davidsohn, I., Norris, H.J., Stejskal, R., Norris, H.Y., Stejskal, R., and Lill, P.: Metastatic squamous cell carcinoma of the cervix: the role of immunology in its pathogenesis, Arch. Pathol. **95**:132, 1973.

207. Derman, H., Koss, L., Hyman, M.P., Penner, D.W., Soule, E., and Hicklin, M.D.: Cervical cytopathology. I. Peers compare performance, Pathologist **35**:317, 1981.

208. DiSaia, P.J., Sinkovics, J.G., Rutledge, F.N., and Smith, J.P.: Cell mediated immunity to human malignant cells: a brief review and further studies with two gynecologic lesions, Am. J. Obstet. Gynecol. **114**:979, 1972.

208a. Dyson, N., Howley, P.M., Munger, K., and Harlow, E.: The human papillomavirus 16 E7 oncoprotein is able to bind to the retinoblastoma gene product, Science **243**:934, 1989.

209. Ehrmann, R.L.: Sebaceous metaplasia of the human cervix, Am. J. Obstet. Gynecol. **105**:1284, 1969.
210. Ferenczy, A., and Winkler, B.: Carcinoma and metastatic tumors of the cervix. In Kurman, R.J., editor: Blaustein's pathology of the female genital tract, ed. 3, New York, 1987, Springer-Verlag N.Y., Inc.
211. Ferry, J.A., and Scully, R.E.: "Adenoid cystic" carcinoma and adenoid basal carcinoma of the uterine cervix, Am. J. Surg. Pathol. **12**:134, 1988.
212. Fluhmann, C.F.: The cervix and its diseases, Philadelphia, 1961, W.B. Saunders Co.
213. Friederich, E.R.: The normal morphology and ultrastructure of the cervix. In Blandau, B.J., editor: The biology of the cervix, Chicago, 1973, University of Chicago Press.
214. Gallagher, H.S., Simpson, C.B., and Ayala, A.G.: Adenoid cystic carcinoma of the uterine cervix: report of four cases, Cancer **27**:1398, 1974.
215. Goodheart, C.R.: Nucleic acid by hydridization and the relationship between cervical cancer and herpes simplex virus type 2, Cancer Res. **33**:1548, 1973.
216. Govan, A.D.T., Haines, R.M., Langley, F.A., Taylor, C.W., and Woodcock, A.S.: The histology and cytology of changes in the epithelium of the cervix uteri, J. Clin. Pathol. **22**:383, 1969.
217. Graham, C.E.: Uterine cervical epithelium of fetal and immature females in relation to estrogenic stimulation, Am. J. Obstet. Gynecol. **97**:1033, 1967.
218. Green, G.H., and Donovan, J.W.: Natural history of carcinoma in situ of the cervix, J. Obstet. Gynaecol. Br. Cwlth. **77**:1, 1970.
219. Gupta, J., Gendelman, H.E., Naghashfar, Z., Gupta, P., Rosenshein, N., Sawada, E., Woodruff, J.D., and Shah, K.: Specific identification of human papillomavirus type in cervical smears and paraffin sections by in situ hybridization with radioactive probes, Int. J. Gynecol. Pathol. **4**:211, 1985.
220. Hall, D.J., Schneider, V., and Gopelrud, D.R.: Primary malignant melanoma of the uterine cervix, Obstet. Gynecol. **56**:525, 1980.
221. Hertig, A.T., and Gore, H.: Tumors of the female sex organ. II. Tumors of the vulva, vagina and uterus. In Atlas of tumor pathology, section IX, fascicle 33, Washington, D.C., 1960, Armed Forces Institute of Pathology.
221a. Iwasaka, T., Yokoyama, M., Hayashi, Y., and Sugimori, H.: Combined herpes simplex virus type 2 and human papillomavirus type 16 or 18 deoxyribonucleic acid leads to oncogenic transformation, Am. J. Obstet. Gynecol. **150**:1251, 1988.
222. Hollinshead, A.C., and Tarro, G.: Soluble membrane antigens of lip and cervical carcinomas: reactivity with antibody for herpes-virus nonviron antigens, Science **179**:698, 1973.
223. Janovski, N.A., and Kasdon, E.J.: Benign mesonephric papillary and polypoid tumors of the cervix in childhood, J. Pediatr. **63**:211, 1963.
224. Jones, H.W., III, Plymate, S., Gluck, F.B., Miles, P.A., and Green, J.F.: Small cell non-keratinizing carcinoma of the cervix associated with ACTH productions, Cancer **38**:1629, 1976.
225. Kaufman, R.H., Garder, H.L., Rawls, W.E., Dixon, R.E., and Young, R.L.: Clinical features of herpes genitalis, Cancer Res. **33**:1446, 1973.
226. Kessler, I.I.: Etiologic concepts of cervical carcinogenesis, Gynecol. Oncol. **12**(suppl.):7, 1981.
227. Kinlen, L.J., and Spriggs, A.L.: Women with positive cervical smears but without surgical intervention, Lancet **2**:463, 1978.
228. Kirkland, J.A., Stanley, M.A., and Cellier, K.M.: Comparative study of histologic and chromosomal abnormalities in cervical neoplasia, Cancer **20**:1934, 1967.
229. Knapp, R.C., and Feldman, G.B.: The problem of optimal management of cervical carcinoma in-situ, Clin. Obstet. Gynecol. **13**:889, 1970.
230. Kolstad, P., and Kelm, V.: Long-term followup of 1121 cases of carcinoma in situ, Obstet. Gynecol. **48**:125, 1976.
231. Kolstad, P., and Stafl, A.: Atlas of colposcopy, Baltimore, 1972, University Park Press.
232. Kraus, F.T.: The biology of carcinoma in situ and microinvasive carcinoma of the cervix. In Norris, H.J., Hertig, A.T., and

Abell, M.R., editors: The uterus, Baltimore, 1973, The Williams & Wilkins Co.
233. Kraus, F.T.: Irradiation changes in the uterus. In Norris, H.J., Hertig, A.T., and Abell, M.R., editors: The uterus, Baltimore, 1973, The Williams & Wilkins Co.
234. Krieger, J.S., and McCormack, L.J.: Graded treatment for *in situ* carcinoma of the uterine cervix, Am. J. Obstet. Gynecol. **101**:171, 1968.
235. Kurman, R.J., Jenson, A.B., and Lancaster, W.D.: Papillomavirus infection of the cervix, Am. J. Surg. Pathol. **7**:39, 1983.
236. Kyriakos, M., Kempson, R.L., and Konikov, N.F.: A clinical and pathologic study of endocervical lesions associated with oral contraceptives, Cancer **22**:99, 1968.
237. LeMoine, N.R., and Hall, P.A.: Epithelial tumors metastatic to the cervix, Cancer **57**:2002, 1986.
238. Levi, M.: Autogenicity of ovarian and cervical malignancies with a view toward possible immunodiagnosis, Am. J. Obstet. Gynecol. **109**:686, 1971.
239. Love, R.R., and Camilli, A.E.: The value of screening, Cancer **48**:489, 1981.
240. Ludwig, M.E., Lowell, D.M., and LiVolsi, V.A.: Cervical condylomatous atypia and its relationship to cervical neoplasia, Am. J. Clin. Pathol. **76**:255, 1981.
241. McDougall, J.K., Galloway, D.A., and Fenoglio, C.M.: Cervical carcinoma: detection of herpes simplex virus RNA in cells undergoing neoplastic change, Int. J. Cancer **25**:1, 1980.
242. McIndoe, W.A., McLean, M.R., Jones, R.W., and Mullins, P.R.: The invasive potential of carcinoma in situ of the cervix, Obstet. Gynecol. **64**:451, 1984.
243. Meisels, A., Fortin, R., and Roy, M.: Condylomatous lesions of the cervix. II. Cytologic, colposcopic, and histopathologic study, Acta Cytol. **21**:379, 1977.
244. Michael, H., Grawe, L., and Kraus, F.T.: Minimal deviation endocervical adenocarcinoma: clinical and histologic features, immunohistological staining for carcinoembryonic antigen, and differentiation from confusing benign lesions, Int. J. Gynecol. Pathol. **3**:261, 1984.
245. Miles, P.A., and Norris, H.J.: Adenoid cystic carcinoma of the cervix: an analysis of 12 cases, Obstet. Gynecol. **38**:103, 1971.
246. Mussey, E., Soule, E.H., and Welch, J.S.: Microinvasive carcinoma of the cervix: late results of operative treatment in 91 cases, Am. J. Obstet. Gynecol. **104**:738, 1969.
247. Naib, Z.M., Nahmias, A.J., Josey, W.E., and Zaki, S.A.: Relation of cytohistopathology of genital herpesvirus infection to cervical anaplasia, Cancer Res. **33**:1452, 1973.
248. Nangle, R., Berger, M., and Levin, M.: Variations in the morphogenesis of squamous carcinoma of the cervix, Cancer **16**:1151, 1963.
249. Newton, C.W., and Abell, M.R.: Iatrogenic fetal implants, Obstet. Gynecol. **40**:686, 1972.
250. Ng, A.B.P., and Atkin, N.B.: Histological cell type and DNA value in the prognosis of squamous cell cancer of the uterine cervix, Br. J. Cancer **28**:322, 1973.
251. Ng, A.B.P., and Reagan, J.W.: Microinvasive carcinoma of the cervix, Am. J. Clin. Pathol. **52**:511, 1969.
252. Niven, P.A.R., and Stansfield, A.G.: Glioma of the uterus: a fetal homograft, Am. J. Obstet. Gynecol. **115**:534, 1973.
253. Paavonen, J., Meyer, B., Vesterinen, E., and Saksela E.: Colposcopic and histological findings in cervical chlamydial infection, Lancet **2**:320, 1980.
254. Paunier, J.P., Delclos, L., and Fletcher, G.H.: Causes, time of death, and sites of failure in squamous cell carcinoma of the uterine cervix on intact uterus, Radiology **88**:555, 1967.
255. Pérez, C.A., Zivnuska, F., Askin, F., Kumar, B., Camel, H.M., and Powers, W.E.: Prognostic significance of endometrial extension from primary carcinoma of the uterine cervix, Cancer **35**:1493, 1975.
256. Pilotti, S., Rilke, F., DePalo, G., Della Torre, G., and Alasio, L.: Condylomata of the uterine cervix and koilocytosis of cervical intraepithelial neoplasia, J. Clin. Pathol. **34**:532, 1981.
257. Qizilbash, A.H.: Papillary squamous tumors of the uterine cervix: a clinical and pathologic study of 21 cases, Am. J. Clin. Pathol. **61**:508, 1974.

258. Qizilbash, A.H.: *In situ* and microinvasive adenocarcinoma of the uterine cervix: a clinical, cytologic, and histologic study of 14 cases, Am. J. Clin. Pathol. **64:**155, 1975.

259. Rapp, F., and Duff, R.: Transformation of hamster embryofibroblasts by herpes simplex viruses types 1 and 2, Cancer Res. **33:**1527, 1973.

260. Rawls, W.E., Adam, E., and Melnick, J.L.: An analysis of seroepidemiological studies of herpesvirus type-2 and carcinoma of the cervix, Cancer Res. **33:**1477, 1973.

261. Reid, R., Laverty, C.R., Coppleson, M., Isarangkul, W., and Hills, E.: Noncondylomatous cervical wart virus infection, Obstet. Gynecol. **55:**476, 1980.

262. Richart, R.M., and Barron, B.A.: A follow-up study of patients with cervical dysplasia, Am. J. Obstet. Gynecol. **105:**386, 1969.

263. Roche, W.D., and Norris, H.J.: Microinvasive carcinoma of the cervix: the significance of lymphatic invasion and confluent patterns of stromal growth, Cancer **36:**180, 1975.

264. Roth, E., and Taylor, H.B.: Heterotopic cartilage in the uterus, Obstet. Gynecol. **27:**838, 1966.

265. Rotkin, I.D., and Cameron, J.R.: Clusters of variables influencing risk of cervical cancer, Cancer **21:**663, 1968.

266. Rubio, C.A., and Lagerlof, B.: Autoradiographic studies of dysplasia and carcinoma *in situ* in cervical cones, Acta Pathol. Microbiol. Scand. **82:**411, 1974.

267. Rutledge, F.N., Galakatos, A.E., Wharton, J.T., and Smith, J.T.: Adenocarcinoma of the uterine cervix, Am. J. Obstet. Gynecol. **122:**236, 1975.

268. Schellhas, H.F., and Heath, G.: Cell renewal in the human cervix uteri: a radioautographic study of DNA, RNA, and protein synthesis, Am. J. Obstet. Gynecol. **104:**617, 1969.

268a. Schneider-Gadicke, A., Kaul, S., Schwarz, E., Gausepohl, H., Frank, R., and Bastert, G.: Identification of the human papillomavirus type 18 E6* and E6 proteins in nuclear protein fraction from human cervical carcinoma cells grown in the nude mouse or in vitro, Cancer Res. **48:**2969, 1988.

269. Scully, R.E.: Definition of precursors of gynecologic cancer, Cancer **48:**531, 1981.

270. Selim, M.A., So-Bosita, J., and Neuman, M.R.: Carcinoma in situ of cervix uteri, Surg. Gynecol. Obstet. **139:**697, 1974.

271. Sherrick, J.C., and Vega, J.G.: Congenital intramural cysts of uterus, Obstet. Gynecol. **19:**486, 1962.

271a. Shibata, D., Yao, S.F., Gupta, J.W., Shah, K.V., Arnheim, N., and Martin, J.W.: Detection of human papillomavirus in normal and dysplastic tissue by the polymerase chain reaction, Lab. Invest. **59:**555, 1988.

272. Shingleton, H.M., Richart, R.M., Weiner, J., and Spiro, D.: Human cervical intraepithelial neoplasia: fine structure of dysplasia and carcinoma in situ, Cancer Res. **18:**695, 1968.

273. Silverberg, E., and Lubera, J.A.: Cancer statistics, 1988, CA **38:**5, 1988.

274. Silverberg, E., and Holleb, A.I.: Major trends in cancer: 25 year survey, CA **25:**2, 1975.

275. Silverberg, S.G.: Adenomyomatosis of the endometrium, Am. J. Clin. Pathol. **64:**192, 1975.

276. Silverberg, S.G., and Hurt, G.W.: Minimal deviation adenocarcinoma ("adenoma malignum") of the cervix: a reappraisal, Am. J. Obstet. Gynecol. **121:**971, 1975.

277. Singer, A.: The uterine cervix from adolescence to the menopause, Br. J. Obstet. Gynaecol. **82:**81, 1975.

278. Sorensen, H.M., Petersen, O., Nielson, J., Bang, F., and Koch, F.: The spontaneous course of premalignant lesions on the vaginal portion of the uterus, Acta Obstet. Gynecol. Scand. **43**(suppl. 7):103, 1964.

279. Spriggs, A.I., Bowey, E., and Cowdell, R.H.: Chromosomes of precancerous lesions of the cervix, Cancer **27:**1239, 1971.

280. Stamler, T., Fields, C., and Andelman, S.L.: Epidemiology of cancer of the cervix. I. The dimensions of the problem: mortality and morbidity from cancer of the cervix, Am. J. Pub. Health **57:**791, 1967.

281. Steiner, G., and Friedell, G.H.: Adenosquamous carcinoma *in situ* of the cervix, Cancer **18:**807, 1965.

282. Stoddard, L.D.: The problem of carcinoma in situ with reference to the human cervix uteri. In McManus, J.F.A., editor: Progress in fundamental medicine, Philadelphia, 1952, Lea & Febiger.

283. Taylor, H.B., Irey, N.S., and Norris, H.J.: Atypical endocervical hyperplasia in women taking oral contraceptives, JAMA **202:**637, 1967.

284. Thompson, B.H., Woodruff, J.D., Davis, H.J., Julian, C.G., and Silva, F.G.: Cytopathology, histopathology, and colposcopy in the management of cervical neoplasia, Am. J. Obstet. Gynecol. **114:**329, 1972.

285. Watson, A.A., and Cochran, A.J.: Sebaceous glands of the cervix uteri and buccal mucosa, J. Pathol. Bacteriol. **98:**87, 1969.

286. Wentz, W.B., and Reagan, J.W.: Survival in cervical cancer with respect to cell type, Cancer **12:**384, 1959.

287. Wentz, W.B., Reagan, J.W., Fu, Y.S., Heggie, A.D., and Anthony, D.D.: Experimental studies of carcinogenesis of the uterine cervix in mice, Gynecol. Oncol. **12**(suppl.):90, 1981.

288. Willis, R.A.: The borderland of embryology and pathology, ed. 2, Washington, D.C., 1962, Butterworth & Co., Inc.

289. Woodruff, J.D., Braun, L., Cavalieri, R., Gupta, P., Pass, F., and Shah, K.U.: Immunological identification of papillomavirus antigen in paraffin-processed condyloma tissue from the female genital tract, Obstet. Gynecol. **56:**727, 1980.

289a. Woodworth, C.D., Bowden, P.E., Doniger, J., Pirisi, L., Barnes, W., Lancaster, W.D., and DiPaolo, J.A.: Characterization of normal human exocervical epithelial cells immortalized in vitro by papillomavirus types 16 and 18 DNA, Cancer Res. **48:**4620, 1988.

290. Worth, A.J., and Boyes, D.A.: A case control study of the possible effects of birth control pills on pre-clinical carcinoma of the cervix, J. Obstet. Gynaecol. Br. Cwlth. **79:**673, 1972.

291. zur Hausen, H.: Human genital cancer: synergism between two virus infections or between a virus infection and initiating events, Lancet **2:**1370, 1982.

291a. zur Hausen, H.: Papillomaviruses in human cancer, Cancer **59:**1692, 1987.

Endometrium

292. Ackerman, L.V., and Rosai, J.: Surgical pathology, St. Louis, 1974, The C.V. Mosby Co.

293. Aikawa, M., and Ng, A.B.P.: Mixed (adenosquamous) carcinoma of the endometrium: electron microscopic observations, Cancer **31:**385, 1973.

294. Aksel, S., and Jones, G.S.: Etiology and treatment of dysfunctional uterine bleeding, Obstet. Gynecol. **44:**1, 1974.

295. Anderson, G.D.: *Listeria monocytogenes* septicemia in pregnancy, Obstet. Gynecol. **461:**02, 1975.

296. Andrews, W.C.: Luteal phase defects, Fertil. Steril. **32:**501, 1979.

297. Arias-Stella, J.: Gestational endometrium. In Norris, H.J., Hertig, A.T., and Abell, M.R., editors: The uterus, Baltimore, 1973, The Williams & Wilkins Co.

298. Armenia, C.S.: Sequential relationship between endometrial polyps and carcinoma of the endometrium, Obstet. Gynecol. **30:**524, 1967.

299. Armstrong, E.M., More, E.M., McSeveney, D., and Carty, M.: The giant mitochondrion–endoplasmic reticulin unit of the endometrial glandular cell, J. Anat. **116:**375, 1973.

300. Armstrong, E.M., More, I.A., McSeveney, D., and Chatfield, W.R.: Reappraisal of the ultrastructure of the human endometrial glandular cell, J. Obstet. Gynaecol. Br. Cwlth. **80:**446, 1973.

301. Arronet, G.H., and Arrata, W.S.M.: Dysfunctional uterine bleeding: a classification, Obstet. Gynecol. **29:**97, 1967.

302. Baggish, M.D., and Woodruff, J.D.: The occurrence of squamous epithelium in the endometrium, Obstet. Gynecol. Surv. **22:**69, 1967.

303. Barwick, K.W., and LiVolsi, V.S.: Malignant mixed müllerian

tumors of the uterus: a clinicopathologic assessment of 34 cases, Am. J. Surg. Pathol. **3**:125, 1979.

304. Blum, R.H., Corson, J.M., Wilson, R.E., Greenberger, J.S., Canellos, G.P., and Frei, E., III.: Successful treatment of metastatic sarcomas with cyclophosphamide, Adriamycin, and DTIC, Cancer **46**:1722, 1980.

305. Blythe, J.G., and Ali, Z.: Endometrial adenocarcinoma: in estrogen, oral contraceptive, and nonhormone users, Gynecol. Oncol. **7**:199, 1979.

306. Bosio, B.B., and Taylor, E.S.: *Bacteroides* and puerperal infections, Obstet. Gynecol. **42**:271, 1973.

307. Boutselis, J.G.: Histochemistry of the normal endometrium. In Norris, H.J., Hertig, A.T., and Abell, M.R., editors: The uterus, Baltimore, 1973, The Williams & Wilkins Co.

308. Braun, P., and Druckman, E.: Public health rounds at the Harvard School of Public Health, N. Engl. J. Med. **295**:264, 1976.

309. Cadena, D., Cavanzo, F.J., Leone, G.L., and Taylor, H.B.: Chronic endometritis: a comparative clinicopathologic study, Obstet. Gynecol. **41**:733, 1973.

310. Cavazos, F., and Lucas, F.V.: Ultrastructure of the endometrium. In Norris, H.J., Hertig, A.T., and Abell, M.R., editors: The uterus, Baltimore, 1973, The Williams & Wilkins Co.

311. Centers for Disease Control: Surgical sterilization surveillance: hysterectomy in women aged 15-44, 1970-1975, Atlanta, 1980.

312. Chambers, T.J., Merino, M., Kohorn, E.I., Perschel, R.E., and Schwartz, P.E.: Uterine papillary serous carcinoma, Obstet. Gynecol. **69**:109, 1987.

313. Chamlian, D.L., and Taylor, H.B.: Endometrial hyperplasia in young women, Obstet. Gynecol. **36**:659, 1970.

314. Chorlton, I., Karnei, R.F., Jr., King, F.M., and Norris, H.J.: Primary malignant reticuloendothelial disease involving the vagina, cervix, and corpus uteri, Obstet. Gynecol. **44**:735, 1974.

315. Chuang, J.T., Van Velden, D.J.J., and Graham, J.B.: Carcinosarcoma and mixed mesodermal tumor of the uterine corpus: review of 49 cases, Obstet. Gynecol. **35**:769, 1970.

316. Clement, P.B., and Scully, R.E.: Uterine tumors with mixed epithelial and mesenchymal elements, Semin. Diagn. Pathol. **5**:199, 1988.

317. Craig, J.M.: The pathology of birth control, Arch. Pathol. **99**:233, 1975.

318. Crum, C.P., Richart, R.M., and Fenoglio, C.M.: Adenoacanthosis of the endometrium: a clinicopathologic study in premenopausal women, Am. J. Surg. Pathol. **5**:15, 1981.

319. Czernobilsky, B., Katz, Z., Lancet, M., and Gaton, E.: Endocervical-type epithelium in endometrial carcinoma: a report of 10 cases with emphasis on histochemical methods for differential diagnosis, Am. J. Surg. Pathol. **4**:481, 1980.

320. Dallenbach-Hellweg, G.: Histopathology of the endometrium, New York, 1975, Springer-Verlag, N.Y., Inc.

321. deLouvois, J., Blades, M., and Harrison, R.F.: Frequency of mycoplasma in fertile and infertile couples, Lancet **1**:1073, 1974.

322. deMoraes-Ruehsen, M.D., Jones, G.S., Burnett, L.S., and Baramki, T.A.: The aluteal cycle: a severe form of the luteal phase defect, Am. J. Obstet. Gynecol. **103**:1059, 1969.

323. Dutra, F.R.: Intraglandular morules of the endometrium, Am. J. Clin. Pathol. **31**:60, 1959.

324. Fechner, R.E.: Endometrium with the pattern of mesonephroma: report of a case, Obstet. Gynecol. **31**:485, 1960.

325. Fechner, R.E., and Kaufman, R.H.: Endometrial adenocarcinoma in Stein-Leventhal syndrome, Cancer **34**:444, 1974.

326. Ferenczy, A., and Richart, R.M.: Female reproductive system: dynamics of scan and transmission electron microscopy, New York, 1974, John Wiley & Sons, Inc.

327. Friederich, E.R.: Effects of contraceptive hormone preparations on the fine structure of the endometrium, Obstet. Gynecol. **30**:201, 1967.

328. Ganem, K.J., Parsons, L., and Friedell, G.H.: Endometrial ossification, Am. J. Obstet. Gynecol. **83**:1592, 1962.

329. Gompel, C., and Silverberg, S.G.: Pathology in gynecology and obstetrics, ed. 2, Philadelphia, 1977, J.B. Lippincott Co.

330. Good, R.G., and Moyer, D.L.: Estrogen progesterone relationships in the development of secretory endometrium, Fertil. Steril. **19**:37, 1968.

331. Gore, H.: Hyperplasia of the endometrium. In Norris, H.J., Hertig, A.T., and Abell, M.R., editors: The uterus, Baltimore, 1973, The Williams & Wilkins Co.

332. Gore, H., and Hertig, A.T.: Carcinoma in situ of the endometrium, Am. J. Obstet. Gynecol. **94**:134, 1966.

333. Hammond, C.B., Jelopsek, F.R., Lee, K.L., Creasman, W.T., and Parker, R.T.: Effects of long-term estrogen replacement therapy. II. Neoplasia, Am. J. Obstet. Gynecol. **133**:537, 1979.

334. Harris, N.L., and Scully, R.E.: Malignant lymphoma and granulocytic sarcoma of the uterus and vagina: a clinicopathologic analysis of 27 cases, Cancer **53**:2530, 1984.

335. Hendrickson, M.R., and Kempson, R.L.: Endometrial epithelial metaplasias: proliferations frequently misdiagnosed as adenocarcinoma: report of 89 cases and proposed classification, Am. J. Surg. Pathol. **4**:525, 1980.

336. Hendrickson, M.R., Ross, J.C., and Kempson, R.L.: Toward the development of morphologic criteria for well-differentiated adenocarcinoma of the endometrium, Am. J. Surg. Pathol. **7**:819, 1983.

337. Hertig, A.T.: Gestational hyperplasia of endometrium: a morphologic correlation of ova, endometrium, and corpora lutea during early pregnancy, Lab. Invest. **13**:1153, 1964.

338. Hertig, A.T., Sommers, S.C., and Bengloff, A.: Genesis of endometrial carcinoma. III. Carcinoma in situ, Cancer **2**:964, 1949.

339. Horwitz, R.I., Feinstein, A.R., Vidone, R.A., Sommers, S.C., and Robboy, S.J.: Histopathologic distinctions in the relationship of estrogens and endometrial cancer, JAMA **246**:1425, 1981.

340. Israel, S.L., Roitman, H.B., and Clancy, E.: Infrequency of unsuspected endometrial tuberculosis, histologic and bacteriologic study, JAMA **183**:63, 1963.

341. Jones, G.S.: The luteal phase defect, Fertil. Steril. **27**:351, 1976.

342. Kahn, H.S., and Tyler, C.W.: Mortality associated with use of IUD's, JAMA **234**:57, 1975.

343. Kaufman, R.H., Abbot, J.P., and Wall, J.A.: The endometrium before and after wedge resection of the ovaries in the Stein-Leventhal syndrome, Am. J. Obstet. Gynecol. **77**:1271, 1959.

344. Kay, S.: Squamous cell carcinoma of the endometrium, Am. J. Clin. Pathol. **61**:264, 1974.

345. Kempson, R.L., and Bari, W.: Uterine sarcomas: classification, diagnosis and prognosis, Hum. Pathol. **1**:331, 1970.

346. Kempson, R.L., and Hendrickson, M.R.: Pure mesenchymal neoplasms of the uterus: selected problems, Semin. Diagn. Pathol. **5**:172, 1988.

347. Kempson, R.L., and Pokorny, G.E.: Adenocarcinoma of the endometrium in women aged 40 and younger, Cancer **21**:650, 1968.

348. Kistner, R.W.: Endometrial alterations associated with estrogen and estrogen-progestin combinations. In Norris, H.J.: Hertig, A.T., and Abell, M.R., editors: The uterus, Baltimore, 1973, The Williams & Wilkins Co.

349. Kistner, R.W., Duncan, C.J., and Mansell, H.: Suppression of ovulation by tri-*p*-anisylchloroethylene (TACE), Obstet. Gynecol. **8**:399, 1956.

350. Klaer, W., and Holm-Jensen, S.: Metastases to the uterus, Acta Pathol. Microbiol. Scand. **80**:835, 1972.

351. Krumholz, B.A., Lobovsky, F.Y., and Hahtsky, V.: Endolymphatic stromal myosis with pulmonary metastases: remission with progestin therapy; report of a case, J. Reprod. Med. **10**:85, 1973.

352. Kurman, R.J., Kaminski, P.F., and Norris, J.H.: The behavior of endometrial hyperplasia: a long term study of "untreated" hyperplasia in 170 patients, Cancer **56**:403, 1985.

353. Kurman, R.J., and Norris, H.J.: Evaluation of criteria for distinguishing atypical endometrial hyperplasia from well differentiated carcinoma, Cancer **49**:2547, 2559, 1982.

354. Langlois, P.L.: The size of the normal uterus, J. Reprod. Med. 4:220, 1970.

355. Larbig, G.G., Clemmer, J.J., Koss, L.G., and Foote, F.W., Jr.: Plexiform tumorlets of endometrial stromal origin, Am. J. Clin. Pathol. 44:32, 1965.

356. Laros, R.K., and Work, B.A.: Female sterilization. II. A comparison of methods, Obstet. Gynecol. 46:215, 1975.

357. Mazur, M.T.: Atypical polypoid adenomyomas of the endometrium, Am. J. Surg. Pathol. 5:473, 1981.

358. Mazur, M.T., and Kraus, F.T.: Histogenesis of morphologic variations in tumors of the uterine wall, Am. J. Surg. Pathol. 4:59, 1980.

359. Ng, A.B.P., and Reagan, J.W.: Incidence and prognosis of endometrial carcinoma by histologic grade and extent, Obstet. Gynecol. 35:437, 1970.

360. Ng, A.B.P., Reagan, J.W., Storaasli, J.P., and Wentz, W.B.: Mixed adenosquamous carcinoma of the endometrium, Am. J. Clin. Pathol. 59:765, 1973.

361. Nogales, F., Beato, M., and Martínez, H.: Funktionelle Veränderungen des tuberculösen Endometriums, Arch. Gynecol. 203:45, 1966.

362. Norris, H.J., Roth, E., and Taylor, H.B.: Mesenchymal tumors of the uterus. II. A clinical and pathological study of 31 mixed mesodermal tumors, Obstet. Gynecol. 28:57, 1966.

363. Norris, H.J., and Taylor, H.B.: Mesenchymal tumors of the uterus. I. A clinical and pathological study of 53 endometrial stromal tumors, Cancer 19:755, 1966.

364. Noyes, R.W.: Normal phases of the endometrium. In Norris, H.J., Hertig, A.T., and Abell, M.R., editors: The uterus, Baltimore, 1973, The Williams & Wilkins Co.

365. Pérez, C.A., Askin, F., Baglan, R.J., Kao, M.S., Kraus, F.T., Pérez, B.M., Williams, C.F., and Weiss, D.: Effects of radiation on mixed müllerian tumors of the uterus, Cancer 43:1274, 1979.

366. Philippe, E.: Endomètre et séquelles d'avortement, Rev. Fr. Gynecol. 65:413, 1970.

367. Picoff, R.C., and Luginbuhl, W.H.: Fibrin in the endometrial stroma: its relation to uterine bleeding, Am. J. Obstet. Gynecol. 88:642, 1964.

368. Poulsen, H.E., Taylor, C.W., and Subin, L.H.: Histological typing of female genital tract tumors, Geneva, 1975, World Health Organization.

369. Robboy, S.J., and Bradley, R.: Changing trends and prognostic features in endometrial cancer associated with exogenous estrogen therapy, Obstet. Gynecol. 54:269, 1979.

370. Rorat, E., Ferenczy, A., and Richart, R.M.: The ultrastructure of clear cell adenocarcinoma of the endometrium, Cancer 33:880, 1974.

371. Rosai, J.: Ackerman's surgical pathology, ed. 6, St. Louis, 1981, The C.V. Mosby Co.

372. Roth, E., and Taylor, H.B.: Heterotopic cartilage in the uterus, Obstet. Gynecol. 27:838, 1966.

373. Ryan, G.M., Jr., Craig, J., and Reid, D.E.: Histology of the uterus and ovaries after long-term cyclic norethynodrel therapy, Am. J. Obstet. Gynecol. 90:715, 1964.

374. Salm, R.: The incidence and significance of early carcinomas in endometrial polyps, J. Pathol. 108:47, 1972.

375. Shanklin, D.R.: Histologic dating of the endometrium: an invitational symposium, J. Reprod. Med. 3:179, 1969.

376. Sheffield, W.H., Soule, S.D., and Herzog, G.M.: Cyclic endometrial changes in response to monthly injections of an estrogen-progestogen contraceptive drug: a histologic study, Am. J. Obstet. Gynecol. 103:828, 1969.

377. Silverberg, S.G., Bolin, M.G., and DeGeorgi, L.S.: Adenoacanthoma and mixed adenosquamous carcinoma of the endometrium: a clinicopathologic study, Cancer 30:1307, 1972.

378. Silverberg, S.G., and DiGeorgi, L.S.: Clear cell carcinoma of the endometrium, Cancer 31:1127, 1973.

379. Silverberg, S.G., and Makowski, E.L.: Endometrial carcinoma in young women taking oral contraceptive agents, Obstet. Gynecol. 46:503, 1975.

380. Silverberg, S.G., Mullen, D., Faraci, J.A., Makowski, E.L., Miller, A., Finch, J.L., and Sutherland, J.V.: Endometrial carcinoma: clinical-pathologic comparison of cases in post-menopausal women receiving and not receiving exogenous estrogens, Cancer 45:3018, 1980.

381. Smith, D.C., Prentice, R., Thompson, D.J., and Herrmann, W.L.: Association of exogenous estrogen and endometrial carcinoma, N. Engl. J. Med. 293:1164, 1975.

382. Stevenson, C.S.: The endometrium in infertile women: prognostic significance of the initial study biopsy, Fertil. Steril. 16:208, 1965.

383. Tavassoli, F.A., and Kraus, F.T.: Endometrial lesions in uteri resected for atypical endometrial hyperplasia, Am. J. Clin. Pathol. 70:770, 1978.

384. Tavassoli, F.A., and Norris, H.J.: Mesenchymal tumors of the uterus. VII. A clinicopathological study of 60 endometrial stromal nodules, Histopathology 5:1, 1981.

385. Terzakis, J.A.: The nucleolar channel system of human endometrium, J. Cell. Biol. 27:293, 1965.

386. Thom, M.H., White, P.J., Williams, R.M., Sturdee, D.W., Paterson, M.E., Wade-Evans, T., and Studd, J.W.: Prevention and treatment of endometrial disease in climacteric women receiving estrogen therapy, Lancet 2:455, 1979.

387. Tiltman, A.J.: Mucinous carcinoma of the endometrium, Obstet. Gynecol. 55:244, 1980.

388. Ulbright, T.M., and Kraus, F.T.: Endometrial stromal tumors of extra-uterine tissue, Am. J. Clin. Pathol. 76:371, 1981.

389. Vellios, F.: Endometrial hyperplasias, precursors of endometrial carcinoma. In Sommers, S.C., editor: Pathology Annual, vol. 7, New York, 1972, Appleton-Century-Crofts.

390. Weiss, N.S., Ure, C.L., Ballard, J.H., Williams, A.R., and Daling, J.R.: Decreased risk of fractures of the hip and lower forearm with postmenopausal use of estrogen, N. Engl. J. Med. 303:1195, 1980.

391. Wienke, E.C., Lavazos, E., Hall, D.G., and Lucas, F.V.: Ultrastructural effects of norethynodrel and mestranol on human endometrial stromal cell, Am. J. Obstet. Gynecol. 103:102, 1969.

392. Williamson, E.O., and Christopherson, W.M.: Malignant mixed müllerian tumors of the uterus, Cancer 29:585, 1972.

393. Wolff, M., Silva, F., and Kaye, G.: Pulmonary metastases (with admixed epithelial elements) from smooth muscle neoplasms: report of nine cases, including three males, Am. J. Surg. Pathol. 3:325, 1979.

394. Woodruff, J.D., and Julian, C.G.: Multiple malignancy in the upper genital canal, Am. J. Obstet. Gynecol. 103:810, 1969.

395. Young, R.H., Kleinman, G.M., and Scully, R.E.: Glioma of the uterus, Am. J. Surg. Pathol. 5:695, 1981.

396. Zaino, R.J., and Kurman, R.H.: Squamous differentiation in carcinoma of the endometrium: a critical appraisal of adenocarcinoma and adenosquamous carcinoma, Semin. Diagn. Pathol. 5:154, 1988.

397. Zaloudek, C.J., and Norris, H.J.: Adenofibroma of the uterus: a clinicopathologic study of 35 cases, Cancer 48:354, 1981.

398. Zettergren, L.: Glial tissue in the uterus, Am. J. Pathol. 71:419, 1973.

Myometrium

399. Banner, A.S., Carrington, C.B., Emory, W.B., Kittle, E., Leonard, G., Ringus, J., Taylor, P., and Addington, W.W.: Efficacy of oophorectomy in lymphangiomyomatosis and benign metastasizing leiomyoma, N. Engl. J. Med. 305:204, 1981.

400. Barlow, J.J., Piver, M.S., Chuang, J.T., Cortez, E.P., Ohnuma, T., and Holland, J.F.: Adriamycin and bleomycin, alone and in combination, in gynecologic cancers, Cancer 32:735, 1973.

401. Bartsich, E.G., Bowe, E.T., and Moore, J.G.: Leiomyosarcomas of the uterus: a 50 year review of 42 cases, Obstet. Gynecol. 32:101, 1968.

402. Boyce, C.R., and Buddhdev, H.N.: Pregnancy complicated by metastasizing leiomyoma of the uterus, Obstet. Gynecol. 42:252, 1973.

403. Christopherson, W.M., Williamson, E.O., and Gray, L.A.: Leiomyosarcoma of the uterus, Cancer 29:1512, 1972.

404. Cramer, S.F., Meyer, J.S., Kraner, J.F., Camel, M., Mazur, M.T., and Tenenbaum, M.S.: Metastasizing leiomyoma of the uterus: S-phase, fraction, estrogen receptor, and ultrastructure, Cancer **45**:932, 1980.

405. Emge, L.A.: The elusive adenomyosis of the uterus: its historical past and its present state of recognition, Am. J. Obstet. Gynecol. **83**:1541, 1962.

406. Fechner, R.E.: Atypical leiomyomas and synthetic progestin therapy, Am. J. Clin. Pathol. **49**:697, 1968.

407. Ferenczy, A., Fenoglio, J., and Richart, R.M.: Observations on benign mesothelioma of the genital tract (adenomatoid tumor): a comparative ultrastructural study, Cancer **30**:244, 1972.

408. Ferenczy, A., Richart, R.M., and Okagaki, T.: A comparative ultrastructural study of leiomyosarcoma, cellular leiomyoma, and leiomyoma of the uterus, Cancer **28**:1004, 1971.

409. Goodhue, W.W., Susin, M., and Kramer, E.E.: Smooth muscle origin of uterine plexiform tumors, Arch. Pathol. **71**:263, 1974.

410. Idelson, M.G., and Dairds, A.W.: Metastasis of uterine fibromyomata, Obstet. Gynecol. **21**:78, 1963.

411. Jacobs, D.S., Cohen, H., and Johnson, J.S.: Lipoleiomyomas of the uterus, Am. J. Clin. Pathol. **44**:45, 1965.

412. Konis, E.E., and Belsky, R.D.: Metastasizing leiomyoma of the uterus: report of a case, Obstet. Gynecol. **27**:442, 1966.

413. Marcus, C.C.: Relationship of adenomyosis uteri to endometrial hyperplasia and endometrial carcinoma, Am. J. Obstet. Gynecol. **82**:408, 1961.

414. Mathur, B.B.L., Shah, B.S., and Bhende, Y.M.: Adenomyosis uteri, Am. J. Obstet. Gynecol. **84**:1820, 1962.

415. Murphy, E.: Diffuse myometrial sclerosis, Am. J. Obstet. Gynecol. **103**:403, 1969.

416. Norris, H.J., and Parmley, T.: Mesenchymal tumors of the uterus. V. Intravenous leiomyomatosis: a report of 14 cases, Cancer **36**:2164, 1975.

417. Paranjothy, D., and Vaish, S.K.: Polycythemia associated with leiomyoma of the uterus, J. Obstet. Gynaecol. Br. Cwlth. **74**:603, 1967.

418. Parmley, T.H., Woodruff, J.D., Winn, K., Johnson, J.W.C., and Douglas, P.H.: Histogenesis of leiomyomatosis peritonealis disseminata (disseminated fibrosing deciduosis), Obstet. Gynecol. **46**:511, 1975.

419. Perrone, T., and Dehner, L.P.: Prognostically favorable "mitotically active" smooth-muscle tumors of the uterus: a clinicopathologic study of ten cases, Am. J. Surg. Pathol. **12**:1, 1988.

420. Pietila, K.: Hysterography in the diagnosis of uterine myoma: roentgen findings in 829 cases compared with operative findings, Acta Obstet. Gynecol. Scand. **48**(suppl. 5):1, 1969.

421. Rothman, D., and Rennard, M.: Myoma erythrocytosis syndrome: report of a case, Obstet. Gynecol. **21**:102, 1963.

422. Rywlin, A.M., Rechner, L., and Benson, J.: Clear cell leiomyoma of the uterus: report of two cases of a previously undescribed entity, Cancer **17**:100, 1964.

423. Saksela, E., Lampinen, V., and Procope, B.J.: Malignant mesenchymal tumors of the uterine corpus, Am. J. Obstet. Gynecol. **120**:452, 1974.

424. Salm, R.: The histogenesis of uterine lipomas, Beitr. Pathol. **149**:284, 1973.

425. Scharfenberg, J.C, and Geary, W.L.: Intravenous leiomyomatosis, Obstet. Gynecol. **43**:909, 1974.

426. Silverberg, S.G.: Leiomyosarcoma of the uterus: a clinicopathologic study, Obstet. Gynecol. **38**:613, 1971.

427. Silverberg, S.G., Wilson, M.A., and Board, J.A.: Hemangiopericytoma of the uterus: an ultrastructural study, Am. J. Obstet. Gynecol. **110**:297, 1971.

428. Stout, A.P.: Bizarre smooth muscle tumors of the stomach, Cancer **15**:400, 1962.

429. Taubert, H.-D., Wissner, S.E., and Haskins, A.L.: Leiomyomatosis peritonealis disseminata: an unusual complication of genital leiomyomata, Obstet. Gynecol. **25**:561, 1965.

430. Taxy, J.B., Battifora, H., and Oyasu, R.: Adenomatoid tumors: a light microscopic, histochemical, and ultrastructural study, Cancer **34**:306, 1974.

431. Taylor, H.B., and Norris, H.J.: Mesenchymal tumors of the uterus. IV. Diagnosis and prognosis of leiomyosarcomas, Arch. Pathol. **82**:40, 1966.

432. Vardi, J.R., and Tovell, H.M.M.: Leiomyosarcoma of the uterus: clinicopathologic study, Obstet. Gynecol. **56**:428, 1980.

433. Youngs, L.A., and Taylor, H.B.: Adenomatoid tumors of the uterus and fallopian tube, Am. J. Clin. Pathol. **48**:537, 1967.

Fallopian tube

434. Acosta, A.A., Kaplan, A.L., and Kaufman, R.H.: Mixed müllerian tumors of the oviduct, Obstet. Gynecol. **44**:84, 1974.

435. Benjamin, C.L., and Beaver, D.C.: Pathogenesis of salpingitis isthmica nodosa, Am. J. Clin. Pathol. **21**:212, 1951.

436. Dokumov, S., and Dekov, D.: A rare case of precocious pseudopuberty due to a Sertoli-Leydig cell tumor originating from the left fallopian tube, J. Clin. Endocrinol. Metab. **23**:1262, 1963.

437. Ferenczy, A., and Richart, R.M.: Female reproductive system: dynamics of scan and transmission electron microscopy, New York, 1974, John Wiley & Sons, Inc.

438. Flege, J.B.: Ruptured tubal pregnancy with elevated serum amylase levels, Arch. Surg. **92**:397, 1966.

439. Fogh, I.: Primary carcinoma of the fallopian tube, Cancer **23**:1332, 1969.

440. Friberg, J., Confino, E., Suarez, M., and Gleicher, N.: *Chlamydia trachomatis* attached to spermatozoa recovered from the peritoneal cavity of patients with salpingitis, J. Reprod. Med. **32**:120, 1987.

441. Jacobson, L., and Weström, L.: Objectivized diagnoses of acute pelvic inflammatory disease, Am. J. Obstet. Gynecol. **105**:1088, 1969.

442. Keeny, G.L., and Thrasher, T.V.: Metaplastic papillary tumor of the fallopian tube: a case report with ultrastructure, Int. J. Gynecol. Pathol. **7**:86, 1988.

443. Keith, L.G., Berger, G.S., Edelman, D.A., et al.: On the causation of pelvic inflammatory disease, Am. J. Obstet. Gynecol. **149**:215, 1984.

444. Manes, J.L., and Taylor, H.B.: Carcinosarcoma and mixed müllerian tumors of the fallopian tube, Cancer **38**:1687, 1976.

445. Mårdh, P.A., and Weström, L.: Tubal and cervical cultures in acute salpingitis with special reference to *Mycoplasma hominis* and T-strain mycoplasmas, Br. J. Vener. Dis. **46**:179, 1970.

446. Mårdh, P.A., Ripa, T., Svensson, L., and Weström, L.: *Chlamydia trachomatis* infection in patients with acute salpingitis, N. Engl. J. Med. **296**:1377, 1977.

447. Mazzarella, P., Okagaki, T., and Richart, R.M.: Teratoma of the uterine tube: a case report and review of the literature, Obstet. Gynecol. **39**:381, 1972.

448. Nogales-Ortiz, F., Tarancon, I., and Nogales, F.F.: The pathology of female genital tuberculosis: a 31 year study of 1436 cases, Obstet. Gynecol. **53**:422, 1979.

449. Palladino, V.S., and Tousdell, M.: Extrauterine müllerian tumors, Cancer **23**:1413, 1969.

450. Platt, R., Rice, P.A., and McCormack, W.M.: Risk of acquiring gonorrhea and prevalence of abnormal adnexal findings among women recently exposed to gonorrhea, JAMA **250**:3205, 1983.

451. Rees, E., and Annels, E.H.: Gonococcal salpingitis, Br. J. Vener. Dis. **45**:205, 1969.

452. Rivlin, M.E., Meeks, F.R., Cowan, B.D., and Bates, G.W.: Persistent trophoblastic tissue following salpingostomy for unruptured ectopic pregnancy, Fertil. Steril. **43**:323, 1985.

453. Rubin, I.C., Lisa, J.R., and Trinidad, S.: Further observations of ectopic endometrium of fallopian tube, Surg. Gynecol. Obstet. **103**:469, 1956.

454. Schiller, H.M., and Silverberg, S.G.: Staging and prognosis in primary carcinoma of the fallopian tube, Cancer **28**:389, 1971.

455. Sedlis, A.: Primary carcinoma of the fallopian tube, Obstet. Gynecol. Surv. **16**:209, 1961.

456. Siegler, A.M., Wang, C.F., and Westhoff, C.: Management of unruptured tubal pregnancy, Obstet. Gynecol. Surv. **36**:599, 1981.

457. Sweet, R.I., Selinger, H.E., and McKay, D.G.: Malignant teratoma of the uterine tube, Obstet Gynecol. **45**:553, 1975.

458. Swenson, R.M., Michaelson, T.C., Daly, M.J., and Spaulding, E.H.: Anaerobic bacterial infections of the female genital tract, Obstet. Gynecol. **42**:538, 1973.

459. Thadepalli, H., Gorbach, S.L., and Keith, L.: Anaerobic infections of the female genital tract: bacteriologic and therapeutic aspects, Am. J. Obstet. Gynecol. **117**:1034, 1973.

460. Thomas, M.L., and Rose, D.H.: Salpingitis isthmica nodosa demonstrated by hysterosalpingography, Acta Radiol. **14**:295, 1973.

461. Timonen, S., and Nieminen, U.: Tubal pregnancy: choice of operative method of treatment, Acta Obstet. Gynecol. Scand. **46**:337, 1967.

462. Washington, A.E., Johnson, R.E., and Sanders, L.L., Jr.: *Chlamydia trachomatis* infections in the United States. What are they costing us? JAMA **257**:2070, 1987.

463. Woodruff, J.D., and Pauerstein, C.J.: The fallopian tube, Baltimore, 1969, The Williams & Wilkins Co.

464. Wright, N.H., and Laemmle, P.: Acute pelvic inflammatory disease in an indigent population, Am. J. Obstet. Gynecol. **101**:979, 1968.

465. Youngs, L.A., and Taylor, H.B.: Adenomatoid tumors of the uterus and fallopian tube, Am. J. Clin. Pathol. **48**:537, 1967.

Ovary

466. Abel, K.P.: Ovarian apoplexy, Lancet **1**:136, 1964.

467. Abel, M.R., and Holtz, F.: Ovarian neoplasms in childhood and adolescence. II. Tumors of non–germ cell origin, Am. J. Obstet. Gynecol. **93**:850, 1965.

468. Adams, E.C., and Hertig, A.T.: Studies on the human corpus luteum. II. Observation on the ultrastructure of luteal cells during pregnancy, J. Cell. Biol. **41**:716, 1969.

469. Angervall, L., and Knutson, H.: Heterotopic ovarian tissue, Acta Obstet. Gynecol. Scand. **38**:275, 1959.

470. Arey, L.B.: The origin and form of the Brenner tumor, Am. J. Obstet. Gynecol. **81**:743, 1961.

471. Arrata, W.S.M., and deAlvarez, R.R.: Oversuppression syndrome, Am. J. Obstet. Gynecol. **112**:1025, 1972.

472. Asadourian, L.A., and Taylor, H.B.: Dysgerminoma: an analysis of 105 cases, Obstet. Gynecol. **33**:370, 1969.

473. Aure, J.C., Hoeg, K., and Kolstad, P.: Clinical and histologic studies of ovarian carcinoma: long-term follow up of 990 cases, Obstet. Gynecol. **37**:1, 1971.

474. Aure, J.C., Hoeg, K., and Kolstad, D.: Psammoma bodies in serous carcinoma of the ovary: a prognostic study, Am. J. Obstet. Gynecol. **109**:113, 1971.

475. Austin, R.M., and Norris, H.J.: Malignant Brenner tumor and transitional cell carcinoma of the ovary: a comparison, Int. J. Gynecol. Pathol. **6**:29, 1987.

476. Ballas, M.: The significance of alpha-fetoprotein in the serum of patients with malignant teratomas and related germinal neoplasms, Ann. Clin. Lab. Sci. **4**:267, 1974.

477. Ballon, S.C, Donaldson, R.C., Berman, M.L., Swanson, G.A., and Byron, R.L.: Myeloblastoma (granulocytic sarcoma) of the ovary, Arch. Pathol. Lab. Med. **102**:474, 1978.

478. Bardin, C.W., Lipsett, M.B., Edgcomb, J.H., and Marshall, J.R.: Studies of testosterone metabolism in a patient with masculinization due to stromal hyperthecosis, N. Engl. J. Med. **277**:399, 1967.

479. Barwick, K.W., and LiVolsi, V.A.: Malignant mixed mesodermal tumors of the ovary: a clinicopathologic assessment of 12 cases, Am. J. Surg. Pathol. **4**:37, 1980.

480. Behrman, H.R., and Caldwell, B.V.: Role of prostaglandins in reproduction. In Greep, R.O., editor: Reproductive physiology, M.T.P. International Review of Science, vol. 8, Baltimore, 1974, University Park Press.

481. Bjorkholm, E., and Silfverswärd, C.: Prognostic factors in granulosa-cell tumors, Gynecol. Oncol. **11**:261, 1981.

482. Blackwell, W.J., and Dockerty, M.B.: Dermoid cysts of the ovary: their clinical and pathologic significance, Am. J. Obstet. Gynecol. **51**:151, 1946.

483. Block, E.: A quantitative morphological investigation of the follicular system in newborn female infants, Acta Anat. **17**:201, 1953.

484. Case records of the Massachusetts General Hospital: Ovarian hyperthecosis with massive edema, case 24-1971, N. Engl. J. Med. **284**:1369, 1971.

485. Chaitin, B.A., Gershenson, D.M., and Evans, H.L.: Mucinous tumors of the ovary: a clinicopathologic study of 70 cases, Cancer **55**:1958, 1985.

486. Chorlton, I., Norris, H.J., and King, F.M.: Malignant reticuloendothelial disease of the ovary as a primary manifestation: a series of 19 lymphomas and 1 granulocytic sarcoma, Cancer **34**:397, 1974.

487. Clement, P.B.: Histology of the ovary, Am. J. Surg. Pathol. **11**:277, 1987.

488. Clement, P.B., and Scully, R.E.: Extrauterine mesodermal (müllerian) adenosarcoma: a clinicopathologic analysis of five cases, Am. J. Clin. Pathol. **69**:276, 1978.

489. Cocco, A.E., and Conway, S.J.: Zollinger-Ellison syndrome associated with ovarian mucinous cystadenocarcinoma, N. Engl. J. Med. **293**:485, 1975.

490. Cooper, H.E., Spellacy, W.N., and Prem, K.A.: Hereditary factors in the Stein-Leventhal syndrome, Am. J. Obstet. Gynecol. **100**:371, 1968.

491. Crosignani, P.G., Trojsi, L., Attanasio, A., et al.: Hormonal profiles in anovulatory patients treated with gonadotropins and synthetic luteinizing hormone releasing hormone, Obstet. Gynecol. **46**:15, 1975.

492. Cummins, P., Fox, H., and Langley, F.A.: An ultrastructural study of the nature and origin of the Brenner tumor of the ovary, J. Pathol. **110**:167, 1973.

493. Daane, T.A., Lurie, A.D., and Barton, R.K.: Ovarian lutein cysts associated with an otherwise normal pregnancy, Obstet. Gynecol. **34**:655, 1969.

494. deMoraes-Ruehsen, M., Blizzard, R.M., Garcia-Bunuel, R., and Jones, G.S.: Autoimmunity and ovarian failure, Am. J. Obstet. Gynecol. **112**:693, 1972.

495. Díaz-Infante, A., Virutamasen, P., Connaughton, J.F., Wright, K.H., and Wallach, E.E.: *In vitro* studies of human ovarian contractility, Obstet. Gynecol. **44**:830, 1974.

496. Easterling, W.E., Talbert, L.M., and Potter, H.D.: Serum testosterone in the polycystic ovary syndrome: effect of an estrogen-progestin on protein binding of testosterone, Am. J. Obstet. Gynecol. **120**:385, 1974.

497. Ehrlich, C.E., and Roth, L.M.: The Brenner tumor: a clinicopathologic study of 57 cases, Cancer **27**:332, 1971.

498. Eifel, P., Hendrickson, M., Ross, J., Ballon, S., Martínez, A., and Kempson, R.: Simultaneous presentation of carcinoma involving the ovary and uterine corpus, Cancer **50**:163, 1982.

499. Evans, A.T., III, Gaffey, T.A., Malkasian, G.D., Jr., and Annegers, J.F.: Clinicopathologic review of 118 granulosa and 82 theca cell tumors, Obstet. Gynecol. **55**:231, 1980.

500. Falls, J.L.: Accessory adrenal cortex in the broad ligament: incidence and functional significance, Cancer **8**:143, 1955.

501. Feldman, G.B., and Knapp, R.C.: Lymphatic drainage of the peritoneal cavity and its significance in ovarian cancer, Am. J. Obstet. Gynecol. **119**:991, 1974.

502. Fenoglio, C.M., Ferenczy, A., and Richart, R.M.: Mucinous tumors of the ovary: ultrastructural studies of mucinous cystadenomas with histogenetic considerations, Cancer **36**:1709, 1975.

503. Finkler, N.J., Kopnick, S.J., Griffiths, C.T., and Knapp, R.C.: Elevated CA-125 serum levels in epithelial ovarian cancer metastatic to retroperitoneal lymph nodes, Gynecol. Oncol. **29**:356, 1988.

504. Fox, H., Agrawal, K., and Langley, F.A.: A clinicopathologic study of 92 cases of granulosa cell tumor of the ovary with special reference to the factors influencing prognosis, Cancer **35**:231, 1975.

505. Foyle, A., Al-Jabi, M., and McCaughey, W.T.: Papillary peritoneal tumors in women, Am. J. Surg. Pathol. **5**:241, 1981.

506. Gambrell, R.D., Greenblatt, R.B., and Mahesh, V.B.: Inappropriate secretion of LH in the Stein-Leventhal syndrome, Obstet. Gynecol. **42**:429, 1973.

507. Garcia-Bunuel, R., and Morris, B.: Histochemical observations on mucins in human ovarian neoplasms, Cancer **17**:1108, 1964.

508. Gershenson, D.M., del Junco, G., Silva, E.G., Copeland, L.J., Wharton, J.T., and Rutledge, F.N.: Immature teratoma of the ovary, Obstet. Gynecol. **68**:624, 1986.

509. Gillim, S.W., Christensen, A.K., and McLennan, C.E.: Fine structure of the human menstrual corpus luteum at its stage of maximum secretory activity, Am. J. Anat. **126**:409, 1969.

510. Girouard, D.P., Barclay, D.L., and Collins, C.G.: Hyperreactio luteinalis: a review of the literature and report of two cases, Obstet. Gynecol. **23**:513, 1964.

511. Givens, J.R., Wiser, W.L., and Coleman, S.A.: Familial ovarian hyperthecosis: a study of two families, Am. J. Obstet. Gynecol. **110**:955, 1971.

512. Gordon, H., Lipton, D., and Woodruff, J.D.: Dysgerminoma: a review of 158 cases from the Emil Novak Ovarian Tumor Registry, Obstet. Gynecol. **58**:497, 1981.

513. Greenblatt, R.B., and Mahesh, V.B.: Some new thoughts on the Stein-Leventhall syndrome, J. Reprod. Med. **13**:85, 1974.

514. Grogan, R.H.: Accidental rupture of the malignant ovarian cysts during surgical removal, Obstet. Gynecol. **30**:716, 1967.

515. Hammerstein, J.: Regulation of ovarian steroidogenesis: gonadotropins, enzymes, prostaglandins, cyclic-AMP, luteolysins. In Greep, R.O., editor: Reproductive physiology, M.T.P. International Review of Science, vol. 8, Baltimore, 1974, University Park Press.

516. Hart, W.R., and Norris, H.J.: Borderline and malignant mucinous tumors of the ovary, Cancer **31**:1031, 1973.

517. Hay, D.M., and Stewart, D.B.: Primary ovarian carcinoma, J. Obstet. Gynaecol. Br. Cwlth. **76**:941, 1969.

518. Hopkins, M.P., Kumar, N.B., and Morley, G.W.: An assessment of pathologic features and treatment modalities in ovarian tumors of low malignant potential, Obstet. Gynecol. **70**:923, 1987.

519. Hutchinson-Williams, K.A., and DeCherney, A.H.: Pathogenesis and treatment of polycystic ovarian disease, Int. J. Fertil. **32**:421, 1987.

520. Jensen, A.B., and Fechener, R.E.: Ultrastructure of an intermediate Sertoli-Leydig cell tumor: a histogenetic misnomer, Lab. Invest. **21**:527, 1969.

521. Joshi, V.V.: Primary Krukenberg tumor of the ovary: review of the literature and case report, Cancer **22**:1199, 1968.

522. Kalderon, A.E., and Tucci, J.R.: Ultrastructure of a human chorionic gonadotropin and adrenocorticotropin-responsive functioning Sertoli-Leydig cell tumor (type I), Lab. Invest. **29**:81, 1973.

523. Kalstone, C.E., Jaffe, R.B., and Abell, M.R.: Massive edema of the ovary simulating fibroma, Obstet. Gynecol. **34**:564, 1969.

524. Kao, G.F., and Norris, H.J.: Cystadenofibromas of the ovary with epithelial atypia, Am. J. Surg. Pathol. **2**:357, 1978.

525. Katzenstein, A.-L., Mazur, M.T., Morgan, T.E., and Kao, M.S.: Proliferative serous tumors of the ovary: histologic features and prognosis, Am. J. Surg. Pathol. **2**:339, 1978.

526. Kempson, R.L.: Ultrastructure of ovarian stromal cell tumors: Sertoli-Leydig cell tumor and lipid cell tumor, Arch. Pathol. **86**:492, 1968.

527. Keyes, P.L.: Luteinizing hormone: action of the Graafian follicle in vitro, Science **164**:846, 1969.

528. Knapp, R.C., and Friedman, E.A.: Aortic lymph node metastases in early ovarian cancer, Am. J. Obstet. Gynecol. **119**:1013, 1974.

529. Konikov, N., Bleisch, V., and Piskie, V.: Prognostic significance of cytologic diagnosis of effusions, Acta Cytol. **10**:335, 1966.

530. Kottmeier, H.-L.: Surgical management—conservative surgery. In Gentil, F., and Junqueira, A.C.: Ovarian cancer, U.I.C.C. monograph series, vol. II, New York, 1968, Springer-Verlag N.Y., Inc.

531. Kriss, B.R.: Neoplasms of a supernumerary ovary: report of two cases, J. Mt. Sinai Hosp. **14**:798, 1947.

532. Kurman, R.J., Goebelsmann, U., and Taylor, C.R.: Steroid localization in granulosa-theca cell tumors of the ovary, Cancer **43**:2377, 1979.

533. Kurman, R.J., and Norris, H.J.: Malignant germ cell tumors of the ovary, Hum. Pathol. **8**:551, 1977.

534. Kurman, R.J., Andrade, D., Goebelsmann, U., and Taylor, C.R.: An immunohistological study of steroid localization in Sertoli-Leydig cell tumors of the ovary and testis, Cancer **43**:1772, 1978.

535. Lauchlan, S.C.: The secondary Müllerian system, Obstet. Gynecol. Surv. **27**:133, 1972.

536. Lavin, P.T., Knapp, R.C., Malkasian, G., Whitney, C.W., Berek, Y.C., and Bast, R.C., Jr.: CA-125 for the monitoring of ovarian carcinoma during primary therapy, Obstet. Gynecol. **69**:223, 1987.

537. Lindner, D., McCaw, B.K., and Hecht, F.: Parthenogenic origin of benign ovarian teratomas, N. Engl. J. Med. **292**:63, 1975.

538. Long, M.F., and Taylor, H.C.: Endometrioid carcinoma of the ovary, Am. J. Obstet. Gynecol. **90**:936, 1964.

539. Long, R.T.L., Spratt, J.S., and Dowling, E.: Pseudomyxoma peritonei, Am. J. Surg. **117**:162, 1969.

540. Malkasian, G.D., Dockerty, M.D., and Symmonds, R.E.: Benign cystic teratomas, Obstet. Gynecol. **29**:719, 1967.

541. Mansell, H., and Hertig, A.T.: Granulosa-theca cell tumors and endometrial carcinoma: a study of their relationship and a survey of 80 cases, Obstet. Gynecol. **6**:385, 1955.

542. Macqueo, M., Rice-Wray, E., Calderon, J.J., and Goldzieher, J.W.: Ovarian morphology after prolonged use of steroid contraceptive agents, Contraception **5**:177, 1972.

543. Mattingly, R.F., and Huang, W.Y.: Steroidogenesis of the menopausal and postmenopausal ovary, Am. J. Obstet. Gynecol. **103**:679, 1969.

544. Morris, J.M., and Scully, R.E.: Endocrine pathology of the ovary, St. Louis, 1958, The C.V. Mosby Co.

545. Munnell, E.W.: Is conservative therapy ever justified in stage I (IA) cancer of the ovary? Am. J. Obstet. Gynecol. **103**:641, 1969.

546. Nieminen, I., von Numers, C., and Widholm, O.: Struma ovarii, Acta Obstet. Gynecol. Scand. **42**:399, 1964.

547. Nikrui, N.: Survey of clinical behavior of patients with borderline epithelial tumors of the ovary, Gynecol. Oncol. **12**:107, 1981.

548. Norris, H.J., and Taylor, H.B.: Nodular theca-lutein hyperplasia of pregnancy (so-called pregnancy luteoma), Am. J. Clin. Pathol. **47**:557, 1967.

549. Norris, H.J., and Taylor, H.B.: Prognosis of granulosa-theca tumors of the ovary, Cancer **21**:255, 1968.

550. Norris, H.J., and Taylor, H.B.: Virilization associated with cystic granulosa cell tumors, Obstet. Gynecol. **34**:624, 1969.

551. Novak, E.R.: Gynandroblastoma of the ovary: review of eight cases from the tumor ovarian registry, Obstet. Gynecol. **30**:709, 1967.

552. Novak, E.R.: Ovulation after 50, Obstet. Gynecol. **36**:903, 1970.

553. Ober, W.B., Grady, H.G., and Schoenbucher, A.K.: Ectopic ovarian decidua without pregnancy, Am. J. Pathol. **33**:199, 1957.

554. O'Hern, T.M., and Neubecker, R.D.: Arrhenoblastoma, Obstet. Gynecol. **19**:758, 1962.

555. Osborne, B.M., and Robboy, S.J.: Lymphomas or leukemia presenting as ovarian tumors: an analysis of 42 cases, Cancer **52**:1933, 1983.

556. Pearl, M., and Plotz, E.J.: Supernumerary ovary: report of a case, Obstet. Gynecol. **21**:253, 1963.

557. Pedersen, P.H., and Larsen, J.F.: Ultrastructure of a granulosa cell tumour, Acta Obstet. Gynecol. Scand. **49**:105, 1970.

558. Peterson, W.F.: Malignant degeneration of benign cystic teratomas of the ovary: a collective review of the literature, Obstet. Gynecol. Surv. **12**:793, 1957.

559. Piver, M.S., Williams, L.J., and Marcuse, P.M.: Influence of luteal cysts on menstrual function, Obstet. Gynecol. **35**:740, 1970.

560. Polansky, S., dePapp, E.W., and Ogden, E.B.: Virilization associated with bilateral luteomas of pregnancy, Obstet. Gynecol. **45**:516, 1975.

561. Richardson, G.S., Scully, R.E., Nikrui, N., and Nelson, J.H.: Common epithelial cancer of the ovary, N. Engl. J. Med. **512**:415, 474, 1985.

562. Robboy, S.J., Norris, H.J., and Scully, R.E.: Insular carcinoid primary in the ovary: a clinicopathologic analysis of 48 cases, Cancer **36**:404, 1975.

563. Robboy, S.J., and Scully, R.E.: Ovarian teratoma with glial implants on the peritoneum, Hum. Pathol. **1**:643, 1970.

564. Robboy, S.J., Scully, R.E., and Norris, H.J.: Carcinoid metastatic to the ovary: a clinicopathologic analysis of 35 cases, Cancer **33**:798, 1974.

565. Roberts, D.W.T., and Haines, M.: Conserving ovarian tissue in treatment of ovarian neoplasms, Br. Med. J. **2**:917, 1965.

566. Rodenburg, C.H., Cornelisse, C.J., Heintz, P.A.M., Hermans, J.O., and Fleuren, G.J.: Tumor ploidy as major prognostic factor in advanced ovarian cancer, Cancer **59**:317, 1987.

567. Roth, L.M.: Fine structure of the Brenner tumor, Cancer **27**:1482, 1971.

568. Roth, L.M.: The Brenner tumor and the Walthard cell nest: an electron microscopic study, Lab. Invest. **31**:15, 1974.

569. Roth, L.M., Deaton, R.L., and Sternberg, W.H.: Massive ovarian edema: a clinicopathologic study of five cases including ultrastructural observations and review of the literature, Am. J. Surg. Pathol. **3**:11, 1979.

570. Roth, L.M., and Ehrlich, C.E.: Mucinous cystadenocarcinoma of the retroperitoneum, Obstet. Gynecol. **49**:486, 1977.

571. Roth, L.M., and Sternberg, W.H.: Proliferating Brenner tumors, Cancer **27**:687, 1971.

572. Rust, L.A., Israel, R., and Mishell, D.R., Jr.: Individualized graduated therapeutic regimen for clomiphene citrate, Am. J. Obstet. Gynecol. **120**:785, 1974.

573. Rutgers, J.L., and Scully, R.E.: Ovarian müllerian mucinous papillary cystadenomas of borderline malignancy: a clinicopathologic analysis, Cancer **61**:340, 1988.

574. Ryan, K.J., Petro, Z., and Kaiser, J.: Steroid formation by isolated and recombined ovarian granulosa and thecal cells, J. Clin. Endocrinol. **28**:355, 1968.

575. Santesson, L., and Kottmeier, H.L.: General classification of ovarian tumors. In Gentil, F., and Junqueira, A.C., editors: Ovarian cancer, U.I.C.C. monograph series, vol. 11, New York, 1968, Springer-Verlag N.Y., Inc.

576. Schenker, J.G., and Polishuk, W.Z.: Ovarian hyperstimulation syndrome, Obstet. Gynecol. **46**:23, 1975.

577. Scully, R.E.: Stromal luteoma of the ovary: a distinctive type of lipoid cell tumor, Cancer **17**:769, 1964.

578. Scully, R.E.: Gonadoblastoma: a review of 74 cases, Cancer **25**:1340, 1970.

579. Scully, R.E.: Recent progress in ovarian cancer, Hum. Pathol. **1**:73, 1970.

580. Scully, R.E.: Tumors of the ovary and maldeveloped gonads, Washington, D.C., 1979, Armed Forces Institute of Pathology.

581. Scully, R.E., and Barlow, J.F.: "Mesonephroma" of the ovary: tumor of müllerian nature related to the endometrioid carcinoma, Cancer **20**:1405, 1967.

582. Scully, R.E., and Richardson, G.S.: Luteinization of the stroma of metastatic cancer involving the ovary and its endocrine significance, Cancer **14**:827, 1961.

583. Serov, S.F., Scully, R.E., and Sobin, L.H.: Histological typing of ovarian tumours, Geneva, 1973, World Health Organization.

584. Shakfeh, S.M., and Woodruff, J.D.: Primary ovarian sarcomas: report of 46 cases and review of the literature, Obstet. Gynecol. Surv. **42**:331, 1987.

585. Silverberg, E., and Holleb, A.I.: Major trends in cancer: 25 year survey, CA **25**:2, 1975.

586. Silverberg, S.G.: Brenner tumor of the ovary: a clinicopathologic study of 60 tumors in 54 women, Cancer **28**:588, 1971.

587. Silverberg, S.G., and Nogáles-Fernández, F.: Endolymphatic stromal myosis of the ovary: a report of three cases and literature review, Gynecol. Oncol. **12**:129, 1981.

588. Sjöstedt, S., and Wahlen, T.: Prognosis of granulosa cell tumors, Acta Obstet. Gynecol. Scand. **40**(suppl. 6):1, 1961.

589. Starup, J., and Sele, V.: Premature ovarian failure, Acta Obstet. Gynecol. Scand. **52**:259, 1973.

590. Stein, I.F., Sr., and Leventhal, M.L.: Amenorrhea associated with bilateral polycystic ovaries, Am. J. Obstet. Gynecol. **21**:181, 1935.

591. Steiner, M.M., and Hadawi, S.A.: Sexual precocity: association with follicular cysts of ovary, Am. J. Dis. Child. **108**:28, 1964.

592. Sternberg, W.H., and Barclay, D.L.: Luteoma of pregnancy, Am. J. Obstet. Gynecol. **95**:165, 1966.

593. Stevens, V.C.: Comparison of FSH and LH patterns in plasma, urine, and urinary extracts during the menstrual cycle, J. Clin. Endocrinol. **29**:904, 1969.

594. Tavassoli, F.A., and Norris, J.H.: Sertoli cell tumors of the ovary: a clinicopathologic study of 28 cases with ultrastructural observations, Cancer **46**:2281, 1980.

595. Taylor, H.B., and Norris, H.J.: Lipid cell tumors of the ovary, Cancer **20**:1953, 1967.

596. Taymor, M.L., Berger, M.J., Thompson, I.E., and Karam, K.S.: Hormone factors in human ovulation, Am. J. Obstet. Gynecol. **114**:445, 1972.

597. Tazelaar, H.D., Bostwick, D.G., Ballon, S.C., Bostwick, D.G., Ballon, S.C., Hendrickson, M.R., and Kempson, R.L.: Conservative treatment of borderline ovarian tumors, Obstet. Gynecol. **66**:417, 1985.

598. Teilum, G.: Classification of endodermal sinus tumour (mesoblastoma vitellinum) and so-called "embryonal carcinoma of the ovary," Acta Pathol. Microbiol. Scand. **64**:407, 1965.

599. Teilum, G., Albrechtsen, R., and Norgaard-Pedersen, J.: Immunofluorescent localization of alpha-fetoprotein in endodermal sinus tumor, Acta Pathol. Microbiol. Scand. **82**:586, 1974.

600. Thurlbeck, W.M., and Scully, R.E.: Solid teratoma of the ovary; a clinicopathological analysis of nine cases, Cancer **13**:804, 1960.

601. Tyson, J.E., Andreasson, B., Huth, J., Smith, B., and Zacur, H.: Neuro-endocrine dysfunction in galactorrhea-amenorrhea and oral contraceptive use, Obstet. Gynecol. **46**:1, 1975.

602. Ulbright, T.M., Roth, L.M., and Stehman, F.B.: Secondary ovarian neoplasia: a clinicopathologic study of 35 cases, Cancer **53**:1164, 1984.

603. van Wagenen, G., and Simpson, M.E.: Postnatal development of the ovary in *Homo sapiens* and *Macaca mulatta* and induction of ovulation in the macaque, New Haven, 1973, Yale University Press.

604. Wharton, L.R.: Two cases of supernumerary ovary and one of accessory ovary, with an analysis of previously reported cases, Am. J. Obstet. Gynecol. **78**:1101, 1959.

605. Woodruff, J.D., Protos, P., and Peterson, W.F.: Ovarian teratomas: relationships of histologic and ontogenetic factors to prognosis, Am. J. Obstet. Gynecol. **102**:702, 1968.

606. Woodruff, J.D., Murthy, Y.S., Bhaskar, T.N., Bordbar, F., and Tseng, S.S.: Metastatic ovarian tumors, Am. J. Obstet. Gynecol. **107**:202, 1970.

607. Young, R.H., and Scully, R.E.: Ovarian Sertoli-Leydig cell tumors: a clinicopathological analysis of 207 cases, Am. J. Surg. Pathol. **9**:543, 1985.

608. Zaloudek, C., and Norris, H.J.: Sertoli-Leydig tumors of the ovary: a clinicopathologic study of 53 intermediate and poorly differentiated neoplasms, Am. J. Surg. Pathol. **8**:405, 1984.

609. Zaloudek, C.J., Tavassoli, F.A., and Norris, H.J.: Dysgerminoma with syncytiotrophoblastic giant cells: a histologically and clinically distinctive subtype of dysgerminoma, Am. J. Surg. Pathol. **5**:361, 1981.

610. Zanartu, J., Dabancens, A., Rodríguez-Bravo, R., and Schally, A.V.: Induction of ovulation with synthetic gonadotropin-releasing hormone in women with constant anovulation induced by contraceptive steroids, Br. Med. J. **1**:605, 1974.

611. Zondek, L.H., and Zondek, T.: Leydig cells of the foetus and newborn in various complications of pregnancy, Acta Obstet. Gynecol. Scand. **46**:392, 1967.

Placenta

612. Acosta-Sisón, H.: Changing attitudes in the management of hydatidiform mole: a report on 196 patients admitted to the Philippine General Hospital from April 10, 1959, to March 27, 1963, Am. J. Obstet. Gynecol. **88**:634, 1964.

613. Adock, E.W., II, Teasdale, T., August, C.S., Cox, S., Meschia, G., Battaglia, F.C., and Naughton, M.A.: Human chorionic gonadotropin: its possible role in maternal lymphocyte suppression, Science **181**:845, 1973.

614. Altshuler, G., and McAdams, A.J.: The role of the placenta in fetal and perinatal pathology, Am. J. Obstet. Gynecol. **113**:616, 1972.

615. Altshuler, G., Russell, P., and Ermocilla, R.: The placental pathology of small-for-gestational age infants, Am. J. Obstet. Gynecol. **121**:351, 1975.

616. Attwood, H.D., and Park, W.W.: Trophoblast (benign) in lung, J. Obstet. Gynaecol. Br. Cwlth. **68**:611, 1963.

617. Bain, A.D., et al.: Congenital toxoplasmosis simulating hemolytic disease of the newborn, J. Obstet. Gynaecol. Br. Emp. **63**:826, 1956.

618. Baker, C.J., and Casper, D.L.: Correlations of maternal antibody deficiency and susceptibility to neonatal group B streptococcal infection, N. Engl. J. Med. **294**:753, 1976.

619. Baldwin, V.J., Kalousek, D.K., Dimmick, J.E., Applegarth, D.A., and Hardwick, D.F.: Diagnostic pathologic investigation of the malformed conceptus, Perspect. Pediatr. Pathol. **7**:65, 1982.

620. Band, P.R., Masse, S.R., Reid, D.W., and Dossetor, J.B.: Hydatidiform mole metastasizing to the lung, Can. Med. Assoc. J. **114**:813, 1976.

621. Banti, D., Jennison, R.F., and Langley, F.A.: Significance of placental pathology in transplacental haemorrhage, J. Clin. Pathol. **21**:322, 1968.

622. Beacham, W.D., Hearnquist, W.C., Beacham, D.W., and Webster, H.D.: Abdominal pregnancy at Charity Hospital in New Orleans, Am. J. Obstet. Gynecol. **84**:1257, 1962.

623. Beer, A.E.: Immunogenetic determinants of the size of the fetoplacental unit and their modus operandi. In Brosens, I.A., Dixon, G., and Robertson, W.B., editors: Human placentation, Amsterdam, 1975, Excerpta Medica.

624. Benirschke, K.: Abortions and moles. In Naeye, R.L., Kissane, J.M., and Kaufman, N., editors: Perinatal diseases, Baltimore, 1981, The Williams & Wilkins Co.

625. Benirschke, K., and Driscoll, S.G.: The pathology of the human placenta, New York, 1967, Springer-Verlag N.Y., Inc.

626. Benirschke, K., and Kim, C.K.: Multiple pregnancy, N. Engl. J. Med. **288**:1276, 1973.

627. Billington, W.D.: Immunologic aspects of normal and abnormal pregnancy. In Brosens, I.A., Dixon, G., and Robertson, W.B., editors: Human placentation, Amsterdam, 1975, Excerpta Medica.

628. Blanc, W.A.: Vernix granulomatosis of amnion (amnion nodosum) in oligohydramnios, NY J. Med. **61**:1492, 1961.

629. Blanc, W.A.: Pathology of the placenta, membranes, and umbilical cord in bacterial, fungal, and viral infections in man. In Naeye, R.L., Kissane, J.M., and Kaufman, N., editors: Perinatal diseases, Baltimore, 1981, The Williams & Wilkins Co.

630. Bleisch, V.R.: The diagnosis of monochorionic placenta, Am. J. Clin. Pathol. **42**:277, 1964.

631. Boyd, J.D., and Hamilton, W.J.: The human placenta, Cambridge, 1970, W. Heffer & Sons.

632. Braunstein, G.D., Grodin, J.M., Vaitukaitis, J., and Ross, G.T.: Secretory rates of human chorionic gonadotropin by normal trophoblast, Am. J. Obstet. Gynecol. **115**:447, 1973.

633. Breen, J.L.: A 21 year survey of 654 ectopic pregnancies, Am. J. Obstet. Gynecol. **106**:1004, 1970.

634. Breen, J.L., Neubecker, R., Gregori, C.A., and Franklin, J.E.: Placenta accreta, increta and percreta: a survey of 40 cases, Obstet. Gynecol. **49**:43, 1977.

635. Brewer, J.I., and Mazur, M.T.: Gestational choriocarcinoma: its origin in the placenta during seemingly normal pregnancy, Am. J. Surg. Pathol. **5**:267, 1981.

636. Brosens, I.A., Dixon, G., and Robertson, W.B., editors: Human placentation, Amsterdam, 1975, Excepta Medica.

637. Brosens, I.A., Robertson, W.B., and Dixon, H.G.: The role of the spiral arteries in the pathogenesis of pre-eclampsia. In Wynn, R.M., editor: Obstetrics and gynecology annual, New York, 1972, Appleton-Century-Crofts.

638. Burrows, S., Gaines, J.L., and Hughes, F.J.: Giant chorioangiomas, Am. J. Obstet. Gynecol. **115**:579, 1973.

639. Cameron, A.H.: The Birmingham twin survey, Proc. R. Soc. Med. **61**:229, 1968.

640. Carr, D.H.: Chromosome studies in selected spontaneous abortion. III. Early pregnancy loss, Obstet. Gynecol. **37**:750, 1971.

641. Carter, B.: Premature separation of the normally implanted placenta, Obstet. Gynecol. **29**:30, 1967.

642. Carter, J.E., Vellios, F., and Huber, C.P.: Histologic classification and incidence of circulatory lesions of the human placenta, with a review of the literature, Am. J. Clin. Pathol. **40**:374, 1963.

643. Clark, P.B., Gusdon, J.P., and Burt, R.L.: Hydatidiform mole with co-existent fetus: discussion and review of diagnostic methods, Obstet. Gynecol. **35**:597, 1970.

644. Craig, J.M.: The pathology of birth control, Arch. Pathol. **99**:233, 1975.

645. Culp, W.C., Bryan, R.N., and Morettin, L.B.: Placenta membranacea: a case report with arteriographic findings, Radiology **108**:309, 1973.

646. Dehner, L.P., and Askin, F.B.: Cytomegalovirus endometritis: report of a case associated with spontaneous abortion, Obstet. Gynecol. **45**:211, 1975.

647. de Ikonicoff, L., and Cedard, L.: Localization of human chorionic gonadotropic and somatomammotropic hormones by peroxidase immunohistoenzymologic method in villi and amniotic epithelium of human placentas (from 6 weeks to term), Am. J. Obstet. Gynecol. **116**:1124, 1973.

648. Demian, S.D.E., Donnelly, W.H., Frias, J.L., and Monif, G.R.G.: Placental lesions in congenital giant pigmented nevi, Am. J. Clin. Pathol. **61**:438, 1974.

649. Desmonts, G., and Couvreur, J.: Congenital toxoplasmosis: a prospective study of 378 pregnancies, N. Engl. J. Med. **290**:1110, 1974.

650. Douthwaite, R.M., and Urbach, G.I.: In vitro antigenicity of trophoblast, Am. J. Obstet. Gynecol. **109**:1023, 1971.

651. Dreskin, R.B., Spicer, S.S., and Greene, W.B.: Ultrastructure localization of chorionic gonadotropin in human term placenta, J. Histochem. Cytochem. **18**:862, 1970.

652. Driscoll, S.G.: Histopathology of gestational rubella, Am. J. Dis. Child. **118**:49, 1969.

653. Dyke, P.C., and Fink, L.M.: Latent choriocarcinoma, Cancer **20**:150, 1967.

654. Elston, C.W.: Cellular reaction to choriocarcinoma, J. Pathol. **97**:261, 1969.

655. Elson, C.W., and Bagshawe, K.D.: The value of histological grading in the management of hydatidiform mole, J. Obstet. Gynaecol. Br. Cwlth. **79**:717, 1972.

656. Enders, A.C., and King, B.F.: The cytology of Hofbauer cells, Anat. Rec. **167**:231, 1970.

657. Faulk, W.P., Jeannet, M., Creighton, W.D., and Carbonara, A.: Immunological studies of the human placenta: characterization of immunoglobulins on trophoblastic basement membranes, J. Clin. Invest. **54**:1011, 1974.

658. Ferenczy, A., and Richart, R.M.: Scanning electron microscopic study of normal and molar trophoblast, Gynecol. Oncol. **1**:95, 1972.

659. Finn, J.L.: Placenta membranacea, Obstet. Gynecol. **3**:438, 1954.

660. Froehlich, L.A., and Fujikura, T.: Follow-up of infants with single umbilical artery, Pediatrics **52**:6, 1973.

661. Gagnon, R.A.: Transplacental inoculation of fatal herpes simplex in the newborn: report of two cases, Obstet. Gynecol. **31**:682, 1968.

662. Gartner, A., Larsson, L.-I., and Sjöberg, N.-O.: Immunohistochemical demonstration of chorionic gonadotropin in trophoblastic tumors, Acta Obstet. Gynecol. Scand. **54**:161, 1975.

663. Gibbs, R.S., Amstey, M.S., Sweet, R.L., Mead, P.E., and Sever, Y.L.: Management of genital herpes infection in pregnancy, Obstet. Gynecol. **71**:779, 1988.

664. Gleicher, N.X., Deppe, G., and Cohen, C.J.: Common aspects of immunologic tolerance in pregnancy and malignancy, Obstet. Gynecol. **54**:335, 1979.

665. Goldstein, D.P.: Prophylactic chemotherapy of patients with molar pregnancy, Obstet. Gynecol. **38**:817, 1971.

666. Goldstein, D.P., Pastorfide, G.B., Osathanondh, R., and Kosasa, T.S.: A rapid solid-phase radioimmunoassay specific for human chorionic gonadotropin in gestational trophoblastic disease, Obstet. Gynecol. **45**:527, 1975.

667. Gruenwald, P.: The placenta and its maternal supply line, Baltimore, 1975, University Park Press.

668. Gurka, G., Rocklin, R.E.: Reproductive immunology, JAMA **258**:2983, 1987.

669. Hammond, C.B., Borchert, L.G., Tyrey, L., Creasman, W.T., and Parker, R.T.: Treatment of metastatic trophoblastic disease: good and poor prognosis, Am. J. Obstet. Gynecol. **115**:451, 1973.

670. Harwick, H.Y., Iuppa, Y.B., Purcell, R.H., and Fekety, F.R., Jr.: *Mycoplasma hominis* septicemia associated with abortion, Am. J. Obstet. Gynecol. **99**:715, 1967.

671. Haust, M.D.: Maternal diabetes mellitus: effects on the fetus and placenta. In Naeye, R.L., Kissane, J.M., and Kaufman, N., editors: Perinatal diseases, Baltimore, 1981, The Williams & Wilkins Co.

672. Hellman, L.M., and Hertig, A.T.: Pathologic changes in the placenta associated with erythroblastosis of the fetus, Am. J. Pathol. **14**:111, 1938.

673. Hertig, A.T.: Vascular pathology on the hypertensive albuminuric toxemias of pregnancy, Clinics **4**:602, 1945 (quoted by Robertson, Brosens, and Dixon, 1975; see reference 725).

674. Hertig, A.T.: Human trophoblast, Springfield, Ill., 1968, Charles C Thomas, Publisher.

675. Herva, R., Rapola, J., Rosti, J., and Karlson, H.: Cluster of severe amniotic adhesion malformations in Finland, Lancet **1**:818, 1980.

676. Heyderman, E., Gibbons, A.R., and Rosen, S.W.: Immunoperoxidase localization of human placental lactogen: a marker for the placental origin of the giant cells in "syncytial endometritis" of pregnancy, J. Clin. Pathol. **34**:303, 1981.

677. Hibbard, B.M., and Jeffcoate, T.N.A.: Abruptio placentae, Obstet. Gynecol. **27**:155, 1966.

678. Higginbottom, M.C., Jones, K.L., Hall, B.D., and Smith, D.W.: The amniotic band disruption complex: timing of amniotic rupture, and variable spectra of consequent defects, J. Pediatr. **95**:544, 1977.

679. Horne, H.W., Hertig, A.T., Knudsin, R.B., and Kosasa, T.S.: Subclinical endometrial inflammation and T-mycoplasma: a possible cause of human reproductive failure, Int. J. Fertil. **18**:226, 1973.

680. Hreshchyshyn, M.M., Bogen, B., and Loughran, C.H.: What is actual present-day management of the placenta in late abdominal pregnancy? Analysis of 101 cases, Am. J. Obstet. Gynecol. **81**:302, 1961.

681. Hulka, J., and Mohr, K.: Trophoblast antigenicity as demonstrated by altered challenge graft survival, Science **161**:696, 1968.

682. Irving, F.C., and Hertig, A.T.: A study of placenta accreta, Surg. Gynecol. Obstet. **64**:178, 1937.

683. Jacobson, F.J., and Enzen, N.: Hydatidiform mole with "benign" metastasis to lung: histological evidence of regressing lesion in lung, Am. J. Obstet. Gynecol. **78**:868, 1959.

684. Jaffe, R.B.: The endocrinology of pregnancy. In Yen, S.C., and Jaffe, R.B., editors: Reproductive endocrinology, Philadelphia, 1978, W.B. Saunders Co.

685. Jaffe, R.B., Lee, P.A., and Midgley, A.R.: Serum gonadotropins before, at the inception of, and following human pregnancy, J. Clin. Endocrinol. **29**:1281, 1969.

686. Kajii, T., and Oyama, K.: Androgenic origin of hydatidiform mole, Nature **268**:633, 1977.

687. Kaufman, P., Luckhardt, M., Schweikhart, G., and Cantle, S.J.: Cross sectional features and three dimensional structure of human placental villi, Placenta **8**:235, 1987.

688. Kay, M.D., and Jones, W.R.: Effect of human chorionic gonadotropin on in vitro lymphocyte transformation, Am. J. Obstet. Gynecol. **109**:1029, 1971.

689. Khudr, G., Soma, H., and Benirschke, K.: Trophoblastic origin of the X cell and the placental giant cell, Am. J. Obstet. Gynecol. **115**:530, 1973.

690. Kitsmiller, J.L., and Benirschke, K.: Immunofluorescent study of placental bed vessels in pre-eclampsia of pregnancy, Am. J. Obstet. Gynecol. **115**:248, 1973.

691. Klopper, A.: The new placental proteins, Placenta **1**:77, 1980.

692. Kurman, R.J., Main, C.S., and Chen, H.-C.: Intermediate trophoblast: a distinctive form of trophoblast with specific morphologic, biochemical and functional features, Placenta **5**:349, 1984.

693. Kurman, R.J., Scully, R.E., and Norris, H.J.: Trophoblastic pseudotumor of the uterus: an exaggerated form of "syncytial endometritis" simulating a malignant tumor, Cancer **38**:1214, 1976.

694. Labarrere, C.A.: Acute atherosis: a histopathological hallmark of immune aggression? Placenta **9**:95, 1988.

695. Levy, G., Müller, G., and Pigaglio, O.: Grossesses intra-utérines et extra-utérines simultanées, Rev. Fr. Gynecol. Obstet. **82**:729, 1987.

696. Luke, R.K., Sharpe, J.W., and Greene, R.R.: Placenta accreta: the adherent or invasive placenta, Am. J. Obstet. Gynecol. **95**:660, 1966.

697. Marshall, J.R., Hammond, C.B., Ross, G.T., Jacobson, A., Rayford, D., and Odell, W.D.: Plasma and urinary chorionic gonadotropin during early human pregnancy, Obstet. Gynecol. **32**:760, 1968.

698. Mazur, M.T., Lurain, J.R., and Brewer, J.I.: Fatal gestational choriocarcinoma: clinicopathologic study of patients treated at a trophoblastic disease center, Cancer **50**:1833, 1982.

699. McConnell, H.D., and Carr, D.H.: Recent advances in the cytogenetic study of human spontaneous abortions, Obstet. Gynecol. **45**:547, 1975.

700. McCord, J.R.: Syphilis of the placenta: the histologic examination of 1,085 placentas of mothers with strongly positive blood Wassermann reactions, Am. J. Obstet. Gynecol. **28**:743, 1934.

701. McKay, D.G., Goldenberg, V., Kaunitz, H., and Csavossy, I.: Experimental eclampsia: an electron microscope study and review, Arch. Pathol. **84**:557, 1967.

702. Monif, G.R.G.: Infectious diseases in obstetrics and gynecology, New York, 1974, Harper & Row, Publishers, Inc.

703. Monif, G.R.G., and Dische, R.M.: Viral placentitis in congenital cytomegalovirus infections, Am. J. Clin. Pathol. **58**:445, 1972.

704. Naeye, R.L.: Functionally important disorders of the placenta, umbilical cord, and fetal membranes, Hum. Pathol. **18**:680, 1987.

705. Naeye, R.L.: Do placental weights have clinical significance? Hum. Pathol. **18**:387, 1987.

706. Naeye, R.L.: Maternal floor infarction, Hum. Pathol. **16**:823, 1985.

707. Naeye, R.L., and Ross, S.M.: Amnionic infection syndrome, Clin. Obstet. Gynecol. **9**:593, 1982.

708. Naib, Z.M., Nahmias, A.J., Josey, W.E., and Wheeler, J.H.: Association of maternal genital herpetic infection with spontaneous abortion, Obstet. Gynecol. **35**:260, 1970.

709. Naughton, M.A., Merrill, D.A., McManus, L.M., Fink, L.M., Berman, E., White, M.J., and Martínez-Hernández, A.: Localization of the B chain of human chorionic gonadotropin on human tumor cells and placental cells, Cancer Res. **35**:1887, 1975.

710. Nelson, D.M., Smith, C.H., Enders, A.C., and Donohue, T.M.: The non-uniform distribution of acidic components on the human placental syncytial trophoblast surface membrane: a cytochemical and analytical study, Anat. Rec. **184**:15, 1976.

711. Ornoy, A., Segal, S., Nishmi, M., Simcha, A., and Polishuk, W.Z.: Fetal and placental pathology in gestational rubella, Am. J. Obstet. Gynecol. **116**:949, 1973.

712. Page, E.W.: The pathogenesis of pre-eclampsia and eclampsia, J. Obstet. Gynaecol. Br. Cwlth. **9**:883, 1972.

713. Park, W.W.: Choriocarcinoma, Philadelphia, 1971, F.A. Davis Co.

714. Park, W.W.: Possible function of nonvillous trophoblast. In Brosens, I.A., Dixon, G., and Robertson, W.B., editors: Human placentation, Amsterdam, 1975, Excerpta Medica.

715. Peterson, E.P., and Taylor, H.B.: Amniotic fluid embolism: an analysis of 40 cases, Obstet. Gynecol. **35**:787, 1970.

716. Philippe, E.: Morphologie et morphométrie des placentas d'abbération chromosomique léthale, Rev. Fr. Gynecol. **68**:645, 1973.

717. Philippe, E.: Histopathologie placentaire, Paris, 1974, Masson et Cie.

718. Philippe, E., Lefakis, P., Laedlein-Greilsammer, D., and Itten, S.: Endomètre et séquelles d'avortement, Rev. Fr. Gynecol. **65**:413, 1970.

719. Poland, B.J., Dill, F.J., and Styblo, C.: Embryonic development in ectopic human pregnancy, Teratology **14**:315, 1976.

720. Ramsey, E.M., Corner, G.W., and Donner, M.W.: Serial and cineradiographic visualization of maternal circulation in the primate (hemochorial) placenta, Am. J. Obstet. Gynecol. **86**:213, 1963.

721. Rappaport, F., Rabinovitz, M., Toaff, R., and Krochi, K.: Genital listeriosis as a cause of repeated abortion, Lancet **1**:1273, 1960.

722. Redline, R.W., and Abromowsky, C.R.: Clinical and pathologic aspects of recurrent placental villitis, Hum. Pathol. **16**:727, 1985.

723. Rewell, R.E., and Whitehouse, W.L.: Malignant metastasis to the placenta from carcinoma of the breast, J. Pathol. **91**:255, 1966.

724. Reynolds, D.W., Stagno, S., Hosty, T.S., Tiller, M., and Alford, C.A., Jr.: Maternal cytomegalovirus excretion and perinatal infection, N. Engl. J. Med. **289**:1, 1973.

725. Robertson, W.B., Brosens, I.A., and Dixon, G.: Uteroplacental vascular pathology. In Brosens, I.A., Dixon, G., and Robertson, W.B., editors: Human placentation, Amsterdam, 1975, Excerpta Medica.

726. Roche, W.D., Jr., and Norris, H.J.: Detection and significance of maternal pulmonary amniotic fluid embolism, Obstet. Gynecol. **43**:729, 1974.

727. Rocklin, R.E., Kitzmiller, J.L., Carpenter, C.B., Garovoy, M.R., and David, J.R.: Absence of an immunologic blocking factor from the serum of women with chronic abortions, N. Engl. J. Med. **295**:1209, 1976.

728. Rotheram, E.B., and Schick, S.F.: Nonclostridial anaerobic bacteria in septic abortion, Am. J. Med. **46**:80, 1969.

729. Sander, C.H., Kinnane, L., Stevens, N.G., and Echt, R.: Haemorrhagic endovasculitis of the placenta: a review with clinical correlation, Placenta **7**:551, 1986.

730. Schneider, J., Berger, C.J., and Cattell, C.: Maternal mortality due to ectopic pregnancy: a review of 102 deaths, Obstet. Gynecol. **49**:557, 1977.

731. Scott, J.S.: Placenta extrachorialis (placenta marginata and placenta circumvallata); a factor in antepartum hemorrhage, J. Obstet. Gynaecol. Br. Cwlth. **67**:904, 1960.

732. Scully, R.E., and Young, R.H.: Trophoblastic pseudotumor: a reappraisal, Am. J. Surg. Pathol. **5**:75, 1981.

733. Seeliger, H.P.R.: Some new aspects of human listeriosis. In Human histeriosis: its nature and diagnosis, Atlanta, 1957, U.S. Department of Health, Education, and Welfare, Communicable Disease Center.

734. Shanklin, D.R., and Scott, J.S.: Massive subchorial thrombohaematoma (Breus' mole), Br. J. Obstet. Gynecol. **82**:476, 1975.

735. Shanklin, D.R., and Sotel-Avila, c.: The pathogenesis and significance of placenta extrachorialis, Lab. Invest. **15**:1111, 1966.

736. Shurin, P.A., Alpert, S., Rosner, B., Driscoll, S.G., Lee, Y.-H., McCormack, W.M., Santamarina, B.A.G., and Kass, E.H.: Chorioamnionitis and colonization of the newborn infant with genital mycoplasmas, N. Engl. J. Med. **293**:5, 1975.

737. Stagno, S., Pass, R.F., Cloud, G., Britt, W., Henderson, R.E., Walton, P.D., Veren, D.H., Page, F., and Alford, C.A.: Primary cytomegalovirus infection in pregnancy: incidence, transmission to fetus and clinical outcome, JAMA **256**:1904, 1986.

738. Steigrad, S.J., James, R.W., and Osborn, R.A.: Choriocarcinoma with intact pregnancy, Aust. NZ J. Obstet. Gynaecol. **8**:79, 1968.

739. Sweet, R.L., Landers, D.V., Walker, C., and Schachter, J.: *Chlamydia trachomatis* infection and pregnancy outcome, Am. J. Obstet. Gynecol. **156**:824, 1987.

740. Szulman, A.E., Philippe, E., Boué, J.G., and Boué, A.: Human triploidy: association with partial hydatidiform moles and nonmolar conceptuses, Hum. Pathol. **12**:1016, 1981.

741. Taylor, H.B., and Peterson, E.P.: Amniotic fluid embolism: an analysis of 40 cases, Obstet. Gynecol. **35**:787, 1970.

742. Teteris, N.J., Lina, A.A., and Holaday, W.J.: Placenta percreta, Obstet. Gynecol. **47**(suppl.):15s, 1976.

743. Thomson, A.M., Billewicz, W.Z., and Hytten, F.E.: The weight of placenta in relation to birth weight, J. Obstet. Gynaecol. Br. Cwlth. **76**:865, 1969.

744. Tominaga, T., and Page, E.W.: Sex chromatin of trophoblastic tumors, Am. J. Obstet. Gynecol. **96**:305, 1966.

745. Vaitukaitis, J.L.: Human chorionic gonadotropin as a tumor marker, Ann. Clin. Lab. Sci. **4**:276, 1974.

746. Vaitukaitis, J.L., Braunstain, G.D., and Ross, G.T.: A radioimmunoassay which specifically measures human chorionic gonadotropin in the presence of human luteinizing hormone, Am. J. Obstet. Gynecol. **113**:751, 1972.

747. Villee, D.B.: Development of endocrine function in the human placenta and fetus, N. Engl. J. Med. **281**:473, 1969.

748. Vorheer, H.: Placental insufficiency in relation to post term pregnancy and fetal postmaturity, Am. J. Obstet. Gynecol. **123**:67, 1975.

749. Wake, N., Fujino, T., Hoshi, S., Shimkai, N., Sakai, K., Kato, H., Hashimoto, M., Yasuda, T., and Yamada, H.: The propensity to malignancy of dispermic heterozygous moles, Placenta **8**:319, 1987.

750. Wallenburg, H.C.S.: Chorioangioma of the placenta: 13 new cases and a review of the literature from 1939 to 1970 with special reference to the clinical complications, Obstet. Gynecol. Surv. **26**:411, 1971.

751. Wilson, C.B., and Remington, J.S.: What can be done to prevent congenital toxoplasmosis? Am. J. Obstet. Gynecol. **138**:357, 1980.

752. Wilson, C.B., Remington, J.S., Stagno, S., and Reynolds, D.W.: Development of adverse sequelae in children born with subclinical congenital *Toxoplasma* infection, Pediatrics **66**:767, 1980.

753. Wynn, R.M.: Noncellular components of the placenta, Am. J. Obstet. Gynecol. **103**:723, 1969.

754. Wynn, R.M.: Cytotrophoblastic specializations: an ultrastructural study of the human placenta, Am. J. Obstet. Gynecol. **114**:339, 1972.

755. Wynn, R.M., and Harris, J.A.: Ultrastructure of trophoblast and endometrium in invasive hydatidiform mole (chorioadenoma destruens), Am. J. Obstet. Gynecol. **99**:1125, 1967.

756. Young, R.H., Kurman, R.J., and Scully, R.E.: Proliferations and tumors of intermediate trophoblast of the placental site, Semin. Diagn. Pathol. **5**:223, 1988.

757. Zhang, J., Kraus, F.T., and Aquino, T.I.: Chorioamnionitis: a comparative histologic, bacteriologic, and clinical study, Int. J. Gynecol. Pathol. **4**:1, 1985.

758. Zhang, J., and Kraus, F.T.: Placental site trophoblastic tumor (PSTT): immunocytochemical correlations, Lab. Invest. **54**:73A, 1986.

35 Breast

ROBERT W. McDIVITT

Breast disease is less varied than diseases of many other organs in that it is predominantly neoplastic. Congenital anomalies of the breast are uncommon and usually only of cosmetic interest. Inflammatory disease for the most part is limited to mastitis caused by staphylococci or streptococci during pregnancy and lactation. Metabolic disease consists primarily of secondary changes in the breast produced by estrogen and androgen therapy or by abnormalities in the production of these hormones. The symptomatology of breast disease also tends to be uncomplicated. Most breast disease produces a palpable mass unaccompanied by other symptoms.

In view of these facts, one may conclude that were neoplastic disease of the breast not so important both as a public health problem and in providing day-to-day medical care, little attention would be devoted to diseases of the breast in relation to other medical subjects. However, breast disease is extremely common. It is estimated that breast cancer will develop in 1 of every 22 women in the United States and that it accounts for approximately 30,000 deaths in this country each year.[49] Therefore breast disease is an important aspect of every physician's life, regardless of the specialty he or she practices.

This chapter presents an introductory view of the pathology of breast disease and its importance in patient care. Although morphology is emphasized, no attempt to be encyclopedic has been made, since several excellent texts describing the pathology of breast disease are available.[8,44] Instead, the role of morphology as it is related to the epidemiology, natural history, and treatment of breast diseases is emphasized.

STRUCTURE AND FUNCTION

The breast is a modified skin appendage that lies superficial to the deep pectoral fascia and the pectoralis major and minor muscles. Its major lymphatic drainage is into the lymph nodes of the ipsilateral axilla. Secondary lymphatic drainage is medial into lymph nodes of the internal mammary chain that lies subjacent to the sternum. The breast is divided into a dozen or more poorly defined lobes, each having its own ramifying collecting duct system that empties into a lactiferous sinus subjacent to the nipple. As the collecting ducts extend out into the breast lobe from the lactiferous sinus, they branch several times, each branching producing ducts of progressively smaller diameter. The collecting duct system terminates peripherally in a myriad of breast lobules, the secretory units of the breast during lactation (Fig. 35-1). Each lobule comprises between six and 20 small terminal ducts invested in loose areolar connective tissue.

The breast lobules and the collecting duct system are included in the epithelial portion of the breast, which in the mature breast accounts for less than 10% of its total volume. The lobules and collecting ducts are surrounded and supported by large quantities of connective tissue that give the breast its form and shape. In young women this connective tissue is predominantly fibrous, but as women age, it is gradually replaced by fat. The terminal ducts composing breast lobules are lined by a single layer of low cuboidal epithelium, as are many of the smaller ramifications of the collecting duct system. Larger collecting ducts at times appear to have a double-layered epithelial lining, as the lactiferous sinuses do. The portion of lactiferous sinuses nearest the surface of the nipple is lined by squamous epithelium. In addition to epithelial cells, myoepithelial cells may occasionally be seen in histologic sections of collecting ducts of intermediate size. These elongated cells with small, flattened nuclei are immediately adjacent to the duct basement membrane. They are arranged around intermediate-sized ducts in a spiral fashion and are believed to assist in the propulsion of milk to the external surface of the nipple.

The various operative procedures performed on the breast are best understood in terms of breast anatomy. In a simple or total mastectomy the breast is removed along with the nipple, overlying skin, and subcutaneous tissue, but the axilla or underlying pectoral muscles and fascia are not disturbed. In a subcutaneous mastectomy the breast is removed, and an attempt is made to preserve the overlying skin, subcutaneous tissue, and nipple. However, in subcutaneous mastectomy, residual breast tissue usually is left behind. In a modified radical

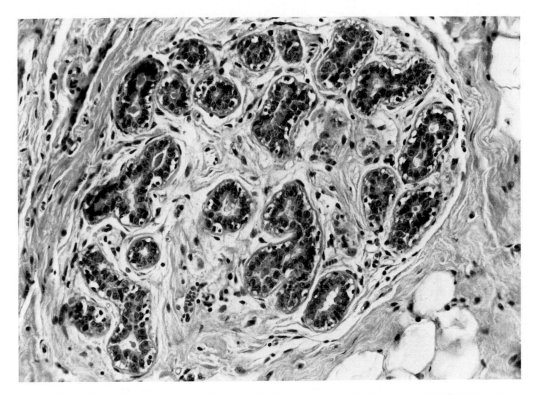

Fig. 35-1. Normal breast lobule. Terminal ducts are surrounded by loose areolar connective tissue demarcating lobule from adjacent stroma. Terminal ducts are lined by single layer of cuboid epithelium.

mastectomy removal of ipsilateral axillary lymph nodes is accomplished in combination with simple mastectomy. The number of axillary lymph nodes removed in a modified radical mastectomy and the extent of the axillary dissection depend on the operative approach and vary in accordance with the disease being treated and the philosophy of the surgeon. In a radical mastectomy the breast along with the overlying skin and nipple, the underlying pectoralis muscles, fascia, and ipsilateral axillary lymph nodes are removed. In an extended radical mastectomy a portion of the chest wall and the subjacent internal mammary lymph nodes are removed in combination with radical mastectomy. An operation that removes a palpable breast lesion along with a margin of grossly normal surrounding breast tissue is referred to as an excisional biopsy. An operation that removes an entire breast quadrant is called a quadrantectomy.

BENIGN BREAST DISEASE

The following outline lists the common benign diseases of the breast:

1. Common benign breast lesions
   a. Cystic disease
   b. Sclerosing adenosis
   c. Fibroadenoma
   d. Mammary duct ectasia
   e. Intraductal papilloma
   f. Epithelial hyperplasia involving lobules
   g. Epithelial hyperplasia involving larger ducts
2. Less common benign breast lesions
   a. Granular cell tumor
   b. Gynecomastia (male)
   c. Juvenile mammary hypertrophy
   d. Lactational mastitis

Although breast disease in children and adult men is much less common than in adult women, a similar spectrum of benign disease is observed, except for epithelial proliferative lesions involving lobules. (In children and in men the lobular apparatus is undeveloped except under unusual circumstances.) Both benign breast disease and carcinoma may occur in adult women of all ages, but benign breast disease tends to occur more commonly in younger women and carcinoma in women who are somewhat older, that is, in the fourth decade extending through the menopausal era. However, there is sufficient overlap in the age distribution of benign and malignant diseases of the breast that age alone cannot be used to predict the nature of any given lesion. Although the incidence of benign breast disease in different populations throughout the world is difficult to estimate, in teaching hospitals in the United States approximately 70% of all breast biopsies performed are interpreted as benign and the remainder are malignant.

Cystic disease

Cystic disease is the most frequent benign breast disease of adult women. Haagensen[28] estimates that about 10% of adult women in the United States have symptomatic fibrocystic disease. Frantz and associates[24] in an autopsy study of women with no history of breast disease have found grossly visible cystic disease in about 20%. Although cystic disease in women in the third and fourth decades of life is not unusual, its peak incidence is in women in the fifth decade. The incidence drops dramatically with menopause, an indication that the cause of cystic disease may somehow be related to estrogen production. Women with this disease usually have a freely movable, palpable mass unassociated with other physical findings or symptoms. However, at times it may cause pain, particularly when women are in the premenstrual phase of the menstrual cycle. The palpable lesion may appear to increase and decrease in size cyclically, usually achieving its maximum size in the premenstrual phase of the menstrual cycle.

Pathologic findings

The characteristic gross pathologic finding is cysts of varying size that are filled with clear or serosanguineous fluid (Plate 6, *A*). The cysts may be solitary and multiple, discrete or multiloculated, and so small as to be almost invisible grossly or 5 to 6 cm in diameter. Ordinarily these cysts are surrounded by rather dense fibrous connective tissue, the normal stromal component of younger women's breasts. The cysts usually are lined with a single or double layer of cuboidal epithelium, though the epithelial lining of larger cysts may be somewhat atrophic and less conspicuous (Fig. 35-2). At times the basement membrane is focally disrupted by dissection of cyst contents out into the adjacent breast stroma, inducing a chronic inflammatory reaction. This may be accompanied by cholesterol clefts and multinucleated giant cells.

Pathogenesis

Although these cysts ordinarily are believed to arise from obstructed collecting ducts, some authors have suggested that smaller cysts may be of lobular origin.[8,61,81] The mechanism of duct obstruction is not clearly understood. Some authors have suggested that localized epithelial hyperplasia may produce duct obstruction, though this is difficult to document in histologic sections.[25] Others suggest that duct obstruction is caused by periductal fibrosis resulting from inspissation and extrusion of duct contents into the adjacent stroma with secondary inflammation and fibrosis. Some suggest that it is caused by an overgrowth of connective tissue

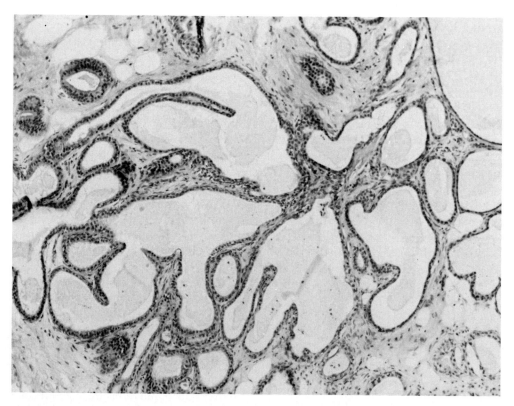

Fig. 35-2. Cystic disease. Numerous ducts are cystically dilated, presumably because of obstruction. They are lined by single layer of flattened, somewhat atrophic epithelium. There is no associated epithelial hyperplasia.

produced by estrogen stimulation.[28] Although most cysts are surrounded by varying amounts of dense fibrous connective tissue, this is a normal stromal component of the mature breast.

Natural history

Most women who have one or more cysts excised from their breasts may expect that additional cysts will appear from time to time until menopause, when the process appears to abate. The question of whether cystic disease increases the risk of subsequent breast cancer has attracted considerable interest. Although some articles have reported an increased breast cancer risk associated with fibrocystic disease, this is probably a false conclusion based on misuse of the pathologic term.[39,46] Cystic disease is frequently accompanied by varying degrees of epithelial hyperplasia in adjacent ducts and lobules. In the past pathologists tended to lump together these two dissimilar disease processes under the single designation "cystic disease," not realizing the precancerous significance of epithelial hyperplastic lesions of the breast. However, several recent pathologic studies have shown that, whereas some types of epithelial hyperplasia are associated with a significant increase in subsequent breast cancer risk, cystic disease itself is not.[14,36,58]

Sclerosing adenosis

Sclerosing adenosis is a benign overgrowth of lobular epithelium, myoepithelium, and stromal connective tissue. Its main importance is that it may be confused with carcinoma by both surgeons and pathologists. It is a common lesion in women during the reproductive years. In most cases involving sclerosing adenosis, a nonpalpable microscopic finding is identified in breast tissue excised for some other reason, usually cystic disease. However, at times sclerosing adenosis may become florid and produce a palpable mass that may mimic carcinoma of the breast both clinically and grossly. On gross pathologic examination, sclerosing adenosis may be firm, white, and stellate though usually not as rock hard as the ordinary scirrhous carcinoma. It rarely exceeds 2 cm in maximum diameter. The pathologist's problems with identifying sclerosing adenosis are compounded because it also may resemble infiltrating carcinoma of the breast microscopically. However, it differs from carcinoma in that its overall pattern as viewed under the scanning lens is whorled and circumferential, whereas carcinoma tends to be linear and stellate (Fig. 35-3). In addition, in adenosis the epithelium lining the small glands often appears somewhat atrophic, being compressed by overgrowth of adjacent myoepithelium and fibrous breast stroma. Often

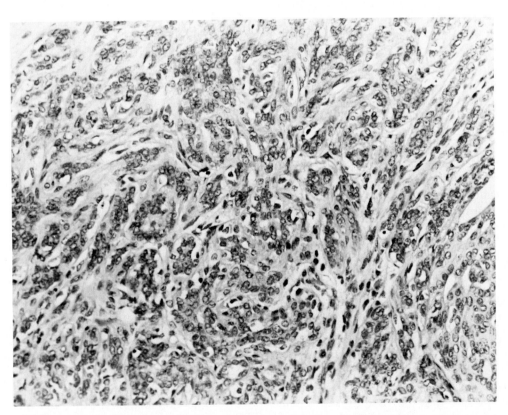

Fig. 35-3. Sclerosing adenosis. Overall pattern is concentric and whorled in contrast to more stellate pattern produced by infiltrating carcinoma. Epithelium appears compressed, and lumens for the most part are absent. Surrounding myoepithelium, which appears homogeneous and dark gray, is prominent.

in sclerosing adenosis, myoepithelial hyperplasia is exuberant, and identification of the rather intensely eosinophilic myoepithelium also aids in differential diagnosis. The cause of sclerosing adenosis is unknown. It is of no known clinical significance, except for its propensity to be confused with breast carcinoma.

Fibroadenoma

Fibroadenoma is a benign overgrowth of periductal stromal connective tissue that tends to compress the entrapped ducts and produce a well-circumscribed or encapsulated mass. Its incidence is less evenly distributed throughout the reproductive years than that of either sclerosing adenosis or cystic disease. It is a disease predominantly of young women and it is the most common cause of a palpable breast mass in women younger than 30 years of age.[28] Clinically, fibroadenomas usually are well circumscribed, freely movable lesions that in most patients are correctly identified preoperatively. In addition, their mammographic appearance is usually quite distinct.

Pathologic findings

On gross pathologic examination fibroadenomas appear as well-circumscribed, spherical lesions that are well demarcated from the surrounding breast stroma (Plate 6, *B*). They vary in size from barely perceptible gross lesions to lesions 15 cm or more in diameter. Their size depends both on their growth rate and on their duration before excision. Blunt dissection may be used to "shell out" fibroadenomas from the adjacent breast tissue. However, they often have small irregular bosselated projections on their external surface that may be amputated by the enucleation procedure. This explains why fibroadenomas may recur locally if enucleated rather than being excised with an adequate margin of adjacent breast tissue. The cut surface of fibroadenomas is firm, rubbery, and light gray. Often the slitlike spaces formed by compressed ducts are obvious grossly. Microscopically, fibroadenomas are easily recognized. Long, attenuated, and compressed ducts lined by a single or double layer of epithelium are surrounded by fibrous connective tissue and stroma (Fig. 35-4).

Fibroadenoma in pregnancy

During pregnancy fibroadenomas may grow rapidly and become relatively large over a short period of time, perhaps of hormone stimulation. At times during a rapid growth phase they may partially or totally infarct, causing acute localized pain in the breast. Infarcted fibroadenomas not removed at this time usually become densely hyalinized and irregularly calcified, producing a distinct mammographic and histologic appearance. During pregnancy fibroadenomas also may assume a

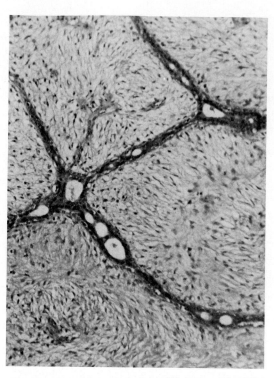

Fig. 35-4. Fibroadenoma. Anastomosing, epithelium-lined intralobar ducts are compressed into slitlike spaces by proliferation of surrounding stromal connective tissue. Stromal cells show no pleomorphism and few mitoses.

histologic appearance different from that of the ordinary fibroadenoma. The lobular epithelium may be sufficiently overgrown to produce a fibroadenoma that appears densely glandular. This epithelium also usually participates in the secretory activity that occurs elsewhere in the breast, giving the fibroadenoma a distinct appearance. Fibroadenomas of this type at times have been designated "lactational adenomas."

Carcinoma in fibroadenomas

Rarely do fibroadenomas contain either in situ or invasive carcinoma of duct or lobular origin.[43] At times carcinomas arise from the epithelium contained in the fibroadenoma; in other cases carcinoma is found to have invaded the fibroadenoma from a primary site in the adjacent breast.

Cystosarcoma phyllodes

The term "cystosarcoma phyllodes" was produced by Müller in 1838 to describe fibroadenoma-like lesions that pursue an aggressive clinical course with local chest wall recurrence or distant metastases.[48] On microscopic examination the stroma of these aggressive tumors appears histologically malignant, explaining the clinical course. In the past, some confusion has been caused by the use of the term "cytosarcoma phyllodes" to describe benign fibroadenomas that are unusually large or that have stroma displaying a modest increase in cellularity. Preferably such lesions are designated "giant fibroadenoma" and "cellular fibroadenoma," respectively, with the term "cystosarcoma phyllodes" being reserved to describe lesions with the potential for aggressive behavior. Cystosarcoma phyllodes is an uncommon tumor of the breast. Treves and Sunderland[76] found only 18 malignant cystosarcomas during a 20-year breast clinic experience at Memorial Hospital in New York, Haagensen[28] states that they comprise about 2% to 3% of fibroadenoma-like lesions seen in the breast clinic at Columbia Presbyterian Hospital in New York. Their clinical presentation is much like that of fibroadenoma. They tend to be totally or partially encapsulated and vary in size from less than 1 cm in diameter to giant lesions that occupy most of the breast.[44] When large, they may ulcerate the skin and become fixed to the underlying chest wall.

Pathologic findings. On gross inspection cystosarcoma phyllodes differs little from fibroadenoma except that it has a greater tendency to show local hemorrhage and necrosis and to become cystic. In addition, the lesion may appear less fully encapsulated with focal areas where the tumor appears to invade the adjacent breast stroma. Microscopically cystosarcoma phyllodes differs from fibroadenoma in that the stroma is more cellular, it displays more cellular pleomorphism, and the stromal cells have an increased mitotic rate. The epithelial portion of the tumor is benign and similar to that of fibroadenoma. In current pathologic practice cystosarcoma phyllodes is divided into two types, those that histologically appear fully malignant (capable of metastasis) and those assigned to a borderline malignant category because it is less clear from histologic examination of the stroma whether the tumor will pursue an aggressive course.[30,31] The stroma of tumors assigned to the fully malignant category displays the characteristics of some other recognized type of sarcoma, such as fibrosarcoma or liposarcoma; in addition eight or more mitotic figures per 10 high-power fields are usually seen. Lesions assigned to the borderline category has less pleomorphism, are less cellular, and have lower mitotic rates. The tendency for malignant cystosarcoma to metastasize appears to depend on size. Overall, approximately 10% of malignant cystosarcomas produce metastases. Metastases usually are first observed in the lungs, though bone and visceral metastases also occur.[35] Regional lymph node metastases also may occur, but this usually happens relatively late in the course of the disease subsequent to or concurrent with pulmonary metastasis. Metastatic lesions show only sarcomatous stroma, not the benign epithelial component of cystosarcoma phyllodes. Cystosarcomas of the borderline histologic type rarely metastasize and usually do so only after having recurred locally one or more times. It is difficult for pathologists to predict from histologic examination which borderline cystosarcomas will produce distant metastases.

Mammary duct ectasia

Mammary duct ectasia is important primarily because it may be confused clinically with carcinoma. It is cured by simple excision. A disease of older women, it is most common among multiparous women who have nursed their children. It affects the larger collecting ducts subjacent to the nipple and may produce a palpable mass and nipple discharge. The pathogenesis of the lesion is not clearly understood. On gross examination, multiple dilated ducts containing inspissated secretions are seen surrounded by varying amounts of dense fibrous connective tissue. By compressing the gross specimen, one may express inspissated secretion from the ducts, a feature that led to the older designation "comedomastitis." Microscopically the ectatic ducts appear to be lined by atrophic epithelium, and their lumens are filled with amorphous debris. The periductal tissue may show rather intense chronic inflammation with scattered foreign-body type of giant cells that have phagocytosed cholesterol debris. In addition, the periductal stroma often shows dense fibrosis. This periductal chronic inflammation with fibrosis is believed to be a reaction to leakage of the inspissated duct secretion into the adjacent tissues.

Benign intraductal papilloma

Pedunculated papillary proliferations composed of a branching central fibrovascular core that is covered externally by one or more layers of epithelium may extend out from the duct walls into the duct lumen. Intraductal papillomas usually are solitary, most frequently are located in large ducts near the nipple, and produce serous or serosanguineous nipple discharge as their most common symptom. They vary in size from lesions that are barely perceptible grossly to those measuring 5 cm or more in diameter. When large, they may partially or totally occlude the duct in which they are located and produce a palpable clinical mass. They occur in women of all ages but are most common in the third and fourth decades of life.

Pathologic findings

Large papillomas and their relationship to the duct wall usually are apparent on inspection of the gross specimen. Small papillomas may be more difficult to locate by random sectioning unless the surgeon has marked the duct in which the papilloma is located. If this is done, the duct can be opened along its course and the anatomic relationship between the papilloma and the duct wall is preserved. Small intraductal papil-

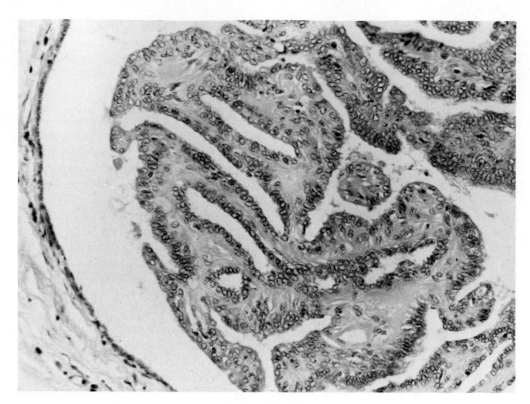

Fig. 35-5. Intraductal papilloma. Central branching fibrovascular stalk is covered by single or double layer of orderly epithelium. Cell polarity is maintained, and there is no epithelial hyperplasia.

lomas usually appear delicate and friable and are attached to the duct wall by a narrow stalk. As papillomas become larger, they tend to become more broadly based, and their anatomic relationship to the duct wall becomes more distorted by fibrosis. Large papillomas frequently contain focal areas of hemorrhage and infarction. Intraductal papillomas that occur in the lactiferous sinuses immediately subjacent to the nipple, sometimes referred to as "adenomas of the nipple," are often multicentric and may be so distorted by fibrosis that their papillary nature and the relationship of the lesion to the sinuses is not obvious on gross examination.[60,73] Lesions of this type produce a firm, poorly circumscribed mass that may resemble carcinoma grossly. Although fibrosis is most often seen with papillomas in the subareolar location, it may occur with papillomas of the more peripheral portions of the duct system, distorting the relationship of the papilloma with the surrounding tissues in such a way as to be suggestive of carcinoma grossly. As mentioned previously, on microscopic examination the typical benign intraductal papilloma is seen to have a central connective tissue core made up of loose areolar connective tissue and small blood vessels (Fig. 35-5). This central stalk branches in treelike fashion to give the papilloma its characteristic structure. The external surface of this central stalk is covered by epithelium

that usually is only one or two layers thick and is arranged along the basement membrane in an orderly fashion. However, at times this relationship is distorted by fibrosis that may result from trauma to the papilloma or from partial duct obstruction with subsequent leakage of duct contents into the adjacent stroma. When this occurs, small nests of epithelium trapped in dense connective tissue give the papilloma a pseudoinfiltrative appearance (Fig. 35-6).

Epithelial proliferative lesions

The epithelium lining the duct system and breast lobules may become hyperplastic independent of any known physiologic stimulus. Epithelial hyperplasia may display varying degrees of atypia (dysplastic changes) such as those described in Chapter 12. Epithelial hyperplasia and dysplasia seem to occur more commonly in the segmental ducts, subsegmental ducts, and terminal ducts composing lobules than in the larger ramifications of the duct system, though the epithelium that lines all portions of the duct system may participate in these changes.

Although epithelial hyperplasia and dysplasia may occur in women of all ages, including prepubertal girls, its incidence increases in the decades when women are at highest risk of breast cancer.[36,58] Most breast biopsy

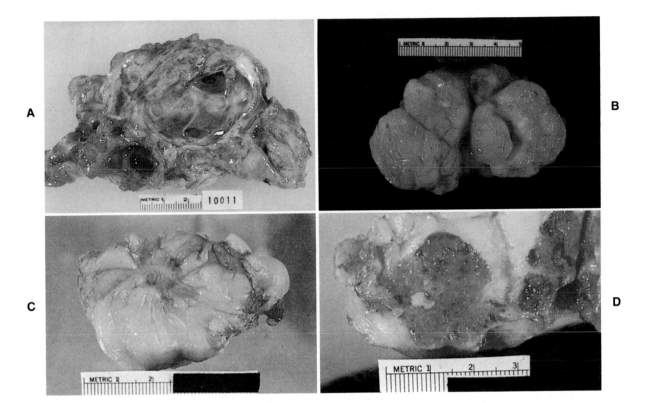

Plate 6

A, Cystic disease. Large cyst, measuring approximately 4 cm in diameter, appears in upper portion of specimen. Anterior cyst wall has been removed to reveal its multiloculation and smooth internal surface. Numerous smaller cysts are seen in lower right-hand portion of specimen. One appears dark red because of its serosanguineous contents.

B, Fibroadenoma. External surface appears well circumscribed. Compressed ducts, which help characterize the lesion microscopically, appear as slitlike spaces on lesion's cut surface.

C, Scirrhous carcinoma. Cut surface is light gray, stellate, and depressed beneath surface of surrounding fat. Notice linear depressions in surrounding fat that radiate out from carcinoma.

D, Medullary carcinoma. In contrast to scirrhous carcinoma in **C,** external surface of this tumor is smooth and convex and appears to push against rather than infiltrate adjacent fat. Cut surface is soft and on the same plane as surrounding fat.

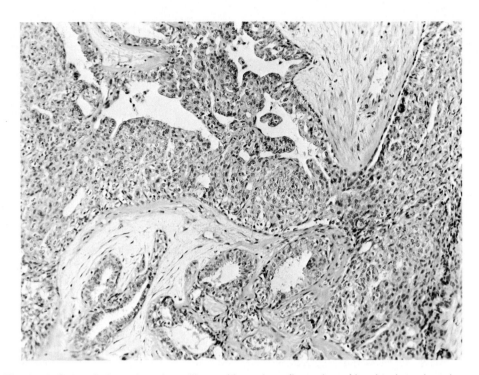

Fig. 35-6. Sclerotic intraductal papilloma. Normal configuration of benign intraductal papilloma has been distorted by dense hyaline connective tissue, trapping small islands of epithelium to produce pseudoinfiltrative appearance.

specimens that contain atypical epithelial hyperplasia are taken from women in the fourth through the sixth decades of life.

The ability of epithelial hyperplasias to produce a mass that can be palpated or appreciated on gross inspection depends primarily on the extent of the proliferative change and secondarily on the portion of the duct system that is involved. Generally, the more peripheral the portion of the duct system involved, the less likely the lesion will be palpable or grossly visible. Because of this, many epithelial hyperplasias and dysplasias are detected first microscopically in the breast biopsy specimens obtained for some other purpose, most commonly because of cystic disease. The microscopic appearance of epithelial hyperplasia and dysplasia also depends to some extent on the portion of the duct system involved. As epithelium proliferates in the small terminal ducts composing lobules, it may rapidly obliterate their lumens with a solid, sheetlike growth of cells that may distend these small ducts. In larger ducts the solid, sheetlike growth pattern may prevail, or the proliferation may be only partly solid, containing microlumens of varying size and shape (Fig. 35-7). At times in larger ducts the pattern may be more papillary, forming small, cellular projections that extend out from various points along the duct wall. This process differs from benign intraductal papilloma in that a central fibrovascular stalk is absent. In larger ducts the epithe-

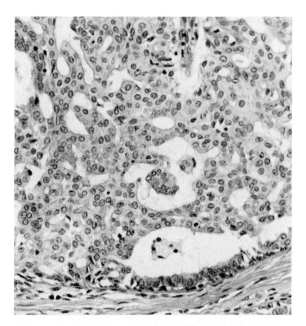

Fig. 35-7. Atypical intraductal epithelial hyperplasia. Proliferating epithelial cells partially fill duct lumen and produce small microglandular spaces that are more irregular in shape than those of intraductal carcinoma. No fibrovascular stroma supports proliferating epithelium. Cell polarity is disrupted, cytoplasmic margins are indistinct, and nuclei are somewhat elongated.

lium that covers benign intraductal papillomas may undergo epithelial hyperplastic change, producing a composite pattern of papilloma and epithelial hyperplasia.

The more closely epithelial hyperplasias of the breast resemble in situ carcinoma, the more atypical they are considered. Therefore in terminal ducts the greater the tendency for cells to lose their basilar orientation, develop indistinct cytoplasmic margins, become loosely cohesive, and develop rounded, monomorphous nuclei, the more they are considered atypical (dysplastic). Similar criteria are usually applied to hyperplastic lesions of larger ducts. In this instance, however, credence also is given to the extent to which the overall configuration of the proliferative lesion resembles one of the recognized patterns of in situ carcinoma. Several recent studies have shown that the risk of subsequent breast cancer is two to six times greater in patients whose breast biopsy specimens contained atypical epithelial hyperplastic (dysplastic) lesions than in comparable women.[14,36,58] Epithelial hyperplastic lesions are the only type of benign breast disease that is associated with a significant increase in subsequent breast cancer risk.

Less common benign breast lesions
Granular cell tumor

Granular cell tumor is an uncommon benign breast lesion that nevertheless represents a bête noire for pathologists because it is easily confused with carcinoma on both gross and microscopic examination. In our review of 110 granular cell tumors, six (5%) were located in the breast.[71] In the world literature an additional 100 granular cell tumors of the breast have been reported, but some of these appear to have been located in the overlying skin rather than in the breast itself.[74] Granular cell tumor may produce skin or deep fascial fixation and may otherwise closely stimulate the clinical presentation of carcinoma of the breast. Also, the gross appearance of the tumor often is indistinguishable from scirrhous carcinoma. Microscopically about 50% of granular cell tumors appear arranged more diffusely infiltrate the breast and induce a stromal response similar to that of scirrhous carcinoma. Diffusely infiltrating granular cell tumors are distinguished from carcinoma cytologically. Their cytoplasm contains coarse, intensely eosinophilic granules, and the nuclei are small, round, and densely basophilic.

Gynecomastia

Gynecomastia may produce either a well-circumscribed breast nodule or diffuse enlargement of one or both breasts. The majority of gynecomastia is idiopathic, transient, and seen in pubertal boys and in men in the fifth and sixth decades of life.[76] Most cases of idiopathic gynecomastia are characterized by a disc-shaped, well-localized subareolar mass. Gynecomastia may also result from diseases that alter endocrine function. The most common of these are testicular neoplasms, hepatic cirrhosis, metastatic lung carcinoma, starvation, adrenocortical neoplasms, and exogenous estrogen or androgen therapy. Microscopically the breast ducts show varying degrees of papillary epithelial hyperplasia and are surrounded by a halo of edematous, loose areolar connective tissue. Beyond this halo zone, the intervening breast stroma is densely sclerotic.

Juvenile mammary hypertrophy

Juvenile mammary hypertrophy, which resembles gynecomastia in microscopic appearance, usually affects girls between 10 and 15 years of age.[42] Like gynecomastia, it may be characterized by a localized nodule, usually subareolar, or by diffuse enlargement of one or both breasts. The disease almost always is idiopathic and self-limited, being corrected by further disease development. When the localized form of the disease occurs in a young girl who has not yet undergone breast development, considerable damage may be done to the subareolar breast bud if an attempt is made to excise it. The damage may result later in a malformed, misshapen breast.

CARCINOMA OF THE BREAST
Factors influencing the risk of developing breast carcinoma

About one of every 11 women in the United States will have breast cancer sometime during her lifetime.[49] Breast cancer is diagnosed in approximately 100,000 women in this country each year, accounting for approximately 30% of all cancers in females.[50]

The incidence of breast cancer varies greatly among geographic regions (Fig. 35-8). Many Western European countries and Canada, Australia, and New Zealand have high breast cancer incidence rates similar to those of the United States, some six times greater than those observed in Asia or among black Africans.[80] The rates in South America and Eastern Europe are intermediate between these two extremes. These geographic differences in breast cancer incidence do not appear to be determined by genetic susceptibility. Black American women have incidence rates similar to those of U.S. white women, and Japanese women who have emigrated to Hawaii and California within a generation or two develop the high incidence rates characteristic of American women.[29] Although at present these geographic differences in breast cancer incidence are not fully understood, evidence indicates that they may be related to nutritional differences, particularly to animal fat and cholesterol consumption.

In addition to these geographic differences, other fac-

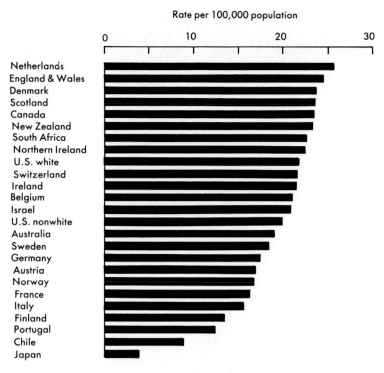

Fig. 35-8. Variation in age-adjusted death rates for breast cancer by country (1964-1965). (Modified from Segi, M.: In Haagensen, C.D.: Diseases of the breast, Philadelphia, 1971, W.B. Saunders Co.)

tors within a given population are associated with increased breast cancer risk. Women who have menarche at an early age,[32] who have menopause relatively late in life,[74] who have their first full-term delivery at a late age, or who are nulliparous[38] have an increased breast cancer risk. It is also increased among women who consume large amounts of fat and high-calorie foods,[6,21] women who use exogenous estrogens for a prolonged period of time at menopause,[34] and women who have a family history of breast cancer.[2,4] For example, women who have menarche before 12 years of age have been estimated to have a 2.8-fold increased risk compared with those who have menarche at 14 years or older.[32] Women who have their first full-term delivery before 20 years of age have about one half the breast cancer risk of nulliparous women.[38] The familial effect on breast cancer incidence is particularly striking in women whose breast cancer occurs at an early age or who have had bilateral breast cancer.[4] Overall there is approximately a twofold to threefold increase in breast cancer among first-degree relatives of women who have had breast cancer; however, among first-degree relatives who have had breast cancer before menopause or who have had bilateral breast cancer, the increase in risk is ninefold. Also, as has been mentioned, women who have had atypical epithelial hyperplastic lesions ex-

cised from their breast have a twofold to sixfold increase in subsequent breast cancer risk.[15,36,58]

In situ carcinoma

In situ carcinoma may develop in any portion of the epithelial lining of the duct system of the breast, including the terminal ducts composing lobules. Because certain clinical and pathologic features of in situ carcinoma involving breast lobules differ from those of in situ carcinoma involving larger ducts, the processes are usually separately designated "in situ lobular carcinoma" and "intraductal carcinoma."

In situ lobular carcinoma

In situ lobular carcinoma does not produce a palpable or grossly visible breast lesion.[42] In the past, it usually was detected microscopically in breast biopsy specimens obtained because of some palpable breast lesion, usually cystic disease. More recently, with the perfection of the mammographic x-ray technique, an appreciable number of in situ lobular carcinomas are being detected by this modality in breasts that contain no palpable abnormality. For example, in a recent breast cancer screening project, 38 of 50 in situ lobular breast cancers were detected by mammography alone.[10]

Pathologic findings. Since in situ lobular carcinoma is

not palpable or grossly visible, the gross pathologic findings of breasts found on biopsy to contain this lesion are those produced by an accompanying palpable breast disease. As is seen in Fig. 35-9, *A,* the microscopic characteristics of in situ lobular carcinoma are easily recognized. The terminal ducts are filled and expanded by rather monomorphous, loosely cohesive tumors cells that have indistinct cytoplasmic margins and small, spherical nuclei. Central terminal duct lumens are obliterated by this epithelial proliferative process.

Natural history. The usual method for studying the natural history of in situ carcinoma of the breasts is to observe the clinical course of patients in whom in situ carcinoma has been found by means of biopsy and in whom further treatment has not been attempted. This of course is an imperfect method, since pathologic

study of mastectomy specimens obtained subsequent to biopsy indicates that the biopsy removes all the in situ carcinoma in 30% to 40% of patients.[19] Fig. 35-10 shows the results of a long-term prospective follow-up study of 42 patients in whom in situ lobular carcinoma was discovered by excisional biopsy and no further treatment was given.[45] Approximately 8% of patients had returned with invasive cancer of the ipsilateral breast at 5 years, 15% after 10 years and 27% after 15 years. Rosen and associates[63] in studying a series of 99 patients similarly treated concluded that patients in whom in situ lobular carcinoma is diagnosed by excisional biopsy have approximately 12 times the subsequent ipsilateral invasive breast cancer risk that would be expected in an otherwise comparable population. They also found the risk of subsequent invasive breast

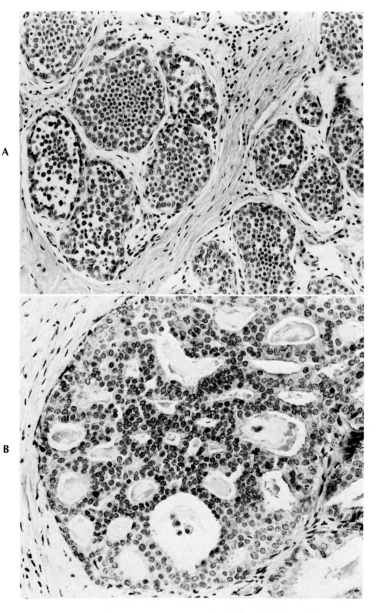

Fig. 35-9. A, In situ lobular carcinoma. Terminal ducts are distended, and their central lumens are obliterated by loosely cohesive tumor cells that have round, monomorphous nuclei and indistinct cytoplasmic margins. No tumor penetration of terminal duct basement membranes is seen. **B,** Cribriform intraductal carcinoma. Proliferating tumor cells produce spherical, smooth-walled microluminal spaces. Nuclei are round, monomorphous, and deeply basophilic. Cytoplasmic margins are indistinct.

cancer to be approximately equal for the ipsilateral and contralateral breasts (Fig. 35-11).

Intraductal carcinoma

Unlike in situ lobular carcinoma, intraductal carcinoma produces a palpable breast mass in 30% to 75% of cases.[82] Ability to produce a mass is related to the bulk of the lesion at the time of discovery and to the portion of the duct system in which the intraductal carcinoma is located. Intraductal carcinoma of the more proximal, larger ducts may expand these ducts and produce a sizable mass before it invades the adjacent stromas; intraductal carcinoma of the smaller, more peripheral portions of the duct system is more likely to be nonpalpable and multicentric. Modern mammographic techniques have proved to be an effective means for detecting nonpalpable intraductal carcinomas, particularly those that produce a partially calcified, central detritus.[10,65] Nipple discharge accompanies intraductal carcinoma in approximately 30% of cases.[28]

Pathologic findings. Gross pathologic findings also depend on the bulk of the lesion and on the portion of the duct system in which the intraductal carcinoma is located. Large intraductal carcinomas in the 3 to 5 cm diameter range often produce gross findings similar to those of large benign intraductal papillomas. They tend to be polypoid and friable and often contain areas of necrosis and scarring. The cystically dilated portion of the duct system that surrounds the intraductal carcinoma usually is easily identified. Intraductal carcinomas that occur in the more peripheral portions of the duct system produce more subtle gross findings that are dif-

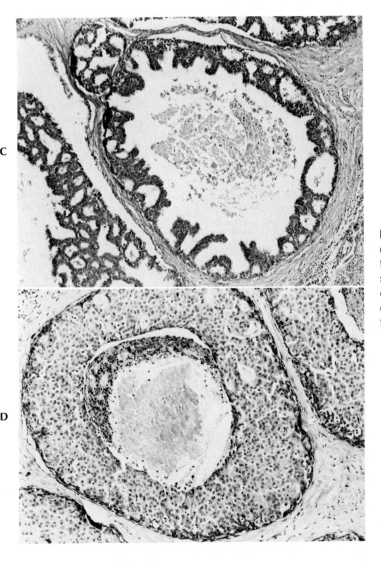

C

D

Fig. 35-9, cont'd. C, Micropapillary intraductal carcinoma. Delicate fronds of tumor cells bridge out from duct basement membrane without supporting stroma. **D,** Comedo intraductal carcinoma. Copious central detritus is surrounded by rim of loosely cohesive tumor cells that show no appreciable tendency toward gland formation.

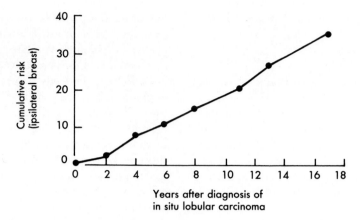

Fig. 35-10. Cumulative risk of ipsilateral invasive breast cancer by year subsequent to excision of in situ lobular carcinoma. (From McDivitt, R.W., et al.: JAMA **201:**94, 1967. Copyright 1967, American Medical Association.)

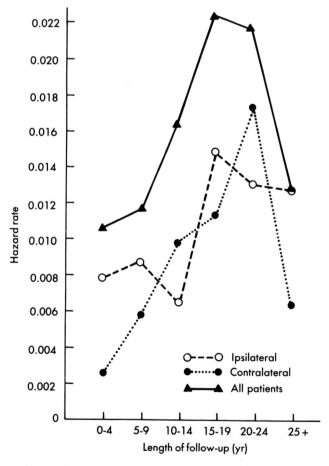

Fig. 35-11. Hazard rates for subsequent carcinoma related to length of follow-up monitoring after excision of in situ lobular carcinoma. Hazard rate indicates risk that subsequent cancer will develop as patient enters given follow-up interval. (From Rosen, P.P., et al.: Am. J. Surg. Pathol. **2:**233, 1978.)

ficult to distinguish from those of cystic disease and benign epithelial hyperplasia. These smaller ducts may appear dilated and partially filled with friable, gray, material. If extensive necrosis has occurred, the gross findings will be similar to those of mammary duct ectasia. Three different microscopic varieties of intraductal carcinoma are recognized: cribriform, micropapillary, and comedo.[36] (Pathologists find these terms useful in describing the varying histologic features of intraductal carcinoma; their use is not meant to imply that there are important differences in behavior.) The cribriform and micropapillary types of intraductal carcinoma occur so often in combination and contain cells that are cytologically so similar that they probably represent variations in a single pattern. Comedo intraductal carcinoma occurs less commonly in combination with the other types and is composed of cells that are cytologically somewhat different. Fig. 35-9, *B*, illustrates the cribriform type of intraductal carcinoma. In contrast to the epithelial hyperplasias, the microlumens formed by the cribriform type of intraductal carcinoma are round and regular and the epithelial cells have lost their polar orientation in relation to the basement membrane. Cytologically the cells are similar in many respects to those of in situ lobular carcinoma, though they may be somewhat larger. Nuclei are round and monomorphous, and cytoplasmic boundaries are indistinct. Fig. 35-9, *C*, illustrates the micropapillary type of intraductal carcinoma, so named because of the pronounced papillarity of the lesion as viewed microscopically. Cytologically the cells are indistinguishable from those of the cribriform type of intraductal carcinoma. Small anastomosing cellular fronds without obvious supporting stroma extend out into the duct lumen. When cut perpendicular to their long axis, these fronds seem to float unattached in the luminal space. A characteristic histologic feature of the comedo type of intraductal carcinoma, as is seen in Fig. 35-9, *D*, is copious necrotic detritus in the center of the duct lumen. Detritus formation of this type and magnitude is of diagnostic importance because it almost never is produced by benign epithelial hyperplasias. In comedo intraductal carcinoma the tumor cells are arranged circumferentially around the central detritus, nearer the duct basement membrane. They are loosely cohesive and may display significantly more cytologic atypia than those of cribriform and micropapillary types of intraductal carcinoma.

Natural history. The natural history of intraductal carcinoma is less well understood than that of in situ lobular carcinoma because no large prospective follow-up study of patients treated by excisional biopsy has been conducted. However, the literature does contain several reports of small numbers of patients with in-

traductal carcinoma followed in this manner. When information from these reports is pieced together to arrive at some sort of composite picture, the impression given is that the chance of invasive carcinoma occurring subsequent to the excision of intraductal carcinoma is similar to or slightly greater than the chance of invasive cancer occurring subsequent to the excision of in situ lobular carcinoma. For example, in a recent series reported from Memorial Hospital in New York, seven of 25 patients who had intraductal carcinoma initially treated by excisional biopsy developed recurrent ipsilateral carcinoma during a follow-up period that averaged just under 10 years.[13] Intraductal carcinoma differs from in situ lobular carcinoma in another important respect. The risk of contralateral breast cancer developing in patients with cribriform or micropapillary intraductal carcinoma is far less than that associated with in situ lobular carcinoma.[13] In contrast, the contralateral breast cancer risk for patients who have comedo type of intraductal carcinoma is approximately equal to that of patients who have in situ lobular carcinoma.[1]

Invasive breast cancer
Pathologic parameters useful in predicting invasive breast cancer prognosis

The clinical course of breast cancer varies considerably from patient to patient; some women have recurrent cancer and die within a year of mastectomy, others are cured by mastectomy, and still others survive for 10 or 15 years after mastectomy with proved metastatic disease. Although it is not possible to predict with certainty how a particular breast cancer will behave in a particular patient, certain parameters are useful in predicting the chance of a woman's being cured or dying of the disease. In discussing these parameters, one must remember that breast cancer is a disease in which total mortality accrues relatively slowly. With some cancers, such as carcinoma of the lung and melanoma, almost all patients who die of the disease will do so within the first few years after primary treatment. In contrast, the mortality from breast cancer accrues steadily during the tenth, fifteenth, and even twenty-fifth postoperative year. Therefore it is possible for a woman to have no clinical evidence of recurrent or metastatic breast cancer for 10 or 15 years after mastectomy and still subsequently die of carcinoma of the breast. Another generalization of equal importance is that the more breast cancer appears favorable in terms of pathologic stage, the more slowly total mortality from the disease will accrue.[1] Therefore the more successful we become in discovering and treating breast cancers of a favorable pathologic stage, the longer we will have to wait to determine the efficacy of our treatment methods.

The median survival of women with untreated breast cancer is 2.7 years, and the 10-year survival subsequent to the onset of symptoms is 3.6%.[16] Overall approximately half of all women who received primary surgical therapy for breast cancer survive for 10 years postoperatively; the remainder die of disease during this interval.[12] If one becomes slightly more sophisticated in characterizing breast cancers according to pathologic stage, one may predict that about 75% of women who have no evidence of regional metastatic disease at the time of primary surgical therapy will be 10-year survivors, whereas only 35% of those whose cancer has spread to axillary lymph nodes will survive for a similar period of time.[12] The chance of 10-year survival of women who have distant metastases at the time of primary treatment is similar to that of untreated breast cancer. Pathologists can make certain additional observations that help characterize the chance of an individual patient's surviving breast cancer. These assume importance in part because they define women at high risk to whom we might wish to give adjuvant chemotherapy. The most important are as follows.

Histologic type of tumor. The rationale for subclassifying breast cancers into various different histologic types lies in the fact that this has an important influence on prognosis (Table 35-1). In a recent analysis of 30-year survivors of invasive breast cancers treated by mastectomy, it was found that 29% of women who had poorly differentiated scirrhous duct cancers and 34% of women who had lobular carcinomas survived for this period of time.[1] In contrast, the chance of 30-year survival among women whose breast cancer was of colloid type was 55% and among women who had medullary type of breast cancer, 58%.[1] Women who had papillary breast cancer had the most favorable 30-year survival of any of the major histologic subtypes, 65%.

Histologic grade. Breast cancers may be characterized in terms of histologic grade as well as histologic type. The most popular method of grading uses three histologic grades of ascending pleomorphism based on degree of gland formation, nuclear atypia, degree of hyperchromatism, and mitotic rate. Twenty-year survival of patients with grade I breast cancer is approximately 40%; 20-year survival for patients with grade II and grade III breast cancers is only 29% and 21%, respectively.

Tumor size. Fig. 35-12 demonstrates an inverse relationship between primary breast cancer diameter at the time of mastectomy and chance of long-term sur-

Table 35-1. Long-term survival of patients with infiltrating breast cancer treated by radical mastectomy

Tumor type	Actuarial survival		
	5 years	10 years	20 years
Scirrhous	59%	47%	38%
Lobular	57%	42%	34%
Medullary	69%	68%	62%
Colloid	76%	72%	62%
Papillary	89%	65%	65%

Modified from McDivitt, R.W., Stewart, F.W., and Berg, J.W.: Tumors of the breast. In Atlas of tumor pathology, Washington, D.C., 1967, Armed Forces Institute of Pathology.

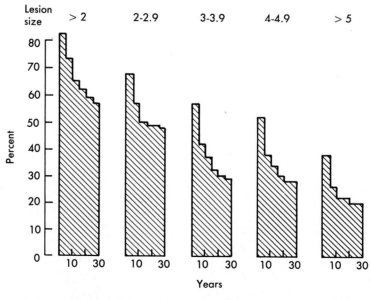

Fig. 35-12. Relationship between primary tumor size and long-term survival. (From Adair, F., et al.: Cancer **33:**1147, 1974.)

vival. Approximately 60% of patients whose breast cancers measured less than 2 cm in diameter were long-term survivors, whereas fewer than half as many patients whose primary tumors measured greater than 3 cm in diameter survived for a similar period of time.[1] Although this relationship between tumor size and survival was particularly noteworthy among patients who had axillary metastases, it was evident among node-negative patients as well. Similarly, in an analysis of 5-year survival of 2000 women with operable breast cancers treated by radical mastectomy, Fisher and associates[23] observed an inverse relationship between tumor size and survival. For tumors less than 1 cm in diameter, 5-year mortality was 18%. For tumors between 1 and 1.9 cm in diameter, it was 22%. The 5-year mortality for tumors measuring between 3 and 6 cm in diameter varied from 37% to 43%. In this study tumor size was also related to probability of axillary metastasis and to extent of axillary nodal involvement by metastatic tumor. The median tumor size of patients who had no axillary lymph node metastases was 2.7 cm; for patients who had between one and three axillary lymph nodes involved by metastatic cancer, the median tumor size was 2.9 cm, and for patients who had more extensive axillary metastatic disease the median tumor size was 3.3 cm.

Axillary lymph node status. In the course of performing mastectomies for breast carcinoma, most often the pathologist removes and examines the axillary lymph nodes. During the course of a complete axillary dissection 20 to 30 lymph nodes may be removed. Lymph nodes that lie near the breast medial to the insertion of the pectoralis minor muscle customarily are designated level I; those under the pectoralis muscle, level II; and those nodes deepest in the axilla, level III. Twenty years after mastectomy, the survival for patients with no axillary metastases is reported by Berg and Robbins[11] as 65%; for patients with metastases at level I only, 38%; for patients with metastases at level II, 30%; and for patients with level III metastases, 12%. Chance of survival also may be calculated according to the number of lymph nodes involved by metastatic disease. About 60% of patients with between one and three lymph nodes involved by metastatic tumor survive 10 years; only 20% of patients with four or more lymph nodes involved by metastatic tumor have a 10-year survival.[64] Survival figures based on counting involved lymph nodes correlate well with survival figures based on level of involvement because metastatic breast cancer usually spreads from the proximal to the distal axilla, progressively involving more lymph nodes.

Other potentially useful parameters. Breast cancers also may be characterized according to whether the tumor cells contain a cytoplasmic protein that binds estrogen, designated estrogen receptor (ERP). Although the presence or absence of ERP has been used primarily to predict which breast cancers will respond to endocrine therapy, evidence indicates that the presence or absence of ERP may correlate with prognosis. Osborne and McGuire[56] have reported that ERP-negative tumors have a higher rate of short-term recurrence after mastectomy than ERP-positive carcinomas do. ERP status, however, has not yet been correlated with chance of long-term breast cancer survival. ERP status correlates to some degree with tumor histology. Invasive lobular carcinomas have a high frequency of ERP positivity (71% to 89%), whereas for medullary carcinomas the rate of ERP positivity is much lower (18%).[66] Meyer and associates[47] also have studied the relationship between ERP status, histologic grade, and breast cancer kinetics, using a tritiated thymidine–labeling index to measure the proportion of cells engaged in DNA synthesis at any given time. They report that tumors of higher histologic grade are more likely to be ERP negative and have higher labeling indices, indicating more rapid cell proliferation. No correlation has been found between ERP status and tumor size or axillary lymph node status.

Interrelationships of prognostic parameters. Alderson and associates[3] in a recent computer-assisted multiple regression analysis of 258 infiltrating breast cancers found axillary lymph node status, tumor size, and histologic grade to be of decreasing order of influence in predicting long-term survival. Other factors such as histologic type were not included in this study, though they are obviously important, in part to predict chance of axillary metastasis. There is also some evidence to suggest that breast cancer cell kinetics may offer the single most useful parameter in predicting the chance of breast cancer survival, though these studies are still incomplete.[46]

Common histologic types of invasive breast carcinoma

The following outline lists the five most common histologic types of invasive breast carcinoma, which in aggregate comprise 90% to 98% of all breast cancers seen in the day-to-day practice of surgical pathology.

A. Common histologic types
  1. Invasive lobular carcinoma
  2. Invasive duct carcinoma
     a. Scirrhous
     b. Colloid
     c. Medullary
     d. Papillary
B. Less common favorable histologic types
  1. Tubular
  2. Secretory
  3. Adenoid cystic
C. Unusual presentations
  1. Paget's disease
  2. Inflammatory carcinoma

Of these, approximately 10% are of lobular origin and the remaining 90% arise from larger ducts.[42] Scirrhous carcinoma comprises approximately 90% of all cancers of duct origin; the remaining 10% are colloid, medullary, or papillary. Invasive breast cancers are subclassified by means of variations in their histologic appearance.

Invasive lobular carcinoma. As is seen in Fig. 35-13, A, invasive lobular carcinoma characteristically produces a linear or single-file pattern of stromal infiltration with very little tendency toward gland formation. At times, infiltrating lobular carcinoma also may distribute itself circumferentially around ducts to produce a bull's-eye or targeting pattern. Individual tumor cells resemble those of in situ lobular carcinoma. They are relatively small, have round nuclei, and have very little pleomorphism. Mitoses are infrequent. Some invasive lobular carcinomas may accumulate considerable cytoplasmic mucus, resembling the signet-ring cells of poorly differentiated carcinomas of gastrointestinal tract origin.[27] This histologic variation appears to be of no prognostic significance.

Scirrhous duct carcinoma. As is seen in Fig. 35-13, B, scirrhous duct carcinoma looks somewhat different histologically from invasive lobular carcinoma. The infiltrating tumor produces small glandular spaces that vary in number and maturity of development in accordance with the pleomorphism of the tumor. In addition, in contrast to invasive lobular carcinoma, the invading ribbons in scirrhous carcinoma usually are

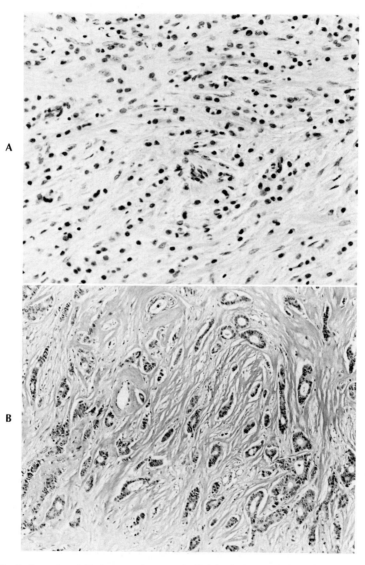

Fig. 35-13. A, Invasive lobular carcinoma. Individual tumor cells infiltrate stroma in linear arrangement without gland formation. **B,** Scirrhous carcinoma. Small clusters of cells, which often form rudimentary glands, infiltrate stroma in haphazard arrangement. Stromal sclerosis is prominent.

several cells thick, and the cells are larger and more pleomorphic. Individual nests of tumor cells are surrounded by copious dense stromal collagen, a feature that gives scirrhous carcinoma its name.

Colloid carcinoma. Colloid carcinoma is characterized by abundant, tumor-produced, extracellular mucus, as is seen in Fig. 35-13, *C*. The mucus is produced by the tumor cells and subsequently extruded into the surrounding stroma. Mucus production may be so abundant that in some histologic sections tumor cells may be difficult to locate. They usually form small clusters and show little pleomorphism. It is useful in the differential diagnosis of colloid carcinoma to remember that no benign breast tumor is capable of producing copious extracellular mucus.

Medullary carcinoma. A medullary carcinoma, as is seen in Fig. 35-13, *D*, is composed of cells that are relatively large and pleomorphic. Mitoses are frequent and often bizarre. Medullary carcinoma produces a sheetlike growth pattern with no appreciable tendency toward gland formation. Desmoplastic stromal reaction is minimal or absent, and an abundant infiltration of mature plasma cells and lymphocytes accompanies approximately 50% of tumors. The presence or absence of mononuclear infiltration is of no prognostic significance.

Papillary carcinoma. Except for stromal invasion, infiltrating papillary carcinoma resembles papillary intraductal carcinoma. The infiltrating carcinoma is arranged in large papillary fronds with varying amounts of stromal fibrosis.

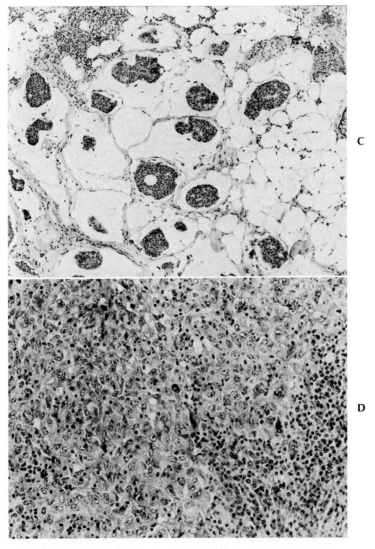

Fig. 35-13, cont'd. C, Colloid carcinoma. Small clusters of tumor cells appear suspended in pool of mucus that is produced by tumor. **D,** Medullary carcinoma. Large pleomorphic tumor cells produce sheetlike growth pattern without obvious gland formation. Mitoses are frequent, and stroma sclerosis is minimal. Mixed infiltration of mature mononuclear cells, seen in the lower right-hand corner, often accompanies medullary carcinoma.

Gross pathologic appearance. Colloid, medullary, and papillary carcinomas produce soft, well-circumscribed, discrete masses that may be lobulated but are generally spherical in contour (Plate 6, *C*). They are sometimes described as having pushing rather than infiltrative margins. The cut surface usually is friable and has a mottled light and dark gray color. The cut surface of colloid carcinomas appears more glistening than the surface of tumors of the other two types and is somewhat sticky. These features help distinguish colloid carcinoma from the medullary and papillary varieties grossly. In contrast, the cut surface of scirrhous carcinoma appears stellate and its margins jagged because of the irregular infiltration of tumor into the adjacent stroma (Plate 6, *D*). The tumor surface usually is depressed in relation to the surrounding breast stroma and is firm, at times rock hard, because of intense desmoplastic stromal collagen production. Radially arranged, dull yellow streaks produced by necrosis may interrupt the otherwise light gray or white appearance of the tumor. The gross appearance of infiltrating lobular carcinoma may be similar to that of scirrhous carcinoma. Alternatively, infiltrating lobular carcinoma may be more subtle, producing no visible gross lesion but only a poorly defined area of localized firmness. However, if one cuts across an area of this type and keeps the knife perpendicular to the surface of the specimen, the edges produced by the cut are firm and sharp rather than rounded and soft as they would be with benign breast disease.

Clinical presentation. The older literature describes the clinical presentation of breast cancer as a firm, palpable mass that is adherent to the surrounding breast tissue and often fixed to the underlying chest wall or overlying skin. Large cancers not infrequently produce dimpling of the overlying skin or nipple retraction and inversion, caused by increased tension on the suspensory ligaments of the breast. At times, skin or nipple ulcerations, caused by direct tumor extension, are observed. These findings are clinical signs of relatively advanced breast cancer. They occur less frequently today because women have learned to seek medical attention as soon as a breast mass is discovered, usually by the woman herself. Since smaller breast cancers may produce no clinical signs or symptoms other than a discrete mass, most surgeons excise any dominant, noncystic breast mass for histologic evaluation. Of course, if invasive breast cancers are sufficiently small, they may be nonpalpable. The diameter at which breast cancers become palpable depends to some degree on the consistency of the tumor and the size and consistency of the breast. However, most breast cancers smaller than 1 cm in diameter are nonpalpable. In a recent breast cancer screening program that employed both physical examination and mammography, 61 of 104 (59%) infiltrat-

ing breast cancers that measured less than 1 cm in diameter were detected by mammography only, not by physical examination.[10] Obviously mammography plays an important role in detecting small cancers of this type.

Prognosis. The rationale for subclassifying infiltrating breast cancers is to identify tumors that vary in their natural history. Table 35-1 shows a similar actuarial survival for patients with infiltrating lobular carcinoma and scirrhous carcinoma treated by radical mastectomy; approximately 45% at 10 years after mastectomy and 35% at 20 years after mastectomy.[44] Ten- and 20-year survival of similarly treated patients with colloid, medullary, and papillary carcinoma is considerably more favorable, varying from 65% to 72% at 10 years, and from 62% to 65% at 20 years.[42] There also are great differences in the chance that carcinoma of the contralateral breast will develop, depending on the histologic type of the first breast carcinoma. Fig. 35-14 shows that during a 30-year follow-up period approximately 25% of patients with infiltrating lobular and comedo types of carcinoma develop contralateral breast carcinoma; the contralateral breast cancer risk is significantly less for tumors of other histologic types.[1]

Less common, favorable histologic types of infiltrating carcinoma

Three additional types of infiltrating carcinoma are noteworthy because they carry a particularly favorable prognosis: tubular, secretory, and adenoid cystic carcinoma.

Tubular carcinoma. Tubular carcinoma is a very orderly type of infiltrating duct carcinoma in which small, nonanastomosing glands lined by a single layer of cells infiltrate the breast stroma (Fig. 35-15). In the majority of cases the infiltrating carcinoma is accompanied by cribriform or micropapillary intraductal carcinoma.[40] Tubular carcinomas tend to be small; in a recent study of 93 tubular carcinomas, tumors were found to vary in diameter from 0.2 to 2.5 cm, with a mean diameter of 0.8 cm.[40] (This small size has led to the speculation that tubular carcinoma may be an early infiltrative growth phase of cribriform and micropapillary intraductal carcinoma, a pattern that is later obliterated by scirrhous overgrowth.) Because tubular carcinomas are small, they are particularly amenable to mammographic detection. Axillary metastases were found in only two of the 93 patients with tubular carcinoma described above. No patient developed disseminated metastatic disease during the follow-up period. Only one patient, initially treated by excisional biopsy, had a local recurrence, and she is currently without evidence of disease subsequent to mastectomy. An additional 17 patients who were treated by procedures less extensive than mastectomy remained without evidence of disease. Al-

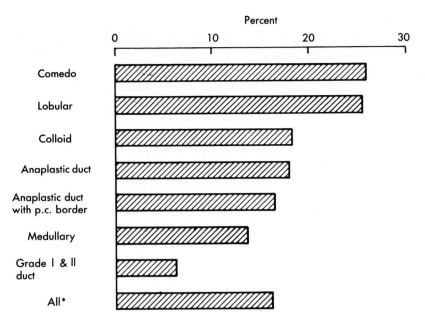

Percent

0	10	20	30

Comedo

Lobular

Colloid

Anaplastic duct

Anaplastic duct
with p.c. border

Medullary

Grade I & II
duct

All*

*Including uncommon types not tabulated.

Fig. 35-14. Risk of contralateral breast cancer by histologic type of first breast cancer during 30-year postmastectomy follow-up period. (From Adair, F., et al.: Cancer **33:**1149, 1974.)

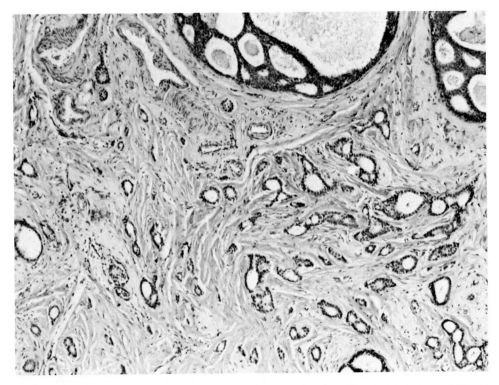

Fig. 35-15. Tubular carcinoma. Small, well-formed glands with patent lumens infiltrate breast stroma. These glands are lined by single layer of tumor cells whose polarity is well maintained. Cribriform type of intraductal carcinoma, seen in the upper right-hand corner, often accompanies tubular cancer.

though previous reports concerning infiltrating carcinomas of relatively large size listed tubular carcinoma as an infrequent variety, more recent studies of infiltrating carcinoma list tubular carcinoma as comprising between 8% to 10% of the total.[10,18]

Secretory carcinoma. Secretory carcinoma is an unusual type of infiltrating duct carcinoma that was first described in children.[41] Although it is the most frequent type of breast cancer seen in children, it comprises less than 1% of lesions excised from children's breasts.[22] Secretory carcinoma may occur in women of any age, but the mean age of patients with secretory carcinoma who seek treatment is only 25 years.[72] The lesion is easily recognized histologically because the tumor produces abundant secretions similar to those seen during lactation. This eosinophilic secretory product is seen both within the cytoplasm of tumor cells and within glandular spaces formed by the tumor. In a recent review of secretory carcinoma, only four of 19 patients were found to have axillary metastases.[72] One patient with axillary metastasis, treated initially by partial mastectomy, had a local recurrence after 8 months but subsequently has remained without evidence of disease after mastectomy. One additional 25-year-old patient in whom eight of 14 axillary lymph nodes were involved by metastatic tumor died of breast carcinoma 8 months later. The remaining 17 patients (90%) have shown no evidence of recurrent or metastatic disease.

Adenoid cystic carcinoma. Adenoid cystic carcinoma is an infrequent type of breast carcinoma comprising from 0.1% to 0.2% of infiltrating carcinomas.[26] The characteristic diphasic histologic growth pattern of the tumor is similar to that of adenoid cystic carcinoma of salivary gland origin (Chapter 27). Approximately 100 adenoid cystic carcinomas of the breast have been reported; none have had axillary metastases.[5] Although three deaths have been attributed to the disease, the details of these case reports are incomplete.[51,54]

Unusual clinical presentation of breast cancer

Paget's disease. In 1874 Sir James Paget observed that an eczematoid lesion of the nipple at times preceded carcinoma of the breast.[59] The nipple lesion that bears Paget's name is caused by tumor cells invading the basilar layers of the epidermis of the nipple after having migrated through the lactiferous sinuses from an underlying carcinoma of the breast (Fig. 35-16). These cells, which are larger and more pleomorphic than the adjacent epidermal cells, form rudimentary glands and stain irregularly with mucicarmine. Most patients with Paget's disease have a crusted, scaling, eczematoid lesion of the nipple; about half have a palpable underlying subareolar mass. However, occasionally Paget's dis-

ease may be discovered by microscopic examination in instances in which gross nipple lesion is absent. Most patients in whom a breast mass is palpated are subsequently proved to have scirrhous carcinoma; however, occasionally an invasive lobular, medullary, or papillary carcinoma produces the nipple lesion. About 70% of patients in whom no breast mass is palpated have intraductal carcinoma; the remainder have small invasive carcinomas, usually scirrhous.[7] The presence of Paget's disease does not alter the excellent prognosis of intraductal carcinoma. The prognosis of patients who have invasive carcinoma accompanied by Paget's disease is slightly less favorable than that of other patients with breast cancer who do not have Paget's disease. The overall 10-year postmastectomy survival of patients with Paget's disease is 60%.[7]

Inflammatory carcinoma. Inflammatory carcinoma is a diffuse erythema of the breast caused by packing of the dermal lymphatics with tumor emboli from an underlying carcinoma of the breast, usually of scirrhous

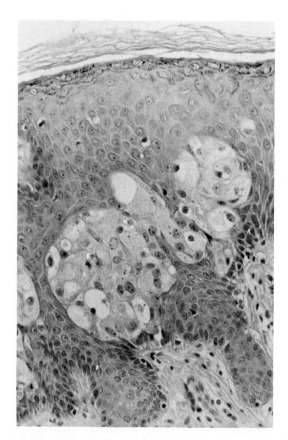

Fig. 35-16. Paget's disease. Small nests of pale-staining tumor cells in basilar region of the epidermis contrast with surrounding squamous epithelium. At times Paget's cells may form rudimentary glands and contain cytoplasmic mucus, behavior characteristics similar to those of underlying breast cancer from which they are derived.

type (Fig. 35-17). This phenomenon accompanies approximately 1% of invasive breast cancers.[62] The mean age of patients with inflammatory carcinoma is the same as that of other breast cancer patients.[70] Most patients have increased warmth and diffuse erythema of the breast, and about 60% have a palpable underlying mass. The prognosis of inflammatory carcinoma is so bleak that most surgeons do not consider it worthwhile to treat patients with this disease by mastectomy.[62] Almost all die within a short time. Occasionally dermal lymphatic emboli are observed microscopically in patients who do not have the clinical stigmas of inflammatory carcinoma. These patients have a similarly poor prognosis.

Breast carcinoma in unusual hosts

Although most discussions of breast carcinoma do not emphasize variations resulting from differences in the host, some special circumstances may modify patterns of breast carcinoma incidence and behavior.

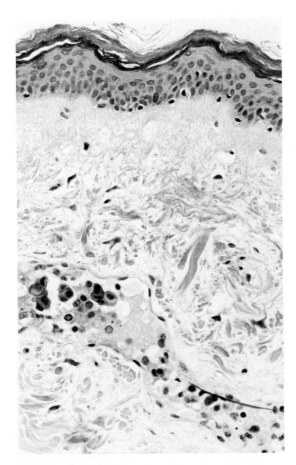

Fig. 35-17. Inflammatory carcinoma. Dermal lymphatics are distended with tumor cells from underlying breast carcinoma. (Notice that there is no inflammatory reaction. "Inflammatory" refers to cutaneous erythema seen clinically.)

Oral contraceptive users

Although the relationship between oral contraceptive use and breast cancer risk remains undetermined, recent studies indicate that long-term oral contraceptive use, particularly in women who have underlying benign breast disease, may increase the chance of subsequent breast carcinoma.[57] Interestingly, other studies have reported a decreased incidence of benign breast disease among long-term oral contraceptive users.[55] LiVolsi and associates[37] have refined this latter observation by showing that oral contraceptive use decreases the incidence of most types of benign breast disease but has no effect on the incidence of atypical epithelial hyperplastic lesions of the breast. It remains to be seen what effect, if any, long-term oral contraceptive use has on breast cancer risk among patients with atypical epithelial hyperplastic lesions.

Perimenopausal exogenous estrogen users

Although most studies investigating the relationship between exogenous estrogen use and breast cancer risk have been poorly controlled. Hoover and associates[34] in a carefully controlled case study showed a 25% excess breast cancer risk among (menopausal) exogenous estrogen users and an even greater risk among women taking high doses of exogenous estrogens for a prolonged period of time.

Males

Breast cancer accounts for 0.2% of male cancers and is approximately 100 times less frequent than carcinoma of the female breast. However, countries, such as Australia, United States, and England, that have high rates of breast cancer in women also have proportionally higher rates in men, and countries, such as Japan, that have low rates of breast cancer in women have proportionally lower rates in men.[68] Gynecomastia does not appear to increase the risk of male breast cancer, whereas Klinefelter's syndrome does by a magnitude of approximately twentyfold.[67,69] Since approximately 4% to 5% of males with breast cancer have Klinefelter's syndrome, appropriate chromosome studies should be done as part of the male breast cancer workup.

Men who seek treatment for breast cancer are on average 10 years older than women, and men delay approximately twice as long as women before seeking medical attention. Most breast cancers in men lie immediately below the areola, 25% are associated with nipple ulceration and retraction, and 10% have associated Paget's disease.[53] With the exception of lobular carcinoma, men develop the same histologic types of breast cancer as women do in approximately the same proportion of each histologic type. Since normally the male breast does not contain lobules, lobular carcinoma of the male breast is not ordinarily seen, except rarely after high doses of estrogen therapy that have induced lobular development.

Because of patient delay in seeking therapy, breast cancer in men tends to be more advanced at the time of primary surgical therapy than breast cancer in women. More than half of all male patients have metastatic carcinoma when first seen. (However, the prognosis of male breast cancer that is developed from studying the size and node is essentially the same as that of the female.) For this reason, the same types of surgical therapies are ordinarily employed. Aside from gynecomastia and carcinoma, breast lesions in men are infrequent.

Malignant mesenchymal tumors

Primary malignant mesenchymal tumors of the breast are infrequent in comparison with carcinoma. At Memorial–Sloan Kettering Cancer Institute between 1926 and 1956, only 86 malignant mesenchymal tumors were indexed by the pathology department. Of these, 47% were diagnosed as malignant cystosarcoma, 29% as stromal sarcoma, 16% as malignant lymphoma, and 8% as angiosarcoma.[39] Aside from these types, an occasional tumor resembling pure liposarcoma or malignant fibrous histocytoma is seen.

Malignant cystosarcoma

Malignant cystosarcoma is discussed in a previous section dealing with fibroadenoma.

Stromal sarcoma

Malignant mesenchymal tumors of the breast that do not contain the elongated ducts characteristic of a fibroadenoma are designated "stromal sarcoma." Stromal sarcomas most often contain a mixture of malignant mesenchymal elements. A fibrosarcomatous component is most frequent; however, about one third also contain areas resembling liposarcoma. Less frequently, malignant bone and cartilage are seen, and areas resembling malignant giant cell tumor also may be present. In Barnes and Pietruszka's review of 100 cases collected from the literature, the average age of patients with stromal sarcoma at initial examination was 52 years, and the median tumor size was 5.3 cm.[9] Stromal sarcomas most often have diffusely infiltrative margins rather than being circumscribed. Their cut surface is usually light gray mottled with areas of hemorrhage and necrosis. At times cystic areas also are seen. Approximately 25% to 30% of patients with stromal sarcoma die of disease, most frequently from pulmonary metastases.[52] Since most patients treated by radical mastectomy who subsequently die of pulmonary metastases were not found to have axillary metastases, it is postulated that metastatic spread is via the bloodstream rather than lymphatic channels. Stromal sarcomas containing malignant bone and cartilage and those with a high mitotic rate (eight to 10 mitoses per 10 high-power fields) are believed to have a particularly poor prognosis.[9,52]

Malignant lymphoma

Although breast involvement by malignant lymphoma most often is a sign of disseminated disease, at times patients have what appears to be primary lymphoma of the breast. The incidence of primary breast lymphoma is estimated to be in the range of 1:500 to 1:1000 malignant breast tumors.[42] The histiocytic type is most common, followed by poorly differentiated lymphocytic lymphoma.[42] Primary Hodgkin's disease of the breast has not been reported. Breast lymphoma is characterized by a well-circumscribed, soft, gray mass that usually is spherical, somewhat resembling the gross appearance of medullary carcinoma. In about 10% of cases there is bilateral breast involvement.[8] Ten-year survival of patients treated with local radiotherapy is about 50%.[20]

Angiosarcoma

Breast angiosarcoma almost always is a relentlessly fatal disease of young women. Although the disease occurs in women of all ages, as well as children, the majority of women are between 20 and 29 years of age at diagnosis. The tumor most frequently is initially seen as a poorly defined area of thickening. During the operation the surgeon may be confronted with little more than a diffusely bloody field that is difficult to control.

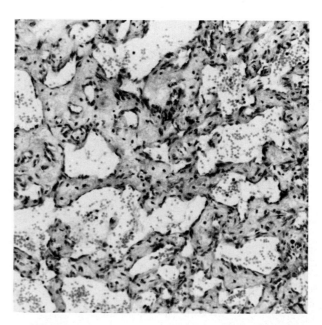

Fig. 35-18. Angiosarcoma. Anastomosing network of small, benign vascular channels, similar to those in hemangioma, may be all that is seen microscopically.

Grossly the biopsy specimen appears hemorrhagic and firm. The histologic features of angiosarcoma often are deceptively bland, resembling those of benign cutaneous hemangioma (Fig. 35-18). In view of this, I hesitate to consider any grossly visible vascular tumor of the breast benign. The 5-year mortality from angiosarcoma of the breast approaches 100%; most patients die within a year of diagnosis. No therapy has proved effective.

REFERENCES

1. Adair, F., Berg, J., Joubert, L., and Robbins, G.F.: Long-term followup of breast cancer patients: the 30-year report, Cancer **33**:1145, 1974.
2. Anderson, D.E.: A genetic study of human breast cancer, J. Natl. Cancer Inst. **48**:1029, 1972.
3. Alderson, M.R., Hamlin, I., and Staunton, M.D.: Relative significance of prognostic factors in breast carcinoma, Br. J. Cancer **25**:646, 1971.
4. Anderson, D.E.: Genetic study of breast cancer: identification of a high risk group, Cancer **34**:1030, 1974.
5. Anthony, P.P., and James, P.D.: Adenoid cystic carcinoma of the breast: prevalence, diagnostic criteria, and histogenesis, J. Clin. Pathol. **28**:647, 1975.
6. Armstrong, B., and Dall, D.: Environmental factors and cancer incidence and mortality in different countries with special reference to dietary practices, Int. J. Cancer **15**:617, 1975.
7. Ashikari, H., Park, K., Huvos, A.G., and Urban, J.A.: Paget's disease of the breast, Cancer **26**:680, 1970.
8. Azzopardi, J.G., Ahmed, A., and Millis, R.R.: Problems in breast pathology, Philadelphia, 1979, W.B. Saunders Co.
9. Barnes, L., and Pietruszka, M.: Sarcomas of the breast, Cancer **40**:1577, 1977.
10. Beahrs, O.H., Smart, C., and Shapiro, S.: Report of the Working Group to Review the National Cancer Institute, American Cancer Society Breast Cancer Detection Demonstration Projects, J. Natl. Cancer Inst. **62**:640, 1969.
11. Berg, J.W., and Robbins, G.F.: Twenty year follow-ups of breast cancer, Acta Unio Int. Cancr. (Louvain) **19**:1575, 1963.
12. Berg, J.W., et al.: Histology epidemiology and end results: the Memorial Hospital Cancer Registry, New York, 1969, Memorial Hospital.
13. Betsill, W.L., Rosen, R.P., Lieberman, R.H., and Robbins, G.F.: Intraductal carcinoma, long-term follow-up after treatment by biopsy alone, JAMA **239**:1863, 1978.
14. Black, M.M., Barclay, T.H.C., Cutler, S.J., Hankey, B.F., and Asire, A.J.: Association of atypical characteristics of benign breast lesions with subsequent risk of breast cancer, Cancer **29**:338, 1972.
15. See reference 14.
16. Bloom, H.J.G.: The natural history of untreated breast cancer, Ann. NY Acad. Sci. **114**:747, 1964.
17. Bloom, H.J.G., and Field, J.R.: Impact of tumor grade and host resistance on survival of women with breast cancer, Cancer **28**:1580, 1971.
18. Carstens, P.H.B.: Tubular carcinoma of the breast, Am. J. Clin. Pathol. **70**:214, 1978.
19. Carter, D.L., and Smith, R.I.: Carcinoma in situ of the breast, Cancer **40**:1189, 1977.
20. Decosse, J.J., Berg, J.W., Fracchia, A.A., and Farrow, J.A.: Primary lymphosarcoma of the breast, Cancer **15**:1264, 1962.
21. Eniq, M.G., Munn, R.J., and Keeney, M.: Dietary fat and cancer trends: a critique, Fed. Proc. **37**:2215, 1978.
22. Farrow, J.H., and Ashikari, H.: Breast lesions in young girls, Surg. Clin. North Am. **49**:261, 1969.
23. Fisher, B.F., Slack, N.H., and Bross, I.D.: Cancer of the breast: size of neoplasm and prognosis, Cancer **24**:1071, 1969.
24. Frantz, V.K., et al.: Incidence of chronic cystic disease in so-called "normal breasts," Cancer **4**:762, 1951.
25. Franzas, F.: Ueber die Mastopathia cystica latenta und andere bemerkenswerte Veränderungen in klinisch symptomfreien weiblichen Brüsten, Arb. a. d. path. Inst. d. Univ. Helsingfors **9**:401, 1936.
26. Friedman, B.A., and Oberman, H.A.: Adenoid cystic carcinoma of the breast, Am. J. Clin. Pathol. **54**:1, 1970.
27. Gad, A., and Azzopardi, J.G.: Lobular carcinoma of the breast: a special variant of mucin-secreting carcinoma, J. Clin. Pathol. **28**:711, 1975.
28. Haagensen, C.D.: Diseases of the breast, ed. 2, Philadelphia, 1971, W.B. Saunders Co.
29. Haenszel, W., and Kurihara, M.: Studies on Japanese migrants. I. Mortality from cancer and other diseases among Japanese in the United States, J. Natl. Cancer Inst. **40**:43, 1968.
30. Hajdu, S.I., Espinosa, M.H., and Robins, G.F.: Recurrent cystosarcoma phyllodes: a clinico-pathologic study of 32 cases, Cancer **38**:1402, 1976.
31. Hart, W.R., Bauer, R.C., and Oberman, H.A.: Cystosarcoma phyllodes: a clinicopathologic study of twenty-six hypercellular periductal stromal tumors of the breast, Am. J. Clin. Pathol. **70**:211, 1978.
32. Henderson, B., Powell, D., Rosario, I., Keys, C., Hanisch, R., Young, M., Casagrande, J., Gerkins, Y., and Pike, M.C.: An epidemiological study of breast cancer, J. Natl. Cancer Inst. **53**:609, 1974.
33. Hirayama, T.: Epidemiology of breast cancer with special reference to the role of diet, Prev. Med. **7**:173, 1978.
34. Hoover, R., Gray, L.A., Sr., Cole, P., and MacMahon, B.: Menopausal estrogens and breast cancer, N. Engl. J. Med. **295**:401, 1976.
35. Kessinger, A., Foley, J.F., Lemon, H.M., and Miller, D.M.: Metastatic cystosarcoma phylloides: a case report and review of the literature, J. Surg. Oncol. **4**:131, 1972.
36. Kidlin, D., Winger, E.E., Morgenstern, N.L., and Chien, U.: Chronic mastopathy and breast cancer, Cancer **39**:2603, 1977.
37. LiVolsi, V.A., Stadel, B.V., Kelsey, J.L., Holford, T.R., and White, C.: Fibrocystic breast disease in oral-contraceptive users, N. Engl. J. Med. **299**:381, 1978.
38. MacMahon, B., Cole, P., Lin, T.M., et al.: Age at first birth and breast cancer risk, Bull. WHO **43**:209, 1970.
39. McDivitt, R.W.: Unpublished data, St. Louis, 1981.
40. McDivitt, R.W., Gersell, D.J., and Boyce, W.H.: Tubular carcinoma of the breast, Lab. Invest. **44**:41, 1981.
41. McDivitt, R.W., and Stewart, F.W.: Breast carcinoma in children, JAMA **195**:388, 1966.
42. McDivitt, R.W., Stewart, F.W., and Berg, J.W.: Tumors of the breast. In Atlas of tumor pathology, series 2, fascicle 2, Washington, D.C., 1967, Armed Forces Institute of Pathology.
43. McDivitt, R.W., Stewart, F.W., and Farrow, J.H.: Breast carcinoma arising in solitary fibroadenomas, Surg. Gynecol. Obstet. **125**:572, 1967.
44. McDivitt, R.W., Urban, J.A., and Farrow, J.H.: Cystosarcoma phyllodes, Johns Hopkins Med. J. **120**:33, 1967.
45. McDivitt, R.W., Hutter, R.V., Foote, F.W., Jr., and Stewart, F.W.: In situ lobular carcinoma, JAMA **201**:96, 1967.
46. Meyer, J.S.: Personal communication, St. Louis, 1982.
47. Meyer, J.S., Bauer, W.G., and Rao, B.R.: Subpopulations of breast cancer defined by S-phase fraction, morphology, and estogen receptor content, Lab. Invest. **39**:225, 1978.
48. Müller, J.: Ueber den feineren Bau und die Farben der krankhaften Geschwulste, Berlin, 1838, G. Reiner.
49. National Cancer Institute Breast Cancer Digest, Pub. no. 80-1691, Bethesda, Md., 1980, National Institutes of Health.
50. National Cancer Institute Cancer Patient Survival Report no. 5 1976, Pub. no. NIH 77-992, Bethesda, Md., 1977, Department of Health, Education and Welfare.
51. Nayer, H.R.: Cylindroma of the breast with pulmonary metastases, Dis. Chest **31**:324, 1957.
52. Norris, H.J., and Taylor, H.B.: Sarcomas and related mesenchymal tumors of the breast, Cancer **22**:22, 1968.
53. Norris, H.J., and Taylor, H.B.: Carcinoma of the male breast, Cancer **23**:106, 1969.

54. O'Kell, R.T.: Adenoid cystic carcinoma of the breast, Mo. Med. **61:**855, 1964.
55. Ory, H., Cole, P., and MacMahon, B.: Oral contraceptives and reduced risk of benign breast diseases, N. Engl. J. Med. **294:**719, 1972.
56. Osborne, C.K., and McGuire, W.L.: Current use of steroid hormone receptor assay in the treatment of breast cancer, Surg. Clin. North Am. **58:**777, 1978.
57. Paffenbarger, R.S., Fasal, E., and Simmons, M.E., et al.: Cancer risk as related to use of oral contraceptives during fertile years, Cancer **39:**1887, 1977.
58. Page, D., Vander Zwaag, R., Rogers, L.W., Williams, L.T., Walker, W.E., and Hartman, W.H.: Relation between component parts of fibrocystic disease complex and breast cancer, J. Natl. Cancer Inst. **61:**1055, 1979.
59. Paget, J.: On disease of the mammary areola preceding cancer of the mammary gland, St. Barth. Hosp. Rep. **10:**86, 1874.
60. Perzin, K.H., and Lattes, R.: Papillary adenoma of the nipple, Cancer **29:**996, 1972.
61. Pullinger, B.D.: Cystic disease of the breast: human and experimental, Lancet **2:**567, 1947.
62. Robbins, G.F., Shah, J., Rosen, P., et al.: Inflammatory carcinoma of the breast, Surg. Clin. North Am. **54:**801, 1974.
63. Rosen, P.P., Kosloff, C., Lieberman, P.H., Adair, F., and Braun, D.W., Jr.: Lobular carcinoma in situ of the breast: detailed analysis of 99 patients with average follow-up of 24 years, Am. J. Surg. Pathol. **2:**225, 1978.
64. Rosen, P.P., and Mike, V.: Prognostic factors in breast cancer. In Hoogstraten, B., and McDivitt, R.W., editors: Breast cancer, Boca Raton, Fla., 1981, CRC Press, Inc.
65. Rosen, P.P., and Snyder, R.E.: Non-palpable breast lesions detected by mammography and confirmed by specimen radiography, Breast **3:**13, 1977.
66. Rosen, P.P., et al.: Estrogen receptor protein (ERP) and the histopathology of human mammary carcinoma. In McGuire, W.L., editor: Hormones, receptors and breast cancer, New York, 1978, Raven Press.
67. Scheike, O., Visfeldt, J., and Peterson, B.: Male breast cancer, Acta Pathol. Microbiol. Scand. **81:**352, 1973.
68. Sergi, M., et al.: An epidemiological study on cancer in Japan, Gan **48**(suppl.):1, 1957.
69. Sirtori, C., and Veronesi, U.: Gynecomastia: a review of 218 cases, Cancer **10:**645, 1957.
70. Stocks, L.H., and Simmons, F.M.: Inflammatory carcinoma of the breast, Surg. Gynecol. Obstet. **143:**885, 1976.
71. Strong, E.W., McDivitt, R.W., and Brasfield, R.D.: Granular cell myoblastoma, Cancer **25:**415, 1970.
72. Tavassoli, F.A., and Norris, H.J.: Secretory carcinoma, Cancer **45:**2404, 1980.
73. Taylor, H.B., and Robertson, A.G.: Adenomas of the nipple, Cancer **18:**995, 1965.
74. Tóth, J.: Das granulärzellige Myoblastom der Mamma, Zentralbl. Allg. Pathol. **115:**366-371, 1972.
75. Treichopoulos, D., MacMahon, B., and Cole, P.: The menopause and breast cancer risk, J. Natl. Cancer Inst. **48:**605, 1972.
76. Treves, N.: Gynecomastia, Cancer **11:**1083, 1958.
77. Treves, N., and Sunderland, D.A.: Cystosarcoma phyllodes of the breast: a malignant and a benign tumor; a clinicopathological study of seventy-seven cases, Cancer **4:**1286, 1951.
78. Veronisi, U., and Pizzocaro, G.: Breast cancer in women subsequent to cystic disease of the breast, Surg. Gynecol. Obstet. **26:**529, 1968.
79. Warren, S.: The relation of "chronic mastitis" to carcinoma of the breast, Surg. Gynecol. Obstet. **71:**257, 1940.
80. Waterhouse, J., et al.: Cancer incidence in five continents. In International Agency for Research on Cancer, vol. 3, no. 15, Lyon, France, 1976, IARC Scientific Publications.
81. Wellings, S.R., Jensen, H.M., and Marcum, R.G.: An atlas of subgross pathology of the human breast with special reference to possible precancerous lesions, J. Natl. Cancer Inst. **55:**231, 1975.
82. Westbrook, K.D., and Gallager, H.S.: Intraductal carcinoma of the breast: a comparative study, Am. J. Surg. **130:**667, 1975.

36 Skin

ARTHUR C. ALLEN

Eight editions ago and since then, the policy of allocating a deservedly and proportionally fair amount of space in this text for a broad coverage of cutaneous pathology was inaugurated. The allocation of this form of increased recognition to cutaneous disorders was soon followed by others. I had hoped that a comprehensive chapter on cutaneous pathology in a text on general pathology would encourage pathologists to acquire a facility with this important discipline. However, I must admit that my initial objective—to help develop among colleagues in general pathology a lively, constant, productive interest, and a workable expertise in dermatopathology—has not been realized. This practical alienation from dermatopathology may be ascribed to several kinds of estrangements, not the least of which is the often inappropriate or rococo terminology of cutaneous disorders. For a random example, an outside observer might be a little intimidated by *pityriasis lichenoides et varioliformis acuta* and bemused to learn that it represents a phase of *lymphoma*. The disinclination to involve general pathologists in this fascinating specialty is particularly costly because, as is becoming better appreciated, valuable clues to systemic disease are overlooked by the limited ability to extract what is available from histologic evaluation of the skin by the prepared observer.

The importance of the immediate diagnostic categorization of the skin biopsy is more fully understood in view of the expanding series of modalities that is being used to confirm, negate, or elucidate the basic histologic analysis. These tests are numerous and include the use of (1) B- and T-cell markers; (2) special bacterial fungal and tissue strains; (3) electron microscopy; (4) monoclonal antibodies and other immunoagents; (5) DNA probes; (6) flow cytometry; (7) immunohistochemistry, immunofluorescence, and immunoperoxidase techniques; (8) determination of oncogene products; (9) tissue culture; and (10) others. Clearly, the greater the pathologist's ability to make solidly based diagnostic judgments of the primitive histology of lesions, the less there will be the likelihood of the kind of indecision and accompanying fear of misdiagnosis, litigation, and so on, that lead to the use often of time-consuming, ex-

pensive tests intended to be primarily supportive or diagnostically contributory. The fact is that they are often employed defensively, with delays in communication and with no transfer of utilizable information to the matter at hand. This is by no means to gainsay the ultimate use and considerable applicability of these tests, though their pitfalls are coming to be known. It is simply to call attention to their common overconsumption or premature use because of a failure to extract all that histology alone could have yielded and thereby expedite the decision to use keratin protein rather than epithelial membrane antigen, or neither, as tumor markers.[68]

Accordingly, this chapter is meant to activate increased interest in this discipline. Surely the pathologist should aim to become as adept at dermatopathology as at renal or hepatic pathology, for example. After all, cutaneous lesions may, as stated, indicate concomitant systemic involvement.

Immunopathology of the skin actually adds another bridging dimension to several disciplines, including rheumatology, hematology, infectious diseases, and therapy. The direct and indirect fluorescent techniques depicting, as they do, the precise localization of antibodies, fibrin, and components of complement, allow a new dynamic insight into the pathogenesis of such dermatoses as the bullous disorders, systemic lupus erythematosus (SLE), porphyrias, psoriasis, vasculitic diseases, and others. Similarly, diagnostic and pathogenic vistas are being opened and rapidly widened by the analysis of HLA (human leukocyte antigens) and their disease-linked genes. These are active in varying degrees in psoriasis, the bullous diseases, lupus erythematosus, atopic dermatitis, lichen planus, granuloma annulare, and many others. Additionally useful is the ability to distinguish individual cells in an infiltrate in a given lesion by the use of tissue homogenates. The indirect peroxidase labeling of anti-HTLA (heterologous human T [or B] cell antiserum) permits this.

In these last 4 to 5 years, major emphasis in cutaneous pathology has been properly and fruitfully placed on the lymphoproliferative diseases and less effectively on previously well analyzed nevi and malignant melanomas. In the instance of lymphomas and pseudolymphomas, the histology, both by dermal pattern and by cellular detail, has long been ripe for the advances of the application of immunohistochemical techniques.

There is a sizable group of dermatoses that have significant morphologic individuality. In many instances the distinguishing features are so clear cut that a diagnosis may be offered on examination merely of the histologic slide. In other cases a small range of diagnoses may be suggested by the section. In the remainder the microscopic changes give no diagnostic help in the absence of a clinical history. Although the size of the last group will obviously be determined by the experience of the examiner, the percentage of cases that falls into it can be made sufficiently low as to spark the lagging interest of the general pathologist. One of the major difficulties in the learning of dermatopathology is that the changes usually are not of the all-or-none or qualitatively distinct variety but are often a matter of weighted quantitative differences. The proper judgment of these differences depends on a knowledge of the normal histologic range of the structures of the skin, as well as on an ability to interrelate and interpret a whole series of aberrations in these structures.

Obviously, only a small segment of cutaneous pathology can be included in this chapter. Accordingly, it would seem to underscore the applicability of dermatopathology best if some of the many lesions diagnosable by histologic characteristics alone were given preference over those less easily recognizable.

STRUCTURE OF NORMAL SKIN

The skin normally varies in color, elasticity, thickness, blood supply, and texture depending on anatomic location, age, state of nutrition, endocrinologic status, and race of the individual. With the unaided eye, fine (Blaschko's) ridges are noted over the skin generally, and coarse folds, allowing for movement, are present, particularly over the joints. Between the ridges are sulci of Heidenhain. The ridges are further marked by delicate crisscross, triangular or polygonal lines. In recent years there has been considerable interest in the science of dermatoglyphics, which deals with the interpretation of detailed patterns of sulci, furrows, and ridges of the palms. Dermatoglyphic abnormalities have been observed in patients with rubella, psoriasis, neurofibromatosis, anonychia, a variety of chromosomal abnormalities, and some disorders otherwise unassociated with cutaneous manifestations.

The ostia of sweat glands, the pores, open into the ridges. The hair also varies in texture, length, density, contour, and color depending on age, race, sex, and so on. The smooth, hairless skin, or the skin with fine vellus hairs, is known as glabrous skin. The epidermis varies from 0.07 to 0.12 mm over most of the body and from 0.8 to 1.4 mm or more on the palms and soles. The cutis has a corresponding range of thickness. The junction of the cutis and the subcutis or subcuticular fat is usually indistinct, except in certain regions such as the forehead, ear, perineum, and scrotum.

Fig. 36-1 is a diagram of normal skin. It is of diagnostic use to bear in mind how the skin varies in different parts of the body. For example, sebaceous glands are particularly prominent about the face, especially in the region of the nose, and so diagnoses of hyperplasia or adenoma of sebaceous glands should take this feature into account. The epidermis is normally thin and the rete ridges are relatively inconspicuous over the tibia, the breasts, and the flexor surfaces of the forearms. This variant should not, therefore, be mistaken for atrophy. Similarly, the dermis over the lower legs is normally much thinner than it is in many other portions of the body, and so, again, the possibility of confusion with atrophy exists. Moreover, the thickness of the papillary and reticular layers varies considerably from one part of the body to another, though inherent in one classification of malignant melanomas is the assumption of its constancy. The elastic tissue of the dermis shows such a large range in its quantity, as well as in the degree of fraying and splintering of the fibers, even in normal tissues, that considerable caution should be used in concluding that abnormalities of elastic tissue are present. Finally, the normally thick stratum corneum of the sole may prompt the diagnosis of keratoderma. These are a few of the examples of the variation in cutaneous histology, an accurate evaluation of which is clearly essential for an appraisal of some of the qualitatively similar pathologic changes.

The objective of the pathologist is to match the dermatologist's clinical observation of erythema, scales, pigmentation, blisters, and patterns of lesions with the pathologist's observation of parakeratosis, acanthosis, edema, epidermal spongiosis or cleavages, vascular alterations, and type and location of inflammatory cells, along with several other ancillary histologic changes. One would hope that these factors, properly weighted and fed into the "clinical-histologic computer," would lead to the appropriate diagnosis. Undoubtedly, when the precise pattern and location of fluorescently revealed immunologic deposits, enzymatic abnormalities, and qualitative, quantitative, and topographic distribution of B- and T-lymphocytes are one day soon added to the input, the composite diagnoses will be refined.

Finally, the assessment of the intradermal cells depends on their patterns, their nature, their source, their correlation with similar cells in the peripheral blood and the regional lymph nodes, their content of immunoglobulins and complement, and their identification with categories, fulminance, and deflorescence of clinical lesions, along with the common antigenicity of these cells and other specific anatomic sites such as the various parts of the epidermis. These are the urgent problems that need to be resolved for better insight

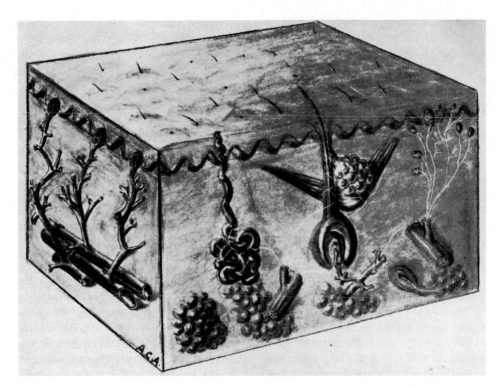

Fig. 36-1. In smaller panel at left are shown arteries, veins, and lymphatic vessels, along with their plexuses within papillae. In reality, plexuses of all three types of vessels overlap in same regions. In larger front panel are included appendages, nerves, and subcutaneous fat. Tubular sweat gland on left reaches surface through duct that, in its course through epidermis, maintains its own epithelial lining. Ductal ostium or sweat pore is independent of hair follicle. In center is pilosebaceous apparatus comprising hair follicle, sebaceous glands, and arrectores pilorum. Nerves and vessels supplying critical papillae are shown at deep portion of follicle. Sebaceous gland is intimately linked to hair follicle, into which its duct empties directly. Arrectores pilorum not only stiffen hair shaft but, as may be surmised from position illustrated, also help, by contraction, to expel contents of sebaceous gland and to constrict superficial vessels. On right are shown nerves and nerve endings—corpuscles of Merkel-Ranvier, Meissner, Ruffini, Krause, and Pacini. Nerve fibers entwined about appendages also are illustrated.

into currently vaguely understood cutaneous disorders. In addition, one of the great deficiencies in dermatopathology is the lack of animal models.

Epidermis

The epidermis is composed of the following layers:
1. Basal cell layer (stratum germinativum)
2. Prickle cell layers (stratum spinosum, rete mucosum, rete Malpighii)
3. Granular layers (stratum granulosum)
4. Stratum lucidum
5. Cornified layer (stratum corneum)

Basal cell layer

The basal cell layer is one cell thick and forms the junction between epidermis and dermis. The nuclei are relatively hyperchromatic, are arranged perpendicularly to the "epidermal basement membrane," and normally contain a few mitoses as evidence of the activity of a layer that serves in part as the progenitor of the remainder of the epidermis. Interspersed in the basal layer are cells with a clear zone separating and often compressing most of the cytoplasm and nucleus away from the cell wall (the so-called *cellule claire*). The cytoplasm may or may not contain melanin, but these cells are likely to be dopa positive and, accordingly, are melanocytes. Not all melanocytes of the basal layer are "clear cells." Ultrastructurally the melanocytes contain melanosomes, but most observers believe that they contain few or no desmosomes or tonofilaments. As a matter of fact, such structures may be noted, albeit often reduced in number, not only in many melanocytes but, more vividly and meaningfully, also in the marginal cells of melanocarcinomas in situ. The fairly universal insistence that keratinocytes lack lysosomes has contributed to the circular reasoning that melanocytes are ipso facto nonkeratinocytes inasmuch as they contain these organelles. A directly contrary observation has recently clearly indicated that keratinocytes are characterized by Odland bodies, which are membrane-coated granules, keratinosomes, or lysosomes.

For a long time it has been accepted, on debatable evidence, that melanocytes are really nerve endings that originated in the neural crest, became incorporated in the epidermis, and later constituted the source of normal pigment in skin as well as of pigmented nevi and melanocarcinomas. It is generally maintained that melanocytes are the same in number in both white and black skin and the pigment is transferred to neighboring keratinocytes, which "nip off" pieces of melanized dendrites attached to scattered, basally located melanocytes.

The simplistic notion that keratinocytes acquire melanosomes by "nipping off" and incorporating tips of dendrites is untenable. The objections to this hypothesis include the following:

1. That the keratinocytic melanosomes usually are not scattered haphazardly in their cytoplasm as they would be in histiocytes or melanophages but usually are located supranuclearly as if produced in situ
2. That the pigmentation or melanosomes are often confined to a single (basal) layer, at times in conjunction with the spinous layer immediately above, unlike the scattered, multilayered distribution to be expected if the sequestration of hydralike dendrites were operative
3. That pigmentation or melanosomes may be uniformly incorporated into keratinocytes within hours after ultraviolet radiation or x radiation, hardly the short time span compatible with the process of dendritic phagocytosis and pigmentary alignment. My opposing theory is that the development of pigment is normally inherent in many keratinocytes. If modulated with certain provocations, such as radiation, drugs, or hormones, they may be induced to express this function.

It is clearly important that these controversial matters be addressed rather than disregarded or presented as if proved.

Another question is how epidermis, regenerated after ulceration, develops basal melanocytes spaced every tenth cell or so. In my opinion the process of conversion of basal cells and keratinocytes into melanocytes normally takes place continuously and may be retarded or eliminated (as in vitiligo) or accelerated (as in sunburn). Actually, as might be anticipated, the numbers of dopa-reactive epidermal melanocytes have been found to be increased after irradiation with ultraviolet rays, though contrary results previously had been reported. In other words, the activation of basal cells and keratinocytes into melanocytes is an in situ conversion and varies in speed and extent with different age groups, races, and stimuli. However, it would be misleading to fail to acknowledge that the concept of neurogenesis of melanocytes, nevi, and melanocarcinomas is the popular one at the moment.

There has been a revival of interest in the nature of the controverted intraepidermal, aurophilic Langerhans cell. To some, it is a worn-out (effete) melanocyte with a possible capacity to manufacture or even to phagocytose melanin. To others, it is a form of intraepidermal neural element with a spectrum of neural enzymes, including adenosine triphosphatase (ATPase) and leucine aminopeptidase. To still others, it is a histiocyte that has wandered into the epidermis and is identical to the histiocytes of histiocytosis X. Ultrastructurally it has been forcefully emphasized that this cell possesses a specific racket-shaped organelle but, as was to be expected, similar organelles have been observed in the cells of other organs, such as the thymus gland. More recently it has been admitted, in a refreshing reversal of opinion, that Langerhans cells are not related to melanocytes, that they are not derived from the neural crest, and that the whole question of their nature, derivation, and function must be regarded from a new perspective.

It now appears clear that this aurophilic, ATPase-positive, antigen-bearing cell with the characteristic racket-shaped (Birbeck) granule is immunologically part of a very much alive migrating population that finds itself not fixed within the epidermis but essentially located wherever macrophages are to be seen. Reality would be better served if this Langerhans cell were regarded as a variety of hematic cell rather than an epidermally derived effete dendritic cell. It is generally affirmed that this cell, far from a melanocyte, is a wandering mononuclear cell related to those of "histiocytosis X."

Prickle cell layer

The prickle cells are several layers thick, their number varying in different parts of the body. The cells are joined by cytoplasmic bridges (spines, prickles, desmosomes), which serve as the most easily recognizable identification of such cells, both in squamous cell neoplasms and in metaplastic processes. The intracellular cytoplasmic tonofilaments are regarded as the precursors of keratin. Glycogen is usually present. The generally accepted absence of lysosomes (keratinosomes) in keratinocytes has been disputed; thus the supposed differences between keratinocytes and melanocytes are narrowed.[37]

Stratum granulosum

The stratum granulosum averages about two layers thick and is composed of cells with blue, round cytoplasmic granules of keratohyalin. The chemical nature of the keratohyaline granules remains essentially obscure. Although superficially resembling nuclear material, they are Feulgen and periodic acid–Schiff negative and contain no protein-bound sulfhydryl groups. They appear as electron-dense bodies and apparently include tonofilaments. The granules are also osmophilic, are digested with elastase, and are presumed to be closely related histogenetically to keratin. Lysosomes are present in abundance in the granular layers, in contrast to their sparse distribution in the basal and squamous cell layers. The stratum lucidum, which is practically confined to the palms and soles, is a clear, homogeneous, acidophilic, anuclear, thin layer of eleidin.

Stratum corneum

The stratum corneum, also normally without nuclei, is made up of various thicknesses of keratin. The stratum corneum, particularly its lower half, is important as the barrier in regulating the transfer of water through the skin. Fat globules may be present in the two uppermost layers.

Periodic acid–Schiff–positive, diastase-resistant mucopolysaccharides are present in the epidermis and are presumed to play a role in binding or cementing the epidermal cells together. Since keratinization normally takes place in the upper layers of epidermis, the acid mucopolysaccharides are presumably degraded, allowing the keratin to be discarded as invisible flakes. With incomplete degradation of the mucopolysaccharides, visible, coherent, parakeratotic nucleated scales occur, as in psoriasis or dandruff.

Basement membrane

There is convincing histologic evidence that a true epidermal basement membrane, equivalent, for example, to the one surrounding glands, does not exist. Basement membranes in other locations, such as those about sweat glands and renal tubules, are argyrophilic. No such continuous epidermal basement membrane is demonstrable with silver strains, though an illusion of one occasionally is created by argyrophilic granules of melanin aligned in the basal layer. On the other hand, stains with the periodic acid–Schiff reagent do reveal what appear to be interrupted segments of a basement membrane. This simulation is caused by the presence of polysaccharides that have been irregularly concentrated by the varying densities of the subepidermal collagen, especially with edema of the upper cutis. In this connection one other fact should be mentioned again. Basal cells do have intercellular bridges (desmosomes) that bind them to the overlying cells of the stratum spinosum and, in their upper portions, to each other. To the corium they are attached by semidesmosomes to an ultrastructurally visible membrane called an adepidermal lamina, visible only electron microscopically and not equivalent to the argyrophilic structures readily detectable even in routine stains, as mentioned. Quite unlike the simple, compact, linearly solid argyrophilic, familiarly known basement membrane that surrounds, as stated, a renal tubule or a coil of a sweat gland, the "epidermal basement membrane" is considered by some to be a complex, multilayered structure. It is now stated to comprise, from its most distal layer downward or proximally to the dermis, (1) plasma membrane with anchoring filaments, (2) subbasal dense plate of hemidesmosomes, (3) lamina lucida, and (4) lamina densa with elastic microfibrils and anchoring fibrils. Whereas, in the past, the locus of linear immunofluorescence at the dermoepidermal area used to be regarded as the basement membrane, it is now more appropriately designated as the "basement membrane zone" (BMZ).

Dermis

The dermis, or corium, is divided into the superficial pars papillaris and the deeper pars reticularis. The papillae of the dermis alternate with projections of epidermis called "rete ridges." The length of the papillae, the thickness of the overlying epidermal plate, the vascularity, the edema, and the direction and consistency of the collagenous fibers of the papillae are all of diagnostic value.

The thickness of the pars papillaris varies considerably, from several to hundreds of micrometers. In the papillary portion the fibers of collagen tend to run vertically. In the deeper part the fibers are rather loosely dispersed in a horizontal direction. Accuracy in evaluating changes in the consistency, tinctorial qualities, and cellularity of the collagen and elastic tissue of the dermis furnishes the basis for many diagnoses. With electron microscopy, elastic fibers show a fibrillar structure within an otherwise almost homogeneous matrix in which the characteristic periodicity of collagen is lacking.[77]

The *cutaneous appendages* include the sweat glands, sebaceous glands, hair follicles, arrectores pilorum, and nails. The sweat glands are coiled glands of two varieties: eccrine and apocrine.

The *eccrine glands* are universally distributed in the skin and are made up of several coils of tubular glands lying deep in the dermis. These glands empty their secretion into tubules traversing the dermis and epidermis, opening into the fine ridges of the skin as pores. The coils are lined by two principal layers of cells: (1) the more superficial, basophilic, dark, granular, mucopolysaccharide-containing cells and (2) the more basilar, acidophilic clear or chief cells. There may be some interdigitation between these cells. A flattened third type of cell, the myoepithelial or basket cell, is interposed between these secretory cells and the basement membrane. A large battery of enzymes is detectable in the eccrine glands, including oxidases, dehydrogenases, phosphorylases, alkaline phosphatases, and glucuronidases. Their presence has been used in defining certain of the neoplasms of sweat glands. The ducts are lined also by two layers of epithelial cells, but the myoepithelium is absent. The inner lining of the ducts of sweat glands is keratinized in their course through the epidermis, and indeed some of the neoplasms of sweat glands show evidence of squamous cell metaplasia. In any case, the inner hyaline membrane of the ducts often serves as a clue to the genesis of these neoplasms.

The apocrine glands occur in the axilla, groin, nipple, umbilicus, anus, and genital region. They are easily recognized by their large lumens, prominence of secretory cytoplasmic granules, and rows of myoepithelial cells longitudinally oriented below the cuboid or columnar secretory cells. The periglandular basement membrane is especially conspicuous. Light yellow, sudanophilic granules, as well as granules of hemosiderin and a minimum of glycogen, are commonly present. Mucin normally is present within the lumen and cells of apocrine glands and is periodic acid–Schiff positive and diastase resistant. Desmosomes, similar to those of keratinocytes, have been noted. The ultrastructural observation of canaliculi, particularly, may help to indicate that an eccrine type as well as an apocrine (that is, apically erosive) type of secretion occurs. Secretory activity varies with the menstrual cycle. The ducts of the apocrine glands usually open in close relationship to the hair follicles but may reach the surface independently, as the eccrine glands do.

The *sebaceous*, or holocrine, glands are racemose structures that serve mainly as appendages to the hair follicles to which they are attached. Each alveolus is rimmed by a basement membrane surrounding one or two layers of squamous cells, internal to which are the characteristic sebaceous cells with small round nuclei and abundant, finely latticed, fatty cytoplasm. The sebaceous cells are pushed toward the duct, wherein they finally rupture and release their fatty contents in the hair follicle. Modifications of sebaceous glands occur in the eyelids and ears, in the areolae of the nipples, and in the male and female genitalia (odoriferous glands). In these regions they are unconnected with hairs or hair follicles. The amount of sebum secreted is about the same in the adolescent boy and girl, shows no appreciable change in the aging woman, and decreases in the aging man. Ectopic sebaceous glands may be found in the salivary glands and in the glans penis. Such ectopic glands of the corona penis are often referred to as Tyson's glands. Actually, Tyson appears to have described a beaded rim of fibroepithelial pearly nodules about the corona.

The *hair* consists of a shaft that at its lower end enlarges into a bulb. The bulb embraces an invaginating dermal papilla, through which the hair receives its blood supply. The intracutaneous portion of the hair shaft and the bulb are enclosed in a hair follicle. The hair shaft is made up of a cuticle, a sheath, and more or less pigmented cortex and medulla, the latter being absent in lanugo hairs.

The *arrectores pilorum* are bands of smooth muscle originating in or near the papillary layers of the dermis and inserting at several points into the outer layer of adjacent hair follicles just above their papillae. The direction of the muscle is at an angle to the hairs so that their contraction causes the hairs to be erected (gooseflesh). At the same time, the superficial vessels are constricted to avoid cooling, and sebaceous secretion is expelled by the preessure of the contracting arrectores pilorum. However, there is some disagreement as to this last function.

The *blood* and *lymphatic vessels* of the skin are arranged in plexuses. The arterial vessels are derived from the subcutaneous arteries, which give off plexuses to the papillary layer, as well as to the reticular layer and the various appendages. It has been suggested that the selective localization of infiltrate to various components of the dermis is related to the pattern of these plexuses. In the skin of certain regions of the body, particularly the fingers, there are normally arteriovenous shunts or glomera that serve to regulate blood flow and surface temperature. The *glomus* is composed of an afferent arteriole, a shunt called the Sucquet-Hoyer canal, and an efferent vein. The canal is lined by layers of rounded glomus cells that have a contractile function. The veins also form plexuses in the papillary, subpapillary, and deep reticular layers, as well as about the appendages.

The lymphatic plexuses are localized principally in the papillae and at the junction of dermis and subcutaneous tissue. The deeper lymphatic vessels have valves.

The *nerves* of the skin are preponderantly medullated. A few are nonmedullated and lead to the blood vessels, smooth muscles, epidermis, hair follicles, and glands. The specialized nerve endings include the corpuscles of Vater-Pacini, which are found in the deep layers of the skin and subcutaneous tissue, in the mucous membranes, and in the conjunctiva and cornea. These structures are particularly numerous in the skin of the nipple and external genital organs. Other nerve endings are the Meissner corpuscles of the papillae of the skin of palms, soles, and tips of fingers and toes, the end bulbs of Krause, which are smaller than but structurally similar to the Meissner corpuscles and are found in the external genitalia, the elongated, dermal corpuscles of Ruffini, and the intraepidermal disclike, tactile Merkel-Ranvier corpuscles, which are identified with silver stains and are present in the epidermis and external root sheath of hairs. The endings are presumably receptors for touch (Merkel-Ranvier and Meissner corpuscles), pressure (pacinian corpuscles), heat (corpuscles of Ruffini), and cold (end bulbs of Krause).

DEFINITIONS
Clinical terms

macule Circumscribed flat area of altered coloration of skin; evanescent or permanent; varies in size from pinhead to several centimeters, in color from red (erythema), brown (ephelis), and the various colors of blood pigment (petechiae and ecchymoses) to white (vitiligo), and in shape from circular, polygonal, or linear to polymorphous varieties of erythema multiforme.

papule Circumscribed elevated area; varies in size from pinhead to about 5 mm, in surface contour from flat, conical, or pointed circular to umbilicated, in color from red, yellow, or white to violaceous, and in shape of base from round to more or less polygonal (such as the papules of lichen planus and psoriasis); the papule, as well as the macule, may provoke pruritus, burning sensation, anesthesia, and pain or may cause no symptoms; both macules and papules may be overlain by scales.

nodule An enlarged papule varying in size from about 0.5 to 2 cm, usually deep seated, involving the lower dermis and subcutaneous fat (for example, the nodules of rheumatoid arthritis and leprosy).

vesicle Circumscribed, single or grouped elevations of the epidermis, beneath or within which are collections containing serum, plasma, or blood; surface may be flat, globoid, or umbilicated (as in smallpox and eczema).

pustule Vesicle containing pus predominantly (for example, impetigo).

bulla (bleb) Similar to vesicle, except that the bullae are larger, varying from 0.5 to more than 8 cm (as in pemphigus).

scale Loosened, imperfectly cornified, parakeratotic superficial layer of skin that is shed as fine, branny, dirty white, yellowish keratinous dust or large pearly-white flakes; distribution may be focal or universal and usually is associated with inflammation of the skin (psoriasis and exfoliative dermatitis) but need not be (as in ichthyosis).

crust Residue of dried serum, blood, pus, and epithelial, keratinous, and bacterial debris; crusts vary in color from yellow to green to dark brown, depending on the admixture of the different ingredients, and in consistency from a thin superficial and watery (as in impetigo) to a thick, bulky and loosely or firmly attached covering of a rupioid syphiloderm; crusts occur after the oozing of serum, blood, or pus in a disrupted, eroded, or ulcerated epidermis (as in eczema, impetigo, smallpox, abrasions, and other conditions).

excoriation (erosion) Superficial erosion and ulceration produced mechanically, usually by the fingernails in scratching pruritic skin or in picking at various lesions (as in neurotic excoriations).

fissure (rhagade) Linear, often crusted, tender, painful defect in continuity of the skin, occurring usually at mucocutaneous junctions at sites where there is normally considerable elasticity of the skin (about the anus, mouth, fingers, palms, and soles) and also in certain diseases (such as syphilis, nonspecific anal fissures, keratoderma, intertrigo, and eczema).

ulcer Defect of the skin, deeper than an erosion or excoriation, extending at least into the dermis; the edges may be ragged, punched out in appearance, undermined, or everted; the floor may be glazed or granular, puriform or hemorrhagic, and shallow or deep; the outline of an ulcer may be circular, serpiginous, crescentic, ovoid, or irregular; ulcers may be painless or exquisitely sensitive; they heal generally by concentric scarring and epithelization (for example, tropical, diphtheritic, and varicose ulcers).

lichenification Thickening of the skin with exaggeration of its normal markings so that the striae form a crisscross pattern; occurs after chronic irritation of pruritic skin.

comedo Keratinous plug, sometimes admixed with bacteria and inflammatory cells, within ducts of sebaceous glands; characteristic of acne.

Histologic terms

acanthosis Thickening through hyperplasia of the rete Malpighii; may exist without hyperkeratosis (Fig. 36-17).

hyperkeratosis Thickening of the keratinized layer, the stratum corneum; generally is associated with a prominent stratum granulosum (Fig. 36-17).

parakeratosis Persistence of nuclei in the stratum corneum, signifying the presence clinically of a loosely adherent scale (such as dandruff); characterized by the absence or striking diminution of the stratum granulosum, except in the stage of healing (Fig. 36-17); with fluorescence microscopy (with acridine orange, rhodamine B, and thioflavine S) hyperkeratosis is reflected by orthochromasia and brilliance, and parakeratosis is reflected by dullness and metachromatic color changes.

spongiosis Intercellular edema of the epidermis, which, when pronounced, progresses to vesiculation (as in eczema) (Fig. 36-6).

acantholysis Separation of individual cells from the stratum spinosum, with loss of prickle cells and consequent isolation within the fluid of a vesicle (for example, pemphigus).

ballooning degeneration One of the diagnostic morphologic phenomena leading to vesiculation in viral diseases; characterized by the isolation of a cell from its neighbors, especially in the lower layers of the epidermis, the withdrawing of its prickles after intracytoplasmic edema and vacuolization, and the amitotic division of its nucleus so as to form a multinucleated giant cells (as in variola, but particularly herpes and varicella) (Fig. 36-11).

reticular colliquation Another characteristic of the cutaneous vesicles caused by viruses; the cytoplasm of several cells becomes edematous, granular, coalescent, and partially disintegrated; the residual cytoplasm forms reticulated septa that partition multiloculated intraepidermal collections of fluid or vesicles; the nuclei become small, pyknotic, or completely karyorrhectic (Fig. 36-11).

dyskeratosis Abnormality of development or distinctive alteration of epidermal cells; two types are distinguished; (1) benign dyskeratosis—such as the molluscum bodies of mulluscum contagiosum, represented by swollen brightly eosinophilic cells, mostly of the stratum granulosum, containing virus elementary bodies, or the corps ronds and grains of the stratum granulosum and stratum corneum, respectively, as noted in Darier's disease; (2) malignant dyskeratosis—anaplastic changes such as hyperchromatism, changes in polarity, increase in mitotic figures, and enlargement of nuclei and nucleoli that signify potential or actual development of carcinoma (Fig. 36-2).

pseudoepitheliomatous hyperplasia Pronounced acanthosis with extensive downgrowth of rete ridges as may occur at the periphery of an ulcer, in bromodermas, and after insect bites; occasionally the exuberant epidermal hyperplasia is mistaken for carcinoma, as in so-called molluscum sebaceum or keratoacanthoma (Fig. 36-38).

liquefaction degeneration Obliteration of the line of demarcation of epidermis and dermis by edema of the basal cells and subepidermal dermis, as well as by the presence of inflammatory cells at this junction (as in lichen planus and lupus erythematosus) (Figs. 36-13 and 36-17).

CUTANEOUS-VISCERAL DISEASE

The cutaneous reflection of visceral disease is finally coming to be accorded the significance it has long merited. Recent surveys show that, because of the increasing awareness of the importance of the association of visceral with cutaneous diseases, graduate students of dermatology are requesting more sophisticated training in internal medicine. A simple listing of some of the cutaneous manifestations of visceral lesions, many of which have become apparent within the past decade, will underscore this often vital relationship:

1. Pigmentations
   a. Acanthosis nigricans of adults ("malignant" type)—commonly associated with visceral adenocarcinoma
   b. Acanthosis nigricans (juvenile)—occasionally associated with congenital lipodystrophy and insulin-resistant diabetes or with Rud's syndrome (tetany, epilepsy, anemia, and mental retardation); also with ichthyosis hystrix
   c. Peutz-Jeghers syndrome—focal mucosal and cutaneous pigmentation with gastrointestinal polyps and, rarely, with carcinomas
   d. Hemochromatosis—with pigmentary cirrhosis of liver and diabetes mellitus
   e. Addison's disease
   f. Incontinentia pigmenti—with neurologic and cardiac abnormalities
   g. Ochronosis—with cardiac disease
   h. Phenylketonuria—with neurologic manifestations
   i. Pellagra
   j. Café-au-lait spots—with von Recklinghausen's disease and fibrous dysplasia
   k. Chediak-Higashi syndrome—with specific leukocytic inclusions and semialbinism
2. Miscellaneous nonbullous dermatoses
   a. Lupus erythematosus—with nephritis, carditis, arthritis, and hypersplenism
   b. Dermatomyositis in adults—with visceral cancer
   c. Ichthyosis in adults—with lymphomas
   d. Alopecia (follicular) mucinosa—with mycosis fungoides
   e. Erythema annulare (gyratum)—with rheumatic fever and cancer; also erythema gyratum repens
   f. Pyoderma gangrenosum—with ulcerative colitis
   g. Sarcoidosis and other granulomatous diseases—with visceral and osseous involvement
3. Vesiculobullous lesions
   a. Zoster—with malignant lymphomas (occasionally dermatitis herpetiformis, pemphigoid, and erythema multiforme bullosum are associated with visceral cancers)
   b. Acrodermatitis enteropathica
   c. Bullous lesions—with porphyrias
   d. Dermatitis herpetiformis—with intestinal disease (spruelike)
   e. Toxic epidermal necrolysis—several instances associated with malignant lymphomas
4. Urticaria
   a. Urticaria pigmentosum—with involvement of bones, liver, spleen, and lymph nodes
   b. Urticaria—with amyloidosis, nerve deafness, and renal disease
5. Diseases of collagen and elastic tissue
   a. Scleroderma—with renal, cardiac, and gastrointestinal lesions
   b. Pseudoxanthoma elasticum—with ocular and cardiac lesions
   c. Ehlers-Danlos syndrome—increased serum hexosamine; involvement of vessels, heart, and gastrointestinal tract
   d. Cutis laxa (with emphysema, cardiopathy, and rectal prolapse)
   e. Necrobiosis lipoidica diabeticorum—with diabetes mellitus
   f. Circumscribed myxedema—with exophthalmic goiter
   g. Amyloidosis (primary and secondary)—with myeloma (primary amyloidosis), chronic infections (secondary amyloidosis)
6. Vascular diseases
   a. Angiokeratoma of Fabry—with renal and vascular lesions
   b. Allergic granulomatosis—with visceral angiitis
   c. Degos's syndrome—thromboangiitis of skin and intestines
   d. Blue rubber-bleb nevus—with intestinal angiomas
   e. Neurocutaneous-vascular syndromes
      (1) Sturge-Weber syndrome—cutaneous angiomatosis and epilepsy
      (2) Ataxia-telangiectasia
      (3) Rendu-Osler-Weber syndrome—with arteriovenous fistulas of lungs, brain
7. Metabolic disorders
   a. Xanthomatoses—with diabetes mellitus, von Gierke's disease, biliary cirrhosis, lipid nephrosis, and essential familial hypercholesterolemia

b. Lipidoses with cutaneous infiltration—reticulohistio-cytic granulomas (lipid dermatoarthritis); lipid pro-teinosis; gangliosidoses and other sphingolipidoses (Fabry's, Tay-Sachs, Gaucher's)

c. Mucopolysaccharidoses—for example, Hurler's syndrome

d. Dysproteinemias—including Waldenström's macro-globulinemia (with malignant lymphomas), cryoglob-ulinemias (with cutaneous infarcts), and multiple my-eloma (with cutaneous infiltration)

8. Cutaneous tumors

a. Arsenical lesions (keratoses, Bowen's disease)—with visceral cancers in limited percentage

b. Kaposi's sarcoma—with malignant lymphomas, AIDS

c. Sebaceous adenomas—with tuberous sclerosis

d. Basal cell nevus syndrome and other neurocutaneous syndromes

DERMATOSES

To be set up as what may possibly be a more work-able and more orderly classification of the dermatoses than seems currently to exist for pathologists, the dis-eases of the skin have been divided primarily into his-tologic categories. Although some overlapping of crite-ria is present, it is hoped that the basis for the classification is sufficiently defined to be of practical value. The diseases discussed are not only those that the pathologist is most likely to encounter but also those that, with minor exceptions, are diagnosable on the basis of histologic changes alone.

Shave biopsy

The shave, or horizontal, biopsy is used commonly by dermatologists. This method is opposed to the ver-tical biopsy performed with a punch instrument or scal-pel. A case for its use has been formally, but uncon-vincingly, made. The advantages listed include the saving of time, supplies, and equipment, the preserva-tion of dermal "hammock" for subsequent curettage, minimal hemorrhage, and good cosmetic results. How-ever, the disadvantages are more serious than generally conceded. The precise histologic diagnosis of many le-sions is jeopardized by a limited, superficial shaving, which of course also fails to disclose the involvement or clearance of the margins.[52]

Diseases principally of epidermis
Hyperplasia

Darier's disease. Clinically, Darier's disease (kerato-sis follicularis, psorospermosis) is recognized by the early development of small, uniform, firm, reddish brown, greasy, keratinous papules that subsequently become coalescent, papillomatous, and crusted and ac-quire an offensive odor. The lesions tend to be located about the face and neck and to spread to the chest, limbs, and loins. The palms and nails may be involved,

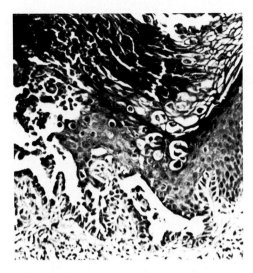

Fig. 36-2. Darier's disease (keratosis follicularis) showing suprabasilar cleavage, corps ronds, grains, and pro-nounced parakeratosis. (Hematoxylin and eosin.)

as may the oral mucosa. The disease occurs predomi-nantly in the second and third decades.

The histologic picture is so distinctive as to be path-ognomonic and consists of the following (Fig. 36-2):

1. Focal, truncated masses of keratin, usually par-tially parakeratinized, especially near the surface, may be located over the ostia of hair follicles or over the interfollicular epidermis. For this reason the term "keratosis follicularis" is inaccurate.

2. Corps ronds, or dyskeratotic cells, practically lim-ited to the stratum granulosum, contain nuclei that are rounded and encircled by a clear cyto-plasmic halo.

3. The "grains" are cells basically similar to the corps ronds, but they occur in the lower portion of the overlying keratinous masses.

4. The suprabasilar cleavage of the epidermis at the junction of the basal layer and the lowermost layer of the stratum spinosum forms a lacuna or small vesicle with a papillary base (Fig. 36-2).

The lesions that may offer some difficulty in differ-entiation are the isolated keratosis follicularis and be-nign chronic familial pemphigus (bullous Darier's dis-ease). Verrucal or isolated keratosis follicularis, originally recorded by me in 1948,[5] is histologically similar to Darier's disease, though the lesions of the latter appear more regular, smaller, and often multiple even in the same section.[5] This verrucal lesion is likely to be single and has a predilection for the scalp. Others have seen an identical histologic picture in the wall of the epidermal inclusion or pilosebaceous cysts.

Acanthosis nigricans. Acanthosis nigricans appears as patches of gray-black warty masses with a predilection for the axilla, groin, submammary region, elbows, knees, and occasionally the oral mucous membranes. Two types are recognized, juvenile and adult. The distinction is based on age rather than any difference in appearance of the lesions.

The juvenile type, unlike the adult form, is rarely associated with cancer, and in some instances it may accompany lipodystrophies and mental retardation.[26] The adult type is associated with visceral cancer in about 50% of patients, particularly in those beyond the fourth decade.[26] In about 65% of patients the associated cancer is a gastric adenocarcinoma. Adenocarcinomas of other viscera, such as the lung and infrequently the uterus, may be found. Occasionally the acanthosis nigricans may appear to antedate the visceral cancer. The association of acanthosis nigricans and abdominal cancer in elderly persons is a very real (if poorly understood) phenomenon. Acanthosis nigricans may also occur after the use of oral contraceptive drugs in the absence of visceral cancer. In addition to adenocarcinomas, acanthosis nigricans has been reported in association with Hodgkin's disease, osteogenic sarcoma, and embryonal carcinoma of the testis.

The histologic picture of acanthosis nigricans is that of a papillary hyperkeratosis, in most areas disproportionately greater than the underlying acanthosis. The epidermis is thrown into folds by its excessive lateral growth and in sections often appears reticulated where rete ridges have joined. The basal layer is densely pigmented with fine argyrophilic melanin granules (Fig. 36-3), and a few chromatophores lie in the upper corium. This folding of a hyperkeratotic epidermis in which the basal layer is diffusely darkened as an almost solid line of melanin is characteristic of acanthosis nigricans. There is no anaplasia of the epidermis even in

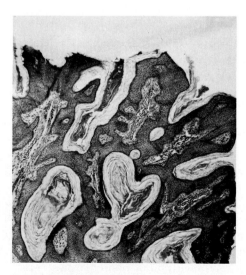

Fig. 36-3. Acanthosis nigricans with melanin pigmentation of basal layer. (Hematoxylin and eosin.)

cases accompanied by abdominal neoplasms. Oral florid papillomatosis may be associated with acanthosis nigricans.

Molluscum contagiosum. Molluscum contagiosum is a mildly contagious autoinoculable disease of the skin, caused by a virus and characterized by pinhead- or pea-sized, waxy, firm, buttonlike, often pruritic papules occurring on the face, trunk, and genital regions particularly and on the feet rarely. The lesions develop slowly over a period of weeks and may remain indefinitely if untreated. The disease appears especially in children and may occur in epidemic proportions in institutions. Molluscum contagiosum may occur in deceptively giant forms and apparently may be transmitted venereally.

The histologic picture should be immediately recognizable. The connective tissue papillae between the lobules are compressed or altogether obliterated, so that the inwardly projecting lobules appear as a bulbous downgrowth. This lobulation of the epidermis is almost as suggestive of the diagnosis as the pathognomonic feature, the molluscum bodies, is and may help to differentiate this lesion from verrucae, particularly when the molluscum bodies are inconspicuous. The molluscum bodies are clustered cells, principally of the stratum granulosum but also of the stratum spinosum, which are enlarged, as are virus-infected cells generally, and contain homogeneously smooth, brightly eosinophilic cytoplasm. The nucleus is inconspicuously flattened to one side of the cell, and keratohyalin granules tend to disappear. The cytoplasm, when studied with vital stains, appears actually to contain many elementary bodies (Lipschütz) embedded in a mucoid matrix. These dyskeratotic cells are enclosed in an eosinophilic, keratin-like membrane that resembles the dense cell membranes of plants. The molluscum bodies have been confused with the brightly eosinophilic cells of the stratum granulosum that are often prominent in verrucae vulgares. The virus seen electron microscopically measures about 300 × 200 × 100 nm, is characteristically brick shaped, and contains a dumbbell-shaped nucleoid. The virus replicates in the cytoplasm rather than in the nucleus.[56] Specific fluorescence staining of the inclusion bodies with tagged antibodies of serum from infected humans and rabbits has been demonstrated.

Vesicles
1. Eczematous vesicles
2. Cleavage vesicles
   a. Dermatitis herpetiformis
   b. Pemphigus
   c. Bullous pemphigoid
   d. Erythema multiforme bullosum
   e. Epidermolysis bullosum
   f. Impetigo
   g. Toxic epidermal necrolysis
   h. Herpes gestationis
3. Viral vesicles

The vesicles of various diseases may closely simulate each other clinically. Inasmuch as the prognosis, even as to fatality, may depend on the exact diagnosis, it is important that the diagnostic histologic features be definitively evaluated. In general, three types of vesicles occur: (1) eczematous, (2) cleavage (such as dermatitis herpetiformis, pemphigus, epidermolysis bullosa, impetigo, and burns), and (3) viral (such as smallpox, chicken pox, and herpes).

Eczema. Eczema may begin as an erythema and evolve through the papular, vesicular, pustular, and exfoliative stages. Some cases of eczema remain in one of the phases (for example, eczema rubrum, eczema squamosum, eczema papulosum), but in most instances the disease passes through the stage of vesiculation. Histologically the vesicle of eczema, whatever the cause, is basically the same whether caused by an external irritant, ingested food, or the product of superficial fungi, as in the epidermophytid. Moreover, the histologic picture of the eczematous vesicle differs sharply from that of cleavage vesicles, such as pemphigus and dermatitis herpetiformis, and the viral lesions of smallpox, chicken pox, and herpes.

The vesicle of eczema begins as foci of spongiosis in the rete Malpighii. The intercellular edema progresses to form microvesicles that coalesce with adjacent vesicles similarly formed. The walls of such vesicles are the compressed epidermal cells that usually are arranged as septa in the large blisters. In addition to the spongiotic vesicles, there may be transepidermal migration of mononuclear cells, upper dermal edema, telangiectasia, and basophils in the acute stages of contact dermatitis. More chronic forms may show acanthosis, parakeratosis, and dermal melanophores.

Histologic changes of this sort occur also in the vesicles of pompholyx, dyshidrosis, acrodermatitis perstans, and other eruptions of unknown cause that are localized chiefly to the hands, as well as in the vesicles of pustular bacterids. These bacterids are usually sterile pustules of the palms and soles and are assumed to be provoked by allergic reactions to bacterial products.

Cleavage vesicles. Some years ago I applied the term "cleavage" to those vesicles formed by the separation or cleavage of the epidermis or dermis through a single horizontal plane.[5] The cleavage may occur at any level of the epidermis and occasionally may split the upper dermis. The precise level of cleavage usually embodies a key diagnostic clue. The following discussion is of representative types of cleavage vesicles.

Dermatitis herpetiformis. The lesions of dermatitis herpetiformis (Duhring's disease) are symmetrically distributed in groups in the scapular regions, on the buttocks, or on the extremities. The lesions may be erythematous macules or papules, but in most cases they are characterized by vesicles that may vary from those detectable only microscopically to large bullae. Oral le-sions in dermatitis herpetiformis are more common than is generally indicated.[36] The disease may be accompanied by mild constitutional symptoms and signs. Itching, burning, and pricking sensations almost always are present. The disease is characterized by spontaneous remissions and relapses. The cause is unknown. The lesions respond curiously in most instances to penicillin and sulfapyridine but usually do not react satisfactorily to other sulfonamides.

Remarkably, the cutaneous lesions of dermatitis herpetiformis can be produced in the susceptible individual with topically applied potassium iodide. The mechanism is unknown.

The microscopic features of the vesicle of dermatitis herpetiformis consist of a collection of serum, fibrin, and a few neutrophilic and eosinophilic leukocytes that have cleaved and lifted the entire epidermis from the corium. The epidermis itself shows no other constant change. Of diagnostic importance is the change in the dermal base of the vesicle—particularly the flattened, edematous papillae that are infiltrated with cells of the same type found in the vesicle itself (Fig. 36-4). Eosinophilic leukocytes are often present in considerable numbers, but their absence by no means precludes the diagnosis of dermatitis herpetiformis. Despite the prominence of the subepidermal extrusions of neutrophils, leukocytoclastic vasculitis, located a bit lower in the dermis, rarely accompanies Duhring's disease. On the other hand, subepidermal foci of neutrophils may appear also with bullous lupus erythematosus and bullous pemphigoid, thereby limiting the differential diagnosis on the basis of this criterion alone.

It has been suggested that dermatitis herpetiformis is attributable to an immunologic disorder linked with

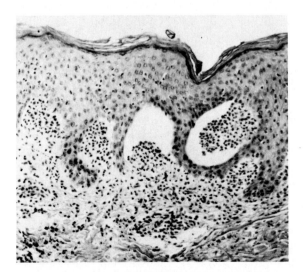

Fig. 36-4. Dermatitis herpetiformis in its early stage showing cleavage of epidermis from dermis by collections of leukocytes. (Hematoxylin and eosin.)

gluten sensitivity. Both the cutaneous and intestinal lesions respond to the withdrawal of gluten. Immunofluorescence studies reveal IgA in granular of fibrillary form, rarely linear, at the dermoepidermal junction. By contrast, in pemphigoid the immunoglobulin is mostly IgG, but it appears in linear form. The third component of complement, C3, is also often present.

Although IgG in the basement membrane zone characterizes bullous pemphigoid, and IgA in granular form in the basement membrane zone is a feature of dermatitis herpetiformis, the two may coexist (including IgA in linear form). This overlapping contribution has suggested to some a relationship between the two entities.[62] The histologic similarity in many instances also points in this direction. Dermatitis herpetiformis may be associated with the nephrotic syndrome, with IgA demonstrable both in the glomerular basement membranes and in the cutaneous basement membrane zone. So-called *benign chronic bullous dermatosis* of childhood appears to have the characteristics of dermatitis herpetiformis, except for the absence of circulating epithelial antibodies.

Pemphigus. Pemphigus refers to a group of bullous diseases of unknown cause that were generally fatal before corticosteroids were available. It is an autoimmune intraepidermal and mucosal disease in which autoantibodies become bound to an intercellular material leading to lower epidermal or epithelial acantholysis and suprabasilar cleavage vesicles. In somewhat more than half of the cases, the lesions originate in the oral cavity and a lapse of several months may occur before the development of the cutaneous disease. Any mucosal surface may become involved.

The prognosis has been dramatically improved with the use of steroids and immunosuppressive agents. The disease involves both sexes equally, affecting mainly those between 40 and 70 years of age. It may take about 5 months for involvement of the glabrous skin after the oral lesions appear. Infection with sepsis (*Staphylococcus aureus*) is the most common cause of death.

Pemphigus occurs in more than one form. The several varieties include *pemphigus vulgaris*, *pemphigus foliaceus*, and *pemphigus vegetans*. These forms are entities primarily on the basis of the acuteness of the disease or the type of lesions accompanying the vesicles, for example, the foul-smelling scales of pemphigus foliaceus and the fungoid papillomatous masses of pemphigus vegetans. *Pemphigus erythematosus* (Senear-Usher syndrome) previously was regarded as a separate entity with a good prognosis. It is now believed that this condition is actually a variant of pemphigus in which the erythematous stage may be prolonged. The incidence of pemphigus vulgaris is about four times that of all other varieties combined. Bullae are observed at some time in the course of pemphigus foliaceus and pemphi-

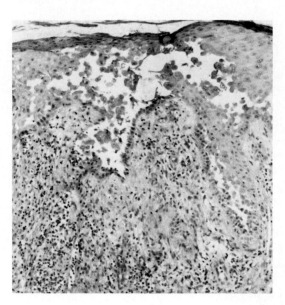

Fig. 36-5. Pemphigus vulgaris with suprabasilar cleavage and isolated clusters of epidermal cells within vesicle. These are acantholytic cells of Tzanck. (Hematoxylin and eosin.)

gus vegetans. The group name is applied also to benign chronic familial pemphigus (Hailey-Hailey disease), but there is reason to believe that this disease is quite distinct from the usually fatal varieties of pemphigus. The actual cause of death in pemphigus uncomplicated by sepsis is not clear, though the loss of proteins and electrolytes in the bullous fluid is probably a significant factor. The prognosis for patients with pemphigus is better if the disease develops before 40 years of age and is treated with steroids early in its course. There is evidence to suggest that a heterogeneity of antigens is involved in pemphigus vulgaris.[82]

The triad of pemphigus, myasthenia gravis, and thymoma has been well documented, as has the association of pemphigus with neoplasms, especially lymphomas.

The histologic picture of the cutaneous lesion of pemphigus is as follows:

1. The typical vesicle or bulla consists of a collection of serous fluid, most often at the suprabasilar layer of the epidermis. As a rule there is little or no reaction in the dermis, though there are many exceptions in which the upper dermis or submucosa is crowded with polymorphonuclear leukocytes admixed with the various mononuclear cells (that is, lymphocytes, plasma cells, and histiocytes). Such a vesicle or bulla characterizes pemphigus vulgaris but may be a part of the picture of other varieties of pemphigus (Fig. 36-5). In addition, rounded epidermal cells loosened by acantholysis (Tzanck cells) frequently are found in the vesicles of pemphigus, but they are not pathognomonic of this dis-

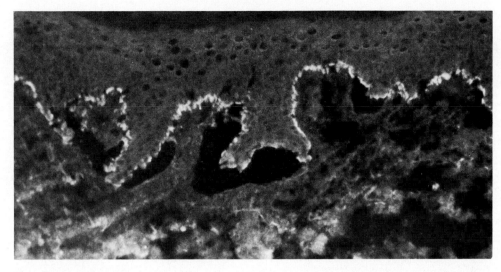

Fig. 36-6. Direct immunofluorescence of IgG in basement membrane zone of bullous pemphigoid. C3, C4, and beta$_{1H}$ globulin also are fixed in this zone in pemphigoid. (Courtesy of Dr. L.P. Pertschuk, Downstate Medical Center, Brooklyn, N.Y.)

ease. These acantholytic cells may be recognized in smears of vesicles stained with hematoxylin and eosin and may be distinguished from cells of viral vesicles, for example. They are characterized by the disintegration of desmosomes and the separation, disorganization, and loss of tonofilaments, a sequence of events accompanying acantholysis not only in other dermatoses such as Darier's disease but also in some epidermal neoplasms, particularly melanocarcinomas. The vulnerability of the desmosomes is regarded as the principal pathogenic basis of pemphigus, a concept reinforced by immunofluorescence demonstration of the fixation of autoantibodies at these intercellular sites.

In pemphigus of whatever variant an IgG antibody is produced against the antigenic epidermal intercellular material. This critical antibody not only binds to the intercellular region but also is detectable in the sera.[1] In bullous pemphigoid the antibodies are localized to the position of the basement membrane zone (Fig. 36-6). Some investigators have noted that the immunoglobulins of bullous pemphigoid are localized between the epidermis and basal lamina, in contrast with the localization deep to the basal lamina in lupus erythematosus.[78]

The histologic differentiation of pemphigus vulgaris from *bullous pemphigoid* is often not as clear as was implied when the latter term was coined. The early mucosal involvement, the relative lack of inflammation, the abundance of acantholysis, and the suprabasilar (versus epidermal-dermal) cleavage are features indicative of pemphigus. The cleavage is attributed to pemphigus antibodies, which induce epidermal cells to activate cellular proteases, with resulting cellular

dyshesion and acantholysis.[81] It has been suggested that the acantholysis is caused by an immunologic reaction between the epidermal cell and the pemphigus antibody, resulting in release of a "pemphigus acantholytic factor."[79] The agent initiating this reaction (such as a virus, toxin, or chemical) is yet to be discerned.

Benign mucosal pemphigoid may involve the conjunctivae, oronasal cavity, larynx, esophagus, and genitalia. The histology is like that of bullous pemphigoid except for the occurrence of cicatrization as a consequence of the submucosal inflammatory reaction. Probably pemphigoid is a variant of erythema multiforme bullosum, as is the *Stevens-Johnson syndrome*. Pemphigoid may, on occasion, be associated with visceral cancer (Fig. 36-7).

Features of dermatitis herpetiformis are granular IgA deposits in the dermal papillae about the bullae and no circulating antibodies. In contrast, bullous pemphigoid shows linear deposition of IgG and complement at the dermoepidermal zone and in the skin uninvolved by lesions, as well as specific antibodies in the serum. Bullae also may result from the use of anticoagulants. These bullae are subepidermal and histologically simulate erythema multiforme.

2. In *pemphigus vegetans*, in addition to the bulla just described, there is an associated diagnostic lesion consisting of pronounced acanthosis with prominent prolongation of the rete ridges, between which are brightly dense collections of eosinophilic leukocytes. The eosinophils may migrate into the epidermis, which may become ulcerated and result in intraepidermal microabscesses. The ulcerations, the intraepidermal abscesses, and the extensive acanthosis with winding re-

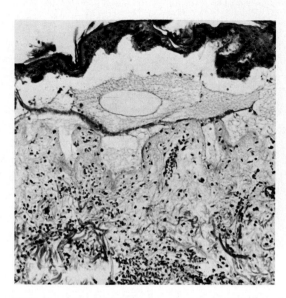

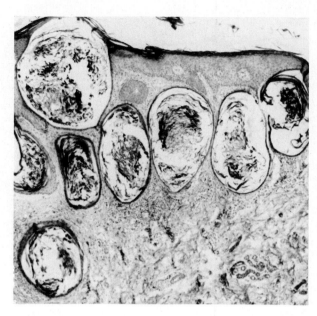

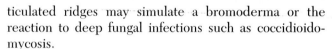

Fig. 36-7. Pemphigoid. Cleavage vesicle between epidermis and dermis with relatively sparse dermal reaction. Tzanck cells are absent. (Hematoxylin and eosin.)

Fig. 36-8. Epidermolysis bullosa with milia (keratinous, sweat gland cysts).

ticulated ridges may simulate a bromoderma or the reaction to deep fungal infections such as coccidioidomycosis.

3. In *pemphigus foliaceus* the typical bulla often is immediately adjacent to a unique acanthosis. Usually the fluid accumulates between layers of the upper part of the rete Malpighii. If the accumulation of fluid is minimal, the cleavage may be sufficient to separate the uppermost portion of the epidermis by crude pressure of the thumb on the patient's skin (Nikolsky's sign). The ridges are rounded and formed in congeries so that in a single section they may appear isolated in the deep dermis, as in early squamous cell carcinoma. This type of acanthosis resembles most the epidermal proliferation commonly seen overlying myoblastomas. The epidermal proliferation usually is accompanied by a polymorphous cellular infiltrate of neutrophilic leukocytes and mononuclear cells. Tzanck cells are present in pemphigus foliaceus and pemphigus vegetans and in lesser numbers in Hailey-Hailey disease and other vesicular dermatoses.

Circulating intercellular antibodies are demonstrable in the serum of patients with pemphigus, and their titers tend to parallel the severity of the disease. Indeed, reappearance of the antibodies may herald the recrudescence of the disease. Immunofluorescence studies of cutaneous biopsy specimens reveal a striking, diffuse, intercellular localization of immunoglobulins in a characteristic polygonal pattern about the keratinocytes. Pemphigus-like antibodies occur in patients with burns, toxic epidermal necrolysis, and several other drug-in-

duced eruptions. In sharp contrast, the results of immunofluorescence studies are negative in Hailey-Hailey (bullous Darier's) disease, in which the acantholysis may present a differential diagnostic problem in routinely stained sections. In bullous and cicatricial pemphigoid, dermatitis herpetiformis, and lupus erythematosus, immunoglobulins may be demonstrated by fluoresceinated sera in the immediate subepidermal region.

Epidermolysis bullosa. Epidermolysis bullosa occurs soon after birth (congenital) or may first appear in the second or third decade (so-called acquired type). There are two varieties of epidermolysis bullosa; simple and dystrophic. In the simple type the lesions occur after slight trauma on any portion of the body and regress, leaving temporary pigmentation but no permanent changes. The dystrophic type is characterized by lesions of the extremities, provoked by minimal trauma and associated with pigmentation, milia (epidermal cysts) (Fig. 36-8), atrophy, destruction of nails, cicatrizations, hypoplasia of dental enamel, and syndactylism. Involvement of extracutaneous stratified epithelium by cleavage vesicles may occur in the eyes, urinary tract, oropharynx, esophagus, anal canal, and respiratory tract. It may be complicated by the development of epidermoid carcinomas both in the skin and in the mucosa of the mouth and esophagus. The pathogenesis may well be related to the associated desmoplasia or scarring as in other situations, such as burns and chronic osteomyelitis. It is known to precede the development of systemic lupus erythematosus, myeloma, diabetes mellitus, and enteritis and to follow penicillamine therapy.

Both the simple and dystrophic types may be congenital or acquired. The histologic features are those of a pressure vesicle with cleavage often at the junction of the stratum corneum and stratum granulosum or between the epidermis and dermis, especially in the dystrophic type (Fig. 36-8). The inflammatory reaction within both the vesicle and the underlying dermis is mild except in regions, such as the feet, that are easily traumatized and infected. Small epidermal inclusions lie in the dermis beneath or at the margins of the vesicles (Fig. 36-8). A congenital disturbance of the dermal elastic tissue is said to occur in the dystrophic type, but the evidence for this is not satisfactory. However, necrosis of upper dermal collagen and elastic tissue may occur in the dystrophic form and may result in severe contractures of the extremities, with bony absorption. Involvement of the conjunctiva, oral mucosa, and esophagus may develop, heralding a poor prognosis. The epidermal inclusion cysts are particularly prone to appear in the dystrophic form and reflect, in part, the dermal isolation of portions of sweat ducts and rete ridges that subsequently form the cysts. The relative lack of inflammatory cellular response within and beneath the vesicles is of diagnostic usefulness in their differentiation from other vesicles with cleavages at corresponding sites. The bullae of dystrophic epidermolysis bullosa have been attributed to the specifically higher local production of collagenase in contrast with pemphigus vulgaris and bullous pemphigoid. A picture simulating epidermolysis bullosa may occur after the administration of penicillamine. Subepidermal cleavage vesicles (along with necrosis of the epithelium of sweat glands and ducts) also may occur, especially over traumatized pressure points and after carbon monoxide or barbiturate poisoning.[15] IgG is localized beneath the basal lamina rather than in the lamina lucida, as occurs in bullous pemphigoid.

Subcorneal pustular dermatosis. Subcorneal pustular dermatosis is considered to be a special vesicular entity. The lesions, which tend to affect particularly middle-aged women, appear as minute gyrate or anular groups of erythematous, superficial vesiculopustules localized chiefly in the intertriginous areas about the breasts, axillae, and groin.

Histologically the changes consist in cleavage vesicles and pustules located immediately beneath the stratum corneum, as the name indicates. Eosinophils are not a part of the picture, though occasionally acantholytic cells may be present. The exudate is usualy sterile—unlike that of impetigo contagiosa, which the lesion otherwise resembles histologically (Fig. 36-9). *Staphylococcus aureus* is the most common offender in impetigo contagiosa; it is often mixed with beta-hemolytic streptococci. Streptococci also may occur alone or in as-

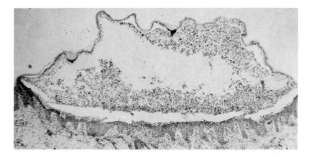

Fig. 36-9. Impetigo contagiosa. Superficial cleavage vesicle with purulent exudate. (Hematoxylin and eosin; AFIP 99848.)

sociation with a variety of organisms. Diphtheroids (*Corynebacterium pyogenes*) are responsible for about 5% of cases.

Intradermal neutrophilic dermatosis. The entity labelled *intraepidermal neutrophilic* (IgA) *dermatosis* is characterized by generalized flaccid vesicles, each with intraepidermal abscesses, with an affinity for IgA. Some state that the already-present IgA attracts the neutrophils.

Transient acantholytic dermatosis. Transient acantholytic dermatosis (TAD, Grover's disease) is characterized by vesicles located on the trunk produced by heat and sweating in susceptible persons.[44] The histologic appearance is that of an intraepidermal cleavage vesicle with loosening of individual keratinocytes (like Tzanck cells) into the vesicle so that the lesion simulates somewhat several other intraepidermal acantholytic vesicular dermatoses.

Toxic epidermal necrolysis (Lyell's disease). Toxic epidermal necrolysis (TEN) is characterized by a tender, painful rash resembling scalded skin, with rapid onset and recovery or rapid death.[58] The exotoxin of *Staphylococcus* organisms is implicated in most cases, but drugs, viruses, and vaccinations (such as those against poliomyelitis, diphtheria, and measles) have also been involved. The drugs linked to this fairly new entity include allopurinol, barbiturates, sulfonamides, penicillin, phenylbutazone, hydantoins, salicylates, and antihistamines.[29] In about 20% of cases no agent can be implicated.

Histologically the epidermal cleavage may develop at one of several levels: dermoepidermal, as in erythema multiforme bullosum; suprabasilar, as in pemphigus; or the upper part of the rete Malpighii. Scattered foci of necrotic keratinocytes are characteristically present, and some of these may occupy the vesicles as acantholytic cells (Fig. 36-10). Few or no dermal inflammatory cells appear unless secondary infection takes place, and so the simulation of erythema multiforme may be strik-

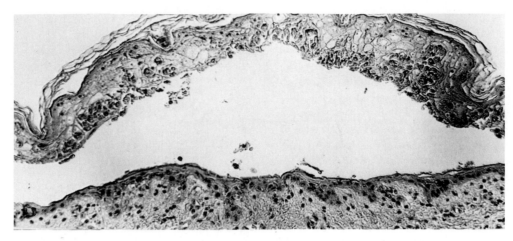

Fig. 36-10. Lyell's disease (toxic epidermal necrolysis) showing bulla with intraepidermal cleavage and necrosis of keratinocytes.

ing. Indeed, some observers regard the disease as a variant of erythema multiforme bullosum. In both there has been occasional association with membranoproliferative glomerulonephritis. In sharp contrast with the good prognosis in small children, the mortality in adults is more than 40%, or, if recovery occurs, it is often protracted for many months.

These days, we are learning to segregate TEN occurring predominantly in adults, and associated with a fulminant reaction to drugs, from the staphylococcic scaling skin syndrome (SSSS) observed mainly in children and, as indicated, attributed to *Staphylococcus*. Actually the scaling in the latter benign designation is more superficial than the deeper angry erosions of TEN. In addition, mucosal involvement (oral, ocular, and genital) is common in TEN and rare in SSSS. The histologic features of the epidermal lesions are similar in the two, both being intraepidermal cleavage vesicles with necrosis of keratinocytes and sparse or absent dermal infiltrate. There is still much to be learned about the pathogenesis of the lesions.

Herpes gestationis. Herpes gestationis is a rare highly pruritic vesiculobullous eruption that is prone to recur in succeeding pregnancies. Approximately 10% of the newborn have the disease, overtly or subclinically. This condition is a rare cleavage type of vesicular rash that appears during or shortly after pregnancy.

"Herpes" in herpes gestationis is derived from the Greek word meaning 'a creeping' and presumably relates to the peripheral extension of the lesions.[80] It does not indicate a viral cause, as in *herpes genitalis;* in fact, the cause of herpes gestationis is still unknown. The differential diagnoses are principally bullous pemphigoid, erythema multiforme, and dermatitis herpetiformis. The immunologic and ultrastructural evidence favors a closer relationship to bullous pemphigoid than to

the others. The disorder is said to be complement-dependent and IgG dependent.[80] The histologic findings also indicate bullous pemphigoid, except for the conspicuous necrosis of cells of the basal layer, even in clinically uninvolved areas. Necrosis of the basal cells over the dermal papillae is said to be characteristic of herpes gestationis. Eosinophils are constantly present in the exudate. Proteases, collagenase, and elastase are found in the blister fluid. The possibility has been offered that such enzymes may play a role in the pathogenesis of the dermoepidermal cleavage vesicles by their action on the dermis with loss of adhesiveness to the epidermis. Others have imputed eosinophils and their release of contained enzymes.

Pyoderma gangrenosum. Pyoderma gangrenosum refers to the ugly, large, purple-rimmed, undermined suppurative ulcerations occurring especially with ulcerative colitis but associated with other diseases, such as rheumatoid arthritis. Its cause and pathogenesis are still problematic, though leukocytoclastic arteriolitis, perhaps as part of a Shwartzman phenomenon, has been suspected.

Viral vesicles. Smallpox (variola), chickenpox (varicella), alastrim, vaccinia (cowpox), herpangina, herpes simplex, and herpes zoster (shingles) are described in Chapter 9. In contrast to the ease with which most of the exanthemas can be differentiated clinically is the difficulty or impossibility of differentiating the vesicles histologically. Nevertheless, there are certain histologic features common to each of these vesicles that at least permit the recognition of each as a vesicle produced by a virus. These features include (1) reticular colliquation, by which the epidermis becomes transformed into multiple locules bounded by a reticulum of drawn-out, stringy, cytoplasmic septa, (2) ballooning degeneration, the formation of multinucleated giant cells in the lower

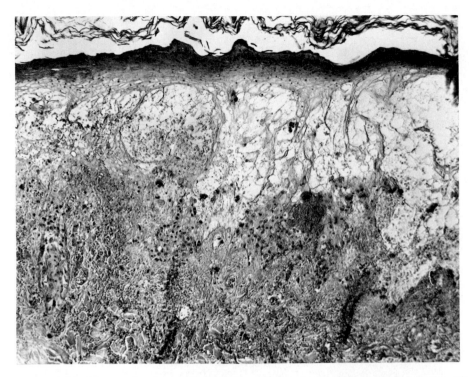

Fig. 36-11. Fatal hemorrhagic smallpox with vesicles showing the reticular colliquation and giant ballooning cells characteristic of viral exanthems. (Hematoxylin and eosin; 145×.) (From Allen, A.C.: The skin, St. Louis, 1954, The C.V. Mosby Co.)

layers of the rete Malpighii, and (3) intranuclear inclusions (Fig. 36-11).

It is stated that in the vesicle of smallpox, reticular colliquation proceeds at a faster pace, particularly at the periphery of the lesion, than does ballooning degeneration, which accounts for the umbilication of this vesicle (Fig. 36-11). In smallpox, Guarnieri bodies are found as eosinophilic, varying-sized, round, cytoplasmic inclusions—especially in cells at the base of the vesicle, including those undergoing ballooning degeneration. In addition, eosinophilic intranuclear inclusions with margination of the nuclear chromatin are common in these cells. In the vesicles of herpes these intranuclear inclusions are referred to as zoster bodies of Lipschütz though they are morphologically similar to the intranuclear inclusions of the other viral vesicles (Fig. 36-12).

The scarring that follows some of these vesicles (such as those of zoster and occasionally of smallpox) is an index of the prior inflammatory destruction of the upper corium. As a rule, edema and infiltrate of inflammatory cells are present in the upper dermis of most vesicles of the various viral diseases. The residual scarring, however, appears to reflect the greater intensity and destructiveness of the process. The virus of zoster appears capable of producing the clinical picture of varicella in susceptible persons. It is suggested that steroids increase this susceptibility.

Relatively recently an entity referred to as herpangina has been described. It is a benign, febrile, self-limited disease of viral etiology, affecting children chiefly and characterized by a sudden onset of grayish white, papulovesicular, oral or pharyngeal lesions with a surrounding red areola. Histologic studies of the vesicles are not available, but it is presumed that they would resemble the vesicles of herpes.

Another controverted disease that now appears clearly virogenic is Kaposi's varicelliform eruption. This disease is actually either disseminated herpes simplex or generalized vaccinia often inoculated in skin made receptive by a preceding dermatosis such as eczema or atopic dermatitis. The diagnosis of viral vesicles is expedited by the use of smears of the vesicular contents. This cytodiagnostic method is particularly useful with the viral vesicles; in other types excessive dependence may be placed on acantholytic cells. It is hypothesized that the virus of varicella-zoster remains latent in sensory ganglia after a preceding varicella and that hematogenous dissemination of the virus occurs with subsequent activation.

Herpesvirus type 2, unlike type 1, tends to disseminate. They may be differentiated by cultural or immunofluorescence studies and, it is said, morphologically by the greater tendency toward ballooning degeneration by type 2 virus.

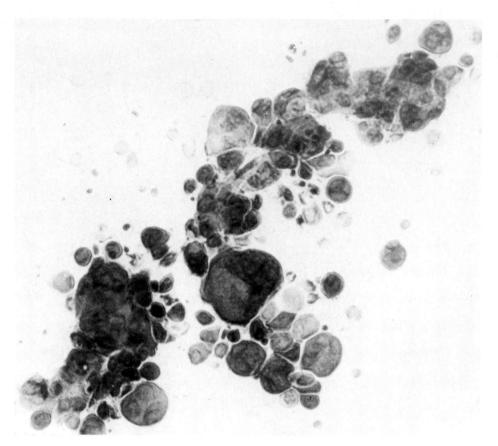

Fig. 36-12. Herpes simplex. Smear of contents of vesicle showing viral inclusions within nuclei of keratinocytes. (Hematoxylin and eosin.)

Superficial mycoses

Superficial mycoses are included in this section because they principally involve the epidermis. The mycoses are separated into the superficial type (ringworm, tinea corporis, and favus) and the deep type (such as blastomycosis, coccidioidomycosis, and actinomycosis). Superficial mycoses are divided, according to the region affected, into tinea capitis, barbae, corporis, cruris, and pedis (or epidermophytosis). Several kinds of fungi may be responsible for the same clinical type of lesion. On the other hand, the form and chronicity of the ringworm may vary considerably with the causative fungus. For example, *Trichophyton* infection of the feet is characterized by a dry, scaly dermatosis, whereas *Epidermophyton* infection appears vesicular and moist. It has therefore been suggested that the cause as well as the anatomic region be indicated in the name, such as tinea corporis trichophytica. However, usage sanctions the retention of additional names for varieties of ringworm infection that have distinguishing features of pattern, color, severity, or chronicity of lesions, for example, favus, kerion (ringworm of scalp complicated by abscesses), tinea imbricata, and tinea versicolor.

Botryomycosis is merely a bacterial infection histo-logically confused with actinomycosis because of the eosinophilic radiate or asteroid formation about the colonies of bacteria. The etiologic agents is usually a *Staphylococcus* organism, but streptococci and *Proteus* organisms also may produce this pattern. Gram stains on histologic sections facilitate the diagnosis.

The fungus may be observed in wet smears of scrapings soaked in sodium or potassium hydroxide, or they may be cultured on special media, such as Sabouraud's agar. However, with the exceptions of tinea versicolor and favus, it is rare to observe the fungus in a routine paraffin section of a lesion of ringworm. Generally, the histologic picture comprises merely the presence of scales or vesicles along with subepidermal hyperemia and slight perivascular cuffing by mononuclear cells. In tinea versicolor the spores and hyphae of *Pityrosporon furfur* are usually abundant and confined to the stratum corneum. In favus the large scutula, or matted scales, contain masses of fungus.

The vesicle of ringworm, no matter where the lesion is located, is eczematous, usually multiloculated, and the morphologic result of excessive spongiosis. This type of vesicle is the picture of the dermatophytid or allergic manifestation of the fungal infection. The dermatophytids are free of fungi and are caused by the cutaneous reaction to the products of fungi transported probably through the blood or lymph. For example, the dermatophytids after ringworm of the feet often occur on the hands. It has been suggested that sensitizing antibiotic therapy with preparations from fungi such as penicillin may be responsible in some measure for the dermatophytids after superficial mycoses. The deep mycoses are described in Chapter 10.

Scabies

Another lesion of the epidermis that is often recognizable in a fortunate histologic section is caused by *Acarus scabiei*. The disease is characterized by the occurrence of intensely pruritic papules, vesicles, pustules, and excoriations usually located in relation to the burrow, cuniculus, or gallery dug by the *Acarus* mite into the epidermis. These lesions tend to occur in the webs of the fingers, on the wrists, in the genital regions, and beneath the breasts. The disease is contagious and in most instances is transmitted by direct body contact with an infected individual. One may make the diagnosis clinically by picking the female mite out of the burrow and identifying it with the low-power lens of the microscope.

Histologically, none of the lesions of scabies is diagnostic except the burrow with the tenant mite. However, the mite often may not be included in the section, but the presence of ova or fecal material of the *Acarus* within the burrow or merely the presence of the gallery itself is strongly presumptive evidence of scabies. The burrow is a superficial epidermal defect extending obliquely through the thickened stratum corneum, which serves as a roof to shelter the *Acarus*.

A form of scabies may be transmitted to man by mites that infest dogs, cats, birds, and monkeys. So-called Norwegian scabies appears to be merely a more fulminant form of ordinary scabies.

Infestation with *Demodex folliculorum*, the acarid commonly found within the keratinous follicular plugs of comedones, has generally been regarded as innocuous, but more recently the harmless nature of the infestation has been questioned. Blepharitis, for example, has been attributed to this arthropod.

DISEASES AFFECTING BOTH EPIDERMIS AND DERMIS

In this discussion are included those histologic entities in which changes in the epidermis and the dermis jointly contribute to the morphologic diagnosis.

Lupus erythematosus

Lupus erythematosus occurs in two principal forms: chronic, or discoid, and acute.

Discoid lupus erythematosus. The discoid variety is fortunately the more common, manifests itself by sta-

tionary or slowly progressive coalescent macules or plaques covered irregularly with fine, whitish or yellowish greasy scales, and is associated with focal gray patches of atrophy and keratotic plugging of follicles. The lesions usually are well defined (hence, discoid) and show a predilection for the malar areas and bridge of the nose distributed in the shape of a butterfly. The process is not limited to this area but may occur also on other parts of the face, the scalp, the neck, extremities, and elsewhere. In any location the lesions are aggravated by exposure to sunlight or other forms of irradiation. The lesions may regress completely, but usually there is residual, rather typical superficial scarring with pigmentation or leukoderma and alopecia. Acute changes also may be superimposed on the discoid lesions. Carcinomatous transformation (squamous cell) may occur in the chronic process, probably for nonspecific reasons similar to those that obtain in some other forms of chronic cicatrizing ulcerations.

The histologic features of the discoid variety of lupus erythematosus are easily recognizable in most cases. They include the following:

1. Alternating acanthosis and atrophy of the epidermis, with the process infrequently progressing to squamous cell carcinoma
2. Liquefaction degeneration of the basal layer
3. Hyperemia or telangiectasis and edema of the papillary and subpapillary layers of the dermis
4. Dense collections of mononuclear cells, principally lymphocytes, in the upper and midportions of the dermis, most concentrated about the appendages, often with atrophy and consequent alopecia (Fig. 36-13)
5. Focal depigmentation of the basal layer along with clusters of melanophages resulting from the subepidermal inflammation

Basophilic "degeneration" of collagen in the upper dermis is a completely unreliable criterion of chronic lupus erythematosus, inasmuch as it is found normally in the skin of the malar regions, especially in older age groups. Changes in vessels, other than telangiectasis, are not part of the picture of discoid lupus erythematosus. The lesions of rosacea may occasionally offer differential diagnostic difficulty because of the presence of keratotic plugs and erythema. The epidermal changes and middermal masses of lymphocytes favor the diagnosis of lupus erythematosus. Occasionally the collections of lymphocytes extend into the underlying panniculus (lupus erythematosus profundus) and may be mistaken for Weber-Christian disease. Lupus erythematosus profundus (lupus erythematosus panniculitis) is characterized by nodular involvement of the subcutis with or without overlying dermal and epidermal involvement. In these instances, there is more likely to be an association with discoid than with systemic lupus erythematosus. This lesion, too, has been attributed to

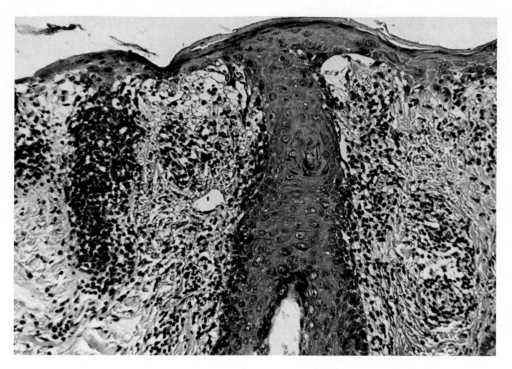

Fig. 36-13. Acute and chronic lupus erythematosus with early vesiculation.

injury caused by immune complexes.[91] Similar dense masses of lymphocytes in the dermis may be confused with a malignant lymphoma, the benign dermal lymphocytosis of Jessner, or the potpourri of lesions labeled Spiegler-Fendt sarcoid.

Acute lupus erythematosus. The acute (or subacute) lupus erythematosus may occur as a focal, transient reaction to sunlight or may be part of the frequently fatal systemization of the disease. These acute lesions may be superimposed on the chronic process or may affect previously uninvolved skin. The chronic lesion is assumed to be complicated by the disseminated form in the rarest instances. However, although this may be the impression clinically, the histologic and recent clinical data belie this impression. Moreover, antinuclear antibodies are stated to be present in over 90% of patients with systemic lupus erythematosus and in 15% to 40% of those with discoid lupus erythematosus. Immunofluorescence studies reveal characteristic often discontinuous bands of immunoglobulins (IgG) and complement at the dermoepidermal junction in both systemic and discoid lupus erythematosus.[27,50] The immunofluorescence is said to be positive occasionally in rosacea and in a few other diseases in which, however, the differential histologic diagnosis may be achieved in sections stained routinely.

Immunoglobulin deposits may be found in clinically uninvolved skin. However, the generally accepted assumption that intact-appearing skin is necessarily normal histologically is not justified. Moreover, no conclusions can be drawn regarding the nature of the antigens or the pathogenesis of the junctional deposition of immunoglobulin. This same facile hypothesis embodying a direct cause-and-effect relationship between the presence of immunoglobulin and the pathogenesis of a lesion of given structures (such as glomeruli, renal tubules, or vessels) is far from proved. There does seem to be greater activity of the disease in patients with IgG at the junctional zone.

In acute cases the skin becomes reddened, edematous, and sometimes purpuric, with patchy macules that may coalesce into an erysipeloid, somewhat mottled malar flush. On the hands the lesions may be erythematous or purpuric and macular or papular. Elsewhere they may take other forms, such as vesicles, bullae, scaling macules, and telangiectases. When the acute process complicates the discoid lesion, fresh superficial or even moderately deep ulcerations may occur, in addition to the other changes mentioned, particularly at the advancing periphery of the old lesion. As stated, the acute cutaneous alterations may be a localized reaction to sunlight without systemic complications. In the disseminated variety, which occurs particularly but by no means exclusively in young women, the constitutional signs and symptoms include fever, thrombocytopenia, leukopenia, excessive gammaglobulinemia, splenomegaly, arthralgias, valvular disease (Libman-Sacks disease), anorexia, vomiting, diarrhea,

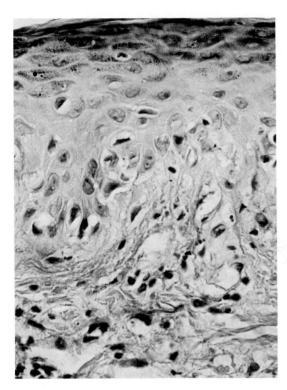

Fig. 36-14. Acute disseminated lupus erythematosus with pronounced liquefaction degeneration at dermoepidermal junction. (Hematoxylin and eosin.)

dysphagia, abdominal pain, and lymphadenitis. The principal causes of death are renal insufficiency, bacterial endocarditis, cardiac failure, sepsis, and pneumonia (see also pp. 652 and 973).

The acute histologic changes in the skin include an exaggeration of the liquefaction degeneration of the basal layer of the epidermis (Fig. 36-14) with eosinophilic swelling of the cytoplasm of the basal cells, edema of the papillary and subpapillary layers, necrobiosis with karyorrhexis and nuclear distortion of inflammatory cells in the upper dermis, telangiectasis, and occasionally fibrinoid degeneration of foci of collagen in this region, as well as in the walls of some of the arterioles. The last change, arteriolar involvement, is inconstant and is surely not responsible for the other cutaneous alterations.

By far the most diagnostically revealing histologic changes occur at the dermoepidermal junction. They are the vacuolization of the basal cells (liquefaction degeneration) and the subepidermal edema with a linear condensation of periodic acid–Schiff–positive material simulating a basement membrane but differing by its discontinuity and nonargyrophilia in the absence of melanin. Direct immunofluorescence studies reveal in this zone an immunofluorescent band reflecting immunoglobulins (IgG, IgM), components of complement (Clq, C3), and fibrin and properdin in both clinically involved and clinically intact skin.[30,50] The presence of the immunofluorescent band in clinically uninvolved skin worsens the prognosis and has been found to be associated with renal disease.[38] Although such skin may appear clinically uninvolved, careful histologic evaluation of even routinely hematoxylin and eosin–stained sections is likely to reveal some evidence of edema in this zone. In patients who have an inherited deficiency of complement there are likely to be an absence of C3 at the dermoepidermal junction and low titers of antinuclear antibodies. Interestingly, systemic lupus erythematosus has been associated with porphyria in more than a fortuitous manner.

Characteristic histologic changes occur in other organs in the disseminated disease. These include the following:

1. Atypical verrucous endocarditis (Libman-Sacks disease)
2. Striking fibrinoid alteration of the interstitial collagen of the myocardium that may but need not be mistaken for Aschoff bodies
3. Concentric dense rings of collagen, apparently thickened reticulum, about the central splenic arterioles (see Fig. 28-28)
4. Focal fibrinoid swelling of the walls of glomerular capillaries ("wire loops")

Viruslike, microtubular cytoplasmic inclusions have been noted in the skin, glomeruli, and other sites. These have provoked much interest, but their presence in patients without systemic lupus erythematosus and even in the vascular endothelium of patients with bullous pemphigoid has dampened the initial enthusiasm for the likelihood that they represent the etiologic virus.

Undoubtedly, one of the most provocative discoveries in the field of cutaneovisceral integration of the last few decades has been the phenomenon of the lupus erythematosus cell. Cytologically the phenomenon is manifested typically by a rosette of neutrophilic leukocytes about a mononuclear cell (apparently a lymphocyte) or, less typically, by a neutrophilic leukocyte with a cytoplasmic vacuole or a cytoplasmic inclusion of a nuclear fragment. Often there is excessive clumping of platelets. The essence of this phenomenon resides in the gamma globulin of the serum of patients with disseminated lupus erythematosus and may be detected not only with cells of the patient's marrow but also with cells of the peripheral blood. It also may be observed with normal cells (human or animal) after mixture with the patient's serum. Similar cells are noted in a cantharides-induced blister in the skin of patients with disseminated lupus erythematosus. It is of interest, but by now not surprising, to see dramatic remissions initiated by cortisone and ACTH in profoundly ill patients. With this improvement the lupus erythematosus cells diminish and may completely disappear. Some instances of a positive lupus erythematosus phenomenon have been recorded in multiple myeloma, leukemia, Hodgkin's disease, rheumatoid arthritis, viral hepatitis, acquired hemolytic anemia, and reactions to drugs (phenylbutazone and hydralazine) and in association with infection or contamination of serum with *Aspergillus niger* or *Trichophyton gypseum*. The lupus erythematosus cell is generally absent in scleroderma and dermatomyositis, which, together with disseminated lupus erythematosus, have been gratuitously linked as diffuse vascular or diffuse collagen disease, notwithstanding this and other discrepancies. Moreover, there is adequate reason to conclude that none of these diseases is either a diffuse vascular disease or a generalized disease of collagen. Review of the histologic findings in even a small number of autopsies in such cases quickly reveals that the involvement of vessels or collagen is, as a rule, neither diffuse nor itself responsible for the clinical picture, except for scleroderma.

Mixed connective tissue disease

Mixed connective tissue disease is a designation applied to a mild form of systemic lupus erythematosus without renal involvement and with high titers of antinuclear antibodies exhibiting a speckled rather than membranous rim of homogeneous nuclear staining with indirect immunofluorescence tests. Features of systemic sclerosis and polymyositis are included.

Dermatomyositis

The purplish red, finely scaly edematous rash located principally about the upper face is fairly diagnostic; the histologic picture of the skin is not. It consists chiefly of spotty parakeratosis, some liquefaction degeneration at the dermoepidermal junction, and edema of the upper dermis. However, the vacuolar sarcolysis, coagulation necrosis, and acute inflammatory changes in the swollen muscle fibers may be strongly suggestive. As stated, the search for vascular alterations is generally fruitless (Fig. 36-15). Widespread calcinosis of the skin, subcutaneous and periarticular tissue, and muscles may occur, along with thickening of arterioles and venules of muscles.

The pathogenic and etiologic spectra of myositides are expanding rapidly and form an intriguing subject dealing with viruses, unresolved relationship to visceral cancer, and lesions of the thymus. It appears evident that some of the confusion related to dermatomyositis occurs because a variety of myositic disorders as well as systemic lupus erythematosus and scleroderma are mistakenly considered to be dermatomyositis. The presence of dermal mucin in a specimen with no specific pattern is stated to be suggestive of dermatomyositis.

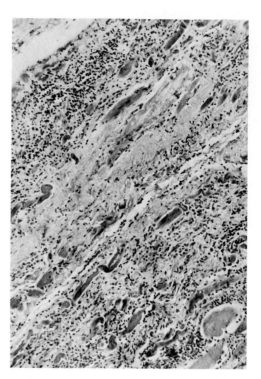

Fig. 36-15. Dermatomyositis with dense inflammatory cells interspersed among atrophic muscle fibers. (Hematoxylin and eosin.)

The cutaneous eruption of dermatomyositis may occur before involvement of muscle is evident clinically or histologically. Direct immunofluorescence studies usually show no abnormalities except globular deposits of IgG, IgM, and IgA in the upper dermis, which are of unknown significance.

Psoriasis

Psoriasis is characterized by reddish brown papules covered with silvery-white micaceous scales with a predilection for symmetric distribution on the extremities, especially on the knees and elbows. Lesions may occur also on the scalp, upper back, face, and genitalia and over the sacrum. The nails often are involved and become thickened, dirty white, irregularly laminated, rigid, and brittle. The disease is notoriously chronic, though remissions may occur spontaneously and after certain therapy, such as x-ray or ultraviolet-ray therapy.

The remarkable, if inconstant, resolution of psoriasis after plasmapheresis or dialysis, as well as its occurrence during dialysis and cardiac disease, must provide pathogenic clues.

Occasionally a widespread erythroderma or exfoliative dermatitis may complicate psoriasis, either spontaneously or, more particularly, after vigorous therapy. Another complication of psoriasis is arthritis, occurring usually in association with the generalized erythro-

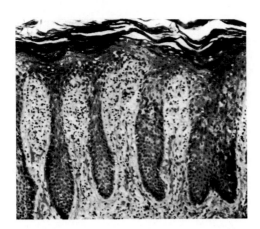

Fig. 36-16. Psoriasis with conspicuous parakeratosis, elongated, clubbed rete ridges, thinned suprapapillary epidermis, and rigid vessels in papillae. (Hematoxylin and eosin.)

derma. Occasionally the arthritis is deforming and persistently ankylotic, as in rheumatoid arthritis.

The use of various qualifying terms, such as psoriasis punctata, psoriasis guttata, psoriasis rupioides, psoriasis follicularis, and psoriasis nummularis, reflects simply the predominant clinical pattern of the lesions.

The histologic features of psoriasis (Fig. 36-16) are as follows:

1. Acanthosis with regular downgrowth of the rete ridges to about the same dermal level
2. Rounded tips of the rete ridges
3. Prolongation of the papillae, frequently with single vessels (venules) extending the length of the papillae as if rigid rather than tortuous
4. Thin epidermal plates over the elongated papillae, which offer so little covering for the dilated vessels of the papillae that bleeding occurs when a scale is lifted (Auspitz's sign)
5. Prominent parakeratosis, usually extending the length of the lesion rather than occurring focally
6. Absence or sparsity of stratum granulosum
7. Microabscesses (of Munro) in the upper rete Malpighii

In addition, there is usually an absence of spongiosis except in the immediate vicinity of the epidermal microabscesses. Intracellular edema in the rete Malpighii is common. The papillae are infiltrated chiefly with lymphocytes and histiocytes. In lesions in the early stage of development, some of these features, such as the rounding of the ridges and the elongation of the papillae with thin epidermal plates, may be absent. Furthermore, as in other dermatoses, recent therapy, trauma, or secondary infection obviously will modify the pattern. However, in patients who have had a superimposed exfoliative dermatitis the basic histologic picture of the psoriatic lesion tends to persist and

thereby may help differentiate it from the exfoliative stage of mycosis fungoides, a problem that occasionally arises. Neurodermatitis may simulate psoriasis so closely as to be histologically indistinguishable. As a rule, however, the psoriasiform features listed previously are irregular or less developed in neurodermatitis, or individual changes are altogether lacking. Ultrastructurally the tonofibrils are abnormal, and a lack of secretion of the adhesive cell surface coat has been noted. As might be anticipated, the lesions of psoriatis plaques are likely to be histologically variable, with chronic centers and acute peripheries. There is also a corresponding change in the concentration of T-helper and T-suppressor cells in the dermis, with the T-suppressor cells being more prominent in the areas undergoing resolution.

Parapsoriasis

Parapsoriasis, despite the name, is not related to psoriasis. The disease is characterized by erythematous macules covered with fine scales and distributed on the trunk and extremities. The lesions are extremely resistant to therapy.

The histologic changes of parapsoriasis are said to be nonspecific and to simulate psoriasis, seborrheic dermatitis, lichen planus, a macular syphiloderm, or the early stage of mycosis fungoides. Although the changes may simulate these other diseases, the specific diagnosis of parapsoriasis may be made with considerable assurance in many cases on the basis of the histologic changes alone. These changes include the spotty, thin areas of parakeratosis, slight to moderate acanthosis, vertical arrangement with some hyperchromatism of the basal layer along with slight liquefaction degeneration, and perhaps most revealing, the localization of inflammatory cells, mostly mononuclear, in the immediately subepidermal zone. The infiltrate hugs the epidermis tightly, and characteristically some of the inflammatory cells are located in the epidermis in their transepidermal migration. The presence of parakeratosis and a minimal stratum granulosum, as well as the shape of the ridges, easily distinguishes parapsoriasis from lichen planus. One of the serious errors of histologic diagnosis is mislabeling as parapsoriasis (en plaque) the early stage of mycosis fungoides. This error is made also clinically.

Lichen planus

Lichen planus is generally easily recognized clinically by the irregular, violaceous, glistening, flat-topped, pruritic papules covered with a thin, horny, adherent film and distributed symmetrically, particularly along the flexor aspects of the wrists, forearms, and legs. The usual form of lichen planus tends to resolve spontaneously after a year or so. On careful examination minute whitish points and lines (Wickham's striae) are seen on the surface of the papules. The disease is chronic, may last from months to years, and is rarely associated with constitutional reaction except in some of the hyperacute cases.

The varieties include lichen planus, lichen planus hypertrophicus, and lichen planus atrophicus. *Actinic* lichen planus affects predominantly children and young adults, especially Oriental persons. The lesions occur in the spring and summer, involving exposed skin and simulating, for example, melasma caused by perfumes, tars, and cosmetics.

The histologic features of lichen planus are strikingly characteristic and are the following:

1. Hyperkeratosis
2. Prominence of the stratum granulosum
3. Acanthosis, with elongated, saw-toothed rete ridges
4. Liquefaction degeneration of the basal layer
5. A mononuclear infiltrate consisting mostly of lymphocytes and histiocytes, sharply limited to the papillary and subpapillary layers of the dermis (Fig. 36-17)

The lesions of lichen planus may be dyschromic or hyperpigmented depending on the numbers and positions of the subepidermal melanophores that have phagocytosed the epidermal melanin released into the dermis. Many of the subepidermal macrophages are laden with melanin from the basal cells, not because these cells are unable to unload their pigment into "damaged" unreceptive neighboring keratinocytes and so spill over into the dermis, but because the subepidermal infiltrate provokes not only the development of the epidermal pigmentation but also its release from

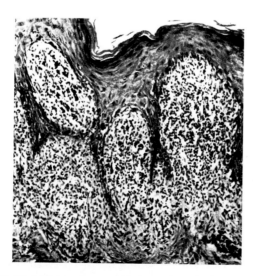

Fig. 36-17. Lichen planus with hyperkeratosis, acanthosis, pointed rete ridges, liquefaction degeneration, and dense subepidermal inflammatory zone. (Hematoxylin and eosin.)

the epidermis into dermal histiocytes. This same phenomenon is observed in other dermatoses, such as mycosis fungoides, Atabrine dermatitis, dermal postinflammatory pigmentation, and lupus erythematosus, in each of which a subepidermal inflammatory or cellular reaction occurs.

In the atrophic form the ridges are flattened, and the dermal infiltrate is sparse and replaced by an increased density of collagen containing somewhat thickened arterioles. Single foci of lesions histologically indistinguishable from the usual lichen planus are labeled "benign lichenoid keratosis" or "solitary lichen planus."

Immunofluorescence reflecting the presence of immunoglobulins and complement is noted in the eosinophilic, clustered, subepidermal globular bodies (Civatte's bodies). Somewhat similar foci and necrotic keratinocytes are seen also in a variety of other dermatoses, but their diagnostic significance in these is inconsequential. Actually, the meaning of these deposits even in lichen planus is not understood. To suggest that they represent an autoimmune process is not warranted at this time. In ulcerated lichen planus of the feet, results of antinuclear-antibody tests may be positive and gamma globulin levels may be elevated, features resulting in confusion with systemic lupus erythematosus.

Keratoderma blennorrhagica

Infrequently, perhaps in 1 in 5000 cases, an ugly eruption develops after the contraction of gonorrheal urethritis. This eruption is called "keratoderma blennorrhagica," or "gonorrheal keratosis," and is associated with a nonsuppurative migrating arthritis and gonorrheal urethritis that persist despite chemotherapy. The cutaneous lesions appear several weeks after the urethritis, do not contain gonococci according to most observers, and clear only after disappearance of the urethritis. The lesions of the skin are identical to those of Reiter's syndrome, which is associated with a presumed nonspecific urethritis, conjunctivitis, and nonsuppurative arthritis. In both the keratoderma and Reiter's syndrome, evolution of the disease is essentially similar. In both the arthritis clears, as a rule, without residual damage to the joints. In the few cases of Reiter's syndrome in which the complement fixation test for gonorrhea was used, results were negative. More recently *Chlamydia trachomatis* and the pleuropneumonia, or L, organisms have been considered responsible for Reiter's syndrome.

The histologic features of keratoderma blennorrhagica are as follows:

1. Prominent parakeratosis with excessive loosening of the scales such that they may be difficult to include in the histologic sections
2. Acanthosis with elongation and rounding of the ends of the rete ridges, much as in psoriasis, such

that pustular psoriasis may be a difficult differential diagnostic problem

3. Elongation of the papillae, but generally not as strikingly as in psoriasis because the overlying epidermal plate usually is not as thinned as it is in the latter disease

4. Numerous polymorphonuclear leukocytes, particularly in the upper part of the rete Malpighii and the scales

DISEASES PRINCIPALLY OF DERMIS
Urticaria pigmentosa

Urticaria pigmentosa is a chronic disease of the skin that begins usually in the first year of life but may start shortly after puberty or in later adult life, particularly in males of light complexion. A significant number of patients with urticaria pigmentosa have a history of asthma or hay fever. The eruption characteristically is made up of oval, 0.5 to 2.5 cm, pigmented, yellowish brown to reddish brown, macular, papular, and even nodular lesions occurring on the back especially but also on the face, scalp, palms, and soles. Infrequently a patient has merely a solitary nodule of urticaria pigmentosa. Solitary mastocytomas generally are detected by the first month of life and comprise about 10% to 15% of all instances of cutaneous mastocytosis. The disseminated cutaneous form usually develops in the next few months. About 25% of cases appear in late teenage or adult life, between 15 and 40 years of age, and occur equally in males and females.

Occasionally the eruptions may be sufficiently yellow to simulate xanthomatosis. The lesions are often intensely pruritic and, when irritated, become reddened, swollen, and urticarial; that is, they show evidence of dermographism. They may persist for years and in many instances disappear spontaneously. When the lesions of urticaria pigmentosa appear in childhood and are confined to the skin, the likelihood of spontaneous resolution during adolescence is great. If the lesions first appear in adolescence or later, the likelihood of their persistence and systemization is considerable. Bullae are common in neonatal mastocytosis.

Systemic involvement (bones, liver, lymph nodes, spleen) occurs in about 10% of patients, mostly in adults, and in about one third of them the equivalent of a mast cell leukemia develops. Uncommonly a solitary nodule or mastocytoma is followed by dissemination to the viscera or to the remainder of the skin. Such dissemination is said not to occur if the nodule remains solitary for approximately 2 months.

The clinical forms of mastocytosis are in summary:

1. Cutaneous
   a. Urticaria pigmentosa
   b. Mastocytoma
   c. Generalized
      (1) Maculopapular
      (2) Telangiectasia macularis
      (3) Erythrodermic, diffuse (papular, "scotch-grain")
2. Systemic

The histologic picture of urticaria pigmentosa is distinctive. In the more striking examples the upper half or two thirds of the dermis is replaced by a compact zone of mast cells that obscure the dermal landmarks (Fig. 36-18). The mast cells should be recognized in sections stained with the routine hematoxylin and eosin, notwithstanding their simulation of ordinary histiocytes and of plasma cells. Frequently, under high

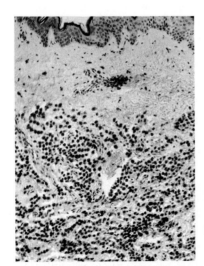

Fig. 36-18. Urticaria pigmentosa with superficial edema of cutis and extensive numbers of mast cells in remainder of dermis. (Hematoxylin and eosin.)

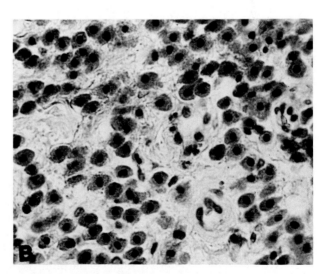

Fig. 36-19. Urticaria pigmentosa showing mast cells recognizable in routine stains of hematoxylin and eosin.

magnification, even with this routine stain the cytoplasmic granules of mast cells may be discerned (Fig. 36-19). These granules are of course more clearly demonstrable in metachromatic stains, such as Giemsa's or toluidine blue.

Mast cells contain heparin, hyaluronic acid, serotonin, and histamine. Indeed, there are isolated reports that these agents are reflected in an increase in the level of serum mucopolysaccharides and in coagulation defects. In some cases mast cells are present in smaller numbers and are dispersed as clumps of 10 to 20 cells about the middermal vessels. In these instances fine judgment may be required to differentiate the presence of mast cells in normal and abnormal numbers. In addition to the mast cells, there often are subepidermal edema (urticaria), chromatophores containing melanin in the upper dermis, and eosinophilic leukocytes scattered among the mast cells. Melanosis of the basal layer of the epidermis also may be present. The full-blown picture of urticaria pigmentosa closely resembles the so-called mastocytoma of dogs. Routine histologic sections of urticaria pigmentosa are commonly mistaken for leukemia, nevi, malignant melanomas, and Letterer-Siwe disease. Acceptance of the teaching that mast cells cannot be detected or strongly suspected with stains of hematoxylin and eosin is in large part responsible for these serious errors.

Simple urticaria may be caused in a variety of ways: by drugs, allergenic foods, infections (melioidosis), ultraviolet irradiation (urticaria solaris), and, fairly commonly, emotional disturbances. Urticaria solaris occurs immediately after exposure to light of sufficient intensity and of proper wavelength, usually in the violet or blue part of the spectrum. The essential histologic picture is that of bland subepidermal edema. In the inherited angioneurotic lesion the edema may extend into the subcutis. The evidence for a deficiency in plasma protease inhibitors (alpha$_1$-antitrypsin) in patients with chronic urticaria has been stressed recently.[28]

Urticarial vasculitis

Urticarial vasculitis appears to be a nonspecific spectrum of clinical, laboratory, and immunopathologic features caused by a variety of agents with variable degrees of severity.[63] The combination of hives and leukocytoclastic, fibrinoid dermal arteriolitis with immune complexes and complement, at times with hypocomplementemia, arthralgias, and glomerulonephritis, may form the background of several diseases, including systemic lupus erythematosus, viral hepatitis, and others.

Leukocytoclastic vasculitis (palpable purpura) represents an activated complement–induced inflammation of the small dermal vessels, chiefly arterioles.

Erysipelas

Erysipelas is described on p. 304.

Diseases of collagen

Keloid. A keloid is a hypertrophic cutaneous scar that develops as a reaction to burns, incisions, insect bites, vaccinations, and other stimuli. Ulcerated keloids are prone to undergo carcinomatous transformation of the epidermis after a long interval, particularly those attributable to burns or associated with chronic sinuses, as in osteomyelitis. The dermal portion of a keloid is not more likely to become sarcomatous than the dermis elsewhere. Rarely, a keloid resolves spontaneously.

The histologic features of a keloid include thick, homogeneously eosinophilic bands of collagen admixed with thin collagenous fibers and large active fibroblasts. The sweat glands, sebaceous glands, follicles, and arrectores pilorum are atrophic, destroyed, or displaced by the scar. The epidermis may be atrophic or only slightly altered by fusion and an irregular pattern of the ridges. The ordinary scar of the skin is more cellular than a keloid and is composed of uniformly thinner collagenous fibers. In both instances elastic tissue is diminished or absent. The keloidal reaction of hypertrophic collagenous bundles and large fibroblasts is characteristic of dermatitis papillaris capillitii (keloidal acne), which occurs particularly in the nuchal region and, with the associated extensive plasmacytic reaction, represents a type of response to folliculitis.

Balanitis xerotica obliterans. Balanitis xerotica obliterans is a disease of collagen that appears clinically as whitish, firm, coalescent papules or a sclerotic plaque of the glans penis and foreskin and often occurs after circumcision. The disease is of some importance because the process tends to extend to the urethral meatus, causing stenosis of the orifice. The lesion is to be differentiated clinically from erythroplasia of Queyrat and circumscribed scleroderma. Balanitis xerotica obliterans is probably a form of *lichen sclerosus et atrophicus*, which tends to occur on the vulva.

The histologic picture is as follows:
1. Atrophic epidermis or epithelium with loss of rete ridges
2. Striking homogenization of the collagen affecting about one third of the upper dermis
3. A more or less dense zone of lymphocytes and histiocytes beneath the homogenized collagen (Fig. 36-20)

The small arteries and arterioles of the upper and middle dermis may show evidence of endoarteritis obliterans, but this process is sufficiently inconstant as not to warrant the use of the qualification "obliterans" in the name of the disease. Furthermore, on the basis of other cutaneous atrophy there is reason to believe

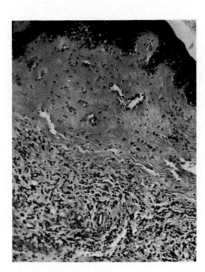

Fig. 36-20. Balanitis xerotica obliterans with homogenization of subepidermal collagen over zone of inflammatory cells. (Hematoxylin and eosin.)

that the vascular change does not initiate the collagenous change but perhaps is an incidental secondary reaction as in other kinds of chronic inflammation (such as chronic gastric ulcer).

Lichen sclerosus et atrophicus. In lichen sclerosus et atrophicus the initial change is a subepidermal edema that subsequently progresses to the characteristically homogenized densely sclerotic collagen in which the elastic fibers are diminished because of their displacement downward. The edema may be so great as to cause actual vesiculation at the dermoepidermal junction. Uncommonly an epidermoid carcinoma develops in the presence of lichen sclerosis et atrophicus. Even though the association is infrequent, the histologic appearance of transition of the two processes indicates that the carcinoma may develop from the sclerosis on more than a chance basis.

Acrodermatitis chronica atrophicans. Acrodermatitis chronica atrophicans involves atrophy of the epidermis and a subepidermal homogenized zone of collagen beneath which is a dense zone of mononuclear cells. There are also loss of dermal elastic tissue and atrophy of appendages.

Acrodermatitis chronica atrophicans begins as erythematous, slightly edematous macules that later become wrinkled, atrophic, and sclerodermatoid. As the prefix *acro-* indicates, the disease tends to select the extremities, particularly the hands and feet and the extensor surfaces of the elbows and knees. The condition occurs predominantly in middle-aged women.

Granuloma annulare and rheumatoid nodule. Granuloma annulare is a chronic eruption made up of pap-ules or nodules grouped in a ringed or circinate arrangement, with a tendency to occur on the dorsa of the fingers and hands and on the elbows, neck, feet, ankles, and buttocks, particularly of children and young adults. The lesions can be palpated intracutaneously rather than subcutaneously, in contrast to rheumatic nodules.

The cause of the disease is unknown. The histologic findings indicate a probable rheumatic or rheumatoid basis for the disease, but clinical evidence is sparse. I have seen cases associated with disseminated allergic granulomatous arteritis. The histologic picture of granuloma annulare has been observed also as a reaction to *Culicoides furans,* a biting gnat.

Histologically granuloma annulare is characterized by an intradermal oval or circular focus of fibrinoid degeneration of collagen. The nodules may occasionally ulcerate and are then categorized as perforating granuloma annulare. These necrotic foci of dermal collagen indicate probable infarcts, though corresponding occlusion of adjacent vessels is not regularly noted. About such a focus are palisaded rows of epithelioid cells or histiocytes, some of which may be vacuolated by fat (Fig. 36-21). It is the combination of fibrinoid alteration of collagen and palisaded histiocytes that indicates a possible rheumatic etiology. In fact, the histologic features of granuloma annulare are identical to those of the rheumatic or rheumatoid nodule—the only difference, as indicated, being the location of the latter in the subcutaneous tissue, adjacent to or within synovial membranes. Certainly the histologic picture is not that of tuberculosis, though the characteristic fibrinoid degeneration of the collagen of granuloma annulare and the rheumatoid nodule has been mistaken for the caseation of tuberculosis, a simulation that usually can be detected easily. There may be considerable difficulty, however, in recognizing early or small lesions of granuloma annulare in which the only clue may be a minimal smudgy fibrinoid swelling of collagen with clumps of a few histiocytes, some vacuolated and others partially palisaded. These minute lesions may be confused with xanthoses, necrobiosis lipoidica diabeticorum, or leprosy. Aschoff bodies are absent in granuloma annulare, as they are in the subcutaneous rheumatic nodule; they are confined to the heart. A protease and a collagenase similar to those of rheumatoid synovial enzymes have been isolated from rheumatoid nodules. The necrosis has been attributed to these, but the greater likelihood is the primacy of *vascular compromise as a cause of the infarctlike necrosis* both in these nodules and in granuloma annulare. These necrotic foci may perforate the epidermis, as stated. The presence of an abundance of T-cells in granuloma annulare has led some observers to attribute the lesion to a cell-mediated immune re-

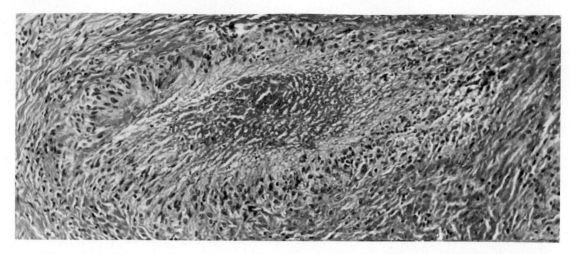

Fig. 36-21. Granuloma annulare with dermal lesion showing central necrosis bordered by histiocytes.

sponse. My own emphasis is to link the characteristic central infarct-like necrosis in granuloma annulare, rheumatic nodules, and others with necrosis from ischemia secondary to arterial compromise in which, possibly, a cell-nucleated response by the vessels may be a factor. Indeed, in a recent contribution, conspicuous arteriolitis was demonstrated at the periphery of the ischemia-like necrosis of papulonecrotic tuberculid and the vascular change was ascribed to an immunogenic response.[95]

Necrobiosis lipoidica diabeticorum. Necrobiosis lipoidica diabeticorum is characterized by oval, circular, firm, sharply defined plaques with yellowish centers and violaceous peripheries, occurring predominantly on the legs but found also on the forearms, palms, soles, neck, and face. The centers of the lesions are prone to ulcerate. Trauma, often inconspicuous, may initiate the lesions. In about 50% to 80% of patients the disease is associated with diabetes. In about 10% the lesions precede the onset of diabetes. In the remainder, diabetes does not develop. Obviously, the recognition of necrobiosis lipoidica diabeticorum can be of prophetic importance. Hyperpigmented, atrophic "shin spots" in diabetics occur chiefly on the extensor surfaces of the lower legs; occasionally they are found also on the forearms and thighs.

Clinically the disease must be differentiated from other such focal diseases of collagen as granuloma annulare, amyloidosis, morphea, and lipid proteinosis, as well as the granulomas of sarcoid and erythema induratum, which tend also to occur on the extremities. The diabetic state in some instances of necrobiosis lipoidica diabeticorum may be missed with the standard glucose tolerance test and discovered with the cortisone glucose tolerance test.

The basic histologic change of necrobiosis diabeticorum consists in ischemia-like degeneration of collagen

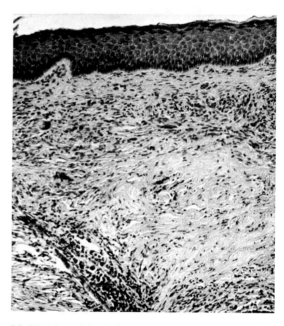

Fig. 36-22. Necrobiosis lipoidica diabeticorum with irregularly homogenized, degenerated dermal collagen and tuberculoid granulomas at periphery. (Hematoxylin and eosin.)

that occurs in irregular patches, especially in the upper dermis. In well-developed foci the altered collagen is swollen and somewhat granular, with loss of fibrils and a diminution in nuclei of fibrocytes. At the periphery of the collagenous alteration are small collections of histiocytes often arranged about Langhans giant cells and simulating sarcoid or tuberculosis (Fig. 36-22). This giant cell reaction occasionally may involve the walls of veins to produce a giant cell phlebitis reminiscent of the reaction in temporal arteritis. Vacuoles may be present in the cytoplasm of the giant cells and histiocytes, but fat is found infrequently within the cells of

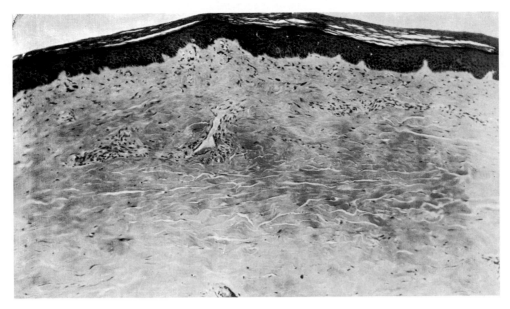

Fig. 36-23. Scleroderma with dense and thickened dermal fibers, atrophy of appendages and epidermis, and melanin pigmentation of basal layer. (Hematoxylin and eosin.)

these lesions, though extracellular fat is detectable about the altered collagen.

Scleroderma. There are two basic varieties of scleroderma, the differentiation of which is of great importance prognostically: (1) morphea, or circumscribed scleroderma, and (2) diffuse scleroderma.

Circumscribed scleroderma occurs as well-delimited, round or oval plaques with whitish, yellowish or ivory-colored centers and violaceous peripheries. Occasionally the plaques correspond in distribution to the innervation of a cutaneous nerve, and so a trophic origin has been suggested. Degeneration and regeneration of dermal nerves are said to occur with characteristic patterns in scleroderma and acrosclerosis. *Morphea guttata,* or white-spot disease, is a modification of circumscribed scleroderma characterized by varying-sized chalky-white patches on the chest and neck. Rarely does circumscribed scleroderma progress into the often fatal diffuse scleroderma. Usually the lesions clear, with a barely noticeable thin atrophic area as a residuum. Linear scleroderma of an extremity may be associated with melorheostosis, or linear hyperostosis of the underlying bone.

Diffuse scleroderma, which affects women twice as often as men, begins insidiously—usually as edema of the hands, other parts of the extremities, or neck—and extends inexorably on to sclerosis that stiffens, binds, and limits the mobility of the affected part. Ulcerations may occur over bony prominences. Calcareous cutaneous deposits and pigmentation, the latter of such a degree as to simulate Addison's disease, are frequent. The normal cutaneous lines become obliterated. Diminution in sweating, hyperesthesias, and pruritus may

occur. Sclerosis limited to the hands in association with the vasospastic symptoms of Raynaud's disease is called "acrosclerosis," or "sclerodactylia." In actuality this symptom complex presents a phase of diffuse scleroderma, though the progress to the fatal disease is not invariable. Diffuse scleroderma has been observed also occurring after silicone augmentation mammoplasty. The mechanism is speculative.

Systemic sclerosis refers to diffuse scleroderma with visceral involvement. Dense fibrosis may affect the myocardium and the esophagus and other portions of the gastrointestinal tract. The lungs may be affected with cystic fibrosis, particularly at the bases. Renal vessels may present the histologic picture of accelerated nephrosclerosis and, if widespread, will indeed be associated with malignant hypertension. The glomeruli may show conspicuous diffuse membranous glomerulonephritis. The cardiac fibrosis or the cystic pulmonary changes may lead to myocardial failure.

The histologic sections of morphea cannot be differentiated from those of diffuse scleroderma. The principal changes involve the collagenous fibers, which become hypertrophied through edema and then atrophy. The atrophic fibers are no longer loosely disposed as in the normal dermis but are compressed into dense, compact collagenous masses, with diminution of fibrocytic nuclei and obliteration of spaces between collagenous bundles so that the thickness of the dermis may in some instances actually be decreased, except in the indurative stage (Fig. 36-23). Inflammatory reaction tends to be absent, except in the early stages, when focal collections of mononuclear cells may be disposed about appendages. The appendages (hair, sweat glands, and sebaceous glands) are atrophic. Elastic fibers may be diminished or distorted, but they represent the least informative alteration and are unduly emphasized in the literature. The epidermis may be normal, but usually it is atrophic, with flattened rete ridges and a hyperpigmented basal layer. Subepidermal melanin-containing chromatophores may be increased. In conjunction with the collagenous change, small arteries and arterioles may become secondarily sclerotic. Calcific or even ossified foci (osteoma cutis) may replace the altered collagen of the dermis and subcutaneous septa. The deposits of calcium may be so extensive as to camouflage the primary diagnosis and be dismissed as calcinosis. Superficial dermal telangiectasia is common, possibly as a consequence of sclerosis of deeper vessels. The dermis of patients in the indurative phase has been found by actual measurement to be thicker and heavier than normal.[75] Mast cells have been shown to increase in the early phases and to decrease in the later phases.[66] It has been suggested that mast cells, perhaps through their histamine, may stimulate the production of collagen.

Eosinophilic fasciitis and *subcutaneous morphea* are considered subsets of scleroderma. In these there are varying degrees of edema, eosinophilia, and sclerosis of the subcutis and fascia. Atrophic myositis may accompany the cutaneous lesions, though uncommonly to the degree found in dermatomyositis or poikilodermatomyositis, in which the inflammatory reaction in the skeletal muscles may be extreme, despite the usual nondescript subepidermal edema and focal liquefaction degeneration in the latter diseases. Here again it is emphasized that neither diffuse vascular nor diffuse visceral collagenous changes occur in dermatomyositis or poikilodermatomyositis any more than they do in the majority of cases of diffuse lupus erythematosus.

CRST refers to a tetrad of findings consisting of calcinosis, Raynaud's phenomenon, sclerodactyly, and telangiectasia. Most patients with CRST eventually develop visceral involvement with esophageal dysmotility.

In view of the association between sclerosis of skin and lung (systemic sclerosis, burns, healed infarcts, and so on) on the one hand and carcinoma on the other, it may be anticipated that carcinoma of the skin would be a complication of diffuse scleroderma. This latter complication is rare and may be a reflection of the duration of the sclerosis. The association of scleroderma with a monoclonal gammopathy (Iq) has been recorded in a significant number of cases.

Scleredema. Scleredema (Buschke's disease) is to be distinguished from scleroderma. Although the entity is commonly known as scleredema adultorum, it does involve children in an appreciable percentage of cases.

Scleredema is usually a self-limited disease characterized by a tough, nonpitting, uniform edema of the head and neck, producing a masklike expression and restricted motion that simulates scleroderma. The periphery of the process is readily palpable. The disease generally runs its course in several months to a year and a half, leaving no residuum. Recurrences have been recorded.

The lesion differs from scleroderma in the rarity of involvement of the hands and feet, and complete resolution with very rare exceptions. The usually self-limited scleredema of Buschke is distinguished from the long-lasting, often extensive scleredema associated with diabetes mellitus.

The histologic picture of scleredema is that of striking edema and hypertrophy of tight collagenous bundles so that, despite the compactness of the bundles, the thickness of the dermis is distinctly increased over normal. The epidermis, vessels, elastic tissue, and muscle show no changes. The changes of *sclerema neonatorum* are altogether different from those of scleredema or scleroderma and consist in the precipitation of fatty acid crystals and foreign-body reaction in the subcutaneous fat, possibly because of a deficiency of olein in the fat, with consequent raising of its melting point. The localized, nodular sclerema, which some believe may result from birth trauma, is also self-limited. The diffuse form, which may involve also visceral (such as periadrenal and perirenal) fat, is a fatal disease. Scleredema and scleroderma are to be differentiated also from myxedema of either the circumscribed or the diffuse type.

Lipid proteinosis. Lipid proteinosis (hyalinosis cutis et mucosae) is another remarkable disease affecting dermal collagen and its vessels. The disorder generally manifests itself in infancy and is characterized by verrucous yellowish plaques, especially on the hands, feet, elbows, and face. The lesions may involve also the mouth and larynx. In the latter location the woody consistency of the lesions may cause a stenosis severe enough to require tracheotomy. Persistent hoarseness is a common symptom. Disturbances in phospholipids are inconstant. A familial tendency toward diabetes mellitus is occasionally present. It does not now appear that the entity is a primary lipidosis but rather that the lipid is normal in composition incidental to other tissue changes, especially those of collagen. One form of lipid proteinosis is light sensitive and occurs with erythropoietic porphyria.

The histologic features of lipid proteinosis are a hyperkeratotic and acanthotic epidermis overlying eosinophilic homogenized collagen in the upper dermis. The walls of arterioles and small arteries of this region are thickened. A fat stain reveals dense sudanophilic deposits in and about their wallls, as well as in the stroma. There are no foam cells such as those found in Fabry's disease (angiokeratoma corporis diffusum). The serum lipids are normal as a rule. It is stated that the fat is

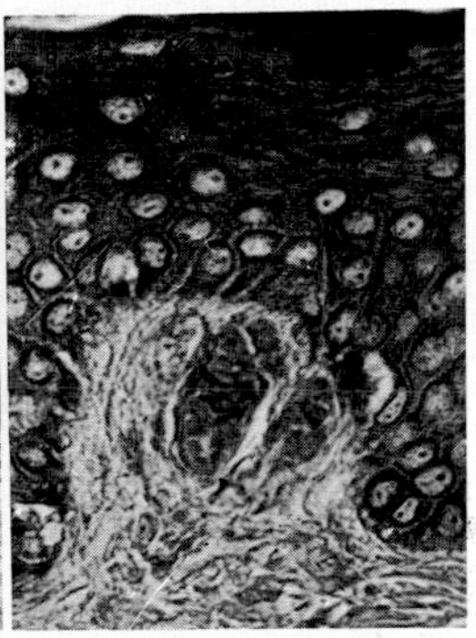

Fig. 36-24. Colloid milium with characteristic nodules of altered collagen. (Hematoxylin and eosin.)

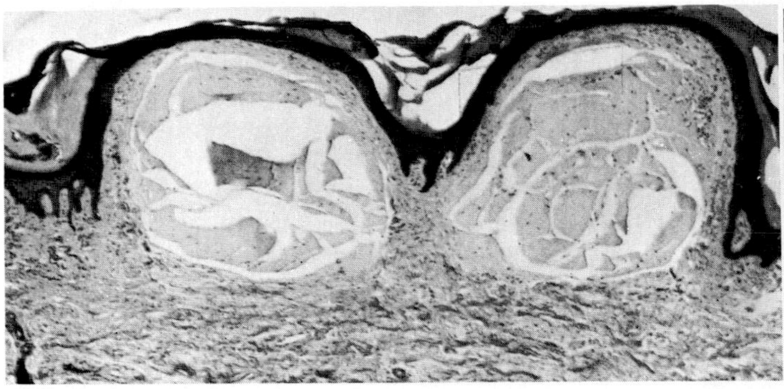

Fig. 36-25. Amyloidosis showing metachromatic focus in papilla. (Toluidine blue stain.)

combined with the protein of the collagen and therefore resists ordinary fat solvents. This property was not borne out in two cases I observed. As might be expected, the hyalinized collagen is a periodic acid–Schiff positive and diastase resistant. Lipid droplets have been noted in the basal cells by ultrastructural examination. Accordingly the entity has been designated a lipoglycoproteinosis.

Amyloidosis. Amyloidosis may be confined to the skin, or the cutaneous lesions may represent part of a systemic process. The eruption is characterized by pruritus and brownish papules, nodules, or plaques occurring particularly on the legs. Histologically there are focal areas of bland homogenization of dense collagen, occasionally scattered in the dermis but often located as subepidermal round masses (lichen amyloidosis) that stain metachromatically with the ordinary stains for amyloid (Figs. 36-24 and 36-25).

The subepidermal nodules of amyloidosis (lichen amyloidosis) tend to be restricted to the skin. The nodular, para-articular masses of amyloid, along with amyloidotic macroglossia, are likely to be a manifestation of primary amyloidosis (para-amyloidosis) and to be associated with myeloma or related plasmacytosis and globulinemias. The cutaneous manifestations of amyloidosis resulting from leprosy, tuberculosis, rheumatoid arthritis, Hodgkin's disease, and chronic suppuration may be detectable only microscopically. The amyloid of primary amyloidosis tends to resist metachromatic stains, in contrast to amyloid of secondary amyloidosis. Rarely, epidermolysis bullosa may overlie secondary amyloidosis of the skin. The notion that dermal amyloid is formed by apoptosis, or the "dropping off," from keratinocytes across the basal lamina is fancifully untenable. Nevertheless, applications of the mechanistic "apoptosis" to pathologic processes are coming to be increasingly popular in the dermatologic literature albeit with questionable justification.

The histologic picture of lichen amyloidosis may closely simulate *colloid milium*, in which there is also a homogeneous alteration, with swelling into nodular masses of the subepidermal collagen (Fig. 36-25). However, the collagen of colloid milium does not stain metachromatically, and the fibers in this disease appear looser, more edematous, and more friable than those of amyloidosis do (Fig. 36-26).

To be distinguished from amyloid are the finely granular, faintly bluish, amorphous, almost diffusely hyaline, dermal deposits or compartments of *cortisone* occurring after injections. Occasionally, birefringent crystals are present and with the granular material simulating urates may provoke an impression of a gouty tophus (Fig. 36-26). Calcification or even ossification may occur in sodium urate powder.

Circumscribed myxedema. Circumscribed or localized myxedema occurs in about 50% of patients with exophthalmic Graves' disease. It appears as a fairly demarcated nonpitting, solidly edematous, usually bilateral plaque of the pretibial region, at times extending to the dorsum of the feet. Rarely it occurs on the face and the dorsum of the hands.

Persistently elevated serum levels of long-acting thyroid stimulator (LATS) are the rule in patients with pretibial myxedema. In some instances LATS has been detected in homogenates of tissue from the affected areas in concentrations significantly higher than in unaffected tissue. It is hypothesized that LATS acts as a specific antibody that, when fixed in tissue, elicts the characteristic local edematous reaction.

Histologically, abundant basophilic mucin is found separating and fragmenting dermal collagenous bundles, without inflammatory reaction other than an occasional increase of mast cells. The diffuse myxedema of hypothyroidism is characterized by swelling of the collagenous bundles by interfibrillary mucin, which in some instances is demonstrable with Alcian or toluidine

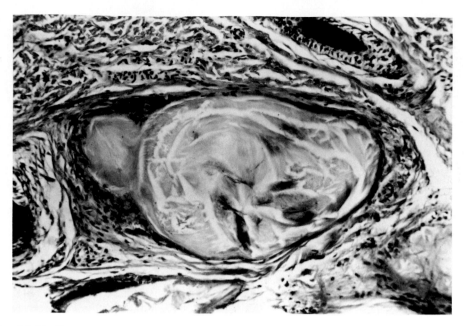

Fig. 36-26. Gout with sodium monourate crystals, mostly granular, in dermis. (Hematoxylin and eosin; 200×.) (From Allen, A.C.: The skin, St. Louis, 1954, The C.V. Mosby Co.)

blue. There is less disruption of the collagenous bundles in diffuse myxedema than in circumscribed myxedema of hyperthyroidism. These lesions are to be distinguished from the nonendocrinogenic subepidermal mucinous papules of *lichen myxedematosis* or *papular mucinosis.*

Mucinous cysts

Mucinous dermal cysts, often loosely referred to as synovial cysts or myxoid cysts, are single, smooth, firm, 5 to 6 mm nodules at the bases of distal phalanges. The overlying epidermis is likely to be slightly thinned but not otherwise significantly altered. The cyst contains a mucinous, clear material quite like that of synovial cysts, and the similarity extends to the histologic structure. The mucin is periodic acid–Schiff negative but contains large amounts of hyaluronic acid as reflected in the positive Alcian blue stain. There is no communication of these cysts with bursae or joint cavities.

Microscopically the cyst is found to be unilocular or multilocular and to be derived from a simple liquefaction of the dermal collagen, and so no mesothelial or endothelial lining is present. Such a lining may be simulated by compressed fibrocytes of the dermal collagenous fibers. Essentially this picture is analogous to that found in what are also loosely called synovial cysts of tendons or ganglions. These, too, do not represent cysts of expanded synovial walls with mesothelial lining but rather foci of mucinous degeneration of collagen of tendon or synovia. The mucinous dermal cyst may become obliterated by fibrosis and calcification.

Diseases of elastic tissue

Although alterations in elastic tissue, especially diminution and fraying, occur in many dermatoses, there are several principal, primary disorders of elastic tissue: (1) cutis hyperelastica (Ehlers-Danlos syndrome), (2) pseudoxanthoma elasticum, (3) senile elastosis, (4) elastoma dorsi, (5) elastosis perforans serpiginosa, and (6) dermatolysis (cutis laxa).

Cutis hyperelastica. Cutis hyperelastica (Ehlers-Danlos syndrome) is a familial disease characterized by hyperelastic velvety skin (rubber skin) associated with hyperlaxity and hyperextensibility of the joints and the tendency of the skin to bleed, tear, and scar after slight trauma. There are at least 10 varieties of this disorder, depending principally on the biochemical defects of both collagen and elastin and possibly also on platelets and on fibronectin, the adhesive glycoprotien that cross-links fibrin and glues it to collagen. The fibronectins are concerned also with the normal aggregation of platelets. The disorder may be associated with skeletal deformities, including arachnodactyly, blue sclerae (as in Löbstein's syndrome), dilatation of viscera (trachea, esophagus, and colon), pulmonary blebs, dissecting aneurysms, scoliosis, and easy bruisability that may be mistaken for battering.

Histologically, abundant compact masses of elastic fibers throughout the dermis are demonstrable by Weigert's stain for elastic tissue (Fig. 36-27). The suggestion that the increase in elastic fibers is illusionary rather than real has not been borne out by my observations. There appears to be no qualitative alteration in these or

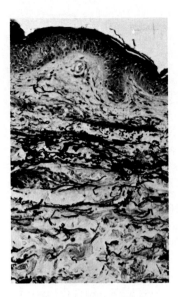

Fig. 36-27. Hyperelastosis cutis. (Weigert–van Gieson.)

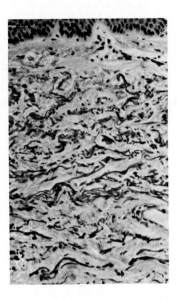

Fig. 36-28. Senile or degenerative elastosis. (Hematoxylin and eosin.)

in the collagenous fibers. The tendency for calcification, as observed in elastic fibers in pseudoxanthoma elasticum and in degenerative arterial diseases, is not apparent in the elastic fibers of Ehlers-Danlos syndrome. Edema of the superficial dermis, with disruption of the normal wavy pattern of the dermal collagenous fibers, may be observed. On the other hand, calcification within the panniculus may be present. Collagen fibrils are said to be arranged in an abnormal wickerwork, allowing for increased distensibility. This disorder has been described in dogs and minks.

Pseudoxanthoma elasticum. Pseudoxanthoma elasticum is a hereditary disease in which yellowish papules and plaques are symmetrically distributed in abnormally lax skin of the neck, axilla, groin, and cubital and popliteal spaces. Other parts of the body are less frequently involved.

In histologic sections the elastic fibers are easily detectable, even in routine preparations stained with hematoxylin and eosin, as masses of basophilic, curved, small, partially calcified fragmented curlicues, with a tendency toward concentration near the mid-dermis. Occasionally there are associated disorganized granulomas of the foreign-body type. About 50% of patients with pseudoxanthoma elasticum have ophthalmoscopically visible angioid streaks in the retina that are said to be similar to the dermal changes histologically and are attributed to cracking of Bruch's elastic membrane of the choroid. The histologic evidence, however, is limited.

Ultrastructurally an elastic fiber appears as a central amorphous core of elastin surrounded by microfibrils. Abnormal fibers show changes in size, shape, and granularity. The presence of calcium and polyanions such as sulfates or pyrophosphates is reported.

Pseudoxanthoma elasticum may be associated with changes in the cardiovascular system, including arterial aneurysms, mitral valve prolapse, and calcification and degeneration of elastic tissue of arteries. Other congenital cardiovascular, gastrointestinal, and genitourinary defects may occur with the syndrome. Rarely, it is associated with cutis hyperelastica and osteitis deformans.

Senile elastosis. Senile elastosis is the loss of elasticity of the skin of elderly people, particularly on the exposed portions of the body such as the face and the dorsum of the hands. In microscopic sections the change is represented by a subpapillary zone of basophilic alteration of swollen elastic fibers. This form of elastosis may or may not be associated with atrophy of the epidermis and appendages (Fig. 36-28). Despite the increase in elastic tissue, such skin is characterized by a loss of elasticity as if the physical properties of these fibers had been altered or as if collagenous fibers had acquired the staining properties of elastic tissue.

A subject of paramount importance, albeit seriously neglected, is dermatogerontology in all of its aspects, with morphology of collagen and elastic tissue being not the least. There is neither the space nor authenticated information to document within this chapter the changes that accompany aging.

Elastofibroma dorsi. Elastofibroma dorsi is an apparently reactive fibrous tumefaction that is localized preponderantly to the scapula and adjacent chest but occurs also near the ischial tuberosity and greater trochanter. It is firm, varies in size from about 2 to 10 cm, and develops over a period of years. The surprising histologic finding is the presence of numerous clusters of thick and fragmented elastic fibers, readily recognizable by their eosinophilia even in sections stained with hematoxylin and eosin. Although these fibers lack the periodicity of collagen and are digested with elastase, there are reasons to suggest origin from denatured collagen. These fibers, which do not contain fat or calcium, exhibit differences from those of the elastic laminae of arteries, elastotic degeneration of the skin, and pseudoxanthoma elasticum.

Elastofibroma dorsi is to be distinguished from the familial fibromas of collagenomas recently described, in which no change in the elastic tissue is noted.

Elastosis perforans serpiginosa. There is a group of disorders that have in common the gross and histologic features of transepidermal extrusion of plugs of keratin, collagen, and elastic tissue. These entities, which are commonly mistaken for one another, are known as reactive perforating collagenosis (RPC), perforating folliculitis, elastosis perforans serpiginosa, and Kyrle's disease. Elastosis perforans serpiginosa is characterized by groups of arciform or circinate, erythematous, acuminate keratotic papules, usually on the face and neck. It has been noted to develop after long courses of penicillamine therapy.

The characteristic histologic feature is compact packets of curled, frayed, thickened basophilic elastic fibers over which the epidermis is acanthotic and hyperkeratotic. The papule or plug is attributable chiefly to the penetration and extrusion of masses of elastic fibers through the epidermis.[60] Lymphocytes and foreign-body type of giant cells surround the lesion. The pattern simulates that of Kyrle's disease (hyperkeratosis follicularis in cutem penetrans), in which the extruded plugs are keratinous rather than elastic tissue. Furthermore, in Kyrle's disease the parakeratotic plug penetrates the dermis through invaginated epidermis. The lesion is not confined to follicles, is not accompanied by pseudoepitheliomatous hyperplasia, and may show a giant cell granulomatous reaction.

Cutis laxa. Cutis laxa (dermatolysis, dermatochalasis, generalized elastolysis) is a disorder of elastic tissue occurring in the heritable (mainly autosomal recessive) and acquired forms. The skin characteristically hangs in loose, nonelastic folds as if too roomy for its contained body. The fully developed lesion may be preceded by erythema, urticaria, or vesicles. The disease may be accompanied by visceral manifestations such as pulmonary emphysema, cardiac abnormalities, rectal prolapse, and diverticula of the urinary bladder. The light microscopic picture reveals strikingly abnormal fragmented, granular, wide-bellied and tapered elastic fibers often enclosing lakes of mucinous material containing acid mucopolysaccharides. The elastic fibers of the involved viscera may show similar changes.

Chondrodermatitis nodularis chronica helicis

Chondrodermatitis nodularis chronica helicis refers to painful nodule of the helix or antihelix of the ear,

characterized by central ulceration with adjacent pseudoepitheliomatous hyperplasia, perichondritis with abundant vascularization about a core of necrotic collagen, which may extrude or "perforate" to the surface. It is generally considered to be caused by persistent pressure such as that produced by telephone operators' earphones, aviators' headpieces or tight-fitting coifs. Irradiation may produce a similar picture. The absence of a fatty subcutis in this region, in which the skin is attached directly to the perichondrium, may lessen the degree of protective cushioning.

Specific granulomas

Of the specific granulomas of the skin the following should be mentioned: those caused by tuberculosis, sarcoidosis, berylliosis, leprosy, brucellosis, leishmaniasis, syphilis, and granuloma inguinale, those caused by atypical acid-fast bacilli, and those from deep fungi, such as sporotrichosis, blastomycosis, coccidioidomycosis, and histoplasmosis.

Tuberculosis cutis. Tuberculosis cutis may assume a large variety of clinical forms of which lupus vulgaris, scrofuloderma, tuberculosis cutis verrucosa, miliary cutaneous tuberculosis, and many kinds of tuberculids are a few examples. Although differing prognostic implications usually make the precise diagnosis of tuberculosis significant, the important service the pathologist is expected to render is to name the overall tuberculous process. In this the problem is complicated by the difficulty with which the sparse tubercle bacilli are demonstrable in paraffin sections of the skin, and so the tubercle is usually the chief basis for the diagnosis. Unfortunately, many agents other than tubercle bacilli are capable of producing tubercles. Moreover, the tubercle often is incompletely formed, and reliance is then placed on such suggestions as epithelioid cells clustered or palisaded in the vicinity or in a matrix of caseated tissue, with or without giant cells. The cutaneous reaction of leishmaniasis, as well as of histoplasmosis and other fungi, is often tuberculoid, but the detection of the respective organisms in histiocytes and giant cells establishes the diagnosis.

Of increasing interest are the cutaneous granulomas produced by atypical acid-fast bacilli or, more accurately, bacilli that although acid fast are basically different from *Myocobacterium tuberculosis* in drug sensitivity as well as in cultural and pathogenic respects. Runyon's classification of these strains into four groups—photochromogens (such as *Mycobacterium balnei*), scotochromogens, Battey strain, and rapid growers—is a workable one. Not all of the granulomas produced by these organisms have a tuberculoid structure histologically. Some appear quite nonspecific.

Sarcoidosis. The histologic diagnosis of Boeck's sarcoid is based on the finding of dermal hyperplastic tubercles, with or without giant cells and Schaumann's or asteroid bodies but in the absence of caseation. Usually the tubercules are surrounded by dense bands of collagenous stroma. No tubercle bacilli are detectable. The term "Darier-Roussy sarcoid" is reserved for an essentially similar histologic process occurring in the deep dermis and subcutaneous fat, thereby resembling erythema induratum. Confusion arises from the simulation of the tuberculous process by the tissue reaction in the tuberculoid form of leprosy, in the syphilitic gumma, and by the tissue response in blastomycosis, coccidioidomycosis, leishmaniasis, and sporotrichosis. Moreover, in some instances of sarcoid a form of fibrinoid degeneration simulating caseation may occur (p. 978).

A diagnostic test for sarcoidosis, called the "Kveim test," consists in injecting intradermally a brei of tissue known to be involved with Boeck's sarcoid and observing the delayed clinical and tuberculoid histologic reaction to the injection several weeks later. Sarcoidosis is rare in children.

Berylliosis and brucellosis. The granulomas of berylliosis (usually acquired by inoculation of the beryllium phosphors from broken fluorescent lamps) and those of brucellosis may be histologically indistinguishable from those of sarcoidosis or tuberculosis. Silica granulomas are distinguished by the presence of birefringent silica crystals within giant cells. Zirconium in stick deodorants may also cause giant cell granulomas.

Other granulomas. The remainder of the granulomatous lesions, including those of leprosy, syphilis and other venereal diseases, the deep mycoses, and parasitic infestation, are discussed in other chapters.

PIGMENTATIONS

The abnormalities of cutaneous pigmentation may be considered under two principal categories: metallic and nonmetallic.

Metallic abnormalities of cutaneous pigmentation

The exogenous pigmentations are chiefly those from metals introduced into the body in a variety of ways, including ingestion, parenteral administration, inunction, and intradermal injection. In general, the metallic pigmentations provoke at least an increased deposition of melanin in the basal layer and in dermal chromatophores. The brown arsenic pigmentation caused particularly by the ingestion of trivalent arsenicals (in Fowler's solution, sodium cacodylate, or arsenic trioxide) often is associated with keratosis of the palms and soles. Histologically there is relative hyperkeratosis with atrophy of the remainder of the epidermis, hyperchromatism, and a tendency toward palisading of the basal cells and increased melanin deposits in these cells as well as in the chromatophores of the upper dermis, which usually is edematous. Late complications include Bowen's disease and squamous and basal cell carcinomas.

Argyria, in which the skin is discolored bluish gray, may occur after the ingestion of silver nitrate, formerly used in the treatment of peptic ulcers, or the application of this drug as well as colloidal silver compounds (Argyrol and Neo-Silvol) to mucous membranes. The pigmentation is particularly noticeable in areas of the skin exposed to light. The black granules of silver are noted especially in the argyrophilic basement membrane of the sweat glands but also in the connective tissue about sebaceous glands and hair follicles and just beneath the epidermis.

Chrysiasis, from the parenteral use of gold preparations, causes an ash-gray or mauve pigmentation characterized histologically by irregular, large granules located chiefly in chromatophores and in the walls of blood vessels. A somewhat similar histologic picture is caused by pigmentation from bismuth and mercury.

In *tattoos* the pigmentation is the result of the deposition of various metallic and vegetable pigments (such as cinnabar or red mercuric sulfide) both within chromatophores and extracellularly in irregularly large clumps sometimes surrounded by foreign-body reaction (Fig. 36-29). *Discoid lupus erythematosus* may selectively involve the red areas of tattoos (mercuric sulfide) and spare the blue. Similarly, persons sensitive to mercury may show allergic reactions in the red portions. In contrast, syphilitic lesions may spare these mercury-impregnated red components of tattoos.

Nonmetallic abnormalities of cutaneous pigmentation

The nonmetallic abnormalities of cutaneous pigmentation include those attributable to hemochromatosis, Addison's disease, pellagra, Peutz-Jeghers syndrome,

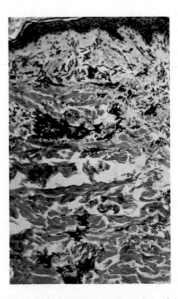

Fig. 36-29. Tattoo with irregular deposits of black-appearing pigment. (Hematoxylin and eosin.)

acanthosis nigricans, chloasma, melanosis of Riehl, ephelides (freckles), sunburn, purpuras, tinea versicolor, and pinta. Several of these entities illustrate once again the cutaneous reflection of visceral disease.

In *hemochromatosis* (bronze diabetes) hemosiderin and, less noticeably, hemofuscin are deposited as brownish granules in melanophores, principally and diagnostically about sweat glands. In addition there is increased melanin in the epidermis and adjacent chromatophores. This cutaneous lesion is commonly associated with deposits of the pigments in the pancreas, liver, and lymph nodes and the development of diabetes mellitus and cirrhosis of the liver. The most deeply pigmented areas are the exposed surfaces but may include also the genital regions and mucous membranes in 10% to 15% of cases.

In *Wilson's disease* (hepatolenticular degeneration) the pigmentation takes the form of epidermal melanosis favoring the anterior portions of the legs.

In *Addison's disease* there is an excessive deposit of melanin in the basal layer of the epidermis and in underlying melanophores. A similar histologic picture is found in the ordinary freckled (ephelis), sunburn, and chloasma (the latter especially during pregnancy).

Melanosis of Riehl, often associated with malnutrition, is characterized by brown macular discoloration of the face, neck, and occasionally hands. Histologically there is irregular pigmentation by melanin of the basal layer and chromatophores, in addition to telangiectasis, varying degrees of hyperkeratosis, liquefaction degeneration of the basal layer, and partial obliteration of the rete ridges. A similar picture is seen in tar melanosis, an occupational dermatosis probably concerned with photosensitization.

The *Peutz-Jeghers syndrome* consists in melanosis of the lips, oral mucosa, and digits in patients with gastrointestinal polyposis and occasional carcinomas.

The association of dermatoses with intestinal disorders is a facet of dermatology that is as intriguing as it is puzzling. A partial list of such dermatoses includes, in addition to the Peutz-Jeghers syndrome, acrodermatitis enteropathica, dermatitis herpetiformis, Fabry's disease, and pyoderma gangrenosum (with idiopathic ulcerative colitis), systemic lupus erythematosus, and systemic sclerosis. In some of the diseases the nature of the relationship is clear but variable for obvious reasons; in others the connection is enigmatic.

Increased pigmentation of the skin follows a variety of cutaneous purpuras: purpura annularis telangiectodes (Majocchi's disease), Schamberg's disease, and pigmented purpuric lichenoid dematitis of Gougerot and Blum. Each of these disorders occurs selectively on the lower extremities. The pigment in these cases is hemosiderin, which is deposited in chromatophores in the upper dermis. Angioma serpiginosum, which is also rather loosely included in the category of cutaneous purpuras, is really an inflammatory telangiectasia and usually shows little or no hemosiderin. In all these purpuras, which are unassociated with systemic disorders, there are inflammatory cells (principally lymphocytes and histiocytes) localized in the upper dermis, especially about arterioles and capillaries, which may have swollen, prominent endothelium. This latter finding is particularly true of Majocchi's disease. There is some question as to whether these conditions are actually different phases of the same basic vascular disease. Occasionally these purpuric lesions, particularly those of Majocchi's disease, may be confused histologically with the vascular changes of polyteritis nodosa or bacterial and rickettsial arteritis. The changes of thromboangiitis obliterans and of thrombophlebitis migrans are discussed elsewhere (pp. 777 and 789).

Achromia should be mentioned among the abnormalities of cutaneous pigmentation. The congenital absence of pigment is referred to as partial or complete albinism, or leukoderma. Vitiligo, or acquired leukoderma, is usually of unknown cause. The depigmented patches may be rimmed by hyperpigmented borders, and the histologic sections reveal the depigmented and hyperpigmented basal layers in the respective portions. Vitiliginous areas may occur also in any lesion in which there is considerable liquefaction degeneration of the basal layer and encroachment onto this layer by inflammatory cells. Pinta and lichen planus are cases in point. In both, the melanin is extracted from the basal layer, phagocytosed by chromatophores, and carried away to regional lymph nodes. Vitiliginous patches occur in patients with tinea versicolor, partly because the areas affected by the fungus prevent absorption of ultraviolet irradiation and partly because the fungus itself actively causes a degree of depigmentation. In skin that has been planed for scars of acne there is a tendency for the unabraded skin to become hyperpigmented and for the abraded epidermis to regenerate with less pigmentation than the original.

Generalized lentiginosis ("leopard syndrome") is an autosomal dominantly inherited disorder that may occur alone or with associated deficiencies such as mental retardation, skeletal defects, short stature, ocular hypertelorism, deafness, pulmonary stenosis, atrial myxomas, and others. There is no clear study of the malignant potential of the lentigines.

DISEASES OF APPENDAGES

Limitations of space permit no more than a brief mention of the nonneoplastic diseases of the cutaneous appendages.

Sweat glands

The disorders of the sweat glands include hyperhidrosis, congenital or acquired hypohidrosis, miliaria (prickly heat and tropical or thermogenic hypohidrosis with plugging of the sweat ducts by hydropic edematous epithelium), bromhidrosis (fetid sweat), chromhidrosis (colored sweat), hidradenitis suppurativa of the apocrine glands, and Fox-Fordyce disease (pruritic papular chronic adenitis of the sweat glands of the axillae, nipples, and pubic and perineal regions).

Sebaceous glands

The diseases of the sebaceous glands include varieties of seborrhea, hyposteatosis or diminished secretion, comedones, acne in its several forms, and rhinophyma.

Hair

The abnormal conditions of the hair are many. Hypertrichosis, the alopecias of the cicatricial types (pseudopelade, folliculitis decalvans, and chronic lupus erythematosus of the scalp) and the noncicatricial types (alopecia areata, ordinary male baldness, fungal infections), fragile hairs (fragilitas crinium), trichorrhexis nodosa, pili torti (twisted hairs), fungal infections such as piedra and trichomycosis nodosa, and trichostasis spinulosa (multiple lanugo hairs in a single follicle) constitute a few of the problems.

One of the more interesting disorders of hair follicles is alopecia mucinosa or follicular mucinosis (Fig. 36-30). Histologically it is characterized initially by intracellular and subsequently extracellular mucin within the hair sheaths, perifollicular inflammatory cells, and loss of hair shafts. The mucin stains with Alcian blue and is periodic acid–Schiff negative. The significant fact concerning this lesion is that in persons over 40 years of age it is strong presumptive evidence of the early stage of mycosis fungoides.[7,10]

Eosinophilic pustular folliculitis is a recently de-

scribed disorder of unknown cause, characterized by erythematous pruritic sterile papules anularly arranged mainly on the trunk, face, and arms; palms and soles may be affected. Histologically abscesses composed of eosinophils with a few mononuclear cells and neutrophils plug the infundibula of the hair follicles and some sebaceous glands involving the epidermis as well. There is also an accompanying peripheral eosinophilia in most patients ranging from 5% to 40%.

Nails

The diseases of the nails are of particular interest not only for the involvement of the nails themselves but also for the accessory information they reflect on systemic disorders. *Beau's lines* are transverse furrows in the nail that date periods of arrested function of the matrix resulting from severe acute illnesses or inflammations near the nail folds.

The discoloration and the thickening of the nail from psoriasis, eczema, or fungi; the spoon nails (koilonychia) associated with trauma, eczema, and the Plummer-Vinson syndrome; the brittleness (onychorrhexis) after the use of certain chemicals or in vitamin A deficiency; the loss of nails (onycholysis) after trauma or systemic diseases such as hypothyroidism; and the whitening of nails (leukonychia) are some of the possible changes.

The yellow nail syndrome is associated with lymphedema and pleural effusions and at times with ascites. The nails not only are discolored yellow but also show transverse ridging, onycholysis, curving, and defective cuticles.

PANNICULITIS

Several diseases of the subcutaneous fat closely simulate each other histologically but have different prognostic and etiologic implications.

Erythema induratum

Erythema induratum appears as chronic, recurring, often ulcerated, bluish red nodules (of the calves of the legs particularly). The lesions generally are found in patients with frank tuberculosis elsewhere. Histologically tubercles, usually of an incomplete or atypical variety, are found in the subcutaneous fat. Caseation may be present. Fat necrosis and fat atrophy associated with nonspecific inflammation of the fibrous septa, fat, and lower dermis are present. Endarterial and endophlebitic inflammation and proliferation are seen commonly. Tubercle bacilli are rarely found in these lesions, though positive results have been reported from guinea pig inoculation of the tissue.

The term "lipomembranous" or "membranocytic" refers to the liquefactive or cystic foci of fat necrosis, attributable to whatever cause, in which the cysts are contained by membranous envelopes of compressed fibrofatty tissue.

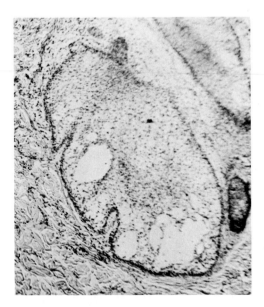

Fig. 36-30. Follicular mucinosis from patient with mycosis fungoides. (Hematoxylin and eosin.)

Factitious panniculitis, which is becoming more frequent, may be induced by the injection of foreign material (feces, milk, drugs, saliva, mineral oil) in accessible sites. The reaction—giant cell, fat necrosis, inflammatory, purpuric—may simulate one of a variety of panniculitides. Still another form of panniculitis is attributable to *alpha_1-antitrypsin deficiency* in which the primary histologic focus is the collagen both of the dermis and the pannicular septa. The dissolution of the collagen may lead to liquefaction necrosis even with transepidermal elimination of some of the necrotic material.

Subacute nodular migratory panniculitis

Subacute nodular migratory panniculitis, which may follow acute infections such as tonsillitis, appears similar to erythema induratum histologically.

Nodular, nonsuppurative, febrile, relapsing panniculitis (Weber-Christian disease)

Nodular, nonsuppurative, febrile, relapsing panniculitis is observed preponderantly in women and is characterized by bluish discoloration of the skin over firm subcutaneous nodules on the extremities and trunk, usually associated with otherwise unexplained fever. Isolated cases have responded to chemotherapy (sulfapyridine and penicillin). Fatalities have occurred in several cases, but autopsy findings were not especially enlightening except for the steatitis in the pretracheal, mediastinal, and retroperitoneal regions. The recently recorded instances of mesenteric panniculitis appear unrelated.

In sections from patients with what are regarded as typical cases, the fat itself is infiltrated chiefly with lymphocytes and histiocytes, but the septa are relatively spared. Wucher atrophy of fat (replacement of atrophied fat by fat-laded histiocytes), foreign-body giant cell reaction, and endophlebitis and endarteritis are also present. However, the septa, though relatively spared, often are infiltrated and edematous. Therefore the involvement of the septa cannot be used as a criterion for excluding the possibility of Weber-Christian disease. If they are free, the evidence is considerable that the panniculitis belongs to this category (Fig. 36-31).

Although "nonsuppurative" is included in the name of the entity, the fact is that sterile abscesses occasionally are noted along with cystic liquefaction necrosis and focal calcification. It has been suggested that Weber-Christian disease has diverse causes and in some instances is attributable to pancreatitis.

Erythema nodosum

Erythema nodosum occurs clinically as tender, pale red to livid nodules, principally on the anterior aspect of the lower extremities. These lesions, unlike those of erythema induratum, do not ulcerate, are transient, lasting only for several weeks on an average, and are not necessarily associated with a tuberculous process elsewhere. The disease may be one manifestation of a variety of unrelated infections, including coccidioidomycosis, leprosy, syphilis, viral diseases (measles, cat-scratch fever), and ringworm, or it may follow lymphomas, the ingestion of drugs, or the administration of a vaccine.

The histologic picture of erythema nodosum is much

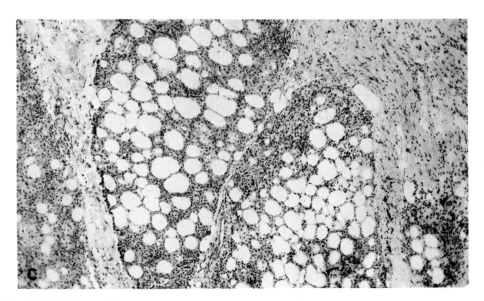

Fig. 36-31. Weber-Christian disease showing lymphocytic infiltration preponderantly of the fat rather than of the interlobular fibrous septa. (Hematoxylin and eosin.) (From Allen, A.C.: The skin, St. Louis, 1954, The C.V. Mosby Co.)

like that of erythema induratum with the addition that there is a greater tendency in erythema nodosum for nonspecific inflammation of the middle and lower dermis, which is usually spared in erythema induratum.

Subcutaneous fat necrosis of the newborn (localized sclerema neonatorum) is a rare entity observed during the first month of life. It has been variously attributed to obstetrical trauma, neonatal asphyxia and maternal diabetes. There appears to be an enigmatic, occasionally lethal, association with hypercalcemia. As in sclerema, the histologic picture is characterized by radially arranged needle-shaped clefts within fat cells along with foreign-body type of giant cells, macrophages, and lymphocytes. Unlike sclerema neonatorum, there are no deposits of calcium, fat necrosis is sparse, and wide fibrous bands are present in the panniculus.

Sclerema neonatorum is an uncommon reaction consisting in diffuse hardening of the panniculus with a serious, debilitating effect on the infant's well-being. The prominent histologic feature consists of needle-shaped clefts within the fat cells. These clefts represent the spaces left by birefringent crystals (in frozen sections) dissolved by the fat solvents (such as xylol) during the processing of the tissue. There is said to be an increased amount of saturated fatty acids in the fat with resultant higher melting and solidification points. Visceral fat (such as perirenal and retroperitoneal) may also be involved.

Lipoatrophy is characterized clinically by well-defined depressions in the skin and histologically by small lipocytes enclaved in eosinophilic myxoid fibrous tissue vascularized by small capillaries with a scarcity of inflammatory cells.

Nodular vasculitis

Nodular vasculitis occurs chiefly in older women and refers to the often recurrent nodosities that are more painful, are of shorter duration, and have less tendency to ulcerate than the lesions of erythema induratum. The histologic picture of nodular vasculitis is the same as that of Bazin's disease (erythema induratum).

Erythema pernio

Erythema pernio ('chilblain') occurs usually on the hands and feet as tender, red, pruritic macules provoked by cold. The histologic picture may closely simulate that of erythema induratum, as may the lesions produced in response to cold allergy.

Miscellaneous forms

Miscellaneous forms of panniculitis include those resulting from trauma, insulin injections, pancreatitis, allergic reactions (including those occurring after insect bites), angiitis, cold agglutinins, and sclerosing lipogranulomas.

Actually the sharp artificial segregation of the panniculitides characteristic of the bulk of the dermatologic literature appears unwarranted by the histologic evidence of transitional merging of supposedly definitive criteria. This statement of confluence of diagnosis applies particularly to acute and chronic erythema nodosum, erythema nodosum migrans, nodular vasculitis, and often erythema induratum. This is so because tuberculoid or foreign-body type of granulomas, phlebitis and arteritis, involvement or lack of involvement of septa or lobules, and the presence of microabscesses may characterize any of these entities. Otherwise, it is the weight given to one or other features, integrated with the clinical details, that leads to more informative diagnoses.

VASCULAR DISORDERS

There is a broad spectrum of vascular disorders in which the skin plays a prominent clinical and at times diagnostic role. A few of these are mentioned in Chapter 17. Additional ones, with probable or clear-cut vascular involvement, include the cutaneous lesions of rheumatic fever, subacute bacterial endocarditis, typhus fevers and other infections, Degos's syndrome, allergenic vasculitides, necrobiosis lipoidica diabeticorum, the vascular changes of diabetes mellitus and hypertension, granuloma annulare, rheumatoid granuloma, Mucha-Habermann disease, urticaria, and the purpuric dermatoses.

Acute, often necrotizing arteriolitis with karyorrhexis of polymorphonuclear neutrophil leukocytes (*leukocytoclasis*), deposition of immune complexes, hypocomplementemia, cryoglobulinemia, and arthralgia have been linked as a syndrome. Immunoglobulins and complement were demonstrable in the vessels of the skin before the infiltration of leukocytes in the development of clinical lesions.[63] Moreover, IgA has been demonstrated in the acutely inflamed dermal arterioles in purpuric hyperglobulinemia of Waldenström. This local finding was associated with elevated circulating levels of IgA and is suggestive of the immunologic pathogenesis (Fig. 36-32).

Immunofluorescence studies of dermal vasculitis promise diagnostic and pathogenic clues. At present IgG, IgM, IgA, and several components of complement have been demonstrated in and about vessels (as in Henoch-Schönlein purpura), but their full significance remains to be determined. Leukocytoclastic vasculitis of the skin may in fact occur in association with hairy leukemia in the absence of leukemic involvement of the skin. Moreover it is being observed increasingly in association with cryoglobulinemia and one or other lymphoma as well as Hodgkin's disease or Waldenström's macroglobulinemia. This is the same lesion provoked by such drugs as thiazides, diuretics, sulfonamides,

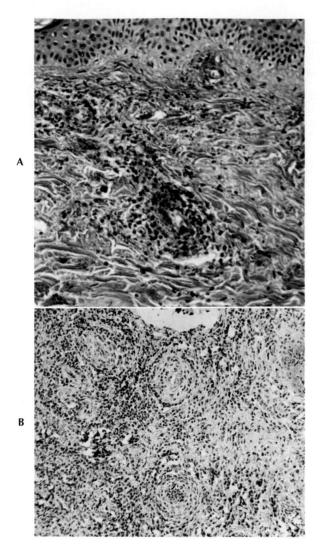

Fig. 36-32. A, Leukocytoclastic arteriolitis in upper dermis. **B,** Chancre showing characteristic acute endarteritis obliterans. (**A** and **B,** Hematoxylin and eosin.) (From Allen, A.C.: The skin, St. Louis, 1954, The C.V. Mosby Co.)

penicillin, and serum in sensitive patients. Leukocytoclastic vasculitis may be associated also with Sjögren's syndrome and attributed to autoantibody systems. The lesion is usually designated "vasculitis" because the identity of the involved vessel is not established. Often it is referred to as "venulitis" when the vessel is cut along its longitudinal axis and is thin-walled, therefore appearing venous. The fact is that in many instances the affected vessels are arterioles and their nature is identifiable by the thicker muscular wall with fibrinoid necrosis (as well as leukocytoclasia). When accompanied by arthritis, gastrointestinal manifestations, and purpura, it is labeled *Henoch-Schönlein purpura* when no cause is found. The lesion is similar to that of the Arthus reaction or Shwartzman phenomenon and attrib-

uted to the deposition of immune complexes. *Cholesterol crystal embolization* (CCE) to the arteries of the skin occurs among the elderly and may manifest itself by cutaneous purpura and ulcers.

Angiolymphoid hyperplasia with eosinophilia (Kimura's disease)

The lesion termed "angiolymphoid hyperplasia with eosinophilia" usually starts as a papule or a cluster of papules in the skin of the head and neck of adults. This lesion is as extraordinary in its behavior as it is in its histologic features. On occasion the lesions may recur after excision or may spread uncontrollably to cover much of the face in the manner of a fulminant angiosarcoma. Histologically the characteristic features include dilated dermal thin-walled vascular sprouts with conspicuously hypertrophic, practically diagnostic endothelial cells with vesicular nuclei and abundant eosinophilic cytoplasm (Fig. 36-33). Often the endothelial cells appear clustered beside or at one end of a vessel that has been cut obliquely and in this pattern simulate masses of histiocytes. The stroma also is characteristically structured with loosely disposed eosinophilic leukocytes, histiocytes, lymphocytes, and mast cells. These cells are strongly positive for adenosine triphosphatase, indoxyl esterase, and nicotinamide adenine dinucleotide but negative for alkaline phosphatase, a pattern characteristic of endothelial cells.[19]

A form of superficial, subcutaneous thrombophlebitis known as "Mondor's disease" is characterized clinically by a linear, cordlike induration with an overlying cutaneous groove extending usually from the axilla toward the nipple. The lesion may be mistaken for a neoplasm clinically.

Thrombocytopenic verrucal angionecrosis (thrombotic thrombocytopenic purpura, TTP)

Of great interest is another truly diffuse vascular disease characterized by thrombocytopenia, purpura, a usually fulminant, fatal course (though rare protracted cases have occurred), and a specific histologic picture of fibrinoid necrosis and platelet-like verrucal thickening of the walls of dilated arterioles and capillaries. In the past the disease has been called "generalized platelet thrombosis" or some variant of this term. However, the histogenesis of the entire lesion from the vascular walls would seem to make the designation "thrombocytopenic verrucal angionecrosis"[5,7,10] more appropriate, as long ago suggested. These cases are rarely diagnosed clinically. Inasmuch as the vascular necrosis occurs in the skin as well as the viscera, a skin, mucosal, marrow, or muscle biopsy is called for in obscure instances of thrombocytopenic purpura. There is strongly impressive clinical and histologic evidence of a factor of hypersensitivity in this primarily diffuse vascular disease. Ac-

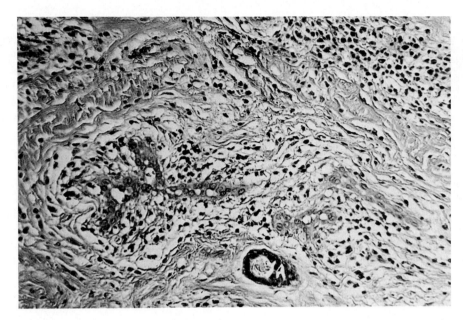

Fig. 36-33. Angiolymphoid hyperplasia with eosinophilia (Kimura's disease). Prominence of endothelium is evident. (Hematoxylin and eosin.)

cordingly, it should be attributed to an immunoreactive response rather than to depletion by so-called generalized thrombosis, which, as already indicated and despite certain immunofluorescence studies, does not occur.

In the syndrome called "disseminated intravascular coagulation" (DIC) the coagulating factors normally residing in the blood are assumed to be depleted by universally distributed clots in small vessels. The widespread presence of such clots has simply not been documented.

POEMS SYNDROME

An unusual multisystemic disorder now referred to as the "POEMS syndrome" is characterized by polyneuropathy, organomegaly, endocrinopathy, M-protein, and skin involvement. The cutaneous lesions include hyperpigmentation, hypertrichosis, thickening of the skin, hyperhidrosis, anasarca, white nails, and capillary *angiomas*.

XANTHOSES

The xanthoses may be classified as follows:
1. Normolipemic
   a. Juvenile xanthoma (or xanthogranuloma)
   b. Xanthoma disseminatum
2. Hyperlipemic
   a. Xanthoma diabeticorum
   b. Xanthoma tuberosum multiplex (Fig. 36-34)
   c. Xanthoma eruptiva (in association with lipid nephrosis, von Gierke's disease, diabetes mel-

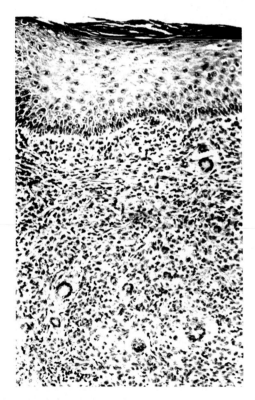

Fig. 36-34. Xanthoma tuberosum with numerous lipid histiocytes, some of which are congregated as Touton giant cells. (Hematoxylin and eosin.)

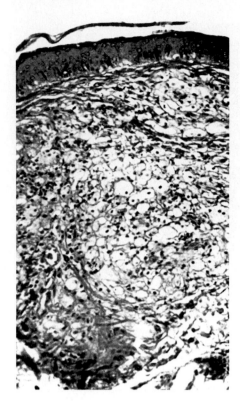

Fig. 36-35. Xanthelasma of eyelid with lipid-filled histiocytes. (Hematoxylin and eosin.)

litus, biliary cirrhosis, hypothyroidism, idiopathic hyperlipemia)

   d. Xanthelasma (approximately 50% with hyperlipemia) (Fig. 36-35)

   e. Xanthoma planum (approximately 50% with hyperlipemia) (in association with biliary cirrhosis, diabetes mellitus, myeloma, and other dysproteinemias)

Other dermatoses characterized by the presence of lipid include lipid proteinosis, angiokeratoma of Fabry, necrobiosis lipoidica diabeticorum, lipid dermatoarthritis (reticulohistiocytoma), Hand-Schüller-Christian disease, and Neimann-Pick disease. These are described elsewhere in this book. It is relevant to record that in 1954 I stressed that Hand-Schüller-Christian disease as well as eosinophilic granuloma are entities basically unrelated to histiocytosis X (malignant histiocytosis), a view that subsequently has been propelled by a few others.[7]

Of course, many patients with xanthoses associated with hyperlipidemia are at increased risk for the development prematurely, some with fatal coronary disease even in childhood. This fact underscores the importance of the definitive recognition of the xanthoses.

Many of the lesions included in this classification are often classified with neoplasms. Actually, none is really a neoplasm in the usual sense of neoplasia. Most are obviously a reflection of disordered metabolism of lipids or lipoproteins, but it would constitute no major contribution to discard the term "xanthoma." The differentiation of these various xanthoses is often important from the prognostic and therapeutic viewpoints, though in many instances the distinction cannot be made on the basis of histology alone. Moreover, several of these types of lesions often are combined in the same patient.

RETICULOHISTIOCYTOMA (RETICULOHISTIOCYTIC GRANULOMA)

The entity "reticulohistiocytoma," which was so named in 1948, produces remarkable lesions, the extent and nature of which are still being investigated.[5,7,10] Because of the association with arthritis, it has more recently been designated "lipid dermatoarthritis."[2] Originally this condition was believed to be limited to the skin and was regarded as a form of ganglioneuroma because of the superficial simulation of ganglion cells by the histiocytes.

Clinically the disease is characterized by cutaneous papules and nodules (rarely solitary) and often by an associated disabling polyarthritis. The nodules may resemble xanthomas, and indeed xanthelasma is present in about one fourth of the patients.

Histologically the cutaneous lesions are characterized by histiocytes with abundant basophilic cytoplasm intermingled with lymphocytes and occasionally scattered eosinophilic leukocytes (Fig. 36-36). The infiltrate tends to be confined to the upper dermis, with resulting moderate atrophy of the overlying epidermis. The cytoplasm of the histiocytes reacts positively with Sudan black B and periodic acid–Schiff stains and is presumed to contain a glycolipid.

ANGIOLIPOMA

There are two types of angiolipomas: (1) noninfiltrating or encapsulated and (2) infiltrating. In both there is likely to be associated pain or tenderness. The infiltrating angiolipomas tend to occur on the extremities and to ramify into the skeletal muscle. They may occur also in the spinal region and cause erosion of portions of vertebrae with resulting neurologic problems. Unlike liposarcomas, the infiltrating angiolipomas lack atypia of the fat cells. Fibrolipomas of infancy commonly show deceptive atypia.

ATYPICAL FIBROXANTHOMA

There has been considerable interest in the past few years in an ulceronodular lesion of the exposed skin (chiefly the ears and cheeks) of elderly people. The lesion has been called "atypical fibroxanthoma" and resembles an anaplastic sarcoma with spindle cells and multinucleated giant cells, as well as bizarre cells with

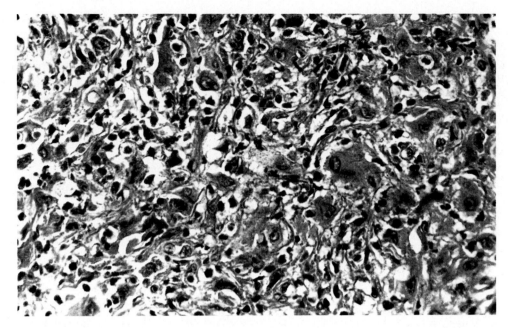

Fig. 36-36. Reticulohistiocytoma, illustrating histiocytes with abundant homogeneous cytoplasm loosely admixed with few lymphocytes and eosinophilic leukocytes. (Hematoxylin and eosin.)

single, large hyperchromatic nuclei, mitoses (often abnormal, tripolar), and some intracellular lipid. The striking feature is the disparity between the histologic anaplasia and the benign course in most instances. Some of these are undoubtedly nonpigmented spindle cell melanocarcinomas. Fat may be present in melanocarcinomas.[7,10]

Although these lesions were originally considered benign, instances of metastasis are accumulating. Undoubtedly more such instances will follow and, in my judgment, for the reason that they represent either spindle cell epidermoid carcinomas or malignant melanomas. The origin from the overlying epidermis may be easily missed because this pivotal evidence is often obscure or minimal in spindle cell epidermoid carcinomas and melanocarcinomas of the ear, in which the epidermis may be thinned or ulcerated. S-100 protein is found sparsely and inconstantly in atypical fibroxanthomas.

Dorfman-Chanarin syndrome

A recently described lipidosis, the Dorfman-Chanarin syndrome, is rare and characterized by generalized ichthyosis with hepatomegaly, splenomegaly, and mental retardation reported, so far, in normolipemic families of Jewish Iraqi origin. Of great interest are the lipid vacuoles in the basal cells of the epidermis. Lipid has been found also in the dermis, muscle, leukocytes in the peripheral blood, and liver. Further biochemical studies are obviously required.

NEOPLASMS OF SKIN

The following classification of neoplasms of the skin is based on the segregation of cutaneous neoplasms with respect to their location and histogenesis from epidermis, dermis and appendages. In the ensuing discussion several of the lesions are taken out of the order of the outline for purposes of clarity of presentation.

   I. Epidermis
     A. Benign
       1. Verruca (including vulgaris, digitata, filiformis, plantaris, and juvenilis)
       2. Seborrheic keratosis
       3. Condyloma acuminatum
       4. Keratoacanthoma
       5. Junctional nevus
       6. Clear cell acanthoma
     B. Precancerous
       1. Senile keratosis
       2. Leukoplakia (with atypia)
       3. Xeroderma pigmentosum
       4. Bowen's disease
       5. Erythroplasia of Queyrat
     C. Malignant
       1. Basal cell carcinoma
       2. Squamous cell carcinoma
       3. Melanocarcinoma (malignant melanoma)
       4. Extramammary "Paget's" disease
       5. Atypical fibroxanthoma
  II. Dermis
     A. Nevus

1. Intradermal nevus (common mole)
2. Compound nevus (dermis and epidermis)
3. Juvenile melanoma (Spitz's nevus) (dermis and epidermis)
4. Blue nevus (Jadassohn-Tièche)

B. Tumors of vessels
   1. Lymphangioma
   2. Hemangioma
   3. Angiokeratoma (dermis and epidermis)
   4. Glomus tumor
   5. Hemangiopericytoma
   6. Kaposi's idiopathic hemorrhagic sarcoma
   7. Postmastectomy lymphangiosarcoma
   8. Sclerosing hemangioma (dermatofibroma lenticulare)
   9. Dermatofibrosarcoma protuberans
   10. Angiosarcoma

C. Fibroma and fibrosarcoma
D. Neurofibroma and neurofibrosarcoma
E. Tumors of muscle
   1. Leiomyoma (arrectores pilorum)
   2. Angiomyoma
   3. Myoblastoma (genesis?)
F. Osteoma
G. Xanthomas (discussed in previous section)
H. Lymphomas and allied diseases
I. Metastatic neoplasms

III. Appendages
A. Sweat glands
   1. Adenoma or epithelioma
      a. Ductal
      b. Glandular
   2. Carcinoma
B. Sebaceous glands
   1. Adenoma
   2. Carcinoma
C. Hair follicles
   1. Brooke's tumor—trichoepithelioma or epithelioma adenoides cysticum
   2. Trichilemmoma
D. Miscellaneous cysts
   1. Dermoid
   2. Epidermoid
   3. Pilosebaceous
   4. Calcifying epithelioma (pilomatricoma, pilomatrixoma)
   5. Trichilemmal cyst

Benign lesions of epidermis
Verruca (wart)

Verrucae, or warts, represent thickenings or projections of epidermis to which are traditionally, if inconsistently, applied one of several adjectives in accordance with the shape, location, or other clinical feature of the lesion: verruca vulgaris, verruca plantaris, verruca digitata, verruca filiformis, verruca plana juvenilis, and verruca senilis.

The verruca vulgaris is the papillary wart common in children and found especially on the fingers, palms, and forearms. They occur singly or in groups. There is some question as to whether these tumors merit inclusion under neoplasms, inasmuch as they may disappear spontaneously or, as in some reported cases, under psychotherapy or with placebos. The possibility that these lesions are caused by viruses is still strongly considered and fortified by evidence from electron microscopy of viral particles. Wart-virus antibodies, measured by immunodiffusion and complement-fixation techniques, are detectable in a high percentage of cases. The warts associated with complement-fixing antibodies seem to disappear more quickly than those with antibodies determined by immunodiffusion techniques. The titers of such antibodies as well as the effects of cell-mediated immunity may be factors in the "spontaneous" regression of warts. The prevention and resolution of warts have been attributed also to cell-mediated immunity.[64]

Exposure to ultraviolet (UV) rays may initiate the development of warts in chronically immunosuppressed patients, in whom the ultraviolet is presumed to act as a cofactor with the human papillomavirus. Genital warts may develop also in patients immunosuppressed in association with renal transplants, in the absence of ultraviolet rays as a cofactor.

Butchers' warts are infected with several kinds of papillomaviruses associated with somewhat varying histologic pictures.

Histologically the verruca vulgaris is characterized by a papillary acanthosis surmounted by friable keratotic material. The cells of the stratum granulosum are often acidophilic and vacuolated. The basophilic intranuclear inclusions of the verrucae are related to the viral particles rather than to the osmiophilic intranuclear eosinophilic material, which is related to keratin. A loose infiltration of various mononuclear cells may be present in the papillae. Carcinomatous transformation of these lesions occurs rarely, if ever, though occasionally a verrucal form of senile keratosis or a squamous cell carcinoma with a prominent papillary hyperkeratotic surface is erroneously regarded as having arisen from a verruca vulgaris.

Condylomata acuminata, or anogenital warts, occur chiefly in the moist skin of the vulva, about the anus, and on the penis. Although initially they appear as soft, small verrucous papules, they may coalesce into bulky cauliflower-like masses. Rarely do they undergo malignant degeneration. Their presence in the prepubertal population is strongly suggestive of child abuse, particularly with the isolation of human papillomavirus (HPV-6) from the lesion, adjacent skin, or mucosa. The histologic features reveal the stratum corneum to be only slightly thickened over a papillomatous and acanthotic rete Malpighii. There is a distinctive perinuclear vacu-olization, hyperchromatism, and mitotic activity within the spinous cells, in some cases looking disturbingly dysplastic. However, proved malignant change is rare, as stated. To confuse the situation further, these may coexist with *bowenoid papulosis* of the genitalia and, indeed, may represent a transformation of one into the other.

Oral florid papillomatosis comprises benign condy-lomatoid verrucal masses covering large portions of the buccal mucosa. These presumably are of viral origin.

An oral and genital lesion histologically similar to condyloma occurs with the entity called "dyskeratosis congenita," which may be associated with a variety of ectodermal and mesodermal changes, including hyper-pigmentation of the skin, reticulated poikilodermatous changes, dystrophic nails, deforming atrophic arthritis, dental dystrophies, cardiovascular lesions, testicular atrophy, and hypersplenism.

Seborrheic keratosis

Seborrheic keratosis is labeled also "verruca senilis" or "pigmented papilloma." The term "verruca senilis" is not well chosen because the lesions often appear in young people and acanthosis is the feature of note. "Seborrheic keratosis" is used by dermatologists and emphasizes the greasy feeling to the touch imparted by the abundant fatty keratinous nests within the lesion. These lesions occur particularly on the trunk and fore-head and are usually dark brown, elevated, and sharply delimited. The sudden appearance of seborrheic kera-toses, along with a rapid increase in their size and num-ber, may herald the presence of a visceral carcinoma, usually an adenocarcinoma. This phenomenon, known as the sign of Leser-Trélat, is inconstant.

The histologic picture is that of abruptly thickened epidermis that encloses nests of laminated keratin re-sulting from focal, irregular maturation of epidermis partially inverted within the core of the lesion. In places the central pearls are incompletely developed and present large mature squamous cells without the keratinous nests (Fig. 36-37). The surrounding cells are usually focally pigmented with fine brown granules of melanin and superficially resemble basal cells. How-ever, close examination often reveals residual intercel-lular bridges that help identify them as squamous cells, despite statements to the contrary. Many of these epi-thelial cells are dopa positive. In my judgment the pig-ment is produced by the tumor cells (that is, the kera-tinocytes). Others assume, on evidence not easily acceptable, that the pigment is inoculated into the tu-mor cells by nonneoplastic melanocytes carried along with the tumor. This same judgment applies to the con-dylomatous, so-called melanocanthoma. Rare cases of

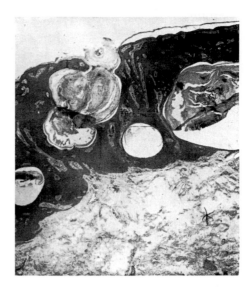

Fig. 36-37. Seborrheic keratosis. (Hematoxylin and eosin.)

malignant transformation of seborrheic keratosis have been recorded.[7,10,11] These have included basal cell car-cinomas and malignant melanomas. Of interest is the high concentration of zinc in seborrheic keratoses.

A lesion that has many of the cellular characteristics of verruca pigmentosum is the so-called inverted pap-illoma, which grows downward rather than outward from the epidermal surface. The inverted papilloma of-ten is associated with an inflammatory reaction of mononuclear cells at its base, much as the senile kara-toses are. The lesion referred to as "eccrine porothe-lioma," or "acrosyringoma," closely resembles the ear-liest stage of seborrheic keratosis.

Clear cell acanthoma

Degos, or *clear cell, acanthoma* also is reminiscent of an initial stage in the development of seborrheic kera-tosis. Clear cell acanthoma occurs about equally in men and women as a slightly raised erythematous plaque or papule, occasionally multiple, measuring about 5 to 10 mm in diameter, usually on lower parts of the legs, es-pecially the calves. The histologic appearance is char-acterized by the presence of an acanthotic epidermis with squamous cells made clear by an abundance of gly-cogen (diastase labile) and sharply marginated from the adjacent normal epidermis. These lesions do not be-come malignant.

A disorder of keratinization, *disseminated spiked hy-perkaratosis,* consists of bland, nonfollicular, nonviral keratosis with minimal underlying acanthosis.[35]

As with the generally benign seborrheic keratosis, other lesions such as linear epidermal nevi and eccrine poromas rarely may lead to basal or squamous cell car-cinomas.

Keratoacanthoma

The problem of pseudoepitheliomatous hyperplasia is directly related to the histologically difficult subject of so-called self-healing squamous cell carcinomas, also more or less equivalently labeled "molluscum sebaceum" and "molluscum pseudocarcinomatosum." Mostly commonly these occur in elderly men, though even adolescents may be affected, especially if there has been contact with oils. The lesions appear as single or multiple nodules that are smooth except for the characteristic umbilication of the central keratin. The nodules often regress spontaneously in about 2 months, leaving little or no scar. Recurrences have been recorded.

Histologically, as already implied, the nodules are not really carcinomas but rather are coalescent comedones or keratinous masses with prominent pseudoepitheliomatous hyperplasia at their bases (Fig. 36-38). Giant keratoacanthomas may become incredibly large, particularly on the face, and may recur after incomplete excision. The well-differentiated, keratoacanthomatous pattern in the rapid recurrence supports the original diagnosis, though considerable self-confidence may be required to maintain it. An important clue is the absence of significant atypia in the epidermis at the margins of the keratoacanthomas. Perineural involvement in keratoacanthomas has been noted without corresponding evidence of malignant biologic behavior.[53]

Despite the occasional recurrences after incomplete removal, these lesions are benign. The attention that has been focused on keratoacanthomas has perforce led to misdiagnosis of squamous cell carcinomas as keratoacanthomas. An analogous problem exists in the erroneous diagnosis of melanocarcinomas as juvenile melanomas.

A variety of the lesion has been designated "generalized eruptive keratoacanthoma." These may be so numerous as to cover most of the body and involve even the oral mucosa.

It is becoming obvious from reports in the literature that prior confidence is being replaced by a nagging uncertainty regarding the differential diagnosis between keratoacanthoma and verrucous, keratinizing squamous cell carcinoma.[7,10] This diagnostic difficulty is expressed in both directions, that is, unnecessarily radical surgical operations for giant keratoacanthomas, including leg amputation, and injudiciously delayed therapy for squamous cell carcinomas mistaken for keratoacanthomas.

Acrochordons (skin tags) are common minute, 1 to 2 mm soft papules occuring chiefly in the region of the head and neck. They tend to be hyperkeratotic, regularly acanthotic, and papillomatous and occasionally include small cysts of keratin. They are often considered to be a type of soft fibroma.

Precancerous lesions of epidermis

The precancerous lesions of the skin include senile keratosis, Bowen's disease, erythroplasia of Queyrat, and the active junctional nevus. Each of these entities is characterized by atypia or dyskeratosis of cells confined to the limits of the epidermis. To such lesions the term "carcinoma in situ" is often applied. *Precancerous* as applied to these lesions connotes, in a crude measure, the relatively high probability that they will undergo malignant degeneration rather than the inevitability of such a complication. Kraurosis valvae, a term that has become unpopular in recent years, had been used diversely either in place of vulval lichen sclerosis et atrophicus, on the one hand, or as equivalent to epidermoid carcinoma in situ on the other.

Senile keratosis

The senile keratoses are irregular brownish patches of epidermis roughened by horny scales, occurring characteristically on the dorsum of the hands of aged people. Histologically similar lesions may occur after irradiation and exposure to arsenic or to the elements of the weather. They may be single or several, or they may occur in great numbers over many parts of the body.

Microscopically they are characterized chiefly by dyskeratosis of the cells of the basal layer and adjacent layers of the rete Malpighii. These cells show hyperchromatism, loss of polarity, increased numbers of mitotic

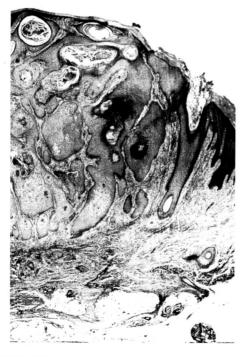

Fig. 36-38. Keratoacanthoma simulating squamous cell carcinoma. (Hematoxylin and eosin.)

figures, and irregularity of size and shape of nuclei. Hyperkeratosis and parakeratosis of varying degrees are responsible for the roughened surface. Inflammatory cells, principally mononuclear, are present in the subepidermal tissue. These cells often encroach onto the epidermis, obscuring the integrity of the "basement membrane" and occasionally prompting the premature and erroneous diagnosis of infiltrating carcinoma. The cutaneous horn in many instances represents a senile keratosis with an accumulation of keratinous material in the form of a projecting spur. The same type of horny projection may be superimposed also on verrucae.

Leukoplakia

"Leukoplakia" is a term that merits discussion of its usage. As applied clinically, or grossly, it refers to whitish patches of mucosa that encompass not only cancerous or precancerous foci, but also those benign patches of mucosa thickened and whitened by mycoses, lichen planus, reaction to dentures, and smoking. Nevertheless, to many (probably most) surgeons and pathologists, leukoplakia connotes a carcinoma in situ or a lesion morphologically approaching an intraepithelial carcinoma. The difficulty is that the diagnosis often is rendered as merely leukoplakia when the pathologist is not certain whether there is sufficient atypia to warrant a designation of leukokeratosis or of carcinoma in situ. This is the situation with lesions of the cervix, when the diagnosis is hedged with such terms as basal cell hyperplasia or dyskaryosis—to the bewilderment of the clinician. Surely there are instances in which the pathologist may not be certain of the malignant potential of such a whitish patch, but it would appear more informative if this uncertainty were indicated rather than concealed euphemistically.

Xeroderma pigmentosum

Xeroderma pigmentosum is a potentially cancerous familial disease of the skin, usually first manifested early in childhood. It is characterized clinically by areas of atrophy, as well as isolated and coalescent scaly patches of keratosis showing varying amounts of pigmentation. A hyper-alpha-2-globulinemia has been found consistently in patients with xeroderma pigmentosum, and it has been hypothesized that this abnormality is related to ceruloplasmin. Some of the patients develop a primary degeneration of Purkinje cells of the cerebellum and pyramidal cells of the cerebrum. The effects of this deneration may simulate the clinical pictures of Friedereich's ataxia, Alzheimer's disease, parkinsonism, and Huntington's chorea.

Histologically the changes in xeroderma pigmentosum are those of irregular atrophy, acanthosis, and hyperkeratosis, with excessive deposits of melanin in the basal layer and lowermost layers of the stratum spinosum, as well as in chromatophores in the upper dermis. Xeroderma pigmentosum may be complicated by junctional nevi, basal cell or squamous cell carcinomas, and melanocarcinomas.

The diagnosis of xeroderma pigmentosum may be established even before the characteristic cutaneous lesions appear, by estimation of the deoxyribonucleic acid excision repair level in cutaneous fibroblasts (after irradiation by ultraviolet rays).[72] This defect in repair of DNA damaged by ultraviolet rays has been detected prenatally with the use of amniotic cells cultured in vitro.[72]

Bowen's disease

Bowen's disease occurs as irregular, scaly, slowly progressive, usually brownish patches on the trunk, buttocks, and extremities. It was estimated that evidence of visceral cancer develops in approximately one third of patients within 6 to 10 years after the initial diagnosis of Bowen's disease. Here again, what was regarded as a proved relationship a few years ago must now be considered moot on the basis of more recent analyses or properly controlled studies.[13,14]

Microscopically the principal feature of the lesions is the presence of isolated dyskeratotic cells scattered haphazardly in all layers of the epidermis. These cells often have large, hyperchromatic single or double nuclei surrounded by cytoplasmic halos. Mitotic figures are numerous in these altered cells. Hyperkeratosis or parakeratosis may be pronounced. The acanthosis is usually uniform, but irregular thickening may be present.

Electron microscopic study of the dyskeratotic cells discloses displaced cytoplasmic fascicular aggregations of tonofilaments and separation of the desmosomal-tonofilament attachments. This desmosomal-tonofilament dissociation would be anticipated not only from the acantholytic appearance of Bowen's cells as seen under light microscopy, but also from the ultrastructural studies of acantholytic cells in other lesions such as Darier's disease and pemphigus vulgaris.[20] As I previously stated, a basically similar retraction of tonofilaments and loss of desmosomes occur in the conversion of keratinocytes to neval and melanocarcinomatous cells.

Erythroplasia of Queyrat

Erythroplasia of Queyrat is the precancerous lesion occurring principally on the glans penis but also on the vulva and on oral mucous membranes.[39] In addition, the acanthotic thickening associated with erythroplasia is often characterized by long rete ridges that are psoriasiform or attached to each other in a reticulated pattern. A cytologic pattern somewhat similar to that of Bowen's disease occurs in the nipple and adjacent areas of the female breast in Paget's disease. However, unlike the lesions just described, Paget's disease is associated with carcinoma of the underlying mammary ducts. As indicated elsewhere, the evidence for the conclusion that so-called *extramammary Paget's disease* is associated with underlying adenocarcinoma of apocrine or eccrine glands is somewhat less than convincing.[7,10] The majority of such lesions are pagetoid melanocarcinomas. The small group of remaining lesions includes epidermoid carcinomas and metastatic mucin-producing carcinomas, principally from the bowel and occasionally from other organs such as the ovaries.[10]

The much emphasized presence of mucopolysaccharides within epidermal cells hardly precludes the possibility that they are keratinocytes. Among several kinds of evidence is the clear fact that under the influence of an excess of vitamin A, keratinocytes are modulated into mucus-secreting cells.[47]

Bowenoid papulosis of the penis

Bowenoid papulosis of the penis refers to the presence of multiple macules and flat papules on the glans with an atypicality reminiscent of condyloma acuminatum or carcinoma in situ. Infrequently virus particles have been noted by electron microscopy. Some lesions with spontaneous regression have been observed on the vulva as well as cervix. From each of these sites, the human papillomavirus (HPV) may be recovered and, indeed, bowenoid papulosis offers a high risk for causing cervical neoplasia.[67] The vulva is less prone to such development. Bowenoid papulosis is characterized by minute papules, 1 to 5 mm in diameter, located on the shaft of the penis, usually sparing the glans, in the perianal area and on the vulva. Their histologic features are generally indistinguishable from that of the solitary lesions of Bowen's disease except for the "wind-swept" pattern of columns of hyperchromatic, almost pyknotic, perinuclearly vacuolated keratinocytes. Mitoses and dysplastic cells are scattered through the rete Malpighii. The sudden appearance and occasional spontaneous regression of these often pigmented lesions are characteristic of bowenoid papulosis in contrast with Bowen's disease. In many instances, there is a preceding history of genital herpes or condyloma acuminatum; the latter may also be concurrent. These lesions do not become invasive. As in Bowen's disease, virus particles are detectable in the stratum corneum, and the presence of human papillomavirus (HPV) of various types is established.

Malignant lesions of epidermis

The malignant lesions of the epidermis include basal cell carcinoma, squamous cell carcinoma, Paget's disease, and melanocarcinoma.

Basal cell carcinoma

The term "carcinoma" is preferred to "epithelioma" in connection with the basal cell tumors that belong to the general group of rodent ulcers. If left untreated, these neoplasms progress, erode, and infiltrate neighboring bone and cartilage in a manner that would seem to merit the designation "cancer" despite the infrequency of metastasis. Over 100 instances of metastasizing basal cell carcinoma have been recorded.[22,32] The term "epithelioma" might best be reserved for the form of basal cell proliferation that does not show these invasive characteristics, that is, the trichoepithelioma (see p. 1834).

Basal cell carcinomas occur predominantly in blond, fair-skinned people in the region of the face bounded by the hairline, ears, and upper lip. The tumor of the skin of the tip of the nose, however, is more likely to be a squamous carcinoma, provided that it is not a keratoacanthoma. Basal cell tumors are not confined to the face but in small numbers may occur in the skin of any part of the body, though there is a tendency to desmoplasia in those located away from the face. Squamous cell carcinomas of the anal canal, which are aggressive, particularly if they are located above the anal verge, may appear deceptively similar to basal cell carcinomas. Indeed, some of them are labeled "basaloid"—to the surgeon's confusion.

The basal cell carcinoma begins as a smooth, slightly elevated papule that may be scaly at first but tends soon to ulcerate centrally as the lesion spreads peripherally beneath the epidermis. Characteristically the ulcer is rimmed by a waxy, smooth firm, rolled border representing the intact epidermis, which is wrapped over but not yet invaded by the underlying and undermining neoplastic nests. If neglected, the tumor may advance to a grotesque erosion of large portions of the soft tissue, as well as the cartilage and bone of the face. Early treatment by irradiation, excision, or the various other means of local destruction is usually adequate. The advantage of treatment of neoplasms by excision is that it then becomes possible to know by histologic examination not only the precise type of tumor present, but also whether the excised tumor is bounded by normal tissue.

Histologically, although there is considerable variability to the pattern of the basal cell carcinomas, there are sufficient characteristics in common to make them recognizable with relative ease. They are made up of nests of closely packed cells of uniform size and oval shape, with dark nuclei separated by a small amount of spineless cytoplasm. The nests often are rimmed by a single layer of similar cells arranged, however, in a neat radial pattern and strongly reminiscent of the more or less vertically arranged basal cells forming the lowermost layer of the normal epidermis or of the hair shafts. Mitotic figures are usually fairly common. Such nests may be observed arising not only from the basal portion of the epidermis but also from the corresponding layer of the hair shaft or from both sources in the same tumor. The presence in these tumors of cells of the same type as those that line both the epidermis and the hair follicle would appear to account for the origin of these neoplasms from either of these structures. This is by no means equivalent to maintaining that embryonic rests of hair matrix, in one or another phase of its development, are the source of basal cell carcinomas. The basal cells of adult epidermis do have a limited range of reaction to carcinogenic stimulation. One major form such a reaction takes is the production of hair matrices in the disheveled manner of a basal cell carcinoma, just as the basal cells in response to normal growth stimuli produce the orderly components of hair. In other words, when carcinogenic agents such as arsenic or x irradiation produce basal cell carcinomas, they do so not by activating embryonic rests of hair follicles but by provoking neoplastic change in previously normally situated adult basal cells. The origin of basal cell carcinomas from any part of the mature pilary complex is demonstrable also in the skin of rats to which anthramine and methylcholanthrene have been applied. Basal cell carcinoma may occur subungually as a pigmented band closely simulating melanoma clinically.

The histologic features of basal cell carcinomas may vary in the following ways:

1. By the presence of edematous stroma rimmed by neoplastic cells to form the alveolar or cystic type
2. By excessive, dense, hyalinized stroma between nests of basal cells to give the morphea type
3. By the presence of foci of squamous cells or pearls, occasionally calcified, in the centers of nests of basal cells

This last modification has been called "basosquamous cell (transitional or metatypical cell) carcinoma." It is stated that the keratin produced by basal cell carcinomas differs from that produced by squamous cell carcinomas in the histochemically demonstrable presence of cystine (hair follicle keratin) in the basal cell cancers. There is, in addition, the comedo type of basal cell carcinoma in which the cores of the masses of basal cells are necrotic.

Basal cell carcinomas, like squamous cell carcinomas, may exhibit focal sebaceous gland differentiation. This process can be distinguished from an original sebaceous gland carcinoma by the presence of abundant alpha-glycerolphosphate dehydrogenase in the latter.

From time to time attempts are made to revive the notion that basal cell carcinomas with foci of squamous cell differentiation represent an intermediate phase in the aggressive deterioration to squamous cell carcinomas. These demonstrations still lack conviction, notwithstanding the invocation of some of the potentials of the basal cells. Despite general belief to the contrary, it has yet to be shown that there is any significant difference in the prognosis of these types. In particular, it is commonly stated that basal cell carcinomas with areas of squamous cells have a more precarious prognosis than the ordinary basal cell carcinomas. However, those few carcinomas in which the deeper margins develop pointed cords of cells, as if aggressively penetrating the stroma, should be viewed as capable of metastasis.

Superficial epitheliomatosis, or multicentric basal cell carcinoma, is a special variety of the basal cell tumors. These lesions occur predominantly on the trunk as either dry and scaly or moist and eczematous, slowly enlarging plaques. Histologically the lesions are small basal cell carcinomas arising from multiple foci in the basal layers of epidermis. The lesion is differentiated from the Jadassohn type of intraepidermal basal cell carcinoma, in which the neoplastic cells appear to be growing upward toward the surface from the basal cell layer instead of into the dermis. In the superficial lesions, as well as in other cutaneous carcinomas in situ, arsenic should be suspected as a possible etiologic factor (Fig. 36-39).

The so-called premalignant fibroepithelial tumor is really part of the spectrum of variants of basal cell carcinomas and hardly merits such segregation.

In situ and, infrequently, superficially invasive basal cell carcinomas may complicate sclerosing angiomas.[41] The existence of these fairly innocuous lesions has been disputed; they are indistinguishable from superficial epitheliomatosis and, probably, they would be so diagnosed if seen without the underlying angioma.

Basal cell nevus syndrome

Basal cell carcinomas, along with a variety of adnexal hamartomas, may occur as a congenital hereditary phenomenon known as the *basal cell nevus syndrome.* These lesions may vary from several on the face to hundreds on the trunk and extremities. The syndrome occurs in children as young as 2 years of age but usually manifests itself in a person between 17 and 35 years of age. The tumors may show the spectrum of variations characteristic of basal cell carcinoma in the absence of the syndrome. The osseous cysts are termed "odontogenic keratocysts" and are lined by thin layers of stratified squamous epithelium. Dermal pits of the hands and feet are practically a hallmark of the syndrome. The pitting is a consequence of the absent or thinned keratinous layer overlying the depressions. The associated lesions or symptom complexes may include pseudohy-

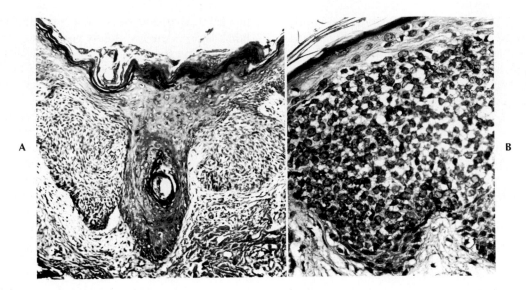

Fig. 36-39. A, Basal cell carcinoma (superficial epitheliomatosis, multicentric basal cell carcinoma). **B,** Intraepidermal basal cell carcinoma (Jadassohn type). (Hematoxylin and eosin.)

poparathyroidism, ovarian fibromas, mesenteric cysts, dental cysts, bifid ribs, spina bifida, hypertelorism, broad nasal root, bridging of the sella turcica, calcification of the falx cerebri, and agenesis of the corpus callosum. Occasionally granulomatous or ulcerative colitis may be present.

Isolated basal cell carcinomas in children occur more often than is generally suspected. As with the tumors of adults, they are present chiefly on the face.[61]

Squamous cell carcinoma

The squamous cell carcinoma may occur in the skin of any part of the body, but there is a predilection for the exposed areas, particularly the face and hands. Certain sources of chronic irritation definitely predispose to squamous cell carcinoma. These include pipe smoking, particularly clay pipes, irritation to the scrotum as incurred by chimney sweeps, the exposure to arsenic, tar, and carcinogenic oils that soak the clothes and abdomen of the mule spinner (in the textile industry), the constant contact of the abdomen with the small charcoal heaters causing the so-called kangri cancers observed in the Kashmir region, the exposure of susceptible blond skins to actinic rays and other elements of the weather, the unexplained cancerous irritant that is present in old scars as from burns or osteomyelitis, the vague irritant of syphilitic leukoplakia, and a variety of others.

The sources of the arsenic include that used therapeutically (Fowler's solution, arsphenamine), orchard sprays, and contaminated water from artesian wells (for example, of Taiwan). In the latter instance the cutaneous manifestations may be endemic and include a broad spectrum comprising benign-appearing keratoses, keratoses with fronds or ridges of early basal cell carcinoma, multicentric in situ and invasive basal cell carcinomas, Bowen's disease in its many variations, epidermoid carcinomas, and combinations of any of these lesions. Scars after vaccination may be complicated infrequently by basal cell carcinomas, squamous cell carcinomas, and melanocarcinomas. The basal and squamous cell carcinomas tend to occur in individuals with the type of skin vulnerable to damage from exposure to ultraviolet rays. However, in most instances of squamous cell carcinoma the source of irritation or stimulation is not apparent.

Clinically the lesion begins as a superficially scaly, slightly indurated areas that bleeds, crusts, and resists casual therapy. With growth the surface becomes ulcerated or cornified and the base indurated. The ulceration may extend to a deforming depth. The sectioned surface is granular and is grayish white flecked with yellow. Usually the limits of the neoplasm may be determined even by gross inspection of the cut surface.

Microscopically these carcinomas are characterized by irregular nests of epidermal cells that have infiltrated the dermis for varying depths. The nests of a squamous cell carcinoma may include cells representing any layer of the epidermis from the basal layer to the stratum corneum. In well-differentiated lesions the intercellular spines and the central keratinous nests, or the epithelial pearls, easily identify the origin of the tumor from squamous epithelium. In highly anaplastic lesions these elements may be altogether lacking. Indeed, the anaplasia may be so extreme in occasional squamous cell carcinomas that they may be almost indistinguishable from spindle cell sarcomas. These spindle cell carcinomas commonly occur after irradiation and are controlled with difficulty. They are not to be confused with the unimportant, focal areas of spindle cells occurring in many basal cell carcinomas or with the spindle cell melanocarcinomas. Another variety characterized by intracellular edema, particularly affecting the central cells of the neoplastic nests that are rimmed by basilar cells, is occasionally mistaken for sebaceous or sweat gland carcinomas, even adamantinomas, or clear cell carcinomas.

Often of greater practical importance than determining the precise type of carcinoma is the decision as to whether an isolated nest of cells represents actual carcinomatous invasion or is merely an obliquely cut rete ridge in an area of pseudoepitheliomatous hyperpasia. In some instances the decision may be most difficult to make. However, the cells of a ridge in hyperplastic epidermis are quite differentiated and tend to resemble very closely the cells of the neighboring, obviously benign ridges and epidermis. The neighboring ridges—elongated, curved, and yet attached to the epidermis and cut perpendicularly—help to indicate that the isolated nest of cells actually represents an obliquely cut ridge rather than cancer. Another problem arises when abundant subepidermal inflammatory cells are present, some of which may have migrated across the basement membrane and lower epidermis, thereby obscuring the integrity of or even actually interrupting the basement membrane. Since disruption of the "basement membrane" is one of the standard (if reliable) criteria for provoking at least the suspicion of carcinoma, it becomes of some limited, importance to judge, particularly by the anaplasia of the epidermal cells involved, whether the disruption is attributed merely to inflammation or to early cancer (Fig. 36-38).

The squamous cell carcinomas of the skin are, as a rule, not as anaplastic as the corresponding lesions of mucous membranes such as the lip or uterine cervix. Accordingly, metastases are considerably more common after squamous cell carcinoma of the mucous membranes than of the skin. Although this difference is the rule, there are conspicuous exceptions. One of the most aggressive imaginable occurred in a scar after a burn of the skin of the leg ("Marjolin ulcer"). The tumor metastasized widely to the viscera. Similarly, anaplastic squamous cell carcinomas have been recorded in familial acne conglobata.[71] Malignant melanomas also have developed from burn scars.

Verrucous carcinoma (carcinoma cuniculatum)

The verrucous carcinoma, an uncommon variant of low-grade squamous carcinoma, occurs principally on the sole of the foot, the leg, buttock, and occasionally hands. The tumor tends to invade deeply even into bone and to metastasize infrequently. They may become bulky, infected, and neglected partly because of confusion with plantar warts, keratoacanthomas, or mere reactive pseudoepitheliomatous hyperplasia.

Effects of ionizing radiation on skin

Ionizing radiation is used therapeutically for a great variety of inflammatory diseases, including acne, psoriasis, eczema, and plantar warts. Such treatment is usually at least temporarily effective for the dermatosis, but sequelae in the form of acute and chronic radiodermatitis occur often enough to warrant serious concern. It is estimated that carcinomas complicate approximately 20% of instances of chronic radiodermatitis.[31] This complication may occur over a wide span of years, from 3 to more than 50, with a median of 12 to 18 years. Because of the great time interval between the induction of therapy and the onset of complications, the frequency of such complications may be underestimated by therapists.

The usual type of cutaneous cancer occurring after radiotherapy is the squamous cell carcinoma, but basal cell carcinomas also may occur, particularly in areas about the face where such tumors are prone to arise spontaneously. As previously mentioned, spindle cell carcinomas are an especially anaplastic variety of squamous cell cancers produced by irradiation.

"Merkel cell" tumor

Recently enthusiasm has been aroused in support of the existence of a Merkel cell, neuroendocrine, or *trabecular carcinoma* of the skin. These are said to occur in various anatomic sites, to be composed of small anaplastic cells, some with neurosecretory granules, capable of aggressive metastatic action, and to be differentiated, often with great difficulty, from metastatic carcinomas and epidermoid carcinomas, including melanocarcinomas. Monoclonal antibodies with specificity for intermediate filaments (IFs) have been given weight, along with S-100 protein (a neuron-specific enolase) and chromogranin, in the segregation of this tumor from anaplastic carcinomas, lymphomas, and melanomas.

The presumed derivation of these tumors from Merkel cells and the presence of neurosecretory granules have persuaded observers that these tumors are individualistic and belong to the APUD system. The finding of neurosecretory granules in a variety of nonneural tumors, such as epidermoid carcinomas and carcinomas of the cervix, prostate, lung, and intestinal tract, as well as the aggressiveness of the Merkel cell tumor, uncharacteristic for a neoplasm of nerve endings, would seem to warrant some reconsideration of the derivation of this neoplasm. For example, no one seems to have wondered why we have seen no evidence of the existence of a benign variant of the so-called Merkel cell tumor. If this lesion is indeed derived from Merkel cells, it is reasonable to anticipate finding evidence of benign neoplasia or, at least, hyperplasia of this nerve ending. It does not appear to be in the nature of nerve endings—Merkel, pacinian, or others—to manifest a malignant potential, especially one as aggressive as the trabecular carcinoma often is.

PIGMENTED NEVI

The term "nevus" is often used by dermatologists to refer to any congenital blemish. Therefore they refer not only to pigmented nevi but also to vascular nevi, sebaceous gland nevi, sweat gland nevi, and others. However, to most, nevus denotes a neoplasm derived from pigmented or at least dopa-positive cells. These nevi and their malignant counterparts are classified as follows:

A. Benign
   1. Junctional nevus
   2. Intradermal nevus
   3. Compound nevus (including halo nevus)
   4. Juvenile melanoma
   5. Blue nevus—cellular blue nevus
B. Malignant
   1. Melanocarcinoma (including superficial spreading, lentigo maligna, and nodular)
      a. In situ
      b. Superficial (including melanotic freckle of Hutchinson)
      c. Deep
   2. Malignant blue nevus

Junctional nevus

The junctional nevus, also known as dermoepidermal or marginal nevus, is of concern because in its active form it is a direct forerunner of the melanocarcinoma. Occasional congenital nevi and, rarely, blue nevi are exceptions to this rule. Happily, this malignant transformation of junctional nevi occurs relatively infrequently.

The uncomplicated (quiescent versus active) junctional nevus appears as a flat, smooth, generally hairless, light brown to dark brown mole. The lesions may be single or multiple. Their smooth appearance may be altered by their combination with an underlying intradermal nevus (compound). *Unfortunately, it is not always possible to diagnose them accurately clinically.* However, one may assume that pigmented moles on the ventral surface of the hands and the feet and on the genitalia are usually junctional nevi or, at least, have a junctional component in the form of a compound nevus.[4-6,10,11]

Histologically the junctional nevus is easily recognized by the clusters of enlarged, rounded, loosened

cells of the basal and adjacent prickle cells of the epidermis. In addition, these cells lose their prickles and cohesion with neighboring cells, and many become powdered with fine granules of melanin. This acantholysis is reflected ultrastructurally in the partial to complete loss of desmosomes and tonofilaments, though residua of these structures are readily noted at the periphery of the junctional or acantholytic focus. If mitotic figures are present and the nuclei show any noteworthy anaplasia, the lesion may be assumed to have been on the verge of melanocarcinomatous transformation. Accordingly, depending on the extent of the atypia, these lesions are designated active junctional nevi, dysplastic (B-K) nevi, or melanocarcinomas in situ.[10,11] The process may be diffuse along a strip of epidermis, or it may be focal, with normal or skipped areas of epidermis intervening between involved portions. The limitation of junctional change or junctional nevus to acantholytic aggregates or nests of intraepidermal nevus cells in the rete ridges is arbitrary. It misses the equivalent contribution of the more diffuse lower epidermal acantholysis between the ridges, as in the Hutchinson freckle. Judgment as to the adequacy of normal margin bordering the lesion must be made with caution, inasmuch as the section may be removed through one of the intervening, unaltered areas (Figs. 36-41 and 36-47).

It is generally assumed that the cells of the junctional nevus are derived from specialized nerve endings intercalated in the basal layer as clear cells. However, it seems that such a restricted view disregards the occurrence of cells of the junctional nevus (many dopa positive) not only in a continuous row in the basal layer, but also as isolated cells high in the prickle cell layers, in the stratum granulosum, and even well into the stratum corneum. This phenomenon would seem to occur not by proliferation of neurogenic cells within the epidermis, as many believe, but rather by the alteration in situ of the preexisting basal cells and spinous keratinocytes, as a few formerly believed.[92]

It was long ago clearly shown that dendrites, which to many seem automatically to connote neurogenesis, may be entirely absent in many of these cells. Actually, when the dendrites of melanocytes are seen with silver stains, they are made evident not because of an intrinsic argyrophilia such as that possessed by cells of true neurons but because of the argyrophilia of the contained granules of melanin. The supranuclear localization of pigment within the prickle cells is, in itself, indicative of an in situ origin rather than by a nipped-off dendrite belonging to a neighboring cell or by the diffusion of tyrosinase from a clear cell.[54] In the latter instance one would expect the granules of pigment to be diffusely or haphazardly deposited as in melanophores or histiocytes.

It is of course well established that the pigment of skin, hair, and feathers may be controlled by the transposition of the embryonic cells of the neural crest. That neural control of many varieties of pigmentation exists is obvious. However, to infer from this that the cells of the neural crest are themselves incorporated in the epidermis as melanocytes is to fail, in effect, to distinguish the artist from his pigments.[10,11]

The addition of these facts, supplemented by evidence from the direct examination of many junctional nevi and melanocarcinomas, indicates that basal cells principally, but also prickle cells or keratinocytes, may become converted to melanocytes and that the junctional nevi are derived from these cells.

Dysplastic (B-K) nevus

Multiple active junctional (or *dysplastic*) *nevi* occur sporadically and in family members with heritable melanoma with a greatly increased risk for the development of malignant melanoma. Clinically, these dysplastic nevi tend to be larger than the usual nevus (over 4 mm) and variably pigmented with irregular scalloped borders. It must be clear that dysplastic nevi do not lend themselves automatically to correct and uniform diagnosis, nor it is apparent that there are more advantages of the term "dysplastic nevus" over the more anatomically specific "active junctional nevus," my original term. The judgmental differences in evaluation of degrees of atypia are as considerable in this setting as they are in the in situ lesions of other organs, such as the cervix. At the time of diagnosis, the familial melanomas tend to be less deeply invasive and are more likely to be multiple than the sporadic nonfamilial tumors.

Intradermal nevus

The intradermal nevus, or common mole, is the ordinary pigmented spot that few people are altogether spared. The mole may be flat or raised, with or without hairs, papillary and keratotic. Intradermal nevi may be present at birth or may develop in later years. They tend to become more prominent at puberty.

Histologically the tumor is composed of nests and cords of cells with round, moderately chromatic nuclei surrounded by an even, easily seen rim of cytoplasm. Melanin pigment, when present, usually is limited to the superficial cells in the upper dermis. Similarly, the cells in the upper part of the lesion are more likely to be dopa positive than the deeper ones are.* Mitotic figures are seen rarely in these nevi in adults. Occasion-

---

*Melanophores are merely phagocytes that engulf and transport melanin. Melanophores are dopa negative. A pigmented neval cell or melanoblast may be dopa negative because its enzyme has been completely utilized at a given time or has never developed. The cells of a nonpigmented (amelanotic) melanoma may be dopa positive. However, not all cells of a pigmented or nonpigmented melanocarcinoma are necessarily dopa positive.

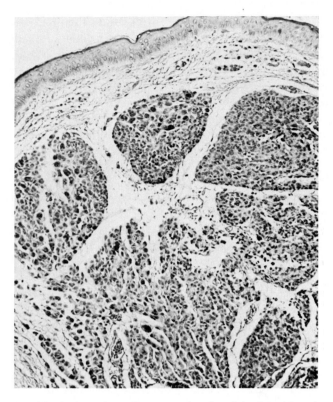

Fig. 36-40. Intradermal nevus showing intact epidermis, that is, without junctional change.

ally hyperchromatism and enlargement of nuclei are simulated by mere agglutination of neval cells. The neval cells characteristically trail off into the depths of the dermis, and rarely into the subcutis, without sharp limitation. The overlying epidermis usually is thinned and may be flat or papillary, with or without hyperkeratosis (Fig. 36-40).

There is impressive histologic basis for the conclusion that the ordinary intradermal mole that is not overlain by a junctional nevus rarely becomes malignant.

The origin of the cells of the common mole is still unsettled. The possibilities include epidermal cells, specialized nerve endings similar to the Merkel-Ranvier corpuscles, and dermal nerves. Those of us who subscribe to the epidermal origin of the intradermal nevus assume, as Unna[92] did, that the altered epidermal cells drop off *(Abtropfung)* and migrate into the dermis. Those who believe in the neurogenesis of pigmented nevi suggest that the neval cells arise from dermal nerves or their sheaths, as well as from the intraepidermal nerve endings or cells that migrated from the neural crest. The frequency with which intradermal nevi are associated with loosened nests of epidermal cells that appear about to drop off (junctional changes) makes the epidermal origin of the common mole (as well as the junctional nevus) the likeliest possibility. This frequent association of the junctional change with the intradermal nevus can hardly be fortuitous, inasmuch as the change is rarely seen with blue nevi and yet is infrequently absent in the moles of children, normally and progressively diminishing in frequency and prominence after puberty. In nevi of the newborn, there is a tendency for the localization of nests of nevus cells within the walls of appendages, the arrectores pilorum, perineural sheaths, and walls of blood vessels in contrast with the positions in acquired nevi.

Balloon cell nevus

Occasional intradermal nevi, called "balloon cell nevi," are characterized by large, coalescent vacuoles within the cytoplasm of nevus cells. These have been shown ultrastructurally to represent altered melanosomes rather than lipid.[42]

Compound nevus

In about 98% of the intradermal nevi occurring before puberty and in about 12% of nevi of adults there is an associated junctional change (Fig. 36-41).[6,11] For lesions with this combination of features the term "compound nevus" was originally introduced by me in 1949.[10,11] It was applied (1) to underscore the morphogenetic interplay between epidermal and dermal neval componens and (2) to create a diagnostically usable classification. It recently has been stated that silver stains are of appreciable help in distinguishing compound nevi from malignant melanomas. This, unfortunately, is not correct.

Clinically, as stated, there is no way to be certain whether an intradermal nevus is compounded with a junctional nevus. This fact emphasizes the importance of histologic examination of all excised nevi. As is indicated in the discussion of melanocarcinomas, the compound nevus has the capacity for undergoing malignant

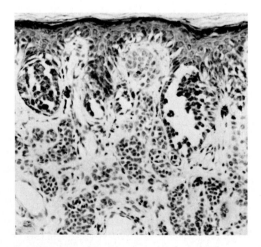

Fig. 36-41. Compound nevus showing junctional and intradermal components. (Hematoxylin and eosin.)

transformation by virtue of its junctional component. This conversion takes place relatively infrequently. The possibility exists that an intradermal nevus may on occasion develop overlying junctional change.

JUVENILE MELANOMAS*

Just a few years ago it was believed that there were lesions of children that were histologically indistinguishable from malignant melanomas. These lesions were designated "benign" because of the arbitrary fact that the individuals were prepubertal. The tumors were accordingly classified as "prepubertal" or "juvenile melanomas." The confidence in such an inferential diagnostic approach was enforced by the generally held impression at the time that metastasizing malignant melanomas did not occur in children. However, because of their histologic resemblance to the melanocarcinomas of adults, it was felt that their removal prior to the onset of puberty was urgent.

This concept of the potential activity of the lesions persisted until 1948. In this year, the juvenile melanomas were for the first time analyzed as a group by Spitz.[85] As a result of her analysis, there was developed a histologic definition of the juvenile melanoma. The enormous practical importance of this definition is now rather universally appreciated.

Clinical features

Our series to date comprises over 600 juvenile melanomas, most of which have been included in our previous reports.[7,8,10-12] Approximately 15 percent of these occurred in adolescents or adults. The oldest patient was a 56-year-old woman. In none was there overt evidence of any endocrinologic disturbance, but no hormonal assays were done. In about half of the cases, the lesions were known to have existed since birth; in the remainder the duration was stated to be either unknown, or several years, months, or weeks. However, the reliability of some of these data, particularly those of short duration, is questionable.

The juvenile melanomas may be found on the skin of any part of the body, with a predilection for the face and lower extremities. None of the personally reviewed lesions has been on mucous membranes and no convincing report of a juvenile melanoma of the mucous membranes has, in my judgment, been recorded as yet, nor, in view of the known occurrence of compound nevi, would any be expected. The suggestion has been made that a juvenile melanoma of the uveal tract may occur, but in the instance which I was permitted to review, the diagnosis of malignant melanoma, rather than juvenile melanoma, seemed justified.

The lesions vary in size from several millimeters to about 3 cm. They are hairless or have few hairs, are smooth or papillary, constantly elevated at least a little above the skin surface, and are often polypoid, resembling the texture, color, and configuration of a granuloma pyogenicum. Ulceration, however, occurs infrequently, having been present in only 8 instances.

Histologic features

There are several key histologic features of the juvenile melanoma. Each is commonly present although none is requisite to the diagnosis. The diagnosis of the juvenile melanoma—as well as of many other lesions of the skin—rests with the recognition of a series of features and becomes difficult to the extent that these features are not fully developed.

Epidermal changes

"Atrophy" and pseudoepitheliomatous hyperplasia. The juvenile melanoma is a variant of what we have chosen to call a *compound nevus*, that is, a nevus composed of both a junctional and a dermal component.[6,11] Rarely, in adults, the lesion presents as an entirely intradermal lesion. In such instances, the junctional component has apparently retrogressed in accordance with the natural evolution of compound nevi. The epidermal pattern may be papillary or smooth, hyperkeratotic or focally parakeratotic. However, these changes are not distinctive. The irregular acanthosis, striking pseudoepitheliomatous hyperplasia and "apparent atrophy" are of some help insofar as they are more characteristic, when all three are present, of the melanocarcinoma rather than of the intradermal or ordinary compound nevus, and to this degree these features narrow the scope of the diagnostic problem. The phrase "apparently atrophy" is used advisedly because the epidermal thinning is not regarded as true atrophy in the sense of pressure or trophic atrophy such as occurs over some dermal tumors.[41] Rather, the thinning is believed to result from the progressive conversion of the epidermis, beginning with the basal layer on upward, into, first, the cells of the junctional and, subsequently, of the intradermal component. These thinned portions may become ulcerated, either accidentally or by active excoriation, especially by children. Ulceration of a pigmented lesion is considered by many as important evidence of malignancy. It is true that ulceration or superficial erosion is commonly noted in melanocarcinomas and, indeed, as just indicated, for a reason fundamentally similar to that for which it occurs with juvenile melanomas although the frequency in the latter is considerably less. The mechanism comprises the epidermal conversion, by acantholytic dissolution, into the tumor cells.

However, in the case of the melanocarcinoma, the epidermis is converted into malignant cells; in the juvenile melanoma, the converted cells are benign. This highly crucial difference is determinable histologically by the application of standard criteria of malignancy, such as nuclear hyperchromasia, pleomorphism, mitoses, and altered cellular polarity. In addition, there is a tendency in the malignant melanoma for the cytoplasm to become swollen and sprinkled with uniformly fine granules of melanin, often with residual blue keratohyaline granules (hematoxylin and eosin) indicating the in situ transformation of cells of the stratum granulosum. These obviously malignant cells may extend to the outermost layers of the stratum corneum as they migrate to the surface with the directional gradient similar to that which transports a normal basal cell to the epidermal surface, there to be sloughed. Unhappily, the malignant cell migrates also downward into the dermis thereby transforming an *in situ* into an invasive melanocarcinoma. As stated, this migration into the dermis occurs from an epidermis that is either thinned, acanthotic, or pseudoepitheliomatous.

When attention was first called to the occurrence of pseudoepitheliomatous hyperplasia in pigmented tumors, several morphogenetic and diagnostic clues were extracted from this phenomenon.[11] Two practical points deserve repetition. First, the pseudoepitheliomatous hyperplasia may be so conspicuous as to be mistaken for a squamous-cell carcinoma. This error is common. Second, if the margins of the bulbous pseudoepitheliomatous ridges are studied in detail, they will frequently reveal in the depths of the dermis not only the existence of diagnostically important junctional change but also the benign or malignant nature of this junctional change that may have been obscured at the surface or entirely obliterated by ulceration.

Junctional alteration. There has been some confusion in the literature concerning the histologic meaning of junctional change. Junctional foci refer to those portions—usually basilar—of the epidermis (or mucosal epithelium) the cells of which show varying degrees of acantholysis or loss of cohesion to each other. Our definition, in contrast with that of others, restricts this change to the epidermis rather than to the epidermis *plus* the upper dermis. The difference in definition is a critical one when the cells are malignant. Often the cells at or near the periphery of the junctional foci may still exhibit traces of stretched or intact intercellular bridges that serve as a landmark of their origin (Figs. 36-42 to 36-45). Their cytoplasm tends to appear more swollen or hydropic than the eosinophilic cytoplasm of the unaltered epidermal cells. These cells may or may not contain fine granules of melanin. The nuclei of the quiescent cells of a junctional focus may be quite like those of other epidermal cells or they may be com-

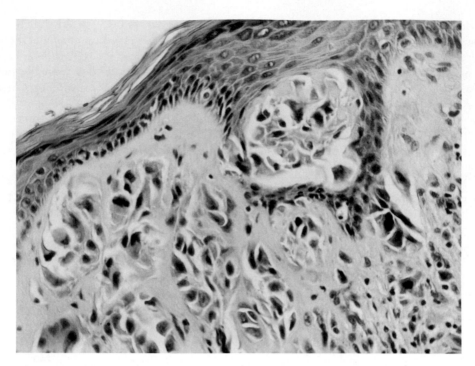

Fig. 36-42. Juvenile melanoma (Spitz's nevus) showing early phase of the formation of "eosinophilic globules" from keratogenic, hyperchromatic, almost pyknotic tumor cells. The globules are in reality necrotic epidermal tumor cells in dermal migration. (Hematoxylin and eosin.)

pressed to one side as in so-called *cellules claires*. The junctional foci of the juvenile melanoma are more commonly localized to the lower or basilar portions of the epidermis of the juvenile melanoma than they are in the malignant melanoma; in the latter, as stated, they are more likely to be found at all levels of the epidermis, either isolated or in clusters of three or four cells. This is not to say that if the junctional change is confined to the lower layers of epidermis, malignancy is ruled out. Contrary to statements occasionally made, the cells of the malignant melanoma need not reach the surface; that is, they may actually lie below the stratum granulosum. A corresponding problem obtains in the evaluation of squamous cell carcinoma in situ of the uterine cervix. Such junctional malignant cells are distinguishable from the corresponding cells of the juvenile melanoma principally by the nuclear qualities already mentioned.

Epidermal cleavage. A striking and, in practice, one of the most revealing clues to the diagnosis of the juvenile melanoma is the abrupt transition from junctional foci to normal or, at most, compressed epidermal cells. It is as if scalloped segments of junctionally altered epidermis were gouged from the unaltered overlying epidermis. The presence of a crescentic space and adjacent flattened epithelial cells may conspire to sim-

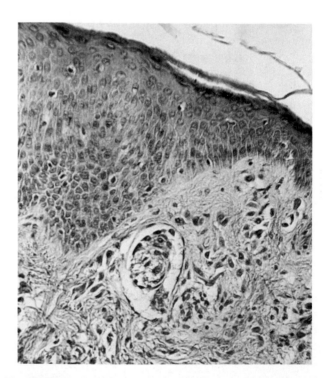

Fig. 36-43. Juvenile melanoma (Spitz's nevus) illustrating pseudoinvasion of dermal vessels produced deceptively by retraction of a partially necrotic cluster of tumor cells in compressed stroma. (Hematoxylin and eosin.) (From Allen, A.C.: The skin, 1954, St. Louis, The C.V. Mosby Co.)

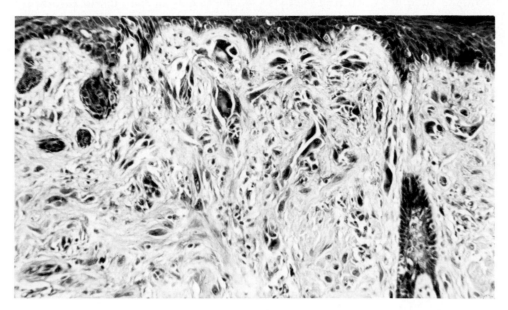

Fig. 36-44. Juvenile melanoma of Spitz. This is from an adult, as reflected by the fibrosis.

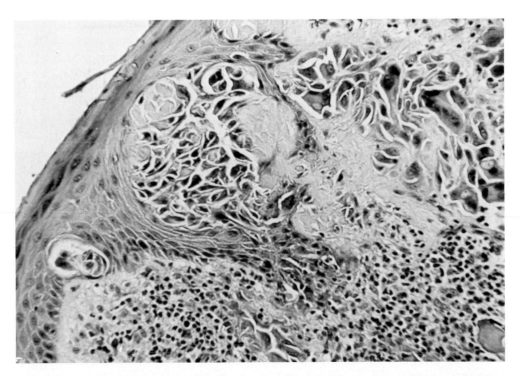

Fig. 36-45. Juvenile melanoma of Spitz showing the compound nevus with characteristic syncytial and myogenous-like nevus cells, necrobiotic nevus, eosinophilic cells, focally homogenized stroma, and a sparsity of melanin.

ulate tumor cells within a lymphatic vessel. It is likely that this cleavage is a kind of meaningful artifact produced by the microtome knife but made possible by a true difference in density between the tumor cells and the neighboring epidermis (Figs. 36-42 to 36-45).

Giant cells. Occasionally some of the cells of the junctional foci of the juvenile melanoma may fuse to form giant cells with single or multiple nuclei. These giant cells constitute the important clue to the diagnosis, as first noted by Spitz.[85] In the mononucleated ones, the cell may resemble a large neoplastic cell of fat or muscle origin with a mass of eosinophilic cytoplasm that tapers off into the underlying edematous stroma. The nuclei of such cells tend to be larger than their neighbors, but usually they are just as vesicular, with sporadic moderately hyperchromatic exceptions. The multinucleated giant cells most closely resemble the Touton cells of juvenile xanthomas, including often the feature of the vacuolization of the otherwise acidophilic cytoplasm. The nucleoli of such cells may be large and eosinophilic, as they commonly are in the more pleomorphic and hyperchromatic cells of malignant melanomas. In instances in which the resemblance of the giant cells of the two lesions is close, the use of other histologic criteria of the juvenile melanoma and of the malignant melanoma is required to establish the differential diagnosis. In my opinion these giant and spindle cells represent modified epidermal tumor cells.

What still is a source of misinterpretation is the frequent failure to distinguish the juvenile melanoma, or Spitz's nevus, from the commonplace, cellular nevus of childhood. The latter does not present the spindle cells with large atypical nuclei often with prominent nucleoli, all in an edematous milieu, not to be confused with malignant lesions.

Dermal changes

Several morphologic features of the dermal component may, when properly evaluated, give substance to the diagnosis of juvenile melanoma. They are (1) ectasia of the superficial thin-walled venules, arterioles, and lymphatic vessels; (2) sparsely nucleated patches of homogenized dermal collagen, especially in the vicinity of these dilated vessels; (3) single and multinucleated giant cells of the type just described under junctional foci, and (4) the presence in the upper dermis of circumscribed packets or nests of cells of the juvenile melanoma that are tightly applied to each other and look tantalizingly like clusters of epidermal cells, which, of course, we believe they are (Fig. 36-45). This resemblance, noted also in ordinary nevi and melanocarcinomas, is particularly striking in the juvenile melanoma. Usually, but by no means always, there is relatively little melanin in either the tumor cells or accompanying

melanophores of the juvenile melanomas. This dearth of pigment in association with ectasia of the vessels is the reason for the pink to reddish-brown color of most of the lesions. However, from the fact that the cells of juvenile melanomas do occasionally manufacture melanin it may be inferred that dopa oxidase and, possibly, tyrosinase activity may also be demonstrable on occasion. For this and other reasons, the use of the demonstration of such activity for the diagnostic elimination of juvenile melanoma is not advised, nor is it suggested that diagnostic reliance be placed on the presence of nonspecific cholinesterase, which is said to characterize juvenile melanomas.

The content of S-100 protein has been found to be inversely proportional to the concentration of melanin, that is, to be high in amelanotic melanomas, intradermal nevi, and juvenile melanomas but low in highly pigmented, blue nevi.[65]

Hazards in the practical diagnostic evaluation of sections of lesions stained for their enzymatic content are (1) the presence of melanin in tumor cells as well as in melanophores interfering with the recognition of enzymes (or their effects), (2) the presence of both benign and malignant cells of nevi and melanocarcinomas in the same lesion, (3) the occurrence of melanocarcinomas in situ, and (4) the absence of enzymes in some of the rapidly growing melanocarcinomas. Although no one would gainsay the academic desirability of investigative pursuit of these enzymes, the diagnosis or morphologically challenging pigmented tumors, as of this date [1989], depends on the nice evaluation of critical histologic changes observed in sections stained with hematoxylin and eosin.

The juvenile melanomas undergo involutional fibrosis or desmoplasia, as other types of nevi do[10] (Fig. 36-44). This desmoplastic variant of the Spitz nevus has been mistaken for a variety of fibrohistiocytic entities, including what has been termed the "fibrous nodule of the tip of the nose."

Ectasia and pseudoectasia of vessels. A prominent feature of the dermis of the juvenile melanoma is edema of the upper dermis along with ectasia, at times cavernous, of subepidermal lymphatics, venules, and arterioles (Fig. 36-43). This degree of dilatation of vessels and the edema are not characteristic of nevi or melanocarcinomas, and the reason for their association with juvenile melanomas is now clear. The picture, which is reminiscent of the effects of interference with vascular drainage, is a major guide to the diagnosis of juvenile melanomas. Of informative practical diagnostic importance is the presence in the upper dermis of tumor cells that appear to be lodged within lymphatics or venules. This feature has repeatedly tripped pathologists into the seriously mistaken diagnosis of "malignant melanoma with lymphatic invasion." In point of fact, this appearance actually is owing to the artifactitious shrinkage or dissolution of several of a cluster of tumor cells with flattening of some of the remaining cells simulating endothelium, and compression of circumscribed collagen so as to resemble thin vascular walls in routinely stained sections. Silver (modified Bielschowsky's) and elastica Van Gieson stains reinforce the impression that the rims of collagen are compressed dermal stroma rather than portions of vascular walls. Further evidence of the nature of these spaces is derived from the observation that although some of the cells lining these cavities are morphologically indistinguishable from endothelial cells, others, often adjacent cells, are unmistakably residual tumor cells, either single or in segments. Occasionally such cells contain granules of melanin.

The simulation of subepidermal lymphatic caverns may be created also by the granular dissolution of clusters of tumor cells so that the eosinophilic debris closely approximates lymph in histologic appearance. Study of the transitional stages in the development of this pattern, particularly of the progressive lysis of these spongiotic clumps of cells, effectively suggests its histogenesis and provides a useful clue in the recognition of the juvenile melanoma.

Mitotic activity. Although most juvenile melanomas do not show evidence of mitotic activity, it is not rare, and a few mitotic figures may be found even in the juvenile melanomas of adults without signifying malignancy. It is appreciated that this latter statement is not in harmony with the impression still retained by many observers. On the other hand, this is not to negate the diagnostic importance of mitoses among questionable nevus cells, but they are not at all necessarily equivalent to malignant change.

Inflammatory reaction. Another impression in need of correction is that an inflammatory reaction provoked by a juvenile melanoma at or near its base constitutes evidence in favor of cancerous change. This notion is quite at variance with our experience. Melanocarcinomas may be free of inflammatory reaction and, counterwise, unmistakably benign juvenile melanomas may commonly be associated with abundant inflammatory reaction. This reaction consists chiefly of lymphocytes, plasma cells, and histiocytes. The inflammatory cells, because of their compactness, may obscure the quality of a dermal nevus or melanocarcinomatous cell. The latter may be mistaken for a histiocyte, especially in superficial melanocarcinomas. If there is some question as to the benign or cancerous nature of a moderately hyperchromatic cell at the advancing deep dermal margin of a lesion, weight should be given to the isolation into relatively widely spaced nests of cells in this peripheral portion of the tumor. The advancing front of a malignant melanoma is much more likely to be a solid mass of cells than a haphazard pattern of cells stringing out singly or in small packets.

Juvenile melanoma of adults

In 1953, as a consequence of the application of the original criteria to the diagnosis of the juvenile melanomas, we discovered that these lesions occurred in fact after puberty, and for the most part retained their identifying characteristics in addition to involutional fibrosis[11] (Fig. 36-44). The oldest patient in our group thus far was 56. These lesions were culled from a large series of what had been previously coded as malignant melanomas, and they were selected without other knowledge of the clinical data. When it was learned that these patients with lesions of the pattern of juvenile melanomas were adults who had never had metastatic cancer, it was appreciated for the first time that the juvenile melanoma could occur in adults and, as a corollary, that in the past these benign lesions had been called malignant and frequently had been so treated for the reason that the patient was postpubertal.[11] This error has by no means been eliminated, and needlessly radical operations are still being performed for these intriguing tumors.

As indicated, the juvenile melanomas of adults may be histologically identical with those of children. As a rule, however, the adult lesions tend to show evidence of involutional fibrosis, so that the cells of the dermal component are likely to be more isolated from each other into small nests or cords (Fig. 36-44). In addition, the deeper, isolated cells have a tendency to be more hyperchromatic, to show more prominent nucleoli, and to extend to a greater dermal depth than the cells of the usual juvenile melanomas of children do. Infrequently, there is a suggestion of the vacuolization of nevus cells of the kind described in association with changes in hormonal status as in pregnancy and at menarche and occasionally noted also in adolescent males.[6,11]

Summary of juvenile melanomas

1. The juvenile melanoma is a benign lesion. It is a variant of a compound nevus and has no greater vulnerability to cancerous transformation than any other compound nevus.
2. Juvenile melanomas occur in adults and should be treated no differently from ordinary compound nevi.
3. The juvenile melanomas of adults may be morphologically identical with those of children but often exhibit an increased fibrosis of the dermal component (Fig. 36-45).

4. The juvenile melanoma may be distinguished from the melanocarcinoma on the basis of histologic pattern alone.

5. The histology of the melanocarcinomas of children is indistinguishable from that of the melanocarcinomas of adults, although there is some tendency toward greater anaplasia in the former.

In summary, the currently applied histologic criteria for the diagnosis of the juvenile melanoma are the same as those originally described by Spitz in 1948. They include (1) the relative superficiality of the essential landmarks of the lesion; (2) the two elements of a compound nevus, junctional and intradermal; (3) edema and telangiectasia of the cutis just below the epidermis; (4) the tendency for single cells or compact nests of spherical or spindled cells to be segregated sharply from adjacent ones; (5) the occurrence of large cells with abundant, usually uniformly basophilic, myogenous-appearing cytoplasm; (6) the superficially located, characteristic giant cells, those with the single large nucleus, as well as the multinucleated ones resembling the pattern either of the giant cells of measles or of Touton giant cells with a complete or incomplete peripheral rim of small nuclei; (7) the generally abrupt transition between the acantholytic, loose junctional cells and the still intact adjacent epidermis; (8) the relative sparsity of pigmentation, so that, in association with the superficial dermal edema and telangiectasis, most of the juvenile melanomas clinically appear purplish-red rather than dark brown; and (9) the progressive fibrosis, increasing with age, of the juvenile melanomas of adults.

Eosinophilic globules in juvenile melanomas

Eosinophilic, diffusely hyalinized, inconsistently periodic acid–Schiff–positive globules, or hyalinized, granular masses have been noted in juvenile melanomas and have been assigned diagnostic significance.[10] Actually, these occur not only in juvenile melanomas, but also in ordinary compound nevi, and infrequently in malignant melanomas they tend to be located at the dermoepidermal junction, both in the lower epidermis and in the clusters of nevus cells in the upper dermis. When present in conspicuous numbers, as others have stated, they represent one of several parameters diagnostically weighted toward Spitz's nevus. They suggest a form of coagulative necrosis that may involve both nucleus and cytoplasm. Indeed, it may produce the necrosis of an almost complete loss of a nest of nevus cells, leaving a space simulating a dilated dermal lymphatic or venule (Fig. 36-45). I have previously referred to these as necrobiotic cells (Figs. 36-42, 36-43, and 36-45).[10] Necrotic or infarcted keratinocytes, reminiscent of these "eosinophilic globules," are seen also in the acral erythema of patients receiving chemotherapy for bone marrow transplantation as well as in the epidermis of some dermatoses, such as erythema multiforme.

BLUE NEVUS

The blue, or Jadassohn-Tièche, nevus appears as a flat or slightly elevated blue or bluish black lesion, occurring particularly on the trunk and extremities and often mistaken clinically for a malignant melanoma. It is structurally essentially the same as the mongolian spot or the nevus of Ota. The former is found in the sacral region. The nevus of Ota occurs in the eye and on the skin of the face. Showers of blue nevi (eruptive) have been observed during pregnancy, at puberty, and in association with bullous dermatoses.

Histologically these nevi are composed of interlacing fasciculi of spindle cells with long cytoplasmic processes and oval fibrocytoid nuclei. The cells are usually much more loosely disposed than those of the blue nevus. If the pigment were not present, the histologic picture of the blue nevus would resemble that of a dermal neurofibroma, and indeed it is possible that the basic morphogenesis of the two is similar. However, many of the cells of the blue nevus and the mongolian spot are dopa positive. Abundant melanin pigment may obliterate the details of most of the cells of the blue nevus. In addition, the neoplastic cells are interspersed with numerous pigment-laden chromatophores. Usually the neval cells lie deep in the dermis; occasionally they are directly apposed to the epidermis. The color of the nevus is, of course, dependent not only on the amount of pigment present but also on the distance of the lesion from the epidermis. Infrequently the blue nevus is combined with the ordinary intradermal nevus (common mole) and with the junctional nevus.

Cellular blue nevus. There is a striking variant of the blue nevus that is frequently incorrectly diagnosed as melanosarcoma. Some years ago I termed this lesion "cellular blue nevus."[6,7,10] It occurs in about 50% of cases in the skin of the buttocks and the dorsum of the hands or feet. The epidermis is unchanged. The cells of this tumor show no significant necrosis or anaplasia, and mitotic figures almost always are absent (Fig. 36-46). Fused nuclei often simulate the hyperchromasia of activity. One of the features that characterize the lesion is the cross sections of fasciculi surrounded by clear zones, giving the illusion that the whorls are metastases in lymphatics when they actually represent artifactitious shrinkage and cleavage of the fasciculi (Fig. 36-46). The melanosomes of the cellular blue nevus are stated to have a distinctive ultrastructure.

Blue nevi undergo malignant change with consoling rarity. I have seen 62 examples of malignant blue nevi arising generally from cellular blue nevi. Although it appears obvious that the diagnosis of sarcomatous trans-

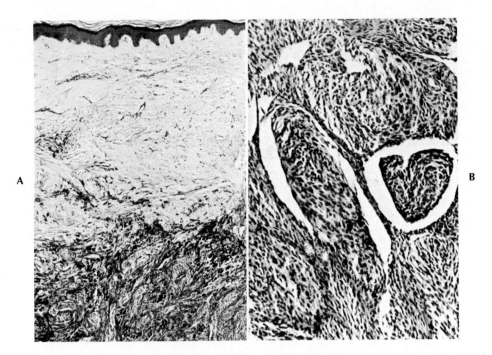

Fig. 36-46. Cellular blue nevus. **A,** Epidermis is intact. **B,** Appearance of invasion of lymphatics is an illusion characteristic of this lesion and results from artifactual shrinkage. (Hematoxylin and eosin.)

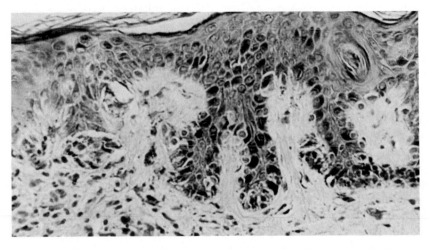

Fig. 36-47. Lentigo with pigmented rete ridges associated with junctional change. (Hematoxylin and eosin.)

formation of a blue nevus is often made unjustifiably, such cancers do occur.

SENILE LENTIGO

The senile lentigo is a common lesion occurring on exposed surfaces in approximately one third of individuals past middle age. It is characterized histologically by hyperkeratosis and parakeratosis and frondlike elon-

gation of the hyperpigmented rete ridges, often showing an increase in basilar clear cells or minimal junctional change (see Fig. 36-47).

MELANOTIC FRECKLE OF HUTCHINSON

Much attention has been given to essentially restatements of information concerning the melanotic freckle of Hutchinson, also known as *la mélanose circonscrite précancéreuse de Dubreuilh,* senile or malignant freckle, precancerous or acquired melanosis, premalignant lentigo, and lentigo maligna. Actually this lesion is characteristically a relatively slow-growing lesion of the face, generally of elderly patients, which evolves from epidermal melanosis to a junctional nevus with varying degrees of activity and finally, if the patient lives long enough, to a superficial and then deep (or nodular) melanocarcinoma. As long ago documented, the melanocarcinomas of the face, especially those of women, tend to be associated with a better prognosis than those of most other regions of the body.[11] Their histogenesis, however, is no different from that of any other junctional nevus or the melanocarcinoma derived therefrom.

HALO NEVUS

Halo nevus (leukoderma acquisitum centrifugum, Sutton's nevus) is the progressive centripetal extension of a zone of depigmentation about a nevus. This perilesional depigmentation may encircle not only benign nevi (intradermal, compound, and blue) but also malignant melanomas, as well as cutaneous metastases. Accordingly, this leukodermatous reaction gives no hint as to whether a given lesion is benign or malignant.

It has been hypothesized that the destruction of the nevus cells may represent an immune response to the antigens of the nevus cells or, on occasion, melanocarcinomatous cells. The eosinophilic globular disintegration of nevus cells that has been noted in juvenile melanomas may reflect a similar immunologic self-destruction. In the instance of juvenile melanomas this reaction may occur in the absence of nearby lymphocytes. The distortion generated by this reaction in both instances—halo nevi and juvenile melanomas—may lead to the mistaken diagnosis of malignant melanomas.

As stated, a spectrum of hypotheses ranging from antigen-antibody reaction to neurotropic disturbance has been suggested to explain the local vitiligo or leukoderma. The most reasonable is that the depigmentation results from the underlying inflammatory reaction similar to the depigmentation that may occur with lichen planus, for example.

MALIGNANT MELANOMAS

In 1953 malignant melanomas were classified as indicated below.[11] Almost two decades later others modified this classification by the addition in effect of more subdivisions indicated by the levels in parentheses[21]:

1. Melanocarcinoma from active junctional nevus (or junctional component of compound nevus)
   a. Melanocarcinoma in situ (level I)
   b. Superficial (level II, some in level III)
   c. Deep (those deeper in level III; IV, reticular; and V, subcuticular)
2. Malignant blue nevus

The essential modification of the parallel classifications involves the subdivision of the deep level into levels III, IV, and V. Actually melanocarcinomas so advanced and neglected as to have directly invaded the panniculus (level V) are rarely seen these days, mostly on the soles where the dermis is especially thin. The debatable contribution therefore centers on deeper levels III and IV[17] (Fig. 36-48). In one large series this subdivision has not proved informative[45] though others disagree somewhat.[93] However, there are several overlooked sources of error inherent in the classification by dermal levels, as follows:

1. Because of the pseudoepitheliomatous hyperplasia frequently associated with malignant melanomas, the rete ridges may extend illusorily deep into the reticular layer (level IV) and still function as a superficial melanocarcinoma.
2. The malignant melanomas have a remarkable propensity for growing outward, or exophytically. Accordingly, the nodular melanocarcinomas may behave the worst and yet not extend below the papillary layer of the dermis (Fig. 36-48). This same nodular lesion eventually complicates or originates from superficially spreading or lentiginous melanocarcinomas.
3. The dermal papillary layer varies considerably in different parts of the body, being particularly thin and superficial in the skin of many areas of the extremities.

In other words, the very premise on which the use of these levels rests is factitious, if only for their great variation in depth in different parts of the body. Hence the arbitrary use of the level of the interface between papillary and reticular layers as a measure of depth of invasion of lesion in various areas is grossly inaccurate. To imply further that the reticular layer is inherently a barrier to spread of the tumor is baseless. Finally, to state that the subdivision of melanoma into five anatomic levels of invasion permits the accurate assignment of prognosis to each case is patently hyperbolic. The behavior of these capriciously aggressive tumors beyond the superficial level cannot be measured predictably by boundaries of highly variable thicknesses, even if they are speciously drawn to the second decimal place. Therefore divisions of dermal invasion, other than superficial and deep, lend little substance to the analysis of these cancers.[11,12] The hard fact is that the least invasive superficial melanocarcinoma in individual instances may be as devastatingly lethal as one that has reached the panniculus. Metastasis to lymph nodes and death may in fact result from melanocarcinomas merely 0.4 to 0.6 mm in depth.[93]

The lack of a relationship between histologic pattern and prognosis is demonstrated frequently in vulval and subungual malignant melanomas, for example. The so-called levels of extension are similarly uninformative in

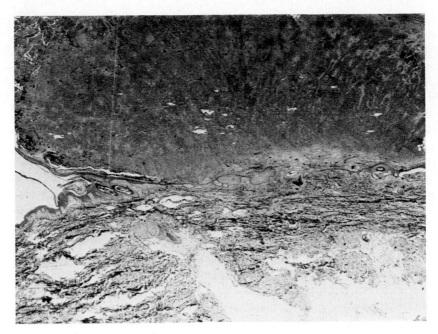

Fig. 36-48. Nodular malignant melanoma. This aggressive lesion does not extend beyond the papillary dermis, or so-called level II.

these areas as well as palms and soles, especially so-called level V.

Directly more consonant with the original categorization of malignant melanomas into superficial and deep types[12] is the popular one of the late Dr. Breslow's derived from the direct measurement of the depth of dermal invasion by the tumor.[17] The critical dermal levels were to be 0.76 mm and 1.51 mm, and these were made the pivotal determinants for surgical therapy (excision of lymph nodes) and prognosis. For a cancer as virulent and as unpredictable as melanocarcinoma, this tissue-thin line of transition would seem to be arbitrarily drawn. Aggressive neoplasms cannot be trusted to follow linearly the behavioral pattern dictated by a finely incremental graduation of the depth of invasion, except crudely as groups of superficial and deep tumors. The prognostic pattern is commonly not sustained in individual melanocarcinomas neither in the prognostically poor nodular melanomas with minimal dermal invasion, nor in the occasional instance of lethal superficially infiltrating melanoma at level II.

The *"thin" melanoma* is defined as measuring less than 0.76 mm. Most observers report that metastases occur rarely in patients with thin melanomas, such as 2%. However, if evidence of focal regression was present, the potential for metastasis was found to be increased.[40]

There is no perceptible advantage to labeling a melanocarcinoma in situ either "superficial spreading melanoma" or "lentigo maligna melanoma." The pivotal point is the presence or absence of dermal invasion

and, if present, whether it is superficial or deep. One of the disquieting consequences of the term "superficial spreading melanoma" is its increasingly facile use as an unwarranted substitute for junctional nevus, dysplastic or active junctional nevus, or melanocarcinoma in situ.

Clinically, malignant melanomas are nevertheless divided by most observers into (1) superficial spreading, (2) lentigo maligna, (3) nodular, and (4) acrolentiginous (Figs. 36-47, 36-48, and 36-50). The malignant melanoma is preceded usually by a flat, hairless mole, pigmented light to dark brown. When such a mole, which may have appeared the same for years, begins to darken, it probably has already undergone at least local malignant transformation. The changes of ulceration, increase in size, and bleeding obviously worsen the prognosis.[6,11] The recently promoted notion that, with few exceptions, mainly congenital, malignant melanomas arise anew, fails to reckon with the duration of the lesions and their histologic composition. These establish the frequent superimposition of malignant melanomas onto long-standing junctional or compound nevi. Malignant melanomas have arisen in burn scars, sites of vaccination, tattoos, severe sunburn, radiation, and an indelible-pencil puncture wound.

A mole that is hairy, elevated, and papillary is uncommonly the site of cancer though the assurance that the lesion is benign is not certain for the histologic reasons to be noted. In some instances the neoplasm appears to arise anew, especially on the scrotum, palms, and soles. In these regions the common (intradermal) mole rarely occurs, but the small, flat, often unnoticed, frecklelike junctional or compound nevus frequently is present. Because the lesions of the soles and genitalia are likely to have a junctional component, tend to escape inspection, and are located in areas that appear to have a proportionately higher incidence of malignant melanomas than other anatomic sites, it would seem reasonable to have such nevi removed electively from these sites when feasible. Some years ago I suggested that the better prognosis for women with malignant melanomas of the face (which are documented statistically) might be related to their greater likelihood of having the unsightly lesions removed earlier than men would.[11] Therefore the lesions would be removed before they had penetrated as deeply as similar lesions in men.

Currently there is an unfortunate tendency to submit for histologic examination the shaved top of a pigmented lesion (shave biopsy). Such a superficial biopsy not only complicates the problems of histologic diagnosis and the determination of clearance of margins, but also leads to recurrences of incompletely removed lesions. Moreover, distortions of their morphologic pattern may foster incorrect diagnoses. Some of the limitations of this technique have recently been emphasized.[24]

Histology and histogenesis

There is considerable variation in the cellular pattern of the melanocarcinomas. The primary lesion may simulate a squamous cell carcinoma, a spindle or basal cell carcinoma, an adenocarcinoma, a neurofibrosarcoma, or other neoplasms. The usual melanocarcinoma is composed of cells arranged as compact masses with some cords and alveoli. The cells are likely to be more or less uniform in size and shape. The nuclei of the primary lesion commonly do not exhibit the classic evidence of anaplasia. Mitotic figures may not be numerous, despite the aggressiveness of the neoplasm. Often the

nuclei are vacuolated and contain large acidophilic nucleoli resembling inclusion bodies, sometimes containing melanin. Melanin pigment may be present or absent without prognostic influence in the human as opposed to the Syrian hamster. In the neoplastic cells the pigment tends to be of a uniform, fine granularity, whereas in the chromatophores the pigment granules are likely to be more irregular in size and shape.

One of the most helpful histologic aids in diagnosis is the active junctional change overlying and continuous with the dermal portion of the cancer. The cells of the rete ridges may be so loosened as to be incorporated in the dermal neoplasm, with consequent partial dissolution of the ridges. Isolated, spherical, haloed cells, often powdered with fine melanin granules, may be found as far up as the stratum corneum (Figs. 36-49 and 36-50, A). Such intraepithelial cells are in my view the source of practically all melanocarcinomas of the skin and mucous membranes (blue nevi excepted) (Fig. 36-50, B). These cancerous cells are not related to Langerhans cells or Merkel-Ranvier corpuscles but actually seem to have been originally cells derived from various layers of the epidermis. Nor is it true, as some believe, that these cells within the epidermis are metastatic from the underlying tumor within the dermis. Evidence for the autochthonous epidermal origin is found not only in the occurrence of such cells within the epidermis alone in early junctional nevi or superficial malignant melanomas but also in their absence in the epidermis overlying a snugly apposed dermal metastasis of a melanoma (Fig. 36-50, C), a criterion that distinguishes the primary from the metastatic melanocarcinoma.

Minimal deviation melanoma

Minimal deviation melanoma is still another in the spate of gratuitous names lately applied to nevi and malignant melanomas. It refers to those melanomas with

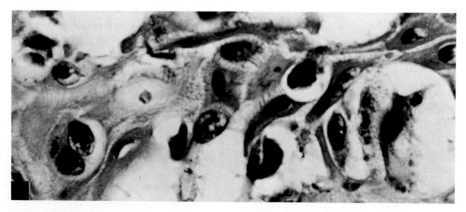

Fig. 36-49. Malignant melanoma in acantholytic, in situ portion, with hyperchromatic, pleomorphic, neoplastic cells, some with residual intercellular bridges denoting keratinocytic origin. (Hematoxylin and eosin.) (From Allen, A.C.: The skin, St. Louis, 1954, The C.V. Mosby Co.)

diffuse or localized foci of well-differentiated malignant cells or "minimally atypical" cells. These are said to occur as nodules in the deeper levels. It is not clear that this designation offers any added information as to prognosis or therapy.

Active junctional nevus (melanocarcinoma in situ)

It is now apparent that when a malignant melanoma appears to be superimposed on a benign intradermal nevus, originally a clinically obvious or latent junctional nevus was present that itself was the source of the malignant melanoma. Routine studies of the epidermis of the primary melanocarcinomas of skin (and mucous membranes, including conjunctivae) demonstrate this junctional change. In other words, the melanocarcinoma arising in the skin would actually seem to be a peculiarly virulent variant of an epidermogenic carcinoma, a view originally expressed by Unna in 1893.[92] Why the malignant melanoma usually behaves more aggressively than other epidermal carcinomas is not yet known. Occasionally it becomes a problem to decide if a given lesion is still in the stage of junctional nevus or has become a melanocarcinoma in situ. The histologic diagnosis of a superficial melanocarcinoma must, in the last analysis, depend on finding evidence of invasion of the upper dermis by the cells of the active junctional nevus (Fig. 36-50, C).[11]

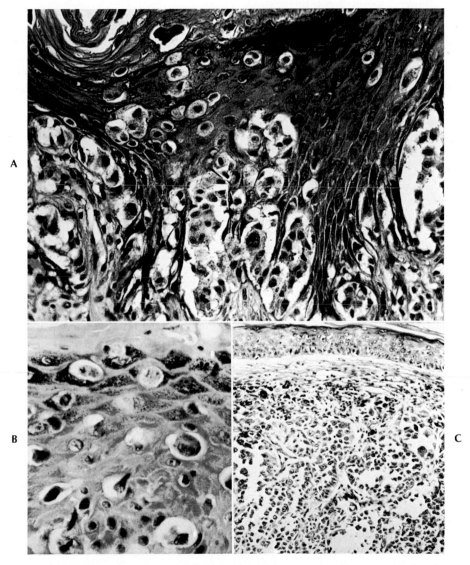

Fig. 36-50. Melanocarcinoma. **A,** Conversion of epidermal cells of pagetoid melanoma into melanocarcinomatous cells. **B,** In situ transformation of epidermal cells into melanocarcinomatous cells. **C,** Metastatic melanocarcinoma to skin showing overlying intact epidermis—criterion for primary versus metastatic melanocarcinoma. (Hematoxylin and eosin.)

Actually, all junctional nevi by definition exhibit a kind of activity or dynamics in the form of varying stages of acantholysis of the intraepidermal cells (Fig. 36-47). However, with this reservation I have in the past applied the term "active junctional nevus" to the one with nuclear atypia and mitotic figures and often with large, pagetoid cells scattered singly or in clumps to various levels of the epidermis.[10-12] Such a lesion is equivalent to melanocarcinoma in situ. The presence of such an active junctional nevus should lead to a painstaking search for dermal invasion with the help of multiple sections. The histologic criteria for the distinction of a superficial melanocarcinoma—from an active junctional nevus on one hand or a deep melanocarcinoma on the other—are essentially similar to those used for distinguishing a superficial squamous cell carcinoma from leukoplakia and from a deeply infiltrating carcinoma. Incidentally, the high degree of pseudoepitheliomatous hyperplasia so commonly associated with melanocarcinomas is largely responsible for mistaking these neoplasms for squamous cell carcinomas.[11] Patients with a melanocarcinoma appear to have a systemic diathesis for activation of junctional nevi, which in a percentage of cases (3.5%) leads to multiple primary melanocarcinomas. The activation of nevi in patients with malignant melanoma, first noted in 1953,[11] has been recently confirmed and its significance appreciated.[90]

Dysplastic nevi

It became clear to me that what was termed the "active junctional nevus" in 1953 was in some instances an intermediate phase in the development of what was soon designated as "melanocarcinoma in situ." Actually, many of the lesions now called "dysplastic nevi" belong to these categories. Mostly, they are active junctional nevi, whether familial (B-K) or nonfamilial with moderate or pronounced dysplasia with bands of concentric or lamellar fibrosis enveloping rete ridges made bulbous by junctional changes.

Local, piecemeal, incomplete regression of malignant melanomas has been repeatedly noted. However, complete regression of the local malignancy may occur.[84] I have seen a patient with inguinal node metastases from a primary melanocarcinoma of the heel of the foot with local residuum only of melanophores and focal minimal junctional change. The humoral attack on melanomas has thus far not provided fruitful, though their spontaneous regression, albeit rare, is suggestive of further study. Cell-mediated and humoral antitumor reactions have been noted in patients with melanomas, but their effect on the clinical course has not been shown. Malignant melanoma assays may exhibit positive estrogen receptors.[89]

Evidence of focal regression within a malignant mel-

anoma is arbitrarily defined as an area of subepidermal fibrosis underlying a flattened epidermis, absence of tumor cells, and a variable amount of melanophages, lymphocytes, and telangiectasia. It is clear that an excessive correlation regarding potential for metastasis or survival has been inferred from this kind of evidence of regression. The pathogenesis of "spontaneous" regression obviously is not known. In harmony with the current trend, the regression is attributed to a local immunologic event akin to that occurring in the halo nevus or perhaps a local change in immunoreactivity linked with an effect from some humoral alteration.

Bathing trunk nevi

These giant congenital nevi may be associated with leptomeningeal melanocytosis and often take the pattern of complex hamartomatous and choristomatous malformations. In addition to all varieties of pigmented nevi and malignant melanomas, they may develop neoplasms of lipoblastic, rhabdomyoblastic, and frankly neural origin (neurofibroma, schwannoma). It is in this type of lesion that the rare malignant melanoma unaccompanied by overlying junctional changes may be found. It is estimated that malignant melanomas develop in approximately 5% to 15% of patients with giant nevi (Fig. 36-51).

Melanocarcinomas of children*

A sizable series of melanocarcinomas or malignant melanomas of children has been collected, although occurrence of this lesion prior to puberty was doubted in the past. The impression that juvenile melanomas cannot be distinguished histologically from the malignant melanomas of children is still widely prevalent. Therefore, knowing that melanocarcinomas do, indeed, occur in children, how is a surgeon to react to a pathologist's report describing a juvenile melanoma as microscopically indistinguishable from a malignant melanoma but that, inasmuch as the patient is a child, the lesion should behave clinically benign? The fact was soon firmly established[11] and adequately confirmed that melanocarcinomas of children, although they may not be differentiable from the melanocarcinomas of adults, can be distinguished histologically from juvenile melanomas. To date [1989] we have been given the opportunity of studying 44 melanocarcinomas of children. Fifteen of those have been fatal; eight others have metastasized; the behavior of the remainder is not known to us. None of these has shown any of the several morphologic landmarks of the juvenile melanoma. This single fact, that is, the absence of features of the juvenile melanoma in

---

*Text from here to "Melanocarcinomas of mucous membranes" is modified from Allen, A.C.: The skin: a clinicopathologic treatise, ed. 2, New York, 1967, Grune & Stratton, Inc.

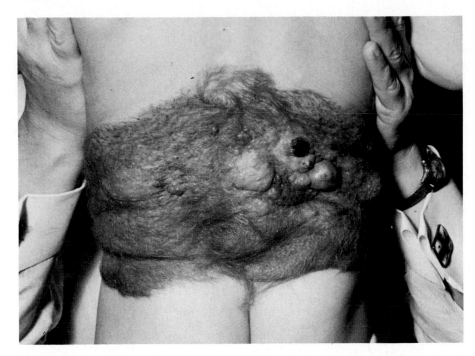

Fig. 36-51. Giant bathing trunk nevus with malignant melanoma, a common complication. (Courtesy Dr. Don Kelley; from Allen, A.C.: The skin, St. Louis, 1954, The C.V. Mosby Co.)

the melanocarcinomas of children, which resemble melanocarcinomas of adults, constitutes the core of the basis for the diagnosis of the tumors. Further to elucidate this criterion would be merely to list the well-known histologic characteristics of the malignant melanomas of adults. In general, it has been our experience thus far that the melanocarcinomas of children appear histologically somewhat more malignant than those of adults, though others seem not to have had this impression from their initial fairly small series. The overall difference in degree of anaplasia obviously cannot be so distinctive, however, as to make possible diagnostic differentiation from the adult cancer in each case.

Inasmuch as we have stated that a melanocarcinoma may occasionally arise from compound nevi including the juvenile melanomas, it is entirely conceivable that an early or small melanocarcinoma from a child may one day be observed in which all the original landmarks of the juvenile melanoma may not have been obliterated by the cancer.[11] This histologic residue of the juvenile melanoma has been noted in melanocarcinomas of adults but, as mentioned, not in those of children thus far. Such a finding does not warrant the statement that some juvenile melanomas are malignant. It merely means that a minute proportion of juvenile melanomas may undergo cancerous transformation, just as a small proportion of mammary fibroadenomas may become cystosarcomas. If a juvenile melanoma is correctly di-

agnosed, its adequate removal is tantamount to cure. To say that a completely resected juvenile melanoma has given rise to metastasis is, in effect, to state that an error in diagnosis has been made and that a malignant melanoma has been mistaken for a juvenile melanoma. There is reason to believe that the juvenile melanoma has essentially the same potentiality for undergoing cancerous change that any other compound nevus has, no greater, no less. This incidence of malignant transformation of compound nevi is extremely low, a fact interpolated from the enormous incidence of compound nevi in the general population in contrast with the relative infrequency of malignant melanomas.

In none of the melanocarcinomas of children was there evidence of the kind of vacuolization of cells that has been associated with pregnancy or menarche.[12] However, in one of the patients personally observed—a 5-year-old Negro—the melanocarcinoma of the buccal mucosa was associated with a functioning adrenocortical carcinoma.

Melanocarcinomas of mucous membranes

Melanocarcinomas of the mucous membranes of the oronasopharynx, larynx, bronchus, esophagus, gallbladder, and genitalia, including the cervix and anorectal region, are almost uniformly fatal. Undoubtedly some of the contributory reasons for their grave prognosis are the delay in detection and in accurate histologic diag-

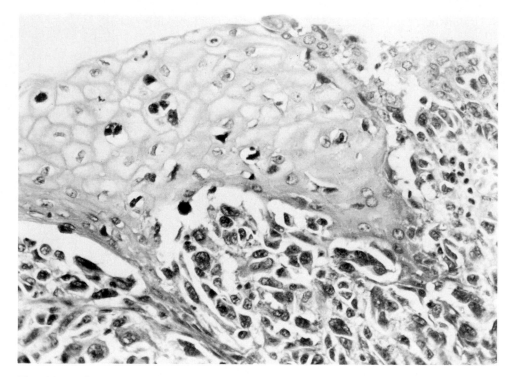

Fig. 36-52. Primary melanocarcinoma of bronchus illustrating the junctional change in the squamous epithelium, diagnostic of the primary site. (Hematoxylin and eosin.)

nosis, the frequent injudicious therapy, the difficulties in adequate operative removal, and possibly such extraneous factors as chronic infection and repeated trauma. In approximately 15% of 337 patients in one study the tumors arose in these various mucous membranes (exclusive of the conjunctiva).[11] The ulceration of the junctional change and the absence of appreciable amounts of pigment in about 50% of the melanomas of mucous membranes increase the difficulties of histologic diagnosis. Melanocarcinomas of mucous membranes may arise in any mucosa lined by either normally present or metaplastic stratified squamous epithelium (Fig. 36-52).[7,10,11]

The occurrence of "acral melanomas," those on the hands and feet, is particularly high among Japanese and African blacks in contrast with their presence on the trunk and face, the more common occurrence in whites.

TUMORS OF VESSELS
Lymphangioma

The number of histologic and clinical variants, as well as the difficulty in distinguishing neoplasia of lymphatic vessels from ectasias, anomalies, and proliferations attributable to stasis, has led to the application of needlessly confusing names. The same situation exists with respect to the angiomas, but in both instances it has existed so long that scrapping of terminology at this point would add to the confusion.

The *lymphangioma simplex* is a soft, compressible, grayish pink nodule. The nodules are often multiple and grouped irregularly. Although the skin of the genitalia is the common site for these tumors, they are found also on the lips and tongue and may be associated with macroglossia or macrocheilia. They are composed of varying-sized, endothelium-lined, thin-walled vessels, either empty or containing lymph with occasional leukocytes. Some of the channels may contain a few red blood cells. There is an abundant proliferation of endothelial cells in a proportion of tumors, to which the designation *lymphangioma tuberosum multiplex* or *lymphangioendothelioma* has been applied.

Lymphangioma cutis circumscriptum occurs in the skin of the face, chest, or extremities in the form of a single tumor or multiple projecting, somewhat papillary, verrucose nodules. They may resemble opalescent vesicles, and there may be an associated telangiectasis. Histologically they are composed of dilated lymphatic vessels in the upper dermis and are so closely linked to the epidermis as to appear incorporated in it. The overlying epidermis may be irregularly atrophied and acanthotic as well as hyperkeratotic in a papillary manner so as to simulate the angiokeratomas (see also p. 1820).

The *lymphangioma cavernosum* may be small and circumscribed, or it may ramify diffusely over an extensive area, causing macrodactylia, for example. Histologically the lymphatic channels are greatly dilated and may penetrate fat and muscle, as the so-called infiltrating angiomas do. The unencapsulated extensions are in neither instance evidence of malignant transformation, but they do complicate local removal.

The *lymphangioma cysticum coli,* or hygroma, is a congenital lesion that arises usually in the neck and submaxillary regions and is histologically similar to the lymphangioma cavernosum in both structure and extension. The hygroma may also ramify widely upward to the parotid area, downward as far as the mediastinum, and inward to lie precariously close to the trachea and adjacent structures. The lymphangioma cysticum may occur too in the region of the sacrum (p. 799).

Hemangioma

The problems of the pathogenesis and terminology of tumors of blood vessels are even more complicated than those of lymphangiomas. Theoretically a true hemangioma is to be differentiated from a simple dilatation of blood vessels by its independence from the adjacent normal circulatory channels. A hemangioma enlarges, therefore, by growth of its own elements rather than by incorporation of nearby vessels. In practice, however, these criteria are seldom applied, and accordingly many ectasias, hyperemias, and hyperplasias are included as neoplasias. The hemangiomas may be classified simply as capillary, cavernous, or mixed (p. 794).

The *capillary angioma* corresponds clinically to the familiar *port-wine stain* on the face and neck, but it exists also as simple small vascular nevi or birthmarks. In infants, such angiomas may be composed of compact masses of endothelial cells in which the capillary lumens are obscured in many areas. These proliferations often extend from the dermis into the subcutaneous tissue. The extension of the lesion beyond the dermis and its rich cellularity may provoke the erroneous diagnosis of angiosarcoma.[86] However, such angiomatous formations are usually sufficiently characteristic to make possible the diagnosis of benign infantile angioma on the basis of histologic appearance alone. The capillary angioma may be confused histologically also with *granuloma pyogenicum,* particularly if the former is ulcerated and inflamed, as the latter usually is. The granuloma pyogenicum, however, is characteristically polypoid, generally has been present for no longer than 1 to 3 months, and bleeds easily and repeatedly. The histologic features of granuloma pyogenicum are identical with those of the so-called *pregnancy tumor* that occurs in the oral mucosa during gestation. Thrombocytopenia may be associated with giant vascular tumors. The remission of the thrombocytopenia after removal of the hemangioma indicates that the tumor may occasionally serve as a reservoir for the platelets.

The *sclerosing hemangioma* appears to be a special variety of capillary angioma, though few dermatologists subscribe to this interpretation. They prefer to regard the lesion as a dermatofibroma lenticulare, histiocy-

toma, or merely subepidermal fibrosis. The lesions occur chiefly on the extremities and appear clinically as single, firm, and slightly elevated intracutaneous nodules, averaging several millimeters to a centimeter in diameter. Their sectioned surface is smooth and yellow.

Histologically, more or less of the dermis is replaced by spindle cells, arranged generally in tight curlicues, though in some areas these cells appear to enclose tiny spaces suggestive of the lumens of capillaries.

Occasionally the vascular luminal component is predominant, and the cavernous channels are characteristically associated with abundant hemosiderin and numerous lipid-filled macrophages. This aneurysmal feature has no significance other than reflecting the vascular histogenesis of the lesion variously termed *fibrous histiocytoma, dermatofibroma, fibroma dura,* and others. It may be associated with pain and tenderness. This histologic variability matches that of the glomangioma, which also may range from a cellular to a cavernous pattern.

Usually the cells are vacuolated by lipid, and in some cases the fat content is the most striking feature. Dark brown granules of hemosiderin are often present in many of the cells. At times the iron pigment may be so abundant that some observers, confusing the pigment with melanin, have made the serious error of labeling the lesion a malignant melanoma. The overlying epidermis may be normal, atrophied, moderately acanthotic, or the site of a superimposed basal cell carcinoma[41] (Fig. 36-53). In some instances a sharply delimited subepidermal zone of the dermis is spared. A similar free zone is seen in the dermal neurofibroma, though perhaps not so frequently. The sclerosing hemangioma may sometimes be justifiably confused with the neurofibroma when, as not infrequently occurs, the deeper portion of the lesion is composed of fasciculi of spindle cells such as characterize the neurifibroma. The impression gained by light microscopy of the hemangiomatous origin of these lesions is confirmed by the observation of Weibel-Palade bodies with the electron microscope. These are intracytoplasmic tubular structures, presumably derived from the Golgi apparatus and apparently specific for endothelial cells.

Occasionally a fibrotic tumor resembling the sclerosing hemangioma, particularly of the trunk, recurs locally with formation of satellite nodules. Usually such tumors originally extended into the subcutaneous fat and were removed incompletely. These tumors, called "dermatofibrosarcoma protuberans," give rise to distant metastases in rare instances.

The *cavernous (aneurysmal) hemangiomas* are histologically similar to the cavernous lymphangiomas except for the presence of blood in the congeries of vessels. The vessels may ramify progressively in the subcutaneous fat, fascia, and intermuscular septa. The extensions may be so wide and inaccessible as to make sur-

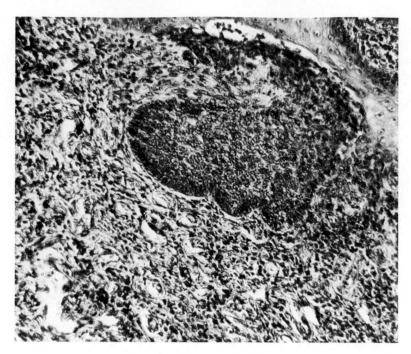

Fig. 36-53. Sclerosing angioma with overlying nest of basal cell carcinoma in situ. (Hematoxylin and eosin.)

gical removal exceedingly difficult. The term "infiltrating angioma," is more aptly applied to such tumors than "angiosarcoma" is. The papillary form of an intravenular organized thrombus has been called "vegetant intravascular hemangioendothelioma" and mistaken even for an angiosarcoma.

Clinically the cavernous hemangiomas appear on the skin surface as purple, single, globular or multilobular tumors or as the flat or slightly elevated strawberry nevus of infants. The angiomas may be multiple and may cause, or at least be associated with, enlargement and distortion of an area of the body in the vicinity of the tumors. The distortion from edema and hypertrophy of an arm (Weber syndrome) may be so great as to require amputation because of the sheer weight of the extremity.

Other syndromes associated with anomalies of blood vessels include the Sturge-Weber syndrome (nevus flammeus of the face, cerebral angiomatosis, hemiplegia, and mental retardation), Maffucci's syndrome (angiomas with dyschondroplasia), and heredofamilial angiomatosis (Rendu-Osler-Weber disease). Cutaneous angiomas also may be part of the complex of multiple congenital angiomas found in the viscera, particularly in the cerebellum and retina, and known as Hippel's disease. The blue rubber-bleb nevus appears to be a form of venous hamartoma involving both skin and gastrointestinal tract. It is characterized by pain, sweating, and a sensation of dermal herniation.[74]

The *angiokeratoma*, or telangiectatic wart, represents a variety of cavernous hemangioma that is structurally similar to the lymphangioma cutis circumscriptum. The dilated blood channels are high in the papillae and are so intimately associated with the epidermis as to appear actually within it in many places. The overlying epidermis is usually papillary, acanthotic, and hyperkeratotic. Clinically the lesions are dark purplish red, firm, the size of a pinhead or split pea, and located in the scrotum, ears, fingers, and toes. The lesions often are associated with some circulatory disturbance such as might follow chillblains and varicosites. This type that tends to occur on the extensor surface of the extremities is known as the Mibelli type of angiokeratoma as opposed to Fordyce's type without associated pernio. The angiokeratoma of Fabry may be associated with lesions of viscera, particularly the kidneys and vessels with characteristic foam cells. Patients with angiokeratoma of Fabry may excrete increased amounts of the glycoproteins ceramide trihexoside and dihexoside. Examination of the urine for these glycoproteins may aid in the detection of the disorder in members of the families of patients.

Spider angiomas, which are really small telangiectases, possibly with arteriovenous shunts, occur with chronic hepatic damage as in Laënnec's cirrhosis, as well as in pregnancy. They are believed to be an effect of excess of estrogenic hormones.

The term "hemangioendothelioma," as previously indicated, is hedgingly applied to hemangiomas in which there is a relative prominence of endothelial cells with or without atypia. The implication in its use is that the neoplasm shows greater activity and therefore presents more likelihood of local recurrence than the ordinary hemangioma. The evidence for this presumption is questionable. A similar situation exists with respect to the use of "lymphangioendothelioma." Unfortunately, the name "hemangioendothelioma," rather than "angiosarcoma," is sometimes applied to the frankly malignant tumor.

Cutaneous meningioma

The cutaneous meningioma occurs as an isolated dysembryogenetic subcutaneous nodule with occasional dermal involvement, or as an ectopic extension into soft tissue corresponding in distribution to cranial and spinal nerves. The latter may cause signs and symptoms reflective of the associated nerves or those of a tumor mass such as proptosis, nasal polyp, or soft-tissue mass. The histologic picture is that of a meningothelial cell tumor or sclerosing angioma with characteristic psammoma bodies.[55]

Angiosarcoma

Primary solitary angiosarcoma of the skin, exclusive of Kaposi's hemorrhagic sarcoma, is rare. However, there have been recorded several cases in which visceral metastases have occurred. The metastases tend to be more cellular and anaplastic than the original growth. As stated, others have been reported as malignant vascular tumors of skin under the title "hemangioendothelioma," but in most instances evidence of origin from dermis, as well as of the cancerous characteristics, is not convincingly presented. It has been suggested that the presence of lymphocytes within and at the periphery of the tumor is more closely correlated with the likelihood of metastasis or survival than other parameters, such as mitoses and anaplasia, are. Knowledge of the rarity of such tumors is of practical importance because of its tempering effect on the tendency to call sarcomatous those nonmetastasizing angiomas with abundant endothelial cells or those that have infiltrated into the subcutaneous fat and beyond into the muscles. Kaposi's sarcoma, on the other hand, represents a process of vastly different significance.

Kaposi's idiopathic hemorrhagic sarcoma

Classical Kaposi's sarcoma begins as purplish brown, discrete or grouped, painful, tender nodules varying from 1 to 2 mm in size to about 1 cm. They occur particularly on the hands and feet, though they may start in the skin of any part of the body. The incidence is about 10 times greater in men than in women, and the disease is seen especially in elderly patients, though it has been described in children. The surface of the nodules may be telangiectatic, but often it is verrucose. Local purpura and bullae may be associated with the lesions. Lymphatic blockage with elephantiasis of the extremities is common and is reminiscent of the edema associated with postmastectomy lymphangiosarcoma. The course of the disease is slow, the nodules often involuting, with resultant atrophic scarring and pigmentation. The condition may last from 1 to fully 25 years, though the average duration is from 5 to 10 years. Apart from patients with AIDS, the disease is found chiefly in Italian and Jewish people.

The lesions may involve extensive areas of the skin and nearly every organ of the body. The gastrointestinal tract, mesenteric nodes, liver, and lungs are the most common sites, though even the osseous and central nervous systems may be affected. The question is unsettled as to whether these lesions are truly metastases or actually multicentric foci of a neoplasm. The intestinal lesions of Kaposi's sarcoma, unlike most other metastatic lesions, have a predilection for the inner coats rather than the serosa. In this location the tumors give rise to profuse hemorrhage. This difference in location in the intestinal tract between Kaposi's sarcoma and other metastatic tumors is evidence in favor of the multicentric origin of the former. Visceral tumors histologically identical to Kaposi's sarcoma have been found infrequently without cutaneous involvement. Patients with Kaposi's sarcoma die of hemorrhage from an intestinal lesion, intercurrent infection, extensive visceral involvement, or complicating malignant lymphomas.

Kaposi's sarcoma is a form of angiosarcoma that is so varied histologically that there is frequently difficulty in the interpretation of a given slide. In one phase, perhaps the earliest, the picture is that of a simple hemangioma or of foci of hyperemic, nonspecific granulation tissue characterized by clusters of capillaries placed close together, with or without a sprinkling of mononuclear cells and histiocytes containing hemosiderin in the intervening and often edematous stroma. At this stage the endothelial cells may be quite regular, without mitotic figures or other evidence of anaplasia. The important histologic clue is the disposition of these vascular foci not only near the epidermis, but also isolated about appendages, muscles, and nerves in the deeper layers of the dermis. The presence of such vascular foci at a distance from the surface of the skin is suspiciously unlike the ordinary pattern of the response of skin inflammation. In more advanced lesions there occurs proliferation of spindle cells and fibroblasts in association with scattered lymphocytes and histiocytes. The cells appear to form abortive capillaries, and in the actively growing lesions these cells are large and hyperchromatic and contain mitotic figures. In the later stages there is a tendency toward focal necrosis of the neoplastic tissue and subsequent fibrosis. These variegated pictures may be observed not only at different stages of the disease but often within a single lesion. Clusters of lymphocytes, histiocytes, and reticulum cells may be interspersed throughout the lesion. Indeed, there is an increasing number of reports in the literature of the simultaneous occurrence of Kaposi's sarcoma with one or another of the malignant lymphomas, including Hodgkin's disease, lymphatic leukemia, lymphosarcoma, and mycosis fungoides. For both statistical and histologic reasons (the latter comprising evidence of transition of the two processes within the same lesion), the association is not considered coincidental.[7,10]

Acquired immunodeficiency syndrome

In 1980 the United States, and later the world, was jolted by the outbreak of hundreds of instances of a dreaded form of Kaposi's sarcoma with a fulminance previously unknown, as part of a heart-breaking symptom complex now known as AIDS (acquired immunodeficiency syndrome). Kaposi's sarcoma occurs in about one third of the cases. Involvement also of lymph nodes, spleen, and gastrointestinal tract is not uncommon. Other cutaneous disorders in AIDS include herpes simplex, herpes zoster, fungal infections, granuloma annulare, varicella, molluscum contagiosum, impetigo, folliculitis, ichthyosis, seborrheic dermatitis, and infection with *Mycobacterium avium-intracellulare.*

As of this writing approximately 85,000 cases have been recorded in the United States and 300,000 worldwide, with a relentless mortality close to 40% within 2 years and almost twice that rate beyond 2 years. The patients have been concentrated in New York City, with a predilection among male homosexuals, users of intravenous drugs, hemophiliacs and other blood recipients, and Haitian immigrants. Adding a frightening new epidemiologic dimensions are the recent discoveries that the disease may be transmitted heterosexually and among prison populations. Fear of the unknown has caused landlords to evict tenants with this disease. It is estimated that 1 in 200 persons in the general population have antibodies to the HIV.

The incubation period is highly variable, and the etiologic factors thus far are unknown. In these immunologically deficient individuals, complication by rampaging opportunistic organisms (for example, *Pneumocystis carinii,* cytomegalovirus, *Mycobacterium avium-intracellulare,* deep fungi, and rarely the organisms causing botryomycosis) is naturally frequent and lethal (Fig. 36-54). The histologic characteristics of cutaneous Kaposi's sarcoma parallel the spectrum of the more slowly evolving counterpart. Although no causative organisms have yet been implicated in these nodules themselves, it is of ancillary interest that verruga peruana, the cutaneous form of bartonellosis, appears histologically as an angiomatoid lesion in which the tiny organisms are harbored within the endothelial cytoplasm, much as rickettsiae and cytomegalovirus are harbored. This observation has been recently reemphasized by others, but up to now an etiologic agent has not been revealed in the endothelial cells of Kaposi's sarcoma.

The more than fortuitous relationship of the indolent,

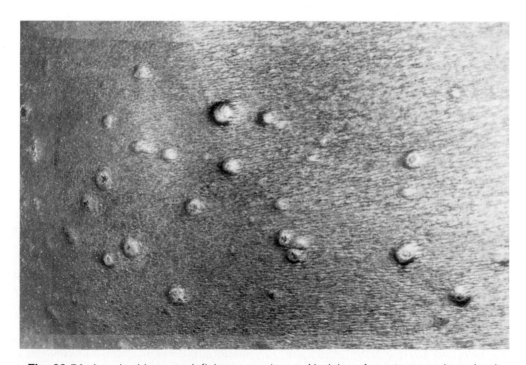

Fig. 36-54. Acquired immunodeficiency syndrome. Nodules of cryptococcosis on back.

rare, old form of Kaposi's sarcoma to various types of malignant lymphomas may be related to the immunologic problem in AIDS. For example, in AIDS the normal 2:1 ratio of helper-to-suppressive T-cells is reversed. The helper cells are also misshapen, a feature further supporting the concept of immunologic compromise presumably triggered by intracellular viral infection. Lymph nodes and spleens show a depletion of lymphocytes. The Kaposi's sarcoma of equatorial Africa (Kenya, Zaïre, Tanzania) is more akin to that of AIDS in that it is virulent and attacks the young. But evidence of immunologic deficiency in the traditional form of torpid Kaposi's sarcoma has not been forthcoming.

Opportunistic cancers other than Kaposi's sarcoma may occur with AIDS, such as B-cell lymphomas and basal and squamous cell carcinomas of the mouth and anus. These are attributed to the failure of immune surveillance to recognize virally transformed target cells.[70] Indeed, it has been hypothesized that the aggressive or metastasizing capacity may be related to the specific deficiency in immune surveillance in patients with AIDS.[83]

Postmastectomy lymphangiosarcoma

In 1948 an entity described as lymphangiosarcoma was recorded[88] as a complication of postmastectomy lymphedema of the upper extremity.[78] The lymphangiosarcoma in the skin of the edematous arm developed 6 to 24 years after the mastectomy, with the lymphedema having existed during the entire latent period. In one instance the tumor of the breast was benign. There was no relationship between the use of radiation and the development of the lymphangiosarcoma. As originally suspected, lymphangiosarcoma may complicate chronic edema, including congenital lymphedema of extremities unassociated with mammary carcinoma or its treatment.

Histologically the sarcoma has a range of variation quite equal to that of Kaposi's sarcoma, and indeed in many sections it is impossible to be certain that the neoplasic elements are lymphatic vessels rather than blood sinuses. The tumor is capable of metastasizing. Rare instances of lymphangiosarcoma as a complication of the lymphedema of filariasis have been recorded. The mechanism of cancerogenesis in the cases of lymphedema is obscure.

Glomus tumor

In the corium of the skin of the fingertips, particularly in the nail beds, around the joints of the extremities, and over the scapulae and coccyx, there are normally arteriovenous shunts, or glomera. These are composed of an afferent artery, the Sucquet-Hoyer canal or shunt, and an efferent vein. The artery is surrounded by several layers of small, spherical uniform glomus cells that superficially resemble the cells of the intradermal nevus and that are presumed to control the flow of blood by their contractility. Nonmedullated nerves and bundles of smooth muscle are intimately associated with the shunt. Tumors of this structure are called glomangiomas, angiomyoneuromas, glomus tumors, or neuromyoarterial aneurysms. They are most common in the nail bed but occur elsewhere on the extremities and trunk and even beneath the skin in muscles and joints, as well as in viscera. No instance of tumor occurring in the coccygeal glomus has been observed.

Glomus tumors appear as purplish red spots several millimeters in diameter, which are often clinically diagnosable by a characteristically lancinating pain, remarkably severe in view of the small size of the tumors. Not all glomangiomas, however, are associated with this characteristic symptom, which occasionally is simulated by dermal angiomyomas.

Histologically the glomus tumors range from compact masses of uniform glomus cells with few vascular channels to cavernous skeins of vessels cuffed by these cells. The vessels of the tumors tend to be small, especially in the nail bed. The identifying features are the several rows of peritheliomatously arranged glomus cells in which mitotic figures are rare or absent. These cells may be so numerous as to obliterate vascular lumens and to resemble a basal cell tumor or a variety of sweat gland adenoma. Nonmedullated nerves usually are discerned, but there appears to be no apparent relationship between the pain and the number or location of these nerves. Occasionally, glomus tumors are called simply "hemangiomas," or "glomangioid tumors," because of the presence of only two or three perivascular rows of glomus cells. However, such tumors have been observed with the typical symptoms of glomangiomas. Ultrastructural studies reveal masses of cytoplasmic fibers suggestive of a transition from smooth muscle cells.

TUMORS OF MUSCLE

Two varieties of tumors of dermal muscle are described: leiomyoma (arising from arrectores pilorum) and angiomyoma.

Leiomyoma cutis

The leiomyoma cutis occurs singly or in groups of as many as dozens of firm, usually pea-sized nodules, which are often tender and painful. Histologically they are composed of interlacing sheets of smooth muscle that may resemble a haphazard compact collection of arrectores pilorum. Infrequently the nuclei are large, irregular in size and shape, and hyperchromatic so as to merit the terms "leiomyosarcoma cutis," or "dermatomyosarcoma."

Leiomyosarcomas, primarily originating in the skin and less frequently in the subcutaneous tissue, occur rarely; approximately 80 such cases have been documented.[33] In these persons they appeared as painful or tender nodules, most commonly on the extremities of middle-aged persons. None of the cutaneous leiomyosarcomas metastasized, whereas almost 50% of the subcutaneous lesions, even though initially circumscribed, metastasized or behaved aggressively.

Angiomyoma

The angiomyoma is a small nondescript nodule that, microscopically, is made up of circular masses of smooth muscle strongly reminiscent of the media of arteries. The residual arterial lumen is discernible in the core of many of the masses of muscle. These lesions remain benign. Occasionally they may be found in the subcutaneous fat or even more deeply in the fascia or intermuscular septa of the extremities. As stated, they may cause the sharp pain generally associated with glomangiomas.

Myoblastoma

The granular cell myoblastoma is found as a nodule in the skin of various parts of the body, as well as on the mucous membranes, particularly of the tongue and isolated sites such as the larynx, thyroid gland, breast, gallbladder, esophagus, stomach, appendix, pituitary gland, and uvea.

Histologically the tumors are composed of nests and alveoli of large cells with small, centrally placed nuclei in cytoplasm loosely stippled with eosinophilic granules, occasionally replaced by polyhedral crystalloids. These periodic acid—Schiff–positive granules appear to contain lipoprotein or glycolipid and ultrastructurally

may be amorphous, vesicular, vacuolar, or particulate. The cells closely resemble those of a xanthoma, but fat stains are negative. Close examination shows that the cytoplasm is not actually vacuolated, as lipid histiocytes are. The loose dispersion of granules that simulate vacuoles has been believed to represent embryonic fibrils of striated muscle cells. Such a hypothesis is open to question, inasmuch as these tumors are present in the corium and other sites where striated muscle does not occur. The same objection may be leveled at the hypothesis that these cells represent degenerated adult striated fibers, though in sites where striated muscle is normally present, such as the tongue, this kind of transition occasionally is suggested. In addition, the evidence for the neurogenesis is not adequate. The concept of a fibroblastic origin has been advanced and appears far more convincing. In any event, whether or not these tumors are proved eventually to be fibroblastic, it is clear that they are easily recognizable histologic entities that rarely if ever metastasize. Some of the so-called malignant granular cell myoblastomas are, in reality, unrelated rhabdomyosarcomas in which a few of the cells happen to be granular.

One of the remarkable and distinctive features of many of the myoblastomas is the characteristic epithelial or epidermal acanthosis that overlies the lesion. This feature is not present in association with frank cutaneous leiomyomas. As a rule, dermal neoplasms leave the epidermis essentially unaltered or cause its atrophy through compression. The myoblastomas, on the other hand, appear to provoke a degree of acanthosis that may simulate squamous cell carcinoma. It is as if some epidermal irritant were present in the cells of the

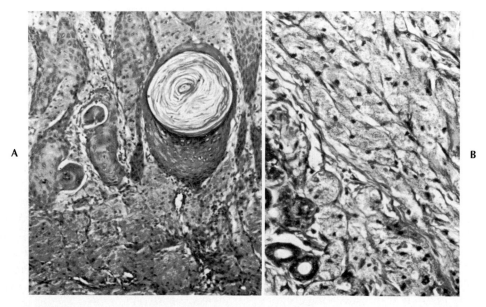

Fig. 36-55. Myoblastoma. **A,** Characteristic pseudoepitheliomatous hyperplasia. **B,** Granular cytoplasm and uniform small nuclei. (Hematoxylin and eosin.)

myoblastoma (Fig. 36-55). An analogous epidermal proliferation overlies many of the sclerosing angiomas, as previously mentioned.

CUTANEOUS FIBROMA

The diagnosis of cutaneous fibroma is usually found on careful review to include dermatofibroma lenticulare or sclerosing hemangioma, neurofibroma, leiomyoma, keloids, and other scars. This confusion does not apply to the pedunculated soft lipofibromas (fibroma molle) in which the fibrous component closely simulates the normal dermal collagen. Undoubtedly some of the spindle-shaped squamous cell carcinomas and melanocarcinomas have been mistaken for fibrosarcomas and atypical fibroxanthomas of the skin.

DIGITAL FIBROUS TUMORS OF CHILDHOOD

A form of well-differentiated, occasionally locally recurrent fibroma of childhood occurs on all digits but the thumb and great toe. Histologically they appear to be cellular fascial or dermal fibromas. They are characterized by a single, paranuclear, eosinophilic *cytoplasmic inclusion* attributed to a metabolic derangement.[25]

NEUROFIBROMA

Neurofibroma may occur in the skin as a single tumor or as multiple nodules. In the latter condition the entity is classified as neurofibromatosis, or von Recklinghausen's disease, and may be associated with café-au-lait pigmented spots and neurofibromas of the sympathetic system, as well as of motor and sensory nerve trunks. The tumors of the skin may be so numerous as to cover almost the entire body from scalp to feet.

The histogenesis of the tumors is complex. The axons, as well as the nerve sheaths (neurilemma) and endoneurium, participate to a varying extent, and so the histologic picture may be altered accordingly. The tumor derived predominantly from nerve sheaths (neurilemoma) tends to manifest more obvious palisading of cells (Antoni A structure), degenerating, edematous microcystic foci (Antoni B), and hyaline Verocay bodies. Occasionally the neurilemoma presents pronounced central necrosis and such excessive telangiectasis that it can be mistaken for an angioma. An examination of the periphery of these degenerated tumors usually reveals the telltale palisading of the neurilemoma. A small percentage of the cutaneous neurofibromas show sufficient hyperchromatism and irregularity in size and shape of nuclei to suggest sarcomatous degeneration. Here, too, however, metastases from these neoplasms of the skin are rare, though local recurrence is fairly frequent. On the other hand, malignant changes in the visceral neurofibromas are common and may take the form of extensive, fatal, local infiltrations or metastases. The benign neurilemoma (schwannoma) undergoes malignant change with extreme rarity. They are presumed not to have developed from a benign neurilemoma but to have been malignant from the start.

OSTEOMA

Osteoma cutis, an example merely of heterotopic bone, represents a metaplastic change of dermal collagen rather than true neoplasia. The lesion occurs as small nodules, as a rule, in scleroderma or syphilis, in association with acne or intradermal nevi, with hyperparathyroidism, and after trauma or cystotomies—the last because of the osteogenic potentialities of urinary tract epithelium—or without apparent reason.

The histologic picture may include fat and even marrow cells in addition to the bony trabeculas.

LYMPHOMAS AND ALLIED DISEASES

The lymphomas and allied diseases of the skin include mycosis fungoides, Hodgkin's disease, lymphosarcoma, and leukemia. Cutaneous lesions characterized by lymphocytic or lymphocytic-histiocytic dermal infiltrates may be among the most difficult to judge. As the following paragraphs indicate, the fact is that many reactive infiltrates may closely simulate neoplastic lesions.

Mycosis fungoides

There has been renewed interest in the histogenesis, histology, and natural history of the entity long ago and still uncomfortably labeled "mycosis fungoides." It is a lymphomatous disease in which the cutaneous component is characterized clinically by three stages: (1) premycotic, (2) infiltrative, and (3) fungoid tumefaction.

The premycotic stage is characterized by eczematoid, severely pruritic, erythrodermic, scaly, well-defined patches or by a generalized erythroderma. The eruption in this phase may simulate erythroderma. The eruption in this phase may simulate eczema, psoriasis, parapsoriasis, seborrheic dermatitis, or a nonspecific exfoliative dermatitis. This stage may persist for months or years and may be impossible to diagnose with assurance either clinically or microscopically. In the second or infiltrative stage, firm, slightly elevated, bluish red plaques arise in both the previously involved and the uninvolved areas. Partial or incomplete loss of hair from the scalp and other regions may occur. The last or fungoid stage follows the infiltrative period by several months (Fig. 36-56). Rarely, nodules of dystrophic xanthomatosis may be the presenting sign. Isolated instances of the disorder beginning in childhood or adolescence have been reported.

The tumors vary in diameter up to 10 cm or larger and are prone to ulcerate. In each of the stages spontaneous remissions may be noted, but these are temporary. Of interest in this respect is the regression, albeit temporary, of cutaneous lesions of mycosis fungoides occurring after reactions of delayed hyper-

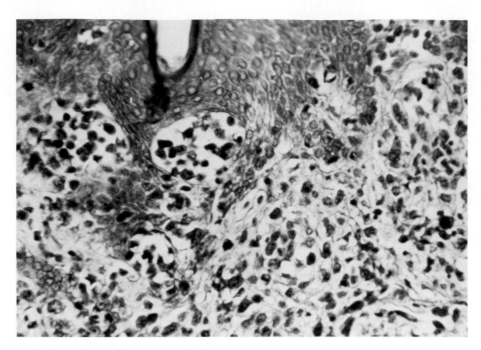

Fig. 36-56. Mycosis fungoides with Pautrier-Darier abscesses and characteristic subepidermal infiltrate. (Hematoxylin and eosin.)

sensitivity provoked directly in the lesions. The diagnosis in the few reported instances of cure must be questioned. In some cases the preliminary two stages do not develop. This form is called "mycosis fungoides d'emblée" (from French 'at the first onset'). True instances of mycosis fungoides d'emblée must be exceedingly rare. Undoubtedly, most of the recorded cases are, in reality, examples of Hodgkin's disease, reticulum or histiocytic cell sarcoma, or leukemia.

Sézary syndrome, or reticulosis, is a variant of mycosis fungoides consisting of erythroderma and Sézary cells in the peripheral blood, marrow, and lymph nodes. The likelihood is that the Sézary cells and the atypical cells of mycosis fungoides, with indented, convoluted, or cerebriform nuclei, are identical and represent T-lymphocytes.[56,57] Similar cells have been noted in normal persons, in patients with benign dermatoses, and after stimulation of lymphocytes with mitogens.[97] Actually, mycosis fungoides is being regarded as a response to antigenic persistence with malignant lymphoma developing as a consequence of immunologic imbalance. Perhaps related in principle is the occurrence of reticulum cell sarcoma in recipients of renal transplants with immunosuppressive therapy, as others have suggested.

The histologic picture of the first or premycotic stage of mycosis fungoides is usually not diagnostic and may resemble one of the many conditions simulated clinically. However, even in this phase of the disease there is a tendency for the infiltrate to be confined as a zone in the upper dermis and for the epidermis to appear

psoriasiform. Occasionally, large single or binucleated hyperchromatic cells are observed, as well as a rare infiltrative cell in mitosis, affording a clue. In the subsequent stages the infiltrate, still selecting the upper dermis principally, becomes dense and polymorphous. In this variegated infiltrate the presence of eosinophilic leukocytes and cells that simulate the Reed-Sternberg cell of Hodgkin's disease and often an abundance of small and large (Marschalko) plasma cells constitute the evidence for mycosis fungoides. In addition, there is a tendency toward scattered clumping of cells of the infiltrate. The epidermis tends to be moderately acanthotic and hyperkeratotic with focal spongiosis and small intraepidermal "microabscesses" of Darier-Pautrier. These "microabscesses" are actually foci of tumor cells that have extended into the epidermis. Their absence does not preclude the diagnosis (Fig. 36-56). The quality of the infiltrate may be indistinguishable from that of Hodgkin's disease. The cutaneous infiltrate of Hodgkin's disease tends to be irregularly distributed in parts of the dermis. The critical point is that the histologic changes even in the premycotic erythrodermatous stage are usually of the pattern and quality that, if properly evaluated, permit the diagnosis to be made.

Potentially the most revealing and yet most disputed morphologic clues to the nature of mycosis fungoides are the findings at autopsy. Recent reports indicate visceral involvement in about 70% of cases in contrast with our finding some years ago of approximately 20%.[73] However, a good deal of this involvement consists of scattered microscopic foci of atypical cells. This applies especially to the lung, which may be involved microscopically in about two thirds of cases.[96] It has been suggested that the lower incidence in our material may reflect the longer survival in later series because of supportive measures not previously available. The peripheral lymph nodes often are enlarged because of their drainage of pigment and other material from the infiltrated skin. Such nodes, now called "dermatopathic lymphadenopathy," show partial obliteration of their architecture by reticulum cell hyperplasia, deposits of melanin and fat, and—an especially common and presumptive clue in mycosis fungoides—numerous plasma cells. Similar plasma cells are generally in the bone marrow and spleen and occasionally contain even Russell bodies. These nonspecifically altered lymph nodes of Pautrier and Woringer may be mistaken for those of Hodgkin's disease. The presence of numerous plasma cells warrant electrophoretic studies in all cases of mycosis fungoides.

Pagetoid reticulosis

Pagetoid reticulosis (Woringer-Kolopp disease) is regarded by some as an epidermotrophic variant of mycosis fungoides, but the absence of focal Pautrier microabscesses and of abnormal Lutzner-like cells in the dermis in pagetoid reticulosis has served to distinguish it from mycosis fungoides.

Hodgkin's disease, lymphosarcoma, leukemia

The criteria for the histologic recognition in the skin of Hodgkin's disease, lymphosarcoma, and the various leukemias are the same as those used for the visceral lesions. Additional clues are offered by the almost constant denseness of the infiltrate, immediately noted with low-power magnification, and the selectivity of the infiltrate for the upper dermis in some instances of leukemia (Fig. 36-56). An important deceptive feature of the lymphomas is the occurrence also of quite nonspecific cutaneous reactions in which neoplastic cells are absent. These reactions may take the clinical form of toxic erythema, excoriated pruritic exfoliative erythroderma, generalized pigmentation, urticaria, and herpes zoster. Severe nonspecific cutaneous reactions lead to dermatopathic lymphadenopathy, changes in the regional lymph nodes that may become so enlarged as to be clinically indistinguishable from lymphomas. Among the most difficult neoplasms to evaluate from a biopsy specimen of skin are Letterer-Siwe disease of infancy and the related malignant histiocytoses of childhood, that is, the so-called reticuloendothelioses, histiocytosis X, or lipid and nonlipid histiocytoses. The crux of the problem is the decision as to whether the cutaneous lesion indicates visceral involvement and a fatal prognosis or merely a local histiocytosis or variant of xan-

thomatosis. In general, the degree of anaplasia and the compactness of the infiltrate of the monocytoid cells in the upper dermis are of great importance in suggesting the grave nature of the disease. However, remarkable disparities have been noted by Spitz.[86]

Another source of clinical and histologic confusion is the entity known as "Spiegler-Fendt sarcoid," which is characterized by grouped, local or disseminated, bright red nodules. The histologic diagnosis is based principally on the finding of mature lymphocytes, as well as reticulum cells either scattered or as germinal centers of follicles. Anaplasia of the infiltrate or histologic evidence of appreciable activity is lacking. It is obvious that differentiation of this lesion from lymphosarcoma must, at times, require a great nicety of judgment. Indeed, some of the cases originally but erroneously considered to be Spiegler-Fendt sarcoid have been recorded as having terminated in lymphosarcoma. Further confusion results from the use of the term "benign lymphocytoma," which is popular in dermatologic literature. This lesion, which may be single or multiple, resembles Boeck's sarcoid, leukemic infiltration, or discoid lupus erythematosus clinically. Histologically it consists essentially of dense masses of mature lymphocytes that may be arranged in follicles with germinal centers. As might be anticipated, the lesions are highly radiosensitive.

Lymphomatoid granulomatosis

Lymphomatoid granulomatosis is a focal, scattered, largely lymphocytic infiltration of the lung concentrated about vessels, both adventitially and intramurally. Since this disorder was first described in 1972, there has been confusion as to the malignant potential of the process. The nature of the lymphocytic infiltrate made it seem likely that the disease might develop in other organs. Indeed, the skin has been found to be involved by a similar infiltrate in about 40% of patients.[49]

The dispersed nodular dermal and subcutaneous infiltrate may include rare multinucleated giant cells and polymorphonuclear leukocytes as well as plasma cells, eosinophils, mature lymphocytes, and distinctly atypical lymphoreticular cells or histiocytes. In one series malignant lymphoma developed in eight of 44 patients within months after the initial diagnosis, often similar to the class of immunoblastic sarcoma.[49] The specific diagnosis of cutaneous lymphomatoid granulomatosis is largely dependent on the association with systemic signs such as neuropathy, arthropathy, and pulmonary lesions.

Lymphomatoid papulosis

Lymphomatoid papulosis is another disease made nosologically enigmatic because of the confusion regarding whether it is inflammatory or neoplastic.[59] As with the reactions to arthropod bites, it has two components, epidermal and dermal. The epidermal reaction commonly but not always consists of acanthosis, spongiosis with microvesiculation and neutrophilic crusting, and the transepidermal migration of cells from the dermal infiltrate. The last consists prototypically of small and large lymphocytes and histiocytes, with a variable admixture of neutrophils and, at times, eosinophils. The infiltrate tends to hug the epidermis in lichenoid fashion and to extend diminishingly toward the subcutis. The disturbing feature is the large hyperchromatic lymphocytes, occasionally in mitosis, that encourage the diagnosis of malignant lymphoma. Indeed, at this point approximately 10% of patients appear actually to develop malignant lymphoma; in the remainder the lesions tend to appear in crops and defloresce with fibrosis. The epidermal changes are not an integral part of the lesion. Rather, they appear ischemogenic, possibly related to the common endarteritis and phlebitis of the appertaining upper dermal vessels. Similar epidermal reactions are seen as a result of primary vascular diseases, including microembolization.

Diagnostically the most impressive cell is the atypical large lymphocyte, suggestive of a relationship between lymphomatoid papulosis and the eventual development of a malignant lymphoma. That these atypical cells reflect a stage in the progression toward malignant lymphoma is highly likely, as was indicated previously and as is now being progressively affirmed with immunohistochemical techniques.[94] Accompanying cells include small lymphocytes, eosinophils, and intradermal, intravascular, and intraepidermal neutrophils. This lesion, along with mycosis fungoides and Sézary syndrome, is of T-cell nature.[98] Actually most cutaneous lymphomas are composed of T-cells, but occasionally B-cell tumors do occur.

Lymphomatoid papulosis has been observed with glomerulonephritis, rheumatoid arthritis, and a mycosis fungoides–like picture and in immunosuppressed patients. The papules develop in crops over a period of weeks on the extremities and trunk. The mononuclear cell infiltrate may be concentrated about blood vessels throughout the dermis along with lower epidermal necrosis and scattered atypical large T-lymphocytes so atypical as to make it difficult to believe that the process will not eventuate as a malignant lymphoma.[23,30] The benign lymphocytic infiltrates tend preferentially to include the upper part of the dermis, and the solitary lymphomatoid papule is likely to have a prominent intraepidermal component. Germinal centers within the dermal infiltrates favor hyperplasia. Interestingly, dense lymphocytic infiltration (mainly T-cells) of the dermis, strikingly similar to that of true lymphoma,

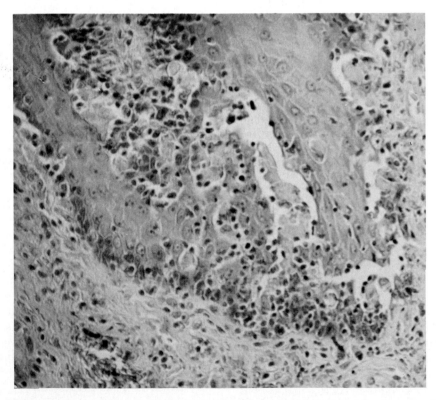

Fig. 36-57. Graft versus host reaction showing transepidermal migration of lymphocytes, liquefactive separation of dermoepidermal junction, and eosinophilic degeneration of keratinocytes.

may be induced by gold earrings.[46] In general, pseudolymphoma is characterized by a polymorphous infiltrate including lymphocytes, plasma cells, macrophages, and eosinophils.

Graft versus host disease

Graft versus host disease occurs after the increasing use of allogeneic bone marrow transplantation as therapy for aplastic anemia, leukemia, and genetic dysfunction of the marrow. The skin and other organs, such as the liver and gastrointestinal tract, may participate in the reaction. The skin shows an angry liquefaction degeneration at the dermoepidermal junction, with infiltration of lymphocytes and piecemeal eosinophilic necrosis of keratinocytes and with a predilection for hair follicles (Fig. 36-57). Sclerodermatous changes may develop in the more chronic reactions.

REACTIONS TO ARTHROPODS

In 1948 I called attention to the remarkable diagnostically troublesome biphasic cutaneous reactions to the arthropods, or insect bites.[4] These reactions involve the epidermis and the dermis. The dermal lesion is commonly mistaken for one of the lymphomas. The reaction usually consists of eosinophilic leukocytes, histiocytes, plasma cells, and reticulum cells, with the last occasionally binucleated and even in mitosis. In some lesions there are also prominent lymphoid follicles with germinal centers. Often such an innocuous reaction has been given the grave diagnosis of Hodgkin's disease, mycosis fungoides, or lymphosarcoma. Part of the reason for the error is that it is not generally appreciated that the reaction to arthopods may persist for many months. The presence of only a single lesion is suggestive evidence, in doubtful cases, of an insect bite. However, an isolated lesion may occur also in the neoplastic conditions.

A similar pseudolymphomatous cutaneous reaction may occur after injection of antigens for hyposensitization. The other deceptive reaction to the venom of insects and ticks is the pseudoepitheliomatous hyperplasias that may be mistaken for squamous cell carcinoma (Figs. 36-58 and 36-59).

Eosinophilic granulomas and *Jessner's lymphocytosis* of the skin of the face also may be erroneously misinterpreted as forms of malignant lymphomas. *Lethal midline* granuloma refers to a fulminant, destructive ulceration of the nose and paranasal tissues often resulting from Wegener's granulomatosis or one of the malignant lymphomas. The abundant necrosis, along with secondary vascular involvement, commonly obscures the precise histologic diagnosis.

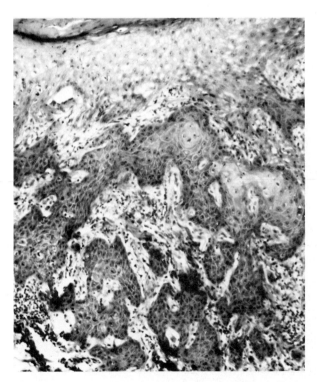

Fig. 36-58. Tick bite with pseudoepitheliomatous hyperplasia simulating squamous cell carcinoma. (Hematoxylin and eosin.)

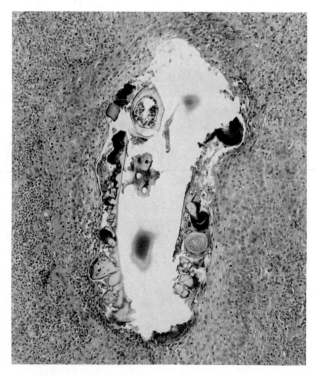

Fig. 36-59. Tick "bite" with inoculated epidermis forming cyst including palp parts of tick. (Hematoxylin and eosin; 115×.) (From Allen, A.C.: The skin, St. Louis, 1954, The C.V. Mosby Co.)

KAWASAKI DISEASE

Kawasaki disease (mucocutaneous lymph node syndrome) occurs in children under 10 years of age and is characterized by fever, pharyngitis, an exanthem, edema, and erythema of the hands followed by desquamation of the fingertips, and nonpurulent cervical lymphadenopathy. Death in 1% to 2% of instances is predominantly the result of coronary arteritis.[51] The cause is unknown.

METASTATIC NEOPLASMS

Cancerous metastases reach the skin by direct invasion or through the lymphatics or blood vessels. The most common metastases include those from carcinomas of the breast, uterus, lung, gastrointestinal tract, pancreas, thyroid gland, and prostate gland, in addition to those from melanocarcinomas, epidermoid carcinomas and lymphomas, and sarcomas of bone, muscle, and fascia.

There is generally little difficulty in recognizing the metastatic character of a tumor in the skin except of course in the case of the lymphomas and in Kaposi's sarcoma. In both of these instances the possibility of autochthonous multicentric origin is to be considered. Plasma cell myeloma occasionally involves skin. A nodule of malignant melanoma usually may be recognized as metastatic by the presence of an overlying intact epidermis showing no evidence of junctional change. Occasionally a metastatic focus of adenocarcinoma is mistaken for a primary cutaneous carcinoma of sweat gland origin, or so-called extramammary Paget's disease.[10]

TUMORS OF DERMAL APPENDAGES

Following is a classification of benign tumors of the sweat apparatus:

1. Ductal (syringal)
   a. Eccrine
      (1) Inverted, papillary syringoma (eccrine poroma, intraepidermal or dermal or both)
      (2) Lobular syringoma (eccrine spiradenoma)
      (3) Lobular hyalinized syringoma (cylindroma)
      (4) Diffuse syringoma
   b. Apocrine
      (1) Syringocystadenoma papilliferum
2. Glandular
   a. Eccrine cystadenoma with chondral metaplasia
   b. Apocrine cystoma or cystadenoma
   c. Hamartoma

Sweat glands

There is obviously an abundance of histologic variants of tumors of sweat gland or duct origin. As a result, a great number of terms that often are used ambiguously and applied inconsistently have arisen. It would seem that no practical purpose would be denied if all the neoplasms of sweat glands were labeled simply as solid or cystic syringadenoma or syringocarcinoma. However, the range of histologic variation is so great as to lead not infrequently to serious diagnostic errors, such as the mistaking of a sweat gland adenoma for a basal or a squamous cell carcinoma, malignant melanoma, or even synovioma. It may be worthwhile therefore at least to mention and illustrate the various sweat gland

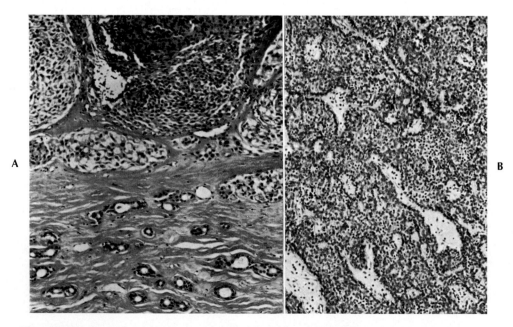

Fig. 36-60. A, Syringadenoma—usually labeled myoepithelioma on questionable evidence. **B,** Lobular syringadenoma (so-called eccrine spiradenoma). (Hematoxylin and eosin.)

tumors. Despite their histologic variations, in almost all instances there are foci of cells that indicate their source by their resemblance to sweat glands or ducts. In many instances of the solid syringadenoma, the hard, smooth, hyalinized, collagenous stroma is a clue to the nature of the tumor. In others, large cells with abundant acidophilic cytoplasm—cells that some observers (on insecure evidence) believe to be myoepithelial—are suggestive of an origin from sweat ducts (Fig. 36-60). In a considerable number of the cystic syringadenomas the stratified epithelium is papillated and the individual cells are vacuolated with glycogen (Fig. 36-61, *D*).

The inverted papillary syringoma *(eccrine poroma)* occurs as a single, slightly raised or pedunculated tu-

mor predominantly on the soles, insteps, and palms.[69] The lesion extends downward into the dermis from the stratum corneum as papillary, reticulated bands of compact, uniform, rarely pigmented, nonkeratinizing, phosphorylase-positive cells suggestive of an origin from the sweat duct. Often there is a fairly sharp demarcation from the adjacent epidermis. A similar lesion, composed apparently of thickened, winding masses of ductal origin, may be confined to the dermis. The so-called clear cell hidroadenoma—the lesion that was once labeled "myoepithelioma"—is probably a partially cystic variant of the papillary syringoma in which abundant glycogen is present in the proliferating ductal cells. One might anticipate that the underlying sweat

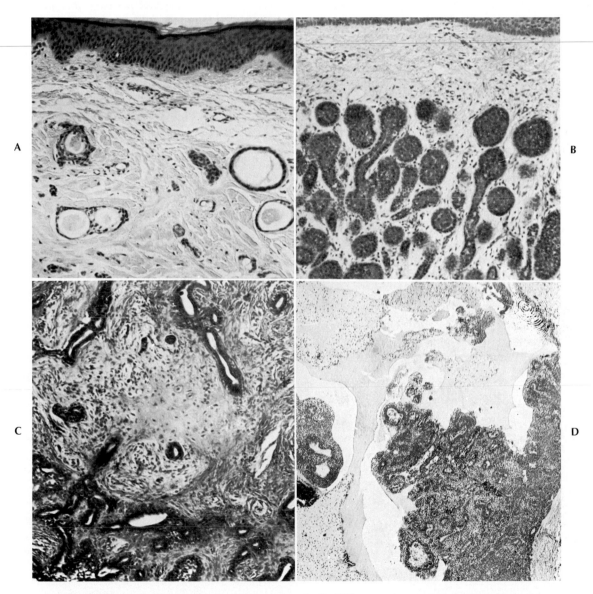

Fig. 36-61. A, Syringadenoma (hidrocystoma). **B,** Diffuse syringoma (spiradenoma). **C,** Syringadenoma with chondral metaplasia (mixed tumor) such as occurs in salivary and lacrimal glands. **D,** Syringocystadenoma. (Hematoxylin and eosin.)

glands would be dilated as a consequence of these presumably obstructive lesions and even manifesting grossly visible cyst formation in the sweat glands subtending this type of syringoma. Rarely do eccrine poromas undergo malignant change.

The terms "eccrine poroepithelioma" (or poroma) and "acrospiroma" also have been applied to what are believed to be intraepidermal proliferations of sweat duct origin (acrosyringium) of patterns somewhat different from the syringoma.

The *lobular syringoma (eccrine spiradenoma)* is usually a solitary firm nodule that is occasionally painful. The tumor is characteristically lobulated and composed of compact acini with predominant proliferation of the outer darker, lymphocytoid-appearing epithelial cells, as distinct from the lighter, larger inner cells that often lie beneath a residual cuticle-like structure. The origin of these tumors from the sweat duct is vividly demonstrable in the early or incompletely developed lesion.

A variant of the lobular syringoma is characterized by conspicuous, hyalinized bands of collagen surrounding and intertwining among the lobules and its cells (Fig. 36-62). This lesion *(turban tumor, cylindroma)* tends to be multiple and may be so extensive as to cover the scalp. Both types of lobular syringoma remain benign.

The *diffuse syringoma* usually occurs as multiple, small, soft yellowish papules on the chest, back, and face. The overlying epidermis is intact or may appear glistening. Histologically the lesion is composed of minute cysts scattered through the upper dermis (hence diffuse rather than lobular syringoma). The cysts are dilated sweat ducts containing inspissated secretion and occasionally keratin and characterized by epithelial spurs coming off the outer walls.

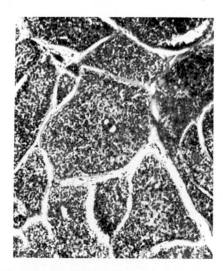

Fig. 36-62. Lobular hyalinized syringoma (turban tumor). (Hematoxylin and eosin.)

The *syringocystadenoma papilliferum* tends to occur as a solitary lesion of the scalp or forehead in patients of all ages. The overlying epidermis may be smooth or ulcerated. The histologic picture is easily recognizable by the cystic, papillary lesion projecting onto the surface from the upper dermis. The papillary components are lined by two layers of cells, a deeper layer of small cuboid cells and an outer layer of tall columnar cells. The luminal secretion of the latter at times is mistaken for cilia, and such tumors in the cervical region have been mistaken for odd branchiogenic fistulas. Frequently the lining is altered focally by squamous cell metaplasia that extends into underlying sweat ducts and glands. There is often considerable surrounding inflammatory reaction and a common association with hamartomas of sebaceous glands, pilary structures, and small basal cell carcinomas.

The term "hidradenoma papilliferum" is applied to the corresponding tumor of the labia majora or adjacent region that also simulates the papilloma of the subareolar mammary ducts.

The *eccrine* and *apocrine cystadenomas* occur on the face as solitary small translucent nodules and are easily identified by their lining epithelium. Some of these are regarded as retention cysts and are called "hidrocystomas." Chondral metaplasia may occur in eccrine or apocrine cystadenomas. As I indicated many years ago, the genesis of such cartilage is epithelial, as it is in corresponding tumors of the salivary, lacrimal, and mammary glands.[7,10] These chondroid syringomas may also contain pilary components.

Eccrine adneoma. Eccrine enzymes include phosphorylase, succinic dehydrogenase, and leucine aminopeptidase. There is little or no concentration of these enzymes in the clear cell syringomas.

Cystic syringadenoma. The clear cell, solid, or partially cystic syringadenoma or hidradenoma (unsupportably labeled "myoepithelioma") tends to be single, with a predilection for middle-aged and older women, and to occur in any region of the body. The tumors are likely to be sharply delimited and usually occur in the dermis but occasionally extend to the subcutis. In some instances the lesions are in direct contact with the epidermis, often thickened by pseudoepitheliomatous hyperplasia. The tumor cells are arranged in solid or cystic masses, the latter lined by stratified or papillary epithelium of characteristically clear, grossly vacuolated, large polyhedral cells. These cells contain abundant glycogen.

In some instances there are tubular lumens lined by cuboid cells and scattered through the lesion. Portions of the walls of the cysts may be lined by double layers of cuboid cells, also suggestive of their origin from sweat glands. These tumors contain abundant phosphorylase, esterases, and respiratory enzymes characteristic of tissue derived from sweat glands. The stroma commonly is focally homogenized and, as long emphasized, is in itself suggestive of the syringadenomatous nature of these tumors.

Syringocarcinoma

There is a tendency to diagnose sweat gland adenomas as malignant not because of anaplasia of the cells but because of the irregular ramification of nests of cells into adjacent dermis. On the other hand, some of the basal and squamous cell carcinomas characterized by small, discrete nests of cells are mistaken for sweat gland tumors—as are adenocarcinomas metastatic to skin, as well as melanocarcinomas. As a rule the uncommon sweat gland carcinomas are of a low grade of virulence, as carcinomas of appendages are generally. There have been notable exceptions.

A smoldering form of syringocarcinoma with a predilection for the upper lip of women has been reemphasized recently. It is being called "microcystic adnexal carcinoma" (MAC). Histologically, its pattern is syringomatous with haphazard nonencapsulated extension into the deep dermis and apparent involvement of perineural lymphatics. The individual units show squamous or basal cell differentiation with the formation of small keratinous cysts. The epithelial cells show no significant atypia or mitotic activity. The cells stain positively for glycogen and for S-100 protein.

Diagnosis. The diagnosis of tumors of the sweat ducts or glands is usually made without difficulty with the light microscope. Electron microscopic and histochemical studies offer supplementary information. However, electron microscopic and histochemical criteria that appear decisive in the recognition of normal structures of the sweat apparatus are apparently not always applicable to neoplasms. The widely prevalent notion that the validity of conclusions parallels the magnification needs reexamination. In general, amylophorylase, branching enzyme, succinic dehydrogenase, and leucine aminopeptidase are regarded as indicative of eccrine ducts and glands, whereas acid phosphatase and beta-glucuronidase are said to be characteristic of apocrine glands. And yet, the lobular hyalinized syringoma (cylindroma), for example, which is clearly of eccrine origin, has been found by some investigators histochemically to have suggestive apocrine rather than eccrine origin.

Adenoid cystic carcinoma

Cases of primary cutaneous adenoid cystic carcinoma matching the well-known cribriform histologic pattern as well as prognosis of the cribriform tumor (adenoid cystic carcinoma) of salivary glands are being reported.

It is difficult to escape the impression that these in reality owe their origin to an undiscovered lesion in the salivary glands.

Sebaceous gland tumors

Adenomas of sebaceous glands occur as small yellowish papules principally about the nose, cheeks, and forehead. In many cases of multiple adenomas, there are associated verrucae, neurofibromas, subungual fibrosis, and shagreen patches. These lumbosacral patches in tuberous sclerosis are nodules or elevated masses of skin produced by the proliferation and sclerosis of dermal collagen. This sclerosis may easily be mistaken histologically for scleroderma. The overlying epidermis may be normal or acanthotically reticulated. In some cases the patients develop tuberous sclerosis of the cerebral cortex and present the triad of sebaceous adenoma, mental deficiency, and epilepsy (see p. 2176). These patients also may have visceral tumors, such as renal angiolipomas. Peliosis, café-au-lait spots, fibroepithelial tags, and hemangiomas also may be associated with this entity. The sebaceous adenomas are likely to have developed during the first few years of life.

The histologic picture is that of an overgrowth of sebaceous glands without apparent linkage to the hair apparatus. Often it is difficult to be sure that the process is not simple hyperplasia rather than neoplasia. There is another histologic form of sebaceous adenoma, characterized by a proliferation of the basal cells lining the sebaceous glands interspersed with isolated sebaceous cells. Rarely there develops a metastasizing sebaceous gland carcinoma in which at least a few scattered sebaceous cells help to identify the source.

The term "nevus sebaceous of Jadassohn" is applied to hamartomatous or dysembryogenetic papular or nodular tumefactions of sebaceous glands or the pilosebaceous apparatus. Such malformations may be associated with other ectodermal or mesodermal malformations. Overlying or adjacent verrucal epidermal hyperplasia, a variety of sweat or lacrimal gland adenomas, focal alopecia, dermoids, dermal lipomas, angiomas, or basal cell carcinomas may accompany the lesion. Occasionally it may be combined with ocular and cerebral lesions, with mental retardation and convulsions, as a form of neurocutaneous syndrome. Sebaceous gland hyperplasia, adenomas, and carcinomas have been reported in association with multiple visceral carcinomas.

Carcinomas of the *sebaceous glands* occur rarely and are of particular interest because of their common association with visceral cancers, an association referred to as the "Torre or Muir-Torre syndrome." The involved viscera have included colon, ampulla of Vater, duodenum, larynx, and more recently breast, urinary, and female genital tracts. Bowen's disease of the vulva has given rise to a sebaceous gland carcinoma with an accompanying colonic carcinoma.[48]

Hair follicle tumors

There is a divergence of opinion as to the types of neoplasms that may arise from hair follicles. Many observers believe that basal cell carcinomas are derived from embryonic hair follicles. However, as previously stated, the histologic evidence favors the view that basal cell carcinomas arise from the mature bassal cells whereever they lie—at the base of the epidermis, at the periphery of sebaceous glands, or in the outermost layer of the hair follicles. The tumors that arise from hair follicles come in a variety of forms and are listed below:

Hair follicle–related tumors
  Trichofolliculoma (primary hair follicle with deep keratinous cyst and secondary radiating hair follicles)
  Trichodiscoma
  Trichoepithelioma (solitary and desmoplastic) (Fig. 36-63)
  Trichoadenoma
  Trichohamartoma (generalized)
  Pilomatricoma (proliferating trichilemmoma)
  Trichilemmoma
    Solitary
    Multiple (Cowden's syndrome with visceral carcinomas)

Superficial infundibular proliferation. The developing hair has many morphologic opportunities to go awry and to form a variety of combinations of its components for each of which an individual name has been applied, as indicated. The practical point is that this disruption of the normal growth patterns of the hair be recognized by the pathologist as of hair follicle rather than of other more serious nature. Similarly the effects of dysembryogenesis of the hair follicle may combine hamartomatously with sebaceous glands and other components of the skin to form bizarre solitary or multiple papules (Fig. 36-63).

Trichilemmal cysts. Trichilemmal cysts occur mainly in the scalp and are commonly mistaken for squamous cell carcinomas both because of the disheveled inward proliferation of the lining and the presence of atypical squamous cells. Sharp circumscription favors the benign lesion. As in pilomatricomas, calcification, at times ossification, and foreign-body reaction to keratin are conspicuous, but the characteristic dense trichilemmal keratinization is absent. A given trichilemmal cyst may show both solid and cystic areas.[18]

Histologically, unlike most basal cell carcinomas, the tumor is overlain by intact epidermis. The lesion is made up of varying-sized units of cysts filled with keratin and lined with stratified squamous epithelium, from which nests of basal cells proliferate. The trichoepithelioma is benign, unlike the basal cell "epithelioma."

Trichilemmoma. Trichilemmoma is an acanthosis of

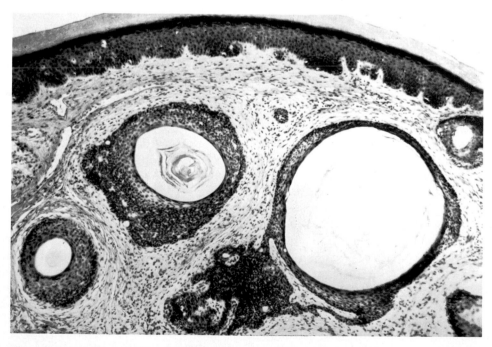

Fig. 36-63. Trichoepithelioma (Brooke's tumor, epithelioma adenoides cysticum). (Hematoxylin and eosin.)

lobulated clear cells (glycogenated) often oriented about a hair follicle and reminiscent of the outer root sheath. A follicle may be present near the center of the lesion, which may contain whorled squamous eddies. The periphery of the lobules is sharply delimited by a vitreous zone of polarized basaloid cells and, indeed, the lesions may be mistaken for basal cell carcinomas. A few observers regard the trichilemmoma as a clear cell variant of a verruca. This may well be true of a few trichilemmomas.

Cowden's syndrome. Trichilemmomas occur in Cowden's syndrome and may reflect visceral involvement in the form of Cowden's syndrome. (Cowden represents the name of the original patient, Rachel Cowden.) Other features of this syndrome include adenoid facies, hypoplasia of the mandible, prominent forehead, a high-arched palate, breast and thyroid carcinomas, and a variety of soft-tissue neoplasms.

Pilomatricoma. The calcifying epithelioma is an exaggeration of this process of proliferation, which frequently is misinterpreted as cancer. Histologically this lesion is usually a sharply circumscribed mass of disheveled fragments of epithelium, many of which are necrotic and often partially calcified. The epithelial cells have a basaloid character, though it is likely that they are predominantly of prickle cell origin. This pattern has been suggestive to some observers that cells with the ever-invoked pluripotentiality attempt to form abortive hair, and so it has been labeled "pilomatrixoma." "Pilomatricoma" or trichomatricoma" would be more suitable or correct. Infrequently these are pigmented with melanocytes as might be expected if their source was hair matrix.

Actual cancerous transformation of the lining of cysts is an infreqeunt occurrence. The incidence of 1% to 6% quoted in the literature is high.

Dermoid cysts

The dermoid cyst is a congenital cutaneous inclusion occurring usually in the skin of the forehead, especially in the supraorbital region or midline. Epidermoid cysts also may be congenital and familial, particularly steatocystoma multiplex, but commonly they are the result of trauma (including insect bites) or inflammatory downgrowth, and separation and eventual isolation and encystment of a fragment of epidermis. Several originate from obstructed sweat ducts or hair follicles rather than from implantation by trauma. As previously indicated, "sebaceous cyst" is the term loosely applied to cysts that are derived from the entire pilary or pilosebaceous apparatus rather than from the sebaceous gland alone.[7] These keratinous cysts are lined by ordinary stratified squamous epithelium with, rarely, some residual sebaceous cells in one segment of the lining. Usually the sebaceous cells have been obliterated in the mature cyst. Accordingly, they are labeled "pilosebaceous cysts," though "pilary cysts" might be even more appropriate.

Grossly the dermoid cysts cannot be differentiated from pilosebaceous and epidermoid cysts. Histologically the wall of the cyst is actually skin with all its appendages, often with a prominence of sebaceous glands. The epidermoid and sebaceous cysts differ from the dermoid cysts in that the former lack the appendages and their walls are made up of stratified squamous epidermis surrounded by fibrous tissue. As a rule it is impossible to distinguish the epidermoid from the pilosebaceous cyst. Infrequently, evidence of the relation of the cyst to a contiguous sebaceous gland may persist. The criteria that have been set up for the differentiation are unreliable. The epithelium of both tends to be nonpigmented.

The contents of each of the cysts are predominantly a beige greasy keratin, representing the stratum corneum, which in these instances cannot be shed but accumulates in the epidermal enclosures. There is also much fat within the laminated keratin, which either may not be demonstrable in routine sections or may be seen as cholesterin slits. In the dermoid cysts, hairs may be included. Occasionally the lining epithelium may proliferate as papillary buds, either externally or inward toward the lumen of the cyst. Because of the irregularity of these proliferations and perhaps because of their superficial resemblance to the carcinomas of epidermis, there is a tendency to classify these hyperplasias or benign proliferations as cancer—a tendency not warranted by their behavior.

REFERENCES

1. Ahmed, R.A.: Pemphigus: current concepts, Ann. Intern. Med. **92**:396, 1980.
2. Albert, J., Bruce, W., and Allen, A.C.: Lipoid dermatoarthritis, Am. J. Med. **28**:661, 1960.
3. Allen, A.C., and Spitz, S.A.: A comparative study of rickettsial diseases, Am. J. Pathol. **21**:603, 1945.
4. Allen, A.C.: Reaction to arthropods, Am. J. Pathol. **24**:367, 1948.
5. Allen, A.C.: Survey of pathology of cutaneous disease of World War II, Arch. Dermatol. **57**:19, 1948.
6. Allen, A.C.: Reorientation on histogenesis of nevi and malignant melanomas, Cancer **2**:28, 1949.
7. Allen, A.C.: The skin: a clinicopathologic treatise, St. Louis, 1954, The C.V. Mosby Co.
8. Allen, A.C.: Juvenile melanomas, Surg. Gynecol. Obstet. **104**:753, 1957. (Editorial.)
9. Allen, A.C.: Juvenile melanomas, Ann. NY Acad. Sci. **100**:29, 1963.
10. Allen, A.C.: The skin: a clinicopathologic treatise, ed. 2, New York, 1967, Grune & Stratton, Inc.
11. Allen, A.C., and Spitz, S.: Malignant melanomas: criteria for diagnosis and prognosis, Cancer **6**:1, 1953.
12. Allen, A.C., and Spitz, S.: Clinico-pathologic correlation of nevi and malignant melanomas, Arch. Dermatol. **69**:150, 1954.
13. Anderson, S., Nielsen, A., Reymann, F., et al.: Bowen's disease and visceral cancer, Arch. Dermatol. **108**:367, 1973.
14. Arbesman, H., and Ransohoff, D.F.: Is Bowen's disease a predictor for the development of internal malignancy? JAMA **257**:23, 1987.

15. Bandy, S., and Ackerman, G.B.: Cutaneous lesions in drug-induced coma, JAMA **213**:253, 1970.
16. Barr, R.J., Morales, R.V., and Graham, J.H.: Desmoplastic nevus, Cancer **46**:557, 1980.
17. Breslow, A.: Thickness, cross-sectioned areas, and depth of invasion in the prognosis of cutaneous melanomas, Ann. Surg. **172**:902, 1970.
18. Brownstein, M.H., and Arbuk, D.J.: Proliferating trichilemmal cyst, Cancer **48**:1207, 1981.
19. Castro, G., and Winkelmann, R.K.: Angiolymphoid hyperplasia, Cancer **34**:1696, 1974.
20. Caulfield, J.B., and Wilgram, G.F.: Ultrastructure of acantholysis, J. Invest. Dermatol. **41**:57, 1963.
21. Clark, W.H., Jr.: Melanomas, Cancer Res. **29**:705, 1969.
22. Coletta, D.F., Haentze, F.E., and Thomas, C.C.: Metastasizing basal cell carcinomas, Cancer **22**:879, 1968.
23. Cormane, R.H., and Hamerlinck, F.: B and T lymphocytes, Ann. NY Acad. Sci. **254**:592, 1975.
24. Cott, R.E., Wood, M.G., and Johnson, B.L.: Use of curettage and shave excision in office practice, J. Am. Acad. Dermatol. **16**:1243, 1987.
25. Crus, T.S., and Reiner, C.B.: Recurrent digital fibroma of children, J. Cutan. Pathol. **5**:339, 1978.
26. Curth, H.O., Hilberg, A.W., and Machacek, G.F.: Acanthosis nigricans, Cancer **15**:364, 1962.
27. Davis, P., Atkins, B., and Hughes, G.R.V.: Antibodies to DNA in discoid lupus erythematosus, Br. J. Dermatol. **91**:175, 1974.
28. Douglas, H.M.G., and Bleumink, E.: Lymphosarcoma and congenital lymphedema, Arch. Dermatol. **11**:608, 1974.
29. Ellman, M.H., Fretzin, D.F., and Olson, W.: Toxic epidermal necrolysis and allopurinol, Arch. Dermatol. **111**:986, 1975.
30. Evans, H.L., and Winkelmann, R.K.: Differential diagnosis of malignant and benign cutaneous infiltrates, Cancer **44**:699, 1979.
31. Fajardo, L.F., and Berthrong, M.: Radiation injury in surgical pathology, Am. J. Surg. Pathol. **5**:279, 1981.
32. Farmer, E.R., and Helwig, E.B.: Metastatic basal cell carcinoma, Cancer **46**:748, 1980.
33. Fields, J.P., and Helwig, E.B.: Leiomyosarcoma of the skin and subcutaneous tissue, Cancer **47**:156, 1981.
34. Flaxman, S.A., and Maderson, P.E.A.: Growth and differentiation of skin, J. Invest. Dermatol. **67**:8, 1976.
35. Frank, E., Mevorah, B., and Leu, F.: Disseminated spiked hyperkeratosis, Arch. Dermatol. **117**:412, 1981.
36. Fraser, N.G., and Kerry, N.W., and Donald, D.: Oral lesions in dermatitis herpetiformis, Br. J. Dermatol. **89**:439, 1973.
37. Gazzolo, L., and Prunieras, M.: Lysosomes and keratinocytes, J. Invest. Dermatol. **51**:186, 1968.
38. Gilliam, J.N., Cheatum, D.E., Hurd, E.R., Stastny, P., and Ziff, M.: Immunofluorescent band and renal disease in S.L.E., J. Clin. Invest. **53**:1434, 1974.
39. Graham, H.J., and Helwig, E.B., Erythroplasia of Queyrat, Cancer **32**:1396, 1973.
40. Gromet, M.A., Epstein, W.L., and Blois, M.S.: Regressing thin melanoma, Cancer **42**:2282, 1978.
41. Halpryn, H.J., and Allen, A.C.: Epidermal changes overlying sclerosing angiomas, Arch. Dermatol. **80**:160, 1959.
42. Hashimoto, K., and Bale, G.F.: Balloon cell nevi, Cancer **30**:530, 1973.
43. Headington, J.T.: Tumors of the hair follicle, Am. J. Pathol. **85**:480, 1976.
44. Hu, C., Michel, B., and Farber, E.: Transient acantholytic disease, Arch Dermatol. **121**:1439, 1985.
45. Huvos, A.G., Lucas, J.C., Jr., and Foote, F.W., Jr.: Melanomas, Am. J. Pathol. **71**:33, 1973.
46. Iwatsuka, K., Yamada, M., Tagikawa, M., Inoue, K., and Matsumoto, K.: Benign lymphoplasia of the earlobes induced by gold earrings, J. Am. Acad. Dermatol. **16**:83, 1987.
47. Jackson, S.F., and Fell, H.B.: Mucus-producing keratinocytes, Dev. Biol. **7**:394, 1963.
48. Jacobs, D.M., Sandler, L.G., and Leboit, P.E.: Sebaceous carcinoma arising from Bowen's disease of the vulva, Arch. Dermatol. **122**:1191, 1986.

49. James, W.D., Odom, R.B., and Katzenstein, A.A.: Cutaneous manifestations of lymphomatoid granulomatosis, Arch. Dermatol. **117**:196, 1981.
50. Jordon, R.E., Schroeter, A.L., and Winkelmann, R.K.: Dermoepidermal deposition of complement components and properdin in S.L.E., Br. J. Dermatol. **92**:263, 1975.
51. Kahn, G.: Mucocutaneous lymph node syndrome (Kawasaki's disease), Arch. Dermatol. **114**:948, 1978.
52. Kopf, A.W., and Popkin, G.L.: Shave biopsies, Arch. Dermatol. **110**:637, 1974.
53. Lapins, W.A., and Helwig, E.B.: Perineural invasion by keratoacanthoma, Arch. Dermatol. **116**:791, 1980.
54. Lever, W.F., and Schaumberg-Lever, G.: Histopathology of skin, ed. 5, Philadelphia, 1975, J.B. Lippincott Co.
55. López, M.R.: Cutaneous meningiomas, Cancer **34**:728, 1974.
56. Lutzner, M.A.: Molluscum bodies, Arch. Dermatol. **87**:436, 1963.
57. Lutzner, M.A.: Sézary cells, J. Natl. Cancer Inst. **50**:1145, 1973.
58. Lyell, A.: Toxic epidermal necrolysis, Br. J. Dermatol. **68**:355, 1956.
59. MacCauley, W.L.: Lymphomatoid papulosis, Arch. Dermatol. **97**:23, 1968.
60. Mehregan, A.H.: Perforating elastosis, Arch. Dermatol. **97**:381, 1968.
61. Milston, E.B., and Helwig, E.B.: Basal cell carcinomas in children, Arch. Dermatol. **108**:523, 1973.
62. Miyagawa, S., Kiriyama, Y., Shirai, T., Ohi, H., and Sakamoto, K.: Chronic bullous disease with coexistent circulating IgG and IgA antibasement membrane zone antibodies, Arch. Dermatol. **117**:349, 1981.
63. Monroe, E.W.: Urticarial vasculitis: an updated review, J. Am. Acad. Dermatol. **5**:88, 1981.
64. Morrison, W.L.: Viral warts and immunity, Br. J. Dermatol. **92**:625, 1975.
65. Nakajima, T., Watanabe, S., Sato, Y., Kameya, T., Shimosato, Y., and Ishihara, K.: Demonstration of S-100 protein in malignant melanoma and pigmented nevus, Cancer **50**:912, 1982.
66. Nishioka, K., Kobayashi, Y., Katayama, I., and Takijiri, C.: Mast cell numbers in diffuse scleroderma, Arch. Dermatol. **123**:205, 1987.
67. Obalek, S., Jablonka, S., Beaudenon, S., Walczak, L., and Orth, G.: Bowenoid papulosis of male and female genitalia, J. Am. Acad. Dermatol. **14**:433, 1986.
68. Pinkus, G.B., Etheridge, C., and O'Conner, E.M.: Are keratin proteins a better tumor marker than epithelial membrane antigen? Am. J. Clin. Pathol. **85**:269, 1986.
69. Pinkus, H., Rogin, J.R., and Goldman, P.: Eccrine poromas, Arch. Dermatol. **74**:51, 1956.
70. Purtilo, D.T.: Opportunistic cancers in immunodeficiency syndromes, Arch. Pathol. **111**:1123, 1987.
71. Quintal, D., and Jackson, R.: Aggressive squamous cell carcinoma arising in familial acne conglobata, J. Am. Acad. Dermatol. **14**(2 Pt. 1):207, 1986.
72. Ramsay, C.S., and Gianelli, F.: Erythemal action spectrum and DNA repair synthesis in xeroderma pigmentosum, Br. J. Dermatol. **92**:49, 1975.
73. Rappaport, H., and Thomas, L.B.: Mycosis fungoides: the pathology of extracutaneous involvement, Cancer **34**:1198, 1974.
74. Rice, J.S., and Fischer, D.S.: Blue rubber-bleb nevus, Arch. Dermatol. **86**:503, 1962.
75. Rodman, G.P., Lipinski, E., and Luksick, L., Jr.: Skin thickness and collagen content in progressive systemic sclerosis, Arthritis Rheum. **22**:130, 1979.
76. Sams, W.B., Jr.: Immunofluorescence in dermatology, Yearbook of dermatology, Chicago, 1973, Year Book Medical Publishers, Inc.
77. Sandberg, L.B., Soskel, N.T., and Leslie, J.G.: Elastin structure, biosynthesis, and relation to disease states, N. Engl. J. Med. **304**:566, 1981.
78. Schaumberg-Lever, G., Rule, A., Schmidt-Ulrich, B., and Lever, W.F.: Immunoglobulins in pemphigoid and lupus erythematosus, J. Invest. Dermatol. **64**:47, 1975.

79. Schiltz, J.R., Michel, B., and Papay, R.: Appearance of "pemphigus, acantholysis factor" in human skin cultured with pemphigus antibody, J. Invest. Dermatol. **73**:575, 1979.
80. Shornick, J.K.: Herpes gestationis, J. Am. Acad. Dermatol. **17**:536, 1987.
81. Singer, H., Sawka, N.J., Samowitz, H.R., and Lazarus, G.S.: Protease activation: a mechanism for cellular dyshesion in pemphigus, J. Invest. Dermatol. **74**:363, 1980.
82. Sison-Fonacier, L., and Bystryn, J.C.: Heterogeneity of pemphigus vulgaris antigens, Arch. Dermatol. **123**:1507, 1987.
83. Sitz, K.V., Kepper, M., and Johnson, D.F.: Metastatic basal cell carcinoma in AIDS-related complex, JAMA **257**:340, 1987.
84. Smith, J.L., and Stehlen, J.S., Jr.: Spontaneous regression of primary malignant melanomas with regional metastases, Cancer **18**:1399, 1965.
85. Spitz, S.: Melanomas of childhood, Am. J. Pathol. **24**:591, 1948.
86. Spitz, S.: Cutaneous tumors of childhood, J. Am. Med. Wom. Assoc. **6**:209, 1951.
87. Srebrnik, A., Tur, E., Perluk, C., Elman, M., Messer, G., Ilie, B., and Krakowski, A.: Dorfman-Chanarin syndrome, J. Am. Acad. Dermatol. **17**:801, 1987.
88. Stewart, F.W., and Treves, N.: Postmastectomy lymphangiosarcoma, Cancer **1**:64, 1948.
89. Suter, L., Brüggen, J., Vakilzadeh, F., Kövary, P.M., and Macher, E.: Human malignant melanoma: assay of tumor-associated antigens, J. Invest. Dermatol. **75**:235, 1980.
90. Tucker, S.B., Horstmann, J.P., Hertel, B., Aranha, G., and Rosai, J.: Activation of nevi in patients with malignant melanoma, Cancer **46**:822, 1980.
91. Tufanelli, D.L.: Lupus erythematosus panniculitis, Arch. Dermatol. **103**:231, 1971.
92. Unna, P.: Epithelial origin of melanocarcinomas, Berl. Klin.-Therap. Wochenschr. **30**:14, 1893.
93. Wanebo, H.J., Woodruff, J., and Fortner, J.G.: Clinicopathologic analysis of malignant melanomas, Cancer **35**:666, 1975.
94. Weiss, L.M., Wood, G.S., Ellison, L.W., Reynolds, T.C., and Sklar, J.: Clonal T-cell proliferations in pityriasis lichenoides et varioliformis acuta (Mucha-Huberman disease), Am. J. Pathol. **126**:417, 1987.
95. Wilson-Jones, E., and Winklemann, R.K.: Papulonecrotic tuberculid, J. Am. Acad. Dermatol. **14**:815, 1986.
96. Wolfe, J.D., Trevor, E.D., and Kjeldsberg, C.R.: Pulmonary manifestation of mycosis fungoides, Cancer **46**:2648, 1980.
97. Yeckley, J.A., Weston, W.L., Thorne, E.G., and Krueger, G.G.: Production of Sézary cells from normal lymphocytes, Arch. Dermatol. **111**:29, 1975.
98. Zackheim, H.S.: Cutaneous T-cell lymphomas, Arch. Dermatol. **117**:295, 1981.

37 Tumors and Tumorlike Conditions of the Soft Tissue

MICHAEL KYRIAKOS

In this chapter a diverse and fascinating group of lesions that arise from the supporting soft tissues of the body is discussed. These soft tissues include all the nonepithelial extraskeletal tissues except for the central nervous system glia and the components of the reticuloendothelial system.[32] Included are lesions composed or derived from fat, fibrous tissue, smooth muscle, skeletal muscle, blood vessels, and lymphatics, all of which have origin from the embryonic mesoderm.

The benign tumors are designated by a prefix indicating the tissue of origin or type of differentiation of the lesion, followed by the suffix -oma, such as "leiomyoma," for the benign tumor of smooth muscle and "lipoma," for the benign tumor of adipose tissue. The malignant mesenchymal lesions are designated as "sarcomas." For many of these the name of the specific tumor is formed by adding the suffix sarcoma to the histogenic or differentiation prefix applicable to that tumor, such as "leiomyosarcoma," as the designation for the malignant tumor of smooth muscle, and "liposarcoma," for the malignant tumor of adipose tissue. In others, however, either because the histogenesis is unknown or because of long-term convention, the name applied to the tumor follows no apparent rule, such as alveolar soft-part sarcoma, epithelioid sarcoma, and malignant fibrous histiocytoma, so that one must learn the applicable terms by rote.

From the above, it should not be construed that the malignant tumors necessarily arise from their benign counterparts. Indeed, with rare exceptions, sarcomas arise ad initium and not from spontaneous malignant transformation of a preexisting benign tumor.[32,33,50] Instead, current dogma implicates a primitive undifferentiated mesenchymal cell having the capacity to differentiate along a variety of cell pathways, as the mother cell of most sarcomas.[31] Whether true or not, this is a convenient way of explaining the wide variety of histopathologic patterns in some of the more pleomorphic sarcomas, as well as the overlap in the type of cells present in the various sarcomas at the fine-structural level.[60,110]

Tumors of peripheral nerve, the components of which are derived from the neurectoderm, are also included within the category of soft-tissue lesions because of their frequent occurrence in the soft tissues. Many of the tumor and tumorlike lesions that arise in the soft tissue are also found within the viscera, but these represent specific problems and are discussed in the appropriate chapters of this book.

Perhaps in no other field of diagnostic pathology has there been such a proliferation of newly described histologic entities as there has been in the area of soft-tissue pathology within the past 10 to 20 years. The student of pathology is now faced with a host of diagnostic entities that number well over 100 and for which there are about 300 synonyms.[1,32,44] However, many are so rare that they fall outside the experience not only of most general physicians, but also of most pathologists. Even large referral centers may have only one or two examples of many of these soft-tissue lesions in their files. This chapter then should not be considered an encyclopedic survey of the entire field of soft-tissue pathology. Only the more common lesions, or those of special interest, are presented. Reference should be made to the more general and encompassing publications in the bibliography for lesions not discussed and for those for which greater detail is sought.[23,31,33,44,53,87,103]

Soft-tissue tumors and tumorlike conditions are uncommon, and comprise probably only 2% or less of all surgical pathology case material.[74] Data on the incidence of the benign tumors are difficult to come by because the emphasis in the literature has been on the malignant tumors. Some idea of their relative frequency, however, is given by the data from the Laboratory of Surgical Pathology, Columbia University, where in a 45-year period only 8700 soft-tissue tumors were accessioned, with the benign outnumbering the malignant in a ratio of about 5:1 (7300 benign and 1400 malignant).[103] However, other institutions report benign-to-malignant ratios that vary from 18.5:1 to 100:1.[1,33,45,74] It has been estimated that approximately

500,000 benign soft-tissue tumors occur per year in the United States.[45] The American Cancer Society placed the estimated number of new soft-tissue cancers in the United States for 1988 at approximately 5500 out of a total of 985,000 new cancers in all sites, exclusive of nonmelanoma skin cases and cases of carcinoma in situ. Approximately 2900 deaths per year were caused by these tumors out of a total of some 495,000 cancer deaths.[100]

It is the very rarity of these soft-tissue tumors that creates both their fascination and their problems. The wide variation that many of them exhibit in their histopathologic patterns extends the pathologist's diagnostic ability to the limit. However, since few pathologists, other than those at large referral medical centers, come into contact with many of these lesions, the fortuitous encounter not infrequently leads to misdiagnosis and disaster for the patient. In a survey of cases in the Swedish Tumor Registry, 10% of the lesions diagnosed as sarcoma were, on review, benign reactive proliferative lesions.[22] In other studies, approximately 6% to 7% of cases initially diagnosed as sarcoma were found, on review, to represent either carcinomas or lymphomas.[85,92] However, even in those cases where it was established that the lesions were sarcomatous, disagreement among pathologists as to the type of sarcoma occurred in from 27% to 39% of cases.[14,85,92]

Contributing to this dramatic diagnostic variance is the fact that many of the soft-tissue tumors and tumorlike lesions have a fibroblastic component, and if the lesion is not sufficiently sampled, it may be misdiagnosed as a malignant fibrous tumor (fibrosarcoma). Further confusing the histologic situation is the variety of cellular constituents and histomorphologic patterns in many sarcomas. At times the histologic pattern may vary not only from tumor to tumor, but even from area to area within a single tumor. Therefore proper sampling with numerous sections may be required before specific diagnostic features are found. In many pleomorphic sarcomas, evaluation of small biopsy specimens may be enigmatic and only suggestive of the true cell type of the lesion. In a large national survey, a difference was found between the diagnosis made on biopsy material and the ultimate diagnosis of the resected tumor in 25% of cases, and in almost three fourths of these cases there was a major variance in the final tumor typing.[62]

Despite these unsettling statistics, most well-differentiated sarcomas are easily diagnosed by light microscopy. Such well-differentiated tumors are composed of cells whose phenotype closely approximates either the proposed cell of origin or the normal type of cell toward which the tumor has differentiated; that is, a well-differentiated leiomyosarcoma is composed of cells that morphologically approach, on a light and electron mi-

croscopic level, normal smooth muscle cells. However, there are other sarcomas whose histogenesis is unclear, such as epithelioid sarcoma, clear cell sarcoma, and alveolar soft-part sarcoma, and whose cells do not resemble any "normal" counterpart. Here, "well differentiated" is a misnomer and is used merely to indicate how closely the tumor resembles its classically described histologic pattern. As a sarcoma becomes less differentiated, its cells lose specific features until few if any clues remain to allow one to classify it by light or electron microscopy. Thus, even when examined by an experienced pathologist, from 5% to 15% of sarcomas will remain "unclassified" in light of present knowledge.[19,29,33,54,61,75,107,108]

Electron microscopy may be helpful in either establishing or supporting a diagnosis reached by light microscopy. However, electron microscopy is frequently of little aid in establishing a diagnosis in poorly differentiated tumors, precisely those tumors that are so difficult to diagnose at the light microscopic level, either because of the sampling problems inherent in electron microscopy or because the tumor cells lack morphologically specific structures.[33,35,52,60,89,110] Electron microscopy has proved of value in helping distinguish among the various small round cell tumors of children, such as primitive rhabdomyosarcoma, Ewing's sarcoma, and neuroepithelioma, and in separating pleomorphic sarcomas from carcinomas, melanomas, and lymphomas.[1,35,89]

In the last edition of this book, mention was made of the first glimmerings of what has now become a revolution in the diagnosis and classification of tumors by means of immunohistochemical techniques. Perhaps nowhere else have these methods found such a fertile field as in soft-tissue pathology. An avalanche of studies using these methods has engulfed pathology journals to the point that it is increasingly difficult to find a current paper on soft-tissue tumors that does not mention the use of some immunohistochemical tumor marker. It cannot be denied that these techniques have greatly aided pathologists in their approach to difficult diagnostic problems. However, as with many a revolution, too much is expected and extreme views are expressed on what these methods can accomplish.[65] Immunohistochemical reagents are expensive and their indiscriminate use is wasteful of resources. More important, however, is that the results of these tumor-marker studies must be interpreted within the context of the clinical situation and the morphology of the lesion.[39] To classify in a child a small round cell malignant tumor of soft tissue that stains positively with an epithelial marker as a carcinoma, despite light morphologic evidence of skeletal muscle differentiation, is obviously foolish. It should be remembered that the best diagnostic tool available to the pathologist is his or her own intelligence and that the evaluation of conventionally stained sections remains the bulwark of diagnostic pathology.[39]

An ever-expanding list of useful tumor markers has developed in the past several years. Antibodies to the intermediate cytoskeleton filament proteins, vimentin, desmin, cytokeratin, neurofilament, and glial fibrillary acidic protein have been those most extensively used in soft-tissue tumor diagnosis.* In theory, cytokeratin is found only in epithelial cells; vimentin in mesenchymal cells; desmin in parenchymal smooth muscle cells, some vascular smooth muscle cells, and skeletal and cardiac muscle; neurofilament in neurons; and glial fibrillary acidic protein in astrocytes and some ependymal cells. Tumors derived from these cells were supposed to retain the same intermediate filament protein composition so that epithelial tumors could be distinguished from mesenchymal tumors because of the presence of cytokeratin in the former and the presence of vimentin in the latter.[71,81,91] Although occasional tumors could coexpress two different intermediate filament proteins, this was believed to be rare and that in all such instances vimentin was always one of the proteins present.[34,81] With more extensive experience it has become evident that there are exceptions to this neat outline.[38] There are sarcomas that express cytokeratin† and carcinomas that express vimentin.‡ Tumors may also coexpress more than two intermediate filaments,§ and in some of these vimentin is absent.[34,38,40]

Other markers that have been used for soft-tissue tumor diagnosis include S-100 protein,[26,34,48,77,114] myoglobin,[10,18,73] muscle-specific actin and myosin,[67,97,109] alpha₁-antichymotrypsin and alpha₁-antitrypsin,[27,58] neuron-specific enolase,[43,56,98,106,112] epithelial membrane antigen,[82,102] type IV collagen and laminin,[6,68,79] factor VIII–related antigen, and *Ulex europaeus* agglutinin I.[11,34,69,80,86] However, disparate results using these markers are reported. Factors such as the type of tissue fixation used, the type and specificity of the antibody used, and the manner in which the tissue sections are processed are of critical importance in determining the type of results obtained and may explain some of the differences in results reported in the literature. Space precludes discussion of each useful marker, and one is referred to the extensive literature that exists on their use and results.[3,6,7,24,99,105,115] However, in the appropriate sections of this chapter reference is made to the results of immunohistochemical studies applicable to specific tumor types.

Another reason for the interest that sarcomas engender is that many of them affect children and young adults. Indeed, sarcomas are the fifth leading form of cancer in children.[104,116] Their anatomic location, frequently in the extemities, and the radical and at times mutilating surgical procedures required for their removal have created a natural interest in them that belies both their prevalence and clinical significance as a major cause of cancer deaths. Finally, recent advances in the use of adjuvant chemotherapy and radiation therapy have made dramatic inroads in the mortality of some of the childhood sarcomas to the point where patients with tumors previously almost uniformly fatal are now being cured.[104]

The clinical symptoms and signs produced by most soft-tissue tumors are nonspecific. Both the benign and malignant tumors usually develop as enlarging, painless masses, frequently located in an extremity, though either may be associated with pain.[36,45,94,96] Tumors arising in areas such as the retroperitoneum or the thigh may grow to a large size before becoming clinially evident. In general, sarcomas grow fairly rapidly, but exceptions exist where the tumor develops only slowly over a period of many months to years. Although benign soft-tissue lesions are characteristically slow growing, some may develop within a few weeks. Some tumors, which might have been very slowly enlarging or even stationary, may suddenly rapidly increase in size over a few days to weeks because of either intralesional hemorrhage or a change in the hormonal status of the patient as during pregnancy.[1,33,36]

Benign soft-tissue tumors are usually located in the skin or subcutaneous tissue above the superficial fascia, with only approximately 1% arising in the deep soft tissues or muscle,[74,94] whereas from 60% to 88% of sarcomas arise in the latter sites.[63,74,75,94,108] Most benign soft-tissue tumors (95%) rarely exceed 5 cm, but from 50% to 90% of sarcomas exceed this size.[1,63,74,94] In general, large deeply located soft-tissue lesions are more likely to be malignant than small, superficial tumors that are freely movable above the fascia.

Clinical inspection of the tumor, or even its gross pathologic appearance, usually fails to provide any clues to its nature. Benign lesions, though frequently well circumscribed or even encapsulated, may have an aggressive appearing infiltrative pattern as in nodular fasciitis or any of the various fibromatoses. Similarly, it is the rule, rather than the exception, for sarcomas to appear grossly well circumscribed or even encapsulated.[1,32,33,36] This appearance has led many a surgeon to attempt to "shell out" a sarcoma because it "looked benign." Microscopy, however, shows that sarcomas always infiltrate the surrounding normal tissue and that no true capsule exists. Areas of cystic degeneration, necrosis, and hemorrhage are frequent in sarcomas, especialy in the larger ones, but such areas may also occur in perfectly benign tumors such as neurilemomas. Furthermore, except for tumors that grossly arise

---

*References 34, 37, 57, 70, 71, 76, 81, 86, 91.
†References 12, 13, 17, 55, 72, 78, 113.
‡References 4, 13, 20, 21, 34, 38, 57, 71, 86.
§References 13, 15, 25, 38, 40, 51, 111.

within a large nerve trunk; the yellow, greasy appearance of some fatty tumors; and the grapelike clusters of botryoid rhabdomyosarcoma, there is such an overlap in the appearance of soft-tissue tumors that a specific tumor diagnosis is not possible from its gross appearance.

Since clinical appearance cannot be used as a definitive guide for distinguishing benign from malignant lesions and because the type of therapy required depends on the nature of the lesion, a well-planned biopsy is a basic requirement for correct management.[16,35,61,62,89,101] This may be either an *incisional biopsy* or, with small superficial lesions, a wide *excisional biopsy* that includes a border of normal tissue.[89] The plans for such a biopsy should take into consideration the possible need for a future radical excision or for radiation therapy; the placement of the biopsy should be such so as to avoid creating potential anatomic problems in the use of these further modalities of treatment.[35,62] Biopsy specimens should include the growing edge of the tumor, with central necrotic zones being avoided. Frozen-section examination of the biopsy material may be useful in order to assure that adequate tissue is obtained, but the surgeon must realize that it may not be possible with frozen-section material to accurately diagnose the tumor.[35,89,101] In all cases subjected to frozen-section analysis it is important that nonfrozen biopsy material also be obtained and routinely fixed in formalin so that permanent histologic sections may be produced that lack tissue-freezing artifacts. At the same time, depending on the type of tumor suspected, tissue may be fixed for immunohistochemical and electron microscopic studies.

Biopsy material of only a few millimeters from large tumors may be misleading, since, as mentioned previously, sarcomas may have a variety of histologic patterns even from area to area within the same tumor. Similarly, benign tumors such as some neurilemomas or pseudosarcomatous fibrous tumors may contain focal cellular areas that mimic a malignancy. Therefore, as generous a biopsy specimen as possible should be obtained. In this light I believe that *core-needle* biopsy specimens have only a limited role in the diagnosis of soft-tissue tumors,[35,89,101] and I discourage the use of *needle aspiration cytology* for the primary diagnosis of these lesions.

Sarcomas occur more frequently in male patients, who account for from 55% to 60% of cases,[19,75,96,107,108] and are most common in patients older than 40 years of age, with median ages between 45 and 62 years.[19,63,75,96,107,108] Although sarcomas occur in all anatomic sites, the extremities are involved in from 50% to 85% of cases, with the lower extremity, especially the thigh, accounting for the majority of cases.[19,54,63,75,96,107,108] The trunk accounts for roughly 20% of cases, the retroperitoneum for 12% to 15% of

cases, and the head and neck area for 4% to 9% of cases.[19,54,107,108] However, these general statistics are of limited value, since most of the major types of sarcoma have a predilection for certain anatomic regions and age groups. For instance, embryonal rhabdomyosarcoma occurs most frequently in the head and neck region of young children and is rarely found in adults, whereas liposarcoma occurs most frequently in the deep soft tissue of the lower extremity of adults and is rarely found in the subcutaneous tissue or in children. Hence such clinical information as the patient's age and size and the location of the tumor are critical pieces of information for the pathologist to have in order to arrive at a correct histologic diagnosis, and hence the clinician should supply and the pathologist must insist on receiving all pertinent clinical information. A pathologist who interprets tissue slides without recourse to the clinical setting does a disservice to his patient.

Most sarcomas grow by spreading along fascial planes, nerve trunks, and tendon sheaths and metastasize through the bloodstream, with the lungs, bones, liver, and skin the common sites involved.[54,63,103] Most metastases develop within 2 years of therapy though with some varieties of sarcoma 10 to 20 years may elapse before metastases become manifest.[31,36,59,63] As a rule, lymph nodes are not commonly involved, with average incidence figures varying from 1.4% to 12%.[54,66,90] However, certain sarcomas including synovial sarcoma, rhabdomyosarcoma, epithelioid sarcoma, clear cell sarcoma, and alveolar soft-part sarcoma have a higher frequency of lymph node metastases.[35,66]

Surgical management is the mainstay for the treatment of both benign and malignant soft-tissue tumors. The type of surgical excision, whether intralesional, marginal, wide, or radical,[30] greatly influences the local recurrence rate.[63,88,94] Local excision of sarcomas results in recurrence rates of from 75% to 90%, and even radical excision or amputation is followed by local recurrence in from 20% to 30% of cases.[59] Most recurrences take place within 3 years of therapy.[94,95] Newer surgical approaches involve the use of less radical therapy with conservative limb salvage procedures combined with postoperative radiation therapy and chemotherapy, with local control results equivalent to those obtained with more radical excisions or amputations.[8,15,16,59] However, in approximately 25% to 30% of patients distant metastases unassociated with local recurrence develop. Hence, microscopic metastatic foci must exist in such patients and require the use of adjuvant chemotherapy to be eradicated. However, despite remarkable success with the use of adjuvant chemotherapy in the treatment of certain sarcomas, notably rhabdomyosarcoma, Ewing's sarcoma, and osteosarcoma, the overall effectiveness of chemotherapeutic agents against most sarcomas has been disappointing in terms of overall survival benefits.[2,28,41,84]

Attempts have been made to establish staging and grading systems for soft-tissue sarcomas and to correlate these with prognosis. Three such staging systems have been proposed, ostensibly applicable to all sarcomas regardless of histologic type. All of these use the grade of the sarcoma as a parameter in establishing the stage of the tumor.[30,44,93] A variety of other studies have used grade alone to provide prognostic information, with some authors employing a three-grade system[19,75,107] and others a four-grade system.[63,96] The criteria used to establish a sarcoma's grade varies in each of these studies, but such factors as degree of anaplasia and pleomorphism, degree of cellularity, mitotic activity, amount of necrosis, and degree of tumor differentiation are the factors that are most commonly employed.[1,19,35,44,63,75,96,107] The problem with all such systems is that they are highly subjective, they are poorly reproducible from pathologist to pathologist, and the precise criteria used are poorly defined.[9,35,96] To say that a tumor's "cellularity" was assessed gives the reader no clear idea of the criteria used to distinguish between a moderately cellular lesion and a highly cellular one. In some studies, the majority of the sarcomas were graded from biopsy material alone.[19] As stated previously, the highly heterogeneous nature of some sarcomas points out the sampling problems inherent in the use of biopsy material. Unfortunately, whereas some sarcomas, such as fibrosarcoma, lend themselves well to grading, others, such as epithelioid sarcoma, clear cell sarcoma, and alveolar soft part sarcoma, have a histopathologic pattern that belies their clinical behavior. Although most grading studies show a direct correlation between tumor grade and survival—that is, the higher the grade, the worse the prognosis[63,75,94-96,107]—there are no universally accepted grading criteria that apply equally to all sarcomas.[1,8,35] This limits the applicability of such systems from institution to institution. Additionally, some use the term "high grade" to refer to the clinical *aggressivity* of a tumor and not its *histopathology*. These are not necessarily synonymous concepts. Tumors such as epithelioid sarcoma or alveolar soft part sarcoma may be histologically "low grade" but are clinically aggressive tumors. A serious defect in many grading studies is the arbitrary assignment of a sarcoma to a "high-grade" category, regardless of its histopathologic pattern, because the tumor is known to be clinically aggressive.[19,30,75,93,96] This is intellectually invalid. A grading system should be based on a tumor's histomorphology and as such is a pure pathology concept. To classify some sarcomas on this basis but grading others on clinical parameters converts the system to a clinicopathologic one. Although the latter may, if rigidly tested by statistical analysis, have some value, at present it is artificial, and for pathologist and clinician alike creates more confusion than illumination. We agree

with those who urge that grade not be used in staging systems.[8] We doubt that an effective grading system that is applicable to all sarcomas is possible, based on present knowledge. Instead, efforts should be directed to individual sarcomas in determining what histologic features, if any, are statistically valid when applied to estimating prognosis. Currently, the grading of sarcomas by pathologists is infrequent, with only approximately 25% of cases graded.[47] Clinicians and radiologists who request a sarcoma grade should realize that what they receive is, in most cases, a fiction.

Aside from an overall tumor grade, other factors such as mitotic activity,[9,75,107,108] degree of tumor necrosis,[9,19,107] depth of the tumor,[108] local recurrence,[63,95] and lymph node metastases[90] have been found to be prognostically important. The effect of tumor size on ultimate survival has been found to be prognostically important by some[54,83,89] and not by others.[15,63,107,108]

Sarcomas may develop after radiation therapy, or in patients with a compromised immune system, such as those with acquired immunodeficiency syndrome in whom Kaposi's sarcoma is relatively frequent. Exposure to phenoxyacetic acid herbicides is believed by some to produce an increased risk for sarcoma development,[5,46] but this association is denied by others.[42,49]

FIBROUS-TISSUE LESIONS
Fibrosarcoma

Despite electron miroscopic studies that have shown occasional myofibroblasts in fibrosarcoma,[118,124] fibrosarcoma remains the prototypical tumor of fibroblasts. Although formerly considered to be the most common of the sarcomas, the number of soft-tissue tumors now diagnosed as fibrosarcoma has been dramatically reduced by the exclusion of other tumors and tumorlike conditions that have been better defined, such as malignant fibrous histiocytoma, nodular fasciitis, and the benign fibromatoses. Indeed, in some series approximately one third to one half of cases previously classified as fibrosarcoma were reassigned to other diagnostic categories based on current classifications.[122,126] Today, fibrosarcomas comprise only 5% to 10% of all sarcomas.[63,96,107,108,119,123,126]

Fibrosarcoma occurs in all age groups but most commonly affects adults between 40 and 70 years of age.[117,122,126,128] Approximately 60% of cases occur in male patients.[117,126] In children, the tumors are usually found during the first year of life, 40% to 50% being congenital.[53,117,128]

Fibrosarcoma develops as a slowly enlarging mass that usually is present for 2 to 3 years before medical attention is sought, though in some patients the clinical history is as short as 2 weeks or as long as 25 years.[122,126] Pain is not a prominent symptom, though in one report slightly over one half of the patients had pain.[126] Large tumors may be tender and cause pressure symptoms. Fibrosarcomas tend to arise in the external soft tissue, only rarely occurring in the retroperitoneum, mesentery, omentum, or mediastinum.[103] They originate from the fascial connective tissues or the deep subcutaneous tissue.[126] In adults, 90% occur in the extremities, mostly in the lower extremity (50% to 60%) where the thigh is the most common site.[33,126] Less common locations include the upper extremity, trunk, and head and neck.[122,129] In children the anatomic location varies somewhat, with the distal portions of the lower extremity, the ankle and foot, being more frequently involved than the thigh and a higher proportion of the tumors being situated in the shoulder and pelvic girdles.[53,117,128]

Grossly, fibrosarcomas are gray white, firm, lobulated masses that may have such good circumscription that they appear encapsulated.[126] Foci of necrosis and hemorrhage are present in the more poorly differentiated tumors. Tumors in children are often softer, more friable, and less well circumscribed than those in adults.[117,122] Tumor size averages about 3 to 4 cm, but in some sites tumors larger than 10 cm are not uncommon.[117,122,126,128] In infantile cases the tumor may involve the entire distal portion of an extremity.[117]

Histologically, fibrosarcomas are composed of spindle-shaped fibroblasts arranged in intersecting fascicles, which, in the better differentiated tumors, produce the typical "herringbone" pattern[122,126,128] (Fig. 37-1). Nuclei are usually uniform, with tapered rather than rounded ends, and the cytoplasm tends to be ill defined with poorly formed cell borders. Reticulin and collagen production is best seen in well-differentiated lesions, where there is an abundant network of reticulin fibers that surround and run parallel to the long axis of each cell.[122,128] In the less well-differentiated tumors there is an increase in the overall cellularity, with nuclei that are plumper and rounder and have more variation in size and shape. There is also increased mitotic activity and less reticulin and collagen formation.[122,128] Foci of necrosis, degeneration, and hemorrhge are frequent in the more poorly differentiated fibrosarcomas. This basic microscopic pattern also holds true for infantile fibrosarcomas, though there is a tendency for such tumors

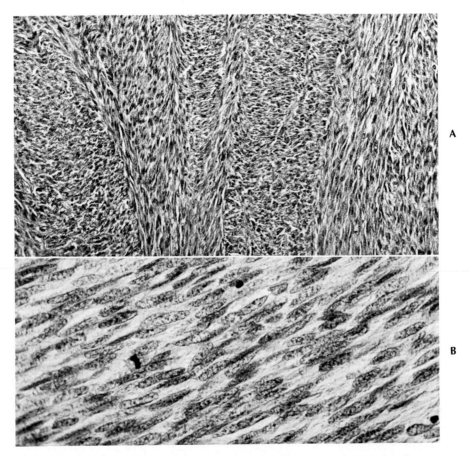

Fig. 37-1. A, Fibrosarcoma. Interlacing fascicles of spindle-shaped fibroblasts produce typical herringbone pattern of well-differentiated fibrosarcoma. **B,** Closely packed fibroblasts with ill-defined cytoplasmic borders. Mitotic figure is present to left of center. (**A,** 120×; **B,** 480×.)

to be less differentiated, with loss of the herringbone pattern, and to be more vascular.[117,122] They also may contain areas of primitive-appearing mesenchymal cells.[117,122] Fibrosarcomas lack the pleomorphism of other sarcomas,[33,122,126,128] and the presence of many large bizarre tumor cells, including tumor giant cell forms, excludes the dignosis of fibrosarcoma.

Despite the occasional presence of myofibroblasts in some electron microscopic studies of fibrosarcoma,[118,124] the dominant cells show the features of fibroblasts.[60,124,129] Studies of some infantile fibrosarcomas have also shown the presence of cells with the morphology of histiocytes.[120,121] Immunohistochemical studies indicate that fibrosarcomas contain vimentin intermediate filament protein.[57,70,81]

Fibrosarcoma is one of the few sarcomas that lends itself well to grading systems based on the differentiation of the tumor. The tumors may be described as either well differentiated, moderately differentiated, or poorly differentiated, or assigned a numerical grade of I to IV, with grade IV the least differentiated category. This grading system has prognostic significance, since it correlates well with survival in adults; the better differentiated the tumor, the better is the long-term survival rate.[126] Most fibrosarcomas tend to be moderately differentiated grade II to III tumors.

It is important to remember that spindle-cell fibroblastic areas may be found in a variety of soft-tissue sarcomas such as synovial sarcoma, malignant fibrous histiocytoma, malignant nerve sheath tumors, and rhabdomyosarcoma, and small biopsy specimens from these sarcomas may easily be misinterpreted as fibrosarcoma. Indeed, even with an apparently adequate amount of tissue, the light microscopic differential diagnosis between fibrosarcoma and such tumors as synovial sarcoma, neurofibrosarcoma, and rhabdomyosarcoma with a fibrosing pattern may be impossible and depend on either immunohistochemical or electron microscopic studies.

A further histologic problem is the difficulty in distinguishing some of the benign fibromatoses from fibrosarcoma. An indeterminate area exists between cellular fibromatosis and well-differentiated fibrosarcoma, especially in young children. Whether a fibrous lesion is too cellular and has too many mitotic figures to be considered benign is often a matter of subjective opinion.

Fibrosarcomas are treated surgically by either wide local excision or, if necessary, amputation. There is some indication that infantile fibrosarcomas may be responsive to chemotherapy.[121,125] In adults, there is a good correlation between the tumor's histologic features and the rate of local recurrence, metastases, and survival. Survival statistics in the literature must be viewed with some caution since older studies include cases of "pleomorphic" fibrosarcomas that today would be considered malignant fibrous histiocytomas. In general, recurrences after wide local excision occur in 60% of patients, and approximately 50% of patients develop distant metastases.[126] The metastases are virtually all blood borne with regional lymph nodes being only rarely involved. Current 5- and 10-year survival rates of 50% to 60% are reported with few deaths because of tumor after 10 years.[126]

Unlike the adult form, the clinical course of childhood fibrosarcoma cannot be predicted on the basis of the tumor's histologic features.[117,128] In general, childhood fibrosarcomas have a more favorable prognosis than the adult forms,[53,103,117] with survival rates of greater than 85% despite local recurrence rates of close to 50% after wide local excision.[117,128] Few patients with a diagnosis of childhood fibrosarcoma have died of metastatic disease.[103,117,127,128] Children younger than 5 years of age may be treated less radically than adults and still have an excellent prognosis.[128] This may reflect the possibility that some childhood fibrosarcomas are in reality benign, locally aggressive, nonmetastasizing fibromatoses that cannot be histologically distinguished from true fibrosarcoma. Older children, however, have the less favorable survival rate of adults.[128]

Fibromatoses

The fibromatoses are a group of lesions, each specific in its own right but all sharing common histologic features. A fibromatosis has been defined as "an infiltrating fibroblastic proliferation showing none of the features of an inflammatory response and no features of unequivocal neoplasia,"[135] or more broadly "a group of non-metastasizing fibroblastic tumors which tend to invade locally and recur after attempted surgical excision."[130] Neither of these definitions is totally accurate, since inflammatory cells are seen in some of the fibromatoses, though to a minimal degree, and some have little or no tendency to recur. In addition, these "fibroblastic" lesions have been found to be composed not only of fibroblasts, but also of cells with electron microscopic features of both fibroblasts and smooth muscle cells, the so-called myofibroblasts.[133,136] Both definitions, however, characterize the general nature of all these lesions and emphasize their most salient feature, that is, that although in rare instances they may prove fatal because of their local aggressiveness they do not metastasize.

The fibromatoses occur in a wide variety of anatomic locations and in all age groups, though some are found exclusively or predominantly in infants and young children. These are broadly grouped as the juvenile or infantile fibromatoses and include fibrous hamartoma of infancy, fibromatosis colli, diffuse infantile fibromatosis, aggressive infantile fibromatosis (congenital fibrosarcoma-like fibromatosis), juvenile aponeurotic fibroma, digital fibrous tumor of childhood, congenital generalized fibromatosis, congenital solitary fibromatosis, hereditary gingival fibromatosis, juvenile nasopharyngeal angiofibroma, and fibromatosis hyalinica multiplex juvenilis.[130,131,137] Several of these lesions are quite cellular, have mesenchymal cells of the primitive type, and grow with an infiltrative pattern to such a degree that they are diagnosed as some form of sarcoma. Indeed, the histologic distinction between the so-called aggressive fibromatosis of children and a true fibrosarcoma may be impossible in some cases, the final truth being determined only by the patient's clinical course.[137] In most fibromatoses, however, careful attention to histologic detail will permit ready recognition of the entity.

In the adult category of fibromatoses, that is, those seen primarily in older patients, are the various forms of the Dupuytren's type of fibromatoses, which include the palmar and plantar fibromatoses and Peyronie's disease, and the various types of the desmoid fibromatoses.[130] As a group, the adult fibromatoses are more common than the juvenile forms, some of which are so exceedingly rare that they are outside the experience of most pathologists.

I agree with those who caution against the use of the term "fibroma" as a designation for any of these lesions or for any fibroblastic lesion occurring in the deep soft tissues.[134] Such a diagnosis implies a well-circumscribed or encapsulated lesion, composed of bland, well-differentiated fibroblasts, that will not recur or become aggressive after attempts at surgical removal. The experience of many diagnostic pathologists has proved that such deep lesions may, despite their gross and microscopic appearance, prove locally aggressive. For fibroblastic lesions in the deep soft tissues the term "fibroma" should not be used.

In this section only a few of the fibromatoses are discussed; refer to several of the excellent reviews of the subject for more extensive coverage.[33,130,132,134,135,137]

Palmar and plantar fibromatoses

Palmar and plantar fibromatoses are the most common and best known of the fibromatoses.[130] Although each has certain specific characteristics, they share a common histomorphology and are considered together. They are members of what has been termed the "Dupuytren-like fibromatoses," which also includes such other entities as knuckle pads and Peyronie's disease.[130]

These lesions affect patients over a broad age range, but in general the palmar lesions are seen in older patients and are uncommon in children, with most patients in the sixth decade of life.[33,130,139,141,143] Plantar fibromatosis is more frequent in younger patients and does occur in children.[33,130,137,143] Palmar lesions occur four to eight times more frequently in male than in female patients,[134,137,141,143] whereas plantar lesions have a more equal sex distribution.[137,143] There is a higher incidence of these fibromatoses

among patients with alcoholism, cirrhosis, long-standing epilepsy, and diabetes.[130,140,142] They apparently are rare in black patients.[140-142] Familial cases occur.[33,130,142] Either palmar or plantar fibromatoses may be bilateral.[134,137,141,143]

The palmar lesion manifests itself as a painless nodule that usually develops on the ulnar side of the palm at the distal palmar skin crease. The lesion arises from the palmar fascia and may extend into the dermis. With time, it extends into the fingers as a longitudinal cord-like band that may eventually cause a flexion contracture (Dupuytren's contracture) of the fingers, with the ring and little fingers being the most frequently involved.[33,141-143] Plantar lesions, which are less common than the palmar forms, usually develop in the medial aspect of the plantar arch and do not cause contractures as frequently as the palmar lesions do.[33,130,143] Both types of fibromatoses may develop in the same patient.[130,140]

The evolution of the individual lesion is divided into three histologic stages—proliferative, involutional, and residual. The diagnostic pattern of the proliferative phase consists in fibrovascular nodules that are composed of plump, tightly packed fibroblasts, at times with a high mitotic rate, surrounding a central small blood vessel. The fibroblasts have round to oval nuclei, with prominent nucleoli, that show distinct transverse nuclear lines because of nuclear folds.[143] As the lesion ages or involutes, there is a progressive increase in the amount of collagen within it and the fibroblasts align themselves into fascicles along lines of stress. In the residual phase one finds a dense collagenized stroma containing only a few fibroblasts that now are slender rather than plump. This fibrosis may extend into the soft tissue of the palm, thus creating the contracture, which histologically is nonspecific scar tissue.[130,134,137,141,143] Electron microscopic studies show the presence of myofibroblasts in both the palmar and plantar lesions,[138-140] and their presence has been proposed as the reason for the development of the contractures.[138]

Both plantar and palmar lesions may remain stationary at the nodular stage, progress, or spontaneously regress. After operative procedures, both may recur, with recurrences more common in younger patients.[130] Plantar lesions are particularly prone to recur after local excision, with recurrence rates as high as 60% to 85%.[130] Radical excision for their complete removal, however, is contraindicated, since they may involute spontaneously.

Desmoid fibromatoses

Historically the desmoid fibromatoses (desmoids) are divided into those of the abdominal wall—the *abdominal wall desmoids*—and those located elsewhere—the *extra-abdominal desmoids*.[130,134] This is an arbitrary division, since the lesions are histologically similar. These lesions are also known as "musculoaponeurotic fibromatoses."[147] They are not common; a survey of the Finnish population yielded an incidence of 2.4 to 4.3 per million population.[165]

Desmoids occur in patients of all ages but are more frequent in the third and fourth decades of life.* It is rare to find abdominal desmoids in patients younger than 20 years of age, but extra-abdominal forms do occur in young children.[130,135,144,165,167] Desmoids are more frequent in female than in male patients, especially the abdominal form, which has a predilection for parous women.[135] The sexual difference in the extra-abdominal desmoids is not so dramatic as in the abdominal type, and in some series the sex ratio is about equal.†

Desmoids are usually slowly growing, firm to hard masses that may be tender or painful, though most are painless.[145–147,156,160,167] Desmoids in the head and neck region, however, may grow rapidly.[145,163] There is an increased incidence of desmoid tumors, particularly those located intra-abdominally at the root of the small bowel mesentery, in patients with familial polyposis coli, especially those with Gardner's syndrome. Here, the desmoids either precede or develop subsequent to the intestinal polyps, though most often some form of colonic resection predates the appearance of the desmoid lesion.[155,158,166] Desmoids also arise in surgical scars and in sites that have been irradiated.[33,130,144] Rare familial cases are reported.[171] A history of trauma is reported in from 30% to 60% of extra-abdominal lesions,[147] and the trauma of delivery has been postulated to explain the occurrence of abdominal wall desmoids in parous women. An increased incidence of radiologic skeletal abnormalities is found in patients with desmoids, even in those lacking any manifestation of Gardner's syndrome.[152,153]

Desmoids arise from fascia or aponeuroses and involve the underlying muscle; invasion of bone is rare.[151] Abdominal wall desmoids primarily affect the rectus abdominis muscle, whereas extra-abdominal desmoids are widely distributed as to site, with the upper arm and shoulder girdle, chest wall, back, lower extremity, and buttocks being the most commonly involved sites.[33,135,144,147,154,167] The head and neck regions account for from 10% to 20% of cases, with the neck being the most common location.[130,135,145,146,154,163] Multicentric desmoids occur in less than 10% of cases; in these cases most are confined to a single limb.[148,165,167,168,169] Intra-abdominal desmoids located at the root of the small bowel mesentery are associated with Gardner's syndrome.[155]

On gross inspection, desmoids, especially the extra-abdominal forms, are large, often exceeding 20 cm.* They infiltrate muscle, usually along its long axis, producing ill-defined masses that have a grayish-white, whorled, and trabeculated cut surface that is unlike the more homogeneous appearance of fibrosarcoma.[130,146,147] They may also extend along the fascia and involve the subcutaneous tissue. The histologic extent may be several centimeters beyond the visible gross margins.[135] It may be impossible to distinguish grossly between scar tissue and tumor tissue.

Microscopically, desmoids show a uniform appearance of long, slender, spindle-shaped fibroblasts arranged in bands and fascicles surrounded by varying amounts of collagen. The cells characteristically lack pleomorphism.[130,147,154,163] The fibroblastic proliferation separates, pushes aside, and replaces the muscle fibers, many of which appear atrophic. (Fig. 37-2) The degree of cellularity varies from area to area, with hypocellular hyalinized foci alternating with compact cellular zones. Mitoses are notably scarce or absent. Electron microscopy shows the presence of myofibroblasts, which may be the predominant cells.[149,164]

Although the absence of pleomorphism and mitotic activity are features that distinguish desmoids from fibrosarcomas, it must be admitted that this distinction is easier on paper than it is in actual practice. The difference between a cellular fibromatosis with occasional mitoses and a well-differentiated fibrosarcoma with only minimal cellular atypia may be blurred.[137]

Desmoids treated by surgical excision have a high rate of local recurrence that has varied from 19% to 77%, with frequent multiple recurrences.† Desmoids of the head and neck are more prone to local recurrence than desmoids in other locations, a probable indication of the inability of surgeons to perform wide excision in this area.[163] Indeed, recurrence rates in general reflect the adequacy of the original resection, with simple marginal local excision yielding recurrences in up to 90% of patients.[160,167] However, even with wide local resections, recurrences may develop in 19% to 50% of patients.[145,146,160,167] Abdominal wall lesions have a lower rate of recurrence, whereas young patients and those with large lesions have a higher incidence of local recurrence.[130,147] Most recurrences manifest themselves within 2 years of the initial therapy.[156,162,167] Despite their lack of metastases, desmoids cause severe morbidity because of their aggressive local behavior with their tendency to invade neurovascular bundles. Intra-abdominal and head and neck desmoids have caused death by virtue of their involvement of vital structures.[130,144,146,155,163,166] A useless limb or the relief of pain may require amputation. Such a therapeutic pro-

---

*References 130, 134, 146, 147, 156, 157, 160, 167.
†References 130, 134, 135, 147, 165, 167.

*References 134, 146, 147, 155, 156, 160, 162.
†References 130, 135, 144, 146, 147, 154, 156, 160, 163, 167.

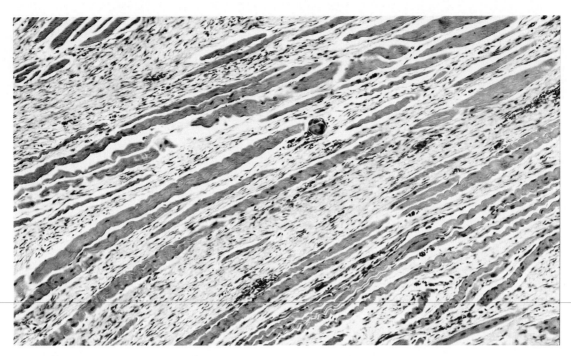

Fig. 37-2. Desmoid fibromatosis. Diffuse infiltration of skeletal muscle by bands of well-formed slender fibroblasts. (90×.)

cedure, however, should be a last resort, since desmoids may stabilize in their growth and some, exceptionally, have even regressed.[130,147]

Despite the high rate of local recurrence, patients can be cured by surgical excision. Indeed, the majority of patients are cured or have persistent tumors that either stabilize or slowly regress without causing physical disability.[135,144,147,162,167] Although previous reports did not indicate great success with the use of radiation therapy,[147] more recent accounts indicate a high rate of success with the use of high-dose radiation therapy even in patients whose tumors are deemed unresectable. The effect of the radiation, other than causing an initial softening of the tumor, may take many months, with ultimate complete disappearance of the lesion in some patients.[150,157,162] This has led to the use of less than radical operative therapy where this would lead to mutilating results and the substitution of simple excision followed by radiation therapy.[156,167] Desmoids have been successfully treated with drug therapy including the use of anti-inflammatory agents, ascorbic acid, progesterone, and antiestrogen agents such as tamoxifen.[155,158,159,161,170]

Fibrous hamartoma of infancy

Fibrous hamartoma of infancy occurs in infants and young children, with almost all lesions appearing during the first 2 years of life.[130,174,175] It has not been reported in adults. Boys are more commonly affected than girls in a ratio of 2:1 to 3:1.[137,174] The lesions occur as palpable masses beneath the skin, with two thirds of cases found in the region of the axilla, shoulder, or upper arm, with the axillary fold being the most common site.[130,137] Other reported locations include the forearm, abdomen, neck, scalp, chest wall, perianal region, foot, pharynx, inguinal region, vulva, and scrotum.[33,137,175-177,179]

As their original designation of "subdermal 'fibromatous tumors' of infancy"[178] indicates, these lesions occur in the lower dermis or the subcutaneous tissue. They grossly appear as round, smooth, or bosselated masses that are usually unencapsulated and blend into the subcutaneous fat or are attached to the superficial fascia.[173,174,176] An infiltrative gross pattern may also be found.[172] The lesions are firm, with a cut surface that shows fibrous bands admixed with streaks of yellow fat.[172-174,176] Most fibrous hamartomas are 3 to 4 cm,[175] though those as large as 15 cm have occurred.[33] Despite its well-accepted name, most authors consider fibrous hamartoma as a fibromatosis and include it within the broad category of the congenital or juvenile fibromatoses.[130,135,137] Others suggest the possibility that it is a true benign neoplasm of uncertain histogenesis.[175]

Fibrous hamartoma has a highly characteristic and uniform microscopic appearance.[174,175,178] The diagnosis depends on finding a combination of mature fat cells, mature fibroblasts arranged in fibrocollagenous bundles, and foci of immature appearing round, oval, or

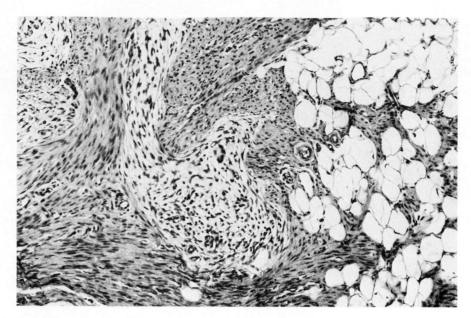

Fig. 37-3. Fibrous hamartoma. Mixture of fat, bundles of mature fibroblasts, and pale edematous-appearing nodules of primitive mesenchymal cells. (120×.)

stellate cells embedded in a loose myxoid matrix. These latter cells are considered to be primitive mesenchymal cells. The proportions of the three elements vary, but they are always intimately admixed with one another (Fig. 37-3). The mesenchymal foci stand out as paler, edematous, ball-like areas within or surrounded by the denser fibrocollagenous bands. Occasionally, dense hyalinized keloidlike areas are present. The fibrous bundles with their myxoid areas may simulate the appearance of a neurofibroma, but the presence of the admixed fat cells helps to distinguish these two lesions.

Histochemical studies have found the presence of hyaluronic acid, chondroitin sulfate, and keratin sulfate within different portions of the lesion.[175] Immunohistochemical stains for S-100 protein, other than in the fat component, are negative, as are those for desmin, cytokeratin, myoglobin, and factor VIII–related antigen.[175] The results of the few electron microscopic studies show the presence of fibroblasts and, in some cases, myofibroblasts, as well as fat cells and preadipose fibroblasts.[137,176,177] From these studies, it was suggested that the lesion appears to recapitulate the fetal development of blood vessels and fat.[176]

The ultimate clinical evolution of these lesions if left untreated is unknown, since they are all locally excised. Although a few have recurred requiring reexcision, they have no aggressive potential.[137,174,175]

Aponeurotic fibroma

Aponeurotic fibroma, also variously termed juvenile aponeurotic fibroma, calcifying juvenile aponeurotic fibroma, and calcifying fibroma,[180,182] is a rare lesion, with less than 100 reported cases.[33,185] Although originally described in young children,[182] it has also occurred in adults, some of whom are in the seventh decade of life,[181,184,185] so that the appellation "juvenile" is no longer appropriate. However, such cases are unusual, and aponeurotic fibroma is predominantly found in patients younger than 20 years of age,[181,185] with about half the patients being less than 10 years of age.[180,181,185] Congenital cases also occur.[137] The lesion is more than twice as common in male as in female patients.[137,185]

Aponeurotic fibroma usually develops as a slowly developing soft-tissue mass present for months or years.[181,184,185] Approximately one half to three fourths of the lesions are located in the hand or wrist, with the majority in the palm about the thenar and hypothenar eminences.[137,180,181,185] Other sites include the fingers, the forearm, thigh, popliteal fossa, trunk, leg, foot, and abdominal wall.

Aponeurotic fibromas are small, usually 2 to 3 cm,[137,180] though those located outside the hands or feet may be up to 8 cm.[185] They are almost always located in the subcutaneous tissue or in close relation to aponeuroses, tendon sheaths, or joint capsules.[135,137,180,184,185] Grossly, they appear as either sharply demarcated nodular masses or they have a distinctly infiltrative pattern.[180,181,183,184] The cut surface, which may be gritty because of the presence of focal calcification, is gray white and may have a vague cartilaginous appearance.[183]

Histologically the lesion is highly cellular and composed of fibroblasts, with plump to round nuclei and ill-defined cytoplasmic borders, that infiltrate the subcutaneous fat, muscle, and neurovascular structures. Occasional osteoclast-like giant cells may be found. Mitoses are scarce and normal. Characteristically the fibroblasts orient themselves to form a syncytium-like appearance of parallel rows that appear to flow out into the adjacent normal tissue to form nodular aggregates. These nodules frequently have central foci of calcification associated with dense hyalinized collagen. The cells adjacent to these calcified foci have a chondroid appearance, lying in lacunae, and appear to differentiate toward fibrocartilage.[135,137,180-184] This cartilaginous appearance has caused the lesion to be considered by some as the cartilage analog of the fibromatoses[184] despite the fact that the plump appearance of the fibroblasts, their streaming in rows, and the presence of calcification and chondroidlike foci are unique and not found in any of the other fibromatoses.

After excision, local recurrence occurs in about half the patients, with some having multiple recurrences.[137,180,181] Younger patients appear more prone to local recurrence.[180] However, there is no metastatic potential, and conservative management is indicated.[130,137,180]

Myofibromatosis (congenital generalized fibromatosis, infantile myofibromatosis)

Myofibromatosis is a rare condition, with fewer than 150 well-documented cases reported in the English medical literature.[137,189,191] This lesion was originally designated as "congenital generalized fibromatosis" because of the congenital presence of numerous fibrous lesions that involved multiple anatomic sites, including the subcutaneous tissue, muscle, and viscera.[203] However, patients were subsequently found without visceral involvement, as well as those with only solitary nodules.[196-198] By electron microscopy, the dominant cells in these lesions had the morphologic features of both fibroblasts and smooth muscle cells (myofibroblasts). For this reason, "infantile myofibromatosis" was introduced as the designation for these lesions. However, rare examples of these lesions are reported in older children and even adults.[33,191,193,195,198] We in the field prefer to use "myofibromatosis" as the general diagnostic term for these lesions, with the modifiers congenital, infantile, juvenile, or adult as the situation dictates.

Authors have used terms such as multiple, diffuse, or generalized to refer either to the number or distribution of the lesions or to cases in which there is visceral involvement. Here we use "multiple" to refer to those multicentric lesions that affect the skin, subcutaneous tissue, muscle, or bone, and "visceral" for those lesions that also involve other organ systems. These are designated by others as "type I and type II lesions."[137] Occasional cases are familial, but there is debate as to whether this disease is genetically an autosomal recessive or an autosomal dominant with reduced penetrance.[187,191,195]

Myofibromatosis is almost always congenital, but new lesions may continue to develop after birth.[33,137,190,191] Although approximately 90% of lesions are recognized within the first 2 years of life,[191,193,195] older children and adults are occasionally affected.[33,191,193,195,198] Visceral lesions, however, apparently occur only in newborns or neonates. Overall, male patients are more commonly affected than female patients, but multicentric lesions occur slightly more frequently in female patients.[137,189-191]

By definition, multiple myofibromatosis involves either the skin, subcutaneous tissue, muscle, or bone, whereas the generalized or visceral form of the disorder may additionally affect any other organ system. In either form, the skin and subcutaneous tissue are the most frequently involved sites, with a predilection for the head and neck, trunk, and lower extremities, though any portion of the body may be involved.[130,137,190,191,193] Bone lesions, which are found in the majority of patients, are radiologically osteolytic metaphyseal defects that may have sclerotic borders.[137,189] Any bone may be involved, but the long bones are those most frequently affected.[189,191,194]

Grossly, the lesions usually consist of well-delimited nodules, though at times an infiltrating pattern is found. The nodules are firm to rubbery and their cut surface may show central necrosis, cystic degeneration, or calcification.[130,137,191] The number of nodules in those patients with multicentric lesions varies from a few to as many as 100.[137] The nodules are usually smaller than 3 cm, but those as large as 9 cm are recorded.[130,190,193,197,199,201] Visceral lesions may be found in any organ including the central nervous system.[130,137,186,189,191,192] Solitary lesions occur in the skin, subcutaneous tissue, muscle or bone,[197-199] but a case of a solitary lesion involving another organ system has not been reported. The solitary form of myofibromatosis is more common than the multiple form.[191]

Histologically, myofibromatosis is characterized by a distinct zonal pattern of growth. The periphery of the nodules is composed of spindle-shaped fibroblastic cells and plumper fusiform smooth muscle–like cells arranged in bands, whorls, or fascicles. The cells may merge with the smooth muscle in the walls of adjacent blood vessels. Hyalin-like or chondroid-like hypocellular foci may alternate with more cellular areas. The central portions of the nodule frequently show bland necrosis and focal or diffuse calcification. In addition, these central regions may have a prominent vascular pattern that has a distinct hemangiopericytomatous appearance. Polypoid protrusion of tumor tissue into the vascular spaces is sometimes found. Mitotic figures are either scarce or frequent, but not atypical.[33,130,137,190,191,193,198,199,204]

By electron microscopy the cells have the combined features of fibroblasts and smooth muscle cells.[188,195,199,200] Immunohistochemically the tumor cells give positive reactions with anti–smooth muscle myosin, anti–smooth muscle antibody, and desmin.[188,193,200] Although most authors accept the tumor cells as being myofibroblasts, others suggest that they are primitive smooth muscle cells.[193]

The mortality for patients with visceral involvement is approximately 80%,[189] whereas patients with pulmonary involvement have an extremely poor prognosis.[137,189,202] Most who die do so soon after birth, most within the first week of life,[130,137,189] though survival for as long as 5 months before death is recorded.[189] The cause of death is attributed to the complications produced by the anatomic location of the lesion such as intestinal obstruction or respiratory failure. A patient with multiple myofibromatosis in which there was isolated colonic involvement has survived for over 5 years.[191] Patients with solitary lesions are cured by simple excision. In the multicentric form without visceral involvement the prognosis is also excellent, since spontaneous regression of the lesions, including the osseous lesions, takes place.[130,137,187,190,191] Only rare local recurrences are recorded after surgical excision of a superficial lesion.[190,191]

Pseudosarcomatous fibrous lesions

Many benign soft-tissue lesions may, because of their cellularity or the presence of atypical-appearing cells, be mistaken for sarcomas and in that sense may be considered "pseudosarcomas." However, in this section the discussion is restricted to those reactive lesions whose main feature is a proliferation of fibrous elements: nodular fasciitis, proliferative fasciitis, and proliferative myositis.

Despite these lesions having been well defined, with excellent descriptions of their histopathology, there are still cases received in consultation that carry the diagnosis of some form of sarcoma and for which radical surgery is contemplated but on review represent one of these reactive fibrous conditions. The magnitude of the problem is illustrated by the fact that in one large cancer registry slightly over 10% of the lesions diagnosed as sarcoma were, on review, reclassified as benign,[209] and in this latter group about 60% of the cases represented one of these three pseudosarcomatous fibrous lesions. Because of their rapid growth, infiltrative growth pattern, cellularity, and high mitotic rate they may be misinterpreted by the pathologist as some form of fibrosarcoma, malignant fibrous histiocytoma, or malignant neurogenous tumor. It should be remembered that very rapid growth and an infiltrative gross pattern are not features of most sarcomas.

Nodular fasciitis

Since its original description as "subcutaneous pseudosarcomatous fibromatosis,"[221] nodular fasciitis has been known by a variety of synonyms, including infiltrative fasciitis, pseudosarcomatous fasciitis, and proliferative fasciitis.[205,220,223] This last term has also been applied to another of the fibrous pseudosarcomas,[207] and I prefer to use "nodular fasciitis" as the designation for the lesion discussed here to avoid any possible confusion. Over 80% of the "sarcomas" reclassified as benign conditions in the study mentioned above were examples of nodular fasciitis.[209]

Nodular fasciitis is the most frequent of the pseudosarcomatous fibrous lesions and occurs at all ages, with patients ranging in age from 2 weeks to 85 years.[206,211,212,220,223,227] However, the usual patients are young adults with mean and median ages between 30 and 40 years.[209,211,212,217,223] Two anatomic variants of nodular fasciitis, cranial fasciitis and intravascular fasciitis, most frequently occur in infants and young children.[222,225] Male patients are slightly more commonly affected than female patients,[223] but this sex difference is not great, with some reports indicating an approximately equal sex distribution.[33,211,227]

Nodular fasciitis develops most frequently as a rapidly growing nodular mass, which is occasionally painful or tender, present for days or a few weeks,[205,212,217,223,227] but some have a slower evolution.[211,217,225,227]

Although originally described in the subcutaneous tissue, nodular fasciitis also occurs in the deep somatic soft tissues and has been reported in such diverse sites as the parotid gland, breast, esophagus, trachea, vagina, labia, and periosteum.[205,216,229] However, approximately half the cases occur in the upper extremity, where the forearm is by far the most common site. The trunk and head and neck region each account for about 20% of cases, with the lower extremity less commonly involved.* In children the head and neck region accounts for about half the cases.[212] Small to medium-sized arteries and veins (intravascular fasciitis) may also be sites of origin.[225]

In the soft tissue the lesion grows from the superficial fascia into the subcutaneous tissue as a round to oval nodule that is usually well circumscribed but may appear poorly delimited and infiltrative.[205,212,223] They tend to be small, rarely exceeding 5 cm, with most between 1 and 3 cm,[205,211,223,225,227] though those up to 10 cm occur.[33,222] Occasionally the process extends along the fascia and downward into the muscle.[212,223] In cranial fasciitis, the lesion may erode the bone and extend to the dura.[222,226]

Microscopically, nodular fasciitis has a wide range of

---

*References 33, 205, 212, 217, 220, 222, 223, 227.

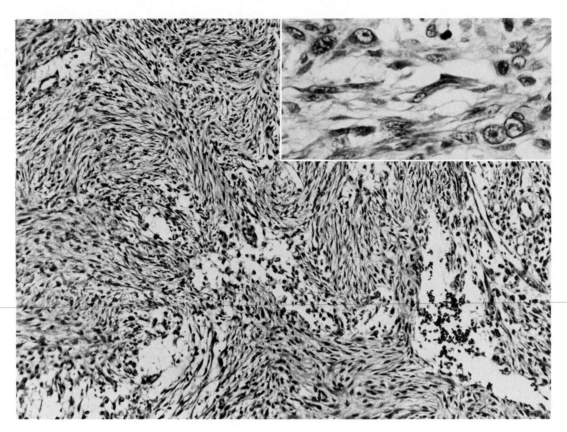

Fig. 37-4. Nodular fasciitis. Whorled pattern of fibroblasts with microcystic spaces containing red blood cells. (150×.) *Inset,* Mild nuclear atypia is present in some cells with round nuclei having prominent nucleoli. (600×.)

morphologic patterns; one report mentions 11 histologic variants.[205] Fortunately, most lesions have mixed patterns, and all share a common set of features. Spindle-shaped fibroblast-like cells are arranged in long fascicles described as having curved, whorled, or S-shaped patterns. The fascicles are loosely arranged, separated by a myxoid stroma, which, at least focally, gives the lesion a characteristic edematous appearance.[205,212,223,227] Cells may vary from the usual spindle-shaped forms to those that are plumper and have prominent nucleoli (Fig. 37-4). Although some cellular atypia occurs, bizarre pleomorphic cells are not present, and mitoses, though numerous, are not atypical.[53,205,212,217,227] Another frequent finding is the presence of extravasated red blood cells either insinuating between the stromal cells or located in clusters within microcystic spaces or clefts.[53,205,223] In sections stained with hematoxylin and eosin, these spaces have a blue-gray appearance and, along with the myxoid stroma, contain hyaluronidase-sensitive acid mucopolysaccharide.[33,53,212] Although its name implies inflammation, inflammatory cells, chiefly lymphocytes, are never very numerous in the clinical experience.[205,211,223] Osteoclastic giant cells may be present.[205,211,227] At times the myxoid stroma is less prominent, and the cells are more compact and ar-

ranged in a storiform pattern similar to that in fibrous histiocytoma.[53,206,227] Some examples of nodular fasciitis, presumably older forms, have zones of increased collagenization that may simulate a fibromatosis. Some also may contain foci of osteoid or cartilage.[217] Areas with the histomorphology of nodular fasciitis are also found in the other two pseudosarcomas—proliferative myositis and proliferative fasciitis.[210] Electron microscopic studies show the majority of the spindle cells to be myofibroblasts.[164,231]

Nodular fasciitis is quite vascular, with capillaries arranged in fanlike or radial arrays especially at the periphery of the nodules.[205,223] A multinodular, serpentine growth pattern is found in those cases of intravascular fasciitis, and elastic stains are frequently necessary to discern that the origin of the lesion is from blood vessels.[225] The histologic distinction of nodular fasciitis from malignant spindle cell tumors rests principally upon the lack of significant cell pleomorphism and atypical mitotic figures in nodular fasciitis.

Local excision is curative in almost all cases of nodular fasciitis, even when the lesion is incompletely excised.[205,211,217,223,227] Recurrences are reported, but this happens in less than 5% of cases.[205,223,225] In one series of supposed recurrent cases of nodular fasciitis reexamination of the original lesions showed that all were some other lesion that had been misdiagnosed as nodular fasciitis.[206]

Proliferative myositis and proliferative fasciitis

Proliferative myositis and proliferative fasciitis are discussed together because their histologic features are similar. They are both less common than nodular fasciitis. The term "proliferative fasciitis" was used in the past as a synonym for "nodular fasciitis" but should be restricted to the lesion discussed here.

Unlike nodular fasciitis, which occurs in children and young adults, both proliferative myositis and proliferative fasciitis occur in older patients with average and median ages of from 50 to 55 years and have not been reported in children.[207,209,213,218,219,224] Both are slightly more frequent in women and, as with nodular fasciitis, are characterized by a rapid clinical evolution over a period of only a few weeks.[207,213,218,219,224] Proliferative myositis develops within muscles, usually of the upper arm and shoulder, but also in the thigh, neck, face, back, and chest wall.* It is a poorly demarcated lesion with the appearance of scarlike tissue within the muscle. It varies in size from 1 to 7 cm.[209,213,218] Proliferative fasciitis involves the extremities in three fourths the cases, with the forearm and thigh being the most common sites.[207] Other sites include the chest, groin, neck, and face.[209,219,228,230] The lesion develops in the region between the muscle and the subcutis where it runs along the superficial fascia in an infiltrative fashion. Mixed forms between proliferative myositis and proliferative fasciitis occur where there is involvement of both muscle and the adjacent fascia and subcutis.[209,228]

Histologically, proliferative myositis shows a proliferation of spindle-shaped fibroblast-like cells that separate the muscle into bundles and infiltrate between individual muscle fibers (Fig. 37-5). Characteristically, the muscle does not show significant necrosis or regenerative phenomena, but there may be individual muscle fiber atrophy.[213,214,218,228] Associated with the spindle cells are prominent large cells having an abundant basophilic cytoplasm, at times granular, and one or two nuclei with prominent basophilic nucleoli.[209,213,218,228] These cells frequently have a ganglion cell–like appearance or resemble rhabdomyoblasts. However, they lack the Nissl substance of ganglion cells and the eosinophilic cytoplasm and cross-striations of rhabdomyoblasts, and they lack myoglobin.[219,228,230] These larger cells are also found in proliferative fasciitis, as the fibroblast-like spindle cells are. Here the cells proliferate along the fascia and fibrous septa of the subcutaneous tissue.[207,209,219] A myxoid stroma surrounds the cells, giving the lesion an edematous appearance much like

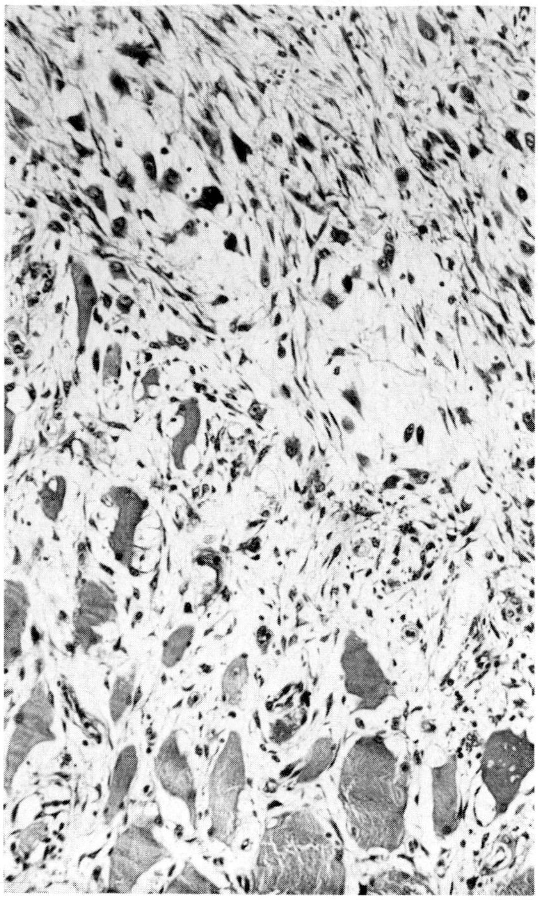

*References 208, 210, 213, 215, 218, 224, 230.

Fig. 37-5. Proliferative myositis. Fibroblasts and ganglion-like cells, embedded in a pale myxoid stroma, infiltrate between skeletal muscle fibers. (150×.)

that in nodular fasciitis. Osteoid, mature bone, and cartilage may occur in both proliferative myositis and fasciitis.[207,209,210,213,218,228] Mitotic activity may be frequent in both lesions. Since focal areas similar to nodular fasciitis may be found in both proliferative fasciitis and proliferative myositis, these entities may all be variants of the same disorder.[209,210]

Electron microscopic studies indicate that the large cells of these two lesions are fibroblastic with the features of myofibroblasts, as the majority of the smaller spindle cells are.[164,208,218,228,230] Immunohistochemical studies show the presence of factor XIIIa, a marker for fibroblasts, in the giant cells.[230]

Despite their histologic appearance, proliferative myositis and proliferative fasciitis are benign and self-limited, with no tendency to recur after local excision.[207,209,213,218,219,224]

FIBROHISTIOCYTIC TUMORS

During the past several years lesions of fibrohistiocytic differentiation, especially the malignant varieties, have held center stage in the field of soft-tissue tumor pathology. From virtual obscurity these malignant tumors, which were not even mentioned in the lists of the common sarcomas 10 to 20 years ago, now comprise from 12% to 33% of all sarcomas.* At the Armed Forces Institute of Pathology, malignant fibrohistiocytic tumors are the commonest sarcomas of older adults,[247,319] and in some institutions they are the most common soft-tissue sarcoma.[29,75,96,108]

Fibrohistiocytic tumors, both benign and malignant, share common light microscopic features characterized by the presence, in varying proportions, of cells with histiocytic and fibroblastic characteristics. There is a histomorphologic spectrum within the group, with some tumors exhibiting a predominantly histiocytic pattern, others a predominantly fibroblastic pattern, but most commonly an equally mixed composition. This has led to a multitude of designations for both the benign and malignant forms of these lesions, including fibroxanthoma, fibrous xanthoma, histiocytoma, malignant histiocytoma, malignant fibrous xanthoma, malignant fibrous histiocytoma, fibroxanthosarcoma, and xanthosarcoma. The general term "fibrous histiocytoma" is used to designate any of these tumors with individual and more specific names applied to the various morphologic subtypes.[268]

As the concept and diagnostic criteria for these tumors evolved,[267,268,306,319] it became evident that many pleomorphic soft-tissue tumors previously diagnosed as pleomorphic fibrosarcoma, pleomorphic liposarcoma, or pleomorphic rhabdomyosarcoma were in reality malignant fibrohistiocytomas.[247,267] Caution should be exercised, however, in the use of "malignant fibrous histiocytoma" as a diagnosis. The current frequency with which these tumors are diagnosed may reflect the increasing use of less stringent histologic criteria by pathologists. Unfortunately, malignant fibrous histiocytoma is in danger of becoming a "wastebasket" diagnosis for every spindle cell or pleomorphic soft-tissue sarcoma.[251,255] It is well to remember that some sarcomas cannot be definitively classified, and to diagnose such tumors as fibrous histiocytomas does violence to the criteria established for their histologic diagnosis,[267,268,271,306,318] and such indiscriminate use detracts from the clinical and pathologic significance of the diagnosis.

Benign fibrous histiocytomas include such diverse entities as subepidermal nodular fibrosis (sclerosing hemangioma, dermatofibroma), atypical fibroxanthoma of skin, juvenile xanthogranuloma (nevoxanthoendothelioma), giant cell tumor of tendon sheath (nodular tenosynovitis), pigmented villinodular synovitis, xanthogranuloma, and plasma cell granuloma.[268] The low-grade malignant cutaneous tumor, dermatofibrosarcoma protuberans, is also considered to be a fibrohistiocytic

lesion. Although malignant fibrous histiocytomas occur in diverse anatomic locations including the skeletal system and a variety of visceral organs, its most common site of origin is the soft tissues, and it is these tumors that are discussed here.

Malignant fibrous histiocytoma

The histologic classification of malignant fibrous histiocytoma is still in a state of flux, since several authors use slightly different terminologies and classifications,[87,247,267,268,273,283,319] and a variety of subtypes have been identified. We classify malignant fibrous histiocytoma into a conventional or fibroxanthosarcoma form,[268] which comprises the majority of these lesions, and myxoid,[318] inflammatory,[271] and angiomatoid varieties.[248] The conventional form is further divided by some into storiform and pleomorphic subtypes,[319] but we do not find this subdivision particularly useful, because most conventional malignant fibrous histiocytomas have a mixture of both fibrous and histiocyte-like elements demonstrating cell pleomorphism and, in the majority of cases, possess at least a focal storiform pattern. Malignant giant cell tumor of soft parts is also considered by most authors to be a subtype of malignant fibrous histiocytoma; however, we prefer not to so designate it and detail this tumor elsewhere in this chapter.

Malignant fibrous histiocytoma occurs more frequently in male than in female patients in a ratio of approximately $1.5:1$[236,246,267,283,319] and most commonly affects patients in the fifth to seventh decades of life with median ages between 60 and 65 years.[246,267,268,283,284,319] However, patients of all ages are affected, with roughly 5% of cases occurring in children.[267,293,310,319] The angiomatoid variety of malignant fibrous histiocytoma occurs in a significantly younger population than conventional malignant fibrous histiocytoma, with most patients being less than 30 years of age; the mean age in the largest single series was 13 years.[248] In 42 reported cases of inflammatory fibrous histiocytoma in which the age and sex of the patients was given, the sex distribution was similar to that for conventional malignant fibrous histiocytoma, but the patients were younger, with the median age being 48 years. However, this was mainly attributable to the female patients whose median age was 37.5 years versus the 59.5 years for the male patients. Whether this age discrepancy is valid must await further reports.

Most malignant fibrohistiocytomas develop as painless enlarging masses that are usually present for less than a year,[267,319] though approximately one fourth of the patients have some pain associated with the mass.[267,268] The angiomatoid variety may clinically resemble a cutaneous hemangioma or a hematoma because of its bluish tint. Patients with the angiomatoid variety may also have associated systemic effects of weight loss, anemia, and fever.[248] Patients with the in-

---

*References 19, 29, 54, 75, 96, 107, 108, 123.

flammatory variant may have an elevation of their peripheral leukocyte count producing in some a leukemoid reaction.[271,297,314] Malignant fibrous histiocytomas may develop secondary to radiation therapy.[291,311]

Two thirds to three fourths of malignant fibrous histiocytomas occur in the extremities, most commonly the lower extremity where the thigh is the most common site, accounting for one third of the cases.* Distal portions of the extremities, the hands and feet, are rarely involved.[236,246,256,319] Other locations include the trunk, shoulder region, and the retroperitoneum. The tumors are usually deeply seated, arising in muscle and the deep fascia, though about 20% to 30% arise in the subcutaneous tissue or lower dermis.[246,267,306,318,319]

The superficial tumors tend to be small, 2 to 4 cm, but deeply situated tumors are usually greater than 5 cm and may reach a large size in the retroperitoneum.[236,246,268,284,306,319] The tumors have a nonspecific gross appearance as either a nodular or multinodular, well-circumscribed firm or fleshy mass. Depending on their cellular composition, they have a gray, white, or yellowish cast, the last caused by a high cellular fat content. Myxoid tumors have a translucent or mucoid cut surface.[284,317] Unlike other malignant fibrous histiocytomas, the angiomatoid variety is almost always located in the subcutaneous tissue, is usually less than 5.0 cm, and on gross inspection contains irregular blood-filled cystic spaces and hemorrhagic zones.[248,266,307,315]

Inflammatory fibrous histiocytoma[271] has an anatomic distribution slightly different from that of conventional malignant fibrous histiocytoma. In 42 reported cases, the retroperitoneum was the site of origin in 36%, the extremities in 26%, with the head and neck and chest wall each accounting for 14% of the cases. Grossly they may have a yellowish or yellow-white cut surface because of the frequent presence of fat within the tumor cells.

The histomorphology of fibrohistiocytomas is characterized by extreme cellular variability not only from tumor to tumor, but also from area to area within the same tumor and even between the original tumor and recurrences and metastases.† Examination of a small biopsy specimen or only a few sections from one of these tumors is insufficient to appreciate their overall pattern. Usually there is an admixture of spindle-shaped fibroblast-like cells and mononuclear, round to oval, histiocyte-like cells, the latter frequently showing phagocytic activity with engulfed red blood cells or hemosiderin pigment.

A histologic characteristic of the fibrohistiocytic tumors, both benign and malignant, is the presence of a storiform pattern, best seen in those tumors composed principally of spindle-shaped fibroblasts, as in derma-

tofibrosarcoma protuberans. This storiform pattern consists of a cartwheel or nebula arrangement of the spindle cells intersecting about a central focus with the cells appearing to radiate or spin outward from this central region (Fig. 37-6). Three-dimensional analysis of this pattern has shown that it is formed by the junction of the peripheral portions of adjacent groups of proliferating cells. The center apparently does not have a consistent relationship to blood vessels as was previously believed.[280] This storiform pattern is found in more than 80% of malignant fibrous histiocytomas, though at times it is only focally present and found only after an extensive search.[236,268,282,283,306] As the histiocytic cell component increases, along with the degree of cellular anaplasia, the storiform pattern becomes less obvious and may be absent. However, metastases from such tumors may demonstrate a storiform pattern. A storiform pattern is not, however, diagnostic of fibrous histiocytoma, since it may also be seen in tumors such as melanomas, epidermoid carcinomas, and sarcomatoid renal cell carcinomas, as well as in benign conditions such as nodular fasciitis. It may also focally be present in other sarcomas such as osteosarcoma, leiomyosarcoma, and malignant nerve sheath tumors. Purely reactive benign lesions may also have prominent storiform regions.[304,320]

The degree of nuclear atypia in the cells of malignant fibrous histiocytoma varies considerably, such that tumors are encountered in which only a few cells are found demonstrating any nuclear atypia. Such may be the case in the early stages of inflammatory fibrous histiocytoma.[271] However, most malignant fibrous histiocytomas show a highly pleomorphic appearance characterized by the presence of significant cellular anaplasia with numerous large bizarre tumor giant cells, many of which are multinucleated (Fig. 37-7). These giant cells have an abundant glassy eosinophilic cytoplasm and may show phagocytic activity. Malignant-appearing spindle-shaped cells and mononuclear histiocyte-like cells are present either haphazardly arranged or in a storiform pattern. Large periodic acid–Schiff–positive, diastase-resistant hyaline globules are found within the cytoplasm of some tumor cells.[268,290] Glycogen, however, is usually not present in the tumor cells. Mitotic activity is abundant, with many abnormal mitotic figures. Necrosis is also frequent and at times widespread. Fibrosis may be minimal or quite extensive, with broad hyalinized regions present. Islands of bland-appearing foam cells (xanthoma cells) may be found among the tumor cells, as are lymphocytes, plasma cells, and eosinophils. Focal hemangiopericytomatous areas are found in some tumors.* Metaplastic bone and cartilage is occasionally found.[236,237,289] Although this bone and cartilage is usually present at

---

*References 236, 246, 256, 267, 268, 279, 306, 319.
†References 246, 247, 249, 256, 267, 268, 279, 283, 319.

*References 236, 246, 247, 267, 268, 283, 306, 318.

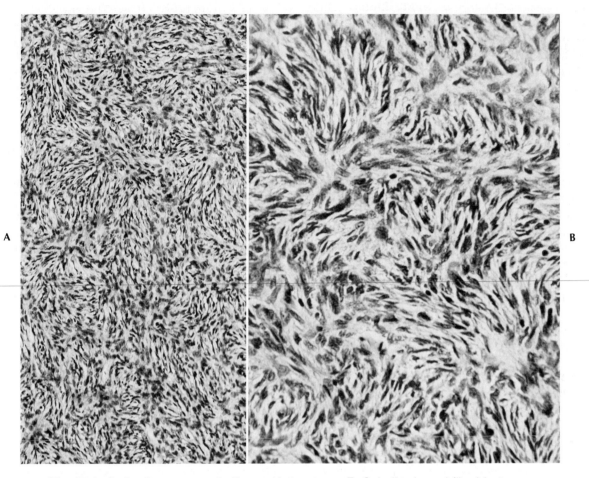

Fig. 37-6. A, Storiform pattern in fibrous histiocytoma. **B,** Spindle-shaped fibroblasts arranged in a whorling cartwheel fashion. This storiform pattern is characteristic but not diagnostic of fibrous histiocytoma. (**A,** 150×; **B,** 350×.)

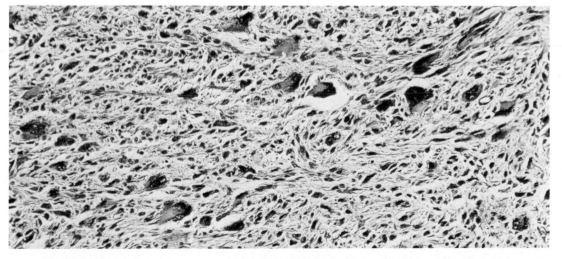

Fig. 37-7. Fibroxanthosarcoma. Bizarre, pleomorphic, multinucleated tumor giant cells with abundant eosinophilic cytoplasm within a fibrous stroma. (150×.)

the periphery of the tumor, or within fibrous septa, occasional small osteoid foci, surrounded by tumor cells, are found within the substance of the lesion, such that a distinction between extraosseous osteosarcoma and malignant fibrous histiocytoma may be difficult.[236,237,241,289]

Rarely, some tumors are composed solely of polygonal histiocyte-like cells. These cells may either have distinct cytoplasmic borders and be arranged in compact nodules, or their cytoplasm may merge to form a syncytium. The cells have large vesicular nuclei with an irregular chromatin distribution and one or two prominent nucleoli. The tumor lacks a storiform pattern. This *malignant histiocytoma*, or histiocytic variant of malignant fibrous histiocytoma, histologically may mimic a lymphoma but differs from the latter by the absence of reticulin fibers about individual cells.[236,243,264,290,306]

Conventional malignant fibrous histiocytoma (fibroxanthosarcoma) with its assortment of pleomorphic and anaplastic cells, is the tumor type that in the past was diagnosed as a pleomorphic form of either fibrosarcoma, liposarcoma, or rhabdomyosarcoma. Although a fascicular arrangement of the tumor cells as found in fibrosarcoma may occasionally be found in malignant fibrous histiocytoma, the pronounced degree of cell pleomorphism and the presence of tumor giant cells precludes a diagnosis of fibrosarcoma. The lack of cells with cross-striations by light microscopy is helpful in distinguishing pleomorphic rhabdomyosarcoma from malignant fibrous histiocytoma, but more frequently immunohistochemical or electron microscopic[314] studies are required to definitively separate these two entities. Pleomorphic liposarcoma has an abundant number of lipoblasts and lacks a storiform pattern. There are, however, occasional malignant tumors where the basic histologic pattern is fibrohistiocytic but in which lipoblast-like cells are found.[247,302,319] In the presence of storiform foci and only a few such lipoblast-like cells, such cases are arbitrarily assigned to the malignant fibrous histiocytoma category. It is well to remember that recurrences of some typical liposarcomas may take on the appearance of malignant fibrous histiocytoma ("dedifferentiated liposarcoma").[305]

The inflammatory variant of malignant fibrous histiocytoma, which accounts for approximately 2% to 4% of these tumors[236,246,267] has, in addition to atypical anaplastic histiocytes and fibroblasts, an intense polymorphonuclear cell infiltrate that is unassociated with tissue necrosis.[265,271,285] Reed-Sternberg–like and ganglion-like cells are also present. Although chronic inflammatory cells are found, sometimes in abundance, any of the malignant fibrohistiocytic tumors may contain chronic inflammatory cells. It is only those that demonstrate a diffuse acute inflammatory component that satisfy the definition of inflammatory fibrous histiocy-

toma.[271] In most inflammatory histiocytomas the histiocytic type of cells are the major cellular component, but spindle-cell fibroblast-like cells arranged in a storiform pattern are seen in almost all cases, and the acute inflammatory component may also be found within the purely fibrous areas of the tumor unassociated with any obvious xanthomatous (histiocytic) component.[271] In its "early" stage of development, inflammatory fibrous histiocytoma may be composed of bland-appearing fibroblasts, histiocytes, and many foam cells, with only a few of the cells showing nuclear atypia. This, combined with the acute inflammatory component, causes them to be diagnosed as "benign reactive lesions" or a form of "xanthogranuloma" (Fig. 37-8). Unfortunately, some[247,249] equate the lesions of inflammatory fibrous histiocytoma with tumors of the retroperitoneum designated as "xanthosarcoma" or "malignant xanthogranuloma."[263] In our view this is incorrect because these latter lesions do not have an acute inflammatory component, ganglion-like cells, Reed-Sternberg–like cells, or, in most cases, a storiform fibrous component.[271] The use of "xanthogranulomatous" or "xanthomatous malignant fibrous histiocytoma" as synonyms for inflammatory fibrous histiocytoma is, in our view, inappropriate.[246,247,256]

Areas of myxoid change are not uncommon in conventional malignant fibrous histiocytoma; however, when the myxoid component comprises at least one half the lesion, it is then classified as a myxoid malignant fibrous histiocytoma,[318] or by some as myxofibrosarcoma.[234,270,284] It is the second most common type of malignant fibrous histiocytoma, accounting for 8% to 17% of cases,[236,246,266] and is composed of hypocellular areas in which the tumor cells, both histiocyte-like and fibroblast-like, are separated by a clear to basophilic mucinous matrix having a high content of hyaluronic acid. The cells vary from well-differentiated to highly pleomorphic, and lipoblast-like cells are also found. More compact cellular areas of conventional malignant fibrous histiocytoma are found adjacent to the myxoid foci (Fig. 37-9). Mitotic figures are common and frequently abnormal. Within the myxoid areas is a prominent capillary network that may be arranged in a plexiform pattern. Myxoid malignant fibrous histiocytoma is easily confused with myxoid liposarcoma. However, myxoid liposarcoma lacks the cellular pleomorphism, mitotic activity, and storiform pattern of malignant myxoid fibrous histiocytoma, and the mucin pools of myxoid liposarcoma do not occur in myxoid malignant fibrous histiocytoma.[233]

Angiomatoid malignant fibrous histiocytoma, of which only relatively few cases have been reported,[248,266,315] is characterized by solid nodular masses of fibroblastic and histiocyte-like cells that surround hemorrhagic foci or blood-filled cystlike spaces.

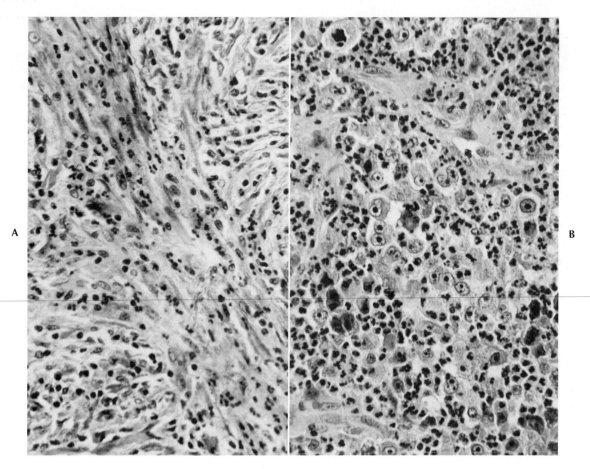

Fig. 37-8. A, Inflammatory fibrous histiocytoma, fibrous pattern. Portion of storiform area showing diffuse infiltration by polymorphonuclear leukocytes. **B,** Inflammatory fibrous histiocytoma, histiocytic pattern. Malignant-appearing histiocyte-like cells, with prominent nucleoli, surrounded by polymorphonuclear leukocytes. (350×.)

There is a prominent lymphocytic and plasmacytic component that is usually found at the periphery of the nodules. The lymphoid component may have germinal follicles thereby simulating a lymph node and creating the impression of a metastatic tumor in a lymph node. The tumor cells are fairly uniform and may be quite bland in appearance, lacking the extreme pleomorphism and anaplasia of conventional malignant fibrous histiocytoma. Mitoses are not common. Hemosiderin pigment is abundant and may be found within the cytoplasm of the tumor cells. Dense, hyalinized fibrous zones exist between the nodules. Foam cells and a storiform pattern are rare.[248,266,315] A benign cutaneous counterpart to this tumor, aneurysmal or angiomatoid fibrous histiocytoma, has been described, but it lacks nodularity and an inflammatory component.[301]

Some tumors diagnosed as malignant fibrous histiocytoma are in all likelihood some other tumor type, since cases of pleomorphic carcinoma, leiomyosarcoma, and malignant nerve sheath tumors have presented with a light microscopic pattern indistinguishable from malignant fibrous histiocytoma, and only by electron microscopic or immunohistochemical studies was the true nature of the lesion determined.[240,257,262,299] I frankly admit, however, that given a patient in the right age group who has a deep-seated soft-tissue tumor in an extremity that has the histologic features of malignant fibrous histiocytoma, I do not routinely call for further diagnostic procedures before applying the diagnosis of "malignant fibrous histiocytoma." However, such a tumor arising in a visceral organ should be investigated fully to rule out the possibility that one is not dealing with a sarcomatoid carcinoma.

As expected from their heterogeneous cell population by light microscopy, a similar variety of cell types is noted by electron microscopy, since there is no one specific morphologic feature for malignant fibrous histiocytoma.* In general, fibroblastic and histiocytic types

---

*References 232, 242, 252, 253, 272, 279, 309, 312.

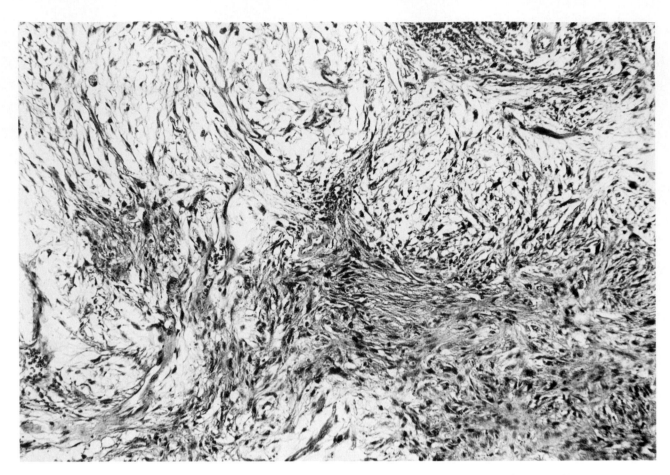

Fig. 37-9. Malignant fibrous histiocytoma, myxoid variant. Hypocellular myxoid area with atypical stromal cells adjacent to a more compact cellular focus at lower right. (150×.)

of tumor cells are the principal cells present, along with transitional forms having features of both fibroblasts and histiocytes. Myofibroblasts are found in the majority of cases but never as a major component. Multinucleated osteoclastic giant cells, xanthoma cells, and inflammatory cells are also seen. Undifferentiated primitive mesenchymal cells are reported in the majority of studies. The presence of these last cells has led to the concept that rather than being a histiocytic tumor, malignant fibrous histiocytoma is derived from primitive mesenchymal cells that differentiate along fibrocytic or histiocytic lines.[232,253,254] Despite the apparent electron microscopic features of histiocytes in many of the tumor cells, Langerhan's granules, considered a specific morphologic marker for histiocytes, have been found in only one case of malignant fibrous histiocytoma.[311]

Although the various subtypes of malignant fibrous histiocytoma are described here as distinct and separate histologic entities, transitions between them do occur, such that either recurrent or metastatic lesions may take on the appearance of another subtype, such as an inflammatory or myxoid form assuming a conventional morphology.[246,249,256,271] The diagnosis of malignant fibrous histiocytoma is further complicated by the fact that not only may other soft-tissue sarcomas contain focal areas of a storiform pattern, but they may also "dedifferentiate" into foci of malignant fibrous histiocytoma and thus express two phenotypes within a single lesion.[239] This has led to speculation that malignant fibrous histiocytoma may be the result of soft-tissue tumor progression. However, this concept was based on the occurrence of alpha$_1$-antichymotrypsin within these "dedifferentiated" foci and its specificity as a marker for fibrohistiocytic tumors,[239,244] a specificity that has recently been questioned.[275,276]

Since malignant fibrous histiocytoma was long considered a tumor of histiocytic origin, or at least one that demonstrated histiocytic features, immunohistochemical studies for the presence of alpha$_1$-antitrypsin and alpha$_1$-antichymotrypsin, both of which are found in normal and neoplastic histiocytes as well as other tissues, have been frequently used as markers for fibrohistiocytic tumors. However, results using these markers have been quite variable; alpha$_1$-antitrypsin is found in from 21% to 100% of malignant fibrous histiocytomas,* and alpha$_1$-antichymotrypsin in from 38% to 100% of cases.† Even in the positive cases, however, the number and the intensity of the positively stained cells varies greatly from case to case. Lysozyme, another histiocytic marker, is less frequently found in these tumors, with positive results in from 0% to 46% of cases.‡ Other markers such as ferritin and various lectins are found in from 11% to 83%[294,313] and 25% to 54%[269,277] of cases respectively. The tumors are also strongly positive for various lysosomal enzymes.[246,287] The intermediate filament protein vimentin is present in all malignant fibrous histiocytomas,[274] but desmin and smooth muscle myosin have also been found in a few tumors, supposedly because of their content of myofibroblasts.[286,300] Surprisingly, cytokeratin, not normally expected in soft-tissue sarcomas has been found in a few malignant fibrous histiocytomas.[274,317] Although the presence of either desmin or cytokeratin in these tumors is a relatively rare event, the fact that they are present at all raises potential diagnostic problems in differentiating some malignant fibrous histiocytomas from leiomyosarcoma or pleomorphic carcinoma, and so electron microscopy may have to be used to arrive at a definitive diagnosis.

Despite the light-microscopic histiocytic appearance of the cells in angiomatoid malignant fibrous histiocytoma, which caused it to be placed in the general category of the fibrohistiocytic tumors, there is some controversy as to their nature. Whereas some electron microscopic studies support a histiocytic origin for these tumors,[315] others suggest either an endothelial origin[266,308] or one from primitive mesenchymal cells capable of differentiating into a variety of cellular elements including vascular endothelium and muscle cells.[279] However, immunohistochemical studies, using markers for endothelial cells have shown negative results in the few cases so far studied.[267,315]

In recent years, a blizzard of reports have ensued attempting to elucidate the histogenesis of malignant fibrous histiocytoma. Originally proposed as a histiocytic lesion whose spindle cells were histiocytes acting as facultative fibroblasts,[259,264,288,290] subsequent electron microscopic studies cast doubt upon this concept.[232,252,253,258,309,311] The focus of controversy has now shifted to the arena of tissue culture, animal transplantation, and immunologic marker studies. A review of this work yields evidence and opinion for§ and against‖ a histiocytic origin or histiocytic differentiation

of these lesions, with diametrically opposed results reported from different laboratories.[261,274,295,303,307,321] It should be remembered that the presence or absence of immunologic markers for either fibroblasts or histiocytes in these tumors may have no bearing on the actual cell of origin, because tumor cells may lose differentiation markers in the course of malignant transformation and what is actually being studied with the use of these markers is the present state of the tumor's differentiation.[251] What can be said is that by light microscopy malignant fibrous histiocytoma is a tumor whose component cells *resemble* either fibroblasts or histiocytes.

Unfortunately, there are few histologic criteria that permit one to predict the clinical course of malignant fibrohistiocytic tumors.[267,268,319] Indeed, metastases may develop from fibrohistiocytic tumors that show no cellular atypia in either the primary tumor or the metastases.[298] One should not apply the term "benign" to any fibrohistiocytic tumor located in the deep soft tissue, since they may all be capable of producing metastases. When cellular atypia is lacking, which is a rare occurrence, they are simply reported as fibrous histiocytomas with an explanation to the clinician of the potential for aggressive behavior. The designation "malignant" is reserved for those tumors with clear cellular anaplasia of the stromal cells.

Approximately 40% to 50% of malignant fibrous histiocytomas recur after excision,* with radical excision or amputation yielding the lowest rate of recurrence.[236] Metastases develop in from 14% to 75% of cases,† with most developing within 2 years of the original diagnosis. The principal site of metastases is the lungs. Some variation is reported on the involvement of regional lymph nodes, with some authors reporting a relatively low incidence of from 2% to 17%[237,247,267] whereas others report an approximately 40% incidence.[273] Large tumors and those that are deeply situated have the highest metastatic rates.[236,318,319] Five-year survival rates are roughly 30% to 50%.[236,247,267] The histologic features of conventional malignant fibrous histiocytoma are not correlated with survival. However, the myxoid variant is reported to have a better prognosis,[236,246,283,284,318] though some find no difference in outlook for this tumor type.[267] The inflammatory variant usually pursues an aggressive course.[265,271,285] Whereas the initial reports of this tumor type indicated a high recurrence and metastatic rate with uniformly fatal results, some long-term survivors have subsequently

---

*References 244, 259, 269, 274, 277, 294, 313.
†References 239, 244, 276, 283, 294, 313.
‡References 244, 259, 269, 274, 277, 283, 313.
§References 259, 261, 287, 303, 306, 312, 321.
‖References 238, 251, 260, 274, 294-296, 321.

---

*References 236, 245, 246, 267, 268, 279, 283, 319.
†References 236, 245, 267, 268, 273, 283, 319.

been reported.[235,236,252] The angiomatoid variant appears to be the least aggressive subtype.[248] Deeply situated malignant fibrous histiocytomas, especially those in the retroperitoneum, have a poorer prognosis than those in the subcutaneous soft tissue.[246,267,283,319] Children may have a better prognosis than adults.[310]

SMOOTH MUSCLE TUMORS

Neoplasms that differentiate toward cells with smooth muscle characteristics may be either benign (leiomyoma) or malignant (leiomyosarcoma). Although this is easily stated, in practice differentiating clearly between these entities may be one of a diagnostic pathologist's most difficult and frustrating tasks. Indeed, in some cases the pathologist must be resigned to awaiting the decision of time on whether the tumor is benign or malignant.

Smooth muscle tumors are far more frequent in organ systems, such as the gastrointestinal tract and female genital system, than in the somatic soft tissue.[103] The visceral lesions present special clinical and pathologic features of their own and are described in the appropriate chapters of this textbook. The basic histopathologic features of smooth muscle tumors are, however, similar regardless of anatomic location.

Leiomyoma

Within the soft tissue, leiomyomas are usually confined to the superficial subcutaneous tissue and skin, only rarely occurring in the deep soft tissues, and arise from structures in these areas that normally contain smooth muscle such as the arrectores pilorum, the tunica dartos, the errector muscles of the nipple, and the media of large and small blood vessels.[358,368] Leiomyomas occur almost exclusively in adults, rarely being found in children,[325,349,376] and show no sex predominance.[368] However, leiomyomas in the skin and subcutaneous tissue may be quite vascular and well innervated and produce paroxysms of pain,[103,338,368]; these *angioleiomyomas* occur most commonly in women.[338] Superficial leiomyomas are found in any location but are most common in the extremities, the trunk, and head and neck regions.[338,368] Angioleiomyomas occur in the extremities in approximately 90% of the cases, with the majority in the lower extremity.[338] In the more deeply located leiomyomas the retroperitoneum, omentum, mesentery, round and broad ligaments of the uterus, and the walls of large blood vessels are the common sites of origin.[103,367,373,377] A mediastinal location is rare, with most of the lesions reported as examples of smooth muscle tumors in this location in reality probably being neurogenous.[356]

Microscopically, one finds interlacing bands and bundles of elongate spindle-shaped cells whose nuclei, in contrast to the tapered nuclei of fibroblasts, are usually blunt-ended giving them the "cigar shape" so frequently mentioned (Fig. 37-10). The nuclei are usually bland without obvious nucleoli. It is not uncommon, however, to find some cells with two to three nuclei, as well as some that exhibit nuclear hyperchromasia and irregular shapes. This nuclear atypia should not be taken as evidence of malignancy when there is no associated mitotic activity. Fine cytoplasmic myofibrils course the length of the cells producing a fibrillar appearance. These fibrils are best seen with the use of phosphotungstic acid–hematoxylin or trichrome stains. The tumor cells may so arrange themselves that their nuclei are aligned in rows creating palisades. This pattern can cause some diagnostic confusion with neurilemomas whose cell nuclei are also frequently aligned in palisades.[103,341,368] There is an abundant network of reticulin fibers that individually surround and run parallel to the long axis of each cell. Many leiomyomas are quite vascular and may, in focal regions, take on the appearance of a glomus tumor or a hemangiopericytoma. Superficial angioleiomyomas have been divided into solid, cavernous, and venous types, with the former being the most common.[338] Necrosis in a leiomyoma is rare, and its presence should indicate the possibility of a leiomyosarcoma and further tissue should be submitted for study.[103,368]

By electron microscopy, the cells of leiomyomas have the same features as normal smooth muscle cells: intracytoplasmic bundles of thin filaments, considered to be actin, dense bodies distributed among these filaments, pinocytotic vesicles, and the presence of a basement membrane around the cells. Unlike the cells of leiomyosarcoma, these fine-structural features are usually easily found in each cell.[352,353]

A histologic variant of leiomyoma is the *epithelioid leiomyoma*, also called bizarre leiomyoma, round cell leiomyoma, and leiomyoblastoma. Originally described in the stomach,[366] its most common location, eipthelioid leiomyoma is also found in a variety of extragastric sites including the uterus, mesentery, omentum, and retroperitoneum.[347,367,373,377] Rather than being elongate, the cells of this tumor are round or polygonal and frequently have a cytoplasmic clear zone about the nucleus creating a clear cell appearance.[103,366] These clear cells may so dominate the histologic pattern that the question of an epithelial tumor is raised. The clear zones do not contain glycogen, fat, or mucin.[360] Transitions between these epithelioid cells and conventional spindle-shaped smooth muscle cells occur, and electron microscopy has confirmed their smooth muscle nature.[329,360] It has been demonstrated that the clear zones are actually formalin-fixation artifacts, since they are not found in tumors rapidly fixed for electron microscopy or when frozen sections are used.[360] Despite the common presence of these clear cells, the diagnosis

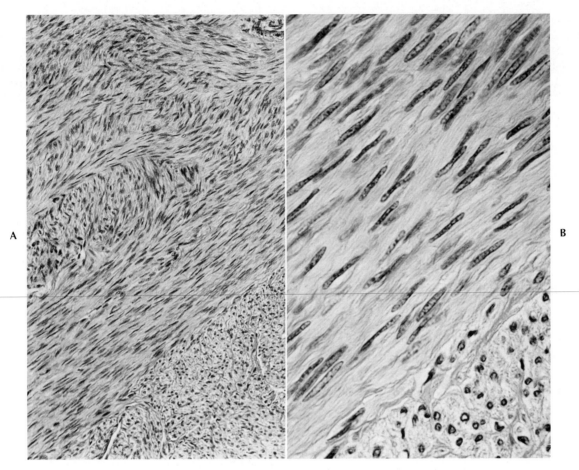

Fig. 37-10. A, Leiomyoma. Bands of smooth muscle cells in longitudinal and cross section. **B,** Higher magnification of area seen in Fig. 39-10. *A,* Cigar-shaped, bland-appearing nuclei of smooth muscle cells in longitudinal array. At lower right cells are seen in cross section. (**A,** 150×; **B,** 600×.)

of epitheliod leiomyoma may be made in their absence based on the presence of the numerous round or polygonal cells.[329] Malignant forms of this tumor, epitheliod leiomyosarcoma, also occur.[323]

A dramatic proliferation of smooth muscle, leiomyomatosis peritonealis disseminata consists of numerous nodules involving the peritoneal surfaces of the pelvis, omentum, mesentery, serosa of the small intestine, uterine serosa, and the uterine adnexa and may be mistaken grossly for metastatic carcinoma. It occurs in women who are or have recently been pregnant or in those taking oral contraceptives, though it is also found in women without this background. Microscopically, the nodules contain smooth muscle cells that, in pregnant patients, may be mixed with decidual cells. The nodules are located beneath a covering mesothelium. By electron microscopy, one may find a combination of smooth muscle cells, fibroblasts, myofibroblasts, and decidual cells. The condition usually spontaneously remits, but cases are reported where it has persisted. The

lesions are believed to arise from metaplasia of subperitoneal mesenchymal stem cells.[331,369] A case of malignant transformation has been reported.[359]

When a smooth muscle tumor lacks mitotic activity, it will in almost every case act in a benign fashion.[325,368] However, most pathologists have encountered large, deep-seated smooth muscle tumors that have pursued an aggressive course with metastases despite the lack of significant mitotic activity.[103,325] Fortunately, this is rare. The use of mitotic counts as an aid in the differential diagnosis between benign and malignant smooth muscle tumors is discussed in the section on leiomyosarcoma.

Leiomyosarcoma

Leiomyosarcomas account for from 2% to 12% of soft-tissue sarcomas.[19,29,75,96,107,108,123] They are one fourth to one fifth as common as leiomyomas.[330,334,339,340,366,368] Their anatomic distribution is as varied as it is for their benign counterparts, and, as with the latter, they are rare in the somatic soft tissue, being more prevalent in the gastrointestinal and female genital tracts.[103,330,358] Deep-seated leiomyosarcomas are rare tumors,[103,364] and when they occur in the soft tissue, they are most commonly found in the superficial subcutaneous tissue and skin.[330,334,358,368,375] Here over 85% arise in the proximal aspect of the extremities, most frequently the lower extremity.[330,334,335,339] Other sites include the head and neck region and trunk.[368] In the deep soft tissues the retroperitoneum is the most common site; other locations include the mesentery, the omentum, the deep soft tissues of the neck, and the region between large muscle groups.[33,103,335,340,357,364,374] Major arteries and veins are also sites of origin,[324,339,348,371] with veins approximately five times more frequently involved than arteries, the inferior vena cava accounting for over half the cases.[327,337,343]

Although patients of all ages are reported, including infants and children,[325,346,368] leiomyosarcomas have their highest incidence in adults in the fifth to sixth decades of life, with the median patient age being 55 to 60 years.[330,339,340,363,374] The male-to-female ratio appar-

ently depends on tumor location, with retroperitoneal leiomyosarcomas and those arising from major blood vessels more common in female patients,* whereas those in the skin and subcutaneous tissue are more common in male patients.[330,334,374,375] Symptoms also depend on tumor location, with superficial leiomyosarcomas developing as slowly growing nodules.[339] Unlike leiomyomas, superficial leiomyosarcomas are not painful;[368] however, a recent report of a large number of patients indicated that spontaneous pain, or pain on pressure, was present in close to 90% of cutaneous and 77% of subcutaneous leiomyosarcomas.[334] Pressure symptoms and abdominal distension are frequent in those patients with retroperitoneal tumors.[364] Leiomyosarcomas of the inferior vena cava produce symptoms of venous obstruction, the pattern of which reflects the level along the vessel where the tumor is located.[327,343]

Grossly, leiomyosarcomas appear well circumscribed and may even "shell out," but as usual with sarcomas they are microscopically always infiltrative.[103] The su-

*References 33, 327, 337, 340, 343, 364, 374.

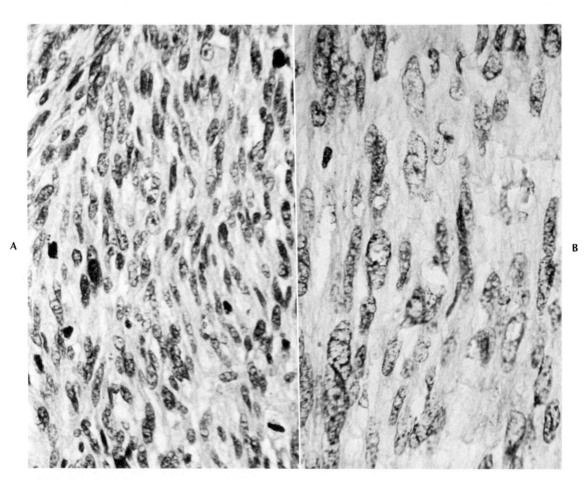

Fig. 37-11. A, Leiomyosarcoma. Spindle and oval cells with vesicular nuclei and some hyperchromasia. Several mitotic figures are present. **B,** Plump atypical vesicular nuclei of leiomyosarcoma. Some cells are multinucleated. (**A,** 350×; **B,** 600×.)

perficial tumors tend to be small, usually less than 2 cm, whereas the deeper tumors are commonly bulky, multinodular lesions, frequently greater than 10 cm,[33,334,340,357,364,374] with some as large as 30 to 35 cm.[33,327] The histologic features that establish a diagnosis of leiomyosarcoma are not clearly defined.[335,346,357,364] Essentially, the microscopic pattern parallels that seen in leiomyomas, with intersecting bundles of spindle-shaped cells having a fibrillar cytoplasm and blunt-ended nuclei (Fig. 37-11). Leiomyosarcomas tend to be more cellular, with a conspicuous increase in the number of cells showing atypical nuclear features, hyperchromasia, and multinucleation.[103,335,357,368,374] Foci with a storiform pattern may be present, as well as areas in which the nuclei are arranged in a palisading pattern.[33,335,339,340,364] A prominent vascular component may be present with large gaping vascular structures.[339,340,364]

Leiomyosarcomas vary from those composed almost entirely of well-differentiated spindle cells to those with many atypical cells, only a few of which have features suggestive of smooth muscle. Tumor cells may assume round or oval shapes resembling epithelioid cells (Fig. 37-12); at times the majority of the tumor is composed of such cells, the tumors being designated as "epithelioid leiomyosarcomas."[33,323,339,340,347,364] Unlike its rar-

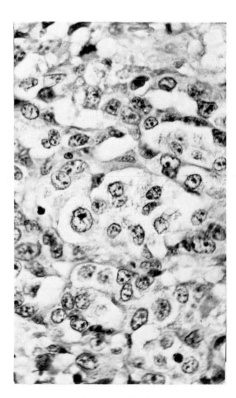

Fig. 37-12. Epithelioid (clear cell) leiomyosarcoma. Atypical nuclei are surrounded by clear zones or halos. (480×.)

ity in leiomyoma, necrosis is frequent in leiomyosarcoma, and such a finding is important in differentiating benign from malignant smooth muscle tumors.[357] Hyalinized areas and edematous myxoid regions are also found.[339,340,374] Occasionally, this hyaluronidase-sensitive myxoid material may so dominate the pattern that the term "myxoid leiomyosarcoma" is used. Here the cells may have intracytoplasmic vacuoles that give them a signet-ring appearance that resembles univacuolated lipoblasts.[328,344,361] The cells of leiomyosarcoma contain glycogen, and this serves as a useful diagnostic point in differentiating leiomyosarcoma from other spindle cell tumors with which it may be confused such as fibrosarcoma, malignant fibrous histiocytoma, and neural sheath tumors that lack glycogen.

Vimentin intermediate filament protein is present in leiomyosarcomas.[332,363] The reported frequency with which the intermediate filament protein desmin is found in malignant smooth muscle tumors varies in different studies, with some authors reporting only rare positive cases[33] whereas others reporting a very high frequency of positive tumors.[339,350,351,363] The location of the tumor appears to determine whether desmin is found, with leiomyosarcomas of the stomach and small intestine frequently lacking this protein.[332,362] HHF-35, a monoclonal antibody to muscle actin, stains virtually all smooth muscle tumors[350,351,370] but is not specific, since rhabdomyosarcomas[370] and some pleomorphic mesenchymal tumors also yield positive results with this antibody.[350] A surprising finding is the positive staining for cytokeratin protein in some leiomyomas and leiomyosarcomas.[326,336,351,355] Whether this cytokeratin-like activity reflects the actual presence of cytokeratin in these tumors is unclear,[355] but such a result emphasizes the need for caution in interpreting the results of immunohistochemical stains when used for the diagnosis of spindle-cell soft-tissue sarcomas.[326,351,355]

Electron microscopy has not been very rewarding in confirming the suspicion that a pleomorphic spindle cell tumor is of smooth muscle origin. Unlike leiomyomas, all the fine structural characteristics of smooth muscle cells may be absent or incompletely developed in leiomyosarcomas, and those that are present may be found in only some cells.[345,352,353,363,372] Because of the inherent sampling problem of electron microscopy, the absence of such cellular features does not eliminate the possibility that the tumor in question is of smooth muscle origin.[345,353,372] In some studies only one half to two thirds of cases considered to be leiomyosarcomas by light microscopy could be established as such by electron microscopy.[353,372]

The principal histologic difference between leiomyoma and leiomyosarcoma is the usual occurrence of a high mitotic rate in the latter. The use of mitotic counts as a means of establishing the malignancy of a soft-tissue smooth muscle tumor evolved from studies on uterine smooth muscle tumors where mitotic indices are prognostically accurate.[341] However, the criteria used for uterine tumors may not be directly applicable to extrauterine smooth muscle tumors.[33,342,357] Indeed, the reliability of mitotic counting has itself been called into question, since there may be a pronounced variability in the results of mitotic counts made by different pathologists on the same tumor.[365] Atypical hyperchromatic nuclei in poorly prepared sections may easily be misinterpreted as mitotic figures.[354] In addition, the cellularity of the tumor and the frequency of mitoses varies in different regions of the same tumor such that failure to obtain an adequate number of sections and to perform the counts in areas containing the greatest number of mitoses will lead to dramatically different results.[365] In large, deeply placed tumors a rule of thumb should be that one histologic section be taken for every centimeter of tumor.[357] All pathologists with experience in evaluating smooth muscle tumors have encountered those that lack the usual parameters of malignancy but behave aggressively.[325,357,364,368] Fortunately these are rare, and a smooth muscle tumor without mitoses, necrosis, or cellular atypia will, in most cases, be benign.[103,368] Those tumors with high mitotic rates (5 or more mitoses per 10 high-power fields), necrosis, and significant anaplasia may be expected to behave aggressively.[33,357,368] This leaves a gray zone in which the pathologist is distinctly uncomfortable with his ability to reasonably predict the clinical course of the tumor. Large tumors (over 5 cm), with or without nuclear atypia, in which necrosis is lacking and for which mitotic figures are absent or infrequent (one or two per 10 high-power fields) present such a problem. I do not diagnose such indeterminate smooth muscle tumors as benign or malignant but explain to the clinician the diagnostic problem and the need for close clinical follow-up observation of the patient. Myxoid leiomyosarcomas may have low mitotic rates, belying their aggressive character.[344,361]

From what has been said concerning the difficulties in distinguishing between benign and malignant smooth muscle tumors, it is obvious that survival statistics are influenced by the inclusion of what are actually leiomyomas among those tumors considered leiomyosarcomas. With this in mind, recurrences are reported in from 40% to 60% of all leiomyosarcomas, with blood-borne metastases, most commonly to the lungs and liver, developing in approximately 30% to 60% of patients.[330,334,364,368,374] Of prognostic importance in soft-tissue leiomyosarcoma is tumor size, anatomic location, and depth of the lesion.[33,332,339,340,364,374,375] Retroperitoneal and mesenteric leiomyosarcomas have a poor prognosis, with over 90% of patients dying of either metastases or local invasion of adjacent structures.[340,357,364,374] Despite a 40% local recurrence rate, patients with cutaneous tumors do well after wide excision of the tumor without the development of metastases.[334,375] Indeed, some advocate labeling these dermally situated tumors as "aggressive leiomyomas" rather than "leiomyosarcomas" because of their potential for local recurrence rather than for metastases.[375] In contrast, subcutaneous leiomyosarcomas are fully malignant with a high rate of local recurrence and metastases.[330,334] Patients with large (over 5 cm) and deep tumors also do poorly.[330,368,374,377] Extragastric epithelioid leiomyosarcomas behave in an aggressive fashion, with over half the patients dying of their tumor.[347] The prognosis for leiomyosarcomas of venous origin is unclear,[324,348] though leiomyosarcomas of the vena cava do poorly.[327] Myxoid leiomyosarcomas are aggressive tumors.[361] There is some difference of opinion in the assessment of the outcome in children with malignant smooth muscle tumors. Some deny that the usual criteria of malignancy for smooth muscle tumors are applicable to tumors in children, claiming that these patients do well,[376] whereas others claim that there is no prognostic difference in children and adults.[325,346]

SKELETAL MUSCLE TUMORS
Rhabdomyosarcoma

Within the past decade, rhabdomyosarcoma is the sarcoma that has stimulated the most clinical interest. Among the factors contributing to this are the highly aggressive nature of this tumor and its propensity to affect children and young adults with all the emotional impact that such a situation engenders among both parents and physicians alike. In addition, improved methods in radiation therapy and chemotherapy have resulted in a dramatic increase in survival rates such that the previous grim prognosis attached to this disease has been replaced by the expectation that the majority of affected patients may now be cured.[419,451]

Rhabdomyosarcoma is the most common sarcoma of childhood, representing more than half of all such cases.[383,451] It accounts for between 4% and 8% of all malignant disease in children younger than 15 years of age, with its incidence among all soft-tissue sarcomas ranging from 5% to 15%.* A familial association with other malignancies is found in patients with rhabdomyosarcoma.[415] A greater incidence of soft-tissue sarcomas is found in the siblings of these patients, and an increased incidence of breast cancer, brain tumors, and adrenocortical carcinoma in their relatives.[415,420,426] There is also some evidence for an increased incidence of rhabdomyosarcomas in patients with neurofibromatosis, at least some of which are malignant peripheral nerve sheath tumors with rhabdomyosarcomatous

---

*References 23, 29, 75, 96, 107, 108, 246, 410, 412, 421.

change (malignant *Triton* tumors, named after a genus of salamander).[422]

Rhabdomyosarcomas are divided into four principal histologic subtypes—embryonal, alveolar, pleomorphic, and botryoid, with the last subtype essentially an embryonal rhabdomyosarcoma with a characteristic gross appearance.[408] Since the embryonal, alveolar, and botryoid types occur predominantly in young children, some use the general term "juvenile rhabdomyosarcoma" for these and "adult rhabdomyosarcoma" for pleomorphic rhabdomyosarcoma, the form found almost exclusively in adults.[103,382] However, any of these subtypes may occur in patients of any age, and they exhibit sufficient clinical and pathologic differences to justify their discussion as separate entities.

Approximately two thirds of patients with childhood rhabdomyosarcomas are younger than 10 years of age,[381,402,405,411,419,451] with even newborns and infants less than 1 month of age reported.[381,405,411,438] Boys are affected more commonly than girls in a ratio of approximately 1.5:1.* Black patients are less commonly affected than white patients.[394,401,418,437]

Among the several hundred childhood cases of rhabdomyosarcoma accessioned by the Intergroup Rhabdomyosarcoma Study Group,[418] the embryonal variety accounted for 57% of the cases, the alveolar 19%, the botryoid 6%, and the pleomorphic variety 1%. Although the specific percentage distribution of the various subtypes varies somewhat in other reports, the embryonal form constitutes the majority of cases in all reports.[381,402,405,411,432] A special histologic group of tumors was culled from the tumors submitted to the Intergroup Rhabdomyosarcoma Study Group. These were composed of cells that resembled the large and small cell types of Ewing's sarcoma, and they accounted for 7% of the total accessioned cases.[421] Such tumors are not considered as specific subtypes of rhabdomyosarcoma but represent tumors that, like childhood rhabdomyosarcomas, are composed of small, round, poorly differentiated tumor cells. These tumors may be histologically difficult to distinguish from rhabdomyosarcoma, but they respond to the same therapeutic modalities as rhabdomyosarcoma does.[432] Another 10% of the tumors in the Intergroup Rhabdomyosarcoma Study consisted of undifferentiated mesenchymal cells that could not be satisfactorily placed into one of the other diagnostic categories, and they were classified as "type indeterminate." Such tumors have been designated by other authors as "sarcoma of undetermined histogenesis" and in some reports represent slightly more than one fourth of all cases originally diagnosed as childhood rhabdomyosarcoma.[404] This indicates the difficulty and inappropriateness of classifying all small cell malignant tumors in childhood as rhabdomyosarcoma.[398] The distribution of the major rhabdomyosarcoma subtypes in these studies is only slightly different from that noted at the Armed Forces Institute of Pathology for patients of all ages. Here, embryonal tumors made up 69%, alveolar 19%, and the pleomorphic forms 11% of the total cases.[390]

Understanding the histology and evolution of malignant skeletal muscle tumors is aided by a knowledge of normal myogenesis.[388,398,429,436] At 1 to 9 weeks of embryonic development, small, primitive-appearing stellate mesenchymal cells proliferate, elongate, and accumulate cytoplasm in which microfilaments develop. These microfilament-containing mononuclear cells, called "myoblasts," soon fuse, forming a syncytium around a hollow core, and their nuclei move peripherally creating the so-called hollow myotube stage. The amount of cytoplasm then increases associated with a further accumulation of cytoplasmic filaments. These filaments soon split into thick (12 to 15 nm) filaments of myosin and thin (6 to 8 nm) filaments of actin. Together these filaments form the myofibrils of skeletal muscle. The position of the filaments relative to each other creates the banded pattern of skeletal muscle seen by light microscopy. These cross-striations first appear at about 10 weeks of embryonic development but are not prominent until 14 weeks of gestation. The Z-bands are the first of the various bands to develop. By electron microscopy, the primitive developing myogenic cells cannot be distinguished from cells that are destined to differentiate into other cell types until the stage is reached where both actin and myosin filaments are present.

From this highly simplified version of myogenesis, it is clear that skeletal muscle cells originate from a proliferation of undifferentiated mesenchymal cells. Since such cells may be located anywhere in the soft tissues, this helps explain the occurrence of rhabdomyosarcomas in such areas as the middle ear, the bile ducts, bladder, and brain where skeletal muscle is not present, as well as the occurrence of tumor cells with skeletal muscle differentiation in heterologous tumors of the uterus and kidney.[33,449]

By light microscopy, the diagnosis of rhabdomyosarcoma is aided by the finding of rhabdomyoblasts. These cells take on a variety of forms including small round cells, strap-shaped cells with nuclei arranged in tandem, racquet-shaped or tadpole-shaped cells with a single nucleus at one end and a long tail-like extension of cytoplasm, multinucleated giant cells, long spindle-shaped cells, and cells with multiple cytoplasmic vacuoles creating so-called spider-web cells. All, however, are characterized by a highly eosinophilic granular or fibrillated cytoplasm. The occurrence and number of these rhabdomyoblasts varies with the apparent differentiation of the tumor, being uncommon in the more

---

*References 383, 402, 419, 421, 426, 436, 451.

primitive tumors and more frequent in the more mature or so-called well-differentiated forms. Thus the degree of "differentiation" of a rhabdomyosarcoma is determined by some authors in accordance with the number and size of the rhabdomyoblasts present such that the tumors are designated as primitive or poorly differentiated, intermediate or moderately differentiated, and well differentiated.[392,445] Most rhabdomyosarcomas, however, are composed of undifferentiated-appearing cells mixed with a variety of rhabdomyoblast forms.[398]

The finding of cells with unequivocal cross striations in a malignant-appearing small cell tumor of soft tissue is sufficient evidence for a diagnosis of rhabdomyosarcoma given the proper clinical setting and that one has eliminated the possibility that the cells represent entrapped residual normal skeletal muscle cells. The operative word here is "unequivocal." An extensive search of many sections may be necessary before such striated cells are found. Care must be taken, however, in evaluating such cells for it is a common experience that cytoplasmic artifacts, combined with a ready mind, can cause wonderous cross striations to appear in direct proportion to the pathologist's desire to prove that the tumor is a rhabdomyosarcoma. It should be made clear, however, that for the embryonal, alveolar, and botryoid tumors the light microscopic identification of cross striations is not required for the diagnosis of rhabdomyosarcoma as long as the correct tumor pattern is present.[378,404,418,424,436,447]

Recently, there have been attempts by the Intergroup Rhabdomyosarcoma Study Group to reclassify rhabdomyosarcomas, based upon their cytologic features, into anaplastic, monomorphous round cell, and mixed types.[378,405,434,435] The *anaplastic* tumor is characterized by large, bizarre mitotic figures and diffuse hyperchromatic and pleomorphic nuclei. The *monomorphous* variety is composed of uniform-sized round cells with "constant" cytologic features. These two tumor forms accounted for approximately 20% of all the childhood rhabdomyosarcoma cases, whereas the *mixed* type consisted of all other rhabdomyosarcoma subtypes. The anaplastic and monomorphous types were considered to be prognostically unfavorable, being associated with a decreased survival.[434,435] This classification scheme is currently still under investigation, and the cytologic parameters used to classify the tumors have not been illustrated.

Electron microscopy may be helpful in arriving at a specific diagnosis of rhabdomyosarcoma when the light microscopic diagnosis is in doubt.[385,388,423,424,429,447] There are differences of opinion among authors as to the minimal electron microscopic criteria necessary for establishing skeletal muscle differentiation in tumor cells, especially in the more primitive cells. Some re-

quire the presence of more than one specific morphologic feature,[385] whereas others are less stringent.[398,423] In brief, the finding of parallel thick and thin myofilaments in alternating or hexagonal array, the presence of either Z-band material or Z-band densities, or a single-file alignment of ribosomes associated with myosin filaments (myosin-ribosome complex) has been used as unequivocal evidence of skeletal maturation.[385,404,423] Other features of rhabdomyosarcoma cells include nuclear indentations, prominent nucleoli, external lamina, monoparticulate (beta) glycogen granules, and rudimentary cell junctions.[378,398] However, the failure to find specific features by electron microscopy should not necessarily deter one from the diagnosis of rhabdomyosarcoma.[110,404,429] The sampling problems inherent in electron microscopy may yield such features in one half or less of cases in which the light microscopic cellular morphology is consistent with rhabdomyosarcoma.[405,424,429]

A variety of immunohistochemical markers have been used in attempts to establish the diagnosis of rhabdomyosarcoma. Among these are desmin,* myoglobin,† the MM isoenzyme of creatine kinase,[393,409] myosin,[454] fast myosin,[391,393,400] Z-protein,[430] specific muscle actin,[350,370,392,393,447] beta-enolase,[443] and antimuscle antibody.[433] These markers may be present even when myogenic differentiation is not present by electron microscopy,[387,423,425] but the results using these markers have varied considerably. For myoglobin and desmin, the two most extensively studied markers, positive results have been found in from 37% to 89% of rhabdomyosarcomas stained for myoglobin and from 32% to 100% of cases using desmin. Such a disparity in results probably reflects differences in the type of tissue fixation employed, the quality of the antibody used, and the type of immunohistochemical method. The differentiation of the tumor is generally correlated with the immunohistochemical results in that cells with more abundant cytoplasm usually stain more commonly than the smaller more primitive cells do. In general, myoglobin has usually been found in the more "mature" cells and desmin in the more primitive cells, but even here exceptions exist.‡ Care must also be exercised in the interpretation of immunohistochemical stains for muscle differentiation when there is tumor invasion and destruction of normal skeletal muscle. Nonspecific adsorption or ingestion of myoglobin by tissue macrophages adjacent to necrotic skeletal muscle has been noted,[384,399] and nonmyogenous tumor cells, such as those of breast carcinoma, melanoma, and lymphoma, have also given positive results for myoglobin when in-

---

*References 379 to 381, 386, 400, 423, 425, 432.
†References 381, 384, 386, 387, 391, 392, 400, 423, 431, 454.
‡References 385, 392, 393, 400, 431, 443, 445, 454.

filtrating skeletal muscle.[399] A new monoclonal antibody to muscle-specific actin, HHF-35, though yielding positive results in smooth muscle tumors and some non-muscle tumors,[350] stains virtually all rhabdomyosarcomas of all types in which it has so far been used.[350,370,446] It apparently also stains a greater number of tumor cells than desmin does.[370,446] One encounters rare rhabdomyosarcomas that stain positively for S-100 protein[386,446] and coexpress cytokeratin.[386]

Rhabdomyosarcoma has a predilection for certain anatomic sites. In the Intergroup Rhabdomyosarcoma Study of over 1600 childhood cases, the commonest locations were the head and neck region, which accounted for 35% of cases, with the orbit being the most common site; the genitourinary system was involved in 21%, with the bladder, prostate and paratesticular region being the most common locations; and the extremities in 19%, the trunk 9%, pelvis 6%, and the retroperitoneum 5%.[432] The frequency of involvement of the head and neck region and the genitourinary tract has been noted in other studies as well.[378,382,402,411] Rhabdomyosarcomas in adults, however, are located mainly in the extremities and only uncommonly arise in the head and neck region.[417]

Embryonal rhabdomyosarcoma

The most common of the rhabdomyosarcomas, the embryonal form occurs predominantly in children who are usually less than 12 years of age, with mean ages ranging from about 5 to 8 years.[33,414,432,451,453] Adults are only occasionally affected.[394,417,450] The most common locations in children are in the head and neck region (where the orbit is the most frequent single location), the urogenital tract, and the retroperitoneum.[212,394,451,453] Most authors consider the occurrence of embryonal rhabdomyosarcomas in the extremities to be uncommon, though in one series the extremities and limb girdles accounted for 20% to 25% of cases.[450] Patients with extremity involvement tend to be older, with average ages between 25 and 30 years. In general, adults with embryonal rhabdomyosarcoma more frequently have the tumor located in the extremities or trunk than in the head and neck.[417]

Embryonal rhabdomyosarcoma frequently has no direct relationship to skeletal muscle, growing instead between muscle groups or in the deep subcutaneous tissue.[383] They produce bulging masses that characteristically grow rapidly so that symptoms are usually present for less than a year before medical attention is sought.[394,414,450] Most exceed 5 cm.[405,417,432]

Nothing distinguishes the gross appearance of most embryonal rhabdomyosarcomas from other soft-tissue malignancies, except for the botryoid variety that grows close to the mucosal surfaces of hollow viscera or body cavities and produces edematous, smooth-appearing grape-like masses that protrude into the hollow cavities.[103,408,436] Botryoid rhabdomyosarcoma is most commonly found in the urogenital tract, nasal cavity, common bile duct, auditory canal, nasal cavity, paranasal sinuses, and nasopharynx.[33,381,395,401,408,418]

The histomorphology of embryonal rhabdomyosarcomas varies and has been likened to the pattern found in the embryonic stage of skeletal muscle development present between the third and tenth weeks of gestation.[103,404,408,436,450] The tumors usually consist of a mixture of small, spindle-shaped cells, with tapering bipolar cytoplasmic extensions, and small, round to oval cells about the size of lymphocytes or small monocytes, with little cytoplasm (Fig. 37-13). The latter cells may accumulate more cytoplasm that is usually intensely eosinophilic and granular to fibrillar. The finding of such eosinophilic rhabdomyoblasts is an important clue to the diagnosis (Fig. 37-14). They may assume a variety of shapes including oval, round, spindle, racquet, or straplike forms. Most embryonal rhabdomyosarcomas are predominantly composed of small cells with little or no cytoplasm mixed with a variable number of cells with a more abundant amount of cytoplasm.[381,382,397]

The tumor cells frequently reside in a loose myxoid stroma, and mitoses are frequent. The spindle cells may be arranged in broad fascicles or bands creating a pattern mimicking that of a leiomyosarcoma or fibrosarcoma.[382,383] Cross striations are found in from 30% to 60% of cases.* At times, the cells are more uniformly round and compact and, since they also contain glycogen, may resemble the cells of extraskeletal Ewing's sarcoma. However, the cells of embryonal rhabdomyosarcoma are less uniform than those of Ewing's sarcoma, with more nuclear irregularity in size, shape, and chromatin content.[381]

The botryoid variant of rhabdomyosarcoma represents an exaggeration of the usual myxoid matrix of embryonal rhabdomyosarcoma. It has a hypocellular to acellular myxoid central region, with the majority of the tumor cells, most of which are small and round to oval, located in a narrow band beneath the overlying mucosa of the affected viscus. This "cambium" layer is characteristic of botryoid rhabdomyosarcoma[103,408] (Fig. 37-15).

Alveolar rhabdomyosarcoma

Alveolar rhabdomyosarcoma is more common in older children, teenagers, and young adults than embryonal rhabdomyosarcoma is. The mean age is between 15 and 20 years, and although the tumor occasionally occurs in older adults, it is rare in those older than 50 years.[33,53,396,397,436]

---

*References 33, 381, 408, 414, 417, 436, 437.

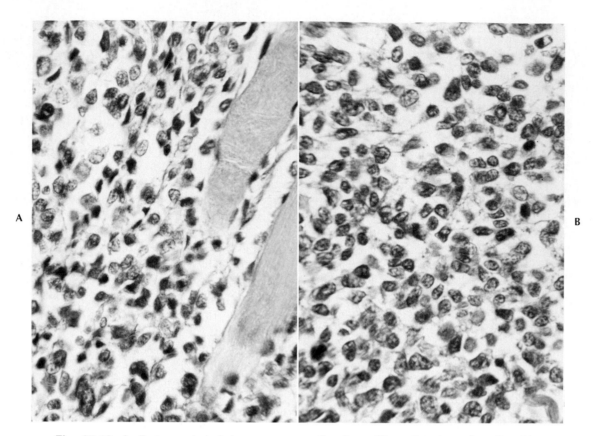

Fig. 37-13. A, Embryonal rhabdomyosarcoma. Small, undifferentiated tumor cells with little or no visible cytoplasm. Skeletal muscle fibers are infiltrated by tumor cells. **B,** Embryonal rhabdomyosarcoma tumor cells with little variation in size or shape of their nuclei. (**A** and **B,** 600×.)

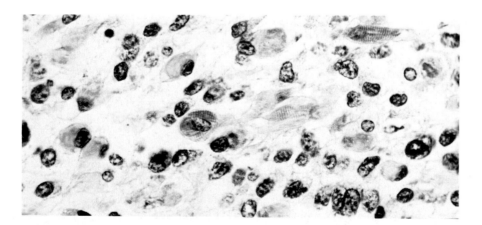

Fig. 37-14. Embryonal rhabdomyosarcoma. In addition to undifferentiated tumor cells, more mature rhabdomyoblasts are present with distinct cross striations. Large, round cells with abundant eosinophilic cytoplasm, but without striations, are also present. (480×.)

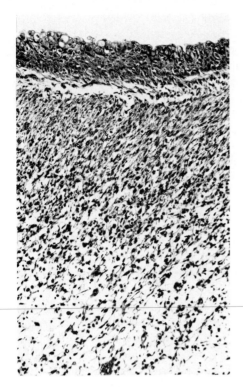

Fig. 37-15. Botryoid rhabdomyosarcoma of vagina. Concentration of tumor cells beneath vaginal mucosa creates cambium layer characteristic of this tumor. (120×.)

Unlike embryonal rhabdomyosarcoma, the alveolar form is commonly located in the extremities (60% to 70% of cases), where it develops as a rapidly growing mass that may reach 20 cm.[397,403,407,432,450] Also, unlike the embryonal form, it grossly appears to arise from within muscle.[396] The forearm, hand, and trunk are common sites of origin but, unlike the embryonal form, less than 20% of cases involve the head and neck region.[53,394,397,403,452]

In its classic form, alveolar rhabdomyosarcoma has a characteristic histologic pattern characterized by the tendency of the tumor cells to be arranged in ill-defined groups and nests in which the central cells are loosely cohesive, forming spaces that mimic, at low-power microscopic examination, pulmonary alveolar spaces[378,396,397,404] (Fig. 37-16). Fibrous trabeculae form the periphery of the cell nests, and the adjacent tumor cells attach themselves to these trabeculae by tapered cytoplasmic strands with their nuclei oriented toward the lumen of the spaces. Cells within the alveolar spaces vary in shape, are from 15 to 30 μm in size, and are frequently seen floating free within the spaces. Multinucleated giant cells, up to 200 μm in diameter, with their nuclei in a wreathlike arrangement within a granular eosinophilic cytoplasm, are commonly found within the alveolar spaces. These giant cells do not

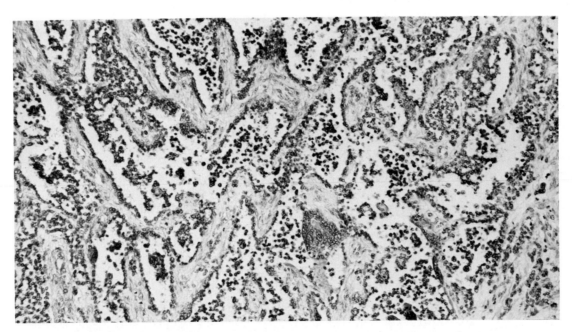

Fig. 37-16. Alveolar rhabdomyosarcoma. Fibrous septa are lined by tumor cells. Central cells are loosely cohesive and appear to float within alveolar spaces. A large multinucleated giant cell is present. (150×.)

show cross striations.[397] Smaller tumor cells, similar to those of the embryonal form, are also present, as may be larger round cells with eccentric nuclei and abundant bright eosinophilic cytoplasm. Solid areas composed of cells similar to those of embryonal rhabdomyosarcoma and lacking an alveolar arrangement are also found. Larger strap- and tadpole-shaped rhabdomyoblasts with bright eosinophilic cytoplasm are also found, but they are less common than in embryonal rhabdomyosarcoma. Some of the larger round cells have peripheral vacuolization of their cytoplasm, giving them a spider-web appearance. The occurrence of cells with cross striations depends on the diligence for which they are sought, with about 30% of the tumors containing such cells, but even in these tumors they are sparse.[53,396,397,409] Mitoses are easily found. There are rhabdomyosarcomas that contain various proportions of both embryonal and alveolar elements and these are diagnosed as "mixed" rhabdomyosarcomas or designated as either embryonal or alveolar depending on the dominant pattern that is present.[381,396] Others diagnose such mixed forms as alveolar rhabdomyosarcoma even if it is not the dominant pattern.[445]

In the past, to some the alveolar pattern was suggestive of the myotube stage of myogenesis in which the cells form a cytoplasmic syncytium around a hollow core. However, electron microscopic studies show that the cells lining the alveolar spaces are not in a syncytium but possess a basement membrane, or remnants of a basal lamina, between the fibrous septa and the cell cytoplasm. These findings negate a myotube hypothesis.[388,447] Recently, a consistent chromosomal translocation involving chromosomes 2 and 13 was described in alveolar rhabdomyosarcoma.[456]

Pleomorphic rhabdomyosarcoma

Formerly considered to be the most common form of rhabdomyosarcoma,[410] pleomorphic rhabdomyosarcoma now ranks as the least frequent.[382,390,381,402,401,432] This reduced frequency has resulted because of a greater awareness on the part of pathologists of the histologic parameters for the diagnosis of embryonal and alveolar rhabdomyosarcoma, as well as the fact that many pleomorphic sarcomas previously diagnosed as rhabdomyosarcoma are now considered to be malignant fibrous histiocytomas.[319,428] The latter tumor also occurs in a similar anatomic location, the extremities, as pleomorphic rhabdomyosarcoma does. Indeed, the very existence of pleomorphic rhabdomyosarcoma has been brought into question.[319] A nonneurogenic pleomorphic sarcoma in an adult in which cells with unequivocal cross striations were present has never been seen. Others are more successful in diagnosing these tumors.[36] Since many of these tumors arise within the substance of the muscle, it is at times difficult to distinguish de-

generative muscle cells, which may have quite atypical-appearing nuclei and may retain their cross striations, from actual tumor cells. The diagnosis of pleomorphic rhabdomyosarcoma should be restricted to those tumors whose cells show cross striations, or in which immunohistochemical or electron microscopic studies demonstrate evidence of skeletal muscle differentiation. If pleomorphic rhabdomyosarcoma exists, it is an extremely rare neoplasm in my experience. The data presented here, which are based on older studies, should be viewed with some skepticism, since at a minimum they probably reflect the result of including tumors other than true rhabdomyosarcomas.

In contrast to the other forms of rhabdomyosarcoma, pleomorphic rhabdomyosarcoma occurs overwhelmingly in older adults, with less than 10% of cases in children.[402,419] The mean patient age is between 50 and 55 years.[410,416,436] Nearly all the tumors arise within large muscles as circumscribed soft masses.[103,212] They are most common in the extremities, with the lower extremity accounting for about half the cases and the thigh being the most common site. The upper extremity, trunk, and head and neck region account for most of the other cases, with occasional tumors being found in the retroperitoneum and the viscera. Pain is associated with these tumors in up to one fourth of patients.[410,416]

Histologically, pleomorphic rhabdomyosarcoma is composed of anaplastic cells, with many having bizarre configurations[382,408,410,416,432] Numerous large, multinucleated cells with deeply eosinophilic cytoplasm are present (Fig. 37-17). Some tumor cells assume racquet or tadpole shapes with a single large nucleus at one end and a tapering cytoplasmic tail, or they form large strap or ribbon shapes with several nuclei in tandem. Small round cells with eccentric nuclei and bright eosinophilic cytoplasm are also common. Cross-striated cells are reported in from 7% to 100% of cases.[381,408,410,416] Areas of necrosis are common, as are mitoses that are frequently abnormal. Glycogen stains are positive.[432] Other than the presence of tumor cells with cross striations, this histomorphology is similar to fibroxanthosarcoma (conventional malignant fibrous histiocytoma). The histologic criteria for a diagnosis of pleomorphic or adult rhabdomyosarcoma have varied among authors. Some equate pleomorphic rhabdomyosarcoma to a "large cell type" in which the tumor contains large cells with round to oval nuclei, sometimes bilobed with occasional nucleoli, and a granular cytoplasm containing fibrils and cross striations. Pronounced multinucleation of tumor giant cells is absent. These tumors also lack spindle cells or fibrosis.[385] Others define pleomorphic rhabdomyosarcoma as a tumor in which 70% or more of the lesion is composed predominantly of differentiated broad straps, or cells with bulky eosinophilic cytoplasm.

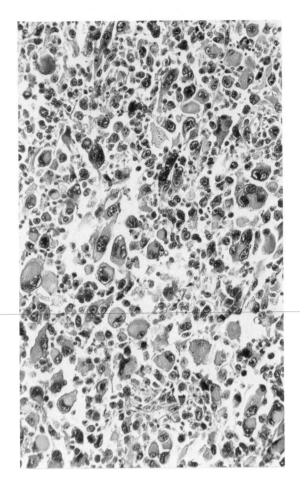

Fig. 37-17. Pleomorphic rhabdomyosarcoma. Anaplastic tumor cells with variety of shapes. Larger cells have abundant densely eosinophilic cytoplasm. Similar cells may be found in other pleomorphic sarcomas such as liposarcoma and malignant fibrous histiocytoma. (150×.)

Some of these so-called "pleomorphic" tumors are actually composed of cells that are uniform in size and shape.[382] This is in sharp contrast to the usual concept of pleomorphic rhabdomyosarcoma as a tumor composed of numerous anaplastic cells.

The Intergroup Rhabdomyosarcoma Study Group developed a relatively simple clinical staging classification that is useful in coordinating and comparing the results of therapy from different institutions.[420,421] This classification consists of four broad groupings that are based upon the extent of the tumor and whether it is totally resected. In brief, group I patients are those with localized tumors that are completely resected; group II contains patients whose tumors were grossly completely resected but where there is microscopic evidence of residual tumor; group III includes patients where gross tumor was still present after resection; and group IV patients are those with distant metastases at initial presentation. Roughly 15% of patients are in group I, 25%

in group II, 40% in group III, and 20% in group IV.[419]

Before the introduction and use of radiation therapy and multidrug chemotherapy, rhabdomyosarcoma had a poor prognosis, with survival rates of only 10% to 35% depending on the type of rhabdomyosarcoma involved.[378,382,402,451,453] However, these treatment modalities have dramatically improved the prognosis, such that survival rates as high as 85% to 95% are now reported depending on the anatomic site involved. Chemotherapy may cause cellular maturation of the tumor.[427] Survival is most strongly correlated with the stage and location of the tumor.[381,382,402,419,440] For clinical groups I to IV, the estimated 5-year survival rates are approximately 95%, 70%, 50%, and 20% respectively, with 5-year disease-free survival rates of 75%, 65%, 45%, and 15%. For all patients, the estimated 5-year survival rates are about 50% to 55%.[402,419] Most patients who die do so within 2 years of diagnosis, the majority of them within 1 year, with only a few deaths or relapses after 3 to 4 years.[381,411,419] Patients who relapse after therapy have an extremely poor prognosis despite the use of further intensive chemotherapy.[411,419,439] High relapse rates are associated with rhabdomyosarcomas involving the perineum and anal area, the retroperitoneum and pelvis, and the extremities.[390,407,439,448] Most patients who die do so with both local and distant disease, with the lungs, lymph nodes, bones, liver, and brain being the commonest sites for metastases.[403,448] Extremity and urogenital tract rhabdomyosarcomas have the highest incidence of lymph node metastases.[413,421,451]

Orbital and genitourinary tract tumors have the best prognosis,[378,411,419,440,441,452] whereas retroperitoneal, pelvic, extremity, trunk, and parameningeal tumors have poorer survival rates.[390,411,419,442,448] Patients who develop bone marrow metastases, half of whom have alveolar rhabdomyosarcoma, also have a poor prognosis.[444] Alveolar rhabdomyosarcoma has the worst survival, with an increased incidence of metastases and local relapse rates.* The "intermediate" type of tumor also has a poor survival rate, whereas botryoid rhabdomyosarcomas have the best overall prognosis.[432]

Rhabdomyoma

Rhabdomyoma of soft tissue is a benign, nonaggressive tumor that accounts for approximately 1% to 2% of all skeletal muscle tumors, with the remainder being rhabdomyosarcomas.[461] Less than 100 cases have been reported.[463]

Soft-tissue rhabdomyoma should not be confused with the glycogen-containing lesion of the heart, also designated as "rhabdomyoma," that is probably a hamartomatous lesion and not a true tumor. It is this car-

---

*References 403, 406, 411, 432, 439, 444, 448, 455.

diac lesion and not the soft-tissue tumor that is associated with the tuberous sclerosis syndrome.[470]

Rhabdomyomas are divided histologically into adult and fetal types, with roughly equal numbers of each being reported. Despite the fact that these tumors are, in most cases, histologically distinct from rhabdomyosarcoma, they are still occasionally misdiagnosed as the latter with horrendous consequences to the patient.

Adult rhabdomyoma occurs almost exclusively in older patients, the mean patient age being approximately 50 years, and only rarely does it occur in children.[462,466,472] Fetal rhabdomyoma, however, affects patients over a broader age range, from newborns to adults, with the mean patient age some 20 to 30 years younger than for the adult type.[462,468] The adult form is four to five times more frequent in male than in female patients, whereas the fetal type has an approximately equal sex distribution.[462,466,472]

Adult rhabdomyomas are predominantly located in the head and neck, with the larynx and pharynx being the most common sites.[462,463] Other locations include the lip, hypopharynx, nasopharynx, tongue, soft palate, floor of mouth, orbit, submandibular region, and the muscles of the neck. Sites outside the head and neck area include the thoracic wall, stomach, finger, abdominal wall, retroperitoneum, mediastinum and anus.[457,462,463,473] Rare multicentric synchronous or metachronous rhabdomyomas, all of which have been located in the head and neck region, are reported.[467,471,472]

Fetal rhabdomyomas principally occur in the subcutaneous tissue of the head and neck, with the posterior auricular region being the most common site.[53,461,462,465,472] Other reported locations include the tongue, larynx, nose, nasopharynx, soft palate, parotid region, orbit, axilla, chest and abdominal wall, stomach, and anus.[462,465,466,468,472] They also occur in the female genital tract, arising in the vulva, vagina, and ectocervix.[462] Multicentric fetal rhabdomyomas also occur.[460,464]

Adult rhabdomyomas grow slowly and may be present for many years, some for over 50 years.[462,467,470] Cell-labeling studies indicate an approximate duration of 10 years before the lesion achieves a size of 1 cm.[472] It may be well-circumscribed or even encapsulated[457,460] and varies in size from a few millimeters to 15 cm.[457,460,462,468] The fetal form is less well defined and may even appear infiltrative.[53,461,462,466,468]

Histologically, adult rhabdomyoma is easily recognized. It consists of large, oval to round cells that have an abundant, distinctly granular eosinophilic cytoplasm that is frequently vacuolated, creating spider web–like cells.[459,462,467,470] The cells have an abundant amount of glycogen.[459,470] Nuclei are uniform and either central or eccentric (Fig. 37-18). Cross striations, though uncommon, are found in at least some of the cells. Mitotic

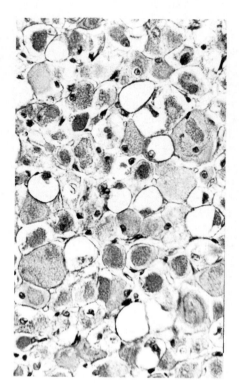

Fig. 37-18. Adult rhabdomyoma. Large cells with abundant granular eosinophilic cytoplasm mixed with cells having vacuolated cytoplasm. Nuclei are bland and central or eccentric in location. (280×.)

figures are rare. Cytoplasmic crystalline-like granules or particles are present and best demonstrated with phosphotungstic acid–hematoxylin stains.[459,466,470,471] By electron microscopy, these granules represent hypertrophic Z-band material that resembles that seen in nemaline myopathy. Thick and thin myofilaments are present as well as enlarged, sometimes atypical, mitochondria. Intranuclear and intramitochondral inclusions have been found, as has basal lamina.[458,459,468,469,471,472,473,474]

Adult rhabdomyoma may be histologically confused with a granular cell tumor whose cells also have a similar granular-appearing cytoplasm. However, the cells of granular cell tumor lack cross striations, contain periodic acid–Schiff–positive cytoplasmic material that is diastase resistant, and by electron microscopy lack the mixture of actin and myosin filaments present in the cells of rhabdomyoma.[458,459,470] Immunohistochemically, granular cell tumors contain S-100 protein, which is not present in rhabdomyomas, and they lack the reactivity for myosin, myoglobin, and desmin that is found in rhabdomyomas.[469,473]

Fetal rhabdomyomas are histologically more heterogeneous than their adult counterparts. They are composed of immature-appearing skeletal muscle fibers, in various stages of differentiation, admixed with mesenchymal cells that vary from small, oval to round cells to large cells with bipolar tapering cytoplasmic extensions.[460-462] The most mature cells are found at the periphery of the lesion, but cells with cross striations are difficult to find.[461] The background stroma is myxomatous, with the tumor cells being loosely arranged within it and giving the lesion an edematous appearance.[461,462] Significantly, the tumor cells lack pleomorphism or necrosis and mitoses are scarce. In the female genital tract rhabdomyomas the stroma is more abundant and the muscle cells appear more mature.[466] There is described a "cellular" variant of fetal rhabdomyoma in which the stroma is either sparse or inconspicuous and in which there is a predominance of thin, elongate spindle cells arranged in a herringbone or palisading pattern.[462] Occasional ribbon and strap cells are present, but cross striations are difficult to find. Although nuclear atypism is present in occasional cells, mitoses are absent or rare. This "fetal cellular" variant is less common than the "fetal myxoid" type. Some fetal rhabdomyomas have a blend of both patterns.[465] Thick and thin myofilaments and basal lamina are found by electron microscopy but, unlike adult rhabdomyomas, no mitochondrial inclusions or hypertrophic Z-band material is present.[460,468,473]

Although adult rhabdomyoma is easily differentiated histologically from rhabdomyosarcoma, fetal rhabdomyoma may be confused with embryonal rhabdomyosarcoma. Indeed, the histologic distinction between these two tumors may be quite subtle.[461] The lack of necrosis, cellular pleomorphism, nuclear hyperchromasia, and significant mitotic activity in fetal rhabdomyoma, as well as its superficial location and gross circumscription, are features that support a benign diagnosis.[460-462]

After surgical excision, occasional patients with adult rhabdomyomas develop local recurrences, some even multiple recurrences.[457,459,472] There has been only one report of a recurrent fetal rhabdomyoma.[468] In neither tumor variety has there been evidence of local aggressiveness or metastases.

The nature of rhabdomyomas is still unclear; some authors have suggested that they may be hamartomas.[460,461] However, since some rhabdomyomas occur in locations such as the vocal cord, ectocervix, and stomach, where skeletal muscle is not normally found, they do not fit the classic definition of a hamartoma, and are considered true tumors.

TUMORS OF ADIPOSE TISSUE
Liposarcoma

Liposarcoma is one of the most common of the adult soft-tissue sarcomas, with a reported incidence that varies from 10% to 25% of all soft-tissue sarcomas.* With the recognition of malignant fibrous histiocytoma as a

distinct entity and the application of this diagnosis to some lesions previously designated as "pleomorphic liposarcoma," malignant fibrous histiocytoma has equaled or surpassed liposarcoma as the most common sarcoma in some institutions.[29,75,96,108,246] Furthermore, with the recent characterization of spindle-cell and pleomorphic variants of lipoma (see p. 1879), some tumors previously designated as well-differentiated or myxoid liposarcoma would now probably be reclassified as one of these benign entities.[489] That the histologic diagnosis of liposarcoma is not sacrosanct is evidenced by the fact that in some series close to half the lesions so designated were, on review, reassigned to other diagnostic categories.[488,493,495] Despite its frequency among the sarcomas, liposarcoma is still a rare tumor, being about 100 times less common than benign lipoma.[74,475]

Liposarcoma is classically considered to be a tumor of lipoblasts. However, the number of lipoblasts varies greatly among the various histologic subtypes of this tumor and, in some, lipoblasts may be scarce. Lipoblasts, or cells that by light microscopy are indistinguishable from lipoblasts, are also found in reactive conditions involving fat as well as in benign adipose tumors such as lipoblastomas.[475] In addition, some pleomorphic sarcomas, such as malignant fibrous histiocytoma and osteosarcoma, may also contain cells that resemble lipoblasts. Hence the presence of lipoblasts or lipoblast-like cells is not by itself an indication of liposarcoma, since the diagnosis of liposarcoma depends equally on the overall histologic pattern of the lesion. With this having been stated, it must be admitted that what constitutes a lipoblast by light microscopy, or even electron microscopy, is still open to some debate since what to one pathologist is a lipoblast may be a multivacuolated histiocyte to another.[475,501] It is at times easier to describe a lipoblast than it is to point one out, with assurance, under the microscope.

Depending on the number of fat vacuoles in their cytoplasm, lipoblasts are divided into univacuolated and multivacuolated varieties[475] (Fig. 37-19). In the univacuolated form the cells are smaller than mature fat cells and assume a signet-ring appearance caused by the presence of a large and sharply delimited cytoplasmic vacuole that pushes the nucleus to one side, giving it a demilune shape.[53,475] Such cells may resemble the signet-ring cells of a mucin-producing adenocarcinoma. Although the nucleus may be hyperchromatic and bizarre, this is usually not the case, and mitotic figures are rarely found in these cells.

In contrast, multivacuolated lipoblasts have a centrally placed nucleus that is frequently large, bizarre in shape, and hyperchromatic. These cells vary greatly in size and may reach 300 to 400 μm in diameter. The cytoplasmic vacuoles may be large or small, are characteristically sharply defined, and indent the margins of the nucleus, giving it a scalloped appearance. Frequent

---

*References 19, 29, 75, 96, 107, 108, 123, 246, 488, 493.

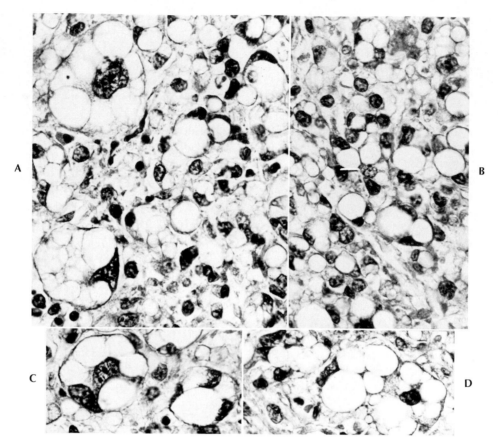

Fig. 37-19. A, Liposarcoma. Univacuolated and multivacuolated lipoblasts. Notice compression of nuclei by fat vacuoles. **B,** Signet-ring lipoblasts are shown. **C,** Multinucleated, multivacuolated lipoblasts. **D,** Single-nucleated, multivacuolated lipoblasts. (480×.)

and abnormal mitotic figures are commonly found in these cells. Both univacuolated and multivacuolated lipoblasts may be multinucleated, though this is more common among the multivacuolated cells.

Histologically, liposarcomas are divided into four major types: well-differentiated, which is further subclassified into lipoma-like and sclerosing forms; myxoid; round-cell; and pleomorphic.[487,495] Mixed forms occur in various combinations, that is well-differentiated areas mixed with pleomorphic areas or myxoid forms with round cell areas. Recently an additional "dedifferentiated" tumor category has been proposed. These latter tumors consist of areas of well-differentiated liposarcoma in combination with some form of specific or undifferentiated spindle-cell sarcoma.[488,505]

In contrast to what might be expected, fat stains are of little help in the diagnosis of liposarcoma. Some liposarcomas lack significant fat content, whereas other pleomorphic sarcomas may stain positively for fat because their cells undergo degeneration and accumulate cytoplasmic lipid.

Myxoid liposarcoma is the most common histologic type and accounts for 35% to 50% of all cases.[475,487,488,493] It is composed of widely separated, monomorphic fusiform or stellate cells that have indistinct cell borders, lying in a mucoid stroma rich in hyaluronic acid. Hypocellular pools or lakes of this mucoid matrix are frequently present (Fig. 37-20). When the mucoid matrix is abundant, there may be diagnostic confusion with a myxoma. However, another component not found in myxoma is always present and obvious in myxoid liposarcoma, that is, a delicate plexiform capillary network. The cells of myxoid liposarcoma are not especially hyperchromatic or atypical. Indeed, pleomorphism and significant mitotic activity are not part of this tumor, and such findings eliminate it from the pure myxoid category.[475,487,488,493] Lipoblasts may be scarce and are usually univacuolated. Myxoid liposarcoma is diagnosed more on the basis of its overall pattern than on the finding of numerous lipoblasts.

Lipoma-like and sclerosing well-differentiated liposarcomas constitute 20% to 30% of all liposarco-

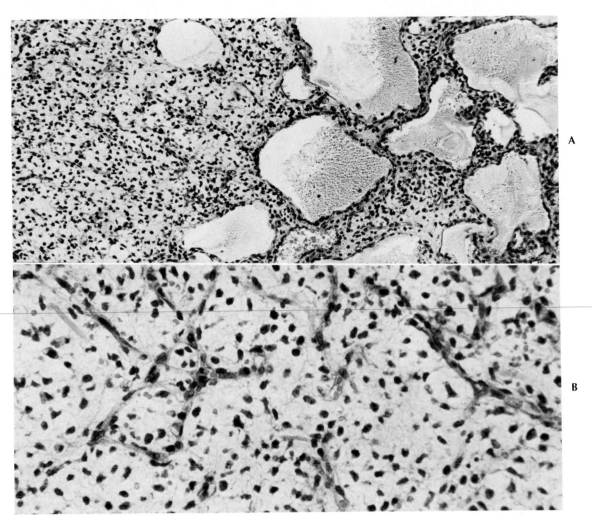

Fig. 37-20. A, Myxoid liposarcoma. Hypocellular pools of mucinous matrix within stellate cellular stroma. **B,** Widely separated round and stellate cells embedded in myxoid stroma. Cells are fairly uniform without pleomorphism. Notice abundant plexiform capillary network. (**A,** 150×; **B,** 600×.)

mas.[475,488,493,495] The lipoma-like variety is, as its name implies, composed principally of mature-appearing fat cells but in which focal regions exist where hyperchromatic and bizarre lipoblasts are found. These lipoblasts tend to be multivacuolated and multinucleated. It is this variety of liposarcoma that may be mistaken for a benign lipoma if sufficient sections are not examined, since the atypical cellular foci may be few and widely separated[495] (Fig. 37-21). In deeply situated fatty tumors, sections should be taken from any areas having increased firmness or whitish discoloration, or from any regions with obvious necrosis. The sclerosing type of well-differentiated liposarcoma is more common than the lipoma-like form and is characterized by broad fibrous zones containing atypical and bizarre lipoblasts, frequently multivacuolated, alternating with areas of mature adipose tissue (Fig. 37-22). In neither of these subtypes of liposarcoma is mitotic activity prominent.[475,495] Zones of lipoma-like and sclerosing forms of liposarcoma are frequently found together within the same tumor.[487]

Both forms of well-differentiated liposarcoma may contain floret type of cells as found in pleomorphic lipomas.[476,489,493,502] The histologic distinction between pleomorphic (atypical) lipoma[502] and well-differentiated liposarcoma may be difficult if not impossible, and the diagnosis may rest more upon the location of the tumor than upon its histomorphology. Retroperitoneal well-differentiated fatty tumors with cellular atypia frequently behave as locally aggressive malignant tumors, whereas superficially located tumors with similar histologic features rarely do so.[476,489,502] Well-differen-

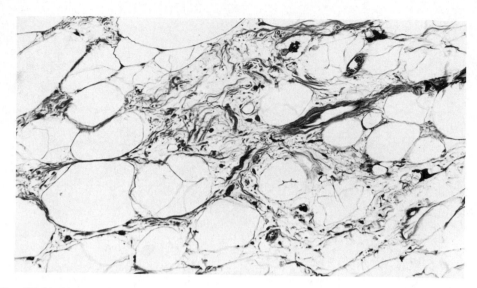

Fig. 37-21. Lipoma-like liposarcoma. Focal region with increased fibrous tissue in which fat cells with atypical nuclei are present. Multinucleated lipoblast is at upper center of the field. Superficial tumors with this pattern have been termed "pleomorphic lipomas." (150×.)

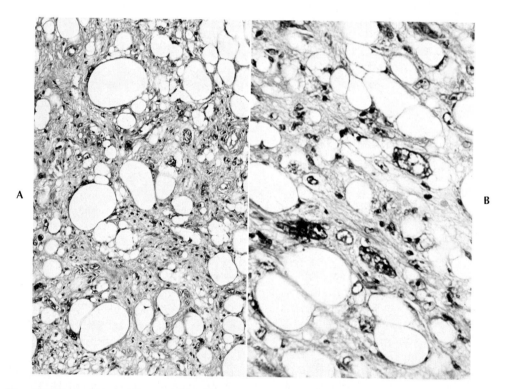

Fig. 37-22. A, Sclerosing liposarcoma. Dense fibrous tissue contains anaplastic tumor cells and lipoblasts. **B,** Higher magnification showing hyperchromatic malignant stromal cells. A few signet-ring lipoblasts are present. (**A,** 120×; **B,** 280×.)

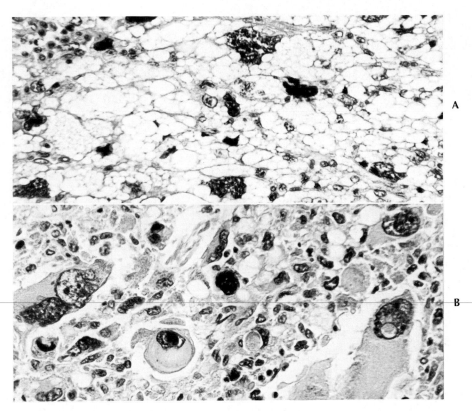

Fig. 37-23. A, Pleomorphic liposarcoma. Numerous multivacuolated lipoblasts with bizarre nuclei are shown. **B,** Another region from pleomorphic liposarcoma shows large bizarre tumor giant cells with abundant, densely eosinophilic cytoplasm. A few signet-ring lipoblasts are at upper right. (280×.)

tiated liposarcomas may be associated with an undifferentiated spindle-cell sarcomatous component, for which the term "dedifferentiated" liposarcoma has been used.[488,505]

Pleomorphic liposarcoma is the most anaplastic of the liposarcomas and accounts for 10% to 25% of cases.[475,487,495] It is characterized by an abundance of large tumor giant cells, many having a dense eosinophilic cytoplasm, and numerous bizarre lipoblasts with frequent and abnormal mitotic figures (Fig. 37-23). Spindle-cell areas are frequent such that distinction from fibroxanthosarcoma (pleomorphic malignant fibrous histiocytoma) or pleomorphic rhabdomyosarcoma may be difficult.[53,487,488] However, the tumor giant cells lack the cross striations of rhabdomyosarcoma cells, and the storiform pattern of malignant fibrous histiocytoma is not usually present in liposarcoma. There are cases, however, that have features or both liposarcoma and malignant fibrous histiocytoma, and so distinction between them at the light microscopic level may be impossible.[53,247,302,319,486] The presence of S-100 protein, which is found in all varieties of liposarcoma, and its absence in malignant fibrous histiocytoma as well as the

different electron microscopic features of these two tumors are useful in resolving this diagnostic problem.[483,492,508]

Round cell liposarcoma comprises approximately 10% to 15% of all liposarcomas[475,487,495] but is considered by some to be a variant of myxoid liposarcoma rather than as a separate histologic type, though myxoid foci are seen in less than half the cases.[476,488] Microscopically the tumor is composed of uniform round to oval cells having a fine multivacuolated cytoplasm and a central round nucleus that may be hyperchromatic but not usually greatly atypical (Fig 37-24). Such cells may resemble those of a hibernoma. Signet-ring lipoblasts are found but not in great numbers. The number of mitotic figures varies, but they are usually not common. Round cell liposarcoma may resemble a signet-ring adenocarcinoma but can be distinguished from it by means of mucin stains.

Liposarcoma is a disease of adults, with most patients in the fourth to sixth decades of life; the mean patient age is about 50 years.[580,487,493,495] Patients with myxoid liposarcoma tend to be younger,[475,488,493,495] whereas those with well-differentiated tumors, especially those

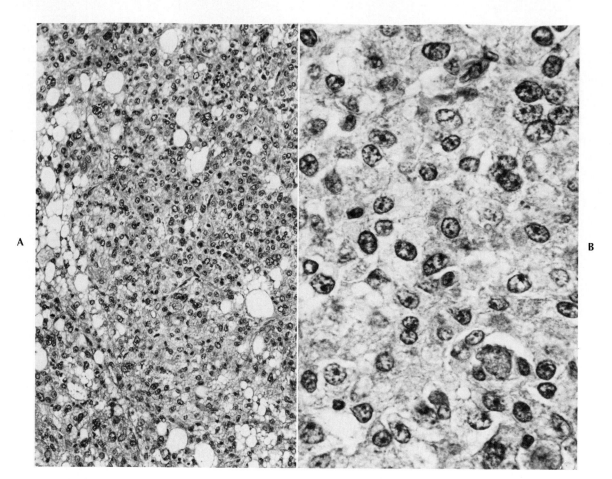

Fig. 37-24. A, Round cell liposarcoma. A few lipoblasts are mingled with uniform round cells. **B,** Higher magnification shows cells with mildly atypical nuclei and finely vacuolated granular cytoplasm. (**A,** 150×; **B,** 600×.)

with retroperitoneal tumors, tend to be among the most elderly of patients.[53,475,488,495] Male patients account for 55% to 60% of cases.[103,487,493,495,500]

Liposarcomas are rare in children.[481,503] Although congenital cases are reported,[481] most childhood cases occur in children over 10 years of age.[503] However, most reported cases of liposarcoma in younger children, especially in those patients less than 3 years of age, are probably examples of lipoblastoma and not liposarcoma.[481,482,503] As in adults, myxoid liposarcoma is the most common childhood histologic type.[503] A multinodular myxoid lesion that affects the omentum and mesentery of infants and that may be confused with myxoid liposarcoma has been reported and termed "myxoid hamartoma."[491]

Unlike lipomas, liposarcomas usually arise from the deep soft tissue and only rarely from the subcutaneous tissue.[475,498] With very rare exceptions, liposarcomas arise anew and not from preexisting lipomas.[494] Liposarcomas are usually located between major muscle groups, with the most frequent sites being the medial area of the thigh and popliteal fossa; the retroperitoneum, especially about the kidney; the shoulder region; the buttocks; and the inguinal and paratesticular areas. They are extremely rare in the hands and feet.[53,103,480,487] Whereas the myxoid and round cell tumors are most frequent in the lower extremities, the well-differentiated and pleomorphic varieties are more common in the retroperitoneum,[53,488,493,495] though there is some variation reported in this general scheme.[496] Paratesticular tumors tend to be of the sclerosing form.[475]

Depending on their anatomic location, liposarcomas usually manifest themselves as painless masses.[475,487,493] Retroperitoneal tumors cause abdominal distension or pressure symptoms.[495]

Grossly, liposarcomas appear as nodular masses, usually greater than 5 cm,[493] that appear well-circumscribed but are always infiltrative. The retroperitoneal tumors may attain enormous size, weighing many kilograms.[103,487,506] The well-differentiated variety may grossly resemble a benign lipoma but frequently has areas of increased firmness or foci of necrosis. The myxoid variety may be brainlike in consistency with a grayish white translucent surface that is slimy. Mucoid material may drip from small cystic spaces on its cut surface.[475,495] The round cell and pleomorphic tumors have no gross characteristics that distinguish them from other soft-tissue sarcomas.

Most electron microscopic studies of liposarcoma have, until recently, dealt mainly with the myxoid variety. Although some have indicated that such tumors may arise from brown fat,[497] the predominance of evidence indicates that the development of these tumors recapitulates the embryonic development of white fat[477-479,484,490,509] Characteristic electron microscopic morphologic features include the presence of cells with non–membrane bound cytoplasmic lipid droplets, micropinocytotic vesicles, and a basal lamina. Poorly differentiated mesenchymal cells, pericytes, and nonspecific perivascular cells are also found.[477-479,490,501,508,509]

Recent cytogenetic observations of a few cases of liposarcoma indicate the occurrence of a reciprocal chromosome translocation in myxoid liposarcoma but not within other liposarcoma subtypes.[504,507]

The prognosis in liposarcoma depends on several factors, paramount of which is the histologic type and the location of the tumor.[475,487,489,500] In general, myxoid and well-differentiated liposarcomas have excellent 5-year survival rates that range from 75% to 100% and 10-year survival rates about 10% to 15% lower.[487,488,493,495] Pleomorphic liposarcoma has a significantly poorer prognosis, with 5-year survival rates of 21% or less and a further decline in overall survival at 10 years. Survival rates with round cell liposarcoma have varied from 18% to 27% at 5 years to less than 10% at 10 years.[475,487,488,495]

Despite their overall good survival rates, both myxoid and well-differentiated liposarcomas have high local recurrence rates that range from 50% to 100% in some series.[475,487,488,495,500] As one would expect, the more aggressive round cell and pleomorphic liposarcomas also yield high local recurrence rates of from 75% to 80%.[487,488,495] Metastatic rates for these latter two sarcomas are also higher than for the other subtypes.[53,488,495] Metastases from liposarcomas are almost all blood borne, usually to the lungs, with only rare involvement of the regional lymph nodes. Well-differentiated tumors tend to recur locally before there is evidence of distal spread. Indeed, metastases from well-differentiated liposarcomas are extremely rare,[487,488,495] whereas approximately 20% to 30% of myxoid liposarcomas metastasize.[476,488,495]

Retroperitoneal liposarcomas have a lower survival, type for type, than liposarcomas in the extremities do.[475,495,496] This probably reflects the adequacy of the type of surgical resection that can be done in these anatomic sites. Radiotherapy may improve survival, with the myxoid and well-differentiated tumors responding best.[480,485] Children have a much better prognosis than adults do, with a lower incidence of recurrences, metastases, and death from tumor, and a survival rate of approximately 80%.[481,503]

Recurrent or metastatic liposarcoma may occur as another histologic subtype, or "transform" into a spindle cell sarcoma with features of malignant fibrous histiocytoma, hemangiopericytoma, malignant schwannoma, or undifferentiated sarcoma.[480,493,505] This "dedifferentiation" most frequently occurs in those retroperitoneal liposarcomas of initially well-differentiated type.[476,488]

Lipoma

Perhaps because familiarity tends to breed contempt, lipoma of soft tissue, despite its position as the commonest soft-tissue tumor,[33,44,511] has suffered from benign neglect by pathologists. Usually interest is aroused only when the lipoma occurs in esoteric locations outside the soft tissue such as the brain or gastrointestinal tract.[512] It is, after all, difficult for diagnostic pathologists to become excited over a histologic expanse of mature fat cells. However, with the recent publication of an excellent monograph describing over 40 varieties of benign mesenchymal lesions in which adipose tissue is a prominent or major component, as well as reports dealing with lipomas whose histologic features can mimic malignant tumors, there has been a renewed interest in lesions of adipose tissue. Lipomas alone account for almost half of all benign soft-tissue tumors.[74,94]

Lipomas usually occur as a single, painless mass that may be present for many years. They either become stationary after achieving their usual size of from 1 to 5 cm,[94] or some continue to grow slowly to achieve a size of 50 to 60 cm.[475] Most patients seek medical treatment when the lesion either becomes cosmetically distracting or reaches such a size that it impinges upon vital structures.

Lipomas tend to occur in obese patients or those with recent weight gain.[510] It has been claimed that the fat within a lipoma is not metabolically available to the body, since in starvation states lipomas do not disappear and may actually increase in size.[103]

Although in some reports of solitary lipomas female patients account for 60% to 70% of cases,[475,510,511,518] in others male patients are more frequent in ratios of 1.2:1 to 1.8:1.[94,519,524,526] Lipomas most often occur in patients in the fifth to sixth decades of life; the mean patient age is between 40 and 50 years[94,475,510,511,524,526]; lipomas are uncommon in the first two decades of life and rarely occur in children.[53,94,103,528]

Lipomas are soft, freely movable masses that almost always arise superficially in the subcutaneous tissue[475,512,528] though deeper intramuscular and intermuscular lipomas occur.[53,94,475,516,522,525] Although any site in the body may be involved, lipomas most frequently occur in the neck, shoulders, arms and trunk.[94,511,524,526,528] The hands, feet, leg, scalp, and face are only rarely affected.[94,510-512,526] Lipomas arising in peripheral nerve, with rare exceptions almost always the median nerve, are associated with enlargement of the digits (macrodystrophia lipomatosa). Described as intraneural or perineural lipomas, these are considered by others to be hamartomas.[525]

Grossly, lipomas are smooth, encapsulated, round to oval, well-circumscribed masses that on cut section are soft, yellow to orange, and greasy, Microscopically, one sees lobules of mature adipose cells separated by thin, delicate, fibrous septa. The tumor is surrounded by a thin fibrous capsule that serves to distinguish lipoma from a simple aggregation of fat. At times myxoid areas replace some of the fat lobules, and there may be evidence of fat necrosis resulting from trauma.[511] Electron microscopy has demonstrated that the lipoma cells are morphologically identical to the cells of normal mature white adipose tissue.[517,521,526] Recent cytogenetic analysis of lipomas indicates a nonrandom reciprocal chromosome translocation involving chromosomes 3 and 12.[520,527] Although biochemical analysis of lipomas have shown no significant differences between their lipid content and that of mature fat, some studies have noted a pronounced increase in lipoprotein lipase activity in lipomas in men.[526]

In deeply located fatty tumors, such as those in the retroperitoneum, atypical-appearing gross foci should be assiduously looked for and many sections taken before one accepts it as a simple lipoma, since some will prove to be well-differentiated liposarcomas. It is just such cases, inadequately sampled perhaps, that result in reports of malignant degeneration in benign lipomas. As a general rule, liposarcomas arise anew and not from lipomas.[494] If not totally removed, lipomas may rarely recur, probably in from 1% to 2% of cases.[53,475,510]

Multiple lipomas occur in from 1% to 7% of patients[475,510,524,526,528] with some patients having over 100 lesions.[523] There is a pronounced male prevalence in patients with multiple lipomas; many also have a positive family history of tumor.[523,524,526] However, many patients with supposed multiple simple lipomas prove to actually have multiple angiolipomas instead (see p. 1883).[475] Multiple lipomas occur in patients with neurofibromatosis and in those with the multiple endocrine adenoma syndrome.[475,511,512]

Infiltrating (intermuscular, intramuscular) lipoma

Unlike their more common subcutaneous counterparts, infiltrating lipomas arise in the deeper soft tissues, either between large muscle groups (intermuscular lipoma) or within muscle (intramuscular lipoma). They comprise roughly 2% of all adipose tumors.[516] Although patients of all ages are affected, with some congenital examples reported,[522] these tumors occur mainly in patients older than those with subcutaneous lipomas, with most patients being adults in the fifth to seventh decades of life; 80% are over 40 years of age.[94,475,513,514,517,521]

Although in some series these tumors are much more common in male patients,[475,514] in others female patients have predominated.[94,516] They are slowly growing tumors that may be present for many years before the patient seeks medical attention.[514,522] The tumors are painless and may become clinically obvious only upon contraction of the involved muscle when they become round and firm.[522] They are usually larger than their subcutaneous counterparts,[94] but despite reaching large size, up to 35 cm, they rarely produce dysfunction of the involved muscle.[513,516,522] Roentgenograms show a sharply circumscribed radiolucent defect within the muscle, and angiographic studies show that, unlike soft-tissue sarcomas, they are poorly vascularized.[522] Approximately two thirds of the tumors occur in the thighs, shoulders, and arms, with the thigh accounting for almost 50% of cases. Less common locations include the chest wall, back, and head and neck area.[514,516,522] However, in one large series the trunk, head and neck region, and upper limb were the sites most frequently involved, with the thigh accounting for only 9% of the cases. The reason for this disparity in anatomic distribution is unclear.[516]

On gross examination the tumor infiltrates and replaces large portions of muscle, or infiltrates between muscles or adjacent tendons.[514,516] Histologically, most of these lipomas are composed of mature fat cells lacking atypicality or mitotic activity.[514,522] The cells infiltrate between muscle fibers, replacing them and causing pressure atrophy and degeneration of adjacent fibers[516] (Fig. 37-25). Recently, intramuscular pleomorphic lipomas have been described.[515] Intramuscular lipomas may be histologically confused with intramuscular hemangioma, a vascular tumor that may be accompanied by a prominent fatty component. The number and type of the blood vessels in the latter lesion, however, differs from the blood vessels found in intramuscular lipomas.[516]

Reported recurrence rates after local excision have ranged widely from 3% to 62.5%, with some patients having multiple recurrences.[475,513,514,516] These disparate recurrence rates probably reflect the adequacy of the initial excision rather than any inherent aggressiveness of these tumors.[516,522] With adequate excision local recurrence rates should be between 3% and 15%.[514,516,522] Metastases are not reported, and patients have remained well on extended follow-up study. As

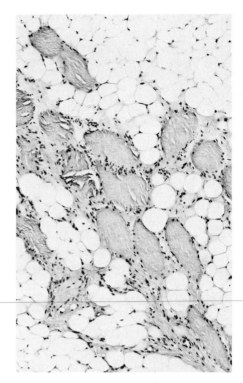

Fig. 37-25. Infiltrating intramuscular lipoma. Mature fat cells infiltrate around and between skeletal muscle fibers. (72×.)

with any fatty tumor, the distinction between these deeply situated lesions and liposarcoma is important.[514,516] The infiltrative pattern of lipoma rather than the expansile growth of liposarcoma, the absence of lipoblasts, and the bland appearance of the fat cells in lipoma serve to differentiate it from well-differentiated liposarcoma.[516]

Spindle cell lipoma

Recently described as a histologic variant of lipoma,[531] spindle cell lipoma accounts for approximately 1.5% of all adipose tumors.[532] Unlike the usual lipoma where women predominate, 90% of spindle cell lipomas occur in men.[531,532] The mean patient age is between 55 to 60 years with an age range of 20 to 81 years; over 80% of patients are older than 40 years of age.[529,531,532]

Almost all spindle cell lipomas occur in the superficial subcutaneous tissue of the posterior neck, the upper back, and the shoulder,[475,531,532] with others reported in the head, the extremities, and perianal region.[475,530-533] The tumors range from 1 cm to 14 cm, with most between 4 cm and 5 cm in diameter,[475,529,531,532] and they usually appear well-circumscribed though infiltrative patterns occur.[475,529,531]

Microscopic examination shows a variable proportion of four elements: bland-appearing, bipolar, elongate spindle cells; mature fat cells; bundles of birefringent collagen; and a myxoid stroma[475,531,532] (Fig. 37-26). In some tumors the spindle cells compose only a small portion of the lesion, with mature fat cells dominating the pattern. In others the fat cells are scarce with the lesion composed almost entirely of spindle cells.[529] The latter are usually haphazardly arranged, but at times they are grouped in such a way that their nuclei produce a palisading pattern suggestive of neurilemoma. The myxoid stroma, in combination with the strands of collagen, may also produce a pattern suggestive of neurofibroma.[514,530] On the whole, the vascular component is not prominent, but it may be so within the more myxoid regions.[532] Mast cells are sometimes numerous.[514,532] Some spindle cell lipomas have focal areas containing multivacuolated cells with hyperchromatic atypical nuclei similar to the cells found in pleomorphic (atypical) lipomas.[514,534] Despite these occasional atypical cells, which might indicate the possibility of liposarcoma, the distinction between spindle cell lipoma and the sclerosing and myxoid forms of liposarcoma is based on the absence in spindle cell lipoma of lipoblasts, nuclear pleomorphism, mitotic activity, a diffuse plexiform capillary network, and pools of mucinous material. The superficial location of spindle cell lipoma is also in sharp contrast to the usual deep location of liposarcoma.[475,529,532]

Histochemically, the fat cells show S-100 protein positivity, but the spindle cells are S-100 negative.[532] A few cases of spindle cell lipoma have been studied by electron microscopy, with conflicting results. Some suggest that the spindle cells are fibroblasts or fibroblast-like cells,[531] whereas others indicate that they are analogous to the stellate mesenchymal cells of developing primitive fat lobules.[530]

Spindle cell lipoma is cured by local excision with only rare local recurrences.[475,532]

Pleomorphic (atypical) lipoma

Fatty tumors histologically containing cells that have atypical nuclei and monovacuolated or multivacuolated cytoplasm have, in the past, all too often received the automatic diagnosis of liposarcoma with all the consequences that such a diagnosis implies. With the recent recognition of subcutaneous and intramuscular fatty tumors composed of such cells but which pursue a benign clinical course,[514,536,537,541] it is hoped that needless radical surgical procedures will be done less frequently as pathologists become familiar with these tumors for which the terms "pleomorphic" or "atypical lipoma" are used. Although some differences of opinion exist as to which lesions should be so designated,[537,541] their general histologic features are well described.[537,538,541]

As with liposarcoma, pleomorphic lipoma occurs almost exclusively in older adults who are usually between 50 and 70 years of age, with the mean patient age being about 60 years,[536,537,541] and it rarely occurs

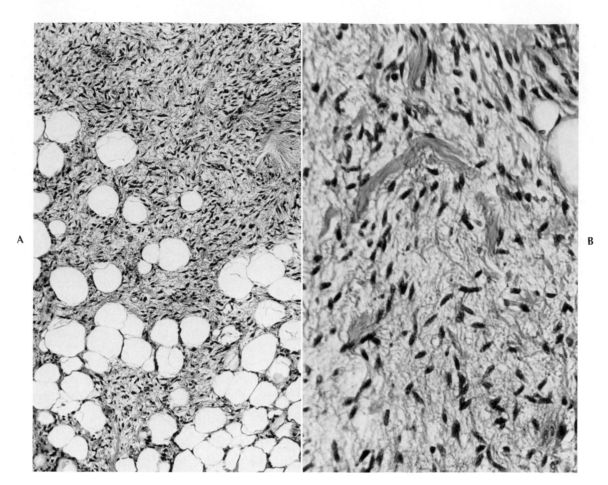

Fig. 37-26. A, Spindle cell lipoma. Mixture of mature fat cells and stellate spindle cells. **B,** Higher magnification shows spindle cells in myxoid stroma. Bundles of thick collagen fibers are present. (**A,** 90×; **B,** 350×.)

in patients less than 40 years of age.[536,537] Approximately 60% to 80% of cases occur in men.[536,537,540,541] In most patients there is a history of a slowly enlarging mass that develops over a course of months to years; it is not unusual for the mass to be present for 10 or more years.[536,537,541] In some patients, however, the mass develops rapidly within a period of only a few weeks.[537] Approximately 80% of pleomorphic lipomas occur in the subcutaneous tissue of the neck, especially the posterior aspect, the shoulder, and the upper back.[541] Other sites include the extremities, face, tongue, axilla, buttocks, and retroperitoneum.[536,537,539,542] In the few reported intramuscular cases the thigh is the most common site.[537,540] In the subcutaneous tissue the lesions are well-circumscribed and partly or completely encapsulated; the intramuscular lesions may be either well circumscribed or infiltrative. In either site, the tumors may achieve a size of 10 cm or more though the subcutaneous ones are usually smaller,[514,537] being 5 cm or less in maximum size.[536,537,540,541]

Atypical lipomas are characterized by the presence of mononuclear cells with pleomorphic nuclei, and a cytoplasm that may be vacuolated, admixed with hyperchromatic multinucleated cells.[536,541] The latter cells may have an appearance that is described as "floret like."[541] Their cytoplasm is eosinophilic, with and without vacuolization, and their multiple nuclei are arranged in a peripheral wreathlike pattern. The nuclei overlap and are smudged together much as the petals of a flower, hence their name. The number of these floret cells varies, being abundant in some cases and rare in others.[536,541] Whereas some believe that their presence is essential for the diagnosis,[475] others report such cells in only one third of cases.[537] Interspersed within the tumor are mature fat cells and "ropy" bands of thick, birefringent collagen (Fig. 37-27). Mast cells and scattered lymphocytes are also present. Focal areas of spindle cell lipoma are reported in up to one fourth of cases.[541] Although classic lipoblasts are found in these tumors, they are rare and never as frequent as in sclerosing or pleomorphic liposarcoma. Myxoid foci, either within the collagen bands or interspersed between

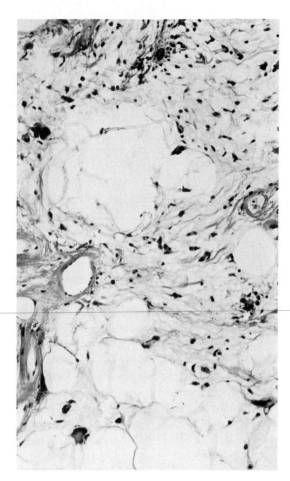

Fig. 37-27. Pleomorphic (atypical) lipoma. Hyperchromatic atypical cells within myxoid area. At lower left is floretlike cell. (150×.)

the cells, are frequent. Mitotic figures are rare to non-existent.[536,537]

The histologic differential diagnosis between pleomorphic lipoma and well-differentiated liposarcoma may at times be difficult to establish. The location of the lesion in the subcutaneous tissue, its sharp circumscription and encapsulation, and the presence of thick collagen bundles are indications of a benign lipoma rather than a liposarcoma.[541] Before making a diagnosis of subcutaneous liposarcoma, one should remember the extreme rarity of liposarcomas in this location. Liposarcomas also have a more even distribution of abnormal cells unlike that of pleomorphic lipoma where mature fat and myxoid foci are interspersed with zones containing atypical cells. The more numerous lipoblasts, the more frequent mitotic activity, and the presence of necrosis in liposarcoma also help to distinguish the two lesions. However, these histologic distinctions may be artificial in some cases, since retroperitoneal fatty tumors with a similar morphology to pleomorphic lipoma frequently behave as fully aggressive malignant tu-

mors.[476,488] Floret cells may also occur in well-differentiated liposarcomas.[476,488,493]

Some studies of subcutaneous pleomorphic lipomas indicate only rare recurrences after local excision, with patients alive and well despite even less than total excision of the tumor.[535-537,541] However, others have noted high recurrence rates in these subcutaneous tumors.[538] Metastases from pleomorphic subcutaneous lipomas are unknown. Pleomorphic lipomas involving the deep soft tissue or muscle have recurrence rates of 33% to 70%.[535,537,540] These high rates may reflect the lack of completeness of the excision and not any inherent aggressiveness of these more deeply located tumors.[537] Others disagree, claiming that such recurrences may be histologically less differentiated and clinically malignant and believe that these intramuscular lesions should be considered as low-grade liposarcomas rather than pleomorphic lipomas.[541] Retroperitoneal fatty tumors with a cellular morphology similar to pleomorphic lipoma may become "dedifferentiated" and cause death of the patient by local extension.[535,537] Despite some opinion to the contrary,[542] such retroperitoneal tumors should be considered as well-differentiated liposarcomas despite their morphologic similarity to pleomorphic lipoma.[535,537]

Angiolipoma

Angiolipoma, a histologic variant of lipoma, accounts for 5% to 17% of all benign fatty tumors.[546] They almost never develop before puberty, with the usual average patient age being between 17 and 21 years,[475,545,546] though in one series the average age was 41.7 years.[544] Men are affected more commonly than women; a familial tendency has been noted.[475] A recent report suggests the possible increased occurrence of angiolipomas in homosexual men.[548]

Most patients seek medical treatment because of single or multiple, painful or tender cutaneous nodules, usually less than 4 cm, that are located on the extremities in 70% of cases, most commonly the upper extremity. The abdomen and back are also common sites of involvement, accounting for 20% of cases.[475,545,546] The pain is usually not sharp or radiating as is that produced by glomus tumors.[545] Patients may develop additional nodules over a period of several years.

The tumor is located subcutaneously as encapsulated red-yellow nodules. Microscopically, angiolipomas are composed of mature fat cells intermixed with a proliferation of delicate thin-walled capillaries (Fig. 37-28). The proportions of these two components vary somewhat—one may find lesions composed primarily of capillaries with only a small amount of associated fat, or those with an abundance of fat and only a few capillaries.[544,545] The blood vessels are predominantly located at the periphery of the tumor beneath the capsule and

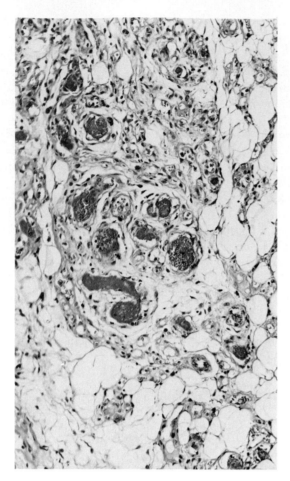

Fig. 37-28. Angiolipoma. Thin-walled blood vessels of capillary type are mixed with mature fat cells. Fibrin thrombi are visible in vessels just below center. (150×.)

proliferate centrally accompanied by fine fibrous septa that extend centrally from the capsule.[475,545,546] The fat cells lack atypia or mitotic activity. Fibrin thrombi are frequently present within the capillary lumens.[544,545] Foci of "undifferentiated" mesenchymal cells may occur, but these are not numerous.[545] Simple excision is curative, with no tendency for recurrence.[475,545,546]

An infiltrating form of angiolipoma is described that is less common than its subcutaneous counterpart and that affects patients over a broader age range,[475,546] with patients' ages varying from 2 to 67 years with an average age between 30 to 35 years.[543,546] Unlike the subcutaneous variety, infiltrating angiolipoma occurs in young children. There is no sex predilection.[543,546] The lesion involves the muscles of the lower extremity, neck, and shoulder region, and it is not usually painful.[543,546] Histologically, infiltrating angiolipoma resembles intramuscular hemangioma with its combination of blood vessels and fat. For this reason, some suggest that the term "angiolipoma" be used to designate all infiltrating hemangiomas of the deep soft tissue and muscle.[475] However, I prefer, as do others,[547] to desig-

nate those intramuscular tumors that have a mixture of vascular and fatty elements as "intramuscular hemangiomas," a description of which is given elsewhere in this chapter. Many of the so-called infiltrating angiolipomas involving the deep soft tissues of children probably represent diffuse angiomatosis rather than angiolipoma.[33]

In an electron microscopic study of angiolipoma, a decrease in the number of Weibel-Palade bodies in the capillary endothelial cells was found. It was suggested that since such a sparsity of Weibel-Palade bodies is also found in other vascular tumors there is a possible relationship between these bodies and the functional state of the endothelial cell. It was further suggested that the fibrin thrombi so frequently present in angiolipomas may be attributable to the occurrence of fibrinogen deposits that are found in the endothelial cells.[544]

Lipoblastoma

The importance of lipoblastoma, which occurs exclusively in children, resides not in what it is, but rather in what it is not. Because of the presence of lipoblasts, a myxoid stroma, and occasionally an infiltrative growth pattern, it has at times been misdiagnosed as a myxoid liposarcoma with drastic consequences for the patient.[514,556]

Approximately 90% of lipoblastomas are diagnosed in patients before 3 years of age, with the majority occurring within the first 2 years of life. The age range in one large series was from 5 days to 7 years.[550] Boys are involved more frequently than girls.[475,550] About three fourths of the tumors occur in the extremities, principally the lower extremity, but other locations include the neck, trunk, mediastinum, retroperitoneum, buttocks, and labia.[475,514,550,555] Two thirds of the lesions occur as circumscribed, encapsulated, lobular masses within the subcutaneous tissue,[514] whereas the remaining one third are deeply situated, infiltrating lesions that grow between and into muscles. Most lipoblastomas range from 3 to 5 cm, but retroperitoneal lesions may be as large as 35 cm.[550,551]

It has been suggested that the term "lipoblastoma" be reserved for the superficially located and well-circumscribed lesion and "lipoblastomatosis" be used to designate the deeper and more diffusely infiltrating lesion.[550] I prefer the single term "lipoblastoma" for both forms of the lesion. Unfortunately, some authors use "lipoblastoma" to refer to hibernoma, the benign tumor of brown fat.[553] This results in unnecessary confusion in the literature; the term "lipoblastoma" should be used only as the diagnostic label for the childhood tumor of white fat discussed here.

The microscopic pattern of lipoblastoma is dominated by the presence of small lobules formed by fibrous connective tissue septa that may be quite thick. Within the lobules are univacuolated and multivacuolated lipo-

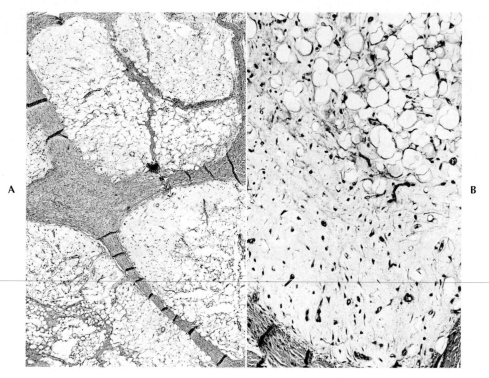

Fig. 37-29. A, Lipoblastoma. Lobules formed by fibrous septa. Notice myxoid foci adjacent to septa. **B,** Central portion of the lobule, with mature fat cells, is at top. Foci containing a few signet-ring lipoblasts, as well as stellate cells embedded in myxoid stroma, are present toward periphery of field *(bottom)*. (**A,** 26×; **B,** 120×.)

blasts that are intermingled with immature-appearing stellate and spindle-shaped mesenchymal cells and mature fat cells. There is a myxoid stroma that is especially well seen at the periphery of the lobules and in areas where the cells are less mature. Some lobules are composed entirely of mature fat cells, whereas immediately adjacent lobules may consist entirely of lipoblasts and stellate cells. In lobules with a mixture of mature and immature cells, the central portions more commonly contain the mature fat cells, giving the impression of a maturation sequence from the periphery to the center (Fig. 37-29). Cells with central nuclei and a finely vacuolated cytoplasm, resembling brown fat cells, are also occasionally present. The fibrous septa contain numerous capillaries that extend into the lobules in a plexiform pattern. Mitoses are infrequent.[475,490,514,550,552,556]

Electron microscopic studies have shown a variety of cells including immature mesenchymal cells, fibroblasts, lipoblasts, mature fat cells, and transitional intermediate cell forms. The cells resemble those in the maturation phases of white fat development, and they lack the fine-structural features of brown fat.[490,549,552,554]

Although lipoblastoma has been histologically confused with myxoid liposarcoma, its lobular character, fibrous septa, apparent zones of cell maturation within the lobules, and the absence of large mucinous pools are not characteristic of myxoid liposarcoma.[475,556] In

this regard, it is well to remember the rarity of liposarcoma in a subcutaneous location and its virtual nonoccurrence in children under 5 years of age.[481,503,550] Most cases reported in the literature as liposarcomas in infants and young children are probably examples of lipoblastomas.

Local recurrences after excision of lipoblastoma develop in up to 20% of cases, but metastases are unknown.[514,550]

Hibernoma

In contrast to tumors arising from white adipose tissue, which are the most common of all soft-tissue lesions, those originating from brown fat are among the rarest human tumors, with less than 100 case reports in the English medical literature as of 1972.[415,563,564] The name "hibernoma" derives from the tumor's histologic similarity to the brown fat of hibernating animals, but whether human brown fat is totally analogous to that of other animals is unclear.[563] Morphologically, human fetal brown fat cells and hibernoma cells are similar.[561]

Human brown fat occurs in only a few anatomic areas. In infants it is found in the interscapular area, the axilla, mediastinum, neck, posterior abdominal wall, and about the kidneys, adrenals, and pancreas. In adults, brown fat persists in the neck, axilla, mediastinum, and periadrenal and perirenal areas.[465,563,565]

Hibernomas develop in most of these same areas, with the majority occurring in the interscapular region. However, they are also found in areas that do not normally contain brown fat such as the buttock, thigh, popliteal fossa, and spermatic cord.[465,560,563,565]

Although hibernomas occur in infants as well as adults in their sixties, most patients are in the third and fourth decades of life.[465,558,563-565] The tumor develops as a painless mass that grows slowly but occasionally enlarges rapidly. Some patients have their tumors for up to 30 years.[463,563]

Grossly, hibernomas are encapsulated, soft, tan-brown to yellow-gray, lobulated subcutaneous masses. Occasional tumors develop within muscle or the retroperitoneum, where they may exceed 20 cm.[465,562-564] Histologically, the tumor cells are arranged in small lobules formed by delicate, well-vascularized, fibrous septa. The lobules themselves have a well-developed capillary network[557,561,563] and are composed of three types of round to polygonal cells—those with a diffuse granular eosinophilic cytoplasm, those with a fine multivacuolated cytoplasm, and univacuolated mature-appearing adipocytes. The proportion of these cells varies from tumor to tumor (Fig. 37-30). The multivacuolated cells, which are the most common cells present, have nuclei that are either central or eccentric, appear bland, and may contain a prominent nucleolus. The cytoplasmic vacuoles are small and delicate, giving the cells a foamy or bubbly appearance. Brown intracytoplasmic lipofuscin pigment is present in many cells. Mitoses and cellular pleomorphism are absent.[465,561,563] Cholesterol, unsaponifiable fat, and adrenal steroid hormones are found in some hibernomas.[557]

Electron microscopic studies show a similarity between hibernoma cells and those of animal brown fat cells.[561,563,565] A characteristic finding is the presence of moderately pleomorphic mitochondria having transverse cristae and plasmalemmal densities and invaginations.[557,559,561,563,565]

Hibernomas apparently have no malignant potential and are cured by simple local excision.[465,563-565] Some consider the round cell liposarcoma to be the malignant counterpart of this tumor, but there is no good evidence to support this view.[465]

VASCULAR TUMORS
Intramuscular hemangioma

Although the common benign vascular tumors, capillary and cavernous hemangioma, and benign hemangioendothelioma occur in the soft tissue, they are more frequently cutaneous lesions. Similarly, with rare exceptions, as in patients with long-standing lymphedema that occurs after radical mastectomy, the malignant vascular tumors—angiosarcoma and malignant heman-

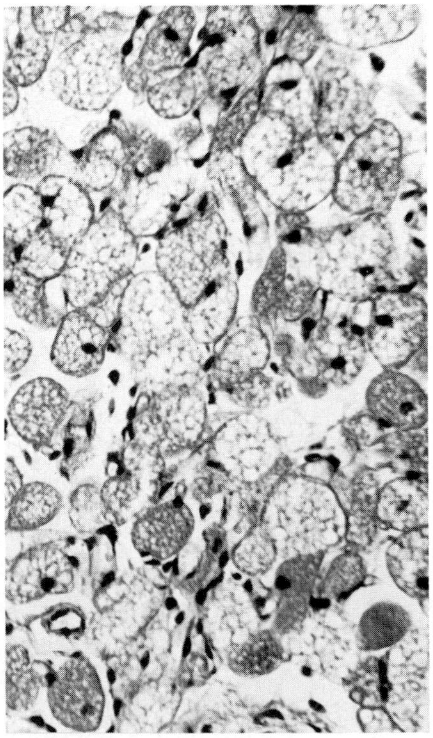

Fig. 37-30. Hibernoma. Cells with multivacuolated cytoplasm are mixed with cells having a less vacuolated, granular, darker, eosinophilic cytoplasm. (280×.)

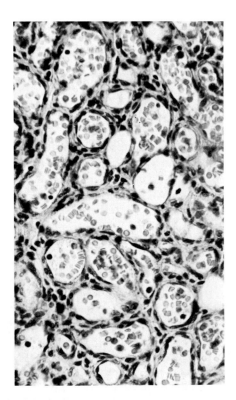

Fig. 37-31. Capillary hemangioma. Closely packed thin-walled blood vessels with small lumens containing red blood cells. (280×.)

gioendothelioma—also occur more commonly in the skin than in the soft tissues. These and other vascular tumors are described in more detail in Chapter 17.

Briefly, capillary hemangioma consists of a proliferation of small thin-walled vessels with well-defined lumens.[33,44,103] The endothelial cells are bland and usually flat (Fig. 37-31). At times, however, they round up and proliferate to such a degree, with obvious increased mitotic activity, that the vascular lumens become obscured creating solid nests and sheets of cells. This is the pattern of benign hemangioendothelioma.[103] The cavernous hemangioma is also composed of thin-walled vessels, but these are larger than in the capillary form and are dilated with gaping lumens filled with red blood cells (Fig. 37-32). Frequently both types of vessels are seen in the same lesion.

In the deep soft tissues, especially in skeletal muscle, these vascular tumors may occur as infiltrating lesions and be misdiagnosed as angiosarcoma. Histologically, few of these intramuscular lesions are of pure type, and they are categorized as either small vessel (capillary), large vessel (cavernous), or mixed types depending on which of the two types of vessels dominate the histologic pattern.[566]

Intramuscular hemangiomas occur in patients of all ages but are most frequent in young adults. Those predominantly of small vessel type occur with more or less equal frequency in the muscles of the trunk, head and neck region, and upper limbs and somewhat less frequently in the lower extremity. The large vessel type occurs more frequently in the muscles of the lower extremity, whereas the mixed type has a propensity to occur in the trunk. However, any of these forms may occur in any muscle. When the small vessel type is present, it may take on the features of a hemangioendothelioma, such that an angiosarcoma is considered. This possibility is further enhanced by the frequent presence of mitoses and apparent invasion of perineural spaces. However, the lesion lacks the bizarre cells, necrosis, multilayering of cells, and extensive pattern of intercommunicating vascular channels of angiosarcoma.[566] When evaluating such lesions one should remember that intramuscular angiosarcoma is an exceedingly rare neoplasm both in absolute terms and relative to the occurrence of intramuscular hemangioma.

In addition to the presence of blood vessels infiltrating between muscle fibers, there is frequently an abundance of adipose tissue, especially in the large vessel and mixed types of intramuscular hemangioma (Fig. 37-

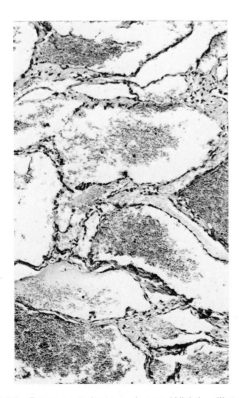

Fig. 37-32. Cavernous hemangioma. Widely dilated, thin-walled vessels containing red blood cells. (280×.)

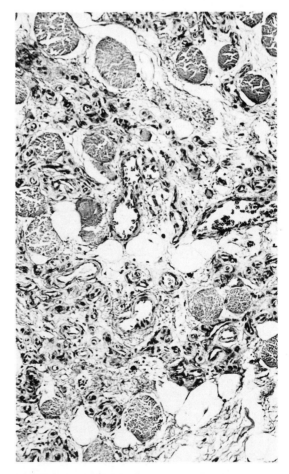

Fig. 37-33. Intramuscular hemangioma. Skeletal muscle infiltrated by blood vessels, mainly of small size. Scattered mature fat cells are present. (150×.)

33). The amount of fat may reach such a degree that it overshadows the vessels, and the lesion appears to be a lipoma or an angiolipoma.[516,566] Indeed, because of the frequent presence of fat cells, "angiolipoma" is now preferred by some as the more appropriate designation for all intramuscular hemangiomas.[465] I, as well as others, do not subscribe to this characterization.[516]

As a group, intramuscular hemangiomas recur in about 20% of cases after local excision, with the mixed pattern having a slightly higher incidence of recurrence. The lesions do not metastasize.[566]

Hemangiopericytoma

Since its original description in 1942,[590] hemangiopericytoma has been a much abused diagnosis, frequently used as a convenient histologic label for any vascular soft-tissue tumor that does not easily fit into another of the major diagnostic tumor categories. In one cancer registry series, only six of 42 cases originally diagnosed as hemangiopericytoma were acceptable as such upon histologic review.[568]

Hemangiopericytoma is uncommon, comprising from 1% to 4% of all malignant soft-tissue tumors.[19,29,75,107] In reports from two large referral institutions, only 60 and 106 cases in the soft tissues were seen in 57 and 43 years respectively.[578,584] The tumor occurs in all age groups, from newborns to adults over 90 years of age,[570] but approximately 80% to 90% occur in patients older than 20 years of age.[576,578] The mean and median patient ages are between 40 and 50 years.[568,576,578,591] In adults, male and female patients are approximately equally affected, whereas in children and infants the tumor appears to be more common in boys.[569,570,578,583,584]

Most patients seek treatment within a year of noting a lump or mass, which may be tender or painful, but others have symptoms for many years.[576,578,584] The pain is typically described as dull, a type that distinguishes it from the sharp pain of a glomus tumor with which hemangiopericytoma may be confused histologically.[578,584]

Hemangiopericytoma is a ubiquitous tumor found in virtually any location including the brain, various viscera, bones, and the soft tissues.[570,572,583,584] The most common sites include the lower extremity, where the thigh is the commonest site, the retroperitoneum and pelvic regions, the head and neck, and the trunk.[570,578,584,591,593] In adults, the tumors are typically located in the deep soft tissue, either within muscle or along fascial planes.[570,578] In infants and children, however, they usually arise in the superficial subcutaneous tissue.[567,573,577,578] Preoperative angiographic studies in hemangiopericytoma show a distinctive pattern that is not found in other vascular lesions.[594]

Grossly, hemangiopericytoma is usually well defined and may appear encapsulated. Despite its vascularity, it is often firm and rubbery with a gray, white, or tan cut surface rather than soft, spongy, and dark red or brown as might be expected.[570,578,583,591] Areas of necrosis and hemorrhage may be present. Tumor size varies from a few millimeters to 25 cm; however, most average over 5 cm.[578,579,583,591] Occasional patients have multiple tumors,[573,577,583,589,593] and rare familial cases are reported.[588]

The histopathologic pattern of hemangiopericytoma is complex and varies considerably from tumor to tumor depending on the compactness of the tumor cells. Common to all, however, are ramifying vascular spaces surrounded by closely packed, plump to spindle-shaped cells having indistinct cytoplasmic margins and oval to round, sharply defined, vesicular nuclei.[578,583,584,591] Mitotic activity is usually sparse.[578,583] The vascular channels, which are lined by flattened endothelial cells, vary in size from large sinusoidal spaces to narrow capillary-sized slits (Fig. 37-34). The angles at which the vascular channels branch create a staghorn- or antler-like effect when the histologic sections are viewed at low-power magnification.[578,591] In some cases the tumor cells compress the channels to such a degree that the tumor appears to be composed only of solidly packed cells without a vascular component.[583,591] The vascular pattern, however, can be dramatically demonstrated by the use of reticulin stains, which show an abundance of reticulin fibers distributed around each vessel and surrounding each tumor cell but absent around the lining endothelial cells.[578,583] Stains for factor VIII antigen show positive results only in the endothelial cells and not in the adjacent tumor cells,[585,591] though one study has shown weak positivity for this antigen in the tumor cells.[581]

At times, the tumor cells are arranged in a storiform pattern suggestive of fibrous histiocytoma.[576,578,591] Areas with this pattern may be so prominent that the distinction between hemangiopericytoma and fibrous histiocytoma cannot, with a reasonable degree of certainty, be made by light microscopy. Indeed, a diagnosis of hemangiopericytoma should only tentatively be made when one is dealing with small biopsy material, since hemangiopericytoma-like areas are found in a variety of other soft-tissue tumors in addition to fibrous histiocytoma, including mesenchymal chondrosarcoma, synovial sarcoma, infantile fibrosarcoma, malignant nerve sheath tumors, and leiomyosarcoma. However, unlike hemangiopericytoma, the pericytoma-like pattern in these tumors is only focally present, and hemangiopericytoma lacks a fasciculated spindle cell pattern as occurs in several of these other tumors.[578,591] A benign hemangiopericytoma-like lesion has been described in the nasal and paranasal region and should be clearly distinguished from a true hemangiopericytoma.[574,575]

Based upon electron microscopic evidence, it is now

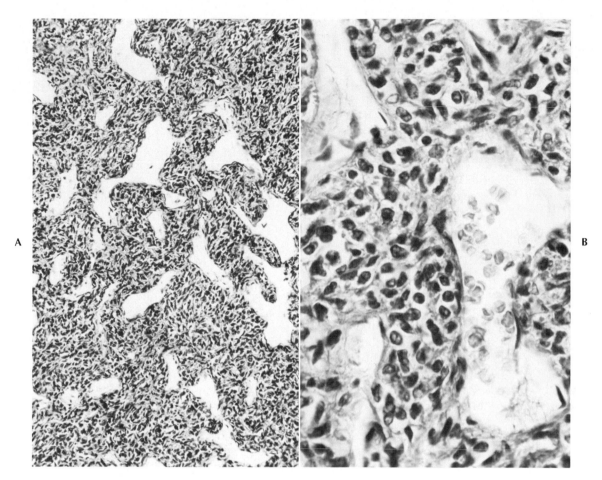

Fig. 37-34. A, Hemangiopericytoma. Vascular channels are surrounded by closely packed small cells. **B,** Higher magnification shows vessels, lined by flat endothelial cells, surrounded by pericytes. (**A,** 150×; **B,** 600×.)

generally agreed that the pericyte is the cell of origin of hemangiopericytoma. Pericytes are normally present wrapped around capillaries and postcapillary vessels and are believed to serve a contractile function.[571,577,578,584] Transitions between pericytes, endothelial cells, and smooth muscle cells in the walls of large blood vessels have been found.[571,577,584,587] The fine structure of pericytes include such features as basal lamina, pinocytotic vesicles, and cytoplasmic microfilaments.[587] Although there are some differences in the reported electron microscopic features of these cells in different studies, electron microscopy may help confirm the diagnosis when the light microscopic pattern is suggestive of hemangiopericytoma.[567,587,592]

Hemangiopericytomas are placed into benign and malignant categories based on their cellularity, degree of anaplasia, mitotic activity, and the presence or absence of necrosis. As one would expect, borderline lesions exist where a definite conclusion cannot be reached with regard to the benignity or malignancy of a particular lesion.[568,576,578,583,584] An aggressive course with metastases is reported in from 12% to 57% of he-

mangiopericytomas.[578,584] The clinical course appears to roughly correlate with the histologic pattern.[578,584] Tumors that are highly cellular, with or without anaplasia, and have a high mitotic rate have a poor prognosis. Similarly, those tumors with a low mitotic rate but with a significant degree of cellular anaplasia or necrosis are also likely to pursue a malignant course. In contrast, patients with tumors that lack these features have 10-year survival rates of 80% to 90%. However, although most hemangiopericytomas that are composed of bland cells and lack mitoses or necrosis behave in a benign fashion, rare tumors with this pattern have recurred and metastasized.[568,576]

Hemangiopericytomas are treated with wide local or radical excision as they are believed to be radioresistant[578,584]; however, some studies indicate that radiation therapy may be useful as adjuvant therapy.[579,582,586] Patients with malignant hemangiopericytomas have a survival rate of approximately 30%.[584] Patients who develop local recurrences after excision of a malignant hemangiopericytoma have a poor prognosis.[578] Recurrences and metastases, however, may be delayed for many years, and even a 15-year survival may not be indicative of a cure.[576,584] Patients may have a prolonged survival of many years despite the presence of metastatic disease.[580]

Hemangiopericytomas in infants apparently behave differently from those in adults. Microscopically these tumors show a proliferation of both endothelial cells and pericytes such that transitions between the pattern of hemangiopericytoma and hemangioendothelioma are found.[567,583] Despite the presence of necrosis and significant mitotic activity within these infantile tumors, they are reported to have a benign course.[570,573,577,578,583]

NEUROGENOUS TUMORS

The terminology of the peripheral neurogenous tumors is somewhat confused by the use of the term "schwannoma" as an appellation for both of the two major benign peripheral nerve sheath tumors, neurofibroma and neurilemoma.[602] Although the Schwann cell is present in both of these tumors,[595,599,610,626] in most cases the two are sufficiently distinct to be easily differentiated. In practice, the term "schwannoma" is used as a synonym for "neurilemoma," but only the latter term will be used here to avoid any possibility of confusion. Tumors of the sympathetic nervous system are not discussed in this chapter.

Since Schwann cells are believed to be a major cellular component of these tumors, they are considered to be neuroectodermal in origin. However, some believe that the mesodermally derived perineurial cells are the actual cells of origin of these tumors or at least take part equally with Schwann cells in their formation.[595,599,614,615] Both cell types are believed to be pleuripotential and capable of forming collagen, bone, cartilage, adipose tissue, and muscle.[595,630] This pleuripotentiality is seen most clearly in the malignant neurogenous tumors where a variety of heterogeneous tissues occur.

Neurilemoma and neurofibroma must be distinguished from the peripheral neuroma that is composed of a tangle of regenerating axons interwoven with Schwann cells, within a fibrous stroma.[595,610] (Fig. 37-35). These "traumatic" neuromas arise subsequent to some injury, be it surgical or blunt trauma, and develop as a firm, rubbery, and usually painful or tender mass at the site of the injury. They are not true tumors but rather represent an exaggeration of the normal repair process in nerve regeneration, much in the fashion of exuberant fracture callus after poor alignment of bone. They produce symptoms only after reaching large size. A variant of this process, Morton's neuroma, arises from one of the interdigital plantar nerves and forms a painful mass near the heads of the metatarsal bones. Approximately 90% are located between the third and

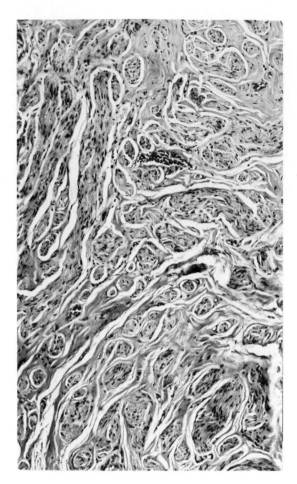

Fig. 37-35. Neuroma. Tangle of nerve bundles of various size within fibrous stroma. (90×.)

fourth toes. Morton's neuroma is probably caused by repeated trauma to this area, leading to reactive overgrowth of connective tissue that disrupts the nerves.[598,609] They are most frequent in women between 30 and 60 years of age.[610]

Neurilemoma

Neurilemomas arise from the neural sheaths of the peripheral motor, sensory, and cranial nerves, except for the optic and olfactory nerves that lack Schwann cell sheaths and are part of the central nervous system.[610,629] Neurilemomas are usually solitary painless lesions, but when large, they can produce pressure symptoms with paresthesia or local tenderness.[599,602,610,629] Neurilemomas also develop in areas that have received radiation therapy.[622] Although no age group is exempt, most patients are older than 40 years of age, with median reported ages being approximately 48 to 52 years.[601,608,613] Male and female patients are affected about equally,[33,601,608] though in some reports male patients are more prevalent[613] and in others female patients are slightly more common.[602]

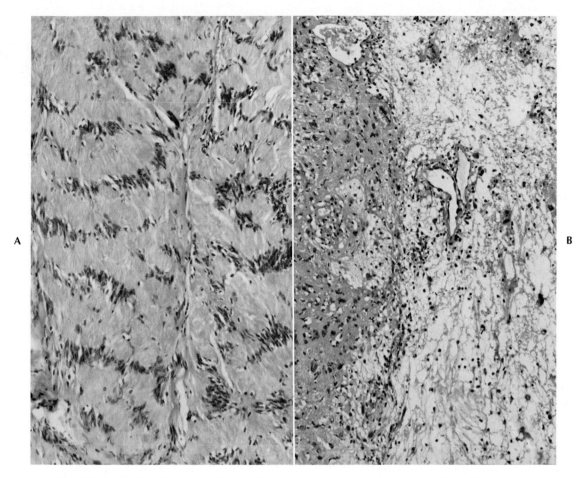

Fig. 37-36. A, Neurilemoma. Antoni A area is composed of spindle cells with tapering cytoplasmic extensions. Nuclei are aligned, creating characteristic palisading pattern. **B,** Antoni B area is present at far right with edematous stroma. More cellular Antoni A area is at left. Several blood vessels are present. (150×.)

Neurilemomas occur anywhere in the soft tissue or the viscera, but the more common locations include the soft tissue of the head and neck, especially the lateral aspect of the neck, the extremities, trunk, mediastinum, and retroperitoneum.[595,601,602,613,629] The acoustic nerve is the cranial nerve most commonly involved.[599,610] Neurilemomas are fusiform, round or oval masses that are sharply circumscribed and encapsulated.[595,599,601,610] In the more superficial soft tissue one may not be able to recognize a nerve of origin. When arising in large nerve trunks, they appear as pedunculated or bulbous masses. Although a plexiform, multinodular gross pattern is most commonly associated with neurofibromas that occur in patients with von Recklinghausen's disease, rare neurilemomas may also have this growth pattern.[606,611,632]

Neurilemomas are usually less than 5 cm, but those in the mediastinum or retroperitoneum may be as large as 20 cm.[601,602,607] On cut surface they are tan-gray to white and have a watery or slimy consistency. Larger lesions frequently have cystic and hemorrhagic foci.[599,601,610] In those that arise in large nerve trunks it may be possible to cleanly dissect the tumor off the nerve, since the nerve fibers do not course through the lesion. Occasionally, patients have multiple neurilemomas, and in patients with acoustic nerve tumors these may be bilateral. Such patients frequently also have associated multiple neurofibromas[600,610] (von Recklinghausen's disease; see Chapter 42).

Histologically, neurilemomas are most frequently biphasic tumors composed of compact cellular areas, which historically have been called "Antoni A regions," and loosely arranged hypocellular areas, known as "Antoni B regions"[595,599,601,610] (Fig. 37-36). The cells of the Antoni A areas are bipolar spindle cells with oval to elongate nuclei and eosinophilic fibrillar cytoplasm. The cells form interweaving fascicles or are so arranged that their nuclei are aligned in rows creating a palisading pattern. Although these nuclear palisades are a frequent finding, one should remember that other tumors, especially those of smooth muscle origin, may also show prominent palisades and so their presence is not diagnostic of a neurilemoma. By electron microscopy, the spindle cells have long, tapering fibrillar cytoplasmic processes. At the light microscopic level, these processes may fuse to form hyalin-like masses. At times, these hyalin-like masses are found between two parallel rows of palisaded nuclei, creating organoid structures, Verocay bodies, that simulate the appearance of tactile corpuscles.[595,603,610] These Verocay bodies are virtually pathognomonic of neurilemoma.[631] Mitotic figures are not common, but their occurrence in a neurilemoma has no clinical significance, unlike the situation in neurofibromas where the finding of more than an occasional mitotic figure is suggestive of the possibility of malignant degeneration.

In the Antoni B areas the cells are widely separated by a loose textured, watery matrix that stains poorly or not at all with stains for acid mucopolysacchride in contrast to the matrix of neurofibroma, which yields a strongly positive reaction. Microcystic spaces are also found in these Antoni B regions. Macrophages and lymphocytes are present in both A and B areas, but mast cells are infrequent. The proportions of A and B regions vary, and one or the other may dominate the pattern, but both are usually found in most neurilemomas. Another characteristic of these tumors is their abundant vascularity, with numerous small blood vessels throughout the lesion. Larger vessels with dense hyalinized walls are common and characteristic of neurilemomas. Some vessels have fibrous mural thrombi with associated evidence of recent and old hemorrhage in the adjacent stroma. Neurites (axons) are not found within the substance of the tumor, unlike their occurrence within neurofibromas.[595,599,610,623]

The role of the perineurial cell in the formation of neurilemoma has received considerable attention.[595,599,610] The relationship between the Schwann cell and the perineurial cell is still debated, with some believing that they are actually functional variants of the same cell. Indeed, rare neural tumors composed entirely of perineurial cells are reported.[615,625,627] However, electron microscopic studies of neurilemomas show that they are composed almost entirely of Schwann cells.[604,608,623] One gastric neurilemoma, studied by electron microscopy, contained cytoplasmic crystals whose morphology was similar to the crystals found in alveolar soft-part sarcoma.[616]

The cells of virtually all neurilemomas are stained by antibodies to S-100 protein. Almost all the cells in the Antoni A regions are strongly stained, whereas there is a more variable staining of cells in the Antoni B areas.[608,613,618,623,628] The finding of S-100 protein positivity in a spindle-cell soft-tissue lesion is of great help in allowing one to distinguish neurogenous tumors from fibrohistiocytic and smooth muscle tumors with which they may be confused. All neurilemomas express the intermediate filament protein vimentin[608,613] and some also coexpress glial fibrillary acidic protein.[608,611,613] Laminin and type IV collagen, both components of the basement membrane, are found in neurilemomas, corresponding to the electron microscopic presence of a complete basal lamina about the Schwann cells.[617,620]

Occasionally one finds neurilemomas whose cells are hyperchromatic and have bizarre nuclear configurations with some multinucleation. These *ancient neurilemomas* are benign, with the cellular changes reflecting degenerative phenomena.[596,600] Cellular pleomorphism in neurogenous tumors is not in itself evidence of malignancy. A form of neurilemoma has recently been described as a *cellular schwannoma*.[607,631] As the name implies, the lesion is more cellular than the usual neurilemoma, with compact spindle cells arranged in interlacing fascicles. A storiform pattern may be present but, significantly, Verocay bodies are absent. Islands of foamy histiocytes and prominent lymphoid aggregates are frequent. Although Antoni B areas may be found, they make up no more than 10% to 20% of the tumor. Because of its cellularity, the occasional occurrence of nuclear pleomorphism, and frequent mitotic activity, these cellular spindle cell neurilemomas are mistaken for other tumors, especially fibrohistiocytic or smooth muscle tumors, and some have been misdiagnosed as being malignant. Electron microscopy, however, shows the tumor cells to be Schwann cells, and by immunoperoxidase studies the cells contain S-100 protein.[607,631]

Rare neurilemomas contain glandular structures,[603,605] though whether these are actually true glands in all such cases is not clear.[605] Mesenchymal elements including fat, bone, cartilage, and angiomatous tissue also occur in neurilemomas.[612]

Upon local excision, solitary neurilemomas only rarely recur and for all practical purposes never undergo malignant degeneration,[595,599] there being only a few such cases ever reported.[494,633]

Neurofibroma

Neurofibromas occur slightly more frequently than neurilemomas and tend to occur in younger patients.[33,597,619] Male and female patients are affected equally. Neurofibromas may be solitary or multiple and in the latter form are part of the von Recklinghausen's disease complex[610] (see p. 2172). They occur as small, 2 to 4 cm nodules in the skin and subcutaneous tissue of the extremities, trunk, and head and neck region but are also found in the deep soft tissues and viscera where they grow to a large size.[595,597,610,613] Neurofibromas also arise in areas that have received prior irradiation.[622] In some patients neurofibromas are associated with local subcutaneous tissue hypertrophy and gigantism of all or part of an affected limb.[595] In patients with von Recklinghausen's disease, the skin lesions may produce protuberant, sagging disfiguring masses. In the superficial soft tissues, neurofibromas are usually ill-defined unencapsulated lesions, whereas in the deeper soft tissues they are often better circumscribed and may appear encapsulated.[595,599,609] When arising from large nerve trunks, they produce multiple irregular fusiform swellings along the nerve, creating a tangled wormlike mass. The finding of this "plexiform" neurofibroma is tantamount to a diagnosis of von Recklinghausen's disease.[610]

On gross examination neurofibromas tend to be softer than neurilemomas and have a gray-white glistening surface that has a distinctly gelatinous appearance and feels slimy. This mucoid appearance may be so noticeable as to be suggestive of a myxoma.[597,610] If the tumor arises in a well-defined large nerve, the nerve runs through the lesion such that it cannot, as with a neurilemoma, be dissected free from the tumor.

Microscopic examination of neurofibroma shows a mixture of elements.[595,597,599,610] Spindle-shaped or stellate cells with elongate and, at times, wavy or twisted nuclei are associated with scattered lymphocytes and mast cells. Collagen fibers or thick collagen bundles are present throughout the tumor, arranged in short lengths or in nodular arrays (Fig. 37-37). Unlike neurilemomas, neurofibromas contain neurites, though they are often difficult to find without the use of silver stains. The background stroma is edematous, and the tumor cells are widely separated within it. This stroma stains strongly for acid mucopolysaccharide, unlike the weak or negative reaction noted in neurilemoma.[597,610] Plexiform neurofibromas show large areas of normal nerve admixed with the spindle cells and the myxoid stroma. Alternating Antoni A and B areas are usually absent, as are the conspicuous blood vessels seen in neurilemomas. However, areas that resemble neurilemoma may occur; indeed some solitary neurofibromas have these foci to such a degree that a clear distinction between the two tumors is at times impossible.[597,610]

In the usual neurofibroma, mitoses are rare, and if more than an occasional mitotic figure is noted in several high-power fields, the possibility of malignant change should be considered. At times, as in neurilemoma, there may be cells that show nuclear pleomorphism.[597,610] However, in the absence of mitotic activity and focal necrosis, this finding is not an indication of malignancy.[33]

Unlike neurilemoma, where electron microscopic studies show that almost all the tumor cells are Schwann cells, neurofibroma has a more varied cell composition. Although Schwann cells are present, many if not most of the component cells have the morphologic characteristics of perineurial cells.[604,608] In addition, cells with features intermediate between classic fibroblasts and perineurial cells are found.[604] As with neurilemoma, S-100 protein is present in virtually all neurofibromas.[608,618,624,628] However, unlike neurilemoma, the intensity of the staining reaction for S-100 protein is not so intense[608,628] and not all cells are stained[618,624,628] presumably because the nonstaining cells represent perineurial cells. Laminin, type IV collagen, and vimentin are, as with neurilemoma, also present in neurofibroma.[613,617,620] Glial fibrillary acidic protein is rarely present in neurofibroma, unlike its more common occurrence in neurilemoma.[613] Rare and unusual forms of neurofibroma are described with a va-

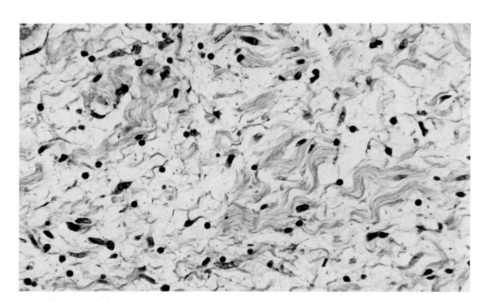

Fig. 37-37. Neurofibroma. Schwann cells within myxoid background intermixed with short, wavy collagen bundles. (350×.)

riety of histologic patterns and cell content, and these are detailed elsewhere.[33,610,621]

Solitary neurofibromas have a low incidence of recurrence after local excision as well as a low incidence of malignant degeneration, especially in those located superficially.[610] However, patients with multiple neurofibromas do have a significant risk of developing malignant neural tumors, and this risk is discussed in the next section.

Malignant nerve sheath tumor (neurosarcoma, malignant schwannoma)

The most common term used to designate malignant tumors of peripheral nerve origin is "malignant schwannoma." This usage creates some semantic difficulty, since we use the term "schwannoma" as a synonym for "neurilemoma," a tumor that virtually never undergoes malignant change.[494] Although most electron microscopic studies of malignant neural tumors do support a Schwann cell derivation,[638,639,665,667] others indicate a possible origin from perineurial cells or fibroblasts.[604] Indeed, some malignant peripheral nerve sheath tumors have histologic features of fibrosarcoma and for this reason have been termed "neurofibrosarcomas."[664] However, many malignant nerve sheath tumors do not show by light microscopy either definitive Schwann cell differentiation or the pattern of fibrosarcoma, being undifferentiated pleomorphic tumors that may contain a variety of mesenchymal and epithelial-like elements.

In the last edition of this book I used the term "neurosarcoma" to designate malignant neural tumors. Although short, easily said, and consistent with the mesenchymal appearance of many of these tumors, the term does not account for the rare epithelioid malignant neural tumors or those that contain glandular elements, and the suffix "sarcoma" ignores the neuroectodermal origin of these malignancies.[604] Currently the nonspecific term "malignant peripheral nerve sheath tumor," or "malignant nerve sheath tumor," is used to encompass all these neurogenous tumors, with more specific terms being used for the various subtypes. In this section, I use the latter appellation.

Unfortunately, regardless of the terms used, the diagnosis of a soft-tissue sarcoma as some form of neurogenic tumor has been used as a convenient way out by diagnostic pathologists faced with a spindle cell or pleomorphic sarcoma that does not obviously fit into another classification niche. I believe that the diagnosis of malignant nerve sheath tumor should be restricted to a tumor that either can be identified as clearly arising within a nerve, has histologic areas of benign neurofibroma within it, develops in an area of a previously excised neurofibroma, arises in a patient with von Recklinghausen's disease (multiple neurofibromatosis), or has electron microscopic or immunohistochemical features consistent with a neural origin. If these criteria

are used, malignant nerve sheath tumors are not common, constituting approximately 5% to 12% of all sarcomas.* They are much less common than benign nerve sheath tumors, constituting only from 2% to 12% of all nerve sheath tumors.[653,666]

Malignant nerve sheath tumors arise in patients with or without von Recklinghausen's disease.[640,641,651] Those that develop in the absence of von Recklinghausen's disease are somewhat more frequent though this depends upon how stringently the criteria for the clinical diagnosis of von Recklinghausen's disease are applied. As a group, however, patients with von Recklinghausen's disease have a higher incidence of these malignant tumors.[651] Estimates of this risk vary, with incidence figures that range from 5% to 30%,[602,641,651] but no long-term prospective study has been done to assess the true risk. In one series, malignancy developed in 19% of patients with von Recklinghausen's disease by 40 years of age, and in 53% of the patients whose multiple neurofibromas appeared between 16 and 25 years of age, a malignant neurogenous tumor developed within 5 to 8 years of the appearance of the neurofibromas.[645]

Malignant nerve sheath tumors occur in patients of all ages but are usually found in middle-aged adults with mean ages between 34 and 52 years.[635,651,661,666,667] Children are involved in approximately 15% of cases.[650] Those malignant nerve sheath tumors arising in association with von Recklinghausen's disease develop in younger patients, with a mean age of approximately 30 years, whereas patients who develop spontaneous malignant nerve sheath tumors are about 10 to 15 years older.† Female patients are somewhat more frequently affected than male patients,[651,653,663,667] though in those with von Recklinghausen's disease male patients are slightly more common.[33,641,655]

The most common initial symptom is of a swelling or mass that is painful in over half the cases.[640,641,654,667] Paresthesia, muscle atrophy, or weakness may be present if a major nerve trunk is involved.[640,641,651,654] Patients with von Recklinghausen's disease may have such a mass for many years, but this probably reflects the presence of the previous neurofibroma rather than the actual malignant tumor that develops within it.[641] The sudden onset of pain or of rapid growth in such a preexisting mass, or of a mass that rapidly develops anew in these patients is highly suspicious for malignancy. Malignant nerve sheath tumors also develop in areas that have been irradiated.[648,651,663]

Malignant nerve sheath tumors are most frequently located in the extremities, the trunk, or paravertebral areas.‡ The head and neck region is not so frequently involved as it is for benign neurogenous tu-

---

*References 19, 29, 75, 96, 107, 108, 123, 635.
†References 604, 640, 641, 651, 654, 655, 663.
‡References 53, 635, 641, 651, 653, 654, 664, 667.

mors.[33,635,640,651] Patients with von Recklinghausen's disease tend to have tumors that are centrally located on the trunk, shoulder region, and pelvic area, with few located on the distal aspect of the extremities.[651,654,663] The tumors frequently involve major nerve trunks where they form fusiform or nodular swellings that infiltrate the nerve proper.* Their cut surface commonly shows areas of necrosis and hemorrhage. In patients with von Recklinghausen's disease the tumors may arise in the soft tissue adjacent to a major nerve or in an area where a major nerve cannot be grossly identified.[641] Malignant nerve sheath tumors tend to be large, commonly exceeding 10 cm.[635,651,653,654]

Schwann cells, or perineurial cells, are considered to have the ability to produce a variety of tissue elements including collagen.[638,657] It is not surprising therefore that malignant nerve sheath tumors may have well-differentiated fibrosarcomatous foci composed of spindle cells arranged in interlacing fascicles in a herringbone pattern.† Indeed, without knowledge that the lesion originated within a nerve, these neurofibrosarcomas may be indistinguishable from their soft-tissue counterparts. Tumor cell nuclei vary from elongate forms with wavy or irregular configurations to those that are round

---

*References 53, 640, 641, 651, 654, 667.
†References 609, 640, 651, 654, 661, 667.

and plump with hyperchromasia and various degrees of pleomorphism (Fig. 37-38). The stroma may be fibrotic or myxomatous, with highly cellular spindle-cell areas frequently admixed with looser, hypocellular zones. In some cases the spindle cells are arranged in a storiform or cartwheel pattern that is indistinguishable from that of malignant fibrous histiocytoma.[656,661,665]

Mitoses are frequent, usually one or more per every high-power field, as are foci of hemorrhage and necrosis.[53,609,653,654,661,667] Some neurofibrosarcomatous tumors may be so well differentiated that only the finding of significant mitotic activity serves as a clue to their malignant nature. Most malignant nerve sheath tumors, especially those arising in von Recklinghausen's disease, show some benign neurofibromatous foci.[651] Undifferentiated pleomorphic sarcomas composed of bizarre giant cells and polygonal mononuclear tumor cells with irregular hyperchromatic nuclei also arise within nerves; patients with von Recklinghausen's disease have a tendency to develop these pleomorphic tumors.[641,651,653]

Metaplastic elements, including malignant osteoid, cartilage, fat, and rhabdomyosarcomatous foci, are found in approximately 15% of malignant nerve sheath tumors.[610,649,650,657] Those with rhabdomyosarcomatous elements are referred to as malignant *Triton* tumors.[637,642,646,671] Care must be exercised, however, in

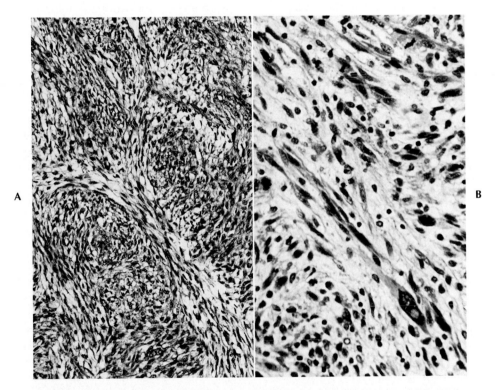

Fig. 37-38. A, Malignant nerve sheath tumor. Cellular nodules of spindle cells. **B,** Higher magnification shows pleomorphic cells in elongate shapes. Mitotic figures are present at top and at left of center. Lymphocytes are scattered among the tumor cells. (**A,** 120×; **B,** 280×.)

making this diagnosis, since normal skeletal muscle fibers may become entrapped by the tumor. In addition, there are rare benign neural sheath tumors that contain benign skeletal muscle elements.[634,636,660]

Malignant nerve sheath tumors composed of cells with epithelioid features and melanocytic differentiation are found,[647,659,661] as well as those with gland formation, the latter of which may have goblet cell or endocrine differentiation.[610,652,668,670] Neurogenous tumors with ganglion cells or neuroblastomatous tissue in combination with one or more malignant mesenchymal elements, most commonly rhabdomyosarcoma, are termed "malignant ectomesenchymomas" and are predominantly found in infants.[657,658]

There are neurilemomas that, because of their cellularity, occasional foci with nuclear pleomorphism, and mitotic activity, may be confused with a malignant nerve sheath tumor.[607,631] These *cellular schwannomas* are described on p. 1892.

By electron microscopy, the better differentiated spindle cell malignant nerve sheath tumors are composed of cells with intertwining cytoplasmic processes in which may be found intermediate and microfilaments, microtubules, and, in some cells, dense core granules. Intercellular junctions are also found. A basal lamina is usually found but may be only focally present and incomplete in the less differentiated or pleomorphic tumors.[604,608,638,639,665,667] Others have found a wide spectrum of morphologic features in these tumors, with Schwann cell, fibroblastic, fibrohistiocytic, histiocytic undifferentiated, and perineurial type of cells present.[604,655]

Immunohistochemical studies have demonstrated S-100 protein in from 50% to 90% of malignant nerve sheath tumors.[628,635,643,655,661,669] Vimentin is present in over 90% of cases.[669] Type IV collagen is also present and may be helpful in distinguishing spindle-cell malignant nerve sheath tumors from fibrohistiocytic lesions, which lack type IV collagen.[620]

Malignant nerve sheath tumors are highly aggressive lesions. Recurrences occur after local excision in from 45% to 80% of patients.* The prognosis is poor for those patients with associated von Recklinghausen's disease where 5-year survival rates range from 15% to 30% versus 50% to 75% for those patients with tumors arising anew.† It is not uncommon, however, for recurrence and metastases to develop 5 to 10 years after therapy.[653,654] The development of local recurrence in patients with associated von Recklinghausen's disease portends a grave prognosis, with almost all patients dying of their disease.[663] Small tumors (less than 5 cm) have a better prognosis than larger lesions.[651] Centrally

located tumors have a poorer prognosis than those on the distal aspect of the extremities. This may reflect the propensity for central tumors to grow to a large size before therapy. Malignant *Triton* tumors, those with glandular differentiation, and radiation-induced tumors also carry a poor prognosis.[637,642,646,648,662,670,671]

Children with malignant nerve sheath tumors do poorly,[650,662] but this may reflect the extent of the surgical resection, since those patients with completely resected tumors have a better prognosis than those in whom there is gross evidence of residual tumor.[662]

MISCELLANEOUS TUMORS
Myxoma

Myxomas are benign tumors that occur in a variety of locations, including the heart, bones, skin, subcutaneous and aponeurotic tissue, genitourinary tract, and skeletal muscle.[103,680,683,686] Myxoma of skeletal muscle is the lesion that mainly concerns us here, since its gross infiltrative pattern causes it to be occasionally misdiagnosed as one of the myxoid-appearing sarcomas.[53,672,677,679] Several tumors and tumorlike conditions of the soft tissues have a mucinous stroma that so dominates the histologic picture they resemble myxoma.[672,677] Indeed, it is probable that some previously reported myxomas were actually other lesions.[103,675]

Although myxomas occur in children, some even in newborns,[675] the intramuscular myxoma is unusual in patients less than 20 years of age.[53,677-681,684] It most frequently occurs in adults, with a mean age of 50 to 55 years,[676,678,679,684] with women being more commonly affected than men.[676,679,684]

Myxomas develop as masses that either tend to grow slowly or are stationary for long periods before suddenly enlarging.[677,686] Most are painless[677,679] and present for an average of 2 to 4 years before treatment.[680,686] However, some patients have their lesions for as long as 10 years, whereas others note their lesions to develop in only a few weeks.[677-680,686] There is no apparent relationship between the size of the myxoma and the duration of its presence.[678,679]

Some myxomas develop subcutaneously or arise from fascial planes and neurovascular sheaths.[103,675,680,686] The intramuscular myxomas tend to involve large muscles, especially those of the thigh, buttocks, upper arm, and shoulder.[676,677,679-681,683] Myxomas also occur in the head and neck, hand, lower leg,[677,679,681] pelvic girdle,[680,684] chest wall,[679,681] axilla, and the clavicular and scapular areas.[684]

On physical examination, the tumor is movable when the involved muscle is relaxed but becomes fixed upon contracture of the muscle.[681] Computerized tomographic and angiographic studies show a homogeneous, low-density, and hypovascular mass that does

---

*References 640, 641, 651, 653, 663, 664, 667.
†References 635, 637, 640, 641, 653, 654, 661, 663.

not become enhanced after intravenous contrast agents. These findings are in contrast to what is found in myxoid liposarcoma, a tumor that may be confused with intramuscular myxoma both clinically and pathologically. Myxoid liposarcoma is hypervascular and shows tomographic enhancement with contrast agents.[676,679,681,683,684]

Grossly, myxomas appear sharply circumscribed and when in the superficial soft tissue may be encapsulated.[680] Intramuscular myxoma, however, lacks a true capsule, and histologically infiltrates the involved muscle.[53,678,680,681] It may also attach itself to the periosteum of adjacent bone or to the overlying fascia.[677,679] Although most myxomas have an average size of from 4 to 6 cm.,[676,677,679,684] those in muscle may exceed 15 cm.[679,680,683] Their consistency may be soft, firm, or even hard.[679,684] The cut surface has a grayish-white to snow-white, glistening, gelatinous appearance and is slimy; mucinous material may drip from its surface. Fibrous septa or trabecular strands traverse the lesion, and millimeter-sized cysts may be present.

Microscopic examination shows a sea of hyaluronidase-sensitive acid mucopolysaccharide myxoid material[672,677,679] in which reside widely separated stellate, oval, or spindle-shaped cells having an ill-defined cytoplasm and nuclei that may contain small vacuoles. Some cells seem to consist of only a hyperchromatic, degenerated nucleus embedded in the mucoid stroma (Fig. 37-39). Although the cellularity of individual tumors varies, most are sparsely cellular.[53,672,677,679,680,684] Within the stroma is a network of reticulin fibers and thin collagen fibers that course in various directions[672,675,677,679,687] but do not surround individual cells as they do in liposarcoma. Microcystic areas are sometimes present,[679,684] and amorphous stromal calcification is reported.[683] Of significance, especially in the differential diagnosis between myxoma and myxoid sarcomas, is the fact that myxomas are poorly vascularized and lack any mitotic activity.[53,677-680,684] Within muscle the tumor expands and infiltrates between muscle fibers causing their atrophy and necrosis.[677,679,684]

Immunohistochemical studies show the presence of vimentin in the tumor cells and the absence of S-100 protein, desmin, and markers for endothelial cells.[679,684] The cells also lack glycogen. Electron microscopically, the majority of the tumor cells have fibroblastic features,[678,679] though myofibroblast-like cells[684] and primitive mesenchymal cells[679] are also found. Current evidence favors the concept that myxomas originate from primitive mesenchymal cells that differentiate as fibroblasts that have lost their capacity to produce collagen and instead produce excess amounts of hyaluronic acid.[677,680]

It is the infiltrative character of myxoma, combined

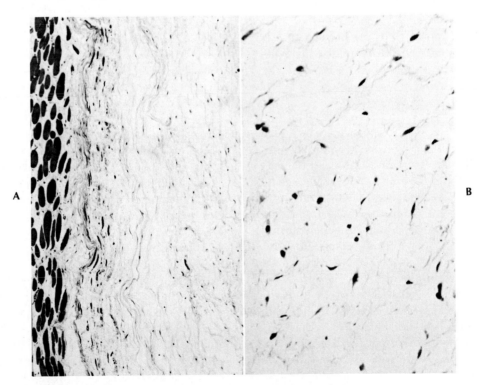

Fig. 37-39. A, Intramuscular myxoma. Pale, relatively hypocellular area, with pushing type of border, within skeletal muscle. **B,** Higher magnification shows small hyperchromatic oval to spindle-shaped nuclei in loose stroma. Notice lack of blood vessels. (**A,** 72×; **B,** 280×.)

with its myxoid stroma, that has caused it to be confused with malignant tumors, especially myxoid liposarcoma and myxoid malignant fibrous histiocytoma.[53,672,677,679,686] Myxoid liposarcoma, though having foci of hypocellular mucinous pools, is more cellular than myxoma and in addition has lipoblasts, and its cells contain glycogen and S-100 protein. Most important, however, is the prominent and diffuse plexiform capillary network of liposarcoma that is absent in myxoma. Myxoid malignant fibrous histiocytoma is easily distinguished from myxoma because of its pleomorphic cells and numerous mitotic figures.

Rarely, some patients develop multiple intramuscular myxomas; such patients have a notable incidence of associated fibrous dysplasia of bone. The myxomas develop many years after the appearance of the bone lesions, most of which are polyostotic. The myxomas seem to occur in the vicinity of the most severely affected bones.[674,680,687] Albright's syndrome is also noted with this clinical combination,[672] which may be associated with the occurrence of hypophosphatemic osteomalacia.[674,682]

Recently, a locally aggressive myxoid tumor that is histologically similar to a myxoma but contains a prominent vascular component has been reported. The tumor, termed "aggressive angiomyxoma," occurs predominantly in women and involves the genital tract, pelvis, and perineum.[673,685] It has a significant recurrence rate after local excision and may account for some previous reports that indicated recurrences in deeply situated myxomas. In contrast, intramuscular myxomas are cured by simple local excision and do not recur locally.[53,677-681,684]

Synovial sarcoma

Synovial sarcoma accounts for approximately 5% to 15% of all sarcomas.* Although no age group is exempt, this tumor principally affects young adults, with almost three fourths of the patients being younger than age 40 years[723] with the mean patient age ranging from 30 to 35 years.[691,696,712,720,723,724] In most series male patients are affected more commonly than female patients in ratios of 1.4:1 to 2:1,[692,702,712,723] but in some studies the sex incidence has been either roughly equal or female patients have been more frequent.[691,696,720,724]

By light microscopy, synovial sarcoma, as its name implies, has some semblance to synovial tissue, with spindle and epithelial cell elements. From this, one might expect that the tumor originates from synovial membranes. This type, however, is the exception rather than the rule, with only about 10% to 20% of the tumors actually involving joint structures,[87,103,212,720,723] since the tumor is usually found

only in the vicinity of large joints and bursae.

Approximately 75% to 95% of synovial sarcomas occur in the extremities, with the lower extremity involved in 40% to 70% of cases.[690,712,714,720,723,724] Principal locations include the thigh in the area of the hip joint, the knee, the ankle, the shoulder, and the wrist.[103,690,692,720,724] Synovial sarcoma is also found in regions where synovial tissue is not present as in the anterior abdominal wall, the pelvis, the anterolateral aspect of the neck, the orofacial area, including the tongue and soft palate, the paravertebral connective tissue from the base of the skull to the hypopharynx, and the wall of the femoral vein.[690,704,707,711,713,717] Such extrasynovial sites of origin, combined with electron microscopic and immunohistochemical studies of synovial sarcoma that show differences from normal synovial tissue (see p. 1900) has convinced some that the term "synovial sarcoma"is a misnomer that should be eliminated in favor of "carcinosarcoma of soft tissue."[698,701,709] Despite the evidence indicating a lack of origin from synovial tissue, there is no advantage in changing the name of this lesion, especially since synovial sarcoma is a term that is so well ingrained in the literature.

Unlike most soft-tissue sarcomas, synovial sarcoma is frequently associated with pain that in about 25% of cases is not related to a palpable mass, the pain being of the referred type.[670,692,723] The pain, either localized or referred, may exist for several years before the appearance of a mass.[690] The duration of symptoms is variable, averaging approximately 2½ years, but some patients have symptoms for as long as 20 years.[103,691,723] It is not uncommon, however, for a mass to be present for only a few months before the patient seeks treatment.[692,723]

Roentgenographic examination shows tumor calcification in from 20% to 40% of cases.[692,723] This finding, combined with the presence of a painful mass near a major joint in a young person, is highly suggestive of synovial sarcoma. The tumor has no characteristic gross appearance and varies in size from 1 to 30 cm,[720,723] with most being at least 5 cm.[720,723,724]

Histologically, "classic" synovial sarcoma is characterized by a biphasic pattern consisting of a fibrosarcoma-like proliferation of spindle cells, arranged in sheets or fascicles, in which are scattered pale or eosinophilic epithelial-like cells that either line cleftlike spaces, occur as small islands surrounded by swirls of spindle cells, or are arranged in true glandular formation[53,103,690,702,723,724] (Fig. 37-40). The spindle cells may be plumper or more oval and have rounder nuclei than the usual fibroblast.[690,702,720,723] The glands are composed of cuboidal to columnar cells, and their lumens are filled with a hyaluronidase-resistant mucinous secretion that stains positively with periodic acid–Schiff, mucicarmine, and Alcian blue stains.[696,699,713,723,724] Hy-

---

*References 19, 29, 75, 96, 107, 108, 690, 697, 700, 720.

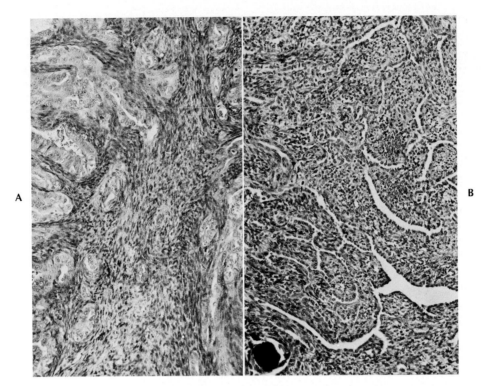

Fig. 37-40. A, Synovial sarcoma. Classic biphasic pattern is composed of glandlike spaces, formed by pale-staining cuboidal to columnar cells, residing in spindle cell stroma. **B,** Another synovial sarcoma. Here spaces are slitlike and resemble vascular channels. However, they are lined by cuboidal cells. Fragment of calcium is present at lower left. (150×.)

aluronidase-sensitive stromal mucosubstance is present in the spindle cell areas.[713] Reticulin fibers are present about the spindle cells but absent within the epithelial or glandular foci.[53,103,720] Hypocellular, loose myxoid regions may alternate with compact cellular areas much like the pattern found in malignant nerve sheath tumors.[724] The proportion of spindle and epithelial-like cells that are present varies not only from tumor to tumor, but even within different areas of the same tumor.[702] The spindle cell component is usually dominant, such that at times numerous sections must be examined before one finds any epithelial-like elements.[699,702] However, occasional synovial sarcomas have such an abundance of epithelial tumor, with only a minor portion of the tumor containing spindle cells, that metastatic adenocarcinoma is suggested.[703] Pleomorphism of either the spindle or epithelial-like cells is not a feature of synovial sarcoma.[690] Squamous differentiation or metaplasia of the glandular foci may rarely occur.[710] Synovial sarcoma is usually highly vascular, with the spindle cells surrounding and abutting narrow vascular slits or dilated vascular channels producing areas suggestive of hemangiopericytoma.[53,696,699,720,724] Mast cells are abundant.[696,713,720,724] In some cases, broad, hyalinized, scarlike zones and bands of collagen

are found.[53,696,720,724] Microscopic calcification, sometimes quite extensive, is found in from 30% to 60% of cases.[690,713,720,722,724]

A "monophasic" form of synovial sarcoma that is composed entirely of spindle cells or, more rarely, of epithelial-like cells is reported. Indeed, the authors of such reports indicate that in their experience the classic biphasic pattern is actually found in a minority of synovial sarcomas.* It should be noted that virtually no report on monophasic synovial sarcoma gives any indication of the number of sections that were obtained from such tumors in an attempt to discover an epithelial component. I suspect that at least some so-called monophasic synovial sarcomas would, upon more extensive examination, prove to have a biphasic pattern. I agree with those who believe it unwise to diagnose a tumor as synovial sarcoma by routine light microscopy in the absence of a biphasic pattern.[53,103,702] Given the cluster of clinical findings mentioned above, a spindle-cell tumor of soft tissue must be examined diligently for the presence of a biphasic pattern, and if this is not found, I do not believe that more should be read into the sections than is there. This diagnostic problem, however,

---

*References 688, 694, 696, 697, 699, 700, 724.

may be resolved by the use of immunohistochemical methods. Stains for cytokeratin and epithelial membrane antigen are positive in the epithelial components of biphasic tumors, whereas vimentin is present in the spindle cells. There is some question in the literature as to whether the epithelial-like cells also contain vimentin.[701,707,719] Of more importance, however, is the finding of cytokeratin and epithelial membrane antigen positivity within the spindle cells though the number of such cells that stain for these antigens may be as few as 5% to 10% of the total cells present.[688,694,697,707,708] However, the mere presence of an epithelial marker such as cytokeratin in a spindle cell tumor should not be taken as prima facie evidence that the lesion is a synovial sarcoma, since other sarcomas may show cytokeratin positivity, including such spindle-cell tumors as leiomyosarcoma and malignant fibrous histiocytoma.[274,317,326,351,355] *Ulex europaeus* I, a marker for endothelial cells, has been found in the epithelial-like cells of the biphasic tumors.[688,709]

Perhaps the best evidence for the existence of a monophasic variant of synovial sarcoma is the electron microscopic data that show evidence of epithelial differentiation in the spindle cells of both the monophasic and biphasic tumors. Tight cellular junctions and even desmosomes are found, along with intercellular spaces containing microvillous cell projections, and basement membrane material (basal lamina) that is present about both the epithelial-like and spindle cells of biphasic tumors. Although basal lamina is also found about the spindle cells of monophasic tumors, it is usually only focally present and not so frequent as about the spindle cells of the biphasic tumors.[688,693,695,697,700,705] These electron microscopic features, as well as the immunohistochemical findings noted above, help serve to distinguish the spindle cell component of synovial sarcoma from those of fibrosarcomas or malignant nerve sheath tumors, though the rare occurrence of glandular differentiation in the latter tumor may result in a pattern that, by morphologic features alone, may be impossible to distinguish from synovial sarcoma.

Basement membranes and cellular junctions are not found in the type A and type B cells that are the components of normal synovial membranes, and normal synovial lining cells stain positively for vimentin protein but not for cytokeratin,[707,709,715] further evidence that synovial sarcomas do not arise from synovial tissue.[695,698,705,716] Current opinion concerning the histogenesis of these tumors is that they originate from undifferentiated mesenchymal cells that can differentiate into spindle and epithelial-like cells.[702,711,713] Whether true or not, this is a convenient explanation for the occurrence of synovial sarcomas in areas such as the abdominal wall, tongue, soft palate, and neck where synovial tissue is not present.

Cytogenetic studies of a few synovial sarcomas have discovered an apparently consistent translocation involving the X-chromosome and chromosome 18.[689,718,721]

Prognostically, synovial sarcomas may pursue a protracted course, with metastases developing as late as 20 years after treatment.[53,103,212,690,700] The average duration of survival is from 5 to 6 years, and long-term survival is possible even in the presence of metastases.[53,690] Local recurrences after excision develop in from 30% to 75% of patients.* There is a wide scatter in the reported 5-year survival rates that range from 3% to 58%.† However, most recent studies indicate 5-year survival rates of approximately 40% to 50%,[712,720,723,724] with 10-year survival rates uniformly lower, reflecting the emergence of late metastases.[53,690,692,700,720,723] Indeed, some believe that metastases are to be expected to develop in most patients if they are followed for a sufficient time and that no real cures are achieved, since survival curves never come to parallel expected life curves.[103,723] Metastases are primarily blood borne, with the lungs and bones the most commonly involved sites.[690,696,712,714,723] Metastases to regional lymph nodes usually occur in less than 10% of cases[712,714,723] but in some series occur in 20% or more of the cases.[87,690,723] Whereas metastases from biphasic tumors may have either a biphasic or a monophasic pattern, metastases from monophasic tumors apparently remain monophasic.[696,699,700]

Synovial sarcomas containing extensive calcification have a significantly better prognosis than those without calcification,[722] as do those with a dominant glandular component, those with a low mitotic rate, and those that are smaller than 5 cm.‡ In studies that separate monophasic from biphasic tumors, the monophasic variety has an increased incidence of local recurrence and a lower 5-year survival rate.[699,700,724]

Epithelioid sarcoma

Epithelioid sarcoma has only recently been well defined as a specific soft-tissue tumor.[732,734] It comprises less than 2% of all sarcomas.[29,96,107,108,123] An important aspect of this tumor is that in its early stages its clinical and histologic features may cause it to be confused with an inflammatory process, and only after repeated local recurrences is the suggestion of malignancy finally raised.[734] This delay does nothing to enhance the patient's chance for survival.

Epithelioid sarcoma most often occurs in male patients, the male-to-female ratio being approximately 2:1.[729,744] Although reported in patients ranging in age

---

*References 691, 692, 696, 700, 702, 712, 723, 724.
†References 53, 212, 690, 692, 699, 700, 702, 713.
‡References 691, 696, 699, 710, 712, 723, 724.

from 2½ to 90 years, approximately 60% to 70% of patients are between 10 and 40 years of age, with mean ages of approximately 30 to 35 years.[727,729,732,734,744,745]

The tumor develops as a painless, subcutaneous, or dermal nodule that slowly enlarges over months to years.[727,734,745] Although the average duration of symptoms ranges from 1 to 3 years, some patients have their lesions for more than 25 years.[727,729,732,745] In from 20% to 70% of cases there is a history of previous trauma to the site of the tumor.[729,732]

About 90% to 95% of epithelioid sarcomas arise in the extremities, usually in the distalmost aspect of the extremity. Slightly over half the cases arise in the hand and forearm, with the most common sites being the volar aspect of the fingers, the palm, and the extensor surfaces of the forearm.[727,732,734,744,745] In the lower extremity the ankle and foot are the most common sites.[727,744] Other locations include the scalp,[725,734] penis,[735,742] vulva,[748] pelvis,[747] buttocks,[732] abdominal wall,[726] and the sternocleidomastoid muscle and neck.[732,745,749]

Epithelioid sarcoma arises in the subcutaneous tissue and superficial fascia and occasionally from tendons and tendon sheaths.[728,734,747] It appears as nonencapsulated firm nodules, which may be woody hard, that eventually become confluent.[729,732] Ulceration of the skin over the tumor may occur, leading to the clinical impression that the lesion is inflammatory.[734] Sinus tracts between the nodules and the overlying ulcerated skin may be present.[729] In some cases, especially with recurrences, multiple separate nodules develop along the length of the extremity.[728] The gross extent of the tumor is usually greater than suspected clinically, since the tumor tends to microscopically grow along tendons, fascia, and nerve trunks.[727,732,733,744,748] The more superficially located tumors are usually less than 2 cm, but deeply located tumors are larger, with some as large as 15 cm.[728,729,732,734,745]

Histologically, the dominant tumor cells are large, polygonal, and mononuclear, with vesicular nuclei and prominent nucleoli. The cytoplasm is characteristically abundant and deeply eosinophilic, giving the cells their epithelioid appearance.[729,732,734,747] The more deeply eosinophilic of these cells may resemble rhabdomyoblasts,[729,732] or rhabdoid cells.[733] Although occasional binucleate and multinucleated giant cells are present,[729,745,747] pleomorphism is not prominent.[737,740] Signet-ring cells, which may be mistaken for adenocarcinoma cells or lipoblasts, may be found.[729,741] Mixed with these cells and showing transitional forms with them are fusiform fibroblast-like cells.[729,732,747] Special stains show the presence of lipid and glycogen within the tumor cells and the absence of mucin.[729,732,741,748] Mitotic activity may or may not be conspicuous.[737,734,740] The tumor cells are frequently arranged in

nodules that commonly show central areas of degeneration and necrosis (Fig. 37-41). In other areas the cells grow as diffuse masses.[729] Microscopic calcification or ossification is found in approximately 30% of cases.[729]

Between the tumor nodules there is a prominent desmoplastic stroma of densely hyalinized collagen.[729,732,734,746] The collagen is frequently infiltrated by tumor cells, creating small nests and cords that simulate the pattern of an infiltrating carcinoma.[732,748] The overlying skin may be ulcerated by tumor, but it is otherwise normal.

Numerous electron microscopic studies, most of which are of single cases, have shown a variety of morphologic cell characteristics including tight cellular junctions, lipid droplets, glycogen, interdigitating filopodia, occasional pseudoacini, and whorled intermediate cytoplasmic filaments that are usually in a perinuclear location.*

Although the above microscopic description would appear to make the histologic diagnosis of epithelioid sarcoma fairly straightforward, in practice there may be considerable diagnostic difficulty, especially when only biopsy material is in hand.[729,737] The presence of centrally necrotic nodules surrounded by epithelioid cells has caused diagnostic confusion with necrobiotic granulomas.[729,732,734,737,749] In addition, the focal infiltrating pattern, combined with tumor ulceration of the skin, has resulted in mistaken diagnoses of either epidermoid carcinoma or malignant melanoma.[732,734,746]

Immunohistochemical studies show an epithelial differentiation with positive staining reactions in the epithelioid cells for cytokeratin and epithelial membrane antigen.[730,735,740,743,747,749] The degree and uniformity of the latter reactions, however, varies greatly from tumor to tumor, and only rare staining of the spindle cells is noted. The tumor cells also show concomitant positivity for vimentin protein.[735,740,743,747] Alpha$_1$-antitrypsin and alpha$_1$-antichymotrypsin are also found in the majority of the tumors.[729,743] Occasional cases in which S-100 protein is present in the tumor cells are reported,[729,740,747] so that the distinction between epithelioid sarcoma and malignant melanoma depends on the presence of cytokeratin or epithelial membrane antigen in the former. The occasional cytoplasmic vacuolization of the epithelioid cells in epithelioid sarcoma may simulate primitive vascular lumens and cause diagnostic confusion with epithelioid hemangioendothelioma.[729,750] The cells of both these tumors are positive for *Ulex europaeus* I, whereas factor VIII antigen is present in the cells of epithelioid hemangioendothelioma but absent in those of epithelioid sarcoma.[750]

The propensity of epithelioid sarcoma to spread along fascial planes, tendon sheaths, and blood vessels results

---

*Reference 729, 731, 732, 735, 738, 739, 741, 744, 748.

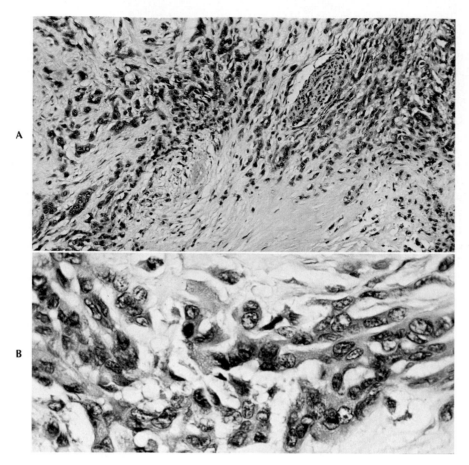

Fig. 37-41. A, Epithelioid sarcoma. Nodule with fibrotic center surrounded by strands and clusters of tumor cells. **B,** Higher magnification of tumor cells with epithelioid appearance. Cells have abundant eosinophilic cytoplasm. They may be arranged in long infiltrating strands. (**A,** 120×; **B,** 480×.)

in local recurrence rates of from approximately 65% to 80% after surgical excision.[729,744-747] Metastases, which usually develop only after repeated local recurrences, occur in 40% to 45% of cases,[729,732,734,744] with the lungs, lymph nodes, skin of the scalp, and bones being the most frequently involved sites.[727,729,745] Five-year survival rates are between 60% to 70%[727,729,745]; however, the clinical course may be quite protracted, with some patients dying of tumor 15 to 20 years after initial therapy[727,729,732] and so 5-year survival rates are no indication of cure. Age, sex, tumor size, location, and microscopic pattern all have prognostic value. The best prognosis is found in young patients, female patients, those whose tumors are located in the distal parts of the extremities, and those whose tumors are less than 2 cm. Patients with deeply located tumors and those with tumors that show vascular invasion, extensive necrosis, and lymph node metastases have a poor prognosis.[727,729,745]

The histogenesis of epithelioid sarcoma remains cloaked behind a variety of conflicting opinions that are based mainly on electron microscopic studies, with almost as many opinions as there are studies.[735] Whereas some claim that the tumor originates from undifferentiated mesenchymal cells that differentiate along synovial, histiocytic, or epithelial lines,[726,734,735,743] others believe that it is a variant of synovial sarcoma,[731,736] or a histiocytic,[744] myofibroblastic,[725] or fibrohistiocytic tumor.[732]

Clear cell sarcoma

In most series, clear cell sarcoma accounts for from 0.5% to 2% of all soft-tissue sarcomas.* Prior to its description as a distinct tumor type, clear cell sarcoma was frequently diagnosed as some other tumor type, especially synovial sarcoma.[757] Despite its infrequent occurence, clear cell sarcoma has stimulated a great deal of interest because of its unusual morphology and possible histogenesis.

Although patients from 7 to 83 years of age are re-

---

*References 19, 29, 75, 96, 107, 108, 123, 756, 764, 767.

ported,[754] clear cell sarcoma primarily affects young adults, the majority of whom are less than 30 years of age[754,755]; mean patient ages vary from 28 to 36 years.[754,755,759] There is a slight preponderance of cases in female patients.[754,755] As with most sarcomas, the presence of a mass or swelling is the dominant symptom, with associated pain or tenderness present in up to one half of patients.[754,755] The duration of symptoms has ranged from several weeks to 20 years, with an average of approximately 2 to 2.5 years, indicating the rather slow growth of most of these tumors.[754-756,759]

The extremities are the most frequent sites involved, accounting for over 90% of cases, with from 60% to 75% of the tumors in the lower extremities.[754,755,759] Although tumors in the region of the knee or thigh occur, most clear cell sarcomas develop about the foot and ankle.[754,755] Other rare sites of involvement include the back,[754,762] the scapular region,[764] the head and neck,[754,759] the masseter, sternocleidomastoid, and paravertebral muscles,[755] the perineum,[767] and the penis.[766]

The tumors are firm, circumscribed nodular masses unattached to the skin but usually fixed to underlying tendons and aponeuroses.[755,757] Although the tumors are usually grayish white, it is not uncommon for the cut surface to show tan to black areas.[752,754,763,665] Most clear cell sarcomas are less than 5 cm, though those as large as 10 to 15 cm occur.[754,757,759]

In primary tumors the microscopic pattern is fairly distinctive, consisting of nests and tight clusters of fairly uniform, round to fusiform cells having a pale, clear, or granular cytoplasm that contains glycogen.[757] Nuclei are round and uniform, lacking any significant degree of pleomorphism. Characteristically, they have prominent nucleoli that are highly basophilic. Mitotic activity is scarce. The cell groups are separated from each other by fibrous septa that are well demonstrated by the use of reticulin stains. These septa appear continuous with that of adjacent tendons and aponeurotic tissue to which the tumors are attached. With invasion of these structures the tumor cells are frequently aligned in a cordlike fashion and surrounded by a dense desmoplastic stroma.[754,755,757,759] Bland, multinucleated giant cells are present in from one half to two thirds of cases.[754,755,759] Recurrent or metastatic lesions may be less orderly and develop a significant pleomorphic appearance such that little if any semblance to the primary tumor remains.[754,757,759,760]

The cells of clear cell sarcoma are noted for their pigment content. In the original description of this tumor, iron stains were positive in all cases in which they were used, with the iron pigment being both intracellular and extracellular, and melanin stains were positive in about half the cases.[757] However, the positive melanin reaction was not abolished by bleaching procedures,

and the same melanin-positive pigment also stained weakly for iron. This raised doubts as to whether the cells contained true melanin. Subsequent reports, however, indicated the presence of melanin in from 13% to 70% of cases, with and without associated iron pigment.[752,754,755,758-760,765] The wide variation in the percentage of cases in which melanin is found may reflect the use of the more sensitive Warthin-Starry stain for melanin by some investigators rather than the usual Fontana-Masson method.[754] The distribution of these pigments within the tumor is uneven, and they may be only focally present. Their presence also varies from recurrence to recurrence.[758,760] Immunoperoxidase stains for S-100 protein are positive in from 70% to 100% of cases[753,754,759,761]; stains for cytokeratin are negative.[761]

Electron microscopy has shown premelanosomes and melanosomes in the tumor cells, even in the absence of positive melanin stains by light microscopy.[752,753,762,765,767] The cells show cytoplasmic processes, cell junctions but no true desmosomes, a basal lamina, cytoplasmic intermediate filaments, and cytoplasmic glycogen.[753,759,761,762] Although it was suggested that clear cell sarcomas are of synovial origin,[767] most investigators believe that the tumor derives from the neural crest[754,759,661] and should be considered as a "melanoma of soft parts."[752,754,765] Others believe that it represents a poorly differentiated or dedifferentiated melanotic malignant schwannoma.[751,753,762,763] Against the latter interpretation, however, is the lack of association of clear cell sarcoma with neurofibromatosis, the lack of nerve bundles within the tumor, and the lack of Schwann cell features by electron microscopy.[754,755,761]

The clinical course after surgical excision may be protracted and characterized by a local recurrence rate of 40% to 85%.[754,755,767] These recurrences may develop many years after initial therapy[755] with an average interval of 4 years.[754] Metastases occur in 50% to 70% of patients[754,759,767] with a high incidence of regional lymph node involvement, as well as pulmonary and skeletal metastases.[754,755,759,764] Such metastases may first manifest themselves after many years.[759] Short-term tumor mortality is about 45% to 60%,[754,759,767] but because of late tumor recurrence and metastasis, 5-year survival is not necessarily an indication of cure.

Alveolar soft part sarcoma

Histologically one of the most distinctive of all the soft-tissue malignant tumors, alveolar soft part sarcoma, has unfortunately been incorrectly interpreted as a malignant granular cell myoblastoma or a malignant nonchromaffin paraganglioma, lesions with which it has no relation.[782,791] The term "alveolar soft part sarcoma" was originally coined as a purely descriptive one, since its histogenesis was unknown.[769] Up to now our ignorance has withstood the test of time. An understanding of this tumor is hampered by its infrequent occurrence, since it accounts for only 1% or less of all sarcomas.* Some institutions report no primary cases in over 20 years, and even cancer referral centers may treat only one or two cases per year.[769] Few reports exist that deal with any appreciable number of patients, with only an estimated 200 cases so far reported.[787]

Although patients from 1 to 74 years of age are reported,[768, 775] the tumors primarily affect children and young adults with approximately two thirds of patients between 11 and 30 years of age[787]; mean ages are from 23 to 30 years.[768,773,775,778,779,786] Some reports of alveolar soft part sarcoma indicate a predominance in female patients with a ratio of approximately 2:1 to 3:1[775,779]; however, others show an equal or near-equal sex distribution.[768,773,786]

Most alveolar soft part sarcomas arise in the deep tissues of the extremities, usually within skeletal muscle or along musculofascial planes.[53,769,773,778,779,786] They occur most commonly in the lower extremity, with 60% located in the thigh or buttock region.[53,787] However, there is a wide anatomic distribution,[103,768,773,779] with cases in the head and neck region, where the orbit[775] and tongue are common sites,[53,789] the retroperitoneum, perineum, female genital tract, trunk, and abdominal wall.[769,774,777,787] The tumors tend to be well circumscribed, pink to reddish brown, and well vascularized.[770,775] They range in size from 2 to 23 cm[770,773] with the majority exceeding 5 cm.[768,773,787] Some reports indicate a predilection for the right side of the body,[778,779,787] but others have not shown this predilection.[768,773,775]

Although some patients have symptoms for only a few weeks,[773,775] most complain of an otherwise asymptomatic mass that may be present for many years, some for 10 or more years.[773,778,785] Pulmonary metastases may be the initial manifestation of the disease.[768,778,779,787]

Microscopically the tumor is characterized by round, ball-like aggregates of cells at the periphery of which are delicate thin-walled blood vessels and fine fibrous septa, the latter well demonstrated by reticulin stains. The cells in the center of the clusters frequently lose their cohesiveness and fall away, leaving the more peripheral cells lining the fibrous septa. This produces the organoid or pseudoalveolar pattern so characteristic of this tumor[670] (Fig. 37-42). The tumor cells appear relatively bland and characterized by a fine, granular, well-defined eosinophilic cytoplasm and a vesicular nucleus containing one or two distinct nucleoli.[53,103,770,775] Mi-

toses are infrequent; pleomorphic foci with high mitotic activity are only rarely seen.[773,786] Tumor invasion of the fine vascular channels is common.[53,768,770] The most distinctive cytologic features of these tumors are the almost universal presence of intracytoplasmic periodic acid–Schiff–positive, diastase-resistant granules, and needlelike crystals arranged in sheaves and clusters. These crystals are found in from 20% to 85% of cases,[53,775,779,788] and by electron microscopy are rhomboid or rod shaped with a distinct periodicity.* These crystals are unique, not being found in other soft-tissue sarcomas, though similar crystals have been reported in a supposed gastric wall schwannoma[780] (Fig. 37-42).

Immunohistochemical studies show the absence of cytokeratin, S-100 protein, neuron-specific enolase, peripheral myelin protein, glial fibrillary acidic protein, and neurofilament protein.[768,782-786] Most of the tumors contain vimentin,[768,784,785] and studies have demonstrated staining for the myogenic markers muscle-specific actin,[785,786] Z-protein, betla-enolase,[783] and desmin,[768, 783-786] though some investigators have been unable to show the presence of desmin or vimentin.[768,786] Despite the immunohistochemical evidence of possible myogenic differentiation, all studies up to now have indicated the absence of myoglobin in these tumors.[768,776,783-786] The presence of significant amounts of renin in the cells of alveolar soft part sarcoma has been claimed by some workers[771] and denied by others.[782]

Aside from the crystalline structures, electron microscopic studies show the presence of glycogen, lipid droplets, basal lamina, and cell junctions but no true desmosomes, sparse numbers of intermediate filaments, and dense-core granules.[771,777,781,790,791] The tumor cells have been characterized as showing the features of Schwann cells[781] or modified smooth muscle cells.[771]

Opinions as to the histogenesis of alveolar soft part sarcoma are multiple and divergent. It has been considered as either a variant of paraganglioma, a neural tumor, a skeletal muscle tumor, or a modified smooth muscle tumor.† What is certain, however, is that the issue of histogenesis remains unsettled.[768,782]

Despite their bland histomorphology, alveolar soft part sarcomas are among the most malignant of sarcomas. Local recurrence rates after excision vary from 20% to 30%.[768,773,779] Metastases are present at the time of diagnosis in from 13% to 25% of patients[768,779,787] and eventually develop in from 40% to 70% of them.[768,770,773,779,787] Metastases may occur as late as 20 or more years after initial diagnosis.[768,775,779] Although the presence of metastases is an ominous

---

*References 19, 29, 75, 96, 107, 108, 123, 772, 787.

*References 53, 771, 772, 775, 786, 788, 791.
†References 103, 771, 776, 781, 783-786, 790, 791.

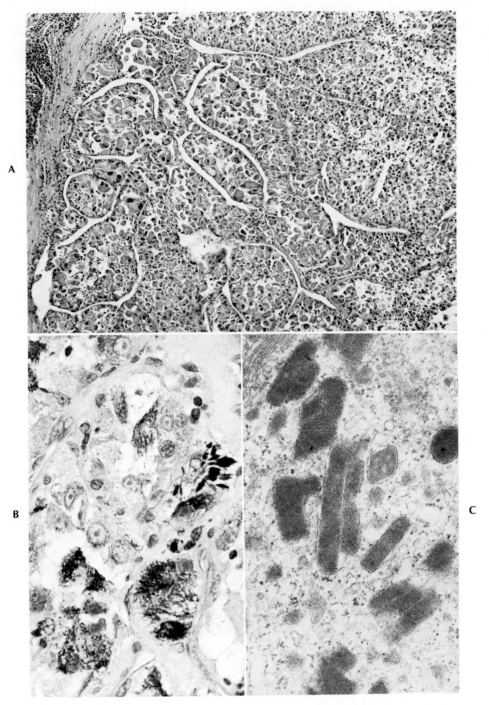

Fig. 37-42. Alveolar soft part sarcoma. **A,** Typical organoid pattern formed by ball-like clusters of cells having granular eosinophilic cytoplasm. Thin-walled vascular channels are present at periphery of clusters. Even at this low magnification, some nuclear atypia can be seen. **B,** Section shows thick intracytoplasmic crystals, as well as sheaves of needlelike crystals. **C,** Electron micrograph shows electron-dense, membrane-bound cytoplasmic structures of variable size and shape. Rhomboids have crystalline substructure of distinctive periodicity. (**A,** 72×; **B,** periodic acid–Schiff; 480×; **C,** 51,200×; courtesy Dr. Katherine De Schryver-Kecskeméti, Case Western Reserve University, Cleveland, Ohio.)

sign, with most patients dying within 18 months,[787] some patients live for many years with known metastases.[768,778] The lungs, bone, and brain are the most common sites of metastases; lymph nodes are infrequently involved.[779,787] Five-year survival rates are approximately 40% to 60%, with a lower 10-year survival rate attributable to the late appearance of metastases.[53,770,773,779] Indeed, there appears to be a cumulative increase in the incidence of metastases over time, with a corresponding cumulative decline in survival.[779] The prognosis may be better in patients under 20 years of age and in those with tumors less than 5 cm.[773,779,787] The type of surgical procedure does not appear to influence the survival rate.[773,787]

Giant cell tumor of soft tissue

Giant cell tumor of soft tissue is a tumor whose histomorphology closely resembles that of giant cell tumor of bone[795,797] (see Chapter 39). Both benign[797] and malignant varieties of giant cell tumor of soft tissue are reported.[792,793,795,796,798] Only a few of these tumors have been reported, with some grouped within studies of malignant fibrous histiocytoma, since many consider malignant giant cell tumor of soft parts as a histologic variant of malignant fibrous histiocytoma. In such studies, the giant cell tumor comprises from 3% to 15% of the malignant fibrous histiocytomas.[236,246,267,306] Giant cell tumors of soft tissue must be distinguished from giant cell tumors of tendon sheath (see p. 2092).

Giant cell tumors of soft tissue occur in patients ranging in age from 1 to 87 years,[793,795-797] but there may be some differences in the ages of patients with the benign and those with the malignant forms of the tumor. In the two largest series of patients with malignant giant cell tumor of soft parts,[793,795] the mean patient ages were 56 and 68 years with approximately 85% to 90% of patient's being over 40 years of age. In the report with the largest number of patients with the benign variety, the mean patient age was 46 years.[797] However, these age differences may simply be attributable to the small number of patients so far reported. Male patients were more frequent in the malignant group, and female patients were more frequent in the benign category, but, especially in the latter study, only a few patients are considered.

Most patients relate a history of having a painless mass present for weeks to months but usually for less than 1 year and frequently for less than 6 months. Some patients, however, had their tumor for periods of up to 15 years.[793,795,797]

Approximately 80% to 90% of the giant cell tumors are located in the extremities, with about 80% of these in the lower extremity, the thigh being the most common site.[792,793,795] Other tumor locations include the face, the abdominal wall, shoulders, neck, and retroperitoneum.[792,793,795] The tumors are either superficially located in the subcutaneous tissue and superficial fascia, or deeply situated in muscle and the deep fascia and adherent to tendon sheaths.[792,793,795] Superficial tumors tend to be smaller than the deeply placed tumors, which may reach up to 15 cm.[793,795] The gross appearance is nonspecific; in the malignant variety hemorrhage and necrosis are common.[793]

The microscopic pattern of the benign tumors consists of multiple nodules composed of a varied mixture of bland-appearing histiocytic and fibroblastic cells, admixed with numerous multinucleated giant cells of osteoclast type. The nodules are separated by dense fibrous septa.[797] Reactive bone or osteoid may be present. In the malignant tumors the cells show varying degrees of anaplasia with mononuclear pleomorphic giant cells present in most cases (Fig. 37-43). The fibroblastic cells produce fibrosarcomatous foci, especially at the periphery of the lesions. Numerous giant cells of the osteoclast type are diffusely distributed within the nodules. These giant cells have bland uniform nuclei, which may number up to 100, and a cytoplasm that may be vacuolated. Phagocytic activity is sometimes seen in these cells, as is the occasional presence of asteroid bodies, an indication that these giant cells may be histiocytes.[793,795,796] Significantly, in up to half the malignant cases, osteoid and, more rarely, malignant-appearing chondroid material, has been found, usually at the periphery of the tumor, but occasionally also more centrally located.[793,795,798] Such foci raise problems in the classification of these tumors. A malignant tumor composed of a sarcomatous stroma that produces osteoid is, by definition, an osteosarcoma. Furthermore, conventional osteosarcomas of bone, as well as extraskeletal osteosarcomas,[794] may also have areas of fibrohistiocytic proliferation, and in about 10% of the intraosseous cases they contain a significant number of osteoclastic giant cells. Indeed, the distinction between a malignant giant cell tumor of soft tissue with osteoid production, a conventional malignant fibrous histiocytoma in which bone and cartilage are present,[236,237,241,289] and extraskeletal osteosarcoma may be difficult.[794] I believe that at least some tumors categorized as malignant giant cell tumor of soft tissue would, if adequately sampled, prove to be extraskeletal osteosarcomas.

Electron microscopic studies of giant cell tumor of soft tissue have been limited to only a few cases.[792,793,798] From these it was concluded that the lesion resembles both the true giant cell tumor of bone and the giant cell reparative granuloma.[792] Some believe that the tumor arises from primitive mesenchymal cells that differentiate along fibroblastic and histiocytic lines and that therefore the tumor is rightly a variant of fibrous histiocytoma.[306,792,793] However, in one study, although the mononuclear cells were interpreted to represent poorly

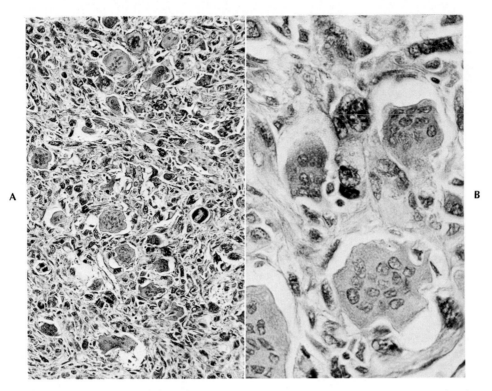

Fig. 37-43. A, Malignant giant cell tumor of soft tissue. Multinucleated, osteoclastic giant cells within fibrous stroma containing anaplastic stromal cells. **B,** Higher magnification shows bland nuclei of the giant cells and atypical stromal cells. (**A,** 120×; **B,** 480×.)

differentiated mesenchymal cells, other tumor cells had chondroblastic and osteoblastic features.[798] It is my view that until further cases are reported and clearly separated from osteosarcoma the question of histogenesis remains open and, because of its unique histopathology, giant cell tumor of soft tissue is not to be included within the fibrohistiocytic category of tumors.

The prognosis for giant cell tumors of soft tissue has varied considerably. In the one report where the histologic features of the lesions lacked any suggestion of malignancy, none of the 10 patients died of tumor and all but one were alive and well at the time of the report.[797] On the other hand, the malignant tumors have in most cases pursued an aggressive course, with local recurrences and metastases; 5-year survival rates have been about 30%.[246,267,792,793,795,796] Patients whose tumors are small and superficially located have a better prognosis than those with larger more deeply situated tumors.[793,795]

Extraskeletal Ewing's sarcoma

Ewing's sarcoma, a tumor composed of small, round, undifferentiated cells, is one of the most aggressive and malignant primary tumors of bone and is found almost

exclusively in young children (see Chapter 39). Only recently has it been recognized that tumors with a similar morphology may originate within the soft tissues,[799,827] where they may be difficult to distinguish histologically from other small cell malignant tumors such as embryonal rhabdomyosarcoma, peripheral neuroepithelioma, peripheral neuroblastoma, malignant lymphoma, and metastatic small cell carcinoma.

Extraskeletal Ewing's are rare tumors accounting for less than 1% of all sarcomas.[29,96,108,123] They occur in patients from newborns to those over 80 years of age but are most common in adolescents and young adults, with reported mean ages ranging from 19 to 26 years and median ages of 16 to 20 years.[799,807,809,812,815,826] In general, most patients are older than those with intraosseous Ewing's sarcoma, and male patients are more often affected than female patients (55% to 45%).[824,826]

Clinically, the tumors grow rapidly, with symptoms of an enlarging mass, which may be associated with pain or tenderness, usually present for only a few months.[799,809,815] Although the trunk, especially the paravertebral region, and the extremities are the most common locations for extraskeletal Ewing's tumors, a wide variety of other soft-tissue sites have been involved, including the retroperitoneum, pelvis, head and neck, mediastinum, and pleura.[799,809,812,821,823] The majority of these tumors arise from the deep soft tissue, usually within or between the skeletal muscles,[799,809,815] though some do arise in the superficial cutaneous or subcutaneous soft tissue.[799,804,809,820] The paravertebral tumors frequently involve the epidural space.[801,812,814,827] Deeply situated extremity tumors may become attached to the periosteum of adjacent bone,[809,815,822] causing a periosteal reaction that may be seen on roentgenograms, thus suggestive of a possible origin of the tumor from the bone. Before a diagnosis of extraskeletal Ewing's tumor is made, careful examination of the adjacent bone by computerized tomography and magnetic resonance imaging techniques should be done to rule out primary origin from within the bone.[802,822]

As the rapid growth and undifferentiated nature of the tumor cells would indicate, these tumors are grossly usually soft and friable with a gray to gray-white cut surface having areas of necrosis and hemorrhage.[799,809,815] The tumors range in size from 1 to 19 cm, with most exceeding 5 cm.[799,809,812]

By routine light microscopy, the morphology of extraskeletal Ewing's tumor is identical to that of its intraosseous counterpart[799,807,809,812,815] and consists of abundant closely packed small, oval to round cells arranged in broad fields separated by fibrous septa. The cytoplasm, which is scanty with ill-defined borders, may be pale or vacuolated. Nuclei are monotonously uniform with a fine evenly dispersed chromatin pattern, at times containing a small uniform nucleolus. In areas of necrosis, which are frequent, pale ghost cell remnants are characteristically found. The tumor is quite vascular, and in necrotic zones the cells that are still viable are found in a cufflike fashion about the blood vessels. Irregularly distributed throughout the tumor are smaller darker cells whose nuclei are less round and more hyperchromatic. Although originally considered as degenerating forms of the more abundant or "principal" tumor cells, the abundant cell organelles, including mitochondria, found in these "dark" cells by electron microscopy has cast doubt on this interpretation. Despite the rapid clinical evolution of these tumors, the number of mitotic figures is variable, with some tumors having few, whereas in others they are numerous. Occasional cell rosettes are found, but these are not frequent and usually not so well developed as those found in conventional neuroblastoma or peripheral neuroepithelioma. Extraskeletal Ewing's tumors contain glycogen, lack reticulin fibers about the tumor cells,* and stain positively for vimentin intermediate filament protein.[817]

Electron microscopy of these soft-tissue tumors has demonstrated fine-structural features that are similar to those of intraosseous Ewing's sarcoma. The "principal" cells show diffuse nuclear chromatin, cytoplasmic glycogen frequently arranged in pools, and a scarcity of cytoplasmic organelles giving the tumor cells an undifferentiated appearance. Occasional rare microfilaments and intermediate filaments may be found. Primitive cell junctions, some desmosome-like, are present, but basement membrane material is absent. The "dark" cells show a denser cytoplasm with a greater number of organelles, including free ribosomes and mitochondria, and a more clumped nuclear chromatin than the "principal" cells.*

Although the above-described light microscopic description of Ewing's tumor would appear to easily distinguish it from other soft-tissue tumors with small cells, doing so is not always possible.[33,809] Indeed, recent studies of both intraosseous and extraosseous Ewing's tumor has caused a remarkable reappraisal not only of the histogenesis of these tumors, but also of the criteria for their diagnosis. There exist, in both anatomic locations, tumors that have the morphologic pattern of "classic" Ewing's tumor but, by either immunohistochemistry, cytogenetics, or electron microscopy, are found to have neural, myogenic, and even epithelial differentiation.[810,811,816,824,826,829] Tumors whose cells contain neuron-specific enolase, a marker for neuroectodermal lesions, are described in both intraosseous and extraosseous locations.[811,816,824,829] Cells from classic Ewing's sarcoma of bone grown in tissue culture can be induced to develop morphologic and immunohistochemical features of neural differentiation.[803] The small cell tumor of the thoracopulmonary soft tissues that occurs in childhood and resembles Ewing's tumor histologically[800] also demonstrates neural features and is now considered to be a neuroectodermal tumor.[808,813,829] A reciprocal 11:22 chromosomal translocation has been found in Ewing's tumors, peripheral neuroepithelioma, and the small cell thoracopulmonary tumors of childhood.[803,829] There is accumulating evidence therefore that many if not most extraskeletal Ewing's tumors actually represent primitive neuroectodermal tumors.[811,816,824,829] Indeed, in one recent study of 14 extraskeletal Ewing's tumors, 13 were shown to have some form of neural differentiation.[824] There is much in the recent suggestion that Ewing's tumor may represent a blastoma that has the potential to differentiate along a variety of morphologic pathways.[816]

It is obvious from the above that by light microscopy alone a definitive diagnosis of soft-tissue Ewing's tumor is not possible. This diagnosis is confined to those small cell tumors that have the appropriate light microscopic features and by electron microscopy contain glycogen

---

*References 33, 799, 801, 809, 815, 820, 824.

*References 801, 804, 805, 809, 811, 812, 814, 821, 824, 828.

and are primitive appearing with no evidence of neural, myogenic, or epithelial differentiation and immunohistochemically fail to demonstrate neural or mesenchymal markers.[806,823]

Whether these histogenetic studies have any practical importance is still to be resolved. In one of the largest initial reports on extraskeletal Ewing's tumors, over 60% of the patients died, usually within a year after diagnosis, with metastases to lungs and bone.[799] In the Intergroup Rhabdomyosarcoma Study, extraskeletal Ewing's tumors, which had originally been submitted as examples of rhabdomyosarcoma, were separated into type I and type II groups that differed from each other only in that the cells of group II were more irregular in shape and slightly larger and had a less hyperchromatic nucleus than that of the cells of group I.[825] Patients with these tumors were treated with the same chemotherapy drug regimens as those used for patients with embryonal rhabdomyosarcoma, and they responded as well as the latter patients did, with an estimated 75% surviving at least 3 years.[819,824,825] There was no difference in prognosis for patients whose tumors were actually found to show neural differentiation, though the number of such patients was small.[824] In another study, again with relatively few patients, over 70% of the patients were disease free at 3 to 7 years after treatment with the same chemotherapy drug regimen as that used to treat patients with Ewing's sarcoma of bone.[812] The prognosis for extraskeletal Ewing's tumors of the extremities may be better than that for such tumors of the trunk.[805,812]

ADDITIONAL READING

Various other tumor and tumorlike conditions of the soft tissues are of interest because of either their distinctive histopathologic features or because they may be confused with other lesions. I briefly mention here a few of these conditions, some of which have only recently been reported, for interest and for which the appended references serve to supply greater detail.

Fibroma of tendon sheath is a benign, well-circumscribed, often lobulated tumorlike condition that mainly affects tendons and tendon sheaths of the fingers, hand, and wrist. It is histologically characterized by a dense fibrocollagenous matrix in which slitlike vascular spaces exist. Electron microscopy shows the presence of fibroblasts and myofibroblasts. After local excision, recurrences develop in approximately 25% of patients.[830-832]

Giant cell fibroblastoma is a tumor of childhood first described in 1982.[836] It arises in the subcutaneous tissue and consists of a proliferation of irregular sinusoidal spaces lined by spindle cells and multinucleated giant cells. The spindle cells may show atypical nuclear features, and this pattern, combined with the tendency of the lesion to locally recur after excision, has caused

giant cell fibroblastoma to be considered malignant by some. However, it is benign and believed to possibly represent a form of fibromatosis.[833-836]

Low-grade fibromyxoid sarcoma has only recently been described in two patients. It consists of benign-appearing fibroblastic cells in a whorled pattern. In parts of the tumor, cells reside in a pale myxoidlike matrix. Despite its overall bland appearance, the tumor is capable of producing metastases and causing death.[837]

Extraskeletal myxoid chondrosarcoma may resemble a variety of soft-tissue myxoid sarcomas and was originally designated as "chordoid sarcoma" because of its histologic resemblance to chordoma. Histologically, it consists of lobules in which loosely arranged tumor cells are found in cords or strands. The tumor cells stain positively for S-100 protein and are cytokeratin negative. By electron microscopy the cells have cartilaginous features. The tumor is considered to be a myxoid variant of chondrosarcoma not related to chordoma, and it has a relatively good prognosis.[838-842]

Extraskeletal osteosarcoma is a rare tumor of soft tissue that may at times be confused with giant cell tumor of soft tissue because some of these tumors contain, in addition to the usual features of conventional osteosarcoma, numerous osteoclast-like giant cells.[236,237,289,794] The tumor has a poor prognosis.[794,843]

Malignant rhaboid tumor of soft tissue is a highly malignant tumor of childhood. Histologically, it is composed of cells that are similar to those of malignant rhabdoid tumors of the kidney and characterized by hyalin-like globular perinuclear inclusions that by electron microscopy consist of closely packed intermediate filaments. Immunohistochemically the tumor cells coexpress cytokeratin and vimentin. The tumor is highly malignant, with a high rate of metastases and a poor prognosis.[844-848] Similar cells of the rhabdoid type may occur in other soft-tissue sarcomas, including epithelioid sarcoma, synovial sarcoma, and extraskeletal myxoid chondrosarcoma; the cells have also been confused with rhabdomyoblasts.[849]

Myxoid hamartoma is a recently described lesion of infants that, because of its myxoid background and component of plump mesenchymal cells, has been confused with other myxoid lesions, especially myxoid liposarcoma. The lesion, however, is benign and considered probably to be hamartomatous.[900]

Finally, there has been described a group of polymorphic mesenchymal tumors, which arise in bone and soft tissue, that are associated with the production of osteomalacia or rickets. These *"phosphaturic mesenchymal tumors"* when they arise in the soft tissue are highly vascular and usually contain multinucleated osteoclast-like giant cells. The tumors are frequently very small and easily overlooked, such that patients may suffer their biochemical effects for many years before the tumors are discovered.[851]

REFERENCES
General

1. Angervall, L., Kindblom, L.-G., Rydholm, A., and Stener, B.: The diagnosis and prognosis of soft tissue tumors, Semin. Diagn. Pathol. 3:240, 1986.
2. Antman, K.H., and Elias, A.D.: Chemotherapy of advanced soft-tissue sarcomas, Semin. Surg. Oncol. 4:53, 1988.
3. Azar, H.A.: Pathology of human neoplasms: an atlas of diagnostic electron microscopy and immunohistochemistry, New York, 1988, Raven Press.
4. Azumi, N., and Battifora, H.: The distribution of vimentin and keratin in epithelial and nonepithelial neoplasms: a comprehensive immunohistochemical study on formalin- and alcohol-fixed tumors, Am. J. Clin. Pathol. 88:286, 1987.
5. Balarajan, R., and Acheson, E.D.: Soft tissue sarcomas in agriculture and forestry workers, J. Epidemiol. Community Health 38:113, 1984.
6. Battifora, H.: Recent progress in the immunohistochemistry of solid tumors, Semin. Diagn. Pathol. 1:251, 1984.
7. Battifora, H., and Kopinski, M.: The influence of protease digestion and duration of fixation on the immunostaining of keratins: a comparison of formalin and ethanol fixation, J. Histochem. Cytochem. 34:1095, 1986.
8. Benjamin, R.S.: Limb salvage surgery for sarcomas: a good idea receives formal blessing, JAMA 254:1795, 1985.
9. Boddaert, A., Trojani, M., Contesso, G., Coindre, J.M., Rouessé, J., Bui, N.B., Genin, J., de Mascarel, A., Goussot, J.F., David, M., Bonichon F., Lagarde C., et al.: Soft tissue sarcomas of adults: study of pathological variables and definition of a histopathological grading system. In van Oosterom, A.T., and van Unnik, J.A.M., editors: Management of soft tissue and bone sarcomas, New York, 1986, Raven Press.
10. Brooks, J.J.: Immunohistochemistry of soft tissue tumors: myoglobin as a tumor marker for rhabdomyosarcoma, Cancer 50:1757, 1982.
11. Burgdorf, W.H.C., Mukai, K., and Rosai, J.: Immunohistochemical identification of factor VIII–related antigen in endothelial cells of cutaneous lesions of alleged vascular nature, Am. J. Clin. Pathol. 75:167, 1981.
12. Chase, D.R.: Keratin in epithelioid sarcoma: an immunohistochemical study, Am. J. Surg. Pathol. 8:435, 1984.
13. Coindre, J.-M., de Mascarel, A., Trojani, M., de Mascarel, I., and Pages, A.: Immunohistochemical study of rhabdomyosarcoma: unexpected staining with S100 protein and cytokeratin, J. Pathol. 155:127, 1988.
14. Trojani, M., Contesso, G., David, M., Rouessé, J., Bui, N.B., Bodaert, A., de Mascarel, I., de Mascarel, A., and Goussot, J.-F.: Reproducibility of a histopathologic grading system for adult soft tissue sarcoma, Cancer 58:306, 1986.
15. Collin, C., Hajdu, S.I., Godbold, J., Friedrich, C., and Brennan, M.F.: Localized operable soft tissue sarcoma of the upper extremity: presentation, management, and factors affecting local recurrence in 108 patients, Ann. Surg. 205:331, 1987.
16. Consensus Conference: Limb-sparing treatment of adult soft-tissue sarcomas and osteosarcomas, JAMA 254:1791, 1985.
17. Corson, J.M., Weiss, L.M., Banks-Schlegel, S.P., and Pinkus, G.S.: Keratin proteins and carcinoembryonic antigen in synovial sarcomas: an immunohistochemical study of 24 cases, Hum. Pathol. 15:615, 1984.
18. Corson, J.M., and Pinkus, G.S.: Intracellular myoglobin—a specific marker for skeletal muscle differentiation in soft tissue sarcomas: an immunoperoxidase study, Am. J. Pathol. 103:384, 1981.
19. Costa, J., Wesley, R.A., Glatstein, E., and Rosenberg, S.A.: The grading of soft tissue sarcomas: results of a clinicohistopathologic correlation in a series of 163 cases, Cancer 53:530, 1984.
20. Dabbs, D.J., and Geisinger, K.R.: Common epithelial ovarian tumors: immunohistochemical intermediate filament profiles, Cancer 62:368, 1988.
21. Dabbs, D.J., Geisinger, K.R., and Norris, H.T.: Intermediate filaments in endometrial and endocervical carcinomas: the diagnostic utility of vimentin patterns, Am. J. Surg. Pathol. 10:568, 1986.
22. Dahl, I., and Angervall, L.: Pseudosarcomatous lesions of the soft tissues reported as sarcoma during a 6-year period (1958-1963), Acta Pathol. Microbiol. Scand. 85A:917, 1977.
23. Das Gupta, T.K.: Tumors of the soft tissues, Norwalk, Conn., 1983, Appleton-Century-Crofts.
24. DeLellis, R.A.: Advances in immunohistochemistry, New York, 1988, Raven Press.
25. Doglioni, C., Dell'Orto, P., Coggi, G., Iuzzolino, P., Bontempini, L., and Viale, G.: Choroid plexus tumors: an immunocytochemical study with particular reference to the coexpression of intermediate filament proteins, Am. J. Pathol. 127:519, 1987.
26. Drier, J.K., Swanson, P.E., Cherwitz, D.L., and Wick, M.R.: S100 protein immunoreactivity in poorly differentiated carcinomas: immunohistochemical comparison with malignant melanoma, Arch. Pathol. Lab. Med. 111:447, 1987.
27. du Boulay, C.E.H.: Demonstration of alpha-1-antitrypsin and alpha-1-antichymotrypsin in fibrous histiocytomas using the immunoperoxide technique, Am. J. Surg. Pathol. 6:559, 1982.
28. Elias, A.D., and Antman, K.H.: Adjuvant chemotherapy for soft-tissue sarcoma: a critical appraisal, Semin. Surg. Oncol. 4:59, 1988.
29. Enjoji, M., and Hashimoto, H.: Diagnosis of soft tissue sarcomas, Pathol. Res. Pract. 178:215, 1984.
30. Enneking, W.F.: A system of staging musculoskeletal neoplasms, Clin. Orthop. 204:9, 1986.
31. Enterline, H.T.: Histopathology of sarcomas, Semin. Oncol. 8:133, 1981.
32. Enzinger, F.M., Lattes, R., and Torloni, H.: Histological typing of soft tissue tumours, World Health Organization, International Histological Classification of Tumors, no. 3, Geneva, 1969, World Health Organization.
33. Enzinger, F.M., and Weiss, S.W.: Soft tissue tumors, St. Louis, 1988, The C.V. Mosby Co.
34. Erlandson, R.A.: Diagnostic immunohistochemistry of human tumors: an interim evaluation, Am. J. Surg. Pathol. 8:615, 1984.
35. Fine, G., Hajdu, S.I., Morton, D.L., Eilber, F.R., Suit, H.D., and Weiss, S.W.: Soft tissue sarcomas: classification and treatment (a symposium), Pathol. Annu. 17(pt. 1):155, 1982.
36. Fine, G., Ohorodnik, J.M., and Horn, R.C., Jr.: Soft-tissue sarcomas: their clinical behavior and course and influencing factors, Proc. Seventh National Cancer Conference, Philadelphia, 1973, J.B. Lippincott Co.
37. Gabbiani, G., Kapanci, Y., Barazzone, P., and Franke, W.W.: Immunochemical identification of intermediate-sized filaments in human neoplastic cells: a diagnostic aid for the surgical pathologist, Am. J. Pathol. 104:206, 1981.
38. Gould, V.E.: The coexpression of distinct classes of intermediate filaments in human neoplasms, Arch. Pathol. Lab. Med. 109:984, 1985. (Editorial.)
39. Gould, V.E.: Histogenesis and differentiation: a re-evaluation of these concepts as criteria for the classification of tumors, Hum. Pathol. 17:212, 1986.
40. Gown, A.M., Boyd, H.C., Chang, Y., Ferguson, M., Reichler, B., and Tippens, D.: Smooth muscle cells can express cytokeratins of "simple" epithelium: immunocytochemical and biochemical studies in vitro and in vivo, Am. J. Pathol. 132:223, 1988.
41. Greenall, M.J., Magill, G.B., DeCosse, J.J., and Brennan, M.F.: Chemotherapy for soft tissue sarcoma, Surg. Gynecol. Obstet. 162:193, 1986.
42. Greenwald, P., Kovasznay, B., Collins, D.N., and Therriault, G.: Sarcomas of soft tissue after Vietnam service, J. Natl. Cancer Inst. 73:1107, 1984.
43. Haimoto, H., Takahashi, Y., Koshikawa, T., Nagura, M., and Kato, K.: Immunohistochemical localization of γ-enolase in normal human tissues other than nervous and neuroendocrine tissues, Lab. Invest. 52:257, 1985.
44. Hajdu, S.I.: Pathology of soft tissue tumors, Philadelphia, 1979, Lea & Febiger.
45. Hajdu, S.I.: Benign soft tissue tumors: classification and natural history, CA 37:66, 1987.
46. Hardell, L., and Eriksson, M.: The association between soft tissue sarcomas and exposure to phenoxyacetic acids: a new case—referent study, Cancer 62:652, 1988.

47. Henson, D.E.: The histological grading of neoplasms, Arch. Pathol. Lab. Med. **112:**1091, 1988.

48. Herrera, G.A., Turbat-Herrera, E.A., and Lott, R.L.: S-100 protein expression by primary and metastatic adenocarcinomas, Am. J. Clin. Pathol. **89:**168, 1988.

49. Hoar, S.K., Blair, A., Holmes, F.F., Boysen, C.D., Robel, R.J., Hoover, R., and Fraumeni, J.F., Jr.: Agricultural herbicide use and risk of lymphoma and soft-tissue sarcoma, JAMA **256:**1141, 1986.

50. Huvos, A.G.: The spontaneous transformation of benign into malignant soft tissue tumors (with emphasis on extraskeletal osseous, lipomatous, and schwannian lesions), Am. J. Surg. Pathol. **9:**7, 1985.

51. Kasper, M., Goertchen, R., Stosick, P., Perry, G., and Karsten, U.: Coexistence of cytokeratin, vimentin and neurofilament protein in human choroid plexus: an immunohistochemical study of intermediate filaments in neuroepithelial tissues, Virchows Arch [A] **410:**173, 1986.

52. Kaye, G.I.: The futility of electron microscopy in determining the origin of poorly differentiated soft tissue tumors. In Fenoglio, C.M., and Wolff, M., editors: Progress in surgical pathology, vol. 3, New York, 1981, Masson Publishing USA, Inc.

53. Lattes, R., and Enzinger, F.M.: Soft tissue tumors, Proc. Thirty-Ninth Annual Anatomic Pathology Slide Seminar of the American Society of Clinical Pathologists, Chicago, 1973.

54. Lawrence, W., Jr., Donegan, W.L., Natarajan, N., Mettlin, C., Beart, R., and Winchester D.: Adult soft tissue sarcomas: a pattern of care survey of the American College of Surgeons, Ann. Surg. **205:**349, 1987.

55. Lawson, C.W., Fisher, C., and Gatter, K.C.: An immunohistochemical study of differentiation in malignant fibrous histiocytoma, Histopathology **11:**375, 1987.

56. Leader, M., Collins, M., Patel, J., and Henry, K.: Antineuron specific enolase staining reactions in sarcomas and carcinomas: its lack of neuroendocrine specificity, J. Clin. Pathol. **39:**1186, 1986.

57. Leader, M., Collins, M., Patel, J., and Henry, K.: Vimentin: an evaluation of its role as a tumour marker, Histopathology **11:**63, 1987.

58. Leader, M., Patel, J., Collins, M., and Henry, K.: Anti-α1-antichymotrypsin staining of 194 sarcomas, 38 carcinomas, and 17 malignant melanomas: its lack of specificity as a tumour marker, Am. J. Surg. Pathol. **11:**133, 1987.

59. Lindberg, R.D., Martin, R.G., Romsdahl, M.M., and Barkley, H.T., Jr.: Conservative surgery and postoperative radiotherapy in 300 adults with soft-tissue sarcomas, Cancer **47:**2391, 1981.

60. Mackay, B.: Electron microscopy of soft tumors. In M.D. Anderson Hospital and Tumor Institute: Management of primary bone and soft tissue tumors, Chicago, 1977, Year Book Medical Publishers, Inc.

61. MacKay, B., and Ordóñez, N.G.: The role of the pathologist in the evaluation of poorly differentiated tumors, Semin. Oncol. **9:**396, 1982.

62. Mankin, H.J., Lange, T.A., and Spanier, S.S.: The hazards of biopsy in patients with malignant primary bone and soft-tissue tumors, J. Bone Joint Surg. **64A:**1121, 1982.

63. Markhede, G., Angervall, L., and Stener, B.: A multivariate analysis of the prognosis after surgical treatment of malignant soft-tissue tumors, Cancer **49:**1721, 1982.

64. Martin, R.G., Lindberg, R.D., Sinkovics, J.G., and Butler, J.J.: Soft tissue sarcomas. In Clark, R.L., and Howe, C.D., editors: Cancer patient care at M.D. Anderson Hospital and Tumor Institute, The University of Texas, Chicago, 1976, Year Book Medical Publishers, Inc.

65. Mason, D.Y., and Gatter, K.C.: The role of immunocytochemistry in diagnostic pathology, J. Clin. Pathol. **40:**1042, 1987.

66. Mazeron, J.-J., and Suit, H.D.: Lymph nodes as sites of metastases from sarcomas of soft tissue, Cancer **60:**1800, 1987.

67. Miettinen, M.: Antibody specific to muscle actins in the diagnosis and classification of soft tissue tumors, Am. J. Pathol. **130:**205, 1988.

68. Miettinen, M., Foidart, J.-M., Ekblom, P.: Immunohistochemical demonstration of laminin, the major glycoprotein of base-ment membranes, as an aid in the diagnosis of soft tissue tumors, Am. J. Clin. Pathol. **79:**306, 1983.

69. Miettinen, M., Holthofer, H., Lehto, V.-P., Miettinen, A., and Virtanen, I.: *Ulex europaeus* I lectin as a marker for tumors derived from endothelial cells, Am. J. Clin. Pathol. **79:**32, 1983.

70. Miettinen, M., Lehto, V.-P., Badley, R.A., and Virtanen, I.: Expression of intermediate filaments in soft-tissue sarcomas, Int. J. Cancer **30:**541, 1982.

71. Miettinen, M., Lehto, V.-P., and Virtanen, I.: Antibodies to intermediate filament proteins in the diagnosis and classification of human tumors, Ultrastruct. Pathol. **7:**83, 1984.

72. Moll, R., Lee, I., Gould, V.E., Berndt, R., Roessner, A., and Franke, W.W.: Immunocytochemical analysis of Ewing's tumors: patterns of expression of intermediate filaments and desmosomal proteins indicate cell type heterogeneity and pluripotential differentiation, Am. J. Pathol. **127:**288, 1987.

73. Mukai, K., Rosai, J., and Hallaway, B.E.: Localization of myoglobin in normal and neoplastic human skeletal muscle cells using an immunoperoxidase method, Am. J. Surg. Pathol. **3:**373, 1979.

74. Myhre-Jensen, O.: A consecutive 7-year series of 1331 benign soft tissue tumours: clinicopathologic data: comparison with sarcomas, Acta Orthop. Scand. **52:**287, 1981.

75. Myhre-Jensen, O., Kaae, S., Madsen, E.H., and Sneppen, O.: Histopathological grading in soft-tissue tumours: relation to survival in 261 surgically treated patients, Acta Pathol. Microbiol. Immunol. Scand. [A] **91:**145, 1983.

76. Nagle, R.B., McDaniel, K.M., Clark, V.A., and Payne, C.M.: The use of antikeratin antibodies in the diagnosis of human neoplasms, Am. J. Clin. Pathol. **79:**458, 1983.

77. Nakajima, T., Watanabe, S., Sato, Y., Kameya, T., Hirota, T., and Shimosato, Y.: An immunoperoxidase study of S-100 protein distribution in normal and neoplastic tissue, Am. J. Surg. Pathol. **6:**715, 1982.

78. Norton, A.J., Thomas, J.A., and Isaacson, P.G.: Cytokeratin-specific monoclonal antibodies are reactive with tumours of smooth muscle derivation: an immunocytochemical and biochemical study using antibodies to intermediate filament cytoskeletal proteins, Histopathology **11:**487, 1987.

79. Ogawa, K., Oguchi, M., Yamabe, H., Nakashima, Y., and Hamashima, Y.: Distribution of collagen type IV in soft tissue tumors: an immunohistochemical study, Cancer **58:**269, 1986.

80. Ordóñez, N.G., and Batsakis, J.G.: Comparison of *Ulex europaeus* I lectin and factor VIII–related antigen in vascular lesions, Arch. Pathol. Lab. Med. **108:**129, 1984.

81. Osborn, M., and Weber, K.: Biology of disease: tumor diagnosis by intermediate filament typing: a novel tool for surgical pathology, Lab. Invest. **48:**372, 1983.

82. Pinkus, G.S., and Kurtin, P.J.: Epithelial membrane antigen—a diagnostic discriminant in surgical pathology: immunohistochemical profile in epithelial, mesenchymal, and hematopoietic neoplasms using paraffin sections and monoclonal antibodies, Hum. Pathol. **16:**929, 1985.

83. Potter, D.A., Kinsella, T., Glatstein, E., Wesley, R., White, D.E., Seipp, C.A., Chang, A.E., Lack, E.E., Costa, J., and Rosenberg, S.A.: High-grade soft tissue sarcomas of the extremities, Cancer **58:**190, 1986.

84. Presant, C.A., Lowenbraun, S., Bartolucci, A.A., Smalley, R.V., and the Southeastern Cancer Study Group: Metastatic sarcomas: chemotherapy with adriamycin, cyclophosphamide, and methotrexate alternating with actinomycin D, DTIC, and vincristine, Cancer **47:**457, 1981.

85. Presant, C.A., Russell, W.O., Alexander, R.W., and Fu, Y.S.: Soft-tissue and bone sarcoma histopathology peer review: the frequency of disagreement in diagnosis and the need for second pathology opinions: the Southeastern Cancer Study Group experience, J. Clin. Oncol. **4:**1658, 1986.

86. Roholl, P.J.M., De Jong, A.S.H., and Ramaekers, F.C.S.: Application of markers in the diagnosis of soft tissue tumours, Histopathology **9:**1019, 1985.

87. Rosai, J.: Ackerman's surgical pathology, ed. 6, St. Louis, 1981, The C.V. Mosby Co.

88. Rosenberg, S.A., Tepper, J., Glatstein, E., Costa, J., Baker, A., Brennan, M., DeMoss, E.V., Seipp, C., Sindelar, W.F.,

Sugarbaker, P., and Wesley, R.: The treatment of soft-tissue sarcomas of the extremities: prospective randomized evaluation of (1) limb-sparing surgery plus radiation therapy compared with amputation and (2) the role of adjuvant chemotherapy, Ann. Surg. **196**:305, 1982.

89. Ross, J., Hendrickson, M.R., and Kempson, R.L.: The problem of the poorly differentiated sarcoma, Semin. Oncol. **9**:467, 1982.

90. Ruka, W., Emrich, L.J., Driscoll, D.L., and Karakousis, C.P.: Prognostic significance of lymph node metastasis and bone, major vessel, or nerve involvement in adults with high-grade soft tissue sarcomas, Cancer **62**:999, 1988.

91. Rungger-Brändle, E., and Gabbiani, G.: The role of cytoskeletal and cytocontractile elements in pathologic processes, Am. J. Pathol. **110**:361, 1983.

92. Russell, W.O.: The pathologic diagnosis of cancer: a crescendo of importance in current and future therapies, Am. J. Clin. Pathol. **73**:3, 1980.

93. Russell, W.O., Cohen, J., Enzinger, F., Hajdu, S.I., Heise, H., Martin, R.G., Meissner, W., Miller, W.T., Schmitz, R.L., and Suit, H.D.: A clinical and pathological staging system for soft tissue sarcomas, Cancer **40**:1562, 1977.

94. Rydholm, A.: Management of patients with soft-tissue tumors: strategy developed at a regional oncology center, Acta Orthop. Scand. **54**(suppl. 203):1, 1983.

95. Rydholm, A., Berg, N.O., Gullberg, B., Persson, B.M., and Thorngren, K.-G.: Prognosis for soft-tissue sarcoma in the locomotor system: a retrospective population-based follow-up study of 237 patients, Acta Pathol. Microbiol. Immunol. Scand. [A] **92**:375, 1984.

96. Rydholm, A., Berg, N.O., Gullberg, B., Thorngren, K.-G., and Persson, B.M.: Epidemiology of soft-tissue sarcoma in the locomotor system: a retrospective population-based study of the inter-relationships between clinical and morphologic variables, Acta Pathol. Microbiol. Immunol. Scand. [A] **92**:363, 1984.

97. Saku, T., Tsuda, N., Anami, M., and Okabe, H.: Smooth and skeletal muscle myosins in spindle cell tumors of soft tissue: an immunohistochemical study, Acta Pathol. Jpn. **35**:125, 1985.

98. Seshi, B., True, L., Carter, D., and Rosai, J.: Immunohistochemical characterization of a set of monoclonal antibodies to human neuron-specific enolase, Am. J. Pathol. **131**:258, 1988.

99. Sheibani, K., and Tubbs, R.R.: Enzyme immunohistochemistry: technical aspects, Semin. Diagn. Pathol. **1**:235, 1984.

100. Silverberg, E., and Lubera, J.A.: Cancer statistics, 1988, CA **38**:5, 1988.

101. Simon, M.A.: Biopsy of musculoskeletal tumors, J. Bone Joint Surg. **64A**:1253, 1982.

102. Sloane, J.P., and Ormerod, M.G.: Distribution of epithelial membrane antigen in normal and neoplastic tissues and its value in diagnostic tumor pathology, Cancer **47**:1786, 1981.

103. Stout, A.P., and Lattes, R.: Tumors of the soft tissues. In Atlas of tumor pathology, series 2, fascicle 1, Washington, D.C., 1967, Armed Forces Institute of Pathology.

104. Sutow, W.W.: Malignant solid tumors in children: a review, New York, 1981, Raven Press.

105. Taylor, C.R.: Immunomicroscopy: a diagnostic tool for the surgical pathologist, Major Problems in Pathology, vol. 19, Philadelphia, 1986, W.B. Saunders Co.

106. Thomas, P., Battifora, H., Manderino, G.L., and Patrick, J.: A monoclonal antibody against neuron-specific enolase: immunohistochemical comparison with a polyclonal antiserum, J. Clin. Pathol. **88**:146, 1987.

107. Trojani, M., Contesso, G., Coindre, J.M., Rouesse, J., Bui, N.B., deMascarel, A., Goussot, J.F., David, M., Bonichon, F., and Lagarde, C.: Soft-tissue sarcomas of adults: study of pathological prognostic variables and definition of a histopathological grading system, Int. J. Cancer **33**:37, 1984.

108. Tsujimoto, M., Aozasa, K., Ueda, T., Morimura, Y., Komatsubara, Y., and Doi, T.: Multivariate analysis for histologic prognostic factors in soft tissue sarcomas, Cancer **62**:994, 1988.

109. Tsukada, T., McNutt, M.A., Ross, R., and Gown, A.M.: HHF35, a muscle actin-specific monoclonal antibody II: reactivity in normal, reactive, and neoplastic human tissues, Am. J. Pathol. **127**:389, 1987.

110. van Haelst, U.J.G.M.: General considerations on electron microscopy of tumors of soft tissues. In Fenoglio, C.M., and Wolff, M., editors: Progress in surgical pathology, vol. 2, New York, 1980, Masson Publishing USA, Inc.

111. Van Muijen, G.N.P., Ruiter, D.J., and Warnaar, S.O.: Coexpression of intermediate filament polypeptides in human fetal and adult tissues, Lab. Invest. **57**:359, 1987.

112. Vinores, S.A., Bonnin, J.M., Rubinstein, L.J., and Marangos, P.J.: Immunohistochemical demonstration of neuron-specific enolase in neoplasms of the CNS and other tissues, Arch. Pathol. Lab. Med. **108**:536, 1984.

113. Weiss, S.W., Bratthauer, G.L., and Morris, P.A.: Postirradiation malignant fibrous histiocytoma expressing cytokeratin: implications for the immunodiagnosis of sarcomas, Am. J. Surg. Pathol. **12**:554, 1988.

114. Weiss, S.W., Langloss, J.M., and Enzinger, F.M.: Value of S-100 protein in the diagnosis of soft tissue tumors with particular reference to benign and malignant schwann cell tumors, Lab. Invest. **49**:299, 1983.

115. Wick, M.R., and Siegal, G.P.: Monoclonal antibodies in diagnostic immunohistochemistry, New York, 1988, Marcel Dekker, Inc.

116. Young, J.L., Jr., and Miller, R.W.: Incidence of malignant tumors in U.S. children, J. Pediatr. **86**:254, 1975.

Fibrous-tissue lesions
Fibrosarcoma

117. Chung, E.B., and Enzinger, F.M.: Infantile fibrosarcoma, Cancer **38**:729, 1976.

118. Churg, A.M., and Kahn, L.B.: Myofibroblasts and related cells in malignant fibrous and fibrohistiocytic tumors, Hum. Pathol. **8**:205, 1977.

119. Enjoji, M., Hashimoto, H., Tsuneyoshi, M., and Iwasaki H.: Malignant fibrous histiocytoma: a clinicopathologic study of 130 cases, Acta Pathol. Jpn. **30**:727, 1980.

120. Gonzalez-Crussi, F., Wiederhold, M.D., and Sotelo-Avila, C.: Congenital fibrosarcoma: presence of a histiocytic component, Cancer **46**:77, 1980.

121. Grier, H.E., Perez-Atayde, A.R., and Weinstein, H.J.: Chemotherapy for inoperable infantile fibrosarcoma, Cancer **56**:1507, 1985.

122. Iwasaki, H., and Enjoji, M.: Infantile and adult fibrosarcoma of the soft tissues, Acta Pathol. Jpn. **29**:377, 1979.

123. Krall, R.A., Kostianovsky, M., and Patchefsky, A.S.: Synovial sarcoma: a clinical, pathological, and ultrastructural study of 26 cases supporting the recognition of a monophasic variant, Am. J. Surg. Pathol. **5**:137, 1981.

124. Lagacé, R., Schürch, W., and Seemayer, T.A.: Myofibroblasts in soft tissue sarcomas, Virchows Arch. [A] **389**:1, 1980.

125. Ninane, J., Gosseye, S., Panteon, E., Claus, D., Rombouts, J.-J., and Cornu, G.: Congenital fibrosarcoma: preoperative chemotherapy and conservative surgery, Cancer **58**:1400, 1986.

126. Pritchard, D.J., Soule, E.H., Taylor, W.F., and Ivins, J.C.: Fibrosarcoma—a clinicopathologic and statistical study of 199 tumors of the soft tissues of the extremities and trunk, Cancer **33**:888, 1974.

127. Rosenberg, H.S., Stenback, W.A., and Spjut, H.J.: The fibromatoses of infancy and childhood. In Rosenberg, H.S., and Bolande, R.P., editors: Perspectives in pediatric pathology, vol. 4, Chicago, 1978, Year Book Medical Publishers, Inc.

128. Soule, E.H., and Pritchard, D.J.: Fibrosarcoma in infants and children, Cancer **40**:1711, 1977.

129. Weiner, J.M., and Hidayat, A.A.: Juvenile fibrosarcoma of the orbit and eyelid: a study of five cases, Arch. Ophthalmol. **101**:253, 1983.

Fibromatoses

130. Allen, P.W.: The fibromatoses: a clinicopathologic classification based on 140 cases, Am. J. Surg. Pathol. **1**:255, 305, 1977.

131. Enzinger, F.M.: Fibrous hamartoma of infancy, Cancer **18**:241, 1965.

132. Enzinger, F.M.: Fibrous tumors of infancy. In Tumors of bone and soft tissue, Chicago, 1965, Year Book Medical Publishers, Inc.

133. Lipper, S., Kahn, L.B., and Reddick, R.L.: The myofibroblast, Pathol. Annu. **15**(pt. 1):409, 1980.
134. Mackenzie, D.H.: The differential diagnosis of fibroblastic disorders, Oxford, Eng., 1970, Blackwell Scientific Publications.
135. Mackenzie, D.H.: The fibromatoses: a clinicopathological concept, Br. Med. J. **4:**277, 1972.
136. Navas-Palacios, J.J.: The fibromatoses: an ultrastructural study of 31 cases, Pathol. Res. Pract. **176:**158, 1983.
137. Rosenberg, H.S., Stenback, W.A., and Spjut, H.J.: The fibromatoses of infancy and childhood. In Rosenberg, H.S., and Bolande, R.P., editors: Perspectives in pediatric pathology, vol. 4, Chicago, 1978, Year Book Medical Publishers, Inc.

Palmar and plantar fibromatosis

138. Gabbiani, G., and Majno, G.: Dupuytren's contracture: Fibroblast contraction? An ultrastructural study, Am. J. Pathol. **66:**131, 1972.
139. Iwasaki, H., Müller, H., Stutte, H.J., and Brennscheidt, U.: Palmar fibromatosis (Dupuytren's contracture): ultrastructural and enymze histochemical studies of 43 cases, Virchows Arch. [A] **405:**41, 1984.
140. James, W.D., and Odom, R.B.: The role of the myofibroblast in Dupuytren's contracture, Arch. Dermatol. **116:**807, 1980.
141. Larsen, R.D., and Posch, J.L.: Dupuytren's contracture: with special reference to pathology, J. Bone Joint Surg. **40A:**773, 1958.
142. Pojer, J., Radivojevic, M., and Williams, T.F.: Dupuytren's disease: its association with abnormal liver function in alcoholism and epilepsy, Arch. Intern. Med. **129:**561, 1972.
143. Ushijima, M., Tsuneyoshi, M., and Enjoji, M.: Dupuytren type fibromatoses: a clinicopathologic study of 62 cases, Acta Pathol. Jpn. **34:**991, 1984.

Desmoid fibromatoses

144. Cole, N.M., and Guiss, L.W.: Extra-abdominal desmoid tumors, Arch. Surg. **98:**530, 1969.
145. Conley, J., Healey, W.V., and Stout, A.P.: Fibromatosis of the head and neck, Am. J. Surg. **112:**609, 1966.
146. Das Gupta, T.K., Brasfield, R.D., and O'Hara, J.: Extra-abdominal desmoids: a clinicopathological study, Ann. Surg. **170:**109, 1969.
147. Enzinger, F.M., and Shiraki, M.: Musculo-aponeurotic fibromatosis of the shoulder girdle (extra-abdominal desmoid): analysis of thirty cases followed up for ten or more years, Cancer **20:**1131, 1967.
148. Fletcher, C.D.M., Stirling, R.W., Smith, M.A., Pambakian, H., and McKee, P.H.: Multicentric extra-abdominal 'myofibromatosis': report of a case with ultrastructural findings, Histopathology **10:**713, 1986.
149. Goellner, J.R., and Soule, E.H.: Desmoid tumors: an ultrastructural study of eight cases, Hum. Pathol. **11:**43, 1980.
150. Greenberg, H.M., Goebel R., Weichselbaum, R.R., Greenberger, J.S., Chaffey, J.T., and Cassady, J.R.: Radiation therapy in the treatment of aggressive fibromatoses, Int. J. Radiat. Oncol. Biol. Phys. **7:**305, 1981.
151. Griffiths, H.J., Robinson, K., and Bonfiglio, T.A.: Aggressive fibromatosis, Skeletal Radiol. **9:**179, 1983.
152. Häyry, P., Reitamo, J.J., Tötterman, S., Hopfner-Hallikainen, D., and Sivula, A.: The desmoid tumor. II. Analysis of factors possibly contributing to the etiology and growth behavior, Am. J. Clin. Pathol. **77:**674, 1982.
153. Häyry, P., Reitamo, J.J., Vihko, R., Jänne, O., Scheinin, T.M., Tötterman, S., Ahonen, J., Norio, R., and Alanko, A.: The desmoid tumor. III. A biochemical and genetic analysis, Am. J. Clin. Pathol. **77:**681, 1982.
154. Hunt, R.T.N., and Morgan, H.C., and Ackerman, L.V.: Principles in the management of extra-abdominal desmoids, Cancer **13:**825, 1960.
155. Jones, I.T., Jagelman, D.G., Fazio, V.W., Lavery, I.C., Weakley, F.L., and McGannon, E.: Desmoid tumors in familial polyposis coli, Ann. Surg. **204:**94, 1986.
156. Khorsand, J., and Karakousis, C.P.: Desmoid tumors and their management, Am. J. Surg. **149:**215, 1985.
157. Kiel, K.D., and Suit, H.D.: Radiation therapy in the treatment of aggressive fibromatoses (desmoid tumors), Cancer **54:**2051, 1984.
158. Kinzbrunner, B., Ritter, S., Domingo, J., and Rosenthal, C.J.: Remission of rapidly growing desmoid tumors after tamoxifen therapy, Cancer **52:**2201, 1983.
159. Klein, W.A., Miller, H.H., Anderson, M., and DeCosse, J.J.: The use of indomethacin, sulindac, and tamoxifen for the treatment of desmoid tumors associated with familial polyposis, Cancer **60:**2863, 1987.
160. Kofoed, H., Kamby, C., and Anagnostaki, L.: Aggressive fibromatosis, Surg. Gynecol. Obstet. **160:**124, 1985.
161. Lanari, A.: Effect of progesterone on desmoid tumors (aggressive fibromatosis), N. Engl. J. Med. **309:**1523, 1983.
162. Leibel, S.A., Wara, W.M., Hill, D.R., Bovill, E.G., Jr., De Lorimier, A.A., Beckstead, J.H., and Phillips, T.L.: Desmoid tumors: local control and patterns of relapse following radiation therapy, Int. J. Radiat. Oncol. Biol. Phys. **9:**1167, 1983.
163. Masson, J.K., and Soule, E.H.: Desmoid tumors of the head and neck, Am. J. Surg. **112:**615, 1966.
164. Navas-Palacios, J.J.: The fibromatoses: an ultrastructural study of 31 cases, Pathol. Res. Pract. **176:**158, 1983.
165. Reitamo, J.J., Häyry, P., Nykyri, E., and Saxén, E.: The desmoid tumor. I. Incidence, sex-, age- and anatomical distribution in the Finnish population, Am. J. Clin. Pathol. **77:**665, 1982.
166. Richards, R.C., Rogers, S.W., and Gardner, E.J.: Spontaneous mesenteric fibromatosis in Gardner's syndrome, Cancer **47:**597, 1981.
167. Rock, M.G., Pritchard, D.J., Reiman, H.M., Soule, E.H., and Brewster, R.C.: Extra-abdominal desmoid tumors, J. Bone Joint Surg. **66A:**1369, 1984.
168. Sanders, R., Bennett, M., and Walton, J.N.: A multifocal extra-abdominal desmoid tumour, Br. J. Plast. Surg. **36:**337, 1983.
169. Sundaram, M., Duffrin, H., McGuire, M.H., and Vas, W.: Synchronous multicentric desmoid tumors (aggressive fibromatosis) of the extremities, Skeletal Radiol. **17:**16, 1988.
170. Waddell, W.R., Gerner, R.E., and Reich, M.P.: Nonsteroid anti-inflammatory drugs and tamoxifen for desmoid tumors and carcinoma of the stomach, J. Surg. Oncol. **22:**197, 1983.
171. Zayid, I., and Dihmis, C.: Familial multicentric fibromatosis—desmoids: a report of three cases in a Jordanian family, Cancer **24:**786, 1969.

Fibrous hamartoma of infancy

172. Albukerk, J., Wexler, H., Dana, M., and Silverman, J.: A case of fibrous hamartoma of infancy, J. Pediatr. Surg. **14:**80, 1979.
173. Baarsma, E.A.: Juvenile fibrous hamartoma of the pharynx, J. Laryngol. Otol. **93:**75, 1979.
174. Enzinger, F.M.: Fibrous hamartoma of infancy, Cancer **18:**241, 1965.
175. Fletcher, C.D.M., Powell, G., van Noorden, S., and McKee, P.H.: Fibrous hamartoma of infancy: a histochemical and immunohistochemical study, Histopathology **12:**65, 1988.
176. Greco, M.A., Schinella, R.A., and Vuletin, J.C.: Fibrous hamartoma of infancy: an ultrastructural study, Hum. Pathol. **15:**717, 1984.
177. Mitchell, M.L., di Sant'Agnese, P.A., and Gerber, J.E.: Fibrous hamartoma of infancy, Hum. Pathol. **13:**586, 1982.
178. Reye, R.D.K.: A consideration of certain subdermal "fibromatous tumours" of infancy, J. Pathol. Bacteriol. **72:**149, 1956.
179. Robbins, L.B., Hoffman, S., and Kahn, S.: Fibrous hamartoma of infancy: case report, Plast. Reconstr. Surg. **46:**197, 1970.

Aponeurotic fibroma

180. Allen, P.W., and Enzinger, F.M.: Juvenile aponeurotic fibroma, Cancer **26:**857, 1970.
181. Goldman, R.L.: The cartilage analogue of fibromatosis (aponeurotic fibroma): further observations based on 7 new cases, Cancer **26:**1325, 1970.
182. Keasbey, L.E.: Juvenile aponeurotic fibroma (calcifying fibroma): a distinctive tumor arising in the palms and soles of young children, Cancer **6:**338, 1953.
183. Keasbey, L.E., and Fanselau, H.A.: The aponeurotic fibroma, Clin. Orthop. **19:**115, 1961.

184. Lichtenstein, L., and Goldman, R.L.: The cartilage analogue of fibromatosis: a reinterpretation of the condition called "juvenile aponeurotic fibroma," Cancer 17:810, 1964.

185. Specht, E.E., and Konkin, L.A.: Juvenile aponeurotic fibroma: the cartilage analogue of fibromatosis, JAMA 234:626, 1975.

Myofibromatosis (congenital generalized fibromatosis, infantile myofibromatosis)

186. Altemani, A.M., Amstalden, E.I., and Filho, J.M.: Congenital generalized fibromatosis causing spinal cord compression, Hum. Pathol. 16:1063, 1985.

187. Baird, P.A., and Worth, A.J.: Congenital generalized fibromatosis: an autosomal recessive condition? Clin. Genet. 9:488, 1976.

188. Benjamin, S.P., Mercer, R.D., and Hawk, W.A.: Myofibroblastic contraction in spontaneous regression of multiple congenital mesenchymal hamartomas, Cancer 40:2343, 1977.

189. Brill, P.W., Yandow, D.R., Langer, L.O., Breed, A.L., Laxova, R., and Gilbert, E.F.: Congenital generalized fibromatosis: case report and literature review, Pediatr. Radiol. 12:269, 1982.

190. Briselli, M.F., Soule, E.H., and Gilchrist, G.S.: Congenital fibromatosis: report of 18 cases of solitary and 4 cases of multiple tumors, Mayo Clin. Proc. 55:554, 1980.

191. Chung, E.B., and Enzinger, F.M.: Infantile myofibromatosis, Cancer 48:1807, 1981.

192. Dimmick, J.E., and Wood, W.S.: Congenital multiple fibromatosis, Am. J. Dermatopathol. 5:289, 1983.

193. Fletcher, C.D.M., Achu, P., van Noorden, S., and McKee, P.H.: Infantile myofibromatosis: a light microscopic, histochemical and immunohistochemical study suggesting true smooth muscle differentiation, Histopathology 11:245, 1987.

194. Gold, R.H., and Mirra, J.M.: Case report 339: congenital multiple fibromatosis, Skeletal Radiol. 14:309, 1985.

195. Jennings, T.A., Duray, P.H., Collins, F.S., Sabetta, J., and Enzinger, F.M.: Infantile myofibromatosis: evidence for an autosomal-dominant disorder, Am. J. Surg. Pathol. 8:529, 1984.

196. Kauffman, S.L., and Stout, A.P.: Congenital mesenchymal tumors, Cancer 18:460, 1965.

197. Kindblom, L.-G., and Angervall, L.: Congenital solitary fibromatosis of the skeleton: case report of a variant of congenital generalized fibromatosis, Cancer 41:636, 1978.

198. Kindblom, L.-G., Termén, G., Säve-Söderbergh, J., and Angervall, L.: Congenital solitary fibromatosis of soft tissues, a variant of congenital generalized fibromatosis: 2 case reports, Acta Pathol. Microbiol. Scand. [A] 85:640, 1977.

199. Liew, S.-H., and Haynes, M.: Localized form of congenital generalized fibromatosis: a report of 3 cases with myofibroblasts, Pathology 13:257, 1981.

200. Mizobuchi, K., Yoshino, T., Ikehara, I., Kawabata, K., Tsutsumi, A., Ogawa, K., and Saku, T.: Infantile myofibromatosis: Report of two cases, Acta Pathol. Jpn. 36:1411, 1986.

201. Modi, N.: Congenital generalised fibromatosis, Arch. Dis. Child. 57:881, 1982.

202. Roggli, V.L., Kim, H.-S., and Hawkins, E.: Congenital generalized fibromatosis with visceral involvement: a case report, Cancer 45:954, 1980.

203. Stout, A.P.: Juvenile fibromatoses, Cancer 7:953, 1954.

204. Walts, A.E., Asch, M., and Raj, C.: Solitary lesion of congenital fibromatosis: a rare cause of neonatal intestinal obstruction, Am. J. Surg. Pathol. 6:255, 1982.

Pseudosarcomatous fibrous lesions

205. Allen, P.W.: Nodular fasciitis, Pathology 4:9, 1972.

206. Bernstein, K.E., and Lattes, R.: Nodular (pseudosarcomatous) fasciitis, a nonrecurrent lesion: clinicopathologic study of 134 cases, Cancer 49:1668, 1982.

207. Chung, E.B., and Enzinger, F.M.: Proliferative fasciitis, Cancer 36:1450, 1975.

208. Craver, J.L., and McDivitt, R.W.: Proliferative fasciitis: ultrastructural study of two cases, Arch. Pathol. Lab. Med. 105:542, 1981.

209. Dahl, I., and Angervall, L.: Pseudosarcomatous lesions of the soft tissues reported as sarcoma during a 6-year period (1958-1963), Acta Pathol. Microbiol. Scand. 85A:917, 1977.

210. Dahl, I., and Angervall, L.: Pseudosarcomatous proliferative lesions of soft tissue with or without bone formation, Acta Pathol. Microbiol. Scand. 85A:577, 1977.

211. Dahl, I., Angervall, L., Magnusson, S., and Stener, B.: Classical and cystic nodular fasciitis, Pathol. Eur. 7:211, 1972.

212. Enzinger, F.M.: Recent trends in soft tissue pathology. In Tumors of bone and soft tissue, Chicago, 1965, Year Book Medical Publishers, Inc.

213. Enzinger, F.M., and Dulcey, F.: Proliferative myositis: report of thirty-three cases, Cancer 20:2213, 1967.

214. Gokel, J.M., Meister, P., and Hübner, G.: Proliferative myositis: a case report with fine structural analysis, Virchows Arch. [A] 367:345, 1975.

215. Heyden, R., Hägerstrand, I., Linell, F., Nordén, G., Akesson, B.-A., and Östberg, G.: Proliferative myositis: report of two cases, Acta Pathol. Microbiol. Scand. [A] 78:33, 1970.

216. Hutter, R.V.P., Foote, F.W., Jr., Francis, K.C., and Higinbotham, N.L.: Parosteal fasciitis: a self-limited benign process that simulates a malignant neoplasm, Am. J. Surg. 104:800, 1962.

217. Hutter, R.V.P., Stewart, F.W., and Foote, F.W., Jr.: Fasciitis: a report of 70 cases with follow-up proving the benignity of the lesion, Cancer 15:992, 1962.

218. Kern, W.H.: Proliferative myositis: a pseudosarcomatous reaction to injury, Arch. Pathol. 69:209, 1960.

219. Kitano, M., Iwasaki, H., and Enjoji, M.: Proliferative fasciitis: a variant of nodular fasciitis, Acta Pathol. Jpn. 27:485, 1977.

220. Kleinstiver, B.J., and Rodríguez, H.A.: Nodular fasciitis: a study of forty-five cases and review of the literature, J. Bone Joint Surg. 50A:1204, 1968.

221. Konwaler, B.E., Keasbey, L., and Kaplan, L.: Subcutaneous pseudosarcomatous fibromatosis (fasciitis), Am. J. Clin. Pathol. 25:241, 1955.

222. Lauer, D.H., and Enzinger, F.M.: Cranial fasciitis of childhood, Cancer 45:401, 1980.

223. Meister, P., Bückmann, F.-W., and Konrad, E.: Nodular fasciitis (analysis of 100 cases and review of the literature), Pathol. Res. Pract. 162:133, 1978.

224. Orlowski, W., Freedman, P.D., and Lumerman, H.: Proliferative myositis of the masseter muscle: a case report and a review of the literature, Cancer 52:904, 1983.

225. Patchefsky, A.S., and Enzinger, F.M.: Intravascular fasciitis; a report of 17 cases, Am. J. Surg. Pathol. 5:29, 1981.

226. Ringsted, J., Ladefoged, C., and Bjerre, P.: Cranial fasciitis of childhood, Acta Neuropathol. (Berlin) 66:337, 1985.

227. Shimizu, S., Hashimoto, H., and Enjoji, M.: Nodular fasciitis: an analysis of 250 patients, Pathology 16:161, 1984.

228. Stiller, D., and Katenkamp, D.: The subcutaneous fascial analogue of myositis proliferans: electron microscopic examination of two cases and comparison with myositis ossificans localisata, Virchows Arch. [A] 368:361, 1975.

229. Stout, A.P.: Pseudosarcomatous fasciitis in children, Cancer 14:1216, 1961.

230. Ushigome, S., Takakuwa, T., Takagi, M., Koizumi, H., and Morikubo, M.: Proliferative myositis and fasciitis: report of five cases with an ultrastructural and immunohistochemical study, Acta Pathol. Jpn. 26:963, 1986.

231. Wirman, J.A.: Nodular fasciitis, a lesion of myofibroblasts: an ultrastructural study, Cancer 38:2378, 1976.

Fibrohistiocytic tumors

232. Alguacil-García, A., Unni, K.K., and Goellner, J.R.: Malignant fibrous histiocytoma: an ultrastructural study of six cases, Am. J. Clin. Pathol. 69:121, 1978.

233. Allen, P.W.: Myxoid tumors of soft tissues, Pathol Annu. 15(pt. 1):133, 1980.

234. Angervall, L., Kindblom, L.-G., and Merck, C.: Myxofibrosarcoma: a study of 30 cases, Acta Pathol. Microbiol. Scand. 85A:127, 1977.

235. Asirwatham, J.E., and Pickren, J.W.: Inflammatory fibrous histiocytoma: case report, Cancer 41:1467, 1978
236. Bertoni, F., Capanna, R., Biagini, R., Bacchini, P., Guerra, A., Ruggieri, P., Present, D., and Campanacci, M.: Malignant fibrous histiocytoma of soft tissue: an analysis of 78 cases located and deeply seated in the extremities, Cancer 56:356, 1985.
237. Bhagavan, B.S., and Dorfman, H.D.: The significance of bone and cartilage formation in malignant fibrous histiocytoma of soft tissue, Cancer 49:480, 1982.
238. Brecher, M.E., and Franklin, W.A.: Absence of mononuclear phagocyte antigens in malignant fibrous histiocytoma, Am. J. Clin. Pathol. 86:344, 1986.
239. Brooks, J.J.: The significance of double phenotypic patterns and markers in human sarcomas: a new model of mesenchymal differentiation, Am. J. Pathol. 125:113, 1986.
240. Chen, K.T.K., Brittin, G., and Phillips, J.R.: Metastatic carcinoma simulating primary malignant fibrous histiocytoma of bone, Arch. Pathol. Lab. Med. 104:548, 1980.
241. Chung, E.B., and Enzinger, F.M.: Extraskeletal osteosarcoma, Cancer 60:1132, 1987.
242. Churg, A.M., and Kahn, L.B.: Myofibroblasts and related cells in malignant fibrous and fibrohistiocytic tumors, Hum. Pathol. 8:205, 1977.
243. Cozzutto, C., Bronzini, E., Bandelloni, R., Guarino, M., and DeBernardi, B.: Malignant monomorphic histiocytoma in children, Cancer 48:2112, 1981.
244. du Boulay, C.E.H.: Demonstration of alpha-1-antitrypsin and alpha-1-antichymotrypsin in fibrous histiocytomas using the immunoperoxidase technique, Am. J. Surg. Pathol. 6:559, 1982.
245. Ekfors, T.O., and Rantakokko, V.: An analysis of 38 malignant fibrous histiocytomas in the extremities, Acta Pathol. Microbiol. Scand. [A] 86:25, 1978.
246. Enjoji, M., Hashimoto, H., Tsuneyoshi, M., and Iwasaki, H.: Malignant fibrous histiocytoma: a clinicopathologic study of 130 cases, Acta Pathol. Jpn. 30:727, 1980.
247. Enzinger, F.M.: Recent developments in the classification of soft tissue sarcomas. In M.D. Anderson Hospital and Tumor Institute: Management of primary bone and soft tissue tumors, Chicago, 1977, Year Book Medical Publishers, Inc.
248. Enzinger, F.M.: Angiomatoid malignant fibrous histiocytoma: a distinct fibrohistiocytic tumor of children and young adults simulating a vascular neoplasm, Cancer 44:2147, 1979.
249. Enzinger, F.M.: Malignant fibrous histiocytoma 20 years after Stout, Am. J. Surg. Pathol. 10(suppl. 1):43, 1986.
250. Ferrell, H.W., and Frable, W.J.: Soft part sarcomas revisited: review and comparison and a second series, Cancer 30:475, 1972.
251. Fletcher, C.D.M.: Malignant fibrous histiocytoma? Histopathology 11:433, 1987.
252. Fletcher, C.D.M., and Lowe, D.: Inflammatory fibrous histiocytoma of the penis, Histopathology 8:1079, 1984.
253. Fu, Y.-S., Gabbiani, G., Kaye, G.I., and Lattes, R.: Malignant soft tissue tumors of probable histiocytic origin (malignant fibrous histiocytomas): general considerations and electron microscopic and tissue culture studies, Cancer 35:176, 1975.
254. Fukuda, T., Tsuneyoshi, M., and Enjoji, M.: Malignant fibrous histiocytoma of soft parts: an ultrastructural quantitative study, Ultrastruct. Pathol. 12:117, 1988.
255. Gilkey, F.W.: Changing MFH to FHS, Hum. Pathol. 18:1301, 1987.
256. Hashimoto, H., and Enjoji, M.: Recurrent malignant fibrous histiocytoma: a histologic analysis of 50 cases, Am. J. Surg. Pathol. 4:753, 1981.
257. Herrera, G.A., Reimann, B.E.F., Salinas, J.A., and Turbat, E.A.: Malignant schwannomas presenting as malignant fibrous histiocytomas, Ultrastruct. Pathol. 3:253, 1982.
258. Hoffman, M.A., and Dickersin, G.R.: Malignant fibrous histiocytoma: an ultrastructural study of eleven cases, Hum. Pathol. 14:913, 1983.
259. Inoue, A., Aozasa, K., Tsujimoto, M., Tamai, M., Chatani, F., and Ueno, H.: Immunohistological study on malignant fibrous histiocytoma, Acta Pathol. Jpn. 34:759, 1984.
260. Iwasaki, H., Isayama, T., Johzaki, H., and Kikuchi, M.: Malignant fibrous histiocytoma: evidence of perivascular mesenchymal cell origin: immunocytochemical studies with monoclonal anti-MFH antibodies, Am. J. Pathol. 128:528, 1987.
261. Iwasaki, H., Kikuchi, M., Takii, M., and Enjoji, M.: Benign and malignant fibrous histiocytomas of the soft tissues: functional characterization of the cultured cells, Cancer 50:520, 1982.
262. Jabi, M., Jeans, D., and Dardick, I.: Ultrastructural heterogeneity in malignant fibrous histiocytoma of soft tissue, Ultrastruct. Pathol. 11:583, 1987.
263. Kahn, L.B.: Retroperitoneal xanthogranuloma and xanthosarcoma (malignant fibrous xanthoma), Cancer 31:411, 1973.
264. Kauffman, S.L., and Stout, A.P.: Histiocytic tumors (fibrous xanthoma and histiocytoma) in children, Cancer 14:469, 1961.
265. Kay, S.: Inflammatory fibrous histiocytoma (? xanthogranuloma): report of two cases with ultrastructural observations in one, Am. J. Surg. Pathol. 2:313, 1978.
266. Kay, S.: Angiomatoid malignant fibrous histiocytoma: report of two cases with ultrastructural observations of one case, Arch. Pathol. Lab. Med. 109:934, 1985.
267. Kearney, M.M., Soule, E.H., and Ivins, J.C.: Malignant fibrous histiocytoma: a retrospective study of 167 cases, Cancer 45:167, 1980.
268. Kempson, R.L., and Kyriakos, M.: Fibroxanthosarcoma of the soft tissues: a type of malignant fibrous histiocytoma, Cancer 29:961, 1972.
269. Kindblom, L.-G., Jacobsen, G.K., and Jacobsen, M.: Immunohistochemical investigations of tumors of supposed fibroblastic-histiocytic origin, Hum. Pathol. 13:834, 1982.
270. Kindblom, L.-G., Merck, C., and Angervall, L.: The ultrastructure of myxofibrosarcoma: a study of 11 cases, Virchows Arch. [A] 381:121, 1979.
271. Kyriakos, M., and Kempson, R.L.: Inflammatory fibrous histiocytoma: an aggressive and lethal lesion, Cancer 37:1584, 1976.
272. Lagacé, R.: The ultrastructural spectrum of malignant fibrous histiocytoma, Ultrastruct. Pathol. 11:153, 1987.
273. Lattes, R.: Malignant fibrous histiocytoma: a review article, Am. J. Surg. Pathol. 6:761, 1982.
274. Lawson, C.W., Fisher, C., and Gatter, K.C.: An immunohistochemical study of differentiation in malignant fibrous histiocytoma, Histopathology 11:375, 1987.
275. Leader, M.: Letter to the editor, Am. J. Surg. Pathol. 11:820, 1987.
276. Leader, M., Patel, J., Collins, M., and Henry, K.: Anti-α1-antichymotrypsin staining of 194 sarcomas, 38 carcinomas, and 17 malignant melanomas: its lack of specificity as a tumour marker, Am. J. Surg. Pathol. 11:133, 1987.
277. Lentini, M., Grosso, M., Carrozza, G., and Risitano, G.: Fibrohistiocytic tumors of soft tissues: an immunohistochemical study of 183 cases, Pathol. Res. Pract. 181:713, 1986.
278. Leu, H.J., and Makek, M.: Angiomatoid malignant fibrous histiocytoma: case report and electron microscopic findings, Virchows Arch. [A] 395:99, 1982.
279. Limacher, J., Delage, C., and Lagacé, R.: Malignant fibrous histiocytoma: clinicopathologic and ultrastructural study of 12 cases, Am. J. Surg. Pathol. 2:265, 1978.
280. Magnusson, B., Kindblom, L.-G., and Angervall, L.: Enzyme histochemistry of malignant fibroblastic histiocytic tumors: a light and electron microscopic analysis, Appl. Pathol. 1:223, 1983.
281. Meister, P., Höhne, N., Konrad, E., and Eder, M.: Fibrous histiocytoma: an analysis of the storiform pattern, Virchows Arch. [A] 383:31, 1979.
282. Meister, P., Konrad, E., and Höhne, N.: Incidence and histological structure of the storiform pattern in benign and malignant fibrous histiocytomas, Virchows Arch. [A] 393:93, 1981.
283. Meister, P., Konrad, E.A., Nathrath, W., and Eder, M.: Malignant fibrous histiocytoma: histological patterns and cell types, Pathol. Res. Pract. 168:193, 1980.
284. Merck, C., Angervall, L., Kindblom, L.-G., and Odén, A.: Myxofibrosarcoma: a malignant soft tissue tumor of fibroblastic-

histiocytic origin, Acta Pathol. Microbiol. Immunol. Scand. [A] **91**(suppl. 282):1, 1983.

285. Merino, M.J., and LiVolsi, V.A.: Inflammatory malignant fibrous histiocytoma, Am. J. Clin. Pathol. **73**:276, 1980.

286. Miettinen, M., Lehto, V.-P., and Virtanen, I.: Antibodies to intermediate filament proteins in the diagnosis and classification of human tumors, Ultrastruct. Pathol. **7**:83, 1984.

287. Nakanishi, S., and Hizawa, K.: Enzyme histochemical observation of fibrohistiocytic tumors, Acta Pathol. Jpn. **34**:1003, 1984.

288. O'Brien, J.E., and Stout, A.P.: Malignant fibrous xanthomas, Cancer **17**:1445, 1964.

289. Ohmori, T., Arita, N., Sano, A., Uraga, N., Tabei, R., Sato, M., Sakai, K., and Watanabe, Y.: Malignant fibrous histiocytoma showing cytoplasmic hyaline globules and stromal osteoids: a case report with light and electron microscopic, histochemical, and immunohistochemical study, Acta Pathol. Jpn. **36**:1931, 1986.

290. Ozzello, L., Stout, A.P., and Murray, M.R.: Cultural characteristics of malignant histiocytomas and fibrous xanthomas, Cancer **16**:331, 1963.

291. Pinkston, J.A., and Sekine, I.: Postirradiation sarcoma (malignant fibrous histiocytoma) following cervix cancer, Cancer **49**:434, 1982.

292. Poon, M.-C., Durant, J.R., Norgard, M.J., and Chang-Poon, V.Y.-H.: Inflammatory fibrous histiocytoma: an important variant of malignant fibrous histiocytoma highly responsive to chemotherapy, Ann. Intern. Med. **97**:858, 1982.

293. Raney, R.B., Jr., Allen, A., O'Neill, J., Handler, S.D., Uri, A., and Littman, P.: Malignant fibrous histiocytoma of soft tissue in childhood, Cancer **57**:2198, 1986.

294. Roholl, P.J.M., Kleyne, J., Elbers, H., Van Der Vegt, M.C.D., Albus-Lutter, Ch., and Van Unnik, J.A.M.: Characterization of tumour cells in malignant fibrous histiocytomas and other soft tissue tumours in comparison with malignant histiocytes. I. Immunohistochemical study on paraffin sections, J. Pathol. **147**:87, 1985.

295. Roholl, P.J.M., Kleijne, J., Van Basten, C.D.H., van der Putte, S.C.J., and van Unnik, J.A.M.: A study to analyze the origin of tumor cells in malignant fibrous histiocytomas: a multiparametric characterization, Cancer **56**:2809, 1985.

296. Roholl, P.J.M., Kleyne, J., and Van Unnik, J.A.M.: Characterization of tumor cells in malignant fibrous histiocytomas and other soft tissue tumors, in comparison with malignant histiocytes. II. Immunoperoxidase study on cryostat sections, Am. J. Pathol. **121**:269, 1985.

297. Roques, A.W.W., Horton, L.W.L., Leslie, J., and Buxton-Thomas, M.S.: Inflammatory fibrous histiocytoma in the left upper abdomen with a leukemoid blood picture, Cancer **43**:1800, 1979.

298. Rosas-Uribe, A., Ring, A.M., and Rappaport, H.: Metastasizing retroperitoneal fibroxanthoma (malignant fibroxanthoma), Cancer **26**:827, 1970.

299. Roth, J.A., Carter, H., and Costabile, D.: An unusual multifocal leiomyosarcoma of the stomach: a light and electron microscopic study, Hum. Pathol. **9**:345, 1978.

300. Saku, T., Tsuda, N., Anami, M., and Okabe, H.: Smooth and skeletal muscle myosins in spindle cell tumors of soft tissue: an immunohistochemical study, Acta Pathol. Jpn. **35**:125, 1985.

301. Santa Cruz, D.J., and Kyriakos, M.: Aneurysmal ("angiomatoid") fibrous histiocytoma of the skin, Cancer **47**:2053, 1981.

302. Shimoda, T., Yamashita, H., Furusato, M., Kirino, Y., Ishikawa, E., Miyagawa, A., and Ubayama, Y.: Liposarcoma: a light and electron microscopic study with comments on their relation to malignant fibrous histiocytoma and angiosarcoma, Acta Pathol. Jpn. **30**:779, 1980.

303. Shirasuna, K., Sugiyama, M., and Miyazaki, T.: Establishment and characterization of neoplastic cells from a malignant fibrous histiocytoma: a possible stem cell line, Cancer **55**:2521, 1985.

304. Snover, D.C., Phillips, G., and Dehner, L.P.: Reactive fibrohistiocytic proliferation simulating fibrous histiocytoma, Am. J. Clin. Pathol. **76**:232, 1981.

305. Snover, D.C., Sumner, H.W., and Dehner, L.P.: Variability of histologic pattern in recurrent soft tissue sarcomas originally diagnosed as liposarcoma, Cancer **49**:1005, 1982.

306. Soule, E.H., and Enriquez, P.: Atypical fibrous histiocytoma, malignant fibrous histiocytoma, malignant histiocytoma, and epithelioid sarcoma: a comparative study of 65 tumors, Cancer **30**:128, 1972.

307. Strauchen, J.A., and Dimitriu-Bona, A.: Malignant fibrous histiocytoma: expression of monocyte/macrophage differentiation antigens detected with monoclonal antibodies, Am. J. Pathol. **124**:303, 1986.

308. Sun, C.-C.J., Toker, C., and Breitenecker, R.: An ultrastructural study of angiomatoid fibrous histiocytoma, Cancer **49**:2103, 1982.

309. Taxy, J.B., and Battifora, H.: Malignant fibrous histiocytoma: an electron microscopic study, Cancer **40**:254, 1977.

310. Tracy, T., Jr., Neifeld, J.P., DeMay, R.M., and Salzberg, A.M.: Malignant fibrous histiocytomas in children, J. Pediatr. Surg. **19**:81, 1984.

311. Tsuneyoshi, M., and Enjoji, M.: Postirradiation sarcoma (malignant fibrous histiocytoma) following breast carcinoma: an ultrastructural study of a case, Cancer **45**:1419, 1980.

312. Tsuneyoshi, M., Enjoji, M., and Shinohara, N.: Malignant fibrous histiocytoma: an electron microscopic study of 17 cases, Virchows Arch. [A] **392**:135, 1981.

313. Ueda, T., Aozasa, K., Yamamura, T., Tsujimoto, M., Ono, K., and Matsumoto, K.: Lectin histochemistry of malignant fibrohistiocytic tumors, Am. J. Surg. Pathol. **11**:257, 1987.

314. Vilanova, J.R., Burgos-Bretones, J., Simón, R., and Rivera-Pomar, J.M.: Leukaemoid reaction and eosinophilia in "inflammatory fibrous histiocytoma," Virchows Arch. [A] **388**:237, 1980.

315. Wegmann, W., and Heitz, Ph.U.: Angiomatoid malignant fibrous histiocytoma: evidence for the histiocytic origin of tumor cells, Virchows Arch. [A] **406**:59, 1985.

316. Weiss, L.M., and Warhol, M.J.: Ultrastructural distinctions between adult pleomorphic rhabdomyosarcomas, pleomorphic liposarcomas, and pleomorphic malignant fibrous histiocytomas, Hum. Pathol. **15**:1025, 1984.

317. Weiss, S.W., and Bratthauer, G.L., and Morris, P.A.: Postirradiation malignant fibrous histiocytoma expressing cytokeratin: implications for the immunodiagnosis of sarcomas, Am. J. Surg. Pathol. **12**:554, 1988.

318. Weiss, S.W., and Enzinger, F.M.: Myxoid variant of malignant fibrous histiocytoma, Cancer **39**:1672, 1977.

319. Weiss, S.W., and Enzinger, F.M.: Malignant fibrous histiocytoma: an analysis of 200 cases, Cancer **41**:2250, 1978.

320. Weiss, S.W., Enzinger, F.M., and Johnson, F.B.: Silica reaction simulating fibrous histiocytoma, Cancer **42**:2738, 1978.

321. Wood, G.S., Beckstead, J.M., Turner, R.R., Hendrickson, M.R., Kemison, R.L., and Warnke, R.A.: Malignant fibrous histiocytoma tumor cells resemble fibroblasts, Am. J. Surg. Pathol. **10**:323, 1986.

322. Yumoto, T., and Morimoto, K.: Experimental approach to fibrous histiocytoma, Acta Pathol. Jpn. **30**:767, 1980.

Smooth muscle tumors

323. Appelman, H.D., and Helwig, E.B.: Gastric epithelioid leiomyoma and leiomyosarcoma (leiomyoblastoma), Cancer **38**:708, 1976.

324. Berlin, Ö., Stener, B., Kindblom, L.-G., and Angervall, L.: Leiomyosarcomas of venous origin in the extremities: a correlated clinical, roentgenologic, and morphologic study with diagnostic and surgical implications, Cancer **54**:2147, 1984.

325. Botting, A.J., Soule, E.H., and Brown, A.L., Jr.: Smooth muscle tumors in children, Cancer **18**:711, 1965.

326. Brown, D.C., Theaker, J.M., Banks, P.M., Gatter, K.C., and Mason, D.Y.: Cytokeratin expression in smooth muscle and smooth muscle tumours, Histopathology **11**:477, 1987.

327. Bruyninckx, C.M.A., and Derksen, O.S.: Leiomyosarcoma of the inferior vena cava: case report and review of the literature, J. Vasc. Surg. **3**:652, 1986.

328. Chen, K.T.K., Hafez, G.R., and Gilbert, E.F.: Myxoid variant of epithelioid smooth muscle tumor, Am. J. Clin. Pathol. **74**:350, 1980.

329. Cornog, J.L., Jr.: Gastric leiomyoblastoma: a clinical and ultrastructural study, Cancer **34**:711, 1974.

330. Dahl, I., and Angervall, L.: Cutaneous and subcutaneous leiomyosarcoma: a clinicopathologic study of 47 patients, Pathol. Eur. **9**:307, 1974.
331. Dreyer, L., Simson, I.W., Sevenster, C.B.v.O., and Dittrich, O.C.: Leiomyomatosis peritonealis disseminata: a report of two cases and a review of the literature, Br. J. Obstet. Gynaecol. **92**:856, 1985.
332. Evans, D.J., Lampert, I.A., and Jacobs, M.: Intermediate filaments in smooth muscle tumours, J. Clin. Pathol. **36**:57, 1983.
333. Evans, H.L.: Smooth muscle tumors of the gastrointestinal tract: a study of 56 cases followed for a minimum of 10 years, Cancer **56**:2242, 1985.
334. Fields, J.P., and Helwig, E.B.: Leiomyosarcoma of the skin and subcutaneous tissue, Cancer **47**:156, 1981.
335. Fletcher, C.D.M., and McKee, P.H.: Sarcomas—a clinicopathologic guide with particular reference to cutaneous manifestation II. Malignant nerve sheath tumour, leiomyosarcoma and rhabdomyosarcoma, Clin. Exp. Dermatol. **10**:201, 1985.
336. Gown, A.M., Boyd, H.C., Chang, Y., Ferguson, M., Reichler, B., and Tippens, D.: Smooth muscle cells can express cytokeratins of "simple" epithelium: immunocytochemical and biochemical studies in vitro and in vivo, Am. J. Pathol. **132**:223, 1988.
337. Griffin, A.S., and Sterchi, J.M.: Primary leiomyosarcoma of the inferior vena cava: a case report and review of the literature, J. Surg. Oncol. **34**:53, 1987.
338. Hachisuga, T., Hashimoto, H., and Enjoji, M.: Angioleiomyoma: a clinicopathologic reappraisal of 562 cases, Cancer **54**:126, 1984.
339. Hashimoto, H., Daimaru, Y., Tsuneyoshi, M., and Enjoji, M.: Leiomyosarcoma of the external soft tissues: a clinicopathologic, immunohistochemical, and electron microscopic study, Cancer **57**:2077, 1986.
340. Hashimoto, H., Tsuneyoshi, M., and Enjoji, M.: Malignant smooth muscle tumors of the retroperitoneum and mesentery: a clinicopathologic analysis of 44 cases, J. Surg. Oncol. **28**:177, 1985.
341. Hendrickson, M.R., and Kempson, R.L.: Surgical pathology of the uterine corpus, Philadelphia, 1980, W.B. Saunders Co.
342. Kempson, R.L.: Mitosis counting—II, Hum. Pathol. **7**:482, 1976. (Editorial.)
343. Kevorkian, J., and Cento, D.P.: Leiomyosarcoma of large arteries and veins, Surgery **73**:390, 1973.
344. King, M.E., Dickersin, G.R., and Scully, R.E.: Myxoid leiomyosarcoma of the uterus: a report of six cases, Am. J. Surg. Pathol. **6**:589, 1982.
345. Knapp, R.H., Wick, M.R., and Goellner, J.R.: Leiomyoblastomas and their relationship to other smooth-muscle tumors of the gastrointestinal tract: an electron-microscopic study, Am. J. Surg. Pathol. **8**:449, 1984.
346. Lack, E.E.: Leiomyosarcomas in childhood: a clinical and pathologic study of 10 cases, Pediatr. Pathol. **6**:181, 1986.
347. Lavin, P., Hajdu, S.I., and Foote, F.W., Jr.: Gastric and extragastric leiomyoblastomas: clinicopathologic study of 44 cases, Cancer **29**:305, 1972.
348. Leu, H.J., and Makek, M.: Intramural venous leiomyosarcomas, Cancer **57**:1395, 1986.
349. Lubbers, P.R., Chandra, R., Markle, B.M., Downey, E.F., Jr., and Malawer, M.: Case report 421: calcified leiomyoma of the soft tissues of the right buttock, Skeletal Radiol. **16**:252, 1987.
350. Miettinen, M.: Antibody specific to muscle actins in the diagnosis and classification of soft tissue tumors, Am. J. Pathol. **130**:205, 1988.
351. Miettinen, M.: Immunoreactivity for cytokeratin and epithelial membrane antigen in leiomyosarcoma, Arch. Pathol. Lab. Med. **112**:637, 1988.
352. Morales, A.R.: Electron microscopy of human tumors. In Fenoglio, C.M., and Wolff, M., editors: Progress in surgical pathology, vol. 1, New York, 1980, Masson Publishing USA, Inc.
353. Morales, A.R., Fine, G., Pardo, V., and Horn, R.C., Jr.: The ultrastructure of smooth muscle tumors with a consideration of the possible relationship of glomangiomas, hemangiopericytomas, and cardiac myxomas, Pathol. Annu. **10**:65, 1975.
354. Norris, H.J.: Mitosis counting—III, Hum. Pathol. **7**:483, 1976. (Editorial.)
355. Norton, A.J., Thomas, J.A., and Isaacson, P.G.: Cytokeratin-specific monoclonal antibodies are reactive with tumours of smooth muscle derivation: an immunocytochemical and biochemical study using antibodies to intermediate filament cytoskeletal proteins, Histopathology **11**:487, 1987.
356. Pachter, M.R., and Lattes, R.: Mesenchymal tumors of the mediastinum. I. Tumors of fibrous tissue, adipose tissue, smooth muscle, and striated muscle, Cancer **16**:74, 1963.
357. Ranchod, M., and Kempson, R.L.: Smooth muscle tumors of the gastrointestinal tract and retroperitoneum: a pathologic analysis of 100 cases, Cancer **39**:255, 1977.
358. Rosen, L., Payson, B.A., and Mori, K.: Leiomyosarcoma of the superficial soft tissues, Mt. Sinai J. Med. **46**:181, 1979.
359. Rubin, S.C., Wheeler, J.E., and Mikuta, J.J.: Malignant leiomyomatosis peritonealis disseminata, Obstet. Gynecol. **68**:126, 1986.
360. Salazar, H., and Totten, R.S.: Leiomyoblastoma of the stomach: an ultrastructural study, Cancer **25**:176, 1970.
361. Salm, R., and Evans, D.J.: Myxoid leiomyosarcoma, Histopathology **9**:159, 1985.
362. Saul, S.H., Rast, M.L., and Brooks, J.J.: The immunohistochemistry of gastrointestinal stromal tumors: evidence supporting an origin from smooth muscle, Am. J. Surg. Pathol. **11**:464, 1987.
363. Schürch, W., Skalli, O., Seemayer, T.A., and Gabbiani, G.: Intermediate filament proteins and actin isoforms as markers for soft tissue tumor differentiation and origin. I. Smooth muscle tumors, Am. J. Pathol. **128**:91, 1987.
364. Shmookler, B.M., and Lauer, D.H.: Retroperitoneal leiomyosarcoma: a clinicopathologic analysis of 36 cases, Am. J. Surg. Pathol. **7**:269, 1983.
365. Silverberg, S.G.: Reproducibility of the mitosis count in the histologic diagnosis of smooth muscle tumors of the uterus, Hum. Pathol. **7**:451, 1976.
366. Stout, A.P.: Bizarre smooth muscle tumors of the stomach, Cancer **15**:400, 1962.
367. Stout, A.P., Hendry, J., and Purdie, F.J.: Primary solid tumors of the great omentum, Cancer **16**:231, 1963.
368. Stout, A.P., and Hill, W.T.: Leiomyosarcoma of the superficial soft tissues, Cancer **11**:844, 1958.
369. Tavassoli, F.A., and Norris, H.J.: Peritoneal leiomyomatosis (leiomyomatosis peritonealis disseminata): a clinicopathologic study of 20 cases with ultrastructural observations, Int. J. Gynecol. Pathol. **1**:59, 1982.
370. Tsukada, T., McNutt, M.A., Ross, R., and Gown, A.M.: HHF35, a muscle actin-specific monoclonal antibody. II. Reactivity in normal, reactive, and neoplastic human tissues, Am. J. Pathol. **127**:389, 1987.
371. Varela-Duran, J., Oliva, H., and Rosai, J.: Vascular leiomyosarcoma: the malignant counterpart of vascular leiomyoma, Cancer **44**:1684, 1979.
372. Weiss, R.A., and Mackay, B.: Malignant smooth muscle tumors of the gastrointestinal tract: an ultrastructural study of 20 cases, Ultrastruct. Pathol. **2**:231, 1981.
373. Wellmann, K.F.: "Bizarre leiomyoblastoma" of the retroperitoneum: report of a case, J. Pathol. Bacteriol. **94**:447, 1967.
374. Wile, A.G., Evans, H.L., and Romsdahl, M.M.: Leiomyosarcoma of soft tissue: a clinicopathologic study, Cancer **48**:1022, 1981.
375. Wolff, M., and Rothenberg, J.: Dermal leiomyosarcoma: a misnomer? Prog. Surg. Pathol. **6**:147, 1986.
376. Yannopoulos, K., and Stout, A.P.: Smooth muscle tumors in children, Cancer **15**:958, 1962.
377. Yannopoulos, K., and Stout, A.P.: Primary solid tumors of the mesentery, Cancer **16**:914, 1963.

Skeletal muscle tumors
Rhabdomyosarcoma

378. Agamanolis, D.P., Dasu, S., and Krill, C.E., Jr.: Tumors of skeletal muscle, Hum. Pathol. **17**:778, 1986.
379. Altmannsberger, M., Osborn, M., Treuner, J., Hölscher, A.,

Weber, K., and Shauer, A.: Diagnosis of human childhood rhabdomyosarcoma by antibodies to desmin, the structural protein of muscle specific intermediate filaments, Virchows Arch. [B] **39**:203, 1982.

380. Altmannsberger, M., Weber, K., Droste, R., and Osborn, M.: Desmin is a specific marker for rhabdomyosarcomas of human and rat origin, Am. J. Pathol. **118**:85, 1985.

381. Bale, P.M., Parsons, R.E., and Stevens, M.M.: Diagnosis and behavior of juvenile rhabdomyosarcoma, Hum. Pathol. **14**:596, 1983.

382. Bale, P.M., Parsons, R.E., and Stevens, M.M.: Pathology and behavior of juvenile rhabdomyosarcoma. In Finegold, M., editor: Pathology of neoplasia in children and adolescents, Philadelphia, 1986, W.B. Saunders Co.

383. Bale, P.M., and Reye, R.D.K.: Rhabdomyosarcoma in childhood, Pathology **7**:101, 1975.

384. Brooks, J.J.: Immunohistochemistry of soft tissue tumors: myoglobin as a tumor marker for rhabdomyosarcoma, Cancer **50**:1757, 1982.

385. Bundtzen, J.L., and Norback, D.H.: The ultrastructure of poorly differentiated rhabdomyosarcomas: a case report and literature review, Hum. Pathol. **13**:301, 1982.

386. Coindre, J.-M., DeMascarel, A., Trojani, M., DeMascarel, I., and Pages, A.: Immunohistochemical study of rhabdomyosarcoma: unexpected staining with S100 protein and cytokeratin, J. Pathol. **155**:127, 1988.

387. Corson, J.M., and Pinkus, G.S.: Intracellular myoglobin—a specific marker for skeletal muscle differentiation in soft tissue sarcomas: an immunoperoxidase study, Am. J. Pathol. **103**:384, 1981.

388. Churg, A., and Ringus, J.: Ultrastructural observations on the histogenesis of alveolar rhabdomyosarcoma, Cancer **41**:1355, 1978.

389. Crist, W.M., Raney, R.B., Tefft, M., Heyn, R., Hays, D.M., Newton, W., Beltangady, M., and Maurer, H.M.: Soft tissue sarcomas arising in the retroperitoneal space in children: a report from the Intergroup Rhabdomyosarcoma Study (IRS) Committee, Cancer **56**:2125, 1985.

390. Dehner, L.P., and Enzinger, F.M.: Fetal rhabdomyoma: an analysis of nine cases, Cancer **30**:160, 1972.

391. de Jong, A.S.H., van Vark, M., Albus-Lutter, Ch.E., van Raamsdonk, W., and Voûte, P.A.: Myosin and myoglobin as tumor markers in the diagnosis of rhabdomyosarcoma: a comparative study, Am. J. Surg. Pathol. **8**:521, 1984.

392. de Jong, A.S.H., van Kessel-van Vark, M., Albus-Lutter, Ch.E., van Raamsdonk, W., and Voûte, PA.: Skeletal muscle actin as tumor marker in the diagnosis of rhabdomyosarcoma in childhood, Am. J. Surg. Pathol. **9**:467, 1985.

393. de Jong, A.S.H., van Kessel-van Vark, M., Albus-Lutter, Ch.E., and Voûte, P.A.: Creatine kinase subunits M and B as markers in the diagnosis of poorly differentiated rhabdomyosarcomas in children, Hum. Pathol. **16**:924, 1985.

394. Dito, W.R., and Batsakis, J.G.: Rhabdomyosarcoma of the head and neck: an appraisal of the biologic behavior in 170 cases, Arch. Surg. **84**:582, 1962.

395. Dito, W.R., and Batsakis, J.G.: Intraoral, pharyngeal, and nasopharyngeal rhabdomyosarcoma, Arch. Otolaryngol. **77**:123, 1963.

396. Enterline, H.T., and Horn, R.C., Jr.: Alveolar rhabdomyosarcoma: a distinctive tumor type, Am. J. Clin. Pathol. **29**:356, 1958.

397. Enzinger, F.M., and Shiraki, M.: Alveolar rhabdomyosarcoma: an analysis of 110 cases, Cancer **24**:18, 1969.

398. Erlandson, R.A.: The ultrastructural distinction between rhabdomyosarcoma and other undifferentiated "sarcomas," Ultrastruct. Pathol. **11**:83, 1987.

399. Eusebi, V., Bondi, A., and Rosai, J.: Immunohistochemical localization of myoglobin in nonmuscular cells, Am. J. Surg. Pathol. **8**:51, 1984.

400. Eusebi, V., Ceccarelli, C., Gorza, L., Schiaffino, S., and Bussolati, G.: Immunocytochemistry of rhabdomyosarcoma: the use of four different markers, Am. J. Surg. Pathol. **10**:293, 1986.

401. Feldman, B.A.: Rhabdomyosarcoma of the head and neck, Laryngoscope **92**:424, 1982.

402. Flamant, F., and Hill, C.: The improvement in survival associated with combined chemotherapy in childhood rhabdomyosarcoma: a historical comparison of 345 patients in the same center, Cancer **53**:2417, 1984.

403. Gaiger, A.M., Soule, E.H., and Newton, W.A., Jr.: Pathology of rhabdomyosarcoma: experience of the Intergroup Rhabdomyosarcoma Study, 1972-78, Nat. Cancer Inst. Monogr. **56**:19, 1981.

404. Gonzalez-Crussi, F., and Black-Schaffer, S.: Rhabdomyosarcoma of infancy and childhood: problems of morphologic classification, Am. J. Surg. Pathol. **3**:157, 1979.

405. Hawkins, H.K., and Camacho-Velasquez, J.V.: Rhabdomyosarcoma in children: correlation of form and prognosis in one institution's experience, Am. J. Surg. Pathol. **11**:531, 1987.

406. Hays, D.M., Newton, W., Jr., Soule, E.H., Foulkes, M.A., Raney, R.B., Tefft, M., Ragab, A., and Maurer, H.M.: Mortality among children with rhabdomyosarcomas of the alveolar histologic subtype, Pediatr. Surg. **18**:412, 1983.

407. Hays, D.M., Soule, E.H., Lawrence, W., Jr., Gehan, E.A., Maurer, H.M., Donaldson, M., Raney, R.B., and Tefft, M.: Extremity lesions in the Intergroup Rhabdomyosarcoma Study (IRS-I): a preliminary report, Cancer **48**:1, 1982.

408. Horn, R.C., Jr., and Enterline, H.T.: Rhabdomyosarcoma: a clinicopathological study and classification of 39 cases, Cancer **11**:181, 1958.

409. Kahn, H.J., Yeger, H., Kassim, O., Jorgensen, A.O., MacLennan, D.H., Baumal, R., Smith, C.R., and Phillips, M.J.: Immunohistochemical and electron microscopic assessment of childhood rhabdomyosarcoma: increased frequency of diagnosis over routine histologic methods, Cancer **51**:1897, 1983.

410. Keyhani, A., and Booher, R.J.: Pleomorphic rhabdomyosarcoma, Cancer **22**:956, 1968.

411. Kingston, J.E., McElwain, T.J., and Malpas, J.S.: Childhood rhabdomyosarcoma: experience of the Children's Solid Tumour Group, Br. J. Cancer **48**:195, 1983.

412. Koh, S.-J., and Johnson, W.W.: Antimyosin and antirhabdomyoblast sera: their use for the diagnosis of childhood rhabdomyosarcoma, Arch. Pathol. Lab. Med. **104**:118, 1980.

413. Lawrence, W., Jr., Hays, D.M., and Moon, T.E.: Lymphatic metastasis with childhood rhabdomyosarcoma, Cancer **39**:556, 1977.

414. Lawrence, W., Jr., Jegge, G., and Foote, F.W., Jr.: Embryonal rhabdomyosarcoma: a clinicopathological study, Cancer **17**:361, 1964.

415. Li, F.P., and Fraumeni, J.F., Jr.: Rhabdomyosarcoma in children: epidemiologic study and identification of a familial cancer syndrome, J. Natl. Cancer Inst. **43**:1365, 1969.

416. Linscheid, R.L., Soule, E.H., and Henderson, E.D.: Pleomorphic rhabdomyosarcomata of the extremities and limb girdles: a clinicopathological study, J. Bone Joint Surg. **47A**:715, 1965.

417. Lloyd, R.V., Hajdu, S.I., and Knapper, W.H.: Embryonal rhabdomyosarcoma in adults, Cancer **51**:557, 1983.

418. Masson, J.K., and Soule, E.H.: Embryonal rhabdomyosarcoma of the head and neck: report on eighty-eight cases, Am. J. Surg. **110**:585, 1965.

419. Maurer, H.M., Beltangady, M., Gehan, E.A., Crist, W., Hammond, D., Hays, D.M., Heyn, R., Lawrence, W., Newton, W., Ortega, J., et al.: The Intergroup Rhabdomyosarcoma Study—I: a final report, Cancer **61**:209, 1988.

420. Maurer, H.M.: Rhabdomyosarcoma in childhood and adolescence, Curr. Probl. Cancer **2**:1, 1978.

421. Maurer, H.M., Moon, T., Donaldson, M., Fernandez, C., Gehan, E.A., Hammond, D., Hays, D.M., Lawrence, W., Jr., Newton, W., Ragab, A., Runey, B., Soule, E.M., Sutow, W.W., and Tefft, M.: The Intergroup Rhabdomyosarcoma Study: a preliminary report, Cancer **40**:2015, 1977.

422. McKeen, E.A., Bodurtha, J., Meadows, A.T., Douglass, E.C., and Mulvihill, J.J.: Rhabdomyosarcoma complicating multiple neurofibromatosis, J. Pediatr. **93**:992, 1978.

423. Mierau, G.W., Berry, P.J., and Orsini, E.N.: Small round cell

neoplasms: can electron microscopy and immunohistochemical studies accurately classify them? Ultrastruct. Pathol. 9:99, 1985.

424. Mierau, G.W., and Favara, B.E.: Rhabdomyosarcoma in children: ultrastructural study of 31 cases, Cancer 46:2035, 1980.

425. Miettinen, M., Lehto, V.-P., Badley, R.A., and Virtanen, I.: Alveolar rhabdomyosarcoma: demonstration of the muscle type of intermediate filament protein, desmin, as a diagnostic aid, Am. J. Pathol. 108:246, 1982.

426. Miller, R.W.: Contrasting epidemiology of childhood osteosarcoma, Ewing's tumor, and rhabdomyosarcoma, Natl. Cancer Inst. Monogr. 56:9, 1981.

427. Molenaar, W.M., Oosterhuis, J.W., and Kamps, W.A.: Cytologic "differentiation" in childhood rhabdomyosarcomas following polychemotherapy, Hum. Pathol. 15:973, 1984.

428. Molenaar, W.M., Oosterhuis, A.M., and Ramaekers, F.C.S.: The rarity of rhabdomyosarcomas in the adult: a morphologic and immunohistochemical study, Pathol. Res. Pract. 180:400, 1985.

429. Morales, A.R., Fine, G., and Horn, R.C., Jr.: Rhabdomyosarcoma: an ultrastructural appraisal, Pathol. Annu. 7:81, 1972.

430. Mukai, M., Iri, H., Torikata, C., Kageyama, K., Morikawa, Y., and Shimizu, K.: Immunoperoxidase demonstration of a new muscle protein (Z-protein) in myogenic tumors as a diagnostic aid, Am. J. Pathol. 114:164, 1984.

431. Mukai, K., Rosai, J., and Hallaway, B.E.: Localization of myoglobin in normal and neoplastic human skeletal muscle cells using an immunoperoxidase method, Am. J. Surg. Pathol. 3:373, 1979.

432. Newton, W.A., Jr., Soule, E.H., Hamoudi, A.B., Reiman, H.M., Shimada, H., Beltangady, M., and Maurer, H.: Histopathology of childhood sarcomas, Intergroup Rhabdomyosarcoma Studies I and II: clinicopathologic correlation, J. Clin. Oncol. 6:67, 1988.

433. Om, A., and Ghose, T.: Use of anti–skeletal muscle antibody from myasthenic patients in the diagnosis of childhood rhabdomyosarcomas, Am. J. Surg. Pathol. 11:272, 1987.

434. Palmer, N.F., and Foulkes, M.: Histopathology and prognosis in the Second Intergroup Rhabdomyosarcoma Study (IRS-II), Proc. Am. Soc. Clin. Oncol. 2:229, 1983. (Abstract.)

435. Palmer, N., Sachs, N., and Foulkes, M.: Histopathology and prognosis in rhabdomyosarcoma (IRSI), Proc. Am. Soc. Clin. Oncol. 1:170, 1982. (Abstract.)

436. Patton, R.B., and Horn, R.C., Jr.: Rhabdomyosarcoma: clinical and pathological features and comparison with human fetal and embryonal skeletal muscle, Surgery 52:572, 1962.

437. Porterfield, J.F., and Zimmerman, L.E.: Rhabdomyosarcoma of the orbit: a clinicopathologic study of 55 cases, Virchows Arch. [A] 335:329, 1962.

438. Ragab, A.H., Heyn, R., Tefft, M., Hays, D.N., Newton, W.A., Jr., and Beltangady, M.: Infants younger than 1 year of age with rhabdomyosarcoma, Cancer 58:2606, 1986.

439. Raney, R.B., Jr., Crist, W.M., Maurer, H.M., and Foulkes, M.A.: Prognosis of children with soft tissue sarcoma who relapse after achieving a complete response: a report from the Intergroup Rhabdomyosarcoma Study I, Cancer 52:44, 1983.

440. Raney, R.B., Jr., Donaldson, M.H., Sutow, W.W., Lindberg, R.D., Maurer, H.M., and Tefft, M.: Special considerations related to primary site in rhabdomyosarcoma: experience of the Intergroup Rhabdomyosarcoma Study, 1972-76, Natl. Cancer Inst. Monogr. 56:69, 1981.

441. Raney, R.B., Jr., Tefft, M., Lawrence, W., Jr., Ragab, A.H., Soule, E.H., Beltangady, M., and Gehan, E.A.: Paratesticular sarcoma in childhood adolescence: a report from the Intergroup Rhabdomyosarcoma Studies I and II, 1973-1983, Cancer 60:2337, 1987.

442. Raney, R.B., Jr., Tefft, M., Newton, W.A., Ragab, A.H., Lawrence, W., Jr., Gehan, E.A., and Maurer, H.M.: Improved prognosis with intensive treatment of children with cranial soft tissue sarcomas arising in nonorbital parameningeal sites: a report from the Intergroup Rhabdomyosarcoma Study, Cancer 59:147, 1987.

443. Royds, J.A., Variend, S., Timperley, W.R., and Taylor, C.B.: An investigation of β enolase as a histological marker of rhabdomyosarcoma, J. Clin. Pathol. 37:904, 1984.

444. Ruymann, F.B., Newton, W.A., Jr., Ragab, A.H., Donaldson, M.H., and Foulkes, M.: Bone marrow metastases at diagnosis in children and adolescents with rhabdomyosarcoma: a report from the Intergroup Rhabdomyosarcoma Study, Cancer 53:368, 1984.

445. Schmidt, D., Reimann, O., Treuner, J., and Harms, D.: Cellular differentiation and prognosis in embryonal rhabdomyosarcoma: a report from the Cooperative Soft Tissue Sarcoma Study 1981 (CWS 81), Virchows Arch. [A] 409:183, 1986.

446. Schmidt, R.A., Cone, R., Haas, J.E., and Gown, A.M.: Diagnosis of rhabdomyosarcomas with HHF35, a monoclonal antibody against muscle actins, Am. J. Pathol. 131:19, 1988.

447. Seidal, T., and Kindblom, L.-G.: The ultrastructure of alveolar and embryonal rhabdomyosarcoma, Acta Pathol. Microbiol. Immunol. Scand. [A] 92:231, 1984.

448. Shimada, H., Newton, W.A., Jr., Soule, E.H., Beltangady, M.S., and Maurer, H.M.: Pathology of fatal rhabdomyosarcoma: report from Intergroup Rhabdomyosarcoma Study (IRS-I and IRS-II), Cancer 59:459, 1987.

449. Smith, M.T., Armbrustmacher, V.W., and Violett, T.W.: Diffuse meningeal rhabdomyosarcoma, Cancer 47:2081, 1981.

450. Soule, E.H., Geitz, M., and Henderson, E.D.: Embryonal rhabdomyosarcoma of the limbs and limb-girdles: a clinicopathologic study of 61 cases, Cancer 23:1336, 1969.

451. Sutow, W.W.: Childhood rhabdomyosarcoma. In Sutow, W.W., editor: Malignant solid tumors in children: a review, New York, 1981, Raven Press.

452. Sutow, W.W., Lindberg, R.D., Gehan, E.A., Ragab, A.H., Raney, R.B., Jr., Ruymann, F., and Soule, E.H.: Three-year relapse-free survival rates in childhood rhabdomyosarcoma of the head and neck: report from the Intergroup Rhabdomyosarcoma Study, Cancer 49:2217, 1982.

453. Sutow, W.W., Sullivan, M.P., Ried, H.L, Taylor, H.G., and Griffith, K.M.: Prognosis in childhood rhabdomyosarcoma, Cancer 25:1384, 1970.

454. Tsokos, M., Howard, R., and Costa, J.: Immunohistochemical study of alveolar and embryonal rhabdomyosarcoma, Lab. Invest. 48:148, 1983.

455. Tsokos, M., Miser, A., Pizzo, P., and Triche, T.: Histologic and cytologic characteristics of poor prognosis childhood rhabdomyosarcoma, Lab. Invest. 50:61A, 1984. (Abstract.)

456. Turc-Carel, C., Lizard-Nacol, S., Justrabo, E., Favrot, M., Philip, T., and Tabone, E.: Consistent chromosomal translocation in alveolar rhabdomyosarcoma, Cancer Genet. Cytogenet. 19:361, 1986.

Rhabdomyoma

457. Agamanolis, D.P., Dasu, S., and Krill, C.E., Jr.: Tumors of skeletal muscle, Hum. Pathol. 17:778, 1986.

458. Battifora, H.A., Eisenstein, R., and Schild, J.A.: Rhabdomyoma of larynx: ultrastructural study and comparison with granular cell tumors (myoblastoma), Cancer 23:183, 1969.

459. Czernobilsky, B., Cornog, J.L., and Enterline, H.T.: Rhabdomyoma: report of a case with ultrastructural and histochemical studies, Am. J. Clin. Pathol. 49:782, 1968.

460. Dahl, I., Angervall, L., and Säve-Söderbergh, J.: Foetal rhabdomyoma: case report of a patient with two tumors, Acta Pathol. Microbiol. Scand. 84A:107, 1976.

461. Dehner, L.P., and Enzinger, F.M.: Fetal rhabdomyoma: an analysis of nine cases, Cancer 30:160, 1972.

462. Di Sant'Agnese, P.A., and Knowles, D.M., II: Extracardiac rhabdomyoma: a clinicopathologic study and review of the literature, Cancer 46:780, 1980.

463. Gale, N., Rott, T., and Kambič, V.: Nasopharyngeal rhabdomyoma: report of case (light and electron microscopic studies) and review of the literature, Pathol. Res. Pract. 178:454, 1984.

464. Gardner, D.G., and Corio, R.L.: Multifocal adult rhabdomyoma, Oral Surg. 56:76, 1983.

465. Gardner, D.G., and Corio, R.L.: Fetal rhabdomyoma of the tongue, with a discussion of the two histologic variants of this tumor, Oral Surg. 56:293, 1983.

466. Gold, J.H., and Bossen, E.H.: Benign vaginal rhabdomyoma: a light and electron microscopic study, Cancer **37**:2283, 1976.

467. Goldman, R.L.: Multicentric benign rhabdomyoma of skeletal muscle, Cancer **16**:1609, 1963.

468. Konrad, E.A., Meister, P., and Hübner, G.: Extracardiac rhabdomyoma: report of different types with light microscopic and ultrastructural studies, Cancer **49**:898, 1982.

469. Lehtonen, E., Asikainen, U., and Badley, R.A.: Rhabdomyoma: ultrastructural features and distribution of desmin, muscle type of intermediate filament protein, Acta Pathol. Microbiol. Immunol. Scand. [A] **90**:125, 1982.

470. Moran, J.J., and Enterline, H.T.: Benign rhabdomyoma of the pharynx: a case report, review of the literature, and comparison with cardiac rhabdomyoma, Am. J. Clin. Pathol. **42**:174, 1964.

471. Schlosnagle, D.C., Kratochvil, F.J., Weathers, D.R., McConnel, F.M.S., and Campbell, W.G., Jr.: Intraoral multifocal adult rhabdomyoma: report of a case and review of the literature, Arch. Pathol. Lab. Med. **107**:638, 1983.

472. Scrivner, D., and Meyer, J.S.: Multifocal recurrent adult rhabdomyoma, Cancer **46**:790, 1980.

473. Whitten, R.O., and Benjamin, D.R.: Rhabdomyoma of the retroperitoneum: a report of a tumor with both adult and fetal characteristics: a study by light and electron microscopy, histochemistry, and immunochemistry, Cancer **59**:818, 1987.

474. Wyatt, R.B., Schochet, S.S., Jr., and McCormick, W.F.: Rhabdomyoma: light and electron microscopic study of a case with intranuclear inclusions, Arch. Otolaryngol. **92**:32, 1970.

Tumors of adipose tissue
Liposarcoma

475. Allen, P.W.: Tumors and proliferations of adipose tissue: a clinicopathologic approach, New York, 1981, Masson Publishing USA, Inc.

476. Azumi, N., Curtis, J., Kempson, R.L., and Hendrickson, M.R.: Atypical and malignant neoplasms showing lipomatous differentiation: a study of 111 cases, Am. J. Surg. Pathol. **11**:161, 1987.

477. Battifora, H., and Nunez-Alonso, C.: Myxoid liposarcoma: study of ten cases, Ultrastruct. Pathol. **1**:157, 1980.

478. Bolen, J.W., and Thorning, D.: Benign lipoblastoma and myxoid liposarcoma: a comparative light- and electron-microscopic study, Am. J. Surg. Pathol. **4**:163, 1980.

479. Bolen, J.W., and Thorning, D.: Liposarcomas: a histogenetic approach to the classification of adipose tissue neoplasms, Am. J. Surg. Pathol. **8**:3, 1984.

480. Brasfield, R.D., and Das Gupta, T.K.: Liposarcoma, CA **20**:3, 1970.

481. Castleberry, R.P., Kelly, D.R., Wilson, E.R., Cain, W.S., and Salter, M.R.: Childhood liposarcoma: report of a case and review of the literature, Cancer **54**:579, 1984.

482. Chung, E.B., and Enzinger, F.M.: Benign lipoblastomatosis: an analysis of 35 cases, Cancer **32**:482, 1973.

483. Cocchia, D., Lauriola, L., Stolfi, V.M., Tallini, G., and Michetti, F.: S-100 antigen labels neoplastic cells in liposarcoma and cartilaginous tumours, Virchows Arch. [A] **402**:139, 1983.

484. Desai, U., Ramos, C.V., and Taylor, H.B.: Ultrastructural observations in pleomorphic liposarcoma, Cancer **42**:1284, 1978.

485. Edland, R.W.: Liposarcoma: a retrospective study of fifteen cases, a review of the literature and a discussion of radiosensitivity, Am. J. Roent. Rad. Therapy Nucl. Med. **103**:778, 1968.

486. Enzinger, F.: Management of primary bone and soft tissue tumors, Chicago, 1977, Year Book Medical Publishers, Inc, p. 455.

487. Enzinger, F.M., and Winslow, D.J.: Liposarcoma: a study of 103 cases, Virchows Arch. **335**:367, 1962.

488. Evans, H.L.: Liposarcoma: a study of 55 cases with a reassessment of its classification, Am. J. Surg. Pathol. **3**:507, 1979.

489. Evans, H.L., Soule, E.H., and Winkelmann, R.K.: Atypical lipoma, atypical intramuscular lipoma, and well-differentiated retroperitoneal liposarcoma: a reappraisal of 30 cases formerly classified as well-differentiated liposarcoma, Cancer **43**:574, 1979.

490. Fu, Y.S., Parker, F.G., Kaye, G.I., and Lattes, R.: Ultrastructure of benign and malignant adipose tissue tumors, Pathol. Annu. **15**(pt. 1):67, 1980.

491. Gonzalez-Crussi, F., de Mello, D.E., and Sotelo-Avila, C.: Omental-mesenteric myxoid hamartomas, Am. J. Surg. Pathol. **7**:567, 1983.

492. Hashimoto, H., Daimaru, Y., and Enjoji, M.: S-100 protein distribution in liposarcoma: an immunoperoxidase study with special reference to the distinction of liposarcoma from myxoid malignant fibrous histiocytoma, Virchows Arch. [A] **405**:1, 1984.

493. Hashimoto, H., and Enjoji, M.: Liposarcoma: a clinicopathologic subtyping of 52 cases, Acta Pathol. Jpn. **32**:933, 1982.

494. Huvos, A.G.: The spontaneous transformation of benign into malignant soft tissue tumors (with emphasis on extraskeletal osseous, lipomatous, and schwannian lesions), Am. J. Surg. Pathol. **9**(suppl.):7, 1985.

495. Kindblom, L.-G., Angervall, L., and Svendsen, P.: Liposarcoma: a clinicopathologic, radiographic and prognostic study, Acta Pathol. Microbiol. Scand. **253**(suppl.):1, 1975.

496. Kinne, D.W., Chu, F.C.H., Huvos, A.G., Yagoda, A., and Fortner, J.G.: Treatment of primary and recurrent retroperitoneal liposarcoma, Cancer **31**:53, 1973.

497. Lagacé, R., Jacob, S., and Seemayer, T.A.: Myxoid liposarcoma: an electronmicroscopic study: biologic and histogenetic considerations, Virchows Arch. [A] **384**:159, 1979.

498. McKee, P.H., Lowe, D., and Shaw, M.: Subcutaneous liposarcoma, Clin. Exp. Dermatol. **8**:593, 1983.

499. O'Connor, M., and Snover, D.C.: Liposarcoma: a review of factors influencing prognosis, Am. Surg. **49**:379, 1983.

500. Reitan, J.B., Kaalhus, O., Brennhovd, I.O., Sager, E.M., Stenwig, A.E., and Talle, K.: Prognostic factors in liposarcoma, Cancer **55**:2482, 1985.

501. Rossouw, D.J., Cinti, S., and Dickersin, G.R.: Liposarcoma: an ultrastructural study of 15 cases, Am. J. Clin. Pathol. **85**:649, 1986.

502. Shmookler, B.M., and Enzinger, F.M.: Pleomorphic lipoma: a benign tumor simulating liposarcoma: a clinicopathologic analysis of 48 cases, Cancer **47**:126, 1981.

503. Shmookler, B.M., and Enzinger, F.M.: Liposarcoma occurring in children: an analysis of 17 cases and review of the literature, Cancer **52**:567, 1983.

504. Smith, S., Reeves, B.R., and Wong, L.: Translocation t(12;16) in a case of myxoid liposarcoma, Cancer Genet. Cytogenet. **26**:185, 1987.

505. Snover, D.C., Sumner, H.W., and Dehner, L.P.: Variability of histologic pattern in recurrent soft tissue sarcomas originally diagnosed as liposarcoma, Cancer **49**:1005, 1982.

506. Takagi, H., Kato, K., Yamada, E., and Suchi, T.: Six recent liposarcomas including largest to date, J. Surg. Oncol. **26**:260, 1984.

507. Turc-Carel, C., Limon, J., Cin, P.D., Rao, U., Karakousis, C., and Sandberg, A.A.: Cytogenetic studies of adipose tissue tumors. II. Recurrent reciprocal translocation t(12;16)(q13;p11) in myxoid liposarcomas, Cancer Genet. Cytogenet. **23**:291, 1986.

508. Wess, L.M., and Warhol, M.J.: Ultrastructural distinctions between adult pleomorphic rhabdomyosarcomas, pleomorphic liposarcomas, and pleomorphic malignant fibrous histiocytomas, Hum. Pathol. **15**:1025, 1984.

509. Wetzel, W., and Alexander, R.: Myxoid liposarcoma: an ultrastructural study of two cases, Am. J. Clin. Pathol. **72**:521, 1979.

Lipoma and infiltrating lipoma

510. Adair, F.E., Pack, G.T., and Farrior, J.H.: Lipomas, Am. J. Cancer **16**:1104, 1932.

511. Brasfield, R.D., and Das Gupta, T.K.: Soft tissue tumors: benign tumors of adipose tissue, CA **19**:3, 1969.

512. Das Gupta, T.K.: Tumors and tumor-like conditions of the adipose tissue, Curr. Probl. Surg. **60**:1, 1970.

513. Dionne, G.P., and Seemayer, T.A.: Infiltrating lipomas and angiolipomas revisited, Cancer **33**:732, 1974.

514. Enzinger, F.M.: Benign lipomatous tumors simulating a sarcoma. In M.D. Anderson Hospital and Tumor Institute: Management of primary bone and soft tissue tumors, Chicago, 1977, Year Book Medical Publishers, Inc.

515. Evans, H.L., Soule, E.H., and Winkelmann, R.K.: Atypical lipoma, atypical intramuscular lipoma, and well-differentiated retroperitoneal liposarcoma: a reappraisal of 30 cases formerly classified as well-differentiated liposarcoma, Cancer **43**:574, 1979.
516. Fletcher, C.D.M., and Martin-Bates, E.: Intramuscular and intermuscular lipoma: neglected diagnoses, Histopathology **12**:275, 1988.
517. Fu, Y.S., Parker, F.G., Kaye, G.I., and Lattes, R.: Ultrastructure of benign and malignant adipose tissue tumors, Pathol. Annu. **15**(pt. 1):67, 1980.
518. Geschickter, C.F.: Lipoid tumors, Am. J. Cancer **21**:617, 1934.
519. Hatziotis, J.C.: Lipoma of the oral cavity, Oral Surg. **31**:511, 1971.
520. Heim, S., Mandahl, N., Kristoffersson, U., Mitelman, F., Rööser, B., Rydholm, A., and Willén, H.: Reciprocal translocation t(3;12)(q27;q13) in lipoma, Cancer Genet. Cytogenet. **23**:301, 1986.
521. Kim, Y.H., and Reiner, L.: Ultrastructure of lipoma, Cancer **50**:102, 1982.
522. Kindblom, L.-G., Angervall, L., and Stener, B.: Intermuscular and intramuscular lipomas and hibernomas: a clinical, roentgenologic, histologic, and prognostic study of 46 cases, Cancer **33**:754, 1974.
523. Leffell, D.J., and Braverman, I.M.: Familial multiple lipomatosis: report of a case and a review of the literature, J. Am. Acad. Dermatol. **15**:275, 1986.
524. Rydholm, A., and Berg, N.O.: Size, site and clinical incidence of lipoma: factors in the differential diagnosis of lipoma and sarcoma, Acta Orthop. Scand. **54**:929, 1983.
525. Silverman, T.A., and Enzinger, F.M.: Fibrolipomatous hamartoma of nerve: a clinicopathologic analysis of 26 cases, Am. J. Surg. Pathol. **9**:7, 1985.
526. Solvonuk, P.F., Taylor, G.P., Hancock, R., Wood, W.S., and Frohlich, J.: Correlation of morphologic and biochemical observations in human lipomas, Lab. Invest. **51**:469, 1984.
527. Turc-Carel, C., Cin, P.D., Rao, U., Karakousis, C., and Sandberg, A.A.: Cytogenetic studies of adipose tissue tumors. I. A benign lipoma with reciprocal translocation t(3;12) (q28;14), Cancer Genet. Cytogenet. **23**:283, 1986.
528. Wakeley, C., and Somerville, P.: Lipomas, Lancet **2**:995, 1952.

Spindle cell lipoma

529. Angervall, L., Dahl, I., Kindblom, L.-G., and Säve-Söderbergh, J.: Spindle cell lipoma, Acta Pathol. Microbiol. Scand. **84A**:477, 1976.
530. Bolen, J.W., and Thorning, D.: Spindle-cell lipoma: a clinical, light- and electron-microscopical study, Am. J. Surg. Pathol. **5**:435, 1981.
531. Enzinger, F.M., and Harvey, D.A.: Spindle cell lipoma, Cancer **36**:1852, 1975.
532. Fletcher, C.D.M., and Martin-Bates, E.: Spindle cell lipoma: a clinicopathological study with some original observations, Histopathology **11**:803, 1987.
533. Robb, J.A., and Jones, R.A.: Spindle cell lipoma in a perianal location, Hum. Pathol. **13**:1052, 1982.
534. Shmookler, B.M., and Enzinger, F.M.: Pleomorphic lipoma: a benign tumor simulating liposarcoma: a clinicopathologic analysis of 48 cases, Cancer **47**:126, 1981.

Pleomorphic (atypical) lipoma

535. Azumi, N., Curtis, J., Kempson, R.L., and Hendrickson, M.R.: Atypical and malignant neoplasms showing lipomatous differentiation: a study of 111 cases, Am. J. Surg. Pathol. **11**:161, 1987.
536. Azzopardi, J.G., Iocco, J., and Salm, R.: Pleomorphic lipoma: a tumour simulating liposarcoma, Histopathology **7**:511, 1983.
537. Evans, H.L., Soule, E.H., and Winkelmann, R.K.: Atypical lipoma, atypical intramuscular lipoma, and well-differentiated retroperitoneal liposarcoma: a reappraisal of 30 cases formerly classified as well-differentiated liposarcoma, Cancer **43**:574, 1979.
538. Fechner, R.E.: Pathologic quiz, case one, Arch. Otolaryngol. **110**:820, 1984.

539. Guillou, L., Dehon, A., Charlin, B., and Madarnas, P.: Pleomorphic lipoma of the tongue: case report and literature review, J. Otolaryngol. **15**:313, 1986.
540. Kindblom, L.-G., Angervall, L., and Fassina, A.S.: Atypical lipoma, Acta Pathol. Microbiol. Immunol. Scand. **90A**:27, 1982.
541. Shmookler, B.M., and Enzinger, F.M.: Pleomorphic lipoma: a benign tumor simulating liposarcoma: a clinicopathologic analysis of 48 cases, Cancer **47**:126, 1981.
542. Zhang, S.Z., Yue, X.H., Liu, X.M., Lo, S.L., and Wang, X.Z.: Giant retroperitoneal pleomorphic lipoma, Am. J. Surg. Pathol. **11**:557, 1987. (Use of following personal names was cataloging error: Shouzhu, Z., Xinhua, Y., Xumin, L., Shulian, L., and Xianzhi, W.)

Angiolipoma

543. Dionne, G.P., and Seemayer, T.: Infiltrating lipomas and angiolipomas revisited, Cancer **33**:732, 1974.
544. Dixon, A.Y., McGregor, D.H., and Lee, S.H.: Angiolipomas: an ultrastructural and clinicopathological study, Hum. Pathol. **12**:739, 1981.
545. Howard, W.R., and Helwig, E.B.: Angiolipoma, Arch. Dermatol. **82**:924, 1960.
546. Lin, J.J., and Lin, F.: Two entities in angiolipoma: a study of 459 cases of lipoma with review of literature on infiltrating angiolipoma, Cancer **34**:720, 1974.
547. Pribyl, C., Burke, S.W., Roberts, J.M., Mackenzie, F., and Johnston, C.E., II: Infiltrating angiolipoma or intramuscular hemangioma? A report of five cases, J. Pediatr. Orthop. **6**:172, 1986.
548. Weldon-Linne, C.M., Rhone, D.P., Blatt, D., Moore, D., and Monitz, M.: Angiolipomas in homosexual men, N. Engl. J. Med. **310**:1193, 1984.

Lipoblastoma

549. Bolen, J.W., and Thorning, D.: Benign lipoblastoma and myxoid liposarcoma: a comparative light- and electron-microscopic study, Am. J. Surg. Pathol. **4**:163, 1980.
550. Chung, E.B., and Enzinger, F.M.: Benign lipoblastomatosis: an analysis of 35 cases, Cancer **32**:482, 1973.
551. Dudgeon, D.L., and Haller, J.A., Jr.: Pediatric lipoblastomatosis: two unusual cases, Surgery **95**:371, 1984.
552. Gaffney, E.F., Vellios, F., and Hargreaves, H.K.: Lipoblastomatosis: ultrastructure of two cases and relationship to human fetal white adipose tissue, Pediatr. Pathol. **5**:207, 1986.
553. Gibbs, M.K., Soule, E.H., Hayles, A.B., and Telander, R.L.: Lipoblastomatosis: a tumor of children, Pediatrics **60**:235, 1977.
554. Greco, M.A., García, R.L., and Vuletin, J.C.: Benign lipoblastomatosis: ultrastructure and histogenesis, Cancer **45**:511, 1980.
555. Mahour, G.H., Bryan, B.J., and Isaacs, H., Jr.: Lipoblastoma and lipoblastomatosis: a report of six cases, Surgery **104**:577, 1988.
556. Vellios, F., Baez, J., and Shumacker, H.B.: Lipoblastomatosis: a tumor of fetal fat different from hibernoma, Am. J. Pathol. **34**:1149, 1958.

Hibernoma

557. Allegra, S.R., Gmuer, C., and O'Leary, G.P., Jr.: Endocrine activity in a large hibernoma, Hum. Pathol. **14**:1044, 1983.
558. Bonifazi, E., and Meneghini, C.L.: A case of hibernoma in a child, Dermatologica **165**:647, 1982.
559. Fleishman, J.S., and Schwartz, R.A.: Hibernoma: ultrastructural observations, J. Surg. Oncol. **23**:285, 1983.
560. Fletcher, C.D.M., Cole, R.S., Gower, R.L., and Heyderman, E.: Hibernoma of the spermatic cord: the first reported case, Br. J. Urol. **58**:99, 1986.
561. Gaffney, E.F., Hargreaves, H.K., Semple, E., and Vellios, F.: Hibernoma: distinctive light and electron miscroscopic features and relationship to brown adipose tissue, Hum. Pathol. **14**:677, 1983.
562. Kindblom, L.-G., Angervall, L., and Stener, B.: Intermuscular and intramuscular lipomas and hibernomas: a clinical, roentgenologic, histologic, and prognostic study of 46 cases, Cancer **33**:754, 1974.

563. Levine, G.D.: Hibernoma: an electron microscopic study, Hum. Pathol. 3:351, 1972.

564. Rigor, V.U., Goldstone, S.E., Jones, J., Bernstein, R., Gold, M.S., and Weiner, S.: Hibernoma: a case report and discussion of a rare tumor, Cancer 57:2207, 1986.

565. Seemayer, T.A., Knaack, J., Wang, N.-S., and Ahmed, M.N.: On the ultrastructure of hibernoma, Cancer 36:1785, 1975.

Vascular tumors
Intramuscular hemangioma

566. Allen, P.W., and Enzinger, F.M.: Hemangioma of skeletal muscle: an analysis of 89 cases, Cancer 29:8, 1972.

Hemangiopericytoma

567. Alpers, C.E., Rosenau, W., Finkbeiner, W.E., and DeLorimier, A.A., and Kronish, D.: Congenital (infantile) hemangiopericytoma of the tongue and sublingual region, Am. J. Clin. Pathol. 81:377, 1984.

568. Angervall, L., Kindblom, L.-G., Nielsen, J.M., Stener, B., and Svendsen, P.: Hemangiopericytoma: a clinicopathologic, angiographic and microangiographic study, Cancer 42:2412, 1978.

569. Atkinson, J.B., Mahour, G.H., Isaacs, H., Jr., and Ortega, J.A.: Hemangiopericytoma in infants and children: a report of six patients, Am. J. Surg. 148:372, 1984.

570. Backwinkel, K.D., and Diddams, J.A.: Hemangiopericytoma: report of a case and comprehensive review of the literature, Cancer 25:896, 1970.

571. Battifora, H.: Hemangiopericytoma: ultrastructural study of five cases, Cancer 31:1418, 1973.

572. Brockbank, J.: Hemangiopericytoma of the oral cavity: report of case and review of the literature, J. Oral Surg. 37:659, 1979.

573. Chen, K.T.K., Kassel, S.H., and Medrano, V.A.: Congenital hemangiopericytoma, J. Surg. Oncol. 31:127, 1986.

574. Compagno, J.: Hemangiopericytoma-like tumors of the nasal cavity: a comparison with hemangiopericytoma of soft tissues, Laryngoscope 88:460, 1978.

575. Compagno, J., and Hyams, V.J.: Hemangiopericytoma-like intranasal tumors: a clinicopathologic study of 23 cases, Am. J. Clin. Pathol. 66:672, 1976.

576. Croxatto, J.O., and Font, R.L.: Hemangiopericytoma of the orbit: a clinicopathologic study of 30 cases, Hum. Pathol. 13:210, 1982.

577. Eimoto, T.: Ultrastructure of an infantile hemangiopericytoma, Cancer 40:2161, 1977.

578. Enzinger, F.M., and Smith, B.H.: Hemangiopericytoma: an analysis of 106 cases, Hum. Pathol. 7:61, 1976.

579. Gerner, R.E., Moore, G.E., and Pickren, J.W.: Hemangiopericytoma, Ann. Surg. 179:128, 1974.

580. Hart, L.L., and Weinberg, J.B.: Metastatic hemangiopericytoma with prolonged survival, Cancer 60:916, 1987.

581. Hultberg, B.M., Daugaard, S., Johansen, H.F., Mouridsen, H.T., and Hou-Jensen, K.: Malignant haemangiopericytomas and haemangioendotheliosarcomas: an immunohistochemical study, Histopathology 12:405, 1988.

582. Jha, N., McNeese, M., Barkley, H.T., Jr., and Kong, J.: Does radiotherapy have a role in hemangiopericytoma management? Report of 14 new cases and a review of the literature, Int. J. Radiat. Oncol. Biol. Phys. 13:1399, 1987.

583. Kauffman, S.L., and Stout, A.P.: Hemangiopericytoma in children, Cancer 13:695, 1960.

584. McMaster, M.J., Soule, E.H., and Ivins, J.C.: Hemangiopericytoma: a clinicopathologic study and long-term followup of 60 patients, Cancer 36:2232, 1975.

585. Miettinen, M., Holthofer, H., Lehto, V.-P., Miettinen, A., and Virtanen, I.: *Ulex europaeus* I lectin as a marker for tumors derived from endothelial cells, Am. J. Clin. Pathol. 79:32, 1983.

586. Mira, J.G., Chu, F.C.H., and Fortner, J.G.: The role of radiotherapy in the management of malignant hemangiopericytoma: report of eleven new cases and review of the literature, Cancer 39:1254, 1977.

587. Nunnery, E.W., Kahn, L.B., Reddick, R.L., and Lipper, S.: Hemangiopericytoma: a light microscopic and ultrastructural study, Cancer 47:906, 1981.

588. Plukker, J.T., Koops, H.S., Molenaar, I., Vermey, A., ten Kate, L.P., and Oldhoff, J.: Malignant hemangiopericytoma in three kindred members of one family, Cancer 61:841, 1988.

589. Seibert, J.J., Seibert, R.W., Weisenburger, D.S., and Allsbrook, W.: Multiple congenital hemangiopericytomas of the head and neck, Laryngoscope 88:1006, 1978.

590. Stout, A.P., and Murray, M.R.: Hemangiopericytoma: a vascular tumor featuring Zimmermann's pericytes, Ann. Surg. 116:26, 1942.

591. Tsuneyoshi, M., Daimaru, Y., and Enjoji, M.: Malignant hemangiopericytoma and other sarcomas with hemangiopericytoma-like pattern, Pathol. Res. Pract. 178:446, 1984.

592. Waldo, E.D., Vuletin, J.C., and Kaye, G.I.: The ultrastructure of vascular tumors: additional observations and a review of the literature, Pathol. Annu. 12(pt. 2):279, 1977.

593. Walike, J.W., and Bailey, B.J.: Head and neck hemangiopericytoma, Arch. Otolaryngol. 93:345, 1971.

594. Yaghmal, I.: Angiographic manifestations of soft-tissue and osseous hemangiopericytomas, Radiology 126:653, 1978.

Neurogenous tumors
Neurilemoma, neurofibroma

595. Abel, M.R., Hart, W.R., and Olson, J.R.: Tumors of the peripheral nervous system, Hum. Pathol. 1:503, 1970.

596. Ackerman, L.V., and Taylor, F.H.: Neurogenous tumors within the thorax: a clinicopathological evaluation of forty-eight cases, Cancer 4:669, 1951.

597. Allen, P.W.: Myxoid tumors of soft tissues, Pathol. Annu. 15(pt. 1):133, 1980.

598. Ariel, I.M.: Tumors of the peripheral nervous system, CA 33:282, 1983.

599. Asbury, A.K., and Johnson, P.C.: Pathology of peripheral nerve, Philadelphia, 1978, W.B. Saunders Co.

600. Dahl, I.: Ancient neurilemmoma (schwannoma), Acta Pathol. Microbiol. Scand. 85A:812, 1977.

601. Dahl, I., Hagmar, B., and Idvall, I.: Benign solitary neurilemoma (schwannoma): a correlative cytological and histological study of 28 cases, Acta Pathol. Microbiol. Immunol. Scand. [A] 92:91, 1984.

602. Das Gupta, T.K., Brasfield, R.D., Strong, E.W., and Hadju, S.J.: Benign solitary schwannomas (neurilemomas), Cancer 24:355, 1969.

603. Dible, J.H.: Verocay bodies and pseudo-Meissnerian corpuscles, J. Pathol. Bacteriol. 85:425, 1963.

604. Erlandson, R.A., and Woodruff, J.M.: Peripheral nerve sheath tumors: an electron microscopic study of 43 cases, Cancer 49:273, 1982.

605. Ferry, J.A., and Dickersin, G.R.: Pseudoglandular schwannoma, Am. J. Clin. Pathol. 89:546, 1988.

606. Fletcher, C.D.M., and Davies, S.E.: Benign plexiform (multinodular) schwannoma: a rare tumour unassociated with neurofibromatosis, Histopathology 10:971, 1986.

607. Fletcher, C.D.M., Davies, S.E., and McKee, P.H.: Cellular schwannoma: a distinct pseudosarcomatous entity, Histopathology 11:21, 1987.

608. Gould, V.E., Moll, R., Moll, I., Lee, I., Schwechheimer, K., and Franke, W.W.: The intermediate filament complement of the spectrum of nerve sheath neoplasms, Lab. Invest. 55:463, 1986.

609. Ha'Eri, G.B., Fornasier, V.L., and Schatzker, J.: Morton's neuroma—pathogenesis and ultrastructure, Clin. Orthop. 141:256, 1979.

610. Harkin, J.C., and Reed, R.J.: Tumors of the peripheral nervous system. In Atlas of tumor pathology, series 2, fascicle 3, Washington, D.C., 1969, Armed Forces Institute of Pathology.

611. Iwashita, T., and Enjoji, M.: Plexiform neurilemoma: a clinicopathological and immunohistochemical analysis of 23 tumours from 20 patients, Virchows Arch. [A] 411:305, 1987.

612. Kasantikul, V., Brown, J., and Netsky, M.G.: Mesenchymal differentiation in trigeminal neurilemmoma, Cancer 50:1568, 1982.

613. Kawahara, E., Oda, Y., Ooi, A., Katsuda, S., Nakanishi, I., and

Umeda, S.: Expression of glial fibrillary acidic protein (GFAP) in peripheral nerve sheath tumors: a comparative study of immunoreactivity of GFAP, vimentin, S-100 protein, and neurofilament in 38 schwannomas and 18 neurofibromas, Am. J. Surg. Pathol. **12**:115, 1988.

614. Lassmann, H., Jurecka, W., Lassmann, G., Gebhart, W., Matras, H., and Watzek, G.: Different types of benign nerve sheath tumors: light microscopy, electron microscopy and autoradiography, Virchows Arch. [A] **375**:197, 1977.

615. Lazarus, S.S., and Trombetta, L.D.: Ultrastructural identification of a benign perineural cell tumor, Cancer **41**:1823, 1978.

616. Marcus, P.B., Couch, W.D., and Martin, J.H.: Crystals in a gastric schwannoma, Ultrastruct. Pathol. **2**:139, 1981.

617. Miettinen, M., Foidart, J.-M., and Ekblom, P.: Immunohistochemical demonstration of laminin, the major glycoprotein of basement membranes, as an aid in the diagnosis of soft tissue tumors, Am. J. Clin. Pathol. **79**:306, 1983.

618. Nakajima, T., Watanabe, S., Sato, Y., Kameya, T., Hirota, T., and Shimosato, Y.: An immunoperoxidase study of S-100 protein distribution in normal and neoplastic tissues, Am. J. Surg. Pathol. **6**:715, 1982.

619. Oberman, H.A., and Sullenger, G.: Neurogenous tumors of the head and neck, Cancer **20**:1992, 1967.

620. Ogawa, K., Oguchi, M., Yamabe, H., Nakashima, Y., and Hamashima, Y.: Distribution of collagen type IV in soft tissue tumors: an immunohistochemical study, Cancer **58**:269, 1986.

621. Reed, R.J., and Harkin, J.C.: Tumors of the peripheral nervous system, series 2, fascicle 3 (supplement), Washington, D.C., 1983, Armed Forces Institute of Pathology.

622. Shore-Freedman, E., Abrahams, C., Recant, W., and Schneider, A.B.: Neurilemomas and salivary gland tumors of the head and neck following childhood irradiation, Cancer **51**:2159, 1983.

623. Sian, C.S., and Ryan, S.F.: The ultrastructure of neurilemoma with emphasis on Antoni B tissue, Hum. Pathol. **2**:145, 1981.

624. Stefansson, K., Wollmann, R., and Jerkovic, M.: S-100 protein in soft-tissue tumors derived from Schwann cells and melanocytes, Am. J. Pathol. **106**:261, 1982.

625. Ushigome, S., Takakuwa, T., Hyūga, M., Tadokoro, M., and Shinagawa, T.: Perineurial cell tumor and the significance of the perineurial cells in neurofibroma, Acta Pathol. Jpn. **36**:973, 1986.

626. Waggener, J.D.: Ultrastructure of benign peripheral nerve sheath tumors, Cancer **19**:699, 1966.

627. Weidenheim, K.M., and Campbell, W.G., Jr.: Perineurial cell tumor: immunocytochemical and ultrastructural characterization: relationship to other peripheral nerve tumors with a review of the literature, Virchows Arch. [A] **408**:375, 1986.

628. Weiss, S.W., Langloss, J.M., and Enzinger, F.M.: Value of S-100 protein in the diagnosis of soft tissue tumors with particular reference to benign and malignant Schwann cell tumors, Lab. Invest. **49**:299, 1983.

629. Whitaker, W.G., and Droulias, C.: Benign encapsulated neurilemoma: a report of 76 cases, Am. Surg. **42**:675, 1976.

630. Woodruff, J.M., Chernik, M.L., Smith, M.C., Millett, W.B., and Foote, F.W., Jr.: Peripheral nerve tumors with rhabdomyosarcomatous differentiation (malignant "Triton" tumors), Cancer **32**:426, 1973.

631. Woodruff, J.M., Godwin, T.A., Erlandson, R.A., Susin, M., and Martini, N.: Cellular schwannoma: a variety of schwannoma sometimes mistaken for a malignant tumor, Am. J. Surg. Pathol. **5**:733, 1981.

632. Woodruff, J.M., Marshall, M.L., Godwin, T.A., Funkhouser, J.W., Thompson, N.J., and Erlandson, R.A.: Plexiform (multinodular) schwannoma: a tumor simulating the plexiform neurofibroma, Am. J. Surg. Pathol. **7**:691, 1983.

633. Yousem, S.A., Colby, T.V., and Urich, H.: Malignant epithelioid schwannoma arising in a benign schwannoma: a case report, Cancer **55**:2799, 1985.

Malignant nerve sheath tumor

634. Azzopardi, J.G., Eusebi, V., Tison, V., and Betts, C.M.: Neurofibroma with rhabdomyomatous differentiation: benign 'Triton' tumour of the vagina, Histopathology **7**:561, 1983.

635. Bojsen-Møller, M., and Myhre-Jensen, O.: A consecutive series of 30 malignant schwannomas: survival in relation to clinicopathological parameters and treatment, Acta Pathol. Microbiol. Immunol. Scand. [A] **92**:147, 1984.

636. Bonneau, R., and Brochu, P.: Neuromuscular choristoma: a clinicopathologic study of two cases, Am. J. Surg. Pathol. **7**:521, 1983.

637. Brooks, J.S.J., Freeman, M., and Enterline, H.T.: Malignant "Triton" tumors: natural history and immunohistochemistry of nine new cases with literature review, Cancer **55**:2543, 1985.

638. Chen, K.T.K., Latorraca, R., Fabich, D., Padgug, A., Hafez, G.R., and Gilbert, E.F.: Malignant schwannoma: a light microscopic and ultrastructural study, Cancer **45**:1585, 1980.

639. Chitale, A.R., and Dickersin, G.R.: Electron microscopy in the diagnosis of malignant schwannomas: a report of six cases, Cancer **51**:1448, 1983.

640. D'Agostino, A.N., Soule, E.H., and Miller, R.H.: Primary malignant neoplasms of nerves (malignant neurilemomas) in patients without manifestations of multiple neurofibromatosis (von Recklinghausen's disease), Cancer **16**:1003, 1963.

641. D'Agostino, A.N., Soule, E.H., and Miller, R.H.: Sarcomas of the peripheral nerves and somatic soft tissues associated with multiple neurofibromatosis (von Recklinghausen's disease), Cancer **16**:1015, 1963.

642. Daimaru, Y., Hashimoto, H., and Enjoji, M.: Malignant "Triton" tumors: a clinicopathologic and immunohistochemical study of nine cases, Hum. Pathol. **15**:768, 1984.

643. Daimaru, Y., Hashimoto, H., and Enjoji, M.: Malignant peripheral nerve-sheath tumors (malignant schwannomas): an immunohistochemical study of 29 cases, Am. J. Surg. Pathol. **9**:434, 1985.

644. Das Gupta, T.K., and Brasfield, R.D.: Solitary malignant schannoma, Ann. Surg. **171**:419, 1970.

645. Das Gupta, T.K., and Brasfield, R.D.: Von Recklinghausen's disease, CA **21**:174, 1971.

646. Dewit, L., Albus-Lutter, C.E., De Jong, A.S.H., and Voûte, P.A.: Malignant schwannoma with a rhabdomyoblastic component, a so-called Triton tumor: a clinicopathologic study, Cancer **58**:1350, 1986.

647. DiCarlo, E.F., Woodruff, J.M., Bansal, M., and Erlandson, R.A.: The purely epithelioid malignant peripheral nerve sheath tumor, Am. J. Surg. Pathol. **10**:478, 1986.

648. Ducatman, B.S., and Scheithauer, B.W.: Postirradiation neurofibrosarcoma, Cancer **51**:1028, 1983.

649. Ducatman, B.S., and Scheithauer, B.W.: Malignant peripheral nerve sheath tumors with divergent differentiation, Cancer **54**:1049, 1984.

650. Ducatman, B.S., Scheithauer, B.W., Piepgras, D.G., and Reiman, H.M.: Malignant peripheral nerve sheath tumors in childhood, J. Neuro-oncol. **2**:241, 1984.

651. Ducatman, B.S., Scheithauer, B.W., Piepgras, D.G., Reiman, H.M., and Ilstrup, D.M.: Malignant peripheral nerve sheath tumors: a clinicopathologic study of 120 cases, Cancer **57**:2006, 1986.

652. Fletcher, C.D.M., Madziwa, D., Heyderman, E., and McKee, P.H.: Benign dermal schwannoma with glandular elements—true heterology or a local 'organizer' effect? Clin. Exp. Dermatol. **11**:475, 1986.

653. Ghosh, B.C., Ghosh, L., Huvos, A.G., and Fortner, J.G.: Malignant schwannoma: a clinicopathologic study, Cancer **31**:184, 1973.

654. Guccion, J.G., and Enzinger, F.M.: Malignant Schwannoma associated with von Recklinghausen's neurofibromatosis, Virchows Arch. [A] **383**:43, 1979.

655. Herrera, G.A., and Pinto de Moraes, H.: Neurogenic sarcomas in patients with neurofibromatosis (von Recklinghausen's disease): light, electron microscopy and immunohistochemistry study, Virchows Arch. [A] **403**:361, 1984.

656. Herrera, G.A., Reimann, B.E.F., Salinas, J.A., and Turbat, E.A.: Malignant schwannomas presenting as malignant fibrous histiocytomas, Ultrastruct. Pathol. **3**:253, 1982.

657. Karcioglu, Z., Someren, A., and Mathes, S.J.: Ectomesenchymoma: a malignant tumor of migratory neural crest (ectomesen-

chyme) remnants showing ganglionic, schwannian, melanocytic and rhabdomyoblastic differentiation, Cancer **39**:2486, 1977.

658. Kawamoto, E.H., Weidner, N., Agostini, R.M., Jr., and Jaffee, R.: Malignant ectomesenchymoma of soft tissue: report of two cases and review of the literature, Cancer **59**:1791, 1987.

659. Lodding, P., Kindblom, L.-G., and Angervall, L.: Epithelioid malignant schwannoma: a study of 14 cases, Virchows Arch. [A] **409**:433, 1986.

660. Markel, S.F., and Enzinger, F.M.: Neuromuscular hamartoma—a benign "Triton tumor" composed of mature neural and striated muscle elements, Cancer **49**:140, 1982.

661. Matsunou, H., Shimoda, T., Kakimoto, S., Yamashita, H., Ishikawa, E., and Mukai, M.: Histopathologic and immunohistochemical study of malignant tumors of peripheral nerve sheath (malignant schwannoma), Cancer **56**:2269, 1985.

662. Raney, B., Schnaufer, L., Ziegler, M., Chatten, J., Littman, P., and Jarrett, P.: Treatment of children with neurogenic sarcoma: experience at the Children's Hospital of Philadelphia, 1958-1984, Cancer **59**:1, 1987.

663. Sordillo, P.P., Helson, L., Hajdu, S.I., Magill, G.B., Kosloff, C., Golbey, R.B., and Beattie, E.J.: Malignant schwannoma: clinical characteristics, survival, and response to therapy, Cancer **47**:2503, 1981.

664. Storm, F.K., Eilber, F.R., Mirra, J., and Morton, D.L.: Neurofibrosarcoma, Cancer **45**:126, 1980.

665. Taxy, J.B., Battifora, H., Trujillo, Y., and Dorfman, H.D.: Electron microscopy in the diagnosis of malignant schwannoma, Cancer **48**:1381, 1981.

666. Trojanowski, J.Q., Kleinman, G.M., and Proppe, K.H.: Malignant tumors of nerve sheath origin, Cancer **46**:1202, 1980.

667. Tsuneyoshi, M., and Enjoji, M.: Primary malignant peripheral nerve tumors (malignant schwannomas): a clinicopathologic and electron microscopic study, Acta Pathol. Jpn. **29**:363, 1979.

668. Warner, T.F.C.S., Louie, R., Hafez, G.R., and Chandler, E.: Malignant nerve sheath tumor containing endocrine cells, Am. J. Surg. Pathol. **7**:583, 1983.

669. Wick, M.R., Swanson, P.E., Scheithauer, B.W., and Manivel, J.C.: Malignant peripheral nerve sheath tumor: an immunohistochemical study of 62 cases, Am. J. Clin. Pathol. **87**:425, 1987.

670. Woodruff, J.M.: Peripheral nerve tumors showing glandular differentiation (glandular schwannomas), Cancer **37**:2399, 1976.

671. Woodruff, J.M., Chernik, N.L., Smith, M.C., Millett, W.B., and Foote, F.W., Jr.: Peripheral nerve tumors with rhabdomyosarcomatous differentiation (malignant "Triton" tumors), Cancer **32**:426, 1973.

Miscellaneous tumors
Myxoma

672. Allen, P.W.: Myxoid tumors of soft tissues, Pathol. Annu. **15**(pt. 1):133, 1980.

673. Bégin, L.R., Clement, P.B., Kirk, M.E., Jothy, S., McCaughey, W.T.E., and Ferenczy, A.: Aggressive angiomyxoma of pelvic soft parts: a clinicopathologic study of nine cases, Hum. Pathol. **16**:621, 1985.

674. Blasier, R.D., Ryan, J.R., and Schaldenbrand, M.F.: Multiple myxomata of soft tissue associated with polyostotic fibrous dysplasia: a case report, Clin. Orthop. **206**:211, 1986.

675. Dutz, W., and Stout, A.P.: The myxoma in childhood, Cancer **14**:629, 1961.

676. Ekelund, L., Herrlin, K., and Rydholm, A.: Computed tomography of intramuscular myxoma, Skeletal Radiol. **9**:14, 1982.

677. Enzinger, F.M.: Intramuscular myxoma: a review and follow-up study of 34 cases, Am. J. Clin. Pathol. **43**:104, 1965.

678. Feldman, P.S.: A comparative study including ultrastructure of intramuscular myxoma and myxoid liposarcoma, Cancer **43**:512, 1979.

679. Hashimoto, H., Tsuneyoshi, M., Daimaru, Y., Enjoji, M., and Shinohara, N.: Intramuscular myxoma: a clinicopathologic, immunohistochemical, and electron microscopic study, Cancer **58**:740, 1986.

680. Ireland, D.C.R., Soule, E.H., and Ivins, J.C.: Myxoma of somatic soft tissues: a report of 58 patients, 3 with multiple tumors and fibrous dysplasia of bone, Mayo Clin. Proc. **48**:401, 1973.

681. Kindblom, L.-G., Stener, B., and Angervall, L.: Intramuscular myxoma, Cancer **34**:1737, 1974.

682. Lever, E.G., and Pettingale, K.W.: Albright's syndrome associated with a soft-tissue myxoma and hypophosphataemic osteomalacia: report of a case and review of the literature, J. Bone Joint Surg. **65B**:621, 1983.

683. McCook, T.A., Martinez, S., Korobkin, M., Ram, P.C., Bowen, J.H., Breiman, R.S., Harrelson, J.M., and Gehweiler, J.A., Jr.: Intramuscular myxoma: radiographic and computed tomographic findings with pathologic correlation, Skeletal Radiol. **7**:15, 1981.

684. Miettinen, M., Höckerstedt, K., Reitamo, J., and Tötterman, S.: Intramuscular myxoma: a clinicopathological study of twenty-three cases, Am. J. Clin. Pathol. **84**:265, 1985.

685. Steeper, T.A., and Rosai, J.: Aggressive angiomyxoma of the female pelvis and perineum: report of nine cases of a distinctive type of gynecologic soft-tissue neoplasm, Am. J. Surg. Pathol. **7**:463, 1983.

686. Stout, A.P.: Myxoma, the tumor of primitive mesenchyme, Ann. Surg. **127**:706, 1948.

687. Wirth, W.A., Leavitt, D., and Enzinger, F.M.: Multiple intramuscular myxomas: another extraskeletal manifestation of fibrous dysplasia, Cancer **27**:1167, 1971.

Synovial sarcoma

688. Abenoza, P., Manivel, J.C., Swanson, P.E., and Wick, M.R.: Synovial sarcoma: ultrastructural study and immunohistochemical analysis by a combined peroxidase–antiperoxidase/avidin-biotin-peroxidase complex procedure, Hum. Pathol. **17**:1107, 1986.

689. Bridge, J.A., Bridge, R.S., Borek, D.A., Shaffer, B., and Norris, C.W.: Translocation t(X;18) in orofacial synovial sarcoma, Cancer **62**:935, 1988.

690. Cadman, N.L., Soule, E.H., and Kelly, P.J.: Synovial sarcoma: an analysis of 134 tumors, Cancer **18**:613, 1965.

691. Cagle, L.A., Mirra, J.M., Storm, F.K., Roe, D.J., and Eilber, F.R.: Histologic features relating to prognosis in synovial sarcoma, Cancer **59**:1810, 1987.

692. Cameron, H.U., and Kostuik, J.P.: A long-term follow-up of synovial sarcoma, J. Bone Joint Surg. **56B**:613, 1974.

693. Cooney, T.P., Hwang, W.S., Robertson, D.I., and Hoogstraten, J.: Monophasic synovial sarcoma, epithelioid sarcoma and chordoid sarcoma: ultrastructural evidence for a common histogenesis, despite light microscopic diversity, Histopathology **6**:163, 1982.

694. Corson, J.M., Weiss, L.M., Banks-Schlegel, S.P., and Pinkus, G.S.: Keratin proteins and carcinoembryonic antigen in synovial sarcomas: an immunohistochemical study of 24 cases, Hum. Pathol. **15**:615, 1984.

695. Dische, F.E., Darby, A.J., and Howard, E.R.: Malignant synovioma: electron microscopical findings in three patients and review of the literature, J. Pathol. **124**:149, 1978.

696. Evans, H.L.: Synovial sarcoma: a study of 23 biphasic and 17 probable monophasic examples, Pathol. Annu. **15**(pt. 2):309, 1980.

697. Fisher, C.: Synovial sarcoma: ultrastructural and immunohistochemical features of epithelial differentiation in monophasic and biphasic tumors, Hum. Pathol. **17**:996, 1986.

698. Ghadially, F.N.: Is synovial sarcoma a carcinosarcoma of connective tissue? Ultrastruct. Pathol. **11**:147, 1987.

699. Hajdu, S.I., Shiu, M.H., and Fortner, J.G.: Tendosynovial sarcoma: a clinicopathological study of 136 cases, Cancer **39**:1201, 1977.

700. Krall, R.A., Kostianovsky, M., and Patchefsky, A.S.: Synovial sarcoma: a clinical, pathological, and ultrastructural study of 26 cases supporting the recognition of a monophasic variant, Am. J. Surg. Pathol. **5**:137, 1981.

701. Leader, M., Patel, J., Collins, M., and Kristin, H.: Synovial sarcomas: true carcinosarcomas? Cancer **59**:2096, 1987.

702. Mackenzie, D.H.: Monophasic synovial sarcoma: a histological entity? Histopathology **1**:151, 1977.

703. Majeste, R.M., and Beckman, E.N.: Synovial sarcoma with an overwhelming epithelial component, Cancer **61**:2527, 1988.

704. Mamelle, G., Richard, J., Luboinski, B., Schwaab, G., Eschwege, F., and Micheau, C.: Synovial sarcoma of the head and neck: an account of four cases and review of the literature, Eur. J. Surg. Oncol. **12**:347, 1986.

705. Mickelson, M.R., Brown, G.A., Maynard, J.A., Cooper, R.R., and Bonfiglio, M.: Synovial sarcoma: an electron microscopic study of monophasic and biphasic forms, Cancer **45**:2109, 1980.

706. Miettinen, M., Santavirta, S., and Slätis, P.: Intravascular synovial sarcoma, Hum. Pathol. **18**:1075, 1987.

707. Miettinen, M., Lehto, V.-P., and Virtanen, I.: Keratin in the epithelial-like cells of classical biphasic synovial sarcoma, Virchows Arch. [B] **40**:157, 1982.

708. Miettinen, M., Lehto, V.-P., and Virtanen, I.: Monophasic synovial sarcoma of spindle-cell type: epithelial differentiation as revealed by ultrastructural features, content of prekeratin and binding of peanut agglutinin, Virchows Arch. [B] **44**:187, 1983.

709. Miettinen, M., and Virtanen, I.: Synovial sarcoma—a misnomer, Am. J. Pathol. **117**:18, 1984.

710. Mirra, J.M., Wang, S., and Bhuta, S.: Synovial sarcoma with squamous differentiation of its mesenchymal glandular elements: a case report with light-microscopic, ultramicroscopic, and immunologic correlation, Am. J. Surg. Pathol. **8**:791, 1984.

711. Nunez-Alonso, C., Gashti, E.N., and Christ, M.L.: Maxillofacial synovial sarcoma: light- and electron-microscopic study of two cases, Am. J. Surg. Pathol. **3**:23, 1979.

712. Rajpal, S., Moore, R.H., and Karakousis, C.P.: Synovial sarcoma: a review of treatment and survival in 52 patients, NY State J. Med. **84**:17, 1984.

713. Roth, J.A., Enzinger, F.M., and Tannenbaum, M.: Synovial sarcoma of the neck: a follow-up study of 24 cases, Cancer **35**:1243, 1975.

714. Ryan, J.R., Baker, L.H., and Benjamin, R.S.: The natural history of metastatic synovial sarcoma: experience of the Southwest Oncology Group, Clin. Orthop. **164**:257, 1982.

715. Salisbury, J.R., and Isaacson, P.G.: Synovial sarcoma: an immunohistochemical study, J. Pathol. **147**:49, 1985.

716. Schmidt, D., and Mackay, B.: Ultrastructure of human tendon sheath and synovium: implications for tumor histogenesis, Ultrastruct. Pathol. **3**:269, 1982.

717. Shmookler, B.M., Enzinger, F.M., and Brannon, R.B.: Orofacial synovial sarcoma: a clinicopathologic study of 11 new cases and review of the literature, Cancer **50**:269, 1982.

718. Smith, S., Reeves, B.R., Wong, L., and Fisher, C.: A consistent chromosome translocation in synovial sarcoma, Cancer Genet. Cytogenet. **26**:179, 1987.

719. Tsujimoto, M., Ueda, T., Nakashima, H., Hamada, H., Ishiguro, S., and Aozasa, K.: Monophasic and biphasic synovial sarcoma: an immunohistochemical study, Acta Pathol. Jpn. **37**:597, 1987.

720. Tsuneyoshi, M., Yokoyama, K., and Enjoji, M.: Synovial sarcoma: a clinicopathologic and ultrastructural study of 42 cases, Acta Pathol. Jpn. **33**:23, 1983.

721. Turc-Carel, C., Cin, P.D., Limon, J., Li, F., and Sandberg, A.A.: Translocation X;18 in synovial sarcoma, Cancer Genet. Cytogenet. **23**:93, 1986.

722. Varela-Duran, J., and Enzinger, F.M.: Calcifying synovial sarcoma, Cancer **50**:345, 1982.

723. Wright, P.H., Sim, F.H., Soule, E.H., and Taylor, W.F.: Synovial sarcoma, J. Bone Joint Surg. **64A**:112, 1982.

724. Zito, R.A.: Synovial sarcoma: an Australian series of 48 cases, Pathology **16**:45, 1984.

Epithelioid sarcoma

725. Blewitt, R.W., Aparicio, S.G.R., and Bird, C.C.: Epithelioid sarcoma: a tumour of myofibroblasts, Histopathology **7**:573, 1983.

726. Bloustein, P.A., Silverberg, S.G., and Waddell, W.R.: Epithelioid sarcoma: case report with ultrastructural review, histogenetic discussion, and chemotherapeutic data, Cancer **38**:2390, 1976.

727. Bos, G.D., Pritchard, D.J., Reiman, H.M., Dobyns, J.H., Ilstrup, D.M., and Landon, G.C.: Epithelioid sarcoma: an analysis of fifty-one cases, J. Bone Joint Surg. **70A**:862, 1988.

728. Bryan, R.S., Soule, E.H., Dobyns, J.H., Pritchard, D.J., and Linscheid, R.L.: Primary epithelioid sarcoma of the hand and forearm: a review of thirteen cases, J. Bone Joint Surg. **56A**:458, 1974.

729. Chase, D.R., and Enzinger, F.M.: Epithelioid sarcoma: diagnosis, prognostic indicators, and treatment, Am. J. Surg. Pathol. **9**:241, 1985.

730. Chase, D.R., Enzinger, F.M., Weiss, S.W., and Langloss, J.M.: Keratin in epithelioid sarcoma: an immunohistochemical study, Am. J. Surg. Pathol. **8**:435, 1984.

731. Cooney, T.P., Hwang, W.S., Robertson, D.I., and Hoogstraten, J.: Monophasic synovial sarcoma, epithelioid sarcoma and chordoid sarcoma: ultrastructural evidence for a common histogenesis, despite light microscopic diversity, Histopathology **6**:163, 1982.

732. Dąbska, M., and Koszarowski, T.: Clinical and pathologic study of aponeurotic (epithelioid) sarcoma, Pathol. Annu. **17**(pt. 1):129, 1982.

733. Daimaru, Y., Hashimoto, H., Tsuneyoshi, M., and Enjoji, M.: Epithelial profile of epithelioid sarcoma: an immunohistochemical analysis of eight cases, Cancer **59**:134, 1987.

734. Enzinger, F.M.: Epithelioid sarcoma: a sarcoma simulating a granuloma or a carcinoma, Cancer **26**:1029, 1970.

735. Fisher, C.: Epithelioid sarcoma: the spectrum of ultrastructural differentiation in seven immunohistochemically defined cases, Hum. Pathol. **19**:265, 1988.

736. Gabbiani, G., Fu, Y.S., Kaye, G.I., Lattes, R., and Majno, G.: Epithelioid sarcoma: a light and electron microscopic study suggesting a synovial origin, Cancer **30**:486, 1972.

737. Heenan, P.J., Quirk, C.J., and Papadimitriou, J.M.: Epithelioid sarcoma: a diagnostic problem, Am. J. Dermatopathol. **8**:95, 1986.

738. Machinami, R., Kikuchi, F., and Matsushita, H.: Epithelioid sarcoma: enzyme histochemical and ultrastructural study, Virchows Arch. [A] **397**:109, 1982.

739. Mackay, B., Rashid, R.K., and Evans, H.L.: Case 9: epithelioid sarcoma, Ultrastruct. Pathol. **5**:329, 1983.

740. Manivel, J.C., Wick, M.R., Dehner, L.P., and Sibley, R.K.: Epithelioid sarcoma: an immunohistochemical study, Am. J. Clin. Pathol. **87**:319, 1987.

741. Mills, S.E., Fechner, R.E., Bruns, D.E., Bruns, M.E., and O'Hara, M.F.: Intermediate filaments in eosinophilic cells of epithelioid sarcoma: a light-microscopic, ultrastructural and electrophoretic study, Am. J. Surg. Pathol. **5**:195, 1981.

742. Moore, S.W., Wheeler, J.E., and Hefter, L.G.: Epithelioid sarcoma masquerading as Peyronie's disease, Cancer **35**:1706, 1975.

743. Mukai, M., Torikata, C., Iri, H., Hanaoka, H., Kawai, T., Yakumaru, K., Shimoda, T., Mikata, A., and Kageyama, K.: Cellular differentiation of epithelioid sarcoma: an electron-microscopic, enzyme-histochemical, and immunohistochemical study, Am. J. Pathol. **119**:44, 1985.

744. Padilla, R.S., Flynn, K., and Headington, J.T.: Epithelioid sarcoma: enzymatic histochemical and electron microscopic evidence of histiocytic differentiation, Arch. Dermatol. **121**:389, 1985.

745. Prat, J., Woodruff, J.M., and Marcove, R.C.: Epithelioid sarcoma: an analysis of 22 cases indicating the prognostic significance of vascular invasion and regional lymph node metastases, Cancer **41**:1472, 1978.

746. Santiago, H., Feinerman, L.K., and Lattes, R.: Epithelioid sarcoma: a clinical and pathologic study of nine cases, Hum. Pathol. **3**:133, 1972.

747. Schmidt, D., and Harms, D.: Epithelioid sarcoma in children and adolescents: an immunohistochemical study, Virchows Arch. [A] **410**:423, 1987.

748. Ulbright, T.M., Brokaw, S.A., Stehman, F.B., and Roth, L.M.: Epithelioid sarcoma of the vulva: evidence suggesting a more aggressive behavior than extra-genital epithelioid sarcoma, Cancer **52**:1462, 1983.

749. Wick, M.R., and Manivel, J.C.: Epithelioid sarcoma and isolated necrobiotic granuloma: a comparative immunocytochemical study, J. Cutan. Pathol. **13**:253, 1986.

750. Wick, M.R., and Manivel, J.C.: Epithelioid sarcoma and epithelioid hemangioendothelioma: an immunocytochemical and lectin-histochemical comparison, Virchows Arch. [A] **410**:309, 1987.

Clear cell sarcoma

751. Azumi, N., and Turner, R.R.: Clear cell sarcoma of tendons and aponeuroses: electron microscopic findings suggesting Schwann cell differentiation, Hum. Pathol. **14**:1084, 1983.
752. Bearman, R.M., Noe, J., and Kempson, R.L.: Clear cell sarcoma with melanin pigment, Cancer **36**:977, 1975.
753. Benson, J.D., Kraemer, B.B., and Mackay, B.: Malignant melanoma of soft parts: an ultrastructural study of four cases, Ultrastruct. Pathol. **8**:57, 1985.
754. Chung, E.B., and Enzinger, F.M.: Malignant melanoma of soft parts: a reassessment of clear cell sarcoma, Am. J. Surg. Pathol. **7**:405, 1983.
755. Eckardt, J.J., Pritchard, D.J., and Soule, E.H.: Clear cell sarcoma: a clinicopathologic study of 27 cases, Cancer **52**:1482, 1983.
756. Ekfors, T.O., and Rantakokko, V.: Clear cell sarcoma of tendons and aponeuroses: malignant melanoma of soft tissues? Report of four cases, Pathol. Res. Pract. **165**:422, 1979.
757. Enzinger, F.M.: Clear-cell sarcoma of tendons and aponeuroses: an analysis of 21 cases, Cancer **18**:1163, 1965.
758. Hoffman, G.J., and Carter, D.: Clear cell sarcoma of tendons and aponeuroses with melanin, Arch. Pathol. **95**:22, 1973.
759. Kindblom, L.-G., Lodding, P., and Angervall, L.: Clear-cell sarcoma of tendons and aponeuroses: an immunohistochemical and electron microscopic analysis indicating neural crest origin, Virchows Arch. [A] **401**:109, 1983.
760. Mackenzie, D.H.: Clear cell sarcoma of tendon and aponeuroses with melanin production, J. Pathol. **114**:231, 1974.
761. Mukai, M., Torikata, C., Iri, H., Mikata, A., Kawai, T., Hanaoka, H., Yakumaru, K., and Kageyama, K.: Histogenesis of clear cell sarcoma of tendons and aponeuroses: an electron-microscopic, biochemical, enzyme histochemical, and immunohistochemical study, Am. J. Pathol. **114**:264, 1984.
762. Ohno, T., Park, P., Utsunomiya, Y., Hirahata, H., and Inoue, K.: Ultrastructural study of a clear cell sarcoma suggesting schwannian differentiation, Ultrastruct. Pathol. **10**:39, 1986.
763. Parker, J.B., Marcus, P.B., and Martin, J.H.: Spinal melanotic clear-cell sarcoma: a light and electron microscopic study, Cancer **46**:718, 1980.
764. Pavlidis, N.A., Fisher, C., and Wiltshaw, E.: Clear-cell sarcoma of tendons and aponeuroses: a clinicopathologic study: presentation of six additional cases with review of the literature, Cancer **54**:1412, 1984.
765. Raynor, A.C., Vargas-Cortes, F., Alexander, R.W., and Bingham, H.G.: Clear-cell sarcoma with melanin pigment: a possible soft-tissue variant of malignant melanoma, J. Bone Joint Surg. **61A**:276, 1979.
766. Saw, D., Tse, C.H., Chan, J., Watt, C.Y., Ng, C.S., and Poon, Y.F.: Clear sarcoma of the penis, Hum. Pathol. **17**:423, 1986.
767. Tsuneyoshi, M., Enjoji, M., and Kubo, T.: Clear cell sarcoma of tendons and aponeuroses: a comparative study of 13 cases with a provisional subgrouping into the melanotic and synovial types, Cancer **42**:243, 1978.

Alveolar soft part sarcoma

768. Auerbach, H.E., and Brooks, J.J.: Alveolar soft part sarcoma: a clinicopathologic and immunohistochemical study, Cancer **60**:66, 1987.
769. Chapman, G.W., Benda, J., and Williams, T.: Alveolar soft-part sarcoma of the vagina, Gynecol. Oncol. **18**:125, 1984.
770. Christopherson, W.M., Foote, F.W., and Stewart, F.W.: Alveolar soft-part sarcomas: structurally characteristic tumors of uncertain histogenesis, Cancer **5**:100, 1952.
771. De Schryver-Kecskemeti, K., Kraus, F.T., Engleman, W., and Lacy, P.E.: Alveolar soft-part sarcoma—a malignant angioreninoma: histochemical, immunocytochemical, and electron-microscopic study of four cases, Am. J. Surg. Pathol. **6**:5, 1982.
772. Ekfors, T.O., Kalimo, H., Rantakokko, V., Latvala, M., and

Parvinen, M.: Alveolar soft part sarcoma: a report of two cases with some histochemical and ultrastructural observations, Cancer **43**:1672, 1979.
773. Evans, H.L.: Alveolar soft-part sarcoma: a study of 13 typical examples and one with a histologically atypical component, Cancer **55**:912, 1985.
774. Flint, A., Gikas, P.W., and Roberts, J.A.: Alveolar soft part sarcoma of the uterine cervix, Gynecol. Oncol. **22**:263, 1985.
775. Font, R.L., Jurco, S., III, and Zimmerman, L.E.: Alveolar soft-part sarcoma of the orbit: a clinicopathologic analysis of seventeen cases and a review of the literature, Hum. Pathol. **13**:569, 1982.
776. Foschini, M.P., Ceccarelli, C., Eusebi, V., Skalli, O., and Gabbiani, G.: Alveolar soft part sarcoma: immunological evidence of rhabdomyoblastic differentiation, Histopathology **13**:101, 1988.
777. Gray, G.F., Jr., Glick, A.D., Kurtin, P.J., and Jones, H.W., III: Alveolar soft part sarcoma of the uterus, Hum. Pathol. **17**:297, 1986.
778. Hurt, R., Bates, M., and Harrison, W.: Alveolar soft-part sarcoma, Thorax **37**:877, 1982.
779. Lieberman, P.H., Foote, F.W., Jr., Stewart, F.W., and Berg, J.W.: Alveolar soft-part sarcoma, JAMA **198**:1047, 1966.
780. Marcus, P.B., Couch, W.D., and Martin, J.H.: Crystals in a gastric schwannoma, Ultrastruct. Pathol. **2**:139, 1981.
781. Mathew, T.: Evidence supporting neural crest origin of an alveolar soft part sarcoma: an ultrastructural study, Cancer **50**:507, 1982.
782. Mukai, M., Iri, H., Nakajima, T., Hirose, S., Torikata, C., Kageyama, K., Ueno, N., and Murakami, K.: Alveolar soft-part sarcoma: a review on its histogenesis and further studies based on electron microscopy, immunohistochemistry, and biochemistry, Am. J. Surg. Pathol. **7**:679, 1983.
783. Mukai, M., Torikata, C., Iri, H., Mikata, A., Hanaoka, H., Kato, K., and Kageyama, K.: Histogenesis of alveolar soft part sarcoma: an immunohistochemical and biochemical study, Am. J. Surg. Pathol. **10**:212, 1986.
784. Ogawa, K., Nakashima, Y., Yamabe, H., and Hamashima, Y.: Alveolar soft part sarcoma, granular cell tumor, and paraganglioma: an immunohistochemical comparative study, Acta Pathol. Jpn. **36**:895, 1986.
785. Ordóñez, N.G., Hickey, R.C., and Brooks, T.E.: Alveolar soft part sarcoma: a cytologic and immunohistochemical study, Cancer **61**:525, 1988.
786. Persson, S., Willems, J.-S., Kindblom, L.-G., and Angervall, L.: Alveolar soft part sarcoma: an immunohistochemical, cytologic and electron-microscopic study and a quantitative DNA analysis, Virchows Arch. [A] **412**:499, 1988.
787. Shen, J.-T., D'Ablaing, G., and Morrow, C.P.: Alveolar soft part sarcoma of the vulva: report of first case and review of literature, Gynecol. Oncol. **13**:120, 1982.
788. Shipkey, F.H., Lieberman, P.H., Foote, F.W., Jr., and Stewart, F.W.: Ultrastructure of alveolar soft part sarcoma, Cancer **17**:821, 1964.
789. Spector, R.A., Travis, L.W., and Smith, J.: Alveolar soft part sarcoma of the head and neck, Laryngoscope **89**:1301, 1979.
790. Unni, K.K., and Soule, E.H.: Alveolar soft part sarcoma: an electron microscopic study, Mayo Clin. Proc. **50**:591, 1975.
791. Welsh, R.A., Bray, D.M., III, Shipkey, F.H., and Meyer, A.T.: Histogenesis of alveolar soft part sarcoma, Cancer **29**:191, 1972.

Giant cell tumor of soft tissue

792. Alguacil-Garcia, A., Unni, K.K., and Goellner, J.R.: Malignant giant cell tumor of soft parts: an ultrastructural study of four cases, Cancer **40**:244, 1977.
793. Angervall, L., Hagmar, B., Lindblom, L.-G., and Merck, C.: Malignant giant cell tumor of soft tissues: a clinicopathologic, cytologic, ultrastructural, angiographic, and microangiographic study, Cancer **47**:736, 1981.
794. Chung, E.B., and Enzinger, F.M.: Extraskeletal osteosarcoma, Cancer **60**:1132, 1987.
795. Guccion, J.G., and Enzinger, F.M.: Malignant giant cell tumor of soft parts: an analysis of 32 cases, Cancer **29**:1518, 1972.

796. Robins, R.E., Johnstone, F.R.C., Worth, A., and Fris, R.J.: The importance of recognizing malignant giant cell tumor of soft parts, Am. J. Surg. **136:**102, 1978.

797. Salm, R., and Sissons, H.A.: Giant-cell tumours of soft tissues, J. Pathol. **107:**27, 1972.

798. van Haelst, U.J.G.M., and de Haas van Dorsser, A.H.: Giant cell tumor of soft parts: an ultrastructural study, Virchows Arch. [A] **371:**199, 1976.

Extraskeletal Ewing's sarcoma

799. Angervall, L., and Enzinger, F.M.: Extraskeletal neoplasm resembling Ewing's sarcoma, Cancer **36:**240, 1975.

800. Askin, F.B., Rosai, J., Sibley, R.K., Dehner, L.P., and McAlister, W.H.: Malignant small cell tumor of the thoracopulmonary region in childhood: a distinctive clinicopathologic entity of uncertain histogenesis, Cancer **43:**2438, 1979.

801. Berthold, F., Kracht, J., Lampert, F., Millar, T.J., Müller, T.H., Reither, M., and Unsicker, K.: Ultrastructural, biochemical and cell-culture studies of a presumed extraskeletal Ewing's sarcoma with special reference to differential diagnosis from neuroblastoma, Cancer Res. Clin. Oncol. **103:**293, 1982.

802. Bignold, L.P.: So-called "extraskeletal" Ewing's sarcoma, Am. J. Clin. Pathol. **73:**142, 1980.

803. Cavazzana, A.O., Miser, J.S., Jefferson, J., and Triche, T.J.: Experimental evidence for a neural origin of Ewing's sarcoma of bone, Am. J. Pathol. **127:**507, 1987.

804. Chen, K.T.K., and Padmanabhan, A.: Extraskeletal Ewing's sarcoma, J. Surg. Oncol. **23:**70, 1983.

805. Dickman, P.S., and Triche, T.J.: Extraosseous Ewing's sarcoma versus primitive rhabdomyosarcoma: diagnostic criteria and clinical correlation, Hum. Pathol. **17:**881, 1986.

806. Erlandson, R.A.: The ultrastructural distinction between rhabdomyosarcoma and other undifferentiated "sarcomas," Ultrastruct. Pathol. **11:**83, 1987.

807. Gillespie, J.J., Roth, L.M., Wills, E.R., Einhorn, L.H., and Willman, J.: Extraskeletal Ewing's sarcoma: histologic and ultrastructural observations in three cases, Am. J. Surg. Pathol. **3:**99, 1979.

808. Gonzalez-Crussi, F., Wolfson, S.L., Misugi, K., and Nakajima, T.: Peripheral neuroectodermal tumors of the chest wall in childhood, Cancer **54:**2519, 1984.

809. Hashimoto, H., Tsuneyoshi, M., Daimaru, Y., and Enjoji, M.: Extraskeletal Ewing's sarcoma: a clinicopathologic and electron microscopic analysis of 8 cases, Acta Pathol. Jpn. **35:**1087, 1985.

810. Jaffe, R., Santamaria, M., Yunis, E.J., Tannery, N.H., Agostini, R.M., Jr., Medina, J., and Goodman, M.: The neuroectodermal tumor of bone, Am. J. Surg. Pathol. **8:**885, 1984.

811. Kawaguchi, K., and Koike, M.: Neuron-specific enolase and leu-7 immunoreactive small round-cell neoplasm: the relationship to Ewing's sarcoma in bone and soft tissue, Am. J. Clin. Pathol. **86:**79, 1986.

812. Kinsella, T.J., Triche, T.J., Dickman, P.S., Costa, J., Tepper, J.E., and Glaubiger, D.: Extraskeletal Ewing's sarcoma: results of combined modality treatment, J. Clin. Oncol. **1:**489, 1983.

813. Linnoila, R.I., Tsokos, M., Triche, T.J., Marangos, P.J., and Chandra, R.S.: Evidence for neural origin and PAS-positive variants of the malignant small cell tumor of thoracopulmonary region ("Askin tumor"), Am. J. Surg. Pathol. **10:**124, 1986.

814. Mahoney, J.P., Ballinger, W.E., Jr, and Alexander, R.W.: So-called extraskeletal Ewing's sarcoma: report of a case with ultrastructural analysis, Am. J. Clin. Pathol. **70:**926, 1978.

815. Meister, P., and Gokel, J.M.: Extraskeletal Ewing's sarcoma, Virchows Arch. [A] **378:**173, 1978.

816. Mierau, G.W.: Extraskeletal Ewing's sarcoma (peripheral neuroepithelioma), Ultrastruct. Pathol. **9:**91, 1985.

817. Miettinen, M., Lehto, V.-P., and Virtanen, I.: Histogenesis of Ewing's sarcoma: an evaluation of intermediate filaments and endothelial cell markers, Virchows Arch. [B] **41:**277, 1982.

818. Moll, R., Lee, I., Gould, V.E., Berndt, R., Roessner, A., and Franke, W.W.: Immunocytochemical analysis of Ewing's tumors: patterns of expression of intermediate filaments and desmosomal proteins indicate cell type heterogeneity and pluripotential differentiation, Am. J. Pathol. **127:**288, 1987.

819. Newton, W.A., Jr., Soule, E.H., Hamoudi, A.B., Reiman, H.M., Shimada, H., Beltangady, M., and Maurer, H.: Histopathology of childhood sarcomas, Intergroup Rhabdomyosarcoma studies I and II: clinicopathologic correlation, J. Clin. Oncol. **6:**67, 1988.

820. Peters, M.S., Reiman, H.M., and Muller, S.A.: Cutaneous extraskeletal Ewing's sarcoma, J. Cutan. Pathol. **12:**476, 1985.

821. Pontius, K.I., and Sebek, B.A.: Extraskeletal Ewing's sarcoma arising in the nasal fossa: light- and electron-microscopic observations, Am. J. Clin. Pathol. **75:**410, 1981.

822. Rose, J.S., Hermann, G., Mendelson, D.S., and Ambinder, E.P.: Extraskeletal Ewing sarcoma with computed tomography correlation, Skeletal Radiol. **9:**234, 1983.

823. Schmidt, D., Harms, D., and Burdach, S.: Malignant peripheral neuroectodermal tumours of childhood and adolescence, Virchows Arch. [A] **406:**351, 1985.

824. Shimada, H., Newton, W.A., Jr., Soule, E.H., Qualman, S.J., Aoyama, C., and Maurer, H.M.: Pathologic features of extraosseous Ewing's sarcoma: a report from the Intergroup Rhabdomyosarcoma Study, Hum. Pathol. **19:**442, 1988.

825. Soule, E.H., Newton, W., Jr., Moon, T.E., and Tefft, M.: Extraskeletal Ewing's sarcoma: a preliminary review of 26 cases encountered in the Intergroup Rhabdomyosarcoma Study, Cancer **42:**259, 1978.

826. Stuart-Harris, R., Wills, E.J., Philips, J., Langlands, A.O., Fox, R.M., and Tattersall, M.H.N.: Extraskeletal Ewing's sarcoma: a clinical, morphological and ultrastructural analysis of five cases with a review of the literature, Eur. J. Cancer Clin. Oncol. **22:**393, 1986.

827. Tefft, M., Vawter, G.F., and Mitus, A.: Paravertebral "round cell" tumors in children, Radiology **92:**1501, 1969.

828. Wigger, H.J., Salazar, G.H., and Blanc, W.A.: Extraskeletal Ewing sarcoma: an ultrastructural study, Arch. Pathol. Lab. Med. **101:**446, 1977.

829. Yunis, E.J.: Ewing's sarcoma and related small round cell neoplasms in children, Am. J. Surg. Pathol. **10**(suppl.):54, 1986.

ADDITIONAL READING

830. Chung, E.B., and Enzinger, F.M.: Fibroma of tendon sheath, Cancer **44:**1945, 1979.

831. Hashimoto, H., Tsuneyoshi, M., Daimaru, Y., Ushijima, M., and Enjoji, M.: Fibroma of tendon sheath: a tumor of myofibroblasts: a clinicopathologic study of 18 cases, Acta Pathol. Jpn. **35:**1099, 1985.

832. Lundgren, L.G., and Kindblom, L.-G.: Fibroma of tendon sheath: a light and electron-microscopic study of 6 cases, Acta Pathol. Microbiol. Immunol. Scand. [A] **92:**401, 1984.

833. Abdul-Karim, F.W., Evans, H.L., and Silva, E.G.: Giant cell fibroblastoma: a report of three cases, Am. J. Clin. Pathol. **83:**165, 1985.

834. Barr, R.J., Young, E.M., Jr., and Liao, S.-Y.: Giant cell fibroblastoma: an immunohistochemical study, J. Cutan. Pathol. **13:**301, 1986.

835. Dymock, R.B., Allen, P.W., Stirling, J.W., Gilbert, E.F., and Thornbery, J.M.: Giant cell fibroblastoma: a distinctive, recurrent tumor of childhood, Am. J. Surg. Pathol. **11:**263, 1987.

836. Shmookler, B.M., and Enzinger, F.M.: Giant cell fibroblastoma: a peculiar childhood tumor, Lab. Invest. **46:**76A, 1982.

837. Evans, H.L.: Low-grade fibromyxoid sarcoma: a report of two metastasizing neoplasms having a deceptively benign appearance, Am. J. Clin. Pathol. **88:**615, 1987.

838. Enzinger, F.M., and Shiraki, M.: Extraskeletal myxoid chondrosarcoma: an analysis of 34 cases, Hum. Pathol. **3:**421, 1972.

839. Fletcher, C.D.M., Powell, G., and McKee, P.H.: Extraskeletal myxoid chondrosarcoma: a histochemical and immunohistochemical study, Histopathology **10:**489, 1986.

840. Hachitanda, Y., Tsuneyoshi, M., Daimaru, Y., Enjoji, M., Nakagawara, A., Ikeda, K., and Sueishi, K.: Extraskeletal myxoid chondrosarcoma in young children, Cancer **61:**2521, 1988.

841. Martin, R.F., Melnick, P.J., Warner, N.E., Terry, R., Bullock, W.K., and Schwinn, C.P.: Chordoid sarcoma, Am. J. Clin. Pathol. **59:**623, 1973.

842. Weiss, S.W.: Ultrastructure of the so-called "chordoid sarcoma": evidence supporting cartilagenous [*sic*] differentiation, Cancer **37**:300, 1976.

843. Sordillo, P.P.: Extraosseous osteogenic sarcoma: a review of 48 patients, Cancer **51**:727, 1983.

844. Dervan, P.A., Cahalane, S.F., Kneafsey, P., Mynes, A., and McAllister, K.: Malignant rhabdoid tumor of soft tissue: an ultrastructural and immunohistochological study of a pelvic tumour, Histopathology **11**:183, 1987.

845. Frierson, H.F., Jr., Mills, S.E., and Innes, D.J., Jr.: Malignant rhabdoid tumor of the pelvis, Cancer **55**:1963, 1985.

846. Gonzalez-Crussi, F., Goldschmidt, R.A., Hsueh, W., and Trujillo, Y.P.: Infantile sarcoma with intracytoplasmic filamentous inclusions: distinctive tumor of possible histiocytic origin, Cancer **49**:2365, 1982.

847. Sotelo-Avila C., Gonzalez-Crussi, F., deMello, D., Vogler, C., Gooch, W.M., III, Gale, G., and Pena, R.: Renal and extrarenal rhabdoid tumors in children: a clinicopathologic study of 14 patients, Semin. Diagn. Pathol. **3**:151, 1986.

848. Tsuneyoshi, M., Daimaru, Y., Hashimoto, M., and Enjoji, M.: Malignant soft tissue neoplasms with the histologic features of renal rhabdoid tumors: an ultrastructural and immunohistochemical study, Hum. Pathol. **16**:1235, 1985.

849. Tsuneyoshi, M., Daimaru, Y., Hashimoto, H., and Enjoji, M.: The existence of rhabdoid cells in specified soft issue sarcomas: histopathological, ultrastructural and immunohistochemical evidence, Virchows Arch. [A] **411**:509, 1987.

850. González-Crussi, F., deMello, D.E., and Sotelo-Avila, C.: Omental-mesenteric myxoid hamartomas: infantile lesions simulating malignant tumors, Am. J. Surg. Pathol. **7**:567, 1983.

851. Weidner, N., and Santa Cruz, D.: Phosphaturic mesenchymal tumors: a polymorphous group causing osteomalacia or rickets, Cancer **59**:1442, 1987.

38 Metabolic and Other Nontumorous Disorders of Bone

MICHAEL D. FALLON
HARRY A. SCHWAMM

The skeleton is composed of cartilage and bone. Cartilage serves a role in bone development during the periods of growth and repair. In the adult the chief role of cartilage is in the articular skeleton, facilitating the motion of joints. This chapter deals with the nonneoplastic diseases of the skeleton. The tumor and tumor-like conditions of bone are discussed in Chapter 39, whereas articular disorders and diseases of the joints are discussed in Chapter 40.

The spectrum of nonneoplastic diseases that may afflict the skeleton is wide and usually encompasses disorders of specific bone cells or cellular functions, as outlined in Table 38-1. Other, organ nonspecific processes, such as inflammation, infection, and infarction, will produce characteristic pathologic changes in bone because of the particular physiologic constraints imposed by the skeleton. For these reasons, an under-standing of normal skeletal physiology is an important prerequisite to the understanding of nonneoplastic skeletal disease.

STRUCTURAL ORGANIZATION AND COMPOSITION OF BONE

Bone is a specialized connective tissue composed predominantly of a mineralized extracellular collagenous matrix and by comparison a relatively small number of hormone-responsive cells. The skeleton not only functions to provide mechanical support and protection, but also serves as a mineral reservoir for calcium homeostasis. The organization of bone may be functionally divided into a cortical (or compact) and trabecular (or cancellous) component (Fig. 38-1). Structural stability is provided by the cortical bone, which composes 80% of the skeleton. Within the cortex are haversian canals

Table 38-1. Diseases of bone

Disorders	Examples
Skeletal growth, modeling, and development	The osteochondrodystrophies Osteogenesis imperfecta Osteopetrosis
Bone-remodeling activity	The osteoporotic syndromes
Mineralization	Rickets-osteomalacia
Mechanical lesions of bone	Fractures
Bone repair	Fracture nonunions
Infectious diseases of bone	Osteomyelitis Tuberculosis Syphilis
Inflammatory diseases of bone	Paget's disease of bone (osteitis deformans) Sarcoidosis of bone
Degenerative/vascular diseases of bone	Bone infarction Idiopathic osteonecrosis Avascular necrosis

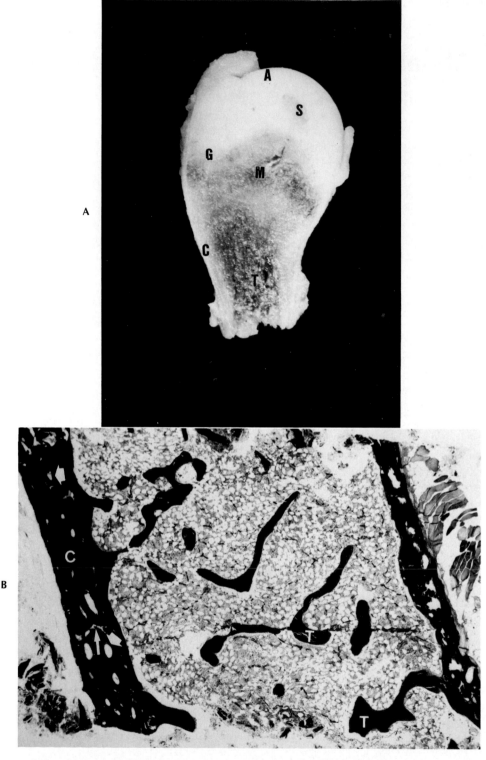

Fig. 38-1. A, Organization of skeleton. Hemisection of a neonatal proximal humeral head. *A,* Articular cartilage; *C,* cortical bone; *G,* epiphyseal growth plate; *M,* medullary cavity of metaphysis; *S,* secondary ossification center; *T,* trabecular bone. **B,** Microscopic organization of skeleton. *C,* Cortical bone; *T,* trabecular bone.

through which longitudinally oriented blood vessels pass and horizontally arranged Volkmann's canals containing vascular offshoots. Surrounding each haversian canal is a series of concentric, lamellar, mineralized collagen bundles, forming the osteon, the structural and remodeling unit of cortical bone (Fig. 38-2). Osteons are joined together by cement lines, which are best demonstrated by the use of a metachromatic stain. Cancellous bone, consisting of bars and plates of trabeculas, traverse the marrow space. Although trabecular bone composes only 20% of the skeleton, the three-dimensional arrangement of the trabecular network provides

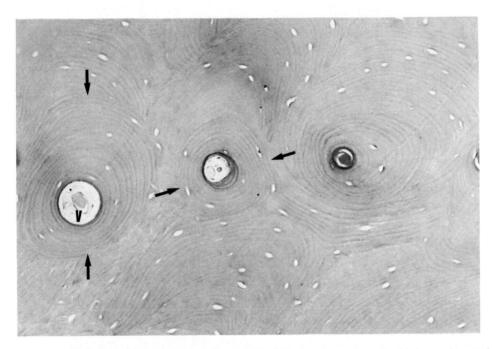

Fig. 38-2. Osteons, the structural unit of cortical bone, examples of which are located between the arrows, contain a central vascular channel, V.

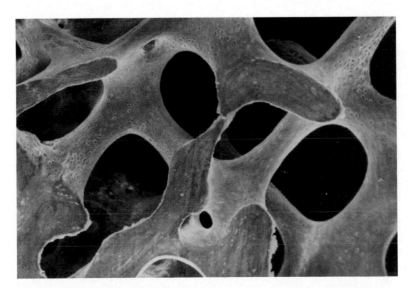

Fig. 38-3. Scanning electron micrograph of trabecular bone after removal of marrow. All trabeculas are joined in complicated meshwork. Small holes on surface are osteocytic lacunae. (57×.)

an enormous surface area (Fig. 38-3). Trabecular bone therefore is well suited to its metabolic role in mineral homeostasis.[179]

Bone matrix and bone cells

Bone consists of a relatively small number of metabolically active cells, associated with a vast quantity of organic and inorganic extracellular matrix. There are three main types of bone cells: osteoblasts, osteocytes, and osteoclasts.[20]

Bone matrix is synthesized by osteoblasts, and the microscopic appearance of osteoblasts in general reflects their metabolic (protein-synthesizing) activity (Fig. 38-4). When bone matrix synthesis is rapid, osteoblasts are cuboid and contain abundant ribonuclear

protein, rendering them basophilic. The prominent Golgi zone results in the formation of a perinuclear clear zone. As the rate of bone formation falls, there is a progressive flattening and attenuation of the osteoblasts, until they are transformed into a fusiform cell that lines the bone surface (Fig. 38-4, *B*). These membrane-appearing cells probably do not participate in the formation of bone at this point but most likely regulate calcium transport between the bone fluid compartment and the extracellular space.[80,175] Active osteoblasts are rich in the cytoplasmic membrane–bound ectoenzyme alkaline phosphatase,[12] which plays a role in the subsequent mineralization of the newly synthesized bone matrix (Fig. 38-5). Bone-related alkaline phosphatase that appears in the circulation has been utilized as a

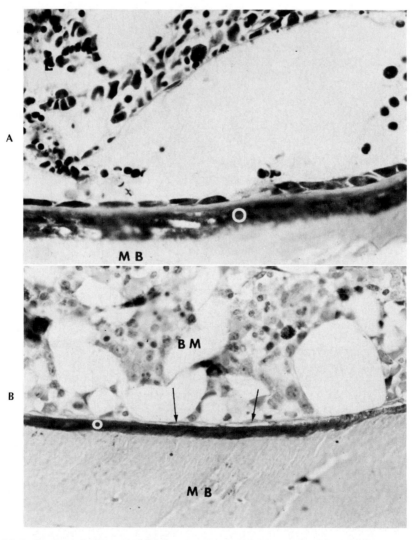

Fig. 38-4. A, Osteoblasts lining osteoid seam, *O. MB,* Mineralized bone. **B,** Syncytium of fusiform cells, *arrows,* covering bone surface, which probably functionally separates bone from general extracellular fluid. *BM,* Bone marrow; *MB,* mineralized bone; *O,* osteoid. (**A** and **B,** Undecalcified, Goldner's stain; 250×.)

marker of osteoblastic activity. For example, the circulating level of alkaline phosphatase normally rises during puberty during the period of rapid skeletal growth, that is, the growth spurt. The serum alkaline phosphatase level may also be elevated in pathologic conditions associated with stimulated osteoblastic activity such as fracture repair and Paget's disease of bone.[173]

Osteocytes represent those osteoblasts that have be-come trapped and incorporated into the bone matrix as it is synthesized. Osteocytic cellular contact is maintained by way of delicate cellular processes transversing the mineralized bone through canalicular spaces (Fig. 38-6). Cellular communication across tight junctions is believed to play a role in the regulation of calcium transfer between the bone surface and the extracellular fluid.[175] The number and configuration of the osteo-

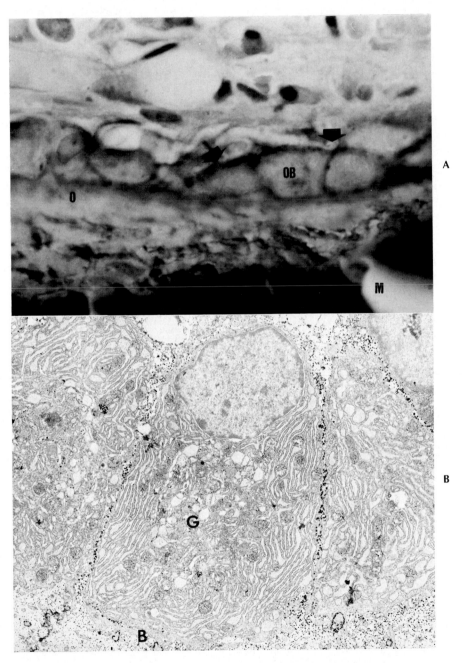

Fig. 38-5. A, Alkaline phosphatase histochemistry of bone. Alkaline phosphatase enzyme reaction product, *arrows,* surrounds the osteoblasts, *OB.* Osteoblasts line the osteoid seam, *O,* over mineralized bone, *M.* **B,** Osteoblasts on bone matrix. Notice abundant endoplasmic reticulum and prominent Golgi body, *G. Black dots,* Alkaline phosphatase reaction product. (**B,** 7400×; courtesy Dr. Stephen Doty, New York, N.Y.)

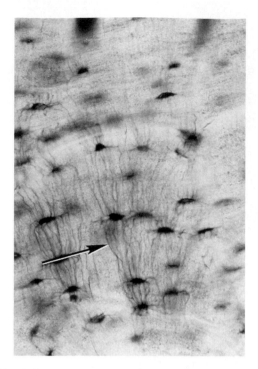

Fig. 38-6. Canaliculae, *arrow*, extending from osteocytic lacuna to osteocytic lacuna in fresh, unembedded ground section. (Villanueva bone stain; 250×.)

cytes is related to the surrounding collagen-fiber orientation, which in turn is a direct function of the rate of bone formation. The spatial distribution of the osteocytic lacunae is a reliable criterion for distinguishing between lamellar and woven bone. Immature, rapidly deposited woven bone contains a greater number of osteocytes, and the osteocytic lacunar spaces are larger than the osteocytes present in lamellar bone (Fig. 38-7). In addition, because the long axes of the osteocyte lacunae are oriented in the direction of the collagen fibers, the lacunae are parallel to one another in lamellar bone. In woven bone, the relative disarray of collagen fibers leads to a randomization of the lacunar pattern. The size of the osteocytic lacunae also reflects the rate of bone formation.[179]

Osteoclasts are the large multinucleated cells responsible for bone resorption.[80] When engaged in bone resorption, the osteoclasts are juxtaposed to the bone surface in resorption bays, or Howship's lacunae (Fig. 38-8). Since there is no satisfactory method of determining osteoclastic activity in a single biopsy specimen, these lacunae merely indicate that resorption has taken place, at that location, and does not provide information regarding the rate of matrix degradation. The ultrastructural features of the osteoclast are, however, closely correlated with osteoclastic functional activity.[78] Actively resorbing osteoclasts exhibit a complex enfolded

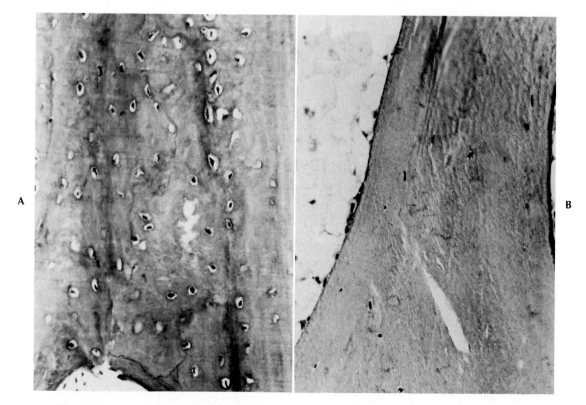

Fig. 38-7. A, Numerous large osteocytic lacunae characterizing woven bone as compared with normal lamellar bone, **B.** (Undecalcified, Goldner's stain; 250×.)

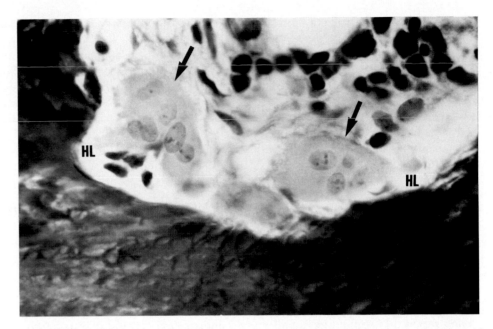

Fig. 38-8. Osteoclasts, *arrows*, resorbing bone, resulting in the formation of a Howship lacunar space, *HL*.

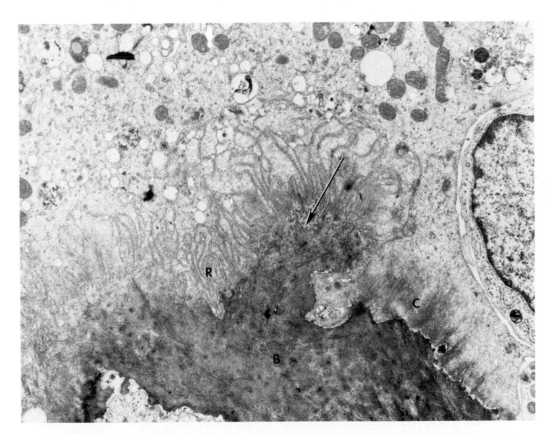

Fig. 38-9. Electron micrograph of osteoclast. Cell is attached to bone, *B*, by actin-rich clear zone, *C*. Resorption is taking place at ruffled border, *R*, as evidenced by presence of demineralized collagen fibers, *arrow*. (Nondecalcified; 2000×; from Teitelbaum, S.L., and Bullough, P.G.: The pathophysiology of bone and joint disease, Bethesda, Md., 1979, The American Association of Pathologists.)

cytoplasmic membrane, termed the "ruffled border" (Fig. 38-9). The complexity and extent of the ruffled border increases with increasing bone degradative activity.

The organic matrix of bone is 90% collagen and composes 25% of the dry weight of bone. Bone collagen is exclusively type I collagen. Because over a half of the body's collagen resides in bone and collagen contains virtually all the hydroxyproline and hydroxylysine of the body, urinary excretion of these amino acids is a useful marker of bone resorption.[141] The architecture of the bone collagen reflects the rate at which it is synthesized. Nonfetal bone collagen is normally deposited in a lamellar fashion, characterized by the parallel, relatively uniform bundles of collagen, which are best appreciated by polarized light or scanning microscopy (Fig. 38-10). The architecture of fetal bone collagen is in contrast "woven." The bundles vary in size and are randomly arranged. In normal skeletal development and repair, woven bone serves as a scaffold for lamellar bone deposition and is eventually resorbed by osteoclasts. Woven bone therefore is not normally found in persons older than 4 years of age. Woven bone in the adult skeleton represents a pathologic process, perhaps

secondary to states characterized by accelerated bone synthesis, such as fracture repair or high bone turnover. The noncollagenous proteins of bone compose only 10% of the organic matrix. The most abundant protein is a vitamin K–dependent gamma-carboxylated calcium-binding protein termed "bone GLA protein," or "osteocalcin."[75] It is synthesized by osteoblasts and becomes incorporated into the bone matrix. Although the physiologic function of osteocalcin is unknown, circulating serum levels of this protein appear to reflect the rate of bone formation.[96,97]

BONE GROWTH AND DEVELOPMENT
Limb bud development

Limb buds are first seen as a slight rounded prominence on the lateral body wall of the 4-week embryo. Limb buds develop from the unsegmented mesoderm (the somatopleure) of the lateral body wall, and each bud consists of an ectodermal covering and a central condensation of mesoderm.[70] Differentiation of the limb structures proceeds in a proximal-to-distal fashion, with the shoulder, forearm, and hand developing sequentially. In addition, lower limb bud development begins about 1 week later than upper limb develop-

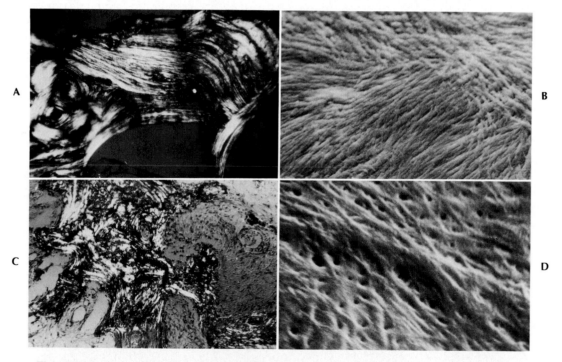

Fig. 38-10. A, Lamellar bone collagen as viewed under polarized light. Fibers are of uniform diameter and arranged in parallel fashion. **B,** Scanning electron micrograph of lamellar bone. **C,** Woven bone collagen viewed under polarized light. There is random directionality of fibers. **D,** Scanning electron micrograph of woven bone. Architectural arrangement and dimensions of collagen bundles are varied. (**A,** Decalcified; **A** and **C,** hematoxylin and eosin; 100×; **B** and **D,** 1000×.)

ment. This craniocaudal lag in skeletal development persists throughout gestation. The apical ridge ectoderm is essential to the subsequent development of the mesenchyme. Poisoning of the epithelium, for example, by thalidomide, phenytoin, or radiation, interrupts continued epithelial development and consequently further mesenchymal development. The portion of the skeletal system that would be altered or arrested can therefore be predicted if one knows the timing of the insult, relative to limb differentiation in the craniocaudal and proximodistal axes.

Ossification

Cartilage is an avascular tissue that originates as clusters of primitive mesenchymal cells differentiating into chondroblasts, which in turn produce a matrix rich in proteoglycans. Like bone, cartilage may grow appositionally, by the maturation of perichondrial cells into chondrocytes. The ability of cartilage to grow interstitially however enables it to serve as a skeletal growth plate and as a model or scaffolding for bone growth. Interstitial growth consists in the expansion of the cartilage mass by the internal proliferation of chondrocytes and the subsequent secretion of ground substance by each of these new cells. In the 8-week embryo, the future skeleton is composed initially as a template of cartilage (Fig. 38-11).

Skeletal development occurs by either endochondral or intramembranous ossification.[3] The former entails the partial replacement of a preexisting cartilage model, or template, by bone, with the residual cartilage serving as the growth plate and articular surface. The majority of the bones in the skeleton form and grow longitudinally by endochondral ossification. Intramembranous ossification consists in bone formation utilizing a collagen template and begins with the differentiation of primitive mesenchymal cells directly into osteoblasts and the production of bone collagen in the absence of cartilage scaffolding.[58] The skull vertex, clavicle, mandible, and other facial bones develop in this fashion. In addition, the progressive thickening of the diaphyseal shafts of long bones by appositional bone growth from the outer periosteum is by this collagen-model process.

Primary ossification center

Endochondral ossification is heralded in the late embryonic period by the development of the primary ossification center within these cartilaginous templates. The initial formation of bone consists of a sleeve, or periosteal collar (the ring of Ranvier), formed directly from the mesenchymal connective tissue of the future periosteum, which surrounds the cartilage model (Fig. 38-12). As the cartilaginous skeleton enlarges, distinct zones are recognized.[3] The cells in the central portion proliferate, secrete matrix, hypertrophy, and degener-

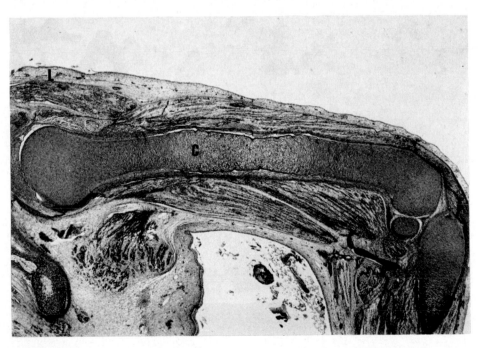

Fig. 38-11. Future skeleton within the 8-week-old embryo is composed entirely of cartilage, C.

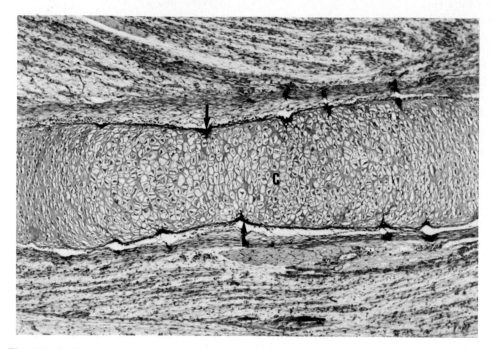

Fig. 38-12. Endochondral ossification. The primary ossification center is initiated by the formation of a periosteal collar of bone, *arrows.*

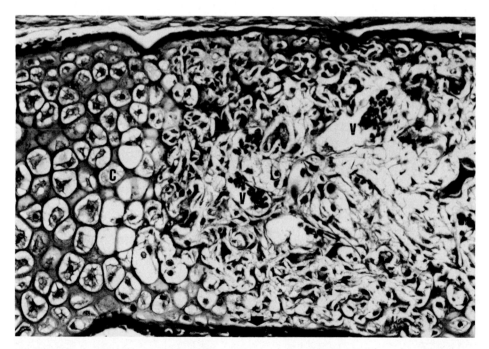

Fig. 38-13. Endochondral ossification. Central portion of the cartilaginous, *C,* template is invaded by blood vessels, *V,* which allow osteoclasts to enter and resorb the cartilage.

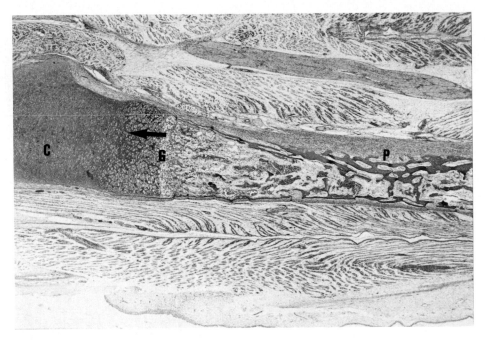

Fig. 38-14. Ossification process. *Arrow,* Direction of cartilage replacement of bone. *C,* Cartilage; *G,* growth plate; *P,* periosteum.

ate. The secreted matrix becomes calcified and provides the latticework upon which bone formation occurs. The dead cartilage in the central portion of the bone is invaded by vascular endothelial cells[159] (Fig. 38-13). Cellular debris is removed by osteoclasts, and osteoid is formed on the remaining cartilage by osteoblasts, which have differentiated from mesenchymal cells that accompanied vascular invasion. The combination of the sleeve of bone and the calcified cartilage matrix is known as the "primary ossification center," and once initiated, the process of cartilage replacement by bone progresses toward the ends of each cartilage limb (Fig. 38-14). By birth, most long bones have ossified through the major portion of their length.

Secondary ossification center

The development of the primary ossification center results in the formation of a shaft of bone with a cartilaginous cap at either end. At different times for each bone the epiphyseal maturation of the cartilage occurs by a process identical to that described for the primary ossification center: The epiphyseal cartilage cells begin to secrete matrix, hypertrophy, and ultimately die, followed by calcification of the residual cartilaginous matrix, subsequent vascular invasion,[159] and ultimately bone formation. Invasion begins from blood vessels located at the periphery, as well as from vessels located within the cartilage, that were previously trapped and incorporated into the canals within the enlarging carti-

laginous mass. Bone is deposited upon the scaffolding of the calcified cartilage. This ossification center, which develops for the epiphysis, is termed the "epiphyseal center," or "secondary ossification center." As a rough guide for estimating gestational age, at birth, the full-term fetus usually displays centers of ossification for the calcaneus, talus, and distal femoral epiphysis. The sequence of appearance of the postnatal ossification centers is predictable, and normal values and standards for comparisons have been published.[84]

The secondary ossification center continues to expand until it is surrounded by a thin strip of articular cartilage at the surface and a thin band of cartilage separating the epiphysis from the metaphysis. This well-defined layer becomes organized into the distinct zones of the growth plate (epiphyseal plate, or physis), which is an efficient mechanism for the dramatic process of rapid longitudinal bone growth in the postnatal period.

Epiphyseal growth plate

A recognizable growth plate, or physis, is formed as the process of cartilage removal approaches the ends of the limbs by the fourteenth week (Fig. 38-14). The physis consists of four distinct zones (Fig. 38-15). A zone of resting chondrocytes gives rise to a proliferative zone, characterized by vertical columns of chondrocytes that expand the growth plate interstitially until they enter the hypertrophic zone, where they enlarge and exclude the cartilaginous matrix into longitudinal col-

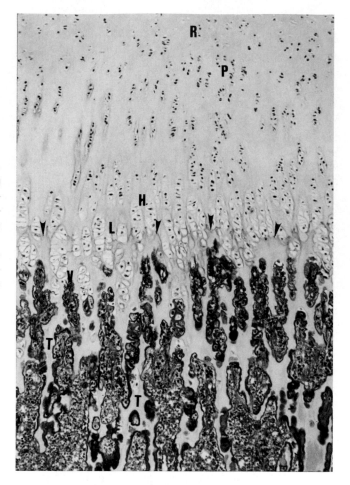

Fig. 38-15. Zones of epiphyseal growth plate. The resting cartilage, *R,* gives rise to the proliferating zone of chondrocytes, *P,* recognized by the vertical orientation of the cartilage cells. *H,* Hypertrophic chondrocyte zone. Expanding cells force the cartilage matrix into longitudinal columns, *L.* This cartilage matrix calcifies in the zone of provisional calcification, *arrowheads,* and is soon invaded by blood vessels, *V. T,* Primary trabeculum, consisting of cartilage bars surrounded by bone matrix.

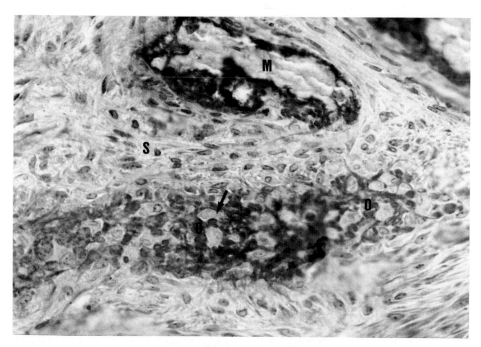

Fig. 38-16. Membranous ossification. Stromal mesenchymal cells, *S,* give rise to osteoblasts, *arrow,* which begin to secrete osteoid matrix, *O. M,* Mineralized bone spicule.

umns. At the zone of calcification the expanded hypertrophic cells appear to degenerate or die and the matrix calcifies. Calcified cartilage is then invaded by an ingrowth of vessels. Horizontal bars of matrix are degraded by osteoclasts, and osteoblasts line up along the inner walls of the acellular longitudinal septa. These calcified cartilaginous septa serve as the scaffolding for osteoid matrix deposition. The resulting bone spicule formed by endochondral ossification below the physis is referred to as a "primary trabecula" and consists of a central calcified core of cartilage surrounded by mineralizing woven bone. Deeper in the metaphysis, these primary spicules are resorbed by osteoclasts and replaced by lamellar bone. These second-generation trabecular bone spicules are referred to as "secondary spongiosa."

Membranous ossification

The ossification centers of those bones that form without a preexisting cartilaginous template (facial bones, mandible, clavicle, and calvarium) are characterized by a cluster of mesenchymal cells, which differentiate into large osteoblasts, capable of secreting osteoid matrix (Fig. 38-16). Coincident with the appearance of alkaline phosphatase, the matrix calcifies.[12] The osteoblasts align themselves along the surface of the trabecula and continue to secrete osteoid. In this manner, the trabecula enlarges peripherally in an appositional fashion by the deposition of successive layers of calcified matrix.

The periosteal collar of new bone formed in long bone development actually takes place by this process of membranous ossification. For practical purposes therefore most bone growth occurs by a combination of endochondral and membranous ossification.

MODELING

Modeling is the shaping of the growing bone such that it maintains its genetically predetermined configuration, typical of the adult skeleton. As the diaphysis elongates, a new sleeve of bone continues to develop adjacent to the growth plate, at the level of the hypertrophic cartilage zone (Fig. 38-17). This sleeve-bone extension, the "ring of Ranvier," ensures the correct directional growth of cartilage. For longitudinal growth, the hypertrophic cells are directed downward toward the growth plate. In addition, this peripheral assembly also serves as a source of proliferating chondrocytes in the form of a perichondrial ring, which accounts for the lateral growth and progressive enlargement of the physis. Because the diameter of the growth plate is larger than the diameter of the diaphyseal shaft, modeling (that is, shaping) of the metaphysis must occur to achieve the reduction in diameter. This process of funnelization is accomplished by osteoclastic activity and

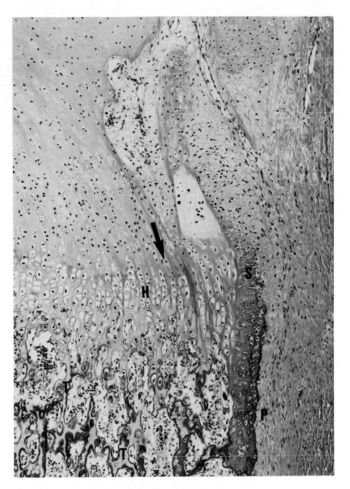

Fig. 38-17. Modeling of bone at fibrocartilaginous ring of Ranvier. Sleeve of bone, *S*, contains the hypertrophic chondrocytes from lateral displacement. *Arrow,* Downward direction of path of cartilage cells. *P,* Periosteum.

removal of the outer circumference of bone until the narrow diaphyseal diameter is established. At the same time, in order to maintain structural support, osteoblastic activity must take place on the inner surface of the shaft to reinforce the cortical bone.[179]

Bone structure

The growth process that occurs at the epiphyseal ends of long bones is responsible for longitudinal growth (that is, growth in length) of the skeleton. The major mass of bone, however, in the adult skeleton is produced by the lateral growth of bone from the shaft in the periosteal region of the diaphysis (that is, growth in width). The cortical bone contains trapped blood vessels within canals, as bone is progressively deposited, between the radiating periosteal spicules of membranous formed trabeculas. This inlay bone is deposited as concentric layers, or lamellae, around the developing vascular haversian canal, creating primary osteons. This

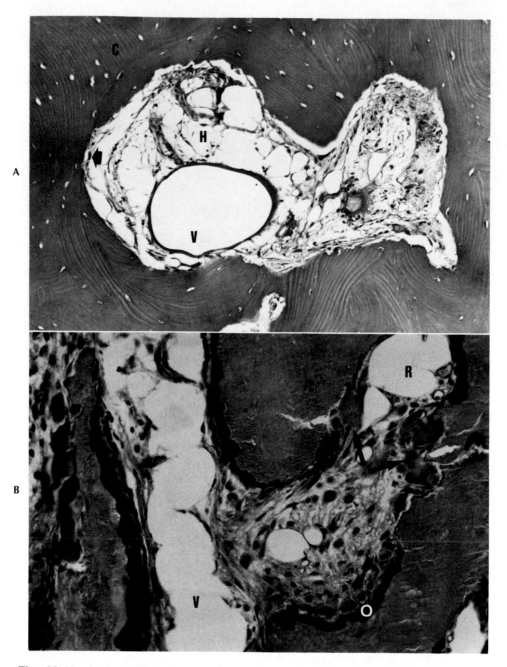

Fig. 38-18. A, Formation of secondary osteons. Vascular channels, *V,* of the central haversian canal, *H,* are expanded by the progressive resorption of cortical bone, *C,* by osteoclasts, *arrows.* **B,** Detailed histologic changes occurring during cortical bone modeling. Osteoclasts, *arrows,* create a resorption cone, *R.* Osteoclastic activity is followed by a wave of osteoblastic *(arrowheads)* activity, resulting in the formation of osteoid, *O. V,* Vascular channel.

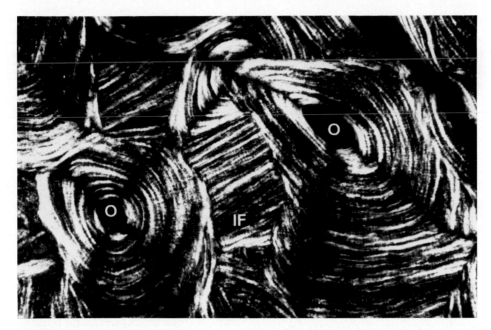

Fig. 38-19. Cortical bone modeling. The creation of new generations of osteons, *O,* results in the formation of interstitial fragments of lamellar cortical bone, *IF.* Notice that each osteon is composed of concentric layers of lamellar bone.

osteonal system is the basic structural and metabolic unit of mature cortical bone. To accommodate stresses and strain transmitted within the bone, new osteons, or secondary osteons, are created (Fig. 38-18). The existing bone is first removed by a wave of osteoclastic activity, resorbing bone along the course of a blood vessel and enlarging the vascular channel, which now has the appearance of a cone. The cavity of this cutting cone is filled in by a secondary wave of osteoblasts, which secrete osteoid matrix in parallel successive layers inward, toward the central vessel. A cement line marks the extent of previous resorption and subsequent concentric bone formation. During adult life physical forces will continue to vary, and replacement of existing osteonal structures will continue. These newly activated cutting cones may cross preexisting osteonal boundaries and remove portions of several adjacent osteons. After this most recent generation of osteons is completed, small interstitial fragments of earlier generations of osteons that are not connected to any haversian system become apparent (Fig. 38-19). After several waves of remodeling activity, the number of interstitial fragments increases. The age of the skeleton may be approximated by the number of interstitial osteonal fragments as well as by the number of rings or lamellar layers within the completed osteons. Younger individuals have fewer interstitial fragments and more osteonal rings.

BONE REMODELING

The cellular processes of growth and modeling cease after closure of the growth plates. Bone however is a dynamic organ, and the remaining skeletal tissue, even though it is composed predominantly of extracellular matrix, will be continually modified by the two groups of hormonally responsive bone cells: osteoblasts and osteoclasts. The linked activation of osteoclasts and osteoblasts termed "coupling" is the cellular basis of bone turnover, or remodeling, the continuous skeletal activity related to the maintenance of mineral homeostasis.[43] In contrast to the structural modification associated with modeling, remodeling is characterized by the anatomic and sequential coupling of osteoclast and osteoblast activity. Remodeling units are initiated by the appearance of osteoclasts, which resorb a packet of bone, creating a scalloped resorption bay (Howship's lacunae) in trabecular bone (Fig. 38-20) or a cutting cone in cortical bone. After osteoclastic activity a reversal phase of varying duration ensues. A densely staining metachromatic line, the reversal line or cement line, is formed at the limits of the resorption focus. The appearance of osteoblasts marks the end of the reversal phase as lamellar bone matrix is deposited in an appositional fashion, filling in the resorptive defect. As a result of this remodeling process, the skeleton in actuality consists of many small pieces of bone that are asynchronously formed and resorbed. The individual pieces are delin-

REMODELING

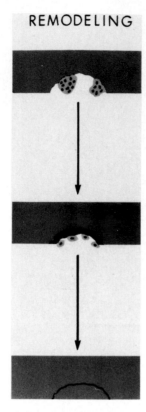

Fig. 38-20. Remodeling is initiated by osteoclastic resorption of packet of bone followed by osteoblastic bone formation in same location. Completed remodeling unit is permanently circumscribed by cement line.

Table 38-2. Regulation of bone remodeling activity

	Bone resorption	Bone formation
Parathyroid hormone	+ +	+
Calcitonin	−	0
1,25-$(OH)_2$-vitamin D	+	0
Cortisol	−	−
Estrogen	−	0
Calcium	−	0
Thyroxine	+	+
Disuse	+	−
Fluoride	−	+

+, Stimulator; −, inhibitor; 0, no effect.

as the renal substrate for further hydroxylation. This active dihydroxylated metabolite of vitamin D stimulates intestinal calcium absorption and at supraphysiologic levels stimulates osteoclastic bone resorption.[146]

REGULATION OF BONE MASS

Once peak bone mass has been attained by the middle of the fourth decade, net bone mass remains relatively constant throughout early adulthood.[153] Bone however is a dynamic vital organ that is constantly turning over and renewing itself in response to metabolic demands and physical forces. This is accomplished by the linked activation of its bone cells, such that in a normal skeleton bone formation equals bone resorption, that is, a zero skeletal balance. If net bone resorption exceeds net bone formation, bone mass declines, that is, a negative skeletal balance.[43] Bone turnover is influenced by a variety of physical forces, endocrine agents, and dietary factors[44] (Table 38-2).

BONE MINERALIZATION

The newly deposited bone matrix is unmineralized and is termed "osteoid." The osteoid layer found along trabecular bone surfaces is termed an "osteoid seam." Mineralization of osteoid in an orderly process that begins with the deposition of amorphous calcium phosphate at the interface between the osteoid seam and the mineralized bone (the so-called mineralization front). These nascent mineral precipitates subsequently mature into the hydroxyapatite crystals of adult bone. The binding affinity of the autofluorescent tetracycline antibiotics for the immature mineral deposits and not the mature crystal enables the identification of calcification foci and subsequently permits the determination of the rate of bone formation.[59] Bound tetracycline is thereby incorporated into the hydroxyapatite crystalline lattice and remains as a permanent marker of mineralization unless removed by osteoclastic resorption or decalcification.

eated by a cement line and hence are easily recognized as either an osteon in cortical bone or a packet in the trabecular bone. Bone remodeling serves to meet the long-term demands of calcium homeostasis: calcium is liberated during the resorptive phase and calcium is deposited, for storage in bone, during the formation phase.

REGULATION OF BONE AND MINERAL HOMEOSTASIS

Mineral homeostasis is determined by a variety of calcium-regulating hormones[22,104] (Fig. 38-21). During states of calcium deficiency, parathyroid hormone is secreted and osteoclast activity is augmented, liberating calcium and phosphate. At the same time, the renal tubular reabsorption of calcium is stimulated, and the urinary excretion of phosphate is enhanced. Elevated parathyroid hormone is also a stimulus for increased 1,25-dihydroxyvitamin D production by the kidney.[145] Parent vitamin D, either produced in the skin by photoactivation or obtained by dietary sources, circulates in the blood and is converted to 25-hydroxyvitamin D by hepatic hydroxylase enzymes. 25-OH-vitamin D serves

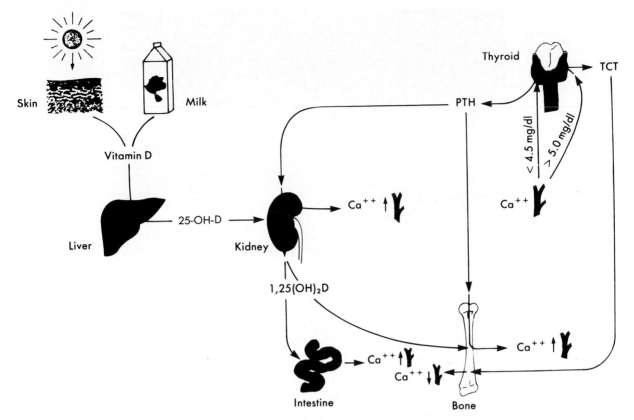

Fig. 38-21. Fundamental aspects of calcium homeostasis. Parathyroid hormone, *PTH*, secretion is stimulated by fall in blood ionized calcium, Ca^{++}. PTH in turn directly mobilizes Ca^{++} from bone and promotes resorption of Ca^{++} from renal tubule. It also promotes conversion of 25-hydroxyvitamin D (25-OH-D) to 1,25-dihydroxyvitamin D, $1,25(OH)_2D$. The latter enhances intestinal absorption of calcium and acts synergistically with PTH to stimulate bone resorption. Calcitonin, *TCT*, which inhibits bone resorption, is secreted when serum Ca^{++} increases.

TETRACYCLINE AS AN IN VIVO BONE MARKER

Tetracycline antibiotics are utilized as biologic markers of mineralization. Tetracycline is administered in two courses for the purpose of labeling the bone-forming sites at two different time points in order to measure the rate of bone mineralization of a subsequent single biopsy specimen. During the first labeling course, tetracycline (1 g/day) is administered for 3 days. After a 14-day drug-free hiatus, a second course of tetracycline is given over another 3-day interval. The bone biopsy sample is obtained 1 to 4 days later. Tetracycline fluorescence is evaluated on an unstained, nondecalcified tissue section by ultraviolet radiation (Fig. 38-22). The first course of tetracycline appears as a discrete fluorescent band within the mineralized bone. The second, more recently administered course of tetracycline is located at the current mineralization front (that is,

the junction between the osteoid seam–mineralized bone interface). The distance between the two bands or labels represents the amount of new bone synthesized and mineralized over the 2-week interval.[108]

REGULATION OF BONE MINERALIZATION

Mineralization is promoted by optimum ambient calcium and phosphorus concentrations, the levels of which are maintained by the aforementioned hormones. It is unclear whether vitamin D metabolites play a direct role in osteoid synthesis, osteoid maturation, and mineralization, or whether they promote mineralization secondarily by maintaining the optimum serum calcium and phosphorus levels. Mineralization is facilitated by the calcification enzyme alkaline phosphatase, which appears to function by removing local inhibitors of mineralization, such as ATP and pyrophosphates.[53] Other exogenous agents such as fluoride,

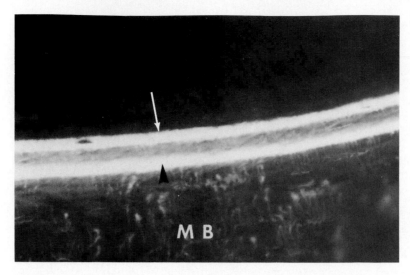

Fig. 38-22. Fluorescent micrograph of bone after administration of two courses of tetracycline. Label, *arrowhead,* deepest in mineralized bone, *MB,* represents first dose. Second label, *arrow,* represents dose administered 2 weeks later. Cellular rate of mineralization is determined by measuring distance between these labels and dividing that distance by interdose duration. (Undecalcified and unstained; 500×.)

synthetic diphosphonates, and aluminum appear to act as crystallization poisons and thereby inhibit mineralization. The factors that regulate mineralization are summarized below:

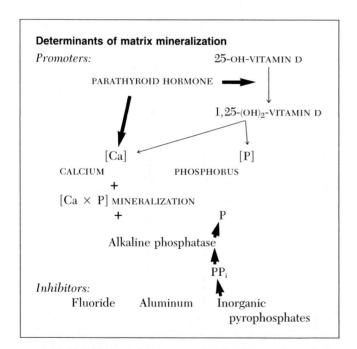

geneous group of heritable connective tissue diseases that result in abnormalities in the size and shape of the bones of the skeleton, such that there is usually a disproportionately short stature. In 1964 Rubin published his classic monograph on the classification of bone dysplasias.[157] He regarded these various abnormalities as expressions of disorders of normal growth and development that could be classified based upon the anatomic site of the potential lesion: epiphyseal, metaphyseal, and diaphyseal. This concept has had a tremendous impact on the subsequent classification of these disorders. As new technology has been applied to the clinical, radiologic, and pathologic investigation of skeletal dysplasias, the classification and terminology of these heterogeneous diseases have been refined. This evolving nomenclature and advances in pathogenesis have been the topics of two international meetings and several excellent recent reviews.[198] A complete discussion of these disorders is obviously beyond the scope of this chapter, but utilizing the basic approach of Rubin, we will discuss representative diseases. The clinicopathologic alterations that may result from a disorder at a particular step in the epiphyseal growth plate can be predicted, based upon a knowledge of normal growth and development presented above (Table 38-3).

DISORDERS OF BONE GROWTH AND DEVELOPMENT

The disorders of bone growth and development, collectively referred to as the "osteochondrodystrophies," are part of the broad spectrum of diseases termed "skeletal dysplasias." These dysplasias are actually a hetero-

ACHONDROPLASIA

Achondroplasia is the most common of the chondrodystrophies and is the most frequent cause of disproportionate short stature. The term originally was applied to all cases of short-limb dwarfism, but it is now reserved for a well-delineated, distinct entity.[160] It oc-

Table 38-3. Growth plate disorders

Cells involved	Chondroblasts	Osteoblasts	Osteoclasts	Mineralization
Disease name	*Achondroplasia*	*Osteogenesis imperfecta*	*Osteopetrosis*	*Fetal rickets*
Result of cellular defect	No growth of epiphyseal cartilage	No bone production	No matrix removal	No matrix calcification
Level of cell defect	Proliferating cartilage	Collagen synthesis	Resorption	Vessel invasion
Site of histologic changes	↓ Cartilage plate	↓ Primary spongiosa, trabecular and cortical bone	↑ Bone mass, calcified cartilage	↑ Hypertrophic chondrocytes, poor transition to primary spongiosa
Clinical changes	↓ Bone length, ↑ bone width	Fracture deformity, thin fragile bones	↑ Bone volume, ↓ marrow	Soft bone, deformity
Disorder	Growth	Growth	Modeling	Growth and remodeling
RESULT	Dwarfism	Short stature	Failure to thrive	Short stature

curs in 1 out of 40,000 live births and is inherited as an autosomal dominant trait. Because of the physical and social difficulties of reproduction, 80% of the cases are sporadic. Homozygous achondroplasia is not compatible with life beyond the first weeks or months after birth.

The characteristic appearance of the achondroplastic patients reflects the failure of normal endochondral ossification at the level of the proliferating and maturing cartilage. Therefore only those bones performed in cartilage (endochondral ossification) will be affected. Bone formation is normal. The limbs are short (Fig. 38-23). Although the spine is involved, truncal length is relatively normal. The calvarium of the skull is normal, since it is formed by membranous ossification. Those portions of the skull preformed in cartilage however are abnormal. The base of the skull is therefore hypoplastic, and combined with a normal-sized calvarium, the characteristic facial appearance of frontal bossing is produced. The nose is saddle shaped because of midface hypoplasia.

There is considerable controversy concerning the appearance of the growth plate in achondroplasia. Rimoin and co-workers, who view the chondrodystrophies as those with normal well-ordered endochondral ossification and those in which endochondral ossification is histologically disordered, believe that achondroplastic cartilage is well ordered and that the resulting dysfunctions are probably related to the rate of cartilage production, rather than the result of any gross cartilaginous abnormality.[154,155] They have stated that the reports of disordered cartilage in achondroplasia are actually observations of other chondrodystrophies, particularly thanatophoric and metatropic dwarfism, as well as achondrogenesis.[155]

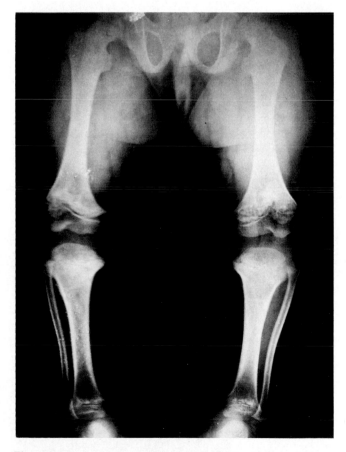

Fig. 38-23. Achondroplastic dwarf. Radiographs of lower extremeties showing broad but shortened lower limb bones because of an attenuation of diaphyseal length with preservation of normal width. The metaphyses are characteristically flared.

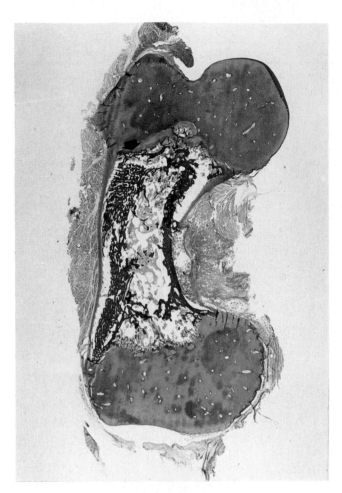

Fig. 38-24. Macrosection of achondroplastic bone. Lack of cartilage maturation results in a greatly decreased length of the long bones. Normal periosteal bone growth with narrowed growth plate is seen with an infolding and apposition of the periosteum and perichondrium at the level of the perichondrial rim, *arrow.*

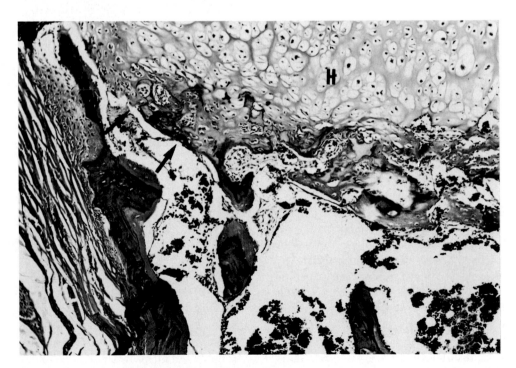

Fig. 38-25. Histologic appearance of similar zone depicted by region of arrow in Fig. 38-24. Notice the narrow and disorganized hypertrophic growth zone, *H,* and the infolding of the periosteal bone *(arrows)* impeding normal endochondral growth.

In contrast, other investigators report striking abnormalities of achondroplastic growth plates.[106,140,172] The hypertrophic zone is attenuated, and the number of chondrocytes is diminished (Fig. 38-24). The cartilage cells present are distributed in short columns or clusters. A broad horizontal plate of trabeculas is also found juxtaposed to the nests of growth plate cartilage at the region of the perichondrial ring because of infolding and apposition of the periosteum (Fig. 38-25).

OSTEOPETROSIS

Osteopetrosis comprises two phenotypically distinct diseases of increased skeletal mass (osteosclerosis) caused by an osteoclast dysfunction. The autosomal recessive form (malignant infantile osteopetrosis) manifests in infancy and is invariably fatal within the first decade of life.[16] The more common form, which is transmitted as an autosomal dominant trait, is not life threatening and is often diagnosed in otherwise healthy adults when a radiograph obtained for other reasons shows osteosclerosis.[85] Although most adult patients are asymptomatic, pathologic fractures may occur because the dense skeleton is composed of brittle calcified cartilage and bone. Although the bone is dense, the marrow is normal, the osteoclasts appear morphologically unremarkable, and marrow fibrosis is not seen (Fig. 38-26).

The hallmark of infantile malignant osteopetrosis is complete failure of normal osteoclast activity, which may be demonstrable by a variety of hematologic, neurologic, radiographic, histologic, and metabolic abnormalities. Defective osteoclastic bone resorption, despite continued bone formation and endochondral ossification, results in a pronounced increase in calcified skeletal tissue, which appears radiographically dense (Fig. 38-27). At the growth plate, the primary spongiosa cannot be removed and converted to the more mature trabecular bone. Thus the central calcified bars of cartilage surrounded by woven bone persist down into the metaphysis. This calcified skeletal tissue often occupies the majority of the available medullary space to the exclusion of the normal marrow elements (Fig. 38-28). This leads to hepatosplenomegaly with extramedullary hematopoiesis and resultant myelophthisic anemia, thrombocytopenia with bleeding, and leukoerythroblastosis. Insufficient osteoclast activity hinders skeletal modeling such that the cranial nerve foramina and sinuses are poorly developed, resulting in nerve entrapment and subsequent optic atrophy with blindness, nasal obstruction, and deafness. Despite the increased density of the skeleton, there is an increased susceptibility toward fractures because of the poor structural support provided by this abnormally dense bone. Metabolically, hypocalcemia is often encountered because defective osteoclast function impairs mineral homeostasis by preventing the release of calcium from bone under the influence of parathyroid hormone. Chronic hypocalcemia results in biochemical evidence of secondary hyperparathyroidism; however the osteoclasts are unable to respond appropriately. Nevertheless marrow fibrosis may occur, and advanced peritrabecular fibrosis of osteitis fibrosa further reduces the

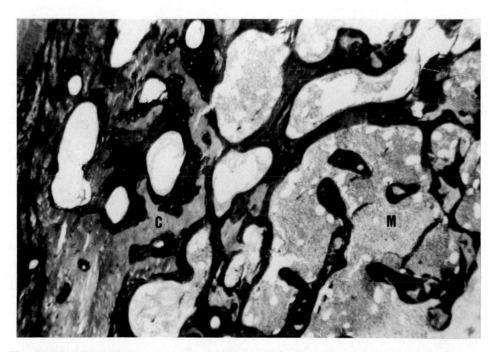

Fig. 38-26. Histologic appearance of adult osteopetrosis. The bone is sclerotic because of the accumulation of cartilage cores. Notice that the marrow, *M,* is preserved and that fibrosis is absent.

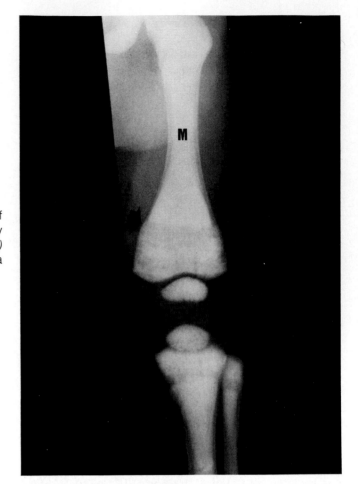

Fig. 38-27. Infantile malignant osteopetrosis, radiograph of the lower extremity. Notice the sclerosis of the medullary canal, *M,* and the lack of metaphyseal modeling *(arrows)* caused by defective osteoclast function and resulting in a broad, flask-shaped bone end.

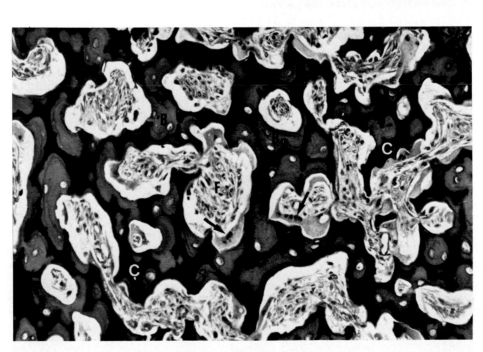

Fig. 38-28. Histologic appearance of infantile malignant osteopetrosis. The bone is sclerotic because of the preservation of the primary spongiosa, which consists of calcified cartilage bars, *C,* surrounded by bone, *B.* The marrow is fibrotic, *F.* The osteoclast morphology is abnormal, *arrows.*

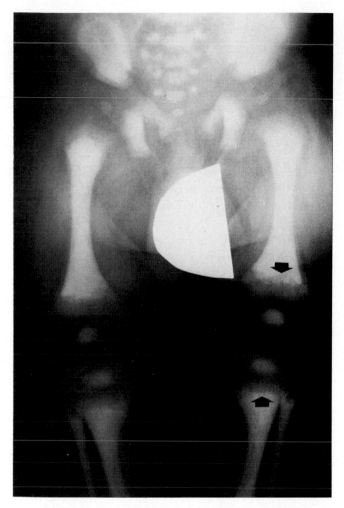

Fig. 38-29. Malignant infantile osteopetrosis with rachitic changes of the growth-plate regions shown radiographically by the presence of irregular, widened epiphyses, *arrows*.

available marrow space (Fig. 38-28). Hypocalcemia in the setting of an actively growing skeleton, which requires large amounts of calcium to ensure mineralization of the osteoid matrix, can result in the development of rickets and defective mineralization because of a subnormal calcium phosphate product (Fig. 38-29).

The number of osteoclasts is usually increased, despite their failure to function normally (Fig. 38-28). Histologically osteoclasts often appear dysplastic with bizarre cellular shapes and irregular nuclei. At the ultrastructural level the ruffled border is either poorly formed or absent—electron microscopic evidence of defective osteoclastic activity (Fig. 38-30).

Virtually all the insights into the pathogenesis and treatment of this rare disorder rest on the pioneering work of Walker. In a series of elegant experiments Walker was able to cure a rodent model of osteopetrosis by bone marrow transplantation or by supplying the os-

teoclast progenitor cell.[187-189] These findings have been extended to the treatment of human osteopetrosis [27,89] (Fig. 38-31).

OSTEOGENESIS IMPERFECTA

Osteogenesis imperfecta, once considered only a disease of bones, is a generalized disorder of connective tissue that becomes manifest by a predisposition toward multiple fractures.[168] Although significant overlap occurs, there are two general phenotypes—congenita and tarda. Infants with the autosomal recessive, most severe, congenital form of the disease, present with multiple fractures at birth and subsequently develop crippling deformities (Fig. 38-32). The scleras are only mildly blue or white. Failure to grow is the hallmark as bones become foreshortened and the spine becomes curved. The teeth are often opalescent, and deafness is less common than in the tarda form.[169] Children and adults with osteogenesis imperfecta tarda exhibit less incapacitating disease, which is usually transmitted as an autosomal dominant trait. Although fractures may appear at birth, clinical evidence of disease often does not appear until some time after the perinatal period. The bones become slender with growth, and bowing may occur (Fig. 38-33). The blue scleras are a prominent feature, but the teeth may be normal or opalescent. Hearing problems may develop in later adolescence. Although the bones are prone to fracture, they heal normally with exuberant callus formation.

The skeletal manifestations of osteogenesis imperfecta are caused by defective osteoblasts. Regardless of the phenotype, the mass of cortical and trabecular bone is reduced.[50] The most advanced changes are seen in the bones of infants who die at birth. The growth plate cartilage is normal, but the cartilaginous bars formed by vascular invasion at the metaphysis do not become enveloped by bone (Fig. 38-34). Cortical bone is almost nonexistent (Fig. 38-35). Osteoblasts are present, but matrix production is drastically retarded. In the less severe forms of the disease (osteogenesis imperfecta tarda) there is a striking increase in the number of osteocytes per unit volume of bone tissue, which may be explained by a decrease in the volume of bone synthesized by the individual osteoblasts before they are incorporated into the bone matrix (Fig. 38-36). There is a failure of normal modeling such that the bony architecture remains immature with a failure of the transformation of cancellous into cortical bone (Fig. 38-37). The trabeculas are irregular, and the cortex remains porous and shows little evidence of osteon formation. Perhaps the most consistent pathologic finding is related to the abnormality in collagen structure. Woven bone, which normally disappears by 4 years of age, is usually present in adult patients with clinically evident osteogenesis imperfecta.[50] At the ultrastructural level,

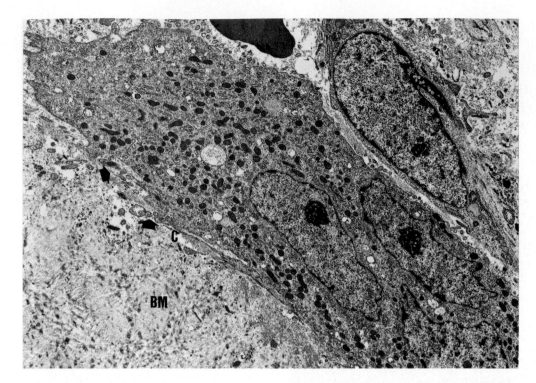

Fig. 38-30. Ultrastructural changes in an abnormal osteoclast from a patient with infantile malignant osteopetrosis. This multinucleated cell has a contact region, *C*, with the underlying bone matrix, *BM*, but the ruffled border zone, *arrows*, is poorly developed.

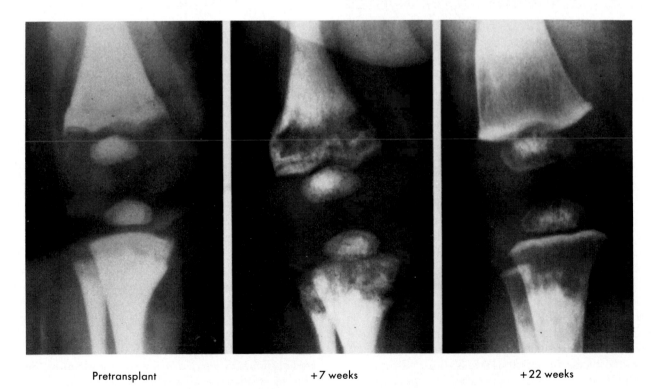

Pretransplant   +7 weeks   +22 weeks

Fig. 38-31. Radiographs of patient with malignant osteopetrosis before and 7 and 22 weeks after bone marrow transplantation. Notice progressive resorption of osteopetrotic bone. (From Coccia, P., et al. Reprinted by permission of The New England Journal of Medicine **302**:701, 1980.)

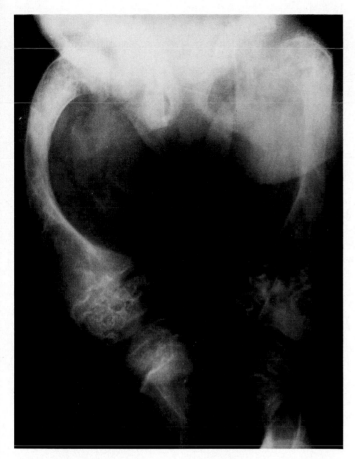

Fig. 38-32. Osteogenesis imperfecta congenita, radiographic changes showing the typical bowing deformities and severe osteopenia of the bones.

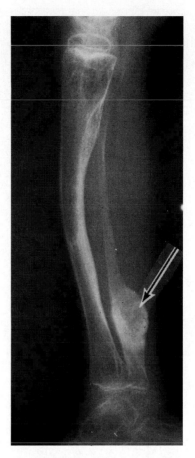

Fig. 38-33. Severely osteopenic and distorted tibia and fibula of child with osteogenesis imperfecta. Healing fracture exhibits abundant callus formation, *arrow*. (Courtesy Dr. James W. Debnam, Jr., Chesterfield, Mo.) .

patients with osteogenesis imperfecta do not aggregate bone collagen into adequately thick fibers (Fig. 38-38). These morphologic abnormalities may reflect the failure of normal collagen cross-linking in this disease.[180] Because of the ubiquity of type I collagen, osteogenesis imperfecta may exhibit varied extraskeletal manifestations. Patients will frequently have ligamentous laxity, the severity of which often parallels the severity of the skeletal disease. Many will ultimately develop umbilical and inguinal hernias and exhibit fragile, easily bruised skin. The thinned scleras appear blue.

In light of these numerous extraskeletal manifestations, studies on skin fibroblast cultures have afforded insights into the pathogenesis of osteogenesis imperfecta. Some laboratories, for example, have demonstrated a decrease in the ratio of type I–to–type III collagen production by these cells.[174] It is also of interest to note that, whether or not abnormalities in collagen synthesis can be demonstrated, the appearance and configurational packing of this collagen is abnormal (Fig. 38-38).

CHONDRODYSTROPHIA CALCIFICANS CONGENITA

The rare disorder of skeletal growth chondrodystrophia calcificans congenita may be thought of as representing a defect in vascular invasion and resorption of the calcified cartilage of the secondary ossification centers. Consequently the calcified cartilage of the secondary ossification centers persists and radiographically results in the designation "stippled epiphyses." The calcifications of the epiphyses are best appreciated in the epiphyseal ends of the long tubular bones (Fig. 38-39). The primary ossification centers and growth plates are normal. In addition, portions of the skeleton formed from membranous ossification will not exhibit calcifications (cranial vault and face).

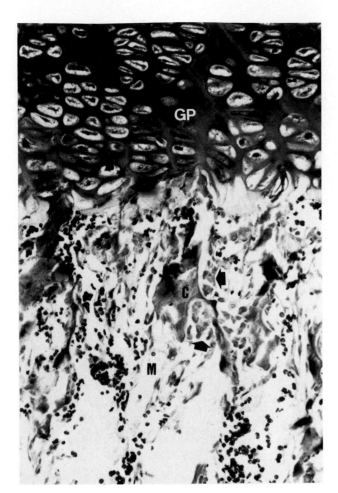

Fig. 38-34. Histologic appearance of osteogenesis imperfecta congenita, fatal case. The growth plate, *GP,* is normal with normal cartilage development. The calcified cartilage bars, *C,* however, do not become enveloped by bone. In the metaphysis, *M,* osteoblasts *(arrows)* are present, but bone collagen deposition is absent.

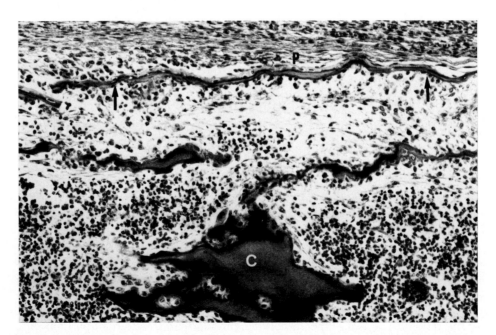

Fig. 38-35. Osteogenesis imperfecta congenita, fatal case. Cortical bone is virtually absent. The periosteum, *P,* contains only a thin ribbon of poorly formed bone, *arrows. C,* Calcified cartilage.

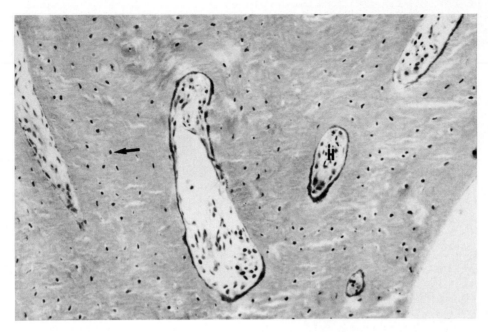

Fig. 38-36. Osteogenesis imperfecta tarda, histologic appearance. Notice the increased number of osteocytes *(arrows)* and poorly developed haversian canals, *H.*

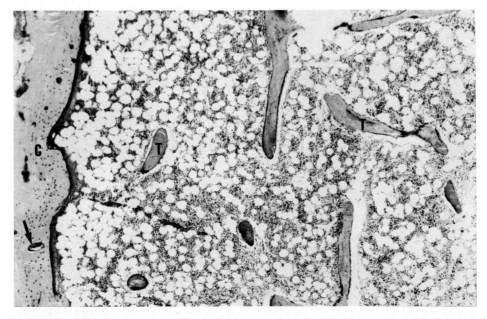

Fig. 38-37. Osteogenesis imperfecta tarda. The histologic organization of the bone is immature, as revealed by the poorly formed cortical bone, *C,* with minimal incorporation of the trabecular bone, *T,* into the cortex. Cortical bone osteons, *arrow,* are also rudimentary.

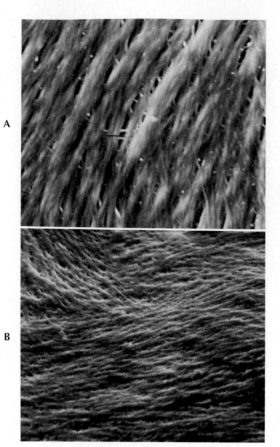

Fig. 38-38. A, Scanning electron micrograph of osteoid of normal 11-year-old child. Notice thick interweaving fiber bundles. **B,** Scanning electron micrograph of 11-year-old patient with osteogenesis imperfecta. Fibers fail to aggregate into bundles of normal width. (2200×; from Teitelbaum, S.L., et al.: Calcif. Tissue Res. **17:**75, 1974.)

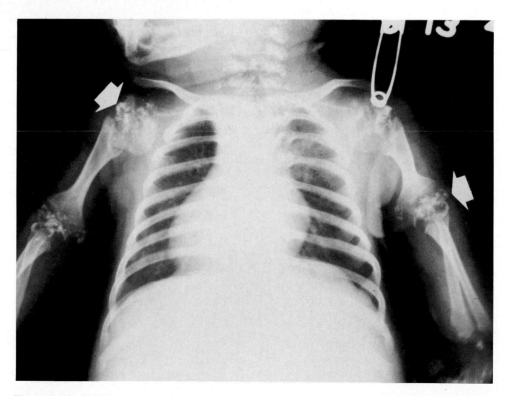

Fig. 38-39. Radiographic appearance of chondrodystrophia calcificans, or stippled epiphyses. Calcified globules of cartilage of the epiphyseal ends of the bones is seen, *arrows.*

MULTIPLE EPIPHYSEAL DYSPLASIA

Multiple epiphyseal dysplasia is characterized by an abnormality in the development and growth of the ossification centers for the epiphyses. In any given case, few or several of the various ossification centers may be involved. A hereditary transmission of this nonfatal disorder with an autosomal dominant mode of transmission has been reported. The hip, shoulder, and ankle joints are the most frequent sites of involvement. The affected ossification centers are chronologically delayed in their appearance and are initially irregular in outline and density. The epiphyses will ultimately appear fragmented (Fig. 38-40). Patients are often normal at birth, and clinically apparent disease is usually not identified until shortness of stature is eventually recognized some years later. Adult patients may come to attention when degenerative arthritis develops in the involved joint, usually the hips (Fig. 38-41).

DISORDERS OF MINERALIZATION AND BONE REMODELING ACTIVITY
The metabolic bone diseases

The ability of the skeleton to provide structural support depends on the skeletal mass (the amount of bone tissue) as well as the quality of that tissue (the degree of mineralization). The amount of bone tissue is determined primarily by the location and extent of bone removal and formation during the remodeling cycle.[43] Because the mineralization processes and the level of bone remodeling activity are influenced by several systemic factors, disorders of these activities result in generalized skeletal disease. Thus a metabolic bone disease is defined as any generalized disorder of the skeleton regardless of cause. For example, diffuse skeletal disease is not strictly limited to the traditionally held "metabolic" conditions, that is, hormonal or nutritional imbalances. In addition to these endocrine disorders, the skeleton may be uniformly affected in hereditary diseases such as osteogenesis imperfecta or osteopetrosis. Osteoporosis and osteomalacia are the two major metabolic bone disease categories. Osteoporosis is not a single disease but a syndrome or group of diseases characterized by a deficiency of bone tissue, resulting in a reduction of bone mass.[7,150] In this quantitative defect, the remaining bone is chemically normal. Osteomalacia, on the other hand, is a group of diseases characterized by bone that is qualitatively abnormal because of an impaired state of matrix mineralization. The total amount of bone tissue (mineralized bone and osteoid) may be low, normal, or high. "Osteopenia" is a generic term that refers to a generalized reduction in bone mass. By radiographic examination the skeleton would appear washed out or demineralized. A patient with osteopenia therefore may suffer from osteoporosis or osteomalacia. The bone biopsy and histologic examination of bone has become important in the differential diagnosis of these metabolic bone disease syndromes.

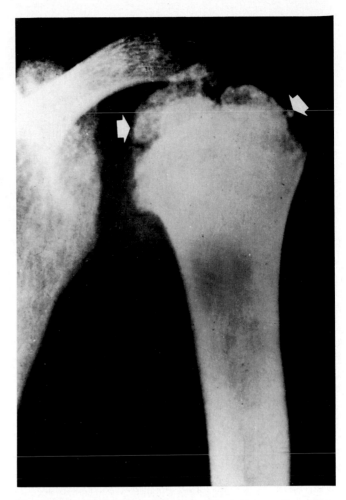

Fig. 38-40. Multiple epiphyseal dysplasia, radiographic findings. The development of the secondary centers of ossification is abnormal and results in the formation of irregular fragmented bone, *arrows*.

Morphologic methods of diagnosis
Iliac crest bone biopsy

The concept that metabolic bone diseases are diffuse skeletal disorders is an important one because it implies that a small sample of bone obtained from any osseous site should be representative of the entire skeletal disease process. The iliac crest is an easily accessible, standardized biopsy site, and histologic alterations in this site reflect changes that may be occurring in the more clinically relevant sites—the spine, hip, and wrist.[144] By examination of the iliac crest bone, the level of bone remodeling activity and the rate of bone mineralization may be determined.[44]

Processing the biopsy specimen. Because the differentiation between the two major metabolic bone dis-

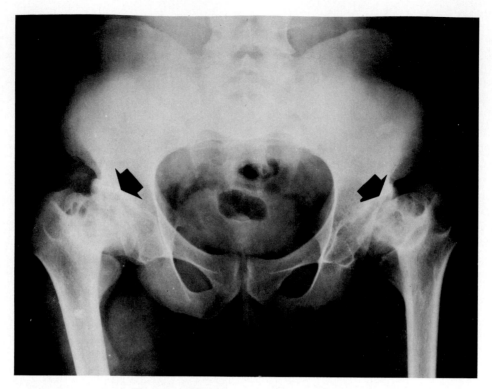

Fig. 38-41. Multiple epiphyseal dysplasia, long-term findings in a young adult. There is severe degenerative joint disease of the hips, *arrows.*

ease syndromes, osteoporosis and osteomalacia, is based in part upon the quality and quantity of bone mineral, the ability to distinguish between calcified and undecalcified bone matrix (osteoid) is critical. The traditional processing procedures (acid decalcification and paraffin embedding) requires that the inorganic matrix be removed to facilitate sectioning and therefore prevents the subsequent determination of the degree of skeletal mineralization. Because the techniques designed to demonstrate the presence of bone mineral and tetracycline markers requires the examination of undecalcified tissue, specialized embedding and sectioning techniques have been developed.[42] For obtainment of undecalcified tissue sections, bone is embedded in a methacrylate plastic without prior demineralization. Histologic sections are obtained either with a heavy-duty sledge microtome or by glass-knife microtomy.

Histomorphometric analysis

Bone histomorphometry is the quantitative analysis of undecalcified bone in which the parameters of skeletal remodeling and mineralization are expressed in terms of volumes, surfaces, and cell numbers.[109-111] To obtain this information in a two-dimensional format, one uses the principles of stereology to reconstruct the third dimension. This principle, described by the French mineralogist Delesse in 1888, is based upon the theory that if measurements are made on extremely thin sections the ratio of the areas is equal to the ratio of the volumes.

Osteoporosis
General features

With the introduction of noninvasive radiographic techniques to measure bone density, osteoporosis may be defined clinically as a mass per unit volume of normally mineralized bone that falls below a population-defined threshold for spontaneous fracture.[150] This structural weakness of bone is associated with a loss of trabecular bone volume, enlargement of the medullary space, cortical porosity, and reduction in cortical thickness. This reduction in bone mass is associated with an increased risk of fractures, which in turn results in pain and deformity. Because bone loss is the general nonspecific response to almost any form of skeletal injury, osteoporosis should be thought of as a disease syndrome that may result from a variety of causes in a variety of clinical settings. Traditionally osteoporosis is classified on a clinical basis into two major groups: primary and secondary osteoporosis. Primary osteoporosis implies that osteopenia is the fundamental disease. In other instances, osteoporosis may be attributed to an underlying clinical disease, medical condition, or medication,

Table 38-4. Histomorphometric correlates of bone remodeling

Parameter	Normal	Examples
Bone mass	20%	Total bone volume = Percentage of biopsy tissue composed of bone tissue (mineralized and non-mineralized)
Bone formation	Up to 4%	Osteoid volume = Percentage of bone tissue that is nonmineralized
	20%	Osteoid surface = Fraction of trabecular bone lined by osteoid seams
	12 to 24 μm or less than 3 or 4 collagen lamellae thick	Osteoid seam width = Average thickness of osteoid seam
	20%	Osteoblast surface = Fraction of trabecular bone lined by osteoblasts
Tetracycline labeling	20%	Tetracycline-labeled surface = Fraction of trabecular bone surface lined by normal single or double tetracycline labels
	80% to 100%	Labeled osteoid surface = Fraction of osteoid seams that contain either a single or a double tetracycline label
	1 μm/day	Mineralization rate = Amount of new bone matrix synthesized and calcified per day
		Represents distance between the two tetracycline labels; normal = 14 μm
Bone resorption	Less than 2 per section (<0.15/mm^2)	Osteoclast number = Number of osteoclasts in biopsy specimen
	<5%	Resorption surface = Fraction of trabecular bone lined by Howship's lacunae

that is known to be associated with the development of an osteopenic state, that is, secondary osteoporosis. The two groups are listed below:

Clinical classification of osteoporosis

I. Primary osteoporosis
  1. Involutional
    a. Postmenopausal
    b. Senile
  2. Idiopathic
    a. Juvenile
    b. Young adults
II. Secondary osteoporosis
  1. Acromegaly
  2. Anticonvulsant drug related
  3. Chronic anemias with erythroid hyperplasia
  4. Disuse-weightlessness
  5. Hemochromatosis
  6. Hepatic disease
    a. Alcohol associated
    b. Cholestatic liver disease—biliary cirrhosis
  7. Hypercortisolism
  8. Hyperparathyroidism
    a. Primary
    b. Secondary
  9. Hypogonadism
  10. Hypoparathyroidism
  11. Pseudohypoparathyroidism
  12. Mastocytosis, including the heparin-associated type
  13. Postgastrectomy and partial gastrectomy
  14. Starvation
    a. Anorexia
    b. Inanition
    c. Malignancy associated
  15. Thyrotoxicosis

Histopathology of osteoporosis

The histologic appearance of the osteoporotic syndromes may be classified into two major subgroups, based upon the level of bone-remodeling activity (accelerated bone turnover versus reduced bone turnover).[18,26,196] By definition, mineralization of bone is normal, whereas defective mineralization, revealed by the pattern of tetracycline label deposition, would be diagnostic of osteomalacia.[46] Histologic evidence of increased bone resorption and increased bone formation (that is, accelerated turnover) is termed "active osteoporosis," whereas suppressed bone cell activity (that is, reduced turnover), with minimal bone formation and reduced but nevertheless continued bone resorptive activity, is referred to as "inactive osteoporosis."

Table 38-4 lists the histomorphometric correlates of bone-remodeling activity that are utilized in the differential diagnosis of the two histologic forms of osteoporosis. The histologic features of active osteoporosis are summarized in Table 38-5 and are illustrated in Figs. 38-42 to 38-46. Histologic correlates of increased bone formation include increased quantities of osteoid with an increase in the percentage of the trabecular bone surface lined by osteoid seams (Fig. 38-42, *A*). Normally about 20% of the trabeculas are lined by osteoid (Fig. 38-42, *B*). This osteoid in turn is of normal width, 12 to 24 μm in thickness. Because the thickness of osteoid seams may be artifactually augmented by an oblique plane of sectioning, it is often helpful to count the number of lamellae which compose that seam. Nor-

mally, an osteoid seam should contain no more than three or four collagen layers. Greater than four collagen layers, or lamellae, is often an indication of osteomalacia. The bone surfaces will also contain plump, prominent-appearing osteoblasts (Fig. 38-43). Generally the fraction of bone surface lined by osteoblasts is equal to that lined by osteoid seams (20%). By tetracycline fluorescence, the bone surfaces will contain double labels or bands of tetracycline (Fig. 38-44). The distance between the double labels should be about 14 μm, reflecting a mineralization rate of about 1 μm/day. As the level of bone turnover increases, both the percentage

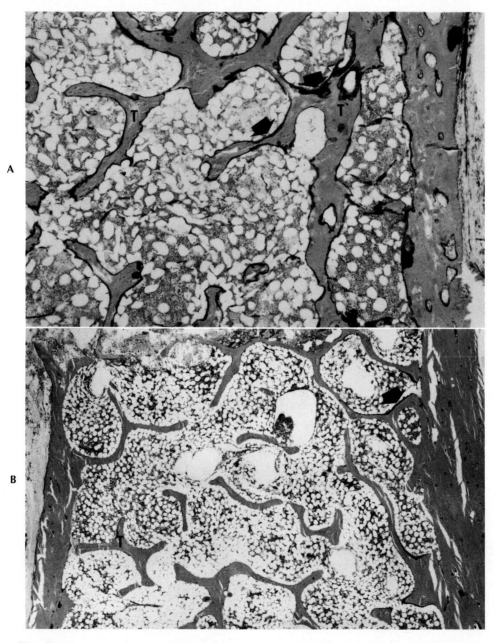

Fig. 38-42. Histologic appearance of active osteoporosis in **A,** compared to a normal control bone specimen in **B.** *T,* Trabecular bone; *arrows,* osteoid.

of the osteoid-covered surfaces and double tetracycline-labeled surfaces increases, perhaps up to 30% of the trabecular bone surface. As a result the fraction of osteoid seams that will bear a tetracycline label by fluorescent microscopy will remain normal; that is, at least 80% of the osteoid seams will contain tetracycline. In addition, the mineralization rate, that is, the distance between the labels, may be increased as the synthetic activity of the individual osteoblasts increases. Increased resorptive activity is manifested as an increase in the number of osteoclasts as well as by the fraction of trabecular bone surface engaged in resorption, resulting in the presence of Howship's lacunae (Fig. 38-45). In a normal 2 to 8 mm diameter core biopsy specimen of iliac crest bone there are only one or two osteoclasts present in the entire tissue section. More than three osteoclasts per biopsy section is suggestive of increased osteoclastic resorption. The clustering of osteoclasts, such that they are found in groups of two to four is diagnostic of an abnormally high osteoclast number. Normally the trabecular bone surfaces are smooth and will contain only an occasional resorption bay. These crenated resorption surfaces should occupy less than 5% of the trabecular bone surfaces.

The presence of peritrabecular fibrous tissue is also diagnostic of rapid bone turnover and is referred to as osteitis fibrosa (Fig. 38-46). Osteitis fibrosa is a generic term, and is not pathognomonic of hyperparathyroidism but may be seen in any state of accelerated turnover, such as idiopathic osteoporosis and thyrotoxicosis.[179] Skeletal mass is reduced in states of accelerated turnover despite the fact that a normal or even excessive rate of bone formation is seen. Because of the coupling of bone formation to bone resorption, there is a compensatory increase in bone formation, but formation is nevertheless exceeded by an even greater degree of resorptive activity, resulting in a net loss of bone.[43]

Histologically, states of reduced bone turnover show little evidence of either bone formation or bone resorption (Table 38-6), illustrated in the series of Figs. 38-47 to 38-49. By low-power examination, very little osteoid is present (Fig. 38-47). These osteoid seams are thin and scanty, osteoblasts are flattened, and osteoclasts are reduced in number (Fig. 38-48). By tetracycline fluorescence, few labels are present, a finding consistent with the amount of osteoid seen by light microscopy. This results in a reduction in the total fraction of trabecular bone lined by fluorescent labels. Few double labels will be seen because as the rate of bone matrix apposition decreases, the distance between the labels is also reduced. When the bone formation rate falls less than 0.5 μm/day, the spatial separation of the dual bands of tetracycline may be impossible, resulting in the fusion, or overlap, of the two labels to produce one single thin band (Fig. 38-49).

In inactive osteoporosis, the low bone mass is the result of suppressed osteoblastic activity, with a reduced level of bone formation, in the face of a normal or slightly reduced level of bone resorptive activity, again resulting in a net loss of bone tissue.

The histologic changes that occur in the skeleton of an aging woman include increased cortical porosity and diminished trabecular bone mass. Numerous small islands of cancellous bone are present in biopsy specimens from symptomatic osteopenic women. In fact, the trabecular bone mass of patients with vertebral crush fractures is invariably less than 16% of the total marrow space. In addition, there is a change in the trabecular

Table 38-5. Histology of active osteoporosis

Parameter	Examples
Bone formation	Increased quantity of osteoid
	Increased osteoid surfaces
	Normal osteoid seam width
	Increased osteoblastic surface
Tetracycline labels	Increased fraction of tetracycline-labeled surfaces
	Double labels predominate
	Normal to increased mineralization rate
	Fraction of osteoid seams labeled is maximal
Bone resorption	Increased osteoclast number
	Increased resorption surfaces
	Peritrabecular fibrosis

Table 38-6. Histology of inactive osteoporosis

Parameter	Examples
Bone formation	Normal to reduced amounts of osteoid
	Decreased osteoid surface
	Normal to decreased osteoid seam width
	Reduced osteoblastic surfaces
Tetracycline labels	Decreased fraction of tetracycline-labeled trabecular bone
	Single labels predominate
	Reduced mineralization rate and fused labels
Bone resorption	Decreased osteoclast number
	Decreased resorption surfaces

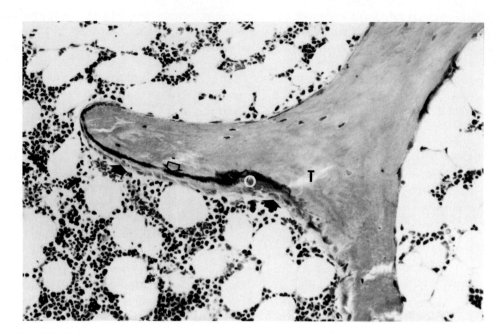

Fig. 38-43. Active osteoporosis, histologic findings of bone-forming surfaces with a trabecular bone spicule, *T,* lined by osteoblasts *(solid arrows)* secreting osteoid matrix *(open arrows* and *O).*

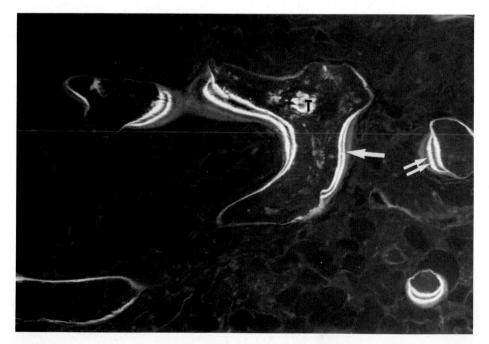

Fig. 38-44. Active osteoporosis, histologic appearance of active bone-forming surfaces by tetracycline fluorescence. Notice the increase in the surface of trabecular bone, *T,* lined by double labels *(arrow)* and those surfaces exhibiting an increased distance between the labels *(double arrows)* indicating an increase in the bone appositional rate.

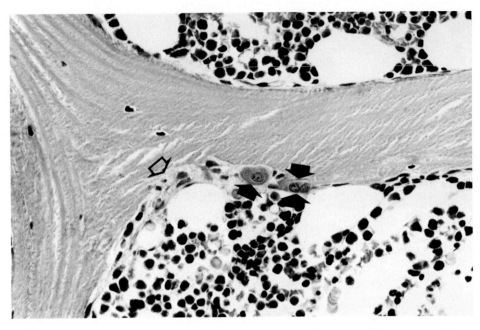

Fig. 38-45. Active osteoporosis. Histologic appearance of increased bone resorptive activity with increased numbers of osteoclasts *(solid arrows),* resulting in the formation of resorption bays, or Howship's lacunae *(open arrows).*

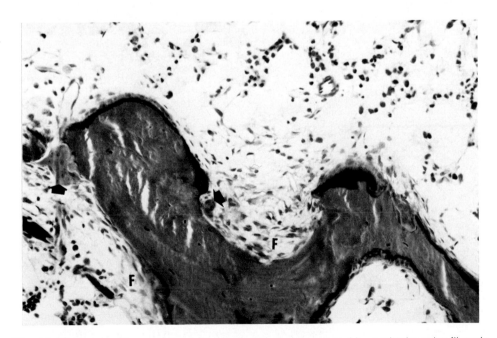

Fig. 38-46. Osteitis fibrosa. Histologic appearance represented by peritrabecular fibrosis, *F,* and increased numbers of osteoclasts, *arrows.*

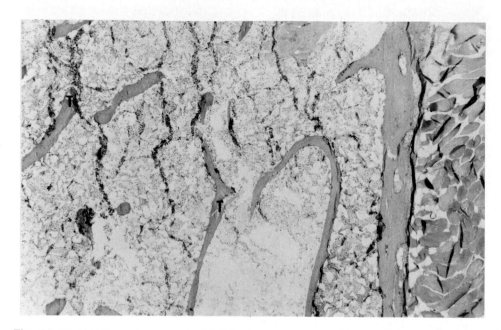

Fig. 38-47. Inactive osteoporosis. Histologic appearance of bone at low-power examination. Notice the relative lack of osteoblastic and osteoclastic activity at this magnification.

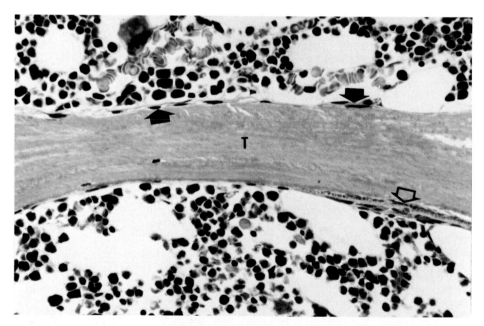

Fig. 38-48. Inactive osteoporosis. Histologic appearance of an inactive, smooth trabecular, *T,* bone surface, with a minimal osteoid lining, *open arrow,* and covered only by flattened lining cells, *solid arrows*.

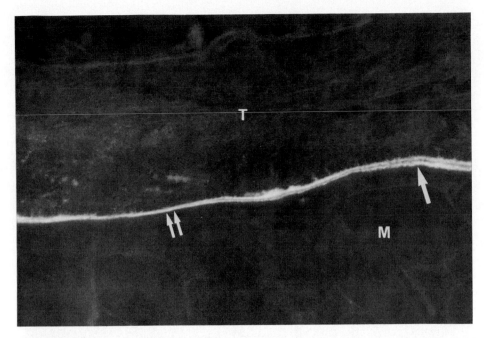

Fig. 38-49. Inactive osteoporosis. Histologic expression of reduced bone synthesis by tetracycline fluorescence. Notice that the double labels when present are narrowly placed *(single arrow)* and are often fused, resulting in the formation of a single thin label *(double arrow)*. *M,* Marrow; *T,* trabecular bone.

bone microstructure. For example, the mean trabecular plate density, an index of the number of the structural elements, is also reduced.[131] Subsequently, individual trabeculas appear as rods or bars widely separated from one another, instead of interconnecting trabecular network. The pattern of cortical and trabecular bone loss that may be observed in iliac crest bone biopsy specimens is shown in Fig. 38-50.

Primary osteoporosis

Primary osteoporosis is traditionally divided into idiopathic and involutional (see the classification on p. 1959). Idiopathic osteoporosis is an uncommon form of primary osteoporosis found in children, adolescents, and young adults, in whom the pathogenesis remains obscure. Involutional osteoporosis is the most common form of bone disease that attends aging and that in women is accelerated by the withdrawal of estrogens at menopause.[149] Of approximately 1 million fractures occurring annually in the United States in women at least 45 years of age, 700,000 are associated with osteopenia. Although aging and menopause are important factors contributing to the observed bone loss, the mechanisms involved are poorly understood, and hence this form of osteoporosis is thought of as a primary bone disease. On the basis of several clinical and pathologic features, involutional osteoporosis has been subdivided, by Riggs and Melton,[148] into two distinct syndromes: type I osteoporosis, formerly postmenopausal osteoporosis, and type II osteoporosis, formerly senile osteoporosis. The pathogenesis of the bone loss associated with the aging process is probably complex and poorly understood, but several nutritional, endocrinologic, and physiologic (risk) factors are believed to play a role,[61,88,95] as shown below.

Risk factors for osteoporosis
Clinical features
   Recently postmenopausal (within 20 years)
   White or Asian
   Positive family history
   Lean, short stature
   Low calcium intake
   Inactivity
   Smoking
   Alcohol use
   Gastric or small bowel disease or resection
   Liver disease
   Hypercortisolism
   Hyperparathyroidism
   Thyrotoxicosis
   Long-term glucocorticoid use
   Anticonvulsant drug use—phenytoin, phenobarbitol
Laboratory findings often normal
Radiographic findings
   Diffuse osteopenia

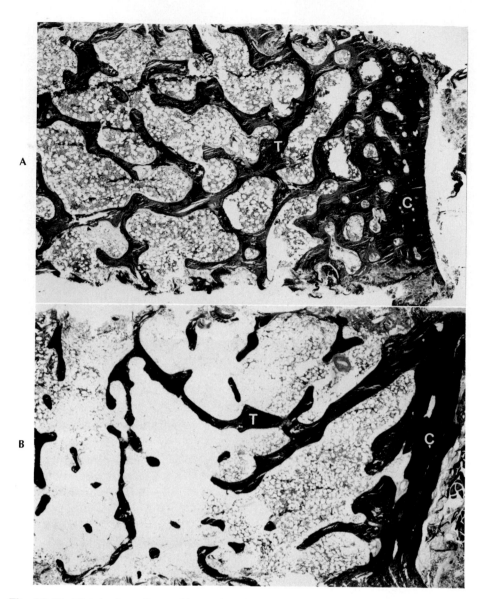

Fig. 38-50. Histologic pattern of bone loss in osteoporosis. **A,** Increased bone remodeling activity of the cortex, *C,* resulting in increasing cortical porosity, *arrow*. Notice that the trabecular bone, *T,* consists of an interconnecting network of cancellous material. **B,** Further bone loss in the medullary space with thinning of the trabecular bone, *T,* resulting in the formation of ribbons of trabeculas.

Low quantitative bone-density measurement
Osteoporotic fractures
    Vertebral crush fracture
    Hip fracture
    Wrist fracture

Involutional forms

Type I osteoporosis. Type I osteoporosis is the traditional form of osteoporosis, which was described in 1940 by Albright and co-workers.[2] Classically it affects women between 15 and 20 years after menopause, but although less common, it can occur in middle-aged men, who have an identical pattern of bone loss. These patients have been shown to lose trabecular bone at a rate three times higher than normal men and women.[151] As a result, bones that are composed predominantly of trabecular bone, that is, the vertebral body, the distal forearms, and the mandible, are most likely to exhibit the disease. These sites account for the typical clinical presentations of vertebral crush fracture, Colles' fracture, and edentulism. It is postulated that this brisk rate of osteolysis will suppress parathyroid hormone secretion, which in turn leads to decreased activity of the renal 1α-hydroxylase system, with pro-

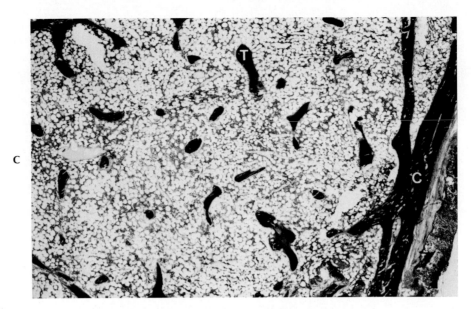

Fig. 38-50, cont'd. C, Osteoporosis is fully developed with a loss of cortical bone thickness, *C,* and trabecular bone volume, such that the trabeculas are reduced to small islands of bone.

portionately less metabolic bioactivation of vitamin D. The resulting decreased circulating concentration of 1,25-dihydroxyvitamin D results in impaired intestinal calcium absorption, which may further increase bone loss by promoting a negative calcium balance. The association of bone loss in women with the menopause indicates that estrogen deficiency may be an etiologic factor.[147] Estrogen is believed to protect the skeleton from parathyroid hormone, blunting the bone resorptive activity of this hormone. With the withdrawal of estrogens, the unopposed action of parathyroid hormone is postulated to result in the accelerated rate of bone resorption and hence bone loss.

Type II osteoporosis, or senile osteoporosis. Type II osteoporosis is seen in men and women 75 years of age and older. In contrast to type I osteoporosis, this bone disease is manifested by a predominant loss of cortical bone, resulting primarily in fractures of the cortical bones: hip, proximal humerus, tibia, and pelvis. Bone-density measurements from these sites are lower than the values in age- and sex-matched normal controls. The rate of loss of trabecular and cortical bone, however, appears to equal the rate of bone loss seen in the normal population.[151] As age-related bone loss continues, a greater number of men and women will have bone-density measurements below the fracture threshold, and those with the lowest bone mass values will have the greatest risk of fracture. The pathogenesis of the bone loss in type II osteoporosis is believed to reflect an age-related defect in osteoblastic bone formation and the skeletal consequences of secondary hy-

perparathyroidism. With age, osteoblastic vigor diminishes, such that less bone is formed than is resorbed at each individual bone remodeling focus.[35] Secondly, because of an age-related decrease in gastrointestinal absorption of calcium, there is a compensatory increase in parathyroid hormone secretion.[130] Calcium absorption decreases with age as a result of reduced renal conversion of 25-OH-vitamin D to 1,25-diOH-vitamin D in the elderly.

Clinical manifestations of involutional osteoporosis. There is usually a prolonged latent period that precedes the clinical symptoms or the complications of osteoporosis. Abnormal skeletal remodeling may have existed for years, resulting in a slowly progressive negative skeletal balance. Once bone mass is sufficiently compromised, the skeletal framework can no longer withstand normal gravitational stresses and skeletal failure may ensue. Although the entire skeleton is at risk from a remodeling imbalance and is therefore susceptible to age-related and postmenopausal bone loss, regions of high trabecular bone remodeling such as the thoracic and lumbar vertebrae, ribs, proximal area of the femur and humerus, and the distal area of the radius sustain the most damage.[122,131] One of the earliest symptoms of osteoporosis is acute back pain associated with thoracic and lumbar vertebral compression fracture, which is often precipitated by routine activity, such as bending, standing, or minor lifting. With increasing episodes of segmental vertebral collapse there is progressive kyphosis and loss of height (Fig. 38-51).

Laboratory and radiographic findings in involutional

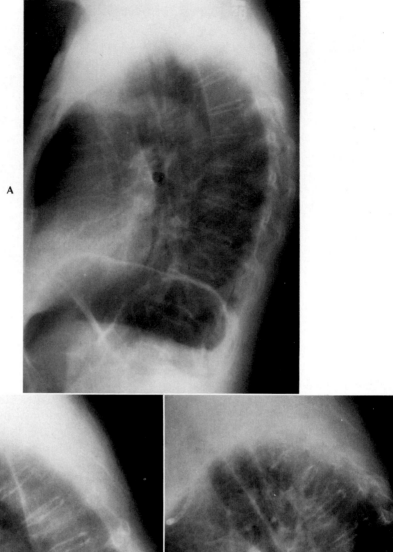

Fig. 38-51. Pattern of progressive bone loss in the spine. **A,** Osteopenia revealed by washed-out appearance of the vertebrae with an accentuation of the prominence of the vertebral end plates. **B,** Wedge deformity of one of the vertebrae, *W*. **C,** Complete horizontal collapse of the vertebrae, also referred to as the crush-fracture (*).

osteoporosis. Laboratory studies in primary osteoporosis usually show normal results. The serum and urine values for the parameters of bone and mineral metabolism usually remain within the normal range. The alkaline phosphatase level may be elevated if there has been a recent fracture. Radiographically osteoporosis often presents with osteopenia, that is, the general impression of a paucity of bone. The amount of bone that must be lost before osteopenia is appreciated varies, but in general 30% to 50% of the bone mass must be lost before a decrease in bone tissue is recognized radiographically. Therefore more sensitive noninvasive densitometric screening techniques are being employed for the early detection of osteopenia. The horizontal trabeculas are preferentially resorbed first, leading to a early accentuation of the vertical trabeculas (Fig. 38-52). Before the collapse of the vertebrae, the vertebral column appears washed out (Fig. 38-53). The vertebral bodies become biconcave as the subchondral bone weakens, and the intervertebral disc expands, the so-called codfish vertebrae. The biconcave central compression is the most commonly seen in the lumbar spine and represents the central compression or collapse of the vertebrae at the concavity (Fig. 38-54). Other types of fractures are the anterior wedge compression and the symmetric transverse collapse, or "crush," vertebrae (see Fig. 38-51).

Histologic findings in involutional osteoporosis. The histologic manifestations of involutional osteoporosis are heterogeneous.[113,196] The histomorphometric analysis of the cellular events of the remodeling cycle indicate three basic changes that may be encountered in iliac crest bone biopsy specimens from osteopenic postmenopausal women. Approximately 30% of untreated women show features of accelerated turnover, such as numerous osteoclasts, resorption bays, abundant osteoid, and occasionally peritrabecular fibrosis, and therefore would be designated as active osteoporosis. An additional 20% will have histologic evidence of reduced bone turnover or inactive remodeling osteoporosis. The remaining 50% of the women have diminished bone mass in the face of normal indices of bone remodeling. The relationship of these histologic features to the mechanism of bone loss is still unclear, particularly since the level of bone-remodeling activity is not reliably predicted by the accompanying biochemical changes.[196] However, it is probable that the rapid-turnover group represents a situation in which both resorption and formation are accelerated but the degradation of bone is more rapid than its synthesis. Alternatively, the slow turnover or inactive osteoporosis probably reflects the original hypothesis by Albright and co-workers that postmenopausal osteoporosis is a disorder of osteoblast function. In these circumstances, the rate of

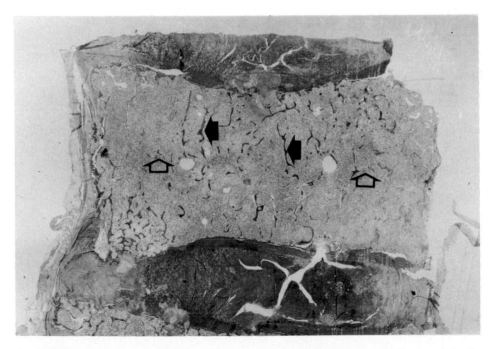

Fig. 38-52. Histologic appearance of bone loss in vertebral body, whole mount. Notice the relative accentuation of the vertical trabeculas *(solid arrows)* and the resorption and loss of the horizontal trabecular bone spicules *(open arrows).*

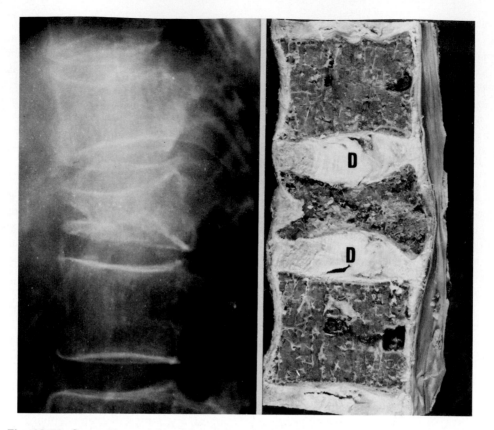

Fig. 38-53. Comparison of the collapsed wedge-shaped vertebrae in the radiograph on the left with the gross appearance of the vertebral specimen on the right. *D*, Intervertebral disc.

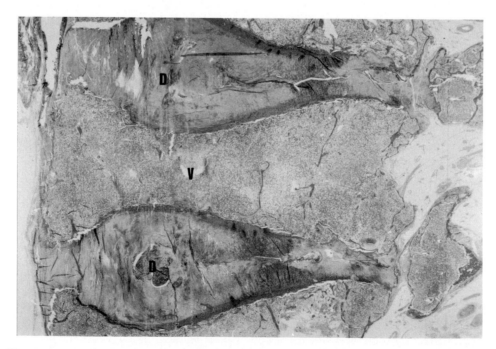

Fig. 38-54. Histologic appearance of the "codfish" deformity of the osteoporotic vertebral body. Histologic whole-mount preparation shows the ballooning of the intervertebral discs, *D*, into the center of the collapsing vertebral body, *V*.

remodeling is reduced, but the absolute amount of bone formed is reduced and is still less than that quantity resorbed. The osteoporotic patients with histomorphometric bone-remodeling parameters that fall within the normal range are more problematic. Perhaps these women develop less bone than normal at maturity, such that the adult peak bone mass is below normal. Although their rate of bone loss is not greater than the rate of loss for normal women, their skeletal mass enters the fracture threshold earlier.

Other forms of primary osteoporosis

Idiopathic juvenile osteoporosis. Idiopathic juvenile osteoporosis is a rare self-limiting form of osteoporosis in prepubertal children.[87] Subsequently over 50 patients with this rare disorder have been reported. It occurs in healthy children between 8 and 14 years of age. The disease runs an acute course, of variable severity, that extends over a period of 2 to 4 years. During this time there is growth arrest, and multiple fractures of the axial and appendicular skeleton may occur. Serum chemistry results are normal, but there may be a mild increase in the alkaline phosphatase. Bone biopsy findings have shown an uncoupling of bone remodeling with increased resorption and reduced bone formation. The most remarkable feature of this disease is the invariable spontaneous remission. From a clinical standpoint, it is important to exclude other causes of juvenile osteoporosis such as Cushing's syndrome, acute leukemia, or osteogenesis imperfecta. Patients with mild to moderate disease may be left with only mild scoliosis, short stature, or bony deformity because of previous fracture.

Idiopathic osteoporosis in young adults. Osteoporosis occurring in young adults is more common than juvenile osteoporosis, yet it is still relatively infrequent compared to involutional osteoporosis. The disorder involves males and female equally and most likely represents a heterogeneous group of ill-defined osteopenic syndromes. Osteopenia in young males, for example, is accompanied by hypercalciuria, and on bone biopsy, histologic evidence of accelerated bone turnover is often encountered.[136] Mild disease may reflect those persons who failed to achieve their peak adult bone mass or represent a genetic predisposition of some patients for a subnormal constitutional bone mass.

Secondary osteoporosis

The term "secondary osteoporosis" may be used when osteopenia is associated with underlying clinical disorders and medical diseases that are known to be, or at least to be potentially, responsible for bone loss. These specific clinical diseases may be the major cause of bone loss in some patients, but often a combination of concurrent medical conditions appear to impact on the skeleton independently of one another, yet their influence on bone physiology appears to be additive as well as cumulative. It has been suggested therefore that these conditions should be thought of as risk factors for the development of osteoporosis, which may aggravate the naturally occurring involutional bone loss. The more common conditions associated with the development of secondary osteoporosis are discussed below and summarized in the list on p. 1959. It must be stressed that the histopathologic findings in a bone biopsy sample will not distinguish the primary from the secondary osteoporoses, or one particular clinical form of osteoporosis from another (such as postmenopausal versus senile, or primary hyperparathyroidism versus thyrotoxicosis). These more specific clinical classifications for osteopenia require the integration of the pathologic findings with the clinical history, laboratory results, and radiographic information. The biopsy information however is very important, since the presence of osteomalacia will be excluded, and the level of bone remodeling activity may shed light on the pathogenesis of the bone loss and thereby indicate more selective forms of therapy.[18,129,192] For example, active osteoporosis may be more effectively treated by agents that inhibit osteoclastic activity, such as estrogen, calcitonin, diphosphonates, or supplemental calcium. Inactive osteoporosis, on the other hand, would not be expected to benefit from these therapeutic agents, since bone resorptive activity is not abnormally high. Osteopenia of inactive osteoporosis is attributable most probably to the greatly suppressed level of bone formation activity. Therefore agents that stimulate osteoblastic activity, such as sodium fluoride, would be more effective.[101] The level of bone-remodeling activity most often associated with the various clinical forms of osteoporosis is listed as follows:

Bone remodeling associated with specific osteoporotic disorders

A. Active osteoporosis
  1. Primary osteoporoses
     a. Idiopathic osteoporosis of young men
     b. Postmenopausal osteoporosis
     c. Senile osteoporosis
  2. Secondary osteoporoses
     a. Anticonvulsant drug related
     b. Chronic anemias with erythroid hyperplasia
     c. Hemochromatosis
     d. Hyperparathyroidism
     e. Hyperthyroidism
     f. Postgastrectomy
     g. Small intestinal disease
     h. Mastocytosis

B. Inactive osteoporosis
  1. Primary osteoporosis
     a. Postmenopausal
     b. Senile
  2. Secondary osteoporoses
     a. Glucocorticoid associated
     b. Hypercortisolism
     c. Hepatic disease—alcohol associated; biliary cirrhosis
     d. Inanition
     e. Starvation, anorexia

For example, one would predict that osteoporosis associated with hyperparathyroidism or thyrotoxicosis would be of the active variety, exhibiting accelerated turnover, because of the known stimulatory effect these hormones have on bone remodeling activity. Idiopathic postmenopausal osteoporosis, as well as senile osteoporosis of aging men and women, may be either active or inactive. Because the current noninvasive tests available do not distinguish between inactive and active osteoporosis, the bone biopsy is still the most reliable manner in which to establish the level of bone-remodeling activity.[183,197]

Acromegaly

The elevation in serum concentrations of growth hormone that is evident in acromegaly causes increased bone turnover, though the frequency of osteoporosis or fractures does not appear to be increased.[152] Bone mass may actually be elevated, with increased thickness of cortical bone and augmentation of the trabecular bone volume. Growth hormone activates bone remodeling sites and may increase bone formation more than bone resorption.[73] In acromegaly, elevations in the active metabolite of 1,25-dihydroxyvitamin D are reported and are believed to result from growth hormone–induced stimulation of the renal 25-hydroxyvitamin D 1α-hydroxylase activity. As a result, intestinal calcium absorption is augmented, promoting hypercalciuria and possibly hypercalcemia.[72] Bone biopsy specimens have shown features of active remodeling.

Anticonvulsant drug-induced osteopathy

Prolonged use of anticonvulsant drugs (phenytoin, phenobarbital), particularly when taken in high doses or in combination, is associated with decreased serum ionized-calcium concentrations and reduced bone mass. Double tetracycline–labeled bone biopsy specimens in ambulatory patients with epilepsy reveal increased quantities of osteoid (related to an increase in the total osteoid surface with osteoid seams of normal width), rapid bone mineralization, and, frequently, histologic evidence of secondary hyperparathyroidism.[193] Low concentrations of vitamin D metabolites and subsequent osteomalacia found in institutionalized patients receiving antiepileptic drugs may be attributable primarily to limited vitamin D intake and reduced solar exposure.

Chronic anemias with erythroid hyperplasia

Skeletal changes that accompany disorders of hemoglobin synthesis, such as thalassemia, are predominantly a result of the compensatory erythroid hyperplasia associated with the anemia.[121] If frequent transfusions are necessary, there may be the additional factor of iron overload. In young children, severely ineffective erythropoiesis leads to abnormal bone modeling, skeletal fragility, and growth retardation. Mineral, electrolyte, and vitamin D metabolism usually is normal. Histologically, increased activity of bone remodeling with increased osteoclastic resorption and increased quantities of osteoid is evident.[194] Often iron deposits may be demonstrated at the mineralization fronts (mineralized bone-osteoid seam interfaces) (Fig. 38-55). With the use of tetracycline kinetic markers, however, widely spaced fluorescent labels are found at these same mineralization fronts, an indication that osteoid excess is a result of increased matrix production and, furthermore, that the presence of iron does not impair the mineralization process.[194]

Disuse osteoporosis

Osteopenia in immobilized portions of the skeleton is a universal phenomenon. It is observed not only in association with bed rest, paralysis, and plaster casting, but also with a weightless environment, as observed with space travel. Astronauts, for example, may lose 4 g of calcium per month during space flight. This remarkable degree of bone mobilization may become the limiting factor in prolonged space exploration.[118,195] Disuse osteoporosis is common in degenerative lower motor neuron disease and in paraplegia and quadriplegia resulting from spinal cord injury.

Disuse osteopenia develops primarily because of accelerated bone resorption without a compensatory increase in bone formation.[117] Osteolysis resulting from osteoclastic overactivity may result in elevated serum calcium levels. Hypercalcemia and hypercalciuria may be so severe as to be life threatening in the immobilized patient. Movement alone does not protect against the development of osteoporosis because actual weight-bearing activity is necessary to maintain skeletal mass. Application of electrical forces prevents loss of bone experimentally in an immobilized limb, an indication that alterations in piezoelectricity may be therapeutically important.

Hemochromatosis

The cause of the osteopenia that frequently attends hemochromatosis is probably complex. Liver disease

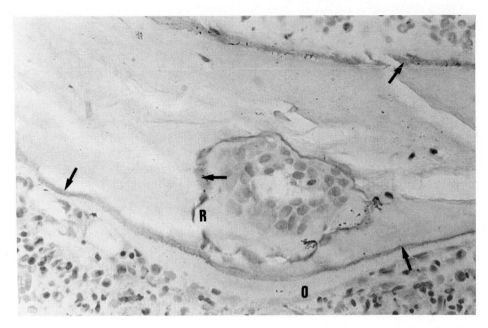

Fig. 38-55. Secondary osteoporosis associated with erythroid hyperplasia of chronic anemia, requiring multiple blood transfusions, and with hemosiderosis. A Prussian blue stain of bone showing the deposition of iron along the interface of the osteoid, *O,* and mineralized bone, *arrows.* Bone resorption is accelerated forming a resorption cone, *R,* an expression of active osteoporosis.

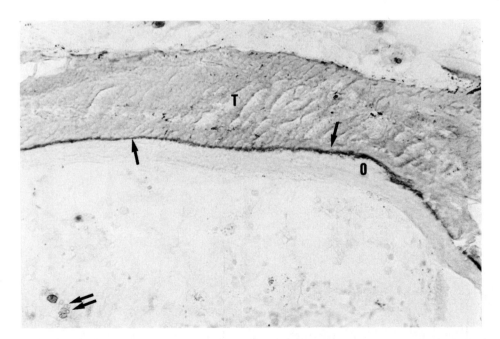

Fig. 38-56. Hemochromatosis with active osteoporosis. The Prussian blue stain reveals the deposition of iron, *arrows,* at the osteoid seam–trabecular bone, *T,* interfaces. Notice the marrow iron, *double arrows.*

and hypogonadism may affect the skeleton indirectly. Bone biopsy documents the presence of osteoporosis, thereby excluding a mineralization defect. A direct effect of iron on bone cell metabolism may occur; iron deposits in the osteoid seam interfaces may be demonstrable by histochemical stains (Prussian blue reaction, Fig. 38-56). Iron deposition in bone tissue often is associated with features of active bone turnover with normal mineralization. In contrast, a small number of patients with chronic renal failure receiving multiple blood transfusions may develop an acquired iron-overload state, which has been associated with the presence of a mineralization defect.[138] Even in the absence of concomitant aluminum deposition, the skeletal abnormalities in these few patients with hemosiderosis improve after chelation therapy with deferoxamine (desferrioxamine B), an agent that removes aluminum as well as iron.

Hepatic osteodystrophy

Alcohol-associated liver disease. Alcohol is the most common risk factor associated with osteoporosis in young men.[171] Although fractures in alcoholic persons generally occur after trauma, it appears likely that chronic alcoholism disrupts calcium homeostasis and predisposes the skeleton to fracture. Several studies have shown a reduction in bone mass in alcoholic persons, especially in areas that have a high proportion of trabecular bone, such as the iliac crest, femoral neck, and calcaneus. Two histologic studies of bone in alcoholic patients confirmed the presence of osteomalacia (increased osteoid volume), though the kinetics of bone remodeling using double tetracycline labeling were not reported.[134,186] A recent study of eight men with a 10-year history of alcohol abuse showed a reduction in vertebral trabecular bone mass with preservation of appendicular cortical bone. Histologically a reduction of active bone formation was seen without evidence of osteomalacia.[10] Several explanations could account for a reduction in bone mass in the alcoholic person, including nutritional deficiencies of calcium and vitamin D, malabsorption of calcium and vitamin D secondary to pancreatic or liver disease, abnormal metabolism of vitamin D secondary to cirrhosis, abnormal parathyroid hormone secretion, and a direct toxic effect of ethanol on calcium absorption.

Cholestatic liver disease. There is general agreement that the metabolic bone disease most commonly associated with cholestatic liver disease is osteoporosis.[105] It is manifested by bone pain, fractures, and reduced bone volume. Even in the investigations that reported a high frequency of osteomalacia in cholestatic liver disease, 50% or more of the patients with cholestasis who had radiographic evidence of osteopenia were shown histologically to have a reduction in mineralized bone and osteoid. Although low serum levels of 25-dihy-

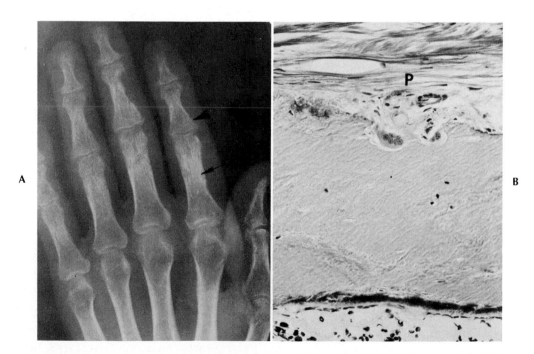

Fig. 38-57. A, Radiograph of a hand of patient with severe skeletal disease caused by hyperparathyroidism. Intracortical striations, *arrow,* are present, as is subperiosteal resorption, *arrowhead.* **B,** Osteoclasts resorbing subperiosteal bone in hyperparathyroidism. *P,* Periosteum. (**A,** Courtesy Dr. James W. Debnam, Jr., Chesterfield, Mo.; **B,** undecalcified, Goldner's stain; 100×.)

droxyvitamin D are found in this disease, histomorphometric analysis of bone fails to reveal evidence of osteomalacia. Hyperosteoidosis is absent, as determined by measurements of fractional osteoid surface, osteoid volume, or fractional osteoid volume. In addition, rates of mineral apposition and bone formation also are normal. These findings indicate that vitamin D deficiency does not contribute significantly to the osteodystrophy that is observed in patients with primary biliary cirrhosis.

Hypercortisolism

Endogenous (Cushing's syndrome) and exogenous (iatrogenic) hypercortisolism is a well-recognized risk factor for fractures.[68] There is a propensity for a greater loss of trabecular bone as compared to cortical bone in states of chronic corticosteroid excess. Thus there is a disproportionate deleterious effect on the axial skeleton with vertebral crush fractures, with a sparing of the appendicular skeleton and few cortical bone fractures. Both endogenous and exogenous hypercortisolism are associated with increased bone resorption and decreased bone formation. Decreased bone formation may result from the direct inhibition of osteoblastic collagen synthesis by cortisol.[135] The increase in bone resorption is believed to be an indirect effect because of the direct inhibition of intestinal calcium absorption by this hormone-promoting secondary hyperparathyroidism with increased bone resorption.[69]

Primary hyperparathyroidism

The clinical manifestations of hyperparathyroidism are protean.[1] In the past, patients usually manifested either renal or skeletal complications of excess parathyroid hormone. Since the advent of multiphasic chemical screening however, most patients are now diagnosed on the basis of asymptomatic hypercalcemia, and only 20% exhibit radiographic skeletal changes. On the other hand, approximately one half of all patients retain increased quantities of bone-seeking isotope tracers, making radionuclide scanning a sensitive method of detecting skeletal involvement. Bone disease when symptomatic may be striking.[142] Not only do pain and fractures develop, but also deformities particularly produced by cystic lesions may be crippling. The radiographic changes of primary hyperparathyroidism are usually first evident in the phalanges and metacarpals (Fig. 38-57). Properly prepared hand radiographs, particularly with magnification viewing techniques, often show resorption of the subperiosteal bone of the radial aspect of the fingers. Intracortical striations, reflecting increased cortical porosity, also appear early but are a nonspecific sign of bone loss. Radiographic evidence of more advanced skeletal involvement includes the cystic lesions of von Recklinghausen's disease of bone, loss of the lamina dura of the alveolar bone of the jaws, and resorption at sites of tendon insertions, resulting in tendon avulsions.

The net effect of primary hyperparathyroidism on

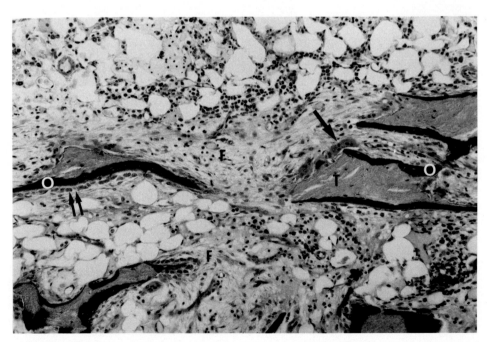

Fig. 38-58. Histologic appearance of osteitis fibrosa of secondary hyperparathyroidism. Notice the deposition of fibrous tissue, *F*, the increased osteoclastic activity *(arrows)*, and the increased osteoblastic activity *(double arrows)*. Osteoid, *O*, is increased therefore along the trabecular bone surface, *T*.

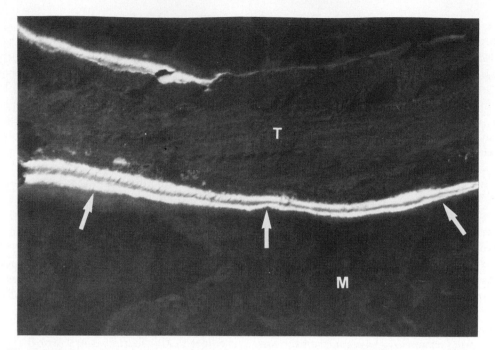

Fig. 38-59. The complex tetracycline-label pattern of hyperparathyroidism. Although the linear extent of double tetracycline labels *(arrows)* over the trabecular bone surface, *T*, may be increased, the distance between the labels is often normal or reduced. *M,* Marrow.

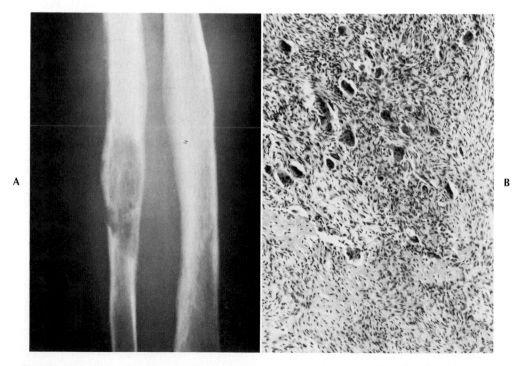

Fig. 38-60. A, Osteitis fibrosa cystica (brown tumor) of ulna. **B,** Osteitis fibrosa cystica (brown tumor). Numerous giant cells are present in cellular stroma. (**A,** Courtesy Dr. James W. Debnam, Jr., Chesterfield, Mo.; **B,** hematoxylin and eosin; 100×.)

skeletal mass is heterogeneous and controversial. Bone-density studies demonstrate osteopenia, particularly with a loss of trabecular bone; however, histologically quantitated cortical and trabecular bone volumes may be normal. Virtually all patients with primary hyperparathyroidism have histologic evidence of accelerated bone remodeling,[120] the magnitude of which correlates with the degree of hypercalcemia. Generally an increase in the number of osteoclasts as well as osteoblasts is seen. Osteoclastic activity appears increased as resorption bays and cutting cones are conspicuous (Fig. 38-58). The quantity of osteoid is often increased but the cellular rate of mineralization, as determined by double tetracycline labeling, is decreased, an indication that although more osteoblasts than normal are present in hyperparathyroid bone the rate of activity of each cell is diminished (Fig. 38-61). The overall rate of bone formation is, however, increased because many more osteoblasts are taking part in this process.[181]

Osteitis fibrosa is a generic term often used to describe the microscopic features of hyperparathyroidism. However, osteitis fibrosa is a histologic entity that may occur in any state of accelerated bone turnover, including secondary hyperparathyroidism, hyperthyroidism, and involutional osteoporosis. In addition to the increased osteoblastic and osteoclastic activity, osteitis fibrosa is characterized by peritrabecular fibrous tissue deposition (Fig. 38-59). In contrast, the fibrosis of idiopathic myelofibrosis is diffusely distributed throughout the marrow, without predilection to the trabecular architecture. The cystic lesions of von Recklinghausen resemble giant cell tumors of bone. There is osteoclast proliferation in a cellular fibrous stroma, characteristically associated with hemosiderin pigment deposition, hence the term "brown tumor" (Fig. 38-60). Unlike giant cell tumors, these lesions generally occur in the diaphyses of long bones and in the jaw and skull. If a giant cell lesion appears in a location other than the usual juxta-epiphyseal region of a long bone, hyperparathyroidism should be considered.

Secondary hyperparathyroidism

In contrast to the primary condition, bone disease associated with secondary hyperparathyroidism is more prevalent. The associated clinical disorders are those that are commonly associated with the development of osteomalacia—renal failure, anticonvulsant medication, gastrectomy, and intestinal malabsorption. Any condition associated with the production of hypocalcemia, regardless of the mechanism, will evoke a compensatory reaction in the form of secondary secretion of parathyroid hormone.[133] Histologically the changes of parathyroid hormone action on bone are identical to those described under primary hyperparathyroidism. Bone loss

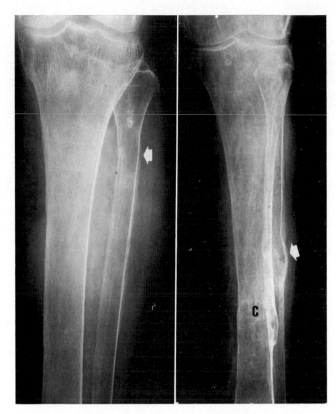

Fig. 38-61. Radiographic appearance of severe bone loss in secondary hyperparathyroidism, resulting in the loss of cortical bone and trabecular bone in these lower extremity long bones. Notice the cytic change, *C,* and the presence of pathologic fractures, *arrows.*

may be substantial, and the development of osteopenia may therefore precede the development of osteomalacia in the conditions mentioned[133] (Fig. 38-61).

Hypogonadism

Hypogonadism in both men and women is associated with an increased risk of osteoporosis. Bone mass is reduced in ovarian agenesis (Turner's syndrome), as well as in women with premature ovarian failure and amenorrheic women with hyperprolactinemia.[17,93] Hypothalamic hypogonadism results in amenorrhea in female athletes and is accompanied by excessive but potentially reversible bone loss. Acquired hypogonadism most commonly results from oophorectomy. Surgical menopause is now recognized as an important risk factor for osteoporosis in young adult women. Although men do not undergo an equivalent hormonal withdrawal, androgen function declines with age. Testosterone deficiency is associated with abnormal calcium metabolism and vertebral fractures. Bone-remodeling activity is suppressed resulting in inactive osteoporosis.

Hypoparathyroidism

Hypoparathyroidism is an uncommon disorder characterized by hypocalcemia, hypocalciuria, and hyperphosphatemia because of a deficiency of parathyroid hormone.[14,127,128] The most frequent cause of hypoparathyroidism is damage to the parathyroid tissue during surgical exploration of the neck. Hypoparathyroidism may rarely be the result of autoimmune disease, congenital absence of the parathyroid glands and thymus (that is, DiGeorge's syndrome), iron-storage diseases, or glandular metastases. Bone turnover is decreased because of the interruption of the effect of parathyroid hormone on the proliferation of osteoprogenitor cells. Increased cortical thickness and trabecular bone volume may be found in hypoparathyroidism, resulting in osteosclerosis. Patients with idiopathic hypoparathyroidism are more likely to exhibit clinical musculoskeletal abnormalities than those patients with iatrogenic disease. It is not uncommon to encounter changes traditionally associated with pseudohypoparathyroidism in these patients. These features include soft-tissue calcification and ossification, abnormal dentition, and osteosclerosis. Intracranial calcifications and ankylosing spondylitis may also complicate idiopathic hypoparathyroidism.

Pseudohypoparathyroidism (PHP)

The syndrome of pseudohypoparathyroidism (PHP) consists of a host of phenotypes inherited as a sex-linked dominant trait. Affected patients are usually short and obese with a characteristic moon-shaped facies. Their dentition is abnormal, and the bones of the hands and feet, particularly the fourth and fifth metacarpals and metatarsals are short (Fig. 38-62). The long bones are often curved, and soft-tissue calcification and ossification are common, as are cataracts and basal ganglia calcifications (Fig. 38-63). As a consequence, mental retardation and seizure disorders are common. The major physiologic defect in these patients is the absence of renal excretion of phosphorus in response to parathyroid hormone. Most commonly, as in type I, this is associated with defective cyclic AMP generation by the kidney when exogenous parathormone is administered.[24] Patients with type II PHP retain the ability to synthesize nephrogenous cAMP in response to parathyroid hormone, but like their type I counterparts, they cannot generate a phosphaturic response.[36] Because of the failure to excrete phosphorus, PHP patients are hyperphosphatemic and have secondary hyperparathyroidism. Attendant hypocalcemia is in part attributable to hyperphosphatemia and low levels of 1,25-dihydroxyvitamin D, secondary to defective renal metabolism of the parent sterol. The calcemic response to parathyroid hormone is blunted in the setting of vitamin D deficiency but is reversible. Therefore the skeletal resistance to parathyroid hormone in PHP is not attributable to end-organ unresponsiveness. Although the bone density in patients with PHP is often normal,

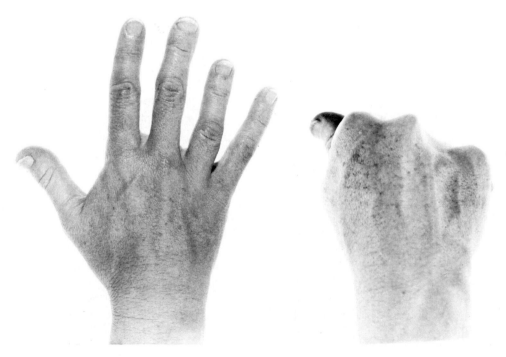

Fig. 38-62. Short fourth metacarpal of patient with pseudohypoparathyroidism. (Courtesy Dr. Susie Humphrey, Baltimore, Md.)

a few exhibit osteopenia, with evidence of subperiosteal resorption and histologic changes of osteitis fibrosa.[55]

Mastocytosis

Mastocytosis is a generic term used to describe the spectrum of disorders characterized by a proliferation of tissue mast cells. Mastocytoma and urticaria pigmen-tosa (Fig. 38-64) generally refer to the unifocal and multifocal accumulation of dermal mast cells, respectively, whereas systemic mastocytosis denotes proliferation of mast cells in the viscera (especially the liver, spleen, lymph nodes, and gastrointestinal tract) and bones.

Approximately 70% of the patients with systemic mastocytosis develop radiographically detectable bone

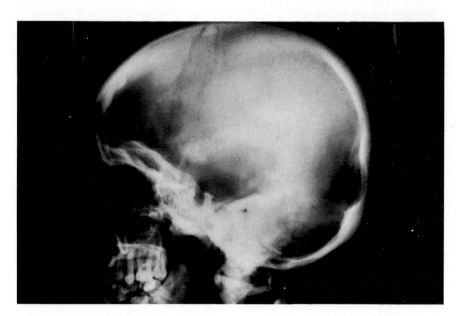

Fig. 38-63. Pseudohypoparathyroidism. Skull radiograph showing basal ganglia calcifications.

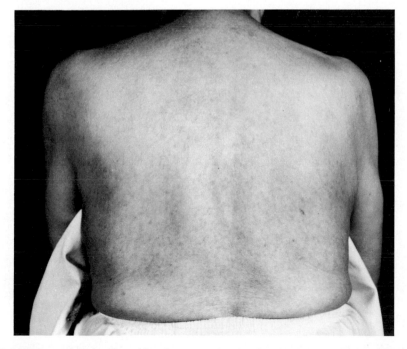

Fig. 38-64. Mastocytosis. The skin changes of urticaria pigmentosa. These brownish lesions with the characteristic hypersensitivity symptoms may be associated with a form of secondary osteoporosis.

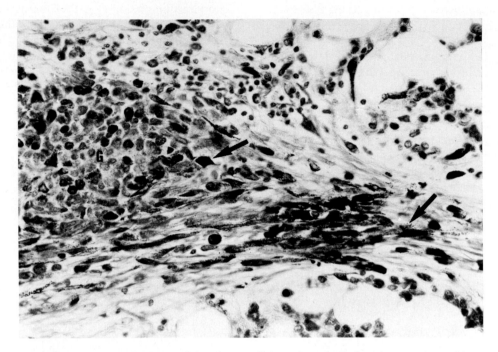

Fig. 38-65. Histologic findings of the mast cell granulomas, *G*, in a bone marrow biopsy specimen from a patient with systemic mastocytosis. The arrows point to the mast cells stained by Giemsa stain, revealing the presence of the hyperchromatic cytoplasmic granules.

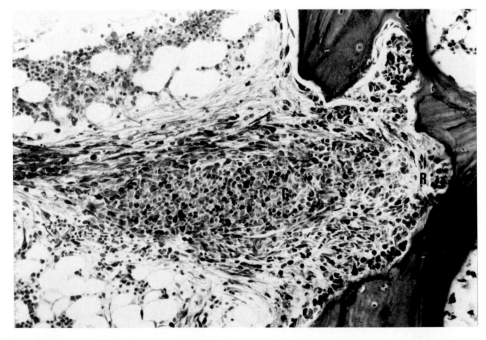

Fig. 38-66. Bone changes in mastocytosis. The marrow granuloma, *G*, is inducing bone resorption of the adjacent trabecular bone, *R*.

lesions. The most common abnormality has been reported to be diffuse, poorly demarcated, sclerotic, and lucent areas involving the axial skeleton. Circumscribed lesions, especially of the skull and extremities, are also well documented. Although generalized osteopenia alone has been reported, it is believed to be a less common radiographic finding.

Because the histologic evaluation of osseous involvement in systemic mastocytosis generally is limited to bone-marrow aspiration and not bone biopsy, the pathologic correlates of the skeletal radiographic abnormalities are poorly characterized. Nondecalcified transiliac crest biopsy specimens from patients with systemic mastocytosis and diffuse osteopenia with vertebral crush fractures exhibit a characteristic pattern of marrow involvement.[49] Distinctive mast cell aggregates, as revealed by metachromatic staining, are present and may mimic granulomas (Fig. 38-65). Histomorphometric analysis of trabecular bone reveals accelerated bone remodeling characterized by osteoidosis, peritrabecular fibrosis, increased numbers of osteoblasts and osteoclasts, and an increase in osteoclastic resorbing surfaces (Fig. 38-66).

The osteolytic foci and diffuse osteopenia associated with mastocytosis may be mediated by the chemical products of mast cells. Heparin is a potent in vitro bone-resorbing agent,[65] and osteopenia has resulted from long-term heparin therapy.[66] Furthermore, there is evidence that mast cells may play a role in the pathogenesis of senile osteoporosis.[48,54]

Partial gastrectomy

Dietary deficiency, impaired absorption of calcium, and malabsorption of vitamin D with steatorrhea may be seen in patients after undergoing gastrectomy.[39,62] The histologic nature of the skeletal disease is therefore variable and depends on the relative contributions of malabsorption of minerals versus vitamin D. In contrast to those persons with small bowel resection, most patients who have undergone partial gastrectomy develop osteoporosis (with features of high turnover and osteitis fibrosa) rather than osteomalacia.

Starvation

Bone formation may be affected not only at the level of mineralization, but also during the earlier stages of synthesis and secretion of organic matrix.[162] General inhibition of cellular protein synthetic capacity may be associated with inanition, starvation, or chronic systemic disease. Anorexia nervosa has been associated with inactive or low-turnover osteoporosis.[90]

Thyrotoxicosis

Endogenous hyperthyroidism has a profound effect on bone and mineral metabolism. Typically, affected

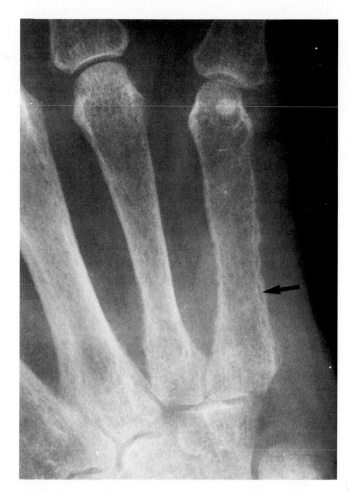

Fig. 38-67. Radiographic changes of the cortical striations that may be produced by thyrotoxicosis.

patients show an accelerated rate of bone-remodeling activity, which in some persons leads to osteopenia and fractures.[112] Excessive administration of thyroid hormone may be associated with active osteoporosis identical to that of endogenous hyperfunction.[45] The primary abnormality in these circumstances is a pronounced osteoclastosis of the trabecular and cortical bone. The rate of bone formation is also increased because of the normal sequential coupling of bone formation to previous bone resorption, with resorption exceeding formation, favoring a net loss of bone mass. Previous studies have noted the particularly severe involvement of the cortical bone in thyrotoxicosis, compared to other catabolic states such as hyperparathyroidism.[107] Radiographs of the hands using fine-grain film have demonstrated the presence of cortical striations (Fig. 38-67), and histologic sections of the cortical bone of the iliac crest have exhibited noticeable porosity and a reduction of cortical width. Often the features of accelerated bone turnover with osteoclastosis in the cortex are paralleled by similar changes in the subjacent trabecular bone. These findings however are nonspecific because these histologic features may also occur in postmenopausal osteoporosis as well as in primary hyperparathyroidism. The biochemical features of thyroid hormone excess include elevated serum levels of alkaline phosphatase, which may represent either hepatic or bone isoenzyme fractions, or a combination of both. Patients with endogenous hyperthyroidism frequently have a tendency toward hyperphosphatemia and hypercalcemia with hypercalciuria. The increased calcium and phosphate levels reflect osteolysis, with osteoclast-mediated bone resorption acting to suppress parathyroid hormone secretion.

Other agents and factors influencing bone metabolism

Vitamin A. Both an excess as well as a deficiency of vitamin A may lead to pathologic skeletal changes. Chronic hypervitaminosis A occurs in children ingesting large quantities of fish oil or chicken liver, in Eskimos eating polar bear liver, and in some food faddists ingesting excessive vitamin supplements.[99,156,158] Excess vitamin A stimulates osteoclasts, particularly those involved in modeling, and as a result gross skeletal deformities may arise in the region of the metaphyseal cutback zone. Osteoid proliferation also develops in juxtaposition to exaggerated bone resorption. There is

characteristically well-developed periosteal new bone formation associated with hypervitaminosis A (Fig. 38-68). The most common skeletal manifestation of toxicity is a proliferation of tender, moundlike periosteal calcifications and exostoses, with thickening of the periosteal connective tissue and calcifications of the tendons and ligaments.[19,56,137]

Vitamin A deficiency has received increased attention because of its association with total parenteral nutrition.[81] In hypovitaminosis A, bone remodeling virtually ceases, osteoclastic activity disappears, and appositional new periosteal bone formation occurs, resulting in an overgrowth of the entire skeleton because of this periostitis. In addition, there is a retardation of endochondral ossification with a failure of the chondrocytes to proliferate and an arrest of chondro-osseous transformation. As a result the bones of a vitamin A–deficient person are short and thick because of arrested longitudinal growth, coupled with continued periosteal bone apposition.

Vitamin C. Clinical scurvy rarely occurs in Western society and is therefore largely of historical interest.[77] However, the dietary deficiency of alcoholic patients may produce a scorbutic syndrome. The essential role of vitamin C in skeletal metabolism is related to collagen formation. It promotes hydroxylation of both pro-

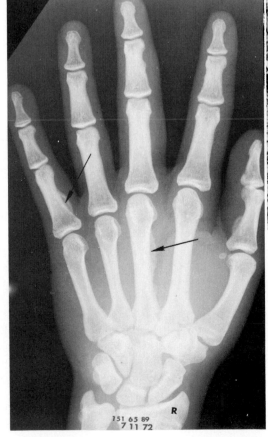

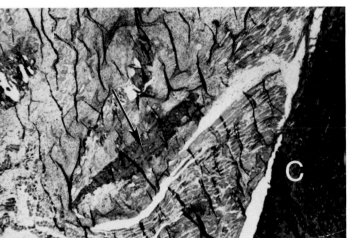

Fig. 38-68. A, Periosteal calcifications *(arrows),* which characterize hypervitaminosis A. **B,** Histologic correlate of **A.** Bone, *arrow,* has formed within periosteal soft tissues in rat with vitamin A toxicity. *C,* Cortex of tibia. (**A,** Courtesy Dr. Boy Frame; from Frame, B., et al.: Ann. Intern. Med. **80:**44, 1974; with permission of publisher; **B,** undecalcified, modified Masson's trichrome stain; 40×.)

line and lysine, and collagen synthesis will cease in the absence of vitamin C, thereby inhibiting osteoid matrix production.[13,51] Defective collagen formation also involves the other connective tissues, resulting in fragile blood vessels, a tendency for bleeding, and easy bruising. Subperiosteal hemorrhage results in the separation and elevation of the periosteum from the underlying cortex. In the growing skeleton, failure to form normal mineralized osteoid results in the persistence of the provisional zone of calcified cartilage at the growth plate. Primary trabeculas are therefore not formed. The calcified cartilage is brittle, and with continued weight bearing and motion, microfractures occur in the metaphysis. This combined instability of the growth plate can result in the lateral slippage of the epiphysis (Fig. 38-69). Because the ring of Ranvier also depends on normal osteoid production, the perichondrial ring is not well formed and the growth-plate cartilage tends to grow laterally. The resultant radiographic features of scurvy are characteristic and well described. The settling epiphysis onto the metaphysis gives the appearance of a spur formation at the margin of the growth plate (Fig. 38-70).

Osteomalacia and rickets

Osteomalacia is a group of metabolic bone diseases resulting from defective mineralization of trabecular and cortical bone matrix.[102,103,176] Rickets refers to the presence of defective mineralization of the epiphyseal growth-plate cartilage. Skeletal disease in children therefore will exhibit a combination of rickets and osteomalacia, provided that the growth plate remains open. In contrast, adults may manifest osteoid (bone) changes only after epiphyseal closure. The resulting bone mass may be decreased, normal, or increased (that is, osteosclerosis). The most common forms of osteomalacia and rickets are associated with a decreased serum calcium-phosphate product (Ca × P), such that mineralization is not supported. Consequently, defective mineralization of skeletal matrices may result directly from disorders that influence calcium homeostasis or phosphate metabolism. Indirectly, calcium and phosphate deficiency may be mediated by secondary mechanisms such as deficiencies in vitamin D or other agents that regulate mineral metabolism. The box on p. 1946 summarizes the determinants of bone matrix mineralization.

Classification of osteomalacia and rickets

The clinical classification of the osteomalacic diseases is based upon the recognition of the underlying abnormality interfering with the mineralization of the bone matrix (Table 38-7). The most common form of osteomalacia in adults is that from secondary vitamin D deficiency, that is, vitamin D–deficiency states secondary to an abnormality of vitamin D metabolism despite ad-

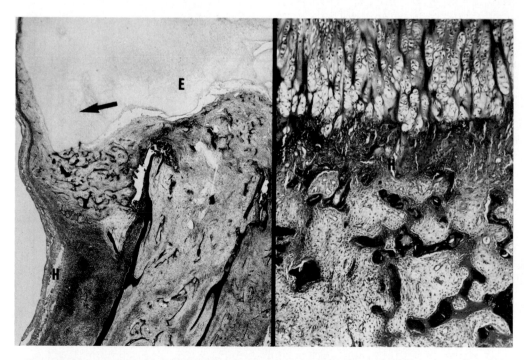

Fig. 38-69. Scurvy. Characteristic histologic features. *Left,* Lateral slippage of the epiphysis, *E,* in the direction of the arrow. Notice the presence of the periosteal hematoma formation, *H. Right,* Growth-plate changes, with extensive hemorrhage, *H,* below the hypertrophic zone of chondrocytes caused by rupture of the penetrating vessels.

equate vitamin D intake. Thus osteomalacia may be further subclassified upon the basis of the abnormality in vitamin absorption or bioactivation. In postmenopausal women presenting with osteopenia, as many as 20% will be found to have osteomalacia, not osteoporosis. In this group, chronic gastrointestinal malabsorption is the clinical condition most often associated with the development of vitamin D–deficiency osteomalacia.

Rickets: general considerations

Clinical manifestations of rickets. In children with mineralization disorders, growth is impaired and height is consequently below the third percentile. The head is abnormal because the skull is soft and may deform (craniotabes). There is prominence of the frontal bones resulting in frontal bossing. The chest examination shows flaring and deformity of the ribs with nodular swelling of the costochondral junctions resulting in the rachitic rosary appearance. In addition to pectus excavatum, there may be an indentation of the thorax at the insertion of the diaphram into the lower ribs referred to as "Harrison's groove." Because of structural compromise of the thorax, frequent respiratory infections and a chronic cough are likely. Along with the chest

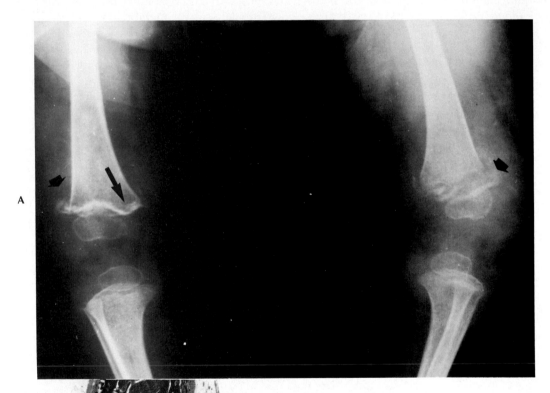

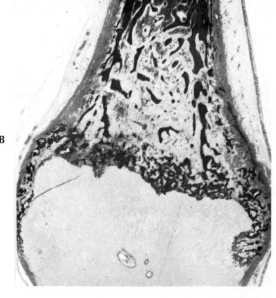

Fig. 38-70. A, Radiographic changes of scurvy at the knee joints. Notice the prominent zone of provisional calcification, which appears sclerotic, with a line of radiolucency that forms in the metaphysis *(long arrow),* which correlates with the collapse of the weakened region of the growth plate where the primary spongiosa fails to form. **B,** Classic histologic features of well-advanced scurvy. Bone shows evidence of osteoporosis and marrow spaces filled with loosely textured and edematous connective tissue in which some hemorrhage has occurred. Metaphyseal end of bone is widened and made up of irregularly arranged spicules of heavily calcified matrix. (**B,** 10×.)

Table 38-7. Clinical classification of osteomalacia

Vitamin D deficiency	Hepatobiliary disease
Primary	Small bowel disease
Secondary	Pancreatic insufficiency
Vitamin D dependency types I and II	
Hypophosphatemic states	X-linked hypophosphatemia (vitamin D–resistant rickets)
	Sporadic hypophosphatemia
	Antacid-induced hypophosphatemia
	Oncogenic osteomalacia
Drugs	Aluminum disposition
	Sodium fluoride toxicity
	Diphosphonate toxicity
Chronic renal failure and renal osteodystrophy	
Hypophosphatasia	

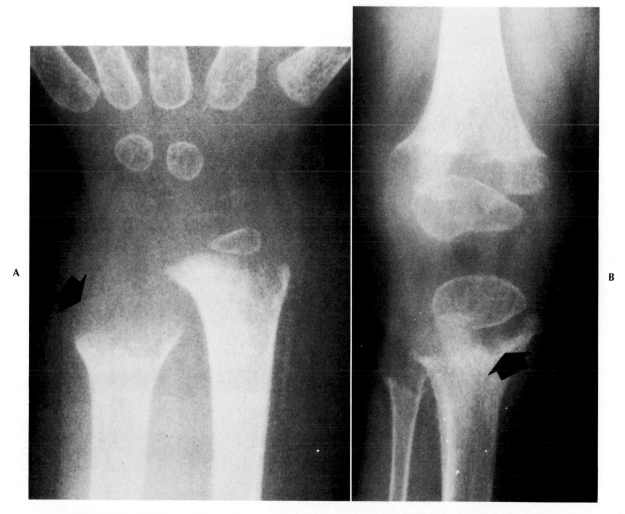

Fig. 38-71. Radiographic appearance of rickets. **A,** The cupping of the distal forearm growth plates, *arrow,* is apparent on this radiograph of the wrist. **B,** Also there is irregularity and flaring of the metaphyses of the bones around the knee, *arrow.*

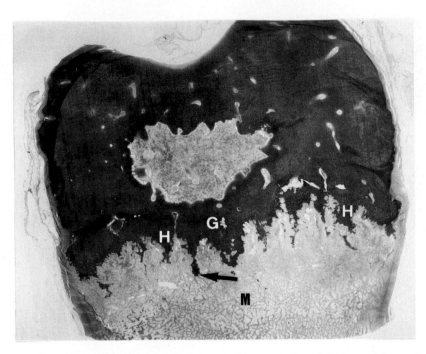

Fig. 38-72. The histologic findings in rickets, whole mount of a distal femoral growth plate from a case of neonatal rickets. The growth-plate, *G,* region is abnormal, with an elongation of the columns of hypertrophic chondrocytes caused by failure of mineralization of the cartilage. Because the matrix is uncalcified, it cannot be resorbed by the penetrating vascular endothelial cells and osteoclasts, resulting in long tongues of cartilage, *arrow,* extending into the metaphysis, *M.*

abnormality, there is deformity of the spine resulting in thoracic kyphosis, which in turn produces a protuberant abdomen, or so called rachitic potbelly. The rapidly growing regions of the extremities also manifest the changes of defective mineralization with symmetric enlargement or swelling of the elbows, wrists, and knees. The legs may be bowed (genu varum) or less frequently exhibit knock-knee (genu valgum).

Radiographic features of rickets. The radiographic changes reflect the underlying pathologic changes. The cortices are thin, and the medullary space is rarefied because of indistinct markings of the poorly calcified trabecular bone. The radiologic hallmarks however are the widened growth plates and poorly defined zone of provisional calcification, which is normally identifiable as a radiodense white line separating the growth plate from the metaphysis. Cupping and flaring of the ends of the bones are a result of the softening of the skeletal tissue (Fig. 38-71).

Histologic features of rickets. The histologic appearance of the growth-plate cartilage is characteristic. The rachitic growth plate is wide and irregular, and the architecture is abnormal (Fig. 38-72). The columnar arrangement of the hypertrophic chondrocytes is lost, and

the zone of provisional calcification disappears. Cartilage extends deep into the metaphysis, where it becomes surrounded by osteoid, which fails to mineralize (Fig. 38-73). In affected children, cup-shaped growthplate indentations and bowed legs develop because of the structural weakness of the widened physes and osteomalacic bone.

Osteomalacia: general considerations

Clinical features of osteomalacia. Adults with osteomalacia complain of generalized weakness, diffuse bone pain, easy fatigability, and malaise. The physical findings may be minimal, in contrast to rickets; they are bony tenderness and a waddling gait attributable to a proximal muscle myopathy, producing a characteristic abductor-lurch type of gait, the so-called Trendelenburg gait. Curvature of the long bones and spine may occur, resulting in bowing with coxa vara and kyphosis.

Radiographic features of osteomalacia. The radiographic signs may be subtle and consist of either increased bone density (osteosclerosis) (Fig. 38-74) or diffuse osteopenia, mimicking primary or secondary osteoporosis. Pseudofractures (also called Looser's zones, or Milkman's syndrome) are generally consid-

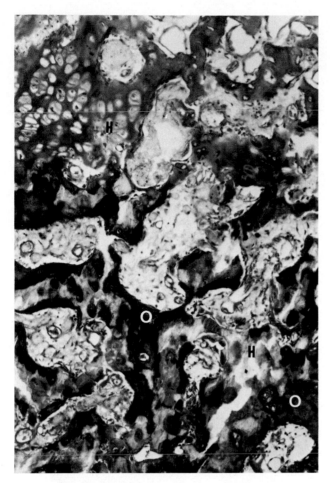

Fig. 38-73. Detailed histologic appearance of rickets. Disorganization of the lower zones of the growth plate is apparent, with irregular columns of hypertrophic chondrocytes, *H,* and cartilage that has failed to mineralize. The bone that is deposited upon this cartilage is unmineralized as well and appears therefore as an increased quantity of osteoid, *O.*

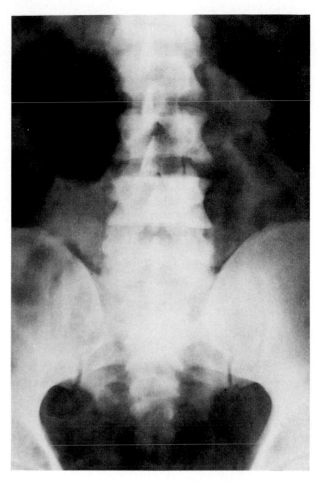

Fig. 38-74. Radiographic appearance of osteomalacia in lumbar area of spine and pelvis. An increase in the bone density has resulted in diffuse osteosclerosis.

ered pathognomonic of osteomalacia. These ribbonlike radiolucencies represent stress fractures that have healed by the deposition of uncalcified osteoid, producing a narrow cortical defect at right angles to the long axis of the bone (Fig. 38-75). They are usually painless and are often bilaterally symmetric, involving the concave side of long bones, the medial femoral neck, the pubic rami, the clavicle, ribs and axillary border of the scapula.

Osteomalacia may be suspected in a patient with a potential metabolic bone disease by identifying risk factors for osteomalacia (by a thorough history and physical examination), characteristic radiographic changes, and a pattern of abnormal laboratory tests (Table 38-8). In contrast to the typical patient with idiopathic osteopo-

rosis, the patient with osteomalacia will often exhibit diffuse bone pain and tenderness, generalized muscle weakness or a proximal myopathy, bowing deformities of the long bones, or other rachitic changes. There may be a history of unusual dietary habits, avoidance of sunlight, vitamin D restriction, or use of medications that interfere with vitamin D metabolism.[8,40,170] Gastrointestinal diseases with malabsorption and steatorrhea and chronic renal insufficiency are major clinical disorders that may be complicated by the development of osteomalacia. The presence of pseudofractures or a pathologic fracture through the midshaft of a long bone is very suggestive of osteomalacia and is only infrequently encountered in the osteoporotic patient. Hypocalcemia, hypophosphatemia, phosphaturia, hypocal-

Table 38-8. Risk factors for osteomalacia

Clinical features	Deformity or rachitic change Diffuse bone pain and tenderness Generalized muscle weakness Vitamin D restriction Avoidance of sunlight Unusual dietary habits Malabsorption and steatorrhea Renal insufficiency Drugs—fluoride, diphosphonates
Laboratory findings suggestive of osteomalacia	Hypocalcemia Hypophosphatemia Increased alkaline phosphatase Low vitamin D levels Decreased 24-hour urinary excretion of calcium Elevated parathyroid hormone levels
Radiographic findings suggestive of osteomalacia	Bilaterally symmetric pseudofractures Pathologic fracture through midshaft of a major bone Bone mass—low, normal, or increased (osteosclerosis)

Table 38-9. Histology of osteomalacia

BONE FORMATION PARAMETERS

Osteoid excess common
Increased osteoid surfaces
Increased osteoid seam width

BONE-REMODELING ACTIVITY STATUS

	Pure osteomalacia	Mixed osteomalacia and osteitis fibrosa
Osteoblasts	Reduced	Normal-increased
Osteoclasts	Normal-decreased	Normal-increased
Resorption	Normal-decreased	Normal-increased
Fibrosis	Absent	Present

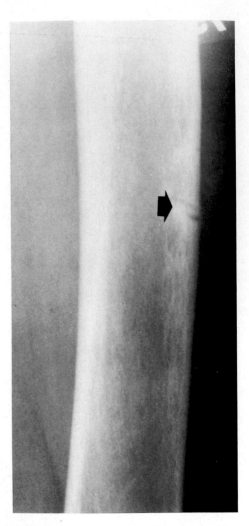

Fig. 38-75. Pseudofractures of the lateral aspect of the femur, *arrow,* shown in this radiograph are another characteristic radiographic change of osteomalacia.

ciuria, secondary hyperparathyroidism, and low levels of 25-OH-vitamin D should raise the possibility of osteomalacia. The diagnosis of osteomalacia may then be confirmed by biopsy.

Histologic features of osteomalacia. Histologically osteomalacia is usually characterized by excessive quantities of osteoid because of the failure of matrix calcification, despite continued matrix synthesis by the osteoblasts (Table 38-9 and Fig. 38-76). Pronounced increases in the thickness of the osteoid seams is characteristic, such that the seams are often greater than 24 μm in width, or as a rough guide, the seams exceed 4 collagen lamellae in thickness (Fig. 38-77). In addition to an increased width of seams, the total quantity of osteoid (that is, the osteoid volume) may be increased as a result of an increase in the osteoid surfaces, that is, the fraction of trabecular bone surfaces lined by osteoid. In severe cases of osteomalacia, the osteoid surface may exceed 60% and may even reach 100%, with the total trabecular surface enveloped by osteoid seams of abnormal thickness. Although osteomalacia is usually characterized by osteoid excess, osteomalacia may be associated with normal or even reduced quantities of osteoid. Because active osteoporosis is associated with increased quantities of osteoid, it may be indistinguishable from those milder cases of osteomalacia. In contrast to the static variables of bone formation (that is, osteoid surface, osteoid seam width, osteoblastic sur-

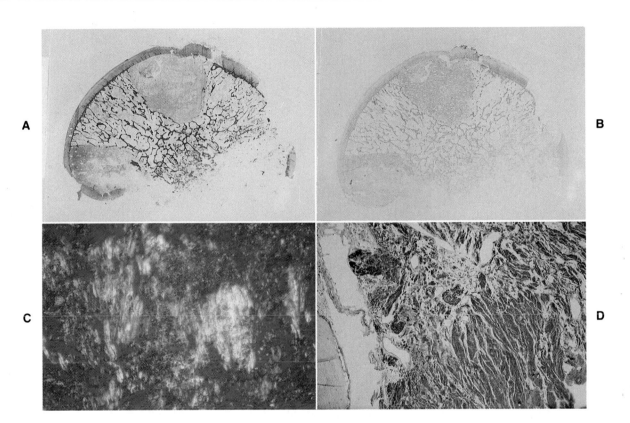

Plate 7. Beta₂-microglobulin amyloidosis of bone in chronic renal failure.

    A, Whole-mount section of resected femoral head for fracture of the femoral neck in a patient on chronic hemodialysis. The homogeneous pale areas represent amyloidomas of bone. (Hematoxylin and eosin stain.)

    B, Same section stained by the Congo Red technique for amyloid. The eosinophilic material seen on the hematoxylin and eosin stain in **A** is Congo Red positive.

    C, Polarized-light examination of the Congo Red–positive material from the femoral head exhibits the characteristic apple-green birefringence of amyloid.

    D, Immunoperoxidase stain for beta₂-microglobulin, the brown reaction product. The amyloid material reacts with antibodies directed against beta₂-microglobulin, resulting in the deposition of the brown reaction product.

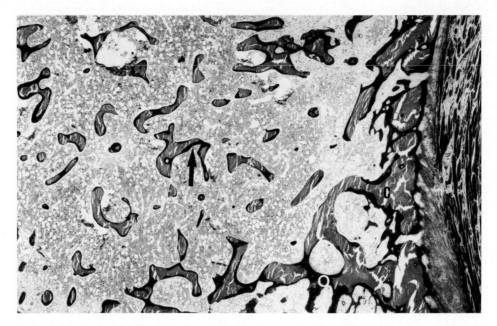

Fig. 38-76. Histologic features of osteomalacia. By low-power examination the quantity of dark-staining osteoid, *O,* is increased, *arrow.* Osteoid seams of increased thickness line the majority of the cortical, *C,* and trabecular bone surfaces.

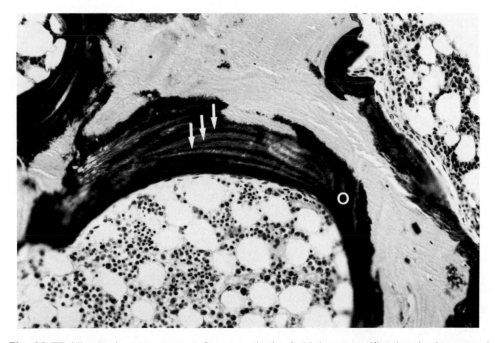

Fig. 38-77. Histologic appearance of osteomalacia. At higher magnification the increased thickness of the osteoid seams, *O,* is more apparent. Notice that the seam is greater than three or four collagen lamellae wide, *arrows.*

face), the interpretation of the in vivo bone marker tetracycline permits the evaluation of kinetic parameters of formation, which are the fraction of double tetracycline–labeled trabecular bone surface, the fraction of osteoid-labeled surfaces, and the rate of bone-matrix mineralization. As the degree of the mineralization defect increases, the percentage of the osteoid seams that bear normal tetracycline labels decreases (often below 20% to 40%). This is recognized by fluorescent microscopy either as osteoid surfaces that fail to assimilate tetracycline or as seams that are diffusely fluorescent (Fig. 38-78). Usually normal double tetracycline labels are absent, such that the fraction of double tetracycline–labeled trabecular bone surfaces is zero. In any double labels that may be recognized, the distance between the labels is reduced; that is, there is a reduction in the mineralization rate.

In summary, the static and dynamic parameters that characterize osteomalacia include an increase in the amount of osteoid and a reciprocal decrease in the rate of mineralization respectively. These two components allow one to distinguish osteomalacia from osteoporotic disorders in which the level of bone-remodeling activity produces an abnormal quantity of osteoid. In low-turnover states, such as inactive osteoporosis, the mineralization rate may be low (less than 0.5 μm/day or thin, discrete "single labels"), but the quantity of osteoid is appropriately reduced. If the mineralization rate is *not* found to be low (that is, more than 1 μm/day, or well-separated parallel bands of tetracycline, "double labels") the presence of a mineralization defect is unlikely, despite the presence of excess amounts of osteoid. (See Table 38-10.)

Although osteomalacia is usually associated with low bone-remodeling activity (that is, pure osteomalacia), there may be features of osteoblast activation, osteoclast proliferation, and peritrabecular fibrosis—all indicative of accelerated turnover. Histologically, osteomalacia may therefore be seen in the context of a mixed bone lesion, that is, defective mineralization coexisting with osteitis fibrosa, usually attributable to secondary hyperparathyroidism (Fig. 38-79). Osteomalacia may then be categorized morphologically as pure osteomalacia or mixed osteomalacia–osteitis fibrosa. The clinical conditions associated with these morphologic types of osteomalacia are shown in the list below:

Histology of specific osteomalacic diseases
I. Mixed osteomalacia
   1. Primary vitamin D deficiency
   2. Secondary vitamin D deficiency states
      a. Malabsorption states with steatorrhea
   3. Renal osteodystrophy
II. Pure osteomalacia
   1. Hypophosphatemic states
      a. X-linked hypophosphatemia
      b. Sporadic hypophosphatemia
      c. Oncogenic osteomalacia
   2. Hypophosphatasia
   3. Aluminum-associated osteomalacia
   4. Osteomalacia of fluorosis

One would predict that conditions that produce the mineralization defect by a mechanism that does not result in compensatory secondary hyperparathyroidism will appear as pure osteomalacia. These conditions are hypophosphatemic osteomalacia, hypophosphatasia, and drugs such as sodium fluoride (an antiosteoporosis drug) and diphosphonates (utilized in the therapy of Paget's disease of bone), which in excessive doses act as crystallization poisons. As is true with many forms of osteoporosis, the histologic features present in a biopsy specimen do not necessarily permit the morphologic differentiation of one clinical form of osteomalacia from another.

Specific forms of osteomalacia and rickets
Primary vitamin D deficiency

In healthy persons the minimum daily requirement of vitamin D necessary to prevent deficiency is just 10 μg (400 IU) for children and 2.5 μg (100 IU) for adults. Primary deficiency of vitamin D is generally found in persons who because of economic, social, or cultural factors do not receive sufficient exposure to sunlight, 5 to 20 minutes several times weekly, for adequate cutaneous synthesis of vitamin D_3 and whose diets do not contain sufficient foodstuffs fortified with vitamin D. Institutionalized patients, the poor, the elderly, food faddists, and some religious groups (because of diet and dress) are most likely to be affected. Infants who are breast fed generally receive adequate antirachitic sterol; however, babies who are bottle fed with nonfortified milk are likely to become vitamin D deficient.

Secondary vitamin D deficiency

Despite adequate solar exposure and a diet fortified in vitamin D, in some instances a deficiency of vitamin D may develop as a result of a variety of gastrointestinal, pancreatic, or hepatobiliary disorders. The mechanisms responsible for the vitamin D deficiency and deranged mineral metabolism are often complex.

Table 38-10. Histologic differential diagnosis—osteoporosis versus osteomalacia

	Osteoporosis	Osteomalacia
Osteoid volume	<4%	Often >20%
Osteoid seam width	<24 μm	Often >24 μm
	<3 lamellae wide	>4 lamellae wide
Tetracycline	Single and double labels	Unlabeled or diffusely labeled seams

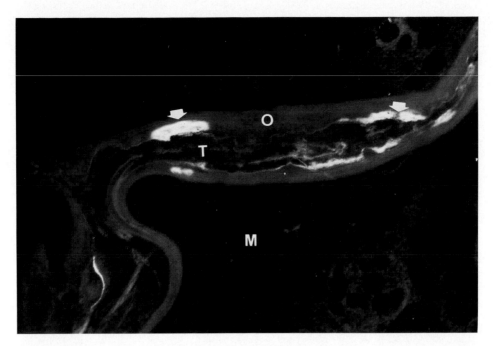

Fig. 38-78. Further histologic manifestations of osteomalacia. The tetracycline fluorescent pattern is abnormal and is diagnostic of osteomalacia. The trabecular bone, *T,* is lined by widened osteoid seams, *O,* which fail to exhibit normal double labels but instead exhibit either diffuse fluorescence, *arrows,* or fail to assimilate tetracycline and are therefore unlabeled.

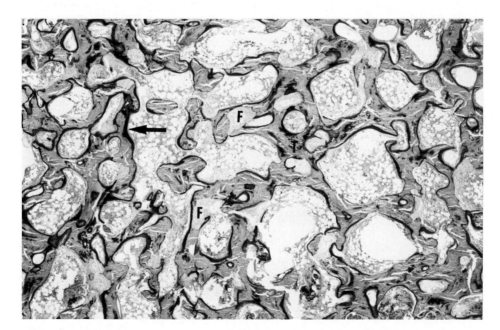

Fig. 38-79. Histologic appearance of mixed osteomalacia–osteitis fibrosa. Osteitis fibrosa is apparent from the presence of fibrous tissue, *F,* that lines the trabeculas, *T.* Also notice that the quantity of osteoid is also increased, *arrow.*

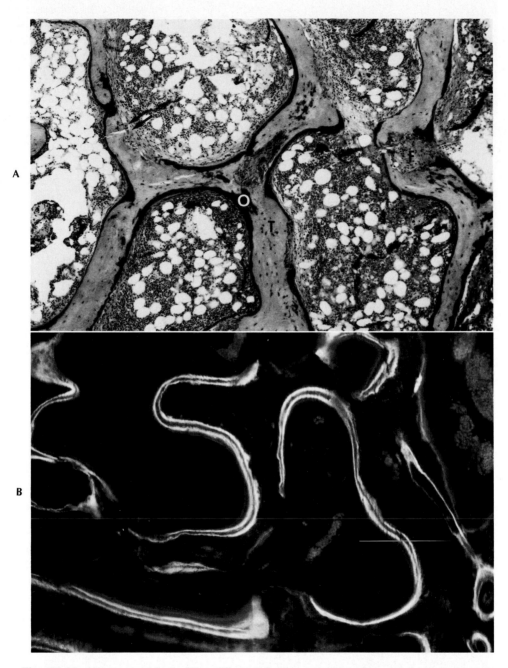

Fig. 38-80. Hyperosteoidosis. The differential diagnosis of accelerated turnover versus osteomalacia. **A,** By low-power examination the bone biopsy specimen exhibits trabecular bone, *T,* which is lined by an increased quantity of osteoid, *O,* and peritrabecular fibrous tissue, *F,* with increased osteoclastic activity, *arrows.* **B,** By fluorescence microscopy, the presence of numerous double tetracycline labels indicates a brisk rate of bone mineralization and therefore excludes the diagnosis of osteomalacia.

Vitamin D and its principle metabolite, 25-OH-vitamin D, are fat-soluble sterols that undergo enterohepatic circulation. Bile salts are necessary for their absorption; hence hepatobiliary disease or short bowel syndrome may result in steatorrhea and both the malabsorption of dietary vitamin D_3 and depletion of endogenous vitamin D_2 and D_3 stores. Malabsorption of vitamin D and calcium may however be selective and may not be reflected by the degree of steatorrhea, amount of small bowel disease, severity of pancreatic insufficiency, or duration of gastrointestinal disease.[63,74,132] Symptomatic osteomalacia in patients with gastrointestinal disease may occur with a paucity of clues. Furthermore in as many as two thirds of these patients there may be a reduction in bone volume (osteoporosis) rather than an increase in osteoid (osteomalacia). In these cases, a nondecalcified bone biopsy specimen of the tetracycline-labeled iliac crest may be required to confirm the presence of a mineralization defect.

Diagnosis of vitamin D deficiency

Measurement of circulating 25-OH-vitamin D, the lipid-soluble storage form of the vitamin, is useful when a diagnosis of vitamin D deficiency is not readily apparent from the routine medical history, physical examination, or biochemical and radiographic studies. Blood levels less than 6 ng/ml (normal 10 to 50 ng/ml) are considered diagnostic of vitamin D deficiency. The associated biochemical findings in classic vitamin D deficiency include a near-normal serum calcium and low serum phosphorus, both reflecting bone resorption and the renal phosphaturic effect of parathyroid hormone. In the face of falling serum calcium concentrations, homeostatic mechanisms attempt to preserve the normal extracellular calcium level at the expense of the skeleton. Histologically the bone exhibits a combination of osteomalacia and osteitis fibrosa, though the histologic changes may be variable and reflect the degree and duration of vitamin D deficiency. Milder forms of vitamin D deficiency may appear as high-turnover osteoporosis and not as osteomalacia because the mineralization defect may be ameliorated by compensatory secondary hyperparathyroidism (Fig. 38-80).

Impaired 25-hydroxylation related to anticonvulsant drug

Rickets and osteomalacia have been reported in institutionalized subjects with seizure disorders who are receiving anticonvulsant medication. This observation led to extensive studies of the effects of anticonvulsant drugs on mineral homeostasis. It was subsequently found that defective mineralization could be attributed to primary vitamin D deficiency caused by poor diets and lack of solar exposure. Double tetracycline–labeled bone biopsy specimens in ambulatory patients with epilepsy on chronic anticonvulsant therapy often fail to document osteomalacia and instead reveal evidence of secondary hyperparathyroidism. The unique direct effects of anticonvulsant drugs in decreasing target-organ responsiveness to calcium-regulating hormones results in drug-induced hypocalcemia.[67]

Impaired 25-hydroxylation with hepatic disease

Severe hepatic disease is usually not associated with osteomalacia. Low levels of 25-OH-vitamin D are probably attributable to nutritional vitamin D deficiency, limited sunlight exposure, or interruption of the enterohepatic circulation of vitamin D metabolites. Patients with primary biliary cirrhosis and alcoholic cirrhosis usually exhibit normal 25-hydroxylation capacity if supplied with adequate amounts of vitamin D substrate.

Vitamin D–dependent rickets, type I

Type I vitamin D–dependent rickets, a form of vitamin D resistance, is an autosomal recessive inborn error of vitamin D biosynthesis with defective conversion of 25-OH- to 1,25-$(OH)_2$-vitamin D. Physiologic doses of 1,25-$(OH)_2$-vitamin D cures the mineralization defect.[57]

Vitamin D–dependent rickets, type II

Type II vitamin D–dependent rickets, the true form of vitamin D resistance, is attributable to a defect in the target-organ sensitivity to 1,25-$(OH)_2$-vitamin D.[41,98,185] Sometimes associated with alopecia, this rare disorder may be sporadic or exhibit autosomal recessive inheritance. Therapy requires extremely high doses of calcitriol, 1,25-$(OH)_2$-vitamin D, which must surpass the endogenous serum levels to overcome the defective receptor binding.

Hypophosphatemic osteomalacia
X-linked hypophosphatemia

Familial hypophosphatemia is the most common cause of rickets in Western society. The disease is generally transmitted as an X-linked dominant trait, though approximately one third of the cases are sporadic.[30,32,34] The availability of the HYP mouse, an animal model of human hypophosphatemic osteomalacia, has provided insight into the pathogenesis and treatment of this disease.[114] The fundamental abnormality is defective renal conservation of phosphorus. Hence the diagnosis is generally based on the presence of diminished tubular reabsorption of phosphorus, despite low circulating levels. The clinical manifestations of familial hypophosphatemia often appear within the second year of life, with growth failure and bowing deformities of the legs. In

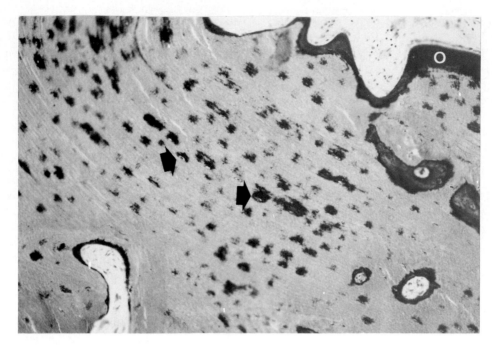

Fig. 38-81. Characteristic histologic appearance of the mineralization defect of vitamin D–resistant osteomalacia (X-linked hypophosphatasia). The quantity of osteoid is increased, *O*, but the accumulation of osteoid around osteocytic lacunae, *arrows*, is characteristic. (Goldner trichrome stained, undecalcified section.)

contrast to other forms of rickets, muscle weakness is uncommon, probably because the sarcolemmal intracytoplasmic phosphorus concentrations remain normal, despite phosphorus depletion. Radiographically, typical rachitic changes are present in the extremities, whereas the axial skeleton is relatively spared. With time osteosclerosis develops. Histologically the mass of mineralized trabecular bone is normal, whereas the quantity of osteoid is greatly increased. Tetracycline labeling confirms the presence of defective mineralization when the characteristic fluorescent patterns of osteomalacia are present. Osteomalacia is present without evidence of osteitis fibrosa, in the absence of associated secondary hyperparathyroidism, that is, pure osteomalacia. Although all these morphologic changes may occur in any form of osteomalacia, there is one specific histologic finding characteristic of X-linked hypophosphatemia. These patients exhibit a peculiar halo effect about the osteocytic lacunae (Fig. 38-81). This abnormality has been shown to reflect a defect in the mineralization of the most recently deposited periosteocytic osteoid.[25] Patients with X-linked hypophosphatemia appear to have a defect in the synthesis of the active metabolite of 1,25-$(OH)_2$-vitamin D, such that therapy with phosphorus and vitamin D improves the defective mineralization of the cartilage but does not alter the mineralization of osteoid. To reverse the component of osteomalacia in these patients, therapy with the 1,25-$(OH)_2$-metabolite of parent vitamin D and phosphorus is required.[64] The non–X linked forms of hypophosphatemic osteomalacia usually do not become apparent until adolescence, and therefore there is no history of rickets.[60] Unlike the X-linked counterpart, adult onset or sporadic hypophosphatemia is often associated with muscle weakness and aminoaciduria.

Oncogenic osteomalacia

Urinary phosphate wasting and osteomalacia are associated with a variety of benign and malignant neoplasms.[191] Like the X-linked form of hypophosphatemia, the levels of 1,25-dihydroxyvitamin D are usually low. Resection of the neoplasm will cure the mineralization defect and restore the serum phosphorus and sterol levels to normal.

Antacid-induced osteomalacia

Chronic consumption of excess aluminum-containing phosphorus-binding antacids can cause hypophosphatemic osteomalacia.[23,29] Bone pain and muscle weakness may be incapacitating, but the excessive use of antacids may be overlooked by the physician. Phosphorus depletion is characterized by hypophosphatemia, hypophosphaturia, hypercalciuria, and nephrolithiasis,[94] with increased intestinal calcium absorption mediated by increased 1,25-$(OH)_2$-vitamin D levels. The serum calcium level may be borderline elevated, and

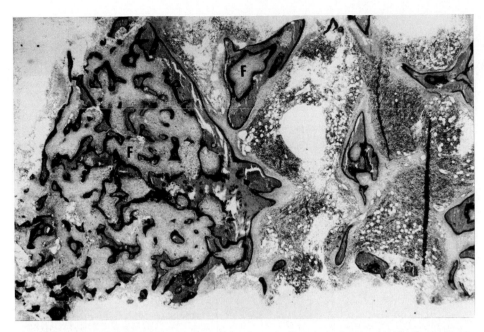

Fig. 38-82. Histologic appearance of mixed osteitis fibrosa–osteomalacia of renal osteodystrophy. Notice that the architecture is disrupted by the presence of advanced fibrous tissue deposition, *F*. In addition the quantity of dark-staining osteoid is also increased and nearly lines the majority of the bone surfaces.

the parathyroid hormone levels reciprocally lowered. Osteomalacia, as in other phosphate-depletion mineralization defects, is not accompanied by secondary hyperparathyroidism.

Renal osteodystrophy

Renal osteodystrophy is the generic term referring to the variety of skeletal and mineral abnormalities that attend chronic uremia. Before the advent of maintenance hemodialysis, the azotemic complications of renal failure overshadowed its skeletal effects. Now, however, virtually all uremic patients maintained on life-support systems have histologic evidence of bone disease. The prevalence and incidence of clinically evident or symptomatic bone disease is variable however.

The pattern of bone involvement in symptomatic patients with renal osteodystrophy may be categorized by histologic examination of bone tissue into three basic groups—pure osteomalacia, mixed osteomalacia–osteitis fibrosa, and pure osteitis fibrosa.[100,161,177]

Mixed osteomalacia–osteitis fibrosa

The pattern of bone disease called "mixed osteomalacia–osteitis fibrosa" is probably the most common histologic manifestation of renal osteodystrophy.[163] The pathogenesis of the mixed bone lesion is complex but probably results from aberrations of vitamin D metabolism with loss of production of the potent 1,25-dihy-

droxyvitamin D metabolite, phosphate retention resulting in hyperphosphatemia, hypocalcemia, and ultimately secondary hyperparathyroidism.[38,166,167] The advanced bone disease seen in symptomatic patients consists of severe disorganization of the trabecular bone architecture because of pronounced osteitis fibrosa (Fig. 38-82). Perhaps because of concurrent hypovitaminosis D, there may be a component of osteomalacia revealed by the presence of thick, broad osteoid seams, reflecting defective mineralization. However, since accelerated bone formation often exists with the osteitis fibrosa of secondary hyperparathyroidism, it may be difficult to predict how much of the osteoid within a sample of bone actually represents defective mineralization.[178] For this reason the interpretation of tetracycline fluorescent labels is critical. By fluorescent microscopy, the combination of osteomalacia and active bone formation is recognized by the coexistence of abnormal tetracycline labels (diffuse fluorescence or nonfluorescent osteoid seams) with normal double labels in osteoid seams in adjacent trabecular bone spicules (Fig. 38-83).

The presence of osteitis fibrosa in this patient group may be detected radiographically by the typical resorptive and cystic changes of hyperparathyroidism just discussed. The serum markers of bone metabolism, parathyroid hormone and alkaline phosphatase, also roughly correlate with the severity of osteitis fibrosa, but the

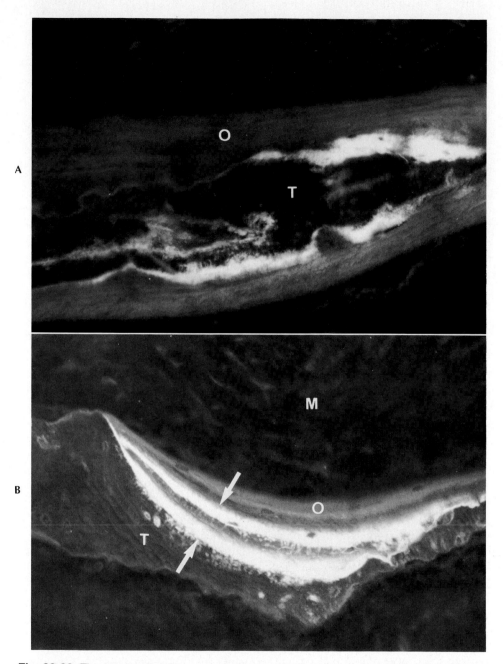

Fig. 38-83. The tetracycline fluorescent pattern of mixed form of renal osteodystrophy. **A,** Osteomalacia. Osteoid, *O,* lines the trabecular bone, *T,* and the deposition of tetracycline is abnormal, an indication of defective mineralization, that is, osteomalacia. **B,** Accelerated bone-remodeling activity. The trabecular bone, *T,* is lined by increased quantities of osteoid, *O;* however, these surfaces are undergoing normal mineralization, as revealed by the presence of double tetracycline labels, *arrows.*

degree of osteomalacia is difficult to establish without the aid of bone biopsy specimens.[82,182] Therapy for this form of renal bone disease is directed at reduction of the degree of secondary hyperparathyroidism, induced by hypocalcemia and hyperphosphatemia. Because parathyroidectomy may be required, establishing the correct diagnosis of this heterogeneous bone disease is critical.

Pure osteitis fibrosa

The osteitis fibrosa predominant form of renal osteodystrophy results from the metabolic complications of secondary hyperparathyroidism. Histologically there is little evidence of osteomalacia, since a mineralization defect may be confidently excluded by the presence of double tetracycline fluorescent label patterns.

Pure osteomalacia

The pure form of osteomalacia of renal osteodystrophy has been associated with the accumulation of aluminum in bone.[31,37] The retention of aluminum is attributable to the inability to excrete this metal in chronic renal insufficiency. Additionally, patients are simultaneously receiving orally administered aluminum-based phosphate-binding medications to minimize the dietary absorption of phosphate. Although the gastrointestinal absorption of aluminum is small, long-term therapy, coupled with the inability to excrete this ion, results in a steady accumulation of total body aluminum and the possible deposition of this ion in bone tissue. Utilizing special stains, one may see aluminum deposited at the mineralization fronts, the interface between the osteoid seam and the mineralized bone surface, and may somehow prevent subsequent calcification of the matrix. In addition aluminum has been found to suppress osteoblastic activity and directly inhibit the secretion of parathyroid hormone from the parathyroid glands.[4,165]

The most important bone biopsy finding is decreased mineralization with osteoid accumulation and the demonstration of aluminum deposition (Fig. 38-84). Although peritrabecular fibrosis is frequently seen in dialysis patients with secondary hyperparathyroidism, it is less common in those with aluminum-associated bone disease for the reasons already discussed. Deferoxamine, the iron-chelating agent, will also bind aluminum and has been successfully used in the treatment of this form of osteomalacia.[5,125] As aluminum is removed from the bone, normal bone mineralization can be demonstrated after chelation therapy.

Osteosclerosis of renal osteodystrophy

Osteosclerosis, an increased matrix volume per unit volume of whole bone, is also a very common but usually clinically silent form of renal osteodystrophy.[21] Ra-

diographically, osteosclerotic patients exhibit a "rugger-jersey spine" caused by the alternating bands of bone with increased and normal density (Fig. 38-85). Pathologically the trabeculas are widened and covered by thick osteoid seams (Fig. 38-86).

Hypophosphatasia

Hypophosphatasia, a rare heritable metabolic bone disease, is characterized by subnormal circulating alkaline phosphatase activity, increased blood and urine levels of the enzyme substrates phosphoethanolamine and pyrophosphate, dental abnormalities, and defective skeletal mineralization that can present as rickets in children and osteomalacia in adults. Depending on the age at which skeletal disease is first noted, hypophosphatasia is classified into three forms—infantile, childhood, and adult.[47,196]

Infantile hypophosphatasia manifests before 6 months of age. Clinical problems are severe and include growth failure and rachitic skeletal deformities. Deformities of the thorax predispose affected infants to recurrent pneumonia, and skull involvement results in synostosis with complications of increased intracranial pressure. Hypercalcemia caused by the failure of the skeleton to deposit mineral leads to hypercalcemia, hypercalciuria, nephrocalcinosis, and renal insufficiency. This form is inherited as an autosomal recessive trait and is often fatal.

Childhood hypophosphatasia may present after 6 months of age with a variable but generally more benign clinical course than the infantile form. Premature loss of deciduous teeth because of poor calcification of the developing tooth and alveolar bone is the most consistent clinical sign and may be associated with rachitic skeletal defects, which may show spontaneous improvement. The pattern of inheritance is less well defined, but studies have suggested either autosomal recessive or autosomal dominant transmission.

Adult hypophosphatasia is the least severe form. Clinically affected patients may give a history of premature loss of deciduous teeth, rachitic deformity, or both, in childhood. Usually the disorder begins with the loss of adult teeth and is followed by recurrent fractures secondary to osteomalacia. Autosomal dominant inheritance with variable penetrance has been described.

The combination of low circulating alkaline phosphatase activity and deficient osteoblast alkaline phosphatase activity by histochemical staining, coupled with the presence of abnormal mineralization, provides strong circumstantial evidence for a role of alkaline phosphatase in normal skeletal mineralization. In adult hypophosphatasia the magnitude of the mineralization defect is proportional to the deficiency of enzyme activity. De-

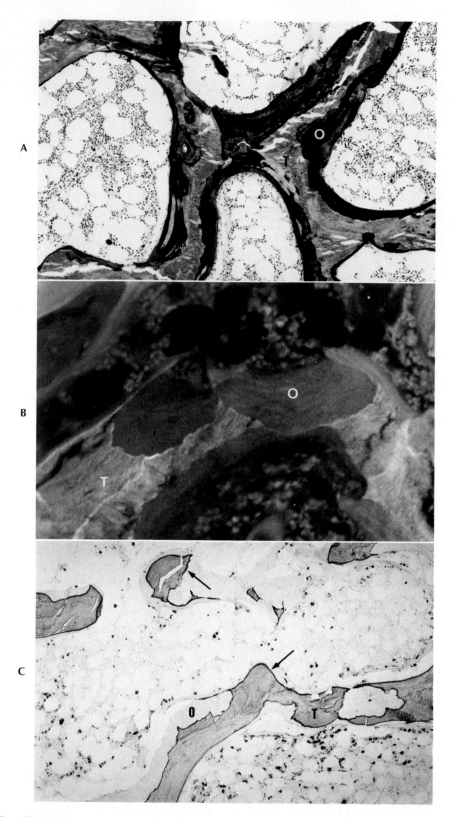

Fig. 38-84. Pure osteomalacia of renal osteodystrophy, aluminum associated. **A,** The trichrome-stained section of bone shows osteomalacia without evidence of osteitis fibrosa. The trabecular bone, *T,* is lined by a vast quantity of dark-staining osteoid, *O.* **B,** The tetracycline fluorescence micrograph demonstrates trabecular bone, *T,* containing large quantities of osteoid, *O,* which fail to assimilate normal tetracycline labels, resulting in an absence of fluorescence. **C,** Positive aluminum-staining reaction. The aluminum reaction product, *arrows,* binds at the osteoid seam, *O,* and trabecular bone, *T,* interface.

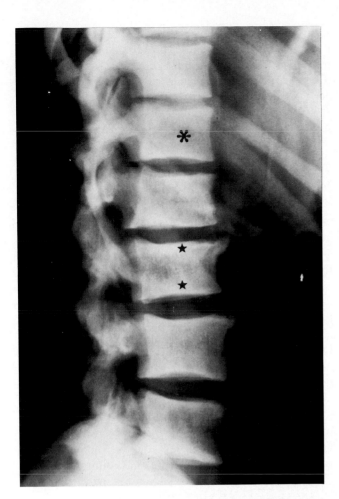

Fig. 38-85. Characteristic radiographic appearance of osteosclerotic renal osteodystrophy is shown on this lateral lumbar spine radiograph. The typical "rugger-jersey" spine is created by the impression of alternating dense (★) and lighter, more radiolucent (*) bands of bone.

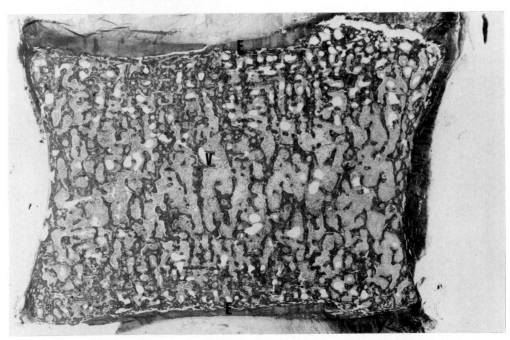

Fig. 38-86. Histologic correlate of the rugger-jersey spine of osteosclerotic renal osteodystrophy. This whole-mount histologic section of a lumbar vertebra shows an accumulation of denser bone toward the end plates of the vertebral body, E, with a relative sparing of the central vertebral, V, area. Notice that the marrow is almost completely replaced by fibrous tissue, an indication of a component of osteitis fibrosa.

fective mineralization may involve the failure of alkaline phosphatase to hydrolyze inorganic pyrophosphates and other endogenous inhibitors of bone mineralization. Progressive failure of the skeletal tissues to mineralize in infantile hypophosphatasia results in the typical rachitic deformities, edentia, and hypercalcemia.

Beta₂-microglobulin amyloid bone disease in chronic hemodialysis

Several of the musculoskeletal complications of long-term (over 10 years) hemodialysis—nerve-entrapment syndromes, synovitis, bursitis, and destructive arthropathies—have been attributed to the deposition of a new type of dialysis-associated amyloid, which has been shown to be beta₂-microglobulin.[6] Amyloid bone lesions, however, are relatively uncommon but have previously been associated with plasma cell dyscrasias and rarely in association with secondary amyloidosis.

Beta₂-microglobulin is an 11,800-dalton protein that is noncovalently associated with the human lymphocyte class I antigens on the cell surface. It possesses a beta structure believed to be essential for amyloid formation and has a significant structural homology with the IgG constant region. The protein circulates in monomer form and is freely filtered at the glomerulus, resorbed, and degraded in the renal tubules. This protein, however, is not cleared from the blood during conventional hemodialysis, and greatly elevated levels may be seen in patients chronically on hemodialysis. Recently pathologic fractures through long bones and containing amyloid deposits have been reported. The fracture sites have been found to contain Congo Red–staining, amorphous material that produces the characteristic apple-green birefringence upon polarized-light examination. These marrow mass–occupying lesions can be shown to be composed of beta₂-microglobulin by immunoperoxidase-staining techniques (Plate 7).

TRAUMA
Fracture repair

In response to trauma, the skeleton attempts to restore functional and anatomic integrity. The general principles of the repair process are not unique to bone, and as for any injured tissue, bone also requires that the adult tissue revert to the basic undifferentiated mesenchymal tissue, the blastema, with subsequent wound closure and scar formation. What is unusual for bone, however, is the fact that the scar tissue of bone is bone, and, as such, repair of any skeletal tissue may be thought of as a recapitulation of many of the steps of normal bone development and growth. Fracture repair may be thought of as a microcosm of endochondral and membranous bone formation occurring within the stabilizing skeletal wound tissue, referred to as "callus," which is ultimately modeled into normal bone.[71] Analogous to growing bone, the callus is dynamic and undergoes structural change rapidly. Callus is composed of fibrous tissue, woven bone, and cartilage (Fig. 38-

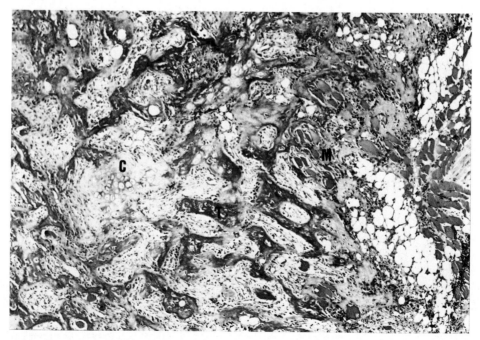

Fig. 38-87. Early fracture repair with immature callus formation. A rich mesenchymal proliferation with trilineage differentiation, which includes cartilage, *C*, mineralized trabecular bone, *T*, and fibrous tissue. *M*, Trapped skeletal muscle.

87). All these components are derived from a common endosteal or periosteal progenitor cell. Mechanical stress and oxygen tension are important in determining whether these cells differentiate into osteoblasts or chondroblasts. For example, intermittent stress favors cartilage formation.[9] Suitably immobilized fractures exhibit predominantly membranous bone formation, whereas endochondral bone formation occurs in free fractures. Fracture healing may be divided into three general phases: inflammatory, reparative, and modeling. The inflammatory phase begins after the moment of trauma, and as for other inflammatory processes occurring elsewhere in the body, cellular and vascular events are recognized. Trauma sufficient to cause a fracture of bone also damages the overlying muscle, tendon, periosteum, associated blood vessels, and marrow, resulting in hematoma formation. During the first 5 days, the necrotic and damaged tissue generates an inflammatory cellular response. Surviving cells and new mesenchymal cells brought in by the ingrowth of granulation tissue create the blastema. The granulation tissue invades and eventually replaces ("organizes") the hematoma. A rich vascular network develops around the fracture zone. Peripherally, reactive hyperemia is present as blood flow around the fracture increases. Centrally in the region of injury, dilated capillary spaces become engorged with blood, and with stasis passive congestion develops. In the congested central region osteoid secretion is stimulated by osteoblasts arising from the blastema. Immature woven bone is deposited, and the first signs of mineralization are visible radiographically after 14 days. The development of this primitive tissue from the blastema represents the primary callus.

Reparative phase

The second stage of fracture healing is characterized by the more orderly secretion of callus, the removal and replacement of the immature woven bone by more mature bone through the process of cartilage differentiation, and endochondral ossification. Several types of callus have been identified and named, primarily by their location in the healing bone, and should not be considered as separate entities with distinct functions. A buttressing callus is adjacent to the outer cortical surface and is formed by the periosteum and skeletal muscle. A sealing callus fills the medullary cavity, and the cellular elements arise from the marrow in order to seal the fracture site. A bridging callus unites the gap between the two buttressed ends. The uniting callus joins the cortical portions of the fractured bone. Clinical union is achieved when the callus is sufficiently developed to allow weight bearing or similar stress, usually at around 4 weeks after injury. The fracture will continue to strengthen during the modeling phase.

Modeling phase

The modeling phase involves the realignment and mechanical shaping of the bone and callus along lines of stress. Extra bone is deposited in stress lines, and bone is removed in areas in which stress is not applied according to the postulates of Wolff's law. This final stage of fracture healing results in the restoration of the medullary cavity and bone marrow. Clinical healing will precede anatomic reconstitution. Extensive modeling will occur for years, and anatomic reconstitution will usually occur as a consequence of extensive osteoclastic resorption and osteoblast formation of bone according to the mechanical demands of that bone. Exact replacement of the fractured bone fragments is not required for complete healing therefore.

The sequence of events in the healing of a fracture are of practical consequence in the subsequent management of patients with fractures. Although the hematoma is not essential for fracture healing, the hematoma plays a metabolic role in inducing granulation tissue formation. The greater the degree of hematoma formation, the greater the response in inducing a more cellular and robust callus. The hematoma therefore should not be disturbed. Large necrotic bone fragments will have to be removed by osteoclastic activity and may impede callus formation. Large sequestered bone fragments may require surgical removal. The injury itself induces a vascular response, which results in the increased vascularity to the damaged area, and, by the subsequent metabolic changes, promotes callus formation. Skeletal muscle is richly vascular and contributes extensively to the development of the callus. Injured soft tissue therefore should not be disturbed. Poor fracture healing, in fact, occurs in those superficial bones with little or no adjacent musculature, such as the tibia.

Complications of fracture healing

Nonunions. The healing times for the majority of patients with fractures is suprisingly uniform. When fractures require longer than the usual time to heal but show signs of progressive healing, a delayed union is said to exist. A nonunion is present when the fracture remains unhealed and shows no signs of further healing (Fig. 38-88). There are numerous factors that may contribute to delayed or nonunion, such as location of the fracture, soft-tissue damage, tissue interposition, bone loss, and wound contamination or infection. The incidence of delayed union is unknown, but the incidence of nonunion is estimated at 5% of all long bone fractures. Bones of the axial skeleton, the skull, ribs, vertebrae, scapulae, and pelvis rarely exhibit nonunion.

Fibrous union. Bones with relatively poor blood supply and little associated subcutaneous tissue and muscle, such as the distal pretibia and carpal navicular bone, have difficulty in establishing the normal vascular

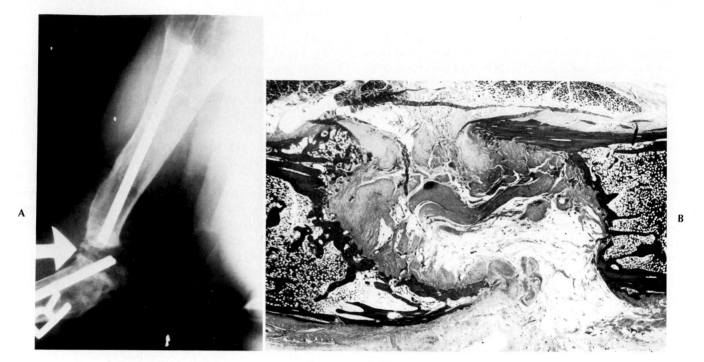

Fig. 38-88. A, Nonunion of fracture of humerus. **B,** Fracture site has resulted in fibrous union, and no evidence of reparative changes remains. Medulla of each fractured bone end is enclosed by osseous plate into which dense connective tissue bundles insert. (**A,** Courtesy Dr. Jerome Gilden, St. Louis, Mo.; **B,** 9×.)

network at the fracture zone. Poor blood supply to a fracture site promotes primitive scar tissue rather than callus. The bridge between the two fractured bone fragments is consequently filled by an avascular fibrous connective tissue rather than the usual bone and cartilage elements of a callus. Electrical stimulation to the fracture site has had a dramatic improvement in response to treatment of these fibrous nonunions.[15]

Pseudarthrosis. If a fracture is not adequately immobilized, motion between the two fractured ends persists, and the small blood vessels that do grow into the fracture zone are often sheared. The callus is therefore poorly vascularized, and the lower oxygen concentration favors cartilage differentiation, rather than bone. Continued motion results in myxoid degeneration and liquefaction of the callus cartilage, with the formation of a pseudojoint cavity, which often exhibits a synovial lining. The pseudarthrosis, or false joint, can only be reversed by refracture of the area, removal of the cartilage, and reestablishment of the vascular network, with new callus formation.

INFLAMMATORY DISORDERS OF THE SKELETON

Inflammation is the general protective response of the body toward injury. In response to biologic, chemical, or physical agents, a stereotyped response involv-

ing cellular, humoral, and vascular responses occurs, aimed at destroying or removing the injurious agent and repairing the damaged tissue. With increased vascular permeability and blood flow, transudation of plasma proteins occurs, resulting in edema. Cellular infiltration of the fluid by leukocytes occurs, and degenerating cellular debris contributes to the formation of an exudate. The acute inflammatory response is followed by a more prolonged proliferative phase of chronic inflammation, characterized by the replacement of the polymorphonuclear leukocytes by lymphocytes, monocytes, plasma cells, and fibrous tissue. The inflammatory response in bone is basically similar to that in other tissues; however there are factors peculiar to bone that alter the usual course of the inflammatory process.

Infection is a subtype of inflammation produced when tissue is invaded by biologic agents—viruses, bacteria, fungi, or protozoa. Infection of the bone (*osteo-*) and marrow (*myelo-*) is termed "osteomyelitis." Osteomyelitis may be classified according to several factors, including (1) the duration—acute, subacute, or chronic; (2) nature of the exudate—hemorrhagic, purulent, or nonsuppurative; (3) location—bone, periosteum, or epiphysis; and (4) etiologic agent—*Staphylococcus aureus, Mycobacterium tuberculosis,* and so on.

Inflammation in bone, as elsewhere, begins by an in-

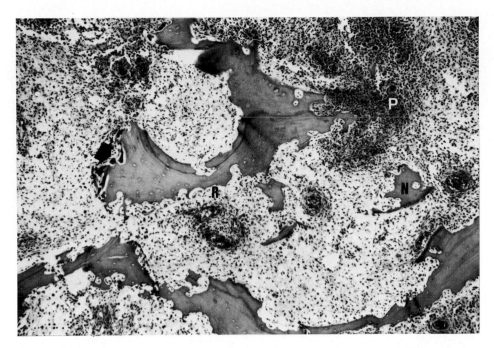

Fig. 38-89. Osteomyelitis, histologic appearance. Necrotic bone, *N*, and bone undergoing extensive resorption, *R*, by osteoclasts, *arrow*, is adjacent to the purulent, *P*, inflammatory infiltrate of the infectious process.

sult to the tissue and is followed by vascular and cellular responses. This process is modified by the rigid wall of the bony cortex and by the baffle system created by the trabeculas of the cancellous bone. Increased tissue pressure cannot be dissipated into the soft tissue, and consequently the traditional swelling, or "tumor," component of the inflammatory triad is lacking. As a result of increased intramedullary pressure there is compression of the capillaries and sinusoids of the marrow, producing infarction of the marrow fat, hematopoietic elements, and bone. At the edge of the infarction, there is active hyperemia. This increased blood flow is associated with increased osteoclastic activity, resulting in the removal of bone and localized osteoporosis (Fig. 38-89). An inflammatory exudate will gather at the margin of the infarcted zone. The inflammatory process penetrates through the cortex into the subperiosteal area through Volkmann's canals. In infants and older children the periosteum has very few anchoring fibers (Sharpey's fibers), and consequently the periosteum is readily stripped from the bone surface by increased periosteal pressure. This results in the disruption of the periosteal component of the blood supply to the cortex, producing cortical bone infarction. The cortical bone infarction results in the formation of the classical sequestrum. The isolated or sequestered bone will retain its original radiographic density until revascularization takes place and osteoclastic activity may ensue. A rim of reactive new bone, or involucrum, will be formed by

the periosteum around the dead (sequestered) fragment (Fig. 38-90).

Histologically, acute osteomyelitis will exhibit the features typically associated with acute inflammation (Fig. 38-89). The most sensitive indicator of skeletal disease will be the loss of the normal marrow tissue architecture. Normal hematopoietic elements and fat are replaced by the leukocytic infiltrate. The nature of the leukocytic infiltrate may vary with the type of infection, but generally polymorphonuclear leukocytes are found. A fibrous wall will be created to sequester the infarcted areas and a chronic inflammatory cell infiltrate will ultimately predominate. Small collections of polymorphonuclear leukocytes however will persist as microabscesses, and on a histologic basis the designation of acute versus chronic osteomyelitis is not meaningful.

The goals of therapy are to reduce the intraosseous pressure and to prevent infarction. In principle, this is accomplished by drainage and specific therapy against the particular etiologic agent. Antibiotics however have a limited effectiveness against organisms harbored within either abscess cavities or infarcted tissue. Despite rigorous antibiotic therapy, recurrent infections are the rule, particularly with *Staphylococcus aureus* infections. Ultimately the osteomyelitis heals, and because the scar tissue of bone is bone, fibrous tissue is replaced by dense bone. The disease process may be chronic from the outset, with a sharply localized reaction to the inflammatory stimulus and without the usual

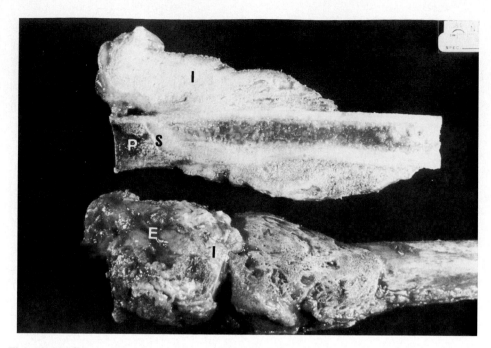

Fig. 38-90. Gross appearance of osteomyelitis. The cut surface, *above,* and the external surface, *below,* of a tibia removed for chronic infection are shown. *E,* Exudate, which is draining from sinus tracts to the surface of the bone; *I,* involucrum, composed of sclerotic, dense reactive new bone; *S,* sequestrum of the retained necrotic bone fragment adjacent to the purulent exudate, *P.*

abscess formation. In these rare instances, the only findings are dense, scarred bone with few clinical symptoms. This silent condition with radiographic evidence of new bone formation is termed "chronic sclerosing osteomyelitis of Garré." Osteomyelitis may also be sharply limited to one site with the formation of an abscess cavity surrounded by a rim of sclerotic bone, a condition referred to as a Brodie's abscess.

Mechanism of infection

Direct bone infection. The incidence of osteomyelitis attributable to direct bone infection has increased recently because of the great rise in the number of traumatic accidents and by the use of more invasive orthopedic procedures (intramedullary rods, open reduction, and prosthetic devices).[143] Osteomyelitis of the lower extremity in peripheral vascular disease, mostly of elderly patients with diabetes, now accounts for a large fraction of the cases of adult osteomyelitis.

Hematogenous osteomyelitis. The pattern of hematogenous osteomyelitis varies significantly with the age of the patient, in part because of the well-recognized age-dependent vascular patterns of bone throughout life.[184]

Infantile osteomyelitis. Infantile and neonatal osteomyelitis has been increasing in frequency as current an-

tibiotic therapy has prevented mortality from neonatal sepsis but has not necessarily prevented some of the sequelae. The cortical bone of the neonate and infant is thin and loose, consisting predominantly of woven bone, which permits the escape of pressure but promotes the rapid spread of the infection directly into the subperiosteal region. The large sequestrum formation is therefore not produced because extensive infarction of the cortex will not occur. Nevertheless, a generous involucrum of reactive bone forms around the subperiosteal abscess.

Childhood osteomyelitis. Classical hematogenous osteomyelitis occurs during the years of rapid skeletal growth and not unexpectedly localizes primarily within the metaphysis of the long bones. Because the metaphyseal cortex is very thin during the growth period, infection extends to the adjacent periosteum.[119]

Adult osteomyelitis. Acute hematogenous osteomyelitis of the long bone of an adult is uncommon. Adult osteomyelitis localizes within the cancellous bones, particularly the lumbar and thoracic areas of the spine. The infectious process, as in tuberculosis, starts in the vertebral body near an intervertebral disc. The disc soon becomes involved and radiologically appears narrowed.[91]

Bacterial osteomyelitis. The etiologic agent for all

types of osteomyelitis is coagulase-positive *Staphylococcus* (60% to 90%). The second most common organism, particularly among infants, is *Streptococcus. Pneumococcus, Escherichia coli, Klebsiella, Salmonella,* and *Bacteroides* are also occasionally isolated in instances of hematogenous osteomyelitis. In postoperative and osteomyelitis contracted by contiguous spread, *Staphylococcus, Streptococcus, Pseudomonas, Proteus,* and *E. coli* are often encountered.

Salmonella osteomyelitis. Osteomyelitis occurring after typhoid fever may arise in about 1% of those patients. The most important association however exists between *Salmonella* osteomyelitis and patients with hemoglobinopathies. In sickle cell anemia, focal necrosis and infarction of bone is common after a sickle cell crisis. The exact mechanism and reason for the *Salmonella* bacteremia however remains unclear. For some reason, *Salmonella* organisms have an unusual predilection for the bone marrow in these patients. The hand-and-foot syndrome consists in the infarction of the small bones of the hands and feet, followed by *Salmonella* osteomyelitis. In some instances, *Salmonella* organisms appear to inhibit the systemic granulocyte response, producing leukopenia. Within bone the lack of polymorphonuclear leukocytes combined with a pronounced lymphocytic-plasmacytic response, the inflammatory response, may be mistaken for multiple myeloma.

Fungal osteomyelitis. In contrast to bacterial osteomyelitis, fungal osteomyelitis is rare. However, when systemic dissemination of a fungal infection occurs, the skeleton may be seeded. The portal of entry is usually the respiratory tract, and organisms reach the bone through the circulation. Although any bone may be involved, there is a predilection for the small bones of the hands and feet. The tissue response is a chronic suppurative inflammation with granuloma formation. Since the granulomatous reaction is nonspecific, identification of the organism is essential for confirming the diagnosis. Organisms that have been associated with fungal osteomyelitis produce the following pathoses: coccidioidomycosis, blastomycosis, paracoccidioidomycosis, cryptococcosis, histoplasmosis, sporotrichosis, mucor, actinomycosis, and nocardiosis.

Syphilis

The incidence of syphilis has decreased steadily during the twentieth century, such that it no longer poses a major public health hazard. The use of penicillin has arrested the disease process early, such that tertiary manifestations in bone are only rarely encountered.

The causative agent is *Treponema pallidum*, which induces an angiitis of vasa vasorum, or small arterioles. This endarteritis produces necrosis of the vessel wall

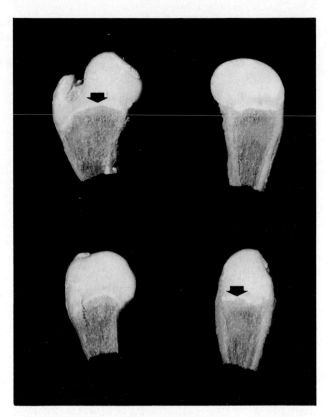

Fig. 38-91. Congenital syphilis of bone, with cut surface of the gross specimens being shown. The calcified cartilage of the growth plates persists because bone fails to form and appears as a dense band, *arrows.*

with subsequent infarction of the tissue supplied by that vessel. The result is a gumma, a focus of coagulative-infarctive necrosis surrounded by an infiltrate of plasma cells and leukocytes. This perivascular distribution of the infiltrate is characteristic of syphilis. Congenital syphilis follows spirochetemia of the mother, resulting in an intrauterine fetal infection. The spirochetes lodge in the metaphysis, within the epiphyseal growth-plate vessels. The normal vascular sprouts are replaced by syphilitic granulation tissue. This inflammatory process interferes with endochondral bone formation, and consequently the primary spongiosa are reduced or absent. The calcified cartilage matrix is deposited but persists as bone fails to form (Fig. 38-91). This type of cartilage will result in the characteristic radiographic appearance of a lucent line in the metaphysis below the densely calcified cartilaginous band at the growth plate.

In congenital as well as acquired syphilis, the periosteum is often involved. A perivascular plasma cell infiltrate, with fibrosis, stimulates reactive new bone formation. The subperiosteal portion of the entire bone shaft becomes progressively thickened, resulting in the formation of so-called saber shins. By a similar mechanism, hyperostosis may also occur in the clavicles and skull.

Tuberculosis

The tubercle bacillus, *Mycobacterium tuberculosis*, is a nonmotile organism that prefers areas of high oxygen pressure. The hematogenously spread organisms therefore commonly lodge in the synovium, producing an erosive deforming arthritis, and, through the common blood supply, involve the associated epiphyseal and metaphyseal portion of the bones on either side of the joint. The granulomatous inflammatory reaction to the organisms with the associated caseating necrosis often involves the subchondral portion of a joint, replacing the trabecular bone support so that destruction of the contiguous articular surface results. With continued inflammatory destruction there is sequestrum formation of the subchondral bone and articular cartilage, which

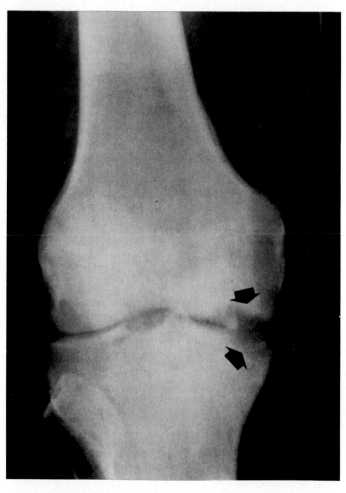

Fig. 38-92. Radiographic appearance of tuberculous arthritis. The medial portions of the bones on either side of this knee joint are involved and result in the formation of "kissing sequestra," *arrows*.

may occur on both sides of the involved joint, resulting in the formation of "kissing sequestrum" (Fig. 38-92). The increased vascularity associated with the inflammatory process results in the formation of localized osteoporosis, a bone loss that is often out of proportion to the degree of associated infection. A very common location for skeletal tuberculosis is involvement of the spine (Pott's disease). The infection is not contained to one vertebral body but rather spreads to involve adjacent discs and the spinal canal and ultimately results in soft-tissue extension and fistula formation.[33,92,124]

Idiopathic inflammatory disease of bone

Sarcoidosis is a noncaseating granulomatous process presenting in the skeleton as small lytic and sclerotic foci in the bones of the hand. Large areas of destruction as seen in tuberculosis are not typically found in sarcoidosis. Sarcoidosis is considered in the differential diagnosis of all granulomatous inflammatory reactions.

Paget's disease of bone, or osteitis deformans

Paget's disease of bone (osteitis deformans) is a common, chronic osteolytic and osteosclerotic disease of uncertain cause that may involve one or more bones and results in pain, skeletal deformities, and occasionally sarcomatous transformation. Over 100 years ago, Sir James Paget described the 20-year clinical course and autopsy findings of a man who suffered from an apparently rare, progressively deforming bone disease.[126]

The increasingly routine application of serum chemical assays (alkaline phosphatase) and widespread availability and utilization of diagnostic radiology has resulted in the frequent detection of patients with limited skeletal involvement and asymptomatic Paget's disease of bone. It became apparent that Paget's disease is not rare and afflicts approximately 3% of the white population over 40 years of age. The incidence increases with age, with males more frequently affected than females. Most patients (80% to 90%) are asymptomatic. Unfortunately one cannot predict which patients will experience progression of their disease.[28] Symptoms include deformity, fracture, deafness, and arthritis. Although many bones may be affected (that is, a polyostotic manifestation), involvement is typically asymmetric, or limited to one bone (that is, monostotic). The hematopoietically active flat bones and acral areas of the long bones (the sacrum, spine, pelvis, skull, femurs, clavicles, tibias, ribs, and humeri) are common skeletal sites of involvement.

There are many reports of familial clustering of Paget's disease, whereby several siblings of one family or various members of several generations of a given family may be affected.

Histopathology

Paget's disease may be divided into three phases—an active resorptive phase, an active formation phase, and a quiescent, inactive phase. Paget's disease is initiated by the replacement of normal marrow by a richly vascular, loose fibrous connective tissue. Isolated clusters of chronic inflammatory cells may be seen. Osteoclasts congregate on the existing bone trabeculas and within the cortex, resulting in the formation of large resorbing fronts (Fig. 38-93). The osteoclasts are morphologically abnormal, with many attaining enormous proportions, and each may contain an excessive number of nuclei, as many as 100 per cell (Fig. 38-94).

After the wave of osteoclastic activity there is an activation of osteoblastic activity. The newly formed bone is woven. Repeated episodes of removal and formation results in innumerable small irregularly shaped bone fragments that appear joined together in a chaotic jigsaw or mosaic pattern, the histologic hallmark of Paget's disease (Fig. 38-95). As the disease progresses, the osteoblastic phase dominates. As excessive formation occurs, bone becomes more compact and dense (Fig. 38-95), but structurally and morphologically this tissue is abnormal. Grossly it resembles the gritty but brittle texture of pumice or lava rock (Fig. 38-96). Radiologically this formation results in a flocculant, radiopaque

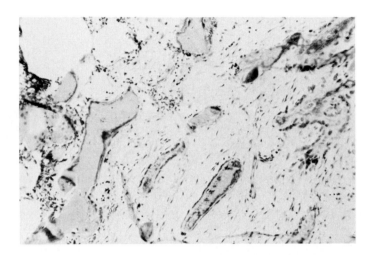

Fig. 38-93. Mixed phase of Paget's disease. There are numerous osteoclasts and osteoblasts. Marrow has myxomatous appearance, and woven bone is present. (Undecalcified, Goldner's stain; 100×.)

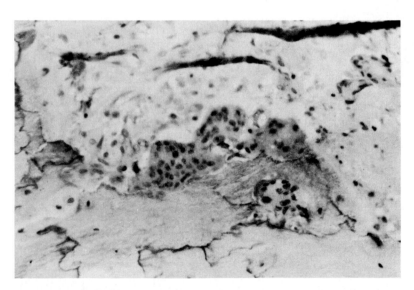

Fig. 38-94. Pagetic osteoclasts containing large numbers of nuclei distributed throughout cytoplasm. (Undecalcified, toluidine blue; 250×.)

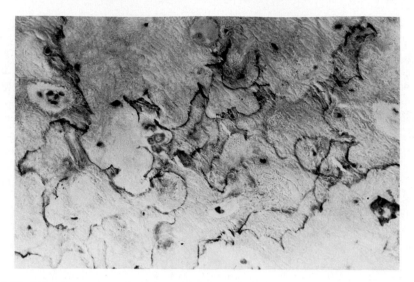

Fig. 38-95. Mosaic pattern of cement lines characteristic of sclerotic phase of Paget's disease. (Undecalcified, toluidine blue; 100 ×.)

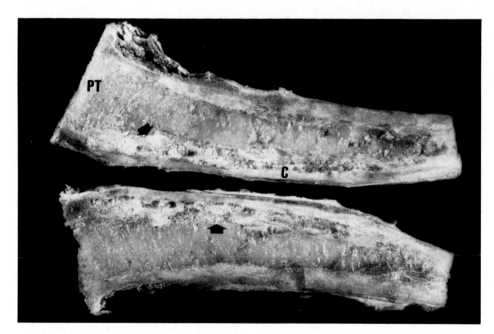

Fig. 38-96. Gross appearance of pagetic bone. The sagittal section of this proximal tibial bone, *PT,* shows dense deposits of new bone with the consistency of lava rock, hence the term "pumice bone," *arrows.* In addition, as is characteristic, the entire bone shaft is enlarged, the cortex is thickened, *C,* and there is anterior bowing.

deposit that has been likened to cotton wool (Fig. 38-97). The remaining trabeculas become thicker, or more dense, since the width of trabecular spicules oriented along lines of stress is augmented. The cortical bone becomes irregularly thickened as the overall size of the bone increases. The cortical trabecular bone junction at the endosteum becomes indistinct. The clinical and radiographic features are easily derived, given this underlying pathologic process. In addition to pain, a common complication of Paget's disease is deformity, manifested as either bowing of a weight-bearing long bone or enlargement of the skull (Fig. 38-98). Hypervascularity with gross dilatation of the superficial vessels in bone was originally described by Paget, and increased blood

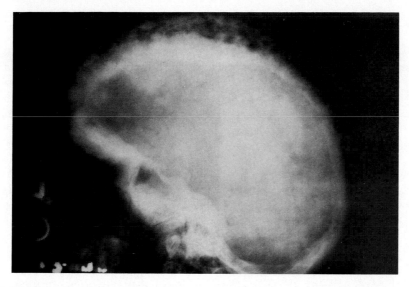

Fig. 38-97. Pagetic skull with characteristic "cotton-ball" appearance. (Courtesy Dr. James W. Debnam, Jr., Chesterfield, Mo.)

flow to an affected extremity with resultant warmth and erythema may be seen.

In long bones the disease is usually initially characterized by the lytic "blade-of-grass" lesion (Fig. 38-99). A wave of osteoclastic activity produces an advancing edge of lysis, which begins at the epiphyseometaphyseal ends of the bone and extends toward the diaphysis. The advancing wedge results in an increased diameter of the long bone because of subsequent periosteal reinforcement of the cortex. Deformities of the long bones are confined to those bones in the lower extremity. Bowing deformity of the femur and tibia may be severe. Nevertheless the involved bone may be weak and be prone to pathologic fracture.

The pelvis is a common site of involvement in Paget's disease. The osteolytic phase of the disorder is not usually appreciated, perhaps because of the asymptomatic nature of this initial phase. The osteoblastic phase may be on occasion confused with metastatic osteosclerotic (blastic) carcinomas. The sclerosis involving the iliopectineal line is frequently seen in patients with Paget's disease and results in the formation of the pelvic brim sign (Fig. 38-100).

Reflecting the elevated level of bone turnover, the serum level of alkaline phosphatase and osteocalcin are both elevated, representing osteoblastic activity. As a measurement of bone resorption, the urinary excretion of hydroxyproline is also elevated.

Paget described malignant transformation in five of his 23 patients. Since Paget's disease involves the osteoblastic, osteoclastic, and fibroblastic cell lines, tumors that arise in this setting not surprisingly are osteosarcomas, fibrosarcomas, and giant-cell malignant fibrous histiocytomas.

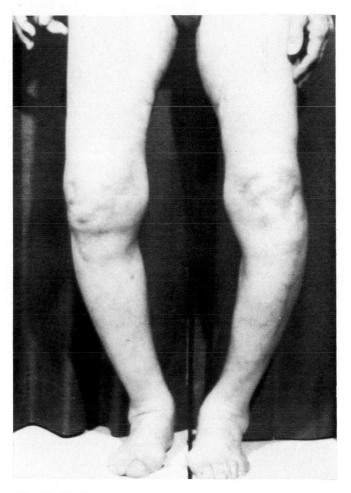

Fig. 38-98. Gross appearance of the typical anterior tibial bowing deformities that may be seen in Paget's disease of bone.

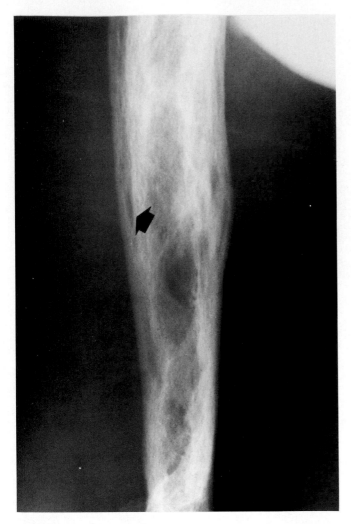

Fig. 38-99. Radiographic appearance of the lytic phase of Paget's disease. This humeral radiograph shows the blade of grass lytic wedge, *arrow*. Notice that the bone shaft is wider and there is a mixed radiographic sclerosis and lucent pattern.

Etiology

Because of the chronic course, lack of generalized but often asymmetric skeletal involvement, and the appearance of an enlarged bone with tenderness, redness, and warmth, many early investigators believed that this disease was the result of a chronic inflammatory process. The earlier speculations regarding an infectious cause for Paget's disease have enjoyed a renaissance in the recent observation of virus like inclusions in osteoclasts from biopsy specimens of pagetic bone[164] (Fig. 38-101). Subsequent immunologic studies have shown *Paramyxovirus* antigens and measles and respiratory syncytial virus in the nuclei and cytoplasm of pagetic osteoclasts.[116] A similar distribution of measle-virus

nucleotide sequences have been identified by in situ DNA hybridization.

DEGENERATIVE DISEASES OF BONE (OSTEONECROSES)

Osteonecrosis is a family of disorders characterized by infarction of bone, typically involving the femoral head. Although all forms of this disorder are characterized by necrotic bone, the natural history and pathologic expression of the various entities may vary.[76]

Although there are many classification schemes, there are three generic categories of osteonecrosis—postfracture, idiopathic, and renal transplantation associated. Most commonly the infarct follows a fracture of the femoral neck, with interruption of the retinacular blood supply. In this setting, osteonecrosis may also be referred to as avascular necrosis of bone.[83] Osteonecrosis may also occur in persons who do not have vascular insufficiency. Although there may be an associated systemic illness in some of these patients, such as alcoholism, hyperlipidemia, or hyperuricemia, the cause of the infarction remains unknown, and this form of the disorder may best be referred to as idiopathic osteonecrosis.[11,86,115] In a third broad category are patients who are receiving immunosuppressive agents, particularly corticosteroids, who sustain osteonecrosis.[52] Patients who are recipients of renal transplants and require multiple immunosuppressive agent therapy are particularly at risk.[139] Although the pathogenesis of the infarction is unknown in the latter two clinical groups, they all may be related by their associated lipid abnormalities.[190] Enlargement of the individual adipocytes within the marrow may increase the intramedullary pressure and occlude sinusoids and blood vessels. Increasing intraosseous pressure is also believed to play a role in the development of osteonecrosis in the miscellaneous marrow-packing disorders, such as Gaucher's disease. In these disorders, marrow infiltration by the foamy histiocytes may produce an intramedullary pressure that exceeds the vascular perfusion pressure.

The earliest histologic change occurring in any of the forms of osteonecrosis is death of the bone and the surrounding hematopoietic and fatty marrow. After a fracture occurs, all the remaining pathologic changes seen in infarction reflect the repair process, and it is by the exuberance of these events that the various clinical forms of osteonecroses differ. For example, idiopathic osteonecrosis, particularly associated with corticosteroid therapy, undergoes a less pronounced repair process, woven bone does not form about the dead trabeculas, and so the degree of bone sclerosis may not be very great. Otherwise, the infarcted tissue incites the same inflammatory response as that seen with any other infarct at any other site in the body. The infarcted tissue

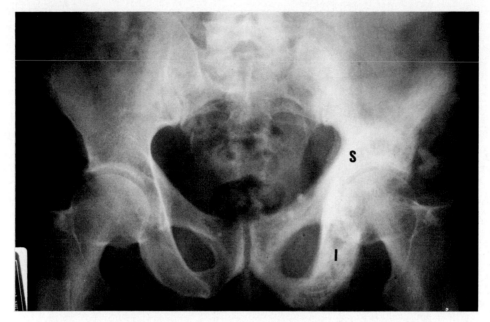

Fig. 38-100. Radiographic appearance of Paget's disease of bone involving the pelvis. The involved left side of this patient's pelvic bone shows sclerosis of the pelvic brim, *S*, and widening of the ischium, *I*. Notice that the disease is focal and only unilateral with sparing of the opposite side.

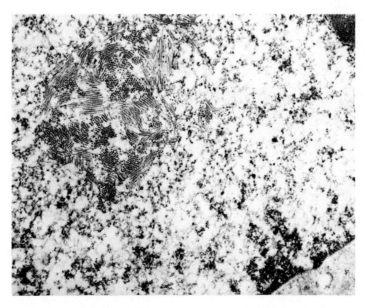

Fig. 38-101. Intranuclear virus-like inclusions in osteoclast of patient with Paget's disease. (31,000×; courtesy Dr. Barbara Mills, Los Angeles, Calif.)

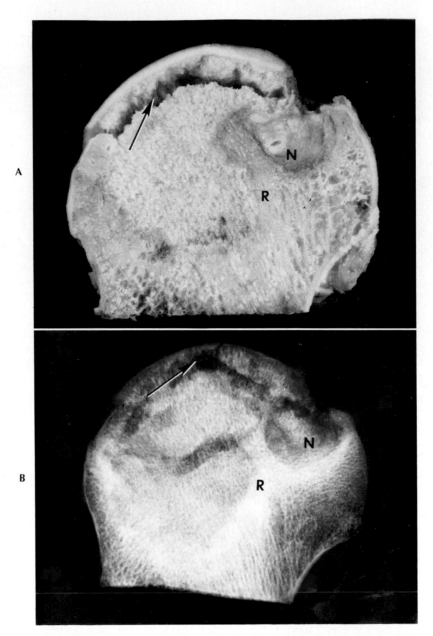

Fig. 38-102. A, Sagittal section and, **B,** radiograph of femoral head excised for advanced avascular necrosis. Notice subchondral lucent zone *(arrow)*, destruction and collapse of the articular cartilage, and sclerotic zone of repair, *R,* surrounding necrotic focus, *N.*

is sharply demarcated from the viable tissue, which has maintained a blood supply. In the immediate vicinity of the infarcted zone, a band of variable width containing ischemic but not infarcted tissue is seen. This ischemic zone is composed of dense fibrous tissue. Outside this zone is a hyperemic reactive zone from which granulation tissue enters the edges of the infarcted regions. Fibroblastic proliferation, accompanied by new blood vessels and osteoclasts, remove dead bone. Osteoblasts differentiate from this connective tissue, and new bone is deposited on top of some of the preexisting necrotic

trabeculas. This removal of old bone and deposition of additional bone on a scaffolding of dead bone is termed "creeping substitution." It is the ability of the granulation tissue to form new bone on the scaffolding of the preexisting bone that is the basis for the success of bone grafts utilized in orthopedic surgery in general and in the core decompression with grafting therapy of avascular necrosis, in particular.

The consequences of infarction may vary from none to severe secondary degenerative joint disease. If the infarct is of limited size and the blood supply can be

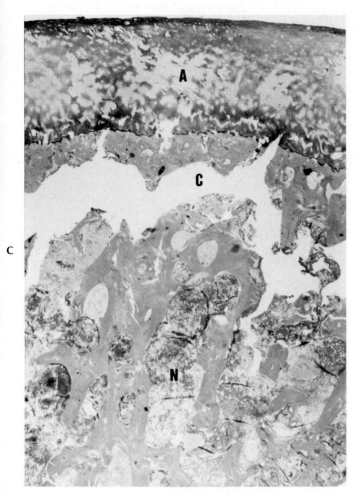

C

Fig. 38-102, cont'd. C, Histologic appearance of avascular necrosis of the femoral head. The articular cartilage, A, is separated from the underlying necrotic bone, N, resulting in a fracture line or the so-called crescent sign, C.

reestablished, recovery will occur without any persistent damage to the structural integrity of the bone. The dead bone cannot resist or transmit stress. Continued use of the affected limb will result in multiple small fractures of the infarcted trabeculas. These small fractures will be of particular importance to the subchondral plate of a major weight-bearing bone such as the femoral head. With continued use, there is impaction of the dead bone, which compresses the trabeculas into a smaller volume, resulting in a relative increase in radiodensity. A separation, or fracture cleft, ultimately forms between the impacted fragments and the overlying subchondral plate, which can be recognized radiographically in the femoral head as the crescent sign.[123] This radiolucent subchondral fracture is often the first diagnostic feature to be recognized on plain film radiographs. At the moment of infarction, however, dead bone will not exhibit any radiographic change. Radio-

graphs will reveal only areas that have undergone secondary structural changes, long after the infarct has occurred. In addition to the crescent sign, the radiographic diagnosis of osteonecrosis is based upon subsequent changes in bone density. In general the density of bone may be increased, decreased, or unchanged. Increased or decreased density are relative concepts, depending on what happens to the adjacent viable bone. The diagnosis of bone infarct is classically made on the basis of the appearance of increased density within the necrotic region. In reality the infarcted bone itself is unchanged. Without a blood supply, there can be no cellular activity and thus no change—increase or decrease—in bone substance.

Once the subchondral bone is resorbed or the necrotic tissue becomes impacted or crushed, the overlying joint surface becomes unstable. This instability leads to femoral head collapse and considerable distortion of the articular cartilage surface, eventuating in degenerative joint disease. The pathologic and corresponding radiographic changes seen in avascular necrosis of the femoral head are reviewed in Fig. 38-102.

REFERENCES

1. Albright, F., Aub, J.C., and Bauer, W.: Hyperparathyroidism, a common and polymorphic condition, as illustrated by seventeen proven cases from one clinic, JAMA **102:**1276, 1934.
2. Albright, F., Bloomberg, E., and Smith, P.H.: Postmenopausal osteoporosis, Trans. Assoc. Am. Physicians **55:**298, 1940.
3. Albright, J.A., and Brand, R.A.: The scientific basis of orthopaedics, ed. 2, Norwalk, Conn./Los Altos, Calif., 1987, Appleton & Lange.
4. Andress, D.L., Maloney, N.A., Coburn, J.W., Endres, D.B., and Sherrard, D.J.: Osteomalacia and aplastic bone disease in aluminum-related osteodystrophy, J. Clin. Endocrinol. Metab. **65:**11, 1987.
5. Andress, D.L., Nebeker, H.G., Ott, S.M., Endres, D.B., Alfrey, A.C., Slatopolsky, E.A., Coburn, J.W., and Sherrard, D.J.: Bone histologic response to deferoxamine in aluminum-related bone disease, Kidney Int. **31:**1344, 1987.
6. Argiles, A., Mourad, G., Berta, P., Polito, C., Canaud, B., Robinet-Levy, M., and Mion, C.: Dialysis-associated amyloidosis in a patient on long-term post-dilutional hemofiltration, Nephron **46:**96, 1987.
7. Avioli, L.V.: Osteoporosis: pathogenesis and therapy. In Avioli, L.V., and Krane, S.M., editors: Metabolic bone disease, vol. 1, New York, 1977, Academic Press, Inc.
8. Backrach, S., Fisher, J., and Parks, J.S.: An outbreak of vitamin D–deficiency rickets in a susceptible population, Pediatrics **64:**871, 1979.
9. Bassett, C.A.L., and Hermann, I.: Influence of oxygen concentration and mechanical factors on differentiation of connective tissues in vitro, Nature **190:**460, 1961.
10. Bikle, D.D., Genant, H.K., Cann, C., Recker, R.R., Halloran, B.P., and Strewler, G.J.: Bone disease in alcohol abuse, Ann. Intern. Med. **103:**42, 1985.
11. Boettcher, W.G., Bonfiglio, M., Hamilton, H.H., et al.: Nontraumatic necrosis of the femoral head. I. Relation of altered hemostasis to etiology, J. Bone Joint Surg. **52A:**312, 1970.
12. Bourne, G.H.: Phosphatase and calcification. In Bourne, G.H., editor: The biochemistry and physiology of bone, New York, 1972, Academic Press, Inc.

13. Bourne, G.H.: The relative importance of periosteum and endosteum in bone healing and the relationship of vitamin C to their activities, Proc. R. Soc. Med. **37**:275, 1944.

14. Breslau, N.A., and Pak, C.Y.C.: Hypoparathyroidism, Metabolism **28**:1261, 1979.

15. Brighton, C.T., Friedenberg, Z.B., Mitchell, E.I., and Booth, R.E.: Treatment of nonunion with constant direct current, Clin. Orthop. **124**:106, 1977.

16. Brown, D.M., and Dent, P.B.: Pathogenesis of osteopetrosis: a comparison of human and animal spectra, Pediatr. Res. **3**:181, 1971.

17. Brown, D.M., Jewsey, J., and Bradford, D.S.: Osteoporosis in ovarian dysgenesis, J. Pediatr. **84**:816, 1974.

18. Brown, J.P., Delmas, P.D., Arlot, M., and Meunier, P.J.: Active bone turnover of the cortico-endosteal envelope in postmenopausal osteoporosis, J. Clin. Endocrinol. Metab. **64**:954, 1987.

19. Caffey, J.: Chronic poisoning due to excess of vitamin A: description of the clinical and roentgen manifestations in seven infants and young children, Am. J. Roentgenol. **65**:12, 1951.

20. Cameron, D.A.: The ultrastructure of bone. In Bourne, G.H., editor: The biochemistry and physiology of bone, vol. 1, Structure, ed. 2, New York, 1972, Academic Press, Inc.

21. Campos, C., Arata, R.O., and Mautalen, C.A.: Parathyroid hormone and vertebral osteosclerosis in uremic patients, Metabolism **25**:495, 1976.

22. Canalis, E., McCarthy, T., and Centrella, M.: Growth factors and the regulation of bone remodeling, J. Clin. Invest. **81**:277, 1988.

23. Carmichael, K.A., Fallon, M.D., Kaplan, F.S., and Haddad, J.G.: Antacid-induced osteomalacia with elevated 1,25-dihydroxyvitamin D levels and increased bone resorption, Am. J. Med. **76**:1137, 1984.

24. Chase, L.R., Melson, G.L., and Aurbach, G.D.: Pseudohypoparathyroidism: defective excretion of 3′,5′-AMP in response to parathyroid hormone, J. Clin. Invest. **48**:1832, 1969.

25. Choufoer, J.H., and Steendijk, R.: Distribution of the perilacunar hypomineralized areas in cortical bone from patients with familial hypophosphatemic (vitamin D–resistant) rickets, Calcif. Tissue Int. **27**:101, 1979.

26. Civitelli, R., Gonnelli, S., Zacchei, F., Bigazzi, S., Vattimo, A., Avioli, L.V., and Gennari, C.: Bone turnover in postmenopausal osteoporosis, J. Clin. Invest. **82**:1268, 1988.

27. Coccia, P.F., Krivit, W., Cervenka, J., Clawson, C., Kersey, J.H., Kim, T.H., Nesbit, M.E., Ramsay, N.K., Warkentin, P.I., Teitelbaum, S.L., Kahn, A.J., and Brown, D.M.: Successful bone-marrow transplantation for infantile malignant osteopetrosis, N. Engl. J. Med. **302**:701, 1980.

28. Collins, D.H.: Paget's disease of bone: incidence and subclinical forms, Lancet **2**:51, 1956.

29. Cooke, N., Teitelbaum, S., and Avioli, L.V.: Antacid-induced osteomalacia and nephrolithiasis, Arch. Intern. Med. **138**:1007, 1978.

30. Costa, T., Marie, P.J., Scriver, C.R., Cole, D.E., Reade, T.M., Nogrady, B., Glorieux, F.H., and Delvin, E.E.: X-linked hypophosphatemia: effect of calcitriol on renal handling of phosphate, serum phosphate, and bone mineralization, J. Clin. Endocrinol. Metab. **52**:463, 1981.

31. Cournot-Witmer, G., Zingreff, J., Bourdon, R., Drüeke, T., and Balsan, S.: Aluminum and dialysis bone-disease, Lancet **2**:795, 1979. (Letter.)

32. Cowgill, L.D., Goldfarb, S., Lau, K., Slatopolsky, E., and Agus, Z.S.: Evidence for an intrinsic renal tubular defect in mice with genetic hypophosphatemic rickets, J. Clin. Invest. **63**:1203, 1979.

33. Davidson, P.T., and Horowitz, I.: Skeletal tuberculosis: a review with patient presentations and discussion, Am. J. Med. **48**:77, 1970.

34. Dent, C.E., and Harris, H.: Hereditary forms of rickets and osteomalacia, J. Bone Joint Surg. **38B**:204, 1956.

35. de Vernejoul, M.C., Bielakoff, J., Herve, M., Gueris, J., Hott, M., Modrowski, D., Kuntz, D., Miravet, L., and Ryckewaert, A.: Evidence for defective osteoblastic function: a role for alcohol and tobacco consumption in osteoporosis in middle-aged men, Clin. Orthop. **179**:107, 1983.

36. Dresner, M., Neelon, F.A., and Lebovitz, H.E.: Pseudohypoparathyroidism type II: a possible defect in the reception of the cyclic AMP signal, N. Engl. J. Med. **289**:1056, 1973.

37. Drüeke, T.: Dialysis osteomalacia and aluminum intoxication, Nephron **26**:207, 1980.

38. Eastwood, J.B., Stamp, T.C., Harris, E., et al.: Vitamin-D deficiency in the osteomalacia of chronic renal failure, Lancet **2**:1209, 1976.

39. Eddy, R.L.: Metabolic bone disease after gastrectomy, Am. J. Med. **50**:442, 1971.

40. Edidin, D.V., Levitsky, L.L., Schey, W., Dumbovic, N., and Campos, A.: Resurgence of nutritional rickets associated with breast-feeding and special dietary practices, Pediatrics **65**:232, 1980.

41. Eil, C., Liberman, U.R., Rosen, J.F., and Marx, S.J.: A cellular defect in hereditary vitamin-D–dependent rickets type II: defective nuclear uptake of 1,25-dihydroxyvitamin D in cultured skin fibroblasts, N. Engl. J. Med. **304**:1588, 1981.

42. Fallon, M.D.: Nontumor pathology of bone. In Spicer, S.S., editor: Histochemistry in pathologic diagnosis, New York, 1987, Marcel Dekker, Inc.

43. Fallon, M.D.: Assessment of bone structure. In Shils, M.E., and Young, V.R., editors: Modern nutrition in health and disease, ed. 3, Philadelphia, 1988, Lea & Febiger.

44. Fallon, M.D.: Bone histomorphology. In Resnick, D., and Niwayama, G., editors: Diagnosis of bone and joint disorders, ed. 2, Philadelphia, 1988, W.B. Saunders Co.

45. Fallon, M.D., Perry, H.M., Avioli, L.V., Droke, D., and Teitelbaum, S.L.: Exogenous hyperthyroidism with osteoporosis, Arch. Intern. Med. **143**:442, 1983.

46. Fallon, M.D., and Teitelbaum, S.L.: The interpretation of fluorescent tetracycline markers in the diagnosis of metabolic bone disease, Hum. Pathol. **13**:416, 1982.

47. Fallon, M.D., Teitelbaum, S.L., Weinstein, R.S., Goldfischer, S., Brown, D.M., and Whyte, M.P.: Hypophosphatasia: clinicopathologic comparison of the infantile, childhood, and adult forms, Medicine **63**:12, 1984.

48. Fallon, M.D., Whyte, M.P., Craig, R.B., and Teitelbaum, S.L.: Mast cell proliferation in post-menopausal osteoporosis, Calcif. Tissue Int. **35**:29, 1983.

49. Fallon, M.D., Whyte, M.P., and Teitelbaum, S.L.: Systemic mastocytosis associated with generalized osteopenia: histopathological characterization of the skeletal lesion using undecalcified bone from two patients, Hum. Pathol. **12**:813, 1981.

50. Falvo, K.A., and Bullough, P.G.: Osteogenesis imperfecta: a histometric analysis, J. Bone Joint Surg. **55A**:275, 1973.

51. Fernández-Madrid, F.: Collagen biosynthesis: a review, Clin. Orthop. **68**:163, 1970.

52. Fisher, D.E., and Bickel, W.H.: Corticosteroid-induced avascular necrosis: a clinical study of seventy-seven patients, J. Bone Joint Surg. **53A**:859, 1971.

53. Fleisch, H., and Bisaz, S.: Mechanism of calcification: inhibitory role of pyrophosphate, Nature **195**:911, 1962.

54. Frame, B., and Nixon, R.K.: Bone marrow mast cells in osteoporosis of aging, N. Engl. J. Med. **279**:626, 1968.

55. Frame, B., Hanson, C.A., Frost, H.M., et al.: Renal resistance to parathyroid hormone with osteitis fibrosa: "pseudohypoparathyroidism," Am. J. Med. **52**:311, 1972.

56. Frame, B., Jackson, C.E., Reynolds, W.A., et al.: Hypercalcemia and skeletal effects in chronic hypervitaminosis A, Ann. Intern. Med. **80**:44, 1974.

57. Fraser, D., Kooh, S.W., Kind, H.P., et al.: Pathogenesis of hereditary vitamin-D–dependent rickets: an inborn error of vitamin D metabolism involving defective conversion of 25-hydroxyvitamin D to 1α,25-dihydroxyvitamin D, N. Engl. J. Med. **289**:817, 1973.

58. Friedenstein, A.J.: Precursor cells of mechanocytes, Int. Rev. Cytol. **47**:327, 1976.

59. Frost, H.M.: Tetracycline-based histological analysis of bone remodeling, Calcif. Tissue Res. **3**:211, 1969.

60. Frymoyer, J.W., and Hodgkin, W.: Adult-onset vitamin-D–resistant hypophosphatemic osteomalacia, J. Bone Joint Surg. **59A**:101, 1977.

61. Gallagher, J.C., and Riggs, B.L.: Current concepts in nutrition, N. Engl. J. Med. **298**:193, 1978.

62. Garrick, R., Ireland, A.W., and Posen, S.: Bone abnormalities after gastric surgery: a prospective histological study, Ann. Intern. Med. **75**:221, 1971.

63. Gertner, J.M., Liliburn, M., and Domenech, M.: 25-Hydroxycholecalciferol absorption in steatorrhoea and postgastrectomy osteomalacia, Br. Med. J. **1**:1310, 1977.

64. Glorieux, F.H., Marie, P.J., Pettifor, J.M., and Delvin, E.E.: Bone response to phosphate salts, ergocalciferol, and calcitriol in hypophosphatemic vitamin D–resistant rickets, N. Engl. J. Med. **303**:1023, 1980.

65. Goldhaber, P.: Heparin enhancement of factors stimulating bone resorption in tissue culture, Science **147**:407, 1965.

66. Griffith, G.C., Nichols, G., Jr., Asher, J.D., and Flanagan, B.: Heparin osteoporosis, JAMA **193**:91, 1965.

67. Hahn, T.J.: Drug-induced disorders of vitamin D and mineral metabolism, Clin. Endocrinol. Metab. **9**:107, 1980.

68. Hahn, T.J., Boisseau, V.C., and Avioli, L.V.: Effect of chronic corticosteroid administration on diaphyseal and metaphyseal bone mass, J. Clin. Endocrinol. Metab. **39**:274, 1974.

69. Hahn, T.J., Halstead, L.R., and Teitelbaum, S.L.: Altered mineral metabolism in glucocorticoid-induced osteopenia, J. Clin. Invest. **64**:655, 1979.

70. Hall, B.K.: Cellular differentiation in skeletal tissue, Biol. Rev. Cambridge Philosophic Soc. **45**:455, 1970.

71. Hall, B.K., and Jacobson, H.N.: The repair of fractured membrane bones in the newly hatched chick, Anat. Rec. **181**:55, 1975.

72. Halse, J., and Haugen, H.N.: Calcium and phosphate metabolism in acromegaly, Acta Endocrinol. **94**:459, 1980.

73. Halse, J., Melsen, F., and Mosekilde, L.: Iliac crest bone mass and remodelling in acromegaly, Acta Endocrinol. **97**:18, 1981.

74. Halverson, J.D., Teitelbaum, S.L., Haddad, J.G., and Murphy, W.A.: Skeletal abnormalities after jejunoileal bypass, Ann. Surg. **189**:785, 1979.

75. Hauschka, P.V., Lian, J.B., and Gallop, P.M.: Direct identification of the calcium-binding amino acid, γ-carboxyglutamate, in mineralized tissue, Proc. Natl. Acad. Sci. USA **72**:3925, 1975.

76. Herndon, J.H., and Aufranc, O.E.: Avascular necrosis of the femoral head in the adult: a review of its incidence in a variety of conditions, Clin. Orthop. **86**:43, 1972.

77. Hess, A.F.: Scurvy past and present, Philadelphia, 1920, J.B. Lippincott Co.

78. Holtrop, M.E., and King, G.J.: The ultrastructure of the osteoclast and its functional implications, Clin. Orthop. **123**:177, 1977.

79. Holtrop, M.E., and Raisz, L.G.: Comparison of the effects of 1,25-dihydroxycholecalciferol, prostaglandin E$_2$, and osteoclast-activating factor with parathyroid hormone on the ultrastructure of osteoclasts in cultured long bones of fetal rats, Calcif. Tissue Int. **29**:201, 1979.

80. Holtrop, M.E., and Weinger, J.M.: Ultrastructural evidence for a transport system in bone. In Talmage, R.V., and Munson, P.L., editors: Calcium, parathyroid hormone, and the calcitonins, Int. Congr. Ser. no. 243, Amsterdam, 1972, Excerpta Medica Foundation.

81. Howard, L., Chu, R., Feman, S., Mintz, H., Ovesen, L., and Wolf, B.: Vitamin A deficiency from long-term parenteral nutrition, Ann. Intern. Med. **93**:576, 1980.

82. Hruska, K.A., Teitelbaum, S.L., and Kopelman, R.: The predictability of the histological features of uremic bone disease by non-invasive techniques, Metab. Bone Dis. Rel. Res. **1**:39, 1978.

83. Jacobs, B.: Epidemiology of traumatic and nontraumatic osteonecrosis, Clin. Orthop. **130**:51, 1978.

84. Jaffe, H.L.: Chronology of postnatal ossification and epiphysial fusion. In Jaffe, H.L.: Degenerative and inflammatory diseases of bones and joints, Philadelphia, 1972, Lea & Febiger.

85. Johnston, C.C., Jr., Lavy, N., Lord, T., et al.: Osteopetrosis: a clinical, genetic, metabolic, and morphologic study of the dominantly inherited, benign form, Medicine **47**:149, 1968.

86. Jones, J.P., and Engleman, E.P.: Avascular necrosis of bone in alcoholism, Arthritis Rheum. **10**:287, 1967.

87. Jowsey, J., and Johnson, K.A.: Juvenile osteoporosis: bone findings in seven patients, J. Pediatr. **81**:511, 1972.

88. Kanis, J.A.: Treatment of osteoporotic fracture, Lancet **1**:27, 1984.

89. Kaplan, F.S., August, C.S., Fallon, M.D., Dalinka, M., Axel, L., and Haddad, J.G.: Successful treatment of infantile malignant osteopetrosis by bone marrow transplantation, J. Bone Joint Surg. **70A**:617, 1988.

90. Kaplan, F.S., Pertschuk, M., Fallon, M.D., and Haddad, J.G.: Osteoporosis and hip fracture in a young woman with anorexia nervosa, Clin. Orthop. Rel. Res. **125**:64, 1986.

91. Kelly, P.J.: Osteomyelitis in the adult, Orthop. Clin. North Am. **6**:983, 1975.

92. Kelly, P.J., and Karlson, A.G.: Musculoskeletal tuberculosis, Mayo Clin. Proc. **44**:73, 1969.

93. Klibanski, A., and Greenspan, S.L.: Increase in bone mass after treatment of hyperprolactinemic amenorrhea, N. Engl. J. Med. **315**:542, 1986.

94. Knochel, J.P.: The pathophysiology and clinical characteristics of severe hypophosphatemia, Arch. Intern. Med. **137**:203, 1977.

95. Kruse, H.P., and Kuhlencordt, F.: Pathogenesis and natural course of primary osteoporosis, Lancet **1**:280, 1980.

96. Lian, J.B., and Gundberg, C.M.: Osteocalcin: biochemical considerations and clinical applications, Clin. Orthop. **226**:267, 1988.

97. Lian, J.B., Hauschka, P.V., and Gallop, P.M.: Properties and biosynthesis of a vitamin K–dependent calcium-binding protein in bone, Fed. Proc. **37**:2615, 1978.

98. Liberman, J.A., et al.: End-organ resistance to 1,25-dihydroxycholecalciferol, Lancet **1**:504, 1980.

99. Mahoney, C.P., Margolis, M.T., Knauss, T.A., and Labbe, R.F.: Chronic vitamin A intoxication in infants fed chicken liver, Pediatrics **65**:893, 1980.

100. Malluche, H.H., Ritz, E., Lange, H.P., et al.: Bone histology in incipient and advanced renal failure, Kidney Int. **9**:355, 1976.

101. Mamelle, N., Meunier, P.J., Dusan, R., Guillaume, M., Martin, J.L., Gaucher, A., Prost, A., Zeigler, G., and Netter, P.: Risk-benefit ratio of sodium fluoride treatment in primary vertebral osteoporosis, Lancet **2**:361, 1988.

102. Mankin, H.J.: Rickets, osteomalacia, and renal osteodystrophy, part I, J. Bone Joint Surg. **56A**:101, 1974.

103. Mankin, H.J.: Rickets, osteomalacia and renal osteodystrophy, part II, J. Bone Joint Surg. **56A**:352, 1974.

104. Martin, T.J.: Drug and hormone effects on calcium release from bone, Pharmacol. Ther. **21**:209, 1983.

105. Matloff, D.S., Kaplan, M.M., Nece, R.M., Goldberg, M.J., Bitman, W., and Wolfe, H.J.: Osteoporosis in primary biliary cirrhosis, effects of 25-hydroxyvitamin D$_3$ treatment, Gastroenterology **83**:97, 1982.

106. Maynard, J.A., Ippolito, E.G., Ponseti, I.V., and Mickelson, M.R.: Histochemistry and ultrastructure of the growth plate in achondroplasia, J. Bone Joint Surg. **63A**:969, 1981.

107. Melsen, F., and Mosekilde, L.: Morphometric and dynamic studies of bone changes in hyperthyroidism, Acta Pathol. Microbiol. Scand. [A] **85**:141, 1977.

108. Melsen, F., and Mosekilde, L.: Tetracycline double-labeling of iliac trabecular bone in 41 normal adults, Calcif. Tissue Res. **26**:99, 1978.

109. Melsen, F., Melsen, B., Mosekilde, L., and Bergmann, S.: Histomorphometric analysis of normal bone from the iliac crest, Acta Pathol. Microbiol. Scand. **86**:70, 1978.

110. Merz, W.A., and Schenk, R.K.: A quantitative histological study on bone formation in human cancellous bone, Acta Anat. **76**:1, 1970.

111. Merz, W.A., and Schenk, R.K.: Quantitative structural analysis of human cancellous bone, Acta Anat. **75**:54, 1970.

112. Meunier, P.J., Bianchi, G., Edouard, C., Bernard, J., Courpron, P., and Vignon, G.: Bony manifestations of thyrotoxicosis, Orthop. Clin. North Am. **3**:745, 1972.

113. Meunier, P.J., Sellami, S., Briancon, D., and Edouard, C.: Histological heterogeneity of apparently idiopathic osteoporosis. In DeLuca, H.F., Frost, H.M., Jee, W.S., Johnston, C.C., and Parfitt, A.M., editors: Osteoporosis: recent advances in pathogenesis and treatment, Baltimore, 1981, University Park Press.

114. Meyer, R.A., Jr., Gray, R.W., and Meyer, M.H.: Abnormal vitamin D metabolism in the X-linked hypophosphatemic mouse, Endocrinology 107:1577, 1980.

115. Mielants, H., Veys, E.M., DeBussere, A., et al.: Avascular necrosis and its relation to lipid and purine metabolism, J. Rheumatol. 2:430, 1975.

116. Mills, B.G., Singer, F.R., Weiner, L.P., and Holst, P.A.: Immunohistological demonstration of respiratory syncytial virus antigens in Paget disease of bone, Proc. Natl. Acad. Sci. USA 78:1209, 1981.

117. Minaire, P., Meunier, P., Edouard, C., et al.: Quantitative histological data on disuse osteoporosis, Calcif. Tissue Res. 17:57, 1974.

118. Morey, E.R., and Baylink, D.J.: Inhibition of bone formation during space flight, Science 201:1138, 1978.

119. Morrey, B.F., and Peterson, H.A.: Hematogenous pyogenic osteomyelitis in children, Orthop. Clin. North Am. 6:935, 1975.

120. Mosekilde, L., and Melsen, F.: A tetracycline-based histomorphometric evaluation of bone resorption and bone turnover in hyperthyroidism and hyperparathyroidism, Acta Med. Scand. 204:97, 1978.

121. Moseley, J.E.: Skeletal changes in the anemias, Semin. Roentgenol. 9:169, 1974.

122. Nordin, B.E.C., Aaron, J., Speed, R., and Crilly, R.G.: Bone formation and resorption as the determinants of trabecular bone volume in post-menopausal osteoporosis, Lancet 2:277, Aug. 8, 1981.

123. Norman, A., and Bullough, P.: The radiolucent crescent line: an early diagnostic sign of avascular necrosis of the femoral head, Bull. Hosp. Joint Dis. 24:99, 1963.

124. O'Connor, B.T., Oswestry, W.M.S., and Sanders, R.: Disseminated bone tuberculosis, J. Bone Joint Surg. 52A:1027, 1965.

125. Ott, S.M., Maldrey, W.A., Coburn, J.W., Alfrey, A.C., and Sherrard, D.: The prevalence of bone aluminum deposition in renal osteodystrophy and its relation to the response to calcitriol therapy, N. Engl. J. Med. 307:709, 1982.

126. Paget, J.: On a form of chronic inflammation of bones (osteitis deformans), Trans. Med. Chir. Soc. Lond. 60:37, 1877.

127. Parfitt, A.M.: The spectrum of hypoparathyroidism, J. Clin. Endocrinol. Metab. 34:152, 1972.

128. Parfitt, A.M.: Surgical, idiopathic, and other varieties of parathyroid hormone–deficient hypoparathyroidism. In Degroot, L.J., editor: Endocrinology, vol. 2, New York, 1979, Grune & Stratton, Inc.

129. Parfitt, A.M.: Morphologic basis of bone mineral measurements: transient and steady state effects of treatment in osteoporosis, Miner. Electrolyte Metab. 4:273, 1980.

130. Parfitt, A.M.: Dietary risk factors for age-related bone loss and fractures, Lancet 2:1181, Nov. 19, 1983.

131. Parfitt, A.M., Mathews, C.H.E., Villanueva, A.R., Kleerekoper, M., Frame, B., and Rao, D.S.: Relationships between surface, volume, and thickness of iliac trabecular bone in aging and in osteoporosis, J. Clin. Invest. 72:1396, 1983.

132. Parfitt, A.M., Miller, M.J., Frame, B., Villanueva, A.R., Rao, D.S., Oliver, I., and Thomson, D.L.: Metabolic bone disease after intestinal bypass for treatment of obesity, Ann. Intern. Med. 89:193, 1978.

133. Parfitt, A.M., Rao, D.S., Stanciu, J., Villanueva, A.R., Kleerekoper, M., and Frame, B.: Irreversible bone loss in osteomalacia, J. Clin. Invest. 76:2403, 1985.

134. Paterson, C.R., and Losowski, M.S.: The bones in chronic liver disease, Scand. J. Gastroenterol. 2:293, 1967.

135. Peck, W.A., Brandt, J., and Miller, I.: Hydrocortisone-induced inhibition of protein synthesis and uridine incorporation in isolated bone cells in vitro, Proc. Natl. Acad. Sci. USA 57:1599, 1967.

136. Perry, H.M., Fallon, M.D., Bergfeld, M., Teitelbaum, S.L., and Avioli, L.V.: Osteoporosis in young men: a syndrome of hypercalciuria and accelerated bone turnover, Arch. Intern. Med. 142:1295, 1982.

137. Persson, B., Tunell, R., and Ekengren, K.: Chronic vitamin A intoxication during the first half year of life: description of 5 cases, Acta Paediatr. Scand. 54:49, 1965.

138. Pierides, A.M., and Myli, M.P.: Iron and aluminum osteomalacia in hemodialysis patients, N. Engl. J. Med. 310:323, 1984.

139. Pierides, A.M., Simpson, W., Stainsby, D., et al.: Avascular necrosis of bone following renal transplantation, Q. J. Med. 44:459, 1975.

140. Ponseti, I.V.: Skeletal growth in achondroplasia, J. Bone Joint Surg. 52A:701, 1970.

141. Prockop, D.J., Kivirikko, K.I., Tuderman, L., and Guzman, N.A.: The biosynthesis of collagen and its disorders (in two parts), N. Engl. J. Med. 301:13, 77, 1979.

142. Purnell, D.C., Smith, L.H., Scholz, D.A., et al.: Primary hyperparathyroidism: a prospective clinical study, Am. J. Med. 50:670, 1971.

143. Putschar, W.G.J.: Osteomyelitis including fungal. In Ackerman, L.V., Spjut, H.J., and Abell, M.R., editors: Bones and joints, International Academy of Pathology Monograph, Baltimore, 1976, The Williams & Wilkins Co.

144. Rao, S.D., Matkovic, V., and Duncan, H.: The iliac crest bone biopsy and its complications, Henry Ford Hosp. Med. J. 28:112, 1980.

145. Rasmussen, H., Wong, M., Bikle, D., et al.: Hormonal control of the renal conversion of 25-hydroxycholecalciferol to 1,25-dihydroxycholecalciferol, J. Clin. Invest. 51:2502, 1972.

146. Reynolds, J.J., Holnick, M.F., and DeLuca, H.F.: The role of vitamin D metabolites in bone resorption, Calcif. Tissue Res. 12:295, 1973.

147. Richelson, L.S., Wahner, H.W., Melton, L.J., and Riggs, B.L.: Relative contributions of aging and estrogen deficiency to postmenopausal bone loss, N. Engl. J. Med. 311:1273, 1984.

148. Riggs, B.L., and Melton, L.J.: Evidence for two distinct syndromes of involutional osteoporosis, Am. J. Med. 75:899, 1983.

149. Riggs, B.L., and Melton, L.J.: Involutional osteoporosis, N. Engl. J. Med. 314:1676, 1986.

150. Riggs, B.L., and Melton, L.J., editors: Osteoporosis, etiology, diagnosis, and management, New York, 1988, Raven Press.

151. Riggs, B.L., Wahner, H.W., Melton, L.J., Richelson, L.S., Judd, H.L., and Offord, K.P.: Rates of bone loss in the appendicular and axial skeletons of women, J. Clin. Invest. 77:1487, 1986.

152. Riggs, B.L., Randall, R.V., Wahner, H.W., et al.: The nature of the metabolic bone disorder in acromegaly, J. Clin. Endocrinol. Metab. 34:911, 1972.

153. Riggs, B.L., Wahner, H.W., Dunn, W.L., Mazess, R.B., Offord, K.P., and Melton, L.J., III: Differential changes in bone mineral density of the appendicular and axial skeleton with aging, J. Clin. Invest. 67:328, 1981.

154. Rimoin, D.L., Hughes, G.N., Kaufman, R.L., et al.: Endochondral ossification in achondroplastic dwarfism, N. Engl. J. Med. 283:728, 1970.

155. Rimoin, D.L., McAlister, W.H., Saldino, R.M., and Hall, J.G.: Histologic appearances of some types of congenital dwarfism, Prog. Pediatr. Radiol. 4:68, 1973.

156. Rodahl, K.: Toxicity of polar bear liver, Nature 164:530, 1949.

157. Rubin, P.: On organizing a dynamic classification of bone dysplasia. In Rubin, P.: Dynamic classification of bone dysplasias, Chicago, 1964, Year Book Medical Publishers.

158. Ruby, L.K., and Mital, M.A.: Skeletal deformities following chronic hypervitaminosis A: a case report, J. Bone Joint Surg. 56:1283, 1974.

159. Schenk, R., Spiro, D., and Weiner, J.: Cartilage resorption in tibial epiphyseal plate of growing rats, J. Cell Biol. 34:275, 1974.

160. Scott, C.I.: Achondroplastic and hypochondroplastic dwarfism, Clin. Orthop. 114:18, 1976.

161. Sherrard, D.J.: Renal osteodystrophy, Semin. Nephrol. 6:56, 1986.

162. Shires, R., Avioli, L.V., Bergfeld, M.A., Fallon, M.D., Slatopolsky, E.A., and Teitelbaum, S.L.: Effect of semi-starvation on skeletal homeostasis, Endocrinology 107:1530, 1980.

163. Shusterman, N.H., Wasserstein, A.G., Morrison, G., Audet, P., Fallon, M.D., and Kaplan, F.: Controlled study of renal osteodystrophy in patients undergoing dialysis, Am. J. Med. 82:1148, 1987.

164. Singer, F.R., and Mills, B.G.: The etiology of Paget's disease of bone, Clin. Orthop. 127:37, 1977.

165. Slatopolsky, E.A.: The interaction of parathyroid hormone and aluminum in renal osteodystrophy, Kidney Int. 31:842, 1987.

166. Slatopolsky, E.A., Cagler, S., Pennell, J.P., et al.: On the pathogenesis of hyperparathyroidism in chronic experimental renal insufficiency in the dog, J. Clin. Invest. 50:492, 1971.

167. Slatopolsky, E.A., Gray, R., and Roams, N.D.: The pathogenesis of secondary hyperparathyroidism in early renal failure. In Norman, A.W., Schaefer, K., and von Herrath, D.: editors: Vitamin D: basic research and its clinical application, New York, 1979, Walter de Gruyter.

168. Smith, R.: Collagen and disorders of bone, Clin. Sci. 59:215, 1980.

169. Smith, R., Francis, M.J.O., and Bauze, R.J.: Osteogenesis imperfecta: a clinical and biochemical study of a generalized connective tissue disorder, Q. J. Med. 44:555, 1975.

170. Soriand, S., Kaplan, F.S., Fallon, M.D., and Haddad, J.G.: Osteomalacia in a night nurse, Clin. Orthop. 205:216, 1986.

171. Spencer, H., Rubio, N., Rubio, E., Indreika, M., and Seitam, A.: Chronic alcoholism: frequently overlooked cause of osteoporosis in men, Am. J. Med. 80:393, 1986.

172. Stanescu, V., Bona, C., and Ionescu, V.: The tibial growing cartilage biopsy in the study of growth disturbances, Acta Endocrinol. 64:577, 1970.

173. Stěpán, J., Pacovský, V., Horn, V., Silinková-Málková, E., Vokrouhlická, O., Konopásek, B., Formánková, J., Hrba, J., and Marek, J.: Relationship of the activity of the bone isoenzyme of serum alkaline phosphatase to urinary hydroxyproline excretion in metabolic and neoplastic bone diseases, Eur. J. Clin. Invest. 8:373, 1978.

174. Sykes, B., Francis, M.J.O., and Smith, R.: Altered relation of two collagen types in osteogenesis imperfecta, N. Engl. J. Med. 296:1200, 1977.

175. Talmage, R.V., and Grubb, S.A.: A laboratory model demonstrating osteocyte-osteoblast control of plasma calcium concentrations, Clin. Orthop. 122:299, 1977.

176. Teitelbaum, S.L.: Pathological manifestations of osteomalacia and rickets, Clin. Endocrinol. Metab. 9:43, 1980.

177. Teitelbaum, S.L.: Progress in pathology: renal osteodystrophy, Hum. Pathol. 15:306, 1984.

178. Teitelbaum, S.L., and Bates, M.: Relationships of static and kinetic histomorphometric features of bone, Clin. Orthop. 156:239, 1980.

179. Teitelbaum, S.L., and Bullough, P.G.: The pathophysiology of bone and joint disease, Am. J. Pathol. 96:283, 1979.

180. Teitelbaum, S.L., Kraft, W.J., Lang, R., et al.: Bone collagen aggregation abnormalities in osteogenesis imperfecta, Calcif. Tissue Res. 17:75, 1974.

181. Teitelbaum, S.L., Hruska, K.A., Shieber, W., Debnam, J.W., and Nichols, S.H.: Tetracycline fluorescence in uremic and primary hyperparathyroid bone, Kidney Int. 12:366, 1977.

182. Teitelbaum, S.L., Russell, J.E., Bone, J.M., Gilden, J.J., and Avioli, L.V.: The relationship of biochemical and histometric determinants of uremic bone, Arch. Pathol. Lab. Med. 103:228, 1979.

183. Teitelbaum, S.L., Whyte, M.P., Murphy, W., and Avioli, L.V.: Failure of routine biochemical studies to predict the histological heterogeneity of untreated post-menopausal osteoporosis. In DeLuca, H.F., Frost, H.M., Jee, W.S., Johnston, C.C., and Parfitt, A.M., editors: Osteoporosis: recent advances in pathogenesis and treatment, Baltimore, 1981, University Park Press.

184. Trueta, J.: The three types of acute haematogenous osteomyelitis, J. Bone Joint Surg. 41B:671, 1959.

185. Tsuchiya, Y.: An unusual form of vitamin D–dependent rickets in a child: alopecia and marked end-organ hyposensitivity to biologically active vitamin D, J. Clin. Endocrinol. Metab. 51:685, 1980.

186. Verbanck, M., Verbanck, J., Brauman, J., Mullier, J.P.: Bone histology and 25-OH vitamin D plasma levels in alcoholics without cirrhosis, Calcif. Tissue Res. 22(suppl.):538, 1977.

187. Walker, D.G.: Congenital osteopetrosis in mice cured by parabiotic union with normal siblings, Endocrinology 91:916, 1972.

188. Walker, D.G.: Experimental osteopetrosis, Clin. Orthop. 97:158, 1973.

189. Walker, D.G.: Osteopetrosis cured by temporary parabiosis, Science 180:875, 1973.

190. Wang, G.J., Sweet, D.E., Reger, S.I., and Thompson, R.C.: Fat-cell changes as a mechanism of avascular necrosis of the femoral head in cortisone-treated rabbits, J. Bone Joint Surg. 59:729, 1977.

191. Weidner, N., and Santa Cruz, D.: Phosphaturic mesenchymal tumors: a polymorphous group causing osteomalacia or rickets, Cancer 59:1442, 1987.

192. Weinstein, R.S.: The histological heterogeneity of osteopenia in the middle-aged and elderly patient. In Feldman, E.B., Spears, R., and Stern, H., editors: Nutrition in the middle and later years, London, 1983, John Wright-PSG, Inc.

193. Weinstein, R.S., Bryce, G.F., Sappington, L.J., King, D.W., and Gallagher, B.B.: Decreased serum ionized calcium and normal vitamin D metabolite levels with anticonvulsant drug treatment, J. Clin. Endocrinol. Metab. 58:1003, 1984.

194. Weinstein, R.S., and Lutcher, C.L.: Chronic erythroid hyperplasia and accelerated bone turnover, Metab. Bone Dis. Rel. Res. 5:7, 1983.

195. Whedon, G.D., Lutwak, L., and Rambout, P.C.: Mineral and nitrogen balance observations: the second manned Skylab mission, Aviat. Space Environ. Med. 47:391, 1976.

196. Whyte, M.P., Teitelbaum, S.L., Murphy, W.A., Bergfeld, M.A., and Avioli, L.V.: Adult hypophosphatasia: clinical, laboratory, and genetic investigation of a large kindred with review of the literature, Medicine 58:329, 1979.

197. Whyte, M.P., Bergfeld, M.A., Murphy, W.A., Avioli, L.V., and Teitelbaum, S.L.: Postmenopausal osteoporosis: a heterogeneous disorder as assessed by histomorphometric analysis of iliac crest bone from untreated patients, Am. J. Med. 72:193, 1982.

198. Yang, S.S., Kitchen, E., Gilbert, E.F., and Rimoin, D.L.: Histopathologic examination in osteochondrodysplasia, Arch. Pathol. Lab. Med. 110:10, 1986.

39 Tumors and Tumorlike Conditions of Bone

JUAN ROSAI

ETIOLOGY AND PREDISPOSING FACTORS

Bone tumors are the oldest form of neoplasia documented in paleopathology; they existed on earth long before human life appeared. In humans, bone neoplasms occur in all races and in all countries. The annual incidence of malignant bone tumors is approximately one case per 100,000 inhabitants.

There are various circumstances, including some benign diseases, that are seen associated with the appearance of bone neoplasms in a significant fashion. However, they account for only a minority of the cases even when considered as a group.

The possibility of trauma predisposing to the development of malignant tumors of bone has been suggested many times but never proved. Major trauma to the bone, such as that resulting from fracture, surgery (particularly amputation), and exodontia, has no statistical relation to bone sarcoma.[146] It is therefore difficult to believe that the relatively insignificant trauma that patients with bone tumors often cite could possibly have been the cause of the neoplasm.

It has been known for many years that various modalities of ionizing radiation can result in the appearance of bone sarcomas. One of the first demonstrations of this occurrence was the production by Lacassagne[120] of a tumor interpreted as fibrosarcoma of the tibia in a rabbit 36 months after irradiation of an abscess near the bone. Osteosarcomas in laboratory animals can be induced with intraperitoneal injections of ^{45}Ca or ^{89}Sr, local inoculation of ^{144}Ce,[59] or intravenous injection of ^{55}Fe.[122] Interestingly, radioactive calcium produces sarcomas chiefly in the spine and pelvis, whereas strontium induces them in the bones of the limb.[12,92]

The most dramatic series of radiation-induced bone sarcomas in humans was the one reported by Martland and Humphries[136] (Fig. 39-1). The victims were young women employed in the painting of clock dials with a luminous compound made of zinc sulfide and 1 part in 40,000 of radium, mesothorium (an isotope of radium), and radiothorium. It was the custom of the workers to moisten the bristles of the brush between their lips,

and this led to the ingestion of a certain amount of radioactive material. Of the 18 patients who died of radium poisoning, five had osteosarcomas.

A large number of osteosarcomas have been seen after the use of thorium in the treatment of tuberculosis and ankylosing spondylitis.[198] A few cases of osteosarcoma have been reported in patients who had undergone angiographic studies with Thorotrast during childhood.[195] Cases of bone sarcomas developing in apparent connection with the local administration of radiation for therapeutic purposes have been reported both in children and in adults from several medical centers.[52,88,216] All bones are susceptible to this complication. The usual interval between the time of irradiation and the clinical appearance of the tumor is between 9 and 15 years. Approximately two thirds of the sarcomas have arisen in preexisting bone lesions, particularly giant cell tumor. The most common types of radiation-induced sarcoma of bone are osteosarcoma, malignant fibrous histiocytoma, and fibrosarcoma.[102,223]

The danger of this complication, though it is of extremely grave consequence, should be viewed in the proper perspective. In most reported cases, the dose of radiation has been 3000 rad or higher, and the patient has received repeated courses. The practical hazard of radiation-induced sarcoma appears to be very remote and should not be a contraindication to the treatment of carcinomas; however, radiotherapy for benign bone tumors should probably be reserved for those not amenable to surgical therapy.

A few reported cases of bone sarcomas arising at the site of foreign bodies (introduced either accidentally or surgically) are on record; their microscopic appearance has varied from case to case.[18,109,124]

It has been well documented that Paget's disease predisposes to the development of bone tumors, especially in men.[97,188] In extensive and advanced cases the rate of malignant transformation is about 10%[62] but the overall incidence is probably less than 1%. This malignant transformation has been attributed to the higher rate of bone turnover seen in Paget's disease, as indicated by the pronounced resorptive and osteoblastic activity. Osteosarcomas predominate, but chondrosarcomas, fibrosarcomas, and giant cell tumors have also been reported.[95,227] The sarcoma developing in Paget's disease usually occurs in areas in which the process is most advanced. The bones involved by sarcoma in patients with Paget's disease, in order of frequency, are

the pelvis, femur, humerus, tibia, skull and facial bones, and scapula. The prognosis for sarcoma arising in Paget's disease is extremely poor; almost 30% of the patients have metastatic disease at the time of diagnosis, and only 8% of the whole group survive for 5 years.[227]

Fibrous dysplasia may also be complicated with bone sarcoma, though the incidence is very low. Most of the cases of fibrous dysplasia in which this complication has supervened have been of the polyostotic type.[191] The tumor is usually on osteosarcoma, though fibrosarcoma and chondrosarcoma can also occur.[100]

An increasing number of malignant bone tumors have been reported at the site of bone infarcts, such as those seen in caisson workers. The types were osteosarcoma, malignant fibrous histiocytoma, and fibrosarcoma.[74,144]

The malignant tumors associated with long-standing osteomyelitis usually take the form of squamous cell carcinoma arising from the draining sinuses. Rarely, fibrosarcoma or angiosarcoma may develop within the inflamed bone as well as in the surrounding soft tissue.

At least three cases of osteogenesis imperfecta associated with osteosarcoma have been reported.[62] In this condition, however, it is much more common to see an exuberant callus at a site of fracture that is confused roentgenographically and even microscopically with an osteosarcoma.

Two polyostotic bone disorders, of either a neoplastic or developmental nature, are associated with an increased occurrence of chondrosarcoma; these are enchondromatosis and osteochondromatosis and are discussed in the section of chondroblastic (cartilage-forming) tumors.

Claims of malignant transformation have been made in isolated cases of benign bone tumors, such as enchondroma, chondroblastoma, chondromyxoid fibroma, nonossifying fibroma, giant cell tumor, and osteoblastoma. Although some of these reports are probably authentic (especially for the last two tumors), it seems likely that many of these cases were initially misdiagnosed as benign or that they represent radiation-induced sarcoma.[197,218]

Fraumeni[72] made the intriguing observation that American youngsters under 18 years of age with osteosarcomas were significantly taller than those in a control group with nonosseous malignant tumors.

Osteosarcomas have been produced by viral inoculations into chickens, mice, and rats[70,158] and by the administration of chemical carcinogens, particularly beryllium salts, into rabbits.[210] There are several clinical and laboratory observations indicating the possibility of a viral cause for human osteosarcoma.[166] The concurrent development of tumors in members of the same family implicates either genetic or infectious factors. This has been documented for osteosarcoma, chondrosarcoma,

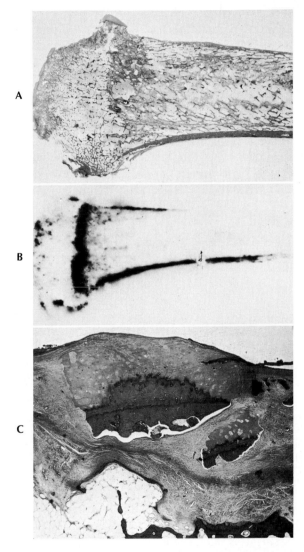

Fig. 39-1. Bone and cartilage changes caused by irradiation. Patient, 46-year-old woman, had worked as watch- and clock-dial painter for 3½ months when 16 years of age. Lower extremity was amputated because of sarcomatous change originating in diseased femur. **A,** Large section of lower segment of femur showing necrosis. **B,** Autoradiogram made from section similar to specimen shown in **A.** Notice evidence of intense radioactivity in region of metaphyseal end of diaphysis, which marks growth zone at time patient was exposed to radioactive material. **C,** As result of radiation injury, articular cartilage and subchondral bone have undergone necrosis and fragmentation.

and Ewing's sarcoma.[87,183] Unusual clustering of bone sarcomas has been seen in small communities.[73,217] Statistical differences in the incidence of osteosarcoma in genetically homogeneous populations depending on geographic location (and presumably caused by environmental factors) have been documented in Malaysia and Kenya. The possibility that human osteosarcomas may be produced by viruses was further raised by the alleged demonstration by immunologic techniques of a high incidence of antibodies to a common antigen of osteosarcoma in the sera of patients with this disease and in members of their immediate families.[148,196] This observation indicate the possibly association of an infectious agent with this neoplasm, which would appear capable of infecting relatives and close associates of the patients.

Another experiment suggesting a viral cause for human osteosarcoma was performed by Finkel and collaborators.[69] They were able to produce osteosarcomas, fibrosarcomas, and benign bone tumors in neonatal hamsters by injecting them with cell-free extracts of human osteosarcomas. These authors also demonstrated with immunofluorescence techniques a reactivity between the serum of human patients with osteosarcoma and sarcoma tissue from hamsters that had been induced with extracts of human osteosarcoma, suggestive of the transmission of a virus in the inoculated extract.

Electron microscopic studies have also lent some support to the viral hypothesis. Thin sections of human bone tumors and of pelleted extracts of these tumors have shown particles that could possibly be associated with DNA,[83] and viral particles of RNA nature (probably corresponding to an oncornavirus) have been detected in murine osteosarcoma.[153]

These studies strongly suggest a relation between a viral infectious agent and human osteosarcoma. However, the fundamental question as to whether this agent is directly related to the tumor cause or is an incidental passenger remains unanswered.

CLASSIFICATION AND DISTRIBUTION

The presence of a large variety of tissues within the skeletal system, the rarity of bone neoplasms, and the uncertainty that still exists regarding their histogenesis have all contributed to the confusion in terminology and classification that for many years has plagued this field of tumor pathology. Fortunately, a satisfactory degree of uniformity in the nomenclature has now been reached. The main contributions for these achievements have been the pioneering work of H.L. Jaffe,[105] the fascicle "Tumors of Bone and Cartilage" of the *Atlas of Tumor Pathology* series,[201] and the booklet by Schajowicz, Ackerman, and Sissons, published under the auspices of the World Health Organization as part of their *International Histological Classification of Tumours* series.[182]

The classification presented in this chapter is based largely on the latter work and is of histogenetic character. Tumors are classified according to the tissue or cell type from which they are presumed to arise, which in turn is deduced mainly from the tissue that the tumor cells are able to manufacture. Thus a bone tumor composed of cells that produce osteoid or bone is presumed to originate from osteoblasts, a tumor composed of cells that produce cartilage (and only cartilage) is presumed to originate from chondroblasts, and so on. In other instances, the histogenetic presumption of origin is derived not from the identification of a manufactured product of the tumor cell but rather from the morphologic similarity of this cell to a given normal cell when studied by light microscopic, histochemical, immunohistochemical, ultrastructural, or any other techniques. For instance, a malignant bone tumor composed of small round cells that morphologically resemble normal lymphocytes is presumed to arise from these cells and is therefore designated "malignant lymphoma." Some terms that have very little histogenetic meaning have remained either to honor the scientist who first recognized them (such as Ewing's sarcoma) or for no reason other than tradition (such as myeloma).

It should be understood that the histogenetic classification of tumors in general and of bone tumors in particular is no more than a useful conceptual framework that might be even misleading if taken too literally. To mention just one example, it is entirely possible and indeed likely that osteosarcoma does not arise from preexisting well-differentiated osteoblasts but rather from primitive and multipotential mesenchymal cells that differentiate toward osteoblasts in the course of neoplastic transformation.

The reader who first scans a classification of bone neoplasms such as the one presented here is likely to wonder what its real practical significance is. This is understandable because there have been in the past (and are even now) classifications of tumors that describe minimal morphologic variations of a basic tumor pattern that have no clinical, surgical, or prognostic significance whatsoever. The reader may be assured that this is not the case with the classification of bone tumors presented here. Each of the entities listed has characteristics of its own; its preference for a given bone, site within the bone, age of the patient, roentgenographic appearance, and behavior are distinctive and allow the clinician to suggest a specific diagnosis, plan therapy, and predict the evolution with a high degree of accuracy.

The basic information regarding these parameters is included in Table 39-1. The data concerning age, sex,

Table 39-1. Characteristics of most common primary bone tumors and tumorlike lesions*

Tumor or tumorlike lesion	Age (yr)	Sex M:F	Bones most commonly affected (in order of frequency)	Usual location within long bone	Behavior
Osteoma	40-50	2:1	Skull and facial bones	—	Benign
Osteoid osteoma	10-30	2:1	Femur, tibia, humerus, hands and feet, vertebrae, fibula	Cortex of metaphysis	Benign
Osteoblastoma	10-30	2:1	Vertebrae, tibia, femur, humerus, pelvis, ribs	Medulla of metaphysis	Benign
Osteosarcoma	10-25	3:2	Femur, tibia, humerus, pelvis, jaw, fibula	Medulla of metaphysis	Malignant; 20% to 40% 5-year survival rate
Juxtacortical (parosteal) osteosarcoma	30-60	1:1	Femur, tibia, humerus	Juxtacortical area of metaphysis	Malignant; 80% 5-year survival rate
Chondroma	10-40	1:1	Hands and feet, ribs, femur, humerus	Medulla of diaphysis	Benign
Osteochondroma	10-30	1:1	Femur, tibia, humerus, pelvis	Cortex of metaphysis	Benign
Chondroblastoma	10-25	2:1	Femur, humerus, tibia, feet, pelvis, scapula	Epiphysis, adjacent to cartilage plate	Practially always benign
Chondromyxoid fibroma	10-25	1:1	Tibia, femur, feet, pelvis	Metaphysis	Benign
Chondrosarcoma	30-60	3:1	Pelvis, ribs, femur, humerus, vertebrae	Central—medulla of diaphysis or metaphysis Peripheral—cortex or periosteum of metaphysis	Malignant; 5-year survival rate—low grade, 78%; moderate grade, 53%; high grade, 22%
Mesenchymal chondrosarcoma	20-60	1:1	Ribs, skull and jaw, vertebrae, pelvis, soft tissues	Medulla or cortex of diaphysis	Malignant; extremely poor prognosis
Giant cell tumor	20-40	4:5	Femur, tibia, radius	Epiphysis and metaphysis	Potentially malignant; 50% recur; 10% metastasize
Ewing's sarcoma	5-20	1:2	Femur, pelvis, tibia, humerus, ribs, fibula	Medulla of diaphysis or metaphysis	Highly malignant; 20%-30% 5-year survival rate in recent series
Malignant lymphoma, large and mixed cell types	30-60	1:1	Femur, pelvis, vertebrae, tibia, humerus, jaw, skull, ribs	Medulla of diaphysis or metaphysis	Malignant, 22%-50% 5-year survival rate
Plasma cell myeloma	40-60	2:1	Vertebrae, pelvis, ribs, sternum, skull	Medulla of diaphysis, metaphysis, or epiphysis	Malignant; diffuse form always fatal; localized form often controlled with radiotherapy
Hemangioma	20-50	1:1	Skull, vertebrae, jaw	Medulla	Benign
Desmoplastic fibroma	20-30	1:1	Humerus, tibia, pelvis, jaw, femur, scapula	Metaphysis	Benign

Slightly modified from Rosai, J.: Ackerman's surgical pathology, ed. 7, St. Louis, 1989, The C.V. Mosby Co.
*It should be emphasized that these data correspond to the typical case and that they should not be taken in an absolute sense. Isolated exceptions to practically every one of these statements have occurred.   *Continued.*

Table 39-1, cont'd. Characteristics of most common primary bone tumors and tumorlike lesions

Tumor or tumorlike lesion	Age (yr)	Sex M:F	Bones most commonly affected (in order of frequency)	Usual location within long bone	Behavior
Fibrosarcoma	20-60	1:1	Femur, tibia, jaw, humerus	Medulla of metaphysis	Malignant; 25% to 50% 5-year survival rate
Chordoma	40-60	2:1	Sacrococcygeal, spheno-occipital, cervical vertebrae	—	Malignant; slow course; locally invasive; 48% distant metastases
Solitary bone cyst	10-20	3:1	Humerus, femur	Medulla of metaphysis	Benign
Aneurysmal bone cyst	10-20	1:1	Vertebrae, flat bones, femur, tibia	Metaphysis	Benign; sometimes follows another bone lesion
Metaphyseal fibrous defect	10-20	1:1	Tibia, femur, fibula	Metaphysis	Benign
Fibrous dysplasia	10-30	3:2	Ribs, femur, tibia, jaw, skull	Medulla of diaphysis or metaphysis	Locally aggressive; rarely complicated by sarcoma
Eosinophilic granuloma	5-15	3:2	Skull, jaw, humerus, rib, femur	Metaphysis or diaphysis	Benign

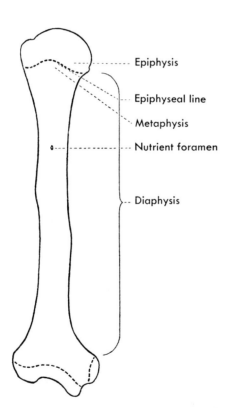

Epiphysis

Epiphyseal line

Metaphysis

Nutrient foramen

Diaphysis

Fig. 39-2. Sketch of long bone (humerus) identifying different anatomic landmarks important for determining location of bone neoplasms.

bone, and bone site most commonly involved are generally not repeated in the text. For a proper understanding of this table, a brief recapitulation of some terms of normal bone anatomy might be helpful. *Medulla* (medullary cavity, or marrow cavity) refers to the inner or central portion of the bone, composed of a network of cancellous (spongy, reticular) bone trabeculas that enclose bone marrow hematopoietic elements, adipose tissue, blood and lymph vessels, and nerves. The *cortex*, composed of compact (dense) bone and essentially devoid of bone marrow and other soft-tissue components, surrounds the medulla in a circumferential fashion. The *periosteum*, which covers the outer surface of the bone, consists of a thick external layer of fibrous connective tissue and a thin osteoblastic layer. Bone tumors in the region of the periosteum, and possibly arising from it, are often designated as periosteal, parosteal, or juxtacortical.

A typical adult long bone is composed of a *diaphysis* which is the central cylindrical shaft; the *epiphyses*, which are two roughly spherical terminal regions covered by the articular cartilage; and the *metaphyses*, two intermediate conelike regions connective the shaft and the articular ends (Fig. 39-2). The metaphysis is particularly important in bone pathology because in the growing person it is adjacent to the cartilaginous *epiphyseal plate*. The latter represents the area of most active bone growth and, perhaps as a result, is the most common site of occurrence of many bone neoplasms.

Definitions of normal bone histologic features that are important to remember in the context of the subject of this chapter include the following.[211] *Osteoid* (preosseous tissue) is the extracellular material produced by the osteoblasts and composed of collagen fibers (largely of type I) and an amorphous protein-poysaccharid matrix. *Bone* refers to the same tissue after calcium salts have been deposited on it. *Woven (membrane or fiber) bone* is the type of bone produced normally in the course of intramembranous ossification and abnormally in a fracture callus, fibrous dysplasia, and a variety of bone neoplasms; it is characterized by the haphazard placement of collagen fibers throughout the osteoid matrix. One can observe this particularly well with polarizing lenses. *Lamellar bone,* on the other hand, is laid down in concentric layers containing collagen in ordered parallel arrays.

The classification* that follows also includes a group of nonneoplastic conditions, mostly of obscure pathogenesis, that can closely resemble a bone neoplasm on roentgenographic and morphologic grounds.

A. Osteoblastic (bone-forming) tumors
  1. Benign
    a. Osteoma
    b. Osteoid osteoma and osteoblastoma
  2. Malignant
    a. Osteosarcoma
    b. Juxtacortical (parosteal) osteosarcoma
B. Chondroblastic (cartilage-forming) tumors
  1. Benign
    a. Chondroma
    b. Osteochondroma
    c. Chondroblastoma
    d. Chondromyxoid fibroma
  2. Malignant
    a. Chondrosarcoma
    b. Mesenchymal chondrosarcoma
C. Giant cell tumor (osteoclastoma)
D. Marrow tumors
  1. Ewing's sarcoma
  2. Malignant lymphoma
  3. Plasma cell myeloma
E. Vascular tumors
  1. Benign
    a. Hemangioma
    b. Lymphangioma
    c. Glomus tumor
    d. Hemangiopericytoma
  2. Borderline
    a. Hemangioendothelioma (histiocytoid or epithelioid)
  3. Malignant
    a. Angiosarcoma
    b. Hemangiopericytoma

F. Fibrous tissue tumors
  1. Benign
    a. Desmoplastic fibroma
  2. Malignant
    a. Fibrosarcoma
G. Other primary tumors
  1. Chordoma
  2. "Adamantinoma" of long bones
  3. Tumors of peripheral nerves
  4. Tumors of adipose tissue
  5. Tumors of alleged histiocytic origin
  6. Tumors of smooth muscle
H. Metastatic tumors
I. Unclassified tumors
J. Tumorlike lesions
  1. Solitary bone cyst
  2. Aneurysmal bone cyst
  3. Ganglion cyst of bone
  4. Metaphyseal fibrous defect (nonossifying fibroma)
  5. Fibrous dysplasia
  6. Myositis ossificans
  7. Histiocytosis X (eosinophilic granuloma, Hand-Schüller-Christian disease, and Letterer-Siwe disease)

DIAGNOSIS, TREATMENT, AND PROGNOSIS

The diagnosis of bone tumors and tumorlike conditions should always be based on a combined clinical, roentgenographic, and pathologic evaluation. In some specific instances, biochemical and hematologic information is also of crucial importance. Laboratory data that are particularly important in this regard include serum levels of calcium, phosphorus, alkaline phosphatase, and acid phosphatase. The tumors and tumorlike conditions in which the knowledge of these data is essential are hyperparathyroidism, Paget's disease, plasma cell myeloma, and metastatic carcinoma. Bone marrow cytology and serum and urinary immunoglobulin determinations are important for the diagnosis of plasma cell myeloma; a thorough hematologic investigation is essential in the evaluation of malignant lymphoma and leukemia of bone; and urinary catecholamine determination is a useful adjunct for the diagnosis of metastatic neuroblastoma.

The most important clinical parameter is the patient's age. Most bone neoplasms show a definite preference for a given age range and are distinctly unusual in another.[199] For instance, a diagnosis of giant cell tumor in a child or of Ewing's sarcoma in an octogenarian should be viewed with great skepticism. Along the same line, a malignant bone tumor composed of uniform small round cells in an infant is likely to be a metastatic neuroblastoma, in a child a Ewing's sarcoma, and in an adult a malignant lymphoma or a metastatic lung carci-

*Modified from Schajowicz, F., Ackerman, L.V. and Sissons, H.A.: Histological typing of bone tumours, International Histological Classification of Tumours, No. 6, Geneva, 1972, World Health Organization.

noma. The sex of the patient, on the other hand, is of little importance in the differential diagnosis of bone tumors, except for some types of metastases.

Symptoms are of importance for the initial detection of the lesion, but are of little consequence in the differential diagnosis; on occasion, they may even be misleading. For instance, a bone tumefaction associated with local pain and redness, fever, and leukocytosis may lead the physician to a diagnosis of osteomyelitis, yet Ewing's sarcoma can result in an identical picture. In general, the larger and more destructive the tumor is, the more likely that it will be malignant. However, one of the largest and most spectacular masses that one can encounter is an aneurysmal bone cyst, which is perhaps not even neoplastic in nature.

The other important information regarding the clinical evaluation pertains to the presence of any of the conditions known to predispose to the appearance of bone tumors, such as Paget's disease, irradiation, bone infarcts, enchondromatosis (Ollier's disease), osteochondromatosis, and fibrous dysplasia.

Radiologic investigation is always of extreme importance. Routine roentgenograms in different views usually provide most of the necessary data for an initial evaluation, but tomograms, xeroradiograms, arteriograms, and particularly the newer techniques of computerized tomography (CT scan) and nuclear magnetic resonance (NMR) imaging provide important additional information.[78,93] Roentgenographic techniques are also useful for guiding the performance of a percutaneous needle biopsy.

The roentgenographic data important for the diagnosis of a bone tumor are the bone involved, precise localization of the lesion (whether medullary, cortical, or juxtacortical and whether diaphyseal, metaphyseal, or epiphyseal if located in a long bone), indication as to whether the lesion has originated in bone or has extended to it from soft tissues, size and shape, margins (whether sharply or ill defined), nature of any changes in the surrounding bone, presence and type of so-called tumor matrix (calcified osteoid or cartilage), and presence and type of periosteal reaction.

On some occasions a tumor that is extensively involving a given bone can hardly be detected by roentgenographic examination. The explanation is that the tumor diffusely permeates the bone marrow spaces without destroying the bone trabeculas (so-called permeative and moth-eaten patterns).

Although a high degree of diagnostic accuracy can be reached on the basis of the roentgenographic examination of the lesion, the final diagnosis on which all prognostic and therapeutic considerations will be made should always be based on a careful pathologic study. I must also emphasize that the relevant clinical and roentgenographic information should always be available to the pathologist before a final diagnosis is made.

This is important because lesions that have a totally different clinical and roentgenographic presentation and are therefore easily distinguished on this basis can have a very similar appearance under the microscope.

Histologic study of a bone tumor usually involves examination of a biopsy specimen, a procedure that should never be omitted when radical surgery, radiotherapy, or chemotherapy is contemplated. The specimen is obtained by either open surgical biopsy (incisional or excisional biopsy) or needle biopsy (aspiration or trochar biopsy).[60,184] Performance of an open surgical biopsy entails a small risk of tumor implantation in the soft tissue, especially in the case of cartilaginous tumors. However, the information obtained by the use of the biopsy far outweighs this potential risk and the procedure should never be omitted. If the tumor proves to be malignant and amenable to surgical ablation, the needle biopsy track is excised in continuity with the tumor mass to prevent a local implantation. Increasingly, the technique of fine-needle aspiration is being used for the diagnosis of malignant bone tumors, particularly osteosarcoma.[226]

The majority of pathologic diagnoses are based on the examination of routinely processed material, that is, tissue that has been subjected to formalin fixation, decalcification if needed, paraffin embedding, and hematoxylin and eosin staining. On occasion, histochemical stains provide additional information of diagnostic significance, such as glycogen identification in Ewing's sarcoma, pyroninophilia of the cytoplasm in plasma cell myeloma, and intense alkaline phosphatase activity in osteosarcoma. Examination of smears of imprints can be useful for the identification of hematopoietic malignancies, such as malignant lymphoma and plasma cell myeloma. Immunohistochemical preparations may permit the precise identification of a cell product, such as factor VIII-related antigen in endothelial cells, lysozyme (muramidase) in histiocytes, or immunoglobulins in plasma cells and their lymphoid precursors. Electron microscopic examination in selected instances has given support for a given diagnosis or has proved of value in the elucidation of the histogenesis of a neoplasm, as in the case of so-called adamantinoma of long bones.

The therapeutic approach to bone tumors varies according to their nature. The three main modalities are surgery, radiotherapy, and chemotherapy. The surgical approach, which is used for most neoplasms, generally consists in curettage (usually followed by packing with bone chips) for benign lesions, block excision for more aggressive but not fully malignant tumors, and more radical operations (such as amputation or disarticulation) for some of the highly malignant neoplasms. Radiotherapy and chemotherapy are particularly important for Ewing's sarcoma and malignant lymphoma.[206] In some instances the combination of these modalities offers better possibilities of cure than when they are given individually. An additional benefit of this approach is that the surgery can be less radical than when it is administered as the only therapy.[108] Indeed, the current trend is decidedly toward a more conservative surgical approach coupled with adjunctive nonsurgical therapy even for highly malignant tumors such as osteosarcoma.[32,168]

From the point of view of behavior, most classifications (including the present one) divide bone neoplasms into a benign and a malignant category. This is very useful for orientation purposes, but it represents a gross oversimplification of the real situation, which is characterized by a whole range of intermediate forms between the perfectly innocuous tumor and the highly invasive and metastasizing neoplasm.

As a general rule the most benign tumors are well circumscribed, have sharply defined outlines, and are surrounded by an area of sclerosis (indicative of slow growth). They may be located within either the medulla or the cortex and show no evidence of soft-tissue extension or periosteal reaction. The most malignant bone tumors tend to be large and poorly circumscribed, often permeate the medullary cavity, extend into the soft tissues, elicit prominent new bone formation from the periosteum, and have the propensity to give distant metastases. The last property is the main criterion for including a bone tumor in the "malignant" category in the classification presented in this chapter. The majority of distant metastases of bone tumors are blood borne and appear in the lungs. Some bone sarcomas, such as Ewing's sarcoma and osteosarcoma, initially located within a single bone, have a tendency to show up later in other bones. Whether these foci represent metastases from the original lesion or multicentric foci of involvement is a moot point.[11] The rarest form of distant metastasis in bone sarcoma is the lymph-borne type. Although instances of lymph node metastases in osteosarcoma and other bone tumors have been reported, the incidence is so low that it can be disregarded when one is planning therapy.

One should understand that local recurrence of a tumor after conservative surgical therapy does not necessarily indicate that it is malignant. The reason for this should be obvious. The most common surgical approach to benign bone tumors consists in unroofing the lesion and removing it in bits with a sharp curette; the space thus formed is then packed with bone chips. No matter how thorough the curettage is, the possibility always exists that a small portion of tumor will remain in situ and provide the nidus for a recurrence.

OSTEOBLASTIC (BONE-FORMING) TUMORS

The common property of the osteoblastic group of bone tumors is the capacity of their constituent cells to produce osteoid or bone, or both, thus fulfilling the criterion of functional osteoblasts. For osteoid or bone for-

mation to be important in this regard, it must be the direct product of the tumor cells. Reactive bone formation by osteoblasts at the periphery of a tumor, or the endochondral ossification that neoplastic cartilage can undergo in the same fashion as normal cartilage, does not necessarily indicate that the tumor associated with them is of osteoblastic origin.

Benign tumors
Osteoma

Osteoma is composed of well-differentiated compact bone of lamellar structure. It has an extremely slow growth rate. It is almost entirely restricted to the skull and facial bones, from which it may grow into the paranasal sinuses.[85] The roentgenographic appearance is that of a dense ivory-like mass. Osteomas can be seen as a component of Gardner's syndrome (intestinal polyposis and soft-tissue tumors).[46] The behavior of this lesion is perfectly benign.

Osteoma of bone is probably not a true neoplasm and perhaps not even a uniform entity. Some cases seem to represent the site of a former injury, such as a subperiosteal hematoma or a localized inflammatory process; others appear to be hamartomas, that is, a the of malformation; still others probably represent the end stage of osteochondroma or fibrous dysplasia.

Osteoid osteoma and osteoblastoma

Osteoid osteoma and osteoblastoma are so closely related that it is better to discuss them together.[89] Their common features include a benign behavior, a preference for children and young adults, and a microscopic appearance characterized by extremely active formation of osteoid and immature bone by plump osteoblasts situated in a highly vascularized stroma (Figs. 39-3 and 39-4). The differences between the two, which are not always clear cut in an individual case, refer to size, presence of pain, location of the lesion, and roentgenographic appearance. Osteoid osteoma is small (usually less than 1 cm), often located in the cortex of a long bone, painful, clearly demarcated, and surrounded by a zone of sclerotic reactive bone[131] (Fig. 39-3). Thus it appears radiographically as a small radiolucent area (the nidus), with or without a minute dense center, in an otherwise sclerotic mass. In the past, it was often confused with a chronic bone abscess or sclerosing osteomyelitis. Osteoblastoma is larger (usually more than 1 cm), painless, located in the vertebrae, in the medulla of long bones, or in the iliac bone, and usually accompanied by a lesser degree of reactive bone formation (Fig. 39-4). It is possible that many of these differences are simply related to the respective sites of the two lesions when they involve a long bone: cortical for osteoid osteoma and medullary for osteoblastoma.[30,61] Examples of osteoid osteoma and osteoblastoma located in the parosteal (juxtacortical) region have been observed.

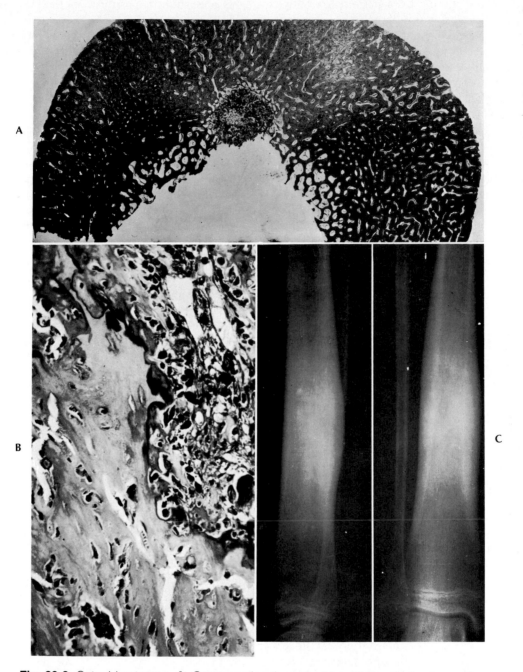

Fig. 39-3. Osteoid osteoma. **A,** Cross section through nidus. Notice thickening and condensation of surrounding cortical bone. **B,** Boundary between highly cellular nidus *(upper right)* and surrounding sclerotized bone. **C,** Lateral and anteroposterior roentgenograms showing typical sclerosis associated with this lesion. Nidus is not well appreciated in this view. (**B,** 180×.)

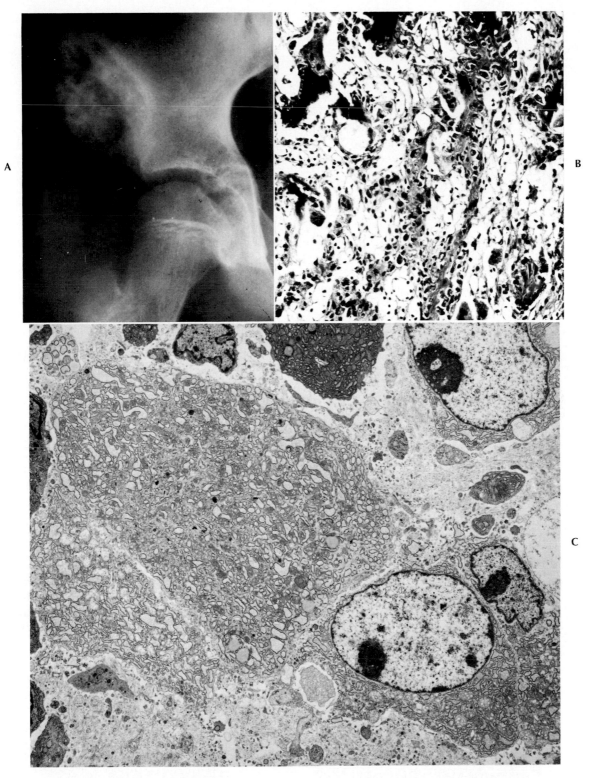

Fig. 39-4. Osteoblastoma. **A,** Roentgenogram showing well-circumscribed lesion in iliac bone, with thin sclerotic border and diffuse ossification. **B,** Microscopic appearance is that of active new osteoid formation by plump fibroblasts. Deposition of calcium salts is evident in upper portion. **C,** Ultrastructurally cells of osteoblastoma show extreme development of granular endoplasmic reticulum. Deposition of interstitial material consistent with osteoid is apparent. (**B,** 160×; **C,** 3950×.)

Very high levels of prostaglandin metabolites have been found in some of these lesions.

Osteoid osteomas and most osteoblastomas are benign. Occasional osteoblastomas behave in an aggressive fashion. This variety has been referred to as aggressive osteoblastoma,[170] malignant osteoblastoma,[187] and osteosarcoma resembling osteoblastoma.[24] Furthermore, an occasional instance of ordinary osteoblastoma developing into osteosarcoma has been recorded.[25]

Malignant tumors
Osteosarcoma

Osteosarcoma is the primary malignant tumor of osteoblasts and is identified microscopically by the direct formation of osteoid or bone, or both, by the neoplastic cells. It is the most common primary malignant tumor of bone, and it is also known as osteogenic sarcoma.[35,55,66,123] Most cases appear in adolescents and young adults. Males are affected more often than females. Many osteosarcomas developing after middle age represent a complication of Paget's disease or irradiation therapy to the area[96] (Fig. 39-5). The classic site of occurrence is the medulla of the metaphysis of long bones, particularly the lower end of the femur, the upper end of the tibia, and the upper end of the humerus. It also occurs in the jaw, where it is associated with a better prognosis.[47] In rare cases there are multiple independent foci throughout the skeleton[162] (Fig. 39-6).

Osteosarcoma is a highly invasive neoplasm. It permeates the medullary cavity and can extend for a long distance from its site of inception (this being one of the causes for the stump recurrences often seen after amputations done too close to the tumor mass)[128]; it also breaks through the cortex, elevates the periosteum, and grows relentlessly into the soft tissues (Fig. 39-7). Only one tissue is able to stop, at least temporarily, the ad-

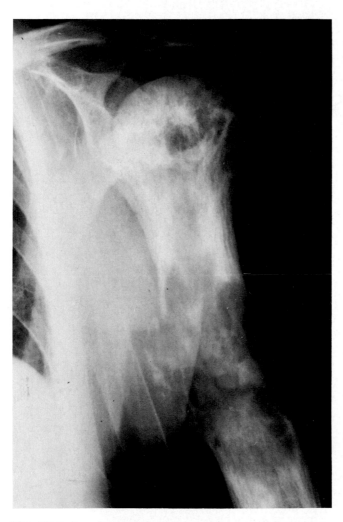

Fig. 39-5. Paget's disease complicated by osteosarcoma and pathologic fracture. Notice thickening of bone resulting from Paget's disease and destructive lytic process in center of figure, corresponding to poorly differentiated osteosarcoma with scanty osteoid formation.

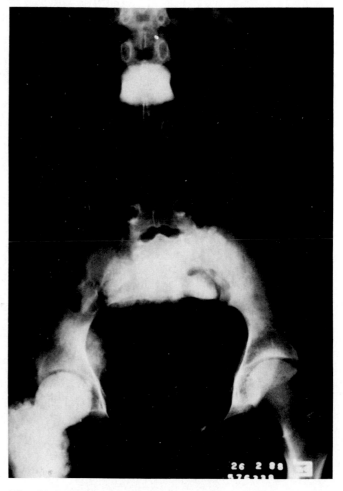

Fig. 39-6. Multicentric osteosarcoma in 14-year-old male. Roentgenogram shows highly blastic foci of tumor in vertebra, pelvis, and femur. (Courtesy Dr. J. Segura, San José, Costa Rica.)

vance of this tumor; it is the cartilage of the epiphyseal plate (Fig. 39-8). Because of this, it is relatively uncommon for osteosarcomas in young persons (when the epiphyseal plate is present) to extend into the epiphyses; once the cartilage from the epiphyseal plate has disappeared, the tumor freely extends into the articular end of the bone and may even penetrate the joint cavity. This remarkable capacity of cartilage to resist the invasion by osteosarcoma cells is also evident in organ-cell culture systems and may be caused by the release of a collagenase inhibitor.[117]

Satellite nodules (known as "skip metastases") may be found proximal to the primary lesion, either in the same bone or into another transarticularly.[67] Distant metastases are common and are the reason for the present high rate of failures in the treatment of this neo-

plasm. They are generally blood borne, and the lungs are the most common site of involvement (Fig. 39-9).

The roentgenographic appearance depends a great deal on the relative amount of bone produced in a particular tumor. A tumor that produces a large amount of osteoid matrix that calcifies will appear as a highly sclerotic lesion; a less-differentiated tumor that produces little or no recognizable bone will occur as a lytic lesion (Fig. 39-10).

The gross appearance of an osteosarcoma depends largely on the relative amounts of osteoid, bone, and cartilage being produced. Tumors with an abundance of these materials have a hard, partially calcified appearance, whereas more undifferentiated tumors are softer and whitish or pink, with frequent areas of necrosis and hemorrhage. Foci of cartilage formation appear as

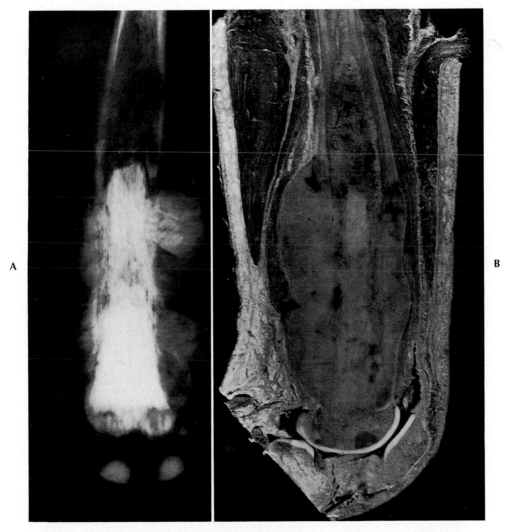

Fig. 39-7. Osteosarcoma. **A,** Roentgenogram of midsagittal slice of femur massively invaded by heavily ossified tumor. Notice condensation and loss of architectural design of affected segment of femur and pronounced osseous tissue growth subperiosteally. **B,** Gross appearance of sectioned surface of osteosarcoma shown in **A.**

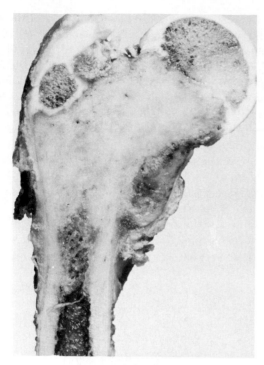

Fig. 39-8. Osteosarcoma of proximal femur in 10-year-old boy. There is extensive involvement of medullary cavity, invasion of cortex and soft tissues, and periosteal elevation. Notice how tumor growth is restrained by epiphyseal cartilage.

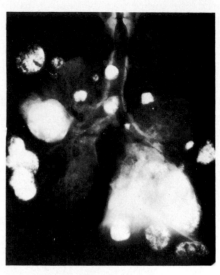

Fig. 39-9. Roentgenogram of lungs removed from patient who died of osteosarcoma. Metastases consist of bone that is heavily mineralized.

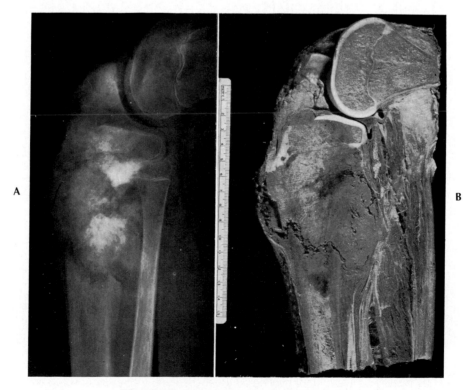

Fig. 39-10. For legend see opposite page.

white, glistening, somewhat mucoid areas. Some osteosarcomas are accompanied by large blood-filled cavities that result in an appearance not unlike that of aneurysmal bone cyst ("telangiectatic osteosarcomas")[101] (Fig. 39-11).

Osteosarcomas show a considerable variation in microscopic pattern.[57] The tumor cells may be small and more or less uniform in size and shape or highly pleomorphic, with bizarre nuclear and cytoplasmic shapes and numerous mitoses[236] (Figs. 39-10 and 39-12). Osteosarcomas predominantly composed of small round cells with little osteoid production can be confused with Ewing's sarcoma.[135] Other intraosseus osteosarcomas are so well differentiated as to simulate fibrous dysplasia.[221]

In addition to osteoid and bone, the tumor cells of osteosarcoma may produce cartilage, fibrous tissue, or myxoid tissue. In fact, in some tumors the production of cartilage or fibrous tissue is even greater than that of osteoid or bone. Other areas may have a totally undifferentiated appearance, without any type of intercellular material being deposited. However, it should be emphasized that as long as a malignant bone tumor is producing osteoid or bone directly from the neoplastic cells it should be designated as "osteosarcoma" regardless of how focal this production may be and regardless of how many other materials (cartilage, fibrous tissue) are being produced elsewhere by the tumor. Some authors have subclassified osteosarcomas into osteoblastic, chondroblastic, and fibroblastic on the basis of the rel-

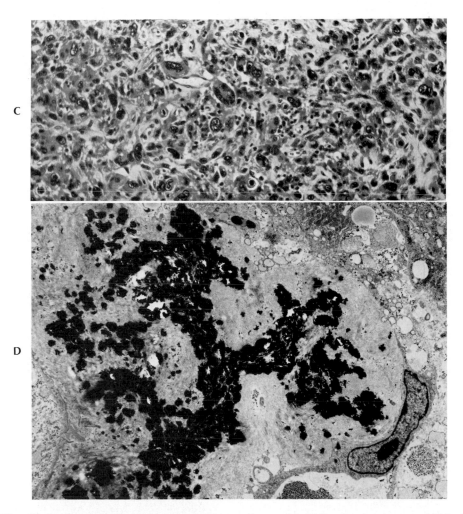

Fig. 39-10. Osteosarcoma. **A** and **B,** Destructive and rapidly growing tumor of tibia that has resulted in pathologic fracture. **C,** Variation in size and shape of cells, bizarre mitoses, and little or no evidence of bone matrix formation are noteworthy features in this lytic form of osteosarcoma. **D,** Electron microscopy shows heavy deposition of interstitial material composed of collagen and acid glycosaminoglycans (osteoid), which is becoming transformed into bone in center through precipitation of darkly staining calcium salts. (**C,** 165×; **D,** 3950×.)

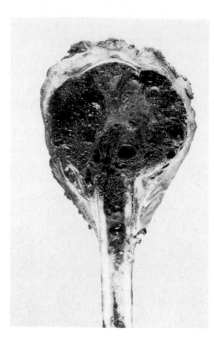

Fig. 39-11. Telangiectatic osteosarcoma of humerus in a 32-year-old male. The presence of large cystic spaces filled with blood results in a gross appearance very similar to that of aneurysmal bone cyst. (Courtesy Dr. J. Costa, Lausanne, Switzerland.)

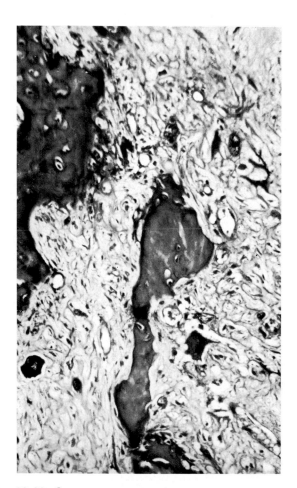

Fig. 39-12. Osteosarcoma. Bizarre cellular pattern and irregular ossification are shown. (230×.)

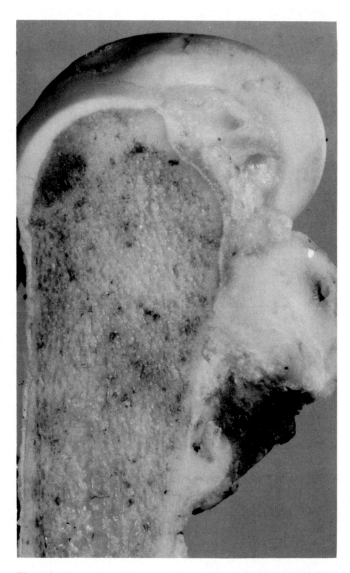

Fig. 39-13. Juxtacortical osteosarcoma in 57-year-old man. Notice periosteal location and lack of intraosseous involvement. Patient remains well over 10 years after amputation.

ative amounts of osteoid, cartilage, and collagen they produce, but there is little if any relationship between these types and the prognosis.[192]

The neoplastic osteoblasts have many of the attributes of their normal counterparts; they contain large amounts of enzymes of the alkaline phosphatase group, produce largely type I procollagen, and have a greatly developed granular endoplasmic reticulum when examined under the electron microscope.[169,193] They also secrete osteonectin, and this can be detected immunohistochemically.[190]

As previously mentioned, most osteosarcomas arise within the medullary cavity. There is, on the other hand, a type of osteosarcoma that originates in a location extrinsic to the cortex, that is, in the periosteal or parosteal region. It is designated as juxtacortical or parosteal osteosarcoma[220] (Fig. 39-13). It is an osteosarcoma in the true sense of the word, in that it produces neoplastic osteoid and bone. However, it should be distinguished from the more common medullary variety because of its distinct form of presentation and better prognosis.[37] It occurs in an older age group, shows no

sex predilection, grows relatively slowly, is circumscribed and sometimes lobulated, and is nearly always located in the lower end of the femur. Roentgenologic examination usually reveals a dense bony mass that, although firmly attached to the bone cortex over a wide base, tends to encircle the shaft as a bulky and heavily calcified growth (Fig. 39-14, A). Microscopically it usually shows a high degree of structural differentiation. It is composed of a mass of bone trabeculas, often mature and lamellar, which merge with the adjacent cortical bone (Fig. 39-14, B). As in the case of the medullary osteosarcoma, fibrous tissue and cartilage may also be present. The tumor cells are often well differentiated, with few mitoses and very little pleomorphism. The diagnosis is often difficult and usually requires a combined evaluation of roentgenographic and microscopic findings. Many of the cases are misdiagnosed as atypical osteochondromas or myositis ossificans. The prognosis is much better than that of the usual osteosarcoma as long as the microscopic pattern remains well differentiated. The few superficially located osteosarcomas that have highly malignant cytologic features behave in a

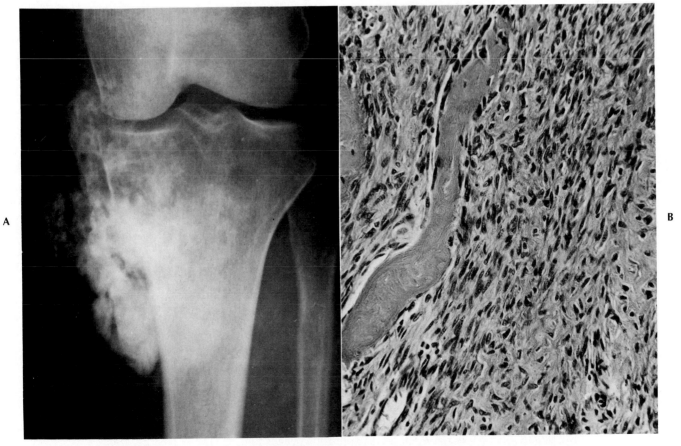

Fig. 39-14. A, Typical juxtacortical osteosarcoma in 40-year-old woman. Notice large exophytic component. **B,** Same lesion shown in **A** demonstrating well-differentiated character of sarcomatous stroma. This lesion has been present for several years. (**B,** 250×.)

correspondingly aggressive fashion.[231] This is also the case for the rare juxtacortical osteosarcoma that undergoes dedifferentiation and acquires the features of a high-grade sarcoma.[232]

Periosteal osteosarcoma (not to be confused with the just-described parosteal variety) is a high-grade tumor that grows on the bone surface (usually in the tibia or femur) and has a prominent cartilaginous component.[84] It is very similar but perhaps not identical to the lesion that other authors designate as juxtacortical chondrosarcoma.[22]

CHONDROBLASTIC (CARTILAGE-FORMING) TUMORS
Benign tumors
Chondroma

Chondroma is a relatively common tumor composed of the elements of mature hyaline cartilage. It typically involves the short tubular bones of the hands and feet and, less commonly, the ribs (particularly at the costochondral junction) and long bones.[209] Chondroma may be solitary or multiple; the latter condition, which is not familial, is referred to as "multiple enchondromatosis." Cases of multiple enchondromatosis with an exclusive or predominant unilateral distribution are known as "Ollier's disease," or "dyschondroplasia." When multiple chondromas are accompanied by multi-

ple soft-tissue hemangiomas, the term *"Maffucci's syndrome"* is used.[127]

Most chondromas are located in the medullary portion of the diaphysis and are therefore referred to as "enchondromas." They result in a well-circumscribed lytic lesion. Calcification, usually present in the form of small punctate areas, may be massive in some cases (Fig. 39-15, *A*). A less common variant of chondroma is seen outside the cortex and is referred to as "juxtacortical or periosteal chondroma"[28,156] (Fig. 39-16).

Grossly and microscopically, chondromas recapitulate the appearance of normal adult hyaline cartilage, though their pattern of orientation is abnormal. They have a characteristic lobulated appearance and may undergo necrosis, calcification, endochondral ossification, and myxoid degeneration. The nuclei of the cartilaginous cells are small, single, and irregular; mitotic figures are absent (Fig. 39-15, *B*). The ultrastructural features are very similar to those of normal cartilaginous cells (Fig. 39-17). Immunohistochemically the tumor cells consistently show nuclear and cytoplasmic reactivity for S-100 protein; this is also true for other types of cartilaginous neoplasms.[157,225] The behavior of both solitary and multiple chondromas is benign. However, chondrosarcomas develop in a small percentage of patients with multiple enchondromatosis or, in Maffucci's syndrome, sometimes multicentrically.[39,129,207] Benign

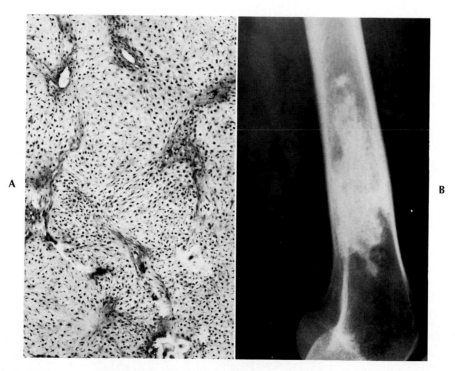

Fig. 39-15. Enchondroma. **A,** Large, benign, cartilaginous tumor of femur exhibiting massive calcification. Lesion was discovered accidentally in 42-year-old woman. It was easily detectable on bone scan because of presence of foci of bone production. **B,** Microscopic appearance of chondroma, showing mature hyaline cartilage growing in lobular arrangement. (**B,** 64×.)

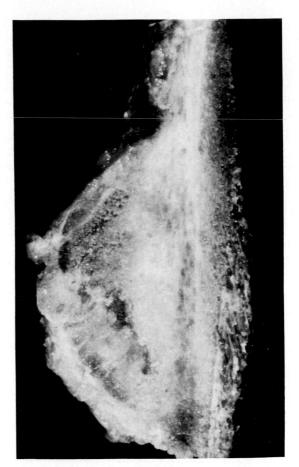

Fig. 39-16. Juxtacortical chondroma of femur. The tumor grows exophytically from the periosteal region. There is no involvement of the underlying cortex.

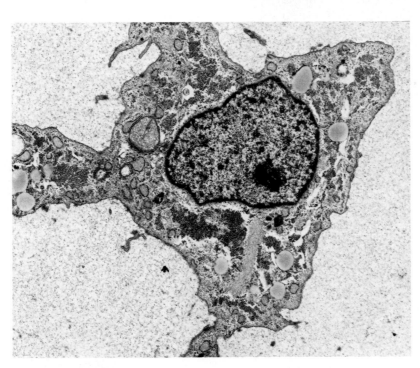

Fig. 39-17. Ultrastructural appearance of cartilaginous cell from patient with enchondroma associated with Maffucci's syndrome. Cytoplasm contains glycogen, lipid vacuoles, scanty mitochondria, and bundles of microfilaments. Cell is surrounded by abundant cartilaginous matrix. (8640×.)

cartilaginous tumors of long and flat bones are very rare; any cartilaginous tumor in these locations should be viewed with suspicion, even if the microscopic features are those of a well-differentiated neoplasm.

Osteochondroma

The typical osteochondroma presents as an exophytic mass protruding from the metaphyseal area of a long bone, invariably pointing in a direction opposite to the articular cavity. It is also referred to as an "exostosis" or "osteocartilaginous exostosis" in the orthopedic literature. It is the most common bone "tumor." As in the case of the osteoma, it is doubtful that osteochondroma is a true neoplasm. It may represent instead a disorder of growth. It is usually solitary, though it may appear as part of a familial condition known as multiple hereditary exostoses (diaphyseal aclasis, hereditary deforming chondrodysplasia) (Fig. 39-18).

Grossly, osteochondromas may have either a broad or a narrow base that is continuous with the cortical bone

(Fig. 39-19). Microscopically they are composed of a center of mature lamellar bone covered by a cartilaginous cap (Fig. 39-20). Active endochondral ossification is seen at the interphase between the two tissues. Eventually, all the cartilage is replaced by bone that contains bone marrow elements between its trabeculas.

It is not clear whether subungual (Dupuytren's) exostosis is a type of osteochondroma or an independent entity, but the latter interpretations is favored. It is often painful and forms beneath the nail of the finger or toe, especially the great toe.[142]

Malignant transformation, usually in the form of chondrosarcoma, is rare with the solitary osteochondroma but is seen with some frequency in patients with multiple hereditary exostoses.[75]

Chondroblastoma

Chondroblastoma is a rare benign cartilaginous tumor that occurs almost exclusively in the epiphyseal ends of long bones, adjacent to the epiphyseal cartilage plate[185] (Fig. 39-21). Occasionally it extends into the adjacent metaphysis. The majority of the patients are under 25 years of age. The roentgenographic appearance is that of a well-circumscribed lytic lesion with multiple small foci of calcification.[202] The gross appearance is not dis-

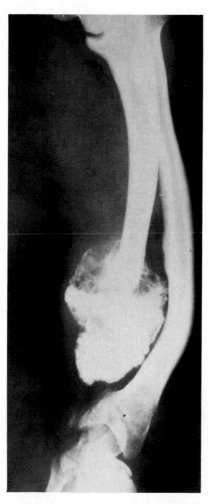

Fig. 39-18. Multiple osteochondromatosis. Large osteochondroma is seen involving distal end of ulna and deforming radius by compression.

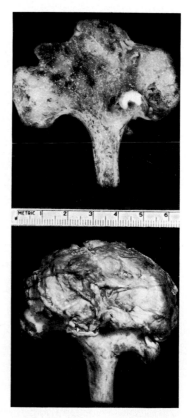

Fig. 39-19. Typical mushroom-shaped osteochondroma.

tinctive. The tumor has a granular texture and a gray to whitish color. Microscopically the first impression is not that of a cartilaginous tumor. What one sees is a polymorphic, highly cellular lesion in which scattered multinucleated cells with the appearance of osteoclasts alternate with much more numerous, small, polygonal or round, mononuclear cells with a histocyte-like appearance. Because of the numerous multinucleated giant cells, this lesion was originally misinterpreted as a var-

iant of giant cell tumor. In this regard, it is important to remember that the mere presence of multinucleated giant cells in a bone tumor is by no means justification to label this neoplasm as a giant cell tumor. One should realize, instead, that giant cells are a common nonspecific accompaniment of a variety of benign and malignant bone tumors and tumorlike nonneoplastic conditions. The important cells are the smaller and more numerous mononuclear elements. In the case of chon-

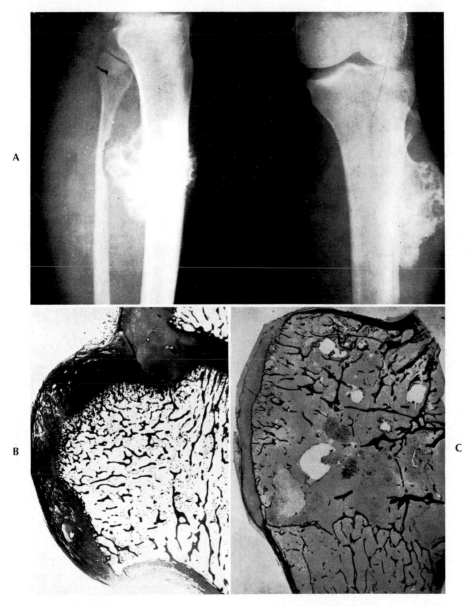

Fig. 39-20. Osteochondroma. **A,** Large, pedunculated mass involved upper tibial metaphysis. Direction of growth has been away from epiphyseal end of shaft. Pressure atrophy of fibula from contact with tumor is apparent in lateral view. **B,** Osteochondroma in early stage of development in young child. Section has been taken through junction of metaphyseal end of tibia *(lower three fourths)* and epiphysis *(upper right).* Relation of tumor to perichondrium is apparent. **C,** Flat osteochondroma of upper end of femur. Notice perichondrial layer, growing cartilage, and irregular trabecular bone that has resulted from imperfect endochondral ossification.

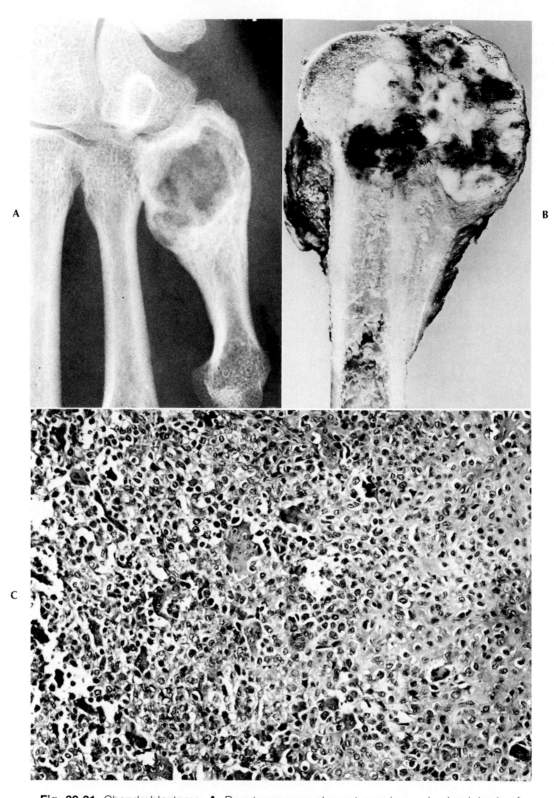

Fig. 39-21. Chondroblastoma. **A,** Roentgenogram shows tumor in proximal epiphysis of fifth metacarpal bone of 17-year-old girl. Lesion is well circumscribed and expansile with sclerotic border, and it exhibits minute foci of calcification. **B,** Gross appearance of well-outlined chondroblastoma involving epiphysis of humerus in young adult. **C,** Microscopic appearance of chondroblastoma is characterized by osteoclast-like giant cells separated by small polygonal cells representing chondroblasts. Deposition of cartilaginous matrix can be appreciated on right side of photograph. (160×.)

droblastoma, these are chondroblasts, as evidence by their electron microscopic appearance, the immunohistochemical positivity for S-100 protein, the lack of histiocytic markers, and the fact that a careful search under the light microscope invariably reveals the presence of small amounts of cartilaginous intercellular matrix with areas of focal calcification.[29,125] In some instances, typical areas of chondroblastoma alternate with large blood-filled vascular spaces reminiscent of aneurysmal bone cysts. These are referred to as "cystic chondroblastomas."

The behavior of chondroblastoma is generally benign. Some tumors recur after curettage, and on occasion they extend into the articular space or the soft tissue.[171] Exceptionally, a tumor that has all the microscopic appearance of chondroblastoma has given rise to distant metastases.[118] This is so uncommon that for purposes of therapy chondroblastoma should be regarded as a benign neoplasm.

Chondromyxoid fibroma

A chondromyxoid fibroma is also a benign tumor of cartilaginous origin, despite its name, which is suggestive of a primarily fibrous derivation. If often occurs in the metaphysis of long bones, and the upper end of the tibia is the single most common area of involvement.[77] The bones of the feet are another site of preferential involvement by this tumor. Roentgenographically, it

appears as an eccentric, sharply outlined, radiolucent area that often causes expansion of the bone (Fig. 39-22, A).[186] Calcification with the lesion is not as common as with other cartilaginous tumors. A thin sclerotic inner border is usually present, as in most benign bone tumors. Grossly it is solid, often lobulated, and yellowish white or tan. Usually there is a quality of translucency, suggestive of cartilaginous derivation. Microscopically a lobulated architecture can be readily observed with low-power examination. The lobules are separated by bands of fibrous tissue lined on the sides by a variable number of multinucleated giant cells with the appearance of osteoclasts (Fig. 39-22, B). The lobules themselves are composed of immature cartilage with a prominent myxoid pattern. Easily identifiable chondroblasts alternate with stellate myxoid cells and scattered large pleomorphic cells. The latter may result in an erroneous diagnosis of malignancy. Mitoses are uncommon. Rarely tumors representing hybrids between chondromyxoid fibroma and chondroblastoma are encountered.[54] This is not surprising in view of the close histogenetic relationship between these neoplasms.

Chondromyxoid fibroma is essentially a benign tumor, yet it may manifest a certain degree of aggressive behavior. The recurrence rate after curettage approaches 25%, and because of this some orthopedic surgeons prefer to treat it with an en bloc excision. Ex-

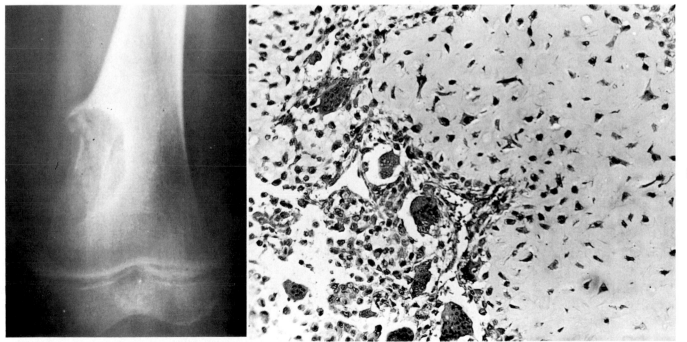

A   B

Fig. 39-22. Chondromyxoid fibroma. **A,** Roentgenogram shows involvement of lower femoral epiphysis by eccentrically located tumor with sharp and sclerotic borders. **B,** Microscopically there is alternation of giant cells, fibroma-like cellular areas, and cartilage. (**B,** 200×.)

tension or implantation into soft tissues has also been seen,[119] but distant metastases have not been encountered so far.

Malignant tumors
Chondrosarcoma

As the name indicates, chondrosarcoma is a malignant tumor of chondroblasts.[19,38] It usually develops in middle age or later. Two major varieties—the central and the peripheral—exist.[90] The central chondrosarcoma originates, presumably anew, in the medullary cavity of the diaphysis or metaphysis. The typical roentgenographic appearance is an osteolytic lesion with splotchy calcification, ill-defined margins, fusiform thickening of the shaft, and perforation of the cortex[139] (Fig. 39-23). The peripheral form, which is cortical in location, can be primary or represent a malignant degeneration in the cartilage of an osteochondroma. Roentgenographically, it is a large tumor, with a heavily calcified center surrounded by a less dense periphery with splotchy calcification. A less common and somewhat controversial variety of chondrosarcoma arises in relation to the periosteum and is known as "juxtacortical chondrosarcoma."

The gross appearance of chondrosarcoma betrays its cartilaginous composition. The tumor is often extremely large and has a lobulated outline (especially in the peripheral variety), firm consistency, and a glistening white or bluish, translucent cut surface (Fig. 39-24). A gelatinous or myxoid quality is often evident. Calcification is often present and may be extreme. Foci of ossification may be encountered. The central chondrosarcoma may be seen pushing into the cortex and eventually reaching the periosteum and surrounding soft tissues.[159]

Microscopically the hallmark of chondrosarcoma is the presence of chondroblasts having atypical cytologic features, situated in a more or less organized cartilaginous matrix (Fig. 39-25). The cytologic signs of malignancy can be very obvious or quite subtle. In the well-differentiated examples the pathologist must rely on minimal morphologic deviations, such as plump nuclei, multinucleated chondroblasts, presence of multiple chondroblasts in a single lacuna, and strikingly accelerated growth activity at the margins of the individual lobules or nodules. In these cases evaluation of the clinical and roentgenographic features is of paramount importance. The just-mentioned minor microscopic characteristics, if present in an invasive tumor of the medullary cavity of a long bone, are diagnostic of chon-

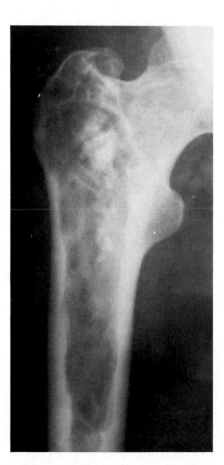

Fig. 39-23. Central chondrosarcoma involving upper metaphysis of femur. Notice splotchy calcification, lobulated contour, and cortical destruction.

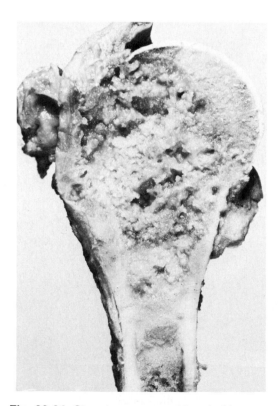

Fig. 39-24. Chondrosarcoma of head of humerus.

drosarcoma but, if present in a small cartilaginous tumor of the hand, are usually of no significance.

On occasion the tumor cells of a chondrosarcoma can have abundant clear cytoplasm, which may lead to confusion with metastatic carcinoma (particularly from the kidney) and chondroblastoma[26] (Fig. 39-26). On other occasions, the tumor has a prominent myxoid appearance; this feature is particularly common in primary chondrosarcomas of soft tissues.

Neoplastic cartilage, like its normal counterpart, may be replaced by bone by a mechanism of endochondral ossification. In this process the cartilage is reabsorbed and new bone is laid down in its place by osteoblasts, that is, cells different from those that produced the cartilage. Presence of endochondral ossification in a neoplastic cartilage is not an indication that the tumor is an osteosarcoma or a reason to call the tumor an osteochondrosarcoma. It is only when the bone or osteoid is produced directly by the neoplastic cells, that is, without the interposition of a cartilaginous phase, that the term "osteosarcoma" should be used. Sometimes it is difficult to decide the nature of the bone present in a tumor that otherwise would qualify as chondrosarcoma; this probably explains why the same tumor is regarded as a juxtacortical chondrosarcoma by some authors and a periosteal osteosarcoma by others.[22,156]

Although both chondromas and osteochondromas (especially the generalized forms) can lead to chondrosar-

coma development, it seems likely that the majority of chondrosarcomas are primary tumors.

The behavior of chondrosarcoma varies a great deal according to the degree of microscopic differentiation.[68,139,178] Well-differentiated (low-grade) neoplasms grow slowly and rarely metastasize. Poorly differentiated (high-grade) tumors invade quickly and are prone to distant metastases, particularly to the lungs. A peculiar feature of chondrosarcoma is its capacity to implant in soft tissues as a result of surgical manipulation. This property is probably attributable to the relatively low need for oxygen that cartilaginous tissue is known to have.[167] In some instances autopsy reveals a continuous intravascular growth of tumor, which may extend to the right side of the heart or even into the pulmonary arteries.

A variant of chondrosarcoma that deserves to be considered separately is the mesenchymal chondrosarcoma.[151] It is more malignant than the conventional variety and more often multicentric. In a significant percentage of cases it arises in the soft tissues.[82] The distinctive microscopic appearance is provided by the alternate arrangements of two greatly different patterns—one of relatively well-differentiated cartilage and the other of highly cellular and vascularized small cells of either round or spindle shape (Fig. 39-27). Although the small cells have some morphologic resemblance to pericytes when viewed with the light micro-

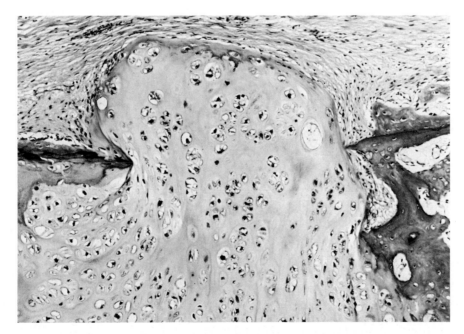

Fig. 39-25. Bizarre and plump nuclei in well-differentiated chondrosarcoma from pelvis. This histologic section also shows tumor protruding through cortical bone into surrounding soft tissues. This feature and lobular pattern seen grossly illustrate danger of enucleating these tumors, which leads almost inevitably to tumor recurrence. (125×.)

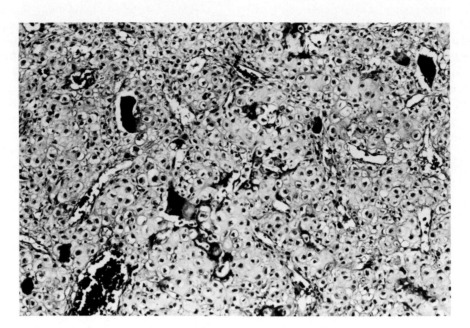

Fig. 39-26. Clear cell chondrosarcoma. The strikingly clear cytoplasmic appearance of the tumor cells may result in a mistaken diagnosis of metastatic carcinoma. Bone spicules are present among the neoplastic cartilaginous lobules.

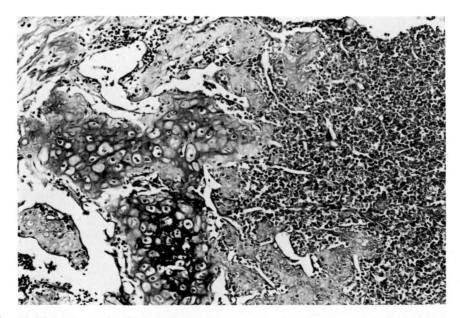

Fig. 39-27. Mesenchymal chondrosarcoma. Lobules of well-differentiated cartilage alternate with foci of undifferentiated small cells growing in a hemangiopericytoma-like pattern. This biphasic appearance is characteristic of this neoplasm.

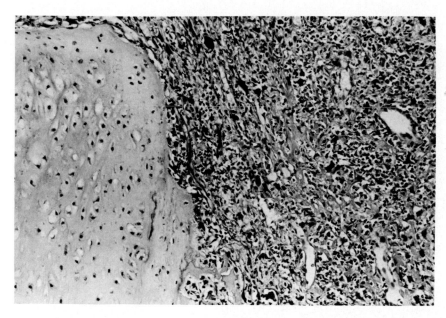

Fig. 39-28. Dedifferentiated chondrosarcoma. The preexisting well-differentiated component is evident at the left, in the form of a well-defined lobule. The dedifferentiated element has the appearance of a high-grade pleomorphic sarcoma.

scope, their fine-structural appearance and relationship with the other component of the tumor indicate that they may instead be poorly differentiated chondroblasts. Jacobson[104] regards mesenchymal chondrosarcoma as the most conspicuous member of a family of neoplasms that arise from primitive multipotential cells and that he likes to call "polyhistiomas."

Another distinctive variant is so-called dedifferentiated chondrosarcoma, in which a long-standing well-differentiated chondrosarcoma is seen to undergo a transformation into a high-grade neoplasm (Fig. 39-28). The latter component may acquire the phenotypical features of osteosarcoma, malignant fibrous histiocytoma, or rhabdomyosarcoma, and is indicative of an extremely aggressive clinical course.[110,213]

GIANT CELL TUMOR (OSTEOCLASTOMA)

The giant cell tumor is in a category by itself in most classifications of bone tumors, mainly because of the uncertainty that still exists regarding its histogenesis. Some investigators even doubt that it constitutes a valid entity. However, the elimination from the category of giant cell tumor of many neoplasms and tumorlike conditions that simulated it because of their high content of giant cells has resulted in the delineation of a lesion with quite definite clinicopathologic features[36,138,150] (Fig. 39-29).

Giant cell tumor is usually a tumor of adults. Although well-documented cases have been recorded in children, one should always keep in mind that if a giant

cell–containing lesion is found in a patient younger than 15 years of age, the chances are overwhelming that it will prove to be something other than a true giant cell tumor.

Giant cell tumor shares with chondroblastoma a predilection for epiphyseal involvement, though in the case of the former there is nearly always also some involvement of the metaphysis, from which the tumor perhaps arises.[36] It may be significant in this regard that the overwhelming number of giant cell tumors occurs after the epiphyses have closed. The lower end of the femur, upper end of the tibia, and lower end of the radius are the most common sites of involvement, in that order of frequency. Pain that is especially severe on weight bearing and motion is usually the first symptom. Later there may be noticeable swelling. A pathologic fracture may supervene. Roentgenographically, giant cell tumor appears as a somewhat lobulated lytic lesion, generally without sclerosis of the borders and usually located eccentrically within the epiphysis, in a condyle. On gross inspection it is well circumscribed and often has a granular hemorrhagic appearance. The expanded portion is partially or completely encased in a thin shell of bone. The neoplastic tissue is firm and friable. It is often grayish, with either a pinkish or a brownish tint. Focal areas of cystic degeneration, of yellow-brown color, and hemorrhagic areas that are red or dark brown, depending on the age of the hemorrhage, are usually present.

The microscopic hallmark of this neoplasm is the

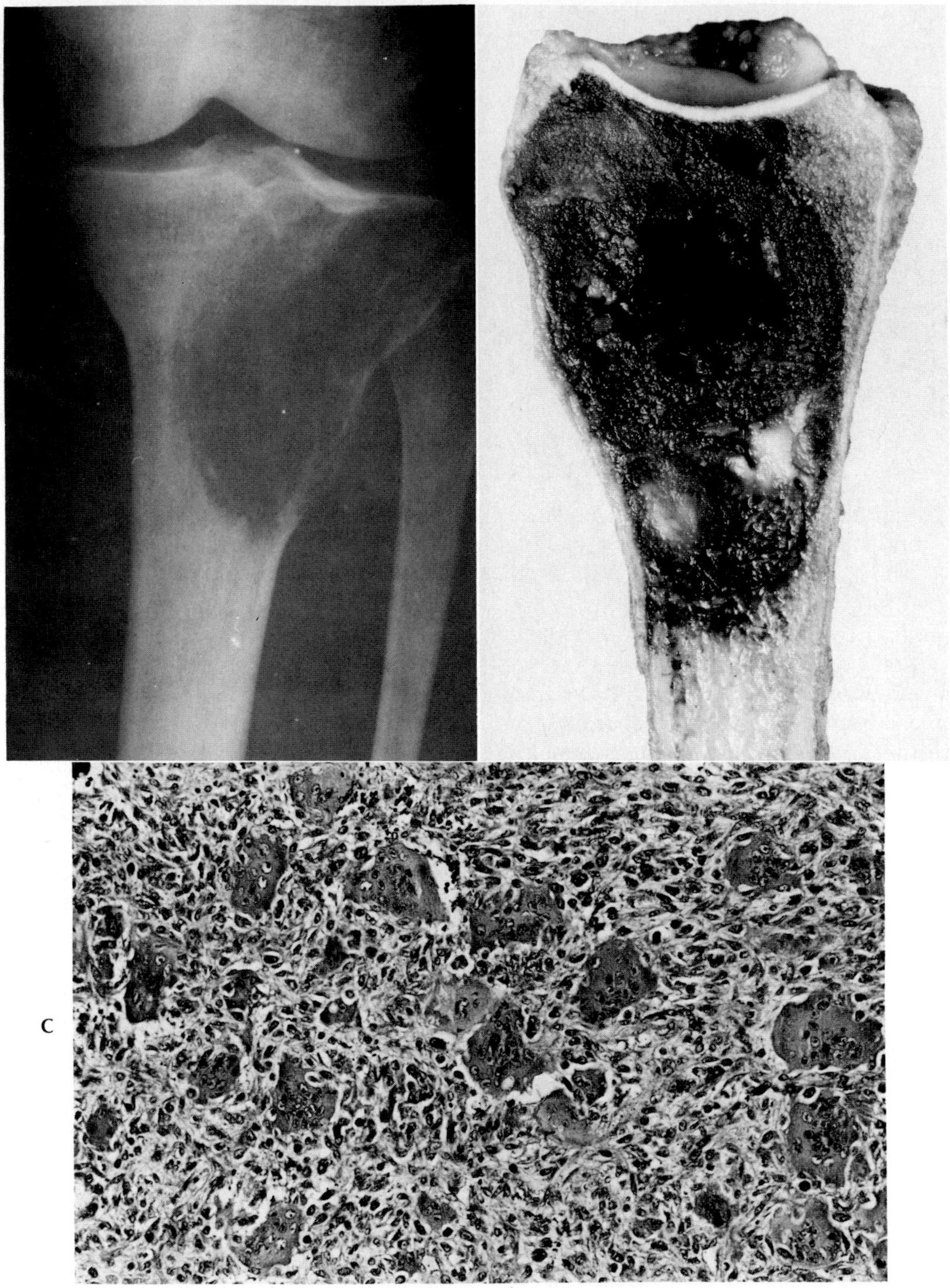

Fig. 39-29. Giant cell tumor. **A,** Typical roentgenographic appearance. Tumor involves upper tibial epiphysis and diaphysis. It is eccentrically located and shows little or no sclerosis of margins. **B,** Gross appearance of giant cell tumor involving upper epiphysis and metaphysis of tibia. Notice granular hemorrhagic appearance and central cystic degeneration. Articular cartilage is intact. **C,** Microscopically, giant cells with features of osteoclasts are seen regularly scattered among smaller mononuclear cells. (**B,** 765×; AFIP 63505.)

presence of a large number of multinucleated giant cells that are *regularly* scattered throughout the tumor mass. This spatial relationship between giant cells and other cellular components is important in the differential diagnosis with the diseases that simulate giant cell tumors. In those, the giant cells are irregularly distributed, often in clumps or surrounding blood vessels, with large tumor areas being devoid of them.

The giant cells of giant cell tumor have an abundant acidophilic cytoplasm and as many as 100 nuclei. Their light microscopic, enzymatic, histochemical, immunohistochemical, and fine-structural features are similar to those of normal osteoclasts.[15,80,181] Thus acid phosphatase activity is very high, and a large number of mitochondria are present in the cytoplasm.[204] Because of these similarities, giant cell tumor of bone is also known as "osteoclastoma."

The second microscopic component of the giant cell tumor is often given the unassuming name "stromal cell." Although far less spectacular than the giant cell when examined under the microscope, it is probably the only real tumor cell. It is certainly more important numerically than the giant cell. The relative number and appearance of these stromal cells correlates with the clinical evolution. In locally aggressive and metastasizing lesions, one often gets the impression that the stromal cell component has taken over the neoplasm. The stromal cells of a typical giant cell tumor are medium sized and oval or spindle shaped, with rather plump nuclei and ill-defined acidophilic cytoplasm. Mononuclear macrophages are also present in large numbers, but they probably are nonneoplastic and an expression of the host reaction to the tumor.[114] The stroma is richly vascularized and contains a small amount of collagen. In about a third of the cases, foci of osteoid or bone formation of reactive appearance are found. Under the electron microscope the stromal cells are seen to contain a well-developed granular endoplasmic reticulum. Their appearance is reminiscent of a fibroblast or an osteoblast.[86]

Giant cell tumors are aggressive lesions. As much as 60% recur after curettage, and about 10% result in distant metastases, usually to the lungs. Metastasis is almost always preceded by a history of repeated curettages and recurrences. Because of this, many authors recommend en bloc excision as the treatment of choice for this neoplasm. It has been suggested that radiotherapy may be influential in triggering the malignant transformation of this tumor.[223] Indeed, in a disproportionately high number of cases of postradiation bone sarcoma the initial lesion was a giant cell tumor.

The microscopic grading systems proposed to allow prediction of the clinical behavior of this tumor have not proved satisfactory, and there is no agreement on specific histologic features that dependably indicate the likelihood of malignant behavior. Indeed, distant metastases have been documented in several microscopically "benign" cases.[172] However, it is safe to assume that the rare giant cell tumors that are cytologically malignant will behave in an aggressive fashion[154] and that most metastasizing giant cell tumors will be histologically malignant.[177]

MARROW TUMORS
Ewing's sarcoma

Ewing's sarcoma, a highly malignant neoplasm first described by Ewing in 1921, usually occurs in patients between 5 and 20 years of age.[116,228] Nearly all cases are in whites.[79] Typically the patient complains of pain in the affected area, sometimes accompanied by swelling. The patient may have a fever, and the leukocyte count and erythrosedimentation rate may be slightly or moderately elevated. These signs and symptoms may lead to an erroneous diagnosis of osteomyelitis. Roentgenographically the lesion is predominantly osteolytic. However, the bond destruction is often associated with patchy reactive periosteal bone formation, which may result in the pattern that radiologists call "onion-skin appearance" (Fig. 39-30, *A*). Grossly the tumor is white and exceedingly soft and friable; large areas of necrosis and hemorrhage are often encountered. The site of origin is the medullary canal of the diaphysis or metaphysis, from which the tumor permeates the cortex and invades the soft tissues. The bone marrow permeation can be quite extensive and still leave the bone trabeculas relatively undisturbed and the tumor may be missed on roentgenographic examination. Distant metastases are common, particularly to the lung, the liver, other bones, and the central nervous system.[212]

Microscopically the tumor tissue has a rather uniform appearance. It is made up of densely packed small cells with round nuclei, frequent mitoses, scanty cytoplasm, and ill-defined cytoplasmic outlines (Fig. 39-30, *B*). The cytoplasm contains a moderate to large amount of glycogen granules, a feature of importance in the differential diagnosis[180] (Fig. 39-30, *C*). Fibrous septa divide the tumor tissue into irregular lobules. Areas of necrosis are frequent; these may be secondarily infiltrated with acute inflammatory cells. Vascularization is usually well developed. The tumor cells may be grouped around blood vessels, producing a false rosette. The fine structural appearance is usually that of primitive cells without signs of differentiation.[132] Focal new bone formation is usually encountered, but this is believed to be of reactive nature. In some cases of Ewing's sarcoma the tumor cells have larger nuclei, with more conspicuous nucleoli than in the usual variety.[155] Tumors morphologically indistinguishable from Ewing's sarcoma are occasionally seen in the soft tissues, particularly in the paravertebral region.[13]

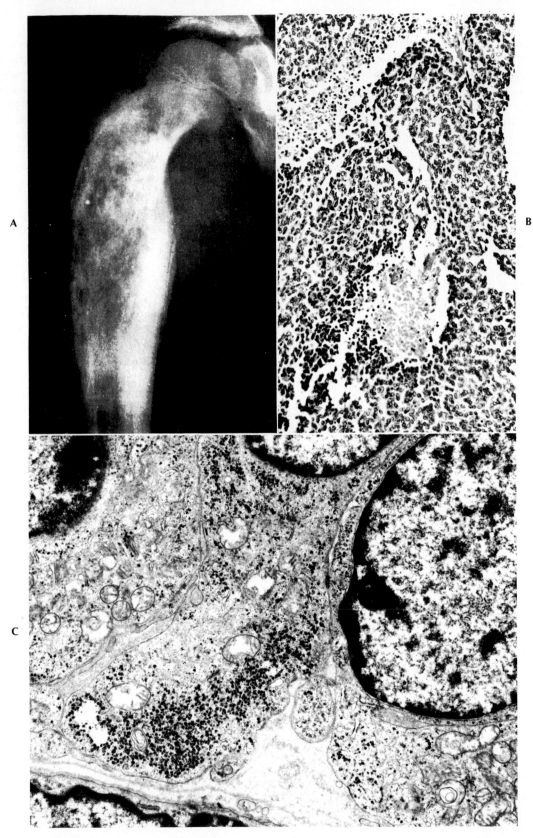

Fig. 39-30. Ewing's sarcoma. **A,** Roentgenographic appearance. Notice irregular areas of bone destruction and production, loss of bone architecture, and multilayered periosteal new bone formation. **B,** Microscopic appearance is that of highly cellular tumor made up of small round or oval cells with scanty cytoplasm. Areas of necrosis are evident. **C,** Ultrastructure of Ewing's sarcoma is that of primitive cells without signs of differentiation. Numerous glycogen particles are seen in cytoplasm. There are several poorly developed cell junctions. Basal lamina in lower left corner belongs to capillary. (**B,** 160×; **C,** 232×.)

The histogenesis of Ewing's sarcoma has been controversial since the tumor was first described. Vascular cells, hematopoietic elements, primitive mesenchymal cells, and neuroectodermal derivatives have all been proposed at one time or another as possible progenitors. Recent ultrastructural and immunohistochemical studies have shown that in at least some of the cases there is evidence of neural differentiation, or that this differentiation can be induced by various agents in tissue culture.[41,107,189] The finding of immunoreactivity for keratin, vimentin, and neuron-specific enolase in some cases demonstrates the potential capacity of these tumor cells for multidirectional differentiation.[145] A cytogenetic abnormality in the form of the reciprocal translocation t(11;22) has been detected in Ewing's sarcoma and other small cell tumors of infancy.[41]

The microscopic differential diagnosis must be made primarily with other "small round cell tumors" of bone—malignant lymphoma, metastatic neuroblastoma, and osteosarcoma of small cell type. Malignant lymphoma affects an older age group, the cells are larger, the nuclei often have a vesicular or indented configuration, glycogen is absent, and reticulin is more prominent. In metastatic neuroblastoma the bone lesions are often multiple and the predilection is for chil-

dren under 3 years of age. Glycogen is not so prominent, and rosettes may be present. When grown in tissue culture, axons form in 24 to 48 hours; levels of urinary catecholamine derivatives are almost always elevated. Osteosarcoma exhibits signs of osteoid formation by the tumor cells.

In the past the prognosis of Ewing's sarcoma was dismal. In most series the 5-year survival rate was less than 5%. This has changed dramatically with the institution of an aggressive combined therapeutic regimen consisting in radiotherapy to the entire bone affected and systemic (and sometimes intrathecal) chemotherapy.[45,175] Even patients with advanced regional and metastatic disease can be saved.[165]

Malignant lymphoma

Any type of malignant lymphoma and leukemia can involve the skeletal system, either as an expression of systemic involvement or as the first manifestation of the disease.[42,134] Hodgkin's disease produces roentgenographically visible bone lesions in about 15% of the cases.[44] The involvement is multifocal in 60%, and the bones most often affected are the vertebrae, pelvis, and ribs. In the vertebrae the lesions often have a striking osteoblastic appearance. Of the four microscopic types

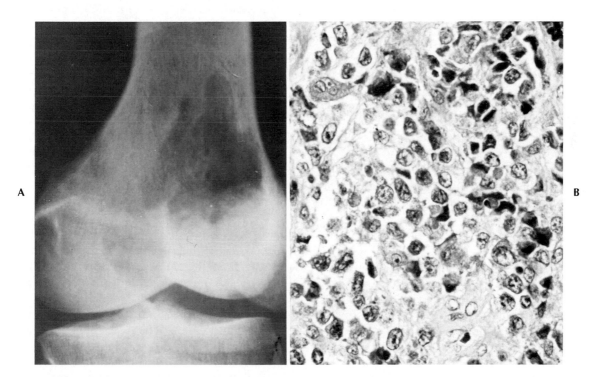

Fig. 39-31. Malignant lymphoma. **A,** Roentgenogram of distal femur showing lytic lesion with irregular outlines, lack of calcification, and absence of periosteal reaction. **B,** Microscopically, large lymphoid cells grow in diffuse fashion. There is associated fibrosis and a residual osteoclast. Tumor cells are larger than those of the usual Ewing's sarcoma. (**B,** 400×.)

of Hodgkin's disease, mixed cellularity and lymphocyte depletion have the greatest tendency to involve bones.

Non-Hodgkin's malignant lymphoma primarily involving bones tends to occur in patients over 30 years of age.[49,160,226] It involves the diaphysis or metaphysis of the bone, producing a roentgenographically ill-defined cortical and medullary destruction (Fig. 39-31, A). It has been observed that the affected patients may remain in good health, even when the tumor has reached a large size, and that dissemination is slow to occur. Grossly the tumor is pinkish gray and granular. It frequently extends into the soft tissues and invades the muscle. Microscopically most bone lymphomas are composed of round cells with relatively large vesicular nuclei, often indented or horseshoe shaped, and prominent nucleoli. Cytoplasmic outlines tend to be well defined, and the cytoplasm is abundant and eosinophilic (Fig. 39-31, B). A rich reticulin framework surrounds individual cells.[133] In the older classifications of malignant lymphoma this tumor was classified as a reticulum cell sarcoma; in Rappaport's classification, most cases were included in the histiocytic category. Immunologic and immunohistochemical observations, have shown that in the bone as well as in other sites most cases of lymphoma composed of large cells actually originate from cells of the lymphocytic line (B-lymphocytes more often than T-lymphocytes). Accordingly, in recently proposed classifications of lymphomas, this type is designated as the large cell type and is further subdivided—if feasible—according to the criteria specified in Chapter 28. By using these guidelines, it was found that most lymphomas of bone belong to the group of large noncleaved cell lymphomas.[65]

Chemotherapy is the treatment of choice in cases with multicentricity or extraosseous involvement. In localized cases, the treatment has traditionally consisted of a combination of surgery and radiation therapy; however, there is evidence that adjunctive chemotherapy is also indicated in this group.[17] The prognosis for primary lymphoma of bone remains substantially better than for Ewing's sarcoma.

Plasma cell myeloma

Plasma cell myeloma is a malignant tumor of plasma cells that can lead to a variety of clinicopathologic expressions[16] (Fig. 39-32). The most common form is generally known as multiple myeloma. It usually occurs between 40 and 60 years of age and is manifested by pain, weakness, weight loss, and osteolytic lesions in the vertebrae, pelvis, rib, sternum, and skull. In rare cases the bone lesions have an osteoblastic roentgenographic appearance.[64] Signs and symptoms referable to pressure on the spinal cord or the spinal nerves may occur. Another complication of the disease is compression fractures of vertebrae or pathologic fractures of other involved bones. Some degree of anemia is usually noted, and examination of the blood often reveals excessive rouleau formation. Roentgenologic examination reveals multiple small and large areas of bone destruction. These have sharp borders ("punched-out" areas) and are unaccompanied by proliferative reactions at the margins unless a fracture has occurred. In advanced cases, extraskeletal spread may be seen, either in the soft tissues adjacent to involved bones or as distant involvement of lymph nodes, spleen, liver, and other organs.[163] Immunoglobulin abnormalities are very common (87% of the cases) and express the functional capability of the neoplastic plasma cells. In a series of 112 patients, increased serum IgG was found in 61%, IgA in 18%, and light chains only (Bence Jones protein) in 9%.[40] The most common finding in the urine of patients with myeloma is the presence of Bence Jones protein, which represents the light chain of the immunoglobulin molecule. Rarely, neoplastic plasma cells are detected in the peripheral circulation. The name "plasma cell leukemia" is sometimes used to designate this phase of plasma cell myeloma.

The other major clinicopathologic form of plasma cell myeloma is represented by the appearance of a solitary tumor mass, either in a bone[51] or in the soft tissues (nasopharynx, nose, tonsil).[229] These are usually not accompanied by immunoglobulin abnormalities. Many of these localized lesions eventually become disseminated in bone, though this may occur many years later and even then may run a more indolent course than the form that is generalized from the beginning.

The gross and microscopic features of the disease are similar in the generalized and localized forms. Grossly the tissue is soft, friable, and hemorrhagic. The focal, slowly growing tumor may have a fairly well-defined border.

Microscopically there is a wide range of differentiation that the neoplastic cells may exhibit. On one extreme there is the tumor that is composed of plasma cells so well differentiated that a confusion with an inflammatory condition may arise; on the other, one sees a highly undifferentiated tumor with formation of tumor giant cells, in which the plasmacytic nature may be missed altogether. The characteristic features of plasma cells, which persist in all but the more undifferentiated neoplasms, include oval cytoplasm, eccentric nucleus with cartwheel distribution of the chromatin, and a distinct perinuclear clear halo. The high ribosomal content of the cytoplasm can be made evident with the methyl green–pyronine stain, which stains cytoplasmic and nucleolar RNA red (pyroninophilic) and nuclear DNA green. By electron microscopy, the most distinctive features are the presence of a highly developed granular endoplasmic reticulum, usually arranged in the form of parallel cisternae, and a prominent Golgi apparatus,

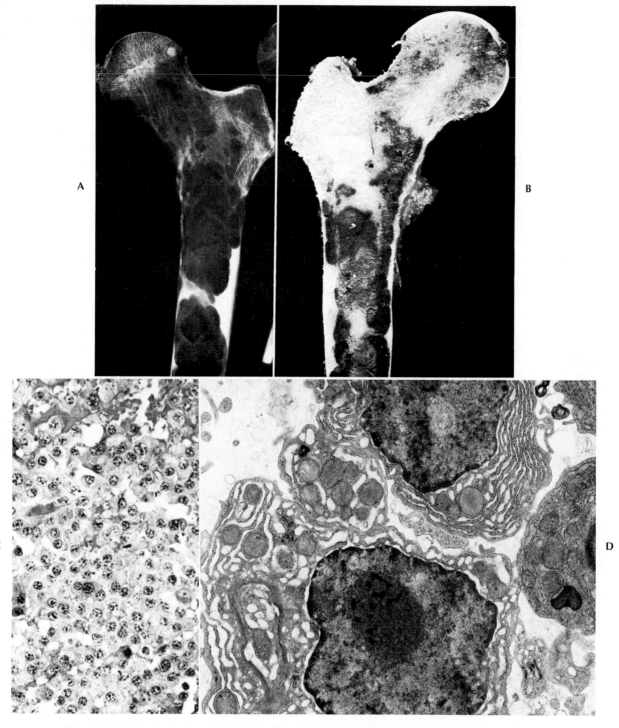

Fig. 39-32. Plasma cell myeloma. **A,** Roentgenogram of hemisection of femur showing extensive bone destruction caused by tumor. Notice absence of reactive bone formation. **B,** Gross specimen from same patient. Myelomatous foci appear as dark granular areas with ill-defined borders. **C,** Microscopic section shows monotonous proliferation of immature plasma cells. Notice clumped chromatin pattern and nuclear peripheralization. **D,** When viewed with electron microscope, neoplastic plasma cells are characterized by well-developed parallel stacks of granular endoplasmic reticulum and prominent Golgi apparatus. (**C,** 400×; **D,** 12,960×.)

the latter corresponding to the perinuclear clear halo of light microscopy.[71]

Immunohistochemically, monoclonal production of cytoplasmic immunoglobulin can be demonstrated.

Osteomyelitis rich in plasma cells (so-called plasma cell osteomyelitis) can be distinguished from plasma cell myeloma by the absence of atypical nuclear forms; no or few binucleated plasma cells; presence of abundant Russell's bodies (intracytoplasmic round eosinophilic bodies that represent inspissated immunoglobulin and are of very rare occurrence in myeloma); presence of other inflammatory components, such as lymphocytes, eosinophils, and neutrophils; and a richer reticular and collagenous background.

In a certain percentage of myeloma cases a deposition of amyloid is observed in the tumor tissue or in other organs; in these cases the amyloid material is made up largely of the immunoglobulin produced by the neoplastic plasma cells.

VASCULAR TUMORS

The most common vascular tumor of bone is the benign tumor of the blood vessel, that is, hemangioma.[230] It is usually of the cavernous variety, in the sense that it is composed of capillaries and venules with thin walls and greatly dilated lumens packed with red blood cells (Fig. 39-33, *A*). The vascular spaces permeate the bone marrow and, if large enough, expand the bone and elicit periosteal new bone formation. In flat bones, particularly the skull, this results in a typical sunburst effect on roentgenographic examination. The most common locations of clinically significant hemangiomas are the skull, vertebrae, and jaw bones. Collections of dilated blood-filled vessels are commonly encountered in the vertebrae at autopsy, but they probably represent malformations rather than true neoplasms.

Bone hemangiomas can be multiple, especially in children; half of these multiple cases are associated with cutaneous, visceral, or soft-tissue hemangiomas.[200]

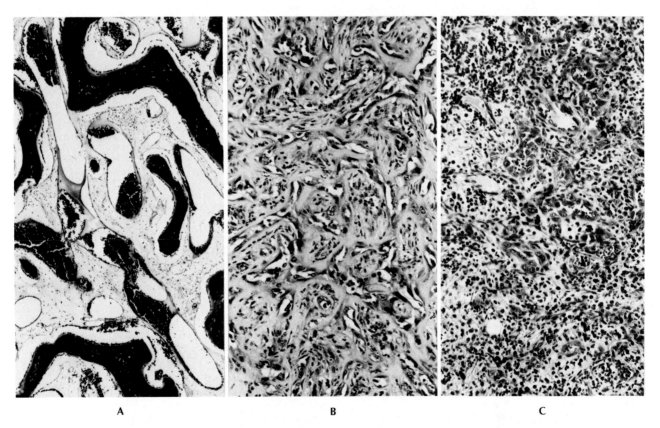

A   B   C

Fig. 39-33. Various types of primary vascular tumors of bone. **A,** Cavernous hemangioma. Greatly dilated blood vessels with thin walls occupy the bone marrow spaces and result in reactive osteoblastic activity of the intervening bone trabeculas. **B,** Angiosarcoma (malignant hemangioendothelioma). Freely anastomosing vascular channels lined by highly atypical endothelial cells are characteristic of this tumor. **C,** Histiocytoid hemangioma (epithelioid hemangioendothelioma). Neoplastic endothelial cells of plump (histiocytoid or epithelioid) appearance form vascular channels separated by a heavy inflammatory infiltrate containing numerous eosinophils.

Massive osteolysis (Gorham's disease) is a disease of unknown cause and pathogenesis characterized by a progressive replacement of the bone structures by heavily vascularized fibrous tissue. This may lead eventually to resorption of a whole bone or several bones.[81]

Three other types of benign vascular tumors that in rare cases involve bone are lymphangioma, glomus tumor, and hemangiopericytoma. Lymphangioma is either solitary or multiple and may be associated with similar lesions in soft tissues.[111] Glomus tumor of bone is invariably located in a terminal phalanx.[30] Most reported cases of hemangiopericytoma of bone have been malignant; as with hemangiopericytomas in other locations, the diagnosis of this tumor type should be made only after exclusion of other tumors that may exhibit a similar vascular pattern.[234]

Angiosarcomas are highly malignant tumors of endothelial cells. They most commonly occur in long bones and have a tendency for multicentricity. Grossly they are cellular, friable, hemorrhagic, and necrotic.[63,233] Microscopically the hallmark of the lesion is the formation of anastomosing vascular channels lined with atypical endothelial cells (Fig. 39-33, *B*). These are often combined with solid, less-differentiated foci. Distant metastases, particularly to the lungs, are common. The differential microscopic diagnosis needs to be made with well-vascularized osteosarcoma and with metastatic carcinoma (particularly from the kidney).

There exists in the skeletal system a vascular tumor that is somewhat intermediate in behavior between the innocuous hemangioma and the highly malignant angio-sarcoma. This is often referred to as "hemangioendothelioma." In some series it has been grouped with the angiosarcoma, but I believe that it represents a distinct entity. A characteristic feature of this tumor is that the neoplastic endothelial cells have a plump, often grooved nucleus and an abundant acidophilic, sometimes vacuolated cytoplasm (Fig. 39-33, *C*). The cells have a somewhat histiocytoid or epithelioid appearance, which has led to the proposal of the term "histiocytoid hemangioma" or "epithelioid hemangioendothelioma" for these tumors.[173] They probably correspond to the grade I (and perhaps some grade II) hemangioendotheliomas described by other authors.[33] These tumors have a strong tendency for multicentricity within the skeletal system and sometimes are seen in association with microscopically similar tumors in the skin or soft tissue. Their behavior, though sometimes locally aggressive, is usually benign; simple curettage cures most lesions.[215]

FIBROUS TISSUE TUMORS
Desmoplastic fibroma

Desmoplastic fibroma is a nonmetastasizing but locally aggressive neoplasm that is characterized microscopically by the presence of mature fibroblasts separated by abundant collagen[76] (Fig. 39-34). Ultrastructurally most of the tumor cells have features intermediate between those of fibroblasts and smooth muscle cells (so-called myofibroblasts).[121] The absence of pleomorphism, necrosis, and mitotic activity distinguishes this tumor from fibrosarcoma. Local recurrences are common. It is likely that desmoplastic fi-

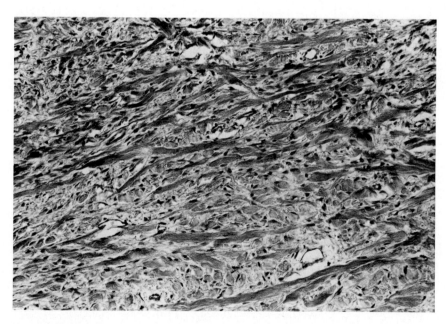

Fig. 39-34. Desmoplastic fibroma of bone. The tumor is poorly cellular, lacks atypia and mitotic activity, and displays abundant collagen fibers, some of which appear hyalinized.

broma represents the osseous counterpart of soft-tissue fibromatosis (so-called desmoid tumor).

Fibrosarcoma is the malignant tumor of fibroblasts.[23,56] In one large series as many as 17% represented radiation-induced neoplasms.[223] Fibrosarcoma usually involves the metaphysis of long bones in adults. It appears roentgenographically as an osteolytic lesion with frequent extension into soft tissues.[99] Most cases arise within the medullary canal (endosteal or medullary fibrosarcomas), but well-documented periosteal examples have also been reported. Grossly the tumor is whitish, firm, and homogeneous (Fig. 39-35, *A*). The microscopic appearance is similar to that of the more common fibrosarcoma of soft tissue and is characterized by atypical spindle cells that form interlacing bundles of collagen fibers *but no cartilage or bone* (Fig. 39-35, *B*). The latter feature is important in the differential diagnosis because both osteosarcoma and chondrosarcoma can have similar spindle cell areas. Fibrosarcomas are less malignant as a group than osteosarcomas are.

OTHER PRIMARY TUMORS
Chordoma

Chordoma is believed to arise from developmental remnants of the notochord. The notochord is the origi-nal axial skeleton that is subsequently replaced by the spine; its remnants are represented by the nucleus pulposus of the intervertebral discs and small clumps of notochordal cells within the verebral bodies. Because of their highly vacuolated cytoplasm, these cells are also known as physaliphorous (*physalis*, 'bubble'; *phoros*, 'bearing').

All true chordomas arise in the axial skeleton. The sacral and spheno-occipital regions are the most common sites,[113,208] with the intervening vertebrae being involved only rarely. Chordomas are slowly growing tumors. They infiltrate adjacent structures and stubbornly recur after excision. Distant metastases are rare and occur late in the course of the disease; skin and other bones are the most common sites.[43] Roentgenographically, chordomas appear as osteolytic or rarely osteoblastic processes. They may encroach on the spine and give rise to symptoms of spinal cord compression. Grossly these tumors are gelatinous and soft and often contain areas of hemorrhage. Microscopically they are formed by cell cords and lobules separated by a variable but usually abundant amount of myxoid intercellular tissue (Fig. 39-36). The tumor cells are quite large, with vacuolated cytoplasm and prominent vesicular nuclei. The cytoplasm contains glycogen and mucosubstances

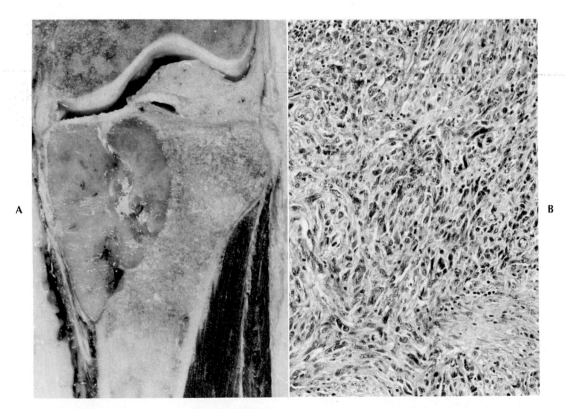

Fig. 39-35. Fibrosarcoma. **A,** Gross appearance of amputation specimen. Well-circumscribed lytic lesion involving epiphysis and metaphysis is seen. **B,** Microscopically a highly cellular proliferation of spindle tumor cells is seen. There is collagen deposition but no evidence of osteoid or bone production. (**B,** 160×.)

but no fat. Areas of cartilage, bone, or fibrous tissue may be present. Some chordomas in the spheno-occipital region have an abundant cartilaginous component; they are known as chondroid chordomas and have a relatively good prognosis.[91]

Immunohistochemically the cells of chordoma are reactive both for cartilaginous (S-100 protein) and epithelial (keratin) markers.[10,141]

Tumors microscopically resembling chordomas (and therefore sometimes known as "chordoid sarcomas") are seen occasionally in the extra-axial skeleton or in soft tissues; they probably represent a morphologic variant of chondrosarcoma.

Adamantinoma of long bones

Adamantinoma of long bones, a mysterious neoplasm that shows a great predilection for the tibia, is so designated because of its microscopic resemblance to the adamantinoma (ameloblastoma) of jawbones[147] (Fig. 39-37). The origin of the latter tumor is the odontogenic tissue, but this can hardly be the case for its long bone counterpart. Three major tissues have been proposed as the origin: epithelial cells, blood vessels, and intraosseous synovial cells. The weight of the evidence favors the epithelial cells. The typical tumor has an obvious epithelial architecture, being formed by lobules with peripheral palisading and a central looser arrangement.[235] By electron microscopy the tumor cells contain tonofibrils and complex desmosomes, two well-known markers of epithelial cells.[235] Immunocytochem-

ical studies have shown the presence of keratin and absence of factor VIII–related antigen.[164,174]

Naturally, the question arises as to how a primary epithelial tumor could arise within a long bone. Significative in this regard is that the most common location is the tibia, which is closer to the skin than any other long bone. Conceivably epithelial cells from the epidermis or its adnexa find their way beneath the periosteum, either as a result of traumatic inclusion or as an abnormality of development, and later undergo a neoplastic transformation. Some support from this interpretation comes from the close morphologic similarity between adamantinoma of long bones and sweat gland carcinoma of skin and also from the occasional occurrence of a tumor morphologically identical to adamantinoma in the soft tissues overlying the tibia.[143] It is also possible that this tumor could arise from primitive intraosseous mesenchymal cells that have retained the capacity to partially differentiate into epithelial tissue.[224]

Long bone adamantinoma produces rounded or oval, sometimes loculated areas of bone destruction that can be seen in roentgenograms and on gross examination. Occasionally it has a fibro-osseous component morphologically similar to that seen in fibrous dysplasia[50]; it is a malignant neoplasm, prone to local recurrence and sometimes leading to distant metastases.[219]

Tumors of peripheral nerves

Peripheral nerve tumors are rare and represented mainly by neurilemoma (schwannoma), a benign tumor

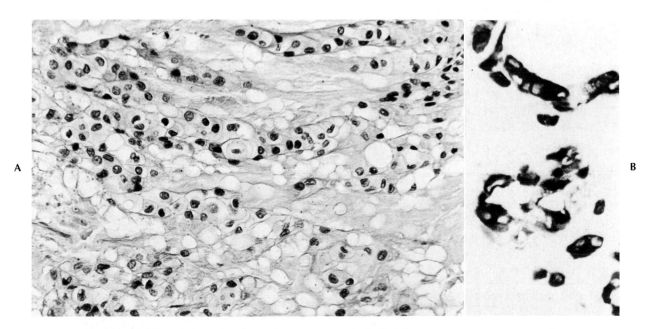

Fig. 39-36. Chordoma of spheno-occipital region. **A,** Cuboid and polyhedral cells with central nucleus form rows and nests among abundant myxoid matrix. (350×.) **B,** Strong immunohistochemical positivity for keratin in the tumor cells (immunoperoxidase technique).

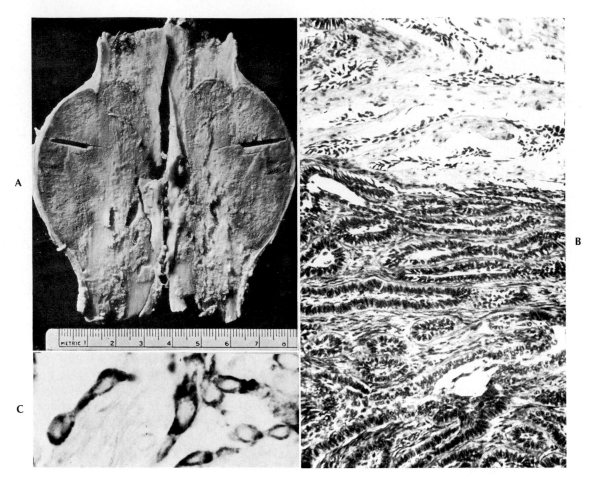

Fig. 39-37. Adamantinoma of tibia. **A,** Large, solitary tumor mass in midportion of tibia had led to sharply defined bone destruction. Neoplasm was dense but moderately cellular and friable. **B,** Alveolar arrangement of tall cylindrical cells with central fusiform and oval cells. Invasion of bone is evident at upper margin. (**B,** 145×.) **C,** Strong immunoreactivity for keratin is evident in the tumor cells (immunoperoxidase technique).

most often located in the mandible.[58] Although von Recklinghausen's disease is often accompanied by skeletal deformities, the occurrence of intraosseous neurofibromas is virtually nonexistent.[94]

Tumors of adipose tissue

Adipose tissue tumors are exceptional and basically represented by the benign lipoma. This is a small to medium-sized nodule of mature fat tissue fairly well demarcated from bone marrow. Primary liposarcomas of bone exist but are rare. Most cases reported in the old literature would probably carry a different diagnosis today.

Tumors of alleged histiocytic origin

It has been postulated that a relatively large number of soft-tissue neoplasms arise from fixed histiocytes (as distinguished from the mobile histiocytes of lymphoid and hematopoietic organs),[115,161] or alternatively from primitive mesenchymal cells that differentiate toward histiocytes. These tumors are designated as "histiocytomas" and "fibrous histiocytomas," the latter having in addition to the histiocytic elements a fibroblastic component, originating either from the histiocytes through a modulating process (facultative fibroblasts) or by divergent differentiation from the same primitive mesenchymal cell that gave rise to the cells with histiocytic features. Each category can be roughly subdivided into a benign and a malignant type. It is becoming evident that similar tumors exist in bone, though their frequency is certainly less than that in soft tissue.[27,112,137] Benign histiocytomas often have a prominent component of fat-containing foamy macrophages (xanthoma cells) and are also referred to as "xanthomas."[48] The rib is the most common location. Malignant fibrous histiocytomas, also known as "fibroxanthosarcomas" and "xanthosarcomas," predominate in long bones, where they tend to involve the medullary portion in the me-

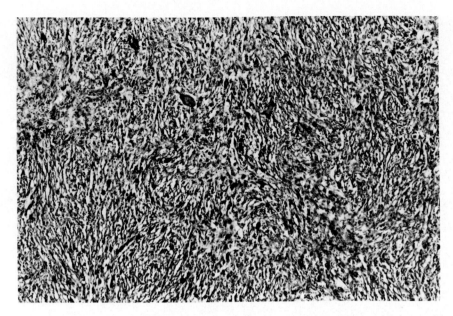

Fig. 39-38. Malignant fibrous histiocytoma of bone. The tumor is highly cellular and lacks bone formation. There are occasional multinucleated tumor cells. A storiform pattern of growth can be appreciated throughout.

taphyseal area. Roentgenographically, they appear as large lytic destructive lesions. The gross appearance is that of a variegated tumor with yellow foci alternating with areas of hemorrhage. Microscopically, spindle cells predominate. They are often arranged around a central point, producing radiating spokes grouped at right angles to each other, a pattern referred to as "storiform." Foamy cells, hemosiderin-laden macrophages, and bizarre giant tumor cells are common[98] (Fig. 39-38).

Some cases of malignant fibrous histiocytomas have been reported as a late complication of bone infarcts[144] and others after radiation therapy.[103]

There is much controversy in the literature concerning the behavior to be expected from this tumor. In most series, however, the prognosis of this neoplasm has proved to be better than that of osteosarcoma.[137]

Tumors of smooth muscle

A few cases of primary leiomyosarcoma of bone have been described.[14] Most of these tumors have appeared in the lower end of the femur in adults.

METASTATIC TUMORS

Metastases to the skeletal system from neoplasms arising in other organs are the most frequent of all malignant neoplasms of bone. Sometimes these metastases represent the first clinical manifestation of the disease, and a fastidious search for the occult primary tumor needs to be undertaken.[194] Carcinomas greatly predominate over sarcomas. The most common types of carcinomas resulting in bone metastases are those that orig-

inate in the breast, prostate, lung, kidney, stomach, and thyroid. Cancers arising in other organs, such as the body and cervix of the uterus, bladder, and testicle, also may spread to bone. Melanomas and adrenal neuroblastomas sometimes give rise to extensive skeletal involvement.

Most skeletal metastases derive from hematogenous spread, but in some specific instances the lymphatic system is involved in their production.[21]

The metastatic foci can be multiple or single. The latter are particularly common with thyroid and renal cancers. In order of frequency, the bones most commonly involved are the spine, pelvis, femur, skull, ribs, and humerus. Metastases to distal bones, such as the bones of forearm, wrist, hand, leg, ankle, and foot, are quite unusual. Roentgenographically, most metastases appear as destructive lytic lesions (Fig. 39-39). Others may be seen as a mixture of lytic and sclerotic changes, and still others may elicit such an exuberant osteoblastic reaction as to produce a roentgenographic sclerotic appearance. Tumors with a particular tendency to produce osteoblastic bone metastases are carcinoma of prostate, carcinoid tumor, and small cell carcinoma of lung.[149,215] Rarely, this feature is also seen with breast and stomach cancer. The mechanism for the osteoblastic stimulation is not known. Metastases from renal and thyroid cancers may pulsate and give rise to an audible bruit because of their pronounced vascularity. Pathologic fracture is often the first evidence that metastasis to a bone has taken place.

The area of long bone most commonly involved by a

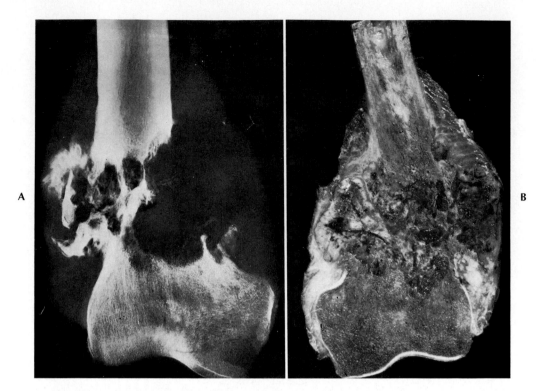

Fig. 39-39. Bone metastasis from renal cell carcinoma. **A,** Roentgenographic appearance of slice of femur showing large destructive lesion with pathologic fracture. **B,** Gross appearance of same specimen.

metastatic process is the metaphysis, presumably by virtue of its greater vascularity.

As mentioned previously, sarcomas metastasize to the skeletal system only rarely. The outstanding exceptions are embryonal and alveolar rhabdomyosarcomas of soft tissues, which are complicated by blood-borne osseous metastases in a large percentage of cases.[31] It should also be mentioned that, among primary bone tumors, Ewing's sarcoma and osteosarcoma have a certain propensity to involve regions of the skeletal system.

Skeletal metastases, which demonstrated in a patient with carcinoma, are obviously of great importance when one is determining prognosis and guiding treatment. Routinely taken bilateral core biopsy samples of the iliac crest are valuable for the early detection of bone metastases.[140] In general, the consequences of such lesions to the patient are pain that is frequently intolerable and disability to the point of complete invalidism until the patient dies of the disease.

TUMORLIKE LESIONS
Solitary bone cyst

Solitary bone cyst is a benign condition, also known as "simple or unicameral bone cyst." It appears as a cavity filled with clear or blood-tinged fluid in the metaphysis of a long bone, particularly the upper ends of the humerus and femur[32] (Fig. 39-40). It may also develop in a short bone such as the calcaneus. Most cases occur in children and adolescents.[205] The pathogenesis is unknown. Microscopically the cavity is lined by a membrane of variable thickness that is formed by loose connective tissue with a scattering of osteoclasts and newly formed trabeculas of reactive nature (Fig. 39-40). Often a layer of organizing fibrin coats the inside of this membrane. Areas of recent or old hemorrhage and cholesterol clefts can sometimes be found, particularly after a fracture of the cyst. The latter is a common event. The treatment consists in curettage followed by packing of the cavity with bone chips.

Aneurysmal bone cyst

Aneurysmal bone cyst, which was often confused in the past with the giant cell tumor, is an expansile mass formed by blood-filled spaces of variable but often large size. Most cases occur in patients under 30 years of age and involve either the shaft of metaphysis of long bones or the vertebral column.[176] Pain and swelling are the main symptoms. The roentgenographic appearance is quite distinctive by virtue of the expansile nature of the mass, resulting in a ballooned-out distension of the periosteum[32] (Fig. 39-41, A). Grossly it forms a spongy hemorrhagic mass that may extend into the soft tissue

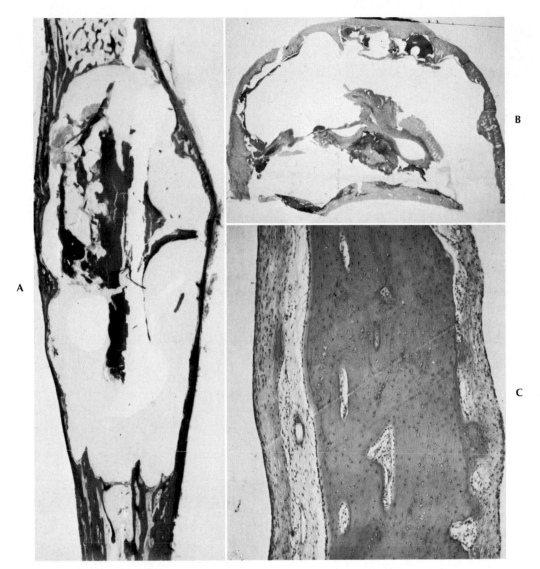

Fig. 39-40. Solitary bone cyst. **A,** Intact cyst included in longitudinal section of bone. Cortex is greatly reduced in thickness and bone shaft is widened. **B,** Cross section illustrating fibrous tissue septa that partially divide such cysts. **C,** Thin bony wall of cyst with fibrous connective tissue lining on left and proliferative changes in subperiosteal layer on exterior surface of expanded bone on right.

and be covered by a thin shell of reactive bone. Microscopically most of the cysts are lined not by endothelial cells but rather by fibrous septa containing osteoid and numerous osteoclast-like multinucleated giant cells (Fig. 39-41, B). The pathogenesis is not clear. Some authors have postulated a persistent local alteration in hemodynamics leading to increased venous pressure and the subsequent development of a dilated and vascular bed within the transformed bone area. Variants of this entity with a predominantly solid appearance attributable to proliferation of fibroblastic, osteoclastic, osteoblastic, and other mesenchymal elements have been seen.[179]

Cystic changes, apparently secondary and closely resembling those of aneurysmal bone cyst, are occasionally found in chondroblastoma, fibrous dysplasia, giant cell tumor, osteosarcoma, and other bone lesions.[126] Therefore it is important to rule out these conditions by careful examination of the entire material when one is confronted with this situation (Fig. 39-42).

Ganglion cyst of bone

Ganglion cyst is a common lesion of soft tissue, where it appears as a mucus-filled cystic mass in a periarticular location. Sometimes a lesion of similar appearance and pathogenesis is found within a bone, usually

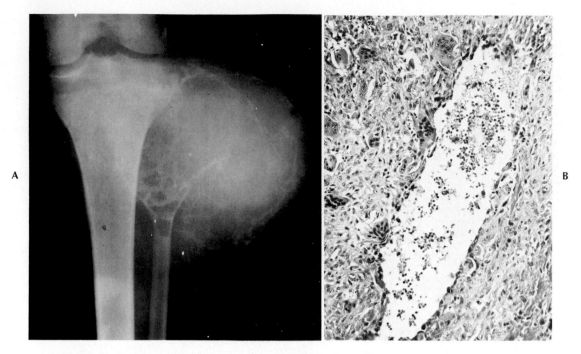

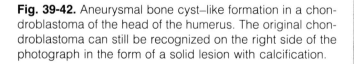

Fig. 39-41. Aneurysmal bone cyst. **A,** Roentgenogram shows ballooned-out expansile lesion of upper end of fibula. Lesion started in metaphysis but now involves entire end of bone. **B,** Microscopic hallmark of lesion is aneurysmal spaces filled with blood and partially lined by osteoclast-like giant cells. (**B,** 160×.)

Fig. 39-42. Aneurysmal bone cyst–like formation in a chondroblastoma of the head of the humerus. The original chondroblastoma can still be recognized on the right side of the photograph in the form of a solid lesion with calcification.

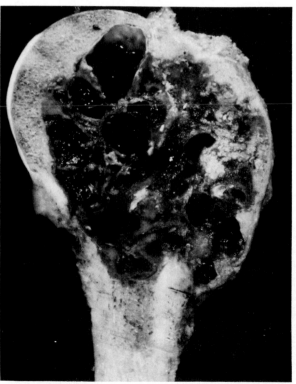

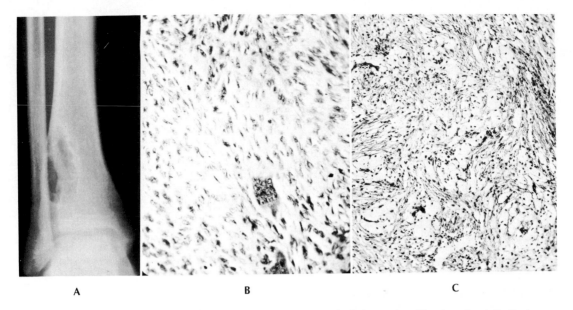

Fig. 39-43. Metaphyseal fibrous defect. **A,** Eccentric lytic area with sharply delimited sclerotic borders in metaphysis. **B,** Cellular lesion composed of plump fibroblasts and scattered giant cells. **C,** Clusters of lipid-laden histiocytes among spindle cells.

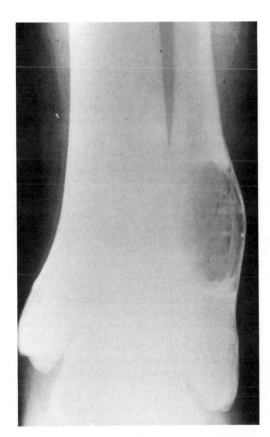

Fig. 39-44. Nonossifying fibroma with superimposed fracture. Lesion, which involves lower metaphysis of tibia, is distinguished from metaphyseal fibrous defect by virtue of its large size and pressure of medullary involvement and bone expansion.

at the lower end of the tibia or humerus.[20] Roentgenographically, it appears as a well-defined osteolytic area with a surrounding zone of osteosclerosis, always close to the joint space. Grossly it is often multiloculated and has a gelatinous content. Microscopically it lacks synovial lining. It has instead a flat fibrous lining, like its soft-tissue counterpart.

Metaphyseal fibrous defect

Metaphyseal fibrous defect is a roentgenographically distinctive benign lesion occurring in the metaphyseal cortex of long bones in children[53] (Fig. 39-43). It is usually solitary but may appear as multiple or even bilaterally symmetric defects. The upper or lower tibia and the lower femur are the sites of predilection. Roentgenographically the lesion is eccentric, has sharply delimited borders, and is centered in the metaphysis. More extensive lesions, involving the medullary canal and resulting in a fusiform expansion of the bone, are sometimes referred to as "nonossifying or nonosteogenic fibromas"[106] (Fig. 39-44). The morphologic appearance of the two lesions is similar, an indication that they are examples of the same entity.[203] Grossly the lesion is granular and brown or dark. Dense bone can be seen around it. Microscopically it consists of cellular masses of fibrous tissue with a storiform pattern of growth, accompanied by scattered osteoclast-like giant cells, hemosiderin-laden macrophages, and foamy cells. The lesion is often asymptomatic and is usually discovered incidentally in a roentgenogram taken for another reason.

The pathogenesis is unknown. The designation "defect" implies that the lesion arises as the result of some developmental aberration at the epiphyseal plate. In favor of this interpretation is the fact that concomitant epiphyseal disorders are not infrequently present. The other possibility, which is currently favored, is that it belongs to the group of tumors described in the discussion of tumors of alleged histiocytic origin. The histologic resemblance to them is certainly pronounced.

Nonossifying fibroma should be clearly separated from ossifying or osteogenic fibroma, a fibro-osseous lesion probably related to fibrous dysplasia, which is also known as "fibro-osseous or osteo-fibrous dysplasia."[152]

REFERENCES
General

1. Dahlin, D.C.: Bone tumors, ed. 4, Springfield, Ill., 1986, Charles C Thomas, Publisher.
2. Fechner, R.E., Huvos, A.G., Mirra, J.M., Spjut, H.J., and Unni, K.K.: A symposium on the pathology of bone tumors, Pathol. Annu. 19(pt. 1):125, 1984.
3. Huvos, A.G.: Bone tumors: diagnosis, treatment and prognosis, Philadelphia, 1979, W.B. Saunders Co.
4. Jaffe, H.L.: Tumors and tumorous conditions of the bones and joints, Philadelphia, 1958, Lea & Febiger.
5. Lichtenstein, L.: Bone tumors, ed. 5, St. Louis, 1977, The C.V. Mosby Co.
6. Mirra, J.M.: Bone tumors: diagnosis and treatment, Philadelphia, 1979, J.B. Lippincott Co.
7. Schajowicz, F.: Tumors and tumor-like lesions of bone and joints, New York, 1981, Springer-Verlag NY, Inc.
8. Schajowicz, F., Ackerman, L.V., and Sissons, H.A.: Histologic typing of bone tumours. In International Histological Classification of Tumours, no. 6, Geneva, 1972, World Health Organization.
9. Spjut, H.J., Dorfman, H.D., Fechner, R.E., and Ackerman, L.V.: Tumors of bone and cartilage. In Atlas of tumor pathology, section 2, fascicle 5, Washington, D.C., 1971, Armed Forces Institute of Pathology.

Specific

10. Abenoza, P., and Sibley, R.K.: Chordoma: an immunohistologic study, Hum. Pathol. 17:744, 1986.
11. Amstutz, H.C.: Multiple osteogenic sarcoma—metastatic or multicentric? Report of two cases and review of literature, Cancer 24:923, 1969.
12. Anderson, W.A.D., Zander, G.E., and Kuzma, J.F.: Cancerogenic effects of Ca^{45} and Sr^{89} on bones of CF$_1$ mice, Arch. Pathol. 62:262, 1956.
13. Angervall, L., and Enzinger, F.M.: Extraskeletal neoplasm resembling Ewing's sarcoma, Cancer 36:240, 1975.
14. Angervall, L., Berlin, O., Kindblom, L.G., and Stener, B.: Primary leiomyosarcoma of bone: a study of five cases, Cancer 46:1270, 1980.
15. Athanason, N.A., Bliss, E., Gatter, K.C., and Heryet, A.: An immunohistological study of giant-cell tumour of bone: evidence for an osteoclast origin of the giant cells, J. Pathol. 147:153, 1985.
16. Azar, H.A.: Plasma-cell myelomatosis and other monoclonal gammopathies, Pathol. Annu. 7:1, 1972.
17. Bacci, G., Jaffe, N., Emiliani, E., Van Horn, J., Manfrini, M., Picci, P., Bertoni, F., Gherlinzoni, F., and Campanacci, M.: Therapy for primary non-Hodgkin's lymphoma of bone and a comparison of results with Ewing's sarcoma: ten years' experience at the Istituto Ortopedico Rizzoli, Cancer 57:1468, 1986.
18. Bagó-Granell, J., Aguirre-Canyadell, M., Nardi, J., and Tallada, N.: Malignant fibrous histiocytoma of bone at the site of a total hip arthroplasty: a case report, J. Bone Joint Surg. 66B:38, 1984.
19. Barnes, R., and Catto, M.: Chondrosarcoma of bone, J. Bone Joint Surg. 48B:729, 1966.
20. Bauer, T.W., and Dorfman, H.D.: Intraosseous ganglion: a clinicopathologic study of 11 cases, Am. J. Surg. Pathol. 6:207, 1982.
21. Berrettoni, B.A., and Carter, J.R.: Mechanisms of cancer metastasis to bone, J. Bone Joint Surg. 68A:308, 1986.
22. Bertoni, F., Boriani, S., Laus, M., Campanacci, M.: Periosteal chondrosarcoma and periosteal osteosarcoma: two distinct entities, J. Bone Joint Surg. 64B:370, 1982.
23. Bertoni, F., Capanna, R., Calderoni, P., Bacchini, P., and Campanacci, M.: Primary central (medullary) fibrosarcoma of bone, Semin. Diagn. Pathol. 1:185, 1984.
24. Bertoni, F., Unni, K.K., McLeod, R.A., and Dahlin, D.C: Osteosarcoma resembling osteoblastoma, Cancer 55:416, 1985.
25. Beyer, W.F., and Kühn, H.: Can an osteoblastoma become malignant? Virchows Arch. [Pathol. Anat.] 408:297, 1985.
26. Bjornsson, J., Unni, K.K., Dahlin, D.C., Beabout, J.W., and Sim, F.H.: Clear cell chondrosarcoma of bone: observations in 47 cases, Am. J. Surg. Pathol. 8:223, 1984.
27. Boland, P.J., and Huvos, A.G.: Malignant fibrous histiocytoma of bone, Clin. Orthop. 204:130, 1986.
28. Boriani, S., Bacchini, P., Bertoni, F., and Campanacci, M.: Periosteal chondroma: a review of twenty cases, J. Bone Joint Surg. 65A:205, 1983.
29. Brecher, M.E., and Simon, M.A.: Chondroblastoma: an immunohistochemical study, Hum. Pathol. 19:1043, 1988.
30. Beyers, P.D.: Solitary benign osteoblastic lesions of bone: osteoid osteoma and benign osteoblastoma, Cancer 22:43, 1968.
31. Caffey, J., and Andersen, D.H.: Metastatic embryonal rhabdomyosarcoma in the growing skeleton: clinical, radiographic, and microscopic features, Am. J. Dis. Child. 95:581, 1958.
32. Campanacci, M., Bacci, G., Bertoni, F., Picci, P., Minutillo, A., and Franceschi, C.: The treatment of osteosarcoma of the extremities: twenty years' experience at the Istituto Ortopedico Rizzoli, Cancer 48:1569, 1981.
33. Campanacci, M., Boriani, S., and Giunti, A.: Hemangioendothelioma of bone: a study of 29 cases, Cancer 46:804, 1980.
34. Campanacci, M., Capanna, R., and Picci, P.: Unicameral and aneurysmal bone cysts, Clin. Orthop. 204:25, 1986.
35. Campanacci, M., and Cervellati, G.: Osteosarcoma: a review of 345 cases, Ital. J. Orthop. Traumatol. 1:5, 1975.
36. Campanacci, M., Giunti, A., and Olmi, R.: Giant-cell tumours of bone: a study of 209 cases with long-term followup in 130, Ital. J. Orthop. Traumatol. 1:249, 1975.
37. Campanacci, M., Picci, P., Gherlinzoni, F., Guerra, A., Bertoni, F., and Neff, J.R.: Parosteal osteosarcoma, J. Bone Joint Surg. 66B:313, 1984.
38. Campanacci, M., Guernelli, N., Leonessa, C., and Boni, A.: Chondrosarcoma: a study of 133 cases, 80 with long term follow up, Ital. J. Orthop. Traumatol. 1:387, 1975.
39. Cannon, S.R., and Sweetnam, D.R.: Multiple chondrosarcomas in dyschondroplasia (Ollier's disease), Cancer 55:836, 1985.
40. Carbone, P.P., Kellerhouse, L.E., and Gehan, E.A.: Plasmacytic myeloma: a study of the relationship of survival to various clinical manifestations and anomalous protein type in 112 patients, Am. J. Med. 42:937, 1967.
41. Cavazzana, A.O., Miser, J.S., Jefferson, J., and Triche, T.J.: Experimental evidence for a neural origin of Ewing's sarcoma of bone, Am. J. Pathol. 127:507, 1987.
42. Chabner, B.A., Haskell, C.M., and Canellos, G.P.: Destructive bone lesions in chronic granulocytic leukemia, Medicine 48:401, 1969.
43. Chambers, P.W., and Schwinn, C.P.: Chordoma: a clinicopathologic study of metastasis, Am. J. Clin. Pathol. 72:765, 1979.
44. Chan, K.W., Rosen, G., Miller, D.R., and Tan, C.T.C.: Hodgkin's disease in adolescents presenting as a primary bone lesion: a report of four cases and review of literature. Am. J. Pediatr. Hematol. Oncol. 4:11, 1982.
45. Chan, R.C., Sutow, W.W., Lindberg, R.D., Samuels, M.L., Murray, J.A., and Johnson, D.A.: Management and results of localized Ewing's sarcoma, Cancer 43:1001, 1979.

46. Chang, C.H.J., Piatt, E.D., Thomas, K.E., and Watne, A.L.: Bone abnormalities in Garnder's syndrome, Am. J. Roentgenol. Radium Ther. Nucl. Med. **103**:645, 1968.

47. Clark, J.L., Unni, K.K., Dahlin, D.C., and Devine, K.D.: Osteosarcoma of the jaw, Cancer **51**:2311, 1983.

48. Clarke, B.E., Xipell, J.M., and Thomas, D.P.: Benign fibrous histiocytoma of bone, Am. J. Surg. Pathol. **9**:806, 1985.

49. Clayton, F., Butler, J.J., Ayala, A.G., Ro, J.Y., and Zornoza, J.: Non-Hodgkin's lymphoma in bone: pathologic and radiologic features with clinical correlates, Cancer **60**:2494, 1987.

50. Cohen, D.M., Dahlin, D.C., and Pugh, D.G.: Fibrous dysplasia associated with adamantinoma of the long bones, Cancer **15**:515, 1961.

51. Corwin, J., and Lindberg, R.D.: Solitary plasmacytoma of bone vs. extramedullary plasmacytoma and their relationship to multiple myeloma, Cancer **43**:1007, 1979.

52. Cruz, M., Coley, B.C., and Stewart, F.W.: Postradiation bone sarcoma, Cancer **10**:72, 1957.

53. Cunningham, J.B., and Ackerman, L.V.: Metaphyseal fibrous defects, J. Bone Joint Surg. **38A**:797, 1956.

54. Dahlin, D.C.: Chondromyxoid fibroma of bone, with emphasis on its morphological relationship to benign chondroblastoma, Cancer **9**:195, 1956.

55. Dahlin, D.C., and Coventry, M.B.: Osteogenic sarcoma: a study of 600 cases, J. Bone Joint Surg. **49A**:101, 1967.

56. Dahlin, D.C., and Ivins, J.C.: Fibrosarcoma of bone: a study of 114 cases, Cancer **23**:35, 1969.

57. Dahlin, D.C., and Unni, K.K.: Osteosarcoma of bone and its important recognizable varieties, Am. J. Surg. Pathol. **1**:61, 1977.

58. De La Monte, S.M., Dorfman, H.D., Chandra, R., and Malawer, M.: Intraosseous schwannoma: histologic features, ultrastructure, and review of the literature, Hum. Pathol. **15**:551, 1984.

59. Delbruck, H.G., Allouche, M., Jasmin, C., Morin, M., Deml, F., Anghileri, L., Masse, R., and Lafuma, J.: Bone tumors induced in rats with radioactive cerium, Br. J. Cancer **41**:809, 1980.

60. DeSantos, L.A., Murray, J.A., and Ayala, A.G.: The value of percutaneous needle biopsy in the management of primary bone tumors, Cancer **43**:735, 1979.

61. de Souza Dias, L., and Frost, H.M.: Osteoid osteoma—osteoblastoma, Cancer **33**:1075, 1974.

62. Dorfman, H.D.: Malignant transformation of benign bone lesions. In Proceedings of the Seventh National Cancer Conference, vol. 7, Philadelphia, 1973, J.B. Lippincott Co.

63. Dorfman, H.D., Steiner, G.C., and Jaffe, H.L.: Vascular tumors of bone, Hum. Pathol. **2**:349, 1971.

64. Driedger, H., and Pruzanski, W.: Plasma cell neoplasia with osteosclerotic lesions: a study of five cases and a review of the literature, Arch. Intern. Med. **139**:892, 1979.

65. Dumont, J., and Mazabraud, A.: Primary lymphomas of bone (so-called "Parker and Jackson's reticulum cell sarcoma"): histological review of 75 cases according to the new classifications of non Hodgkin's lymphomas, Biomedicine (Express) **31**:271, 1979.

66. Enneking, W.F., editor: Osteosarcoma, Symposium Clin. Orthop. **111**:1, 1975.

67. Enneking, W.F., and Kagan, A.: "Skip" metastases in osteosarcoma, Cancer **36**:2192, 1975.

68. Evans, H.L., Ayala, A.G., and Romsdahl, M.M.: Prognostic factors in chondrosarcoma of bone: a clinicopathologic analysis with emphasis on histologic grading, Cancer **40**:818, 1977.

69. Finkel, M.P., Biskis, B.O., and Farrell, C.: Osteosarcomas appearing in Syrian hamsters after treatment with extracts of human osteosarcomas, Proc. Natl. Acad. Sci. USA **60**:1223, 1968.

70. Finkel, M.P., Biskis, B.O., and Jinkins, P.B.: Virus induction of osteosarcoma in mice, Science **151**:698, 1966.

71. Fisher, E.R., and Zawadski, A.: Ultrastructural features of plasma cells in patients with paraproteinemias, Am. J. Clin. Pathol. **54**:779, 1970.

72. Fraumeni, J.F., Jr.: Stature and malignant tumors of bone in childhood and adolescence, Cancer **20**:967, 1967.

73. Frentzel-Beyme, R., and Wagner, G.: Malignant bone tumours: status of aetiological knowledge and needs of epidemiological research, Arch. Orthop. Trauma Surg. **94**:81, 1979.

74. Furey, J.G., Ferrer-Torells, M., and Reagan, J.W.: Fibrosarcoma arising at the site of bone infarcts: a report of two cases, J. Bone Joint Surg. **42A**:802, 1960.

75. Garrison, R.C., Unni, K.K., McLeod, R.A., Pritchard, D.J., and Dahlin, D.C.: Chondrosarcoma arising in osteochondroma, Cancer **49**:1890, 1982.

76. Gebhardt, M.C., Campbell, C.J., Schiller, A.L., and Mankin, H.J.: Desmoplastic fibroma of bone: a report of eight cases and review of the literature, J. Bone Joint Surg. **67A**:732, 1985.

77. Gherlinzoni, F., Rock, M., and Picci, P.: Chondromyxoid fibroma: the experience at the Istituto Ortopedico Rizzoli, J. Bone Joint Surg. **65A**:198, 1983.

78. Ginaldi, S., and de Santos, L.A.: Computed tomography in the evaluation of small round cell tumors of bone, Radiology **134**:441, 1980.

79. Glass, A.G., and Fraumeni, J.F., Jr.: Epidemiology of bone cancer in children, J. Natl. Cancer Inst. **44**:187, 1970.

80. Goldring, S.R., Schiller, A.L., Mankin, H.J., Dayer, J.M., and Krane, S.M.: Characterization of cells from human giant cell tumors of bone, Clin. Orthop. **204**:59, 1986.

81. Gorham, L.W., and Stout, A.P.: Massive osteolysis (acute spontaneous absorption of bone, phantom bone, disappearing bone): its relation to hemangiomatosis, J. Bone Joint Surg. **37A**:985, 1955.

82. Guccion, J.G., Font, R.L., Enzinger, F.M., and Zimmerman, L.E.: Extraskeletal mesenchymal chondrosarcoma, Arch. Pathol. **95**:336, 1973.

83. Györkey, F., Sinkovics, J.G., and Györkey, P.: Electron microscopic observations on structures resembling myxovirus in human sarcomas, Cancer **27**:1449, 1971.

84. Hall, R.B., Robinson, L.H., Malawar, M.M., and Dunham, W.K.: Periosteal osteosarcomas, Cancer **55**:165, 1985.

85. Hallberg, O.E., and Begley, J.W., Jr.: Origin and treatment of osteomas of the paranasal sinuses, Arch. Otolaryngol. **51**:750, 1950.

86. Hanaoka, H., Friedman, B., and Mack, R.P.: Ultrastructure and histogenesis of giant cell tumor of bone, Cancer **25**:1408, 1970.

87. Harmon, T.P., and Morton, K.S.: Osteogenic sarcoma in four siblings, J. Bone Joint Surg. **48B**:493, 1966.

88. Hatcher, C.H.: The development of sarcoma in bone subjected to roentgen or radium irradiation, J. Bone Joint Surg. **27**:179, 1945.

89. Henley, J.H., and Ghelman, B.: Osteoid osteoma and osteoblastoma: current concepts and recent advances, Clin. Orthop. **204**:76, 1986.

90. Healey, J.H., and Lane, J.M.: Chondrosarcoma, Clin. Orthop. **204**:119, 1986.

91. Heffelfinger, M.J., Dahlin, D.C., MacCarty, C.S., et al.: Chordomas and cartilaginous tumors at the skull base, Cancer **32**:410, 1973.

92. Howard, E.B., Clarke, W.J., Karagianes, M.T., et al.: Strontium-90–induced bone tumors in miniature swine, Radiat. Res. **39**:594, 1969.

93. Hudson, T.M.: Radiologic-pathologic correlation of musculoskeletal lesions, Baltimore, 1987, The Williams & Wilkins Co.

94. Hunt, J.C., and Pugh, D.G.: Skeletal lesions in neurofibromatosis, Radiology **76**:1, 1961.

95. Hutter, R.V.P., Foote, F.W., Jr., Frazell, E.L., and Francis, K.C.: Giant cell tumors complicating Paget's disease of bone, Cancer **16**:1044, 1963.

96. Huvos, A.G.: Osteogenic sarcoma of bones and soft tissues in older persons: a clinicopathologic analysis of 117 patients older than 60 years, Cancer **57**:1442, 1986.

97. Huvos, A.G., Butler, A., and Bretsky, S.S.: Osteogenic sarcoma associated with Paget's disease of bone: a clinicopathologic study of 65 patients, Cancer **52**:1489, 1983.

98. Huvos, A.G., Heilweil, M., and Bretsky, S.S.: The pathology of malignant fibrous histiocytoma of bone: a study of 130 patients, Am. J. Surg. Pathol. **9**:853, 1985.

99. Huvos, A.G., and Higinbotham, N.L.: Primary fibrosarcoma of

bone: a clinicopathologic study of 130 patients, Cancer **35**:837, 1975.

100. Huvos, A.G., Higinbotham, N.L., and Miller, T.R.: Bone sarcomas arising in fibrous dysplasia, J. Bone Joint Surg. **54A**:1047, 1972.

101. Huvos, A.G., Rosen, G., Bretsky, S.S., and Butler, A.: Telangiectatic osteogenic sarcoma: a clinicopathologic study of 124 patients, Cancer **49**:1679, 1982.

102. Huvos, A.G., Woodard, H.Q., Cahan, W.G., Higinbotham, N.L., Stewart, F.W., Butler, A., and Bretsky, S.S.: Postradiation osteogenic sarcoma of bone and soft tissues: a clinicopathologic study of 66 patients, Cancer **55**:1244, 1985.

103. Huvos, A.G., Woodard, H.Q., and Heilweil, M.: Postradiation malignant fibrous histiocytoma of bone: a clinicopathologic study of 20 patients, Am. J. Surg. Pathol. **10**:9, 1986.

104. Jacobson, S.A.: Polyhistioma: a malignant tumor of bone and extraskeletal tissues, Cancer **40**:2116, 1977.

105. Jaffe, H.L.: Tumors and tumorous conditions of the bones and joint, Philadelphia, 1958, Lea & Febiger.

106. Jaffe, H.L., and Lichtenstein, L.: Nonosteogenic fibroma of bone, Am. J. Pathol. **18**:205, 1942.

107. Jaffe, R., Santamaria, M., Yunis, E.J., Tannery, N.H., Agostini, R.M., Jr., Medina, J., and Goodman, M.: The neuroectodermal tumor of bone, Am. J. Surg. Pathol. **8**:885, 1984.

108. Jaffe, N., Watts, N., Fellows, K.E., and Yawter, G.: Local en bloc resection for limb preservation, Cancer Treat. Rep. **62**:217, 1978.

109. Jennings, T.A., Peterson, L., Axiotis, C.A., Friedlaender, G.E., Cooke, R.A., and Rosai, J.: Angiosarcoma associated with foreign body material: a report of three cases, Cancer **62**:2436, 1988.

110. Johnson, S., Tetu, B., Ayala, A.G., and Chawla, S.P.: Chondrosarcoma with additional mesenchymal component (dedifferentiated chondrosarcoma). I. A clinicopathologic study of 26 cases, Cancer **58**:278, 1986.

111. Jumbelic, M., Feuerstein, I.M., and Dorfman, H.D.: Solitary intraosseous lymphangioma: a case report, J. Bone Joint Surg. **66A**:1479, 1984.

112. Kahn, L.B., Webber, B., Mills, E., Anstey, L., and Heselson, N.G.: Malignant fibrous histiocytoma (malignant fibrous xanthoma: xanthosarcoma) of bone, Cancer **42**:640, 1978.

113. Kaiser, T.E., Pritchard, D.J., and Unni, K.K.: Clinicopathologic study of sacrococcygeal chordoma, Cancer **54**:2574, 1984.

114. Kasahara, K., Yamamuro, T., and Kasahara, A.: Giant-cell tumour of bone: cytological studies, Br. J. Cancer **40**:201, 1979.

115. Kempson, R.L., and Kyriakos, M.: Fibroxanthosarcoma of the soft tissues: a type of malignant fibrous histiocytoma, Cancer **29**:961, 1972.

116. Kissane, J.M., Askin, F.B., Foulkes, M., Stratton, L.B., and Shirley, S.F.: Ewing's sarcoma of bone: clinicopathologic aspects of 303 cases from the Intergroup Ewing's Sarcoma Study, Hum. Pathol. **14**:773, 1983.

117. Kuettner, K.E., Pauli, B.E., and Soble, L.: Morphological studies on the resistance of cartilage to invasion by osteosarcoma cells in vitro and in vivo, Cancer Res. **38**:277, 1978.

118. Kunze, E., Graewe, T.H., and Peitsch, E.: Histology and biology of metastatic chondroblastoma: report of a case with a review of the literature, Pathol. Res. Pract. **182**:113, 1987.

119. Kyriakos, M.: Soft tissue implantation of chondromyxoid fibroma, Am. J. Surg. Pathol. **3**:363, 1979.

120. Lacassagne, A.: Conditions dans lesquelles ont été obtenus, chez le lapin, des cancers par action des rayons x sur des foyers inflammatoires, C.R. Soc. Biol. **112**:562, 1933.

121. Lagacé, R., Delage, C., Bouchard, H.L., and Seemayer, T.A.: Desmoplastic fibroma of bone: an ultrastructural study, Am. J. Surg. Pathol. **3**:423, 1979.

122. Laissue, J.A., Burlington, H., Cronkite, E.P., and Reincke, U.: Induction of osteosarcomas and hematopoietic neoplasms by ^{55}Fe in mice, Cancer Res. **37**:3545, 1977.

123. Lane, J.M., Hurson, B., Boland, P.J., and Glasser, D.B.: Osteogenic sarcoma, Clin. Orthop. **204**:93, 1986.

124. Lee, Y.-S., Pho, R.W.H., and Nather, A.: Malignant fibrous histiocytoma at site of metal implant, Cancer **54**:2286, 1984.

125. Levine, G.D., and Bensch, K.G.: Chondroblastoma—the nature of the basic cell: a study of means of histochemistry, tissue culture, electron microscopy, and autoradiography, Cancer **29**:1546, 1972.

126. Levy, W.M., Miller, A.S., Bonakdarpour, A., and Aegerter, E.: Aneurysmal bone cyst secondary to other osseous lesions: report of 57 cases, Am. J. Clin. Pathol. **63**:1, 1975.

127. Lewis, R.J., and Ketcham, A.S.: Maffucci's syndrome: functional and neoplastic significance; case report and review of the literature, J. Bone Joint Surg. **55A**:1465, 1973.

128. Lewis, R.J., and Lotz, M.J.: Medullary extension of osteosarcoma: implications for rational therapy, Cancer **33**:371, 1974.

129. Liu, J., Hudkins, P.G., Swee, R.G., and Unni, K.K.: Bone sarcomas associated with Ollier's disease, Cancer **59**:1376, 1987.

130. Mackenzie, D.H.: Intraosseous glomus: report of two cases, J. Bone Joint Surg. **44B**:648, 1962.

131. MacLennan, D.I., and Wilson, F.C., Jr.: Osteoid osteoma of the spine: a review of the literature and report of six new cases, J. Bone Joint Surg. **49A**:111, 1967.

132. Mahoney, J.P., and Alexander, R.W.: Ewing's sarcoma: a light and electron microscopic study of 21 cases, Am. J. Surg. Pathol. **2**:283, 1978.

133. Mahoney, J.P., and Alexander, R.W.: Primary histiocytic lymphoma of bone: a light and ultrastructural study of four cases, Am. J. Surg. Pathol. **4**:149, 1980.

134. Marsh, W.L., Jr., Bylund, D.J., Heath, V.C., and Anderson, M.J.: Osteoarticular and pulmonary manifestations of acute leukemia: case report and review of the literature, Cancer **57**:385, 1986.

135. Martin, S.E., Dwyer, A., Kissane, J.M., and Costa, J.: Small-cell osteosarcoma, Cancer **50**:990, 1982.

136. Martland, H.S., and Humphries, R.E.: Osteogenic sarcoma in dial painters using luminous paint, Arch. Pathol. **7**:406, 1929.

137. McCarthy, E.F., Matsuno, T., and Dorfman, H.D.: Malignant fibrous histiocytoma of bone: a study of 35 cases, Hum. Pathol. **10**:57, 1979.

138. McDonald, D.J., Sim, F.H., McLeod, R.A., and Dahlin, D.C.: Giant-cell tumor of bone, J. Bone Joint Surg. **68A**:235, 1986.

139. McKenna, R.J., Schwinn, C.P., Soong, K.Y., and Higinbotham, N.L.: Sarcomata of the osteogenic series (osteosarcoma, fibrosarcoma, chondrosarcoma, parosteal osteogenic sarcoma, and sarcomata arising in abnormal bone): an analysis of 552 cases, J. Bone Joint Surg. **48A**:1, 1966.

140. Meinshausen, J., Choritz, H., and Georgii, A.: Frequency of skeletal metastases are revealed by routinely take bone marrow biopsies, Virchows Arch. [Pathol. Anat.] **389**:409, 1980.

141. Miettinen, M., Lehto, V.-P., Dahl, D., and Virtanen, I.: Differential diagnosis of chordoma, chondroid, and ependymal tumors as aided by anti-intermediate filament antibodies, Am. J. Pathol. **112**:160, 1983.

142. Miller-Breslow, A., and Dorfman, H.D.: Dupuytren's (subungual) exostosis, Am. J. Surg. Pathol. **12**:368, 1988.

143. Mills, S.E., and Rosai, J.: Adamantinoma of the pretibial soft tissue: clinicopathologic features, differential diagnosis, and possible relationship to intraosseous disease, J. Clin. Pathol. **83**:108, 1985.

144. Mirra, J.M., Bullough, P.G., Marcove, R.C., Jacobs, B., and Huvos, A.G.: Malignant fibrous histiocytoma and osteosarcoma in association with bone infarcts: report of four cases, two in caisson workers, J. Bone Joint Surg. **56A**:932, 1974.

145. Moll, R., Lee, I., Gould, V.E., Berndt, R., Roessner, A., and Franke, W.W.: Immunocytochemical analysis of Ewing's tumors: patterns of expression of intermediate filaments and desmosomal proteins indicate cell type heterogeneity and pluripotential differentiation, Am. J. Pathol. **127**:288, 1987.

146. Monkman, G.R., Orwoll, G., and Ivins, J.C.: Trauma and oncogenesis, Mayo Clin. Proc. **49**:157, 1974.

147. Moon, N.F., and Mori, H.: Adamantinoma of the appendicular skeleton—updated, Clin. Orthop. **204**:215, 1986.

148. Morton, D.L., and Malmgren, R.A.: Human osteosarcomas: immunologic evidence suggesting an associated infectious agent, Science **162**:1279, 1968.

149. Muggia, F.M., and Hansen, H.H.: Osteoblastic metastases in small-cell (oat-cell) carcinoma of the lung, Cancer **30**:801, 1972.

150. Murphy, W.R., and Ackerman, L.V.: Benign and malignant giant-cell tumors of bone, Cancer **9**:317, 1956.

151. Nakashima, Y., Unni, K.K., Shives, T.C., Swee, R.G., and Dahlin, D.C.: Mesenchymal chondrosarcoma of bone and soft tissue: a review of 111 cases, Cancer **57**:2444, 1986.

152. Nakashima, Y., Yamamuro, T., Fujiwara, Y., Kotoura, Y., Mori, E., and Hamashima, Y.: Osteofibrous dysplasia (ossifying fibroma of long bones): a study of 12 cases, Cancer **52**:909, 1983.

153. Nakata, Y., Ochi, T., Kurisaki, E., Okano, H., Hamada, H., Amitani, K., Tanabe, S., Ono, K., and Sakamoto, Y.: Identification of type A and type C virus particles in BF murine osteosarcoma, Cancer Res. **40**:127, 1980.

154. Nascimento, A.G., Huvos, A.G., and Marcove, R.C.: Primary malignant giant cell tumor of bone: a study of eight cases and review of the literature, Cancer **44**:1393, 1979.

155. Nascimento, A.G., Unni, K.K., Pritchard, D.J., Cooper, K.L., and Dahlin, D.C.: A clinicopathologic study of 20 cases of large-cell (atypical) Ewing's sarcoma of bone, Am. J. Surg. Pathol. **4**:29, 1980.

156. Nojima, T., Unni, K.K., McLeod, R.A., and Pritchard, D.J.: Periosteal chondroma and periosteal chondrosarcoma, Am. J. Surg. Pathol. **9**:666, 1985.

157. Okajima, K., Honda, I., and Kitagawa, T.: Imunohistochemical distribution of S-100 protein in tumors and tumorlike lesions of bone and cartilage, Cancer **61**:792, 1988.

158. Olson, H.M., and Capen, C.C.: Virus induced animal model of osteosarcoma in the rat, Am. J. Pathol. **86**:437, 1977.

159. O'Neal, L.W., and Ackerman, L.V.: Chondrosarcoma of bone, Cancer **5**:551, 1952.

160. Ostrowski, M.L., Unni, K.K., Banks, P.M., Shives, T.C., Evans, R.G., O'Connell, M.J., and Taylor, W.F.: Malignant lymphoma of bone, Cancer **58**:2646, 1986.

161. Ozzello, L., Stout, A.P., and Murray, M.R.: Cultural characteristics of malignant histiocytomas and fibrous xanthomas, Cancer **16**:331, 1963.

162. Parham, D.M., Pratt, C.B., Parvey, L.S., Webber, B.L., and Champion, J.: Childhood multifocal osteosarcoma: clinicopathologic and radiologic correlates, Cancer **55**:2653, 1985.

163. Pasmantier, M.W., and Azar, H.A.: Extraskeletal spread in multiple plasma cell myeloma: a review of 57 autopsied cases, Cancer **23**:167, 1969.

164. Perez-Atayde, A.R., Kozakewich, H.P.W., and Vawter, G.F.: Adamantinoma of the tibia: an ultrastructural and immunohistochemical study, Cancer **55**:1015, 1985.

165. Pilepich, M.V., Vietti, T.J., Nesbit, M.E., Tefft, M., Kissane, J., Burgert, E.O., Pritchard, D.: Radiotherapy and combination chemotherapy in advanced Ewing's sarcoma—intergroup study, Cancer **47**:1930, 1981.

166. Pritchard, D.J., Finkel, M.P., and Reilly, C.A.: The etiology of osteosarcoma: a review of current considerations, Clin. Orthop. **111**:14, 1975.

167. Pritchard, D.J., Lunke, R.J., Taylor, W.F., Dahlin, D.C., and Medley, B.E.: Chondrosarcoma: a clinicopathologic and statistical analysis, Cancer **45**:149, 1980.

168. Rao, B.N., Champion, J.E., Pratt, C.B., Carnesale, P., Dilawari, R., Fleming, I., Green, A., Austin, B., Wrenn, E., and Kumar, M.: Limb salvage procedures for children with osteosarcoma: an alternative to amputation, J. Pediatr. Surg. **18**:901, 1985.

169. Reddick, R.L., Michelitch, H.J., Levine, A.M., and Triche, T.J.: Osteogenic sarcoma: a study of the ultrastructure, Cancer **45**:64, 1980.

170. Revell, P.A., and Scholtz, C.L.: Aggressive osteoblastoma, J. Pathol. **127**:195, 1979.

171. Reyes, C.V., and Kathuria, S.: Recurrent and aggressive chondroblastoma of the pelvis with late malignant neoplastic changes, Am. J. Surg. Pathol. **3**:449, 1979.

172. Rock, M.G., Pritchard, D.J., and Unni, K.K.: Metastases from histologically benign giant-cell tumor of bone, J. Bone Joint Surg. **66A**:269, 1984.

173. Rosai, J., Gold, J., and Landy, R.: The histiocytoid hemangiomas: a unifying concept embracing several previously described entities of skin, soft tissue, large vessels, bone, and heart, Hum. Pathol. **10**:707, 1979.

174. Rosai, J., and Pinkus, G.S.: Immunocytochemical demonstration of epithelial differentiation in adamantinoma of the tibia, Am. J. Surg. Pathol. **6**:427, 1982.

175. Rosen, G., Caparros, B., Nirenberg, A., Marcove, R.C., Huvos, A.G., Kosloff, C., Lane, J., and Murphy, M.L.: Ewing's sarcoma: ten-year experience with adjuvant chemotherapy, Cancer **47**:2204, 1981.

176. Ruiter, D.J., van Rijssel, T.G., and van der Velde, E.A.: Aneurysmal bone cysts: a clinicopathological study of 105 cases, Cancer **39**:2231, 1977.

177. Sanerkin, N.G.: Malignancy, aggressiveness, and recurrence in giant cell tumor of bone, Cancer **46**:1641, 1980.

178. Sanerkin, N.G., and Gallagher, P.: A review of the behaviour of chondrosarcoma of bone, J. Bone Joint Surg. **61A**:395, 1979.

179. Sanerkin, N.G., Mott, M.G., and Roylance, J.: An unusual intraosseous lesion with fibroblastic, osteoclastic, osteoblastic, aneurysmal and fibromyxoid elements: "solid" variant of aneurysmal bone cyst, Cancer **51**:2278, 1983.

180. Schajowicz, F.: Ewing's sarcoma and reticulum-cell sarcoma of bone: with special reference to the histochemical demonstration of glycogen as an aid to differential diagnosis, J. Bone Joint Surg. **41A**:349, 1959.

181. Schajowicz, F.: Giant-cell tumors of bone (osteoclastoma): a pathological and histochemical study, J. Bone Joint Surg. **43A**:1, 1961.

182. Schajowicz, F., Ackerman, L.V., and Sissons, H.A.: Histologic typing of bone tumours. In International Histological Classification of Tumours, No. 6, Geneva, 1972, World Health Organization.

183. Schajowicz, F., and Bessone, J.E.: Chondrosarcoma in three brothers, J. Bone Joint Surg. **43A**:1, 1961.

184. Schajowicz, F., and Derqui, J.C.: Puncture biopsy in lesions of the locomotor system: review of results in 4,050 cases, including 941 vertebral punctures, Cancer **21**:531, 1968.

185. Schajowicz, F., and Gallardo, H.: Epiphyseal chondroblastoma of bone: a clinico-pathological study of sixty-nine cases, J. Bone Joint Surg. **52B**:205, 1970.

186. Schajowicz, F., and Gallardo, H.: Chondromyxoid fibroma (fibromyxoid chondroma) of bone: a clinico-pathological study of thirty-two cases, J. Bone Joint Surg. **53B**:198, 1971.

187. Schajowicz, F., and Lemos, C.: Malignant osteoblastoma, J. Bone Joint Surg. **58B**:202, 1976.

188. Schajowicz, F., Santini Araujo, E., and Berenstein, M.: Sarcoma complicating Paget's disease of bone: a clinicopathological study of 62 cases, J. Bone Joint Surg. **65**:299, 1983.

189. Schmidt, D., Mackay, B., and Ayala, A.G.: Ewing's sarcoma with neuroblastoma-like features, Ultrastruct. Pathol. **3**:143, 1982.

190. Schulz, A., Jundt, G., Berghäuser, K.-H., Gehron-Robey, P., and Termine J.D.: Immunohistochemical study of osteonectin in various types of osteosarcoma, Am. J. Pathol. **132**:233, 1988.

191. Schwartz, D.T., and Alpert, M.: The malignant transformation of fibrous dysplasia, Am. J. Med. Sci. **247**:1, 1964.

192. Scranton, P.E., DeCicco, F.A., Totten, R.S., and Yunis, E.J.: Prognostic factors in osteosarcoma: a review of 20 years experience at the University of Pittsburgh Health Center Hospitals, Cancer **36**:2179, 1975.

193. Shapiro, F.: Ultrastructural observations on osteosarcoma tissue: a study of 10 cases, Ultrastruct. Pathol. **4**:151, 1983.

194. Simon, M.A., and Bartucci, E.J.: The search for the primary tumor in patients with skeletal metastases of unknown origin, Cancer **58**:1088, 1986.

195. Sindelar, W.F., Costa, J., and Ketcham, A.S.: Osteosarcoma associated with Thorotrast administration, Cancer **42**:2604, 1978.

196. Singh, I., Tsang, K.Y., and Blakemore, W.S.: Immunologic studies in contacts of osteosarcoma in humans and animals, Nature **265**:541, 1977.

197. Smith, G.D., Chalmers, J., and McQueen, M.M.: Osteosarcoma arising in relation to an enchondroma: a report of three cases, J. Bone Joint Surg. **68**:315, 1986.

198. Spiess, H., Poppe, H., and Schoen, H.: Strahleninduzierte Knochentumoren nach Thorium X-Behandlung, Monatsschr. Kinderheilkd. **110**:198,1962.

199. Spjut, H.J., and Ayala, A.G.: Skeletal tumors in children and adolescents, Hum. Pathol. **14**:628, 1983.

200. Spjut, H.J., and Lindbom, A.: Skeletal angiomatosis: report of two cases, Acta Pathol. Microbiol. Scand. **55**:49, 1962.

201. Spjut, H.J., et al.: Tumors of bone and cartilage. In Atlas of tumor pathology, sect. 2, fascicle 5, Washington, D.C., 1971, Armed Forces Institute of Pathology.

202. Springfield, D.S., Capanna, R., Gherlinzoni, F., Picci, P., and Campanacci, M.: Chondroblastoma: a review of seventy cases, J. Bone Joint Surg. **67A**:748, 1985.

203. Steiner, G.C.: Fibrous cortical defect and nonossifying fibroma of bone, Arch. Pathol. **97**:205, 1974.

204. Steiner, G.C., Ghosh, L., and Dorfman, H.D.: Ultrastructure of giant cell tumors of bone, Hum. Pathol. **3**:569, 1972.

205. Stewart, M.J., and Hamel, H.A.: Solitary bone cyst, South. Med. J. **43**:926, 1950.

206. Suit, H.D.: Role of therapeutic radiology in cancer of bone, Cancer **35**:930, 1975.

207. Sun, T.-C., Swee, R.G., Shives, T.C., and Unni, K.K.: Chondrosarcoma in Maffucci's syndrome, J. Bone Joint Surg. **67A**:1214, 1985.

208. Sundaresan, N.: Chordomas, Clin. Orthop. **204**:135, 1986.

209. Takigawa, K.: Chondroma of the bones of the hand, J. Bone Joint Surg. **53A**:1591, 1971.

210. Tapp, E.: Osteogenic sarcoma in rabbits following subperiosteal implantation of beryllium, Arch. Pathol. **88**:89, 1969.

211. Teitelbaum, S.L., and Bullough, P.G.: The pathophysiology of bone and joint disease, Am. J. Pathol. **96**:283, 1979.

212. Telles, N.C., Rabson, A.S., and Pomeroy, T.C.: Ewing's sarcoma: an autopsy study, Cancer **41**:2321, 1978.

213. Tetu, B., Ordóñez, N.G., Ayala, A.G., and Mackay, B.: Chondrosarcoma with additional mesenchymal component (dedifferentiated chondrosarcoma). II. An Immunohistochemical and electron microscopic study, Cancer **58**:287, 1986.

214. Thomas, B.M.: Three unusual carcinoid tumours, with particular reference to osteoblastic bone metastases, Clin. Radiol. **19**:221, 1968.

215. Tsuneyoshi, M., Dorfman, H.D., and Bauer, T.W.: Epithelioid hemangioendothelioma of bone: a clinicopathologic, ultrastructural, and immunohistochemical study, Am. J. Surg. Pathol. **10**:754, 1986.

216. Tucker, M.A., D'Angio, G.J., Boice, J.D., Jr., Strong, L.C., Li, F.P., Stovall, M., Stone, B.J., Green, D.M., Lombardi, F., Newton, W., Hoover, R.N., and Fraumeni, J.F., Jr.: Bone sarcomas linked to radiotherapy and chemotherapy in children, N. Engl. J. Med. **317**:588, 1987.

217. Turner, R.C.: Unusual group of tumours among schoolgirls, Br. J. Cancer **21**:17, 1966.

218. Unni, K.K., and Dahlin, D.C.: Premalignant tumors and conditions of bone, Am. J. Surg. Pathol. **3**:47, 1979.

219. Unni, K.K., Dahlin, D.C., Beabout, J.W., and Ivins, J.C.: Adamantinomas of long bones, Cancer **34**:1796, 1974.

220. Unni, K.K., Dahlin, D.C., Beabout, J.W., and Ivins, J.C.: Parosteal osteogenic sarcoma, Cancer **37**:2466, 1976.

221. Unni, K.K., Dahlin, D.C., McCleod, R.A., and Pritchard, D.J.: Intraosseous well-differentiated osteosarcoma, Cancer **40**:1337, 1977.

222. Vassallo, J., Roessner, A., Vollmer, E., and Grundmann, E.: Malignant lymphomas with primary bone manifestation, Pathol. Res. Pract. **182**:381, 1987.

223. Weatherby, R.P., Dahlin, D.C., and Ivins, J.C.: Postradiation sarcoma of bone: review of 78 Mayo Clinic cases, Mayo Clin. Proc. **56**:294, 1981.

224. Weiss, S.W., and Dorfman, H.D.: Adamantinoma of long bone: an analysis of nine new cases with emphasis on metastasizing lesions and fibrous dysplasia–like changes, Hum. Pathol. **8**:141, 1977.

225. Weiss, A.-P.C., and Dorfman, H.D.: S-100 protein in human cartilage lesions, J. Bone Joint Surg. **68A**:521, 1986.

226. White, V.A., Fanning, C.V., Ayala, A.G., Raymond, A.K., Carrasco, C.H., and Murray, J.A.: Osteosarcoma and the role of fine-needle aspiration: a study of 51 cases, Cancer **62**:1238, 1988.

227. Wick, M.R., Siegal, G.P., Unni, K.K., McLeod, R.A., and Greditzer, H.G., III: Sarcomas of bone complicating osteitis deformans (Paget's disease): fifty years' experience, Am. J. Surg. Pathol. **5**:47, 1981.

228. Wilkins, R.M., Pritchard, D.J., Burgert, E.O., Jr., and Unni, K.K.: Ewing's sarcoma of bone: experience with 140 patients, Cancer **58**:2551, 1986.

229. Wiltshaw, E.: The natural history of extramedullary plasmacytoma and its relation to solitary myeloma of bone and myelomatosis, Medicine **55**:217, 1976.

230. Wold, L.E., Swee, R.G., and Sim, F.H.: Vascular lesions of bone, Pathol. Annu. **20**(pt. 2):101, 1985.

231. Wold, L.E., Unni, K.K., Beabout, J.W., and Pritchard, D.J.: High-grade surface osteosarcomas, Am. J. Surg. Pathol. **8**:181, 1984.

232. Wold, L.E., Unni, K.K., Beabout, J.W., Sim, F.H., and Dahlin, D.C.: Dedifferentiated parosteal osteosarcoma, J. Bone Joint Surg. **66A**:53, 1984.

233. Wold, L.E., Unni, K.K., Beabout, J.W., Ivins, J.C., Bruckman, J.E., and Dahlin, D.C.: Hemangioendothelial sarcoma of bone, Am. J. Surg. Pathol. **6**:59, 1982.

234. Wold, L.E., Unni, K.K., Cooper, K.L., Sim, F.H., and Dahlin, D.C.: Hemangiopericytoma of bone, Am. J. Surg. Pathol. **6**:53, 1982.

235. Yoneyama, T., Winter W.G., and Milsow, L.: Tibial adamantinoma: its histogenesis from ultrastructural studies, Cancer **40**:1138, 1977.

236. Yunis, E.J., and Barnes, L.: The histologic diversity of osteosarcoma, Pathol. Annu. **21**(pt. 1):121, 1986.

40 Diseases of Joints

RUTH SILBERBERG

NORMAL JOINT STRUCTURE AND FUNCTION
Diarthrodial joints

The joints most commonly affected by disease are the diathrodial or synovial joints. Unlike the serosal cavities of pleurae and peritoneum, joint spaces are not closed or lined by a continuous layer of mesothelial cells. Instead, they are open tissue spaces, communicating directly with the periarticular tissues.

The articulating ends of two bones are held together by the joint capsule, a tubular structure of dense connective tissue inserting at the outer surfaces of the bony shafts. The capsule has an abundant supply of sensory nerve fibers that are highly sensitive to stretching and twisting and that are primarily responsible for the intense pain accompanying many joint lesions. Ligaments and tendons insert at the outer surface of the capsule. The capsule is lined by the synovial membrane, or synovium, which also cover the soft structures within the joints, fat pads, and ligaments and which forms outpouchings (bursae). The bursae communicate with the joint space and are therefore likely to become involved in pathologic processes affecting the joints and vice versa. The articulating surfaces of the bones are covered by bluish glistening hyaline cartilage, which varies in thickness not only in different joints but also within the same joint, with weight-bearing areas usually having a thicker cartilage cover than non–weight bearing areas. The cartilage is supported by a layer of cancellous bone.[123]

A small amount of free viscid fluid is present in the joint space and, by forming a thin layer over the cartilage, acts as a lubricant during joint motion.

Histologically and by electron microscopy, the surface of the articular cartilage is not smooth but shows innumerable roundish pits 20 to 30 μm in diameter, which correspond to the underlying most superficially located cartilage cells. The articular surface proper is entirely composed of matrix with cells. This architecture is of importance to the nutrition of the avascular articular cartilage, since it facilitates the flow of the synovial fluid into the cartilage. The chondrocytes vary in size, shape, and distribution. Three zones are usually distinguishable: a superficial zone characterized by spindle-shaped cells with their long axis oriented circumferentially; an intermediate or midzone of groups or small columns of polygonal cells that are capable of multiplying and are highly active metabolically; and the deepest, the pressure zone, possessing the largest cells, often in perpendicular orientation to the joint surface and separated from the underlying bone by a narrow layer of calcified matrix. By electron microscopy, articular chondrocytes have been shown to possess all the subcellular organelles of cells engaged in active synthesis and secretion—rough endoplasmic reticulum, free ribosomes, a Golgi apparatus, mitochondria, and so on. They produce the intercellular matrix and have been shown to respond readily to changes in the internal environment.[276]

Chondrocytes are also capable of synthesizing degrading enzymes, which may contribute to the eventual destruction of the surrounding matrix.[79] Under normal conditions the matrix seems protected by inhibitors of these enzymes.[125]

The matrix of the articular cartilage is composed of an amorphous phase (the ground substance) and a fibrillar phase (collagen fibrils). The ground substance contains water, electrolytes, and a variety of protein-polysaccharides (glycosaminoglycans or proteoglycans), chiefly chondroitin sulfates A and C and keratan sulfate,[125,251] that are responsible for the elasticity of the cartilage. Ninety percent of the collagen of cartilage is of type II; the remaining 10% is made up of varying amounts of different "minor" collagens. Collagen II is more resistant to degradation than the other collagens are. The collagen fibrils vary in thickness and distribution. Near the suface they are oriented in a circumferential direction, an arrangement that enables the cartilage to resist shearing forces; in the midzone they are meshlike in distribution; and in the deep zone, where they are thicker and more densely packed than elsewhere, they are often perpendicularly oriented to the joint surface. "Arcades," formed by fibers, presumably in conformity with mechanical stresses[127] and visualized at the tissue level, are not apparent on electron micrographs.

The synovial membrane is composed of an outer layer of loose vascular connective tissue and an inner discontinous layer of specialized cells, the synoviocytes.[108]

Vertebral joints

The vertebrae possess two kinds of joints. (1) Small apophyseal joints link the spinal processes and are typically diarthrodial in architecture. Thus anatomic, physiologic, and pathologic principles governing these joints are the same as those applying to all other diarthrodial joints. (2) The articulations between the vertebral bodies are unique insofar as the free joint space is replaced by the intervertebral discs. These cushion the impact of mechanical forces on the vertebrae by virtue of their elasticity and their intrinsic pressure. The discs have a jellylike center, the nucleus pulposus, containing much water and a variety of mucopolysaccharides, and an outer coat of dense connective tissue, the anulus fibrosus. The anulus restrains the nucleus within its boundaries during motion; it inserts at the opposing "end plates" of the vertebral bodies. These end plates are the actual articulating surfaces of the vertebral bodies and are composed of stratified cartilage structured similar to that of the diarthrodial joints. In the course of time, this cartilage may be partly replaced by bone and the anulus becomes inserted into bone rather than into cartilage.

The joints commonly affected by disease are the diarthrodial or synovial joints. The normal functioning of these joints depends on a delicate balance of morphologic, physiologic, and biochemical conditions,* some of which are local but many of which are modifiable by extra-articular factors. By the same token, joint diseases may be purely local in character or may be manifestations of systemic disorders.

CONGENITAL MALFORMATIONS AND DEVELOPMENTAL DEFECTS OF JOINTS

Disregarding traumatic dislocation of joints during birth, congenital deformities occur in about 6% of newborns.[28] Such lesions may result from abnormalities in muscles or capsular connective tissue, or they may be primary in the osseous system. Various chromosomal aberrations may be associated with instability or dislocation of axial or peripheral joints.[75,97]

Generalized joint rigidity, a rare condition, is seen in arthrogryphosis multiplex, which is characterized by clubfeet, clubhands, and contractures of the large joints.[305,313] The cause of the disorder is unknown. The changes have been attributed to primary disorders of

---

*References 27, 104, 108, 123, 151, 161, 187, 202, 259, 276, 283, 307, 333.

the nervous system, particularly of motor neuron or motor end plate. Multiple congenital contractures may be found in a variety of chromosomal aberrations and have thus a heterogeneous genetic background.

Synoviocytes synthesize and secrete hyaluronate, which is given off into the joint space. Two morphologic types of synoviocytes have been described, one rich in endoplasmic reticulum (B-cells) and the other with a prominent Golgi apparatus (A-cells). It is likely that these two types represent different functional states of the same cell. Under pathologic conditions, synovial lining cells are capable of synthesizing immunoglobulins and mediators of inflammation.[133]

The articular cartilage is constantly exposed to mechanical stresses occurring during joint motion and as a result of static loading. The mechanical forces acting on a joint are those of tangential shear and of static pressure, forces that may act with sudden impact or in a protracted fashion. Static forces are brought about by weight and, more important, by the action of muscles and ligaments. Several mechanisms protect the joints from damage by such forces: the elasticity and the surface architecture of the cartilage permit it to absorb some force, and the synovial fluid provides lubrication that is ideally adapted to maintain joint function.[288]

The synovial fluid, or synovia, a term used first by Paracelsus, is a dialysate of plasma. It becomes viscid because of the discharge into it of protein hyaluronate, secreted by the synoviocytes. Under normal conditions the synovial fluid forms a thin film on the cartilaginous surfaces; the total amount of synovial fluid is small, about 3 ml in the adult knee joint. Its lubricating effect is enhanced by changes in viscosity with joint motion. At rest or at slow motion it is more viscid than at high rates of motion. Normal synovial fluid contains about 3.5 mg/g of hyaluronate bound to protein, plasma components, polymorphonuclear and mononuclear leukocytes, and some sloughed off synoviocytes. The fluid acts not only as a lubricant, but also as the main source of nutrients for the articular cartilage into which it penetrates because of a pumping effect created by joint motion.

The biomechanical mechanisms whereby joint lubrication is accomplished are still under discussion. The original concept of simple hydrodynamic action has been supplemented by the concepts of boundary lubrication and weeping lubrication. Boundary lubrication stresses the interaction of small irregularities in the articulating surfaces (as shown by scanning electron microscopy) with extremely thin layers of lubricating fluid in the lubricating process. The concept of weeping lubrication is based on the fact that cartilage acts like a sponge, from which tissue fluid is expressed during stresses on the joint and into which fluid is sucked after release of the stress.[333] Whatever the mechanisms of lubrication, a decrease in lubrication causes increasing friction between the articulating surfaces and leads to tissue damage.

The opposite condition, joint flaccidity, is generalized in the Ehlers-Danlos syndrome, especially in type VII of the disorder.[122] Associated with hyperextensibility of joints, it results in loosening of the joint capsule. This abnormality is often the cause of congenital subluxation of the hip.[54] It is hereditary, transmitted as an autosomal recessive, and results from inadequate cross-linking of the collagen molecule. The basic defect is the inadequate cleavage of the type I procollagen, either because of a defect in the cleaving enzyme *N*-proteinase or because of primary changes in the structure of the collagen I molecule.[236,240]

Clubfoot, a positional abnormality involving flexion of the ankle, inversion of the foot, and medial rotation of the tibia, has been attributed to intrauterine compression, a widely held but poorly substantiated point of view. The increased concordance of the lesion in monozygotic twins (32%) as compared with 2.9% in fraternal twins is suggestive of the presence of a genetic factor.[146] Clubfoot may result from inborn errors of connective tissue metabolism, as discussed in the previous paragraph. It is thus advisable to consider clubfoot as a pathogenetically heterogeneous disorder.

Defective development, dysplasia, of the acetabulum is difficult to diagnose in the newborn but becomes more distinct with increasing age. Inadequate ossification of the roof of the acetabulum prevents the formation of a close-fitting socket for the femoral head. Consequently the femoral head becomes dislocated cranially, posteriorly or laterally, with resulting complete luxation of the hip. Major development defects of the large joints have been noted in children born to mothers who had received thalidomide during pregnancy.[195] Clubfoot and hip dysplasia occur with increased frequency in infants of mothers with untreated or poorly controlled diabetes mellitus during pregnancy.[279]

NONINFLAMMATORY JOINT DISEASES
Joint disorders caused by physical injury

The term "traumatic arthritis," under which joint disorders caused by physical injury are usually classified, is a misnomer. Although physical injury may cause inflammatory changes, as implied in the term, the sequelae of physical injury are most often noninflammatory. All tissue components of the joints may be affected, and most repair processes correspond to those seen in other locations. However, disorders involving the articular cartilage have special significance. Although articular chondrocytes retain some growth potential into old age, the healing tendency of the cartilage is poor. Once the continuity of the surface has been disrupted, it is rarely if ever restored to normal, despite active proliferation and synthetic activity of many of the chondrocytes in the middle and deep layers of the articular covering. Defects that reach as deep as the subchondral bone are repaired by fibrous tissue growing into the defect from the bone marrow. Under the effects of friction and pressure during motion, this "scar" may be transformed into fibrocartilage.[52,184]

Injuries of the joints resulting from physical forces are of two main types: (1) acute injuries, which are usually produced by the action of a single violent force, and (2) chronic injuries, which occur after minor and frequently repeated inflictive forces.

Acute injuries

Any one of the component parts of a joint may be injured by physical force, particularly if the stress is applied suddenly. If a joint is twisted, hyperextended, hyperflexed, or otherwise forced to move beyond the limits permitted by the elasticity of its ligaments, a sprain, subluxation, or dislocation occurs. Such injuries represent varying degrees of single type of damage. Thus, as the result of a twist, blow, or fall, the synovial tissues, the ligaments, or the capsule may be stretched, lacerated, or ruptured. In the knee, menisci may be displaced, detached, or torn. The articular cartilage may be compressed, split, or detached from the underlying bone. More severe injuries include lacerations of ligaments and joint capsules. Despite spontaneous or surgery-aided healing processes, such severely damaged joints may be permanently weakened, unstable, and predisposed to recurrent dislocation. With greater violence the articulating bones may be dislocated or fractured, and there may be a bloody effusion into the joint space.

Usually extravasated blood is completely absorbed. In some instances, however, the blood clot organizes, with the production of fibrous adhesions across the joint space. Portions of bone that are completely detached by the fracture become necrotic, though the cartilage survives. These detached fragments of cartilage and bone remain in the joint as loose bodies ("joint mice") and may cause pain or recurrent locking of the joint. Malalignment of the fracture fragments may cause an uneven joint surface and thus excessive friction. The relation of these factors to secondary osteoarthrosis is discussed in a later section of this chapter.

Open laceration of a joint capsule may lead to secondary infection. In addition, physical injury may trigger recurrence of, or reactivate, an old quiescent lesion such as tuberculosis, gouty arthritis, or pyogenic infections.

Chronic injuries

Injuries from minor repeated forces are of many kinds and grades of severity. They include those incurred in daily activities, those sustained in recreational or occupational pursuits, and mechanical dysfunction induced by abnormal posture, disturbed locomotion, skeletal deformities, or previous acute trauma. The articular changes produced by chronic injury are varied in both kind and extent of involvement. In some instances the lesions are confined to periarticular structures, including ligaments, tendon sheaths, or bursae. More frequently the joint proper is the site of involvement. Effusions of fluid into the bursae, tendon sheaths, or articular cavities occasionally result. Loose bodies may be present within distended bursal or synovial cavities. Occasionally, calcification is found in tendons or bursal walls. Such changes are especially common in the shoulder region and knee.[210,309]

Neuropathic joint disease (Charcot's joint)

The lesions of neuropathic joint disease, usually monarticular, are seen in patients with a variety of neurologic disorders. Originally described by Charcot in 1868, they were attributed chiefly to tabes or syringomyelia; they are now known to be associated with spina bifida, with amyloid infiltration in the course of multiple myeloma,[268] with diabetes mellitus,[281] and with chronic alcoholism.[314] The site of the neurologic lesion determines which joint is affected; with tabes, it is commonly a knee, with syringomyelia the shoulder, with spina bifida the hip, and with diabetes the small joints of the feet and ankles.

An initial nonspecific noninflammatory effusion within the joint space may subside without further damage. Subsequently there are increasing deterioration and erosion of the articular cartilage and sclerosis of the adjacent bone. Eventually the bone also undergoes necrosis and disintegrates, a condition leading to gross disfiguration or even disappearance of the involved epiphysis.

Anesthetization of the joint caused by the disrupted nerve supply has been incriminated as a main contributor to the lesion. The patient suffering no pain is not aware of a disease process and continues to traumatize the joint. However, factors other than purely neurologic dysfunction may be involved in the pathogenesis of some forms of Charcot's joints; diabetic neuropathy especially may be complicated by simultaneous vascular disease, and the disturbed glucose metabolism may directly alter the protein-polysaccharide composition of the cartilage matrix.

Amyloid arthropathy

Generalized amyloidosis can affect multiple joints with deposition of amyloid in the synovium, in cartilage, and in the joint cavity. The shoulder is a site of predilection, but elbows, hands, knees, hips, and temporomandibular and sternoclavicular joints are also commonly involved. Large quantities of amyloid may be free in the joint cavity or deposited in the tissues.[216] Massive deposits of amyloid may develop after long periods of hemodialysis for renal failure.[15] Minute amyloid deposits, on the other hand, were found in knees and sternoclavicular joints in unselected autopsies of aging persons—apparently an articular manifestation of generalized age-linked amyloidosis.[111]

Cartilage containing amyloid is whitish opaque, and infiltrated synovium is stiffened. By electron microscopy typical amyloid fibrils with a 7.5 to 10 nm diameter and a periodicity of two or three per 10 nm length are found extracellularly in the synovium. With special stains, amyloid may be identified as a thin layer on and slightly below the surface of the cartilage. The surface may be smooth or frayed, depending on whether there is associated degradation of the matrix.[86] No amyloid is found within the chondrocytes.[47] The problem of how the amyloid reaches the joint cavity—whether by precipation from the synovial fluid or by discharge of synovial deposits into the free joint space—is unresolved.

Arthropathy associated with ochronosis

The joint disease associated with ochronosis is caused by the intra-articular deposition of polymerized homogentisic acid, a black pigment. The homogentisic acid is the product of incomplete degradation of tyrosine and phenylalanine, occurring because of an inborn absence of the enzyme homogentisic acid oxidase. The joints involved are primarily those of the vertebral column, although later in the course of the disorder, hips, knees, and shoulder joints may become affected.

Grossly the large joints may be distended by effusion, which is usually noninflammatory. The cartilage is stained a deep black to various shades of gray and is fragmented and brittle (Plate 8, A and B). The synovium has hypertrophic folds that contain small fragments of detached deteriorated cartilage.

Microscopically, granular pigment is seen within chondrocytes and synovial lining cells. Calcium pyrophosphate crystals may be associated with the pigmentation.[263] The synovium may show evidence of acute or chronic inflammation. By electron microscopy, amorphous pigment particles have been demonstrated in both the chondrocytes and the surrounding matrix.[171]

Arthropathy associated with hemochromatosis

Joint involvement is seen in about half the cases of primary hemochromatosis, and frequently there is associated chondrocalcinosis. The small joints of the hands are most conspicuously affected, but knees, hips, and the vertebral column also become involved.[48,70]

Grossly the synovium is brownish red. In the presence of chondrocalcinosis, multiple, whitish, chalklike deposits are present in the cartilage, especially in fissures and erosions that appear during the course of the disease.

Microscopically the synovium shows slight hyperplasia with proliferation of fibroblasts, perivascular deposits of hemosiderin in the deep layers, thickening of the vessel walls, occasional microaneurysms, and medial calcification. By electron microscopy the pigment can be demonstrated mainly in synoviocytes.[261] Inflammatory changes are negligible.

Chondrocytes may contain pigment and calcium pyrophosphate or apatite crystals, and crystals may be present without iron deposits. Necrotic chondrocytes, fibrillation of the matrix, and erosions characteristic of chondrocalcinosis are suggestive of the fact that crystal deposition rather than iron deposits play a pathogenetic role in the arthropathy. That similar lesions do not occur in other conditions associated with iron deposition in the joints supports this view.[264] Disturbed proteoglycan synthesis, related to the diabetic imbalance in hemochromatosis, may predispose to crystal deposition in the cartilage.

Arthropathy associated with hemophilia

Adverse joint manifestations eventually develop in 80% to 90% of hemophiliacs with factors VII and IX and, more rarely, factor XIII deficiency because of hemorrhage into the articular cavities and periarticular tissues. A single hemorrhagic episode may be followed by complete resorption and restoration of normal conditions. Repeated hemorrhage, however, sets off a sequela of changes resulting in severe disfiguration and functional impairment of the involved joints.[137,289]

Grossly the synovium takes on a reddish brown color and becomes hypertrophic with polypous folds or diffuse mosslike thickening. With increasing duration of the condition, there is more fibrous thickening of the synovium, as well as of the subsynovial connective tissue, and development of fibrous adhesions between the opposing surfaces of the joint. The cartilage becomes eroded and cystic because of the focal necrosis. The subchondral bone responds with early sclerosis, which may give way to atrophy and breakdown with formation of cysts in the epiphyses. Such cysts enclose organizing blood clot and may communicate with the articular cavity.

Microscopically the synovium contains numerous hemosiderin-laden macrophages, especially in the near-surface layers. By electron microscopy hemosiderin has been found in the cytoplasm of some chondrocytes but not in the extracellular matrix.[142] The lining cells, particularly B-cells, are hyperplastic, as are the fibroblasts of the deep layers. Especially near the insertion of ligaments, ingrowth of synovium into degenerating cartilage may be seen. In advanced cases the cartilage resembles that found in osteoarthrosis.[69,163]

Osteochondroses

Osteochondroses result from aseptic necrosis of the bone underlying the articular cartilage. Since the articular cartilage does not depend on blood vessels for its nutritional supply, the injury to the cartilage is not attributable to nutritional failure. Rather, it is the loss of mechanical support from the underlying bone that causes the cartilage to break down. The ensuing defects may initially be small, but there may be further deterioration of the articular covering and reactive chondrocyte proliferation, resulting in lesions similar to those of osteoarthrosis. Many syndromes associated with osteochondrosis have been described in various skeletal sites (see Chapter 38).

Osteochondrosis dissecans

The formerly used term "osteochondritis" is a misnomer that should be abandoned. The lesion has no inflammatory component, and therefore the suffix "-itis" is inappropriate. The characteristic gross findings in the joints are single or multiple loose or lightly attached bodies composed of cartilage and underlying bone. These bodies, termed "joint mice," are ovoid or roundish and measure 0.5 to 1.5 cm in diameter and several millimeters in thickness (Fig. 40-1). Often a groove in the articular surface indicates the site from which a body has been detached. Microscopically the grooves are covered with fibrous tissue. The cartilage of the fragments may be intact or show various degrees of fibrillation and foci of calcification. The attached bone is usually sclerotic with thickened trabeculas.

The lesions are commonly found in children and adolescents, in boys more often than in girls, and usually involve the knee joint, especially the medial condyle of the femur. However, hip, shoulder, and elbow may also be affected.[242] Mechanical, especially shear, forces acting on normal joint tissue but with local developmental defects have been considered a major cause of the changes; the lesions also develop as a result of aseptic necrosis of subchondral bone. Apparent familial aggregation has been reported.[211,284]

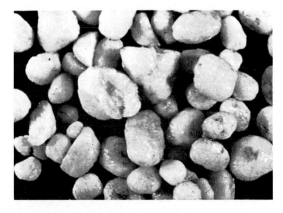

Fig. 40-1. Joint mice removed from shoulder joint. Synovial membrane was studded with small nodules composed of dense fibrous tissue and cartilage. Detachment of these tissue excrescences was apparent source of loose bodies.

Arthropathy associated with sickle cell disease

Sickling and thrombosis occur in small vessels of the articular tissues as in nonskeletal locations. Thrombi composed of dead cells, platelets, and red blood corpuscles occlude vascular lumens; the cartilage becomes involved secondarily because of avascular necrosis of the subchondral bone.[57] Tissue destruction, which may become extensive, thus resembles that seen in aseptic avascular necrosis as well as, in advanced cases, that seen in aseptic necrosis. Microinfarcts may develop in the synovium. The vascular basement membranes are thickened, and perivascular fibrosis is present.[262] The synovium shows low-grade infiltration by mononuclear leukocytes. The joints most commonly involved are hip, shoulder, and knee in the order mentioned.

Arthropathy associated with renal dialysis

"Erosive azotemic arthropathy" occurs in about one third of patients on renäl dialysis for more than one and a half years and apparently is more often in those on peritoneal than on hemodialysis. Hand, shoulder, elbow, knee, and sacroiliac joints may be involved with periarticular calcification as well as deposition of calcium pyrophosphate or apatite in and erosion of the articular cartilage. The synovium reacts with mild lining cell hyperplasia, low-grade mononuclear cell infiltration, and fibrosis.

The pathogenesis of the condition is poorly understood, but it is believed to be related to secondary hyperparathyroidism after renal failure and to the ensuing increased Ca × P product in the serum.[15,56,253]

Hypertrophic osteoarthropathy

The clubbing of fingers and toes characteristic of hypertrophic osteoarthropathy is primarily attributable to periarticular and periosteal hyperemia and fibroblastic proliferation and to overgrowth of bone; joints may become involved, with an increase of synovial fluid that is rich in mucins but has fewer cells than what would be present with an inflammatory lesion. The condition is found in association with circulatory failure as occurs in congenital heart disease, with a variety of digestive disorders, and chiefly with malignant or chronic benign pulmonary disease.

The pathogenetic mechanisms involved in the disorder are unknown. The presence of a vasodilator acting on the arteriovenous anastomoses has been postulated for instances of clubbing in congenital heart disease; in association with pleural or pulmonary disease an interaction with the adrenergic vascular innervation may play a pathogenetic role.[286]

In addition to this secondary type of clubbing, there is a primary form of the disease, pachydermatoperiostosis, that is inherited as a sex-linked dominant trait.[246]

Aging of articular cartilage

The morphologic, biochemical, and physical properties of the articular cartilage change with age. These changes are important pathogenically because they render the cartilage more susceptible to injury.

The growth potential and the cellularity of the articular cartilage decrease progressively from birth to the end of the growth period, but some growth potential persists throughout life.[274] This fact is responsible for lifelong cell renewal, the gradual remodeling of the articular contour,[151] and the resumption of cell proliferation under pathologic conditions, such as osteoarthrosis of old age or of hyperpituitarism. During adulthood the decline in cellularity slows down, and in old age a slight increase in the number of cells may occur.[301] Associated with this increase in cell number is an increase in cellular activity, as indicated by increased uptake of radiosulfate by the articular chondrocytes.[60] An age-linked increase in intracellular lipid apparently does not interfere with the functioning of the chondrocytes.

The matrix likewise changes with advancing age. During growth the ratio of chondroitin-4-sulfate to chondroitin-6-sulfate decreases, and an increase in keratan sulfate is demonstrable in tissue sections and biochemically by a decrease in the galactosamine-to-glucosamine ratio. From early adulthood on, there is a net loss of water and total proteoglycans[4,260,302] and an increase of the protein-to-glucosamine ratio of the proteo-

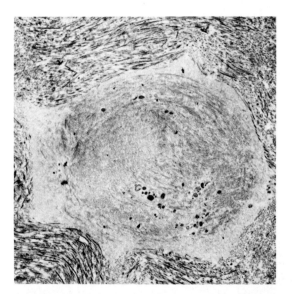

Fig. 40-2. Electron micrograph of "microscar" in aging human articular cartilage of hip joint. Whorls of collagen fibrils with intermingled electron-dense fat globules have replaced disintegrated chondrocyte. Scar is still surrounded by halo of relatively electron-lucent matrix, which surrounded former chondrocyte. There is regular matrix with collagen fibrils at periphery. (Courtesy Dr. Max Spycher, Zurich.)

glycan molecules.[237] In many joints proteoglycan content becomes stabilized thereafter; however, proteoglycan molecules appear less aggregated than those in the joints of young persons.[233] No further changes occur unless additional pathogenic factors become active.

As proteoglycans decrease, the collagen fibrils increase in thickness and become packed more tightly than those in young persons.[295] Focal whorl-like aggregations of collagen fibrils develop at the sites of disintegrated cells (Fig. 40-2). Associated with these changes are impairment of tensile strength, tensile stiffness, and elasticity and an increase in compliance of the articular cartilage.[10,162] The remaining chondrocytes, in an apparent attempt at repair, become temporarily overactive and after this are prematurely exhausted and die; thus a vicious circle is initiated resulting ultimately in osteoarthrosis. The age-linked progressive accumulation of lipid in the matrix results from disintegration of cell components but does not seem to influence subsequent disease processes.

Age changes in capsule, ligaments, and synovial membrane presumably are the same as those in connective tissue in other locations.[321]

Osteoarthrosis

Osteoarthrosis, a noninflammatory disorder of synovial joints, is characterized by regressive changes and proliferation of the articular cartilage and by overgrowth of subchondral and juxta-articular bone and intra-articular soft tissues. The disease is, so far as is known, a strictly skeletal disorder without accompanying changes in the biochemistry of body fluids or in nonskeletal tissues.

In view of the absence of inflammatory changes, synonyms such as osteoarthritis, hypertrophic arthritis, or arthritis deformans are misnomers. The term "degenerative joint disease" is correct only insofar as it denotes general deterioration of the joints; it does not take into account the prominent processes of growth occurring in the course of the disease, and furthermore it disregards the fact that "degeneration" of articular tissues occurs in many other joint disorders.

Prevalence and distribution

Osteoarthrosis is one of the oldest and most widespread diseases known. The characteristic alterations have been observed in the skeletons of prehistoric animals, in many nonmammalian and mammalian species of present-day animals,[288] and in humans. The disease is age linked, starting as subtle biochemical biophysical, and microscopic changes at the beginning of the third decade, becoming roentgenographically noticeable at the end of the fourth decade and giving rise to clinical symptoms some time thereafter. Practically no aging human is spared the development of osteoarthrosis in one or several locations. Particularly severe or early clinical involvement of one joint may be so prominent as to make the disease appear monarticular, though commonly multiple joints are affected to a lesser degree. Pathologic involvement is thus more widespread than clinical symptoms would indicate, and localized monarticular osteoarthrosis should be considered a special occurrence rather than the rule. Reports of a higher incidence of clinical disease in women than in men are not borne out by autoptic and roentgenographic observations. In men the disease develops at least as often and at even earlier ages than in women; however, the advanced lesions of later ages seem to be more common in women than in men.[121,132,157,317]

Osteoarthrosis is most conspicuous in the large joints of the lower extremity, knees, and hips, but the interphalangeal, shoulder, metacarpophalangeal, and sternoclavicular joints are commonly involved. The temporomandibular joints may also be affected by the disease.

Histogenesis

The early stages of the disease merge imperceptibly with the lage aging changes.[21,24,197,198,237] Because of loss of mucopolysaccharides, which normally invest the collagen fibrils, the latter are unmasked and the cartilage appears fibrillated; the fibrils are held together less tightly than normal, and if this process involves the surface layer, they change from the circumferential to a radial orientation as the articular surface becomes frayed and fissured (Fig. 40-3). The chondrocytes respond with proliferation, hypertrophy, and increased synthesis of proteoglycans followed by accelerated disintegration (Fig. 40-4). Changes in water content and in the amount and proportion of proteoglycans observed in osteoarthrotic cartilage[4,30,212] seem to be related to the presence of young chondrocytes and newly formed matrix.[106,220] In reconciling apparently contradictory histologic findings one should realize that the osteoarthrotic process varies (1) in different locations because of differing weight-bearing and non–weight bearing areas and (2) because of the age or state of activity of the process itself.[113,198,311]

Once the continuity of the articular surface has been disrupted, the conditions for smooth joint motion and normal lubrication no longer exist, and mechanical forces contribute to further erosion of the articular surface. The cartilage may show increased calcification, invasion by blood vessels, and progressive ulceration (Fig. 40-5 and Plate 8, *D*). Collagenolysis by collagenase is increased in osteoarthrotic cartilage and most noticeably so in the center of the lesions.[232] The underlying bone is bared and reacts with osteosclerosis; the

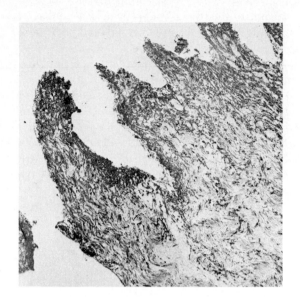

Fig. 40-3. Electron micrograph from osteoarthrotic ulcer at femoral head. Surface of lesion is frayed, and villous projections are composed of short, irregularly clustered collagen fibrils, mainly in radial orientation to joint surface. (Courtesy Dr. Max Spycher, Zurich.)

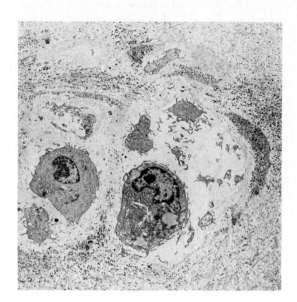

Fig. 40-4. Electron micrograph from osteoarthrotic femoral head. Cluster of chondrocytes indicates proliferation. Two chondrocytes are shown completely; others are sectioned tangentially and only partly shown. Numerous electron-dense granules—some scattered diffusely and others aggregated in crescents—represent lipid derived from disintegrated cells. (Courtesy Dr. Max Spycher, Zurich.)

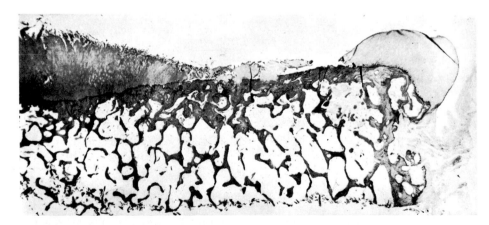

Fig. 40-5. Low-power photomicrograph of cartilage of patellar surface of femur: osteoarthrosis. Fibrillation and splitting of matrix are seen. Fragmentation and detachment of cartilage are evident toward right, where subchondral bone has been denuded. (10×; AFIP 67996.)

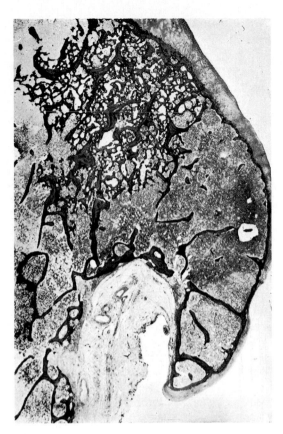

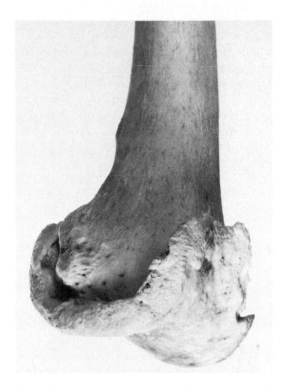

Fig. 40-6. Low-power photomicrograph of joint, showing extensive marginal lipping. "Lip" is extension of epiphyseal end of tubular bone. (AFIP 67998.)

Fig. 40-7. Macerated specimen of lower femur. There is pronounced osteoarthrosis of femoral aspect of knee joint with extensive marginal lipping.

epiphyseal bone marrow often becomes fibrotic and occasionally cystic. The intra-articular soft tissues, synovial villi, and fat pads become hypertrophic, but unlike conditions in inflammatory joint disease, pannus overgrowth is limited in extent and significance; yet the presence of fibronectin in osteoarthrotic cartilage may be related to the tendency of fibrosed synovial tissue to spread out.[202] Fragments of cartilage may be detached into the joint cavity and persist and move about as free bodies. Although destructive processes are prominent in the center regions of the joints, the cartilage at the periphery proliferates, ossifies, and with new periosteal bone forms large, elevated, overhanging outgrowths (Figs. 40-6 and 40-7). This process, described as "lipping," results in further distortion of the articular surface, with considerable functional impairment. However, even in severely altered osteoarthrotic joints, complete immobilization rarely occurs.

Etiology and pathogenesis

Osteoarthrosis is now recognized as being of multifactorial origin, and the earlier simplistic concept of a "wear-and-tear disease" is outdated. From an etiologic point of view, primary and secondary osteoarthrosis may be distinguished, though morphologically the two types are indistinguishable. Secondary osteoarthrosis is posttraumatic in the broadest sense of the term, with trauma being related to (1) action of mechanical force on a joint, as by a single impact or presumably a series of repeated occupational insults (such as those incurred by professional dancers or men working with pneumatic tools); (2) malalignment of joints attributable to congenital malformations, to incongruencies of the opposing articular surfaces, to metabolic or circulatory bone disease, or to superimposition on previous inflammatory disease associated with fibrosis and scarring of the joint capsule; or (3) deposition of extraneous injurious material within the articular tissues. Most experimental models are examples of secondary osteoarthrosis.

Osteoarthrosis is considered primary if none of the foregoing conditions applies. In the absence of unequivocal evidence as to the cause of the disorder, several hypotheses have been advanced in the past, among which the "wear-and-tear" hypothesis was the most widely held. This concept maintained that the microtrauma of daily wear and tear was the basic etiologic factor in the disorder; accordingly, it was postulated that the greater the mechanical stress of weight bearing, the greater would be propensity of a particular joint to become diseased. However, this concept neither clearly distinguished between the traumatic and the primary forms of the disease, nor accounted for the facts that osteoarthrosis is not increased in athletes,[2,241] that the disorder commonly involves non–weight bearing joints,[121,275] and that particularly severe forms of the disease occur in such locations as the interphalangeal joints regardless of the amount of use to which these joints have been subjected before the onset of the disease. Furthermore, the "wear-and-tear" concept disregarded the fact that early changes can involve the non–weight bearing rather than the weight-bearing areas of a joint.[42,197] The modern version of the wear-and-tear hypothesis introduces the concept of fatigue failure of the articular cartilage.[51] However, unlike metal, from which the analogy is derived, cartilage contains living cells, which support maintenance of the matrix and a turnover of proteoglycans and collagen (though turnover of collagen may be extremely slow).

Some of the problems of pathogenesis can be overcome by the concept of variability in tissue susceptibility, which may depend on variations in cellularity and in biochemical and biophysical properties of the matrix. In the presence of high tissue susceptibility, a comparatively low-grade extraneous influence suffices to produce a lesion, whereas more powerful stimuli are required to trigger disease if the tissue is comparatively resistant. The following factors have been shown to determine the susceptibility of the articular cartilage to becoming arthrotic:

1. *Genetic factors.* This is demonstrated by increased familial incidence of a special type of osteoarthrosis of the interphalangeal joints, Heberden's nodes,[299] and of polyarticular osteoarthrosis.[158,159]

2. *Hormonal factors.* This is indicated by the earlier onset and increased severity of osteoarthrosis associated with acromegaly and diabetes.[278,325]

3. *Nutritional factors.* This is shown by the frequent coexistence of osteoarthrosis and obesity. This coexistence is not fortuitous, nor is osteoarthrosis the consequence of the increased weight bearing associated with obesity[90,255] (as demonstrated by the finding that Heberden's nodes are as common in obese as in nonobese men). It appears more likely that both obesity and osteoarthrosis are related to a metabolic disorder involving lipid metabolism.

4. *Biologic age.* The articular changes occurring at a relatively early age are pacemakers for the disease. The rate at which they proceed is decisive for the subsequent pathologic events into which they gradually merge.[24,234]

In addition to these and possibly other systemic factors[1,4] there may be local factors, that is, blood and nerve supply. Local traumatization of a previously diseased joint, as by increased weight bearing, may cause further deterioration of a preexisting lesion. The concept of multiple etiologic factors acting on the joints to produce osteoarthrosis is diagrammed in Fig. 40-8.

Osteoarthrosis associated with acromegaly

In patients with acromegaly, joint lesions develop that are grossly indistinguishable from those of the usual type of osteoarthrosis.[11,277] Microscopically proliferation of chondrocytes may be more pronounced than that in senile osteoarthrosis, especially in the young acromegalic person[92,273]—a quantitative difference not sufficient to prove a specific nature of the arthropathy. The changes that distinguish the arthropathy of acromegaly from the age-linked disorder are associated with extra-articular skeletal manifestations of hyperipituitarism, particularly the resumption of osteogenesis at periosteal surfaces.

Kashin-Beck disesase

Kashin-Beck disease is a special form of severe osteoarthrosis endemic to areas of Siberia. It occurs in

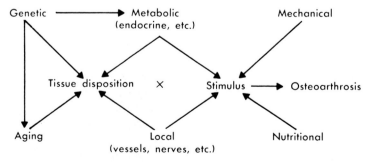

Fig. 40-8. Diagram illustrating the multifactorial etiology of osteoarthrosis. (From Silberberg, R., and Silberberg, M.: Pathol. Microbiol. **27**:447, 1964.)

young children and is associated with pronounced disturbances of skeletal growth. The joint lesions, typically those of osteoarthrosis, have been attributed to the presence of a fungus, *Fusarium sporotrichiella*, in grain used in the diet and to toxic effects of the fungus on cartilage.[217]

Suggestions of an etiologic role of selenium deficiency were not substantiated by results from chondrocyte cultures.[326] A disorder resembling Kashin-Beck disease has recently been found in the African Zululand near the Mozambique border spreading from a mission in Mseleni and therefore termed "Mseleni disease." Osteoarthrotic changes included those of distal radius and ulna, carpal and metacarpal joints, and the acetabulum. No cause has as yet been found.[85]

INFLAMMATORY JOINT DISEASES
Arthritis caused by infectious agents

Infectious arthritis is one of the possible complications of any infectious disease. Although the incidence of infectious joint lesions has decreased with the advent of antibiotic therapy, the disorders still are of considerable clinical importance.

The histogenetic mechanisms active in the development of infectious arthritides are the same as those prevading in other connective tissue spaces, modified by the special anatomic and physiologic conditions prevailing in joints. The infection may be attributable to direct contamination as in open wounds, to extension from the adjacent tissue, or to lymphatic spread, or it may be blood borne (Plate 8, *C*). The process begins acutely with hyperemia and swelling of the synovium, infiltration by polymorphonuclear and mononuclear leukocytes, and development of an effusion in the joint cavity. The exudate may be predominantly serous or fibrinous or purulent, depending on the severity of the infection, the resistance of the host, and the duration of the process. The synovium may be involved diffusely or focally. A predominantly serous effusion or comparatively small amounts of fibrin may disappear completely, the latter after fibrinolysis has occurred. With increasing amounts of fibrin and increasing duration of the infection, however, granulation tissue develops with formation of adhesions between the soft tissues of the joints and between opposing articular surfaces; synovium and subsynovial tissues become thickened and fibrotic. In pyogenic infections this is accompanied by abscess formation, which may involve the entire joint space or more or less isolated pockets. Even after successful surgical intervention, which usually is required to remove the exudate, the increase in fibrous tissue and the subsequent collagenization may result in permanent impairment of joint motion.

The characteristic feature of inflammatory arthritis is the involvement of the articular cartilage. The changes are degenerative rather than inflammatory, which is consistent with the fact that the cartilage contains no blood vessels. With the development of exudate in the joint cavity and granulation tissue in the synovium, the cartilage becomes frayed and eroded. In advanced cases it may disappear completely, and the underlying bones undergo osteosclerosis, or it may become thinned out and eroded by granulation tissue. This tissue may then invade the epiphyseal marrow cavity.

The injury to the cartilage is presumably brought about by lysosomal enzymes, such as cathepsins, collagenase, and hyaluronidase, which attack both the protein and the nonprotein moieties of the matrix. Since chondrocytes contain few lysosomes, one must surmise that the degradative enzymes are chiefly derived from leukocytes of the exudate and the synovium. Yet enzymes produced by chondrocytes may contribute to the destruction of the matrix.[1,172,327]

The pathogenic organisms most commonly found in bacterial arthritis of adults are *Staphylococcus aureus*, hemolytic streptococci.[59,161] *Neisseria gonorrhoeae*,[141,230] and *Haemophilus influenzae*. *Haemophilus influenzae* arthritis in infants and children and *Serratia* arthritis in adults are seen with increasing frequency.[82,217] Pneumococci,[315] *Pseudomonas, Proteus, Salmonella*,[84] *Enterobacter, Bacteroides, Escherichia*, and other intestinal organisms[3] as well as the tick-transmitted spirochete *Borrelia*[152] are among the rarer causes of bacterial arthritis (Plate 8, *C*).[160]

Joint involvement is monarticular more often than polyarticular. The large joints of the lower limbs, knee, and hip are usually affected. In the most instances, predisposing factors are demonstrable, such as oral or local corticosteroid administration, diabetes, or preexisting rheumatoid arthritis.[154]

Viral arthritis

Rubella, mumps, infectious mononucleosis, lymphogranuloma venereum, variola, and other generalized viral infections may be accompanied by episodes of acute arthritis,[73] yet reports of tissue changes are scanty. The findings in mumps-associated arthritis are probably characteristic of viral joint inflammations in general; synovial biopsy specimens show edema, lymphocytic infiltration, and hyperplasia of synoviocytes. A patchy fibrinous exudate completes the picture of a nonspecific synovitis.[335]

With the use of immunohistochemical methods evidence for the presence of virus in synovial tissue can be obtained in arthritis after smallpox or rubella vaccination.[280]

Tuberculous arthritis

Approximately 1% of subjects with tuberculosis have skeletal involvement; in 30%, hips or knees are involved, and in 20% various other joints.[67] Not uncommonly, the skeletal infection remains dormant and without clinical symptoms for many years. Almost invariably tuberculous arthritis results from hematogenous dissemination of the organisms. These may reach the synovial membrane directly or they may involve the joint secondarily, spreading from a focus of tuberculous osteomyelitis close to the articulation. Thus, in the knee of adults, the synovial membrane is frequently the primary site, whereas in children the secondary spread from a focus in the adjacent metaphyseal or epiphyseal bone is the more common occurrence. Regardless of the point of origin, the result of the infection is likely to be the same. the synovial membrane becomes hyperemic and edematous. A grayish yellow exudate is deposited on its surface, and occasionally tubercles can be recognized on gross inspection. In some cases the synovium is transformed into a necrotic mass mixed with a shaggy fibrinous exudate; the joint space contains grayish white "bodies the size and shape of melon seeds and varying amounts of turbid or clear exudate. Occasionally an excessive amount of fluid distends the joint (tuberculous hydrops). The changes in the articular cartilage depend to a considerable extent on the duration of the infection. In early stages the cartilage may merely lose its glistening appearance, a change sometimes accompanied by the extension of tuberculous granulation tissue from the synovium over the cartilaginous surfaces. In more severely affected joints, fragments of cartilage are loosened and detached from the underlying bone, leaving an uneven granular ulcerated base of necrotic bone and exudate.

Microscopically the loosened fragments consist of necrotic cartilage with faintly staining matrix and devoid of cells. The involved areas of bone show caseous necrosis surrounded by tuberculous granulation tissue. The necrotic trabeculas undergo gradual resorption (caries). The synovial membrane contains numerous solitary or conglomerate tubercles.

Healing may occur, with the result depending on the extent of the lesion. If the lesion was confined to the synovial membrane, functional impairment may be limited; advanced involvement of cartilage and bone may result in total destruction of the articulation, with either fibrous or bony union of the articulating bones (ankylosis).

Syphilitic arthritis

The frequency with which joints are involved in syphilis is declining. Arthritis may, however, occur in congenital as well as in acquired forms of the disease.

In congenital syphilis varying degrees of involvement of the joint capsules and epiphyses may accompany the characteristic changes of osteochondritis and periostitis.

Microscopically these joints show hyperemia, edema, lymphoid and plasma cell infiltration, and proliferation of fibroblasts. In addition, there may be small areas of necrosis in cartilage, bone, and capsular tissues.

In older children showing manifestations of congenital syphilis a peculiar form of arthritis, known as Clutton's joint,[58] may develop. One or both knees, and occasionally other joints, are swollen and lax and contain an excessive amount of fluid. The synovial membrane is thickened and appears gelatinous. Microscopically there is edema, diffuse infiltration with lymphocytes and plasma cells, and occasional gummas.[9]

Acquired syphilis

Pathologic investigations of joint tissues in secondary syphilis are notably lacking; however, inflammatory and vascular lesions resembling those found in skin and mucous membranes may produce an acute synovitis, sometimes associated with a transitory effusion. The knee joint is more often affected then other articulations, and the involvement is often bilateral.

In later stages of acquired syphilis the joints may be the site of gumma formation or of a diffuse chronic nonspecific synovitis with more or less pronounced effusion. Gummas may also be found in ligaments, cartilage, and adjacent bone. In addition, gummas may spread by direct extension from the bone marrow and bone to neighboring joints.

As a nonspecific sequela of tabes dorsalis, neuropathic joint disease may ensue.

Arthritis of brucellosis

Arthritis occurs as a complication of *Brucella bovis* or *B. suis* infection in about 10% of affected individuals. Hips, sacroiliac, and the small joints of hands and feet may be the site of acute suppurative synovitis or of chronic synovitis and bursitis.[294] Involvement of the spine is prominent. Subacute osteomyelitis of the vertebral bodies with destruction of cancellous bone and microabscesses is associated with destruction of the end plates, separating the vertebral body from the intervertebral disc, and with breakdown of the discs. There is a tendency to repair, with production of granulomas. Although blood-borne infection of the intervertebral discs has been considered a primary event in the evolution of the lesion, it appears more logical, in the absence of clear-cut evidence, to assume that the process starts as an osteomyelitis and involves the discs secondarily as seen in other chronic infections.[182]

Fungal arthritis

A variety of fungal organisms may lodge in the synovium and give rise to suppurative or granulomatous lesions. The synovium may be the primary site of joint involvement, or the infection may spread from the marrow cavity to the subchondral bone and from there into the articular tissues.[20]

Toxic arthritis

A most unusual form of chronic arthritis, characterized by lymphocyte, plasmocyte, and eosinophilic infiltration of the synovium, with subsequent fibrosis and irreversible immobilization of the affected joints, has been observed after ingestion of a toxic oil.[249]

Arthritis associated with rheumatic fever

The arthritis that occurs in most patients with acute rheumatic fever is characteristically an acute, transient, migratory disorder, involving most commonly the large articulations such as knees, ankles, and wrists. A nonspecific synovitis involves the joint cavity proper as well as bursae and tendon sheaths. The effusion present in the joint cavity is always sterile; initially the inflammatory cells are predominantly polymorphonuclear leukocytes, with varying numbers of eosinophils; at later stages mononuclear cells may predominate. If the occlusive vasculitis characteristic of rheumatic fever is present in synovium or periarticularly, the diagnosis of rheumatic arthritis can be made. The arthritis usually subsides after a few weeks without residual changes.[214]

Rheumatic arthritis is often accompanied by the appearance of subcutaneous nodules in the vicinity of joints. These nodules resemble in some ways the subcutaneous nodules of rheumatoid arthritis on the one hand and the Aschoff bodies of the myocardium on the other. The nodules usually measure several millimeters in diameter. Microscopically they have an acellular center of eosinophilic material, much of which can be identified as swollen or disintegrated collagen, with an admixture of mucopolysaccharides and, more rarely, necrotic tissue elements. This center is surrounded by a rim of lymphocytes, large and small monocytes, multinucleated giant cells, and occasionally eosinophils. Typical rheumatic vasculitis is usually found in the immediate vicinity of the nodules.[23] The nodules may be completely resorbed after a few weeks of existence. Some of the features that distinguish the rheumatic from the rheumatoid nodules seem related to the time factor involved in their pathogenesis: nodules of rheumatic fever come and go quickly and fail to show the extensive necrosis and the granulomatous character of the rheumatoid nodules, which develop and regress in a more chronic fashion.

The pathogenesis of the arthritis of rheumatic fever is unknown, though it has been shown experimentally that streptolysin, injected into the joint cavity, will produce arthritis, probably by disrupting lysosomes and thus liberating enzymes.[327] The possibility that strep-

tococcal debris might also call forth the synovial inflammation has not been ruled out.

Repeated attacks of rheumatic arthritis of the hands or feet may be followed by flexion deformities, particularly striking in metacarpophalangeal joints. The condition, described first by Jaccoud in 1869[147] and therefore termed "Jaccoud's arthritis," is associated with pronounced ulnar deviation of the digits. However, the deformities seem to be attributable to fibrosis of fasciae and tendons rather than to synovitis.[45]

Rheumatoid arthritis

Rheumatoid arthritis (RA) is a chronic progressive inflammatory arthritis of unknown origin involving multiple joints and characterized by a tendency to spontaneous remissions and subsequent relapses.

Arthritis is the most prominent manifestation of rheumatoid disease, a generalized connective tissue disorder that may involve para-articular structures such as bursae, tendon sheaths, and tendons as well as extra-articular tissues such as the subcutis,[290] cardiovascular system, lungs, spleen, lymph nodes, skeletal muscle, central and peripheral nervous system, and eyes.[145]

Rheumatoid disease is often accompanied by characteristic immunoglobulin, called rheumatoid factors (RFs), in affected persons' serum.[222] These factors are of considerable complexity; they are capable of acting as antiglobulins and of forming complexes with abnormal antigenic gamma globulins in vivo and in vitro. With appropriate techniques, such antigens or antibodies or their complexes can be demonstrated in serum, in synovial fluid, in leukocytes of blood and articular exudates, and in the synovial tissues (Fig. 40-9). Several tests have been developed to detect these immune bodies, using the agglutination of antibody on antigen coated particles, such as red blood corpuscles,[175] bacteria,[323] or bentonite particles.[38]

RF is present in 85% to 95% of subjects with rheumatoid arthritis, and a distinction is therefore made be-

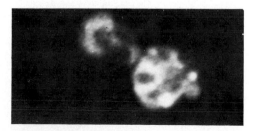

Fig. 40-9. Cell from synovial fluid of patient with rheumatoid arthritis. Cell was treated with serum containing antigammaglobulin. Brightly fluorescent globular inclusion indicates probable presence of rheumatoid factor (RF). (From Zucker-Franklin, D.: Arthritis Rheum. **9:**24, 1966.)

tween seropositive and seronegative forms of the disease. On the other hand, RF may be found in 2% to 7% of patients with connective tissue diseases other than rheumatoid arthritis. Yet the tests are considered useful for diagnostic and prognostic purposes, since there is a positive correlation between the level of the serum titers of RF and the severity of the clinical disease.

Distribution and prevalence

Young adults are frequently affected, but with increasing age an increase in prevalence has been reported.[318] Depending on the criteria used for diagnosis, women are 2½ to 5 times more often affected than men.[228,318] Familial aggregation seems safely established for the severe forms of seropositive disease,

whereas no such aggregation is seen in seronegative or low-grade seropositive forms.[68,177] Geographic distribution, considered significant at one time, has recently been shown to be random.[43,177] A slightly increased incidence is seen in men engaged in occupations requiring physical work as compared with those in professional or managerial positions.[318] The small joints of hands and feet are usually the first and most common to be involved, with lesions of the large joints appearing later in the course of the disease.

Pathologic anatomy

The basic tissue changes of rheumatoid disease are similar, regardless of site. In different locations they are modified in accordance with the properties peculiar to the tissue in which they take place. None of the histo-

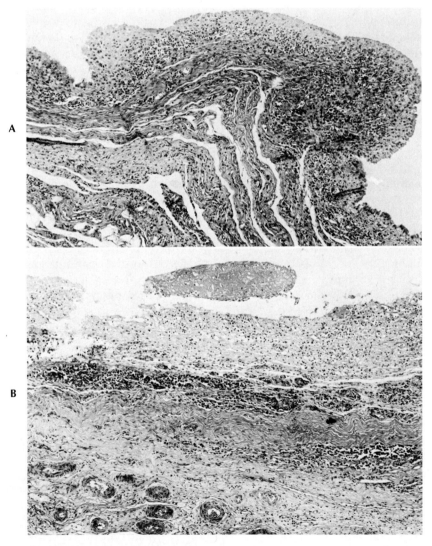

Fig. 40-10. Rheumatoid synovitis. **A,** There is infiltration of synovium by lymphocytes. **B,** Fibrinous exudate is superimposed on inflamed synovium. Superficial layer of synovium is necrotic, and subsynovial tissue is thickened and necrotic.

logic changes is by itself specific; but in combination they give a fairly typical and diagnostically suggestive picture. Similar uncertainties exist in regard to the clinical diagnosis of rheumatoid arthritis.[250]

Several features characterize the rheumatoid lesion:

1. Diffuse or focal infiltration of the tissue by lymphocytes or plasma cells, or both, with development of lymphoid centers
2. Vasculitis with endothelial proliferation, narrowing or occlusion of the lumens, fibrinoid change or necrosis of the walls, and perivascular aggregation of lymphocytes and plasma cells
3. The rheumatoid granuloma, a focal lesion with an amorphous center composed of necrotic tissue, fibrin, and immune complexes[338] surrounded by a band of oblong histiocytes (often in palisade-like radial orientation) and an outer zone of granulation tissue containing a variety of mononuclear leukocytes, capillaries, and fibroblasts; with time the granuloma may undergo resorption or increasing fibrosis and collagenization

In the joints the early changes involve the synovium, which becomes congested, edematous, and infiltrated by small and large lymphocytes, both B-cells and T-cells, plasma cells, plasmoblasts, mast cells,[64,170] and macrophages, indicating the presence of both humoral and cellular immune responses (Fig. 40-10).[167,337] There

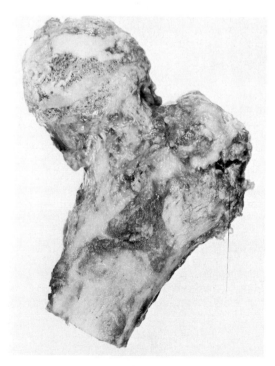

Fig. 40-11. Fresh specimen of proximal femur, showing rheumatoid arthritis with destruction of joint surface by pannus. (WU 49-5578.)

often are small areas of superficial necrosis of synovial lining cells with formation of superficial erosions covered by fibrinoid deposits; these deposits are composed of fibrin and small amounts of gamma globulin and complement components. An exudate containing polymorphonuclear leukocytes, many with ingested immune complexes, accumulates in the joint cavity. Not infrequently, 2 to 3 mm "rice" bodies, composed of fibrin, fibronectin, collagen, and immunoglobulin are present in the joint cavities of seropositive patients.[238] At later stages the synovitis is characterized by plasma cells, lymphoid centers, occasional multinucleated giant cells, and vasculitis. Granulation tissue composed of synovial fibroblasts and capillaries causes grossly recognizable villous thickening of the synovium, whose lining cells become hypertrophic and hyperplastic. In some of these lining cells as well as in lymphocytes and plasma cells of the synovium and in leukocytes of the synovial fluid, rheumatoid factor, gamma globulins, and antigen-antibody complexes can be demonstrated after incubation of smears or of tissue sections with the proper fluorescein-conjugated antigens.[36,41,140] The granulation tissue does not remain localized to the synovium but spreads over the surface of the articular cartilage and produces adhesions between the opposing joint surfaces (Figs. 40-11 to 40-13). This spread is apparently facilitated by the presence within the pannus of fibronectin, which is more abundant in rheumatoid pannus than in normal synovium or in disorders other than rheumatoid arthritis.[192,266] This pannus comes to be interposed between the cartilage and the lumen of the joint cavity and may interfere with the flow of synovial fluid into the cartilage. Thus malnutrition of the cartilage may contribute to its destruction, though most of the destruction is attributed to an extraordinarily complex interaction of degradative processes, including enzymatic collagenolysis, breakdown of proteoglycans, and demineralization and enzymatic degradation of bone.[126,168,331] As the pannus ages, vascularity decreases, and fibrosis and collagenization lead to shrinkage of the capsule, progressive narrowing of the joint space, and displacement or increasing approximation of the ends of the opposing bones. Closely apposing bones may become fused by bony bridges developing in the scar tissue, or they may be telescoped into each other, with complete elimination of the joint (Figs. 40-14 to 40-16). Disuse osteoporosis develops locally in the immobilized bones and becomes generalized in patients totally crippled by the disease and bedridden for long periods of time. The osteopenia may be compounded by prolonged corticosteroid therapy given to alleviate the arthritic symptoms.

The most common extra-articular lesion is the subcutaneous nodule,[25] a granuloma of a few millimeters to several centimeters in size, developing usually in areas

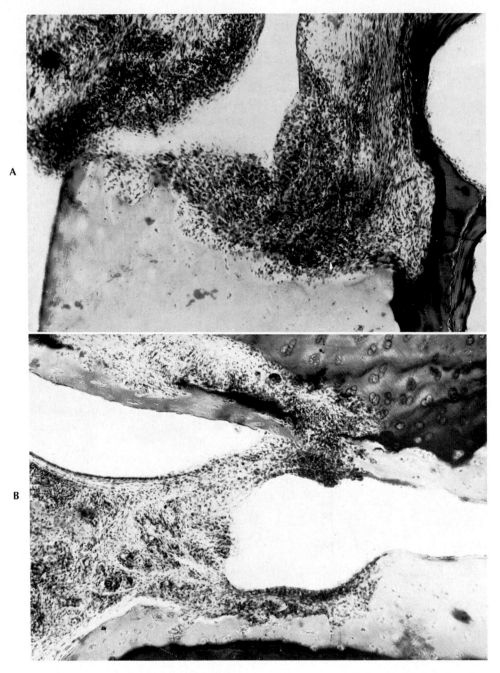

Fig. 40-12. Rheumatoid arthritis. **A,** Early stage of fibrous ankylosis. **B,** Granulation tissue projecting inward from margin of interphalangeal joint has formed adhesion across joint space. Nearly all articular cartilage has disappeared beneath pannus, which is clearly shown in lower half.

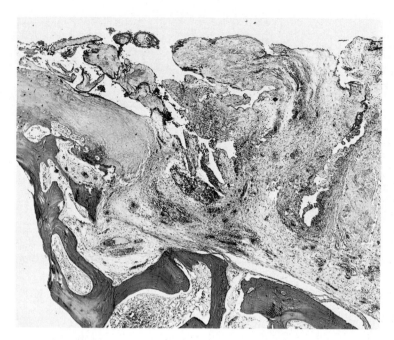

Fig. 40-13. Rheumatoid pannus. Exuberant granulation tissue replaces most of articular cartilage and forms hypertrophic villi projecting into joint space. Some preserved articular cartilage is seen at left.

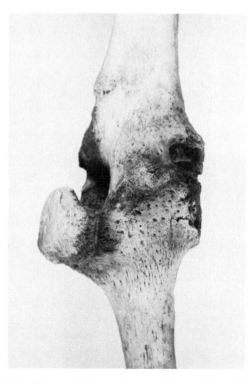

Fig. 40-14. Macerated specimen of knee joint. Advanced rheumatoid arthritis with bony fusion (ankylosis) of patella, femur, and tibia.

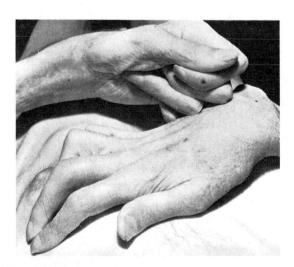

Fig. 40-15. Deformed and stiffened hands in chronic rheumatoid arthritis. Notice evidence of muscular atrophy and smooth glossy skin.

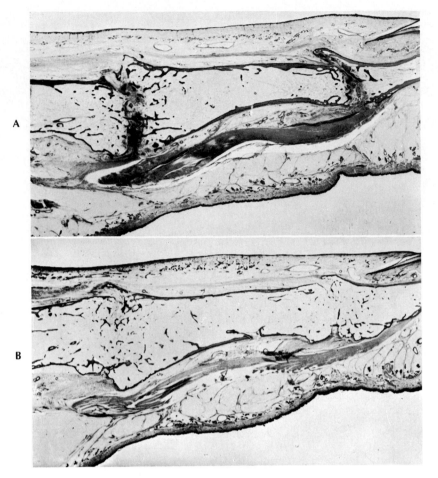

Fig. 40-16. Midline longitudinal sections of second and fourth digits. Atrophy of osseous and dermal tissues is evident in both **A** and **B**. Active chronic inflammation is shown in middle and terminal interphalangeal joints in **A**. All other joints have been destroyed, and bony ankylosis is evident.

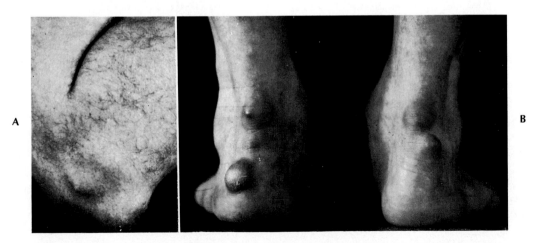

Fig. 40-17. Rheumatoid arthritis. **A,** Large subcutaneous nodule over olecranon process. **B,** Subcutaneous nodules of tendo achillis areas having typical morphologic features of nodule of rheumatoid arthritis. (Courtesy Dr. F.A. Chandler, Atlanta, Ga.)

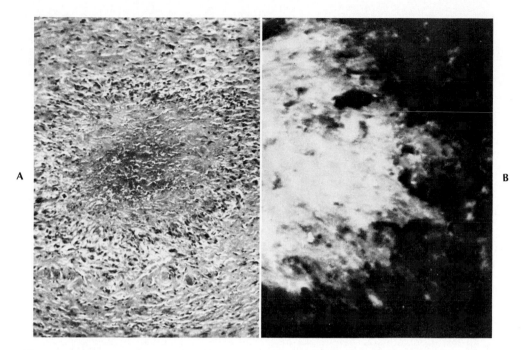

Fig. 40-18. Two consecutive microscopic sections of rheumatoid nodule. **A,** Hematoxylin and eosin stain shows center of fibrinoid necrosis and rim of macrophages with some palisading. **B,** Unstained section treated with fluorescein-conjugated antigammaglobulin. Large fluorescing area indicates presence of gamma globulin in nodule. (From Vázquez, J.J., and Dixon, F.J.: Lab. Invest. **6:**205, 1957.)

close to the joints and subject to minor mechanical insults (Figs. 40-17 to 40-19).

Nodules are more common in seropositive patients and in those with high serum titers of RF than in seronegative persons with low titers of RF. An arteritis is often found close to a nodule and may contribute to the gradual expansion of the necrotic center of the granuloma. Nodules may also be found in bursae and tendon sheaths. In contradistinction to the similar but smaller nodules of rheumatic fever, the rheumatoid nodules develop and regress slowly and are less rich in hydroxyproline than the former nodules are.

Vasculitis associated with deposition of immune complexes in vessel walls is seen especially in patients with high serum titers of IgM-RF complex; occlusion of the vessel may result in ischemia and microinfarcts, characteristically occurring along the nail beds. Occlusion of larger vessels can cause gangrene of the terminal phalanges of fingers and toes.

Cardiac lesions may involve the pericardium, myocardium, and endocardium, with focal accumulation of lymphocytes and plasma cells, vasculitis, granulomas, fibrosis, and amyloidosis.[145]

Pulmonary lesions may be focal and granulomatous or diffuse, interstitial, or intra-alveolar. The result is focal or diffuse fibrosis. In association with pneumoconiosis, especially of coal miners, rheumatoid pneumoconiosis develops (see Chapter 20).[53] Rheumatoid factor has been demonstrated in such lungs.[324] Both pleural effusions containing T-lymphocytes and fibrous adhesions are common.

Lymph nodes, especially those draining the areas of involved joints show hyperplasia and, less commonly, granulomas (Fig. 40-20).

Several types of scleritis and retinopathy have been described in about 1% of patients with rheumatoid disease.[145]

Arteritis and granulomas or inflammatory processes extending from diseased joints nearby may involve the central and peripheral nervous systems. Characteristic complications are degenerative myelopathy resulting from subluxation of the atlanto-occipital joint and the "entrapment" syndromes resulting from pressure on peripheral nerves.[145]

Sjögren's syndrome, a combination of typical, but relatively mild, nondestructive rheumatoid arthritis with keratoconjunctivitis sicca, iridocyclitis, and parotitis, develops in 10% to 15% of patients with rheumatoid arthritis.[271,282]

The association of rheumatoid arthritis with splenomegaly and leukopenia is known as "Felty's syndrome."[16,95,145]

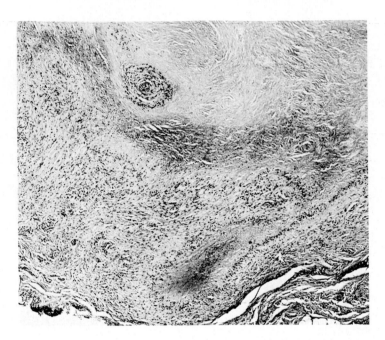

Fig. 40-19. Subcutaneous rheumatoid granuloma with occluded vessel at its periphery.

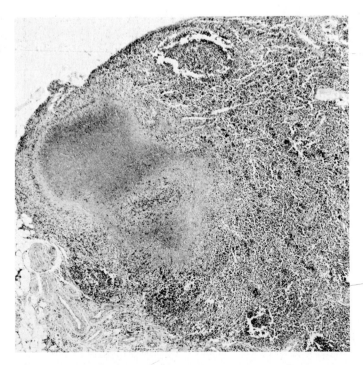

Fig. 40-20. Rheumatoid granuloma in lymph node.

Amyloidosis is a late complication of rheumatoid arthritis with data on the frequency varying from 25% to 60%.[47,310]

Etiology and pathogenesis

Of the factors once believed to play a role in the etiology or pathogenesis of rheumatoid arthritis, several (such as allergy, endocrine imbalance, climate, and "collagen disease") have not withstood tests by strict standards; others (especially infections,[26,124] postinfectious immunopathology,[177] autoimmunity,[189] and heredity[340] are still being actively investigated, as are the effects of psychophysiologic disorders that seem to be related to the onset of attacks.[100,200] No living organism has consistently been found in rheumatoid joints despite widespread search, which in years past was directed mainly toward streptococci[124] and more recently has centered on mycoplasma and diphtheroids,[149] and, on the basis of experimental results in animals, on bacterial cell wall debris.[235] The role of viruses remains controversial.[73,189]

The frequent presence of rubella virus (*Rubivirus*) or of antibodies to rubella and other viruses in the synovial fluid does not necessarily indicate a role of these agents in the initiation of arthritis.[116] Ongoing research into the role of the Epstein-Barr virus indicates less a part in the initiation than possibly in the perpetuation of the disease.[235,340] Yet infection—systemic or localized extra-articularly and often observed clinically some time before an attack[190]—may be responsible for initiating a

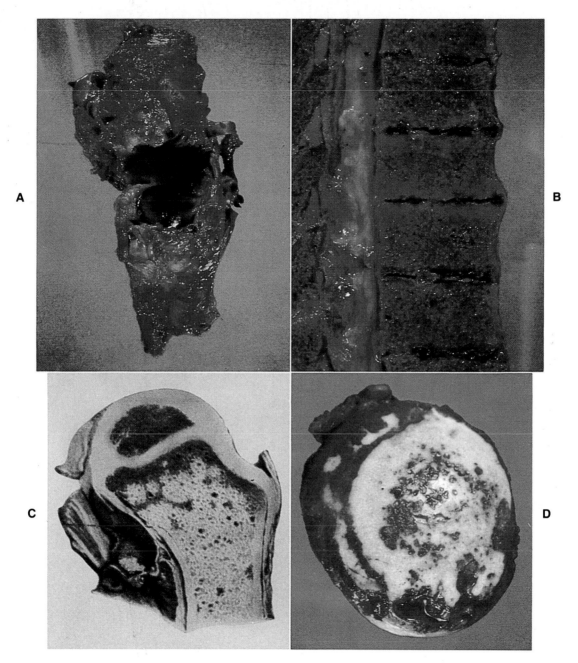

Plate 8

A, Ochronosis of knee joint. Intensely black stain of articular cartilage.

B, Ochronosis of intervertebral discs. Discs are stained deep black.

C, Purulent arthritis developing in course of staphylococcic osteomyelitis. Purulent exudate in both joint capsule and bone marrow. Notice communication between bone marrow and joint space.

D, Osteoarthrosis of femoral head. Pronounced ulceration of articular cartilage and some marginal lipping.

(**A** and **B,** Courtesy Dr. Steven L. Teitelbaum, St. Louis, Mo.; **C,** from Henke, F., and Lubarsch, O., editors: Handbuch der pathologischen Anatomie und Histologie, New York, 1934, Springer-Verlag, vol. 9, chap. 2; **D,** BH 75-1635.)

sequence of immune processes that, in turn, seem involved in the pathogenesis of articular and extra-articular lesions. The absence of an inciting organism from the joint thus need not preclude infection as cause of the disease.

On the basis of available data, two concepts of the nature of rheumatoid arthritis have emerged:

1. A noxious foreign agent may be the primary trigger in the sequence of immunologic, biochemical, and histologic events—some of them specific and others nonspecific—that combine to produce the lesions. It is surmised that the responding immune system is basically normal and that potential changes in the reacting components result secondarily from the action of the invading organism.

2. The alternative hypothesis suggests a primary defect of the immune system, which reacts abnormally to agents that are readily handled and eliminated by a normal immune system. The abnormality may reside in any or several of the effector cells or mediators involved in the immune response.

Regardless of the nature of the primary cause of rheumatoid arthritis, its pathogenesis comprises processes common to other types of acute or chronic inflammation together with those that are characteristic of, though not necessarily specific for, the disease.

The role of immune processes in the development of the rheumatoid lesions is indicated by some observations of patients with the disease:

1. The presence of gamma globulins (in particular, IgG and IgM) in synovial fluid[130,229] and leukocytes,[140] in synovial plasma cells,[319] lymphoid centers,[194] and lining cells,[165] and in subcutaneous nodules and vessel walls[340]; these gamma globulins are not a direct cause of rheumatoid disease, since the disease occurs in persons with agammaglobulinemia[114]

2. The presence of RF in synovial plasma cells and in synovial lining cells, which are capable of synthesizing RF[340]

3. The presence of antigen-antibody complexes (RF plus gamma globulin) in synovial plasma cells[36] and synoviocytes[165]

4. The presence in synovial leukocytes, interstitial connective tissue, and lining cells of complement components[41,340] associated with decreased complement titers in the synovial fluid[131]

5. The presence of IgG, IgA, IgM, and B_{1c} complement in the articular cartilage of patients with classic rheumatoid arthritis, in contradistinction to patients with first- or second-degree osteoarthrosis[61,150]

6. The common association of rheumatoid arthritis with amyloidosis[50,310]

A possible role of autoimmunity is suggested by the following:

1. Presence of antinuclear factor (ANF) in the serum of patients with advanced disease[117]

2. Increased titers of antibodies to type II collagen in the serum of patients with rheumatoid arthritis[304,316]

3. Antigenicity of proteoglycans of human articular cartilage[109]

A role of heredity in rheumatoid arthritis is not inconsistent with that of abnormal immune mechanisms. The propensity to formation of abnormal gamma globulins or to abnormal tissue reactivity to all kinds of challenges may well be under genetic control.[110] The first mentioned possibility is strongly supported by clinical observations: some rheumatoid factors show familial aggregation regardless of the presence or absence of joint disease.[178] The association of rheumatoid arthritis and related disorders with HLA-DW4 or other HLA antigens seems to provide a link between immune processes and genetics in relation to joint disease.[39]

Results of investigations into the role of heredity in rheumatoid arthritis differ with the methods of sampling.[224] When strict criteria have been used (such as inclusion into the surveys of only those patients with severe erosive involvement of multiple joints), familial aggregation has been demonstrated.[177] This aggregation is apparently not attributable to the common environment shared by members of the same family: in pairs of monozygotic twins, rheumatoid arthritis occurred 33 times more often than in pairs of dizygotic twins. The dizygotic twins showed no higher propensity for the disease than what would be expected from a sample of the general population.

On the basis of available histologic and immunologic data, a concept of the histogenesis of rheumatoid arthritis has evolved. An antigen, which could be extraneous (related to infection) or endogenous (related to abnormal gamma globulins), gains access to the joint cavity and elicits an immune reaction that is both humoral and cell mediated and in which polymorphonuclear leukocytes, T- and B-lymphocytes, and macrophages interact. (The histocompatibility between these cells, normally required for recognition and elimination of the antigen, and the potential lack of histocompatibility in disease stress the role of genetic factors in the pathogenesis of rheumatoid arthritis.) Complexes of various immunoglobulins, RF, and complement—some quite large and insoluble—are formed and phagocytosed by cells termed "RA cells," or "rhagocytes"[287,339]; thus the inflammatory process is set in motion, terminating in the formation of granulation tissue and scarring.[143] Lysosomal enzymes from the cells of the exudate and from the pannus participate in the destruction of cartilaginous matrix by degrading both proteoglycans and collagen; they thus play a major role in the deterioration of the joint.

No plausible concept has yet been developed to explain the chronicity of the disease. There is no spontaneous animal analog of the disorder, and numerous attempts to create an animal model with consistent chronicity without the need for repeated challenge have failed[103] (which has reinforced the hypothesis that autoimmunity may be involved in this as well as in other aspects of rheumatoid arthritis).

SERONEGATIVE SPONDYLOARTHROPATHIES

Several arthritides, formerly considered to be variants of rheumatoid arthritis, have more recently been grouped as seronegative spondyloarthropathies. They differ from rheumatoid arthritis in various, expecially immunologic, respects.[35,332] Patients with these types of joint diseases are, as the term implies, seronegative for rheumatoid factor; however, 90% or more of the patients possess HLA-B27 antigens, which show familial aggregation and, when present, multiply many times the risk of developing the disease. Spinal involvement is universally present, and there is male predominance. The group comprises the enteropathic arthropathies, Reiter's disease, Behçet's disease, psoriatic arthritis, Still's disease, ankylosing spondylitis, and possibly others.

Enteropathic arthritis

Included with enteropathic arthritis are the arthritides that are commonly associated with *Yersinia* infection,[3] ulcerative colitis, regional ileitis (Crohn's disease), and intestinal lipodystrophy (Whipple's disease).[35,71] First as well as recurring episodes follow bowel involvement. After surgical removal of the diseased segment of the intestine, arthritis does not recur. The lesions are usually monarticular; the knees are most commonly involved, with the ankle next in order of frequency.

Whipple's disease is no longer considered to be a metabolic disorder; rather, it is now believed to be attributable to an infectious agent. The associated arthritis is a transient, migratory, nonspecific synovitis that subsides without residual changes.[55,160] The rodlike particles seen in large numbers in the intestinal laminae propriae have not been demonstrated in articular tissues.

Reiter's syndrome

Reiter's syndrome was originally described as a combination of conjunctivitis, urethritis, and arthritis. More recently keratoderma, oral ulcerations, and cardiovascular abnormalities have been added to the list of characteristic lesions. The arthritis is polyarticular and asymmetric, involving the knee and ankles and often starting at the heel. The usual subacute stage is char-

acterized by a fibrinopurulent exudate. The synovium is hyperemic and infiltrated by polymorphonuclear leukocytes, lymphocytes, and a few plasma cells. Some extravasation of red blood corpuscles may occur and lead to deposition of small amounts of hemosiderin. Commonly there is no major residual change; a few lymphocytic foci in the synovium may be the only evidence of the earlier involvement.

More rarely the subacute process progresses with development of synovial hypertrophy and proliferation of synovial lining cells and fibroblasts. This pannus spreads over the cartilage and erodes it as well as the subchondral bone. Ultimately the appearance of the joints may be similar to that in rheumatoid arthritis.[169] However, a para-articular ossifying periostitis distinguishes these lesions of Reiter's syndrome from rheumatoid arthritis.

The spondylitis of Reiter's syndrome resembles roentgenographically that of psoriasis in the random distribution of osteophytic outgrowths.[196]

The cause of Reiter's syndrome is unknown; a genetic background has been demonstrated, but its role in the pathogenesis of the disease has not been clarified.

Behçet's syndrome

Behçet's syndrome, a multisystem disorder causing ulcerations of skin, eyes, and mucous membranes, involves large and small joints with a nonspecific, self-limited synovitis in about 90% of patients.[225,320] The changes resemble those of rheumatoid arthritis but are milder and lead only rarely to shallow erosions of the articular cartilage.

Arthritis associated with psoriasis

The association of arthritis and psoriasis is more than coincidental but nevertheless occurs in only 5% to 7% of patients suffering from psoriasis. The lesions involve mainly the distal interphalangeal joints in an asymmetric fashion. Histologically the chronic fibrosing synovitis and subsequent destruction of the joint resemble those of rheumatoid arthritis. In advanced stages osteolysis of the tips (acra) of the phalanges occurs.[19,207] A characteristic finding is terminal convolutions of the nail capillaries in the vicinity of the affected joints, suggestive of a role of decreased vascular supply in the necrotizing process involving the epiphyses of the phalanges. A triggering role has been attributed to mechanical injury. Spondylitis also occurs as a complication of psoriasis; the lesions resemble those of Reiter's syndrome.

Still's disease

Rheumatoid arthritis occurring before 16 years of age has been termed "juvenile rheumatoid arthritis" (JRA) or "Still's disease."[46,300] Morphologically the lesions are identical to those of the adult disorder, but clinically the disease differs from that in adults. Three clinical forms are distinguished depending on systemic involvement with fever, lymphadenopathy, skin rash, pleurisy, pericarditis, or iridocyclitis. Joint involvement may be polyarticular; lesions are found predominantly in the joints of the hands, or a few of the large joints (knees, ankles, and elbows) may be affected. This variability in the distribution of lesions, in their clinical course, and in the results of immunologic tests for rheumatoid and antinuclear factors has suggested to some investigators that JRA is not a single disease entity but a group of heterogeneous disorders.[256] Pairs of monozygotic twins show a high level of concordance for the disorder, whereas dizygotic twins do not.[8,99,209]

Ankylosing spondylitis

Ankylosing spondylitis is discussed in a later section with diseases of the spine (p. 2097).

Arthritis associated with viral hepatitis

Viral hepatitic arthritis occurs in the presence of high serum titers of hepatitis-associated antigen (HAA) and decreased serum levels of the C4 component of complement.[7,226] Although no immune complexes have yet been demonstrated in the articular tissues, it is believed that complexes of HAA, homologous antibody, and early components of complement are causes of the joint lesions.

Arthritis associated with familial Mediterranean fever

A genetic background has been demonstrated for arthritis of familial Mediterranean fever, which occurs mainly in populations of Mediterranean origin. Sephardic Jews, Arabs, and Armenians. The acute, subacute, or chronic synovitis may be accompanied by an effusion that is sterile on culture. After repeated attacks, changes of early osteoarthrosis may develop. One joint at a time is usually involved, but in the course of years, multiple joints may be affected.[257]

Arthritis associated with sarcoidosis

Acute or chronic nonspecific, often symmetric, synovitis can develop in the course of a sarcoid-associated arthritis.[293] Formation of granulomas in the synovium may be followed by erosion of the cartilage, advanced joint destruction, and osteophytic outgrowth at the joint margins. Ankle and knee joints are most commonly affected, but as a rule, joint involvement is less conspicuous than that of adjacent or distant bones.

Arthritis associated with connective tissue diseases

Acute transitory arthritides may be more or less prominent in serum sickness but are particularly common in association with lupus erythematosus, erythema nodosum, and various forms of vasculitis.[17,117] Familial aggregation and increased concordance in monozygotic twins are suggestive of some genetic influences in the propensity of lupus patients to develop arthritis.[34]

Usually no permanent lesions ensue. An exception is the changes seen in progressive systemic sclerosis. In this disorder progressive resorption of the tufts of the terminal phalanges eventually involves the distal interphalangeal joints; because of occlusive disease of the afferent vessels, the subchondral bone and the overlying cartilage undergo avascular necrosis accompanied by fibrinous synovitis and progressive synovial fibrosis.[247,329]

CRYSTAL-DEPOSITION DISEASES

The knowledge of articular or periarticular crystal deposition and of the nature of the crystals deposited has increased rapidly during the past decades. Besides monosodium urate, the oldest known crystal to cause arthritis, calcium pyrophosphate, apatite, calcium phosphate, and calcium oxalate as well as lipid crystals have been demonstrated in joint fluid and tissues.[78,139,243] Crystals act as pathogens on account of their physical structure and not of their chemical composition. The mechanism of initial precipitation is unknown, but it may require some tissue factor as predisposing condition, such as degradation of the cartilage matrix. Once precipitated, the crystals are taken up by phagocytic cells, a process that starts the inflammatory sequence, which in turn causes additional tissue damage.[206]

Gout (crystal-deposition disease, type I)

Gout is a disorder of purine metabolism directly related to serum levels of uric acid and characterized by deposition of monosodium urate monohydrate crystals in various connective tissues. A distinction is usually made between primary or idiopathic gout, developing on the basis of a primary abnormality of purine metabolism, and secondary gout, associated with diseases conducive to "secondary" hyperuricemia. There is no known difference in the tissue changes seen in the two forms of gout.

Historical background

Gout belongs to that group of diseases known and discussed through the ages.[115,127,248] From Hippocrates to Galen and physicians of the Renaissance, the disease was considered to be caused by bad humors, poisoning the body in association with excessive eating, drinking, and generally lecherous living. Paracelsus was the first to attribute the disease to the deposition of an abnormal substance, tartar, derived from food and subsequently altered to form stony material, especially when mixed with "synovia," an egg white–like substance contained in the joints. Sydenham still held onto the concept of ill humors but elaborated specifically on the connection between gout and stone formation and gave a classic description of the disease.

Modern thinking about gout seems to have originated in 1769 with the discovery by Scheele that kidney stones found in patients with gout were made up of an acid, which was also present in the urine. The identification of urates in tophi by Wollaston in 1797[330] and the discovery of hyperuricemia in patients suffering from gout by Garrod in 1848[105] created new directives for all subsequent work dealing with this disorder. Gout is distinctly familial in distribution, with both heredity and environmental factors having been shown to be involved in the pathogenesis.[37,227,267,272]

Distribution and prevalence

The disease usually begins in the third decade. Men are affected more often and at an earlier age than women. The higher the serum level of uric acid, the greater is the likelihood that the disease will develop. Yet the number of persons with hyperuricemia who actually develop gouty arthritis is small, probably not exceeding 2% or 3%[176,179]; one reason for this may be the need for comparatively large amounts of energy for nucleation, which are not available at physiologic temperature, pH, or ionic strength.[308] The mere presence of hyperuricemia at one time or another is a predisposing factor for local manifestations of gout to appear, regardless of the cause of hyperuricemia.

The joint most commonly involved is the metatarsophalangeal joint of the great toe, but knees and ankles, elbows and fingers, and spinal and sternoclavicular joints are commonly affected. Arthritis does not develop in all patients suffering from gout: lesions may be confined to periarticular tissues and extraskeletal sites, such as the outer ear, eyelids, scleras, kidneys, heart valves, blood vessels, and cartilages of the respiratory system.

Pathologic anatomy

The acute lesion is triggered by precipitation of needle-shaped crystals of monosodium urate from serum or synovial fluid. In the joints the crystals produce an acute synovitis accompanied by an effusion with numerous polymorphonuclear leukocytes. These leukocytes may take up as much as 95% of the urates into their cytoplasm or into phagosomes. There is hyperplasia of synoviocytes, some of which are being sloughed off into the effusion. Urate crystals are found in synoviocytes and interstitially in the synovial membrane, where they tend to form clusters.[336] By electron microscopy, crystals measure 10×0.5 nm and consist of dense globular bodies suspended in an electron-lucent matrix.[239,245]

With recurring attacks the lesions become chronic. The deposits enlarge, and urate crystals disposed radially around an amorphous proteinaceous matrix become the center of a foreign-body granuloma with a rim of fibroblasts and multinucleated giant cells (Fig. 40-21). Immunoglobulins IgM, IgG, and IgA have been demonstrated in the granulomas by immunofluorescent techniques.[129] The granuloma is spoken of as tophus (Latin *tophus* or *tofus*, 'porous stone'). Tophi vary in diameter from a few millimeters to several centimeters.

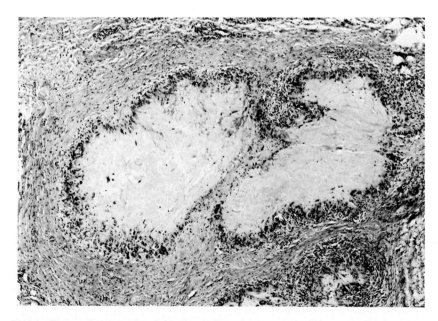

Fig. 40-21. Photomicrograph of portion of gouty tophus in periarticular tissue. Two of several aggregates of which tophus is composed. Urate crystals originally present have been dissolved in processing of tissue, and only proteinaceous matrix is preserved in centers. Latter are surrounded by corona of granulation tissue with numerous multinucleated giant cells. (BH 69-1754.)

If located subcutaneously, they occur as prominent nodules; if on the hands and feet, they may cause conspicuous disfiguration. More or less diffuse fibrosis may develop around tophi as the lesions age. Synovial granulomas may erode the articular cartilage, but crystals are also directly precipitated in the cartilage. Since articular cartilage is avascular, there is no inflammatory reaction to such deposits; urates at first occupy the superficial layers of the cartilage, which undergo necrosis and assume an opaque, whitish, chalky appearance. Incrustation of the deeper layers of the cartilage is seen in association with advanced regression, resembling the changes of early osteoarthrosis (Fig. 40-22).

Pathogenesis

Hyperuricemia may be primary or secondary; one form of primary hyperuricemia is the result of a deficiency of the enzyme hypoxanthine-guanine phosphoribosyltransferase (HGPRT), a defect that inhibits reconversion of hypoxanthine to inosinic acid, one step in purine resynthesis. Consequently, hypoxanthine is further degraded to produce excessive quantities of uric acid.[22,119,134,155,334] In addition, overactivity of the enzyme 5-phosphoribosyl-1-pyrophosphate synthetase contributes to hyperuricemia.[136]

Secondary hyperuricemia is seen when excessive amounts of nuclear material are being degraded as in leukemia or polycythemia, or when renal excretion is impaired as in lead poisoning or renal calcification. Characteristically, in secondary hyperuricemia the pathways of purine degradation are normal.[118]

The mechanism that causes deposition of urates in tissues is complex and is discussed in Chapter 1. Rapid fluctuations in uric acid serum levels as after excessive alcohol consumption, fasting, or the administration of uricosuric drugs[187] are likely to trigger an acute attack in persons predisposed to gout.

Tissues with low oxygen tension are particularly prone to becoming the site of urate precipitation. Moreover, the peak incidence of gouty arthritis coincides with the age at which age-linked loss of mucopolysaccharide from the cartilaginous matrix is maximal.

The irritating effect of urate crystals has long been known to be linked to their physical configuration and not to their chemical composition: a minor inflammatory response is observed after introduction of dissolved sodium urate into tissues, in contradistinction to the intense reaction to crystalline monosodium urate. The crystals induce inflammation by virtue of absorption at their surfaces of numerous proteins, immunoglobulins, fibronectin, fibrinogen and others and mediators of inflammation. These substances interact with receptors on synovial cells, fibroblasts, neutrophils, and thrombocytes, thus initiating the inflammatory process.[193] Agents differing from sodium urate chemically but similar in crystallinity evoke an inflammatory reaction resembling that produced by crystalline sodium urate.[93]

A decrease in pH, as occurs in acute inflammation, promotes crystal deposition[270]; thus a vicious circle that is responsible for self-perpetuation of the lesion may be

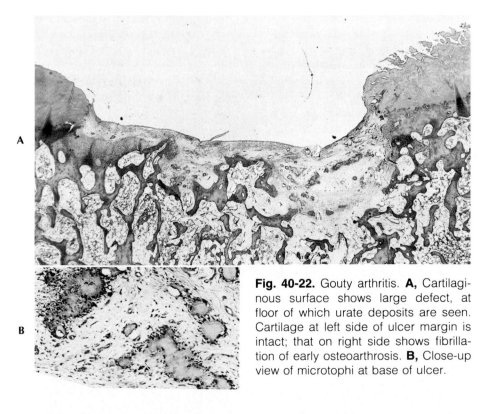

Fig. 40-22. Gouty arthritis. **A,** Cartilaginous surface shows large defect, at floor of which urate deposits are seen. Cartilage at left side of ulcer margin is intact; that on right side shows fibrillation of early osteoarthrosis. **B,** Close-up view of microtophi at base of ulcer.

initiated. The importance of the Hageman factor in the inflammatory sequence of gout has been questioned, since crystals may provoke acute inflammation in the absence of the factor.[292] Similarly, the role played by kinins in the process has been doubted. Complement, however, is still considered to be involved.[155] The mechanism of action of polymorphonuclear leukocytes, by contrast, remains unexplained: in experimentally produced aleukocytosis no attack develops.[269] The role of prostaglandins is being investigated; some experimental evidence indicates that several of the prostaglandins may promote urate crystal–induced inflammation.[72]

Pyrophosphate arthropathy

Among the other names for pyrophosphate arthropathy are pseudogout, articular calcinosis, and crystal-deposition disease type II. This abnormality was recognized after demonstration of calcium pyrophosphate in the synovial fluid of certain inflamed joints, characterized by the presence of calcium pyrophosphate dihydrate crystals in articular cartilage, synovium, articular ligaments, and intervertebral discs. The crystals can be demonstrated by polarized light, electron microscopy, electron probe analysis, and x-ray diffraction.[29,31,174] The disorder differs from true gout not only in the chemical nature of the crystals but also in distribution; in pseudogout the large joints such as knees, hips, and shoulders are preferentially involved rather than the small joints of hands and feet. By electron microscopy, calcium pyrophosphate crystals appear as 0.4 μm rods with a bubbly end and are sometimes arranged in clusters. By electron probe analysis they have a phosphorus-to-calcium ratio of 1.5:1, which is compatible with calcium pyrophosphate.[5] Pyrophosphate arthropathy occurs by itself or in systemic disorders such as hyperparathyroidism, true gout, diabetes, and acromegaly[66] as well as rheumatoid arthritis and osteoarthrosis.[77] The joints show an acute synovitis, often with a large effusion—changes that may subside without residual damage. With repeated recurrences, or insidiously without an acute phase, changes typical of osteoarthrosis develop, and deposits of calcium pyrophosphate are found in the articular cartilage. These deposits are composed of crystals or microspheroliths,[129] are confined to the midzone of the cartilage, and have no apparent relationship to chondrocytes.

Familial aggregation of persons with the disorder points to a genetic background,[322] possibly related to changes in the cartilage matrix.[80]

Apatite arthropathy

Apatite crystals may be deposited in aging articular cartilage in the absence of joint lesions but are more commonly associated with arthropathies from various causes.[265]

Needle-shaped crystals 7.5 × 25 nm have been identified as apatite in the sediment of joint effusions and in synovial cells of patients with acute arthritis. Injection of crystalline apatite into dog knees has produced similar lesions.[265] Besides apatite, other calcium salts are presumed to give rise to crystal-induced arthropathies.[76,258]

Relapsing polychondritis (chronic atrophic polychondritis)

Relapsing polychondritis, which occurs in both men and women, is characterized by degeneration and inflammation of any of the cartilages of the body.[81] The disintegration leads to gross deformities, such as floppy ears, saddle nose, and collapse of the trachea. Involvement of intervertebral discs may lead to spondylitis and, at late stages, to deformities of the spine. In the joints a picture resembling rheumatoid arthritis is seen. The synovium is infiltrated by lymphocytes and plasma cells, and there is an increase in both A- and B- cells. The cartilage matrix loses some of the acid mucopolysaccharides, resulting in decreased staining with Alcian blue and other cationic dyes. The cartilage is infiltrated by lymphocytes, and many chondrocytes disappear from their capsules. Electron microscopy shows that chondrocytes have peculiar bulbous bodies attached to or within the elongated cytoplasmic processes; the cells contain an unusual number of lysosomes and dense bodies, both signs of degeneration. In the cell vicinity, there appear aggregates of granular material from which long spacing bodies are formed.[205] The nature of this material is unknown, but it seems related to degenerative processes in both cells and matrix. The cause of the disorder is likewise unknown; repeated suggestions of a role played by autoimmune processes are controversial.[88,135,199]

Diseases of bursae, tendons, and fasciae
Bursitis

Since bursae are synovial membrane–lined sacs, their reaction to injury may be expected to resemble that of the synovial lining of joints (Fig. 40-23). The common lesions are those occurring after mechanical insults or infection.

Traumatic bursitis may result from a single injury, such as a blow to the elbow (olecranon bursa) or the knee (prepatellar bursa). More commonly, however, it is the repeated injuries from excessive pressure or bruises that initiate the inflammatory changes. This is exemplified by "housemaid's knee," in which the prepatellar bursa becomes enlarged and painful as the result of crawling on floors and closing drawers and doors with the knee.

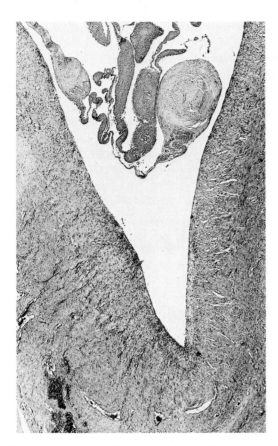

Fig. 40-23. Portion of wall of chronically inflamed bursa. Synovial lining has been replaced by layer of vascular fibrous tissue infiltrated by lymphocytes. Inspissated old exudate is present in bursal lumen.

Purulent inflammation of bursal cavities may be caused by pathogenic microorganisms. This may follow penetrating injuries, be an extension of infection from an adjacent cellulitis or abscess, or result from embolization of blood-borne organisms.

Tendinitis and tenovaginitis

Inflammation of tendons and tendon sheaths may occur after chronic mechanical insults or direct or blood-borne infection. The lesions can assume any form of acute or chronic inflammation with or without effusion, with or without suppuration, with or without calcification,[94] or with development of diffuse granulation tissue or granulomas. A special type of involvement is known as "stenosing tenovaginitis." This lesion develops preferably in places where tendons pass over bony prominences, especially at the wrist. The tendon sheath is narrowed because of the anulus fibrosus of the wall, which inhibits the free motion of the tendon. The tendon distal to the stenosis becomes thickened and at times locked in a certain position, from which it must be unlocked before normal motion is restored.

Dupuytren's contracture

Contracture of the digits of the hand, first observed by Plater in 1614, was recognized as caused by changes in the palmar aponeurosis by Dupuytren[83] and more recently reported as also occurring in the plantar aponeurosis. The lesion results in permanent flexion contracture, with the fifth, fourth, and third digits being usually involved in this order of frequency. Men are more commonly affected than women, and in about half the patients the lesion is bilateral.

Grossly the involvement may be diffuse or nodular. Microscopically three developmental phases have been described[183]: (1) proliferation of fibroblasts, (2) decreasing cellularity and increasing collagenization, and (3) a residual stage, characterized by regression of the nodules, atrophy of the fibrous cords, and almost complete acellularity. The lesions extend into the adjacent subcutaneous fat tissue and into the corium, causing attachment of the aponeurosis to the skin.

The amounts of hexosamine, galactosamine, and type III collagen are increased, not only in the lesions proper, but also in histologically normal fasciae.[40] However the chemical composition of collagen and glycoproteins of the ground substance has been found to be normal.[144] Electron microscopic investigations have disclosed a cytoplasmic fibrillar system and other evidence of contractility in the cells of the lesion.[102] The involved cells thus appear to be myofibroblasts, which have the ability to contract. This property is believed to play a role in the clinical contractures.

The cause of the lesion is unknown. A more than coincidental association with diabetes has been observed,[74,221] and heredity may be involved in some cases.[181]

ARTICULAR CHANGES ASSOCIATED WITH DIABETES MELLITUS

Limited joint mobility attributable to flexor muscle contractures is seen in a high percentage of juvenile and adult-onset diabetics. The lesions correlate with either age or duration of diabetes and often coincide with microvascular disease. An equal incidence of impaired joint mobility in diabetic children and in their nondiabetic sibs points to a genetic background of the condition.

The hands are most commonly affected. The skin over the contracted joints appears tight, thickened, and waxy; microscopically the dermis is thickened and the lower part of the dermis is fibrotic and devoid of sweat glands and hair follicles.[44,62,98,252] The biochemical basis of the disorder has so far been incompletely explored, however, a sharp increase in the glycosylation of collagen has been reported.[252]

CYSTS OF JOINTS AND PARA-ARTICULAR TISSUES
Cysts of ganglion

The lesions are round or ovoid, movable, subcutaneous nodules that may be cystic or semicystic. They occur most commonly on the wrist but also on the dorsal surface of the foot, close to the ankle, or about the knee. They may or may not have a pedicle attachment to or communicate with a tendon sheath or a joint cavity. The cysts are filled with a clear mucinous fluid that by electron microscopy contains flakes or delicate filaments and disintegrated collagen. In some instances the cysts have a more or less continuous lining of cells resembling synovial cells. In others the lining is discontinuous or lacking altogether; the cyst wall then consists of dense connective tissue lined by necrotic cells, cell debris, and disintegrated collagen.[107] Other ganglia contain fragments of tissue resembling synovium incorporated in a loose edematous connective tissue mass.

The histogenesis of the lesion is disputed. Herniation of the synovium into the surrounding tissue, displacement of synovial tissue during embryogenesis, and posttraumatic degeneration of connective tissue have all been incriminated as causes.[291] More recently demonstrated aggregates of cytoplasmic filaments in lining cells have indicated a possible relationship to smooth muscle fibrils. It was therefore suggested that the lesions arise from proliferating pluripotential mesenchymal cells.

Cysts of semilunar cartilage

Cysts of the semilunar cartilages are usually located in the lateral meniscus near its anterior insertion. They contain a number of indistinct locules filled with mucinous or gelatinous fluid. Microscopic sections may reveal bits of synovial lining and diffuse fraying of the fibrocartilage of the meniscus. The fraying probably results from seepage of mucin-containing fluid into the interstices of the dense and relatively acellular tissue of the semilunar cartilage. These lesions have much in common with ganglia of tendon sheath origin and are probably formed in a similar manner.

Bursal cysts connected with the knee joint cavity are not uncommon, particularly in patients with rheumatoid arthritis. In some cases the cysts communicate with the articular space by a long and tortuous duct. The opening may become obliterated by cicatrization. These cysts are usually referred to as "Baker's cysts," though Baker originally described cystic lesions in association with a variety of pathologic conditions of dissimilar etiology.[13,166,328]

Bursal cysts have a dense fibrous wall of variable thickness. The enclosed cavity often is divided partially or completely into two or more chambers by fibrous septa that project inward from the cyst wall. The lumen contains fluid that may be either clear or turbid and either watery or mucinous. At times the fluid is stained with blood pigment. Some cavities contain "melon seed" bodies originating from detached small excrescences or tips of villi projecting into the cavity.

Microscopically synovial membrane may be present, but more frequently the cyst is lined with dense fibrous connective tissue that contains focal and diffuse infiltrates of lymphocytes and hemosiderin-laden phagocytes.

TUMORS AND TUMORLIKE LESIONS OF JOINTS, BURSAE, TENDONS, AND TENDON SHEATHS

Any of the tissue components of the articulations, including bursae, tendons, and tendon sheaths, may give rise to benign or malignant neoplasms. Among the benign tumors are chondromas, osteochondromas, myxomas, angiomas, fibromas, and lipomas. These neoplasms and the malignant tumors derived from corresponding cell types are no different from tumors of the same histologic composition elsewhere in the body. Neoplasms whose origin and behavior are determined by the presence of specialized synovial lining cells, and which are thus peculiar to structures normally lined by such cells, may be benign or malignant.

Xanthofibroma

Included as synonyms for xanthofibroma are villonodular synovitis, giant cell tumor of tendon sheath, and benign synovioma. The lesion has been considered as benign tumorous by some investigators[296] and as granulomatous by others.[148,191] Doubt has been cast on the neoplastic character of the lesions, especially because similar changes may involve the synovium of joints, bursae, and tendon sheaths multifocally or diffusely.

Xanthogranulomas occur most commonly in young adults and are localized on fingers, wrists, ankles, feet, and knees. They grow slowly, with compression and displacement of the adjacent tissues. Where the tendons and other tissues are firmly anchored in bone, the tumors may cause surface erosions or deep rounded depressions in the bone from pressure atrophy.

The gross appearance of these lesions varies within wide limits. They measure from a few millimeters to several centimeters in greatest diameter. They have a dense fibrous covering formed by the compressed surrounding tissues. They are firm and only slightly elastic. Cut surfaces show a gray, dense, inelastic tissue and in many instances yellowish flecks or streaks, proportional to the amount of lipid contained within histiocytes. Because of the yellow color, these lesions have

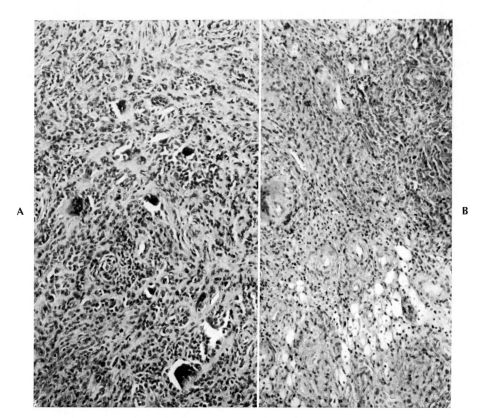

Fig. 40-24. Xanthofibromas of tendon sheath. **A,** Tumor composed of spindle-shaped fibroblasts and giant cells. **B,** Tumor containing many lipid-laden cells. (130×; **A,** AFIP 90662; **B,** AFIP 82251.)

been named "xanthomas" or "xanthofibromas."

Microscopically the lesions are characteristically composed of small oval or spindle-shaped cells, multinucleated giant cells, lipid-laden macrophages, and irregularly placed bundles of connective tissue. The ratio of these elements is exceedingly variable within the same and in different tumors. Some neoplasms are highly cellular and show active cell proliferation. Others are dense and fibrous with few cellular elements. Giant cells may be numerous or few. They contain many small oval nuclei that are usually crowded together in one portion of the cell. The cytoplasm may be scant or abundant, and the shape of the cells is equally variable. The number of lipid-laden phagocytes ("foam cells") is also variable; some tumors are composed chiefly of foam cells, whereas others contain only small aggregates or scattered single such cell (Fig. 40-24).

Some tumors show irregular slitlike cavities lined by oval or flattened cells. Small tufts of these cells may project into the cavities. Cellular tumors with many clefts and tufts may be difficult to distinguish from synovial sarcoma.

The origin and histogenesis of xanthofibroma have been traced to the proliferation of synovial cells resem-

bling histiocytes. These cells are transformed into multinucleated giant cells and macrophages laden with hemosiderin or lipid. The underlying tissue is infiltrated by lymphocytes, a finding of basic significance in support of the view that the nodules are of inflammatory rather than neoplastic origin. As the nodules age, collagenous and often hyalinized matrix is laid down between the cells. The term "villinodular synovitis" is being used to describe the diffuse lesion; benign giant cell tumor of the tendon sheath and villinodular synovitis have been considered to be manifestations of the same underlying process: a chronic granulomatous inflammation with an as yet unknown cause.[148]

Osteochondromatosis

Osteochondromatosis may occur as an isolated lesion or with other forms of joint disease. It is characterized by the development, in the synovial tissues, of cartilaginous nodules that tend to undergo secondary ossification. The synovial lining contains translucent masses of proliferating cartilage projecting from the surface or hanging from narrow pedicles into the joint space (Fig. 40-25). Many of the nodules become detached, and dozens or even hundreds of them float free in the joint

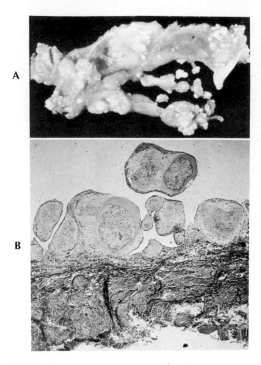

Fig. 40-25. Osteochondromatosis. **A,** Portions of synovial membrane showing numerous attached and superimposed cartilaginous nodules. **B,** Photomicrograph of synovial membrane showing ectopic cartilage forming numerous nodules projecting into joint cavity.

fluid, where they may continue to grow or become inactive.[201] By electron microscopy, transition from regular synovial cells to chondrocytes producing cartilaginous matrix along with deposition of crystals in the collagen fibrils of the matrix can be demonstrated.[6,63]

The cause of the disorder is unknown. Although mechanical injury and inflammation have been implicated, the lesions can occur in the absence of either. Histogenetically two mechanisms must be considered: (1) metaplasia from regular elements of the synovium and (2) development from undifferentiated chondrogenic cells; such cells are to be expected, especially at the reflection of the synovium, where during embryogenesis cells develop into either synoviocytes or chondrocytes.[231]

An uncommon variant of osteochondromatosis has been described as *osteomatosis*. In this disorder multiple osseous bodies develop in the synovial tissue without previous formation of cartilage.[87,215]

Synovioma (synovial sarcoma)

The term "synovioma" was suggested to designate a group of rare malignant tumors involving the regions of diarthrodial joints and once believed to arise from the synovium.[285] However, only 10% of the tumors develop within the joint cavities; the rest arise in tissues close to the articulations and seem to involve the synovium secondarily.[303] The tumor is most often seen in young adults, and the sex ratio is 3:2 (males predominating). The knee joint is the most common site. The survival rate is low, and metastasis occurs more often by the bloodstream than by lymphatics.[186]

Grossly the tumors are usually single, roughly ovoid, and often lobulated and vary from 1 to 18 cm in diameter.[49] They may be sharply delimited but may extend along fascial planes. Growing expansively, they are partially or completely surrounded by a pseudocapsule formed by the compressed or attenuated adjacent nontumorous tissue. On the cut surface the tumors may be firm, focally gritty, or spongy and friable. Homogeneous areas alternate with areas of fibrous, even whorl-like appearance, and hemorrhage, necrosis, or cysts may be present, the cysts containing gelatinous or mucinous material.

Microscopically the tumors are characterized by a biphasic cell pattern: (1) areas resembling fibrosarcoma, composed of fairly uniform spindle-shaped cells with hyperchromatic nuclei and densely packed in bands or sheets, and (2) cells resembling epithelium (synovioblastic cells), arranged in pseudoglandular structures, lining clefts in the fibrosarcomatous stroma or forming papillae (Figs. 40-26 and 40-27). These cells vary in shape from cuboid to tall columnar and may undergo squamous metaplasia.[204] They may secrete a mucopolysaccharide, probably hyaluronic acid, which is also found in the occasional cysts. The cell sheets are surrounded by abundant masses of reticulin, but no fibrils are found between the cells. In addition, there is nonfibrillar eosinophilic material that resembles osteoid and sometimes contains deposits of calcium. In the presence of an old hemorrhage, hemosiderin-laden macrophages or, more rarely, foreign-body giant cells may be found. The number of mitoses varies from moderate to large. The tumor may invade adjacent tissues and blood vessels.

The biphasic pattern of the tumors has been confirmed by electron microscopy.[101,185] Stromal cells have folded nuclei with clumped chromatin at the membrane and prominent nucleoli; the cytoplasm is vesiculated. Endoplasmic reticulum, both rough and smooth, and microfilaments are more prominent than Golgi apparatus of mitochondria. The epithelium-like cells, by contrast, contain many mitochondria. The cells are always in contact with one another; the presence of desmosomes, other junctional zones, and a basement membrane at the junction of stromal and epithelioid cells indicates a comparatively advanced stage of differentiation of a tumor.[96]

The histogenesis of the neoplasm is obscure. The similarity of the cells to the two types found in normal

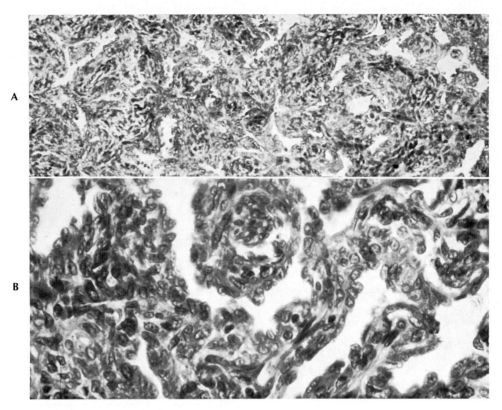

Fig. 40-26. Synovial sarcoma. **A,** Low-power view. **B,** High-power view. (**A** and **B,** AFIP 90623.)

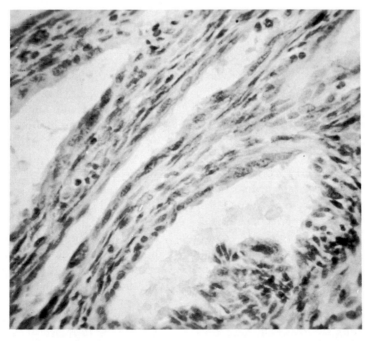

Fig. 40-27. Highly differentiated synovial sarcoma with epithelium-like cells forming surface lining of tissue clefts.

synovium is suggestive of synovial origin. However, the extra-articular origin of the majority of the tumors, the presence of transitional cell types, and the behavior of the tumor cells in tissue culture are not consistent with this hypothesis. It seems more justified to consider a pluripotential undifferentiated mesenchymal cell as the true precursor of the neoplasm.

Clear cell sarcoma of tendon sheaths and aponeuroses

Clear cell sarcoma of tendon sheaths and aponeuroses has been recognized only recently.[33,91] It occurs most commonly in the region of the hands or feet. The spherical smooth or nodular tumors are attached to tendons or aponeuroses; on cut surface they are grayish white, solid, and sometimes gritty, with occasional foci of necrosis or cysts. Microscopically they are not biphasic like the synoviomas but consist of nests of pale, fusiform, epithelioid cells surrounded by delicate fibrous septa. The tumor cells have light-staining nuclei with contrasting prominent nucleoli and do not contain lipid. Multinucleated giant cells are common. By electron microscopy melanosomes have been found in such a tumor.[138]

Miscellaneous malignant lesions

Malignant giant cell tumor of the tendon sheath combines features of clear cell sarcoma and benign giant cell tumor of tendon sheaths. It differs from clear cell sarcoma in that there are transitions between the clear cells and foam cells and the multinucleated giant cells of osteoclastic, or Touton, type. The intercellular substance, which can be removed with bovine hyaluronidase, is closely related to the plasma membrane of the tumor cells, a finding that is suggestive of secretion of the substance by the membrane.[153,223]

Chondrosarcoma of the joint is a rare and highly malignant neoplasm[112] that involves the joint diffusely, simulating benign chondromatosis at the early stages. The tumor may arise from the synovium directly or from previously present chondromatosis.[213] Histologically the neoplasm is characterized by large atypical cells with hyperchromatic nuclei and by large binucleated or multinucleated cells. Myxoid change in synovial chondrosarcoma constitutes a rare occurrence, giving rise to a subtype of chondrosarcoma of the synovium.[164]

Multicentric histiocytic reticulosis may involve multiple or simple joints by development of granulomatous tissue in the synovium. As elsewhere in this disorder, the granulation tissue is characterized by the presence of numerous histiocytes and multinucleated giant cells and forms transitional between the two. All these cells may characteristically have a foamy cytoplasm and, with special stains, can be shown to contain neutral fats and phospholipids.[18] More rarely, lipid may be absent from the cells.[89] The granulation tissue spreads aggressively, and with time there is extensive destruction of the articular cartilage and the adjacent bone, leading to partial or complete loss of joint function.

DISEASES OF THE VERTEBRAL COLUMN
Deformities

The significance of spinal deformities lies in their effects on motor activity, on the integrity of peripheral joints, and on the viscera (such as the heart and lungs, which depend on normal spatial relations for their proper functioning).

Deformities of the spine may be caused by changes in the vertebral bodies (a topic outside the scope of this chapter) or by changes in the intervertebral discs. Three types of deformity involving large segments of the spine exist: (1) kyphosis, characterized by increased convexity in the anteroposterior direction; (2) lordosis, increased concavity in the anteroposterior direction; and (3) scoliosis, lateral deviation from the normal orientation. One of the most common deformities, kyphosis of old age (senile kyphosis), is caused by uneven distribution of degenerative processes in the discs that cause the discs to collapse anteriorly so that the anterior portions of the vertebral bodies tilt toward each other.

Disc disease

Starting in late adolescence and progressing with increasing age, the intevertebral discs can deteriorate.[307] Water is lost from the nucleus, and there are loss of chrondroitin sulfate, increase of keratan sulfate and collagen, and calcification. These changes lead to a decrease in intranuclear pressure and loss of elasticity. The anulus fibrosus likewise loses water, becomes fibrillated and fissured, and loses its tight attachment to the vertebral bone. It thus exerts less than normal restraints on the nucleus during mechanical stress. Sudden or, more commonly, chronic stretching and bending that produce mechanical strain may then force the nucleus out of the confines of the anulus into neighboring structures. If the prolapse occurs into the spinal canal, pressure on and potential damage to neural tissues ensue. Another site of predilection for prolapses is the terminal plates of the vertebrae; disc tissue may penetrate the bone marrow space of the vertebral body and there form globular masses. These structures are termed "Schmorl's nodules"; roentgenographically they superficially resemble metastatic tumors. Prolapsed nuclei undergo further degeneration, such as hyalinization, calcification, and sclerosis. Amyloid may be present in herniated discs as well as in nonherniated discs, since the amyloid is apparently unrelated to herniation.[173]

Spondylosis

Degenerating discs, even if they do not prolapse, may yet assume a role in the initiation of spondylosis deformans, though this disorder can also develop in the absence of disc disease. Spondylosis deformans, or hypertrophic spondylosis, is a disease peculiar to vertebral bodies and their articulating surfaces. It does not involve the small joints of the spinal processes, which are subject to osteoarthrosis like other large diathrodial joints. Spondylosis deformans is an age-linked disorder having its steepest rise in incidence during the fourth to sixth decades, after which age nearly everyone is affected.[259] Men seem to be affected somewhat more severely and at an earlier age than women.[132] The increased incidence of the disorder in miners as compared with that found in factory workers or craftsmen has suggested to some investigators in etiologic role of extraneous mechanical stresses.

The fully developed lesions of spondylosis are characterized by fraying, fibrillation, and chondrocyte proliferation of the cartilage of the terminal plates and by chondro-osseous outgrowths (osteophytes) at the vertebral margins. Osteophytes may bridge the narrowed intervertebral space and overlap the adjacent vertebral edge (Fig. 40-28). Two opposing osteophytes may fuse, causing immobilization of the joint. The origin of the osteophytes is disputed, but one should keep in mind that during development the edge of the vertebral body consists of a cartilaginous ring. Although this ring ossifies in time, the adjacent fibrous tissues still contain cells with a chondrogenic or osteogenic potential that is activated under the effect of stimulating factors. The age-linked loosening of the anulus fibrosus in association with the narrowing of the intervertebral space gives rise to friction, which has long been recognized as a cause of spondylosis. The frequent association with diabetes mellitus[278,279] indicates that metabolic factors may enter into the etiology of the disorder, either by acting on the vertebral end plates directly or by first causing abnormalities in the intervertebral discs.

In ochronosis the intervertebral discs are discolored a deep black; they are softened or calcified and brittle, shrunken, and often prolapsed posteriorly into the spinal canal or anteriorly through the retaining ligaments. With shrinkage of the discs the intervertebral spaces are narrowed, and eventually the vertebral bodies touch and become fused by osseous links (Plate 8, *B*).

Ankylosing spondylitis (Marie-Strümpell-Bekhterev disease)

Ankylosing spondylitis is a chronic progressive inflammation of unknown origin involving primarily the small apophyseal and costovertebral joints of the spine, as well as the sacroiliac joints. The overall incidence of the disorder in the general population is less than 1%; men are affected nine times more frequently than women. The disease usually starts late in the second or in the third decade, progresses to involve several segments or the entire length of the spine, and terminates in ankylosis of individual joints with immobilization of the involved segments of the spine. The histologic and immunohistologic changes seen in both spinal and peripheral joints are basically similar to those seen in rheumatoid arthritis: a nonspecific chronic synovitis with destruction of the cartilage by pannus, adhesions between the opposing surfaces of the joint, and thickening and fibrosis of the joint capsule. In contrast to the situation observed in spondylosis, the intervertebral spaces are not narrowed, but the discs may be partially or completely destroyed by granulation tissue, which undergoes fibrosis, calcification, and ossification.[65,244] The process may extend into ligaments and their insertion at the vertebral bodies[14]; consequently adjacent vertebrae may become fused by osseous bridges that often protrude from under the longitudinal ligament and give rise to the gross appearance of the "bamboo spine."

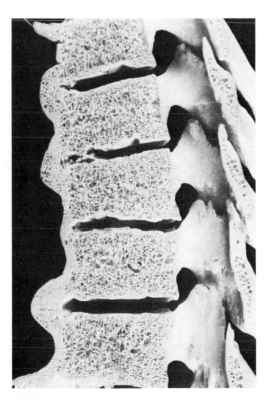

Fig. 40-28. Hyperostotic spondylosis. Anterior fusion of vertebral bodies by osseous bridges. (Courtesy Dr. Max Aufdermaur, Lucerne.)

Etiology

Despite their morphologic similarity, ankylosing spondylitis differs from rheumatoid arthritis. As a member of the group of spondyloarthropathies (see p. 2086), ankylosing spondylitis shares with the other members of that group an unknown cause, a male preponderance, the absence of rheumatoid factors, and the positive association with HLA-B27 antigens, found in 90% of the patients with this disease. This association, however, varies in different populations.[39] Familial incidence is high, especially in fathers of probands who are HLA-B27 positive,[208,219] but identical twins are discordant for ankylosing spondylitis, an observation that points to an etiologic role by environmental factors.

REFERENCES

1. Acheson, R.M., and Collart, A.B.: New Haven Survey of Joint Diseases XVII. Relationship between some systemic characteristics and osteoarthrosis in a general population, Ann. Rheum. Dis. 34:379, 1975.
2. Adams, I.I.: Osteoarthritis and sport, Clin. Rheum. Dis. 2:523, 1976.
3. Akoonen, P.: Human yersiniosis in Finland, Ann. Clin. Res. 4:30, 1977.
4. Ali, S.Y.: New knowledge of osteoarthrosis, J. Clin. Pathol. 31(suppl. 12):191, 1978.
5. Ali, S.Y., et al.: Ultrastructural studies of pyrophosphate crystal deposition in articular cartilage, Ann. Rheum. Dis. 42(suppl.):97, 1983.
6. Allred, C.D., and Gondos, B.: Ultrastructure of synovial chondromatosis, Arch. Pathol. Lab. Med. 106:688, 1982.
7. Alpert E., Isselbacher, K.J., and Schur, P.H.: The pathogenesis of arthritis associated with viral hepatitis, N. Engl. J. Med. 285:185, 1971.
8. Ansell, B.M.: Chronic arthritis in childhood, Ann. Rheum. Dis. 37:107, 1978.
9. Argen, R.J., and Dixon, A.St.J.: Clutton's joint with keratitis and periostitis, Arthritis Rheum. 6:341, 1963.
10. Armstrong, C.G., Bahrani, A.S., and Gardner, D.L.: Alteration with age in compliance of human femoral head cartilage, Lancet 1:1103, 1977.
11. Arnold, J.: Acromegalie, Pachyacrie oder Ostitis? Beitr. Pathol. Anat. 10:1, 1981.
12. Badalamente, M.A., Stern, L., and Hurst, L.C.: The pathogenesis of Dupuytren's contracture: contractile mechanisms of the myofibroblasts, J. Hand Surg. 8:235, 1983.
13. Baker, W.M.: On the formation of synovial cysts in the leg in connection with disease of the knee joint, St. Barth. Hosp. Rep. 13:245, 1877.
14. Ball, J.: Articular pathology in ankylosing spondylitis, Clin. Orthop. 143:30, 1979.
15. Bardin, T., Kuntz, D., Zingraff, J., Voisin, M.C., Zelmar, A., and Lansaman, J.: Synovial amyloidosis in patients undergoing long-term hemodialysis, Arthritis Rheum. 28:1052, 1058, 1985.
16. Barnes, C.G., Turnbull, A.L., and Vernon-Roberts, B.: Felty's syndrome, Ann. Rheum. Dis. 30:359, 1971.
17. Barnett, E.V., North, A.F., Jr., Condemi, J.J., et al.: Antinuclear factors in systemic lupus erythematosus and rheumatoid arthritis, Ann. Intern. Med. 63:100, 1965.
18. Barrow, M.V., Sunderman, F.W., Jr., Hackett, R.L., et al.: Identification of tissue lipids in lipid dermatoarthritis (multicentric reticulohistiocytosis), Am. J. Clin. Pathol. 47:312, 1967.
19. Bauer, W., Bennett, G.A., and Zeller, J.W.: The pathology of joint lesions in patients with psoriasis and arthritis, Trans. Assoc. Am. Phys. 56:349, 1941.
20. Bayer, A., Choi., C., Tillman, D.B., and Guze, L.B.: Fungal arthritis, V, Semin. Arthritis Rheum. 9:218, 1980.
21. Bayliss, M.J., and Ali, S.Y.: Isolation of proteoglycans from human articular cartilage, Biochem. J. 169:123, 1978.
22. Becker, M.A., Meyer, L.J., Wood, A.W., et al.: Purine overproduction in man associated with increased phosphoribosylpyrophophate synthetase activity, Science 179:1123, 1973.
23. Bennett, G.A.: Comparison of the pathology of rheumatic fever and rheumatoid arthritis, Ann. Intern. Med. 19:111, 1942.
24. Bennett, G.A., Waine, H., and Bauer, W.: Changes in the knee joints at various ages with particular reference to the nature of degenerative joint disease, New York, 1943, Commonwealth Fund.
25. Bennett, G.A., Zeller, J.W., and Bauer, W.: Subcutaneous nodules of rheumatoid arthritis and rheumatic fever, Arch. Pathol. 30:70, 1940.
26. Bennett, J.C.: The infectious etiology of rheumatoid arthritis, Arthritis Rheum. 21:531, 1978.
27. Benninghoff, A.: Form und Bau der Gelenkknorpel in ihren Beziehungen zur Funktion, Z. Zellforsch. 2:783, 1925.
28. Bick, E.M.: Congenital deformities of the musculoskeletal system noted in the newborn, Am. J. Dis. Child. 100:861, 1960.
29. Bjelle, A.O.: Morphological study of articular cartilage in pyrophosphate arthropathy, Ann. Rheum. Dis. 31:449, 1972.
30. Bjelle, A.O.: Glycosaminoglycans in human articular cartilage of the lower femoral epiphysis in osteoarthrosis, Scand. J. Rheumatol. 6:37, 1977.
31. Bjelle, A., Crocker, P., and Willoughby, D.: Ultramicrocrystals in pyrophosphate arthropathy, Acta Med. Scand. 207:89, 1980.
32. Bjelle, A.: Cartilage matrix in hereditary pyrophosphate arthropathy, J. Rheumatol. 8:959, 1981.
33. Bliss, B.O., and Reed, R.J.: Large cell sarcomas of tendon sheath, Am. J. Clin. Pathol. 49:776, 1968.
34. Block, S.R., Winfield, J.B., Lockskin, M.D., et al.: Studies of twins with systemic lupus erythematosus, Am. J. Med. 59:533, 1975.
35. Bluestone, R., editor: Seronegative spondyloarthropathies, Clin. Orthop. 143:1, 1979.
36. Bonomo, H., Tursi, A., Trizio, D., Gillardi, V., and Dammaco, F.: Immune complexes in rheumatoid synovitis: a mixed staining immunofluorescence study, Immunology 18:557, 1970.
37. Boyle, J.A., Greig, W.R., Jasani, M.K., et al.: Relative role of genetic and environmental factors in the control of serum uric acid levels in normouricaemic subjects, Ann. Rheum. Dis. 26:234, 1967.
38. Bozicevich, J., Bunim, J.J., Freund, J., and Ward, S.B.: Bentonite flocculation test for rheumatoid arthritis, Proc. Soc. Exp. Biol. Med. 97:180, 1958.
39. Brewerton, D.A.: HLA system and rheumatic disease, J. Clin. Pathol. 31(suppl. 12):117, 1978.
40. Brickley-Parsons, D., Glimcher, M.J., Smith, R.J., Albin, R., and Adams, J.P.: Biochemical changes in collagen of the palmar fascia in patients with Dupuytren's disease, J. Bone Joint Surg. 63A:787, 1981.
41. Britton, M.C., and Schur, P.H.: The complement system in rheumatoid synovitis, II. Intracytoplasmic inclusions of immunoglobulin and complement, Arthritis Rheum. 14:87, 1971.
42. Bullough, P.G., Goodfellow, J., and O'Connor, J.: The relationship between degenerative changes and load bearing in the human hip, J. Bone Joint Surg. 55B:746, 1973.
43. Bunim, J.J., Burch, T.A., and O'Brien, W.M.: Influence of genetic and environmental factors in the occurrence of rheumatoid arthritis and rheumatoid factors in American Indians, Bull. Rheum. Dis. 15:349, 1964.
44. Burton, J.L.: Thick skin and stiff joints in insulin-dependent diabetes mellitus, Br. J. Dermatol. 66:369, 1982.
45. Bywaters, E.G.L.: The relation between heart and joint disease including "rheumatoid" heart disease and chronic posttraumatic arthritis (type Jaccoud), Br. Heart. J. 12:101, 1950.
46. Bywaters, E.G.L.: Pathologic aspects of juvenile chronic polyarthritis, Arthritis Rheum. 20(suppl.):271, 1977.
47. Bywaters, E.G.L., and Dorling, J.: Amyloid deposits in articular cartilage, Ann. Rheum. Dis. 30:294, 1971.
48. Bywaters, E.G.L., and Hamilton, E.B.D.: The spine in idiopathic hemochromatosis, Ann. Rheum. Dis. 30:457, 1971.

49. Cadman, N.L., Soule, E.H., and Kelly, P.J.: Synovial sarcoma: an analysis of 134 tumors, Cancer **18**:613, 1965.
50. Calkins, E., and Cohen, A.S.: Diagnosis of amyloidosis, Bull. Rheum. Dis. **10**:215, 1960.
51. Cameron, H.K., and Fornasier, V.L.: Trabecular stress fractures, Clin. Orthop. **111**:266, 1975.
52. Campbell, C.J.: The healing of cartilage defects, Clin. Orthop. **64**:45, 1969.
53. Caplan, A., Payne, R.B., and Whitey, J.L.: A broader concept of Caplan's syndrome related to rheumatoid factors, Thorax **17**:205, 1962.
54. Carter, C., and Wilkinson, J.: Persistent joint laxity and congenital dislocation of the hip, J. Bone Joint Surg. **46B**:40, 1964.
55. Caughey, D.E., and Bywaters, E.G.L.: The arthritis of Whipple's disease, Ann. Rheum. Dis. **22**:327, 1963.
56. Chalmers, A., Reynolds, W.J., Oreopoulos, D.G., Meema, H.E., Meindok, H., and deVeber, G.A.: The arthropathy of maintenance intermittent peritoneal dialysis, Can. Med. Assoc. J. **123**:635, 1980.
57. Chung, S.M.K., and Ralston, E.L.: Necrosis of femoral head associated with sickle cell anemia and its genetic variant, J. Bone Joint Surg. **51A**:33, 1969.
58. Clutton, H.H.: Symmetrical synovitis of the knee in hereditary syphilis, Lancet **1**:391, 1866.
59. Cohen, A.S., and Kim, I.C.: Acute suppurative arthritis. In Hill, A.S., editor: Modern trends in rheumatology, London, 1966, Butterworth & Co. (Publ.), Ltd., pp. 347-361.
60. Collins, D.H., and McElligott, T.F.: Sulphate $^{35}SO_4$ uptake by chondrocytes in relation to histological changes in osteoarthritic human cartilage, Ann. Rheum. Dis. **19**:318, 1960.
61. Cooke, T.D.V., Richer, S., Hurd, E., et al.: Localization of antigen-antibody complexes in intraarticular collagenous tissues, Ann. NY Acad. Sci. **256**:10, 1975.
62. Costello, P.B., Tambar P.K., and Green, F.A.: The prevalence and possible prognostic significance of arthropathy in childhood diabetes, J. Rheumatol. **11**:62, 1984.
63. Cotta, H., Rauterberg, K., Binzus, G., and Dettmer, U.: Elektronen-optische und biochemische Untersuchungen an der Gelenkkondromatose, Arch. Orthop. Unfallchir. **63**:73, 1968.
64. Crisp, A.J., Chapman, C.M., Kirkham, S.E., Schiller, A.L., and Krane, S.M.: Articular mastocytosis in rheumatoid arthritis, Arthritis Rheum. **27**:845, 1984.
65. Cruikshank, B.: Lesions of cartilaginous joints in ankylosing spondylitis, J. Pathol. Bacteriol. **71**:73, 1956.
66. Currey, H.L.F.: Pyrophosphate arthropathy and calcific periarthritis, Clin. Orthop. **71**:70, 1970.
67. Davidson, P.T., and Horowitz, J.: Skeletal tuberculosis, Am. J. Med. **48**:77, 1970.
68. de Blécourt, J.J.: Hereditary factors in rheumatoid arthritis and ankylosing spondylitis. In Kellgren, J.H., Jeffrey, M.R., and Ball, J., editors: The epidemiology of chronic rheumatism, Philadelphia, 1963, F.A. Davis Co.
69. De Palma, A.F.: Hemophilic arthropathy, Clin. Orthop. **52**:145, 1967.
70. De Sèze, S., Solnica, J., Mitovic, D., Miravet, L., and Dorfmann, H.: Bone and joint disorders and hyperparathyroidism in hemochromatosis, Semin. Arthritis Rheum. **2**:71, 1972.
71. Dekker-Saeys, B.J., Meuwissen, S.G., Van Den Berg-Loonen, E.M., De Haas, W.H., Agenant, D., and Tytgat, G.N.: Ankylosing spondylitis and inflammatory bowel disease. II. Prevalence of peripheral arthritis, sacroiliitis, and ankylosing spondylitis in patients suffering from inflammatory bowel disease, Ann. Rheum. Dis. **37**:33, 1978.
72. Denko, C.W.: Effect of prostaglandins in urate crystal inflammation, Pharmacology **12**:331, 1974.
73. Denman, A.M.: Rheumatoid arthritis: a virus disease, Clin. Pathol. **31**(suppl. 12):132, 1978.
74. Devach, M., and Cabilli, C.: Dupuytren's contracture and diabetes mellitus, Isr. J. Med. Sci. **8**:774, 1972.
75. Diamond, L.S., Lynne, D., and Sigman, B.: Orthopedic disorders in patients with Down's syndrome, Orthop. Clin. North Am. **12**:57, 1981.
76. Dieppe, P.: New knowledge of chondrocalcinosis, J. Clin. Pathol. **31**(suppl. 12):214, 1978.
77. Dieppe, P.A., Alexander, G.J., Jones, H.E., Doherty, M., Scott, D.G., Manhire, A., and Watt, I.: Pyrophosphate arthropathy: a clinical and radiological study of 105 cases, Ann. Rheum. Dis. **41**:371, 1982.
78. Dieppe, P., Doherty, M., and McFarlane, D.: Crystal related arthropathies, Ann. Rheum. Dis. **42**(suppl.):1, 1983.
79. Dingle, J.T.: Catabolin: a cartilage catabolic factor from synovium, Clin. Orthop. **156**:219, 1980.
80. Doherty, M., and Dieppe, P.A.: Multiple microcrystal deposition within a family, Ann. Rheum. Dis. **44**:544, 1985.
81. Dolan, D.L., Lemmon, J.B., Jr., and Teitelbaum, S.L.: Relapsing polychondritis, Am. J. Med. **41**:285, 1966.
82. Donovan, T.L., Chapman, M.W., Harrington, K.D., et al.: *Serratia* arthritis, J. Bone Joint Surg. **58A**:1009, 1976.
83. Dupuytren, C.: [Permanent retraction of the fingers produced by an affection of the palmar fascia], Leçons orales **1**:1, 1883; translated in Classics **4**:142, 1939.
84. Editorial: *Salmonella* bone and joint infections, Infection **6**:107, 1983.
85. Editorial: Mseleni joint disease, Lancet **2**(1):483, 1985.
86. Egan, M.S., Goldenberg, D.L., Cohen, A.S., and Segal, D.: The association of amyloid deposits and osteoarthritis, Arthritis Rheum. **25**:204, 1982.
87. Ehalt, W., Ratzenhofer, M., and Gergen, M.: Die synoviale Osteochondromatose kombiniert mit paraartikulärer cartilaginärer Exostose und die Beziehungen zu einem seltenen Fall primärer Osteomatose, Der Chirurg **40**:464, 1969.
88. Ebringer, R., Rook, G., Swana, G.T., Bottazzo, G.F., and Doniach, D.: Autoantibodies to cartilage and type II collagen in relapsing polychondritis and other rheumatic diseases, Ann. Rheum. Dis. **40**:473, 1981.
89. Ehrlich, G.E., Young, I., Nosheny, S.Z., et al.: Multicentric reticulohistiocytosis (lipoid dermatoarthritis): a multisystem disorder, Am. J. Med. **52**:830, 1972.
90. Engel, A.: Osteoarthritis and body measurements, USPH National Center for Health Statistics, series 11, no. 29, pp. 1-37, Washington, D.C., 1968, United States Public Health Service.
91. Enzinger, F.M.: Clear cell sarcoma of tendons and aponeuroses, Cancer **18**:1163, 1965.
92. Erdheim, J.: Die Lebensvorgänge im normalen Knorpel und seine Wucherung bei Akromegalie: Pathologie in Einzeldarstellungen, Berlin, 1931, Springer.
93. Faires, J.S., and McCarthy, D.J., Jr.: Acute synovitis in normal joints of man and dog produced by injection of microcrystalline sodium urate, calcium oxalate and corticosteroid esters, Arthritis Rheum. **5**:295, 1962.
94. Faure, G., and Dagulsi, G.: Calcified tendinitis: a review, Ann. Rheum. Dis. **42**(suppl.):49, 1983.
95. Felty, A.R.: Chronic arthritis in the adult associated with splenomegaly and leucopenia, Bull. Johns Hopkins Hosp. **35**:16, 1924.
96. Fernández, G.B., and Hernández, F.J.: Poorly differentiated synovial sarcoma: a light and electron microscopic study, Arch. Pathol. Lab. Med. **100**:221, 1976.
97. Finidori, G., Rigault, P., de Grouchy, J., Rodriguez, A., Pouliquen, J.C., Guyonvarch, G., and Fingerhut, A.: Osteoarticular abnormalities and orthopedic complications in children with chromosomal aberrations, Ann. Genet. **26**:150, 1983.
98. Fisher, L., Kurtz, A., and Shipley, M.: Association between cheiroarthropathy and frozen shoulder in patients with insulin-dependent diabetes mellitus, Br. J. Rheumatol. **25**:141, 1986.
99. Førre, Ø., Doubloug, J.H., Høyeraal, H.M., and Thossby, E.: HLA antigens in juvenile arthritis, Arthritis Rheum. **26**:35, 1983.
100. Friedman, H.: Aspects psychosomatiques de la polyarthrite chronique évolutive (PCE) ou polyarthrite rhumatoïde, Acta Psychiatr. Belg. **72**:117, 1972.
101. Gabbiani, G., Kaye, G.I., Lattes, R., et al.: Synovial sarcoma: electron microscopic study of a typical case, Cancer **28**:1031, 1971.

102. Gabbiani, G., and Majno, G.: Dupuytren's contracture: fibroblast contraction? An ultrastructural study, Am. J. Pathol. **66**:131, 1972.

103. Gardner, D.L.: The experimental production of arthritis, Ann. Rheum. Dis. **19**:297, 1960.

104. Gardner, E.: The nerve supply of muscles, joints and other deep structures, Bull. Hosp. Joint Dis. **21**:153, 1960.

105. Garrod, A.B.: The nature and treatment of gout, London, 1859, Walton & Naberly.

106. Gay, S., Müller, P.K., and Lemmen, C.: Immunohistological study on collagen in cartilage-bone metamorphosis and degenerative osteoarthrosis, Klin. Wochenschr. **54**:969, 1976.

107. Ghadially, F.N., and Mehta, P.N.: Multifunctional mesenchymal cells resembling smooth muscle cells in ganglia of the wrist, Ann. Rheum. Dis. **30**:31, 1971.

108. Ghadially, F.N., and Roy, S.: Ultrastructure of synovial joints in health and disease, New York, 1969, Appleton-Century-Crofts.

109. Glaub, T., Czongor, J., and Szucs, T.: Immunopathologic role of proteoglycan antigen in arthritic disease, Scand. J. Immunol. **11**:247, 1980.

110. Glynn, L.E.: Pathogenesis and etiology of rheumatoid arthritis, Ann. Rheum. Dis. **31**:412, 1972.

111. Goffin, Y.A., Thona, Y., and Potvliege, P.R.: Microdeposition of amyloid in the joints, Ann. Rheum. Dis. **40**:27, 1981.

112. Goldman, R.L., and Lichtenstein, L.: Synovial chondrosarcoma, Cancer **17**:1233, 1964.

113. Goldwasser, M., Astley, T., van der Rest, M., and Glorieux, F.H.: Analysis of the type of collagen present in osteoarthritic human cartilage, Clin. Orthop. (167):296, 1982.

114. Good, R.A., and Rotstein, J.: Rheumatoid arthritis and agammaglobulinemia, Bull. Rheum. Dis. **10**:203, 1960.

115. Graham, W., and Graham, K.M.: Martyrs to the gout, Metabolism **6**:290, 1966.

116. Grahame, R., Armstrong, R., Simmons, N., Wilton, J.M.A., Dysen, M., Laurent, R., Miller, R., and Micus, R.: Chronic arthritis associated with the presence of intrasynovial rubella virus, Ann. Rheum. Dis. **42**:2, 1983.

117. Grigor, R., Edmonds, J., Lewkonia, R., Bresnihan, B., and Hughes, G.R.: Systemic lupus erythematosus, Ann. Rheum. Dis. **37**:121, 1978.

118. Gutman, A.B.: Renal mechanisms for regulation of uric acid excretion with special reference to normal and gouty man, Semin. Arthritis Rheum. **2**:1, 1972.

119. Gutman, A.B., and Yu, T.F.: Hyperglutamatemia in primary gout, Am. J. Med. **54**:713, 1973.

120. Haagensen, C.D., and Stout, A.P.: Synovial sarcoma, Ann. Surg. **120**:826, 1942.

121. Hagemann, R., and Ruttner, J.R.: Arthrosis of the sternoclavicular joint, Z. Rheumatol. **38**:27, 1979.

122. Halila, R., Steinmann, B., and Peltonen, I.: Processing of types I and III collagen in Ehlers-Danlos syndrome type VII, Am. J. Hum. Genet. **39**:222, 1985.

123. Ham, A.W., and Cormack, D.H.: Joints. In Histology, ed. 8, Philadelphia, 1979, J.B. Lippincott Co.

124. Hamerman, D.: Evidence for an infectious etiology of rheumatoid arthritis, Ann. NY Acad. Sci. **256**:25, 1975.

125. Hardingham, T.E.: Structure and biosynthesis of proteoglycans, Rheumatology **10**:143, 1986.

126. Harris, E.D., Faulkner, C.S., and Brown, F.E.: Collagenolytic systems in rheumatoid arthritis, Clin. Orthop. **110**:303, 1975.

127. Hartung, E.F.: Historical considerations, Metabolism **6**:196, 1957.

128. Hass, J.: Congenital dislocation of the hip, Springfield, Ill., 1957, Charles C Thomas, Publisher.

129. Hasselbacher, P., and Schumacher, H.R.: Localization of immunoglobulins in gouty tophi by immunohistology and on the surface of monosodium urate crystals by immune agglutination, Arthritis Rheum. **19**(suppl.):802, 1976.

130. Hay, F.C., Nineham, L.J., Perumal, R., and Roitt, I.M.: Intra-articular and circulating immune complexes and antiglobulins (IgG and IgM) in rheumatoid arthritis: correlation with clinical features, Ann. Rheum. Dis. **38**:1, 1979.

131. Hedberg, H.: Studies on the depressed hemolytic complement activity of synovial fluid in adult rheumatoid arthritis, Acta Rheum. Scand. **9**:165, 1963.

132. Heine, J.: Ueber die Arthritis deformans, Virchows Arch. [Pathol. Anat.] **260**:521, 1926.

133. Henderson, B., and Pettipher, E.R.: The synovial lining cell: biology and pathobiology, Semin. Arthritis Rheum. **15**:1, 1985.

134. Henderson, J.F., Rosenbloom, F.M., Kelley, W.N., et al.: Variations in purine metabolism of cultured skin fibroblasts from patients with gout, J. Clin. Invest. **47**:1511, 1968.

135. Herman, J.H., and Dennis, M.: Immunopathologic studies in relapsing polychondritis, J. Clin. Invest. **52**:549, 1973.

136. Hershfield, M.S., and Seegmiller, J.E.: Gout and the regulation of purine biosynthesis, Horiz. Biochem. Biophys. **2**:134, 1976.

137. Hilgartnet, M.W.: Hemophilic arthropathy, Adv. Pediatr. **21**:139, 1974.

138. Hoffman, G.J., and Carter, D.: Clear cell sarcoma of tendons and aponeuroses with melanin, Arch. Pathol. **95**:22, 1973.

139. Hoffman, G.S., Schuhmacher, H.R., Paul, H., Varghese, C., Reed, R., Ramsay, H.G., and Franck, W.A.: Calcium oxalate microcrystalline–associated arthritis in end stage kidney disease, Ann. Intern. Med. **97**:36, 1982.

140. Hollander, J.L., McCarty, D.J., Jr., Astorga, G., et al.: Studies on the pathogenesis of rheumatoid joint inflammation. I. The "R.A. cell" and a working hypothesis, Ann. Inter. Med. **62**:271, 1965.

141. Holmes, K.K., Counts, G.W., and Beatty, H.N.: Disseminated gonococcal infection, Ann. Intern. Med. **74**:979, 1971.

142. Hough, A.J., Banfield, W.G., and Sokoloff, L.: Cartilage in hemophilic arthropathy, AMA Arch. Pathol. **100**:91, 1976.

143. Howie, S., and Feldman, M.: Cellular interaction in antibody production, Clin. Rheum. Dis. **4**:481, 1978.

144. Hunter, J.A.A., Ogden, C., and Norris, M.C.: Dupuytren's contracture. I. Chemical pathology, Br. J. Plastic Surg. **28**:10, 1975.

145. Hurd, E.R.: Extra-articular manifestations of rheumatoid arthritis, Semin. Arthritis Rheum. **8**:151, 1979.

146. Idelberger, K.: Die Ergebnisse der Zwillingsforschung beim angeborenen Klumpfuss, Verh. Dtsch. Ges. Orthop. **33**:272, 1939.

147. Jaccoud, F.S.: Leçons de clinique médicale faites à l'Hôpital de la Charité, ed. 2, Paris, 1869, Delahaye.

148. Jaffe, H.L., Lichtenstein, L., and Sutro, C.J.: Pigmented nodular synovitis, bursitis and tenosynovitis, Arch. Pathol. **31**:731, 1941.

149. Jansson, E.: Isolation of fastidious mycoplasm from human sources, J. Clin. Pathol. **24**:53, 1971.

150. Jasin, H.E.: Autoantibody specificities of immune complexes sequestered in articular cartilage of patients with rheumatoid arthritis and osteoarthritis, Arthritis Rheum. **28**:241, 1985.

151. Johnson, L.C.: Morphologic analysis in pathology. In Frost, H.M., editor: Bone dynamics, 1964, Little, Brown & Co.

152. Johnston, Y.E., Duray, P.H., Steere, A.C., Kashgarian, M., Buza, J., Malawista, S.E., and Askenase, P.W.: Lyme arthritis, Am. J. Pathol. **118**:26, 1985.

153. Kahn, L.B.: Malignant giant cell tumor of the tendon sheath: ultrastructural study and review of literature, Arch. Pathol. **95**:203, 1973.

154. Karten, I.: Septic arthritis complicating rheumatoid arthritis, Ann. Intern. Med. **70**:1147, 1969.

155. Kellermeyer, R.W., and Naff, G.B.: Chemical mediators of inflammation in gout, Arthritis Rheum. **19**:765, 1975.

156. Kelley, W.N., Greene, M.L., Rosenbloom, F.M., et al.: Hypoxanthine-guanine phosphoribosyltransferase deficiency in gout, Ann. Intern. Med. **70**:155, 1969.

157. Kellgren, J.R.: Osteoarthritis in patients and populations, Br. Med. J. **1**:1, 1961.

158. Kellgren, J.R., in discussion of Lawrence, J.L., and Bier, F.: Nodal and non-nodal forms of generalized osteoarthrosis, Ann. Rheum. Dis. **23**:205, 1964.

159. Kellgren, J.H., Lawrence, J.S., and Bier, F.: Genetic factors in generalized osteoarthrosis, Ann. Rheum. Dis. **22**:237, 1963.

160. Kelly, J.J., III, and Weisiger, B.B.: The arthritis of Whipple's disease, Arthritis Rheum. 6:615, 1963.

161. Kelly, P.J., Martin, W.J., and Coventry, M.B.: Bacterial (suppurative) arthritis in the adult, J. Bone Joint Surg. 52A:1595, 1970.

162. Kempson, G.: Relationship between the tensile properties of articular cartilage from the human knee and age, Ann. Rheum. Dis. 41:508, 1982.

163. Key, J.A.: Hemophilic arthritis, Ann. Surg. 95:198, 1932.

164. Kindblom, L.G., and Angervall, L.: Myxoid chondrosarcoma of the synovial tissue: a clinicopathologic, histochemical and ultrastructural study, Cancer 52:1886, 1983.

165. Kinsella, T.D., Baum, J., and Ziff, M.: Immunofluorescent demonstration of an IgG-B$_{1c}$ complex in the synovial lining cells of rheumatoid synovial membrane, Clin. Exp. Immunol. 4:265, 1969.

166. Kogstad, O.: Baker's cyst, Acta Rheum. Scand. 11:194, 1965.

167. Konttinen, Y.T., Reitamo, S., Ranki, A., Häyry, P., Kankaanpää, U., and Wegelius, A: Characterization of the immunocompetent cells of rheumatoid synovium from tissue sections and eluates, Arthritis Rheum. 24:71, 1981.

168. Krane, S.: Mechanisms of tissue destruction in rheumatoid arthritis. In McCarty, D.J., editor: Arthritis and allied conditions, ed. 10, Philadelphia, 1985, Lea & Febiger.

169. Kulka, J.P.: The lesions of Reiter's syndrome, Arthritis Rheum. 5:195, 1962.

170. Kurosaka, M., and Ziff, M.: Immunoelectron microscopic study of the distribution of T cell subsets in rheumatoid synovium, J. Exp. Med. 158:1191, 1983.

171. Kutty, M.K., Iqbal, Q.M., and Teh, E.C.: Ochronotic arthropathy, Arch. Pathol. 96:100, 1973.

172. Lack, C.H.: Lysosomes in relation to arthritis. In Dingle, J.T., and Fell, H.B., editors: The lysosomes, vol. 1. New York, 1968, John Wiley & Sons.

173. Ladefoged, C., Fedders, O., and Petersen, O.F.: Amyloid in intervertebral discs: a histopathological investigation of surgical material, Ann. Rheum. Dis. 44:239, 1986.

174. Lagier, R., Baud, C.A., and Buchs, M.: Crystallographic identification of calcium deposits as regards their pathological nature with special references to chondrocalcinosis. In Fleisch, H., Blackwood, H.J.J., and Gwen, M., editors: Calcified tissues, New York, 1966, Springer Publishing Co.

175. Lamont-Havers, R.W.: Nature of serum factors causing agglutination of sensitized sheep cells and group A hemolytic streptococci, Proc. Soc. Exp. Biol. Med. 88:35, 1955.

176. Lawee, D.: Uric acid: the clinical application of 1000 unsolicited determinations, Can. Med. Assoc. J. 100:838, 1969.

177. Lawrence, J.S.: Heberden oration: Rheumatoid arthritis—nature or nurture? Ann. Rheum. Dis. 29:357, 1970.

178. Lawrence, J.S.: Rheumatoid factors in families, Semin. Arthritis Rheum. 3:177, 1973.

179. Lawrence, J.S., Hewitt, J.V., and Popert, A.J.: Gout and hyperuricemia in the United Kingdom. In Kellgren, J.H., Jeffrey, M.R., and Ball, J., editors: The epidemiology of chronic rheumatism, Philadelphia, 1963, F.A. Davis, Co.

180. Lawrence, J.S., Hewitt, J.V., and Popert, A.J.: Gout and hyperuricemia in the United Kingdom. In Kellgren, J.H., Jeffrey, M.R., and Ball, J., editors: The epidemiology of chronic rheumatism, Philadelphia, 1963, F.A. Davis, Co.

180. Lazarus, G.S., Brown, R.S., Daniels, J.R., et al.: Human granulocyte collagenase, Science 159:1483, 1968.

181. Ling, R.S.M.: The genetic factor in Dupuytren's disease, J. Bone Joint Surg. 45B:709, 1963.

182. Lowbeer, L.: Brucellosis osteomyelitis in man and animals, Am. J. Pathol. 24:723, 1948.

183. Luck, V.: Dupuytren's contracture, J. Bone Joint Surg. 41A:635, 1959.

184. Luck, V.: Articular cartilage: responses to destructive influence. In Basset, C.E., editor: Cartilage, degradation and repair, Washington, D.C., 1967, National Research Council.

185. Luse, S.A.: A synovial sarcoma: studies by electron microscopy, Cancer 13:321, 1960.

186. Mackenzie, M.D.: Synovial sarcoma, Cancer 19:169, 1966.

187. MacLachlan, M.D., and Rodnan, G.P.: Effects of food, fast and alcohol on serum uric acid and acute attacks of gout, Am. J. Med. 42:38, 1967.

188. Mankin, H.J., and Radin, E.: Structure and function of joints. In McCarty, D.J., editor: Arthritis and allied diseases, Philadelphia, 1979, Lea & Febiger.

189. Marmion, B.P.: Infection, autoimmunity and rheumatoid arthritis, Clin. Rheum. Dis. 4:565, 1978.

190. Martenis, T.W., Bland, J.H., and Phillips, C.A.: Rheumatoid arthritis after rubella, Arthritis Rheum. 11:683, 1968.

191. Martens, M., Tanghe, W., Mulier, J.C., et al.: Pigmented villonodular synovitis of joints, tendons and bursae, Acta Orthop. Belg. 38:233, 1972.

192. Matsubara, T., Spycher, M.A., Rüttner, J.R., and Fehr, K.: The localisation of fibronectin in rheumatoid arthritis synovium by light and electron microscopic immunohistochemistry, Rheumatol. Int. 3:153, 1983.

193. McCarthy, D.: Pathogenesis and treatment of crystal induced inflammation. In McCarthy, D.: Arthritis and allied conditions, ed. 10, Philadelphia, 1985, Lea & Febiger.

194. McCormick, J.N.: An immunofluorescence study of rheumatoid factor, Ann. Rheum. Dis. 22:1, 1963.

195. McCredie, J.: Thalidomide and congenital "Charcot joints," Lancet 2:1058, 1973.

196. McEwen, C., Ditata, D., Lingg, C., Porini, A., Good, A., and Rankin, T.: Ankylosing spondylitis accompanying colitis, regional ileitis and Reiter's disease, Arthritis Rheum. 14:291, 1971.

197. Meachim, G.: Age changes in articular cartilage, Clin. Orthop. 64:33, 1969.

198. Meachim, G., and Emery, I.H.: Cartilage fibrillation in shoulder and hip joints in Liverpool necropsies, J. Anat. 116:161, 1973.

199. Meyer, O., Cyna, J., Dryll, A., Cywiner-Golenzer, C., Wassef, M., and Ryckewaert, A.: Relapsing polychondritis: pathogenic role of anti-native collagen type II antibodies, J. Rheumatol. 8:820, 1981.

200. Meyerowitz, S.: The continuing investigation of psychosocial variables in rheumatoid arthritis, Mod. Trends Rheum. 2:92, 1971.

201. Milgram, W.J.: Synovial osteochondromatosis: a histopathological study of 30 cases, J. Bone Joint Surg. 59A:792, 1978.

202. Miller, D.R., Mankin, H.J., Shah, H., and D'Ambrosia, R.D.: Identification of fibronectin in preparations of osteoarthritic human cartilage, Conn. Tiss. Res. 12:267, 1984.

203. Miller, E.J.: A review of biochemical studies on the genetically distinct collagens of the skeletal system, Clin. Orthop. 92:260, 1973.

204. Mirra, J.M., Wang, S., and Bhuta, S.: Synovial sarcoma with squamous differentiation of the mesenchymal glandular elements, Am. J. Surg. Pathol. 8:791, 1984.

205. Mitchell, N., and Shepard, N.: Relapsing polychondritis: an electron microscopic study of synovium and articular cartilage, J. Bone Joint Surg. 54A:1235, 1972.

206. Mitovic, D.R.: Pathology of articular deposition of calcium salts in the relationship to osteoarthrosis, Ann. Rheum. Dis. 42(suppl.):19, 1983.

207. Moll, J.H.M., and Wright, V.: Psoriatic arthritis, Semin. Arthritis Rheum. 3:55, 1973.

208. Møller, P., Vinje, O., and Dale, K., Berg, K., and Kåss, E.: Family studies in Bechterew's syndrome I, Scand. J. Rheumatol. 13:1, 1984.

209. Morling, N., Fries, J., and Pedersen, F.K.: HLA-B27 in juvenile chronic arthritis, J. Rheumatol. 12:119, 1985.

210. Moseley, H.F.: Shoulder lesions, ed. 3, Baltimore, 1969, The Williams & Wilkins Co.

211. Mubarak, S.J., and Carroll, N.C.: Familial osteochondritis dissecans of the knee, Clin. Orthop. 140:131, 1979.

212. Muir, H.: Molecular approach to the understanding of osteoarthrosis, Ann. Rheum. Dis. 36:199, 1976.

213. Mullins, F., Berard, C.W., and Eisenberg, S.H.: Chondrosarcoma following synovial chondromatosis, Cancer 18:1180, 1965.

214. Murphy, E.G.: The histopathology of rheumatic fever: a critical review. In Lewis, L.T., editor: Rheumatic fever, Minneapolis, 1952, University of Minnesota Press.
215. Murphy, F.P., Dahlin, D.C., and Sullivan, C.R.: Articular synovial chondromatosis, J. Bone Joint Surg. **44A:**77, 1962.
216. Nashel, D.J., Widerlite, L.W., and Pekin, T.J.: IgD myeloma with amyloid arthropathy, Am. J. Med. **55:**426, 1973.
217. Nelson, J.A., and Koontz, W.C.: Septic arthritis in infants and children, Pediatrics **38:**966, 1966.
218. Nesterov, A.I.: Clinical course of Kashin-Beck disease, Arthritis Rheum. **7:**29, 1964.
219. Nichol, F.E., and Woodrow, J.C.: Genetics of ankylosing spondylitis, Proc. Ninth Eur. Congr. Rheum., Wiesbaden, p. 196, 1979.
220. Nimni, M., and Dekmush, K.: Differences in collagen metabolism between normal and osteoarthritic human articular cartilage, Science **181:**751, 1973.
221. Noble, J., Heathcote, J.G., and Cohen, H.: Diabetes mellitus in the aetiology of Dupuytren's disease, J. Bone Joint Surg. **66B:**322, 1984.
222. Nowoslawski, A.: Immunopathological features of rheumatoid arthritis. In Müller, W., Harwerth, H.G., and Fehr, K., editors: Rheumatoid arthritis, New York, 1971, Academic Press, Inc.
223. O'Brien, J.E., and Stout, A.P.: Malignant fibrous xanthomas, Cancer **17:**1445, 1964.
224. O'Brien, W.W.: Twin studies in rheumatic diseases, Arthritis Rheum. **11:**81, 1986.
225. O'Duffy, J.D., Carney, J.A., and Deodhar, S.: Behçet's disease: a report of 10 cases, three with new manifestations, Ann. Intern. Med. **75:**561, 1971.
226. Onion, D.K., Crumpacker, C.S., and Gilliland, B.C.: Arthritis of hepatitis associated with Australian antigen, Ann. Intern. Med. **75:**29, 1971.
227. O'Sullivan, J.B.: Gout in a New England town: a prevalence study in Sudbury, Mass., Ann. Rheum. Dis. **31:**166, 1972.
228. O'Sullivan, J.B., and Cathcart, E.S.: The prevalence of rheumatoid arthritis, Ann. Intern. Med. **76:**573, 1972.
229. Panush, R.S., Bianco, N.E., and Schur, P.H.: Serum and synovial fluid IgG, IgA and IgM antigammaglobulins in rheumatoid arthritis, Arthritis Rheum. **14:**737, 1971.
230. Partain, J.O., Cathcart, E.S., and Cohen, A.S.: Arthritis associated with gonorrhea, Ann. Rheum. Dis. **27:**156, 1968.
231. Paul, G.R., and Leach, R.E.: Synovial chondromatosis of the shoulder joint, Clin. Orthop. **68:**130, 1970.
232. Pelletier, J.P., Martel-Pelletier, J., Howell, D.S., Ghandur-Mnaymneh, L., Enis, J.E., and Woessner, J.F., Jr.: Collagenase and collagenolytic activity in human osteoarthritic cartilage, Arthritis Rheum. **26:**63, 1983.
233. Perricone, E., Palmoski, M.J., and Brandt, K.D.: Failure of proteoglycans to form aggregates in morphologically normal aged human cartilage, Arthritis Rheum. **20:**1372, 1977.
234. Peyron, J.C.: Epidemiologic and etiologic approach to osteoarthritis, Semin. Arthritis Rheum. **8:**288, 1979.
235. Philips, P.E.: Infectious agents in the pathogenesis of rheumatoid arthritis, Semin. Arthritis Rheum. **16:**1, 1986.
236. Pinnell, S.R., Krane, S.M., Kenzora, J.E., and Glimcher, M.Y.: A heritable disorder of connective tissue: hydroxylysine-deficient collagen disease, N. Engl. J. Med. **286:**1013, 1972.
237. Poole, A.R.: Changes in the collagen and proteoglycans of articular cartilage in arthritis, Rheumatology **10:**316, 1986.
238. Popert, A.J., Scott, D.L., Wainwright, A.C., Walton, K.W., Williamson, N., and Chapman, J.H.: Frequency of occurrence, mode of development, and significance of rice bodies in rheumatoid joints, Ann. Rheum. Dis. **41:**109, 1982.
239. Pritzker, K.P.H., Zahn, C.E., Nyburg, S.C., Luk, S.C., and Houpt, J.B.: The ultrastructure of urate crystals in gout, J. Rheumatol. **5:**1, 1978.
240. Prockop, D.J., and Kuivaniemi, H.: Inborn errors of collagen, Rheumatology **10:**246, 1986.
241. Puranen, J., Ala-Ketola, L., Peltokallio, P., et al.: Running and primary osteoarthritis of the hip, Br. Med. J. **2:**424, 1975.
242. Reichelt, A.: Beiträge zur Aetiologie der Osteochondrosis dissecans des Hüftgelenks, Arch. Orthop. Unfallchir. **65:**220, 1969.
243. Reginato, A.J., Schumacher, H.R., Allan, D.A., and Rabinowitz, J.L.: Acute monoarthritis associated with lipid liquid crystals, Ann. Rheum. Dis. **44:**537, 1985.
244. Revell, P.A., and Mayston, V.: Histopathology of the synovial membrane of peripheral joints in ankylosing spondylitis, Ann. Rheum. Dis. **41:**579, 1982.
245. Riddle, J.M., Bluhm, G.B., and Barnhart, M.J.: Ultrastructural study of leucocytes and urates in gouty arthritis, Ann. Rheum. Dis. **26:**289, 1967.
246. Rimoin, D.L.: Pachydermoperiostosis: genetic and physiologic considerations, N. Engl. J. Med. **222:**923, 1965.
247. Rodnan, G.P.: The nature of joint involvement in progressive systemic sclerosis (diffuse scleroderma): clinical study and pathologic examination of synovium in twenty-nine patients, Ann. Intern. Med. **56:**422, 1962.
248. Rodnan, G.P.: Early theories concerning etiology and pathogenesis of gout, Arthritis Rheum. **8:**599, 1965.
249. Rodríguez, M., Noguera, E., del Villar, R.S., Vegazo, S., Mulero, J., Cruz, J., and Larrea, A.: Toxic synovitis from denatured rapeseed oil, Arthritis Rheum. **25:**1477, 1982.
250. Ropes, M.W., Bennett, G.A., and Cobb, S.: Revision of diagnostic criteria for rheumatoid arthritis, Ann. Rheum. Dis. **18:**49, 1958.
251. Rosenberg, L.C.: Structure and function of proteoglycans. In McCarty, D.J., editor: Arthritis and allied disease, ed. 9, Philadelphia, 1979, Lea & Febiger.
252. Rosenblum, A.L.: Skeletal and joint manifestations of childhood diabetes, Pediatr. Clin. North Am. **3:**569, 1984.
253. Rubin, L.A., Fam, A.G., Rubenstein, J., Cambell, J., and Saiphoo, C.: Erosive azotemic osteoarthropathy, Arthritis Rheum. **27:**1086, 1984.
254. Rüttner, J.R., and Spycher, M.: Electron microscopic investigations on aging and osteoarthrotic human cartilage, Pathol. Microbiol. **31:**4, 1968.
255. Saville, P.D.: Age and weight in osteoarthrosis of the hip, Arthritis Rheum. **11:**635, 1968.
256. Schaller, J., and Wedgwood, R.J.: Juvenile rheumatoid arthritis: a review, Pediatrics **50:**940, 1967.
257. Schar, E., Pras, M., and Gafni, J.: Familial Mediterranean fever and its articular manifestations, Clin. Rheum. Dis. **1:**195, 1975.
258. Schmidt, K.L., Leber, H.W., and Schuetterle, G.: Arthropathy in primary oxalosis—crystal synovitis or osteopathy? Dtsch. Med. Wochensch. **106:**19, 1981.
259. Schmorl, C., and Junghanns, H.: The human spine in health and disease, English translation by S.P. Wilkins and L.S. Coin, New York, 1959, Grune & Stratton, Inc.
260. Schofield, J.D., and Weightman, B.: New knowledge of connective tissue aging, J. Clin. Pathol. **31**(suppl. 12):174, 1978.
261. Schumacher, H.R., Jr.: Ultrastructure of the synovial membrane in idiopathic hemochromatosis, Ann. Rheum. Dis. **31:**465, 1972.
262. Schumacher, H.R., Jr., Andrews, R., and McLaughlin, G.: Arthropathy in sickle-cell disease, Ann. Intern. Med. **78:**203, 1973.
263. Schumacher, H.R., Jr., and Holdsworth, D.E.: Ochronotic arthropathy. I. Clinico-pathologic aspects, Semin. Arthritis Rheum. **6:**207, 1977.
264. Schumacher, H.R.: Articular cartilage in the degenerative arthropathy of hemochromatosis, Arthritis Rheum. **25:**1460, 1982.
265. Schumacher, H.R., Cherian, P.V., Reginato, A.J., Bardin, T., and Rothfuss, S.: Intra-articular apatite crystal deposition, Ann. Rheum. Dis. **42**(suppl.):54, 1983.
266. Scott, D.L., Wainwright, A.C., Walton, K.W., and Williamson, N.: Significance of fibronectin in rheumatoid arthritis and osteoarthritis, Ann. Rheum. Dis. **40:**142, 1981.
267. Scott, J.T., and Pollard, A.C.: Uric acid excretion in the relatives of patients with gout, Ann. Rheum. Dis. **29:**397, 1970.
268. Scott, R.B., Elmore, S.M., Brackett, N.C., Jr., et al.: Neuropathic joint disease (Charcot joints) in Waldenström's macroglobulinemia with amyloidosis, Am. J. Med. **54:**535, 1973.
269. Seegmiller, J.E., Howell, R.R., and Malawista, S.E.: The inflammatory reaction to sodium urate, JAMA **180:**469, 1973.

270. Seegmiller, J.E., Laster, L., and Howell, R.R.: Biochemistry of uric acid and its relation to gout. III, N. Engl. J. Med. **268**:821, 1963.

271. Shearn, M.A.: Sjögren's syndrome, Philadelphia, 1971, W.B. Saunders Co.

272. Shirahama, T., and Cohen, A.S.: Ultrastructural evidence for leakage of lysosomal contents after phagocytosis of monosodium urate crystals, Am. J. Pathol. **76**:501, 1974.

273. Silberberg, M., and Silberberg, R.: The effects of endocrine secretions on articular tissues and their relation to the aging process. In Slocum, C.H., editor: Rheumatic diseases, Philadelphia, 1952, W.B. Saunders Co.

274. Silberberg, M., and Silberberg, R.: Aging changes in cartilage and bone. In Bourne, G.H., editor: Structural aspects of aging, London, 1961, Pitman Medical Publishers.

275. Silberberg, M., Frank, E.L., Jarrett, S.R., and Silberberg, R.: Aging and osteoarthrosis of the human sternoclavicular joint, Am. J. Pathol. **35**:831, 1959.

276. Silberberg, R.: Ultrastructure of articular cartilage in health and disease, Clin. Orthop. **57**:233, 1968.

277. Silberberg, R.: Obesity and osteoarthrosis, Proc. Int. Conf. on Clinical Complications of Obesity, Naples, March 1979, pp. 301-305, New York, 1979, Academic Press, Inc.

278. Silberberg, R.: The pituitary in skeletal aging and disease. In Everitt, A.V., and Burgess, J.A., editors: Hypothalamus, pituitary and aging, Springfield, Ill., 1976, Charles C Thomas, Publisher.

279. Silberberg, R.: The skeleton in diabetes mellitus: a review of the literature, Diabetes Res. **3**:329, 1986.

280. Silby, H.M., et al.: Acute monoarticular arthritis after vaccination, Ann. Intern. Med. **62**:347, 1965.

281. Sinha, S., Munichovdappa, C.L., and Kozak, G.P.: Neuroarthropathy (Charcot joints) in diabetes mellitus, Medicine **51**:191, 1966.

282. Sjögren, H.: Keratoconjunctivitis sicca and chronic polyarthritis, Acta Med. Scand. **130**:484, 1948.

283. Sledge, C.B.: Structure, development and function of joints, Orthop. Clin. North Am. **6**:619, 1973.

284. Smillie, J.L.: Osteochondritis dissecans: loose bodies in joints; etiology, pathology, treatment, Edinburgh, 1960, E. & S. Livingstone.

285. Smith, L.W.: Synoviomata, Am. J. Pathol. **3**:355, 1927.

286. Sneerson, J.M.: Digital clubbing and hypertrophic osteoarthropathy: the underlying mechanisms, Br. J. Dis. Chest **75**:113, 1981.

287. Snyderman, R., and McCarthy, G.A.: The role of macrophages in the rheumatic diseases, Clin. Rheum. Dis. **4**:499, 1978.

288. Sokoloff, L.: The biology of degenerative joint disease, Chicago, 1969, University of Chicago Press.

289. Sokoloff, L.: Biochemical and biophysical aspects of degenerative joint disease with special reference to hemophilic arthropathy, Ann. NY Acad. Sci. **240**:285, 1975.

290. Sokoloff, L., McCluskey, R.T., and Bunim, J.J.: Vascularity of the early subcutaneous nodule of rheumatoid arthritis, Arch. Pathol. **55**:475, 1955.

291. Soren, A.: Pathogenesis and treatment of ganglion, Clin. Orthop. **48**:173, 1966.

292. Spilberg, J.: Current concepts of the mechanism of acute inflammation in gouty arthritis, Arthritis Rheum. **18**:129, 1975.

293. Spilberg, J., Silzbach, L.E., and McEwen, C.: The arthritis of sarcoidosis, Arthritis Rheum. **12**:126, 1969.

294. Spink, W.W.: The nature of brucellosis, Minneapolis, 1956, University of Minnesota Press.

295. Spycher, M., Moor, H., and Ruettner, J.R.: Electron microscopic investigation on aging and osteoarthrotic cartilage, Z. Zellforsch. **98**:512, 1969.

296. Srinivasa, A., and Vigorita, V.J.: Pigmented villonodular synovitis (giant cell tumor of the tendon sheath and synovial membrane), J. Bone Joint Surg. **66A**:76, 1984.

297. Statsny, P.: Immunogenic factors in rheumatoid arthritis, Clin. Rheum. Dis. **3**:315, 1977.

298. Statsny, P., Rosenthal, M., Andreis, M., and Ziff, M.: Lymphokines in the rheumatoid joint, Arthritis Rheum. **18**:237, 1975.

299. Stecher, R.M.: Heberden oration: Heberden's nodes: a clinical description of osteoarthritis of the finger joints, Ann. Rheum. Dis. **14**:1, 1955.

300. Still, G.F.: On a form of chronic joint disease in children, Med. Chir. Trans. (London) **80**:47, 1897.

301. Stockwell, R.A.: The cell density of human articular cartilage and costal cartilage, J. Anat. **101**:753, 1967.

302. Stockwell, R.A.: Changes in the acid glycosaminoglycan content of the matrix of aging human articular cartilage, Ann. Rheum. Dis. **29**:509, 1970.

303. Stout, A.P., and Lattes, R.: Tumors of soft tissues. In Atlas of tumor pathology, series 2, fascicle 1, Bethesda, Md., 1967, Armed Forces Institute of Pathology.

304. Stuart, J., et al.: Incidence and specificity of antibodies to types I, II, III, IV, and V collagen in rheumatoid arthritis and other rheumatic diseases as measured by ^{125}I radioimmunoassay, Arthritis Rheum. **6**:832, 1983.

305. Swinyard, C.A., and Mayer, V.: Multiple congenital contractures (arthrogryposis), JAMA **183**:23, 1963.

306. Swinyard, C.A., and Bleck, E.E.: The etiology of arthrogryposis (multiple congenital contractures), Clin. Orthop. **194**:15, 1985.

307. Sylven, B., et al.: Biophysical and physiological investigations on cartilage and other mesenchymal tissues. II. The ultrastructure of bovine and human nuclei pulposi, J. Bone Joint Surg. **33A**:333, 1951.

308. Tak, H.K., Cooper, S.M., and Wilcox, W.R.: Studies on the nucleation of monosodium urate at 37° C, Arthritis Rheum. **23**:574, 1980.

309. Tasker, T., and Waugh, W.: Articular changes with internal derangement of the knee, J. Bone Joint Surg. **64B**:486, 1982.

310. Teilum, G., and Lindahl, A.: Frequency and significance of amyloid changes in rheumatoid arthritis, Acta Med. Scand. **149**:449, 1954.

311. Teshima, R., Treadwell, B.V., Trahan, C.A., and Mankin, H.J.: Comparative rates of proteoglycan synthesis and size of proteoglycans in normal and osteoarthritic chondrocytes, Arthritis Rheum. **26**:1225, 1983.

312. Thakker, S., McGehee, W., and Quismorio, F.P.: Arthropathy associated with factor XIII deficiency, Arthritis Rheum. **29**:808, 1986.

313. Thompson, G.H.: Arthrogryposis multiplex congenita, Clin. Orthop. **194**:1, 1984.

314. Thornhill, H.L., Richter, R.W., Shelton, M.L., et al.: Neuropathic arthropathy (Charcot forefeet) in alcoholics, Orthop Clin. North Am. **4**:7, 1973.

315. Torres, J., Rathburn, H.K., and Greenough, W.B.: Pneumococcal arthritis: report of a case and review of the literature, Johns Hopkins Med. J. **132**:234, 1973.

316. Trentham, D.: Immunity to type II collagen in rheumatoid arthritis: a current appraisal, Proc. Soc. Exp. Biol. Med. **176**:95, 1984.

317. U.S. National Center of Health Statistics: Prevalence of osteoarthritis in adults, Public Health Service Publications, series 11, no. 15, 1961-1962.

318. U.S. National Health Service: Rheumatoid arthritis in adults, Public Health Service Publications, series 11, no. 17, 1966.

319. Vaughan, J.H., Barrnett, E.V., Sobel, M.V., et al.: Intracytoplasmic inclusions of immunoglobulins in rheumatoid arthritis and other disorders, Arthritis Rheum. **11**:125, 1968.

320. Vernon-Roberts, B., Barnes, C.G., and Revell, R.A.: Synovial pathology in Behçet's syndrome, Ann. Rheum. Dis. **37**:139, 1978.

321. Verzar, F.: Aging of connective tissue, J. Gerontol. **12**:915, 1964.

322. Vlasik, J., Zitman, D., and Sitaj, S.: Articular chondrocalcinosis. III. Genetic study, Ann. Rheum. Dis. **22**:153, 1963.

323. Waaler, E.: The occurrence of a factor in human serum activating the specific agglutination of sheep blood corpuscles, Acta Pathol. Scand. **17**:173, 1940.

324. Wagner, J.C., and McCormick, J.N.: Immunological investigations of coal workers disease, J. R. Coll. Phys. **2**:49, 1967.

325. Wayne, H., et al.: Association of osteoarthritis and diabetes, Tufts Fol. Med. **7:**13, 1961.

326. Wei, X.Q., Wright, G.C., Jr., and Sokoloff, L.: The effect of sodium selenite on chondrocytes in monolayer culture, Arthritis Rheum. **29:**660, 1986.

327. Weissman, G., Zurier, R.B., Spieler, R.J., and Goldstein, J.M.: Mechanisms of lysosomal enzyme release from leukocytes exposed to immune complexes and other particles, J. Exp. Med. **134:**149s, 1971.

328. Wigley, R.D.: Popliteal cysts: variations on a theme by Baker, Semin. Arthritis Rheum. **12:**1, 1982.

329. Wilde, A., Mankin, H.J., and Rodnan, G.P.: Avascular necrosis of the femoral head in scleroderma, Arthritis Rheum. **13:**445, 1970.

330. Wollaston, W.H.: On gouty and urinary concretions, Philos. Trans. Roy. Soc. London **87:**388, 1797.

331. Wood, G.C., Pryce-Jones, R.H., and White, D.D.: Chondromucoprotein-degrading neutral protease activity in rheumatoid fluid, Ann. Rheum. Dis. **30:**73, 1971.

332. Wright, V.: A unifying concept for the spondyloarthropathies, Clin. Orthop. **143:**8, 1979.

333. Wright, V.A., Dowson, D., and Kerr, J.: The structure of joints, Int. Rev. Conn. Tiss. Res. **6:**105, 1973.

334. Wyngaarden, J.B.: The overproduction of uric acid in primary gout, Arthritis Rheum. **8:**648, 1965.

335. Yanez, J.E., Thompson, G.R., Mikkelsen, W.M., et al.: Rubella arthritis, Ann. Intern. Med. **64:**772, 1966.

336. Zevely, H.A., French, A.J., Mikkelsen, W.M., and Duff, I.F.: Synovial specimens obtained by knee joint punch biopsy, Am. J. Med. **20:**510, 1956.

337. Ziff, M.: Relation of cellular infiltration of rheumatoid synovial membrane to its immune response, Arthritis Rheum. **17:**313, 1974.

338. Ziff, M., et al.: Studies on the composition of the fibrinoid material in the subcutaneous nodule of rheumatoid arthritis, J. Clin. Invest. **32:**1253, 1953.

339. Zucker-Franklin, D.: The phagosomes in rheumatoid synovial fluid leucocytes: a light, fluorescence and electron microscopic study, Arthritis Rheum. **9:**24, 1966.

340. Zwaifler, N.J.: Etiology and pathogenesis of rheumatoid arthritis. In McCarthy, D., editor: Arthritis and allied conditions, ed. 10, Philadelphia, 1985, Lea & Febiger.

41 Diseases of Skeletal Muscle

REID R. HEFFNER, Jr.

NORMAL STRUCTURE

Most striated muscles are partitioned into multiple fascicles, or bundles of fibers, each being surrounded by a connective tissue sheath, the perimysium, through which the intramuscular nerves and blood vessels are conveyed. Intramuscular nerve twigs are especially prominent in the muscle belly at the innervation zone. An individual twig consists of up to 10 myelinated nerve fibers inside a thin coat of perineurial fibrous connective tissue. Within the perimysium, muscle spindles also reside. These mechanoreceptors are present in all muscles, usually in the vicinity of the muscle belly, but are more prevalent in small muscles devoted to finely coordinated movements such as the interossei. The normal muscle spindle is composed of several intrafusal fibers that are enclosed by a lamellar fibrous capsule. The perimysial septa are projections from the epimysium, which in turn encircles groups of fascicles or the entire muscle. Thicker than the perimysial trabeculas and constructed of dense collagen, the epimysium is part of the mesenchymal scaffolding to which the fascia overlying the muscle and the tendons are connected. Each muscle fiber is invested with an endomysial envelope, normally an unobstructive interconnecting meshwork of collagen, reticulin, and elastic fibers that support a rich capillary bed. The muscle fiber is a multinucleated, syncytium-like cell with a shape resembling that of a cylinder. Muscle fibers vary in length but typically extend for several centimeters, traversing the length of a fascicle without interruption or branching. In cross section, the normal adult myocyte is polygonal rather than rounded in configuration. The diameter of fibers measured in the transverse plane depends on several factors. Powerful, large, proximal muscles are composed of fibers with greater mean diameter (85 to 90 μm) than those of slender, distal or ocular muscles (20 μm). In general, muscles designed for precisely coordinated activity like those of the eyes or digits have smaller fibers than muscles involved in less refined or postural movements like the glutei and quadriceps femoris. Fiber size in males exceeds that in females, presumably because of more strenuous physical demands and hormonal factors, though it is well known that exercise induces fiber hypertrophy, regardless of gender. Muscle fibers in infants (mean diameter, 12 μm) and children are smaller than in healthy young adults. Some reduction in fiber size is also a legacy of advancing age. In longitudinal sections, especially paraffin sections stained with phosphotungstic acid–hemotoxylin or resin-embedded sections, striations within the sarcoplasm are visible, reflecting the arrangement of the contractile proteins that is seen better ultrastructurally. In hematoxylin and eosin–stained cross sections, the sarcoplasm has a somewhat granular appearance without evidence of striations, unless the cut is tangential. The sarcolemmal nuclei are peripherally located and number four to six per fiber. These nuclei are oriented parallel to the long axis of the fiber in longitudinal sections, and they are seen at intervals of 10 to 50 μm.

The ultrastructural examination of muscle is optimally conducted on longitudinal sections where any departure from the orderly striated tectology is more easily appreciated than in transverse sections. The plasma membrane measures about 8 nm in width and may be difficult to visualize as a discrete entity. Externally and closely adherent to the plasmalemma is the broader, more conspicuous basement membrane, a moderately electron-dense, amorphous structure with a mean width of 20 to 30 nm. Satellite cells, with scant cytoplasm and devoid of cross striations, are deployed between the basement membrane and the plasmalemma of the muscle fiber. These cells cannot be distinguished from sarcolemmal nuclei in light microscopic sections. Their nuclei represent 5% to 10% of nuclei having a parasarcolemmal location. Satellite cells are considered to be quiescent stem cells with a penchant for responding to muscle fiber injury by participating in the enterprise of regeneration. Each muscle fiber is composed of a myriad of parallel subunits, the myofibrils, which are minute, virgate contractile elements with an average diameter of 1 μm. The myofibril is apportioned into an iterative series of identical segments known as "sarcomeres." The sarcomeres of each myofibril are of equal length and are aligned in register with those in neighboring myofibrils. The cross striations or periodicity of

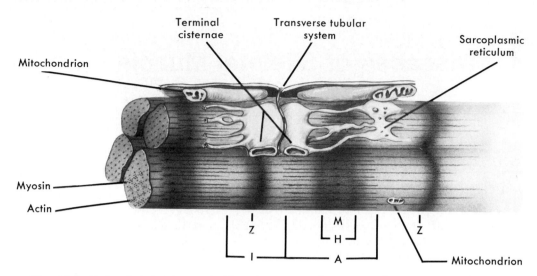

Fig. 41-1. Stylized skeletal muscle fiber. Important ultrastructural components of sarcomere are shown. See text for explanation of structures designated by letters. Not included in the text are the H zone ((*heller* for 'lighter' or 'brighter') and the M zone (*Mittelscheibe* for 'middle disc').

the muscle fiber is a function of the strict regimentation of the sarcomeres. The arrangement of the filaments within the sarcomere is responsible for the concatenation of rectangular bands that are seen. The length of the sarcomeres, 2.5 to 3 μm, is the distance between consecutive Z bands, which constitute the lateral boundaries of the sarcomere (Fig. 41-1). The Z band (*Zwischenscheibe*, meaning 'intermediate disc') is an extremely electron-dense linear disc perpendicular to the long axis of the myofibril. The Z band bisects the I (isotropic) bands of adjacent sarcomeres. Situated medial to the Z discs of a sarcomere, the I bands are more lightly stained and shorter in length than the central A (anisotropic) band. Inside the sarcomere are imbricating parallel filaments in the A and I band regions. The thick filaments, which are chiefly composed of myosin, measure 15 nm in diameter. The thin filaments, containing predominantly actin, have a diameter of 8 nm. The thick filaments, confined to the A band, dictate its length. The thin filaments extend from the Z band, to which they are attached, traverse the I band, where only thin filaments are present, and enter the A band to interdigitate with the thick filaments. The Z band, a major constituent of which is alpha-actinin, exhibits a grid-like or basketweave infrastructure. During muscular contraction, the Z bands are drawn toward the center of the sarcomere. The sarcomere length shortens as the thick and thin filaments slide past each other until the I bands are virtually obliterated. The organelles of the myofiber tend to congregate around the sarcolemmal nuclei and between the myofibrils. Glycogen granules, ranging from 15 to 30 nm in diameter, are found

in greater concentration in type 2 fibers and are more prevalent in the I band regions. Lipid vacuoles and mitochondria are more prominent in type 1 fibers. The majority of mitochondria are ovoid or elliptical in shape with an average diameter of 1.0 μm. They are predictably situated adjacent to the Z bands with their long axes parallel to those of the myofibrils. The sarcotubular complex (SRT), a bipartite system comprising the sarcoplasmic reticulum (SR) and the transverse (T) tubules, is a distinctive ultrastructural component of striated muscle. The T tubules originate as invaginations from the plasmalemma and are distributed at regular intervals along the fiber at the junction of the A and I bands. Coursing in a generally transverse direction, they form a weblike network of tubules that is perforated by the longitudinally oriented myofibrils. Unlike the transverse tubular system, which communicates with the extracellular space, the sarcoplasmic reticulum is a closed, internalized array of vesicles that arborizes in all directions around the myofibrils. In routine electron microscopic sections, the SR and T tubules appear as hollow, membrane-bound profiles. At the A-I band junctions, branches of the SRT come together into triads, composed of a pair of terminal cisternae of the SR between which is a centrally positioned tubule. The physiology of the sarcotubular system is intimately related to muscle contraction. An important early event is the depolarization of the plasma membrane, which causes excitation of the T system throughout the muscle fiber. Under these circumstances, calcium is liberated from the terminal cisterns of the SR, activating the contraction mechanism.

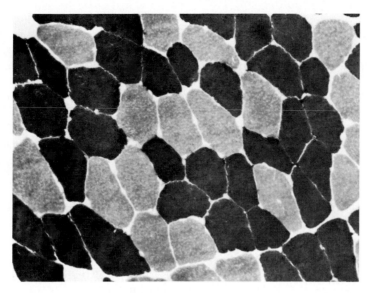

Fig. 41-2. Frozen section of normal skeletal muscle showing the typical checkerboard staining pattern. Type 1 fibers are light, and type 2 fibers are dark. (ATPase, pH 9.4; 175×.)

For a great many years it has been well known that there are physical and biochemical differences among skeletal muscles. For example, in endothermic vertebrates, particularly some avian genera, it is posible to distinguish between red (weight-bearing) and white (alar) muscles. The color of red muscles is bestowed upon them by their richer myoglobin content and increased capillary density. Red muscle, with its larger mitochondrial population and higher rate of blood flow, is more specialized for aerobic respiration and for postural or sustained activity. On the other hand, white muscle, endowed with fewer mitochondria, yet with abundant glycogen stores, is more suited to anaerobic respiration and is thus designed for sudden, intermittent activity. Although in lower vertebrates an entire muscle may be composed of either red or white fibers, human muscles are a mosaic of both fiber types, arranged in a pattern like that of a checkerboard. The proportion of type 1 and type 2 fibers depends on the function and anatomic location of the muscle, but the idealized muscle contains approximately 35% to 40% type 1 fibers and 60% to 65% type 2 fibers. Fiber typing, the demonstration of the histochemical properties of muscle fibers within a tissue sample, is determined through the use of enzyme histochemistry and is not evident in routine hematoxylin and eosin sections. Most laboratories utilize two complementary histochemical reactions carried out on fresh frozen sections for this purpose. Oxidative enzyme reactions, such as NADH-TR or succinic dehydrogenase, display the density of mitochondria within the muscle fiber. With this method, darkly stained fibers are designated as type 1

(oxidative) and lighter fibers as type 2. Most oxidative enzyme reactions further segregate type 2 fibers into two subpopulations, type 2B fibers being most lightly stained and type 2A fibers being intermediately stained. In the ATPase reaction, a spectrum of staining intensities can be achieved by manipulation of the pH during the staining procedure. When the standard or alkaline ATPase reaction is conducted at a pH of 9.4, type 1 fibers appear light and type 2 fibers are dark (Fig. 41-2). Fibers with intermediate staining properties are not apparent in the alkaline ATPase reaction. It is possible to reverse the staining reaction by altering the incubating solution to an acidic pH, usually about 4.6. In the reverse ATPase reaction, type 1 fibers are very darkly stained, type 2A fibers are very lightly stained, and type 2B fibers are intermediate in their staining attributes between the two. Some laboratories employ a histochemical reaction for phosphorylase, which is more abundant in type 2 (glycolytic) fibers, as a means of fiber typing. Although type 2 fibers should theoretically appear dark and type 1 fibers should appear light, in my experience this staining reaction is capricious and unreliable.

MUSCLE BIOPSY[18,29,30]

Our knowledge of neuromuscular diseases has expanded in dramatic fashion during the past 25 years.[21,46,48] Much of this enlightenment has been a product of the application of modern pathologic technology to the study of muscle biopsy samples. Today, with increasing frequency the pathologist is required to process and interpret muscle biopsy specimens that are being utilized as a diagnostic tool in hospitals of all sizes, from smaller community hospitals to large university medical centers.

Unlike neoplasms of muscle, neuromuscular diseases are medical rather than surgical conditions, requiring that the pathologic examination of muscle tissue, which is only one infrangible part of the total diagnostic effort in evaluating the patient, not be divorced from the patient's history, physical examination, and apposite laboratory tests. In the subsequent discussion of individual neuromuscular diseases (p. 2111), the relevance of clinical data will soon become obvious. For example, the temporal profile of disease is often informative, in that a rapid onset of symptoms is suggestive of an infectious or inflammatory myopathy, whereas insidious progression favors muscular dystrophy, metabolic myopathy, or a neurogenic process. The distribution of weakness is frequently an indication of whether the neuromuscular disorder is a primary myopathy, in which weakness tends to be proximal in location, or a denervating disease, in which weakness begins distally. Grossly detectable wasting of muscles is a sign of myotonic dystrophy or a denervating disorder. The past medical record, specifically a familial history of muscle disease, may provide an important clue to the diagnosis of those muscle diseases, such as the congenital myopathies, which are hereditary. Among the most revealing laboratory data is the serum level of a creatine kinase (CK), significant elevations of which are indicative of active muscle destruction and point toward a myopathic rather than an atrophic process. Electromyography (EMG) can be invaluable in demonstrating myotonia or myasthenia and in discriminating between myopathic and denervating disorders. Reports of EMG studies are helpful in putting the pathologic picture into the proper perspective in some cases.

In the collection of the biopsy specimen, certain aspects of the routine should be emphasized.[9] A physician familiar with the patient is obligated to ensure that an appropriate muscle is sampled. It is imperative that the biopsy sample be representative of the disease status. Accordingly, if symptoms are confined to the legs, a biopsy of the upper extremity is not likely to accurately reflect the disease process. The biopsy sample should be obtained from a muscle in which the disease is active rather than from a severely affected muscle in which there is considerable weakness or atrophy, since the latter can be expected to reveal end-stage disease that is difficult to interpret. Muscle subjected to previous trauma, such as needle EMG or intramuscular injections of therapeutic drugs, should not be biopsied. The residua of trauma—fiber necrosis, regeneration, inflammation, and endomysial fibrosis—mimic the stigmas of certain neuromuscular diseases and may confuse the pathologist. The biopsy specimen should be removed from the belly of the muscle at a distance from tendinous insertions where normal histology, specifically extreme variability in fiber diameters and numerous internal nuclei, simulate pathologically involved muscle.

In most laboratories two separate specimens, which are employed for different purposes, are routinely submitted. The first specimen is maintained in an isometric state by its insertion into a muscle clamp. Such a device prevents a contraction artifact that results from excision of the specimen and immersion of it into fixative. Not all surgeons agree on the necessity of using a muscle clamp, but in my experience the instrument has several distinct advantages over any alternative method. Inasmuch as the muscle is placed into the clamp in the longitudinal plane, the specimen is automatically oriented for processing. Moreover, use of a clamp ensures that an adequate sample size is obtained, since the specimen must extend across the width of the instrument. Whether or not a clamp is used, the fixed specimen should measure a minimum of 1 cm in length and 0.5 cm in diameter. The fixed sample is dedicated to the preparation of routine paraffin, 1 to 2 μm resin-embedded, and ultrathin sections. A second specimen ideally measuring $1 \times 0.5 \times 0.5$ cm remains unfixed for the preparation of frozen sections. A variety of special techniques have been advocated for tissue freezing. The most important condition governing the procedure is that it permit extremely rapid freezing. Most laboratories enjoy considerable success using liquid nitrogen as the primary freezing medium. Serial frozen sections are generally subjected to a standard panel of stains including hematoxylin and eosin, rapid Gomori trichrome (RTC), ATPase, and an oxidative enzyme reaction such as NADH-TR or succinic dehydrogenase. As required, additional stains such as periodic acid–Schiff (PAS) for glycogen, Oil Red O or other suitable method for fat, phosphorylase, and additional histochemical reactions may be performed. Frozen tissue may also be utilized in selected cases for immunohistochemical or biochemical analysis.

GENERAL REACTIONS OF MUSCLE TO INJURY[8,11,16,40]
Dysvoluminal changes

One of the fundamental manifestations of disease in skeletal muscle is a variation in fiber size, the basis of which may be atrophy or hypertrophy of fibers. Since the integrity of the muscle fiber is contingent upon neural and other homeostatic influences, any compromise of its milieu may encourage fiber atrophy. The most familiar example of atrophy in neuromuscular disease is that associated with denervation. The maintenance of normal fiber volume is predicated on intermittent, regular muscular contraction. Prolonged bed rest or orthopedic immobilization, which does not allow the muscle to engage in sufficient activity, may engender

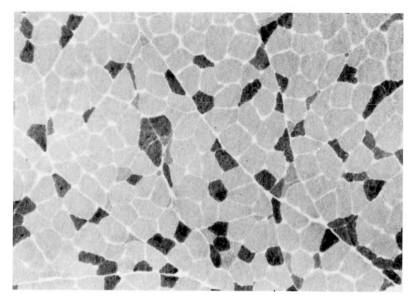

Fig. 41-3. Type 2 fiber atrophy in which the majority of small fibers are darkly stained. (ATPase, pH 9.4; 80×.)

disuse atrophy. Likewise, a reduction in fiber size may represent a complication of malnutrition, aging, or ischemia. Muscle hypertrophy, on the other hand, is principally attributable to increased muscular effort, either from exercise or as a compensatory adjustment of normal intact fibers to the process of atrophy among nearby counterparts. The technique of morphometric analysis may be especially useful when shifts in fiber diameters are minor and equivocal.[6] One can perform morphometry manually by taking measurements directly from a microscopic slide using an eyepiece micrometer or electronically using a computerized apparatus for image analysis. In order to garner statistically significant data, one should record measurements of the lesser diameter of each muscle fiber and the sample should consist of at least 200 fibers. In histochemical preparations, the atrophic or hypertrophic process may be selective, affecting mainly one fiber type, or nonselective, affecting all types.[23] Selective atrophy of type 1 fibers is seen in several of the congenital myopathies but is most commonly encountered in myotonic dystrophy. Type 2 fiber atrophy, in my experience, is most often a sequela of corticosteroid therapy (Fig. 41-3). It is also associated with myasthenia gravis, acute denervation, disuse, and malignancy as a paraneoplastic syndrome.[4] Hypertrophy restricted to type 1 fibers occurs in normal athletes who participate in endurance training programs and in children with Werdnig-Hoffmann disease. Type 2 fiber hypertrophy has been described in sprinters and, as a pathologic incident, in patients with congenital fiber type of disproportion. Nonselective changes in fiber size are quite nonspecific. A large proportion of cases of nonselective atrophy are ascribable to denervation, though nonselective hypertrophy

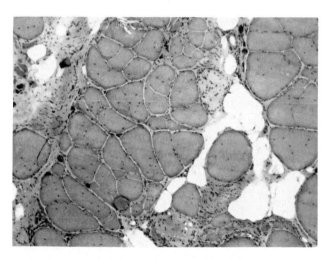

Fig. 41-4. Muscular dystrophy. Increased numbers of internal nuclei and two necrotic muscle fibers are seen. Interstitial fibrosis and fatty infiltration are also evident. (Hematoxylin and eosin, 85×.)

of fibers has also been reported in limb-girdle dystrophy, myotonia congenita, and acromegaly.

Reactions of the sarcolemmal nuclei

Quantitative studies have demonstrated that in cross sections of normal muscle the nuclei are peripheral or subsarcolemmal in 97% of fibers. An augmented population of internalized nuclei are noted in many biopsy specimens from patients with neuromuscular disease (Fig. 41-4). Typically this change affects no more than 10% of fibers. Internal nuclei may be seen in virtually any type of muscle disease, whereas the finding of scores of internal nuclei in the majority of fibers is

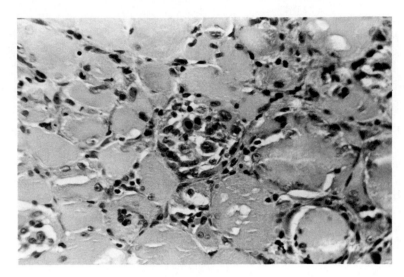

Fig. 41-5. Fiber necrosis in which the large fiber in the center of the field is vacuolated and invaded by macrophages. (Hematoxylin and eosin; 320×.)

highly suspicious for myotonic dystrophy. In contrast to nuclear internalization without compromise to the sarcoplasm, after sarcoplasmic damage the nuclei may no longer remain in a peripheral location. Sarcolemmal nuclei commonly migrate centripetally during the evolution of fiber necrosis and regeneration. Atrophic fibers may also harbor multiple, often pyknotic internal nuclei, which seem to escape significant harm, despite reduction in the sarcoplasmic volume.

Disfigurative changes

Abnormalities of the sarcoplasm, which are usually nonlethal, have been referred to as "disfigurative."[33] Such changes include hyaline, moth-eaten, ragged-red, ring, and target fibers as well as cores, rods, and vacuoles. These are discussed with the individual neuromuscular diseases where they take on the most importance. One of the most common disfigurative alterations is vacuolization of muscle fibers. Vacuolar change after improper freezing of the specimen is a vexing artifact. Vacuoles produced in this way may stimulate bone fide pathologic change, as might be confronted in a vacuolar myopathy, or so distort pathologically affected fibers that accurate morphologic interpretation is impossible. Moreover, vacuoles may also represent abnormal accumulations of glycogen in the glycogenoses or lipid in the rather rare lipid storage diseases.

Fiber necrosis

Fiber necrosis, a minor part of the pathologic reaction in many muscle diseases, is widespread in the muscular dystrophies, particularly Duchenne muscular dystrophy, and in the inflammatory myopathies such as polymyositis and dermatomyositis. In light microscopic

sections stained with hematoxylin and eosin, the first warning of impending necrosis is a departure from the expected color of the sarcoplasm. The acutely necrotic fiber initially assumes a bright eosinophilic tone that is gradually converted to a pale shade of pink. During this interval, the sarcoplasm becomes coarsely granular, vacuolated, and finally fragmented. The sarcolemmal nuclei migrate internally and are pyknotic or karyorrhexic. As necrosis continues, phagocytosis of the dead cellular contents procedes apace (Fig. 41-5). The sarcoplasm is invaded by macrophages, but before the ingestion of all the necrotic debris, the process of restoration has ensued and so myogenesis and phagocytosis may be observed in the same cell simultaneously.

Fiber regeneration

Fiber necrosis seems to serve as a stimulus for subsequent regeneration. Current evidence indicates that the regeneration of fibers may arise by two independent routes. If necrosis is segmental within the fiber, buds of myoplasm from the viable sarcomeres adjacent to the damaged segment are the mediators of the regenerative effort. A second source of regeneration is the satellite cell, which is probably a more important agent in regeneration than sarcoplasmic sprouting.[13] Satellite cells, prompted by cellular injury to transform into myoblasts, have the capacity to synthesize new muscle. Regenerating fibers are rapidly sighted in hematoxylin and eosin sections, wherein the basophilia of their sarcoplasm may be readily appreciated. Ultrastructurally, the regenerating fiber is amply endued with ribosomes, a condition that accounts for its sarcoplasmic basophilia under the light microscope.[36] The nuclei of regenerating fibers are often internalized and numerically increased. They tend to be enlarged and to have dispersed chromatin with prominent nucleoli.

Interstitial reactions

The interstitial compartment surrounding the muscle fibers may also sustain pathologic change. Interstitial inflammatory infiltrates are most often discernible in the immunologically mediated myopathies such as polymyositis-dermatomyositis and in the systemic connective tissue diseases, some of which are stigmatized by vasculitis. Particularly in the setting of chronic neuromuscular disease of either myopathic or neurogenic persuasion, fibrosis and fatty replacement of muscle tend to be prominent (Fig. 41-4). At a point in the disease when they have attained significant proportions, the ardor of an active pathologic process has probably cooled and the likelihood of discovering specific pathologic changes is remote. The biopsy of an end-stage muscle that is not likely to provide relevant diagnostic information should be strongly discouraged.

THE MUSCULAR DYSTROPHIES

The rather unsophisticated term "dystrophy," literally meaning 'poor nourishment,' was popularized at the close of the nineteenth century and has been preserved like the Book of Kells ever since, perhaps in homage to our continuing nescience about the pathogenesis of the muscular dystrophies. Although all the muscular dystrophies, which are collectively similar both clinically and pathologically, have traditionally been considered under a single rubric, this time-honored convention has foundered on such an erroneous oversimplification. In fact, each type of muscular dystrophy is a discrete entity. Nonetheless, in general, these diseases make their debut in childhood or early adulthood. The cardinal symptom is muscular weakness that worsens steadily and unremittingly. Most forms of dystrophy are genetically inherited, and so a family history of neuromuscular difficulties is likely to be elicited in many cases. The pathologic reactions unifying this group of myopathies—fiber necrosis, regenerative activity, and interstitial fibrosis—are more prominent in some types of dystrophy than in others.

Duchenne muscular dystrophy

With a prevalence rate of 3 per 100,000, Duchenne muscular dystrophy (DMD) is the most common member of this disease category. Inherited as an X-linked recessive disorder, in which genetic mapping studies have shown the DMD gene to be situated in band Xp21 on the short arm of the X chromosome,[31] this dystrophy occurs almost exclusively in young boys, the onset in most cases being before 5 years of age. The affected child shows no overt signs of disease at birth, but by the time he begins to ambulate, clumsiness and frequent falling have already become a cause for concern. Weakness, initially in the shoulder, pelvic, and proximal appendicular muscles, is remorselessly progressive and eventually generalized, save for the extraocular, facial, and pharyngeal muscles. Pseudohypertrophy, particularly in muscles of the calves and buttocks, is highly suggestive of DMD. This adventitious enlargement of muscles, which are swollen by fat and fibrous tissue infiltration yet are weak and rubbery, is paradoxical. Cardiac along with striated muscle impairment is not infrequent, giving rise to labile tachycardia and various cardiac arrhythmias. Diminished metal prowess (mean IQ 80) does not correlate with the measure of physical disability and is therefore considered to be an independent component of the disease. The most informative laboratory determination is the serum CK, which soars to very high values prematurely in this condition, preceding detectable pathologic changes in muscle in many cases. Pathologically, the most striking feature of DMD is necrosis and commensurate regeneration of muscle fibers, the intensity of which far surpasses that in other forms of muscular dystrophy. Hyaline or opaque fibers are also more conspicuous than in other dystrophies. These fibers are so named because they are dense and darkly stained in both paraffin and frozen sections. Such fibers tend to be rounded and increased in diameter with smudged, homogeneous cytoplasm. The hyaline appearance has been shown to be secondary to hypercontraction in electron microscopic studies, perhaps incidental to excessive "irritability" of the fiber. The hyaline fiber is believed to represent an nascent phase of cell necrosis.[15] In serial sections of the same fiber, regions of necrosis and phagocytosis can be demonstrated adjacent to hyalinization. Patchy endomysial fibrosis, an expected nonspecific reaction to injury in chronic neuromuscular disease, develops almost from the outset and is disproportionately severe when compared to the destruction of muscle cells.

Facioscapulohumeral dystrophy

Facioscapulohumeral (FSH) dystrophy is a relatively mild disorder principally involving the muscles of the head and neck, shoulders, upper back, and arms. In most pedigrees this dystrophy follows an autosomal dominant mode of inheritance and is equally expressed in males and females. FSH dystrophy starts to exact its toll in the second and third decades. Pseudohypertrophy, mental deficiency, and cardiac dysfunction are not part of the clinical picture. Pathologic review of muscle tissue reveals numerous atrophic and hypertrophic muscle fibers but little fiber necrosis or regeneration. A consistent observation in this disease is the moth-eaten or mottled fiber, which is most convincingly demonstrated in oxidative enzyme reactions. The peculiar uneven staining reaction of fibers is produced by multiple, punctate zones of diminished enzyme activity that are randomly dispersed in the sarcoplasm. The fact that the ultrastructural integrity of the sarcoplasm between zones of mottling is maintained upholds the idea that the mottled fiber represents a form of reversible cell injury. The identification of inflammatory cells, almost exclusively mature lymphocytes, serves to distinguish FSH dystrophy from other dystrophies where inflammation is absent. Inflammatory infiltrates within the endomysium and surrounding perimysial blood vessels are usually only noticeable during the ingravescent states of the illness.

Limb-girdle dystrophy

The hallmark of this disease is a decline in strength in the shoulder and pelvic girdles as well as in the proximal limbs.[14] The clinical course is one of steady deterioration, though the pace is slow, after the first manifestations of myopathy in late adolescence or young adulthood. Most cases are inherited through an autosomal recessive mechanism. Muscular pseudohypertrophy is a significant finding in approximately one third of patients. The pathologic theme in this disorder is epitomized by prominent internalization of sarcolemmal nuclei, fiber atrophy, and often florid fiber hypertrophy associated with widespread fiber splitting. Fiber necrosis and regeneration tend to occur in chronic disease.

Distal myopathy

Distal myopathy is an unusual congener of dystrophy because of its rather atypical clinical features. Enervation and muscle wasting affect primarily the acral muscles of the extremities, generally in males between 40 and 60 years of age. The largest cluster of cases has been reported in the Scandinavian countries where distal myopathy appears to be a dominantly transmitted infirmity. Pathologic examination of muscle shows excessive numbers of internal nuclei, selective atrophy of type 1 fibers, and minimal fiber necrosis and regeneration. In many cases so-called rimmed vacuoles, which ultrastructurally appear to be autophagic vacuoles, have been described.[35]

Myotonic muscular dystrophy

Myotonic muscular dystrophy (MyD) is a common, multisystem disorder that approaches DMD in incidence in certain geographic locations within the United States. MyD is dominantly inherited with variable penetrance, making the age of exordium and the clinical expression somewhat unpredictable. Symptoms become apparent in the average patient during the third or fourth decade. Muscular weakness and tabescence are at first confined to the face and distal portions of the extremities. Hence typical signs are ptosis, a vacant countenance, a slack transverse smile, and difficulty swallowing. Myotonia is an early clue to the patient's

condition and a prerequisite for the diagnosis of MyD. An inability of muscle to relax after contraction, myotonia is a consequence of muscle membrane instability and may be exacerbated during vigorous voluntary muscular contraction or at the bedside by percussion of the muscle with a reflex hammer. Electromyography may be necessary to document myotonia that is clinically silent. The classical systemic semeiology is embodied in ocular cataracts in 90% of patients, testicular atrophy, endocrine disturbances such as hyperinsulinism, cardiomyopathy, and dementia. There may be smooth muscle dysfunction in the esophagus, colon, urinary bladder, or uterus that can be demonstrated with the assistance of appropriate physiologic and roentgenographic studies. In muscle biopsy specimens a multitude of internal nuclei and selective atrophy of type 1 fibers are found initially. Ring fibers, in which a group of peripherally located myofibrils are circumferentially oriented and encircle the normal internal portion of the fiber, are frequently identified without difficulty in MyD. Ring fibers are considered to represent a bona fide pathologic disturbance in MyD, but they may reflect the phenomenon of hypercontractility, since they have been reported in muscle tissue specimens containing contraction artifact. In muscle samples from patients with long-standing disease, the *leitmotif* of dystrophic change—fiber necrosis, regeneration, and reactive fibrosis—is likely to supervene.

CONGENITAL MYOPATHIES

Congenital myopathies are most often manifest in childhood, though not all cases meet the definition of congenital, inasmuch as symptoms are not invariably apparent at birth. Typically the patient exhibits evidence of the floppy infant syndrome—a triad of adaxial weakness, hypotonia, and a poverty of spontaneous activity.[26] Being inherited diseases, the congenital myopathies usually display familial tendencies within a kinship. In contrast to the muscular dystrophies, the clinical course is static, or progressive but at a largo tempo, or sometimes remitting. Conventionally, certain myopathies such as the lipid and glycogen storage diseases and the periodic paralyses, which are congenital disorders, are excluded from this disease category. Although the congenital myopathies are similar from a clinical standpoint, each is distinguished by a characteristic if not a unique morphologic feature. As a result, the muscle biopsy is a valuable tool in the diagnostic evaluation of children with these neuromuscular diseases.

Central core disease

Central core disease was described in a seminal, now-famous publication as a benign, familial, congenital myopathy.[43] This report heralded a new era in which the application of modern techniques, particularly en-

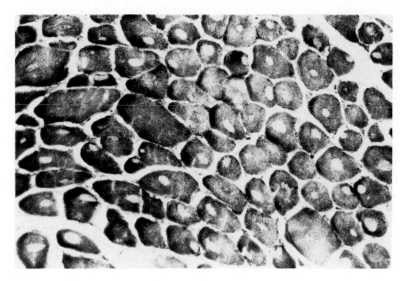

Fig. 41-6. Central core disease. There are numerous focal areas of reduced enzyme activity, which are usually central and singular in the fibers. (NADH-TR; 120×.)

zyme histochemistry and electron microscopy, promoted the discovery of an entire category of neuromuscular disorders. Central core disease is a myopathy of infants and children, causing a delay in the development of motor milestones. Muscle involvement is mild, proximal, and nonprogressive. Within a carefully evaluated family, an autosomal dominant pattern of inheritance usually emerges. In sections of skeletal muscle, cores are visualized as regions of depleted or absent oxidative enzyme activity (Fig. 41-6). Based on ultrastructural appearance, cores may be structured, in which the cross-banding pattern is maintained, or unstructured, in which there is myofibrillar disorganization resulting in an effacement of cross striations.[37] Structured and unstructured cores may coexist in the same specimen. In central core disease, cores are numerous and more prevalent in type 1 fibers. They are likely to be single and centrally positioned inside the fiber. Cores cannot be construed as a totally specific pathologic finding, in light of their occurrence in other diseases, most notably in chronic denervation. Cores, if they are a nonspecific reaction to injury, are confined to only a few fibers and tend to be large, eccentric, and at times multiple within the fiber.

Nemaline (rod) myopathy

Nemaline myopathy may be passed on in accordance with mendelian dominant or recessive precepts and is inexplicably more common in girls. When seen by the pediatrician, the child will lament his or her inability to keep up with peers. During physical examination, a poor motor performance is more pronounced in the facial muscles and proximal muscles of the extremities. The diagnosis may be suspected in patients in whom facial dysmorphism is evident. This peculiar abnormal-

ity is a composite of facial elongation, prognathism of the mandible, and arching of the hard palate. The term "nemaline," derived from the Greek word meaning 'thread' or 'threadlike,' was chosen to underscore the pathologic hallmark of this disease.[44] Rods are difficult to discern in hematoxylin and eosin sections and are ideally detected in rapid Gomori trichrome (RTC) stains on frozen sections and in resin sections (Fig. 41-7). Rods may be haphazardly distributed in the sarcoplasm but more commonly are found as focal subsarcolemmal collections. Electron microscopically, rods are electron-dense and rectangular or cylindrical in shape, having a maximum dimension of 6 to 7 μm. They are in continuity with the Z bands and are believed by many authorities to arise as proliferations of Z band material. Moreover, immunocytochemical studies have demonstrated that rods, like normal Z discs, are partly composed of alpha-actinin. They have a lattice-like ultrastructure, similar to that of the normal Z band,[27] with an axial periodicity of 14 to 20 nm when viewed in the longitudinal plane.[41] After the original description of nemaline myopathy, it has become unavoidably clear that rods are not a unique pathologic attribute. Rods have been reported in many diverse conditions such as muscular dystrophy, polymyositis, peripheral neuropathy, and experimental tenotomy. However, in this context rods are sparse in number and located in only occasional fibers.

Centronuclear myopathy

In transverse microscopic sections, a central or paracentral nucleus is visible within almost every muscle fiber. These abnormally situated nuclei are larger than normal and possess a vesicular chromatin pattern. The sarcoplasm in the immediate vicinity of the nucleus

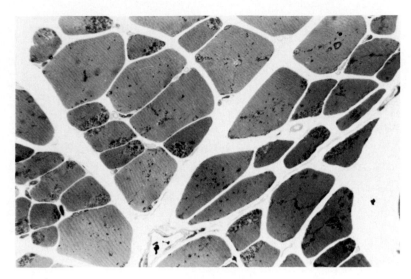

Fig. 41-7. Nemaline myopathy. Large numbers of dark, rod-shaped structures, often in clusters, are present in nearly every fiber. (Resin section, toluidine blue; 320×.)

may be clear, producing a rarefaction or halo that is poorly stained in paraffin sections. This disease, described by Spiro and co-workers as "myotubular myopathy."[45] has been considered by these authors and others to constitute an arrest of muscle maturation because of the resemblance of the muscle biopsy to the fetal myotube stage of muscle development. However, this embryologic explanation has not been widely accepted. Evincing genetic heterogeneity, centronuclear myopathy may be transmitted as a dominant, recessive, or X-linked abnormality. The time of onset is difficult to date and may be delayed until middle age. There is a progression of weakness in some cases, but the extent of eventual disability is unpredictable. Extraocular and facial muscle palsies may accompany the loss of strength in the axial musculature.

Congenital fiber type disproportion

As defined by Brooke,[18] congenital fiber type disproportion has two essential pathologic features—type 1 fiber atrophy and enlargement of type 2 fibers. A predominance of type 1 fibers has been observed in some cases. The genetics in this condition are poorly understood, though congenital fiber type disproportion is presumably inherited in certain families. Both an autosomal recessive and an autosomal dominant mode of inheritance have been suggested. The clinical spectrum ranges from a rapidly fatal disease of infants to an indolent myopathy of midlife adults. Skeletal deformities such as kyphoscoliosis, hip dislocation, joint contractures, high-arched palate, and diminutive stature have been reported in over 50% of patients.[12]

METABOLIC DISEASES
Glycogen storage diseases

Glycogen storage diseases are genetically determined errors of metabolism leading to abnormal cellular accumulations of glycogen. Types II, IV, and VII are routinely associated with polysaccharide storage in skeletal muscle. In such glycogenoses, patients relate a history of muscle fatigue and pain, particularly after exercise or exertion. Because they are unable to break down carbohydrates efficiently, affected individuals cannot generate lactate during ischemic exercise, a deficit that is exploited at the bedside in the ischemic forearm or tourniquet test. A sphygmomanometer cuff is placed on the arm above the elbow and inflated to occlude arterial blood flow. Ischemic exercise of the forearm muscles is induced by instructing the subject to repeatedly squeeze against a standard resistance (that is, an ergometer or similar device) at a rapid rate for a specified period of time, usually 1 to 2 minutes. With exercise, a normal two- to fivefold rise in venous blood lactate fails to occur.

Acid maltase deficiency

The typical clinical presentation of type II glycogenosis is in the guise of the floppy infant syndrome complicated by failure to thrive, macroglossia, cardiomyopathy with cyanosis, hepatomegaly, and intellectual impairment. In late-onset disease during adolescence or adulthood, muscle weakness reminiscent of limb-girdle dystrophy or a congenital myopathy may supersede involvement of other organs.[19] The prognosis is considerably more optimistic than in the fatal infantile form of

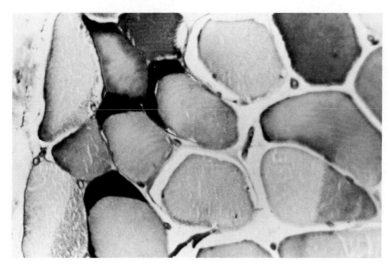

Fig. 41-8. McArdle's disease. Dark, crescentic, strongly PAS-positive regions are evident in several fibers. (PAS; 320×.)

deficiency. Although the natural history is variable, acid maltase deficiency is transcribed by means of a recessive gene in all cases. Pathologic examination of muscle tissue reveals a myriad of vacuoles that disrupt the sarcoplasm of the fibers. The vacuoles are bloated with abundant PAS-positive, diastase-labile granular material that under the electron microscope proves to be membrane-bound collections of glycogen. A deficiency of lysosomal acid maltase or alpha-glucosidase, which cleaves 1,4 and 1,6 glycosidic linkages, cannot be demonstrated histochemically. Therefore a definitive diagnosis depends on biochemical analysis of muscle tissue.

McArdle's disease

Myophosphorylase deficiency, or type V glycogenosis, is a recessively inherited metabolic flaw in which there is a lack of the enzyme responsible for the hydrolysis of alpha-1,4-glycosidic bonds in the glycogen molecule. Beginning in childhood or adolescence, patients complain of muscle weakness, myalgias, and stiffness that are precipitated by exercise. Inspection of the muscle biopsy discloses numerous subsarcolemmal PAS-positive vacuoles that are crescent-shaped or bleb-like, protruding above the surface of the fiber (Fig. 41-8). At the ultrastructural level, masses of glycogen granules are contained within the vacuoles. Histochemical reactions substantiate an absence of phosphorylase activity in fresh-frozen sections.

Phosphofructokinase deficiency

Type VII glycogenosis is transmitted as a autosomal recessive defect and is manifest as a clinical syndrome

closely mimicking McArdle's disease. Pathologically, excess glycogen may be deposited in crescentic vacuoles with a predilection for a subsarcolemmal location. An absence of phosphofructokinase (PFK) can be detected in muscle tissue using histochemical methods. This enzyme facilitates the conversion of fructose-6-phosphate to fructose-1,6-diphosphate in the Embden-Meyerhof pathway. PFK deficiency is not restricted to skeletal muscle and may affect several other cell populations, particularly erythrocytes.

Lipid storage diseases[17]
Carnitine deficiency

In carnitine deficiency, there is insufficient intracellular free L-carnitine, the primary function of which is to shuttle long-chain fatty acids into the mitochondria where they are a major substrate for beta-oxidation. Carnitine is also believed to modulate the intramitochondrial coenzyme A–to–acyl coenzyme A ratio. A derangement in these functions predisposes to an impaired catabolism of fatty acids and clinical symptoms related to poor utilization of fatty acids as an energy source. The syndrome of systemic carnitine deficiency may simulate Reye's syndrome and is typified by acute episodes of encephalopathy, hepatomegaly with hepatic dysfunction, hypoglycemia, cardiac failure, and abnormally low plasma levels of carnitine. Weakness of proximal muscles and myalgias are more profound in the myopathic form of carnitine deficiency where the disease is restricted to skeletal muscle. In both the myopathic and systemic types, symptoms may be noted at any juncture from infancy to middle age, and they fre-

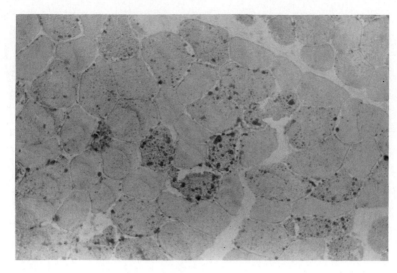

Fig. 41-9. Lipid-storage myopathy. The majority of fibers contain multiple, darkly stained sarcoplasmic vacuoles of varying sizes. (Oil Red O; 125×.)

quently exacerbate with time. In histologic sections, a multitude of lipid droplets, which can be properly identified in fat stains, are seen within muscle fibers (Fig. 41-9). Ultrastructurally, lipid vacuoles do not appear to be membrane bound and are often arranged in parallel rows that distend the intermyofibrillar spaces. Moreover, the mitochondria are enlarged, are atypical in structure, and contain paracrystalline inclusions.

Carnitine palmityltransferase deficiency

Carnitine palmityltransferase (CPT) is an enzyme system with two components, CPT 1 and CPT 2, which promote the coupling of free fatty acids to carnitine in preparation for passage across the mitochondrial membrane. CPT deficiency is associated with exercise-induced cramps and muscle weakness that usually become symptomatic in childhood. A potentially dangerous complication of the disease is recurrent myoglobinuria, often provoked by fasting and prolonged exercise, either alone or in combination. Muscle biopsy specimens between attacks are morphologically unremarkable in most patients. In abnormal biopsy specimens, the extent of lipid accumulation is variable, and the mitochondria display no morphologic alterations.

Mitochondrial myopathies

From both a clinical and biochemical standpoint, those disorders exhibiting mitochondrial abnormalities represent a diverse and heterogeneous group encompassing many pure myopathies in addition to a growing litany of multisystem diseases. Further information addressing this rather confusing subject is cited in the references.[5,47] One way to classify these disorders is to view them as primary or secondary. In the primary disorders, the major focus of pathologic change is on the mitochondria. Often there is a biochemical abnormality that is related to a defect in mitochondrial metabolism. Some of these, like Menkes' syndrome[24] and Zellweger's syndrome,[25] are systemic illnesses that are not limited to skeletal muscle. A preeminent feature of several mitochondrial myopathies is progressive ptosis and external ophthalmoplegia, most notably in the Kearns-Sayre syndrome[7] and oculocraniosomatic neuromuscular disease with ragged-red fibers.[38] In the secondary disorders, however, some underlying clinical condition, such as lipid storage disease or hypothyroidism, appears to foster the mitochondrial changes, which are only a minor element in the overall pathologic process.

The morphologic abnormalities affecting mitochondria are rather stereotyped and qualitatively similar in most of the mitochondrial myopathies. Thus, it is not feasible to devise a classification of the mitochondrial myopathies or base a definitive diagnosis solely upon morphologic criteria. Ragged-red fibers, a sentinel finding, are conveniently identified in frozen sections stained by the RTC method (Fig. 41-10). Such abnormal fibers stand out by virtue of bright red, nodular foci that elevate the sarcolemma and create an irregular, ragged cellular margin. Ragged-red fibers may evince an equally intense reaction in oxidative enzyme stains. Large aggregates of mitochondria appear as dark, coarsely granular deposits that may be subsarcolemmal in location or disseminated throughout the fiber. Ultrastructurally, ragged-red fibers are replete with mitochondria that are enlarged and aberrant in shape. They frequently possess an overabundance of cristae, which are either excessively branched, concentrically arranged, or totally disorganized. A variety of intramito-

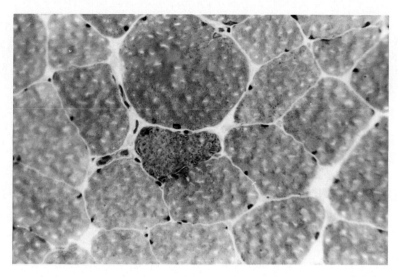

Fig. 41-10. Mitochondrial myopathy. Ragged red fiber with coarsely granular, somewhat darker sarcoplasm and irregular cellular borders. (RTC; 320×.)

chondrial inclusions may be encountered, the most common being lucent vacuoles, floccular matrix densities, glycogen aggregates, myelin-like membranous profiles, and paracrystalline structures. The last are square or rectangular in conformation and grid-like under low magnification. Paracrystalline inclusions are located either in the intracristal spaces or between the inner and outer mitochondrial membranes and are organized into sets of parallel, intersecting osmiophilic membranes separated by narrow clear spaces.

INFLAMMATORY AND IMMUNE-MEDIATED MYOPATHIES
Polymyositis and dermatomyositis complex

The polymyositis and dermatomyositis complex (PM/DM) is the most frequently biopsied myopathy in adults and accounts for 25% of all cases in my files. The majority of patients seek medical attention between 20 and 40 years of age. The incidence in women is approximately twice that in men. Individuals initially experience difficulty in ambulation, particularly with climbing stairs and arising from a chair. Myalgias, muscle tenderness, and dysphagia are also disconcerting. Symptoms are somewhat sudden in their appearance and rapidly advancing in many patients, reaching a crescendo over a period of several weeks. Frequent concomitant problems are fever, arthralgias, Raynaud's phenomenon, and malaise. Remissions and exacerbations occasion a desultory clinical course, even when corticosteroids, which are the treatment of choice for PM/DM, are not administered promptly. The cynosure of DM is a blotchy, erythematous, or tachetic rash involving the eyelids, face, and extensor surfaces of the hands and feet, especially the knuckles. The serum CK

and erythrocyte sedimentation rate are characteristically elevated. Electromyographic evaluation indicates that the motor unit potentials are reduced in amplitude, brief in duration, and polyphasic. A clinical complex indistinguishable from PM or DM may represent a complication of virtually any of the systemic connective diseases. In about 20% of cases, PM/DM is discovered to be a paraneoplastic syndrome that has a greater prevalence in males and in people of both sexes over 50 years of age in whom carcinomas of the lung, colon, and breast are found. Signs and symptoms of a neoplasm may precede the onset of neuromuscular disease or remain occult for months after the diagnosis of PM/DM.

PM/DM is an idiopathic, autoimmune disease in which lymphocytes, presumably T-cells, are in some way sensitized to skeletal muscle, which they come to view as antigenic. This cell-mediated reaction causes necrosis of muscle fibers and the subsequent attempts at repair that are observed histologically as fiber regeneration. The target tissue is invaded by activated lymphocytes, which penetrate the endomysium and surround their prey, necrotic muscle fibers (Fig. 41-11). Some infiltration of intramuscular blood vessels is seen without evidence of true vasculitis. Neutrophils, eosinophils, and plasma cells are excluded from the ensemble of inflammatory elements. In studies employing direct immunofluorescence techniques, deposits of immunoglobulins and complement have been reported in PM/DM,[39] but I have not been impressed by such reactants in PM.[28] As a matter of fact, in my laboratory, the demonstration of immune deposits in skeletal muscle tissue militates against the diagnosis of adult polymyositis.

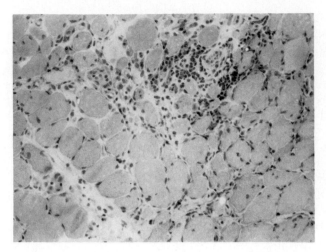

Fig. 41-11. Polymyositis. Collections of lymphocytes in the endomysium surrounding several muscle fibers. (Hematoxylin and eosin; 212×.)

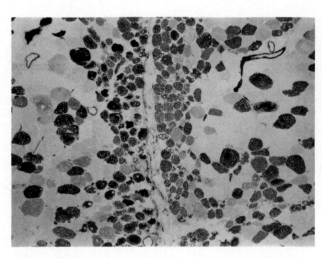

Fig. 41-12. Dermatomyositis. There is selective atrophy of fibers at the periphery of the fascicles. (ATPase, pH 9.4; 85×.)

Childhood dermatomyositis

As opposed to classical adult DM, childhood DM is a systemic disorder with extension beyond skeletal muscle to skin, subcutaneous tissues, alimentary tract, and peripheral nerve.[3] This inflammatory myopathy is most common in girls who are approaching puberty. One is surprised to find more than a modicum of inflammation or fiber necrosis morphologically. For obscure reasons, perifascicular atrophy, in which nearly all small fibers are located at the periphery of the fascicles, is an almost constant observation in this disease (Fig. 41-12). Deposition of immunoglobulins, particularly IgG, and complement can be detected in the walls of intramuscular blood vessels. These deposits are adjudged to be the result of an immunologically mediated vasculopathy that ultimately reduces the size of the muscular capillary bed.[10] Undulating tubular profiles, superficially resembling virions, have been noted in endothelial cells by electron microscopy, but their significance is unknown at present.[2]

Myasthenia gravis

Myasthenia gravis is a chronic, autoimmune disease that has received considerable attention throughout the past decade.[32] Recent research indicates that a humoral mechanism plays a pivotal role in the pathogenesis of myasthenia gravis, in that patients with this disease synthesize circulating antibodies against the postsynaptic receptor protein at the motor end plate (MEP). These antibodies bind to the postsynaptic membrane of the MEP, blocking neuromuscular transmission and initiating the phenomenon of myasthenia. Furthermore, the binding of antibody at postsynaptic sites ac-

tivates the complement cascade and a complement-dependent destruction of the end-plate region ensues.[20] The ultrastructural evidence for this process is the eventual simplification of the junctional folds and a widening of the synaptic clefts at the MEP.[42] In routine muscle biopsy specimens, examination of the MEP region by electron microscopy is generally impractical, since the end plates are primarily localized to the innervation zone of the muscle, which can be properly identified only by electrical stimulation while the biopsy is being performed. Experimentally, the pathogenesis of human myasthenia gravis has been elucidated by injection of animals with purified acetylcholine receptor, resulting in the production of antibodies against the motor end plate and the development of autoimmune myasthenia gravis.

Myasthenia gravis is more prevalent in young adult females with a peak age of onset before 40 years. Patients typically suffer from easy fatigability and muscular fecklessness that is worse at the end of the day. At first, symptoms predominate in the extraocular and facial muscles, prompting complaints of diplopia, dysphagia, and dysarthria. The clinical diagnosis depends heavily upon a salutary response to anticholinesterase agents such as edrophonium and punctilious electromyographic examination during which a decrement in motor-action potentials evoked by repetitive stimulation is documented. In my experience, the muscle biopsy sample is frequently unremarkable or characterized by a nonspecific atrophy. The well-known diagnostic parameter of moderate to severe type 2 fiber atrophy is present in only about 50% of cases. Its immune-oriented pathogenesis notwithstanding, myas-

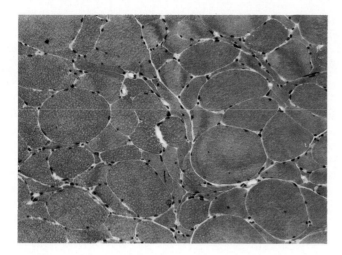

Fig. 41-13. Denervation atrophy. Numerous small, angular fibers are seen. (Hematoxylin and eosin; 212×.)

thenia gravis is not a prototype of inflammatory myopathy. Small focal lymphocytic infiltrates are appreciated in muscle tissue only in exceptional cases.

DENERVATING DISEASES

As mentioned previously, the welfare of the muscle fiber is intimately linked to the preservation of its nerve supply. Any disruption of these neural trophic influences will probably subject the myofiber to adverse dysvoluminal changes. Neurogenic atrophy may stem from disease of the anterior horn cell, exemplified by amyotrophic lateral sclerosis and Werdnig-Hoffmann

disease, or from injury to its myelinated axon, most commonly against a clinical background of peripheral neuropathy. It should be pointed out that, statistically, the most important neuromuscular disorders are neurogenic in origin, more than 80% of which in my experience are attributable to some form of peripheral nerve disease. A consideration of the peripheral neuropathies is a ambitious topic in itself, beyond the pale of the discussion here.

With the exception of Werdnig-Hoffmann disease, the pathologic effects of denervation are essentially the same in all neurogenic atrophies.[1] During acute denervation, atrophic fibers are randomly scattered. Abnormally small fibers are angular or ensiform when cut transversely, with tapered or pointed, rather than gradually curving, edges (Fig. 41-13). At this stage, many or all of the atrophic fibers are glycolytic in type. If denervation continues unabated, the population of atrophic type 1 and type 2 fibers approaches parity. Advanced denervation is typified by a pattern of atrophy that progresses from one of random distribution to one in which there is grouping of affected fibers. Grouped atrophy is usually recognized in the presence of multiple aggregations of five or more small, ensiform fibers in the tissue sample (Fig. 41-14). At the same time, the normal checkerboard staining profile obtained in histoenzymatic reactions is distorted as a consequence of type grouping, denoted by unnaturally large congeries of muscle fibers having identical histochemical properties (Fig. 41-15). Type grouping occurs when residual, intact intramuscular nerve fibers send out collateral sprouts to reestablish innervation to denervated, atrophic fibers.[34] For practical purposes, target fibers

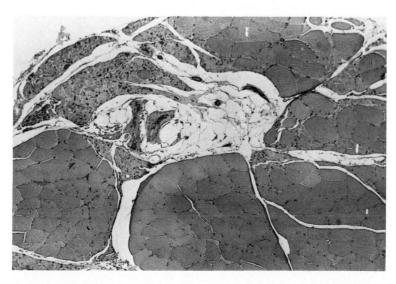

Fig. 41-14. Chronic denervation atrophy. Several groups of atrophic fibers are present in the section. (Hematoxylin and eosin; 60×.)

are pathognomonic of chronic denervation,[22] though they are encountered in fewer than 25% of cases of neurogenic atrophy. Despite certain similarities, targets are not synonymous with cores. In contrast to the core, the target boasts a three-zone architecture (Fig. 41-16). The bull's-eye or central zone, imitative of an unstructured core, is surrounded by an intermediate zone, a rim that is darkly stained in oxidative enzyme reactions. The intermediate zone, not part of the core lesion, is one of the pathologic transition between the severely disrupted center zone and the third zone, which is the outer portion of the fiber composed of intact sarcoplasm.

Amyotrophic lateral sclerosis

Amyotrophic lateral sclerosis (ALS), or motor neuron disease, is a feral disorder in which skeletal muscle is at the mercy of a gradual, inexorable destruction of upper and lower motor neurons in the central nervous system. The illness begins insidiously in adults at the prime of life, who experience an erosion of strength, betrayed by muscle wasting that is more evident distally. Bulbar muscle dysfunction accompanied by dysphagia and dysarthria signify an ominous prognosis. Muscle fasciculations, spasticity, hypertonia and hyperreflexia, and Babinski responses are noteworthy signs in the physical examination. Once a diagnosis is made, ALS pursues a path that renders the victim bedfast in a span of 2 to 5 years.

Werdnig-Hoffmann disease

Infantile spinal muscular atrophy is the commonest neurogenic disease in the pediatric age group. This disorder is typically ushered in as the floppy infant syndrome in which there is sparing of the sensory system and mentation. The tremulous cry, feeble suck, poor head control, and respiratory distress are attributable to pronounced generalized weakness. Fasciculations may be discernible in the tongue but are difficult to appreciate elsewhere. In this familial, recessively inherited condition, as a rule the age of onset determines the natural history of the disease. The sooner the symptoms are diagnosed, the more guarded is the prognosis. Par-

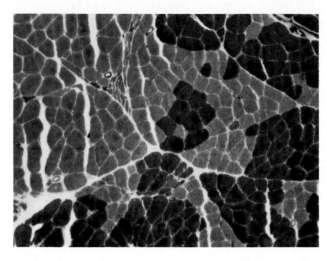

Fig. 41-15. Denervation atrophy with reinnervation. Type-grouping replaces the normal checkerboard staining pattern. (ATPase, pH 9.4; 85×.)

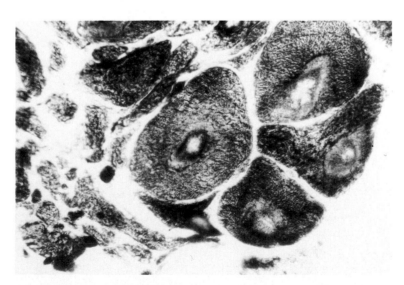

Fig. 41-16. Chronic denervation. Several target fibers are seen. The fiber at the center with a poorly reactive inner zone surrounded by a densely stained rim exhibits a typical three-zone architecture. (NADH-TR; 320×.)

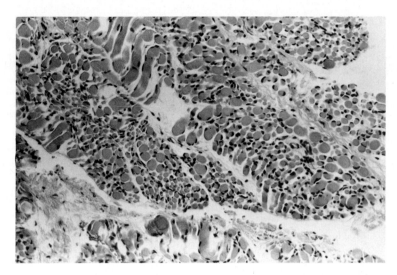

Fig. 41-17. Werdnig-Hoffmann disease. Many fibers within each fascicle are small and rounded in configuration. (Hematoxylin and eosin; 150×.)

ents of children with Werdnig-Hoffmann disease are haunted by the prospect that life expectancy seldom exceeds 18 months. Unlike other denervating conditions, the atrophic process in infantile spinal muscular atrophy, where only lower motor neurons are damaged, is very diffuse, affecting nearly every fascicle. The majority of fibers within each fascicle are small and rounded (Fig. 41-17). Interspersed among the denervated myocytes are variable numbers of fibers that are hypertrophic or normal in size. In some cases, there is selective hypertrophy of type 1 fibers.

REFERENCES

1. Armbrustmacher, V.W.: Skeletal muscle in denervation. In Sommers, S.C., and Rosen, P.P., editors: Pathology Annual, New York, 1978, Appleton-Century-Crofts.
2. Banker, B.Q.: Dermatomyositis of childhood: ultrastructural alterations of muscle and intramuscular blood vessels, J. Neuropathol. Exp. Neurol. **34**:46, 1975.
3. Banker, B.Q., and Victor, M.: Dermatomyositis (systemic angiopathy) of childhood, Medicine **45**:261, 1966.
4. Barron, S.A., and Heffner, R.R.: Weakness in malignancy: evidence for a remote effect of tumor on distal axons, Ann. Neurol. **4**:268, 1978.
5. Bauserman, S.C., and Heffner, R.R.: Mitochondrial myopathies. In Heffner, R.R., editor: Muscle pathology, New York, 1984, Churchill Livingstone.
6. Bennington, J.L., and Krupp, M.: Morphometric analysis of muscle. In Heffner, R.R., editor: Muscle pathology, New York, 1984, Churchill Livingstone.
7. Berenberg, R.A., Pollock, J.N., DiMauro, S., et al.: Lumping or splitting: "ophthalmoplegia-plus" or Kearns-Sayre syndrome, Ann. Neurol. **1**:37, 1977.
8. Bethlem, J.: Myopathies, ed. 2, New York, 1980, Elsevier Science Publications.
9. Bossen, E.H.: Collection and preparation of the muscle biopsy, In Heffner, R.R., editor: Muscle pathology, New York, 1984, Churchill Livingstone.
10. Carpenter, S., Karpati, G., Rothman, S., et al.: The childhood type of dermatomyositis, Neurology **26**:952, 1976.
11. Carpenter, S., and Karpati, G.: Pathology and skeletal muscle, New York, 1984, Churchill Livingstone.
12. Clancy, R.R., Kelts, K.A., and Oehlert, J.W.: Clinical variability in congenital fiber type disproportion, J. Neurol. Sci. **46**:257, 1980.
13. Chou, S.M., and Nonaka, I.: Satellite cells and muscle regeneration in diseased human skeletal muscles, J. Neurol. Sci. **34**:131, 1977.
14. Chutkow, J.G., Heffner, R.R., Jr., Kramer, A.A., and Edwards, J.A.: Adult-onset autosomal dominant limb-girdle muscular dystrophy, Ann. Neurol. **20**:240, 1986.
15. Cullen, M.J., and Fulthrope, J.J.: Stages in fiber breakdown in Duchenne muscular dystrophy, J. Neurol. Sci. **24**:179, 1975.
16. DeGirolami, U., and Smith, T.W.: Pathology of skeletal muscle diseases, Am. J. Pathol. **107**:235, 1982.
17. DiMauro, S., Trevisan, C., and Hays, A.: Disorders of lipid metabolism in muscle, Muscle Nerve **3**:369, 1980.
18. Dubowitz, V., and Brooke, M.H.: Muscle biopsy: a modern approach, Philadelphia, 1973, W.B. Saunders.
19. Engel, A.G., Gomez, M.R., Seybold, M.E., and Lambert, E.H.: The spectrum and diagnosis of acid maltase deficiency, Neurology **23**:95, 1973.
20. Engel, A.G., Lambert, E.H., and Howard, F.M.: Immune complexes (IgG and C3) at the motor end-plate in myasthenia gravis: ultrastructural and light microscopic localization and electrophysiologic correlations, Mayo Clin. Proc. **52**:267, 1977.
21. Engel, A.G., and Banker, B.Q.: Myology, New York, 1986, McGraw-Hill Book Co.
22. Engel, W.K.: Muscle target fibers, a newly recognized sign of denervation, Nature **191**:389, 1961.
23. Engel, W.K.: Selective and nonselective susceptibility of muscle fiber types: a new approach to human neuromuscular diseases, Arch. Neurol. **22**:97, 1970.
24. Ghatak, N.R., Hirano, A., Poon, T.P., and French, J.H.: Trichopoliodystrophy. II. Pathological changes in skeletal muscle and nervous system, Arch. Neurol. **26**:60, 1972.
25. Goldfischer, S., Moore, C.L., Johnson, A.B., et al.: Peroxisomal and mitochondrial defects in the cerebro-hepato-renal syndrome, Science **182**:62, 1973.

26. Greenfield, J.G., Cornman, T., and Shy, G.M.: The prognostic value of the muscle biopsy in the "floppy infant." Brain **81**:461, 1958.
27. Heffner, R.R.: Electron microscopy of disorders of skeletal muscle, Ann. Clin. Lab. Sci. **5**:338, 1975.
28. Heffner, R.R., Barron, S.A., Jenis, E.H., and Valeski, J.E.: Skeletal muscle in polymyositis: immunohistochemical study, Arch. Pathol. Lab. Med. **103**:310, 1979.
29. Heffner, R.R., editor: Muscle pathology, New York, 1984, Churchill Livingstone.
30. Heffner, R.R.: Muscle biopsy in the diagnosis of neuromuscular disease, Semin. Diagn. Pathol. **1**:114, 1984.
31. Hejtmancik, J.F., Harris, S.G., Tsao, C.C., et al.: Carrier diagnosis of Duchenne muscular dystrophy using restriction fragment length polymorphisms, Neurology **36**:1553, 1986.
32. Johns, T.R.: Myasthenia gravis, Semin. Neurol. **2**:193, 1982.
33. Kakulas, B.A., and Adams, R.D.: Diseases of muscle, Philadelphia, 1985, Harper & Row, Publishers.
34. Karpati, G., and Engel, W.K.: "Type grouping" in skeletal muscles after experimental reinnervation, Neurology **18**:447, 1968.
35. Markesbery, W.R., Griggs, R.C., and Herr, B.: Distal myopathy: electron microscopic and histochemical studies, Neurology **27**:727, 1977.
36. Mastaglia, F.L., Dawkins, R.L., and Papadimitriou, J.M.: Morphological changes in skeletal muscle after transplantation: a light and electron-microscopic study of the initial phases of degeneration and regeneration, J. Neurol. Sci. **25**:227, 1975.
37. Neville, H.E., and Brooke, M.H.: Central core fibers: structured and unstructured. In Kakulas, B.A., editor: Basic research in myology, Proc. Second International Congress on Muscle Diseases, Amsterdam, 1973, Excerpta Medica.
38. Olson, W., Engel, W.K., Walsh, G.O., and Einaugler, R.: Oculocraniosomatic neuromuscular disease with "ragged-red" fibers, Arch. Neurol. **26**:193, 1972.
39. Oxenhandler, R., Adelstein, E.H., and Hart, M.N.: Immunopathology of skeletal muscle: the value of direct immunofluorescence in the diagnosis of connective tissue disease, Hum. Pathol. **8**:321, 1977.
40. Pearson, C.M., and Mostofi, F.K., editors: The striated muscle, Baltimore, 1973, The Williams & Wilkins Co.
41. Price, H.M., Gordon, G.B., Pearson, C.M., et al.: New evidence for excessive accumulation of Z-band material in nemaline myopathy, Proc. Natl. Acad. Sci. USA **54**:1398, 1965.
42. Santa, T., Engel, A.G., and Lambert, E.H.: Histometric study of neuromuscular junction ultrastructure. I. Myasthenia gravis, Neurology **22**:71, 1972.
43. Shy, G.M., and Magee, K.R.: A new congenital non-progressive myopathy, Brain **79**:610, 1957.
44. Shy, G.M., Engel, W.K., Sommers, J.E., and Wanko, T.: Nemaline myopathy: a new congenital myopathy, Brain **86**:793, 1963.
45. Spiro, A.J., Shy, G.M., and Gonatas, N.K.: Myotubular myopathy: persistence of fetal muscle in an adolescent boy, Arch. Neurol. **14**:1, 1966.
46. Swash, S., and Schwartz, M.S.: Neuromuscular diseases, New York, 1981, Springer Publishing Co., Inc.
47. Tassin, S., and Brucher, J.M.: The mitochondrial disorders: pathogenesis and aetiological classification, Neuropathol. Appl. Neurobiol. **8**:251, 1982.
48. Walton, J.N., editor: Disorders of voluntary muscle, ed. 4, Edinburgh, 1981, Churchill Livingstone.

42 Pathology of the Nervous System

JAMES S. NELSON

EVOLUTION OF NEUROPATHOLOGY

Neuropathology emerged as a distinct discipline during the latter half of the nineteenth century. Stimulated by the possibility of a clearer understanding and explanation of human actions and behavior, European neuroscientists, particularly in Germany and France, conducted systematic morphologic studies of the diseased human brain. The German approach, led by Weigert, Nissl, and Alzheimer, focused on the anatomic changes in neurons and glia associated with various disease states and the etiologic and pathogenetic insights provided by these phenomena. These scientists, followed by Jakob and Spielmeyer, supplemented the human data with experimental studies. The French school, on the other hand, influenced by Charcot, emphasized the correlation between neurologic signs and symptoms and the anatomic location of lesions. This information formed a basis for inferences regarding the function of tracts, nuclei, and other anatomic components of the human brain.[85] Modern diagnostic neuropathology represents an attempt to combine the French and German goals. Thus the successful practice of diagnostic neuropathology requires not only a detailed knowledge of anatomic pathology, but clinical and neuroanatomic sophistication as well. Furthermore, the growing availability of elegant and dynamic neuro-imaging techniques has not attenuated the need for clinicopathologic skills on the part of the neuropathologist. These studies are a source of valuable information and insight for the neuropathologist because of his ability to integrate readily the newer observations with knowledge of the pathology and pathogenesis of disease states. As a corollary, the neuropathologist can provide his colleagues roaming the "Valley of the Shadows" with a rational basis for interpreting their observations.

In the United States the practice of neuropathology did not become a viable full-time occupation until some time after 1950. Before that, neuropathology needs were met by clinicians, usually neurologists, or by general anatomic pathologists on a part-time basis. Physicians devoting their professional and scientific efforts exclusively to neuropathology could be found in only a very few institutions. The first subspecialty examination in neuropathology was given by the American Board of Pathology in 1948. Two neuropathologists, Dr. Webb Haymaker and Dr. Helena Riggs, were certified.[1] The growth of clinical neurology, neurosurgery, and the basic neurosciences that began after World War II significantly increased the demands for neuropathology skills and influenced the eventual creation of full-time neuropathology positions at major medical institutions. The need for accurate, meaningful, and reliable neuropathologic diagnosis increased with the development of refined, costly, and sometimes hazardous approaches to patient management and therapy. The special requirements for residency training programs in neuropathology were first published in the *1971-1972 Directory of Approved Internships and Residencies*. The first published list of accredited training programs in neuropathology appeared in the directory for 1972-1973.[1] At present the probable course which United States neuropathology will follow remains uncertain. During the initial phase of its growth considerable financial support was derived from the National Institutes of Health chiefly through training grants. With the attenuation of these funds and the highly competitive research grant environment, very few extramural dollars find their way into most neuropathology budgets. Neuropathologic diagnostic efforts, though necessary and time consuming, are not of sufficient volume at any institution to support even one full-time neuropathologist. The extensive teaching contributions chiefly to clinical colleagues and expected by them often lack corresponding financial support. The future development of neuropathology depends on solving the problem of supporting, maintaining, and periodically repopulating a neuropathology cadre commensurate with this country's medical requirements.

GROUND RULES OF NEUROPATHOLOGY

The principles of general anatomic pathology are relevant to neuropathology. The following ground rules, or guidelines, should be considered when one is applying those principles to the pathology of the nervous system.

1. Neurologic diseases may be primary or secondary disorders. Primary diseases, such as multiple sclerosis, are those that develop initially within the parenchymal and supporting elements of the nervous system. Secondary conditions, such as hepatic encephalopathy, are those that arise as complications of extraneural disorders. Admittedly, the application of this distinction may be debated in some cases. The important point to be kept in mind, however, is that neurologic disturbances and lesions may be an indication of either a significant extraneural pathologic condition or intrinsic disease of the nervous system. For the neuropathologist, sorting out these relationships is an important part of the evaluation and interpretation of a brain biopsy specimen or postmortem neuropathologic findings. The assessment is based upon an integration of data from clinical, laboratory, and pathology studies, studies of previous cases, and the neuropathologist's experience.

2. The diagnosis and classification of neurologic diseases are often based upon a combination of clinical and pathologic criteria, including the anatomic distribution of the lesions. There are relatively few instances in which the pathologic findings alone are pathognomonic of a specific disease. The subacute encephalitis with multinucleated cells caused by HIV-1 infection of the brain may be one such example.[168] In contrast, the diagnosis of amyotrophic lateral sclerosis is based on motor neuron loss with astrocytosis and corticospinal tract degeneration as well as the clinical characteristics of the patient's illness.

3. Neurologic signs and symptoms are influenced by the inciting disease, the part of the nervous system affected, and the rate at which the disease evolves. The clinical features of infarction of the spinal cord are very different from those of cerebral infarction. Further, the symptoms of cerebral infarction caused by sudden vascular occlusion, such as embolism, are often different from those produced when the occlusion develops more slowly in the case of thrombosis. These considerations of location and rate of evolution are sometimes emphasized dramatically when a slowly growing tumor such as a meningioma involves a relatively clinically silent part of the brain such as the right subfrontal area. By the time symptoms are recognizable the tumor may, by central nervous system standards, have become enormous. Similarly, the early, subtle indications of a slowly progressive degenerative disease may go unnoticed until its extent causes obvious functional disturbance. If this unmasking happens to coincide with some chance event such as head trauma, or emotional stress etiologic importance may be erroneously attributed to the event.

4. The nervous system is a complex anatomic structure with widely divergent parts. In postmortem studies, in contrast to the comparatively small number of histologic sections required for adequate examination of anatomically homogeneous organs such as liver or kidney, microscopic examination of the major anatomic subdivisions of the nervous system and, if indicated, skeletal muscle is necessary to accomplish satisfactory neuropathologic evaluation. The diagnostic importance of determining the anatomic distribution of lesions has been mentioned previously. The selection of specimens for microscopic examination is guided by the set of neurologic symptoms and the gross examination. In addition, sections of the superior frontal gyrus with the adjacent arterial boundary zone, hippocampus, corpus striatum, midbrain, caudal pons, mid- or caudal medulla, cerebellar hemisphere with dentate nucleus, and cervical, thoracic, and lumbar areas of the spinal cord are examined routinely in cases of neurologic interest. Representative coronal sections of the cerebrum, cross sections of brainstem, sagittal sections of cerebellum, and cross sections of spinal cord are saved in formalin at least until final disposition of the case. When the disease process extends to peripheral nerve and skeletal muscle sections of the brachial and the lumbosacral plexuses, sciatic nerve, sural nerve, and proximal and distal skeletal muscle from the upper and lower extremities are examined. Specimens from the right and left sides of the body should be included to help determine the symmetry and distribution of the lesions. In cerebrovascular disorders attention is directed to the cervical arteries of the anterior and posterior circulation and to the intracranial vascular channels (including the dural venous sinuses).

5. The central and peripheral divisions of the nervous system have different regenerative capacities. In the central nervous system, repair and recovery involves chiefly anatomic reduction of structural defects or organization of damaged parenchyma by proliferation of astrocytes and sometimes fibroblasts. The latter cells are derived mainly from the walls of blood vessels. Proliferation of mature neurons does not occur. Regrowth of disrupted axons and collateral axonal sprouting takes place only to a very limited extent. Thus full functional recovery from larger central nervous system lesions is unlikely. On the other hand, axonal regeneration does take place in the peripheral nervous system and restoration of normal function is observed after recovery from some peripheral neuropathies such as acute idiopathic polyneuritis (Guillain-Barré disease).

6. Selective vulnerability is a concept often used to explain the preferential damage to certain regions or structures in the nervous system observed in generalized metabolic disturbances (hypoxia, intoxications), viral infections, and degenerative diseases. The affected structures may consist of functionally related tracts and nuclei. This pattern of injury is referred to as a "systematized disease." Examples include amyotrophic lateral sclerosis and the spinocerebellar degenerations.

Selective vulnerability may involve discrete nuclei or groups of neurons as is the case with hypoxic damage to the hippocampal cortex or hemorrhagic necrosis of the medial temporal lobes in herpes simplex type 1 encephalitis. The concept may even be extended to subcellular structures, such as the myelin sheath in multiple sclerosis. The basis for the selectivity is often uncertain. In the case of hypoxia or intoxication the vascular supply (distal arterial perfusion bed) or the metabolic characteristics of the tissue (energy reserves, sensitive enzymes) may be influencing factors. The presence or absence of cell receptors may determine the localization of viral lesions.

7. Neurons, astrocytes, axons, myelin sheaths and other structures are unique to the nervous system. The study of neuropathology necessitates familiarity with the normal morphologic variations of these structures and their alterations in response to injury.

MORPHOLOGIC TECHNIQUES USED IN NEUROPATHOLOGY

The autopsy procedure for removal of the brain depends, in part, on whether the cranial sutures are open or closed. The cranial cavity is opened either by cutting along suture lines or sawing off the calverium. The spinal cord may be removed anteriorly after sectioning of the vertebral bodies or posteriorly, after laminectomy. The anterior method is generally more convenient except for dissection of the cervical cord, portions of which are usually left behind when the anterior approach is used. Cranial and spinal nerve roots remain attached to the brain and spinal cord. Sensory ganglia are dissected as required. The presence or suspicion of infectious disease particularly HIV and Creutzfeldt-Jakob disease requires special precautions. In case of Creutzfeldt-Jakob disease these precautions extend to formalin-fixed tissue, which can be used to transmit the disease.[48]

Various fixatives have been used in neuropathology studies most often aimed at enhancing the effects of a particular stain. At present in the United States the best general fixative for routine surgical and autopsy neuropathology studies is 10% neutral buffered formalin. For electron microscopy, specimens are fixed in 3% phosphate-buffered glutaraldehyde or buffered solutions of paraformaldehyde and glutaraldehyde. The best fixation is obtained when intravascular perfusion of the specimen is possible. Most human neural tissue is fixed by immersion though some degree of perfusion fixation can be achieved if postmortem brains are injected with formalin through the major arteries at their base.

Neural tissue may be embedded in either paraffin or celloidin for light microscopic studies. The paraffin method is much faster and permits utilization of a wider range of stains than the celloidin procedure. It is the technique employed most often in the United States. The celloidin method is valuable for the preparation of large specimens, such as a coronal section of cerebrum, to determine patterns of injury, for the study of delicate normal and malformed fetal and neonatal brains, and for morphometric investigations. Electron microscopy specimens are commonly embedded in epon, epon araldite, or Spurr's medium. Fresh or fixed tissues for histochemical studies involving enzymes, lipids, carbohydrates, or antigens (immunohistochemistry) are rapidly frozen in isopentane chilled at least to $-80°$ C and sectioned without embedding in a cryostat.

Both special stains for selective demonstration of neural structures as well as stains for collagen, reticulin, carbohydrates, microorganisms, and so on are used in diagnostic neuropathology. The characteristics of the common stains for neural tissues are summarized in Table 42-1. The array of special stains traditionally associated with neuropathology studies is being supplanted by conventional and immunohistochemical procedures, ultrastructural studies including the use of 1 μm–thick plastic sections stained with alkaline toluidine blue, and by better familiarity with the morphologic features of nervous system injury delineated with routine stains. The immunostains of importance in diagnostic neuropathology apply mainly to tumors and are covered in that section of the chapter. The special procedures used for peripheral nerve examination are briefly summarized in the section concerning diseases of the peripheral nervous system.

DISEASES OF THE CENTRAL NERVOUS SYSTEM
General reactions to injury

The following pathologic conditions that accompany a variety of central nervous system diseases are considered in this section: brain edema, increased intracranial pressure and brain herniations, hydrocephalus, and the reactions of neurons and glia to injury.

Brain edema

Brain edema is defined as an increase in the brain's volume because of an increase in its water and sodium content. A significant degree of brain edema may occur in head injury, stroke, infection, lead encephalopathy, hypoxia, hypo-osmolality, the disequilibrium syndromes associated with dialysis and diabetic ketoacidosis, and some forms of obstructive hydrocephalus.[70] Klatzo[114] has classified brain edema according to its pathogenesis as either vasogenic or cytotoxic. A third type called "intestitial or hydrocephalic edema" is sometimes added to the classification.[69,130]

Vasogenic edema results from increased permeability of the cerebrovascular endothelial blood-brain barrier

Table 42-1. Diagnostic neuropathology stains

Stain and section preparation: paraffin (P), frozen (F)	Used for	Comments
Hematoxylin and eosin (F or P)	General diagnostic neuropathology	Very satisfactory stain for survey and diagnostic purposes. Virtually all the parenchymal and supporting tissues are stained. Individual cellular structures, such as axons, dendrites, glial cell bodies and processes, may be difficult to identify specifically.
Nissl (F or P) Includes cresyl violet thionine, toluidine blue, and gallocyanine methods	Nerve cell bodies	Useful for demonstrating neuronal distribution patterns, such as cerebral cortical layers, or zones of nerve cell loss in thick (>20 μm) sections. Nucleic acids in both nuclei and cell bodies are stained; thus all types of nuclei are demonstrated. Cell bodies rich in nucleic acid are also delineated. In the nervous system those perikarya are almost exclusively neuronal. At the proper pH, gallocyanine binds specifically with nucleic acid.
Bielschowsky (F or P) Bodian (P) Sevier-Munger (P)	Axons, dendrites, neurofibrils, neurofibrillary degeneration, senile plaques	Silver impregnation techniques distinct from those used for glia. The silver deposits appear black or dark brown. Results are similar with all three methods; however, target structures are more clearly and extensively delineated with the Bielschowsky impregnation.
Loyez (P) Mahon (P) Weil (P) Luxol fast blue, LFB (P)	Intact myelin	Intact myelin is stained black by the first three stains listed, which are hematoxylin based. LFB is a copper phthalocyanine dye that stains intact CNS myelin bluish green and PNS myelin deep blue. LFB may be combined with a Nissl or periodic acid–Schiff counterstain to delineate other structures. Loss or absence of myelin is indicated by lack of staining in areas expected to contain myelin. Other lipid membranes, such as erythrocytes, are also stained by these methods.
Marchi (F) Sudan Red dyes (F): Sudan III, Sudan IV Scharlach R Oil Red O	Degenerating myelin black (Marchi) or red (Sudan)	The Marchi stain is rarely used in human neuropathology because of problems with artifacts. The Sudan Red dyes dissolve in and color the later products of myelin breakdown. These sudanophilic breakdown products are not neutral fats. The presence of sudanophilic lipids in areas of demyelination is considered one indication that normal pathways of myelin catabolism are operating.
Hortega silver carbonate (F or P) Cajal gold chloride sublimate (F)	Astrocytes; silver carbonate method can be modified to stain oliodendroglia and microglia.	Metallic impregnation techniques for demonstrating cell bodies and processes of glial cells including protoplasmic astrocytes. Nuclei of cells appear as negative areas of staining in cell body. The metal deposits are black (silver) or reddish brown (gold).
Holzer (P) Phosphotungstic acid–hematoxylin, PTAH (P)	Fibrillary astrocytes	The cell bodies and processes of fibrillary astrocytes are stained blue. The stains are useful but technically demanding. They are not specific for astrocytic processes.

to macromolecules, particularly proteins.[115] Consequently, protein tracers such as Evans blue, trypan blue, or horseradish peroxidase can now enter and accumulate in brain parenchyma after systemic injection. The change in permeability may be the consequence of defects in the tight junctions between endothelial cells, increased vesicular transport across endothelial cells, transendothelial passage through damaged or necrotic cells, or neovascularization.[12,70,166] The last instance could involve incomplete tight junctions in newly formed endothelium or the appearance of fenestrated endothelial cells. The edema fluid biochemically resembles a plasma filtrate with high sodium and serum protein concentrations. The location of the fluid is chiefly in the extracellular spaces of the white matter. The reason why vasogenic edema affects the white matter more severely than gray matter is not known. Possibly, the lower capillary density and cerebral blood flow in white matter are influential.

Clinically, vasogenic edema probably is the most common type of brain edema. It complicates head injury, abscess, tumors, and hemorrhages. Both vasogenic and cytoxic edema occur with ischemic injury including infarction. The edematous regions of brain appear as hypodense areas in the nonenhanced computerized tomographic scan. After contrast enhancement, sites of vasogenic edema are marked by increased densities because the contrast medium leaks across the permeable vascular membrane.[70]

In cytotoxic edema excessive amounts of water enter one or more of the cellular elements in the central nervous system causing them to swell and reduce the volume of the brain's extracellular space. Neurons, glia, endothelial cells, and myelin sheaths may be affected. The shift of water into the cells is brought about by increased cellular concentration of osmotically active solutes. This increase develops because of an injury impairing the cell's capacity to maintain ionic homeostasis or in association with systemic disturbances in fluid and electrolyte metabolism. Biochemically the edema fluid consists of water and sodium. The endothelial barrier to macromolecules including protein is usually unaffected, and plasma proteins are not a component of the cellular edema. The disorder affects both gray and white matter.

Clinically, cytotoxic edema complicates hypoxia and ischemia because of ATP-dependent sodium pump failure in the affected cells. It also occurs in osmotic disequilibrium syndromes associated with hemodialysis or diabetic ketoacidosis and in acute plasma hypo-osmolality states such as water intoxication and inappropriate secretion of antidiuretic hormone. Because the cerebrovascular macromolecular barrier remains intact, cytoxic edema is not contrast enhancing.[70]

Interstitial or hydrocephalic edema refers to the accumulation of cerebrospinal fluid in the extracellular spaces of the periventricular white matter associated with obstructed flow of cerebrospinal fluid in either the ventricular system or the subarachnoid space.[70] As fluid collects within the obstructed ventricles, pressure increases and the cerebrospinal fluid is forced across the ependymal lining into the adjacent extracellular spaces. Although there is an absolute increase in the volume of extracellular fluid, the volume of the periventricular white matter is reduced (presumably because of loss of myelin lipids) and the ventricles become dilated. These changes are reversible, including reestablishment of white matter volume after the obstruction is relieved either spontaneously or by shunting. The recovery mechanisms and their determinants are not fully understood.

Grossly, the edematous areas of brain are swollen and soft. The swelling increases the volume of the intracranial contents leading to compression of the brain surfaces against the inner table of the skull causing flattening of cerebral gyri, narrowing of intervening sulci, and accentuation of foraminal and tentorial markings on the inferior cerebellar and medial temporal surfaces. The cut surfaces may be wet and shiny (Fig. 42-1). If the edema is diffuse and not of the hydrocephalic type, the ventricles are decreased in size. In severe cases they are reduced to slitlike cavities.

Microscopic changes in all forms of brain edema are variable. Routinely processed paraffin sections may appear normal. In the more severe forms of vasogenic edema the parenchyma is pale-staining and vacuolated. The vacuoles may contain cell nuclei or appear to lie between parenchymal elements. In the white matter the distance between adjacent myelin sheaths or axons is increased. Eosinophilic droplets or even lakes of amorphous plasmatic fluid are present around blood

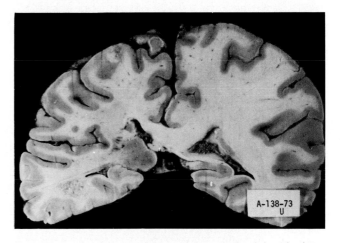

Fig. 42-1. Vasogenic edema, right cerebral hemisphere. The white matter volume is increased; gyral crests are flattened; sulci are narrowed.

vessels (Fig. 42-2). In cases of cytotoxic edema, vacuoles can be seen in the affected parenchyma. These alterations require careful consideration and correlation with other gross and microscopic observations before a definitive diagnosis of edema is made. In particular decreased staining intensity and parenchymal vacuolization can be induced as artifacts through improper fixation, dehydration, embedding, or staining of brain tissue. Morphologic evaluation is somewhat more precise when properly fixed, and stained 1 μm–thick plastic embedded sections are examined by light microscopy or thin sections are studied by electron microscopy. With these methods it is possible to demonstrate, more convincingly, cellular swelling in cytotoxic edema or enlargement of the extracellular space in vasogenic edema. Unfortunately, these procedures are most reliable in this regard when the tissue can be fixed rapidly after separation from its blood supply, as in experimental studies or brain biopsy specimens. Postmortem changes such as swelling of cells and organelles or breakdown of cell membranes begin quickly and can impede conclusive analysis of the observed alterations.

Questions regarding the possible deleterious effects of edema on brain structure or function have not been fully answered. The increases in intracellular or extracellular space caused by the edema could affect the timely availability of critical metabolites and disturb cell function. Biochemical activity could be affected by the elevated sodium levels. Reduced blood volume has

been described in edematous regions of brain.[163] Histologically, occasional lipid phagocytes and a reactive proliferation of astrocytes can be observed in areas of chronic edema. Clinically, changes in consciousness, seizure threshold, and the electroencephalogram accompany brain edema and are reversed by successful treatment. These abnormalities, however, might be caused by the same injury that led to the edema or by the effects of increased intracranial pressure rather than the simple accumulation of water and sodium in the parenchyma. Further studies are required to clarify the mechanisms of cerebral dysfunction in brain edema.

The delineation of vasogenic, cytotoxic, and interstitial forms of edema is based chiefly on controlled experimental studies in previously healthy animals. Within the limits of these experimental protocols, only one type of edema is induced. In humans, however, the pathogenesis of brain edema often involves multiple mechanisms. Patients can have two or more diseases or develop complications of their primary disorder. These factors can lead to the occurrence of more than one type of edema, such as development of acute hydrocephalus in a patient with a brain tumor, would be associated with both vasogenic and interstitial brain edema.

Increased intracranial pressure and brain herniation

After closure of the sutures, the volume of the cranial cavity is fixed by rigid bony walls and compartmentalized by partitions of bone and dura. The normal contents of the cranial cavity (blood, brain, cerebrospinal fluid) are relatively incompressible. Under these conditions an increase in the volume of the cranial contents can cause compensatory, intercompartmental displacement of brain, blood, or cerebrospinal fluid and eventually increased intracranial pressure as well as the gyral flattening, sulcal narrowing, and so on described in association with brain edema.[22,70,184] Expansion of intracranial contents occurs because of diffuse brain edema, increased cerebral blood flow and blood volume (such as chronic pulmonary insufficiency with respiratory acidosis), or the development of space-occupying lesions such as tumors, abscesses, hematomas, or large infarcts accompanied by edema. The effects of space-occupying lesions on intracranial pressure are caused not only by the mass of the lesion, but also by accompanying edema and obstruction of venous or cerebrospinal fluid pathways.

The compensatory displacements of brain from one intracranial compartment to another caused by increases in the volume of cranial contents are called "brain herniations." In general, if the volumetric increase takes place over a long period of time, such as the result of a slowly growing meningioma, a consider-

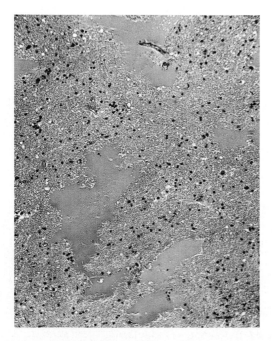

Fig. 42-2. Brain edema. Intercellular lakes of high protein content fluid. (Hematoxylin and eosin; 90×.)

able degree of displacement can develop asymptomatically and without a rise in intracranial pressure. In contrast, more rapid expansion of cranial contents leads quickly to symptomatic brain herniations and increased intracranial pressure. The three herniations commonly encountered in this circumstance are transtentorial herniation of the medial temporal lobe and brainstem, ventral cerebellar herniation into the foramen magnum, and subfalcial herniation of the cingulate gyrus (Figs. 42-3 to 42-5). Less frequently observed are herniations of the orbital gyri into the temporal fossa, the hypothalamus into the hypophyseal fossa, the anterior midline cerebellum upward through the incisura of the tentorium, and portions of the cerebral convexity through surgical or traumatic defects in the calvarium.

Transtentorial herniation is caused by supratentorial space-occupying lesions. It is sometimes separated into two components: (1) central herniation,[172] which refers to the rostrocaudal displacement of the hypothalamus and rostral brainstem through the incisura of the tentorium, and (2) uncal or medial temporal lobe herniation, which involves herniation of the uncus and parahippocampal gyrus over the free edge of the tentorium and through the incisura. Central herniation may be present without associated uncal herniation when both cerebral hemispheres are enlarged equally, such as a result of diffuse cerebral edema. In this circumstance symmetric, prominent tentorial grooves are evident on the inferior surfaces of both unci, the gyri are flattened, and the sulci are narrowed over both cerebral convexities. Midline cerebral structures, however, are not displaced laterally. Portions of the ventral posterior hypothalamus (such as mamillary bodies) and rostral brainstem are displaced caudally. These alterations are often more evident by in situ imaging than by conventional macroscopic examination of the brain.

Uncal herniation is caused chiefly by ipsilateral or asymmetric supratentorial space-occupying lesions. As the medial temporal lobe herniates through the incisura, both the ipsilateral oculomotor nerve and rostral brainstem are compressed, giving rise to pupillary di-

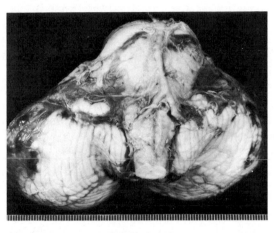

Fig. 42-4. Ventral cerebellar herniation. The cerebellar tonsils are closely opposed to the medulla and a prominent foraminal groove is present.

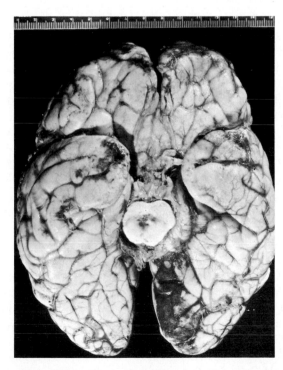

Fig. 42-3. Brain displacement with large right uncal herniation. There is compression of right posterior cerebral artery with hemorrhagic infarct of medial portion of occipital lobe and with overlying subarachnoid hemorrhage. Secondary hemorrhages are in lower midbrain.

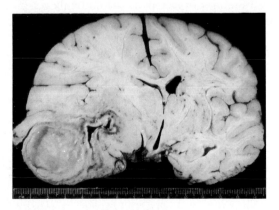

Fig. 42-5. Chronic brain abscesses in temporal lobe and insula. Surrounding brain shows swelling and edema. There is compression and displacement of lateral and third ventricles. Cingulate gyrus and uncal herniations are also present.

latation, disturbed consciousness, and other signs of rostrocaudal deterioration of brainstem function (Fig. 42-3). In addition to the gyral flattening commonly associated with increased intracranial pressure, the brainstem and adjacent basilar cerebral structures are displaced laterally away from the herniating temporal lobe. If the displacement is severe, the rostral brainstem is forced against the edge of the opposite tentorial leaf causing a wedge-shaped lesion in the brainstem involving the cerebral peduncle including descending motor pathways. The lesion is referred to as "Kernohan's notch." Its occurrence is characterized clinically by the development of hemiplegia on the same side as the herniated temporal lobe. The posterior cerebral artery crosses the ventral and medial surface of the temporal lobe. As the medial temporal lobe herniates through the incisura, the posterior cerebral artery is occluded by compression against the tentorial edge causing infarction of the ipsilateral ventromedial occipital lobe (Fig. 42-3). The infarction produces a homonymous hemianopsia that becomes evident should the patient survive. Rostro-caudal displacement of the brainstem also occurs with uncal herniation. The displacement causes stretching and eventually disruption of the intrinsic vasculature (chiefly arterioles) in the pons and midbrain giving rise to midline and lateral hemorrhages (sometimes called "Duret hemorrhages") (Fig. 42-3). These hemorrhages produce profound deterioration of brainstem function and can cause death through destruction or interruption of cardiorespiratory centers and pathways.

Herniation of the cerebellum into the foramen magnum (Fig. 42-4) is most often associated with space-occupying lesions in the posterior fossa. In addition, the herniation can occur with supratentorial midline frontal masses, in association with uncal herniation, and with generalized increases in the volume of cranial contents. The cerebellar displacement is commonly referred to as tonsillar herniation; however, the herniation also includes the biventral lobule as well as the tonsils. Clinical evidence of ventral cerebellar herniation includes head tilt, stiff neck, paresthesias over the shoulders, and eventually respiratory arrest resulting from medullary compression. The pathologic diagnosis of tonsillar herniation is based primarily on macroscopic findings, including identification of an inciting cause, evidence of increased intracranial or posterior fossa pressure, a prominent foraminal groove on the ventral surface of the cerebellum, close approximation of the tonsils and medulla, and edema of the medulla indicated by bulges on the cut surface of the caudal medulla where it was separated from the upper cervical spinal cord during removal of the brain post mortem. In addition, compression of the vascular supply to the ventral cerebellum can cause congestion, focal hemorrhages, and infarction of the tonsillar parenchyma. In some cases

focal necrosis of the caudal medulla and upper cervical cord is demonstrable. The pathologic lesions indicative of tonsillar herniation may be bilaterally symmetric or asymmetric depending on the direction of forces generated by the inciting lesion. In determining whether tonsillar herniation has occurred, the pathologist must be aware of the normal variations in foraminal markings on the ventral cerebellar surface and demonstrate in addition to a prominent foraminal groove other anatomic evidence of tonsillar herniation.

Herniation of the cingulate gyrus beneath the falx (Fig. 42-5) is not associated with any well-defined clinical syndrome, probably because any symptoms produced by the lesion are masked either by the lesion causing the herniation or by the clinical effects of an accompanying uncal herniation. In some cases, however, compression of branches of the anterior cerebral artery against the free edge of the falx produces hemorrhagic infarction of the medial hemispheric surface. Cingulate herniation is caused by ipsilateral, supratentorial space-occupying lesions, especially those involving the upper half of the frontoparietal cerebral convexity. The cingulate gyrus is forced beneath the falx and across the midline. The ipsilateral corpus callosum is pushed ventrally and the adjacent lateral ventricle is compressed.

Hydrocephalus[22,70]

Under normal conditions the rates of cerebrospinal fluid formation and absorption are equal. If the equilibrium is disturbed, by either a decreased rate of absorption or an uncompensated rise in the rate of formation, hydrocephalus develops. This condition is distinguished by an increased volume of cerebrospinal fluid and dilatation of the ventricular system (Fig. 42-6). Hydrocephalus usually results from delayed absorption induced by obstruction of cerebrospinal fluid pathways either within the ventricular system or in the subarachnoid space. Increased production of cerebrospinal fluid causing hydrocephalus has been demonstrated only in cases of choroid plexus papilloma with secretion of the excess fluid by the tumor. In addition to these mechanisms, impaired absorption of cerebrospinal fluid through arachnoid villi and decreased venous drainage after occlusion or venous hypertension have been implicated as contributing factors in some cases of hydrocephalus.

The lesions responsible for obstructive hydrocephalus include tumors and other masses, malformations, and inflammation of the ventricular system or leptomeninges. The obstruction restricts the flow of cerebrospinal fluid, and so the amount reaching absorption sites decreases. Correspondingly, the volume absorbed is reduced. The secretory rate, however, remains relatively constant. With more cerebrospinal fluid produced than absorbed per unit time, both fluid volume and pressure increase proximally to the site of restricted flow, even-

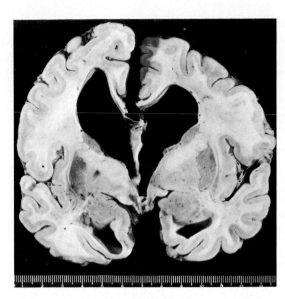

Fig. 42-6. Internal hydrocephalus of lateral and third ventricles caused by obstructive lesion in fourth ventricle (not illustrated).

tually leading to dilatation of the obstructed parts of the ventricular system. The obstruction within the ventricular system is usually located at sites where the fluid pathway narrows, such as the foramina of Monro, aqueduct of Sylvius, exit foramina of the fourth ventricle, or at the third or fourth ventricle when the lumens become filled with tumor or blood clot. Subarachnoid pathways most often become blocked over the cerebral convexities and around the rostral brainstem (incisural block) as a result of inflammation or hemorrhage. In the acute phase, the blood clot or inflammatory exudate forms a barrier to flow. Subsequently, organization of the clot or exudate leads to fibrous obliteration of the subarachnoid space.

Obstructive hydrocephalus is frequently described as "communicating" or "noncommunicating". In communicating hydrocephalus, the obstruction is located in the subarachnoid space, and cerebrospinal fluid passes freely through the entire ventricular system into the subarachnoid space proximal to the obstruction. In noncommunicating hydrocephalus the obstruction is located somewhere between the foramina of Monro and the exit foramina of the fourth ventricle, preventing free flow of cerebrospinal fluid between all or part of the ventricular system and the subarachnoid space. The operational difference between these two types of obstructive hydrocephalus originally was based upon detection of a visible dye in the lumbar cerebrospinal fluid shortly after injection of the dye into the lateral ventricle. The presence of dye indicated communicating hydrocephalus, and the absence of dye indicated noncommunicating hydrocephalus. The distinction between the two types of obstructive hydrocephalus is important in

the determination of the location of surgical shunts used to bypass the obstruction and reduce ventricular size.

Compensatory increase in cerebrospinal fluid volume and ventricular dilatation occurring secondary to loss of brain tissue through atrophy or other primary injuries to brain parenchyma is called "hydrocephalus ex vacuo." In this condition there is no obstruction to the flow of cerebrospinal fluid, and the intracranial pressure is normal.

Clinical evidence of hydrocephalus may be present or absent. If the hydrocephalus is associated with increased intracranial pressure, then mental dullness, headaches, nausea, vomiting, and papilledema may occur. In addition, in children enlargement of the head is noted when hydrocephalus develops before the cranial sutures close. When the obstructive lesion causing the hydrocephalus is not severe and progressive, the hydrocephalic process may stabilize probably through small changes in the rates of formation and absorption of cerebrospinal fluid as well as the development of auxiliary absorption pathways. The cerebrospinal fluid pressure returns to normal limits, but a characteristic triad of clinical findings composed of dementia, gait disorder, and urinary incontinence is present. The term "normal-pressure hydrocephalus" is applied to this condition. Timely and accurate diagnosis of this disorder is a matter of special importance because it is amenable to treatment with surgically placed shunts.

Several alterations in the brain are common to all forms of hydrocephalus. These include dilatation of the ventricular system, reduction of the volume of the white matter, disruption of the ependymal lining, accentuation of the primary, secondary, and tertiary cerebral sulci producing an enriched gyral pattern without true microgyria, and perforation of the septum pellucidum. The lesions associated with congenital and related forms of childhood hydrocephalus are covered in the section on malformations and perinatal brain injuries.

Neurocellular reactions to central nervous system injury

Aside from alterations affecting supporting structures such as blood vessels or meninges, central nervous system cellular changes that have proved to be reliable indicators of nonneoplastic neural parenchymal injury involve neurons, astrocytes, and microglia. Reactions involving one or more of these cells are present in almost every central nervous system disease. Correlation of the characteristics of the cellular response and its anatomic distribution with the clinical findings, in many instances, forms the basis of the neuropathologic diagnosis.

Neurons. Familiarity with the diverse morphology of normal central nervous system neurons is necessary for accurate identification of injured neurons. Nerve cell bodies range in size from very small, such as the lymphocyte-like granule cells of the cerebellar cortex, to large and prominent, such as motor neurons in the precentral gyrus or anterior horns of the cervical and lumbar cord. The neuronal perikaryon may be multipolar, round, oval, pyramidal, or flask shaped. Nissl substance, the histologic counterpart of clumped granular endoplasmic reticulum, appears as large, well-defined bodies in some types of neurons and in others as small granules or dustlike particles spread diffusely throughout the cytoplasm. In Clarke's column the normal concentration of Nissl substance at the periphery of neuronal perikarya is sometimes misinterpreted as chromatolysis, a neuronal reaction to injury. Pigments, such as neuromelanin or lipofuscin, are found in otherwise normal nerve cells. The latter pigment is evident in many neurons throughout the central nervous system of older persons and is sometimes referred to as an age pigment, though it has been observed in the inferior olivary and spinal cord neurons of some very young humans as well as in the inferior olivary, hypoglossal, and trigeminal nuclei of 6-month-old rhesus monkeys unassociated with neurologic disease.[236] The most prominent groups of neurons containing neuromelanin are in the substantia nigra and locus ceruleus; however, the pigment can be seen in other neurons located along the floor of the fourth ventricle. Neuromelanin pigment is not associated with melanomas, is unaffected in cases of albinism, and is ultrastructurally distinct from the melanin formed by melanocytes in the skin, eye, and leptomeninges.

General types of neuronal injury. Neuronal injury causes either lethal or progressive, sometimes reversible, morphologic alterations.

LETHAL INJURY. Nerve cell loss or atrophy and eosinophilic neuronal necrosis are two morphologic indicators of lethal injury.

NEURONAL ATROPHY. The process of neuronal atrophy, which occurs in various degenerative diseases, is characterized grossly by a reduction in the volume of the affected structure and microscopically by reduced neuronal density accompanied by an astrocytic or microglial reaction.

Nerve cell bodies are generally arranged in vaguely defined groups rather than homogeneously in the gray matter of the brain and spinal cord. This grouping gives rise to areas devoid of neurons that may be mistakenly diagnosed as foci of nerve cell loss or developmental absence. Accurate evaluation of these foci can be difficult, particularly in regard to potential developmental disturbances. The use of serial and control sections as well as a careful search for evidence of an astrocytic or microglial reaction will usually resolve this type of problem. The mechanisms responsible for atrophic nerve cell loss are unknown. Dependable morphologic markers for the early stages of the process have not been identified. Occasionally, neuronal phagocytosis is observed apparently representing the final step in the atrophic reaction.

ISCHEMIC (EOSINOPHILIC) NEURONAL NECROSIS. Probably, the most common morphologic expression of lethal neuronal injury in human pathology is ischemic or eosinophilic neuronal necrosis, expressed epigrammatically as: "Red is dead." This lesion is most clearly associated with ischemic disturbances, such as severe systemic hypotension with impaired cerebral perfusion or strokes caused by occlusive vascular disease. In sections stained with hematoxylin and eosin, the cytoplasm of the affected neurons has lost its usual, slightly basophilic color and stains red. The nucleus is shrunken and darkly staining, and internal details are obscured. These changes are evident in experimental animals killed 30 to 90 minutes after the ischemic event.[61] In humans the shortest survival time after the ischemia required for the appearance of unequivocal red neurons is not known precisely. Six to 8 hours is a commonly mentioned interval for the evolution of ischemic neurons in humans; however, such changes can, on occasion, be recognized with confidence after even shorter periods, and these figures should be viewed as approximations rather than irrefutable doctrine.

PROGRESSIVE OR REVERSIBLE INJURIES. Morphologic evidence of progressive, sometimes reversible, neuronal injury includes central chromatolysis, neurofibrillary degeneration, neuronal storage of metabolic products, and inclusion bodies.

CENTRAL CHROMATOLYSIS. The term "central chromatolysis" refers to the changes occurring in the nerve cell body after injury to its axon relatively close to the perikaryon or possibly to the cell body itself. The Nissl substance disappears beginning centrally and extending peripherally. At the same time the nucleus is displaced eccentrically, and the cell body enlarges, causing conversion of its contours from concave to convex. Depending on the severity of the injury and the regenerative capacity of the affected axon, the neuron may eventually recover or degenerate and disappear. This type of alteration can be seen in the anterior horns of the spinal cord in cases of acute idiopathic inflammatory polyneuropathy (Guillain-Barré syndrome) or anterior nerve root compression.

NEUROFIBRILLARY DEGENERATION. Neurofibrils are the argyrophilic linear densities seen by light microscopy in nerve cell bodies, and their processes seen after silver impregnation. Ultrastructural studies have demonstrated that neurofibrils are a light microscopic composite of three types of neuronal fibrous proteins: microtubules (neurotubules), neurofilaments, and microfilaments.[95] Microtubules are long hollow structures measuring 25 nm in diameter. The major protein component is tubulin. Neurofilaments belong to the family of intermediate filaments. They are 10 nm in diameter and contain a distinctive protein composed of three polypeptides with molecular weights of 68,000, 150,000, and 200,000 daltons. Microfilaments range from 5 to 7 nm in diameter and contain actin as their chief protein. The physiologic functions of these fibrous elements are not fully defined but are believed to involve maintenance of cellular shape and intracellular transport of macromolecules and organelles. Increases in the number and changes in the morphology of neurofilaments and microtubules are associated with several human neurologic disorders including Alzheimer's disease, postencephalitic parkinsonism, progressive supranuclear palsy, and the punch-drunk syndrome as well as experimental or therapeutic exposure to aluminum salts and the *Vinca* alkaloids used to treat hematologic malignancies. The term "neurofibrillary degeneration" is applied to the light microscopic appearance of this alteration. Affected neurons contain prominent woven and convoluted masses or tangles of neurofibrils that are most reliably demonstrated with silver impregnation methods. The ultrastructural pattern of the neurofibrillary tangle varies according to the fibrous proteins affected and the morphologic modifications they undergo. Some of these patterns may be characteristically associated with a particular disease or group of disorders, such as paired helical filaments in Alzheimer's disease.

NEURONAL STORAGE. Characteristic morphologic evidence of neuronal damage occurs in some hereditary metabolic diseases caused by enzymatic defects involving synthetic or degradative pathways for lipids or carbohydrates. Interruption of the pathway leads to cytoplasmic accumulation or storage of intermediate substrates and their by-products. The cell body of the neuron enlarges, its contours change from concave to convex, and the nucleus is eccentrically displaced. In several neuronal storage disorders, the cytoplasmic accumulations have distinctive histochemical and ultrastructural features. Identification of these characteristics in biopsy specimens of brain and other tissues has been used as a means of confirming and further categorizing clinically suspected cases of storage disorders.[86] More recently, however, as the underlying metabolic disturbances have been delineated more completely, biochemical tests on blood, leukocytes, and other body fluids have supplanted the use of biopsy in several of these diseases.

INCLUSION BODIES. Intracytoplasmic or intranuclear inclusions are important indicators of neuronal injury. They occur in viral, metabolic, and degenerative diseases. Viral infections associated with intranuclear inclusions include those caused by herpes simplex virus type 1, cytomegalovirus, measles virus (subacute scle-

rosing panencephalitis) and papovavirus (progressive multifocal leukoencephalopathy). Cytoplasmic viral inclusions are seen in rabies (Negri bodies) and occasionally in cytomegalovirus infections. Among the metabolic and degenerative diseases, intracytoplasmic inclusions with characteristic (not necessarily specific) associations are Pick bodies (Pick's disease), Lewy bodies (Parkinson's disease), and Lafora bodies (Lafora's disease). Eosinophilic rods, referred to as Hirano bodies, and granulovacuolar degeneration, one or more cytoplasmic vacuoles each containing basophilic body, are intracytoplasmic neuronal inclusions found chiefly in the pyramidal cell layer of the hippocampus. Although these latter two inclusions occur in older persons without clinical evidence of neurologic disease, they appear more prevalent in certain degenerative disorders such as Alzheimer's disease. Bunina bodies are eosinophilic, nonviral intranuclear inclusions that may be observed in cases of familial or sporadic amyotrophic lateral sclerosis. Other neuronal inclusions that have no known pathologic significance are Marinesco bodies (small, eosinophilic intranuclear inclusions located chiefly in melanin-containing brainstem neurons) and eosinophilic, intracytoplasmic inclusions in hypoglossal and anterior horn neurons. The numbers of both increase with age.

Astrocytes. Two types of astrocytes, protoplasmic and fibrillary, are distinguishable by light microscopy by use of metallic impregnation techniques. Protoplasmic astrocytes are located in gray matter and fibrillary astrocytes chiefly in white matter. Ultrastructural studies have demonstrated that both types contain intermediate filaments (glial fibrils); however, the filaments are more numerous in fibrillary astroctyes. Glial fibrillary acidic protein (GFAP) is a major component of astrocytic intermediate filaments. Immunoperoxidase methods for allowing detection of this astrocytic marker protein are used regularly in diagnostic neuropathology.

The most important reactions of astrocytes to injury are the primary and secondary forms of astrocytosis. Other disease-related astrocytic changes include swelling, necrosis, and inclusions. The terms "astrocytosis," "astrogliosis," and "gliosis" are often used synonymously. Some authors use astrocytosis in reference to increases in the size and number of astrocytes and astrogliosis for increases in astrocytic processes. In this chapter "astrocytosis" refers generically to both reactions, and the term "fibrillary astrocytosis" is used for those reactions in which an increase in number of astrocytic processes is the predominant finding.

Secondary or reactive astrocytosis is one of the most common and important neurocellular reactions to injury. It occurs in a variety of central nervous system diseases ranging from infarction to degeneration. The morphologic characteristics of the reaction cannot be used to identify specific diseases, and in this sense the reaction may be considered nonspecific. Nevertheless, it is a reliable indication that some type of parenchymal damage has taken place in the central nervous system. Artifactual changes in the morphology and staining characteristics of neurons, axons, and myelin sheaths occur commonly in human surgical and postmortem neuropathologic specimens. Evidence of reactive changes involving astrocytes, microglia, or blood vessels provides the neuropathologist with an objective basis for deciding whether subtle histologic alterations reflect disease or artifact.

The early stages of secondary astrocytosis vary according to the acuteness and severity of the parenchymal damage as well as the extent of white matter involvement. If the lesion develops rapidly with necrosis or myelin destruction, the size and number of astrocyte nuclei increase, and small but distinct amounts of cytoplasm become visible with a hematoxylin and eosin stain around these nuclei. Often the nuclei may be side by side in pairs or even larger, even-numbered groups. Mitotic figures with rare exception are not seen in human nonneoplastic astrocytic proliferations. The reasons for their absence has not been fully explained but may be related to the rate of tissue fixation.[40] Traditionally the pairs of astrocyte nuclei in the absence of mitotic figures have been interpreted as evidence of an amitotic astrocytic proliferation. For many reasons amitotic division is an unlikely mechanism for astrocytic multiplication, and the explanation for the lack of mitotic figures in human material lies elsewhere. As the reaction proceeds, the astrocytic cell body becomes larger and more conspicuous with the nucleus displaced toward the periphery. These enlarged astrocytes are often referred to as "hypertrophied astrocytes," "large-bodied astrocytes," "plump astrocytes," or "gemistocytes" (Greek *gemistos* 'laden, full,' based on original German *gemästete Zellen* 'fattened cells'). They are prominent in hematoxylin and eosin preparations because of their enlarged pink-staining cell bodies. Later, as the number of astrocytic processes increase, the cell bodies become more widely separated and reduced in size though hypertrophied astrocytes may persist for months or years within inactive lesions. The term "fibrillary astrocytosis" is applied to this stage of the reaction. The major component of the reaction is a fibrous meshwork consisting of astrocytic cell processes. There is no extracellular deposition of fibers as is the case in scars derived from fibroblasts. Eosinophilic masses called "Rosenthal fibers" can be seen within the processes especially when the lesion involves the white matter.

Astrocytic reactions to parenchymal injuries that evolve slowly without associated tissue necrosis or white matter lesions, as in chronic, degenerative diseases of gray matter, are characterized by an increase in the number of astrocytes without a readily perceptible increase in the size of their perikarya. In other respects the astrocytic reactions to acute and chronic injuries are similar.

Secondary astrocytosis, that is, the astrocytic reaction to injury of other parenchymal elements, is a generally accepted concept and has well-defined morphologic features. In contrast, the occurrence and characteristics of primary astrocytosis, that is, the response of astrocytes when they are the targets of sublethal injury, have not been completely proved and defined.[87] At present the astrocytic changes associated with hepatic encephalopathy and other conditions in which blood ammonia levels are elevated are viewed as a primary astrocytosis. In these disorders the altered astrocytes, referred to as "Alzheimer type II astrocytes," are found chiefly in gray matter. The nuclei are enlarged and vesicular and often contain nucleoli or glycogen inclusions. Their numbers appear increased, though the question of enhanced prominence versus absolute numerical increase is unresolved. The cell body may enlarge slightly but does not become visible with hematoxylin and eosin stains, and there is no increase in astrocytic processes. Changes resembling Alzheimer type II astrocytosis are sometimes seen in metabolic and toxic disorders other than those associated with elevated blood ammonia levels.

Microglia. Modern immunohistochemical, ultrastructural, and autoradiographic studies have uncovered substantial evidence against the traditional concept of the microglia as a single, silver-positive population of small cells, indigenous to the central nervous system but derived from mesoderm, which, when activated, form rod cells or macrophages and give rise to tumors called "microgliomas."[203] The data from these investigations indicate that rod cells and macrophages are derived from cells of the mononuclear phagocyte system that migrate to the central nervous system in response to parenchymal injury. The tumors previously referred to as microgliomas are, in fact, extranodal lymphomas composed mainly of B lymphocytes.[232] The function and cellular relationships of the small, silver-positive, branched cells scattered through the central nervous system is uncertain.

The formation of macrophages and their morphologic characteristics in the central nervous system are similar to those in other organs. Rod cells are elongated spindle-shaped cells that can be recognized in hematoxylin and eosin preparations by the presence of a cigar-shaped nucleus. They develop in response to subacute parenchymal injuries in which necrosis is minimal or absent. In the first part of this century the most common lesion associated with rod cells was general paresis, a type of tertiary neurosyphilis. At present they are seen most often in cases of subacute encephalitis, such as subacute sclerosing panencephalitis (SSPE).

Malformations and perinatal brain injury
Development of the central nervous system[122,157]

The human brain and spinal cord are derived from ectoderm. The basic form of the central nervous system is established between the third and eighth postovulatory weeks. The neural plate, the forerunner of the nervous system, can be recognized during third week. It enlarges and folds dorsally, completing formation of the neural tube by the fourth week. At the same time formation of the neural crest occurs. This structure consists of two columns of cells derived from the neural tube and lies on either side of its dorsal half. The dorsal root ganglia, most of the cranial nerve ganglia, autonomic ganglia, Schwann cells, adrenal medulla, leptomeninges, and melanocytes are neural-crest derivatives. The sensory epithelium and ganglia associated with cranial nerves 1, 5, 7, and 8 to 10 are not derived from the neural crest but originate from a series of ectodermal thickenings called "ectodermal placodes," which are located in the head region.

During the fourth and fifth weeks three vesicles—the prosencephalon (forebrain), mesencephalon (midbrain), and rhombencephalon (hindbrain)—become evident in the rostral end of the neural tube. These developments are accompanied by formation of a primitive but functioning cerebral circulation with identifiable arteries and veins. By the end of the fifth or sixth month the general morphologic features of the adult brain and spinal cord are recognizable in all these components. The prosencephalon forms the telencephalon and diencephalon, from which are derived respectively the cerebral hemispheres (including neostriatum) and the thalamus-hypothalamus. The midbrain develops from the mesencephalon, and the cerebellum, pons, and medulla develop from the rhombencephalon. The spinal cord develops from the neural tube caudal to the rhombencephalon.

Cowan[51] has called attention to an important series of progressive and regressive cellular events he refers to as the primary processes of neurogenesis, which underlie the gross changes in the developing nervous system. In their approximate order of occurrence the progressive events are proliferation, migration, selective cell aggregation, cytodifferentiation, and formation of neuronal connections. During the formation of neuronal connections selective cell death, the regressive phase of neurogenesis, occurs. Up to 50% of the original population of cells in a given region may be eliminated along with their connections. In this sequence the final form and composition of each region arises by the initial accumulation of cells and the establishment of intercellular relationships followed by selective removal of cells and eradication of superfluous cellular relationships.

Characteristics of the normal full-term brain

The brain of a full-term infant weighs between 350 and 420 g. It is softer than the adult brain because water constitutes 90% by weight of the neonatal brain. In contrast 70% to 75% of the adult brain weight is attributable to water.[113] The pattern of cerebral gyri and sulci characteristic of human brain is easily recognizable. Microscopically, cortical layers can be distinguished. The neurons, however, are smaller and more closely packed than in the adult brain. The nuclei are large in relation to the amount of cytoplasm present, and arborization of nerve cell processes has occurred only to a limited extent.

Because myelination is incomplete in the full-term brain, there is no sharp distinction macroscopically between gray and white in many parts of the central nervous system. Nevertheless nuclear groups such as the corpus striatum, thalamus, inferior olivary, and dentate nuclei can be seen grossly. Myelinated axons are found in the spinal and cranial nerve roots, including the optic nerves and tracts. Except for the lateral and anterior corticospinal tracts, the principal ascending and descending spinal cord pathways contain prominent myelinated axons. Within the brainstem there are myelinated axons in the internal arcuate, spinocerebellar, and corticospinal tracts, the medial and lateral lemniscus, and the medial longitudinal fasciculus. Myelinated cerebellar axons are seen in the central and folial white matter and in the peduncles. In the cerebral hemispheres the thalamus, subthalamic nucleus, globus pallidus, and posterior limb of the internal capsule contain myelinated axons. The corpus callosum and fornix are unmyelinated.[120,187]

Difficulties may be encountered when one is identifying reactive astrocytosis in the neonatal brain because of the occurrence of myelination glia. These cells are present in large numbers in myelinating tracts but have not acquired the morphologic features of mature oligodendroglia. At this stage, because they have recognizable, eosinophilic cytoplasm, they may be confused with astrocytes. Myelination glia are accompanied by fatty, sudanophilic droplets, some of which are located in the bodies and processes of the myelination glia, whereas others are present in the neuropil without a definite cellular localization. All the white matter of the central nervous system is affected by this accumulation of droplets; however, the intensity of the process varies from tract to tract. The significance of these fatty droplets is controversial. They have been interpreted both as a pathologic change in the white matter and as a normal feature of myelination. Ultrastructural studies in developing human and primate brain indicate that the lipid droplets occur either in undifferentiated glial cells or in astrocytes. In monkeys the droplets are present in small numbers in normal brain but are greatly increased by hypoxic exposure.[205,226]

The adult pattern of the cerebral vasculature is present in the full-term brain. The arteries forming the major branches of the circle of Willis are considerably smaller in diameter than their adult counterparts. The functional capacity of the blood-brain barrier in the full-term infant has not been fully delineated. Ultrastructural studies, however, have demonstrated tight junctions between endothelial cells in humans and animals very early in development. Further, studies with trypan blue and similar dyes have not demonstrated parenchymal staining in normal full-term human and animal brains.[142,200]

Other features of the normal central nervous system at term include a cavum septi pellucidi and the persistence of small amounts of immature neuroepithelium beneath the ependyma of the lateral ventricles and over the cerebellum as the external granular cell layer. These elements disappear during the 12 to 15 months after birth. The substantia nigra and locus ceruleus are not pigmented macroscopically at birth. Microscopically, however, pigment granules may be detectable as early as midterm.[71,122]

Congenital malformations

Developmental brain injury may result from genetic determinants, chromosomal aberrations, and a variety of environmental factors such as infection, maternal illness, drugs, and chemicals. Often, however, no cause can be identified. The type of lesion induced by the injury varies from major structural derangements to subtle subcellular alterations. Its characteristics are influenced by several factors including the developmental period in which the injury occurred, the duration and severity of the injury, and the nature of the injury (mechanical, metabolic, and so on). In most cases morphologic examination alone will not establish a specific cause. Etiologic associations, however, have been identified for some neural malformations. In these cases the morphologic data are helpful indicators of potential etiologic agents.

Experimental studies demonstrating a correlation between specific types of malformations and the developmental stage at which injury was induced have led to the idea that timetables of developmental events can be used to determine the time at which the teratogenic damage actually occurred. Warkany[245] has reviewed the limitations involved in assigning dates of origin for human malformations based on these timetables. He points out that the developmental data may in some instances establish the termination period or latest time at which a teratogen could have caused a particular malformation but not the exact time the injury actually occurred. Furthermore, termination periods are known for some but not all malformations. There are many, such as microcephaly, hydrocephalus, and porencephaly, without known termination periods, and their inception cannot be established precisely.

Data concerning the frequency of central nervous system malformations varies because of differences in the design of epidemiologic studies, differences in diagnostic methods, and ethnic or geographic differences in incidence or prevalence. Based upon the analysis of several studies, Myrianthopoulos[147] estimates an incidence of 80 to 100 central nervous system malformations per 10,000 births, both live and stillborn. The common lesions are anencephaly, microcephaly, hydrocephalus, spina bifida, and Down's syndrome. If CNS malformations in spontaneous abortions (chiefly exencephaly, encephalocele, and spinal cord defects) are included, the incidence increases to a range of 100 to 130 per 10,000 conceptions and represents 10% of all malformations. The figures refer only to primary CNS malformations and do not include various syndromes and metabolic or chromosomal disorders in which CNS lesions are sometimes found. Reliable data concerning these cases are difficult to acquire. The features of the more important malformations are presented in the remainder of this section.

Neural tube defects (NTD). The neural tube group of malformations is characterized by a complete or regional disturbance in the continuity of neural tube structures and their coverings. Examples include the neurulation, or open, defects—craniorachischises, anencephaly, meningomyelocele—and the postneurulation, or closed, defects—iniencephaly, encephalocele, some forms of hydrocephalus, and various lumbosacral anomalies such as diastematomyelia, occult spina bifida, and lipoma.[121] Neurulation defects are considered to arise between the seventeenth and thirtieth day after conception. The coverings of the nervous system are absent, and the nervous system is open to the amniotic fluid. Alpha-fetoprotein (AFP) leaks from exposed neural vessels into the fluid causing elevated levels. Recognition of this phenomenon has led to the use of amniocentesis and determination of AFP concentrations as part of the procedure for prenatal diagnosis of neurulation defects. In postneurulation defects the nervous system is closed to contact with the amniotic fluid by intact coverings. Consequently lesions of this type are not associated with increased AFP concentration in amniotic fluid.

The most common neural tube defects are anencephaly and meningomyelocele. Many anatomic variants of anencephaly have been described. The basic defects include absence of all (holocrania) or part (mer-

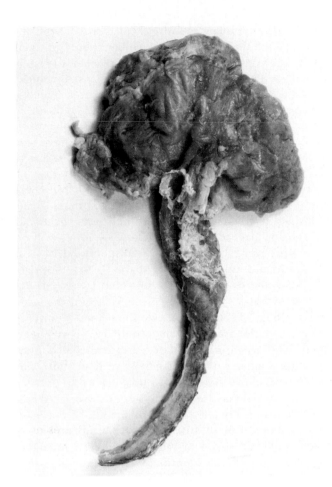

Fig. 42-7. Anencephaly. The brain is replaced by the area cerebrovasculosa, a disorganized collection of blood vessels and neuroepithelial tissues.

ocrania) of the cranial vault and replacement of the cerebrum by a mass composed of thin-walled vascular channels, neural tissue, and structures resembling choroid plexus (Fig. 42-7). The caudal extent of the lesion varies and may extend into the spinal cord. The eyes are well developed and optic nerves are present but may terminate blindly. The lower cranial nerves and spinal nerves can often be identified. The anterior lobe of the pituitary is present, but the posterior lobe may be absent. The adrenal cortex is thin with an absent or reduced fetal zone. Abnormalities of other systemic organs such as thyroid, thymus, and lung may be observed.

Meningomyeloceles may involve any level of the spinal cord but most commonly affect the lower thoracic and lumbar segments. In the vicinity of the lesion the vertebral arches are absent, and a mass of disorganized neural parenchyma, meninges, nerve roots, and connective tissue is evident on the body surface providing a pathway for spread of infection to the central nervous system. (Fig. 42-8). Abnormalities of the spinal cord such as hydromyelia (dilatation of the central canal) frequently occur adjacent to the main defect. Meningomyelocele is also associated with other congenital lesions of the nervous system including the Chiari type II (Arnold-Chiari) malformation causing hydrocephalus. This lesion is discussed in a later section of the chapter. Less severe lesions related to meningomyelocele include meningocele and spina bifida occulta. In the former, a cystic structure composed of meninges without neural parenchyma protrudes through the vertebral defect out to the body surface. In occult spina bifida one or more vertebral arches are missing, and although there may be abnormalities of adjacent neural and der-

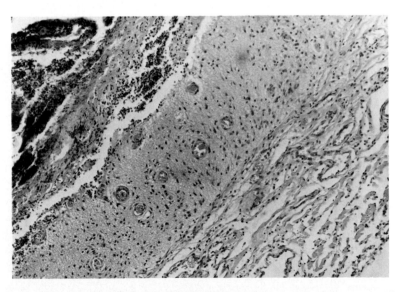

Fig. 42-8. Dorsal wall of meningomyelocele. Band of astrocytic tissue runs diagonally from lower left to upper right. *Upper left corner,* Ulcerated cutaneous surface; *lower right corner,* leptomeninges. (Hematoxylin and eosin; 100 ×.)

mal tissues, the lesion remains asymptomatic for many years or an entire lifetime.

Holoprosencephalies.[74] Holoprosencephalies form a group of malformations that reflect disordered development of telencephalic and diencephalic structures from the prosencephalon. In alobar holoprosencephaly, the most severe of these defects, the forebrain is small, consisting of an undivided spherical structure with irregularly disposed gyri of average to large size on its

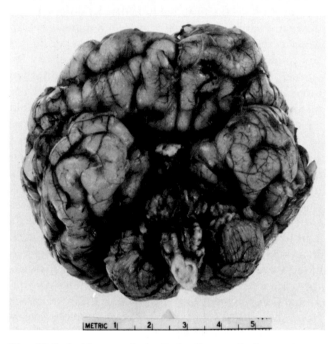

Fig. 42-9. Arrhinencephaly. Both olfactory bulbs and tracts are absent. There is approximation of the frontal lobes.

surface. The olfactory bulbs and tracts are absent, and anomalies of the optic nerves are common. Internally the sphere contains a single cavity in place of the lateral ventricles. The basal ganglia are fused, partially obliterating the third ventricle. Midline structures including the corpus callosum, septum pellucidum, and fornix are absent. Facial and cranial deformities involving the eyes, nose, and mouth accompany the brain lesion. Malformations are also commonly present in other organ systems.

In less severe forms of holoprosencephaly, imprecisely referred to as "arrhinencephaly," the olfactory bulbs and tracts are absent, but other parts of the rhinencephalon have developed (Fig. 42-9). The forebrain is partially separated into two hemispheres by a longitudinal fissure. In the depths of the fissure, however, the hemispheres are closely connected by gray matter or interdigitating gyri. The corpus callosum is absent, and a single ventricle replaces the lateral ventricles. Portions of the isocortex are absent or poorly developed. The accompanying facial and cranial malformations are similar to but less extensive than those associated with alobar holoprosencephaly.

Several etiologic factors have been associated with the holoprosencephalies.[244] These include chromosomal abnormalities especially trisomy 13-15 and trisomy 18 as other chromosomal disorders. Familial and hereditary cases have been identified. Holoprosencephaly is also linked with maternal diabetes.

Migration disorders. Congenital defects categorized as disorders of migration include (1) lesions indicating disturbance in the movement of neurons from their origin along the lumen of the neural tube to the positions they will occupy in the adult nervous system, such as

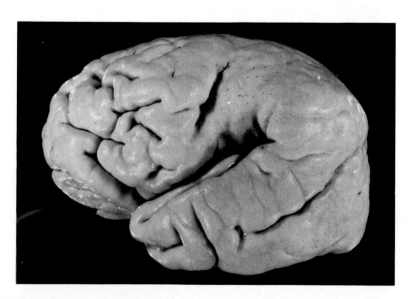

Fig. 42-10. Pachygyria. The gyri are broad and flat. Some primary and few secondary sulci are present.

heterotopic (ectopic) gray matter and glial cells, and (2) lesions indicating disturbance in the orderly arrangement of neurons at their adult locations, such as lissencephaly, pachygyria, and polymicrogyria. The usual sites for islands of heterotopic gray matter and glia are along the margins of the lateral ventricles, the cerebral or cerebellar white matter, and the subarachnoid space. These collections may occur as isolated lesions or in association with other central nervous system malformations, especially polymicrogyria.

Both lissencephaly and pachygyria involve a reduction in the number of cerebral convolutions. In the former condition gyri and sulci are absent from the cerebral hemisphere. The pachygyric cortex consists of occasional, broad flat gyri separated by sulci (Fig. 42-10). In polymicrogyria the surface of the affected cortex has a wrinkled appearance caused by the presence of many small poorly formed gyri (Fig. 42-11). One of the morphologic types of polymicrogyria is believed to be the consequence of neuronal destruction after completion of migration to the cortex rather than the usual mechanism involving the migratory process itself. Microscopically, abnormal lamination of neurons is present in each of the three cortical malformations.

Agenesis of the corpus callosum. The defect agenesis of the corpus callosum may occur in association with other malformations including migrational disorders or as an isolated, asymptomatic lesion. The defect may be complete or partial with absence of the splenium corporis callosi and posterior body. Both sporadic and hereditary forms of the malformation have been recognized.

Porencephaly, hydranencephaly, and multicystic encephalomalacia. These are cavitary lesions of the cerebral hemispheres. Some type of destructive process is involved in their pathogenesis. Porencephaly is used most often in reference to a circumscribed cavitary lesion involving one cerebral hemisphere. Architectural abnormalities of the adjacent cortex may be present if the lesion originated during the earlier stages of cortical development. In hydranencephaly most or all of the cerebral cortex and white matter is replaced by translucent membranous sacs filled with cerebrospinal fluid and composed of leptomeninges and glial tissue. In the less severe cases, gyri at the base of the brain can be identified. The onset is prenatal, though lesions resulting in extensive hemispheric destruction after birth are sometimes referred to as postnatal hydranencephaly. Multicystic encephalomalacia is characterized by the presence of multiple cavitary lesions in both cerebral hemispheres. The cavities are separated to some extent by glial septa containing lipid phagocytes. The lesions occur chiefly in the distribution of the anterior and middle cerebral arteries.

Congenital hydrocephalus. Congenital hydrocephalus may be either communicating or noncommunicating. Common causes include aqueductal obstruction, the Chiari type II (Arnold-Chiari) malformation, and the Dandy-Walker malformation. Less frequently, intrauterine infection, intraventricular hemorrhage, or other malformations underlie the ventricular enlargement. In her landmark study, Dorothy Russell[198] recognized four obstructive lesions of the aqueduct that cause congenital hydrocephalus. Three of these (simple stenosis, forking, and septum formation) were regarded as malformations. The fourth (gliosis of the aqueduct) was believed to be probably caused by an inflammatory process. In practice, however, it may be difficult to distin-

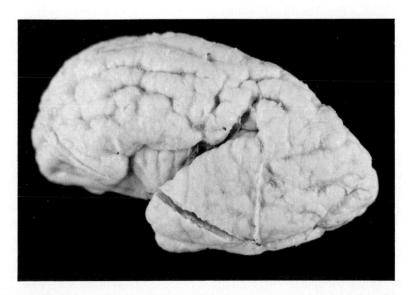

Fig. 42-11. Polymicrogyria. Notice wrinkled appearance of the gyral surfaces.

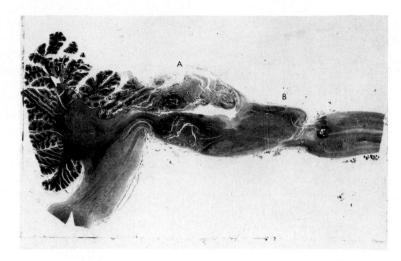

Fig. 42-12. Arnold-Chiari malformation. The vermis, *A*, is caudally elongated. There is dorsal and caudal displacement, *B*, of brainstem on cervical cord. (Loyez stain; 10×.)

guish between these lesions morphologically.[59] Further, experimental studies[108,132] have demonstrated the induction of aqueductal lesions resembling both the presumed developmental and inflammatory human types in suckling laboratory rodents after intracerebral inoculation and aqueductal ependymal infection with myxovirus, paramyxovirus, and reovirus type I. How frequently similar viral infections in humans cause congenital hydrocephalus is unknown. Occasional cases have been reported in children.[221]

Typically in cases of simple aqueductal stenosis, the aqueduct is histologically normal but abnormally small. Forking is characterized by replacement of the normal aqueduct with a dorsal and a ventral ependymal channel separated by normal parenchyma. The channels may communicate with each other, enter the ventricles separately, or end blindly. Septum formation involves the presence of a neurological membrane wholly or partially obstructing the caudal aqueduct. Gliosis of the aqueduct is reduction of the lumen by a distinct collar of fibrillary astrocytosis with remnants of the original ependymal lining located at the periphery of the astrocytic reaction. Ependyma is absent from its neoluminal margin. The aqueduct may be affected segmentally or throughout its length.

Two of the Chiari group of malformations deserve particular attention. The Chiari type II lesion is most common and often referred to as the Arnold-Chiari malformation (Fig. 42-12). In this condition the brainstem is displaced caudally and slightly overrides the rostral spinal cord. An S- or Z-shaped curve is evident in longitudinal section at the cervicomedullary junction. A tongue of cerebellar vermis extends for a variable distance caudally over the dorsal surface of the medulla into the spinal canal. Spina bifida and meningomyelocele are almost always present in Chiari type II malfor-

mations. Other central nervous system anomalies may also occur. The hydrocephalus is caused in some cases by aqueductal obstruction, whereas in others it may be related to blockage of subarachnoid cerebrospinal fluid pathways at the foramen magnum by the displaced cerebellum and brainstem.

The Chiari type I malformation may not cause symptoms until adolescence or adulthood, at which time signs of increased intracranial pressure may appear abruptly. Portions of one or both cerebellar tonsils rather than vermis extend below the plane of the foramen magnum. Syringomyelia and bony deformities of the foramen magnum may coexist with this lesion. Spina bifida and meningomyelocele are rare.

The Dandy-Walker syndrome involves the association of hydrocephalus with a posterior fossa cyst, partial or complete absence of the vermis, and dolichocephaly. The pathogenesis of the condition has been attributed to absence of the fourth ventricular exit foramina. Several studies indicate, however, that the lesion originates as an anomaly of the vermis. Hart and co-workers[91] have suggested the following criteria for neuropathologic diagnosis: hydrocephalus, partial or complete absence of the cerebellar vermis, and posterior fossa cyst continuous with the fourth ventricle.

Syringomyelia. The term "syringomyelia" is frequently applied to any spinal cord lesion that is tubular and cavitary and extends over several segments. When used in this way, the term encompasses lesions of different etiology, pathogenesis, and clinical importance. The condition in which the cavity represents only a distension of the central canal is more precisely termed "hydromyelia." Minor degrees of this lesion are observed in routine autopsies; however, it has an important association with the Chiari type II malformation and meningomyelocele. The cavity is lined by ependymal cells and a meshwork of astrocytic processes. When used in a restricted sense, syringomyelia refers to a cavitary lesion lined by an astrocytic meshwork and devoid of ependymal cells except where the cavity may encroach on remnants of the central canal. The defect extends transversely across the cord and is most extensive in the cervical segments. Caudally the lumbosacral segments are not usually involved. The presence of histologically similar slitlike lesions in the brainstem is termed "syringobulbia." Although the lesion is believed to be a developmental disorder, clinical symptoms often do not appear until the second or third decade. The term "secondary syringomyelia" is sometimes used to designate tubular cavities of obvious cause, such as tumors, trauma, and adhesive arachnoiditis.

Down's syndrome. The disorder called "Down's syndrome" is relatively common, having an incidence of 1 in 600 to 1000 births. It is the first human disease shown to be associated with chromosomal abnormalities, which include trisomy 21, D/G and G/G translocations, and mosaicism. Trisomy 21 is present in 90% to 95% of cases. It is associated with sporadic cases and advancing maternal age (above 35 years).[15] Although there are no structural lesions in the central nervous system specific for Down's syndrome, certain gross abnormalities such as brain weight less than 1200 g, flattened occipital pole, and narrow superior temporal gyrus are often seen in this disorder (Fig. 42-13). Microscopically, reduced numbers of cerebral cortical neurons, morphologic irregularities of cerebral cortical dendrites, and indications of disturbed development of cerebral cortical synapses have been reported,[165,188,230] suggestive of the possibility of an underlying disturbance of cerebral cortical organization. Fibrillary astrocytosis of the cerebral white matter has also been described.[139] Cerebral infarction or abscess may develop as complications of the congenital heart defects commonly present in the Down's patient. Within the last two decades, the frequent occurrence of Alzheimer changes in the brains of Down's syndrome patients over 30 years of age has been recognized.[185]

Fetal alcohol syndrome. The fetal alcohol syndrome comprises a group of congenital disorders observed in the children of mothers who drink regularly during pregnancy. Anomalies include growth retardation, dysmorphic cranial and facial features, malformations of the central nervous system and of the viscera. Clinically, mental retardation and microcephaly are prominent features. The central nervous system lesions are among the most serious components of this syndrome. Neuropathologic changes include neuronal and glial migrational defects, hydrocephalus, schizencephaly, agenesis of the corpus callosum, and neural tube defects[42,43,250] In addition to maternal alcohol consumption, other coexisting factors such as drug abuse, poor nutrition, and smoking can be etiologically related to the syndrome.[111]

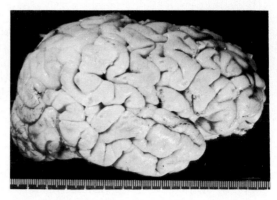

Fig. 42-13. Down's syndrome. Small superior temporal gyrus and blunted occipital lobe.

A recent study, however, addressing this question indicates a definitive, dose-response relationship between prenatal alcohol exposure and the craniofacial abnormalities. A significant but less striking relationship was noted for the systemic anomalies.[64]

Perinatal brain injury

The term "perinatal brain injury" comprises a group of hemorrhagic and necrotic lesions and their sequelae that are believed to have their inception at or near birth (prenatal or postnatal). Mechanical trauma, metabolic disturbances including hypoxia, and intoxications are among the mechanisms implicated in their pathogenesis often on the basis of indirect or circumstantial evidence. Consequently, the influence and importance of these mechanisms remain uncertain and open to debate. The use of new methods for evaluating the fetus and newborn infant such as fetal monitoring, real-time ultrasound scanning, and other types of neuroimaging, evoked potentials, and so forth to evaluate the systemic and neurologic status of the infant before, during, and after delivery will add significantly to the understanding of perinatal brain injuries particularly when these studies are correlated with the results of careful neuropathologic examinations. These data should help resolve some of the controversy surrounding the mechanisms of perinatal brain injury.

Hemorrhage. Both external and internal hemorrhages involving the head are encountered in the neonatal neuropathologic examination. The external lesions are the caput succedaneum, subaponeurotic hemorrhage, and cephalhematoma. Intracranial hemorrhage may be extradural, intradural, subdural, subarachnoid, parenchymal, and periventricular-intraventricular. Among all of these, there are four with major clinical significance: subdural, subarachnoid, intracerebellar, and periventricular-intraventricular hemorrhage.

Subdural hemorrhage. With rare exceptions this type of hemorrhage is caused by intrapartum traumatic compression and distortion of the skull related to one or more of the following risk factors: small, rigid birth canal; prematurity with excessive skull compliance; full-term infants large in relation to the size of the birth canal; precipitous labor with insufficient dilatation of the birth canal; prolonged labor with excessive molding of the head; and difficult deliveries, such as breech, forceps, and rotation. The hemorrhage usually originates from tears in bridging veins that pass between the surface of the brain and the dural venous sinuses. The superior cerebral veins are most commonly affected. Other sources include tentorial lacerations involving the straight or lateral sinuses, laceration of the falx and adjacent venous channels, and occipital osteodiastasis with laceration of the occipital sinus. Blood accumulates in the subdural space around the torn veins forming a hematoma, which may behave as a space-occupying mass. Large posterior fossa hematomas are often fatal, whereas infants with cerebral-convexity hematomas may survive without sequelae.[244] Although most cases of neonatal subdural hemorrhage still occur in full-term infants, the incidence has declined in this group because of improved obstetrical management.

Subarachnoid hemorrhage. The localized or diffuse accumulation of blood in the subarachnoid space as a result of bleeding from leptomeningeal vessels is referred to as "primary subarachnoid hemorrhage." Involvement of the subarachnoid space by extension of subdural, parenchymal, or intraventricular hemorrhage is designated as "secondary subarachnoid hemorrhage." Only primary subarachnoid hemorrhage is considered in this section. Diffuse, primary neonatal subarachnoid hemorrhage varies in quantity from a few thin patches to prominent collections of blood. It occurs in premature and full-term infants. The cause is uncertain; however, both hypoxia and trauma have been implicated. The latter mechanism is associated with occurrence of the hemorrhage in full-term babies and the former with premature infants. Thick, localized neonate subarachnoid hemorrhage usually occurs over the temporal and occipital lobes. It is associated with coagulation disorders and exchange transfusions.[249] The clinical features of neonatal primary subarachnoid hemorrhage are not completely defined. Volpe[244] has tentatively identified three groups of patients: those with minimal or absent neurologic signs, those with seizures, and those with catastrophic neurologic deterioration and a rapidly fatal course. Most of the patients in the first two categories appear to do well with little or no residual neurologic deficit, provided that there is no accompanying major hypoxic or traumatic brain damage.

Parenchymal hemorrhage. Except for periventricular hemorrhage, which is discussed separately, most hemorrhage lesions in the neonatal cerebrum are not primary hematomas but hemorrhagic infarcts associated with either arterial or venous occlusion. Primary he-

matomas occur infrequently and are related to a variety of causes, including coagulation defects, trauma, vascular malformations, and congenital tumors.[190] Hemorrhagic lesions of the neonatal cerebellum may be the result of traumatic lacerations in cases of occipital osteodiastasis, venous infarction, extension from intraventricular or subarachnoid sources, and primary intracerebellar bleeding. The last three conditions account for most cases.[244] Pathogenetic factors include difficult delivery, hypoxic events, and prematurity. The occurrence of hemorrhagic venous infarction of the cerebellum in premature infants ventilated by face mask has been associated with the use of occipital straps or nets to attack the mask.[249] The overall prognosis for intracerebral hemorrhagic lesions is uncertain. With regard to cerebellar lesions of this type, premature infants usually have a fatal outcome, whereas full-term infants may survive.

Periventricular-intraventricular hemorrhage. Periventricular-intraventricular hemorrhage is a major cause of neurologic disability and death in the premature infant. Its prevalence based upon imaging studies is between 35% and 45% among newborns of less than 35 weeks' gestation.[244] In contrast, it occurs in only 2% to 3% of full-term infants.[120,186] The hemorrhage usually develops during the first 72 hours after birth.[244] It has also been reported in utero.[120,186] Commonly the infant also has the respiratory distress syndrome. At autopsy blood clot fills and distends all or part of the ventricular system and may extend through the fourth ventricular foramina into the cisterna magna and subarachnoid space over the cerebellum and brainstem (Fig. 42-14).

In premature infants the intraventricular accumulation of blood most often results from extension of hemorrhage in the subependymal germinal matrix into the

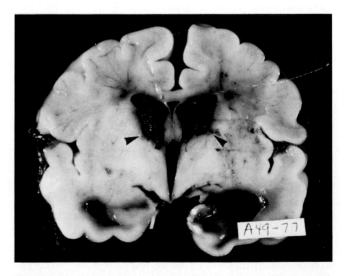

Fig. 42-14. Bilateral periventricular, *arrows,* caudate hemorrhage with intraventricular extension.

ventricular lumen. These matrix hemorrhages may be single or multiple and unilateral or bilateral. They may develop at any site along the ventricular borders where germinal matrix is present such as the lateral margins of the lateral ventricles (including the temporal and occipital horns) or the roof of the fourth ventricle. Characteristically, the matrix hemorrhage, which is the source of the intraventricular hemorrhage, is located either adjacent to the ventral head of the caudate nucleus at the level of the foramen of Monro or along the body of the caudate nucleus.[249] Less frequently, choroid plexus hemorrhage is the source of the intraventricular blood, and in some cases both matrix and choroid plexus lesions are present. Matrix hemorrhages may also occur without associated intraventricular hemorrhage. In full-term infants relatively little of the germinal matrix remains and the intraventricular component of the hemorrhage usually originates from another site, most often the choroid plexus.[58]

The pathogenesis of periventricular-intraventricular hemorrhage appears to be complicated and not fully defined.[244] Several factors, including disturbances in blood flow, pressure, and volume, asphyxia and respiratory distress, coagulation disorders, metabolic vulnerability of the matrix zone, and immaturity and fragility of vascular channels, may be involved.

Clinically, periventricular-intraventricular hemorrhage may be associated with a rapid (minutes to hours) or subacute (up to 24 hours) deterioration of neurologic function, including alterations in consciousness and tone, respiratory disturbances, and seizures. In some cases there is minimal evidence of a neurologic disturbance. The diagnosis is confirmed with an ultrasound scan. The short-term mortality is related to the severity of the hemorrhage and varies from 20% to 60% for moderate to severe grades. Among survivors the frequency of major neurologic sequelae (motor deficits, intellectual retardation) varies from 15% to 40%. In cases with extensive hemorrhagic involvement of the cerebral parenchyma in addition to periventricular-intraventricular hemorrhage, the figure rises to 90%.[244]

The neuropathologic findings in survivors of periventricular-intraventricular hemorrhage have not been extensively documented chiefly because until recently few infants lived more than 1 or 2 days after onset of the hemorrhage. Because of improved medical management, there are now, as noted above, significant numbers of survivors. In an autopsy study, Armstrong and co-workers[7] observed lesions related to periventricular-intraventricular hemorrhage as well as necrotic parenchymal lesions traditionally associated with hypoxia and ischemia. The principal hemorrhagic sequela was hydrocephalus. This form of posthemorrhagic hydrocephalus is usually caused by organization of the subarachnoid extension of the intraventricular hemorrhage with obliteration of the subarachnoid space and foramina of

the fourth ventricle. Less often, the block occurs at the aqueduct because of gliosis induced by intraventricular bleeding.[120] In addition to ventricular dilatation, hemosiderin staining of the ependymal lining and leptomeninges is also apparent. Other hemorrhagic sequelae include hemosiderin-stained subependymal cysts evolved from matrix hemorrhages that did not rupture into the ventricle and destruction of germinal matrix tissue. The clinical and developmental effects of this disruption and loss of matrix tissue are unknown.

Parenchymal necrosis. Hypoxic ischemic necrosis including its sequelae and kernicterus are covered in this section. The former condition ranks with periventricular-intraventricular hemorrhage as a major cause of perinatal neurologic disability and death. The frequency of kernicterus, on the other hand, has declined with the development of methods for controlling hemolytic disease in the newborn.

Hypoxic-ischemic necrosis. The lesions described in this section are widely viewed as developing against the background of a reduced oxygen supply to the brain because of inadequate vascular perfusion (ischemia) or diminished circulatory transport (hypoxemia). These two disturbances, hypoxemia and ischemia, may occur ante partum, intra partum, or post partum. Their principal causes include cardiac or circulatory insufficiency associated with intrauterine asphyxia, recurrent apneic spells, congenital abnormalities of the heart or great vessels, or septic shock; respiratory insufficiency or failure associated with disturbed exchange of respiratory gases across the placenta, the respiratory distress syndrome, or recurrent apneic spells; and severe right-to-left vascular shunts.[244] Although perinatal asphyxial events are recognized as significant risk factors associated with the development of permanent neurologic disability, their occurrence does not lead inevitably to such an outcome. Many infants with documented evidence of perinatal asphyxia escape without lasting neurologic complications.[32] These observations indicate that the evolution of the necrotic lesions regarded as hypoxic-ischemic in origin is a complex process influenced by factors that have not been fully characterized or identified.

Both acute and chronic central nervous system lesions are attributed to hypoxic-ischemic injury. The acute forms are periventricular leukomalacia and gray-matter necrosis, which may involve structures in the cerebrum, brainstem, or cerebellum. Chronic lesions include ulegyria and status marmoratus. At least some cases of the cavitary lesions mentioned previously—hydranencephaly, multicystic encephalomalacia, and porencephaly—may also develop as a consequence of hypoxic-ischemic parenchymal destruction.

PERIVENTRICULAR LEUKOMALACIA. Although periventricular leukomalacia was recognized almost a century ago, this lesion received little attention until

Banker and Larroche[13] published their classic study delineating its pathologic characteristics, including the distinctive anatomic distribution of the lesions. Premature infants are affected most often; however, the disorder also occurs in full-term and stillborn infants.[119,186] The clinical setting most often associated with periventricular leukomalacia includes prematurity, postnatal survival beyond a few days, and cardiorespiratory disturbances associated with various conditions, such as congenital heart disease, shock sepsis, and respiratory distress syndrome.[244]

Macroscopically the typical acute lesions appear as one or more irregular, white or yellow foci in the cen-

trum semiovale near the lateral angles of the ventricles and in the optic or auditory radiations (Fig. 42-15, *A*). Some foci are hemorrhagic. Microscopically, the features are those of coagulation necrosis with swollen axons accompanied by histiocytes, phagocytes, reactive astrocytes, and vascular proliferation according to the age of the lesion. In older lesions fibrillary astrocytosis, mineral deposits, or even cavitation may be evident (Fig. 42-15, *B*).

Pathogenetic studies have focused on ischemia occurring after perfusion failure in arterial boundary zones or end-artery zones of the white matter as a basis for the necrotic lesions.[55,231] Gilles and co-workers[80,81] have

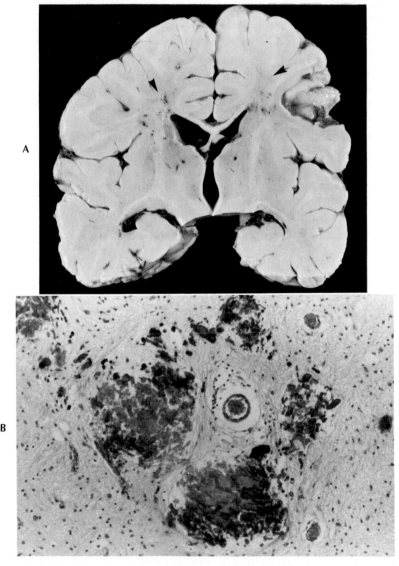

Fig. 42-15. A, Periventricular leukomalacia. Bilateral foci of white matter discoloration and vascular congestion, *arrows,* adjacent to lateral ventricular angles. The child died between 3 and 4 months of age. **B,** Histologic section through periventricular white matter in **A,** with parenchymal loss, fibrillary astrocytosis, vascular congestion, and basophilic foci mineralization. (Hematoxylin and eosin; 250×.)

described a group of white matter changes comprising astrocytosis, amphophilic globules, and acutely damaged glia occurring alone, together, or in combination with necrotic white matter foci in neonatal autopsies. They have suggested the term "perinatal telencephalic leukoencephalopathy" to designate these changes. Clinical and experimental studies indicate that endotoxemia may play an important role in the induction of the alterations. The precise relationship between perinatal telencephalic leukoencephalopathy and periventricular leukomalacia has not been clarified. The former may represent an early stage or less severe variant of the latter.

The clinical characteristics of periventricular leukomalacia in the neonatal period are not yet defined, chiefly because data needed for clinicopathologic correlation are lacking and, until the recent advent of more sophisticated imaging procedures, confirmation of the clinical diagnosis was difficult. The principal long-term neurologic disturbance is spastic diplegia.[244]

GRAY MATTER NECROSIS. Gray matter necrosis is a characteristic finding associated with perinatal asphyxia in full-term infants.[244] It also occurs, at least to some extent, in cases of periventricular leukomalacia.[13] If only a few cells are involved, no gross changes may be evident. In the case of larger lesions, however, acutely affected areas are grossly swollen and soft and appear pale, congested, or hemorrhagic. Histologic changes such as eosinophilic neuronal necrosis occur but may be difficult to recognize because of the small size of the infant's neuronal perikarya and the close packing of neurons in regions such as cerebral cortex. Subsequently, astrocytes and macrophages are activated, dead nerve cells disappear, and the neuropil becomes vacuolated. Necrotic neurons, especially in the thalamus, may have intensely basophilic cell bodies that stain positively with periodic acid–Schiff stain and with methods for iron and calcium. Four anatomic patterns of gray matter necrosis have been described: cerebral cortical, striatal, diencephalic-rhombencephalic, and pontosubicular.[154] These patterns often overlap and should be regarded as regional accentuations of the damage rather than as discrete lesions.

Cerebral cortical lesions may be diffuse, boundary zone, or arterial in their distribution. Microscopically, the necrosis may be focal, laminar, or transcortical. In the hippocampus neurons in the pyramidal cell layer as well as those in the subiculum and presubiculum are commonly affected. Patchy or diffuse neuronal involvement may be seen in the corpus striatum and thalamus. Prominent lesions are found in the subthalamic nuclei, lateral geniculate bodies, inferior colliculi, and cranial nerve nuclei. In the cerebellum neurons in the dentate nucleus, Purkinje cells, and the internal granular layer are most severely affected. Occasionally, necrotic neu-

rons are observed in the anterior horns of the spinal cord.[119]

There are several chronic lesions attributed to hypoxic-ischemic injury including atrophy and astrocytosis of the affected region sometimes accompanied by gross or microscopic cavitation, ulegyria, and status marmoratus. The morphologic evolution of atrophy, astrocytosis, cavitation, and ulegyria from initial injury to end-stage appearance can be traced or reasonably inferred without great difficulty. This analysis, however, can be complicated because infants with these lesions who have survived for months or years may also have acquired during this period of survival additional hypoxic-ischemic damage as a result of repeated seizures, apneic spells, and so on. The application of sophisticated neuroimaging techniques should prove valuable in resolving such problems. On the other hand, the exact nature of the injury that leads to status marmoratus is still obscure.

The atrophic-gliotic lesions are not unlike the changes of similar cause that occur in adults. Because of the higher water content of infant brain or possibly other factors, the degree of cavitation may be greater in the neonate than in older persons.

Ulegyria refers to the groups of atrophic, roughly mushroom-shaped gyri with adjacent widened sulci that characteristically are found in the parietal and occipital convexities. Microscopically, parenchymal loss is greater along sulcal valleys than over the gyral crests, giving rise to the mushroom configuration.

Status marmoratus, or marbling, most often involves the thalamus, neostriatum, or cerebral cortex. It is the name given to the irregular, intersecting bands of myelin and astrocytic processes that develop abnormally in these regions. Their gross and microscopic appearance in myelin-stained sections recalls the variegated patterns seen on marble surfaces. The development of the abnormal myelin appears to be the result of aberrant myelination of astrocytic processes.[26] The precise relationship of this lesion to hypoxic-ischemic injury is unknown. Both ulegyria and marbling may coexist.

Kernicterus. Kernicterus refers to the overt form of bilirubin encephalopathy in which there is selective staining of gray matter and neuronal necrosis. The disorder is caused by relatively high serum levels of unbound, unconjugated bilirubin that develop in the newborn period as a consequence of hemolytic disorders, resorption of large hematomas, congenital and acquired defects in bilirubin conjugation, and so on. A serum bilirubin concentration in excess of 20 mg/dl is considered a clear indication for exchange transfusion to prevent kernicterus. Other factors such as prematurity, low serum albumin concentration, asphyxia, acidosis, and sepsis may lower the serum bilirubin threshold for kernicterus to a range of 10 to 15 mg/dl. Some data indicate that there may be more subtle forms of bilirubin encephalopathy with even lower serum bilirubin levels and without kernicterus; however, this issue is unresolved.

The pathogenesis of kernicterus involves movement of the bilirubin into the brain most likely followed by intoxication and death of neurons. Although the concept of an immature blood-brain barrier permitting bilirubin access to neural parenchyma is no longer accepted, increased permeability of the barrier resulting from endothelial damage caused by asphyxia, intracranial infection, or increases in serum osmolality may facilitate entry of bilirubin, which may bind with phospholipid forming a lipophilic complex, which could readily cross an intact blood-brain barrier.[244] The neuronal toxicity of bilirubin is believed to involve an effect on mitochondria perhaps enhanced by other concomitant neuronal injury, such as hypoxia and hypoglycemia.[104,244] The basis for the selective involvement of specific nuclei and regions of gray matter is uncertain. The explanation may involve vascular factors, binding sites, or biochemical processes at the affected sites.

The chief pathologic features of kernicterus are macroscopic, symmetric bilirubin staining of specific regions of gray matter and neuronal necrosis at those sites. Most commonly affected are the globus pallidus, thalamus, subthalamus, cranial nerve nuclei, inferior olives, gracile and cuneate nuclei, and cerebellar roof nuclei. Less often the hippocampus, putamen, lateral geniculate body, and anterior horns are involved. The yellow color of these structures is readily apparent in the fresh brain and after formalin fixation. Histologically, shrunken neurons with pyknotic nuclei are found at the sites of gross staining. Bilirubin pigment is also discernible even in paraffin sections, possibly reflecting tight binding of the pigment to cell membranes. Evidence of ischemic neuronal necrosis may be superimposed on the pigmentary lesions. In the brains of infants who survive the acute phase of kernicterus and die at a later date, neuron loss and astrocytosis are evident in many of the structures that stained during the acute stage. During their first year such children exhibit hypotonia, brisk deep tendon reflexes, a persistent tonic neck reflex, and slow development of motor skills. Later, the extrapyramidal signs and gaze disturbances generally regarded as characteristic sequelae of kernicterus appear.[244]

Circulatory and vascular disorders

Ischemic necrosis of central nervous system parenchyma and nontraumatic subarachnoid or parenchymal hemorrhage are the two most important neuropathologic lesions caused by this group of diseases. The term "stroke" is used clinically in reference to the neurologic disorder that may accompany certain types of ischemic or hemorrhagic lesions. This topic is discussed more fully at the end of this section.

Ischemic necrosis

As the name implies, ischemic necrosis is a type of lesion that results from ischemia, a condition in which, because of considerable reduction or complete interruption, the blood supply to neural tissue is insufficient to meet metabolic needs. Although the brain can metabolize other energy-yielding substrates, such as ketone bodies, only oxygen and glucose are available in sufficient quantities to sustain the brain's considerable energy requirement. Most of the needed energy is derived from glucose oxidation by the citric acid (Krebs) cycle, which requires oxygen. Moreover, because of the limited stores of energy reserves in neural tissues, the supply of oxygen and glucose must be continuous. Experimental studies, for example, show that these reserves may be consumed in as little as 2 minutes after onset of total tissue ischemia.[125] Energy failure alone, however, does not cause the necrosis. Current evidence indicates that energy failure precipitates several cellular and subcellular reactions such as failure of ionic pumps, formation of free radicals, release of excitatory neurotransmitters, tissue lactic acidosis, and microcirculatory impairment, which may lead ultimately to the development or extension of the necrotic lesion.[77,171,191]

The necrotic lesions are anatomically distributed in two patterns: (1) widespread, affecting many parts of the central nervous system, and (2) discrete and focal, lying within the central nervous system territory supplied or drained by an artery or vein. The pattern is determined by the circumstances of the inciting ischemic episode. The widespread pattern, usually designated as ischemic, hypoxic, or anoxic encephalopathy, develops when blood flow to much or all of the brain is temporarily interrupted or reduced to ischemic levels. The common causes of this type of circulatory crisis are severe systemic hypotension (mean arterial pressure less than 60 mm Hg); cardiac arrhythmias such as ventricular fibrillation; transient cardiac arrest; and sudden, massive increases in intracranial pressure with vascular compression, as in cases of closed head injury. The discrete focal necrotic lesion, customarily referred to as an infarct, is caused by occlusive vascular disease affecting either arteries or veins.

Ischemic (hypoxic, anoxic) encephalopathy. The maximum length of time the central nervous system can survive an ischemic circulatory crisis without incurring irreversible damage (necrosis) is influenced by several factors including the severity of the episode, the presence of cerebrovascular disease, the age of the patient, and body temperature. In the case of cardiac arrest, parenchymal necrosis and permanent neurologic sequelae can be expected when the period of complete ischemia exceeds 5 to 10 minutes in a normothermic adult. This time may be longer in younger children and in the presence of hypothermia. The extent of the necrosis and the severity of the permanent neurologic deficit increase with prolongation of the ischemic period. Clinical disturbances vary from permanent coma with a continuing requirement for cardiorespiratory support in cases of profound ischemia to a mixture of extrapyramidal signs, visual disorders, action myoclonus, amnesia, and dementia in cases of lesser severity.

The neuropathologic findings depend in part on the length of survival after the ischemic episode and the extent to which blood flow is restored to the brain during the resuscitative effort. Gross and microscopic changes except for edema may be slight or absent when the brains of patients dying within a few minutes or hours after the ischemic period are examined by conventional methods. After a range of 6 to 12 hours, neuropathologic alterations are detectable with these techniques. Special procedures including plastic embedding, histochemistry, and electron microscopy can be employed to detect very early lesions; however, because of problems with postmortem artifact usually related to delayed fixation, these methods are used primarily for experimental studies. On the other hand, in cases of severe, generalized ischemic brain injury where the electroencephalogram is devoid of spontaneous activity and the patient has been maintained on external cardiorespiratory support for several days, a group of central nervous system changes collectively designated as "respirator brain" are frequently encountered. The brain is noticeably swollen, soft, friable, and dusky. The cerebellar tonsils are herniated into the foramen magnum because of the increased intracranial pressure induced by the parenchymal swelling. Sometimes, fragments or even larger masses of the easily disrupted cerebellar tissue are forced, like toothpaste from a tube, along the vertebral canal caudally as far as the lumbosacral level. Microscopically, there is widespread eosinophilic neuronal necrosis without accompanying astrocytic, vascular, or inflammatory reactions. The internal granular layer of the cerebellar cortex is pale staining and loose meshed. These changes, which are in part autolytic, occur when brain death precedes somatic death and the devitalized central nervous system tissues remain near normal body temperature but devoid of circulation until somatic death takes place. The mechanism involves severe, extensive ischemic brain injury causing massive brain swelling and a rise in intracranial pressure above the level of systolic blood pressure, effectively cutting off all blood flow to the central nervous system. In the meantime body temperature remains at or near 37° C, while systemic circulation and respiration are maintained with mechanical means. Under these circumstances the phenomenon of respirator brain develops within a few days.

In cases of acute ischemic encephalopathy not of the respirator brain type, gross changes include edema (cytotoxic) indicated by flattened gyri and narrowed sulci over the cerebral convexities, accentuation of tentorial and foraminal markings at the base of the brain, and reduced ventricular lumens. Foci of congestion, or petechiae, are present within the gray matter, especially the cerebral cortex along sulcal valleys or in arterial border zones (the junctions between territories supplied by cerebral arteries; for example, the anterior–middle cerebral artery border zone extends along the superior cerebral convexity, parallel, and a few centimeters lateral to the interhemispheric fissure). Microscopically, the principal change is eosinophilic necrosis of neurons, the parenchymal elements most sensitive to ischemia. Necrotic neurons may be widely distributed, but they are found most often in certain locations including the third and fifth layers of cerebral cortex along sulcal valleys and arterial border zones, Sommer's sector of the hippocampus, and the cerebellar Purkinje layer. The reasons why neurons in these areas are affected more often than those in other areas are not fully known. In some cases this apparent selective vulnerability may be related to the location of the neurons in the most distal regions of an arterial blood supply such as arterial border zones or sulcal valleys. These are the sites at which perfusion failure and ischemia would develop first during a circulatory crisis such as severe systemic hypotension.[29] In other locations neuronal involvement may reflect regional variations in metabolism or even the distribution of neurotransmitters. In severe forms of ischemic encephalopathy, neurons in the corpus striatum, thalamus, brainstem, and dentate nucleus are affected. The lesions are bilateral and more or less symmetric. The term "laminar" or "pseudolaminar necrosis" is applied to cerebral cortical lesions with extensive damage to some but not all the cortical layers. The third and fifth laminae are the usual sites of such extensive damage. Because, however, necrotic neurons are almost always found in the other cortical laminae, the features of the lesion are best described as transcortical neuronal necrosis with laminar accentuation. In the days and weeks after the ischemic period, necrotic tissue is removed by phagocytosis, endothelial proliferation repairs damaged blood vessels, and reactive astrocytosis replaces the lost parenchyma. After several months these reactive changes are complete, and the lesions have acquired their permanent structural features. Grossly, the affected gray matter is reduced in volume and is spongy and yellow (Fig. 42-16). Microscopically it is the site of nerve cell loss and fibrillary astrocytosis.

Infarct. In the central nervous system as well as in other organs an infarct is defined as a localized area of

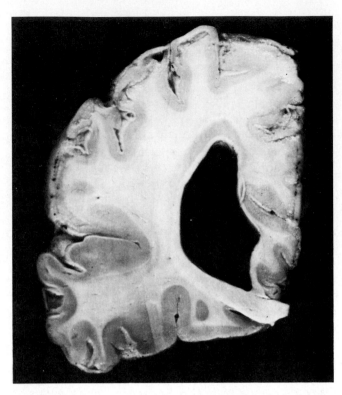

Fig. 42-16. Diffuse, chronic ischemia encephalopathy. The cerebral cortex over the convexity is greatly thinned, and the normal anatomic markings are obscured.

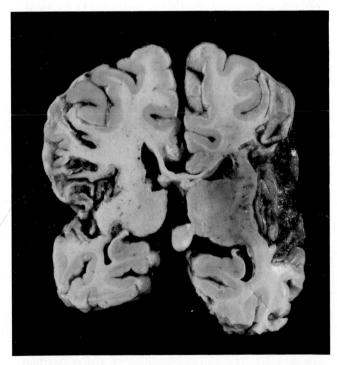

Fig. 42-17. Bilateral old infarcts with middle cerebral artery distribution. The patient was a child with tetralogy of Fallot.

tissue necrosis involving all parenchymal elements, caused by vascular occlusion (venous or arterial), and lying within the territory of the occluded vessel (Fig. 42-17). Occasionally the term "infarct" is applied less restrictively to the more severe types of focal lesions seen in cases of ischemic encephalopathy. At least in the acute stage, the core of necrotic tissue is believed to be surrounded by a zone of nonfunctional but still viable parenchyma called the "ischemic penumbra."[9,10] The pathophysiologic characteristics of this zone are being vigorously explored because it represents brain tissue that may be therapeutically salvaged, thus limiting the extent of any permanent neurologic deficit brought about by the infarct.

Infarcts of the central nervous system may be caused by a variety of occlusive vascular disorders.[76] Because of collateral circulation the size of the infarct is usually smaller than the territory supplied by the occluded vessel. Most often, the occlusive process involves thrombosis or thromboembolism associated with atherosclerosis. Other causes include vasculitis and hematologic disorders such as sickle cell anemia.[189] Occlusions may occur in the intracranial arteries and arterioles or in cervical portions of the carotid and vertebral arteries. Embolic sources include cardiac thrombi associated with myocardial infarction, atrial fibrillation, and endocarditis, as well as atheromatous plaques located within arteries supplying the central nervous system and giving rise embolic fragments. In many cases the exact mechanism responsible for the infarction cannot be proved directly even with sophisticated clinical imaging procedures or careful neuropathologic examination. This problem results in part from the progressive changes in occluding emboli and thrombi, which eventually obliterate either their distinguishing features or even eliminate conclusive evidence of their occurrence.

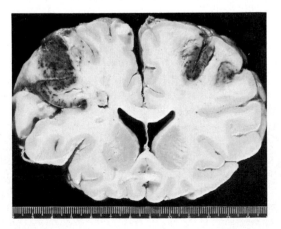

Fig. 42-18. Recent mixed hemorrhagic and anemia infarcts resulting from emboli in middle cerebral arteries.

In addition to the actual precipitating event, attention is also directed toward treatable or preventable conditions that are statistically associated with an increased likelihood of infarctions. Such conditions are referred to as risk factors and include systemic hypertension, diabetes mellitus, heart disease, and cigarette smoking.[46] Venous thrombosis involves one or more of the dural sinuses or their major branches and is usually a complication of dehydration (especially in children), congestive heart failure, hematologic disorders, the puerperium, and pyogenic infections around the nose, mouth, and eyes.[110]

Clinically, an infarct is associated with the development of a localized neurologic deficit. The signs and symptoms depend on the area of the brain affected. If the deficit resolves within 24 hours, the episode is termed a "transient ischemic attack" (TIA). TIAs are commonly attributed to the effects of small emboli arising in the heart or arteries supplying the brain. Permanent parenchymal lesions are small or undetectable. Approximately 30% of patients will experience a major infarct within 5 years after their first TIA.[238] Symptoms persisting more than 24 hours but less than 3 weeks are termed a "reversible ischemic neurologic deficit" (RIND). The combination of infarction and stepwise progression of the neurologic disability is referred to as a "stroke in evolution." When the neurologic disorder becomes stabilized, the condition is termed a "partial nonprogressing stroke" or "completed stroke" depending on the extent of the deficit. The mortality for major brain infarction during the first 30 days after onset is 25% to 30% usually as a result of pneumonia or brain herniation.

Grossly, neuropathologic changes are evident within 6 to 12 hours after the development of neurologic signs. The affected region is swollen and soft. The swelling is the result of edema that is initially cytotoxic. During the first week after the infarct occurs a vasogenic component develops. If the infarct is large, such as one affecting most of a cerebral hemisphere, the swollen tissue behaves as a mass lesion causing herniation of the ipsilateral medial temporal lobe with fatal results. The infarcted tissue may be pale (anemic) or hemorrhagic. Hemorrhagic infarcts are typically associated with embolic occlusion of arterial vessels or venous thrombosis (Figs. 42-18 and 42-19). In the former case, the embolus becomes fragmented and is carried distal to its initial lodgment site bringing about reperfusion of damaged, leaky vessels. With venous obstruction, the continued egress of blood from patent arterial sources into the occluded veins leads to congestion, stasis, and vascular disruption. The possibility of other mechanisms causing hemorrhagic infarction is debated. Hemorrhagic infarction can be distinguished from parenchymal hematomas by demonstration of the predominant perivascular location of the bleeding combined with necrosis of the intervening tissue. Further, in the case of infarction the hemorrhage is confined chiefly to gray matter.

Microscopically, the earliest changes are pallor, vacuolization and eosinophilic neuronal necrosis (Fig. 42-20). During the first week reactive changes including transient inflammatory cell infiltration, astrocytic and vascular proliferation, and phagocyte formation occur. During the next several months necrotic debris is re-

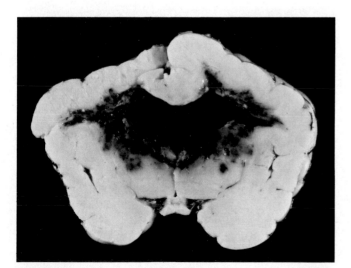

Fig. 42-19. Acute venous infarction in an infant after thrombosis of vein of Galen and straight sinus. The distribution of the lesions is characteristic for occlusions in these venous channels.

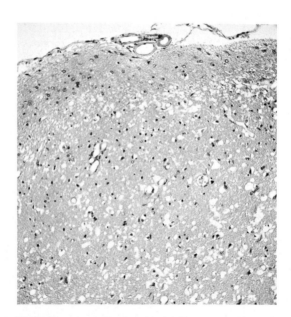

Fig. 42-20. Recent anemic infarct. There is intact outer cortical layer with reactive astrocytosis. Pallor, cellular pyknosis, and microcavitation result from edema in deeper cortical layers. (Hematoxylin and eosin; 90×.)

moved by phagocytosis, and astrocytes proliferate reducing the parenchymal deficit to some extent (Figs. 42-17 and 42-21).

The morphologic evolution of the infarct reaches its end stage after 3 or 4 months, and no further major changes occur. Thus all end-stage infarcts have similar pathologic features. On this basis it is possible to say that a lesion is at least 3 or 4 months old. It is difficult or impossible however to distinguish with certainty, using only morphologic criteria, for example, end-stage infarcts that are 6 months old from those that have been present several years. End-stage lesions are well-demarcated foci of soft, cavitated, yellow, or tan tissue. Microscopically the infarcted neural parenchyma has been replaced by a proliferation of fibrillary astrocytes in which cavities traversed by small blood vessels are present. Small (less than 1.5 cm in maximum dimension) cavitary infarcts are referred to as lacunes ('small lakes') or lacunar infarcts (Fig. 42-22). These lesions are found in greatest numbers in the corpus striatum and thalamus and less often in the striate pons. They are a common complication of systemic hypertension and usually result from occlusive lesions in arterioles between 200 and 400 μm in diameter.[140]

Hemorrhage

The disorders under consideration here are those in which the primary pathologic process is spontaneous (nontraumatic) intracranial bleeding. The resulting lesions vary from petechial to substantial amounts of blood clot that fill ventricular and subarachnoid spaces or form masses (hematomas) within central nervous system parenchyma. Lesions of this type, where the fundamental event is bleeding, need to be distinguished from hemorrhagic infarcts and similar lesions, where bleeding is a secondary phenomenon, because of important etiologic, pathogenetic, and prognostic differences between the two types.

Spontaneous intracranial hemorrhage may be associated with several disorders including cerebrovascular amyloidosis, coagulopathies, vasculitis, primary or metastatic tumors, and certain types of intoxications, such as arsenic. The most common causes of extensive, life-threatening hemorrhage of this type are systemic hypertension and ruptured intracranial aneurysms or vascular malformations.[197,247]

Hypertensive hemorrhage. The primary anatomic sites of these hemorrhages and their approximate frequency at those sites are as follows: cerebrum, 80%; brainstem, 10%; cerebellum, 10%.[223] Lesions greater than 3 cm in diameter in the cerebrum or 1.5 cm in the brainstem are considered large, and those of lesser dimensions at these sites as small. The comparable figure applicable to cerebellar hematomas in probably 3 cm. Among the large fatal hemorrhages (Fig. 42-23), 60% chiefly involve the corpus striatum or thalamus; 10% involve cerebral white matter; 16%, brainstem, chiefly pons; and 12%, cerebellum, chiefly near the dentate nucleus. Those hematomas frequently extend into adjacent parts of the ventricular system, and this blood may eventually leak into the subarachnoid space. Rupture of the hemorrhage directly into the subarachnoid space occurs but is uncommon.

Small, usually nonfatal hypertensive hemorrhages

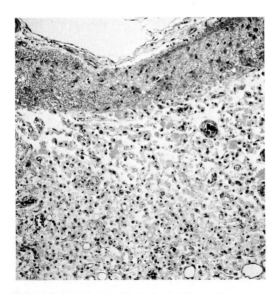

Fig. 42-21. Remote anemic infarct. There is intact outer cortical layer with reactive astrocytosis. Notice scattered macrophages and newly formed capillaries in cavity. (Hematoxylin and eosin; 135×.)

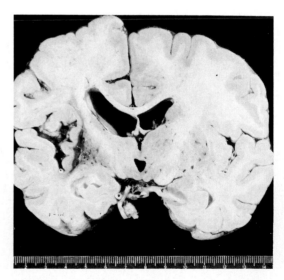

Fig. 42-22. Several small lacunar infarcts are present medial to the larger cavitary infarct adjacent to the insular cortex.

may occur anywhere in the brain. They are probably most frequent in the cerebral white matter and in the putamen.

The clinical findings associated with large hypertensive hemorrhages develop and evolve quickly over a period of minutes or hours. Most patients lose consciousness. Hemispheric, brainstem, or cerebellar signs will be present depending on the location of the lesion. The majority of these patients will die within the first month, frequently during the first 3 or 4 days, after onset of the hemorrhage. Small hemorrhages cause symptoms similar to those of infarcts and before the availability of computerized tomographic scans were often diagnosed as such. Recovery after small hemorrhages is common, and the residual deficit may be minimal especially if the lesion is located in the cerebral white matter.

Grossly and microscopically the large, acute hemorrhage consists of a homogeneous, dark red mass of clotted blood replacing brain parenchyma (Fig. 42-23). In the white matter fiber tracts may be separated rather than destroyed in the path of the blood. The borders of the lesion are sharply defined, though a few, small satellite hemorrhages may be present. A narrow rim of disrupted, partially necrotic parenchyma surrounds the hematoma, but extensive infarction is rare. Often there is fibrinoid necrosis of arterioles adjacent to the hemorrhage. The large hematomas behave as mass lesions causing both increased intracranial pressure and, according to location, uncal, cingulate, or cerebellar herniations with their attendant complications. In addition, cerebellar hematomas may directly compress the brain-

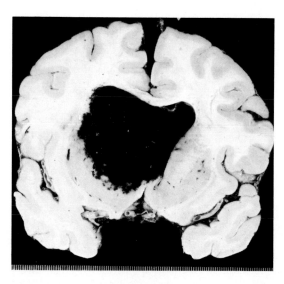

Fig. 42-23. Recent massive hemorrhage in inner striate area, with rupture into lateral ventricle in patient with hypertension. There are remote lacunar infarcts in putamina.

stem. Intraventricular extension of the hemorrhage can abruptly obstruct flow of cerebrospinal fluid, producing acute hydrocephalus and further increasing intracranial pressure.

After several weeks the hematoma appears brick red in color, and its margins are stained yellow or brown with hematoidin and hemosiderin. Microscopically, these pigments lie freely or in phagocytes at the border of the hemorrhage. Some fibroblastic proliferation arising from blood vessel walls and large-bodied, reactive astrocytes are present in the adjacent parenchyma. In smaller lesions the clot is eventually resorbed leaving a narrow cavitary defect stained with blood pigments.

Aside from the importance of systemic hypertension, many of the pathogenetic details involved in development of the hemorrhage are unresolved. Perforating arterioles between 200 and 400 μm in diameter are regarded as the usual source of the bleeding. One of two lesions involving vessels, fibrinoid necrosis, or ruptured miliary aneurysm of Charcot and Bouchard is considered the most likely explanation for the loss of vascular integrity.[47,65,68] The Charcot-Bouchard aneurysm is a microscopic outpouching found on arterioles most commonly but not exclusively in corpus striatum and thalamus of hypertensive patients over 50 years of age.

Hemorrhage from ruptured aneurysms and vascular malformations. The principal types of aneurysmal lesions involving larger caliber intracranial arteries are saccular, or "berry," aneurysms, mycotic aneurysms, and fusiform aneurysms. Of these, saccular aneurysms are most important and common. They are discussed in greater detail after brief descriptions of the other two lesions.

Mycotic aneurysms. Mycotic aneurysm occurs most often as a complication of infectious endocarditis. Microorganisms from impacted, infected emboli invade the arterial wall causing inflammation and necroses leading to dilatation of the weakened mural segment. This type of aneurysm is most often located on the more distal branches of the anterior or middle cerebral artery. The lesions, which may be solitary or multiple, can give rise to small or large hemorrhages.

Fusiform aneurysms. Fusiform aneurysm is an elongated dilatation particularly affecting the basilar or internal carotid arteries. It results from scarring with a loss of elasticity in the blood vessel wall usually caused by atherosclerosis. These aneurysms rarely rupture. Symptoms, if any, arise from compression of adjacent structures by the aneurysm.

Saccular aneurysms. Saccular, or "berry," aneurysms are rounded or lobulated bulges arising at the bifurcations of intracranial arteries (Fig. 42-24). They range in size from a few millimeters to several centimeters in diameter. "Giant" aneurysms are those exceeding 2.5 cm. Saccular aneurysms are rarely if ever present at birth and should not be referred to regularly as congenital. In fact, saccular aneurysms are uncommon before puberty. The approximate frequency after 20 years of age is 5% to 7%.[136,223] Both intact and ruptured aneurysms occur more frequently in women than in men. Unruptured, asymptomatic aneurysms are found incidentally at autopsy in 25% of persons over 55 years of age.[137] Approximately 90% of all saccular aneurysms occur on the arteries of the anterior (internal carotid) circulation. The common sites are the internal carotid artery particularly near the origin of the posterior communicating artery, the bifurcation of the middle cerebral artery, and the anterior communicating artery. The site with the highest frequency varies, according to the study consulted, between the internal carotid–posterior communicating region and the middle cerebral artery bifurcation, according to the study consulted. The remaining 10% of saccular aneurysms occur in the posterior (vertebrobasilar) circulation. The rostral basilar artery is the most common location, but other vessels such as the posterior inferior cerebellar artery are also affected. Saccular aneurysms are multiple and frequently bilateral in 20% to 25% of all affected persons[136,247] (Fig. 42-25).

Microscopically the aneurysmal sac is composed of fibrous tissue and endothelium. An atheromatous plaque is sometimes present near the dome of the sac, and a thrombus may partially or completely fill the lumen. The mouth of the sac is marked by disappearance of the

media and internal elastic lamina of the contiguous artery and by a focus of intimal thickening.

The pathogenesis of saccular aneurysms is unsettled. They are most frequently attributed to progressive enlargement of defects, composed of fibrous tissue, that occur in the wall of intracranial and other arteries. These defects are present in all persons at birth, but some unexplained mechanism is believed to subsequently lead to formation of the aneurysm. This explanation, however, is not universally accepted and many unanswered questions remain.[223] Some studies indicate an increased frequency of saccular aneurysm in patients with polycystic kidney disease, coarctation of the aorta, and other conditions. The statistical validity of these associations has been challenged.[136]

A saccular aneurysm may cause neurologic dysfunction by compressing adjacent areas of the brain. Most often, however, this type of aneurysm becomes symptomatic, suddenly and without warning as a result of rupture and primary subarachnoid hemorrhage (Fig. 42-24). The term "primary" indicates that the bleeding has occurred directly into the subarachnoid space rather than secondarily, such as leakage from the ventricles. Although aneurysms of any size may rupture in patients at any age, the majority of ruptured aneurysms occur between 40 and 70 years of age and measure more than 0.8 to 1 cm in diameter. Systemic hypertension does not appear to be a risk factor for rupture; however, some cases occur in conditions of great physical exertion or emotional excitement. The onset is indicated by sudden, violent headache, stiff neck, evi-

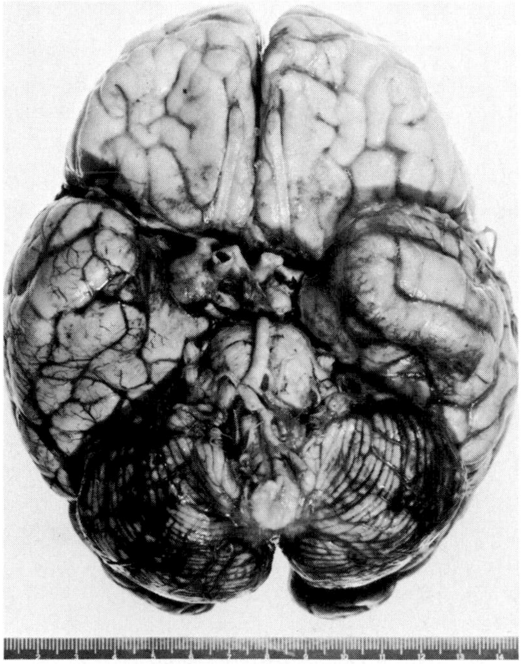

Fig. 42-24. Berry aneurysm at junction of right internal carotid and posterior communicating arteries. Pons is slightly widened and foreshortened, and there is cerebellomedullary herniation.

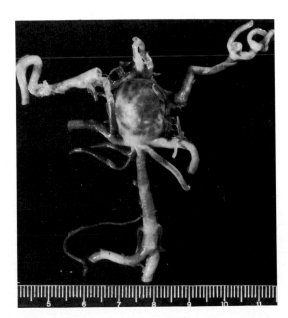

Fig. 42-25. Unruptured berry aneurysms. Larger aneurysm is at terminal portion of basilar artery. Smaller aneurysm is in bifurcation angle of middle cerebral artery on right.

dence of increased intracranial pressure, and loss of consciousness. These disturbances result, in part, from meningeal irritation caused by subarachnoid bleeding and blood clot acting as a mass lesion as well as causing subarachnoid obstruction and acute hydrocephalus. In at least 20% of cases the aneurysm and point of rupture are positioned so that blood not only enters the subarachnoid space but, under arterial pressure, dissects also through brain parenchyma forming a hematoma that gives rise to focal neurologic signs.[155]

Over two thirds of all patients with ruptured saccular aneurysm die or develop a major neurologic deficit even with treatment. In addition to the initial hemorrhage, recurrent hemorrhage and vasospasm with infarction may complicate the patient's subsequent course. Although some patients are successfully treated by surgical occlusion of the aneurysm, a method for preventing the hemorrhage altogether would be the most effective solution to this problem.

Vascular malformations are also a cause of subarachnoid and parenchymal hemorrhage. They are divided into four types according to the structure of their constituent vessels: arteriovenous malformation, venous angioma, cavernous angioma, and capillary telangiectasis.[199] Arteriovenous malformations (AVMs) (Fig. 42-26) are symptomatic more often than any other type of malformation, usually because of hemorrhage or an associated seizure disorder. Among the other vascular malformations, capillary telangiectases rarely bleed and are ordinarily discovered in the striate pons, incidentally at autopsy.

Stroke

The ischemic and hemorrhagic lesions discussed in this section represent the pathologic basis for most cases of the clinical syndrome referred to as a "stroke." The principal clinical features of a stroke include the sudden onset of a focal, nonconvulsive neurologic deficit that reaches its peak within minutes to a few days after onset. Strokes are the most common form of focal, organic neurologic disease among adults and are directly involved in 10% of the annual deaths in the United States.[76] Infarction is the basis of 80% of strokes, with ruptured saccular aneurysm with subarachnoid hemorrhage standing at 10% and intracerebral hemorrhage (chiefly hypertensive) at 10%.

Infections

An extensive, heterogeneous group of pathogens comprising various kinds of bacteria, fungi, viruses, rickettsias, parasites, and the recently recognized "unconventional agents" can cause central nervous system infection.[206] These organisms may reach the central nervous system through the bloodstream, by extension from a contiguous focus such as otitis media, through congenital (such as meningomyelocele) or acquired (such as skull fracture) defects in the bony and meningeal coverings of the central nervous system, and by centripetal migration along or within cranial and spinal nerves. The resulting lesions include epidural abscesses, subdural empyema, septic thrombophlebitis of dural sinuses, septic infarcts, meningitis, brain abscess, and encephalomyelitis.

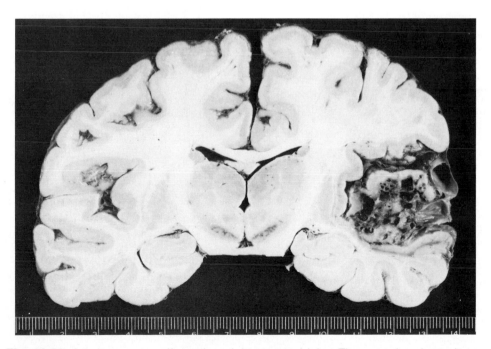

Fig. 42-26. Arteriovenous malformation, right temporal lobe. The vascular channels are seen in cross section.

Epidural abscesses may be located in either the cerebral or spinal extradural space. The cerebral form develops as an extension of adjacent osteomyelitis, paranasal sinusitis, or mastoiditis and can be found with subdural empyema. Spinal epidural abscesses are a consequence of either direct extension of paraspinal lesions or hematogenous spread from more distant sources. Subdural empyema is a collection of pus in the subdural space between the inner surface of the dura and the arachnoid. The lesion is located predominantly in the cranial cavity and in most cases represents extension from a contiguous infection in the cranium, paranasal sinuses, or middle ear. Septic thrombophlebitis of the dural sinuses is also the result of infection spreading from local sites including the skin and subcutaneous tissues about the eyes, nose and mouth, middle ear, and paranasal sinuses as well as extension from intracranial lesions such as subdural empyema. Complications of dural sinus thrombosis include hemorrhagic brain infarction and increased intracranial pressure related to impeded venous drainage. Septic infarcts are caused by infected emboli. They are most often associated with infectious endocarditis. In addition to features of parenchymal necrosis, intravascular clumps of bacteria, necrosis of blood vessel walls, and perivascular inflammation are present within and adjacent to the infarcted area.

Meningitis, brain abscess, and encephalomyelitis are the lesions most frequently caused by infection of the central nervous system.

Meningitis

Meningitis (leptomeningitis) is an acute or chronic inflammatory process chiefly affecting the pia and arachnoid mater and may be caused by bacteria, fungi, or parasites. In the United States purulent meningitis is the most frequent form of this disorder. The common etiologic organisms for this type of meningeal reaction vary according to the age of the patient, as indicated below:

Newborns: *Escherichia coli* and other gram-negative enteric organisms; group B streptococci; *Listeria monocytogenes*

Infants and children: *Haemophilus influenzae, Streptococcus pneumoniae, Neisseria meningitidis*

Adults: *Streptococcus pneumoniae, Neisseria meningitidis*

Important etiologic agents associated with subacute or chronic inflammation of the leptomeninges include the following:

Bacteria: *Mycobacterium tuberculosis, Treponema pallidum*

Fungi: *Cryptococcus neoformans, Coccidioides immitis*

Parasites: *Naegleria fowleri, Acanthamoeba, Cysticercus cellulosae*

In most cases, these bacteria and fungi and even some parasites (*Cysticercus, Acanthamoeba*) reach the central nervous system through the bloodstream. The mechanism and circumstances that permit their passage across the blood–cerebrospinal fluid barrier and invasion of the leptomeninges are unclear. In addition to the pathogenicity of the invading organism, conditions affecting the host, such as malnutrition or immunologic deficits, may increase the likelihood of infection. Clinical features include fever, stiff neck, headache, evidence of increased intracranial pressure, and inflammatory cells in the cerebrospinal fluid.

Acute purulent meningitis. Grossly the brain is swollen, and the subarachnoid vessels are congested. If the swelling is severe, herniation of the medial temporal lobe or cerebellum may occur.[99,228] Approximately 24 hours after inception of the illness, exudate can be seen in the subarachnoid space. Initially it is visible along blood vessels lying in sulci over the cerebral convexities and in cisterns at the base of the brain. Later it becomes confluent and is present about the cerebrum, brainstem, cerebellum, and spinal cord, particularly its posterior surface (Fig. 42-27). The color of the exudate may be white, yellow, or green and is not especially helpful in identifying the causative organism. Microscopically, in cases of purulent meningitis polymorphonuclear leukocytes and fibrin accumulate within the subarachnoid space during the first few days of the illness (Fig. 42-28). Later, mononuclear and plasma cells

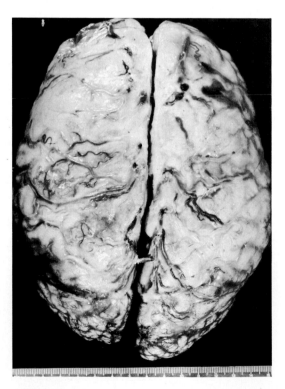

Fig. 42-27. Severe acute purulent leptomeningitis with thrombophlebitis.

appear. Microorganisms may be identified in the exudate with conventional or special stains. Increased numbers of astrocytes and histiocytes as well as inflammatory cells in Virchow-Robin spaces can be seen in the subpial parenchyma. The infection may extend into the ventricular system through the foramina of Magendie and Luschka causing ventriculitis. Involvement of subarachnoid blood vessels leads to vasculitis with infarction. In newborns this type of lesion is especially frequent and an important source of permanent, se-

vere, neurologic deficits[18] (Fig. 42-29). Other complications of meningitis include hydrocephalus resulting from ventricular obstruction or meningeal fibrosis, subdural effusion caused by fluid leading into the subdural space through defects in the arachnoid and occuring most commonly in children, and cranial nerve palsies probably related to inflammatory involvement of nerve roots crossing the subarachnoid space.

Chronic meningitis. Tuberculous and cryptococcal meningitis are two of the most important varieties of chronic meningeal inflammation. Both organisms cause a granulomatous reaction, and both may produce parenchymal lesions.

Tuberculous meningitis. Tuberculous meningitis occurs in children and adults through hematogenous spread to the central nervous system. In children, nervous system involvement takes place during the healing stage of the primary systemic infection. In adults evidence of active tuberculosis in other organ systems is variable, and the tuberculin test may be negative.[209] Infection of the leptomeninges is usually attributed to erosion of a superficial parenchymal granuloma into the subarachnoid space.[180] In most fatal cases a thick exudate is present at the base of the brain. Microscopic features include acute and chronic inflammatory cells, granulomas with and without caseation necrosis, infrequent giant cells, and acid-fast organisms (Fig. 42-30). Vasculitis and small parenchymal infarcts are common occurrences. The pathologic spectrum of neurotuberculosis also includes large parenchymal granulomas referred to as "tuberculomas." These are rare in the United States but are an important form of intracranial space-occupying lesion in those parts of the world where tuberculosis is prevalent.

Cryptococcal meningitis. Cryptococcal meningitis

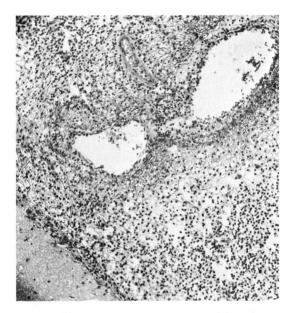

Fig. 42-28. Acute fibrinopurulent leptomeningitis with numerous neutrophils and some fibrin. (Hematoxylin and eosin; 90×.)

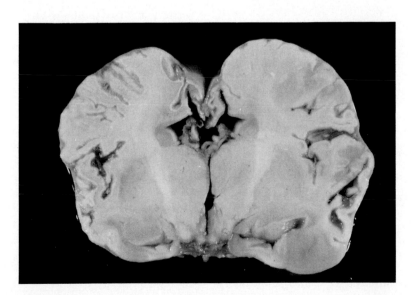

Fig. 42-29. Sequelae of neonatal meningitis. There is extensive cortical and subcortical atrophy. Patient died at 2½ years of age.

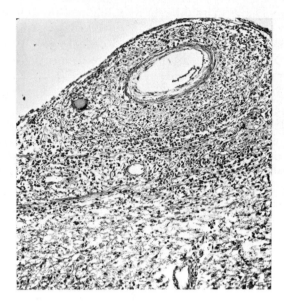

Fig. 42-30. Tuberculous leptomeningitis. Presence of Langhans' type of giant cell is unusual. (Hematoxylin and eosin; 90×.)

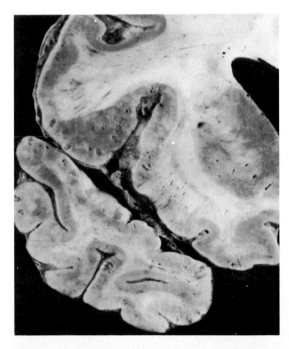

Fig. 42-31. Cryptococcosis with leptomeningeal exudate and many cortical cavities.

may develop in immunocompetent or immunodeficient persons, usually as a result of hematogenous dissemination from a pulmonary lesion. Grossly the exudate is scanty, translucent, and gelatinous. It distends the Virchow-Robin spaces producing small cavities within the parenchyma (Fig. 42-31). Microscopically, lymphocytes, plasma cells, and occasional granulomas are seen. Cryptococci are usually abundant and are easily recognized even without special stains as budding yeast up to 25 μm in diameter. The organism is surrounded by a thick mucopolysaccharide capsule, which is responsible for the gelatinous character of the exudate. Demonstration of the capsule requires special stains. Parenchymal granulomas occur in addition to meningeal lesions.

Neurosyphilis. During the nineteenth and early twentieth centuries syphilitic involvement of the central nervous system was one of the most important causes of chronic meningitis. Development of effective diagnostic and therapeutic procedures and their application during the early stages of the generalized infection has significantly reduced the frequency of neurosyphilis so that, currently, neuropathologists rarely encounter this disorder.

Invasion of the central nervous system by *Treponema pallidum* usually occurs during the first 2 years after the initial systemic infection and is characterized by asymptomatic chronic inflammation of the leptomeninges. This asymptomatic form of neurosyphilis is diagnosed by cerebrospinal fluid examination including serodiagnostic testing. Very little information is available concerning the pathology of asymptomatic neurosyphilis. Even without adequate treatment the meningeal reaction may resolve resulting in a spontaneous cure. In other cases the meningitis progresses over a period of years to symptomatic, tertiary neurosyphilis.[5] Active tertiary neurosyphilis is customarily divided into two clinical forms: meningovascular and parenchymatous, which includes general paresis and tabes dorsalis. Adams and Victor[5] point out, however, that these categories are only convenient abstractions based upon dominant clinical features. At autopsy all forms of tertiary neurosyphilis have several similar features, indicating the common origin of these disorders from a chronic meningitis. These features include fibrosis and chronic inflammation of the leptomeninges with extension of the infiltrate into the Virchow-Robin spaces (Fig. 42-32). In addition, more extensive parenchymal, vascular, or meningeal lesions are present in accordance with the clinical syndrome.[5,85] The reasons why parenchymal lesions are accentuated in some cases and meningovascular lesions in others are unknown.

In meningovascular syphilis there is fibrous thickening and infiltration of the leptomeninges with lympho-

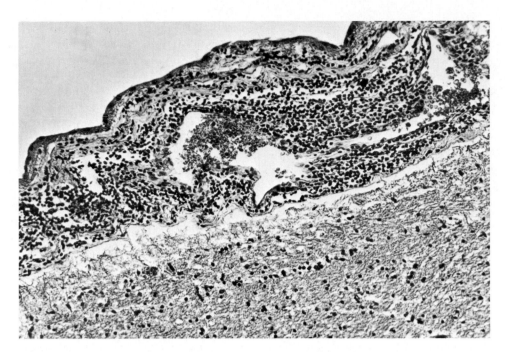

Fig. 42-32. Meningovascular syphilis. Lymphocytes and plasma cells are present in leptomeninges. (Hematoxylin and eosin; 180×.)

cytes and plasma cells. The adventitia and media of arteries and arterioles are involved by the inflammatory process. The term "Heubner's arteritis" is applied to arterial vessels with concentric or eccentric intimal thickening accompanying the chronic inflammatory changes in the outer layers. The intimal lesion is proliferative in character and usually free of inflammatory cells. Nevertheless, it is often referred to as an endarteritis. Regional accentuation of the lesions may occur around the optic nerves or spinal cord. Chronic ventriculitis (granular ependymitis) is a frequent finding in these cases. Focally there is loss of ependymal cells with reactive proliferation of the subependymal glial cells forming small nodules, called "ependymal granulations," that protrude into the ventricular lumen. Patients with meningovascular syphilis may develop infarcts as a result of the vascular lesions and hydrocephalus because of fibrous obliteration of subarachnoid pathways or obstruction of the aqueduct by ependymal granulations.

The lesions of general paresis include meningeal fibrosis and cortical atrophy, which is most severe over the frontal and temporal lobes along with chronic ventriculitis. Microscopically the atrophic cortex is the site of a subacute encephalitis with nerve cell loss, astrocytosis, proliferation of rod-shaped microglia (histiocytes) that contain iron, and lymphocytes and plasma cells within Virchow-Robin spaces. The term "windswept cortex" is used in reference to particularly extensive ce-

rebral lesions. Spirochetes may be demonstrable in the parenchyma with special stains. The cortical lesions are the basis of the cognitive dissolution that occurs in general paresis. Although some patients develop the elaborate psychotic delusions often referred to in classical accounts of this disorder, most exhibit a progressive dementing illness. As the lesions progress, deteriorating cortical function leads to disturbances in gait, posture, muscle tone, and eventually a helpless, bedridden state.[5] At one time an important cause of chronic psychiatric admissions, general paresis is now a rare disorder.

Tabes dorsalis is characterized pathologically by pronounced atrophy of the posterior spinal roots, especially in the lumbosacral region, and degeneration of the posterior columns indicated by flattening of the convex posterior surface of the spinal cord. Microscopically, axons and myelin sheaths are lost in equal numbers from the roots and in the spinal cord chiefly from the posterior columns. There is only slight loss of neurons in the dorsal root ganglia. Chronic inflammatory cells are present in the meninges and Virchow-Robin spaces. The pathogenesis of the parenchymal lesions are still debated. The most likely explanation, however, appears to be an inflammatory reaction involving the posterior roots leading to axonal disruption followed by disintegration of the segments of these axons and myelin sheaths located in the posterior columns distal to the site of the disruption. The mild neuron loss in the ganglia is attributed to occasional retrograde degeneration also arising from the posterior root lesion.[5] Clinically, patients have ataxia, absent deep-tendon reflexes in the lower extremities, impaired vibratory and position sense, and a Romberg sign correlating with the lesions in the posterior roots and columns. Additional disturbances include pupillary abnormalities (usually of the Argyll Robertson variety), lightning pains, visceral crises (attacks of chest or abdominal pain), urinary incontinence, and arthropathic changes affecting hips, knees, or ankles referred to as "Charcot joints."

Brain abscess

Brain abscess develops through three main routes: (1) extension of infections originating in adjacent cranial structures to neural parenchyma presumably by means of retrograde thrombophlebitis, (2) hematogenous dissemination of infected emboli from systemic sources, and (3) direct inoculation usually associated with trauma. The most common source is middle ear infections (otogenic abscess). Paranasal sinuses (rhinogenic abscess) are also important as local sites of origin. Hematogenous abscesses represent at least 20% of cases. These are associated chiefly with infections of the lungs and pleura such as lung abscess, bronchiectasis, or emphema, with acute bacterial endocarditis, and with cyanotic forms of congenital heart disease in children over 2 years of age.[206] In about 10% of cases no source can be identified.

Otogenic abscesses are located in the temporal lobe or cerebellum (Fig. 42-5). Rhinogenic abscesses usually involve the frontal lobes. Hematogenous abscesses may affect any part of the brain but are found most often in the distribution of the middle cerebral artery near the junction of cortex and white matter or in the basal ganglia. Otogenic and rhinogenic abscesses usually occur as solitary lesions; hematogenous abscesses may be single or multiple.

The etiologic agents of brain abscess include many bacteria and fungi. Aerobic and anaerobic streptococci are the most common organisms isolated. Other common bacterial agents include enteric gram-negative organisms such as *Escherichia coli*, *Staphylococcus aureus* in cases of trauma, and *Bacteroides* organisms. Mixed as well as single organisms may be isolated.[78] In immunocompromised patients fungi such as *Candida* or *Aspergillus* may cause abscesses.

The abscess begins as a focal encephalitis or cerebritis. This early type of lesion is not usually encountered in human neuropathology but has been studied in experimental models.[141] Inflammatory infiltrate, bacteria, thrombosed blood vessels, and necrotic parenchyma are the main features of the early lesion. The presence of necrotic tissue may be related in part to ischemia associated with embolic vascular occlusion in the case of hematogenous abscesses or septic thrombophlebitis

with otogenic and rhinogenic abscesses. The occurrence of necrosis is believed to favor the parenchymal invasion and proliferation of the organisms causing the abscess. After 1 or 2 weeks the central part of the abscess consists of pus and necrotic debris. At the periphery, granulation tissue and a fibrocollagenous capsule derived from fibroblasts in walls of neighboring blood vessels are forming. With the passage of time the capsule increases in thickness. External to the capsule the parenchyma is often the site of considerable vasogenic edema and reactive astrocytosis.

Clinically, patients have focal neurologic signs related to the location of the abscess as well as evidence of infection, including transient fever and inflammatory cells in the spinal fluid. The mortality for brain abscess has been high but with earlier diagnosis by computerized tomographic scans is now about 10%.[153] Brain abscesses are a form of space-occupying lesion and can cause death through temporal lobe or cerebellar herniation. In other cases mortality follows rupture of the abscess into the ventricular system with fulminating ventriculitis and meningitis.

Encephalitis

Encephalitis is a form of acute, subacute, or chronic central nervous system inflammation chiefly affecting brain parenchyma. The lesions may be focal, regional, or diffuse. Conditions in which there is concomitant meningeal or spinal cord inflammation are referred to, respectively, as "meningoencephalitis" or "encephalomyelitis." Most cases of encephalitis are caused by viruses. Those that are the common agents for acute encephalitis affecting adults and children in the United States include picornaviruses (coxsackieviruses groups A and B, echoviruses), togaviruses (St. Louis, eastern equine, western equine), herpesviruses (HSV-1 herpes simplex, type 1), paramyxoviruses (mumps), and arenaviruses (lymphocytic choriomeningitis). In parts of Asia, Africa, and Latin America rabies virus would also be included on this list.[41] With the development of an effective vaccine, poliomyelitis (inflammation of the gray matter, especially in the spinal cord) caused by the poliovirus is rare. When the disease does occur, it is either caused by other picorna viruses or represents poliovirus infection in an immunocompromised or nonimmune host. Several of the encephalitogenic viruses such as coxsackie, ECHO, and mumps are also responsible for many cases of the self-limited, nonfatal clinical syndrome referred to as aseptic meningitis.[246]

The severity of the acute encephalitic process and the likelihood of permanent neurologic deficits vary according to the etiologic agent. Those viruses associated with significant mortality or residual neurologic damage are herpes simplex type 1 and the togaviruses, which cause eastern, western, and St. Louis encephalitis.

The epidemiology of these viruses may involve

spread from person to person through hand to mouth and respiratory routes or contact with contaminated fomites or insect vectors. Some agents such as the lymphocytic choriomeningitis virus are transmitted by exposure to dust or food contaminated by infected animals. The togaviruses are transmitted by arthropods, mainly mosquitoes. Encephalitis in the neonate may be the result of transplacental transmission of the virus or infection during labor. In the case of HSV-1 encephalitis the disease may occur as a primary infection or through reactivation of a latent virus.

In humans most of the viruses that cause acute encephalitis reach the central nervous system through the bloodstream. In a few instances such as rabies, they enter peripheral nerves and are carried centrally by retrograde axonal flow. After gaining access to the central nervous system, parenchyma viruses may produce widespread infection affecting all varieties of cells or may selectively involve certain regions, anatomic formations, or cell types. The basis for the selectivity includes the availability of cellular membrane receptors for the virus as well as the capacity of cells to assimilate the virus and provide metabolic support necessary for viral replication.[106,240]

The general morphologic features of acute viral encephalitis are presented in the following paragraph. Acute herpes simplex encephalitis (HSV-1) and the neonatal encephalitides are described in greater detail. Subsequently, rickettsial and slow virus infections are reviewed.

Many of the acute viral encephalitides have similar neuropathologic features despite differences in cause.

Grossly the brain may appear normal or somewhat swollen. Microscopically, diffuse or focal inflammatory infiltrates composed of chiefly monocytes, lymphocytes, and plasma cells are present in gray or white matter and in the Virchow-Robin spaces (perivascular cuffs) (Fig. 42-33). The occurrence of perivascular cuffs alone without parenchymal inflammation is suggestive but not conclusive morphologic evidence of encephalitis. Polymorphonuclear leukocytes may be present in the infiltrate during the early stages of the disease. The extent of frank neuronal or general parenchymal necrosis and vasculitis is variable. In some infections intranuclear (such as HSV-1) or intracytoplasmic (such as rabies) inclusions are seen. The histology and anatomic distribution of the lesions along with epidemiologic, clinical, and laboratory data sometimes provides a rational basis for speculations about which viruses are the more likely etiologic agents in a case of encephalitis. Definitive etiologic diagnosis, however, generally depends on special procedures involving virus isolation, immunologic studies, and diagnostic electron microscopy or immunohistochemistry.

Herpes simplex encephalitis. Herpes simplex virus (HSV) is the most common cause of acute, sporadic, severe encephalitis affecting children and adults in the United States.[107] Although both HSV-1 and HSV-2 may cause encephalitis, HSV-1 accounts for 95% of all cases.[50] HSV-2 is an important cause of neonatal encephalitis, which is discussed later. The pathogenesis of HSV-1 encephalitis remains unsettled. Some studies indicate that up to 30% of cases, especially those in children and young adults, may be the result of primary

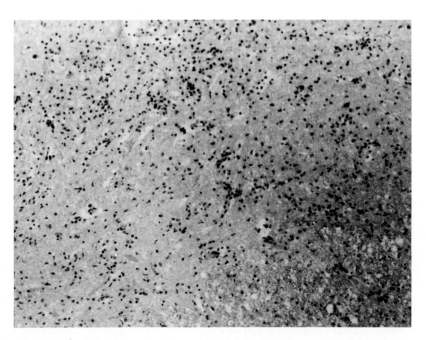

Fig. 42-33. Acute encephalitis. The parenchyma is infiltrated with neutrophils and mononuclear cells. (Hematoxylin and eosin; 100×.)

infection.[50,246] Autopsy studies, however, have demonstrated the occurrence of latent HSV-1 infection of the trigeminal ganglion in most adults without HSV-1 encephalitis.[14] This observation and others including the recurrence of orofacial HSV-1 infection or salivary excretion of the virus in association with dental procedures and trigeminal surgery indicate that HSV-1 encephalitis may also result from reactivation of a latent virus.[50,246] Evidence of latent infection involving other neural tissues including autonomic ganglia and brain lend further support to the reactivation hypothesis.[72,175] The route by which the virus enters the central nervous system is also debated. The characteristic localization of lesions in the medial temporal and orbitofrontal lobes indicated the possibility of spread along the olfactory nerves from the olfactory bulbs. Evidence of olfactory bulb infection, however, is not consistently present. Alternatively, transport of the virus from the trigeminal ganglion along axons extending to the meninges in the anterior and middle fossae has been proposed.

Clinically the illness may develop acutely with fever, headache, delirium, convulsions, and loss of consciousness or subacutely with behavioral changes, memory disturbance, and hallucination. Active HSV-1 infection of other organs usually does not accompany the encephalitis. The cerebrospinal fluid contains increased numbers of cells, chiefly mononuclear leukocytes, and neuroimaging may demonstrate temporal lobe involvement. Confirmation of the diagnosis is problematic. The virus is rarely cultured from the spinal fluid, and serologic testing is often inconclusive or is impractical for use in therapeutic decisions during the acute illness. Brain biopsy with virus isolation and immunohistochemical studies in addition to conventional histologic examination is advocated by many for timely definitive diagnosis and for exclusion of other treatable diseases.[50] The mortality for HSV-1 encephalitis without treatment is 70%, and only 10% of patients recover sufficiently to lead normal lives. The use of the antiviral drugs vidarabine and more recently acyclovir has improved the prognosis to some extent in regard to both mortality and morbidity. In too many cases, however, the infection still leads to a devastating disorder.[94]

There are characteristic gross and microscopic lesions that point to the diagnosis of HSV-1 encephalitis. Grossly, areas of hemorrhagic necrosis involve one or both medial temporal lobes as well as the orbital surfaces of the frontal lobes (Fig. 42-34). The necrosis may extend to the insular cortex and cerebral convexity. The affected temporal lobes are swollen and edematous and may act as space-occupying lesions causing midline shifts and herniations. Microscopically, there is acute hemorrhagic necrosis of gray and white matter accompanied by acute and chronic inflammatory cell infiltration and thrombosis and fibrinoid necrosis of parenchy-

mal vessels. Inflammatory cells are also present in the Virchow-Robin spaces and adjacent leptomeninges. Intranuclear Cowdry type A inclusions are found in astrocytes, oligodendroglia, and neurons. HSV-1 antigen can be demonstrated in infected neurons by the immunoperoxidase technique. Electron microscopy can be used to identify nucleocapsids characteristic of HSV-1 in affected nuclei.

Neonatal encephalitis. The acronym "TORCH" is used to designate an important group of pathogens that cause fetal or neonatal infections (including encephalitis) that have similar clinical findings, such as prematurity, skin petechiae, and hepatosplenomegaly, and require serologic tests for diagnosis. TORCH comprises *T*oxoplasma, *r*ubella, *c*ytomegalovirus, *h*erpes simplex, type 2 (HSV-2), and *other*, such as *Treponema pallidum* and *Listeria monocytogenes*.[149]

The infant's central nervous system becomes infected as a result of transplacental transmission of the organism during subclinical or symptomatic maternal infection or by intrapartum infection. In the latter case the infant becomes contaminated from the maternal urinary tract or birth canal during delivery or through an ascending infection arising in the lower birth canal associated with a prolonged interval between rupture of the membranes and delivery. Except for HSV-2, the TORCH infections occur by transplacental transmission. HSV-2 infection usually takes place during the infant's passage through the birth canal, less often as a consequence of ascending infection, and rarely by the transplacental route.[244] Neonatal infections caused by HSV-1 also occur, but these are acquired postnatally through contact with symptomatic or asymptomatic family members or from nosocomial infection.

The neuropathologic findings in these disorders con-

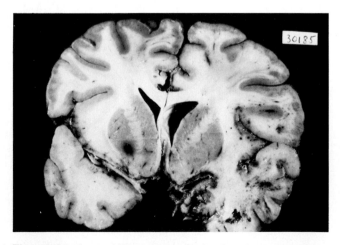

Fig. 42-34. Acute HSV-1 (herpes simplex virus, type 1) encephalitis. Hemorrhagic parenchymal necrosis is most prominent in the right medial temporal lobe.

sist of varying degrees of acute and chronic parenchymal and leptomeningeal inflammation, which, in cases of prenatal infection, may be accompanied by microcephaly. In addition, there may be recent parenchymal necrosis, evidence of older tissue destruction and loss, focal or multifocal calcification, ventricular enlargement, and, in some instances, changes characteristic of specific organisms. Truly malformative lesions are infrequent, except in cases of congenital cytomegalovirus infection.

The associations of specific organisms with distinctive or characteristic neuropathologic alterations are summarized in the following paragraphs.

Cytomegalovirus. Destructive meningoencephalitis with prominent periventricular calcification, polymicrogyria, and large, basophilic, intranuclear neuronal inclusions of viral type (Fig. 42-35).

Toxoplasma. Necrotizing granulomatous encephalitis with cysts containing organisms and multiple, randomly distributed foci of parenchymal calcification.

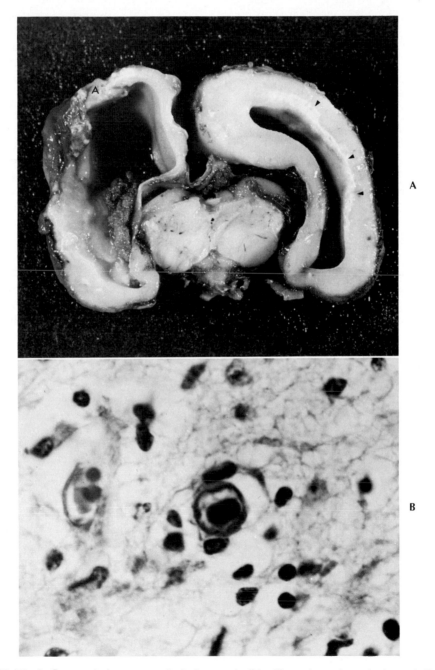

Fig. 42-35. A, Congenital cytomegaloviral encephalitis. There is periventricular calcification, *arrows,* and focal cortical destruction, *A.* **B,** Cytomegaloviral encephalitis. Large intranuclear inclusion body. (Hematoxylin and eosin; 400×).

Rubella. Vasculopathy with mural deposition of periodic acid–Schiff–positive mucopolysaccharide and calcium, focal parenchymal necrosis, and variable inflammation.

Listeria. Granulomatous meningoencephalitis.

Syphilis. Acute or chronic meningitis. Parenchymatous lesions develop later during childhood or adolescence.

Rickettsial infections. Parenchymal inflammation of the central nervous system is also observed in rickettsial infections. Perivascular collections of acute and chronic inflammatory cells and some degree of endothelial proliferation are found in cases of typhus, Rocky Mountain spotted fever, and scrub typhus.

Slow virus infections. Other forms of CNS parenchymal infection are encountered in immunodeficient patients and in association with disorders caused by a group of pathogens referred to as slow viruses, defective viruses, and unconventional agents. Progressive multifocal leukoencephalopathy, one of the opportunistic infections associated with immunodeficiency is covered in the section on demyelinative diseases. Other examples of opportunistic infection are included in the discussion of CNS infection by the human immunodeficiency virus (HIV).

The term "slow virus" is applied to transmissible viral pathogens with prolonged incubation periods. The clinical and pathologic characteristics vary from agent to agent and in some cases resemble degenerative rather than inflammatory disorders.[107,246] Slow virus infections of the human central nervous system include subacute sclerosing panencephalitis (SSPE), AIDS-dementia complex, progressive multifocal leukoencephalopathy (PML), Creutzfeldt-Jakob disease (CJD), and progressive rubella panencephalitis. Three of these—SSPE, AIDS-dementia complex, and CJD—are discussed in this section. PML, as noted previously, is covered in the section on demyelinative disorders.

SSPE. Subacute sclerosing panencephalitis is an insidious form of encephalitis occurring mainly during the first two decades of life. Dementia and myoclonus are accompanied by a characteristic electroencephalogram showing periodic bursts of high-voltage slow and sharp waves with suppressed general activity. Cerebrospinal fluid pressure and cells are not increased; however, there are significant elevations of gamma globulin and measles antibody. There is no specific treatment, and the disease ends fatally in most cases with 1 or 2 years after onset. A few patients may survive 5 or more years.[246]

SSPE is caused by a persistent measles virus that is defective in the accumulation of the matrix protein. The virus cannot be released at the cell surface because of this defect but undergoes intercellular spread in the central nervous system through fusion of cytoplasmic membranes.[27,49,97,219] Many pathogenetic aspects of this disease are unexplained, including the role of immunodeficiency in its development, the mechanism and site of the latent measles virus infection, and the factors that lead to activation.[211]

The currently accepted views regarding the pathology of this condition are based in large measure on correlative studies by Greenfield.[84] His work showed that Dawson's subacute inclusion body encephalitis and van

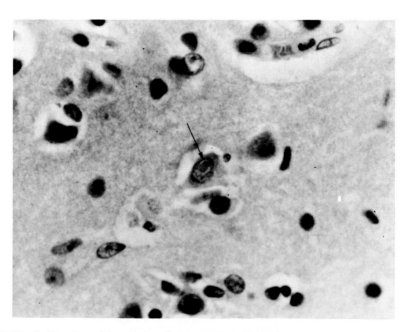

Fig. 42-36. Subacute sclerosing panencephalitis (SSPE). Intranuclear, *arrow*, neuronal inclusion. (Hematoxylin and eosin; 400×.)

Bogaert's subacute sclerosing leukoencephalitis were different morphologic expressions of the same basic disease that Greenfield christened "subacute sclerosing panencephalitis." Subsequently the cases of nodular panencephalitis described by Pette and Döring are also regarded as variants of SSPE.[169]

Grossly the brain may appear normal or atrophic depending on the length of the illness. Microscopically the features of a subacute encephalitis are evident in gray matter with neuron loss, perivascular and parenchymatous infiltration of lymphocytes, and plasma cells, astrocytic proliferation, and rod cell formation. Cowdry type A inclusions are found in glial and neuronal nuclei (Fig. 42-36). Occasionally neuronal cytoplasmic inclusions are also present. Astrocytosis, oligodrendroglia with intranuclear inclusions, and varying degrees of chronic inflammation and demyelination are seen in the white matter. Measles antigen can be demonstrated immunohistochemically in infected cells. Intranuclear tubular nucleocapsids are demonstrable by electron microscopy.

AIDS. Adults and children with the acquired immunodeficiency syndrome (AIDS) caused by the human immunodeficiency virus type 1 (HIV-1) develop a variety of disorders affecting both the central and peripheral nervous system.[39] These include opportunistic infections of the central nervous system by fungi, parasites, viruses, and bacteria as well as primary CNS lymphoma. In one autopsy study cytomegalovirus encephalomyelitis and toxoplasmosis were encountered most often. Less frequently, infections with *Cryptococcus, Aspergillus, Candida, Pneumocystis,* herpes simplex, varicella-zoster, papovavirus (progressive multifocal leukoencephalopathy), and atypical acid-fast or-

ganisms were identified. Primary CNS lymphoma occurred in 6% of the patients, and less than 20% of the patients had either normal brains or a terminal metabolic encephalopathy.[168] Recently, there have been case reports of neurosyphilis developing in HIV-infected patients who had previously been treated by an established regimen for early syphilis.[19,105] In addition to these complicating illnesses, direct infection of the nervous system by HIV-1 occurs commonly during the early stages of AIDS. The infection may be asymptomatic or associated with signs of encephalitis, aseptic meningitis, ataxia, or myelopathy, which resolve over a period of weeks. The neuropathologic counterparts of these disorders are at present unknown.[176]

Many patients, perhaps 75%, usually in the later stages of AIDS develop the AIDS-dementia complex, which is also attributable, at least in part, to direct CNS infection by HIV-1. This disorder usually occurs with systemic manifestations of AIDS but may also develop in the absence of systemic symptoms. The occurrence of the dementia closely correlates[176] with a form of subacute encephalitis with multinucleated cells described by Petito and associates[168] and considered pathognomonic of HIV-1 encephalitis (Fig. 42-37). These lesions are found most often in the cerebral white matter but occur at other sites including the spinal cord. They feature a collection of several multinucleated calls associated with small numbers of lymphocytes, rod cells, macrophages, reactive astrocytes, and focally vacuolated myelin. The multinucleated cells may be small with 3 to 5 nuclei and scanty cytoplasm or appear as giant cells. Some of the macrophages contain brown pigment, which may stain positively for hemosiderin. Similar lesions occur in children with an additional

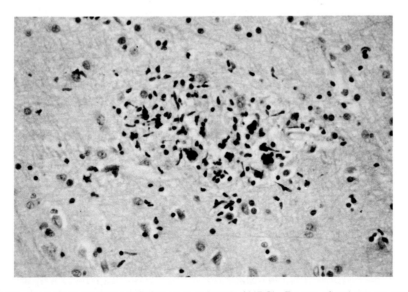

Fig. 42-37. Acquired immunodeficiency syndrome (AIDS). Focus of subacute encephalitis with multinucleated cells. The presence of such lesions has a high correlation with clinical dementia in patients with AIDS. (Hematoxylin and eosin; 50×.)

finding of vascular calcification. Other neuropathologic changes include diffuse pallor of the cerebral white matter and a vacuolar myelopathy. The latter condition is often found in conjunction with dementia and subacute encephalitis with giant cells but may occur in the absence of both. The spinal cord lesion resembles the myelopathy of vitamin B_{12} deficiency. Foci of vacuolated myelin caused by intramyelin swelling involve the posterior and lateral columns. The lesions are most severe in the lower half of the thoracic cord. Axonal degeneration also occurs in more severe cases.[167,168]

The pathogenesis of the AIDS-dementia complex is not fully delineated. The presence of HIV-1 in the multinucleated cells and macrophages of the subacute encephalitis has been demonstrated[176] indicating that the virus may be carried into the brain by infected peripheral macrophages. Alternatively the virus may cross the vascular endothelium or enter through the choroid plexus. The questions of whether other cell types such as neurons and glia also become infected and how the virus injures the brain at present are unanswered.

Creutzfeldt-Jakob disease (CJD). Creutzfeldt-Jakob disease is a rare form of fatal subacute, progressive dementia associated with myoclonus chiefly but not exclusively affecting adults. Most patients die within 1 year of onset. The disease has been transmitted to experimental animals by inoculation with infected tissue. It has also been transmitted inadvertently from human to human by contact with contaminated tissue or tissue extracts (corneal transplant, dura, pituitary extract) and surgical instruments.[246] The etiologic agent is not destroyed by ordinary sterilization procedures including formalin. Special techniques must be employed to disinfect instruments that have come into contact with the tissues and body fluids of affected patients. Furthermore, special precautions are necessary when one is performing autopsies on these patients and is handling surgical or autopsy tissue specimens even after formalin fixation.

From the time the disease was originally described it was regarded as a degenerative disorder. The discovery of its transmissibility along with that of other related disorders such as kuru has significantly changed many of the concepts of infections and degenerative disease and led to speculation concerning the role of atypical infection in other degenerative diseases.[75,108] The etiologic agent for CJD and related human and animal disorders has not been unequivocally identified and characterized. Current interest is focused on a fibrillar protein found in these disorders and referred to as a "prion," a slightly scrambled acronym for "*prot*ein-aceous *in*fectious particle." The biochemical composition of prions and their possible roles as etiologic agents of CJD and other conditions is under active investiga-

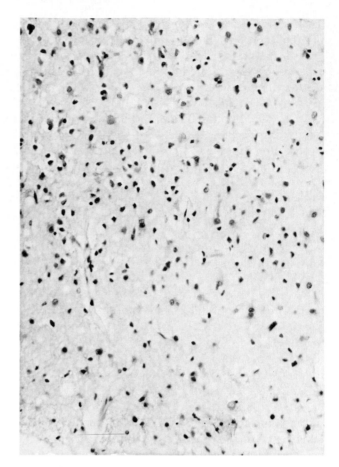

Fig. 42-38. Creutzfeldt-Jakob disease. There are spongiform changes in cerebral cortex and loss of nerve cells with mild reactive astrocytosis. (Hematoxylin and eosin; 157×.)

tion.[66,177] CJD is one of a group of spongiform encephalopathies that include kuru and Gerstmann-Sträussler syndrome in humans and scrapie (in sheep and goats), transmissible mink encephalopathy, and chronic wasting disease of mule deer and elk. The neuropathologic changes in these conditions are similar. Grossly in patients with CJD the brain usually appears normal. Atrophy may be present in long-standing cases. Microscopically the lesions involve the gray matter. The cerebral cortex is consistently the site of nerve cell loss and shows reactive astrocytosis and numerous vacuoles within the neuropil (Fig. 42-38). Characteristically, some of the vacuoles present should measure less than 7 μm in diameter, and others that indent nuclei should be found.[135,210] By electron microscopy the vacuoles are located within the cell bodies and processes of neurons and astrocytes. In addition to the cerebral cortex, spongiform change may also involve the basal ganglia, brainstem, and rarely the white matter.[159]

Tumors

The central nervous system is affected by both primary and metastatic tumors. Approximately 85% of all CNS tumors are intracranial, and 15% intraspinal. The figures include pituitary adenomas, which are covered separately in Chapter 30. Although there are similarities with systemic neoplasms, tumors involving the CNS have the following distinctive characteristics.

Primary CNS tumors rarely metastasize to other organs. Malignancy of the tumor is indicated by rapid growth, invasion of adjacent structures, and direct spread or metastasis to other parts of the CNS along anatomic pathways such as the ventricular system or subarachnoid space. Even slowly growing or apparently benign tumors may cause considerable mortality or death because they involve major blood vessels or other vital structures and cannot be safely excised. Such tumors are referred to as malignant by position.

Both primary and metastatic tumors behave as space-occupying lesions causing compression of neural parenchyma, increased intracranial pressure, and brain herniations. The growth of the tumor may obstruct the circulation of cerebrospinal fluid through the ventricles or subarachnoid space causing hydrocephalus and further increasing intracranial pressure. In very young children, before closure of the cranial sutures the rising intracranial pressure causes widening of the sutures and eventually an increasing head size.

The anatomic location of the tumor is a major determinant of the accompanying neurologic signs and symptoms. A tumor involving major motor pathways, for example, may quickly cause prominent symptoms, whereas one of the same size and type beneath the nondominant frontal lobe may, for many years, give rise to hardly perceptible effects. In the case of intracranial tumors the focal signs may be accompanied by signs of increased intracranial pressure.

Primary tumors of the CNS will account for an estimated 1.5% of new cancer cases in the United States during 1988 and 2.2% of cancer deaths.[38] In children under 15 years of age they are second only to leukemia as a cause of death from cancer. The relative 5-year survival rate is approximately 27%. Even with survival, the morbidity associated with CNS tumors often limits the patient's ability to work and diminishes the quality of life.

The principal location and the frequency of the different types of tumors varies in the CNS according to age and sex.[193] In adults 70% of intracranial tumors are supratentorial, and 30% infratentorial. The most common types are glioblastoma multiforme, metastatic tumors, astrocytoma with atypical or anaplastic foci, meningioma, and schwannomas. The first four occur most often above the tentorium, whereas the schwannoma usually arises from the eighth nerve in the cerebellopontine angle. Three of the tumors—glioblastoma, atypical or anaplastic astrocytoma, and metastatic tumors—are malignant. The percentages for the supratentorial-infratentorial distribution of intracranial tumors in childhood are the reverse of the adult figures—30% supratentorial and 70% infratentorial. In this age group medulloblastoma, astrocytoma, ependymoma, craniopharyngioma, and glioblastoma are the most frequent types. The medulloblastoma and the majority of the astrocytomas occur in the cerebellum. Another common site for astrocytoma is the brainstem. Ependymomas are found above and below the tentorium, most often in the fourth ventricle. Glioblastomas arise in the brainstem and to a lesser extent in the cerebrum. The craniopharyngioma is located at the base of the brain in the parapituitary area. Malignant forms include medulloblastoma, glioblastoma, and some astrocytomas and ependymomas.

The common spinal cord tumors in adults are schwannoma, meningioma, metastatic tumors, and gliomas, chiefly ependymoma and astrocytoma. These tumors have characteristic (but not invariable) anatomic locations. This information can be helpful in the assessment of clinical or imaging studies and in the establishing of the probable type of tumor present before pathologic examination. Most gliomas are intramedullary, located within the spinal cord itself and producing local enlargement. Schwannomas and meningiomas are extramedullary (external to the spinal cord) and intradural, lying between the inner surface of the spinal dura and the cord. Metastatic tumors are generally located in the extradural space. Intramedullary metastases are very rare occurrences. The malignant varieties of spinal cord tumors are the metastatic lesions and occasional astrocytic or ependymal tumors. Glial tumors, such as astrocytoma or ependymoma, in the spinal cord, however, are usually slowly rather than rapidly growing. In children spinal cord tumors are uncommon, and statistics concerning the frequency of individual types vary. In addition to gliomas, schwannomas, meningiomas, and metastases, tumors such as dermoids, teratomas, and lipomas are encountered in children. CNS tumors of all types occur in both men and women; however, gliomas are twice as common in males, whereas meningiomas and acoustic (eighth nerve) schwannomas are at least twice as common in females.

There is no known cause for the majority of primary CNS tumors in humans. These tumors have been induced experimentally in laboratory animals with chemical and viral carcinogens such as the nitrosoureas, Rous sarcoma virus, avian sarcoma virus, and the SV-40 and JC papovaviruses.[199] There is no evidence, however, causally linking environmental chemical carcinogens or viruses with human brain tumors. Although the question is still debated especially in regard to meningiomas, there is as yet no convincing direct demonstration that physical trauma can cause CNS tumors. Such trauma can appear to be causal when it induces hemorrhage within a clinically latent tumor bringing about a rapid increase in size and the appearance of neurologic symptoms. A small number of CNS tumors, chiefly of mesenchymal origin, have developed many years after radiation therapy for intracranial disorders.[199] An increased incidence of CNS tumors, especially primary lymphoma, is observed in patients with immunodeficiency syndromes, including AIDS, and in immunosuppressed transplant recipients as well.[96,195]

Central nervous system neoplasia is an important component of several genetically determined disorders such as von Recklinghausen's neurofibromatosis, tuberous sclerosis, von Hippel-Lindau syndrome, Turcot's familial polyposis syndrome, and the multiple nevoid basal cell carcinoma syndrome.[83,98,134,148,179] Cytogenetic abnormalities and evidence of proto-oncogene amplification have been detected in sporadic primary CNS tumors.[204,217] Malignant gliomas (atypical and anaplastic astrocytoma and glioblastoma multiforme), meningiomas, and CNS schwannomas in patients with one form of neurofibromatosis have been studied most extensively. Among the malignant gliomas gains of chromosome 7, losses of chromosome 10, structural abnormalities especially involving 9p and 19q, and double minutes were observed.[21] Gene amplification occurs in approximately 50% of these malignant gliomas most often involving the epidermal growth factor receptor gene and less often N-*myc*, *gli*, or c-*myc* genes.[20] The most common cytogenetic abnormality in meningiomas is monosomy 22 or deletion of the long arm of chromosome 22.[252] Analysis of genomic DNA from intracranial and intraspinal schwannomas in patients with neurofibromatosis 2 has demonstrated losses of genetic material from chromosome 22 including partial deletion in the long arm of the chromosome or loss of the entire chromosome.[134] The etiologic and pathogenetic significance of the alterations in chromosomal number or structure and the occurrence of gene amplification in these tumors is uncertain. They may reflect molecular oncogenetic mechanisms. In addition they might serve as indicators of neoplastic transformation and subsequent biologic behavior as has been demonstrated by N-*myc* amplification in neuroblastoma.[31]

The pathologic classification and diagnosis of CNS tumors is based upon their microscopic characteristics, particularly cell types and histologic patterns. Much of this information is still obtained by conventional light microscopy. In difficult or equivocal cases, cell types may be determined on the basis of additional information acquired by ultrastructural or immunohistochemical examination. Immunostains that are useful in the diagnosis of CNS tumors are summarized in Table 42-2.

The pathologic characteristics of the more important CNS tumors and three hereditary neoplastic disorders are briefly outlined in the following paragraphs. For detailed treatment of the material, refer to the monographs of Burger and Vogel, Rubinstein, and Russell and Rubinstein.[35,193,199]

Primary tumors

Gliomas. The important tumors of this type are astrocytoma, astrocytoma with atypical or anaplastic features, glioblastoma multiforme, ependymoma, choroid plexus papilloma, oligodendroglioma, and mixed gliomas. Gliomas are the most common group of central nervous system tumors, accounting for 50% of these neoplasms. Astrocytic tumors including glioblastoma represent 80% to 90% of all gliomas. As the name im-

Table 42-2. Immunohistochemical markers for nervous system tumors

Antigen	Used as a marker for these tumors	Expression in other tissues
GFAP (glial fibrillary acidic protein)	Astrocytic tumors, including glioblastoma	Expressed in other glial cells and in extraneural tissues
S-100 protein	Schwannoma Neurofibroma	Expressed by glial cells and in nonneural tissues
Neurofilament antigen	Tumors with cells of neuronal origins	Expressed in neuroendocrine tumors
Neuron-specific enolase	Tumors with cells of neuronal or neuroendocrine origin	Expressed by a variety of neural tissues
Vimentin	Astrocytic tumors (limited value)	Expressed by a large number of cells of various origins

From Perentes, E., and Rubinstein, L.J.: Arch. Pathol. Lab. Med. **111**:796, 1987.[164]

plies, they are composed of tumor cells resembling nonneoplastic glial elements or their relatives (choroid plexus epithelium) in the mature or developing nervous system and are classified on the basis of the predominant cell type present. These tumors are unencapsulated, infiltrate the surrounding neural parenchyma to a varying extent, and are difficult to excise completely. Attempts have been made to correlate the extent of anaplasia in glial tumors with biologic behavior through the use of a three- or four-step grading system in which increasing degrees of anaplasia are indicated by increasing numerical grades between 1 and 3 or 4.[183,227] As an extension of this concept, well-differentiated glial tumors are often referred to generically as low-grade gliomas and the more anaplastic varieties as high-grade gliomas. Although these systems have had some success, they are not widely accepted among neuropathologists in the United States for several reasons, including the use of subjective criteria and the problem of determining whether a surgical specimen includes the most anaplastic portion of the glioma on which the grade is based.[199] The identification of histologic features in gliomas that are of prognostic value is a matter of continuing interest for several reasons, including the need to evaluate accurately new therapeutic approaches to these tumors. Two recent studies have described objective criteria for a three-tiered classification of supratentorial astrocytic tumors and demonstrated their prognostic reliability and practicality.[36,152] This classification is now the basis for the pathology criteria used in most of the National Institutes of Health–sponsored cooperative therapeutic trials involving supratentorial astrocytomas. The histologic and prognostic features of the system are included in the description of astrocytic

tumors. Similar histologic investigations have been extended to oligodendroglial tumors.[34,126,143] It is important to keep in mind that histology is only one of several factors, including age of the patient, extent of surgery, and location of the tumor, that significantly influence the glioma patient's clinical course.[45,150]

Astrocytoma (well differentiated). Astrocytomas are found chiefly in children and young adults. They occur throughout the central nervous system. Overall, the cerebral examples are probably most numerous; however, the cerebellar astrocytoma is one of the most common primary CNS tumors in children. Astrocytomas are composed of morphologically uniform cells closely resembling mature resting or reactive, nonneoplastic fibrillary, or protoplasmic, astrocytes. Fusiform fibrillary astrocytes, also called "piloid or pilocytic astrocytes," are often encountered. Cell density is low to moderate. Mitoses are rare or usually absent entirely. Small or large cysts may be present (Fig. 42-39). Cerebral and brainstem astrocytomas frequently infiltrate brain parenchyma widely and characteristically develop anaplastic foci and aggressive behavior. Juvenile pilocytic astrocytomas are slowly growing partially circumscribed tumors occurring most often in children in the region of the third ventricle or cerebellum (Fig. 42-40). Histologically they are made up of compact bundles of astrocytes longitudinally arranged around blood vessels, adjacent to which are loose-meshed collections of tumor cells. Cerebellar astrocytomas are found characteristically in children. If brainstem involvement is absent, the outlook for long-term survival is good. Anaplastic changes rarely occur in either cerebellar or juvenile pilocytic astrocytomas.

Astrocytoma with atypical or anaplastic foci (ana-

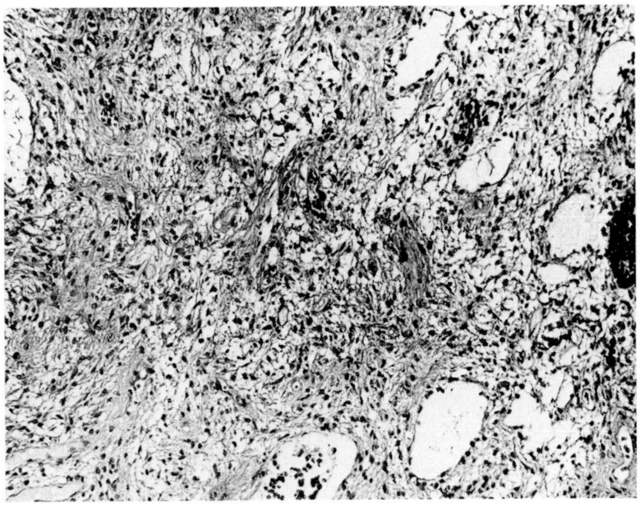

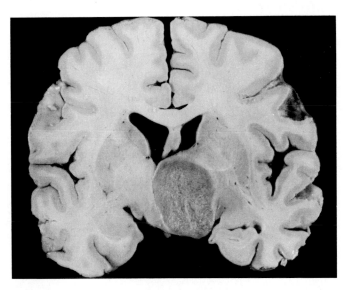

Fig. 42-39. Well-differentiated fibrillary astrocytoma. Astrocytic morphology is easily recognized. Microcysts are present. (Hematoxylin and eosin; 250×.)

Fig. 42-40. Well-circumscribed hypothalamic juvenile pilocytic astrocytoma.

plastic astrocytoma). More than half of the astrocytic tumors appear to be malignant or aggressive. Anaplastic astrocytomas form approximately 20% of this group. They occur most commonly in the cerebral hemispheres of adults between 20 and 50 years of age. There is multifocal or diffuse cellular and nuclear pleomorphism of the tumor astrocytes. Cell density is moderate to high. Mitotic figures are often present. Blood vessels within the tumor appear prominent, and endothelial proliferation is sometimes apparent. *Tumor necrosis is not present* (Fig. 42-41). The median survival for patients from 18 to 39 years of age with supratentorial anaplastic astrocytoma is 48 months and for patients from 40 to 59 years of age, 26 months.[150]

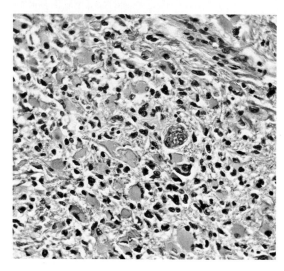

Fig. 42-41. Anaplastic astrocytoma with cellular pleomorphism and increased cell density. (Hematoxylin and eosin; 280×.)

Glioblastoma multiforme. Glioblastomas are tumors composed of cells chiefly of astrocytic lineage. They are the most common type of CNS tumor and thus are also the most common malignant astrocytoma and glioma. They occur most often in the cerebrum of adults over 40 years of age (Fig. 42-42). Histologically their features include all those associated with the atypical or anaplastic astrocytoma *and* one or more foci of coagulation necrosis involving tumor astrocytes. The necrosis may occur in sheets or in the center of tumor cells arranged in pseudopalisades (Fig. 42-43). The median survival for patients from 18 to 39 years of age with supratentorial glioblastoma is 17 months; from 40 to 59 years of age, 9 months; and from 60 to 70 years of age, 6 months.[150] In 2% to 5% of glioblastomas, a sarcomatous component arises within the astrocytic neoplasm. Such tumors are referred to as mixed glioblastoma and sarcoma or simply gliosarcoma. The sarcomatous elements are usually derived from fibroblasts in the walls of hyperplastic blood vessels. The occurrence of the sarcoma does not appear to alter the prognosis.

Ependymoma. Approximately 4% of gliomas are ependymomas. They arise predominantly in children and young adults from ependymal elements along the ventricular system or from ependymal cell clusters in the center of the spinal cord, conus medullaris, and filum terminale. Ependymomas are the most common variety of intraspinal gliomas. The tumor cells are uniform and often arranged radially around blood vessels. In this pattern the nuclei are located away from the blood vessel at one end of an elongated cell body that tapers as it extends to the blood vessel wall (Fig. 42-44). In some cases the cells are columnar or cuboid and form tubules or rosettes with a central lumen (Fig.

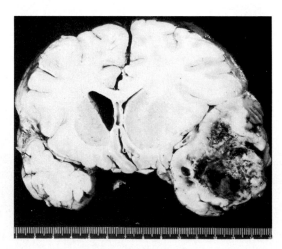

Fig. 42-42. Temporal lobe glioblastoma multiforme with hemorrhage and necrosis.

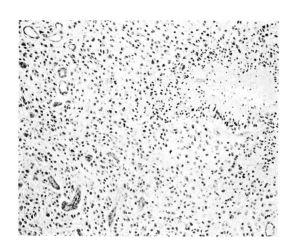

Fig. 42-43. Glioblastoma multiforme. Coagulative tumor necrosis, *upper right,* is present in addition to cellular pleomorphism and increased cell density. (Hematoxylin and eosin; 135×.)

42-45). A linear row of densities referred to as "blepharoplasts" can be seen along the luminal margin of the cells. These structures correspond to basal bodies associated with cilia. Ependymomas tend to be slowly growing; however malignant forms occur. Intracranial ependymomas may seed along ventricular or spinal fluid pathways.

Choroid plexus papillomas. Choroid plexus papillomas are derived from the epithelium of the choroid plexus, a homolog of the ependyma. They may occur at any age but are most common during the first two decades of life. They make up less than 1% of all intracranial tumors. The lateral or fourth ventricles are most often the sites of origin. The tumor appears grossly as a red finely lobulated mass. Microscopically the tumor resembles choroid plexus (Fig. 42-46). Cytologically, malignant forms are uncommon, but even well-differentiated forms may give rise to subarachnoid deposits. Rarely, these tumors secrete excessive cerebrospinal fluid causing internal hydrocephalus.

Oligodendroglioma. Oligodendrogliomas also make up about 4% of gliomas. They occur in children and adults, usually the latter. Typically they are located in the cerebral hemispheres near the cortex, but some examples grow from the ventricular wall into the adjacent lumen. Oligodendrogliomas are composed of small oval or polygonal uniform cells with dark-staining round nuclei, clear cytoplasm, and distinct cell borders. The clear cytoplasm is an artifact but a useful one. Cell density is usually moderate (Fig. 42-47). The tumor cells are often arranged diffusely and subdivided into incomplete lobules by small-caliber thin-walled blood vessels

producing the characteristic "chicken wire" appearance. Foci of calcification are frequently present in or near the tumor. The tumor is often regarded as a slowly growing neoplasm, but aggressive forms with cellular atypia, mitoses, vascular hyperplasia, and even necrosis are recognized.

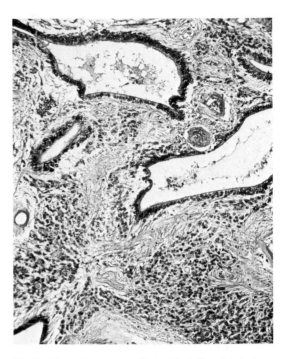

Fig. 42-45. Ependymoma with well-defined tubular structures. (Hematoxylin and eosin; 90×.)

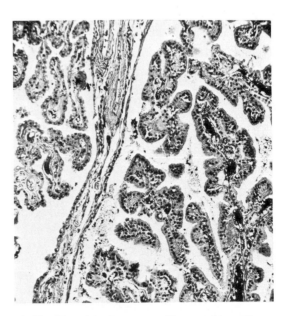

Fig. 42-46. Choroid plexus papilloma with uniform cells. (Hematoxylin and eosin; 90×.)

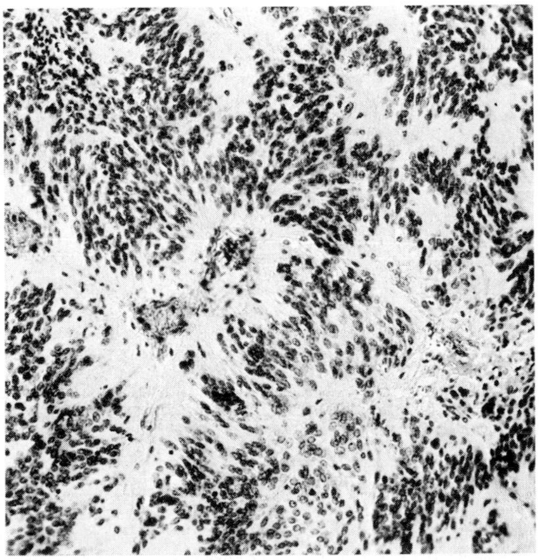

Fig. 42-44. Ependymoma, cellular type, with characteristic perivascular arrangement. (Hematoxylin and eosin; 90×.)

Mixed gliomas. In 4% to 6% of gliomas two or more distinct, mature, neoplastic glial cell types are present in sufficient numbers to warrant a diagnosis of mixed glioma.[92] Such tumors are named according to the cell types present. The most common combination is mixed oligoastrocytoma. The cell types may be intermingled or form adjacent more or less homogeneous groups. In general, moderately cellular and morphologically uniform tumors grow slowly, whereas those with increased cell density and cellular atypia affecting either component grow more rapidly.

Medulloblastoma. Medulloblastomas are located in the midline or lateral cerebellum. In some cases they arise from the external granular layer or nests of primitive cells in the posterior medullary velum.[109] They occur most frequently in children between 5 and 10 years of age with a second peak in adults between 20 and 30 years of age. They are the most common malignant primary CNS tumor in children. Medulloblastomas are highly cellular tumors composed of small, undifferentiated neuroepithelial cells with scanty cytoplasm that may show evidence of glial or neuronal differentiation. The cells are usually arranged in sheets; however, in about 25% of tumors Homer Wright rosettes are pres-

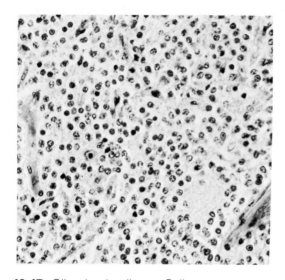

Fig. 42-47. Oligodendroglioma. Cells are compartmentalized by blood vessels. Some cells have nonstaining halos. (Hematoxylin and eosin; 280×.)

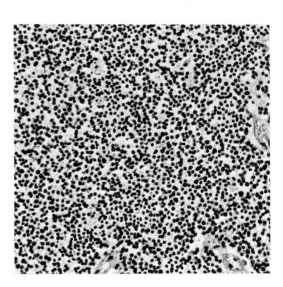

Fig. 42-48. Medulloblastoma. In some areas the cells are arranged in vaguely defined Homer Wright rosettes. (Hematoxylin and eosin; 280×.)

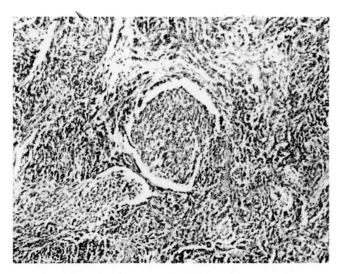

Fig. 42-49. Desmoplastic medulloblastoma with pale cellular islands. (Hematoxylin and eosin; 100×.)

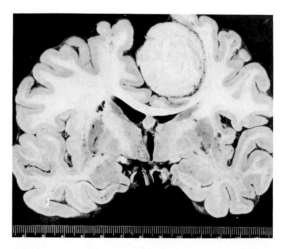

Fig. 42-50. Encapsulated parasagittal meningioma compressing but not invading the medial hemispheric surface.

ent (Fig. 42-48). These structures are composed of cells grouped radially around a central focus that does not contain a lumen. In some cases tumor cells invade the leptomeninges stimulating a reticulin response. Characteristically the tumor cells in the leptomeninges form cords separated by reticulin. Circumscribed foci of reduced cell density and free of reticulin appear as pale islands in the midst of the leptomeningeal deposits (Fig. 42-49). At one time tumors of this type were regarded, because of the reticulin, as mesenchymal tumors and called "circumscribed cerebellar sarcomas." This misapprehension was finally corrected by the study of Rubinstein and Northfield,[196] who suggested the name "desmoplastic medulloblastoma" by which these tumors are now designated. In addition to local parenchymal invasion, there is a significant risk of extensive spread of tumor cells along cerebrospinal fluid pathways from both conventional and desmoplastic medulloblastomas. Although these tumors are malignant, improved therapeutic regimens have increased the 5- and 10-year survivals to 40% and 30% respectively.[23]

Meningioma. Tumors of this type occur chiefly in adults over 30 years of age and account for 10% to 15% of all intracranial tumors and 25% of all intraspinal tumors. Although they are usually attached to the dura, meningiomas actually arise from arachnoidal cell clusters that have become included within the dura. The most common sites for these tumors are frontal parasagittal area, lateral cerebral convexity, base of the cerebrum (sphenoid ridge, olfactory groove, suprasellar area), spinal cord, and occasionally posterior fossa. Rarely meningiomas develop within the ventricles or in ectopic locations. The majority are encapsulated, slowly growing neoplasms that compress rather than invade the neural parenchyma (Fig. 42-50). Microscopically, tumor cells are uniform, oval, or fusiform, and present in moderate numbers. They are characteristically arranged in curving bundles or in concentric layers forming whorls (Fig. 42-51). These latter structures may degenerate and calcify giving rise to psammoma bodies. Many histologic patterns have been described in meningiomas, and most have no consistent relation to the biologic behavior of the tumors. Rarely, malignant changes may be observed in recurrences of previously benign meningiomas. There are, however, certain histologic types of meningiomas and histologic features that are associated with an increased potential for malignant or aggressive behavior. These include the hemangiopericytic variant of angioblastic meningioma, papillary meningioma, histologic evidence of parenchymal invasion, and meningiomas with increased cellularity and atypia, mitotic figures, and necrosis.[199] Except for the malignant or aggressive varieties, most meningiomas can be successfully removed by surgery. Approximately 10% of benign meningiomas recur most often because complete excision has been prevented by proximity of the tumor to vital structures or major blood vessels.[28]

Nerve sheath tumors. Nerve sheath tumors are of two histologic types, schwannoma and neurofibroma. Both are composed of Schwann cells though in the case of neurofibromas, fibroblasts may also be involved. Schwannomas arise from cranial and spinal nerve roots. They account for 10% of all intracranial tumors and 25% of all intraspinal tumors. Neurofibromas are rare in these locations except in cases of von Recklinghausen's disease where they are often in continuity with similar tumors involving spinal nerves outside the vertebral foramina. The schwannoma is an encapsulated tumor that produces eccentric enlargement of the nerve root. Sensory roots are affected most often. Intracranial schwannomas most frequently involve the eighth nerve roots and less often affect the fifth nerve roots. In the spinal cord the tumor may occur at any level but most commonly involves thoracic roots. Microscopically the tumor is composed of compact (Antoni A) and loose-meshed (Antoni B) areas. The compact areas consist of moderate numbers of uniform, fusiform cells in curving, interlacing bundles. Nuclei may be arranged in palisades at the ends of a fibrillar bundle forming a structure referred to as a "Verocay body" (Figs. 42-52 and 42-53). Delicate reticulin fibers are present around the individual tumor cells. The loose-meshed areas are sparsely cellular and composed of roughly stellate cells.

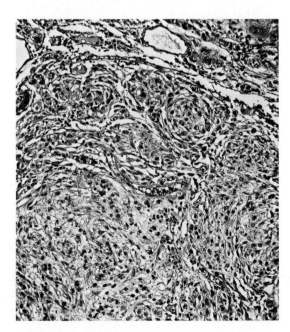

Fig. 42-51. Meningioma with uniform cells in bundles and concentric layers of whorls. (Hematoxylin and eosin; 90×.)

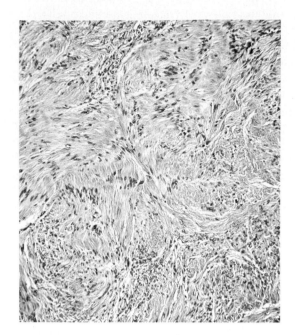

Fig. 42-52. Schwannoma. Portion with interlacing fascicular pattern. (Hematoxylin and eosin; 90×.)

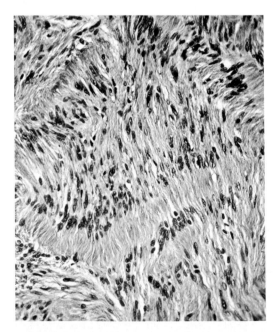

Fig. 42-53. Schwannoma. Verocay body. (Hematoxylin and eosin; 185×.)

A solitary schwannoma is not a feature of von Recklinghausen's disease.[199] They rarely if ever become malignant. Schwannomas can be cured surgically with minimal morbidity if they are diagnosed and treated while they are still small and do not extensively involve adjacent neural structures.

Although solitary neurofibromas occur, most are associated with von Recklinghausen's disease.[199] This hereditary disorder is discussed later in this section. The tumor grows within the nerve causing it to enlarge diffusely rather than eccentrically (Fig. 42-54). When the process extends throughout a segment of nerve and its branches, the lesion is referred to as a "plexiform neurofibroma." Microscopically, the tumor is composed of bundles of fusiform cells usually separated by intervening spaces. Some myelinated axons are preserved and spread apart by the proliferation. They can be identified within the tumor with special stains for axons and

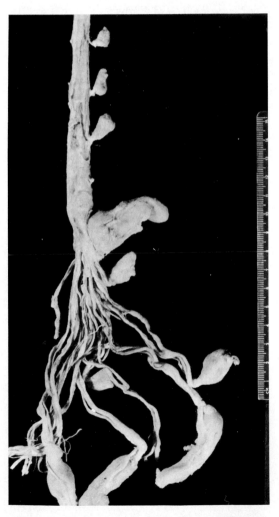

Fig. 42-54. Neurofibromatosis involving cauda equina and spinal ganglia in patient with von Recklinghausen's disease.

myelin sheaths. Neurofibromas can be removed surgically. Because most of these tumors are associated with von Recklinghausen's disease, the prognosis is determined primarily by this disorder.

Malignant nerve sheath tumors, sometimes inappropriately called "malignant schwannomas," may arise from neurofibromas in patients with von Recklinghausen's disease or develop spontaneously in the absence of this condition. The survival with treatment varies depending on the presence or absence of von Recklinghausen's disease.[60]

Craniopharyngioma. Craniopharyngiomas are well-demarcated, slowly growing epithelial tumors that arise at the base of the cerebrum in the vicinity of the tuber cinereum and above the sellar diaphragm. Craniopharyngiomas account for 2% to 3% of all intracranial tumors. They may occur at any age but are most common in children and young adults. Their origin is usually attributed to clusters of squamous cells in the stalk of the pituitary and adjacent infundibulum, which have been regarded as remnants of Rathke's pouch. This view is still debated however, and the histogenesis of craniopharyngioma has not been settled definitively. The tumor does not invade neural parenchyma but is closely attached to it by a dense meshwork of reactive fibrillary astrocytes at the interface of tumor and parenchyma. Gross and microscopic cysts are present and are filled with a viscous, dark brown oily fluid containing cholesterol crystals. The tumor is composed of uniform epithelial cells that form irregular confluent clusters. Columnar cells are present along the borders of these clusters, whereas in the center loosely arranged stellate cells are present (Fig. 42-55). Deposits of keratin, often quite large, are present in the midst of the tumor cells

in addition to cholesterol clefts and focal calcification. A chronic granulomatous inflammatory reaction chemically induced by leakage of cyst contents onto the adjacent meninges may also be seen. Although the tumors are not malignant in the usual sense, they may be difficult to remove surgically because of their close attachment to adjacent parenchyma. The reported recurrence rates for craniopharyngiomas treated by gross total excision vary from 0% to 50%. The 10-year survival rates in these cases range from 50% to 100%. After subtotal excision, recurrence occurs in 50% to 90% of cases, and 50% of patients survive 10 years. A combination of limited surgery and postoperative radiation in those cases where total excision is not feasible appears to produce results comparable to those obtained in cases where total excision could be accomplished.[52]

Hemangioblastoma. Hemangioblastomas are vascular tumors that may occur at any age but are most frequent between 20 and 50 years of age. The most common sites are the cerebellum and spinal cord. They constitute 2% to 3% of all CNS tumors, and in some series they are as frequent as meningiomas in the posterior fossa.[199] Occasionally multiple tumors may be present in the cerebellum or brainstem. The tumor is circumscribed and may be solid or variably cystic with a hemorrhagic or yellow appearance grossly. The tumor is composed of numerous thin-walled endothelium-lined vascular channels between which lie large, oval, or polygonal cells, called "stromal cells," which sometimes contain cytoplasmic lipid vacuoles (Fig. 42-56). Three

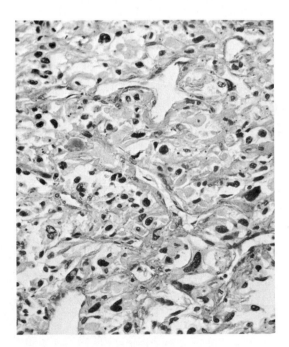

Fig. 42-56. Capillary hemangioblastoma in cerebellum. (Hematoxylin and eosin; 135×.)

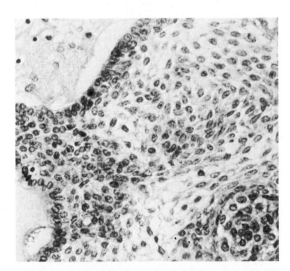

Fig. 42-55. Craniopharyngioma. Interior of islands have stellate cells with cuboid to columnar cells adjacent to stroma.

cell types—endothelial cells, pericytes, and stromal cells—are evident by electron microscopy. The origin of the stromal cells is uncertain.[199] The prognosis for hemangioblastoma is good. Approximately 85% of patients are alive and well 5 to 20 years after surgical excision.[193] Hemangioblastomas occur sporadically or as part of the von Hippel-Lindau syndrome, which is discussed later in this section.

Primary CNS lymphoma. Primary CNS lymphomas, formerly called "microgliomas," are now recognized as extranodal lymphomas arising in the central nervous system.[93,193,232] They are usually of B-cell origin and may be of either diffuse small cell or large cell type, most often the latter.[96] Sporadically occurring primary CNS lymphoma has a peak incidence during the fifth to seventh decades and accounts for 1% of all CNS tumors and 1% of all non-Hodgkin lymphomas.[201,213] Patients with congenital immunodeficiencies, AIDS, and drug-induced immunosuppression after organ transplant are at increased risk of developing primary CNS lymphoma.[96] The tumor usually arises in the parenchyma; however, meningeal infiltrates also occur in some cases. The parenchymal deposits are multiple in up to 50% of cases and occur throughout the central nervous system but are most frequent above the tentorium.[96] Microscopically the larger deposits are formed by confluence of perivascular collections of lymphoma cells. Infiltration of the parenchyma by the neoplastic lymphocytes is associated with a prominent reactive astrocytosis. Characteristically, concentric layers of reticulin separated by collections of tumor cells are present around the blood vessels within the confluent tumor as well as those surrounded by perivascular accumulations of lymphoma cells. Even with treatment few patients live more than 2 to 3 years after diagnosis.[96]

Germ cell tumors. Five histological types of germ cell tumors are found in the nervous system: germinoma, embryonal carcinoma, choriocarcinoma, endodermal sinus tumor, and teratoma. The first four are malignant, the fifth may be either benign or malignant. As the names imply, they are histologic counterparts of germ cell tumors with similar nomenclature arising outside the central nervous system. They occur most often in males during the first three decades of life and are usually located in the midline in the vicinity of the pineal gland or at the base of the brain near the tuber cinereum. The germinoma is the most common type of CNS germ cell tumor and histologically resembles the seminoma of the testis and dysgerminoma of the ovary (Figs. 42-57 and 42-58). In the older literature tumors of this type arising in the pineal region were referred to as "pinealomas" and those originating near the tuber cinereum as "ectopic pinealomas." The term "pinealoma" is now used only for those rare neuroectodermal tumors that are composed of pineal parenchymal cells.[103,194]

Metastatic tumors

Metastatic tumors account for 15% to 25% of all CNS tumors. CNS metastases occur in approximately 24% of all cancer patients and 30% to 50% of patients die of causes related to those metastases.[25,170] Carcinomas of the lung and breast are the most common sources of CNS metastases. Some relatively uncommon tumors such as renal cell carcinoma, melanoma, and choriocarcinoma metastasize with high frequency to the central nervous system. All parts of the central nervous system may be affected, most commonly the cerebrum. The lesions are multiple in at least 70% of cases. The parenchymal deposits are sharply demarcated and often surrounded by a zone of edema. In the cerebrum hema-

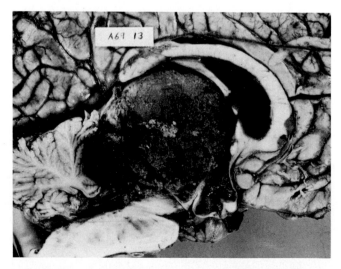

Fig. 42-57. Pineal germinoma. Bulky vascularized tumor has destroyed the middle of the brain and is invading hypothalamus and cerebellum.

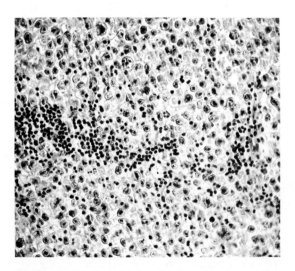

Fig. 42-58. Pineal germinoma. Notice the two cell types. (Hematoxylin and eosin; 135×.)

togenous metastases are found near the junction of cortex and white matter or in the basal ganglia. In the posterior fossa they are usually located in the cerebellar hemispheres in the boundary region between the superior and inferior arterial supply.

In some cases the bulk of the tumor is chiefly confined to and extensively infiltrates the subarachnoid space. This type of involvement referred to as "meningeal carcinomatosis" is often associated with adenocarcinomas arising in various sites such as lung or colon.[67] Intraspinal metastases are as noted previously, usually extradural.

Hereditary neoplastic disorders

Neurofibromatous, tuberous sclerosis, and von Hippel-Lindau disease are genetically determined autosomal dominant disorders in which neoplastic lesions of the central and peripheral nervous system are conspicuous features. Those conditions are often included with other neurocutaneous syndromes in a group of disorders referred to as the phakomatoses.

Neurofibromatosis. At least two distinct forms of this disorder have been established—neurofibromatosis 1 and 2.[134,179] Neurofibromatosis 1 corresponds to the classic disorder described by von Recklinghausen and accounts for 90% of cases of neurofibromatosis.[101] The defining features are multiple café-au-lait spots, peripheral neurofibromas, and pigmented hamartomas of the iris called "Lisch nodules." Approximately a third of the patients with the disease develop complications such as intellectual handicap, plexiform neurofibroma with cosmetic disfigurement, and malignant tumors of the

nerves and viscera. Tumors involving the central nervous system including optic gliomas and other astrocytomas, unilateral acoustic schwannomas, meningiomas, neurofibromas, and other types occur in 5% to 10% of patients and contribute to the morbidity and mortality of the disease.[179] Recent studies cited by Martuza and Eldridge[134] indicate that the gene for this disorder is located on chromosome 17.

Neurofibromatosis 2 is characterized by bilateral acoustic schwannomas. Café-au-lait spots and cutaneous neurofibromas are less common than in neurofibromatosis 2 but do occur as well as plexiform neurofibromas. In addition to bilateral acoustic neuromas, schwannomas of other cranial and spinal nerve roots, meningiomas, and gliomas may involve the central nervous system. The gene for neurofibromatosis 2 is located on chromosome 22.[248]

Tuberous sclerosis. Tuberous sclerosis is a disorder transmitted as a single gene defect with a penetrance of about 80%.[83] The characteristic CNS lesions are multiple, firm hamartomatous masses involving the cortex and ventricles and subependymal giant cell astrocytomas. The cortical lesions, called "tubers," are composed of astrocytes, neurons, and large dysplastic cells resembling both astrocytes and neurons (Figs. 42-59 and 42-60). The ventricular hamartomas called "candle gutterings" are made up of large-bodied astrocytes and their processes as well as foci of calcification. They are located most frequently in the thalamostriate sulcus.[212] Ultrastructural and immunohistochemical studies show that the cells in the ventricular candle gutterings and some of the large dysplastic cells in the cortical tubers

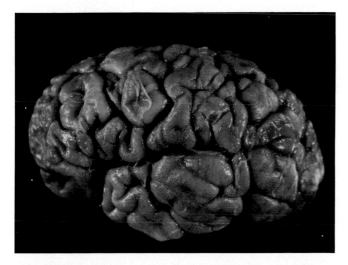

Fig. 42-59. Tuberous sclerosis. Cortical tubers are present in the posterior two thirds of the middle frontal gyrus and the posterior half of the superior and middle temporal gyri. The lesions are sharply demarcated. The surfaces contain shallow sulci, which usually do not communicate with normal secondary sulci.

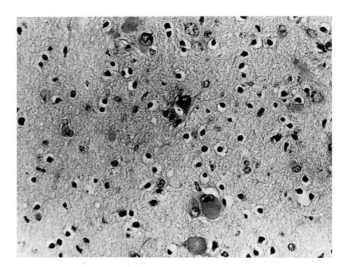

Fig. 42-60. Histologic section of cortical tuber with large, often multinucleated cells, astrocytosis, and distorted cortical lamination. (Hematoxylin and eosin; 250×.)

have features of astrocytic differentiation and stain variably for GFAP.[17] Subependymal giant cell astrocytomas usually arise in the vicinity of the foramen of Monro. They are typically associated with tuberous sclerosis but also occur in the absence of this condition. The tumors are well circumscribed, slowly growing, and composed of large fusiform, piriform, and strap-shaped astrocytes, which stain variably for GFAP. These tumors rarely undergo malignant change.[24] In addition to the CNS lesions, cutaneous and visceral lesions including adenoma sebaceum of the face, cardiac rhabdomyomas, and renal angiomyolipomas occur. Seizures and mental deterioration are present in severe forms of the disease, but milder cases with normal mentation and no seizures are also reported.

Von Hippel-Lindau disease. Hemangioblastoma of the central nervous system is the characteristic lesion in this disorder. The tumors may be single or multiple and are usually found in the cerebellum, spinal cord, or brainstem. Similar tumors are present in the retina in 50% of patients with this condition. Visceral lesions include cysts of the kidneys and pancreas as well as renal adenomas and carcinomas and pheochromocytomas. Cutaneous lesions are absent.[98]

Demyelinative diseases

Loss of myelin occurs in the central and peripheral nervous system. The loss may be through primary or secondary mechanisms or as part of a pathologic process in which all the parenchymal elements are simultaneously and uniformly affected. The term "demyelinative disease" is used only in reference to a central or peripheral nervous system disorder in which primary demyelination is the mechanism causing the loss of myelin. In primary demyelination the myelin sheaths or the myelin-forming cells—oligodendrocytes and Schwann cells—are injured first, most severely, and in greatest numbers. Although oligodendroglial and myelin damage are the dominant features, axonal, neural, or other glial elements in the lesion may be affected less severely or undergo later degenerative changes. In secondary demyelination the myelin disintegrates as a consequence of neuronal or axonal disease leading to loss of the axon whose presence is necessary for maintenance of an intact myelin sheath. This process of axonal and myelin loss distal to the point of injury is also called "wallerian degeneration." It is seen in fiber tracts in degenerative axonopathies, physically induced spinal cord injury, and other conditions. Demyelination may also occur as part of a nonselective injury such as infarction of the white matter. In this situation all the parenchymal elements within the lesion are damaged more or less equally and simultaneously. With appropriate stains mature stabilized white matter infarcts will, of course, appear as demyelinated lesions. Further investigation with axonal stains will demonstrate that both axons and myelin sheaths have been lost in equal numbers and the demyelination is not a primary process. The case is similar for tracts undergoing wallerian degeneration.

In this section the following demyelinative diseases affecting the central nervous system are described: multiple sclerosis, acute disseminated encephalomyelitis, acute hemorrhagic leukoencephalitis, progressive multifocal leukoencephalopathy, central pontine myelinolysis, and the leukodystrophies.

Multiple sclerosis (MS)

The most common of the CNS demyelinative diseases is multiple sclerosis. The usual time of onset is 20 to 40 years of age. Most often, multiple sclerosis follows a chronic relapsing course with remissions or periods of stability and exacerbations over a period of 30 to 40 years. The initial symptoms may involve any part of the central nervous system. Among the most frequent are weakness of one or more extremities, visual disturbances, incoordination, and paresthesias. In subsequent episodes various combinations of signs and symptoms may occur. Clinically, multiple sclerosis is strongly suspected when these episodes are separated by weeks or months and the neurologic disturbances indicate two or more lesions affecting different parts of the central nervous system. Thus the clinical hallmark of multiple sclerosis is the occurrence of lesions disseminated in time and space. The majority of patients have a selective increase of IgG in the cerebrospinal fluid, which is characteristically in the form of oligoclonal bands.[63] None of the laboratory or neuroimaging studies, however, are specific. The diagnosis is based on clinical observation and the exclusion of other conditions. Although steroids may shorten acute attacks, there is no definitive therapy for the disease. Most patients become progressively disabled with time and eventually die from respiratory or urinary tract infection. The cause and pathogenesis of the disease is unknown. Over the years, many hypotheses have been proposed concerning its cause. Most have been disproved and discarded. Currently, multiple sclerosis is widely viewed as an immunologically mediated disorder affecting genetically susceptible persons caused by a virus that either produces a slow persistent infection of the central nervous system or induces autoimmunity and disappears.[63,138]

The characteristic lesion of chronic relapsing multiple sclerosis is a sharply circumscribed area of myelin loss called a "plaque" (Fig. 42-61). Although multiple plaques varying in size and shape are present bilaterally in all parts of the central nervous system, certain sites are regularly affected. In the cerebrum these include the borders of the lateral ventricles around the angles, atria, occipital and frontal horns, and the junction of cortex and white matter. Elsewhere the pons, cerebellar peduncles and central white matter, optic nerves, and spinal cord are frequent sites. Plaques may encroach upon or lie within areas of gray matter because of the presence of myelinated axons in these locations. Macroscopically, chronic plaques appear as well-demarcated, gray semitranslucent foci with slightly sunken surfaces (Fig. 42-62). More recent active plaques have less well-defined borders and are yellowish white in color sometimes with a pink border. Microscopically the active lesions show myelin loss, macrophages containing myelin debris, perivenular mononuclear infiltrates, relative sparing of axons, and astrocytic proliferation. In the early stages of the lesion oligodendroglia are spared because the initial injury is directed toward the myelin membrane.[138] In older plaques the dominant features are a diffuse fibrillary astrocytosis, loss of oligodendroglia within the lesion, and relative preservation of axons (though these may be reduced in number compared with adjacent uninvolved parenchyma) (Fig. 42-62). Thinly myelinated axons suggestive of a limited degree of remyelination are sometimes seen at the plaque borders.[127] Perivascular infiltrates and macrophages are absent.

Other variants of multiple sclerosis include acute multiple sclerosis of Marburg type, Balo's concentric sclerosis, Devic's disease (neuromyelitis optica) and certain cases of Schilder's disease. These conditions differ from chronic relapsing multiple sclerosis in regard to the rate of disease progression and some of the pathologic characteristics of the lesions.[6]

Acute disseminated encephalomyelitis

Acute disseminated encephalomyelitis is an acute monophasic disease characterized by perivenous demyelination accompanied by perivenous mononuclear inflammatory cell infiltration (Fig. 42-63). The lesions are usually bilateral and distributed throughout the brain and spinal cord; however, localized forms of the disease occasionally occur. Acute disseminated encephalomyelitis may develop spontaneously, or after acute viral infections in childhood (especially the exanthemas), or after immunization against smallpox, typhoid, or rabies (Pasteur treatment). The spontaneous form may develop at any age but is most common in young adults. The disease may be fatal or cause severe neurologic deficits; however, most patients recover with little or no sequelae. In view of the similarities with experimental allergic encephalitis, a disease produced by injected susceptible animals with emulsions of homologous brain containing myelin basic protein in Freund's

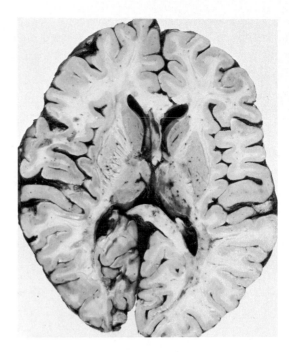

Fig. 42-61. Multiple sclerosis. Plaques are prominent along the ventricular borders.

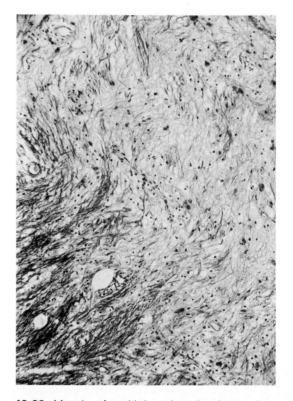

Fig. 42-62. Margin of multiple sclerosis plaque. Intact axons are present in demyelinated area, *upper right*. (Luxol–fast blue–silver nitrate; 135×.)

adjuvant, and the inability to isolate virus from the brains of affected patients, acute disseminated encephalomyelitis is currently regarded as an immune-mediated disorder.

Acute hemorrhagic leukoencephalitis

Rapidly progressive and often fatal, acute hemorrhagic leukoencephalitis is considered to be an immunopathologic disorder similar to but more severe than acute disseminated encephalomyelitis. The disease chiefly affects adults and develops spontaneously or af-

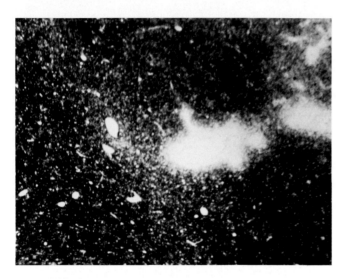

Fig. 42-63. Acute disseminated encephalomyelitis. Perivascular demyelination. (Loyez stain; 100×.)

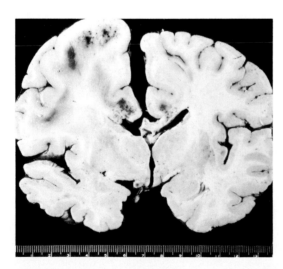

Fig. 42-64. Acute hemorrhagic leukoencephalitis, predominantly unilateral. (Courtesy Dr. J. Langston; from Chason, J.L.: Brain, meninges and spinal cord. In Saphir, O., editor: A text on systemic pathology, vol. 2, New York, 1958, Grune & Stratton, Inc.; by permission.)

ter an upper respiratory illness. Grossly, multiple petechiae are present diffusely or asymmetrically and chiefly involve white matter (Fig. 42-64). Microscopically there is fibrinoid necrosis of venules and arterioles and deposits of fibrin in perivascular spaces. Surrounding these vessels are perivascular zones of demyelination, hemorrhage, and collections of neutrophils.

Progressive multifocal leukoencephalopathy (PML)

In progressive multifocal leukoencephalopathy infection of the brain chiefly affecting oligodendroglia is caused by members of the papovavirus family as a consequence of impaired cell-mediated immunity and results in multiple demyelinative lesions involving the cerebrum and, to a lesser extent, the brainstem and cerebellum. Occasionally, the spinal cord may be affected. Three groups of viruses compose the papova family: *pa*pillomaviruses, *po*lyoma viruses, and simian *va*cuolating virus (simian virus 40, SV40), with the acronym "papova." Among the cases studied by virus isolation, the JC polyoma virus has been recovered from the brain in all but two instances in which the SV40 virus was isolated.[182,214] Asymptomatic JC virus infection is common. By the later teens approximately 75% of persons in the United States have serologic evidence of previous infection.[215] Recent studies indicate that the virus may be carried into the brain by B-lymphocytes from bone marrow and spleen.[100] Originally, PML was chiefly found in cases of leukemia, lymphoma, and other spontaneously occurring disorders associated with deficient immune responsiveness. Subsequently, cases have been reported after the use of immunosuppressive agents in transplant recipients and patients with au-

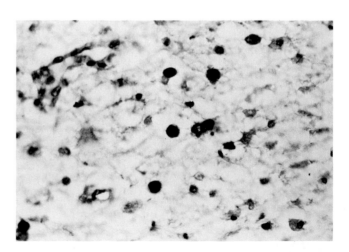

Fig. 42-65. Progressive multifocal leukoencephalopathy. Enlarged, effaced oligodendroglial nuclei. (Hematoxylin and eosin; 400×.)

toimmune disorders. Most recently, PML has been identified as one of the CNS complications of AIDS. The disease affects adults and runs a subacute, progressive, fatal course lasting 3 to 6 months. Grossly, patchy sometimes confluent foci of softened, spongy white matter are seen most readily in the cerebrum. Microscopically within the lesions there is destruction of the myelin sheath, loss of oligodendroglia, accumulation of lipid phagocytes, and relative preservation of axons. Inflammatory cell infiltration is usually absent. Enlarged hyperchromatic oligodendroglial nuclei with an effaced chromatin pattern or recognizable eosinophilic or basophilic inclusions are found at the margins of the lesion (Fig. 42-65). The nuclear changes indicate death of the oligodendrocyte from the cytopathic effects of the virus. It is this destruction of the oligodendroglia that determines the demyelinative characteristics of the lesion.[181] Ultrastructural examination of the nuclei shows filamentous and round virions characteristic of the papovavirus group. In addition to the changes involving the oligodendroglia, there are also striking astrocytic alterations that accompany the lesions. The astrocytes resemble neoplastic forms with hypertrophied cell bodies and one or more enlarged, pleomorphic nuclei. Despite their appearance, these astrocytes do not show other evidence of neoplastic tendencies. It is of interest, however, in this regard that the JC virus is oncogenic. Intracerebral inoculation of newborn hamsters induces a variety of primary CNS tumors.

Central pontine myelinolysis (CPM)

The principal lesion in central pontine myelinolysis is a symmetric focus of demyelination chiefly involving the rostral and middle thirds of the striate pons (Fig. 42-66). The larger lesions may encroach on the tegmentum and extend from the midbrain to the pontomedullary junction. The medulla is rarely affected, and the lesions do not extend to the pial or ventricular surfaces. In occasional cases extrapontine demyelinative lesions may be present.[251] Grossly the lesion appears as a circumscribed area of soft spongy or granular tissue symmetrically involving the striate pons. The smaller lesions are located centrally, whereas the larger lesions extend laterally on both sides of the midline. Microscopically, myelin sheaths and oligodendroglia are lost within the lesion, axons and neurons are spared except toward the center of the lesion, and lipid phagocytes are present. There is no evidence of perivascular demyelination, and inflammatory changes are absent. Characteristically the longitudinally directed myelinated tracts in the ventrolateral striate pons are less severely affected. The original cases of this condition occurred against a background of chronic alcoholism and malnutrition.[4] Subsequently, the disorder has been associated with other conditions, including electrolyte disturbances chiefly involving sodium, and with severe debilitating illnesses in children.[37,251] At present, clinical and experimental evidence indicates that pontine and extrapontine myelinolysis may be induced either by too rapid correction of serum sodium deficits in hyponatremic patients[116,224] or by corrections of excessive magnitude.[11] Currently the debate is unresolved.

Leukodystrophies

Leukodystrophies are a group of progressive disorders involving myelin in the central and, in some cases, the peripheral nervous system. The leukodystrophies usually have their onset during the first decade of life;

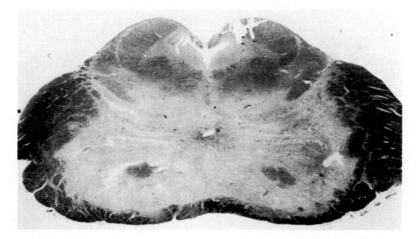

Fig. 42-66. Central pontine myelinolysis. There is symmetric loss of myelin chiefly in the striate portion of the pons with some sparing of corticospinal fibers. (Luxol–fast blue–PAS; 8.5×.)

however, in several of these diseases juvenile and adult varieties have been recognized. In a few instances the underlying biochemical defect or the principal biochemical abnormalities have been identified. The disturbance in myelin associated with the leukodystrophies is sometimes referred to as "dysmyelination" to indicate that disorders of myelin formation as well as myelin breakdown may be involved in the pathogenesis of the lesions. The general gross and microscopic features are similar in most of the leukodystrophies. They are symmetric absence of myelin staining, variable but usually severe loss of axons, and diffuse fibrillary astrocytosis in the cerebrum and cerebellum (Fig. 42-67). The subcortical arcuate fibers are characteristically spared. The lesions usually do not have the sharply defined borders seen in multiple sclerosis plaques, and with some exceptions, perivascular inflammation is minimal or absent. The features of three of the more common leukodystrophies are summarized in the following paragraphs. For further details the review by Stam[222] should be consulted.

Metachromatic leukodystrophy (MLD).   The autosomal recessive disorder metachromatic leukodystrophy is the most common of the leukodystrophies. Late infantile, juvenile, and adult varieties are recognized according to the age of onset. All have similar pathologic features.[129] The basic biochemical defect in the majority of cases is a deficiency of cerebroside sulfatase, a lysosomal enzyme commonly referred to as "arylsulfatase A." In a few cases the activator for arylsulfatase A is absent.[89] As a result of this deficiency sulfatide deposits accumulate in the central white matter, Schwann cells, and epithelial cells of the gallbladder, intrahepatic bile ducts, or renal tubules where they can be demonstrated in frozen sections with the Hirsch-Peiffer acidified cresyl violet stain as foci of brown metachromasia (Fig. 42-68). Formerly, this technique was used on sural nerve biopsy specimens to establish the diagnosis. At present, however, the diagnosis is confirmed by assay of arylsulfatase A in urine, fibroblasts, leukocytes, or serum.

Globoid cell (Krabbe's) leukodystrophy. Globoid cell leukodystrophy is an autosomal recessive disorder usually of infantile onset. The basic biochemical defect is an absence of galactosyl ceramide–beta-galactosidase. Deficiency of this enzyme leads to the accumulation of galactocerebroside in the central white matter; this accumulation provokes the formation of clusters of rounded or globoid cells with one or more nuclei, a characteristic feature of this disease (Fig. 42-69).

Adrenoleukodystrophy (ALD). There are two distinct forms of adrenoleukodystrophy—X-linked ALD and neonatal ALD. The latter condition has an autosomal recessive mode of inheritance.[145] In both conditions adrenocortical atrophy, striated cortical cells with lamellar inclusions, and cerebral perivascular demyelination with perivascular cuffs of lymphocytes are seen.[174] In the neonatal form, however, abnormalities of neuronal migration are also present. The underlying defect in X-linked ALD involves an inability to degrade very long chain fatty acids, a reaction carried out by the peroxisome. Thus X-linked ALD is regarded as one of the peroxisomal disorders. In addition to the degradative defect involving very long chain fatty acids, other biochemical disturbances involving phospholipids, enzymes, and bile acids are present in patients with neonatal ALD and are not found in cases of X-linked ALD.

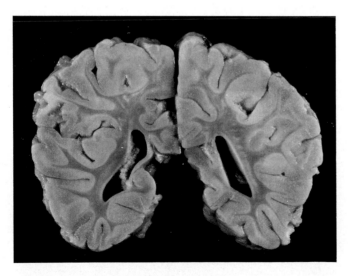

Fig. 42-67. Leukodystrophy. Symmetric uniform involvement of white matter that is gray, firm, and slightly retracted below the cut surface. The optic radiation is barely visible.

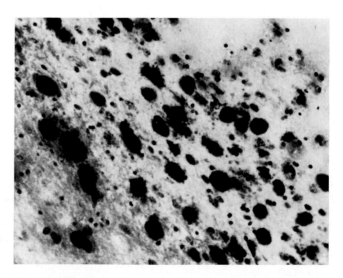

Fig. 42-68. Metachromatic leukodystrophy. Intracellular and extracellular deposits of metachromatic sulfatide. (Hirsch-Peiffer; 250×.)

Degenerative diseases

Degenerative diseases are disorders of unknown cause and pathogenesis characterized pathologically by progressive loss of CNS neurons and their processes accompanied by fibrillary astrocytosis. These changes proceed in the absence of obvious precipitating factors such as metabolic disturbances, vascular disease, nutritional deficiency, or infection. Some of the degenerative diseases are genetically determined, whereas others are not. In certain disorders there is an accentuation of neuron loss in particular anatomic regions, such as the cerebral cortex in Alzheimer's disease. In others, the lesions tend to be systematized, chiefly affecting functionally or anatomically related nerve cells and traits such as the motor neurons and pathways in amyotrophic lateral sclerosis. In virtually all cases, however, the lesions are distributed symmetrically. The classification of the degenerative diseases is based upon clinical and pathologic features. In this regard the anatomic distribution of the lesions is an important consideration, since the histologic features of many of these disorders are similar. In this section five of the more common degenerative diseases—Alzheimer's disease, Huntington's disease, Parkinson's disease, and two forms of motor neuron disease, amyotrophic lateral sclerosis and Werdnig-Hoffmann disease—are discussed. For comprehensive coverage of this entire group of disorders the pertinent reviews[156,208,233,237] should be consulted.

Alzheimer's disease

Alzheimer's disease is a progressive dementing illness occurring chiefly in older adults with the highest incidence in the ninth decade of life.[112] Alzheimer's disease accounts for approximately 50% of all cases of adult dementia and is the most common cause of this condition among elderly persons. Previously, the diagnosis of Alzheimer's disease was often used only in cases where the dementia began before 65 years of age. A similar disorder developing after age 65 was called "senile dementia." The fundamental similarities between Alzheimer's disease and most cases of senile dementia is widely recognized. The term "Alzheimer's disease" is used in reference to cases of senile dementia as well as those cases with onset before 65 years of age.

The cause and pathogenesis of Alzheimer's disease are unknown. In a small number of families an autosomal dominant inheritance pattern has been recognized. Genetic studies, however, are complicated by variations in the age of onset. Chromosome 21 has been implicated in some studies as the Alzheimer gene site in familial cases; however, confirmation of these observations is presently lacking.[202] In experimental studies aluminum salts can induce excessive formation of neurofilaments; however, the ultrastructural characteristics of this change are distinct from those associated with neurofibrillary degeneration in Alzheimer's disease. It

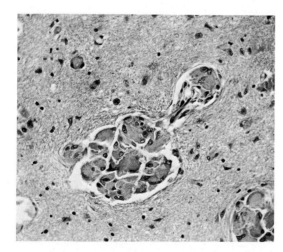

Fig. 42-69. Globoid sclerosis (Krabbe's disease). (Hematoxylin and eosin; 135×.)

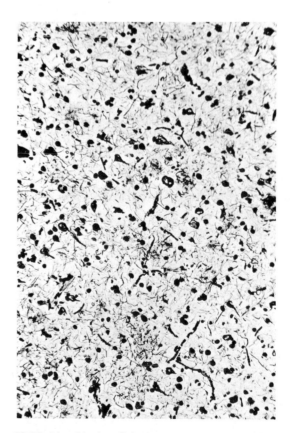

Fig. 42-70. Neuritic (senile) plaques and neurofibrillary tangles in Alzheimer's disease. (Hortega silver carbonate; 135×.)

is interesting, however, that both aluminum and silicon have been found within the neurofibrillary tangles of Alzheimer's disease. There is no evidence that exposure to exogenous sources of aluminum such as antacids and antiperspirants or use of a course of renal dialysis increases the risk of Alzheimer's disease.[112]

Grossly there is evidence of cerebral atrophy with widened sulci and narrowed gyri. The medial temporal lobes are particularly affected. The lateral ventricles are often enlarged, at least to some extent. The principal microscopic findings are neurofibrillary tangles (NFT) and neuritic (senile) plaques (Fig. 42-70). Although both of these structures can be seen on occasion with hematoxylin and eosin stains, silver impregnation techniques or amyloid stains are recommended as the most sensitive and reliable methods for their detection. Neurofibrillary tangles are rounded, elongated, or twisted clusters of argyrophilic fibers found within neurons and distributed widely throughout the cerebral cortex especially in the hippocampus and adjacent temporal lobe. They are also seen in the amygdala and in the gray matter adjacent to the third and fourth ventricles. Ultrastructurally, neurofibrillary tangles are composed of paired helical filaments. Each filament of the pair measures 10 nm in diameter and the twists occur at intervals of 80 nm. This type of structure is also seen in other diseases in which neurofibrillary tangles are present. The neuritic plaques are found throughout the cerebral cortex and are particularly prevalent in the hippocampus. Deep cerebral gray matter and occasionally the cerebellum may be affected. The plaques have a central core composed of amyloid beta protein that is surrounded by abnormal neurites filled with degenerating organelles, lysosomes, and paired helical filaments. Both neurofibrillary tangles and neuritic plaques occur with advancing age in the absence of dementia. In Alzheimer's disease their numbers are dramatically increased. These quantitative differences as well as the fact that dementia is not a regular component of the aging process indicate that Alzheimer's disease is, in fact, a disease and not simply accelerated aging. Other common histologic findings include rod-shaped eosinophilic inclusions (Hirano bodies) or vacuoles containing basophilic inclusions in hippocampal neurons and amyloid deposition in the walls of subarachnoid and parenchymal arterioles. Characteristic neurochemical changes involving decreases in cerebral cortical acetylcholine and somatostatin are also present in Alzheimer's disease. The cholinergic deficit is associated with neuron loss from the basal nucleus of Meynert, the principal source of cholinergic input to the neocortex. The course of Alzheimer's disease varies from 1 to 15 years. Death most commonly is from infection such as pneumonia.

Huntington's disease

Huntington's disease is an autosomal dominant disorder transmitted to a gene localized to chromosome 4. The disease usually begins during the fourth decade and is characterized by involuntary choreiform movements, dementia, and personality disorder.[133] The pathogenesis of the disorder is unknown though several abnormalities of neurotransmitter concentrations including decreased GABA and increased somatostatin have been observed. The most striking pathologic changes involve the corpus striatum (Fig. 42-71). There is pronounced atrophy of the caudate nucleus and to a lesser extent the putamen and globus pallidus.

Microscopically there is considerable nerve cell loss in the neostriatal nuclei and a lesser degree in the globus pallidus. The neuronal atrophy is accompanied by fibrillary astrocytosis. Among the various types of neostriatal neurons, the medium-sized spiny cells (type I) are affected first. Neuron loss is also described in the cerebral cortex, thalamus, and subthalamus. The dementia is customarily attributed to cortical neuronal atrophy; however, this putative loss is frequently difficult to document. The disease runs a chronic course of many years. Death is usually from infection.

Parkinson's disease

The movement disorder Parkinson's disease, characterized by bradykinesia, rigidity, abnormal gait, and resting tremors of the extremities and other parts of the body, has its onset usually during the fifth and sixth decades. Although a small number of familial cases have been recognized, most cases of Parkinson's disease are

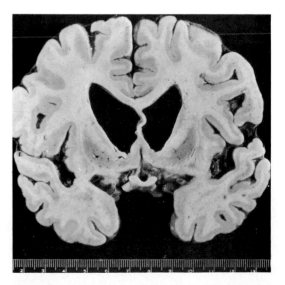

Fig. 42-71. Huntington's disease. There is noticeable bilateral atrophy of the caudate and putamen with ventricular enlargement.

sporadic. The condition referred to as "idiopathic Parkinson's disease," or simply "Parkinson's disease," is clinically similar but etiologically and pathologically distinct from a group of disorders referred to as "parkinsonism." Included in the latter group are conditions such as postencephalitic or arteriosclerotic parkinsonism. As the name suggests, the cause and pathogenesis of idiopathic Parkinson's disease are unknown. The parkinsonian syndrome caused by intoxication with MPTP, a contaminant of synthetic heroin is not associated with the characteristic pathologic features found in Parkinson's disease. The lesions in Parkinson's disease involve brainstem catecholaminergic neurons, most strikingly the substantia nigra and locus ceruleus. Both of these structures may appear grossly depigmented. Microscopically, in the affected nuclei there is nerve cell loss, melanin pigment lying free or within macrophages, reactive fibrillary astrocytosis, and intracytoplasmic neuronal inclusions called "Lewy bodies" (Fig. 42-72). The latter are concentrically laminated structures with an eosinophilic core surrounded by a clear halo. Immunohistochemical evidence indicates Lewy bodies are composed in part of neurofilaments.[82] Although Lewy bodies are a characteristic finding in idiopathic Parkinson's disease, they also occur in other conditions and in persons without overt neurologic disease.[79] Within the

neostriatum dopaminergic axon terminals originating from nigral neurons degenerate along with their parent neurons. Thus dopamine levels are reduced in the caudate and putamen. This reduction plays a role in the symptomatology of Parkinson's disease and its recognition has led to the use of levodopa as a therapeutic measure for the disease. Although dementia may eventually develop in a third of patients, its pathologic basis is uncertain. The disease runs a slow, prolonged, progressive course but does not directly cause death.

Motor neuron disease

Amyotrophic lateral sclerosis (ALS) and Werdnig-Hoffmann disease are the principal forms of motor neuron disease respectively affecting adults and children. Typically, ALS begins in the fifth and sixth decades. Approximately half the patients die within 3 to 5 years after onset. Most cases are sporadic but 10% occur in familial form, a proportion suggestive of autosomal dominant inheritance.[192] The cause and pathogenesis are unknown. Clinically, patients develop progressive motor weakness, muscle atrophy, and corticospinal tract signs. The lesions involve upper and lower motor neurons and the motor pathways. In the spinal cord there is loss of anterior horn neurons with fibrillary astrocytotic corticospinal tract degeneration, loss of axons and myelin sheaths, and atrophy of the anterior nerve roots secondary to the neuron loss. The skeletal musculature undergoes neurogenic atrophy. In the brainstem the hypoglossal nucleus is regularly affected. Other motor nuclei may be less severely affected. Occasionally, neuron loss can be detected in the motor cortex. Loss of axons and myelin sheaths is usually evident in the medullary pyramids and can sometimes be traced rostrally to the pes pedunculi or internal capsule.[231] Death usually occurs from respiratory failure.

Werdnig-Hoffmann disease is one of a group of conditions referred to as spinal muscular atrophy (SMA) that occur chiefly in infants, children, and young adults. In these conditions the lower motor neurons are affected without involvement of the corticospinal tracts. Werdnig-Hoffmann disease (SMA type 1, infantile SMA) is a rapidly fatal autosomal recessive disorder characterized by weakness and hypotonia evident at birth or in the neonatal period. The presence of the disease in utero is sometimes indicated by decreased fetal movements. The cause and pathogenesis are unknown. The pathologic changes are loss of neurons and fibrillary astrocytosis involving the anterior horns of the spinal cord and brainstem motor nuclei. Atrophy of the anterior nerve roots and neurogenic muscular atrophy are also present. The disease follows a subacute course with death from respiratory complications usually within 1 year.[162]

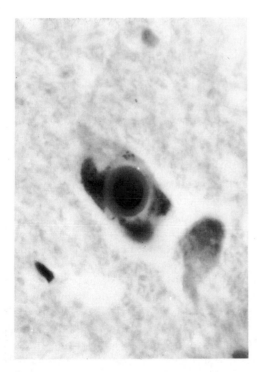

Fig. 42-72. Lewy body in cell of substantia nigra in patients with Parkinson's disease. (Hematoxylin and eosin; 1100×.)

Metabolic diseases

Metabolic diseases result from neurochemical disturbances that are either initiated within the central nervous system by hereditary or toxic mechanisms or induced by systemic disease. Endogenous metabolic diseases of the central nervous system include genetically determined disorders of carbohydrate, lipid, amino acid, and mineral metabolism as well as neurotoxic injuries induced by metals, gases, organic solvents, and drugs. The associated neuropathologic lesions are diverse and may involve edema, neuronal storage phenomena, degenerative changes, and even parenchymal necrosis.[16,62,102,117,118,173,207]

Disruption of CNS metabolism is also produced by the consequences of pathophysiologic disturbances in other organ systems occurring in the course of systemic disease or intoxication.[62,173,207] In this section three of these disorders are discussed: hepatic encephalopathy, acute toxic encephalopathy including Reye's syndrome, and hypoglycemia.

Hepatic encephalopathy (HE)

Hepatic encephalopathy is an acute or chronic, reversible, clinically characteristic neurologic disorder associated with metabolic disturbances caused by hepatocellular diseases such as cirrhosis or massive hepatic necrosis.[3] The term "portal-systemic encephalopathy" is generally synonomous with "hepatic encephalopathy" but also includes cases occurring in the absence of significant liver diseases where hepatic portal blood is shunted into the systemic circulation, as through the surgical creation of an Eck fistula. In addition to these potentially reversible disorders, Victor and associates[242] have characterized a disorder called acquired nonwilsonian hepatocerebral degeneration in which fixed or progressive neurologic deficits develop as a consequence of portacaval shunting. The pathogenesis of these neurologic conditions is incompletely understood. Lockwood[124] has recently reviewed this problem and pointed out the complex relationship between cerebral and hepatic function. Although ammonia is a common focus in pathophysiologic investigations, this substance affects virtually every biochemical and physiologic aspect of brain functions. Thus it is unlikely that a single agent or process is responsible for the development of these encephalopathies.

There are no gross brain changes indicative of hepatic encephalopathy. Microscopically, however, an Alzheimer type II astrocytosis (see description on p. 2134) is characteristically found in the gray matter chiefly of the cerebrum and cerebellum. They are most prominent in the deeper layers of the cerebral cortex. In acute cases the astronuclear changes begin to appear after 2 or 3 days of coma. In nonwilsonian, acquired hepatocerebral degeneration there is multifocal softening and discoloration of the cerebral cortex and lentiform nucleus. Microscopically there is Alzheimer type II astrocytosis in the gray matter as well as spongy degeneration and parenchymal loss at sites corresponding to the grossly softened, discolored lesions.

Reye's syndrome and acute toxic encephalopathy

In 1961 Lyon and co-workers[128] reviewed the clinical and neuropathologic findings in a common, often fatal or disabling neurologic syndrome chiefly occurring in children that they termed "acute toxic encephalopathy" (ATE). Although the cause and pathogenesis of this syndrome were obscure, those authors emphasized the frequency of cerebral edema in their cases and the absence, except where ischemic encephalopathy had supervened, of definite parenchymal lesions. Subsequently, Reye and co-workers[178] called attention to a particular form of ATE that they characterized as acute encephalopathy with fatty degeneration of the viscera. This disorder, now referred to as "Reye's syndrome" (RS), is regarded as a major cause of noninfectious neurologic death after viral disease in children though there is some recent evidence indicating a decline in its frequency.[144] The syndrome has a peak incidence in children from 5 to 15 years of age. It consists of an infectious phase followed by an encephalopathic phase. Influenza B or A and varicella account for most of the infections. About 5 to 6 days after onset of the infection the patient develops episodes of repetitive vomiting followed by altered behavior and eventually coma. Characteristic laboratory findings include a threefold elevation of both glutamic oxaloacetic and glutamic pyruvic acid transaminase activities in serum, prolonged prothrombin time, and increased blood ammonia levels. Blood glucose concentration is frequently normal especially in children over 4 years of age.[57]

Characteristic pathologic changes involve the liver and brain. The liver is enlarged and tan. There is a panlobular accumulation of lipid droplets within hepatocytes. Ultrastructural studies have demonstrated consistent mitochondrial abnormalities including swelling and alterations in the cristae and matrix accompanied by glycogen depletion and increased peroxisomes. Similar mitochondrial changes have been observed in biopsy specimens of brain and skeletal muscle.[160,161,216] In fatal cases there is massive brain swelling as a result of cytotoxic edema with tentorial and cerebellar tonsillar herniations. Ischemic neuronal necrosis, swollen astrocytes and oligodendroglia, and intramyelinic edema are evident histologically or by electron microscopy.[131] Advances in therapy have reduced the mortality from Reye's syndrome from 90% to 10%.[56] The pathogenesis of the disease, however, remains unclear. Since 1980, convincing evidence implicating salicylates in the development of Reye's syndrome has been presented. Strong sanctions against the use of aspirin or other forms of salicylates in children, especially with varicella or influenza-like illness, have been issued.[144]

Hypoglycemia

Brain lesions associated with hypoglycemia in humans have occurred chiefly through the injection or production of excess amounts of insulin. Cases include deaths from insulin shock therapy, accidental insulin overdose in diabetic patients, suicidal attempts with insulin, and islet cell tumors with insulin production, as well as other disorders that may lead to profound hypoglycemia. The neuropathologic findings resemble those found in cases of diffuse ischemic neuronal necrosis associated with hypotension or cardiac arrest.[30] Experimental studies support the view that the structural effects of hypoglycemic and hypoxic-ischemic injuries on the brain are similar.

Nutritional diseases

Malnutrition caused by lack of access to an adequate diet is associated with neurologic disorders in many underdeveloped countries and among underprivileged socioeconomic groups. In some cases the neurologic disturbances may be a direct consequence of inadequate diet; however other factors commonly encountered among poor, ill-fed people, such as infection and unavailability of proper medical care, may also be involved in the development of the disease. In the United States and Western Europe, however, nutritionally induced neurologic disease is found chiefly in association with chronic alcoholism or in patients with a congenital or acquired inability to absorb, transport, or metabolize dietary nutrients. The nutritional diseases discussed in this section are Wernicke's encephalopathy, subacute combined degeneration of the spinal cord, and the spinocerebellar syndrome associated with vitamin E deficiency. Each of these conditions is a crippling neurologic disorder that could be prevented by early diagnosis and treatment.

Wernicke's encephalopathy

Wernicke's encephalopathy is caused by thiamine deficiency and in the United States is encountered chiefly among severe chronic alcoholics. Clinical features include confusion, oculomotor disturbances, ataxia, and Korsakoff's psychosis. The last is actually a form of memory disturbance involving an inability to retain new information. The lesions are located in the mamillary bodies, the gray matter along the third and fourth ventricles and aqueduct, and in up to 50% of cases the superior cerebellar vermis (Fig. 42-73). In most cases atrophy of the mamillary bodies and vermis are the only grossly evident changes. In acute cases, however, pe-

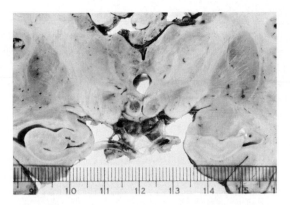

Fig. 42-73. Acute Wernicke's disease with involvement of mamillary bodies, hypothalami, and thalami.

techiae may be present in the affected gray matter. Histologic changes in subacute or chronic lesions involving the mamillary bodies or periventricular gray matter include parenchymal loss and fibrillary astrocytosis. The myelin appears to be affected slightly more severely than other parenchymal elements. Varying degrees of endothelial proliferation and perivascular collections of lipid-laden macrophages may be evident. Hemosiderin is uncommon. The cerebellar lesion involves all the cortical neurons; however, the Purkinje cells are affected most severely. The nerve cell loss is accompanied by fibrillary astrocytosis. A similar cerebellar disorder called "alcoholic cerebellar degeneration" is found in some alcoholic patients without concomitant clinical or pathologic evidence of Wernicke's encephalopathy. In acute cases frank parenchymal necrosis and perivascular hemorrhages may be seen microscopically in the mamillary bodies and to a lesser extent in the periventricular gray matter.[243]

Subacute combined degeneration of the spinal cord

Most cases of this disorder are caused by a deficiency of cobalamin (vitamin B_{12}) resulting from an inability to absorb this vitamin associated with pernicious anemia, gastric atrophy, and lack of intrinsic factor necessary for absorption.[158] Other causes for the inability to absorb the vitamin include gastrectomy, fish-tapeworm infection, and various malabsorption syndromes. Rarely, similar lesions develop in cases of folate deficiency.[44] Clinically, neurologic symptoms usually but not always occur after onset of pernicious anemia and include evidence of posterior column and corticospinal tract dysfunction. The lesions are bilateral but often asymmetric. The cervical and upper thoracic segments of the posterior columns are affected initially and most severely. Later the lateral and even the anterior columns are affected. The lesions at these sites, however, are not confined to specific pathways such as the cortico-spinal tracts but involve other fiber systems as well. The earliest changes involve coalescing foci of vacuolization involving the myelin sheath (Fig. 42-74). Although the earliest changes seem to involve the myelin sheaths, axonal degeneration appears very soon after the myelin changes. These changes are accompanied by fibrillary astrocytosis and the accumulation of lipid-con-

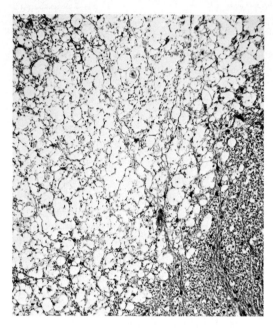

Fig. 42-74. Vacuolated appearance of fasciculus gracilis in patient with vitamin B$_{12}$ deficiency. (Hematoxylin and eosin; 90×.)

taining macrophages. Similar lesions called "Lichtheim plaques" are sometimes present in the cerebral white matter.

Vitamin E deficiency

Within the last two decades experimental and human studies have demonstrated that chronic vitamin E deficiency in humans is regularly associated with a progressive neurologic syndrome comprising areflexia, ataxia, and loss of proprioception and vibration sense.[90,146,151,220] Vitamin E is one of the fat-soluble vitamins with many dietary sources. Deficiency of the vitamin in humans and the development of the neurologic syndrome occurs chiefly in patients with severe, long-standing disorders of lipid malabsorption such as abetalipoproteinemia, cholestatic liver disease, some cases of cystic fibrosis, and intestinal resection. The neuropathologic changes involve a loss of large-caliber myelinated axons chiefly from the posterior columns of the spinal cord and the distal sensory branches of the peripheral nervous system (Fig. 42-75). In advanced cases the spinocerebellar tracts may be affected. The spinal cord lesions are associated with the development of swollen, dystrophic axons in the gracile and cuneate nuclei as well as other afferent nuclei in the lower medulla and spinal cord. Treatment of affected patients with vitamin E will prevent or control the progress of the neurologic disorder.

Trauma[123]

The effects of mechanical forces, either direct or indirect, on the central nervous system, though varied, are frequently predictable. A systematic approach to

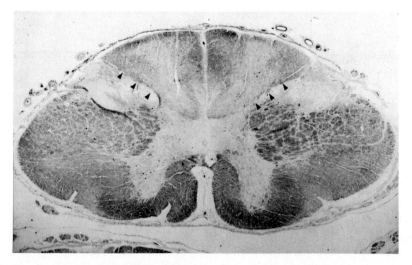

Fig. 42-75. Vitamin E deficiency. Cervical spinal cord of an 8-year-old child with congenital biliary atresia, low serum vitamin E concentration, and a progressive spinocerebellar syndrome. There is loss of axons and myelin sheaths from the posterior columns, *arrows*. (Loyez stain; 8.5×. From Nelson, J.S.: Biology of vitamin E, Ciba Foundation Symposium 101, London, 1983, Pitman Pub., Ltd.)

the structural changes resulting from mechanical forces causing injury, usually begins with lesions of the dura, followed by the lesions that are produced at successively deeper levels.

Epidural hematoma

The dura mater covering the brain is represented by a fused dura and periosteum of the skull. Below the level of the foramen magnum, the two layers are separated by adipose tissue, blood vessels, and nodular accumulation of lymphocytes, sometimes with follicle for-mation. Epidural hematomas from blunt traumatic forces are almost always intracranial (Fig. 42-76). They usually are associated with a recent skull fracture that frees the dura and, in crossing the groove of the middle meningeal artery, tears that artery and often the accom-panying vein as well. Rarely the hematoma may be at-tributable to a tear in the anterior or posterior menin-geal artery or in a vein between the skull and dura. The usual amount of blood found at autopsy in untreated persons varies between 75 and 125 g. This amount is in the same range found in fatal acute subdural hemato-

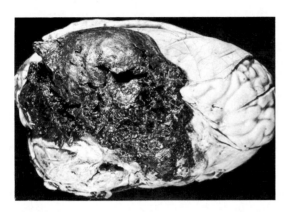

Fig. 42-76. Acute epidural hematoma resulting from skull fracture with tear of middle meningeal artery and vein.

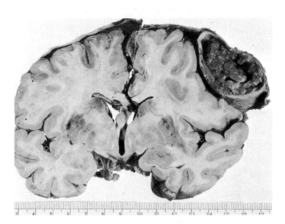

Fig. 42-77. Chronic subdural hematoma with compression of underlying brain and lateral ventricle. Notice bone for-mation in falx and uncal herniation on side of hematoma.

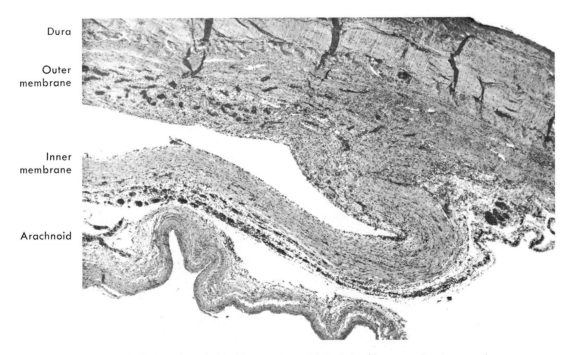

Dura

Outer membrane

Inner membrane

Arachnoid

Fig. 42-78. Wall of chronic subdural hematoma at junction of inner and outer membranes. (Hematoxylin and eosin; 30×.)

mas and intracerebral hypertensive hemorrhages. Death is caused by the effects of brain compression, with brain displacement, herniation, and secondary brainstem hemorrhages.

Subdural hematoma

Subdural hematomas usually result from blunt head injury. They can also occur without direct injury to the skull. This is particularly true in older persons with brain atrophy in whom sudden anterior or posterior movement of the head, as from stumbling, may easily tear one of the bridging veins. On rare occasions, arterial bleeding may be the cause of the hematoma. Acute and chronic types of subdural hematomas are recognized and are based on the interval between the trauma and onset of symptoms.

With the acute subdural hematoma, blood accumulates rapidly after a tear of a bridging vein at the point where the vessel leaves the subdural space (a potential space) to enter the dura. There is little or no evidence of early organization of the acute subdural hematoma on its dural surface or at its margins, nor is there any evidence of organization of the hematoma from the arachnoid membrane except when this membrane is torn.

Organization of subdural blood, which characterizes the chronic subdural hematoma, begins within the first week and is readily identified after 2 weeks. The typical chronic hematoma is encapsulated by highly vascular granulation tissue originating from the dura, forming inner and outer membranes that enclose the blood clot. The outer membrane is attached to the dural surface, and the inner membrane covers the surface of the hematoma adjacent to the brain (Figs. 42-77 and 42-78).

Chronic subdural hematomas may enlarge progressively because of bleeding from vessels in the granulation tissue or other mechanisms and behave as space-occupying lesions associated with brain displacement, herniations, and, when fatal, brainstem hemorrhages.

Subarachnoid hemorrhage

Bleeding into the subarachnoid space has many causes, one of the more common of which is blunt trauma to the skull with or without fracture. Although bleeding can be the sole result of trauma (at least clinically), at postmortem examination the hemorrhages often are associated with other lesions (such as contusions and lacerations). With small hemorrhages the blood may be completely removed by following the cerebrospinal fluid flow into the draining sinuses. In some individuals, particularly those with other traumatic brain lesions, the blood may be trapped by adhesions and then converted to hemosiderin and hematoidin.

Contusion[54,123]

Contusions are foci of necrosis and linear hemorrhages that affect the crests of gyri initially but may en-

large with time. They are separated into two groups based upon whether their anatomic distribution is determined or uninfluenced by the status of the head (resting or moving) at the time of impact. The contusions whose distribution is determined by the status of the head are coup, contrecoup, and intermediate contusions.

Coup contusions occur when the resting head is struck with an object such as a club. They are located beneath the point of impact. Rarely in these circumstances are contusions present opposite to the point of impact.

Contrecoup contusions occur when the moving head strikes a fixed hard object such as the concrete roadway after a person is thrown from a car during an accident. They are located opposite to the point of impact and are found most frequently in the frontal poles, orbital gyri, and temporal poles (Fig. 42-79). In these circumstances there is no contusion beneath the point of impact unless the skull is fractured.

Intermediate contusions also occur when the moving head strikes a fixed object. They are located midway between the impact point and the usual site of the contrecoup lesion. Brainstem contusions are an example of this type of lesion.

Crushing type of head injuries occur when the head is firmly supported and struck by a powerful force or by the impact sustained by the head after a fall from a great height. In these cases the lesions consist of extensive skull fractures, which cause brain lacerations. Contusions are minimal or absent.

The contusions whose distribution is unrelated to the status of the head are fracture contusions, herniation contusions, and gliding contusions.

Fracture contusions are associated with both depressed and undepressed skull fracture. In the latter instance the mechanism is believed to involve transient displacement of the bony edges of the fracture site.

Herniation contusions are caused by transient displacements of brain tissue from one intracranial com-

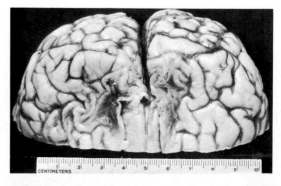

Fig. 42-79. Remote contusions of orbital gyri and olfactory bulbs.

partment to another in response to transmission of traumatic forces through brain parenchyma. The medial temporal lobes and cerebellar tonsils are characteristically affected.

Gliding contusions are rounded or linear foci of hemorrhage in the parasagittal cerebral white matter. They are probably caused by stretching and tearing of veins caused by anteroposterior movement of the brain within the cranial cavity.

Diffuse impact injury

Strich[225] and Adams and co-workers[2] have called attention to the widespread disruption of axons that can occur throughout brain as a consequence of the forces applied to it during blunt head trauma. Thus the axonal lesions develop independently of other traumatic lesions such as contusions or hematomas. Grossly this type of lesion is not readily identifiable. Microscopically, numerous axonal swelling are the characteristic finding. The corpus callosum and brainstem are affected most frequently.

Penetrating injuries to brain

The brain and spinal cord may be penetrated by bullets and fragments of metal and bone sometimes covered by scalp, hair, and other contaminated foreign material. The damage in high-velocity bullet injuries is generalized as well as local. The effects are caused by the sudden increase in intracranial pressure, the shearing and tearing of the tissue, and the intense local heat. There is extensive necrosis and hemorrhage in and about the tract of the missile.

Trauma of spinal cord

The spinal cord of the newborn infant can be injured in breech deliveries by the exertion of too great an extractile force with the hyperextended head. The overstretched cord, usually at the cervicothoracic level, has an hourglass narrowing.

Hematomyelia with necrosis of the cord is usually caused by fractures or dislocations of the vertebrae with compression of the cord. In some cases the lesion appears to follow extreme degrees of hyperextension and hyperflexion at the cervical level with fracture or dislocation. The cord appears to be slightly to moderately narrowed at the level of compression, with bulging and softening above and below caused by necrosis with hemorrhage into the gray matter. This may extend for several levels to either side of the point of initial injury.

DISEASES OF THE PERIPHERAL NERVOUS SYSTEM (PNS)
Morphologic examination of peripheral nerves

Special morphologic techniques are necessary in order to detect and assess accurately the pathologic changes in peripheral nerves. In addition to studies with conventional stains on paraffin sections for cells, axons, and myelin sheaths, 1 μm thick, glutaraldehyde-fixed cross sections of the nerve in questions should be examined by light microscopy after staining with alkaline toluidine blue. In addition, properly fixed samples of peripheral nerve should be set aside for possible morphometric studies of axonal caliber and distribution, electron microscopy to examine unmyelinated as well as myelinated axons, and teased-fiber studies to assess the characteristics of myelin or axonal degeneration. The techniques involved exceed the capacity of most routine histopathology laboratories and require both specialized equipment and trained technicians. The monograph by Asbury and Johnson[8] provides a helpful introduction to these techniques.

Pathologic reactions of the PNS to injury

With few exceptions, such as amyloidosis and leprosy, the pathologic changes in peripheral nerves are not distinctively characteristic for particular diseases. The morphologic examination determines the presence of pathologic changes, the structural elements chiefly affected (axons, myelin sheaths, blood vessels, and so on), and the type of reaction occurring (demyelination, inflammation, axonal degeneration). This information when correlated with the results from clinical and laboratory data provides a rational basis for establishing a diagnosis.

Disorders of the peripheral nervous system can be separated into neuronopathies and neuropathies depending on whether the condition is a result of injury primarily affecting the neurons, which give rise to peripheral nerve axons, or the nerves themselves. The latter case is more common and includes axonopathies, demyelinative neuropathies, and diseases primarily affecting supporting tissues and blood vessels with secondary effects on the axons and myelin sheaths.

Axonopathies. In these disorders the axon disintegrates while the cell body from which it arises remains intact or shows reactive changes (chromatolysis) (Fig. 42-80). The axonal lesions are sometimes further separated into those characterized by wallerian degeneration and those characterized by what is termed "axonal degeneration." In practice the distinction between these two processes on morphologic grounds may be difficult because of similarities between the two processes. Wallerian degeneration occurs after transection of the axon. The transection may involve several destructive processes including knife wounds, compression, traction, and ischemia, which interrupt axonal continuity. Initially, organelles accumulate in the proximal and distal stumps adjacent to the transection site causing swelling of these structures. Subsequently the axon and myelin sheath distal to the transection site undergoes disintegration and phagocytosis. Regenerative

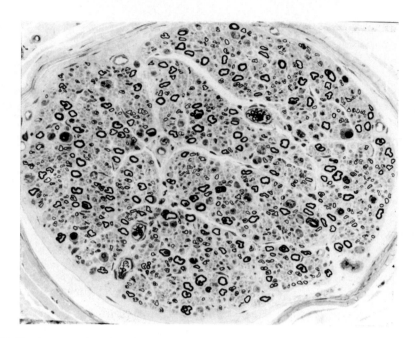

Fig. 42-80. Axonopathy. Sural nerve in vitamin E–deficient monkey. Moderate loss of axons and myelin sheaths. Occasional degenerating axons, macrophages, and proliferating Schwann cells are present. (1.5 μm plastic section, alkaline toluidine blue; 250×. From Nelson, J.S.: Biology of vitamin E, Ciba Foundation Symposium 101, London, 1983, Pitman Pub., Ltd.)

changes in the form of axonal sprouts and proliferating Schwann cells extend distally from the proximal stump. The proliferating columns of Schwann cells are referred to as bands of Büngner. Depending on a number of factors, regeneration may be functionally and anatomically successful in varying degrees, or fail entirely, resulting in formation of a neuroma. If the initial axonal injury is close to the parent neuron, chromatolysis may be present. In axonal degeneration the loss of axonal integrity develops presumably as a result of some primary metabolic disturbance within the axon itself. Changes similar to those seen in wallerian degeneration develop, though the regenerative reaction may be minimal or absent. If the degenerative changes initially involve the distal axonal segment, the process is referred to as a distal or dying back type of axonopathy. Some points of distinction between the morphologic appearances of wallerian and axonal degeneration include selective or isolated axonal involvement with axons in varying phases of disintegration in the latter, whereas wallerian degeneration is associated with groups of uniformly affected axons.

Demyelinative neuropathies. In demyelinative neuropathies myelin sheaths are injured initially or most severely and axons remain relatively intact. The myelin loss results from a disturbance involving Schwann cells or the myelin itself. Myelin breakdown begins segmen-

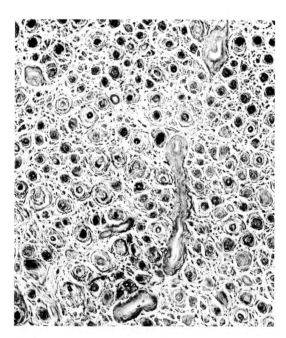

Fig. 42-81. "Onion-bulb" neuropathy. (Hematoxylin and eosin; 90×.)

tally adjacent to the node of Ranvier and proceeds throughout the internode (the segment between two consecutive nodes) leaving a denuded axon segment. Some Schwann cell proliferation accompanies the demyelination. Subsequently, remyelination occurs with one or more Schwann cells forming short internodal myelin segments. Repeated episodes of segmental demyelination and remyelination are associated with concentric proliferation of Schwann cells around axons giving rise to structures referred to as "onion bulbs" (Fig. 42-81).

Neuropathies secondary to injuries involving supporting or vascular tissue. In addition to axonal or wallerian degeneration, changes indicative of the inciting disease process are often present. Examples include amyloid deposits, neoplastic or inflammatory infiltrates, and vasculitis.

For details of the pathologic changes associated with specific neuropathies refer to the review by Thomas and co-workers.[234]

REFERENCES

1. Abell, M.R.: Personal communication, Tampa, Fla., 1988.
2. Adams, J.H., Graham, D.I., Murray, L.S., and Scott, G.: Diffuse axonal injury due to non-missile head injury in humans: an analysis of 45 cases, Ann. Neurol. **12**:557, 1982.
3. Adams, R.D., and Foley, J.M.: The neurological disorder associated with liver disease, Res. Publ. Assoc. Res. Nerv. Ment. Dis. **32**:198, 1953.
4. Adams, R.D., and Victor, M., and Mancall, E.L.: Central pontine myelinolysis, Arch. Neurol. Psychiatry **81**:154, 1959.
5. Adams, R.D., and Victor, M.: Principles of neurology, ed. 3, New York, 1985, McGraw-Hill Book Co.
6. Allen, I.V.: Demyelinating diseases. In Adams, J.H., Corsellis, J.A.N., and Duchen, L.W., editors: Greenfield's neuropathology, ed. 4, New York, 1984, John Wiley & Sons, Inc.
7. Armstrong, D.L., Sauls, C.D., and Goddard-Finegold, J.: Neuropathologic findings in short-term survivors of intraventricular hemorrhage. Am. J. Dis. Child. **141**:617, 1987.
8. Asbury, A.K., and Johnson, P.C.: Pathology of peripheral nerve, Philadelphia, 1978, W.B. Saunders Co.
9. Astrup, J., Klinken, L., and Nedergaard, M.: The ischemic penumbra: a neuropathological study of the peri-infarct zone in the human brain, Acta Neurol. Scand. **73**:88, 1986.
10. Astrup, J., Siesjo, B.K., Symon, L.: Thresholds in cerebral ischemia: the ischemic penumbra, Stroke **12**:723, 1981.
11. Ayus, J.C., Krothapalli, R.K., and Arieff, A.I.: Treatment of symptomatic hyponatremia and its relation to brain damage: a prospective study, N. Engl. J. Med. **317**:1190, 1987.
12. Baker, R.N., Cancilla, P.A., Pollock, P.S., and Frommes, S.P.: The movement of exogenous protein in experimental cerebral edema, J. Neuropath. Exp. Neurol. **30**:668, 1971.
13. Banker, B.Q., and Larroche, J.C.: Periventricular leukomalacia of infancy, Arch. Neurol. **7**:386, 1962.
14. Baringer, J.R.: Herpes simplex virus infection of nervous tissue in animals and man, Prog. Med. Virol. **20**:1, 1975.
15. Barlow, C.F.: Mental retardation and related disorders, Philadelphia, 1978, F.A. Davis Co.
16. Becker, L.E., and Yates, A.: Inherited metabolic disease. In Davis, R.L., and Robertson, D.M., editors: Textbook of neuropathology, Baltimore, 1985, The Williams & Wilkins Co.
17. Bender, B.L., and Yunis, E.J.: Central nervous system pathology of tuberous sclerosis in children, Ultrastruct. Pathol. **1**:287, 1980.
18. Berman, P.H., and Banker, B.Q.: Neonatal meningitis: a clinical and pathological study of 29 cases, Pediatrics **38**:6, 1966.
19. Berry, C.D., Hooton, T.M., Collier, A.C., and Lukehart, S.A.: Neurologic relapse after benzathine penicillin therapy for secondary syphilis in a patient with HIV infection, N. Engl. J. Med. **316**:1587, 1987.
20. Bigner, S.H., Burger, P.C., Wong, A.J., Werner, M.H., Hamilton, S.R., Muhlbaier, L.H., Vogelstein, B., and Bigner, D.D.: Gene amplification in malignant human gliomas: clinical and histopathologic aspects, J. Neuropathol. Exp. Neurol. **47**:191, 1988.
21. Bigner, S.H., Mark, J., Burger, P.C., Mahaley, M.S., Jr., Bullard, D.E., Muhlbaier, L.H., and Bigner, D.D.: Specific chromosomal abnormalities in malignant human gliomas, Cancer Res. **88**:405, 1988.
22. Black, P.M., and Conner, E.S.: Chronic increased intracranial pressure. In Asbury, A.K., McKhann, G.M., and McDonald, W.I., editors: Disease of the nervous system, vol. 2, Philadelphia, 1986, Ardmore-Saunders.
23. Bloom, H.J.G.: Intracranial tumors: response and resistance to therapeutic endeavors, 1970-1980, Int. J. Radiat. Oncol. Biol. Phys. **8**:1083, 1982.
24. Bonnin, J.M., Rubinstein, L.J., Papasozomenos, S.C., and Marangos, P.J.: Subependymal giant cell astrocytoma: significance and possible cytogenetic implications of an immunohistochemical study, Acta Neuropathol. (Berlin) **62**:185, 1984.
25. Borgelt, B., Gelber, R., Kramer, S., Brady, L., Chang, C., Davis, L., Pérez, C., and Hendrickson, F: The palliation of brain metastases: final results of the first two studies by the Radiation Therapy Oncology Group, Int. J. Radiat. Oncol. Biol. Phys **6**:1, 1980.
26. Borit, A., and Herndon, R.M.: The fine structure of plaques fibromyéliniques in ulegyria and status marmoratus, Acta Neuropathol. (Berlin) **14**:304, 1970.
27. Bouteille, M., Fontaine, C., Bédrenne, C., and Delarue, J.: Sur un cas d'encéphalite subaiguë à inclusions: étude anatomo-clinique et ultrastructurale, Rev. Neurol. (Paris) **113**:454, 1965.
28. Boylan, S.E., and McCunniff, A.J.: Recurrent meningioma, Cancer **61**:1447, 1988.
29. Brierley, J.B., and Excell, B.J.: The effects of profound hypotension upon the brain of *M. rhesus*: physiological and pathological observations, Brain **89**:269, 1966.
30. Brierley, J.B., and Graham, D.I.: Hypoxia and vascular disorders of the central nervous system. In Adams, J.H., Corsellis, J.A.N., and Duchen, L.W., editors: Greenfield's neuropathology, ed. 4, New York, 1984, John Wiley & Sons, Inc.
31. Brodeur, G.M., Seeger, R.C., Schwab, M., Varmus, H.E., and Bishop, J.M.: Amplification of N-myc in untreated human neuroblastomas correlates with advanced disease stage, Science **224**:1121, 1984.
32. Brown, J.K., Purves, R.J., Forfar, J.O., and Cockburn, R.F.: Neurological aspects of perinatal asphyxia, Dev. Med. Child Neurol. **16**:567, 1974.
33. Bruce, D.A.: Pathophysiology of intracranial pressure. In Asbury, A.K., McKhann, G.M., and McDonald, W.I., editors: Diseases of the nervous system, vol. 2, Philadelphia, 1986, Ardmore-Saunders.
34. Burger, P.C., Rawlings, C.E., Cox, E.B., McLendon, R.E., Schold, S.C., and Bullard, D.E.: Clinicopathologic correlations in the oligodendroglioma, Cancer **59**:1345, 1987.
35. Burger, P.C., and Vogel, F.S.: Surgical pathology of the nervous system and its coverings, ed. 2, New York, 1982, John Wiley & Sons, Inc.
36. Burger, P.C., Vogel, F.S., Green, S.B., and Strike, T.A.: Glioblastoma multiforme and anaplastic astrocytoma, Cancer **56**:1106, 1985.
37. Cadman, T.E., and Rorke, L.B.: Central pontine myelinolysis in childhood and adolescence, Arch. Dis. Child. **44**:342, 1969.
38. Cancer Statistics, 1988, CA **38**:5, 1988.
39. Carne, C.A., and Adler, M.W.: Neurological manifestations of human immunodeficiency virus infection, Br. Med. J. **293**:462, 1986.

40. Cavanaugh, J.B.: The proliferation of astrocytes around a needle wound in the rat brain, J. Anat. **106**:471, 1970.

41. Chopra, J.S., Banerjee, A.K., Murthy, J.M.K., and Pal, S.R.: Paralytic rabies, a clinicopathologic study, Brain **103**:789, 1980.

42. Clarren, S.K.: Neural tube defects and fetal alcohol syndrome, J. Pediatr. **95**:328, 1979.

43. Clarren, S.K., Alvord, E.C., Sumi, S.M., Streissguth, A.P., and Smith, D.W.: Brain malformations related to prenatal exposure to alcohol, J. Pediatr. **92**:64, 1978.

44. Clayton, P.T., Smith, I., Harding, B., Hyland, K., Leonard, J.V., and Leeming, R.H.: Subacute combined degeneration of the cord, dementia, and Parkinsonism due to an inborn error of folate metabolism, J. Neurol. Neurosurg. Psychiatry **49**:920, 1986.

45. Cohadon, F., Couad, N., Rougier, A., Vital, C., Rivel, J., and Dartigues, J.F.: Histologic and non-histologic factors correlated with survival time in supratentorial astrocytic tumors, J. Neurooncol. **3**:105, 1985.

46. Colditz, G.A., Bonita, R., Stampfer, M.J., Willett, W.C., Rosner, B., Speizer, F.E., and Hennekens, C.: Cigarette smoking and the risk of stroke in middle-aged women, N. Engl. J. Med. **318**:937, 1988.

47. Cole, F.M., and Yates, P.D.: The occurrence and significance of intracerebral microaneurysms, J. Pathol. Bacteriol. **93**:393, 1967.

48. Committee on Health Care Issues, American Neurological Association: Precautions in handling tissues, fluids, and other contaminated materials from patients with documented or suspected Creutzfeldt-Jakob disease, Ann. Neurol. **19**:75, 1986.

49. Connolly, G.H., Allen, I.V., and Hurwitz, L.J.: Measles virus antibody and antigen in SSPE, Lancet **1**:542, 1967.

50. Corey, L., and Spear, P.G.: Infections with the herpes simplex viruses. Parts 1 and 2, N. Engl. J. Med. **314**:686 and 749, 1986.

51. Cowan, W.M.: Development of neurons. In Asbury, A.K., McKhann, W.I., and McDonald, W.I., editors: Diseases of the nervous system, Philadelphia, 1986, Ardmore-Saunders.

52. Danoff, B.F., Cowchock, F.S., and Kramer, S.: Childhood craniopharyngioma: survival, local control, endocrine and neurologic function following radiotherapy, Int. J. Radiat. Oncol. Biol. Phys. **9**:171, 1983.

53. Dawson, J.R., Jr.: Cellular inclusions in cerebral lesions of lethargic encephalitis, Am. J. Pathol. **9**:7, 1933.

54. Dawson, S.L., Hirsch, C.S., Lucas, F.V., and Sebek, B.A.: The contrecoup phenomenon: reappraisal of a classic problem, Hum. Pathol. **11**:155, 1980.

55. DeReuck, J., Chatta, A.S., and Richardson, E.P.: Pathogenesis and evolution of periventricular leukomalacia in infancy, Arch. Neurol. **27**:229, 1972.

56. DeVivo, D.C.: How common is Reye's syndrome? N. Engl. J. Med. **309**:179, 1983. (Editorial.)

57. Diagnosis and treatment of Reye's syndrome, Consensus Conference, JAMA **246**:2441, 1981.

58. Donat, J.F., Okazaki, H., Kleinberg, F., and Reagan, T.J.: Intraventricular hemorrhages in full-term and premature infants, Mayo Clin. Proc. **53**:437, 1978.

59. Drachman, D.A., and Richardson, E.P.: Aqueductal narrowing: congenital and acquired, Arch. Neurol. **5**:552, 1961.

60. Ducatman, B.S., Scheithauer, B.W., Piepgras, D.G., Reiman, H.M., and Astrup, D.M.: Malignant peripheral nerve sheath tumors: a clinicopathologic study of 120 cases, Cancer **57**:2006, 1986.

61. Duchen, L.W.: General pathology of neurons and neuroglia. In Adams, J.H., Corsellis, J.A.N., and Duchen, L.W., editors: Greenfield's neuropathology, ed. 4, New York, 1984, John Wiley & Sons, Inc.

62. Duchen, L.W., and Jacobs, J.M.: Nutritional deficiencies and metabolic disorders. In Adams, J.H., Corsellis, J.A.N., and Duchen, L.W., editors: Greenfield's neuropathology, ed. 4, New York, 1984, John Wiley & Sons, Inc.

63. Ellison, G.W., moderator: Multiple sclerosis, Ann. Intern. Med. **101**:514, 1984.

64. Ernhart, C.B., Sokol, R.J., Martier, S., Moron, P., Nadler, D., Ager, J.W., and Wolf, A.: Alcohol teratogenicity in the human: a detailed assessment of specificity, critical period, and threshold, Am. J. Obstet. Gynecol. **156**:33, 1987.

65. Feigin, I., and Prose, P.: Hypertensive fibrinoid arteritis of the brain and gross cerebral hemorrhage, Arch. Neurol. **1**:98, 1959.

66. Fields, B.N.: Powerful prions? N. Engl. J. Med. **317**:1597, 1987.

67. Fischer-Williams, M., Bosanquet, F.D., and Daniel, P.M.: Carcinomatosis of the meninges: a report of three cases, Brain **78**:42, 1955.

68. Fisher, C.M.: Cerebral miliary aneurysms in hypertension, Am. J. Pathol. **66**:313, 1972.

69. Fishman, R.A.: Brain edema, N. Engl. J. Med. **293**:706, 1975.

70. Fishman, R.A.: Cerebrospinal fluid in diseases of the nervous system, Philadelphia, 1980, W.B. Saunders Co.

71. Foley, J.M., and Baxter, D.: On the nature of pigment granules in the cells of the locus coeruleus and substantia nigra, J. Neuropathol. Exp. Neurol. **17**:586, 1958.

72. Fraser, N.W., Lawrence, W.C., Wróblewska, Z., Gilden, D.H., and Koprowski, H.: Herpes simplex type 1 DNA in human brain tissue, Proc. Natl. Acad. Sci. USA **78**:6461, 1981.

73. Freytag, E.: Fatal hypertensive intracerebral hematomas: a survey of the pathological anatomy of 393 cases, J. Neurol. Neurosurg. Psychiatry **31**:616, 1968.

74. Friede, R.L.: Developmental neuropathology, New York, 1975, Springer-Verlag.

75. Gajdusek, D.C.: Unconventional viruses and the origin and disappearance of kuru, Science **197**:943, 1977.

76. García, J.H.: Circulatory disorders and their effects on the brain. In Davis, R.L., and Robertson, D.M., editors: Textbook of neuropathology, Baltimore, 1985, The Williams & Wilkins Co.

77. García, J.H., and Anderson, M.L.: Physiopathology of cerebral ischemia, CRC Critical Reviews in Neurobiology. (In press.)

78. Garvey, G.: Current concepts of bacterial infections of the central nervous system: bacterial meningitis and bacterial brain abscess, J. Neurosurg. **59**:735, 1983.

79. Gibb, W.R.G.: Idiopathic Parkinson's disease and the Lewy body disorders, Neuropathol. Appl. Neurobiol. **12**:223, 1986.

80. Gilles, F.H.: Perinatal neuropathology. In Davis, R.L., and Robertson, D.M., editors: Textbook of neuropathology, Baltimore, 1985, The Williams & Wilkins Co.

81. Gilles, F.H., Averill, D.R., and Kerr, C.S.: Neonatal endotoxin encephalopathy, Ann. Neurol. **2**:49, 1977.

82. Goldman, J.E., Yen, S.H., Chiu, F.C., and Peress, N.C.: Lewy bodies of Parkinson's disease contain neurofilament antigenes, Science **221**:1082, 1983.

83. Gómez, M.R., editor: Tuberous sclerosis, New York, 1979, Raven Press.

84. Greenfield, J.G.: Encephalitis and encephalomyelitis in England and Wales during the last decade, Brain **73**:141, 1950.

85. Greenfield, J.G., Blackwood, W., McMenemey, W.H., Meyer, A., and Norman, R.M.: Neuropathology, Baltimore, 1958, The Williams & Wilkins Co.

86. Greenwood, R.S., and Nelson, J.S.: Atypical ceroid lipofuscinosis, Neurology **28**:710, 1978.

87. Gregorios, J.B., Mozes, L.W., Norenberg, L.O.B., and Norenberg, M.D.: Morphologic effects of ammonia on primary astrocyte cultures. I. Light microscopic studies, J. Neuropathol. Exp. Neurol. **44**:397, 1985.

88. Gusella, J.F., Wexler, N.S., Conneally, P.M., et al.: A polymorphic DNA marker genetically linked to Huntington's disease, Nature **306**:234, 1983.

89. Hahn, A.F., Gordon, B.A., Feleki, V., Hinton, G.G., and Gilbert, J.J.: A variant form of metachromatic leukodystrophy without arylsulfatase A deficiency, Ann. Neurol. **12**:33, 1982.

90. Harding, A.E.: Vitamin E and the nervous system, CRC Crit. Rev. Neurobiol. **3**:89, 1987.

91. Hart, M.N., Malamud, N., and Ellis, W.G.: The Dandy-Walker syndrome: a clinicopathologic study based on 28 cases, Neurology **22**:771, 1972.

92. Hart, M.N., Petito, C.K., and Earle, K.M.: Mixed gliomas, Cancer **33**:134, 1974.

93. Henry, J.M., Geffner, R.R., Jr., Dillard, S.H., Earle, K.M., and Davis, R.L.: Primary malignant lymphomas of the central nervous system, Cancer 34:1293, 1974.

94. Herpes simplex encephalitis, Lancet 1:535, 1986.

95. Hirano, A.: Neurons, astrocytes, and ependyma. In Davis, R.L., and Robertson, D.M., editors: Textbook of neuropathology, Baltimore, 1985, The Williams & Wilkins Co.

96. Hochberg, F.H., and Miller, D.C.: Primary central nervous system lymphoma, J. Neurosurg. 68:835, 1988.

97. Horta-Barbosa, L., Fuccilo, D.A., Sever, J.L., and Zeman, W.: Subacute sclerosing panencephalitis: isolation of measles virus from a brain biopsy, Nature 221:974, 1969.

98. Horton, W.A., Wong, V., and Eldridge, R.: Von Hippel-Lindau disease, Arch. Intern. Med. 136:769, 1976.

99. Horwitz, S.J., Boxerbaum, B., and O'Bell, J.: Cerebral herniation in bacterial meningitis in childhood, Ann. Neurol. 7:524, 1980.

100. Houff, L.A., Major, E.O., and Katz, D.A.: Involvement of J.C. virus–infected mononuclear cells from the bone marrow and spleen in the pathogenesis of progressive multifocal leukoencephalopathy, N. Engl. J. Med. 318:301, 1988.

101. Huson, S.: The different forms of neurofibromatosis, Br. Med. J. 294:1113, 1987.

102. Jacobs, J.M., and Le Quesne, P.M.: Toxic disorders of the nervous system. In Adams, J.H., Corsellis, J.A.N., and Duchen, L.W., editors: Greenfield's neuropathology, ed. 4, 1984, John Wiley & Sons, Inc.

103. Jennings, M.T., Gelman, R., and Hochberg, F.: Intracranial germ cell tumors: natural history and pathogenesis, J. Neurosurg. 63:155, 1985.

104. Jew, J.Y., and Sandquist, D.: CNS changes in hyperbilirubinemia, Arch. Neurol. 36:149, 1979.

105. Johns, D.R., Turney, M., and Felsenstein, D.: Alteration in natural history of neurosyphilis by concurrent infection with the human immunodeficiency virus, N. Engl. J. Med. 316:1569, 1987.

106. Johnson, R.T.: Selective vulnerability of neural cells to viral infections, Brain 103:447, 1980.

107. Johnson, R.T.: The contribution of virologic research to clinical neurology, N. Engl. J. Med. 307:660, 1982.

108. Johnson, R.T., and Johnson, K.P.: Hydrocephalus as a sequela of experimental myxovirus infections, Exp. Mol. Pathol. 10:68, 1969.

109. Kadin, M., Rubinstein, L.J., and Nelson, J.S.: Neonatal cerebellar medulloblastoma originating from the fetal external granular layer, J. Neuropathol. Exp. Neurol. 29:583, 1970.

110. Kalbag, R.M., and Woolf, A.L.: Cerebral venous thrombosis, New York, 1967, Oxford University Press.

111. Kalter, H., and Warkany, J.: Congenital malformations (part 2), N. Engl. J. Med. 308:491, 1983.

112. Katzman, R.: Alzheimer's disease, N. Engl. J. Med. 314:964, 1986.

113. Katzman, R., and Pappius, H.M.: Brain electrolytes and fluid metabolism, Baltimore, 1973, The Williams & Wilkins Co.

114. Klatzo, I.: Neuropathological aspects of brain edema, J. Neuropathol. Exp. Neurol. 26:1, 1967.

115. Klatzo, I.: Pathophysiological aspects of brain edema, Acta Neuropathol. (Berlin) 72:236, 1987.

116. Kleinschmidt-DeMasters, B.K., and Norenberg, M.D.: Neuropathologic observations in electrolyte-induced myelinolysis in the rat, J. Neuropathol. Exp. Neurol. 41:67, 1982.

117. Krigman, M.R., and Bouldin, T.W.: Intoxications and deficiency diseases. In Rosenberg, R.N., editor: The clinical neurosciences, vol. 3, Neuropathology, New York, 1983, Churchill Livingstone.

118. Lake, B.D.: Lysosomal enzyme deficiencies. In Adams, J.H., Corsellis, J.A.N., and Duchen, L.W., editors: Greenfield's neuropathology, ed. 4, New York, 1984, John Wiley & Sons, Inc.

119. Larroche, J.C.: Developmental pathology of the neonate, Amsterdam, 1977, Excerpta Medica.

120. Larroche, J.C.: Perinatal brain damage. In Adams, J.H., Corsellis, J.A.N., and Duchen, L.W., editors: Greenfield's neuropathology, ed. 4, New York, 1984, John Wiley & Sons, Inc.

121. Lemire, R.J.: Neural tube defects, JAMA 259:558, 1988.

122. Lemire, R.J., Loeser, R.D., Leech, R.W., and Alvord, E.C.: Normal and abnormal development of the human nervous system, Hagerstown, Md., 1975, Harper & Row, Publishers.

123. Lindenberg, R.: Mechanical injuries of the brain and meninges. In Spitz, W.N., and Fisher, R.S., editors: Medicolegal investigation of death, ed. 2, Springfield, Ill., 1980, Charles C Thomas, Publisher.

124. Lockwood, A.H.: Hepatic encephalopathy: experimental approaches to human metabolic encephalopathy, CRC Crit. Rev. Neurobiol. 3:105, 1987.

125. Lowry, O.H., Passonneau, J.V., Hasselberger, F.X., and Schulz, D.W.: Effect of ischemia on known substrates and cofactors of the glycolytic pathway in brain, J. Biol. Chem. 239:18, 1964.

126. Ludwig, C.L., Smith, M.T., Godfrey, A.D., and Armbrustmacher, V.W.: A clinicopathologic study of 323 patients with oligodendrogliomas, Ann. Neurol. 19:15, 1986.

127. Ludwin, S.K.: Remyelination in demyelinating diseases of the central nervous system, CRC Crit. Rev. Neurobiol. 3:1, 1987.

128. Lyon, G., Dodge, P.R., and Adams, R.D.: The acute encephalopathies of obscure origin in infants and children, Brain 84:680, 1961.

129. MacFaul, R., Cavanagh, N., Lake, B.D., Stephens, R., and Whitfield, A.E.: Metachromatic leukodystrophy: review of 38 cases, Arch. Dis. Child. 57:168, 1982.

130. Manz, H.J.: The pathology of cerebral edema, Hum. Pathol. 5:291, 1974.

131. Manz, H.J., and Colon, A.R.: Neuropathology, pathogenesis and neuropsychiatric sequelae of Reye syndrome, J. Neurol. Sci. 53:377, 1982.

132. Margolis, G., and Kilham, L.: Hydrocephalus in hamsters, ferrets, rats, and mice following inoculations with reovirus type I: pathologic studies II, Lab. Invest. 21:189, 1969.

133. Martin, J.B., and Gusella, J.F.: Huntington's disease: pathogenesis and management, N. Engl. J. Med. 315:1267, 1986.

134. Martuza, R.L., and Eldridge, R.: Neurofibromatosis 2 (bilateral acoustic neurofibromatosis), N. Engl. J. Med. 318:684, 1988.

135. Masters, C.L., and Richardson, E.P.: Subacute spongiform encephalopathy (Creutzfeldt-Jakob disease): the nature and progression of spongiform change, Brain 101:333, 1978.

136. McCormick, W.F.: Vascular diseases in the clinical neurosciences. In Schochet, S.S., Jr., editor: Neuropathology, vol. 3, New York, 1983, Churchill Livingstone.

137. McCormick, W.F., and Nofzinger, J.D.: Saccular intracranial aneurysms: an autopsy study, J. Neurosurg. 33:422, 1970.

138. McFarlin, D.E., and McFarland, H.F.: Multiple sclerosis, N. Engl. J. Med. 307:1183 and 1246, 1982.

139. Meyer, A., and Jones, T.B.: Histological changes in brain in mongolism, J. Mental Sci. 85:206, 1939.

140. Mohr, J.P.: Lacunes: progress in cerebrovascular disease, Stroke 13:3, 1982.

141. Molinari, G.F., Smith, L., Goldstein, M.N., and Satran, R.: Brain abscess from septic embolism: an experimental model, Neurology 23:1205, 1973.

142. Mollgard, K., and Saunders, N.R.: Complex tight junctions of epithelial and endothelial cells in early fetal brain, J. Neurocytol. 4:453, 1975.

143. Mørk, S.J., Halvorsen, T.B., Lindegaard, K.-F., and Eide, G.E.: Oligodendroglioma: histologic evaluation and prognosis, J. Neuropathol. Exp. Neurol. 45:65, 1986.

144. Mortimer, E.A., Jr.: Reye's syndrome salicylates, epidemiology and public health policy, JAMA 257:1941, 1987.

145. Moser, H.W., Nardu, S., Kumar, A.J., and Rosenbaum, A.E.: The adrenoleukodystrophies, CRC Crit. Rev. Neurobiol. 3:29, 1987.

146. Muller, D.P.R., Lloyd, J.K., and Wolff, O.H.: Vitamin E and neurological functions, Lancet 1:225, 1983.

147. Myrianthopoulos, N.C.: Epidemiology of central nervous system malformations. In Vinken, P.J., and Bruyn, G.W., editors: Handbook of clinical neurology, vol. 30, Amsterdam, 1977, North Holland Publishing Co.

148. Naguib, M.G., Sung, J.H., Erickson, D.L., Gold, L.H.A., and

Seljeskog, E.L.: Central nervous system involvement in the nevoid basal cell carcinoma syndrome: case report and review of the literature, Neurosurgery **11**:52, 1982.

149. Nahmias, A.J., and Keyserling, H.L.: Neonatal herpes simplex in context of the TORCH complex. In Holmes, K.K., Mårdh, P.A., Sparling, P.F., and Wiesner, P.J., editors: Sexually transmitted diseases, New York, 1984, McGraw-Hill Book Co.

150. Nelson, D.F., Nelson, J.S., Davis, D.R., Chang, C.H., Griffin, T.W., and Pajak, T.F.: Survival and prognosis of patients with astrocytoma with atypical or anaplastic features, J. Neuro-oncol. **3**:99, 1985.

151. Nelson, J.S.: Neuropathological studies of chronic vitamin E deficiency in mammals including humans, Ciba Foundation Symposium 101, Biology of vitamin E, London, 1983, Pitman Books, Ltd.

152. Nelson, J.S., Tsukada, Y., Schoenfeld, D., Fulling, K., Lamarche, J., and Peress, N.: Necrosis as a prognostic criterion in malignant supratentorial astrocytic gliomas, Cancer **52**:550, 1983.

153. New, P.F.J., Kavis, K.R., and Ballentine, H.T., Jr.: Computed tomography in cerebral abscess, Radiology **121**:641, 1976.

154. Norman, M.G.: Perinatal brain damage. In Rosenberg, H.S., and Bolande, R.P., editors: Perspectives in pediatric pathology, vol. 4, Chicago, 1978, Year Book Medical Publishers.

155. Ojemann, R.G., and Heros, R.C.: Spontaneous brain hemorrhage, Stroke **14**:469, 1983.

156. Oppenheimer, D.R.: Diseases of the basal ganglia, cerebellum, and motor neurons. In Adams, J.H., Corsellis, J.A.N., and Duchen, L.W., editors: Greenfield's neuropathology, ed. 4, New York, 1984, John Wiley & Sons, Inc.

157. O'Rahilly, R., and Gardiner, E.: The developmental anatomy and histology of the human central nervous system. In Vinken, P.J., and Bruyn, G.W., editors: Handbook of clinical neurology, vol. 30, Amsterdam, 1977, North Holland Publishing Co.

158. Pant, S.S., Asbury, A.K., and Richardson, E.P.: The myelopathy of pernicious anemia: a neuropathological reappraisal, Acta Neurol. Scand. **44**(suppl. 35):1, 1968.

159. Park, T.S., Kleinman, G.M., and Richardson, E.P.: Creutzfeldt-Jakob disease with extensive degeneration of the white matter, Acta Neuropathol. (Berlin) **52**:239, 1980.

160. Partin, J.C., Schubert, W.K., and Partin, J.S.: Mitochondrial ultrastructure in Reye's syndrome (encephalopathy and fatty degeneration of the viscera), N. Engl. J. Med. **285**:1339, 1971.

161. Partin, J.S., McAdams, A.J., Partin, J.C., Schubert, W.K., and McLauren, R.L.: Brain ultrastructure in Reye's disease. II. Acute injury and recovery processes in three children, J. Neuropathol. Exp. Neurol. **37**:796, 1978.

162. Pearn, J.H.: Infantile motor neuron diseases. In Rowland, L.P., editors: Human motor neuron diseases, New York, 1982, Raven Press.

163. Penn, R.D., and Kurtz, D.: Cerebral edema mass effects and regional blood volume in man, J. Neurosurg. **46**:282, 1977.

164. Perentes, E., and Rubinstein, L.J.: Recent applications of immunoperoxidase histochemistry in human neuro-oncology: an update, Arch. Pathol. Lab Med. **111**:796, 1987.

165. Petit, T.L., LeBoutillier, J.C., Alfano, D.P., and Becker, L.E.: Synaptic development in the human fetus: A morphometric analysis of normal and Down's syndrome neocortex, Exp. Neurol. **83**:12, 1984.

166. Petito, C.K.: Early and late mechanisms of increased vascular permeability following experimental cerebral infarction, J. Neuropathol. Exp. Neurol. **38**:222, 1979.

167. Petito, C.K., Navia, B.A., Cho, E.S., Jordan, B.D., George, D.C., and Price, R.W.: Vacuolar myelopathy pathologically resembling subacute combined degeneration in patients with the acquired immunodeficiency syndrome, N. Engl. J. Med. **312**:874, 1985.

168. Petito, C.K., Cho, E.S., Lemann, W., Navia, B.A., and Price, R.W.: Neuropathology of acquired immunodeficiency syndrome (AIDS): an autopsy review, J. Neuropathol. Exp. Neurol. **45**:635, 1986.

169. Petsche, H., Schinko, H., and Seitelberger, F.: Encephalitides, Proceedings of a symposium at Antwerp, 1959, Amsterdam, 1961, Elsevier Publishing Co.

170. Pickren, J., López, G., Tsukada, Y., and Lane, W.: Brain metastases: an autopsy study, Cancer Treat. Symp. **2**:295, 1983.

171. Plum, F.: What causes infarction in ischemic brain, Neurology **33**:222, 1983.

172. Plum, F., and Posner, J.B.: The diagnosis of stupor and coma, ed. 3, Philadelphia, 1980, F.A. Davis.

173. Powers, J.M.: Metabolic diseases of the nervous system. In Rosenberg, R.N., editor: The clinical neurosciences, vol. 3, Neuropathology, New York, 1983, Churchill Livingstone.

174. Powers, J.M.: Adreno-leukodystrophy (adreno-testiculo-leukomyelo-neuropathic-complex): a review, Clin. Neuropathol. **4**:181, 1985.

175. Price, R.W., Katz, B.J., and Notkins, A.L.: Latent infection of the peripheral ANS with herpes simplex virus, Nature **257**:686, 1975.

176. Price, R.W., Brew, B., Sidtis, J., Rosenblum, M., Scheck, A.C., and Cleary, P.: The brain in AIDS: central nervous system HIV-1 infection and AIDS dementia complex, Science **239**:586, 1988.

177. Prusiner, S.B.: Prions and neurodegenerative diseases, N. Engl. J. Med. **317**:1571, 1987.

178. Reye, R.D.K., Morgan, G., and Baral, J.: Encephalopathy and fatty degeneration of the viscera: a disease entity in childhood, Lancet **2**:749, 1963.

179. Riccardi, V.M.: Von Recklinghausen neurofibromatosis, **305**:1617, 1981.

180. Rich, A.R., and McCordock, H.A.: The pathogenesis of tuberculous meningitis, Bull. Johns Hopkins Hosp. **52**:5, 1933.

181. Richardson, E.P., Jr.: Our evolving understanding of progressive multifocal leukoencephalopathy, Ann. NY Acad. Sci. **230**:358, 1974.

182. Richardson, E.P., Jr.: Progressive multifocal leukoencephalopathy 30 years later, N. Engl. J. Med. **318**:315, 1988.

183. Ringertz, N.: Grading of gliomas, Acta Pathol. Microbiol. Scand. **27**:53, 1950.

184. Ropper, A.H.: Acute increased intracranial pressure. In Asbury, A.K., McKhann, G.M., and McDonald, W.I., editors: Diseases of the nervous system, vol. 2, Philadelphia, 1986, Ardmore-Saunders.

185. Ropper, A.H., and Williams, R.S.: Relationship between plaques, tangles and dementia in Down syndrome, Neurology **30**:639, 1980.

186. Rorke, L.B., and Riggs, H.E.: Myelination of the brain in the newborn, Philadelphia, 1969, J.B. Lippincott Co.

187. Rorke, L.B.: Pathology of perinatal brain injury, New York, 1982, Raven Press.

188. Ross, M.H., Galaburda, A.M., and Kemper, T.L.: Down's syndrome: Is there a decreased population of neurons? Neurology **34**:909, 1984.

189. Rothman, S.M., Fulling, K.H., and Nelson, J.S.: Sickle cell anemia and central nervous system infarction: a neuropathological study, Ann. Neurol. **20**:684, 1986.

190. Rothman, S.M., Nelson, J.S., DeVivo, D., and Coxe, W.: Congenital astrocytoma presenting with intracerebral hematoma, J. Neurosurg. **51**:237, 1979.

191. Rothman, S.M., and Olney, J.W.: Glutamate and the pathophysiology of hypoxic-ischemic brain damage, Ann. Neurol. **19**:105, 1986.

192. Rowland, L.P.: Looking for the cause of amyotrophic lateral sclerosis, N. Engl. J. Med. **311**:979, 1984.

193. Rubinstein, L.J.: Tumors of the central nervous system. In Atlas of tumor pathology, series 2, fascicle 6, Washington, D.C., 1972, Armed Forces Institute of Pathology.

194. Rubinstein, L.J.: Cytogenesis and differentiation of pineal neoplasms, Hum. Pathol. **12**:441, 1981.

195. Rubinstein, L.J., and Herman, M.M.: Recent advances in human neuro-oncology. In Smith, W.T., and Cavanagh, J.B., editors: Recent advances in neuropathology, vol. 1, London, 1979, Churchill Livingstone.

196. Rubinstein, L.J., and Northfield, D.W.C.: The medulloblastoma and the so-called "arachnoidal cerebellar sarcoma": a critical re-examination of a nosological problem, Brain **87**:379, 1964.

197. Russell, D.S.: Discussion: The pathology of spontaneous intracranial hemorrhage, Proc. R. Soc. Med. **47**:689, 1954.

198. Russell, D.S.: Observations on the pathology of hydrocephalus, Medical Research Council Special Rep. Ser. no. 265, London, 1966, Her Majesty's Stationery Office.

199. Russell, D.S., and Rubinstein, L.J.: Pathology of tumors of the nervous system, ed. 4, Baltimore, 1977, The Williams & Wilkins Co.

200. Saunders, N.R.: Ontogeny of the blood-brain barrier, Exp. Eye Res., suppl., p. 523, 1977.

201. Schaumberg, H.H., Plank, C.R., and Adams, R.D.: The reticulum cell sarcoma-microglioma group of brain tumors: a consideration of their clinical features and therapy, Brain **95**:199, 1972.

202. Schellenberg, G.D., Bird, T.D., Wysman, E.M., et al.: Absence of linkage of chromosome 21q21 markers to familial Alzheimer's disease, Science **241**:1507, 1988.

203. Schelper, R.L., and Adrian, E.K., Jr.: Monocytes become macrophages; they do not become microglia: a light and electron microscopic autoradiographic study using 125-iododeoxyuridine, J. Neuropathol. Exp. Neurol. **45**:1, 1986.

204. Schmidek, H.H.: The molecular genetics of nervous system tumors, J. Neurosurg. **67**:1, 1987.

205. Schneider, H., Sperner, J., Droszus, J.U., and Schachinger, H.: Ultrastructure of the neuroglial fatty metamorphosis (Virchow) in the perinatal period, Virchows Arch. [Pathol. Anat.] **372**:183, 1976.

206. Schochet, S.S., Jr.: Infectious disease in the clinical neurosciences. In Schochet, S.S., Jr., editor: Neuropathology, vol. 3, New York, 1983, Churchill Livingstone.

207. Schochet, S.S., Jr.: Exogenous toxic-metabolic diseases including vitamin deficiency. In Davis, R.L., and Robertson, D.M., editors: Textbook of neuropathology, Baltimore, 1985, The Williams & Wilkins Co.

208. Schoene, W.C.: Degenerative diseases of the nervous system. In Davis, R.L., and Robertson, D.M., editors: Textbook of neuropathology, Baltimore, 1985, The Williams & Wilkins Co.

209. Scully, R.E., editor: Case records of the Massachusetts General Hospital, N. Engl. J. Med. **306**:91, 1982.

210. Scully, R.E., editor: Case records of the Massachusetts General Hospital, N. Engl. J. Med. **309**:1440, 1983.

211. Scully, R.E., editor: Case records of the Massachusetts General Hospital, N. Engl. J. Med. **314**:1689, 1986.

212. Scully, R.E., editor: Case records of the Massachusetts General Hospital, N. Engl. J. Med. **315**:1013, 1986.

213. Scully, R.E., editor: Case records of the Massachusetts General Hospital, N. Engl. J. Med. **315**:1079, 1986.

214. Scully, R.E., editors: Case records of the Massachusetts General Hospital, N. Engl. J. Med. **316**:35, 1987.

215. Shah, K.V.: Papovaviruses: biology, pathogenic potential and diagnosis. In De La Maza, L., and Peterson, E., editors: Medical virology, New York, 1987, Elsevier Science Publishing Co.

216. Shapira, Y., Deckelbaum, R., Statter, M., Tennenbaum, A., Aker, M., and Yarom, R.: Reye's syndrome: diagnosis by muscle biopsy? Arch. Dis. Child. **56**:287, 1981.

217. Shapiro, J.R.: Biology of gliomas: heterogeneity, oncogenes, growth factors, Semin. Oncol. **13**:4, 1985.

218. Sharer, L.R., Epstein, L.G., Cho, E.S., and Petito, C.K.: HTLV-III and vacuolar myopathy, N. Engl. J. Med. **315**:62, 1986.

219. Sheppard, R.D., Raine, C.S., Bornstein, M.B., and Udem, S.A.: Measles virus matrix protein synthesized in a subacute sclerosing panencephalitis cell line, Science **228**:1219, 1985.

220. Sokol, R.J.: Vitamin E deficiency and neurologic disease, Annu. Rev. Nutr. **8**:351, 1988.

221. Spataro, R.F., Lin, S.R., Horner, F.A., Hall, C.B., and McDonald, J.V.: Aqueductal stenosis and hydrocephalus: rare sequelae of mumps virus infection, Neuroradiology **12**:11, 1976.

222. Stam, F.C.: Concept, classification and nosology of the leukodystrophies: an historical introductory review. In Vinken, P.J., and Bruyn, G.W., editors: Leukodystrophies and poliodystrophies, Handbook of clinical neurology, vol. 10, Amsterdam, 1970, North Holland Publishing Co.

223. Stehbens, W.E.: Pathology of cerebral blood vessels, St. Louis, 1972, The C.V. Mosby Co.

224. Sterns, R.H., Riggs, J.E., and Schochet, S.S., Jr.: Osmotic demyelination syndrome following correction of hyponatremia, N. Engl. J. Med. **314**:1535, 1986.

225. Strich, S.J.: Diffuse degeneration of cerebral white matter in severe dementia following head injury, J. Neurol. Neurosurg. Psychiatry **19**:163, 1956.

226. Sumi, S.M.: Sudanophilic lipid accumulation in periventricular leukomalacia in monkeys, Acta Neuropathol. (Berlin) **47**:241, 1979.

227. Svien, H.J., Mabon, R.F., Kernohan, J.W., and Craig, W.M.: Astrocytomas, Proc. Staff Meet. Mayo Clin. **24**:54, 1949.

228. Swartz, M.N.: Bacterial meningitis, N. Engl. J. Med. **7**:524, 1980. (Editorial.)

229. Takashima, S., and Tanaka, K.: Development of cerebrovascular architecture and its relationship to periventricular leukomalacia, Arch. Neurol. **35**:11, 1978.

230. Takashima, S., Becker, L.E., Armstrong, D.L., and Chan, F.: Abnormal neuronal development in the visual cortex of the human fetus and infant with Down's syndrome: a quantitative and qualitative Golgi study, Brain Res. **225**:1, 1981.

231. Tandan, R., and Bradley, W.G.: Amyotrophic lateral sclerosis: Part 1. Clinical features, pathology, and ethical issues in management, Ann. Neurol. **18**:271, 1985.

232. Taylor, C.R., Russell, R., Lukes, R.J., and Davis, R.L.: An immunohistological study of immunoglobulin content of primary central nervous system lymphomas, Cancer **41**:2197, 1978.

233. Terry, R.D.: Alzheimer's disease. In Davis, R.L., and Robertson, D.M., editors: Textbook of neuropathology, Baltimore, 1985, The Williams & Wilkins Co.

234. Thomas, P.K., Landon, D.N., and King, R.H.M.: Disease of the peripheral nerves. In Adams, J.H., Corsellis, J.A.N., and Duchen, L.W.: Greenfield's neuropathology, ed. 4, New York, 1984, John Wiley & Sons, Inc.

235. Todd, D.W., Christoferson, L.A., Leech, R.W., and Rudolf, L.: A family affected with intestinal polyposis and gliomas, Ann. Neurol. **10**:390, 1981.

236. Tomlinson, B.E.: The aging brain. In Smith, W.T., and Cavanaugh, J.B., editors: Recent advances in neuropathology, Edinburgh, 1979, Churchill Livingstone.

237. Tomlinson, B.E., and Corsellis, J.A.N.: Aging and the dementias. In Adams, J.H., Corsellis, J.A.N., and Duchen, L.W., editors: Greenfield's neuropathology, ed. 4, New York, 1984, John Wiley & Sons, Inc.

238. Toole, J.F., Janeway, R., Choi, K., Cordell, R., Johnston, F., and Miller, H.S.: Transient ischemic attacks due to atherosclerosis, Arch. Neurol. **32**:5, 1975.

239. Torack, R.M., Terry, R.D., and Zimmerman, H.M.: The fine structure of cerebral fluid accumulation. II. Swelling produced by triethyl tin poisoning and its comparison with that in the human brain, Am. J. Pathol. **36**:273, 1960.

240. Tyler, K.L., and McPhee, D.A.: Molecular and genetic aspects of the pathogenesis of viral infections of the central nervous system, CRC Crit. Rev. Neurobiol. 3:221, 1987.

241. van Bogaert, L.: Une leuco-encéphalite sclérosante subaiguë, J. Neurol. Neurosurg. Psychiatry 8:101, 1945.

242. Victor, M., Adams, R.D., and Cole, M.: The acquired (non-Wilsonian) type of chronic hepatocerebral degeneration, Medicine 44:345, 1965.

243. Victor, M., Adams, R.D., and Collins, G.H.: The Wernicke-Korsakoff syndrome, Philadelphia, 1971, F.A. Davis.

244. Volpe, J.J.: Neurology of the newborn, ed. 2, Philadelphia, 1987, W.B. Saunders Co.

245. Warkany, J.: Congenital malformations, Chicago, 1971, Year Book Medical Publishers.

246. Weiner, L.P., and Fleming, J.O.: Viral infections of the nervous system, J. Neurosurg. 61:207, 1984.

247. Weller, R.D.: Spontaneous intracranial hemorrhage. In Adams, J.H., Corsellis, J.A.N., and Duchen, L.W., editors: Greenfield's neuropathology, ed. 4, New York, 1984, John Wiley & Sons, Inc.

248. Wertelecki, W., Rouleau, G.A., Superneau, D.W., Forehand, L.W., Williams, J.P., Haines, J.L., and Gusella, J.F.: Neurofibromatosis 2: clinical and DNA linkage studies of a large kindred, N. Engl. J. Med. 319:278, 1988.

249. Wigglesworth, J.S.: Perinatal pathology, Philadelphia, 1984, W.B. Saunders Co.

250. Wisniewski, K., Dambska, M., Sher, J.H., and Qazi, Q.: A clinical neuropathological study of the fetal alcohol syndrome, Neuropediatrics 14:197, 1983.

251. Wright, D.G., Laureno, R., and Victor, M: Pontine and extrapontine myelinolysis, Brain 102:361, 1979.

252. Zang, K.D.: Cytological and cytogenetical studies on human meningioma, Cancer Genet. Cytogenet. 6:242, 1982.

Index

Page numbers in *italics* indicate illustrations. Page numbers followed by a *t* indicate tables.

CRST syndrome, 1780; *see also* CREST syndrome
Crush syndrome, 448
Crushing head injuries, 2188
Crust, 1757
Cruveilhier-Baumgarten syndrome, 1250
Cryoglobulinemia, mixed, 769
Cryoimmunoglobulinemia, 826
Crypt cells of intestinal epithelium, 257t
Cryptococcal meningitis, 415, *415*, 2155-2156, *2156*
Cryptococcosis, 394t, 415-416, *416*
    acquired immunodeficiency syndrome and, *1822*
    cerebromeningeal, 415, *415*, 2155-2156, *2156*
    pulmonary, 415
Cryptococcus, 1053
Cryptococcus neoformans, 394t, 410, 415, *415*
    acquired immunodeficiency syndrome and, 1287
    infective endocarditis and, 654
    meningitis and, 2154, 2155-2156
Cryptogenic chronic active hepatitis, 1230-1231
Cryptogenic cirrhosis, 1202, 1209
    hepatitis B virus and, 1212
    hepatocellular carcinoma and, 1295
    nodular, 1227, *1228*
Cryptogenic organizing pneumonitis, 971, *971*
Cryptorchidism, 871, *872*
Cryptosporidiosis, 445, 968, 1167
    cholecystitis and, 1328, 1328t
Crypts
    of Lieberkühn, 557, 1163, 1184
        and irradiation, 272
    of Morgagni, 1168
Crystal-deposition diseases, 2087-2091
Crystalline cholesterol stones, 1323, *1324*
Crystalloids of Reinke, 1687
CSF-1 and CSF-2, 590t
Ctenodactylus gundi, 448
Cuff cells, *1464*, 1464-1465
Culex, 470
Culicoides furans, 1777
Cuneate nuclei bilirubin staining, 2146
Cunninghamella, 395t, 425
Curie, 248, 249
Curling's ulcers, 1160, *1160*
Current, electrical, 140-141
Curvularia geniculata, 392t
Cushing's disease, 1534, 1589, 1592t
Cushing's syndrome, 163, 873, *1590*, 1592t, 1592-1593
    in child, 1585
    hyperadrenocorticism and, *1524*, 1525, *1594*, 1975
    pathophysiologic classification of, 1592t
Cusps, congenital heart disease and, 739
Cut, 114
Cutaneous anaphylaxis, 518, 539t; *see also* Skin
Cutaneous appendages, 1755
Cutaneous larva migrans, 467
Cutaneous reactions, 523
Cutaneous vasculitis, 539t
Cutaneous-visceral disease, 1758-1759
Cutis hyperelastica, 1782-1783
Cutis laxa, 1784
Cyanide poisoning, 193t
Cyanocobalamins, 560

Cyanotic tetralogy in newborn, 743, *744*
Cycasin, 596, 597
Cyclic AMP, 8
Cyclists, injuries to, 118
Cyclophosphamide, 708, 825, 856
    oxygen toxicity and, 180-182
Cyclopia, agenesis of pituitary and, 1526
Cyclops, 473
Cyclosporin
    cholestasis and gallstones and, 1326
    lung transplantation and, 967
    orthotopic liver transplant and, 1300
    toxicity of, 182-183
Cyclotron, 248
Cylindrical cell papilloma in nasal cavity, 1081, *1081*
Cylindroid aneurysm, 778
Cylindroma, 1832
Cyst, 87
    adrenal glands and, 1606
    Baker's, 2092
    Bartholin's gland, 1628
    of Blandin-Nuhn, 1128
    bone, 2056-2057
        ganglionic, 2057-2059
    bronchogenic, 923, 1024
    bursal, 2092
    daughter, 461
    dermoid, 1077, 1835
    of echinococcosis, 461
    of *Entamoeba histolytica*, 433
    enteric, 1024, 1153-1154
    of epididymis, 892
    of fallopian tube, 1669-1670
    fissural, 1077
    Gartner's duct, 1639
    of heart, 700
    hydatid, 662
    intrasellar, 1537
    of jaws, 1117-1120
    of joints and para-articular tissues, 2092
    laryngeal, 1085
    liver, 1293
        congenital, *1297*
    mediastinal, 1024-1025, 1025t
    mesentery and, 1191
    mesonephric, 1669
    mother, 461
    Müllerian, *1626*
    myxoid, 1782
    neck, 1143-1144
    of nose, 1077
    ovarian
        follicular, oral contraceptives and, 165
        nonneoplastic, 1674-1677
        theca-lutein, 1674
    parathyroid, 1577
    of pars plana, 1069
    pericardial, 1024
    pilary, 1835
    pilosebaceous, 1835
    of prostate gland, 902
    salivary gland, 1127-1128
    sebaceous, 1835
    splenic, 1426
    sweat gland, *1764*
    synovial, 1782
    of thymus gland, 1502
    thyroglossal, 1546
    Toxoplasma, 449
    trichilemmal, 1834
    urachal, 867
    of urethra, 899
    of vagina, 1639

Cystadenocarcinoma of pancreas, 1354
Cystadenofibromas of ovary, 1684
Cystadenoma, 610
    bile duct, 1291-1292
    eccrine, 1832
    of epididymis, 892
    of ovary, *1681*
    pancreatic, 1354, *1354*
    of salivary glands, 1134-1135, *1135*
Cystamine, 254, 1233
Cystectomy, *860*
Cysteine, 254
Cystic adventitial disease of popliteal artery, 785-786, *787*
Cystic bile duct, congenital, 1257-1258
Cystic breast disease, *1728*, 1728-1729
Cystic chondroblastoma, 2039
Cystic endometrial hyperplasia, 1657
Cystic fibrosis, 950-951
    gastrointestinal manifestations of, 1172-1173
    liver disease and, 1268
    pancreas and, 1348-1351, *1349*, *1350*
Cystic hygroma
    in mediastinum, 1024
    in neck, 1144
Cystic lung, herbicide toxicity and, 230
Cystic lymphangioma, 799, *799*
Cystic medial necrosis, 783, *784*
Cystic syringadenoma, 1832-1833
Cystic teratoma, *1689*, 1689
Cysticercosis, 459
    cerebral, *459*, 460
    meningitis and, 2154
    of myocardium, *460*
Cystine stones, 854
Cystinosis, cornea and, 1074
Cystitis, 311, 834, 855, 855-857
    bullous, 855
    candidiasis and, 412
    emphysematous, 855
    encrusted, 856
    gangrenous, 856
    interstitial, 856
    irradiation, 856
    polypoid, 857
    tuberculous, 857
Cystitis cystica, 857, *858*
Cystitis glandularis, 458, 857
Cystoprostatectomy, *861*
Cystosarcoma, malignant breast, 1748
Cystosarcoma phyllodes, 1730-1731
Cystothionuria, 559
Cytochrome oxidase, 2, 558
Cytochrome P-450, 5, 16
    drug metabolism and, 1232
Cytogenetics, 45-49, 603, 1624-1627
Cytokeratin, 1012
    leiomyosarcomas and, 1863
    malignant fibrous histiocytomas and, 1859
    soft-tissue tumors and, 1840
Cytokines, 93
Cytology, 12, 610
    neoplastic cells and, 580-581
    in urothelial tumors, 866
    vaginal pathology and, 1638-1639
Cytolysis, 12, 504t, 509, *509*
Cytomegalic inclusion disease; *see* Cytomegalovirus
Cytomegalovirus, 379, *381*
    acquired immunodeficiency syndrome and, 1167, 1286
    alimentary tract and, 1054